MW01040978

SECOND EDITION

Foundations of ANESTHESIA

BASIC SCIENCES FOR CLINICAL PRACTICE

Commissioning Editor: Natasha Andjelkovic
Project Development Manager: Joanne Scott
Project Manager: Anne Dickie
Cover Designer: Jayne Jones
Text Designer: Stewart Larking
Illustration Manager: Mick Ruddy
Illustrator: Antbits Illustration
Marketing Manager(s) (UK/USA): Brant Emery/Emily M Christie

SECOND EDITION

Foundations of ANESTHESIA

BASIC SCIENCES FOR CLINICAL PRACTICE

Hugh C Hemmings, Jr, MD PhD
Professor of Anesthesiology
Professor of Pharmacology
Vice Chair of Research
Department of Anesthesiology
Weill Medical College of Cornell University
New York, New York
USA

Philip M Hopkins, MBBS MD FRCA
Professor of Anaesthesia
Academic Unit of Anaesthesia
St. James's University Hospital
Leeds
UK

MOSBY

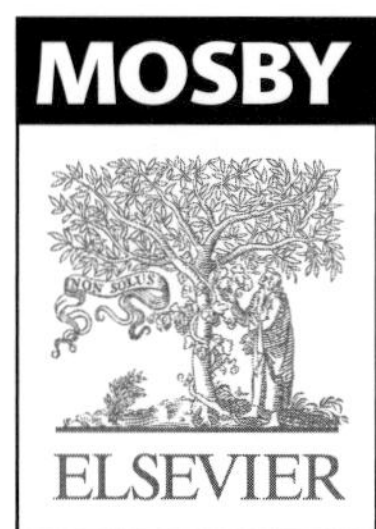

ELSEVIER

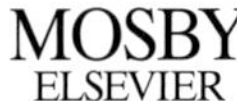

An imprint of Elsevier Limited

First edition 2000

ISBN 0 3230 3707 0

British Library Cataloguing in Publication Data
A catalogue record for this book is available from the British Library

Library of Congress Cataloging in Publication Data
A catalog record for this book is available from the Library of Congress

Notice
Medical knowledge is constantly changing. Standard safety precautions must be followed, but as new research and clinical experience broaden our knowledge, changes in treatment and drug therapy may become necessary or appropriate. Readers are advised to check the most current product information provided by the manufacturer of each drug to be administered to verify the recommended dose, the method and duration of administration, and contraindications. It is the responsibility of the practitioner, relying on experience and knowledge of the patient, to determine dosages and the best treatment for each individual patient. Neither the Publisher nor the authors assume any liability for any injury and/or damage to persons or property arising from this publication.
The Publisher

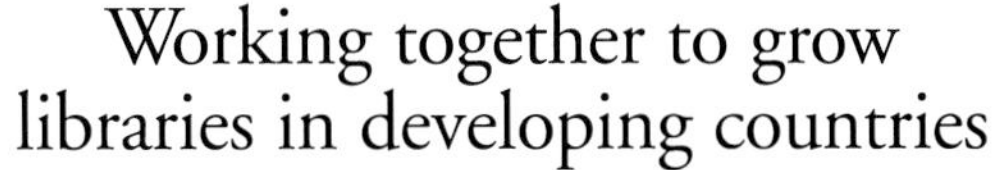

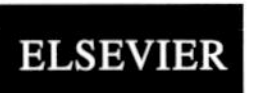

Printed in China
Last digit is the print number: 9 8 7 6 5 4 3 2 1

Contents

Foreword

Drs Hemmings and Hopkins have assembled seventy three chapters written by well-recognized authorities from both sides of the Atlantic. Though the sea of knowledge is never full, they have completed an extraordinary and successful labor in producing a significant tidal surge that will be regarded as the high water mark to be noted by generations of anesthesiologists yet unborn.

Essential to the understanding of this text is the editors' conviction that the successful practice of the art of anesthesia requires a sound understanding of the underlying scientific principles'. This quotation from the invitational letter to each contributor summarizes the philosophy which underlines the entire work. The seventy three chapters are grouped under eight major headings (General Principles, Neurosciences, Cardiovascular system, Respiratory system, Pathological sciences, Renal system, Gastrointestinal system and metabolism, and Adaptive physiology). Within each section of the book, there are chapters that cover the essential basic science information necessary for the understanding of the section's utility in clinical practice.

The amount of basic science information has grown tremendously during my half century in medicine. When I started my training, I was initially taught clinical anesthesia by very skillful nurse anesthetists who were far more concerned with the art of anesthesia. Scientific information was scarce. John Snow's classic monograph on the inhalation of the vapor of ether was one of the first publications to provide a scientific basic for the practice of our art. In 1924, Howard Haggard published five classic papers in the *Journal of Biological Chemistry* on the uptake and elimination of diethyl ether, attributing his failure to effect quantitative recovery to the volatility of ether rather than to the possibility of its metabolism by the body. The importance of water solubility on the speed of anesthetic action was soon elucidated by Seymour Kety. So opened a new era in the scientific understanding of what had previously been largely a clinical art.

When Dr Hemmings honored me by asking me to write this piece, I asked myself not only what to say, but also who might have said it very well in the past. The answer rose immediately to mind: more than 30 years ago, John Severinghaus wrote the foreword for the first edition of John Nunn's classic book on respiratory physiology- a book which, like this one, combined and correlated basic science with clinical practice. He chose the title ' A Flame for Hypos', and illustrated it with a photograph of a lighted candle before the statue of the god of sleep. No one has ever said it so well. Never have I read a more beautiful foreword and append a part of it here with the permission of Dr Severinghaus (who himself has contributed a chapter to this book). So from the work of many minds and hands this book goes forth, that we too, by understanding the process, may better the art.

Alan Van Poznak, M.D.
New York City
1999

The world will little note nor long remember what I say here, but it can never forget what we did here.
Abraham Lincoln, Gettysburg November 19, 1863

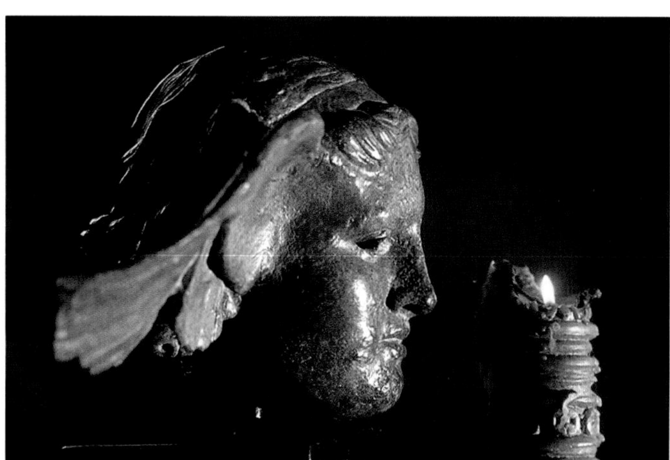

Excerpted from the foreword to the first edition (1969) of *Applied Respiratory Physiology* by John F. Nunn, reprinted with the permission of Butterworth-Heinemann

The lighted candle respires and we call it flame. The body respires and we call it life. Neither flame nor life is substance, but process. The flame is as different from the wick and wax as life from the body, as gravitation from the falling apple, or love from a hormone. Newton taught science to have faith in processes as well as substances–to compute, predict and depend upon an irrational attraction. Caught up in enlightenment, man began to regard himself as a part of nature, a subject for investigation. The web of self-knowledge, woven so slowly between process and substance, still weaves physiology, the process, and anatomy, the substances, into the whole cloth of clinical medicine. Within this multihued fabric, the warp fibres of process shine most clearly in the newest patterns, among which must be numbered anesthesiology.

And what of the god of sleep, patron of anesthesia? The centuries themselves number more than 21 since Hypnos wrapped his cloak of sleep over Hellas. Now before Hypos, the artisan, is set the respiring flame–that he may, by knowing the process, better the art.

John W Severinghaus
San Francisco

Preface

The successful practice of the art of anesthesia, critical care and pain medicine demands a sound understanding of underlying scientific concepts and familiarity with the evolving vocabulary of medical science. This is recognized in the postgraduate examinations in anesthesia in North America, Europe and Australasia, for which a thorough understanding of the relevant basic sciences is required. Furthermore, many trainees in anesthesia come to view learning the basic sciences to the required depth as a necessary chore. This is disappointing to those of us who find the scientific basis for our clinical practice to be a constant source of interest, fascination and, indeed, sometimes excitement. Part of the problem is that basic science texts directed towards anesthetists tend to be fact, rather than concept-oriented, and therefore difficult to read and to learn from.

Foundations of Anesthesia: Basic Sciences for Clinical Practice second edition, provides comprehensive coverage in a single text of the principles and clinical applications of the four major areas of basic science that are relevant to anesthesia practice: molecular and cell biology, physiology, pharmacology, and physics and measurement. The approach is integrated and systems oriented, avoiding the artificial boundaries between the basic sciences. Recognizing that no single author possesses the breadth and depth of understanding of all relevant subjects, each chapter is authored by an expert in that area. These authorities represent many of the finest institutions of North America, the United Kingdom and Europe to take advantage of the globalization of medicine facilitated by electronic communication. This allows an international presentation of current anesthesia science presented by relevant experts at the cutting edge of anesthesia research and education.

Each chapter stresses the scientific principles necessary to understand and manage various situations encountered in anesthesia. Detailed explanations of techniques are avoided since this information is available in many clinical subspecialty anesthesia texts. Nor is this book intended to provide a detailed review of specialized research areas for the scientist. Rather, the fundamental information necessary to understand 'why' and 'how' is stressed, and basic concepts are related to relevant anesthesia situations. The style stresses a conceptual approach to learning, using factual information to illustrate the concepts. Chapters are self-contained with minimal repetition, and include a short list of Key References and suggestions for Further Reading to stimulate further exploration of interesting topics. This style and approach is modeled after the ground-breaking text *Scientific Foundations of Anaesthesia,* edited by Cyril Scurr and Stanley Feldman, updated to cover the revolutionary developments in modern molecular biology and physiology. Recognizing that graphics are the most expressive way of conveying concepts, full-color illustrations facilitate use of the book as a learning aid and make it enjoyable to read.

The second edition of *Foundations of Anesthesia: Basic Sciences for Clinical Practice* includes a number of notable developments. Text boxes are included to highlight important points with particular relevance to clinical implications for the practice of anesthesia. Important key words from the American in-training examination are highlighted in the index. A number of new chapters have been incorporated: Adverse Drug Reactions, Sensory Systems, Physiology of Pain, General Anesthetics: Mechanisms of Action, Consciousness and Cognition, Sleep and Anesthesia, Ischemic Brain Injury, Blood Constituents and Transfusion and Hemostasis and Coagulation. An accompanying CD includes the figures and tables to facilitate teaching from the text and a searchable index. These improvements significantly enhance the use of *Foundations of Anesthesia: Basic Sciences for Clinical Practice* as a tool for learning, teaching and review of the fundamental concepts essential to anesthesiology, pain and critical care medicine.

Hugh C Hemmings Jr and Philip M Hopkins 2005

List of Contributors

John P Adams MB ChB MRCP FRCA
Consultant in Anaesthesia and Intensive Care
Department of Anaesthesia
Leeds General Infirmary
Leeds
UK

Maria G Annetta MD
Assistant Professor
Universita Cattolica
Rome
Italy

James Arden MD PhD
Consultant Anaesthetist
Department of Anaesthesia
King's College Hospital
London
UK

Solomon Aronson MD FRCA
Professor of Anesthesiology
Department of Anesthesiology
Duke University Medical Center
Durham, North Carolina
USA

Helen A Baghdoyan PhD
Professor of Anesthesiology and Pharmacology
Department of Anesthesiology
The University of Michigan
Ann Arbor, Michigan
USA

Jeffrey R Balser MD PhD
Associate Vice Chancellor for Research,
Professor of Anesthesiology and Pharmacology
Vanderbilt University Medicine Center
Nashville, Tennessee
USA

Christofer D Barth MD
Fellow, Cardiothoracic Anesthesia
Cleveland Clinic Foundation
Cleveland, Ohio
USA

Marcus R Beadle MB BS FRCA
Specialist Registrar Anaesthetics
Department of Anaesthesia
St James's University Hospital
Leeds
UK

Paul CW Beatty PhD MSc BSc C Eng FIPEM
Senior Lecturer in Biomedical Engineering
Imaging Science and Biomedical Engineering
University of Manchester
Manchester
UK

Mark C Bellamy MA MB BS FRCA
Professor of Critical Care Anaesthesia
Intensive Care Unit
St James's University Hospital
Leeds
UK

Keith H Berge MD
Assistant Professor of Anesthesiology
Mayo Clinic College of Medicine
Rochester, Minnesota
USA

Thomas JJ Blanck MD PhD
Professor and Chairman of Anesthesiology
Professor of Physiology and Neuroscience
Department of Anesthesiology
NYU Medical Center
New York, New York
USA

Andrew R Bodenham FRCA
Consultant in Anaesthesia and Intensive Care Medicine
Department of Anaesthesia
Leeds General Infirmary
Leeds
UK

Francis Bonnet MD FRCA
Professor of Anesthesiology
Department of Anesthesia Reanimation
Hospital Tenon
Paris
France

Timothy J Brennan PhD MD
Associate Professor of Anesthesia and Pharmacology
Department of Anesthesia
University of Iowa Hospitals and Clinics
Iowa City, Iowa
USA

Marek Brzezinski MD
Anesthesiology Fellow
Department of Anesthesiology
Duke University Medical Center
Durham, North Carolina
USA

Donal J Buggy MB ChB (Hons) MD MSc DME FRCPI FCA (Ire) FRCA
Honorary Senior Lecturer in Anaesthesia
Department of Anaesthesia
National University of Ireland
Mater Misericordiae University Hospital
Dublin
Republic of Ireland

Iain T Campbell MB BS MD FRCA
Consultant Anaesthetist
Department of Anaesthesia
University Hospital of South Manchester
Manchester
UK

Franco Carli MD MPhil FRCA FRCPC
Professor of Anesthesia
Department of Anesthesia
McGilll University Health Centre
Montreal, Quebec
Canada

Surinder PS Cheema MBBCh DA FRCA
Consultant Anaesthesiologist
Dept of Anaesthetics
Bradford Royal Infirmary
Bradford
UK

Andrew T Cohen MBChB DRCOG FRCA
Consultant in Anaesthesia and Intensive Care
Department of Anaesthesia
St James's University Hospital
Leeds
UK

Joan P Desborough MBChB FRCA MD
Consultant Anaesthetist
Anaesthetic Department
Epsom and St Helier NHS Trust
Surrey
UK

Marc L Dickstein MD
Associate Professor of Anesthesiology
Columbia University
New York, New York
USA

Xueqin Ding MD PhD
Research Fellow
Center for Anesthesiology Research
The Cleveland Clinic Foundation
Cleveland, Ohio
USA

James D Dodman MBBS FRCA
Specialist Registrar in Anaesthesia
Department of Anaesthesia
Leeds General Infirmary
Leeds
UK

Mary Doherty MB ChB FCA(Ire)
Specialist Registrar in Anaesthesia
Department of Anaesthesia
Mater Misericordiae University Hospital
Dublin
Republic of Ireland

Marcel E Durieux MD PhD
Professor of Anesthesiology & Neurological Surgery
Department of Anesthesiology
University of Virginia Health System
Charlottesville, Virginia
USA

Thomas J Ebert MD PhD
Professor of Anesthesiology and Staff Anesthesiologist
Department of Anesthesiology
The Medical Center of Wisconsin
Milwaukee, Wisconsin
USA

Simon M Enright MBChB FRCA
Clinical Director, ICU
Pinderfields Hospital
Wakefield
UK

John R Feiner MD
Associate Professor
Department of Anesthesia and Perioperative Care
University of California
San Francisco, California
USA

Gary Fiskum PhD
Professor and Vice-Chair for Research of Anesthesiology
Department of Anesthesiology
University of Maryland School of Medicine
Baltimore, Maryland
USA

Patricia Fogarty-Mack MD
Associate Professor of Clinical Anesthesiology,
Director Neuroanesthesiology
Department of Anesthesiology
Weill Medical College of Cornell University
New York, New York
USA

Manuel L Fontes MD
Associate Professor of Anesthesiology and Critical Care
Department of Anesthesiology
Weill Medical College of Cornell University
New York, New York
USA

Kirsty Forrest MBChB BSc (Hons) FRCA
Lecturer in Anaesthesia
Academic Unit of Anaesthesia
Leeds General Infirmary
Leeds
UK

Helen F Galley PhD FIMLS
Senior Lecturer
Institute of Medical Sciences
University of Aberdeen
Aberdeen
UK

Susan Garwood MBChB FRCA
Associate Professor of Anesthesiology
Department of Anesthesiology
Yale University School of Medicine
New Haven, Connecticut
USA

Kevin J Gingrich MD
Associate Professor of Anesthesiology
NYU School of Medicine
Department of Anesthesiology
New York, New York
USA

Jean-Antoine Girault MD PhD
Director of Research
Laboratory of Signal Transduction and Plasticity in the Nervous System
Institut du Fer à Moulin
Paris
France

Andrew P Gratrix MBChB FCARCSI
Specialist Registrar in Anaesthesia and Intensive Care Medicine
Pinderfields Hospital
Wakefield
UK

Roger Hainsworth MB ChB PhD DSc
Emeritus Professor of Applied Physiology
Institute for Cardiovascular Research
University of Leeds
Leeds
UK

Neil L Harrison BA PhD
Professor of Anesthesiology and Pharmacology
Department of Anesthesiology
Weill Medical College of Cornell University
New York, New York
USA

Paul M Heerdt MD PhD
Associate Professor of Anesthesiology and Pharmacology
Weill Medical College of Cornell University
New York, New York
USA

Hugh C Hemmings Jr MD PhD
Professor of Anesthesiology and Pharmacology
Department of Anesthesiology
Vice Chair of Research
Weill Medical College of Cornell University
New York, New York
USA

Norman L Herman MD PhD
Assistant Professor Anesthesiology (Retired);
Associate Attending Anesthesiology (Retired)
Weill Medical College of Cornell University
New York, New York
USA

Sue A Hill MA (Cantab) PhD (Cantab) FRCA Dip Comp Dip Stats
Consultant Neuroanaesthetist
Shackleton Department of Anaesthesia
Southampton University Hospitals Trust
Southampton
UK

Andrew T Hindle MB ChB BSc(Hons) DA FRCA
Consultant Anaesthetist
Department of Anaesthesia
Warrington Hospital
Warrington
UK

Kirk Hogan MD JD
Professor of Anesthesiology
Department of Anesthesiology
University of Wisconsin Hospitals and Clinics
Madison, Wisconsin
USA

Philip M Hopkins MB BS MD FRCA
Professor of Anaesthesia
Academic Unit of Anaesthesia
St James's University Hospital
Leeds
UK

Simon J Howell MBBS MA (Cantab) MRCP FRCA MSc MD
Senior Lecturer in Anesthesia
Academic Unit of Anaesthesia
Leeds General Infirmary
Leeds
UK

Michael J Hudspith MB BS BSc PhD FRCA
Consultant in Pain Management and Anesthesia
Norfolk & Norwich University Hospital
Norwich
UK

Uday Jain PhD MD
Department of Anesthesia
St Mary's Medical Center
San Francisco, California
USA

Peter M Kimpson MB ChB BSc FRCA
Lecturer in Anaesthesia
Academic Unit of Anaesthesia
St James's University Hospital
Leeds
UK

H Thomas Lee MD PhD
Assistant Professor of Anesthesiology
Department of Anesthesiology
Colombia University Medical Center
New York, New York
USA

Jerrold Lerman MD FRCPC FANZCA
Clinical Professor of Anesthesia
Department of Anesthesiology
Woman and Children's Hospital of Buffalo
Buffalo, New York
USA

Cynthia A Lien MD
Professor of Clinical Anesthesiology
Department of Anesthesiology
Weill Medical College of Cornell University
New York, New York
USA

Martin J London MD
Professor of Clinical Anesthesia
Department of Anesthesia and Perioperative Care
University of California
San Francisco, California
USA

Andrew B Lumb MB BS FRCA
Consultant Anaesthetist
Department of Anaesthesia
St James's University Hospital
Leeds
UK

Ralph Lydic PhD
Bert La Du Professor of Anesthesiology and Associate Chair for Research
Department of Anesthesiology
The University of Michigan
Ann Arbor, Michigan
USA

Ken Mackie MD
Professor of Anesthesiology, Adjunct Professor of Physiology and Biophysics
Department of Anesthesiology
University of Washington
Seattle, Washington
USA

Abhiram Mallick MD FRCA FFARCSI
Consultant in Anaesthesia and ICM
Department of Anaesthesia
Leeds General Infirmary
Leeds
UK

Emmanuel Marret MD
Associate Professor of Anesthesiology
Department of Anesthesia Reanimation
Hospital Tenon
Paris
France

Ian G Marshall BSc PhD
Department of Biomedical Sciences
University of Central Lancashire
Preston
UK

Thomas S McDowell MD PhD
Assistant Professor of Anesthesiology
Department of Anesthesiology
University of Wisconsin
Madison, Wisconsin
USA

Gregory A Michelotti PhD
Assistant Research Professor
Duke University Medical Center
Durham, North Carolina
USA

Salim Mujais MD
Vice President Medical Affairs
Renal Divison
Baxter Healthcare Corporation
McGaw Park, Illinois
USA

Rajesh Munglani MB BS FRCA
Consultant in Pain Management
West Suffolk Hospital
Bury St Edmonds and BUPA Lea Hospital
Cambridge
UK

Paul G Murphy MA MB ChB FRCA
Consultant in Anaesthesia and Intensive Care
Department of Anaesthesia
Leeds General Infirmary
Leeds
UK

Paul A Murray PhD
Carl E Wasmuth Endowed Chair and Director of Anesthesiology Research, Professor of Anesthesiology
Center for Anesthesiology Research
The Cleveland Clinic Foundation
Cleveland, Ohio
USA

Timothy J Ness MD PhD
Simon Gelman Endowed Professor of Anesthesiology
Department of Anesthesiology
University of Alabama at Birmingham
Birmingham, Alabama
USA

Ramona Nicolau-Raducu MD
Instructor of Anesthesiology and Fellow of Hepatic Transplantation Anesthesiology
UPMC Presbyterian/Montefiore
Pittsburgh, Pennsylvania
USA

Daniel Nyhan MD MRCPI
Professor of Anesthesiology and Critical Care Medicine, Chief, Division of Cardiac Anesthesia, Vice Chairman
Department of Anesthesiology and Critical Care Medicine
The Johns Hopkins Hospitals
Baltimore, Maryland
USA

Klaus T Olkkola MD PhD
Professor and Chairman
Department of Anaesthesiology and Intensive Care Medicine
Turku University Hospital
Turku
Finland

Beverley A Orser MD PhD FRCPC
Professor of Physiology and Anesthesia; Canada Research Chair in Anesthesia
Department of Physiology
University of Toronto
Toronto, Ontario
Canada

Gavril W Pasternak MD PhD
Anne Burnett Tandy Chair of Neurology; Member and Attending Neurologist; Head, Laboratory of Molecular Neuropharmacology
Memorial Sloan-Kettering Cancer Center
New York, New York
USA

Misha A Perouansky MD
Associate Professor of Anesthesiology
Department of Anesthesiology
University of Wisconsin Medical School
Madison, Wisconsin
USA

Raymond M Planinsic MD
Director of Hepatic, Intestinal and Multivisceral Transplantation Anesthesiology and Associate Professor of Anesthesiology
UPMC Presbyterian/Montefiore
Pittsburgh, Pennsylvania
USA

Alison J Pittard MBChB MD FRCA
Consultant in Anaesthesia and Intensive Care
Department of Anaesthesia
Leeds General Infirmary
Leeds
UK

Brian J Pollard BPharm MB ChB MD FRCA
Professor of Anaesthesia
Department of Anaesthesia
Manchester Royal Infirmary
Manchester
UK

Ian Power MD FRCA FFPMANZCA FANZCA FRCS Ed FRCP Edin
Professor of Anaesthesia, Critical Care and Pain Medicine
Department of Clinical and Surgical Sciences
The University of Edinburgh
Edinburgh
UK

Christopher B Prior BSc PhD
Senior Lecturer in Pharmacology
Department of Physiology and Pharmacology
University of Strathclyde
Glasgow
UK

Kane O Pryor MD
Instructor in Anesthesiology
Department of Anesthesiology
Weill Medical College of Cornell University
New York, New York
USA

Andrew Quinn MB ChB FRCA
Specialist Registrar in Anaesthesia
Department of Anaesthesia
St James's University Hospital
Leeds
UK

Robert E Rosenthal MD
Professor of Surgery, Program in Trauma; Section Chief Hyperbaric Medicine
R Adams Cowley Shock Trauma Center
University of Maryland School of Medicine
Baltimore, Maryland
USA

David J Rowbotham MBChB MD FRCA MRCP
Professor of Anaesthesia and Pain Management
University of Leicester and University Hospitals of Leicester
Leicester
UK

John J Savarese MD
Professor and Chairman,
Department of Anesthesiology
Weill Medical College of Cornell University
New York, New York
USA

Thomas Schricker MD PhD
Assistant Professor
Department of Anesthesia
McGilll University Health Centre
Montreal, Quebec
Canada

Debra A Schwinn MD
James B Duke Professor of Anesthesiology, Professor of Pharmacology/Cancer Biology & Surgery, Vice-Chairman of Research and Director of Perioperative Genomics and Head of Molecular Pharmacology Laboratories
Duke University Medical Center
Department of Anesthesiology
Durham, North Carolina
USA

Jane E Sellors MBChB FRCA
Consultant Paediatric Anaesthetist
Department of Anaesthesia
St James's University Hospital
Leeds
UK

John W Severinghaus MD
Professor Emeritus
Department of Anesthesia and Perioperative Care
University of California San Francisco School of Medicine
San Francisco, California
USA

Steven L Shafer MD
Professor of Anesthesia, Adjunct Professor of Biopharmaceutical Science
Anesthesiology Service
PAVAHCS
Palo Alto, California
USA

Stanton K Shernan MD
Director of Cardiac Anesthesia
Department of Anesthesiology, Perioperative and Pain Medicine
Brigham and Women's Hospital
Havard Medical School
Boston, Massachusetts
USA

Philip J Siddall MBBS PhD FFPMANZCA
Clinical Senior Lecturer
Pain Management Research Institute
University of Sydney
Royal North Shore Hospital
Sydney, New South Wales
Australia

Jeffrey H Silverstein MD
Vice Chair for Research
Department of Anesthesiology
Mount Sinai School of Medicine
New York, New York
USA

Karen H Simpson MBChB
Consultant in Pain Medicine and Anaesthesia
Pain Management Service
St James's University Hospital
Leeds
UK

Nikolaos Skubas MD
Assistant Professor of Anesthesiology
Department of Anesthesiology
Weill Cornell Medical College
New York, New York
USA

Tod B Sloan MD MBA PhD
Professor of Anesthesiology
Department of Anesthiology
University of Colorado Health Sciences Center
Denver, Colorado
USA

Richard M Smiley MD Ph D
Professor of Clinical Anesthesiology
Columbia University
New York, New York
USA

Ian Smith BSc MD FRCA
Senior Lecturer in Anaesthesia
University Hospital of North Staffordshire
Stoke-on-Trent
UK

Nina J Solenski MD
Associate Professor of Neurology
Department of Neurology
University of Virginia School of Medicine
Charlottesville, Virginia
USA

David F Stowe BA MA MD PhD
Professor of Anesthesiology and Physiology
Medical College of Wisconsin
Milwaukee, Wisconsin
USA

Robert E Study MD PhD
Staff Anesthesiologist
First Colonies Anesthesia Associates
Suburban Hospital
Bethesda, Maryland
USA

Richard Teplick MD
Chief of Staff; Associate Dean for Clinical Affairs
University of South Alabama Hospitals
Mobile, Alabama
USA

Dafydd Thomas MB ChB FRCA
Consultant in Intensive Care
Intensive Therapy Unit
Morriston Hospital
Swansea
UK

Stephen J Thomas MD
Topkins-Van Poznak Distinguished Professor of Anesthesiology
Department of Anesthesiology
Weill Cornell Medical College
New York, New York
USA

Annemarie Thompson MD
Assistant Professor of Anesthesiology and Medicine
Department of Anesthesiology
Vanderbilt University Medical Center
Nashville, Tennessee
USA

Howard M Thompson MD
Consultant in Anesthesia and Pain Management
Pilgrim Hospital
Boston
UK

Simon Turner BSc(Hons) MBChB FRCA
Clinical Lecturer in Anaesthesia
Academic Unit of Anaesthesia
Leeds General Infirmary
Leeds
UK

Robert A Veselis MD
Associate Professor of Anesthesiology,
Director, Neuroanesthesiology Research Laboratory
Department of Anesthesiology/Critical Care Medicine
Memorial Hospital in Memorial Sloan-Kettering Cancer Center
New York, New York
USA

Mladen Vidovich MD
Department of Medicine
Northwestern University
Chicago, Illinois
USA

David O Warner MD
Professor of Anesthesiology
Mayo Clinic College of Medicine
Rochester, Minnesota
USA

Nigel R Webster MBChB PhD FRCA FRCP FRCS
Professor of Anaesthesia and Intensive Care
Academic Unit of Anaethesia and Intensive Care
Institute of Medical Sciences
University of Aberdeen
Aberdeen
UK

Ian G Wilson MBChB FRCA
Consultant Paediatric Anesthetist
Department of Anaesthesia
St James's University Hospital
Leeds
UK

Jay Yang MD PhD
Professor of Anesthesiology, Director of
Neurobiology Research in Anesthesia
Columbia University
College of Physicians & Surgeons
New York, New York
USA

William L Young MD
Professor of Anesthesia
Department of Anesthesia and Perioperative Care
UCSF
San Francisco, California
USA

Michael Zaugg MD DEAA
Head of Cardiovascular Anesthesia Laboratory
Institute of Anesthesiology
University Hospital
Zurich
Switzerland

Acknowledgement

We would like to acknowledge our mentors and students, who have taught us and from whom we continue to learn.

Dedication

To our wives Katherine Albert and Carmel Hopkins, whose countless contributions and support were vital.

SECTION 1

General principles

Chapter 1

Molecular structure and biochemistry

James Arden

TOPICS COVERED IN THIS CHAPTER

- **Properties of atoms and molecules**
  - Atoms
  - Bonding: the basis of molecular structure
  - Special properties
- **Biomolecular structure**
  - Amino acids and proteins
  - Lipids and membranes
  - Nucleic acids
  - Carbohydrates
- **Solution chemistry**
  - Solutions
  - Nonelectrolytes
  - Electrolytes
  - Diffusion and flow
  - Electrochemistry and acid–base chemistry
  - Chelation
  - Surface interactions
- **Enzymes**

In this chapter the fundamental ideas of molecular structure and principles of biochemistry, pharmacology, and physiology relevant to anesthesiology are introduced.

PROPERTIES OF ATOMS AND MOLECULES

Atoms

An atom consists of *elementary particles*: protons, neutrons, and electrons, and approximately 20 *subatomic particles* (mesons, bosons, etc.). The mass of the atom is provided principally by the *protons* and the slightly heavier *neutrons*. *Electrons* are much smaller and lighter, with a mass approximately 0.05% that of a proton. The number of protons (and electrons in an uncharged atom) is the *atomic number* (6, 7, and 8 for carbon, nitrogen, and oxygen, respectively), and the total mass of the protons plus neutrons is the *atomic mass* or *mass number* (12, 14, and 16 for carbon, nitrogen, and oxygen, respectively). Mass numbers are indicated by superscripts before the element symbol (e.g. ^{12}C, ^{14}N, ^{16}O). *Isotopes* are atoms with the same atomic numbers but with different atomic masses. Naturally occurring elements are found as mixtures of isotopes. For hydrogen, the hydrogen atom of atomic number 1 and atomic mass 1 (^{1}H) is about 5000 times more common than its stable isotope deuterium (^{2}H), which has one neutron (atomic number 1, atomic mass 2). The atomic mass of an element is actually the weighted average of the masses of the isotopes of that element. A *mole* of a substance contains as many atoms or molecules as there are atoms in exactly 12 g of ^{12}C (6.023×10^{23}). By analogy to atomic mass, the *molecular mass* of a molecule is described with reference to the mass of ^{12}C, hence the term 'relative' molecular mass.

Bonding: the basis of molecular structure

Atoms interact to form molecules by chemical bonds, which are described by two theories. The *valence bond theory* concentrates on the transfer (ionic bond) or sharing (covalent bond) of electrons and is the basis for traditional organic chemistry. *Molecular orbital theory* considers bonding as a coalescence of the electron orbitals (probabilistic electron density maps) of two atoms to create a new orbital that spreads over the entire molecule. To describe electron orbitals mathematically, electrons are described as waves, rather than as negatively charged points. Like light waves, sound waves, or sine waves, an electron wave is defined by a formula. Because an electron moves in three dimensions, its formula has *x*-, *y*-, and *z*-components; changes along the three axes are described by partial derivatives. As it is hard to freeze electrons in time and space, their location is defined as a probability (ψ). For example, $\partial^2\psi/\partial x^2$ is the derivative of ψ calculated in the *x*-dimension, with the *y*- and *z*-dimensions held constant. An electron has a small mass (m) that is included in energy calculations and, depending on its position, it also has potential energy (V). Adding constants to balance the function mathematically (h), electron energy (E) is defined in probability terms ($E\psi$) by Equation 1.1, the Schrödinger equation.

■ Equation 1.1

$$E\psi = V\psi + [(\partial^2\psi/\partial x^2) + (\partial^2\psi/\partial y^2) + (\partial^2\psi/\partial z^2)]\,(h/2m)$$

The solutions to this differential equation for a single particle are simple equations that can be plotted on a graph to give mathematical pictures of electron densities, called *orbitals*. The orbitals of molecules can be defined by combining the equations for the electron orbitals of individual atoms, which defines three types of molecular orbital (Fig. 1.1):

- those with a high probability of finding electrons (*bonding orbital*, s or p);
- those with a low probability of finding electrons (*antibonding orbital*, s* or p*); and
- those of lower energy, inner shell electrons that do not participate in bonding (*nonbonding*).

'Antibonding' does not refer to a repulsive interaction, but rather to an electron distribution determined from the wave equation that shows a low probability of finding an electron between the nuclei of the bonded atoms.

Special properties

RADICALS

Certain electron configurations are of special interest to physicians. *Radicals* (or free radicals) are molecules or atoms that contain one or more unpaired electrons. 'Pairing' of electrons refers to the orientation (+½ or −½) of the electron 'spin', which is an intrinsic property of electrons (like mass), rather than a spinning movement. Atoms such as Cl and Na (not the ions Na^+ and Cl^-) have unpaired electrons and are radicals.

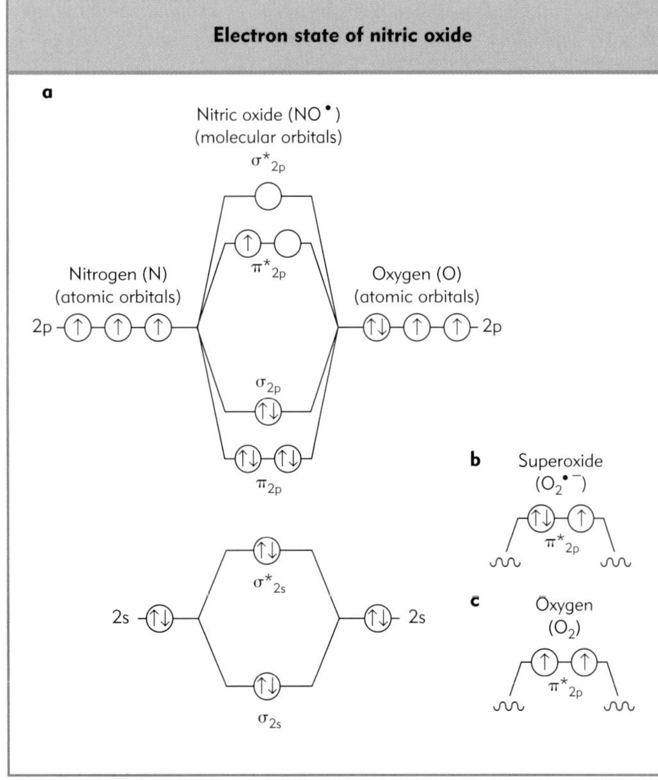

Figure 1.1 Electron diagram of nitric oxide. (a) Oxygen (eight electrons, $8e^-$) and nitrogen ($7e^-$) are the components of nitric oxide (NO). Electrons in the inner shells are not depicted. The remaining 11 electrons are shown for nitrogen (left) and oxygen (right). The molecular orbital model distributes these electrons into bonding and antibonding orbitals in order of increasing energy level: two into σ_{2s}, two into σ^*_{2s}, four into π_{2p}, two into σ_{2p}, and one into π^*_{2p}. The electron in a π^*_{2p} orbital remains unpaired, which defines $NO^\bullet$ as a radical. (b) An electron diagram for superoxide ($O_2^{\bullet-}$) distributes 16 electrons from the two oxygen atoms similarly, except that $3e^-$ are in the π^*_{2p}orbital. (c) Ground state oxygen (O_2) is also formally a radical and has one electron in each π^*_{2p} orbital with spins unpaired.

Nitric oxide ($NO^\bullet$) has an unpaired electron and is thus a radical. It is composed of N (nitrogen), which has seven electrons, and O (oxygen), which has eight electrons (see Fig. 1.1). The radical $NO^\bullet$ has received considerable attention as a diffusible modulator of cell signaling via the cyclic GMP pathway (Chapter 3) and as a direct vasodilator (Chapter 41). Another radical of physiologic interest is the *superoxide radical* ($O_2^{\bullet-}$), generated by the addition of an electron to molecular oxygen (O_2). Excessive production of superoxide induces *oxidative stress* and ultimately cell death. Superoxide is converted into less reactive products (hydrogen peroxide and oxygen) by the enzyme *superoxide dismutase*.

Nitric oxide and superoxide are biologically relevant free radicals.

DIPOLES

Because molecules consist of combinations of charged atoms, an uneven distribution of charge over the molecule can exist when atoms with different atomic numbers are combined. Most biomolecules, which combine N, C, O, H, and a few other atoms, have a complex distribution of charge. The charge of a molecule may also be distorted by an externally applied electric field, which need only be as large as a neighboring molecule with its own uneven charge distribution. When charges on a molecule are separated by a distance they constitute an *electric dipole*. The dipole is represented by a vector (which has magnitude and direction), which by convention points from the negative toward the positive charge, and is called the *dipole moment* (the unit is a Debye, or coulomb meter (Cm) in SI units, i.e. charge X distance). Some molecules are polar and have an *intrinsic* dipole moment. Nonpolar molecules, when placed in an externally applied electric field, can have an *induced* dipole. The dipole moment determines in part the solubility of molecules. A polar molecule with a large dipole moment is difficult to integrate into a nonpolar medium, such as the interior of the plasma membrane of a cell, which results in a slow transfer into the cell interior

MOLECULAR MAGNETISM

A moving charge generates a magnetic field. For molecules, the *electron spin* and *orbital motion* of electrons around the nucleus of each atom result in a molecular *magnetic moment*. When an external magnetic field is applied, molecules become oriented in the field according to their magnetic moment. Three types of interaction occur between the external field and the molecular magnetic moment: *diamagnetism*, *paramagnetism*, and *ferromagnetism*. If the molecular field opposes the external magnetic field, the material is referred to as *diamagnetic*. Diamagnetic molecules (such as N_2) have paired electron spins in the outer shell. If the molecular field augments the applied magnetic field, the molecule is termed *paramagnetic*. Paramagnetic molecules (such as O_2) have unpaired electron spins in the outer shell. In *ferromagnetic* materials, electron spins align in parallel and greatly augment an external magnetic field (by as much as 10^5). Magnetic interactions are the physical basis for oxygen analyzers (paramagnetism) and magnetic resonance imaging (ferromagnetism). Nuclear magnetic resonance manipulates molecular magnetism to define molecular structure.

STEREOCHEMISTRY

Stuctural issomers are molecules that have the same molecular formula but with the atoms arranged differently in space; for example, glucose, galactose, and mannose (all $C_6H_{12}O_6$) or isoflurane and enflurane (both $C_3H_2OF_5Cl$) are structural isomers with distinct structures and properties. In *stereoisomers*, molecules have identical structures except for the arrangement of substituents around one atom (the *stereocenter*), so that the two molecules are not superimposable on one another (e.g. pseudoephedrine is a stereoisomer of ephedrine). If the configuration of atoms around the stereocenter produces a mirror image of the original structure, the compounds are *chiral* and are called *enantiomers*.

Stereochemistry can be described according to three different systems, *optical activity*, *'relative' configuration*, and the *Cahn–Ingold–Prelog system*.

Approximately 60% of drugs used in anesthesia are chiral.

Optical activity is a property of molecules that can rotate plane-polarized light. *Dextrorotary* molecules have a positive (+) angle of rotation and rotate plane-polarized light to the right (or clockwise, as viewed when looking into the beam). *Levorotary* molecules have a negative (–) angle of rotation and rotate plane-polarized light counterclockwise. Molecules that can rotate plane-polarized light have a *chiral* (handed) center, are not superimposable on their mirror images, and are known as enantiomers. Enantiomeric pairs have identical chemical and physical properties (e.g. boiling point, density, solubility, absorption spectrum), but each enantiomer rotates plane-polarized light in the opposite direction. A mixture of equal amounts of enantiomers of a molecule is a *racemic* mixture, which is optically *inactive*. Racemic epinephrine (adrenaline) contains equal amounts of the two enantiomers of epinephrine.

Relative configuration defines the structure of a molecule as either the D or the L form by relating it to the two forms of a standard molecule, glutaraldehyde. Most naturally occurring sugars are of the D-configuration [e.g. D-(+)-glucose]. The optical rotation of a molecule, (+) or (–), is independent of its relative configuration. These two nomenclatures are sometimes confused by the use of the lower case *d* and *l* to denote optical rotation. Thus, *l*-epinephrine (optical rotation) and L-epinephrine (configuration) are not the same enantiomer; only *l*-epinephrine (the D-configuration) is biologically active.

The *Cahn–Ingold–Prelog* system can only be applied if the absolute stereochemistry is known. This system defines the *absolute configuration* based on the atomic mass of the four substituents attached to a chiral carbon center. The three highest mass number substituents at the chiral center are projected on to a triangle (the lowest mass substituent is projected backward behind the triangle) and ranked in order of decreasing mass number, starting with the highest mass at the top of the triangle. If the mass numbers of the substituents follow a clockwise direction from the top, the molecule is in the (*R*)-configuration; if it is counterclockwise, it is in the (*S*)-configuration. The stereochemical standard molecule is (*R*)-glyceraldehyde, which, coincidentally, is the same as D-(+)-glyceraldehyde. *Conformation* refers to the arrangements of a molecule that are achieved by rotation of substituents at a bond (the molecules are superimposable if correctly rotated), whereas the *configuration* (e.g. 'absolute configuration') of a molecule cannot be converted by bond rotation.

About 60% of drugs used in anesthesia are chiral. Chirality influences the actions of intravenous hypnotics: etomidate is administered as a single enantiomer, and the enantiomers of ketamine and thiopental have small differences in pharmacodynamic and pharmacokinetic effects. The volatile anesthetics in current use are racemic mixtures, except sevoflurane, which is achiral. The stereochemistry of local anesthetics is an important clinical consideration: e.g. levobupivacaine, the S-enantiomer of bupivacaine, has less effect on cardiac conduction than the racemic mixture. As synthetic and separation techniques improve, new drugs will be introduced as the single safest and most efficacious enantiomer.

BIOMOLECULAR STRUCTURE

Amino acids and proteins

The 20 common amino acids (Table 1.1) are distinguished by the side chains attached to the α-carbon. The side chains are chemically distinct, and are classified as nonpolar, polar uncharged, acidic, or basic. At neutral pH, amino acids and proteins are mostly in a form with both positive and negative charges (*zwitterions*). Amino acids are almost always of the L-form. Glycine, the simplest amino acid, is the only amino acid that is not chiral, as it has two hydrogens on the α-carbon. Amino acids can have other functions in addition to being components of

Table 1.1 Amino acid classification and abbreviations

Nonpolar	**Abbreviations**	
Aspartate	A	Asp
Cysteine	C	Cys
Phenylalanine	F	Phe
Glycine	G	Gly
Isoleucine	I	Ile
Leucine	L	Leu
Methionine	M	Met
Proline	P	Pro
Valine	V	Val
Tryptophan	W	Trp
Polar uncharged		
Asparagine	N	Asp
Glutamine	Q	Gln
Serine	S	Ser
Threonine	T	Thr
Tyrosine	Y	Tyr
Acidic		
Aspartic acid	D	Asp
Glutamic acid	E	Glu
Basic		
Histidine	H	His
Lysine	K	Lys
Arginine	R	Arg

proteins (for example glutamate and glycine are excitatory and inhibitory neurotransmitters, respectively).

Peptides are short chains of amino acids joined by *peptide bonds* (Fig. 1.2), and proteins are longer *polypeptides* (as long as 8000 amino acids). Both peptides and proteins are broken down by the addition of water (*hydrolysis*), which is catalyzed by enzymes called *proteases*. Proteins contain successive levels of organization, which endows them with complex three-dimensional structures (Fig. 1.3a). The *primary structure* is the sequence of amino acids. Certain *motifs*, or short segments of amino acids, are associated with cellular functions (e.g. NPXY for internalization of the low-density lipoprotein (LDL) receptor, where X is any amino acid) or identified as sites of enzyme action. Certain amino acids can be modified by the addition of a phosphoryl group (on Y, S, or T), carbohydrate chains (on O or N), or lipids (on S or N), thus affecting activity or subcellular location (Chapter 2).

Secondary structure incorporates more information into the protein by organizing some sections along the chain into regular conformations, such as the right-handed α-helix, (10–15 amino acids/turn) and the β-sheet. In the α-helix the polypeptide backbone is closely packed with hydrogen bonds at every fourth residue of the helix. The side chains project outward into the surrounding solution or environment. At a higher level of organization, sequences of approximately 70–100 amino acids are organized into *domains*, which are loosely defined organizational units that do not have distinct structures.

Tertiary structure is the overall pattern of folding or topology. Unlike secondary structure, which consists of repeating patterns, tertiary structure is diverse and results from interaction of the side chains that project from the peptide backbone. Through a variety of interactions, including hydrogen, electrostatic, hydrophobic and disulfide bonds (between the sulfur atoms on cysteine), a complex, energetically favorable conformation is generated. The tertiary structures of most soluble (i.e. neither membrane-bound nor transmembrane) proteins are tightly packed, water excluding, and stable. Tertiary structure is not static, as conformational changes are essential to protein functions such as catalysis, ligand binding, and signal transduction. The tertiary structures of thousands of proteins are known at the atomic level, and have been described by several methods, including *X-ray* and *electron diffraction* of protein crystals (Fig. 1.3b), and *mass spectrometry* and *nuclear magnetic resonance* of small proteins in solution. For example, structural studies of proteins have direct applications in medicine. X-ray diffraction analysis and molecular dynamic calculations of the structure of human immunodeficiency virus (HIV-1) protease have contributed to the rational structure-based development of HIV-1 protease inhibitors, which have dramatically altered the therapy of HIV infection.

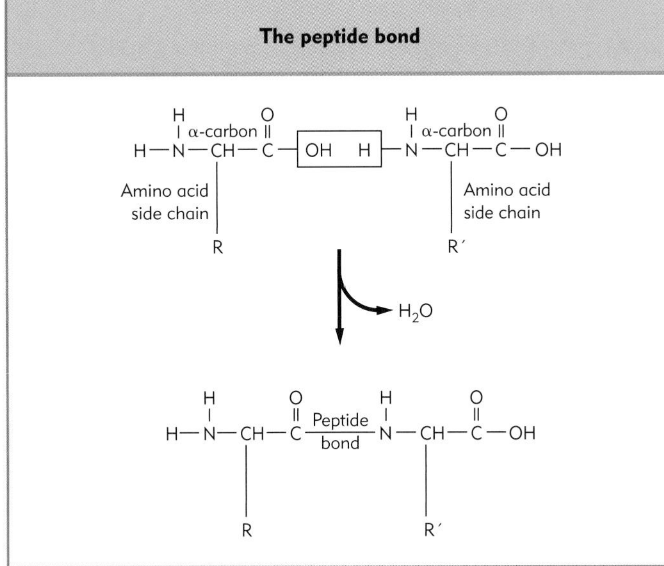

Figure 1.2 The peptide bond. The peptide bond of the polypeptide backbone is an amide bond formed by the condensation of carboxy and amino groups of amino acids. This bond has some double-bond character and acts as a rigid, planar unit. R and R′are linked to the α-carbon and denote the side-chain groups specific to each amino acid. The amino (N) terminus is on the left, and the carboxy (C) terminus is on the right.

Atomic structures of drug targets allow structure-based drug development.

Quarternary structure refers to the grouping of two or more proteins by noncovalent bonds. A well-known example is hemoglobin, which consists of two pairs of subunits (2α, 2β), each with its own tertiary structure. Interactions between the subunits alter their affinity for oxygen through conformational changes. Current experimental evidence favors a protein site of action for general anesthetics (Chapter 24). The lipid membrane had been proposed as the site of action of volatile anesthetics based on the observed correlation between volatile anesthetic potency and lipid solubility (Meyer–Overton hypothesis). The initial hypothesis of a global effect by anesthetic agents on membrane lipids was revised to suggest that the lipids surrounding membrane proteins (boundary lipids) and/or hydrophobic sites in proteins are the sites of anesthetic action. Much recent evidence, such as the existence of a 'cut off' in the length of long-chain hydrocarbons and alcohols which have anesthetic effects, the evidence for stereoselectivity in anesthetic effects, and the ability of point mutations in proteins to alter their sensitivity to anesthetics, strongly favors hydrophobic sites on cell membrane proteins, particularly the ion channels, as the sites of anesthetic action.

Lipids and membranes

The lipids of cell membranes are amphipathic; they have a *nonpolar* (or *hydrophobic*) *hydrocarbon tail* and a *polar* (or *hydrophilic*) *head group*. In the cell membrane lipid bilayer (Chapter 2), the tails are clustered in the interior and the head groups face the aqueous environments. Thus, the cell membrane is dynamic, and the lipids and proteins embedded in the membrane are able to move laterally within it (the fluid mosaic model of cell membrane structure), although specific membrane proteins can be immobilized to particular domains by interactions with anchoring proteins.

The head groups of *phospholipids* are small, charged molecules (e.g. serine, ethanolamine, choline) linked by a phosphate group to the hydrocarbon tail (Fig. 1.4). The hydrocarbon tail usually consists of two long-chain *fatty acids* linked by glycerol. The tail molecules may be of different lengths (14–24 carbons), and may be saturated ($-CH_2-CH_2-$) or unsaturated

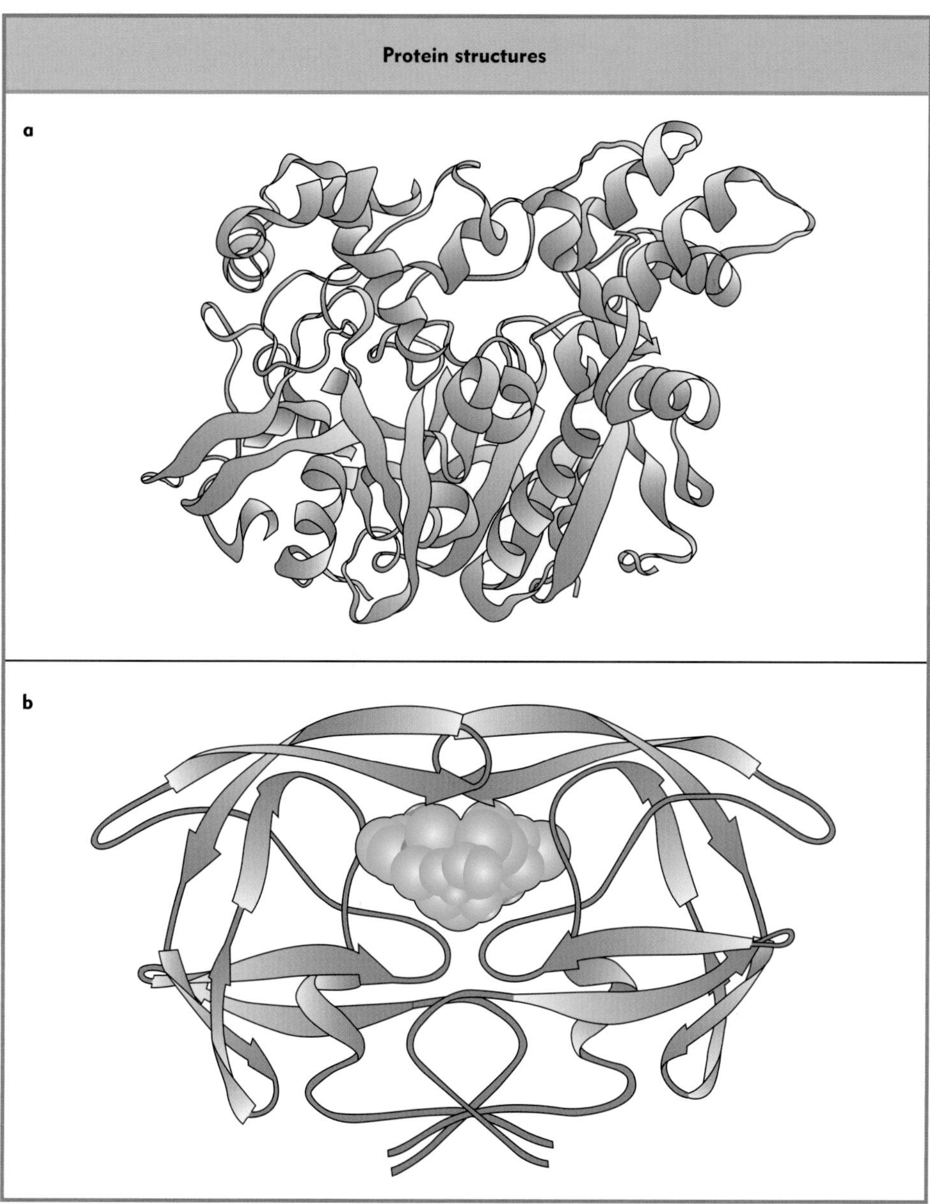

Figure 1.3 Protein structures. (a) In X-ray diffraction, X-rays (wavelength 1.5Å) are scattered by the atoms of the protein crystal. The regular, repeating arrangement of atoms, called a *crystal lattice*, acts like a *diffraction grating* and the X-rays are scattered in a pattern that is the reciprocal of the crystal lattice pattern. The structure of the molecule is calculated mathematically from this diffraction pattern by *Fourier transformation*. Here, a ribbon diagram of acetylcholinesterase from coordinates stored in the Brookhaven Protein Data Bank was generated using RasMol software. The substrate-binding site is within the open area slightly above center. (See Sussman JL, Harel M, Frolow F, *et al*. Atomic structure of acetylcholinesterase from *Torpedo californica*: a prototypic acetylcholine-binding protein. *Science* 1991;253:872–79.) (b) Human immunodeficiency virus (HIV) protease complexed with an inhibitor. The protease dimer is shown in ribbon form. The inhibitor molecule is colored blue. The twofold axis of symmetry of the dimer is vertical, in the plane of the figure. (See Silva AM, Cachau RE, Sham HL, Erickson JW. Inhibition and catalytic mechanism of HIV-1 aspartic protease. *J Mol Biol*. 1996;255;321–46.

(–CH=CH–). Saturated tails are straighter and more flexible than the kinked, unsaturated tails. The hydrocarbon tail is poorly soluble in water. The exclusion of water by collections of hydrocarbon chains allows an energetically more favorable arrangement of the water molecules, which stabilizes the hydrocarbon cluster. This is called the 'hydrophobic' effect, although the arrangement is more a property of water packing than of hydrocarbons excluding water. This water–hydrocarbon separation is the basis for the formation of the lipid bilayer of cell membranes.

The cell membrane is not symmetrical. Instead, the inner and outer leaflets of the membrane may contain different phospholipids. The inner leaflet contains more phosphatidylserine and phosphatidylethanolamine and the outer leaflet contains more phosphatidylcholine and sphingosine. Cholesterol, a planar steroid molecule, is a major component (about 20%) of mammalian plasma membranes. The rigidity of cholesterol helps to 'stiffen' the plasma membrane.

Lipids have functions in addition to membrane structure. *Phosphatidylinositol bisphosphate*, a phospholipid, is involved in G protein-coupled transmembrane signaling cascades (Chapter 3). LDL, a large complex of phospholipids and cholesterol packed together and bound to specific proteins, is a cholesterol storage and transport molecule, the regulation of which is critical in atherogenesis.

Nucleic acids

Nucleotides consist of a nitrogen-containing ring (a base) and a five-carbon sugar (ribose or deoxyribose) linked to a phosphate group. *Nucleosides* are composed of the base and the sugar minus the phosphate. The sugar is a five-carbon ribose ring which has a hydoxyl group (OH) in ribonucleosides or an H (in deoxynucleoside) at the 2′-position of the sugar ring. The bases are planar, aromatic heterocycles that contain carbon and nitrogen, and they are chemically classified as either purines (adenine,

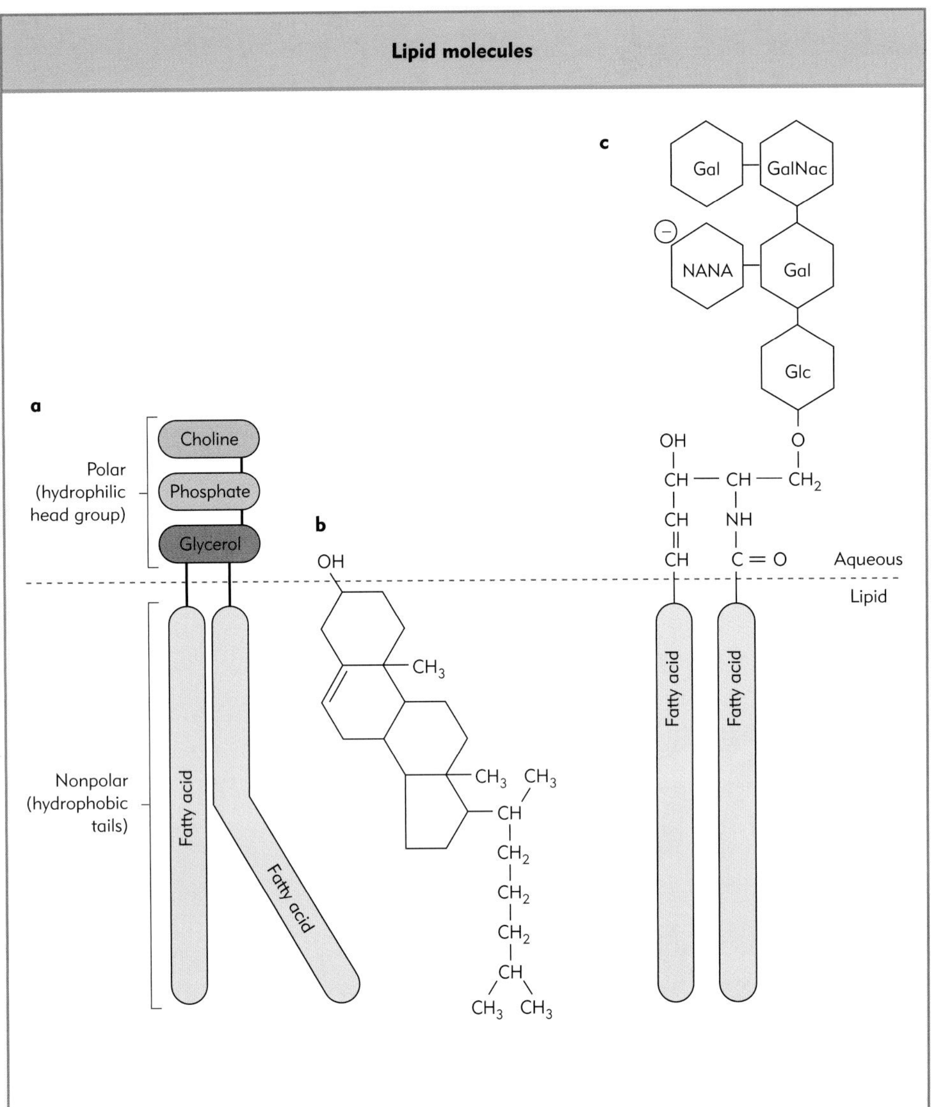

Figure 1.4 Lipid molecule structure. Lipid molecules have the same basic structure, consisting of a polar *head group* and a hydrophobic *tail.* (a) The tail may be extended as in the saturated fatty acid, or bent if double bonds (–C=C–) are present. (b) The head group may be small and the hydrocarbon tail compact as in cholesterol, or (c) the head group may be large and complex as in ganglioside GM_1, which contains several sugars. The overall structural elements are the same for each lipid. (Gal, galactose; Glc, glucose; GalNAc, *N*-acetylgalactosamine; NANA, *N*-acetylneuraminic acid.

A; guanine, G) or pyrimidines (thymine, T; uracil, U; cytidine, C). The bases are synthesized from the amino acids glutamine, glycine, and aspartate by tightly regulated enzymatic pathways.

The nucleotides are widely disseminated throughout the cell and are multifunctional. Encoding genetic information in linear sequences of the different nucleotides in DNA is the most celebrated role for these molecules (Chapter 4). Nucleotides in mRNA and tRNA also mediate the translation of this code into proteins. In addition to reproducing and processing genetic information, nucleotides function at some point in almost all intracellular processes. Nucleotides, especially ATP, are the functional storehouses for chemical energy in the cell. Hydrolysis of phosphate from these nucleotides releases the energy to power thousands of critical cellular reactions. Nucleotides are also components of intracellular signaling pathways (GTP in G proteins, cAMP) and are involved as cofactors (NAD, NADP) in the reactions of catalytic proteins. Volatile anesthetics can affect cyclic nucleotide levels (cGMP, cAMP) in some experimental models. The possibility of toxic interactions of anesthetics with DNA and chromosomes has long been an area of investigation, but so far no relationship has been clearly shown.

Carbohydrates

Sugars have carbons arranged in a straight chain or ring form with the general formula $(CH_2O)_n$, where $n = 3$ (triose), 5 (pentose, e.g. ribose), or 6 (hexose, e.g. glucose). Sugars are generally depicted in their closed ring form (Fig. 1.5). Chains of sugars may be linked together in pairs (e.g. sucrose = glucose–fructose, lactose = galactose–glucose). Longer chains, including branched chains, are *polysaccharides*, and shorter chains are *oligosaccharides*. A number of biologically important molecules are branched-chain polysaccharides, including red cell surface antigens and heparin.

The brain and red cells depend almost completely on glucose for energy. Glycogen, the storage form of glucose, is a polymer of glucose. Glucose is synthesized (*gluconeogenesis*) in the liver to provide an energy source for cells (Chapter 65). Gluconeogenesis and glucose breakdown (*glycolysis*) are not simply reversals of the same reactions. Rather, each pathway has its own energetically favorable reactions, mediated by different sets of enzymes. Gluconeogenesis involves the conversion of pyruvate to glucose via oxaloacetate (Equation 1.2), a molecule

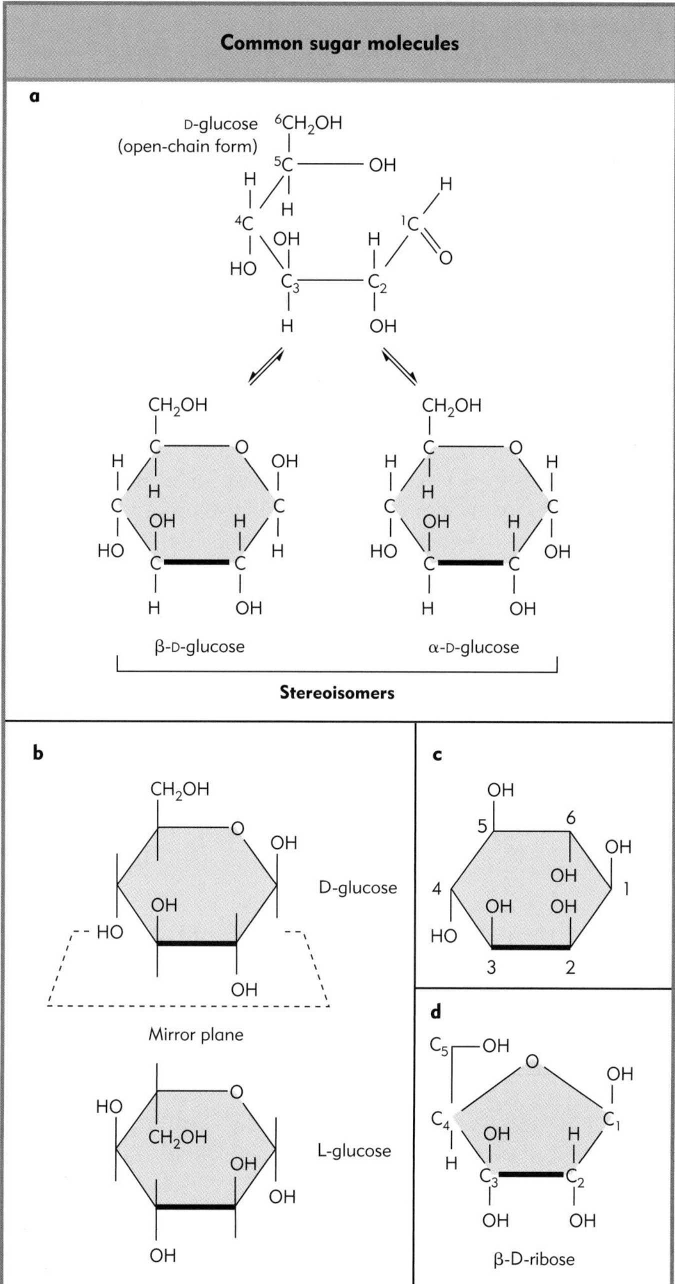

Figure 1.5 Common sugar molecules. (a) Opening the glucose ring and closing it during bonding can result in reconfiguration of the OH group at C1 into an α- or β-linkage. (b) The two enantiomers of glucose. (c) Inositol. Inositol 1,4,5-triphosphate (IP_3) with phosphates (PO_4) at the 1, 4, and 5 positions, is an intracellular signaling molecule. (d) Ribose. In RNA, the phosphate backbone of ribose is attached at the 3- and 5-positions.

from which CO_2 is removed in order to provide a favorable energy balance for glucose synthesis.

■ Equation 1.2

$$\underset{\text{pyruvate}}{C_3H_3O_3} \rightarrow \text{oxaloacetate} \rightarrow \underset{\text{glucose}}{C_6H_{12}O_6}$$

After breakdown, glycerol (derived from fats), and some amino acids, enter the glucose synthetic pathway as pyruvate. Other amino acids enter as other intermediates, which can be converted to pyruvate in the series of reactions referred to as the *citric acid cycle*.

To generate energy, glucose is metabolized (Equation 1.3), during which electrons and protons are removed from glucose and utilized in the two processes of *glycolysis* and *oxidative phosphorylation*, to convert glucose ultimately into CO_2 and water (Chapter 65):

■ Equation 1.3

$$\underset{\text{glucose}}{C_6H_{12}O_6} \rightarrow \underset{\text{pyruvate}}{C_3H_3O_3} \rightarrow CO_2 + H_2O + \text{energy}$$

The removal of an electron is called *oxidation*, hence glucose is *oxidized* during glycolysis. The addition of an electron (a negative charge) is called *reduction*. In the oxidative breakdown of glucose during glycolysis, nicotinamide adenine dinucleotide (NAD^+) is the primary oxidizing agent of glucose, from which it removes electrons and protons, and is itself converted into NADH. Electrons transferred from glucose to NADH then enter the oxidative phosphorylation pathway, where sequential oxidation-reduction steps result in the ultimate reduction of O_2 to H_2O with the release of energy.

Carbohydrates have other cellular functions in addition to storing and releasing metabolic energy. Inositol (Fig. 1.5d) is phosphorylated to different degrees with 1–4 phosphates and acts as an intracellular signaling molecule (Chapter 3). A variety of cellular proteins and lipids are also modified by oligosaccharides, often creating hydrophilic and antigenic sites on cell surface and extracellular matrix proteins.

SOLUTION CHEMISTRY

Solutions

A *solution* is a mixture of two or more components that makes a homogenous dispersion in a single phase. The component in the greater amount is the *solvent* and that in the lesser is the *solute*. As there are three states of components (solid, liquid, and gas), nine solute–solvent combinations are possible. Anesthesia involves solid–liquid, gas–gas, and gas–liquid solutions, which are the usual drug delivery and disposition combinations. Note that a vapor refers to the gaseous form of any substance that is either liquid or solid under normal conditions of temperature and pressure (e.g. isoflurane). The *colligative properties* of a solution depend primarily on the number of solute particles, and include osmotic pressure, vapor pressure lowering, freezing point lowering, and boiling point elevation.

Concentrations of the components of a solution are defined in several ways. *Molarity* is the number of moles of solute per liter of solution (mol/L). Note that the denominator is for the total solution, not the volume of solvent. Molarity is temperature dependent, as the solvent expands or contracts as temperature changes. *Molality* is defined as moles of solute per kilogram (mol/kg) of solvent. Note that the denominator is mass. Molality has experimental advantages because it is not temperature dependent and is useful in examining colligative properties. The *mole fraction* (X_A) is used to calculate partial pressures of gases and in working with vapor pressures, and is defined as '(moles of component A)/(moles of all components)'. In considering the properties of a solution it is valuable to recognize that, as a result of solute interactions, the properties of the solution are not simply the additive sum of the properties of each component.

Nonelectrolytes

Nonelectrolytes do not form ions when placed in water solution. Solutions of nonelectrolytes are defined as either ideal or real. In an ideal solution, made by mixing components with similar properties, no change in component properties (e.g. vapor pressure, refraction of light, viscosity, surface tension) occurs on mixing the components. This implies an absence of attractive forces between molecules in gas mixtures, or a complete uniformity of attractive forces among liquid molecules. In an ideal solution, the properties of the components are equal to the properties of a pure solution of each individual component multiplied by the mole fraction of that component. As an example, consider *vapor pressure*, which is defined as the tendency of molecules of a liquid to escape from the liquid phase into the vapor phase. If the vapor pressure of component A (p_A) in a solution is proportional to the vapor pressure of the pure component (p^*_A) times its mole fraction (X_A), then the solution is an *ideal* solution and $p_A = X_A p^*_A$. This is referred to as Raoult's Law.

When a component is a minor part of a dilute solution, the vapor pressure is no longer directly proportional to the vapor pressure of the pure component, as in an ideal solution. In this case, Raoult's Law is not obeyed and these solutions are called *real* or *nonideal*. In real solutions, the property (e.g. vapor pressure, p_B) of component B is described by an experimentally determined proportionality constant specific to the component (K_B), rather than by the vapor pressure of the pure component. Thus, for the minor component in a real solution, $p_B = X_B K_B$, where X_B is the mole fraction of B. This is Henry's Law, which is usually applied to very low concentrations of gases in liquid solutions, such as anesthetics in solution. Henry's Law describes the pressure of the minor component gas above the solution. The law also describes the remaining amount of the gas, which is dissolved in the solution. The concentration of the gas which is dissolved in the solution at equilibrium defines the *solubility* of the gas. Henry's Law states that the solubility of a gas in a solution increases in direct proportion to the pressure on the gas. A practical application of this law comes from the physiology of diving, where nitrogen, which is in solution in a diver's blood at depth, becomes less soluble and can form bubbles in the blood as pressure decreases upon surfacing.

Electrolytes

When dissolved in water, electrolytes form ions, conduct electric current, and have exaggerated (compared with nonelectrolytes) freezing point depression and boiling point elevation (colligative properties). Electrolytes are classified as strong (e.g. NaCl, HCl) or weak (e.g. acetic acid, ammonium hydroxide). Strong electrolytes are highly dissociated in water solution, but in moderately concentrated solutions the large number of positive and negative charges results in electrostatic attractions between ions. One result of electrostatic attraction is that the ions sometimes form *ion pairs*, rather than being free. The net result of these attractions between ions is that the 'effective' concentration of ions is lower than the actual concentration, which gives rise to the use of *activity*, rather than concentration, to describe ionic solutions.

Diffusion and flow

Diffusion is the transport by random motion of particles down a concentration gradient. *Electrical conduction* is the transport of charge down a potential gradient, and *thermal conduction* is the transport of energy (thermal motion) down a temperature gradient. Somewhat less intuitive than these processes is *viscosity*, which involves the transport of momentum. To approach viscosity, the idea of *flux* must be examined. Flux is a *rate* of movement and is dependent on a *gradient* of the property that is moving. The flux (J) of a particle is its rate of diffusion (in one direction) along its concentration gradient (in the same direction). If C is the concentration along a gradient, $J = -D(\partial C/\partial x)$, where x is a distance along the gradient and D is the diffusion coefficient (the minus sign indicates that movement is toward decreasing concentration). This is Fick's First Law of Diffusion. The usual model for viscosity is a series of liquid plates stacked together and moving along the x-axis. As the top plate moves, it drags the plates beneath it. Successively lower plates are accelerated to a lesser extent, so a *gradient* occurs in the velocity of the plates down the z-direction. The rate of movement in the x-direction (flux, J_x) is proportional to the gradient in velocity (v) down the plates in the z-direction, $J \propto \partial v/\partial z$. A constant can be substituted for the proportionality sign, $J_x = \eta(\partial v/\partial z)$, where η is the viscosity coefficient that describes the amount of drag between the plates. Viscosity is a determinant of gas and liquid flow through a tube, which is described by *Poiseuille's Law* for laminar flow through a cylinder, $\delta V/\delta t = [(P_a - P_b)\pi r^4]/(8\eta l)$, where V is the volume of gas or liquid, P_a and P_b are the pressures at each end, l is the length, and r is the radius.

Electrochemistry and acid–base chemistry

Acid–base chemistry is intimately tied to electrochemistry – the movement of protons (H^+) is the movement of positive charge and results in ionization. The pH of a solution is determined by measuring the *electromotive force*, the potential difference in a reversible electrochemical cell when no current flows. More commonly, pH is defined as the negative logarithm of the proton concentration, $pH = -\log_{10}[H^+]$. The measurement of pH relative to the pH of water (pH = 7.0) leads to the definition of an *acid* as a proton donor, $HA \rightarrow H^+ + A^-$, where A^- is the *conjugate base* of acid HA. A *base* is a proton acceptor, $B^- + H^+ \rightarrow BH$, and BH is the *conjugate acid*. More general definitions also exist: a Lewis acid is an electron-pair acceptor and a Lewis base is an electron-pair donor. The extent of dissociation of the acid HA is quantified by the dissociation constant $K_a = [H^+][A^-]/[HA]$. Separating the proton concentration and taking the negative $\log_{10}$ of both sides gives Equation 1.4, the Henderson–Hasselbach equation.

Equation 1.4

$$pH = pK_a + \frac{\log [A^-]}{[HA]}$$

The pK_a is the pH at which the concentrations of A^- and HA are equal. The pH may be calculated from this equation if the ratio of $[A^-]/[HA]$ is known, but it is only accurate between pH 3 and 11 (beyond this range water ionization must be included).

A *buffer* can be made to attenuate pH changes by combining a weak acid and its conjugate base (i.e. the salt of its conjugate base). Combining a weak base and its conjugate acid also makes a buffer. The buffering capacity is the quantity of acid (or base) that may be added to a buffer to change the pH by one unit. Buffers are most effective (permit the smallest pH change) in the region of their pK_a. Bicarbonate ($pK_a = 6.1$) is the principal buffer in blood.

Bicarbonate, a weak base, is the principle buffer in blood.

Chelation

In general, a *metal* is a substance that conducts heat and electricity, and in each case the conduction is the result of the movement of electrons within the material. Metal ions commonly found in biology include iron, cobalt, and magnesium. If a Lewis base, which was described earlier as an electron pair donor, has two or more groups of electrons available, it may combine with a metal to form a complex called a *chelate*. In biology, naturally occurring chelating compounds are polycyclic molecules such as heme, which complexes iron, and chlorophyll, which complexes magnesium. Drugs that form chelation complexes include EDTA, which chelates iron and copper to prevent oxidation in drug preparations and binds calcium in banked blood; and deferoxamine, which chelates iron.

Surface interactions

The surface at which a phase interaction (between gas–liquid, solid–liquid, etc.) occurs is an *interface*. If a liquid forms an interface with a gas, the cohesive force of the molecules of liquid holds the liquid together. A small attractive force also occurs between the liquid and the gas. The work that must be done (or the energy expended) to counteract this attraction at the interface is the *surface tension*. Surface tension is a critical factor in defining the relationship between the pressure inside a cavity and the cavity curvature (the *Laplace relation*, $P_{in} = P_{out} + 2\gamma/r$, where γ is the surface tension and r is the radius of curvature). Extensions of this relationship to the ventricle and the alveolus are important in cardiac (Chapter 39) and pulmonary physiology (Chapter 47). The units of surface tension are those of energy/area ($ergs/cm^2$) or force/distance (dyne/cm). *Adsorption* refers to the movement of molecules in solution to an interface, which results in an interface concentration higher than that of the solution. Molecules and ions that are adsorbed at interfaces are called *surfactants* (surface-active agents), which are essential to pulmonary alveolar function

ENZYMES

Enzymes *catalyze* chemical reactions, that is, they lower the *activation energy barrier* between products and reactants or substrates (Fig. 1.6). Enzymes are usually proteins, though ribonucleotides can catalyze reactions of RNA (ribozymes). Enzymes can increase the *rate* of a reaction by as much as a billion times over the rate of the spontaneous reaction, but they do not change the equilibrium (ratio of products to reactants) of a reaction, and cannot by themselves drive an energetically unfavorable reaction. A cell has thousands of enzymes. Some enzymes catalyze specific reactions, whereas others facilitate reactions of several related substrates. The large number of enzymes led to the development of an enzyme classification (EC) system. An enzyme is classified as an (1) oxidoreductase, (2) transferase, (3) hydrolase, (4) lyase, (5) isomerase, or (6) ligase. Plasma cholinesterase, also known as butyrylcholinesterase, is a hydrolase that breaks down the ester bond of succinylcholine and other esters.

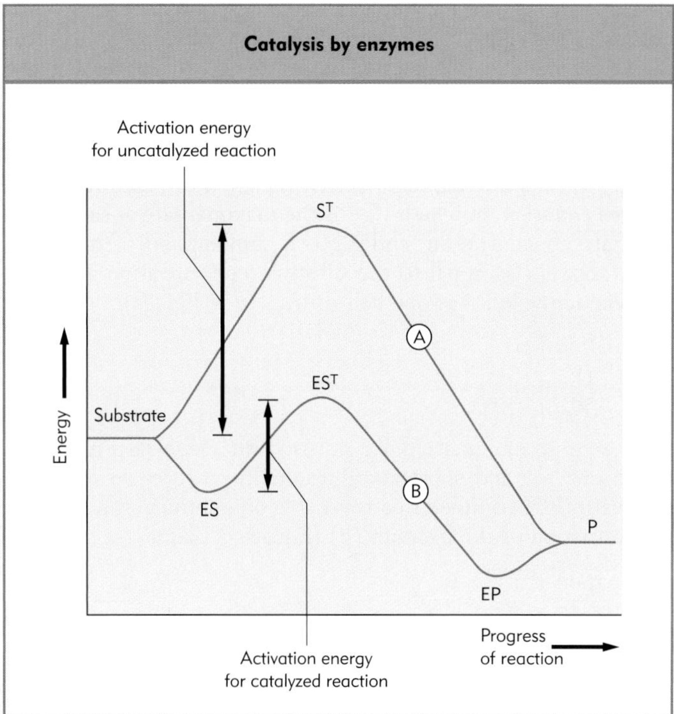

Figure 1.6 Catalysis by enzymes. Enzymes accelerate chemical reactions by decreasing the activation energy. Often both the uncatalyzed reaction (A) and the enzyme-catalyzed reaction (B) go through several transition states. It is the transition state with the highest energy (S^T and ES^T) that determines the activation energy and limits the rate of the reaction.

Enzymes enhance the rate, but do not change the equilibrium, of chemical reactions.

Enzymes catalyze reactions in three basic ways:

- distorting a bond of the substrate;
- proton transfer to or from the substrate; or
- electron donation to or withdrawal from the substrate.

In each case the few amino acid residues involved in catalysis are positioned together from separate parts of the polypeptide chain by precise protein folding to create an *active site* (see Fig. 1.3). The active site usually contains amino acids such as C, H, S, D, E, and K, which have available protons or electrons or can bind with a substrate. Prosthetic groups are also located at active sites, which, as shown by X-ray diffraction studies, are actually pockets or grooves in enzymes where the substrate binds. Most naturally occurring amino acids are of the L-configuration, and it is consistent that enzymes are *stereospecific* in their choice of substrates.

The rate of an enzyme-catalyzed reaction increases with increasing substrate concentration. At high substrate concentrations, the increase in reaction rate attained by increasing the substrate concentration reaches a limit (i.e. the reaction is *saturable*), which is reflected by the hyperbolic shape of the plot of reaction velocity (v) versus substrate concentration [S] (Fig. 1.7a). This curve is described by Equation 1.5, the *Michaelis–Menten equation*, in which V_{max} is the maximal rate at saturating substrate concentration, and K_m is a combination of rate constants that is also equal to the substrate concentration at which the reaction velocity is one half of V_{max} ($v = V_{max}/2$).

■ Equation 1.5

$$v = \frac{(V_{max}\,[S])}{(K_m + [S])}$$

The curve of Equation 1.5 is based on a two-step model in which enzyme and substrate join initially to form an enzyme–substrate (ES) complex in a reversible equilibrium, followed by the formation of the product (P) (Equation 1.6).

■ Equation 1.6

$$E + S \underset{k_{-1}}{\overset{k_1}{\rightleftharpoons}} ES \xrightarrow{k_{cat}} E + P$$

The term k_{cat} describes the maximum number of substrate molecules converted into product per active site per unit time, or how often the enzyme 'turns over'. The k_{cat}/K_m value is a measure of an enzyme's *efficiency* as a catalyst: if $k_{cat}/K_m = k_1$ the enzyme is 100% efficient, and catalyzes a reaction every time it encounters a substrate molecule. In this case, the reaction is *diffusion rate limited*, that is, the reaction proceeds as quickly as substrate and enzyme make contact and product leaves. Acetylcholinesterase is an example of a nearly perfectly efficient enzyme in these terms.

Replotting the velocity–substrate concentration plot as the reciprocals gives a linear plot of 1/[S] versus $1/v$ (Fig. 1.7b). These plots are imperfect, but are useful to describe different enzyme inhibitors (Figs 1.7c–e). In *competitive inhibition*, substrate and inhibitor compete for the substrate-binding site on the enzyme. In *uncompetitive* inhibition, the inhibitor binds to the enzyme–substrate complex but not to the free enzyme. In *noncompetitive inhibition*, the inhibitor binds the enzyme at a site that inhibits both catalysis and substrate binding.

Enzyme action may also be modulated by *allosteric regulation*. A modulator or *regulator* binds to the enzyme at a distinct site and either enhances or inhibits the binding of the substrate with the enzyme or its catalytic efficiency. Many enzymes that are allosterically regulated are composed of two or more protein subunits bound together – one subunit binds the regulator (*regulatory subunit*) and the other contains the active site (*catalytic subunit*). These functions may also be achieved by separate domains of the same protein. These diverse regulatory mechanisms are essential to the adaptability of cellular regulation in response to various normal and pathological conditions.

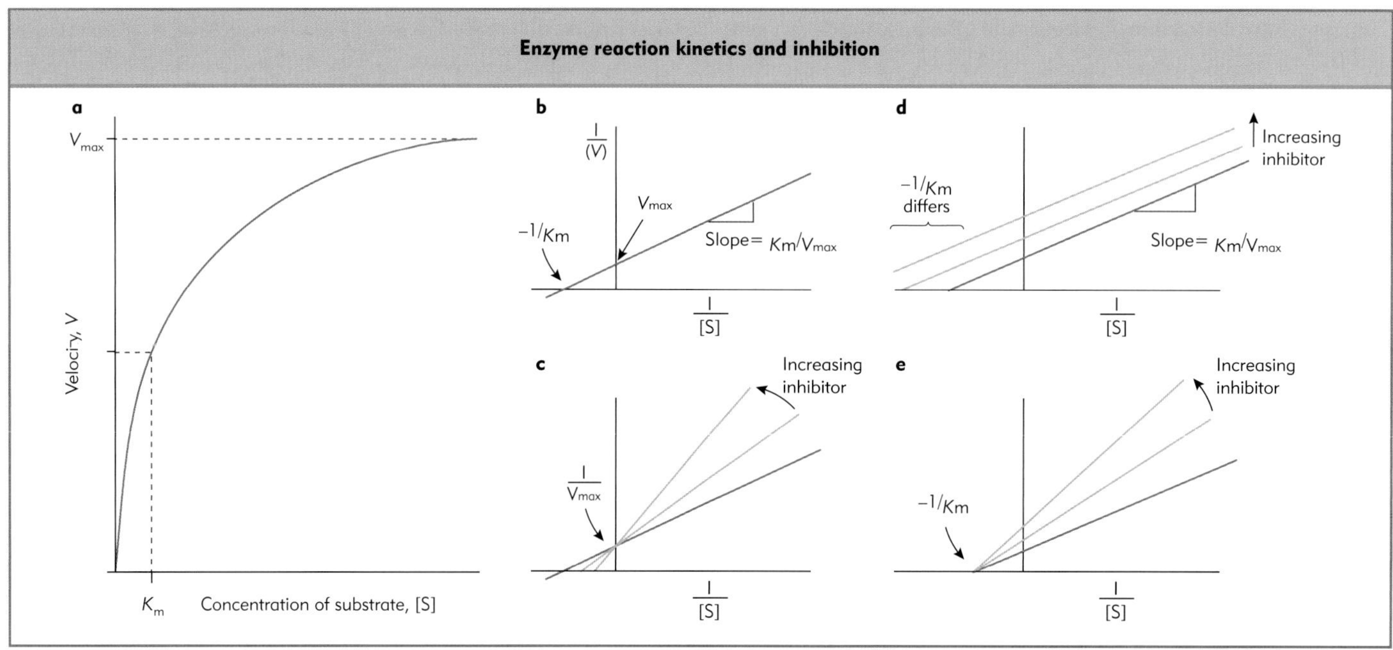

Figure 1.7 Enzyme reaction kinetics and inhibition. (a) Enzyme reaction velocity is described by a plot of velocity (V) versus substrate concentration [S]. (b–e) Different types of enzyme inhibition are described by *double reciprocal plots* of $1/V$ versus 1/[S] – the values of the normal plot (b) are shown in dark blue in each plot. (c) In competitive inhibition, all lines intersect the y-axis at $1/V_{max}$. (d) In uncompetitive inhibition, the slopes (K_m/V_{max}) are parallel. (e) In noncompetitive inhibition, lines intersect the x-axis (1/[S]) at $-1/K_m$.

Key References

Alberts B, Johnson A, Lewis J, Raff M, Roberts K, Walter P. Molecular biology of the cell, 4th edn. New York: Garland Science Publishing; 2002.

Atkins PW. Physical chemistry, 6th edn. New York: Freeman and Co.; 1997.

Creighton TE. Proteins, 2nd edn. New York: Freeman and Co.; 1993.

Ferscht A. Enzyme structure and mechanisms, 2nd edn. New York: Freeman and Co.; 1985.

Martin A. Physical pharmacy principles in the pharmaceutical sciences, 4th edn. New York: Williams & Wilkins; 1993.

Voex D, Voex JG. Biochemistry, 2nd edn. New York: John Wiley; 1995.

Further Reading

Bonner FT. Nitric oxide, Part A: nitric oxide gas. Meth Enzymol. 1996;268:50–7.

Calvey TN. Isomerism and anaesthetic drugs. Acta Anaesth Scand. 1995;39:83–90.

Egan TD. Stereochemistry and anesthetic pharmacology: joining hands with the medicinal chemists. Anesth Analg. 1996;83:447–50.

Halliwell B, Gutteridge MC. Oxygen radicals in biological systems, Part B: Role of free radicals and catalytic metal ions in human disease: an overview. Meth Enzymol. 1990;186:1–85.

Nau C, Strichartz GR. Drug chirality in anesthesia. Anesthesiology 2002;97:497-502.

Chapter 2

Biology of the cell

Misha A Perouansky

TOPICS COVERED IN THIS CHAPTER

- **Cellular death, ageing and immortality**
  - Apoptosis and necrosis
  - Senescence
  - Extending lifespan
  - Immortality – stem cell technology
- **The cell cycle**
  - Cyclins
  - Chromosomes
  - Mitosis and regulation of the cell cycle
  - Oncogenes
  - Benefits of cellular senescence and mortality
  - Meiosis
- **Cell compartments**
  - Membrane structure
  - Nucleus
  - Mitochondria
  - Endoplasmic reticulum
  - Intracellular degredation
- **The cytoskeleton: structure and movement**
  - Actin
  - Myosin
  - Microtubules
  - Filaments
- **Protein synthesis, folding and modification**
- **Protein transport and secretion**

The cell is the fundamental building block of all organisms. It is the closest thing to an autonomous biological unit that exists.

Modern living organisms fall into three lineages, domains or kingdoms (Fig. 2.1). *Prokaryotes*, which lack a defined nucleus and have a simplified internal organization, form two of the lineages – the *bacteria* and the *archeae*. *Eukaryotes* form the third lineage. Prokaryotes have only one chromosome, are haploid (i.e. they have only a single copy of the chromosome) and, from a biological point of view, are potentially immortal. All other forms of life have at least two copies of usually multiple chromosomes (i.e. they are either di- or polyploid). This complexity has enabled eukaryotes to evolve into more complicated multicellular organisms, but has also made them mortal (i.e. subject to ageing and death).

CELLULAR DEATH, AGEING AND IMMORTALITY

Apoptosis and necrosis

Cellular death is defined as the complete absence of active metabolism, and can be initiated in various distinct ways. At the extremes of the spectrum are *apoptosis* (programmed cell death) and *necrosis* (accidental cell death) or *oncolysis*. Neither is necessarily linked to ageing (senescence). Apoptosis is an essential part of life for any multicellular organism. The process of apoptosis is genetically programmed, but is activated only in those cells destined to die. During development, apoptosis is used to sculpt tissues (e.g. embryogenesis, metamorphosis) and to select competent T and B lymphocytes. Later, it is essential for hormone-regulated tissue atrophy as well as the elimination of virally infected or mutated cells. Autoimmune diseases, immunodeficiencies, malignancies, ischemia and other diseases involve the dysregulation of apoptosis.

Apoptosis is a genetically programmed cell death pathway involved in physiologic as well as pathologic processes.

Apoptosis is triggered either by extrinsic receptor-mediated or intrinsic mitochondria-mediated signaling pathways that induce death-associated proteolytic and/or nucleolytic activities (Fig. 2.2). Activation of death receptors in the extrinsic pathway is followed by the formation of a signaling complex that induces cell death via activation of caspases (cysteine-dependent aspartate-specific proteases). In the intrinsic pathway, death signals act either directly or indirectly on mitochondria, causing the release of cytochrome c, which leads to the formation of an apoptosome complex and caspase activation. In both pathways, the dying cell undergoes a characteristic sequence of histologic events: nuclear compaction (karyopyknosis), chromatin condensation, internucleosomal cleavage of DNA, blebbing of the

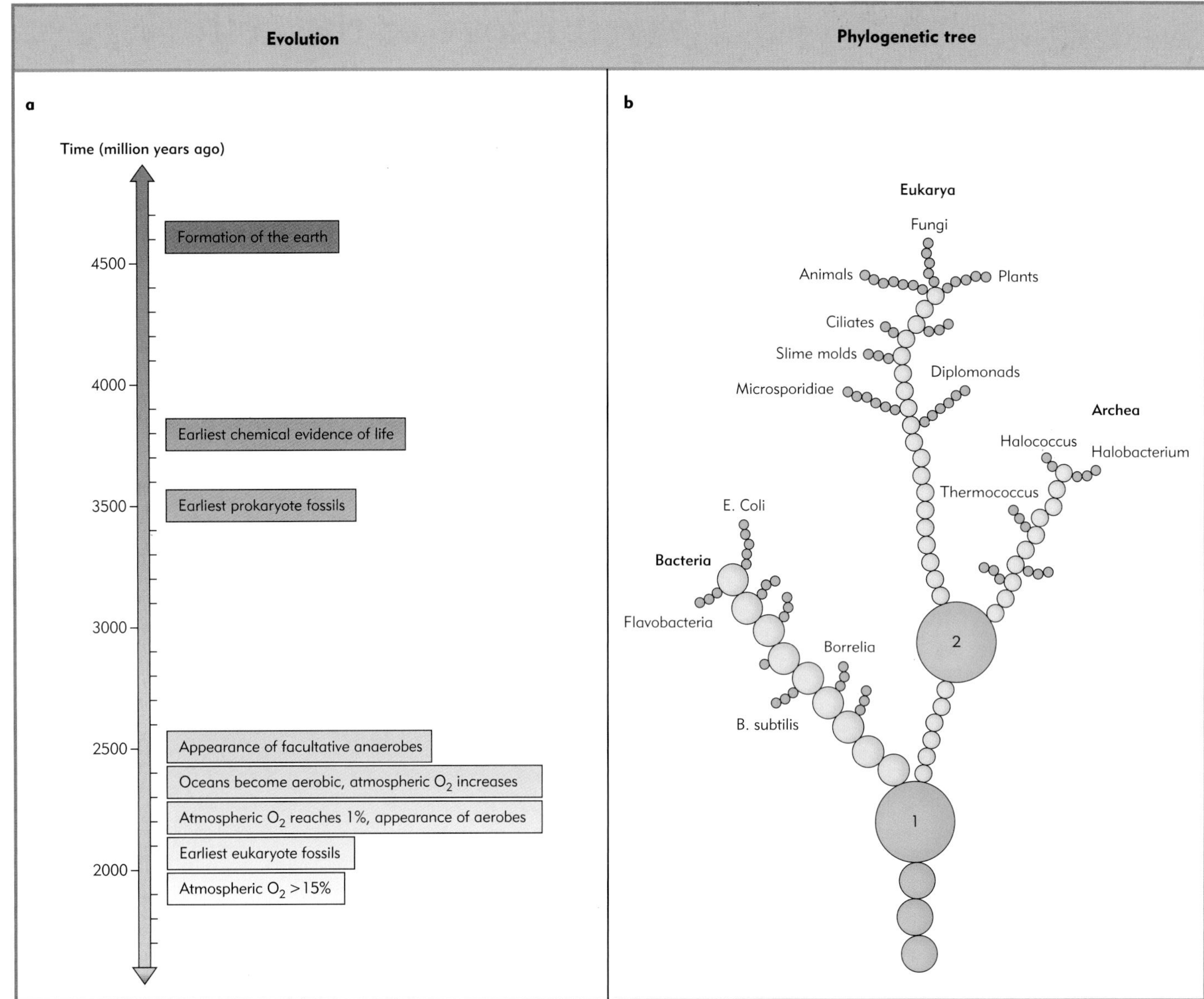

Figure 2.1 Evolution. Geological intervals during the first 4 billion years of the earth's history. (a) By 3900 Myr (million years) ago, liquid water, a prerequisite for life, was present. The atmosphere consisted mostly of water, nitrogen, hydrogen methane, reduced sulfur gases, carbon monoxide and carbon dioxide at 100–1000 times PAL (present atmospheric level). Life may have originated many times, only to be wiped out by meteorite impacts large enough to sterilize the planet's surface. Fossils resembling prokaryotic cyanobacteria have been identified in 3500 Myr-old rocks, and by 544 Myr ago multicellular eukaryotic plants and animals were abundant. (b) **Phylogenetic tree of the three extant kingdoms (domains)**. The last common ancestors of Archea, Bacteria and Eukarya (progenotes) had very high mutation rates, but the primary evolutionary mechanism was lateral gene transfer. As the organisms became more complex, lateral gene transfer became more restricted and mutations were the driving force of evolution. The last common ancestor of the two bacterial kingdoms (Archaea and Bacteria) was a thermophilic, sulfur-dependent anaerobe (1; green field), pointing to deep-sea vents as a potential site for the origin of life. Other types of organisms may have evolved from the universal ancestors and become extinct.

plasma membrane (zeiosis), and disintegration of the cell into multiple vesicles that are taken up by neighboring cells without causing an inflammatory response. This orderly series of events is orchestrated by dozens of genes, including a family of 'inhibitors of apoptosis' genes. The balance between apoptosis-promoting and -inhibiting proteins is often disturbed in human tumors: high expression of antiapoptotic proteins (Bcl-2, Bcl-x_L, Bcr-Abl) and/or inactivation of proapoptotic tumor suppressor proteins (p53, p19^{arf}) are common.

Necrosis is a distinct form of cell death often associated with edema (organelle swelling), vacuolation of the cytoplasm, karyolysis and cell lysis without the formation of vesicles, hence the alternate term oncolysis. Cellular contents are spilled into the extracellular space, damaging neighboring cells and inducing an inflammatory response. Whereas apoptosis typically affects isolated cells scattered throughout the tissue, necrotic cells are usually found in contiguous zones. Necrosis is an important component in a number of neurodegenerative conditions, as well as acute ischemic insults to the myocardium and the brain. Until recently, necrotic cell death was regarded as an unregulated process, too chaotic for underlying biochemical regulatory pathways to be identified. The current model of necrotic cell death

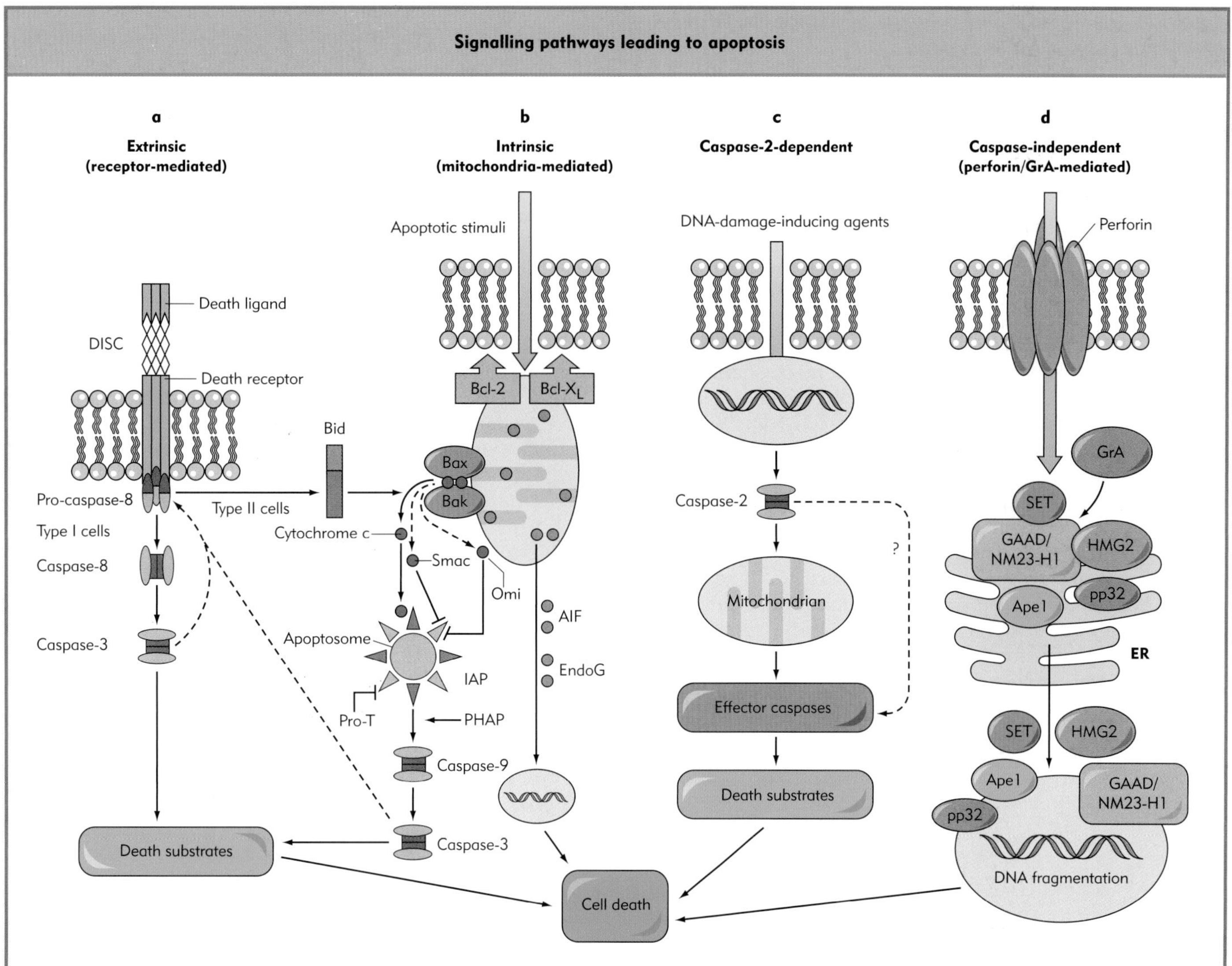

Figure 2.2 Signaling pathways leading to apoptosis. (a) The extrinsic receptor-mediated pathway. Ligation of the death receptor is followed by formation of the death-inducible signaling complex (DISC), which results in the activation of caspase-8. In type I cells, caspase-8 activates caspase-3, which cleaves target proteins, leading to apoptosis. In type II cells, caspase-8 cleaves Bid, which in turn induces the translocation, oligomerization and insertion of Bax and/or Bak into the mitochondrial outer membrane. Subsequent release of several proteins from the mitochondrial intermembrane space, including cytochrome c, forms a cytosolic apoptosome complex with apoptosis activating factor-1 (Apaf-1) and caspase-9 in the presence of d-ATP. This results in the activation of procaspase-9, which leads to the activation of caspase-3. The yellow circle represents a complex of Apaf-1, procaspase-9, and dATP (apoptosome). (b) The intrinsic mitochondria-mediated pathway. Death signals function directly or indirectly on the mitochondria, resulting in the formation of the apoptosome complex. This cell death pathway is controlled by Bcl-2 family proteins (regulation of cytochrome c release), inhibitor of apoptosis proteins (IAPs, inhibition of caspases), second mitochondrial activator caspases (Smac) and Omi (negative regulation of IAPs). Apoptosome function is also regulated by the oncoprotein prothymosin-a (Pro-T) and the tumor suppressor putative HLA-DR-associated protein (PHAP). The intrinsic pathway might also operate through caspase-independent mechanisms, which involve the release from mitochondria and translocation to the nucleus of at least two proteins, apoptosis inducing factor (AIF) and endonuclease G (EndoG). The nuclear location of AIF is linked to chromatin condensation and the appearance of high-molecular-mass chromatin fragments, whereas the role of EndoG is still unclear. (c) Caspase-2-dependent pathway. The activation of caspase-2 by DNA damage leads to the release of cytochrome c and apoptosome formation (as shown for the intrinsic pathway) by an unclear mechanism. (d) Caspase-independent pathway. Recently, a new caspase-independent, granzymeA (GrA)-mediated pathway was described. After being delivered into the target cell cytosol through Ca^{2+}-dependent perforin-mediated pores, GrA triggers a pathway characterized by single-stranded DNA nicks and the appearance of apoptotic morphology. The endonucleases involved in the formation of DNA strand breaks in this system was identified as GAAD (GrA-activated DNase). GAAD activity is inhibited by a specific inhibitor (SET complex), which is located in the endoplasmic reticulum (ER). This complex contains a number of factors (pp32, SET, HMG2 and Ape1). (Reproduced with permission from Orrenius S, Zhivotovsky B, Nicotera P. Regulation of cell death: the calcium–apoptosis link. Nature Reviews Mol Cell Biology 2003;4:552–65. Copyright © 2003 Nature Publishing Group, London. http://www.els.net).

Necrosis, characteristic of ischemia, is associated with cell swelling, lysis and inflammation.

is as follows: severe energy depletion following the destruction of mitochondria causes elevation of intracellular Ca^{2+}. Increased Ca^{2+} activates proteases (calpains) that compromise the integrity of lysosomes, spilling hydrolytic enzymes, including cathepsin proteases, which degrade cellular structures, interfere with normal metabolism, and ultimately cause cell death.

Senescence

Ageing (senescence) is the conversion of a metabolically active cell, through a series of genetically controlled events, to one with impaired metabolic function. Senescence, followed by obligatory death, appeared in evolution when eukaryotes diverged from prokaryotes, and must have offered evolutionary advantages in maximizing reproductive success. Evolution is targeted at maximizing the reproductive success of an individual, not its longevity beyond that. Therefore, genes that negatively affect the survival of an organism after it has had a chance to reproduce will not be selected against, and traits that will keep an individual alive after its optimal reproductive years will not be selected for. Sexual reproduction (i.e. mixing the DNA from two different individuals and recombining it to form a new individual with a genetic make-up slightly different from that of the parents) offered evolutionary advantages and was selected for. Sexual reproduction involves the partitioning of DNA into two types of cell: germ cells and somatic cells. The exclusive function of somatic cells is to optimize the reproductive success of the germline DNA. Once the DNA contained in germ cells has reproduced, somatic DNA becomes dispensable. Until the groundbreaking experiments of Hayflick and Moorhead in 1961, cultured cells were considered to be immortal and senescence was thought to be an in vivo artifact of less than perfect conditions present in the organism as a whole.

Two general forms of cellular senescence can be distinguished: replicative and nonreplicative. Replicative senescence is observed when cells capable of division (e.g. fibroblasts) are cultured in vitro. These cells undergo a certain number of divisions and then stop. The 'life clock' is based on a set number of cell divisions, not on calendar time, as cells that are frozen partway through their set number of cycles and thawed will continue to completion of their program, independently of how long they have been frozen. The number of cell divisions that cultured fibroblasts are capable of correlates with the life expectancy of the species they are taken from: mouse or rat embryo fibroblasts divide about a dozen times, human fibroblasts about 50, and those from the Galapagos tortoise about 120 times.

Most adult cells rarely divide and undergo nonreplicative senescence, mainly due to oxidative damage.

However, the mechanism by which cells enter replicative senescence may differ from species to species. Telomeres are important components of a human cell's 'life clock' and consist of short DNA motifs (TTAGG) repeated multiple times at the tips of chromosomes. Telomeres protect the ends of chromosomes from digestion, and also anchor chromosomes to the nuclear membrane. With each round of cell replication, telomeres shorten by a constant amount (40–100 bp) unless they are restored to their original length by the enzyme telomerase. When a certain degree of shortening of the telomere caps has been reached, a cell cycle checkpoint (termed M1; see Fig. 2.4) is triggered that initiates the terminally nondividing state of replicative senescence. In multicellular eukaryotes, telomerase is present only in ovaries and testes (but not in mature ova or sperm) and in some tissues that continue to divide throughout life, but not in otherwise normal adult tissue. In contrast, telomerase can be found in cells of the early, rapidly dividing embryo (and in over 90% of human tumors). Replicating cells also undergo genome reorganization (e.g. translocation); the ability to detect and respond to these changes diminishes with age, thereby contributing to age-dependent functional impairment.

Most cells in the adult organism rarely divide; instead, they undergo nonreplicative senescence. As cells age they accumulate lipofuscin, which is largely oxidized fat. The amount of oxidized protein increases as a function of cellular age. Cellular damage by oxidative byproducts of metabolism is a major cause of cellular degeneration in ageing. One of the most damaging effects of senescence is mutation of DNA. Mitochondrial DNA is particularly affected, as it lacks both shielding by histones and effective repair mechanisms. Common causes are oxidative metabolites and UV radiation. Although cells are equipped to repair DNA damage, this ability falls off with age, and the resulting alterations in DNA are thought to be a major cause of senescence in both dividing and nondividing cells. Secreted proteins of many cells change with age. For example collagen, the matrix supporting most cells, becomes more rigid. Another protein, amyloid, is secreted by a variety of cells. Once condensed outside the cell to amyloid fibrils, it contributes to dysfunction of a number of organs, e.g. the brain in Alzheimer's disease.

Extending lifespan

Is the maximal lifespan of an organism a predetermined, genetically-controlled, species-specific property? In organisms like roundworms and fruit flies single gene mutations can result in substantial increases in maximal lifespan. Experiments conducted in the 1930s suggested that maximal lifespan might also not be an unalterable quantity in warm-blooded animals. It has been firmly established that caloric restriction (CR; typically to 40–70% of the calories of an unrestricted diet) prolongs life in nearly every species tested so far. Until recently, the proposed explanations centered on reduced oxidative cell damage secondary to reduced availability of cellular 'fuel'. Recently, a link has emerged between CR and two pivotal regulators that robustly extend survival across taxa: forkhead transcription factor FOXO and SIR2 (silencing information regulator 2, which silences transcriptional at repeated DNA sequences) histone deacetylase. In yeast, lifespan extension by CR requires SIR2, a NAD^{+}-dependent enzyme. Similar conclusions came from experiments in *Drosophila* in which upregulation of SIR2 prolonged lifespan while a decrease in SIR2 blocked the lifespan-extending effect of CR (parallel pathways for CR and SIR2 effects on longevity have, however, also been proposed). FOXO is linked to insulin/IGF-1 mediated signal transduction pathways. When insulin signaling is inhibited, unphosphorylated FOXO enters the nucleus where it promotes somatic endurance, stress resistance and longevity by induction of genes linked to detoxification of reactive oxygen species, heat stock, DNA damage repair, growth

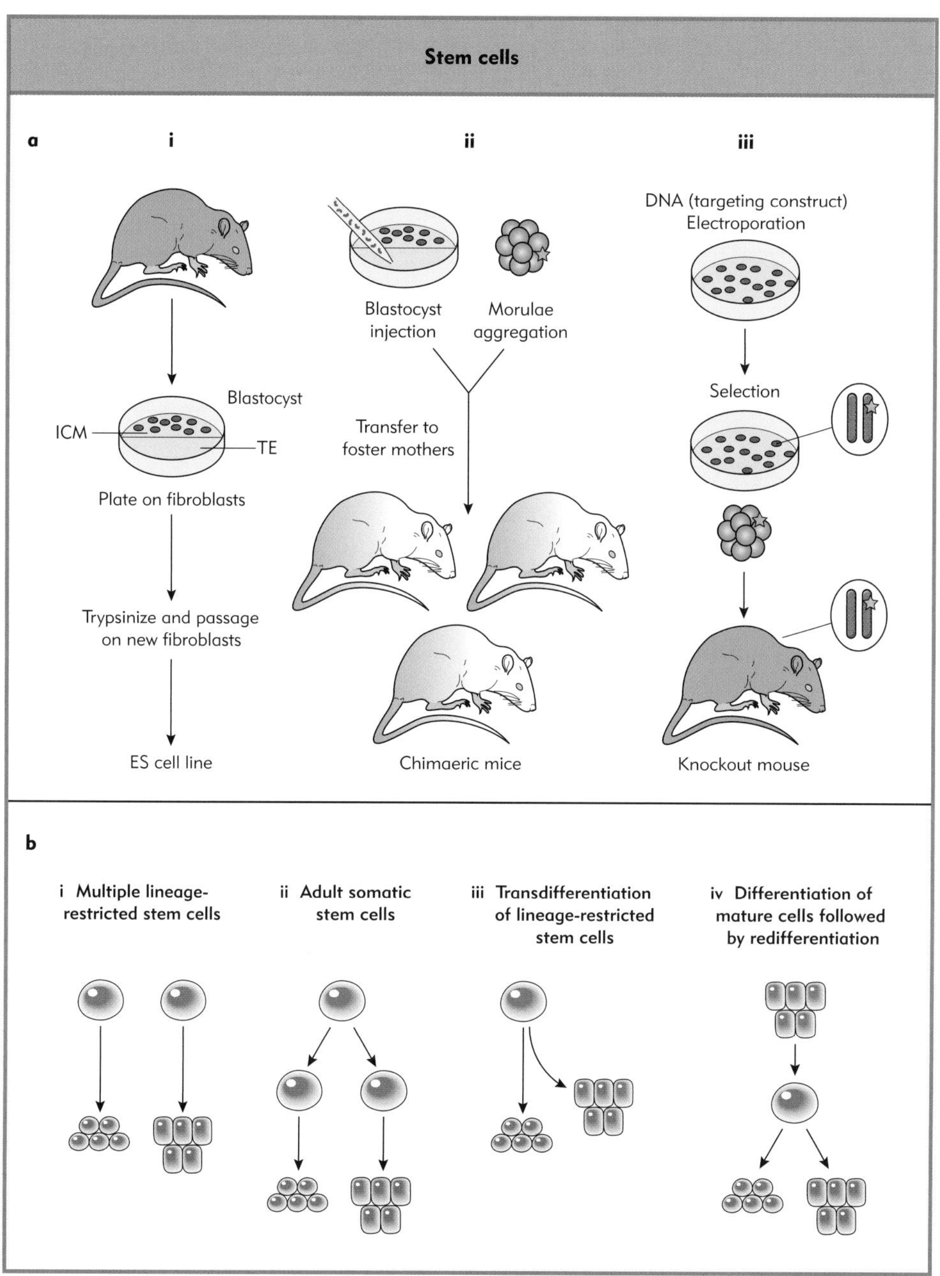

Figure 2.3 Stem cells. (a) Embryonic stem (ES) cell technology. Genetically altered higher organisms can be generated by 'knocking in' or 'knocking out' specific genes from the DNA of ES cells grown in the laboratory, and then reintroducing the genetically altered cells into a normally developing embryo. (i) The establishment of ES cells from the mouse blastocyst. The brown color indicates that the ES cells are isolated from a mouse strain with an agouti coat color which is dominant over albino or black. This allows monitoring of the degree of chimerism by the coat color. (Copyright © 2000 Nature Publishing Group, London. http://www.els.net.) (ii) Generation of chimeric mice by blastocyst injection or morula aggregation. The aggregated embryos are transferred to foster mothers. When the delivered embryos are partially derived from the pluripotent ES cells, the coat color is mixed. These mice are called chimeras. When they are mated to normal wildtype mice they often transmit the ES cell genome to the germline. (Copyright © 2003 Massachusetts Medical Society. All rights reserved. Adapted with permission.) (iii) A typical gene targeting experiment. The construct is electroporated into ES cells. After selection and screening, the positive homologous recombinant clone (blue) is aggregated to wildtype embryos to generate chimeras, which transmit the mutation to the mouse germline. The mutation is indicated in the inset by an asterisk on one chromosome (Reproduced with permission from Mansouri A. Mouse knockouts. In: Nature encyclopedia of life sciences. London: Nature Publishing Group; 2000. http://www.els.net/). (b) Adult (AS) stem cells. Recent data suggest that, contrary to previous assumptions, AS cells are capable of generating differentiated cells beyond their own tissue boundaries. Models for generating solid-organ tissue cells through differentiation of bone marrow-derived and circulating AS cells are shown. In the first model (i), distinct stem cells differentiate, each into its own organ-specific cell (panel a). In the second model (ii), primitive somatic stem cells located in hematopoietic tissue differentiate into various organ-specific cells (iii). In the third model, stem cells, such as hematopoietic stem cells, differentiate along their predetermined pathways. Under certain, probably rare, conditions, tissue injury or another stimulus causes some stem cells to deviate from their predetermined pathway and generate cells of a different tissue – a process known as transdifferentiation. In the fourth model (iv), mature cells dedifferentiate into cells with stem cell-like characteristics and eventually redifferentiate into terminally differentiated cells of their own tissue or a different tissue. (Reproduced with permission from Körbling M, Estrov Z. Adult stem cells for tissue repair – A new therapeutic concept? New Engl J Med. 2003;349:570–82, Massachusetts Medical Society).

control, etc. SIRT1 (the best studied of the seven members of the mammalian SIR2 gene family) may specifically modulate FOXO activity toward maximal survival.

Immortality – stem cell technology

A period of potential cellular immortality exists in ontogeny: the descendents of the first few divisions of the diploid zygote, the embryonic stem (ES) cells, can replicate indefinitely if prevented from differentiating. Mouse ES cell lines can exist for more than a decade without signs of senescence. ES cells offer the opportunity to understand the transition from immortality to mortality, as well as providing a tool to generate genetically altered organisms. After inactivating or inserting specific genes in the genome of cultured ES cells, they can be transferred into an embryo at the blastula stage (approximately 100 cells) where they participate in the formation of tissues and organs, including the gonads. The resulting 'mosaic' individuals (chimeras) can be bred to generate animals that are homozygous for the desired genetic alteration (Fig. 2.3a). In the course of differentiation into more specialized cells, ES cells restrict accessibility to parts of their genome not needed for specific functions of the developing tissue. A current senescence hypothesis postulates that 'senescence repressor genes' are gradually suppressed and the

Stem cell technology has potential clinical applications in tissue repair and replacement.

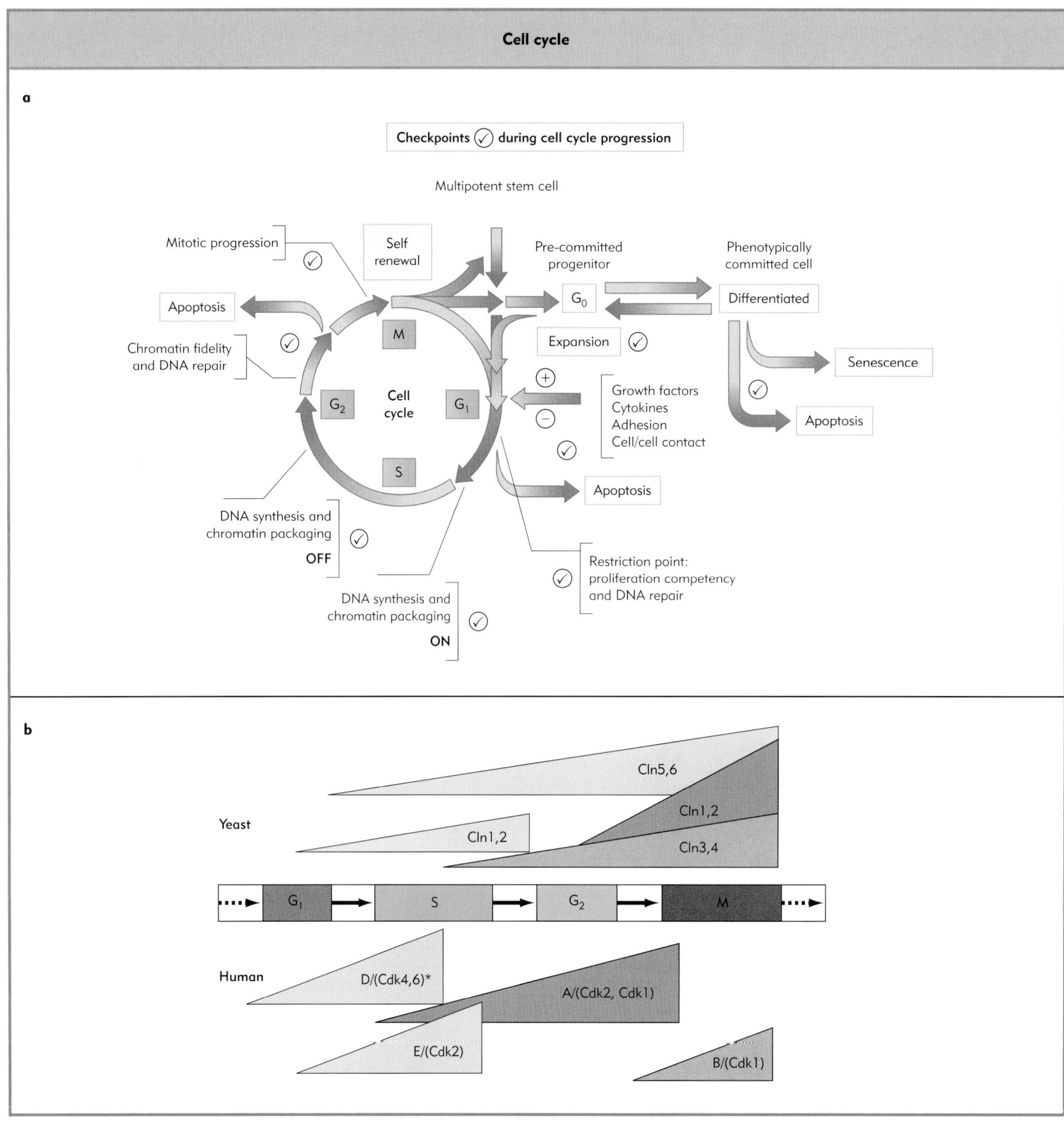

Figure 2.4 The cell cycle. (a) Checkpoints during cell cycle progression. The cell cycle is regulated by several critical cell cycle checkpoints (ticks) at which competency for cell cycle progression is monitored. Entry into and exit from the cell cycle (black lines and lettering) are controlled by growth regulatory factors (e.g. cytokines, growth factors, cell adhesion and/or cell–cell contact) which determine self-renewal of stem cells and the expansion of precommitted progenitor cells. The biochemical parameters associated with each cell cycle checkpoint are indicated by red lettering. Options for defaulting to apoptosis (blue lettering) during G_1 and G_2 are evaluated by surveillance mechanisms that assess the fidelity of structural and regulatory parameters of cell cycle control. (Reproduced with permission from Stein G S, van Wijnen A J, Stein J L, Lian J B, Owen T A. Cell cycle. In: Nature encyclopedia of life sciences. Copyright © 2001 Nature Publishing Group, London. http://www.els.net). (b) Cyclin expression and degradation in the yeast and mammalian (human) cell cycles. Cyclins comprise a large and diverse family of proteins of 50–90 kDa that share weak homology in their amino acid sequences. The combination of both protein level and activity is depicted. D cyclin expression (indicated by *) is induced by mitogenic signals and can be found in the cell during two successive cell cycles, under the constant presence of the signal. The main role of D cyclins is at the G_1/S transition. At the end of mitosis, cyclins are marked for degradation by coupling with ubiquitin and disappear abruptly. (Reproduced with permission from Kitazono A A, FitzGerald J N, Kron S J. Cell cycle: regulation by cyclins. In: Nature encyclopedia of life sciences. Copyright © 1999 Nature Publishing Group, London. http://www.els.net).

'senescence program' is activated. This process begins by the time the embryo implants into the uterine wall, but senescence is not fully expressed until reproductive maturity is reached. Adult stem (AS) cells are intrinsic to various tissues. These cells are capable of maintaining, generating, and replacing terminally differentiated cells within their own tissue, such as those from the hematopoietic lineage. AS cells are not committed to differentiation within their own tissue, but are capable of dedifferentiation and transdifferentiaton (Fig. 2.3b). AS cells derived from bone marrow can differentiate to nonlymphohematopoietic tissues, such as muscle fibers, hepatocytes, micro- and astroglia, and neurons. Hematopoietic AS cells have numerous potential clinical applications for tissue repair and replacement.

THE CELL CYCLE

Cyclins

The cell cycle is the sequence of events that leads to mitosis, in which a parental cell gives rise to two daughter cells, normally identical to the parent. An appropriate growth factor can induce the cell to exit the resting stage (G_0) and enter the replication cycle. Initially the cell enters the G_1 (growth 1) phase of the cycle. Once the cell reaches the restriction point in G_1, it proceeds through the rest of the cell cycle even in the absence of growth factors. However, replication can be stopped at a number of checkpoints throughout the cycle if DNA damage is detected (Fig. 2.4a). The cell is guided through the cell cycle by specialized cyclin proteins and cyclin-dependent kinases (Cdk), synthesized early in G_1, and E2F molecules that guide the cell beyond the restriction point and into the S (synthesis) phase of the cycle, where replication of DNA (duplication of chromosomes) takes place (Fig. 2.4b).

Chromosomes

Chromosomes are linear molecules of DNA, extensively bound to proteins. Histones facilitate packing of the DNA into condensed loops of DNA called nucleosomes. Nucleosomes pack together to form fibers, which in turn form higher-order structures such as loops. Certain gene regulatory proteins can decondense chromosomes, unwind loops, and create nucleosome-free regions. Genes being transcribed are found in decondensed portions of chromosomes, which are termed active chromatin. All chromatin becomes tightly condensed as a prelude to mitosis. As a result of condensation, mitotic chromosomes can be stained to reveal the distinct banding patterns (karyotyping). Most DNA in mammals does not encode proteins; some is used to encode RNA, some is regulatory, but most has no known function (Chapter 4). This could account for the lack of correlation between cellular DNA content and organism complexity. DNA replicates during S phase at multiple replication origins. Active chromatin replicates first, whereas condensed chromatin replicates late in S phase. Because of the unidirectional nature of DNA polymerase, the ends of a chromosome cannot be fully replicated by DNA polymerase. This problem is addressed by the telomeres, which are allowed to shorten with every cell division unless restored by telomerase. Histones are also synthesized in the S phase, and new DNA is assembled into nucleosomes. After completion of S phase the cell (which now has double the amount of DNA) passes into the G_2 phase and, guided by a cyclin-Cdk2 dimer (M-phase promoting factor or MPF), into M (mitosis) phase.

Mitosis and regulation of the cell cycle

During M phase the chromosomes, the nucleus, and finally the cytoplasm are divided between two daughter cells. The first step, prophase, is marked by compaction of the duplicated chromosomes into chromatids (pairs of chromosomes attached at their centromeres) and the formation of the mitotic spindle in the cytoplasm. At prometaphase the nuclear envelope disintegrates into vesicles, and the chromatids attach to the microtubules of the mitotic spindle. Kinetochores are protein complexes that link centromeres to microtubules. During metaphase the chromatids line up in the metaphase plate, separate during anaphase, and move towards the spindle poles. When the chromosomes reach the poles, the cell enters telophase. The nuclear envelope coalesces around the chromosomes, and the nucleolus reappears as RNA synthesis resumes. After mitosis is complete, the cytoplasm and the organelles are separated into two cells.

Certain cells, such as endothelial cells, divide rapidly, whereas in other cells, such as hepatocytes, the cell cycle may last a year. In tissue culture, the cell cycle for many mammalian cell lines lasts about 24 hours (compared to 90 minutes for yeast). Mature neurons do not progress through the cell cycle at all. Deficiencies of cell replication and cell death control (replicative immortality) lie at the root of malignancies. One protein of major importance in cell cycle regulation is p53, which detects damaged DNA. Depending on the severity of the damage, p53 can either stop the cell cycle until the DNA is repaired or direct the cell into apoptosis. p53 exerts control before (to prevent damaged DNA from replicating) and after (to check for integrity of the DNA after replication) the S phase. Defective p53, as in Bloom syndrome and Li–Fraumeni syndrome, leads to a high incidence of malignancies. The retinoblastoma protein (Rb), which is missing or mutated in various cancers, is an important negative regulator of the cell cycle (via interaction with E2F in G_1).

Defects in cell replication and death control underlie malignancy.

Oncogenes

Even if a cell escapes cell cycle control, it will not replicate uncontrollably without stimulation. This stimulus can be provided by mutations in a category of genes that can drive normal cell division toward the development of cancer, called oncogenes. More than 50 oncogenes have been defined in humans, and they are found in many tumors. The products of these genes are involved in receiving, transmitting, and processing growth signals. When an appropriate mutation of an oncogene occurs, the components of the signaling pathway downstream of the mutated oncogene are activated and the cell enters the cell cycle repeatedly. The Philadelphia chromosome is a mutation (via translocation) where the oncogene Abl is activated on chromosome 22, causing chronic myelogenous leukemia. Unless the cell is 'immortalized' most oncogenes induce only a limited number of uncontrolled cell divisions before entering the replicative senescent state incapable of division. The development of full-blown cancer requires a simultaneous mutation in one or more of the guardians of the cell cycle, such as Rb, p53 and p16, which are collectively known as tumor suppressor genes.

Benefits of cellular senescence and mortality

A replicatively senescent cell is unable to respond to growth signals because of safeguards at various stages of the cell cycle. Cells that circumvent these safeguards pose a threat to the organism in the form of malignant cells. Therefore, replicative senescence appears to be a reaction of cells to certain kinds of damage that, in other cells, cause apoptosis. The sophistication of the controls necessary to prevent cells from escaping replicative senescence depends on the life expectancy of the organism. Human cells are approximately 90 000 times more resistant to tumorigenic conversion per unit time than mouse cells, reflecting the different lifespans of the organisms.

Meiosis

Meiosis is a special kind of cell division, taking place only in testicles and ovaries, in which a cell with the full double set of chromosomes (e.g. 46 in humans) divides to form sex cells with a single set of chromosomes (23 in humans). In contrast to mitosis, the homologous chromosomes in each sex cell that results from meiotic division will be slightly different because of the process of crossing over that takes place prior to the first meiotic division. The pairs of homologous chromosomes physically 'cross over' (at sites termed chiasmata) and exchange pieces of DNA, thus increasing the genetic diversity of the sex cells. Whereas in somatic cells each chromosome can be identified as having been inherited from either parent, sex cells have a unique 'recombination' of genes. The first meiotic division results in two diploid sex cells that divide for a second time without DNA replication, forming four haploid gametes.

CELL COMPARTMENTS

Membrane structure

Eukaryotic cells, like prokaryotic cells, are surrounded by a plasma membrane. However, most eukaryotic cells also contain extensive internal membranes that enclose specific compartments (organelles) and separate them from the cytoplasm. Most organelles are surrounded by a single phospholipid bilayer membrane, but several, including the nucleus and the mitochondria, are enclosed by two membranes. These membranes control the ionic composition of organelles and spatially segregate metabolic pathways within the cell. The plasma membrane is a thin (5 nm) bilayer of lipids and proteins. Plasma membrane lipids are chemically diverse, but phospholipids are the most abundant. Phospholipid molecules are amphipathic and spontaneously form bilayers in water. They typically contain either a glycerol (as in phosphoglycerides) or a sphingosine (as in sphingomyelin) backbone. The plasma membrane also contains cholesterol, which confers rigidity. Under physiologic conditions, lipids and integral membrane proteins can diffuse laterally through the membrane leaflet (they do not usually migrate from one leaflet of a bilayer to the other), a concept known as the *fluid mosaic model*. The two sides (faces) of the lipid bilayer have different lipid compositions. Inositol phospholipids, which are substrates for enzymes that create second messengers such as inositol trisphosphate (Chapter 3), tend to be concentrated on the cytoplasmic face. Glycolipids (i.e. lipids with sugars attached to their head groups) are found on the extracellular face. Glycolipids are prominent in the myelin membrane that sheaths axons.

Pure lipid bilayers allow hydrophobic and small uncharged polar molecules to pass through, but largely block the diffusion of ions and larger polar molecules. Biologic membranes contain two major types of membrane transport protein to facilitate selective permeability to ions and large molecules. Carrier proteins have at least two different conformational states, which bind a solute on one side of the membrane and release it on the other. Channel proteins span the membrane and allow the passage of molecules across the membrane. Channel proteins allow more rapid transfer than carrier proteins, but only facilitate the diffusion of certain molecules down electrochemical gradients. Most channel proteins are highly selective for particular molecules or ions. In general, channels are not constantly open, but act as gated pores and open in response to a particular stimulus. Carrier proteins, by comparison, can actively transport compounds; they are often pumps driven by the energy derived from ATP hydrolysis or by the energy stored in ion gradients.

Nucleus

A double nuclear membrane surrounds the largest organelle of eukaryotic cells. In many cells the outer membrane is continuous with the rough endoplasmic reticulum (ER) and the space between the membranes is continuous with the lumen of the rough ER. The inner membrane defines the nucleus itself, physically segregating DNA from cytoplasm. Separation of gene transcription in the nucleus from messenger RNA translation in the cytoplasm may facilitate RNA processing. The nuclear membrane and its associated cytoskeleton may also protect chromosomes from physical stress. Cytoplasmic intermediate filaments surround the outer membrane, and nuclear filaments known as lamins form a mesh underneath the inner nuclear membrane. The two nuclear membranes are bridged by nuclear pores, large protein complexes that regulate molecular traffic into and out of the nucleus. Proteins synthesized in the cytosol that contain nuclear localization signals bind to the nuclear pore and are actively transported into the nucleus. A suborganelle of the nucleus, the nucleolus, is dedicated to the synthesis of ribosomal RNA. Some ribosomal proteins are added to ribosomal RNAs in the nucleolus before export to the cytosol through nuclear pores.

Mitochondria

Mitochondria and chloroplasts probably arose by the incorporation of photosynthetic and nonphotosynthetic bacteria into ancestral eukaryotic cells about 1.5 billion years ago. Like bacteria, they reproduce by fission. The bacterial origin of mitochondria explains the existence of mitochondrial DNA, which is circular and encodes some mitochondrial proteins. Most mitochondrial proteins, however, are derived from nuclear genes. Mitochondria are membrane-delimited organelles that oxidize organic compounds, generate an electrochemical proton gradient across the mitochondrial membrane, and synthesize adenosine triphosphate (ATP) from adenosine diphosphate (ADP) and phosphate. Mitochondria may occupy up to 25% of the volume of the cytoplasm. The outer mitochondrial membrane, composed of about half lipid and half protein, contains large porin channels, which render the outer membrane permeable to molecules <10 kDa. The inner membrane (20% lipid, 80% protein) is a convoluted membrane with a large surface area that surrounds the mitochondrial matrix. Most solutes, such as protons, hydroxyl ions, and other ions, cannot pass freely through the inner mitochondrial membrane, but carrier proteins facilitate the movement of metabolites. The respiratory chain, located in the inner membrane, oxidizes metabolic substrates and establishes an electrochemical proton gradient across the inner membrane. Protons are pumped across the inner membrane out of the matrix. ATP synthase, a large protein complex, uses the proton gradient to drive ATP synthesis as protons return into the matrix. The inner matrix contains enzymes used in intermediary metabolic cycles, mitochondrial DNA, mitochondrial transfer RNAs, and ribosomes for translation of mitochondrial proteins. Matrix enzymes catalyze the tricarboxylic acid cycle (Krebs or citric acid cycle) using acetyl coenzyme A (CoA) to produce high-energy electrons (NADH) used by the respiratory chain to pump protons out of the matrix. The intracellular location of mitochondria is influenced by their association with microtubules. The number of mitochondria per cell is not fixed, and repeated exercise of muscles leads to a large increase in mitochondrial numbers. Mitochondrial inheritance is nonmendelian. Unlike the precise segregation of nuclear genes during meiosis, mitochondrial inheritance is the result of random separation of mitochondria. The ovum has much more cytoplasm than the sperm, and the zygotic mitochondria are descended from maternal mitochondria. Therefore, inheritance of mitochondrial DNA follows the maternal line.

Endoplasmic reticulum

The endoplasmic reticulum is an extensive web of membranes that courses throughout the cytoplasm of eukaryotic cells. In a typical cell, the ER makes up about half of the total cellular membrane and encloses about one-tenth of the cell volume. Synthesis of fatty acids, phospholipids, and steroid hormones takes place in the smooth ER, and most cells have relatively little of it. The hepatic cytochrome P450 system, located in smooth ER, metabolizes many drugs, including volatile anesthetics (in particular halothane and methoxyflurane) (see Chapter 27). Chronic ingestion of certain drugs, such as barbiturates, phenytoin, and ethanol, induces the proliferation of hepatic smooth ER. The sarcoplasmic reticulum of muscle cells is smooth ER specialized for Ca^{2+} sequestration. Synthesis of cell membrane lipids occurs on the outer, cytoplasmic side of the ER. Movement of lipids to the other face is catalyzed by phospholipid translocators that flip lipids from one side of the membrane to the other. Membrane lipids are transported along the secretory pathway by transport vesicles to the Golgi apparatus (a series of flattened sacs located near the nucleus and surrounded by a number of spherical vesicles), where they may undergo further modification (e.g. attachment of polysaccharides), and then to the plasma membrane, endosomes, or lysosomes. Cytosolic phospholipid transfer proteins shuttle lipids from the secretory pathway to other membrane-bound organelles.

The hepatic cytochrome P450 system located in smooth endoplasmic reticulum metabolizes many drugs, including volatile anesthetics.

Intracellular degradation

Eukaryotic cells contain specialized membrane-bound vesicles for the degradation of exogenous and endogenous compounds. A number of hereditary diseases have been linked to defects in these pathways.

Peroxisomes degrade fatty acids and toxic compounds (especially in the liver and kidney) using oxidases and molecular oxygen and generating hydrogen peroxide. Hydrogen peroxide is highly reactive and is degraded by catalase. Oxidation of fatty acids into acetyl CoA occurs in both peroxisomes and mitochondria. In peroxisomes, however, it is not linked to ATP generation. The energy released during peroxisomal oxidation is converted to heat and the acetyl groups are transported into the cytosol, where they are used in the synthesis of cholesterol and other metabolites. Peroxisomes are present in all eukaryotic cells except erythrocytes. Proteins destined for the peroxisome are synthesized in the cytosol with a specific C-terminal signal sequence that triggers uptake into the peroxisome. New peroxisomes are formed by the fission of pre-existing peroxisomes. In X-linked adrenoleukodystrophy, peroxisomal oxidation of very long-chain fatty acids is defective, causing death in late childhood in the severe form. In Zellweger syndrome and related disorders, peroxisomes are unable to take up proteins into the peroxisomal matrix.

Lysosomes are membrane-bound organelles specialized for acidic hydrolysis. Lysosomal degradative enzymes, which are optimally active at acid pH, are physically sequestered within the lysosomes. The pH inside lysosomes is kept at about 5 (versus cytosolic pH of 7.2) by an H^+-ATPase that pumps protons into the lysosome. Molecules can follow several pathways to the lysosome. Lysosomal enzymes receive a specific marker (mannose-6-phosphate) in the Golgi apparatus. Proteins that carry this modification bind to mannose-6-phosphate receptors, which mediate the movement of lysosomal enzymes through transport vesicles to lysosomes. Defects in the function of various lysosomal enzymes cause lysosomal storage diseases such as Tay–Sachs disease.

Proteins, other solutes, and fluids are taken up by cells by endocytosis and enter vesicles called early endosomes. This continuous process is termed pinocytosis and results in the formation of small vesicles at invaginated portions of the plasma membrane. The cytosolic face is coated with clathrin, a protein that mediates pinching-off of clathrin-coated pits into clathrin-coated vesicles. Specific proteins are taken up during pinocytosis by the inclusion of receptors in clathrin-coated pits. Many cells have another type of invagination, termed caveolae or plasmalemmal vesicles, which may function in transcytosis and as subcellular compartments to store and concentrate various signaling molecules. Some endosomes undergo maturation into late endosomes, and the internal pH begins to drop. Transport vesicles containing lysosomal enzymes fuse with late endosomes, creating lysosomes. Other proteins contained in early endosomes, such as cell-surface receptors, do not go to lysosomes but are recycled to the plasma membrane. Specialized cells, such as macrophages or neutrophils, engulf large particles or microorganisms by phagocytosis, creating a large vesicle known as a phagosome. Phagocytosis is triggered after a particle binds to a specific receptor, such as the Fc receptor, which recognizes antibodies. Phagosomes fuse with lysosomes, which degrade the engulfed object. Organelles no longer needed by the cell, such as aged mitochondria, are surrounded by membranes derived from

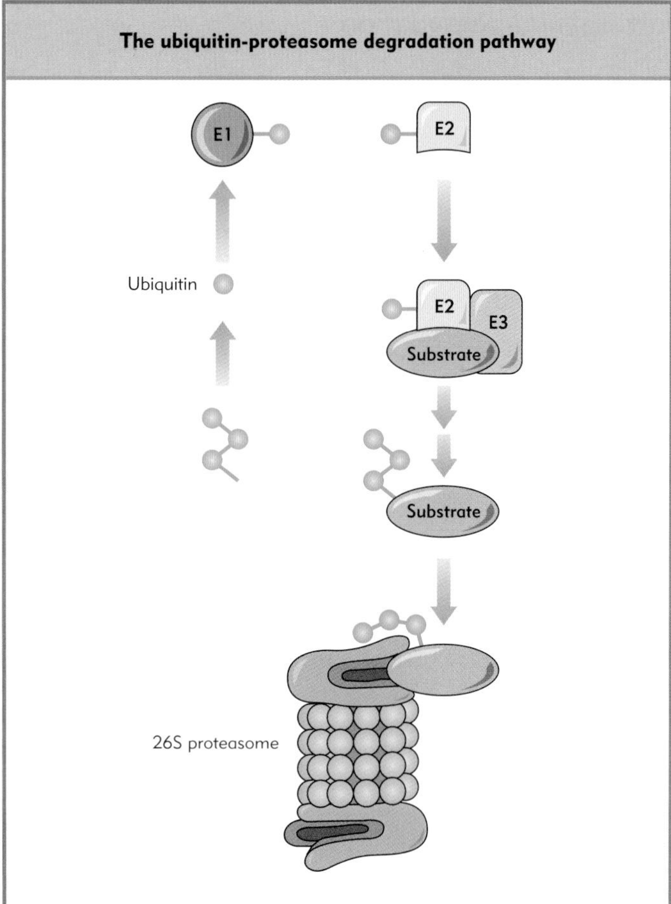

Figure 2.5 The ubiquitin–proteasome degradation pathway. The ubiquitin-activating enzyme E1 forms a thioester linkage with ubiquitin using its C terminus. The activated ubiquitin is transferred to the active cysteine group on the ubiquitin-conjugating enzyme E2. E2, sometimes with the help of ubiquitin ligase E3, transfers ubiquitin to lysine residues on other proteins. Repeated conjugation leads to the formation of multiubiquitin chains. Proteasomes recognize proteins with ubiquitin chains and degrade the labeled proteins. The multiubiquitin chains are released and recycled. (Modified with permission from Hilt W, Wolf DH. Proteasomes: destruction as a programme. Trends Biochem Sci. 1996; 21:96–102. Copyright © 1996, with permission from Elsevier.)

the ER to form autophagosomes. The autophagosome fuses with lysosomes, and the contents are broken down.

The ubiquitin/proteasome pathway is the main nonlysosomal route for intracellular protein degradation in eukaryotes. It is essential for various cellular processes, such as cell-cycle progression, transcription, antigen processing, and apoptosis. Cytosolic proteins can be marked for degradation by covalent linkage with a chain of ubiquitin proteins. Proteins thus marked are broken down by proteasomes, which are large multiprotein cylinders. Proteins at the ends of the cylinders recognize ubiquitinated proteins and pass them into the interior of the cylinder, where degradation occurs (Fig. 2.5). Understanding the multiple roles of the ubiquitin/proteasome system might lead to new therapeutic approaches for human diseases linked to dysregulated apoptosis, for example neurodegenerative diseases such as Alzheimer's and Parkinson's diseases, amyotrophic lateral sclerosis etc., in which apoptosis may be excessive, and autoimmune diseases, cancer, and acquired resistance to chemotherapy, which are instances of downregulated apoptosis.

THE CYTOSKELETON: STRUCTURE AND MOVEMENT

The cytoskeleton is a cytoplasmic web of filamentous proteins. It provides structure to the cell, allows the movement of organelles, and translates energy into force for cell movement. The cytoskeleton consists of three types of fiber: microfilaments (composed of actin polymer along with bound proteins, 7–9 nm in diameter); intermediate filaments (10 nm in diameter, polymers of tissue-specific proteins, such as vimentin); and microtubules (24 nm in diameter). All eukaryotic cells have microtubules and actin; intermediate filaments are present in most cells from multicellular eukaryotes. The nucleus also has a filamentous protein structure, the nuclear lamina, composed of intermediate filament proteins termed lamins.

Actin

Actin is the most abundant protein in many cells. A typical liver cell, for example, has approximately 2×10^4 insulin receptors but approximately 0.5×10^9 actin molecules. Actin exists as a globular monomer called G-actin and a filamentous polymer of G-actin subunits called F-actin. A striking property of G-actin is its ability to polymerize into F-actin; conversely, F-actin can depolymerize into G-actin. Actin filaments are flexible double-stranded helices. Actin cross-linking proteins dictate the structure of actin filaments. Actin filaments are commonly arranged as bundles and networks. Actin bundles form the core of microvilli and filopodia, fingerlike projections of the plasma membrane. Actin networks can be either planar, i.e. two-dimensional (like a net), or three-dimensional (conferring a gel-like property). The cell cortex is an actin-containing gel located beneath the cell membrane. Actin filaments are organized into bundles and networks by a variety of bivalent cross-linking proteins such as filamin in platelets, spectrin in erythrocytes (deficient in hereditary spherocytosis and elliptocytosis), dystrophin in muscle (deficient in Duchenne's muscular dystrophy), and fimbrin and fascin in microvilli. Other cross-linking proteins promote the formation of parallel bundles of actin filaments. α-Actinin is found in stress fibers, which are loosely packed bundles that span large distances in cells. Stress fibers also contain myosin, which produces tension in the fibers. Transmembrane proteins, such as integrins, anchor stress fibers to the extracellular substrate of the cell.

An actin filament is a polar structure; the plus end has a high affinity for free actin molecules and the minus end has a lower affinity. Actin filaments can simultaneously grow by net addition of actin subunits at the plus end and shrink by loss of subunits from the minus end (Fig. 2.6a). Free actin subunits bind ATP, which is hydrolyzed after the subunits are incorporated into actin filaments. At steady state, the filaments undergo treadmilling: the average length of the filaments remains constant, but subunits progress through the filaments by binding to the plus end and passing along the length of the filament until they reach the minus end and dissociate from the filament. Energetically, treadmilling is driven by the hydrolysis of ATP. Normal cell function depends upon the instability of actin. If actin filaments are stabilized by toxins (such as the mushroom toxin phalloidin) or actin polymerization is blocked, cell structure is grossly distorted. Actin-binding proteins control the polymerization and depolymerization of actin filaments. Some of these proteins bind

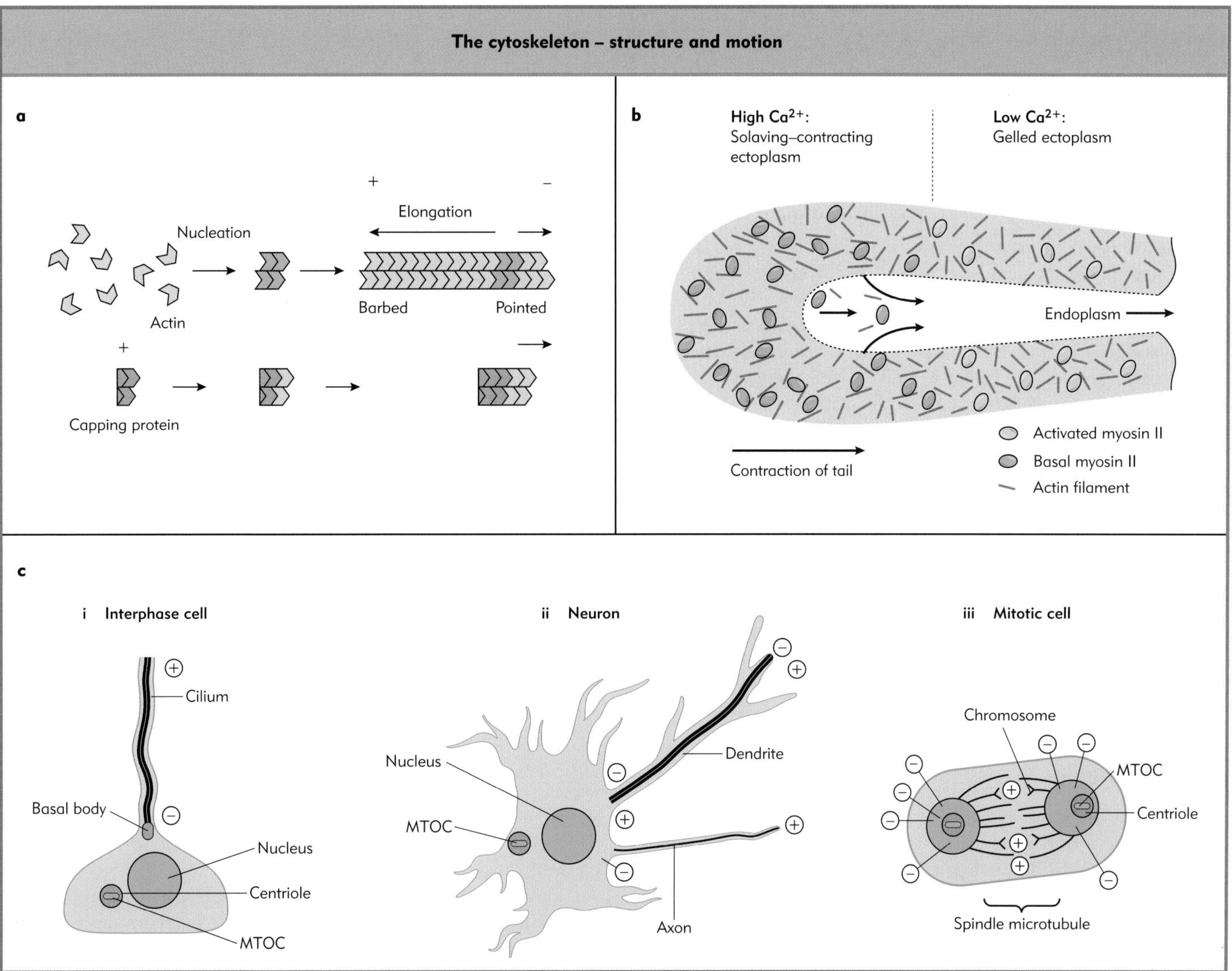

Figure 2.6 The cytoskeleton – structure and motion. (a) Actin filament formation. Actin filaments are unstable in the absence of actin-binding proteins. Capping protein binds the fast-growing, or plus, ends of actin filaments. It blocks further addition or loss of actin monomers from that end. Similarly, other proteins can block the minus end. Capping protein also binds small actin oligomers and thereby promotes the nucleation of new filaments. (b) Ameboid cell movement. The ectoplasm, or the cortical gel layer, consists of actin filaments cross-linked by actin-binding proteins and myosin II motor proteins. It is hypothesized that local increases in Ca^{2+} induce partial solvation of the cortical gel. Ca^{2+} activates proteins that shorten actin filaments, decreases the extent of cross-linking of filaments, and activates myosin (causing local contraction). The combination of solvation and contraction generates hydrostatic pressure, and the contracting tail is pulled forward. (Reproduced from The Journal of Cell Biology 1993;123:345–56, by copyright permission of The Rockefeller University Press.) (c) Orientation of cellular microtubules. (i) In interphase cells the minus ends of most microtubules are proximal to the microtubule organizing center (MTOC). Similarly, the microtubules in flagella and cilia have their minus ends continuous with the basal body, which acts as the MTOC in these structures. (ii) In nerve cells, the minus ends of axonal microtubules are oriented toward the base of the axon. However, dendritic microtubules have mixed polarities. (iii) As cells enter mitosis, the microtubule network rearranges, forming a mitotic spindle. The minus ends of all spindle microtubules point towards one of the two MTOCs, or poles as they are called in mitotic cells. (Adapted from a drawing by Sergey Perouansky.)

actin monomers and sequester them from polymerizing. Others, such as tropomyosin, stabilize and strengthen actin filaments. Capping protein binds the plus end of the filament and blocks elongation. Gelsolin, a Ca^{2+}-activated actin-severing protein, cuts filaments and binds to the plus end, thereby generating shorter filaments that are less likely to extend. By shortening filaments, gelsolin can liquify the cell cortex. Localized transformation of the cell cortex from a gel to a solution plays a role in cell movement and release of the contents of secretory vesicles. Stable actin filaments are found in microvilli, small extensions that greatly increase the surface area of intestinal epithelial cells. Other actin filaments exhibit rapid turnover and reorganization. Changes in actin filaments can alter cell shape by inducing the formation of spikes, invaginations, or sheet-like extension of the cell. Ameboid movement of cells such as leukocytes is mediated by actin filaments (Fig. 2.6b). Following massive cell death, as occurs in fulminant hepatic necrosis and septic shock, actin is released into the bloodstream. In normal circumstances, circulating actin is depolymerized and bound by gelsolin and Gc protein in plasma. If this actin-scavenging system is saturated by excessive amounts of actin, free Gc protein is depleted, which can be fatal. Intravenous injection into rats of large amounts of actin causes pulmonary lesions similar to those found in the lungs of patients who have adult respiratory distress syndrome (ARDS), which suggests a role in the pathogenesis of ARDS (Chapter 49).

Actin, the most abundant protein in many cells, is released into the circulation following massive cell death.

Myosin

Myosins are mechanochemical enzymes capable of transforming chemical into mechanical energy. As they are associated with actin, they are referred to as actin motor proteins. Other motor proteins, associated with microtubules, are kinesin and dynein. Contraction is a special form of movement resulting from actin and myosin interaction. Skeletal muscle cells are giant multinucleated syncytia that contain actin and myosin filaments tightly organized into sarcomeres (Chapter 35). Individual cardiac muscle cells are smaller and have only one nucleus. Cardiac cells are physically tightly linked via binding of actin filaments to desmosomes, and are electrically linked by gap junctions (Chapter 39). Smooth muscle cells have individual nuclei and lack sarcomeres. The loose organization of actin and myosin filaments in smooth muscle cells allows only slow contractions, but permits the cells to stretch or contract through a broad range of lengths (Chapter 38). Myosin and actin also have many important functions in cells other than muscle cells. Myosin generates force for the division of cells, movement of cells, alteration of cell shape, and intracellular movement of some organelles.

Microtubules

Microtubules are large, relatively rigid cylinders with a diameter of 25 nm (Fig. 2.6c). They are heterodimeric polymers of α- and β-tubulin. Like actin filaments, microtubules are polar. One end of a microtubule is often attached to the centrosome, also called the microtubule-organizing center, which is often located near the center of the cell. The end of the microtubule attached to the centrosome is the minus end (i.e. the end of the filament with lower affinity for binding of free tubulin). Free microtubules tend to lose subunits from the minus end and add subunits at the plus end. Assembly and disassembly of microtubules depends on the critical concentration (C_c) of αβ-tubulin subunits. Assembly occurs above and disassembly below the C_c. About half of the tubulin in a typical cell is polymerized into microtubules, and half exists as free tubulin. The tubulin heterodimer is the structural subunit of microtubules. Microtubule arrays grow and shrink rapidly; this dynamic instability is crucial for microtubule function in intracellular transport and cell division.

Certain drugs alter the stability of microtubules. Paclitaxel (Taxol), a tumor chemotherapeutic agent, stabilizes microtubules and causes mitotic arrest in dividing cells. Colchicine, vinblastine, and vincristine all bind tubulin monomers and cause disassembly of microtubules. Microtubule-associated proteins (MAPs) stabilize assemblies of microtubules and link microtubules to other cellular components. Organelles are often associated with microtubules and are propelled along microtubules to other parts of the cell by microtubule-dependent motor proteins, such as kinesins or dyneins. Axons of nerve cells contain microtubules. All microtubules of an axon have the same polarity; the plus end points towards the synapse. This unipolar organization has functional importance, as secretory vesicles use motor proteins to move along microtubules towards the plus end, where the contents are released. The shorter microtubules of dendrites have a mixed polarity. Motor proteins also play essential roles in cell division and the motion of cilia and flagella.

Filaments

Intermediate filaments are structural polymers with a diameter of 10 nm. Intermediate filament proteins are diverse and vary by cell type. Cytopathologists use intermediate filament subtype to determine the tissue of origin of tumors. The fibrous subunits of intermediate filaments are structurally different from the globular subunits of actin and tubulin. Intermediate filaments play a major role in distributing mechanical forces within and across cells. Keratin filaments – intermediate filaments found in epidermal cells – distribute stress between and within cells. Desmosomes, which link cells together, and hemidesmosomes, which fix cells to their substrate, are attached to keratin filaments. The disease epidermolysis bullosa simplex results from a mutation in keratin leading to a fragile epidermis.

PROTEIN SYNTHESIS, FOLDING AND MODIFICATION

A typical mammalian cell contains greater than 10 000 different proteins; proper function depends not only on correct synthesis, but also on localization of each protein to the appropriate cellular membrane or compartment. Some proteins encoded for by mitochondrial DNA are synthesized on ribosomes in the mitochondria and incorporated directly into compartments within the organelle. The majority of mitochondrial proteins and all the proteins encoded for by the nuclear DNA are synthesized on ribosomes in the cytosol (either 'free' or bound to the endoplasmic reticulum [ER]), and are distributed to their correct destinations via sorting signals and multiple sorting events (Fig. 2.7, 2.8). Certain membrane and organelle proteins and virtually all secretory proteins are synthesized and pass through the rough ER. Ribosomes are bound to ER by the nascent peptide chain (and give the ER a 'rough' appearance on electron microscopy). Therefore, rough ER is particularly abundant in cells that produce secreted proteins. As free (cytoplasmic) ribosomes synthesize a secretory protein, the N-terminal signal sequence emerges from the ribosome and is bound by a signal-recognition particle, and this complex binds to the signal-recognition particle receptor on the rough ER. Protein synthesis continues as the nascent protein is translocated into the lumen of the ER through a protein conducting channel, not through the membrane itself. The signal sequence is often removed by signal peptidase. Proteins synthesized on the rough ER pass through the Golgi complex en route to their final destination, which could be lysosomes, endosomes, secretory vesicles, or the plasma membrane. Transmembrane proteins and proteins for many cellular organelles follow the same pathway. Proteins imported into mitochondria or peroxisomes are synthesized in the cytosol and have signal sequences that are different from those that mediate translocation into the ER.

Rapid folding of proteins into secondary structures (e.g. α-helices, β-sheets, and random coils) occurs during and shortly after synthesis. Then the slower process of searching for the final correct protein conformation occurs. For some proteins, this state is reached spontaneously; others require molecular chaperones, which are ATPases that bind nascent or incorrectly

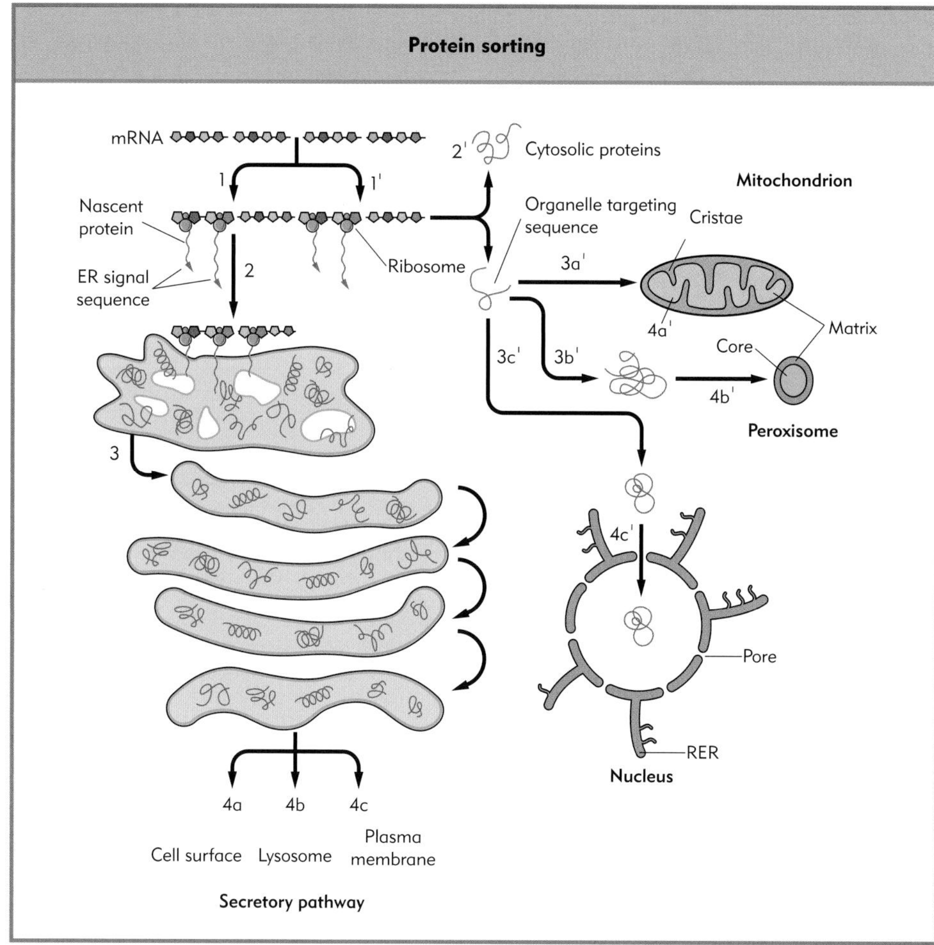

Figure 2.7 Protein sorting. All nuclear-encoded mRNAs are translated on cytosolic ribosomes. Ribosomes synthesizing nascent proteins in the secretory pathway (1) are directed to the rough endoplasmic reticulum (ER) by an ER signal sequence (2). After translation is completed in the ER, these proteins move via transport vesicles to the Golgi complex (3), whence they are further sorted to several destinations (4a–c). After synthesis of proteins lacking an ER signal sequence is completed on free ribosomes (1′), the proteins are released into the cytosol (2′). Those with an organelle-specific uptake-targeting sequence are imported into the target organelle (3a′–c′). Unlike mitochondrial proteins, which are imported in a partially unfolded form (4a′), most peroxisomal proteins cross the peroxisome membrane as fully folded proteins (4b′). Folded nuclear proteins enter through visible nuclear pores (4c′). (Adapted from a drawing by Sergey Perouansky.)

folded proteins to promote correct folding and block unwanted aggregation. Despite these safeguards, some proteins become irreversibly misfolded and are destroyed. Abnormal protein folding can cause diseases; some mutations cause loss of function through abnormal folding of the final protein. Kuru, bovine spongiform encephalopathy (BSE, 'mad cow disease'), Creutzfeld–Jakob disease (all variants), scrapie, fatal familial insomnia and Gerstmann–Straussler–Scheinker syndrome are diseases apparently caused by abnormal protein folding. These diseases, known as transmissible spongiform encephalopathies or prion diseases, are associated with the accumulation of an abnormal form of a host cell protein. In scrapie, for example, the normal protein has an α-helical conformation, whereas its pathological form is β-helical, hydrophobic, neurotoxic, resistant to proteolytic degradation contagious, and tends to polymerize into scrapie-associated fibrils and rods.

Nearly every protein is chemically altered after its synthesis. These alterations fall into two general categories: chemical modifications (may be reversible) and processing (irreversible). *Chemical modifications* include acetylation (the addition of an acetyl group to the N-terminal amino group involves 80% of all proteins, rendering them resistant to intracellular degradation), phosphorylation (regulates function), glycosylation (attachment of linear or branched carbohydrate chains, common in membrane and secreted proteins) and the attachment of lipid (forming lipoproteins). *Protein processing* involves proteolytic cleavage (catalyzed by proteases, a common mechanism of activation/inactivation in the coagulation cascade). Protein degradation can occur in the cytosol, in lysosomes, or in the ER. Reasons for selective degradation of proteins include misfolding, damage, overproduction, or targeted destruction of short-lived proteins such as cyclins. Cytoplasmic proteins can be marked for degradation in proteosomes by covalent linkage with a chain of ubiquitin proteins (Fig. 2.5).

PROTEIN TRANSPORT AND SECRETION

Constitutive exocytosis of proteins is a nonregulated process that occurs in all cells. Transport vesicles involved in the default pathway of secretion have a cytosolic coat of the protein coatamer. A GTPase regulates the assembly and disassembly of coatamer-coated vesicles. The coatamer coat is removed after the vesicle reaches its destination. Many cells, such as neurons, hormone-secreting cells, and other specialized secretory cells, have a regulated secretory system. Secretory vesicles are stored for subsequent release. Proteins and other compounds stored in secretory vesicles are sorted into clathrin-coated vesicles as they leave the Golgi apparatus. As the secretory vesicles mature, they lose the clathrin coat and the contents of the vesicle become concentrated. Further processing of secretory proteins, such as proteolytic cleavage of pro-opiomelanocortin into β-endorphin and adrenocorticotropic hormone, occurs as the secretory vesicle matures. Transport vesicles contain surface proteins that mediate binding to the correct destination. The fidelity of binding is ensured by GTPases known as Rab proteins. Different Rab proteins are associated with different membrane systems.

In neuronal cells, protein-containing secretory vesicles are synthesized in the cell body and transported along microtubules of the nerve axon until they reach the axonal terminal. The vesicles accumulate, and some undergo a modification known as priming that readies them for release of their contents. The next step in release is docking, the close association of vesicles with the plasma membrane. Actual release of vesicular contents occurs after protein-mediated fusion of the two membranes. In nerve cells, an action potential leads to depolarization of the axonal terminal, which causes an influx of Ca^{2+} through Ca^{2+} channels and subsequent secretion (Chapter 20). In other cells regulated secretion is receptor mediated, and binding of a specific hormone can cause a localized increase in intracellular Ca^{2+} that leads to regulated exocytosis. Fusion of the secretory vesicles with the plasma membrane is followed by release of the contents of the vesicle, and rapid recycling of the secretory vesicle and associated membrane proteins by endocytosis.

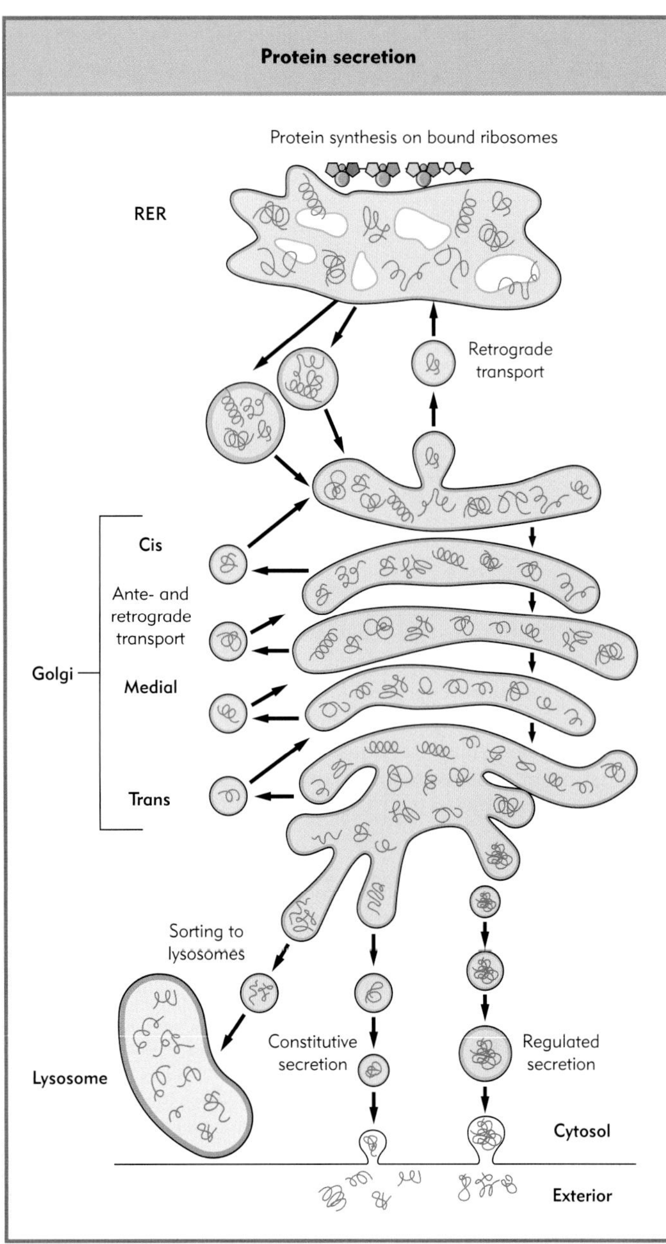

Figure 2.8 Protein secretion. Ribosomes synthesizing proteins bearing an ER signal sequence become bound to the rough endoplasmic reticulum (RER). As translation occurs on the ER, the polypeptide chains are inserted into the ER membrane or cross it into the lumen. Some proteins remain resident in the ER. The remainder move into transport vesicles that fuse together to form new *cis*-Golgi vesicles. Each *cis*-Golgi cisterna and its protein content physically moves from the *cis* to the *trans* face of the Golgi stack (red arrows). As this cisternal progression occurs, many lumenal and membrane proteins undergo modifications, primarily glycosylation by attachment of oligosaccharide chains. Some proteins remain in the *trans*-Golgi cisternae, whereas others move via small vesicles to the cell surface or to lysosomes. Secretion of proteins can be either regulated (in response to a signal) or constitutive. The orientation of a membrane protein, established when it is inserted into the ER membrane, is retained during all the sorting steps: some segments always face the cytosol, and others always face the exoplasmic space (the lumen of organelles or the cell exterior) (Adapted from a drawing by Sergey Perouansky.)

Key references

Blander G, Guarente L. The Sir2 family of protein deacetylases. Annu Rev Biochem 2004; 73:417–35.

Hayflick L, Moorhead P. The serial cultivation of human diploid cell strains. Exp Cell Res. 1961;25:585.

Jesenberger V, Jentsch S. Deadly encounter: ubiquitin meets apoptosis. Nature Reviews Molecular Cell Biology 2002; 3:112–121.

Körbling M, Estrov Z. Adult stem cells for tissue repair – A new therapeutic concept? NEJM 2003; 349:570–82.

Leist M, Jäättelä M. Four deaths and a funeral: from caspases to alternative mechanisms. Naature Reviews Molecular Cell Biology 20001; 2:1–10.

Orrenius S, Zhivotovsky B, Nicotera P. Regulation of cell death: the calcium-apoptosis link. Nature Reviews Molecular Cell Biology 2003; 4:552–565.

Syntichaki P, Tavernakis N. The biochemistry of neuronal necrosis: rogue biology? Nature Reviews Neuroscience 2003; 4:672–684.

Further reading

Clark WR. A means to an end. The biological basis of aging and death. New York: Oxford University Press; 1999.

Dawkins R. The selfish gene, 2nd edn. Oxford: Oxford University Press; 1990.

Lodisch H et al. Molecular cell biology, 4th edn. London: W H Freeman and Co; 2000.

The Encyclopedia of Life Sciences at www.els.net (Macmillan Publishers Ltd, Nature publishing Group) is an excellent resource that offers review articles at the introductory and advanced levels on any topic related to the natural sciences.

Acknowledgements

I would like to thank Sergey Perouansky, computer graphic designer, for drawing Figures 2.6c, 2.7 and 2.8.

Chapter 3

Cell signaling

Hugh C Hemmings, Jr and Jean-Antoine Girault

PRINCIPLES OF CELLULAR SIGNALING

Signal transduction or cell signaling concerns the mechanisms by which biological information is transferred between cells. Functional coordination in complex multicellular organisms requires intercellular communication between a diverse range of specialized cell types in various tissues and organs. Maintaining this coordination requires a constant and dynamic stream of intercellular communication. Adjacent cells can communicate directly by interactions of surface proteins, and through specialized plasma membrane junctions (gap junctions) that allow the direct passage of small cytoplasmic molecules from one cell to the other. Long range cell-to-cell communication is possible through the involvement of extracellular signaling molecules (such as hormones and neurotransmitters) that are synthesized and released by specific cells, diffuse or circulate to target cells, and elicit specific responses in target cells that express receptors for the particular signal. The responses to the extracellular signal are generated by diverse signal transduction mechanisms that frequently involve small intracellular molecules (*second messengers*) that transmit signals from activated receptors to the cell interior, resulting in changes in the expression of genes and the activity of enzymes. These intercellular and intracellular signaling pathways are essential to the growth, development, metabolism, and behavior of the organism.

At the level of individual cells, signaling is crucial in division, differentiation, metabolic control and death. Cell signaling pathways are involved in the pathophysiology of many diseases. Cancer is a disease of signaling malfunction due to inactivation of a growth-inhibiting (tumor suppressor) pathway, or to activation of a growth-promoting (oncogene) pathway by genetic mutation. Diabetes results from defects in insulin signaling involved in blood glucose homeostasis. Cell signaling pathways are also involved in the mechanisms of action of many drugs, including local and general anesthetics. Knowledge of basic cell signaling mechanisms is therefore essential for an understanding of many pathophysiologic and pharmacologic mechanisms. Progress in this area has been enhanced by the completion of a draft sequence of the human genome, which includes at least 3775 genes (~14% of all genes) involved in signal transduction. The new challenge in cell signaling is to understand the temporal and spatial regulation of signaling events in cells.

EXTRACELLULAR SIGNALS

Communication by extracellular signaling is usually classified according to the distance over which the signal acts. In *autocrine* signaling the signaling cell is its own target, as occurs with many growth factors which are released by cells to stimulate their own growth. *Paracrine* signaling involves the release of extracellular signals that affect target cells in close proximity to the signaling cell, as occurs via neurotransmitters in neuromuscular transmission and synaptic transmission. *Endocrine* signaling involves the release of hormones, which are extracellular signals that usually act on distant target cells after being transported by the circulatory system from their sites of release. This classification is not strict, in that many signals function in more than one manner, as both a neurotransmitter and a hormone, for example epinephrine (adrenaline).

The cellular response to an extracellular signal requires its binding to specific receptors (Table 3.1), which are coupled to changes in the functional properties of target cells. The

Table 3.1 Receptor classification

Cell surface receptors
G protein-coupled receptors (GPCRs) – receptors for hormones, neurotransmitters (biogenic amines, amino acids) and neuropeptides
Activate/inhibit adenylyl cyclase
Activate phospholipase C
Modulate ion channels
Ligand-gated ion channels – receptors for neurotransmitters (biogenic amines, amino acids, peptides)
Mediate fast synaptic transmission
Enzyme-linked cell surface receptors
Receptor guanylyl cyclases – receptors for atrial natriuretic peptide, *Escherichia coli* heat-stable enterotoxin
Receptor serine/threonine kinases – receptors for activin, inhibin, transforming growth factor (TGF)-β, müllerian inhibiting substance
Receptor tyrosine kinases – receptors for peptide growth factors
Tyrosine kinase-associated – receptors for cytokines, growth hormone, prolactin
Receptor tyrosine phosphatases – ligands unknown in most cases
Intracellular receptors
Steroid receptor superfamily – receptors for steroids, sterols, thyroxine (T_3), retinoic acid, and vitamin D

particular receptors expressed by target cells determine their sensitivity to various signals and are responsible for the specificity involved in cellular responses to various signals. Receptors can be classified by their cellular localization (Fig. 3.1). The majority of hormones and neurotransmitters are water-soluble (hydrophilic) signaling molecules that interact with *cell surface receptors* that are directly or indirectly coupled to intracellular effector molecules. This includes peptides, catecholamines, amino acids, and their derivatives. Prostaglandins are the major class of lipid-soluble signaling molecule that interact with cell surface receptors. A number of lipid-soluble (hydrophobic) signaling molecules diffuse across the plasma membrane and interact with *intracellular receptors*. Steroid hormones, retinoids, vitamin D, and thyroxine are transported in the blood bound to specific transporter proteins, from which they dissociate and diffuse across cell membranes to bind to specific receptors in the nucleus or cytosol. The hormone-receptor complex then acts as a ligand-regulated transcription factor to modulate gene expression by binding to *cis*-acting regulatory DNA sequences in target genes that alter transcription, and thereby regulates target cell function. A sharp boundary between ligands acting extracellularly and intracellularly may not exist. Recent evidence suggests that receptors for the steroid estrogen also act at the plasma membrane by coupling to G proteins to modulate intracellular Ca^{2+} and cAMP levels. Nitric oxide (NO) and carbon monoxide (CO) are members of a new class of gaseous signaling molecules that diffuse across cell membranes to affect neighboring cells. Nitric oxide, which is unstable and has a short half-life (5–10 s), acts as a paracrine signal as it is able to diffuse only a short distance before being inactivated. Cell surface receptors can also bind to insoluble ligands, such as the extracellular matrix or cell adhesion molecules at the surface of other cells, interactions which are crucial to cell development and migration.

Signal transduction pathways have a number of common properties with important functional implications. *Signal amplification* occurs as a result of sequential activation of catalytic signaling molecules. This enables sensitive physiological responses to small physical (several photons) or chemical (a few molecules of an odorant) stimuli, as well as graded responses to increasingly larger stimuli. *Specificity* is imparted by specific receptor proteins and their association with cell type-specific signaling pathways and effector mechanisms. *Pleiotropy* results from the ability of a single extracellular signal to generate multiple responses in a target cell, for example the opening of some ion channels, the closing of others, activation or inhibition of many enzymes, modification of the cytoskeleton, and/or changes in gene expression. Signal *integration* occurs as the cascades of reactions triggered by different signals interact at multiple levels (*crosstalk*), both positively and negatively, to produce a unique cellular response distinct from that of any single signal. In some instances signaling mechanisms transform a graded stimulus into an all-or-none response (bistability), a mechanism which may be very important for many cellular responses, such as cell division. *Feedback* loops can occur in signaling pathways in which a component can negatively (or positively) influence the activity of an earlier (upstream) component. Activation of signaling pathways can lead to *long-lasting effects* on cellular function as a result of changes in gene expression and receptor trafficking, mechanisms that provide potential molecular bases for learning and memory.

A *modular* organization of signaling proteins is an emerging theme in signal transduction. Modules are domains of proteins that are usually involved in protein interactions. They direct protein interactions through their ability to specifically recognize other modules or molecular targets. Larger proteins can contain multiple modules that appear to impart higher selectivity for a given protein–protein interaction and to provide a scaffold to help bring multiple partners together in a signaling complex. These interactions are important in a number of pathways that involve the *translocation* of signaling proteins to different cellular locations.

Receptors

Signal transduction begins with receptor proteins in the plasma membrane, which sense changes in the extracellular environment. As a result of the interactions between receptors and their ligands, signals are transduced across the plasma membrane (Fig. 3.1). Ligand binding to a receptor protein causes a change in the shape (conformation) of the protein, which is transmitted to the cell interior. This can result in the stimulation of an enzyme activity or function that is intrinsic to the receptor (e.g. protein kinase activation, ion channel opening). Other receptors interact with downstream signaling proteins that couple the change in receptor conformation to a change in the activity of an interacting protein, as illustrated by the G protein-coupled receptors.

Diverse cellular functions are independently regulated, partly by the existence of distinct extracellular signals. Receptors bind the signaling molecule with high affinity and specificity.

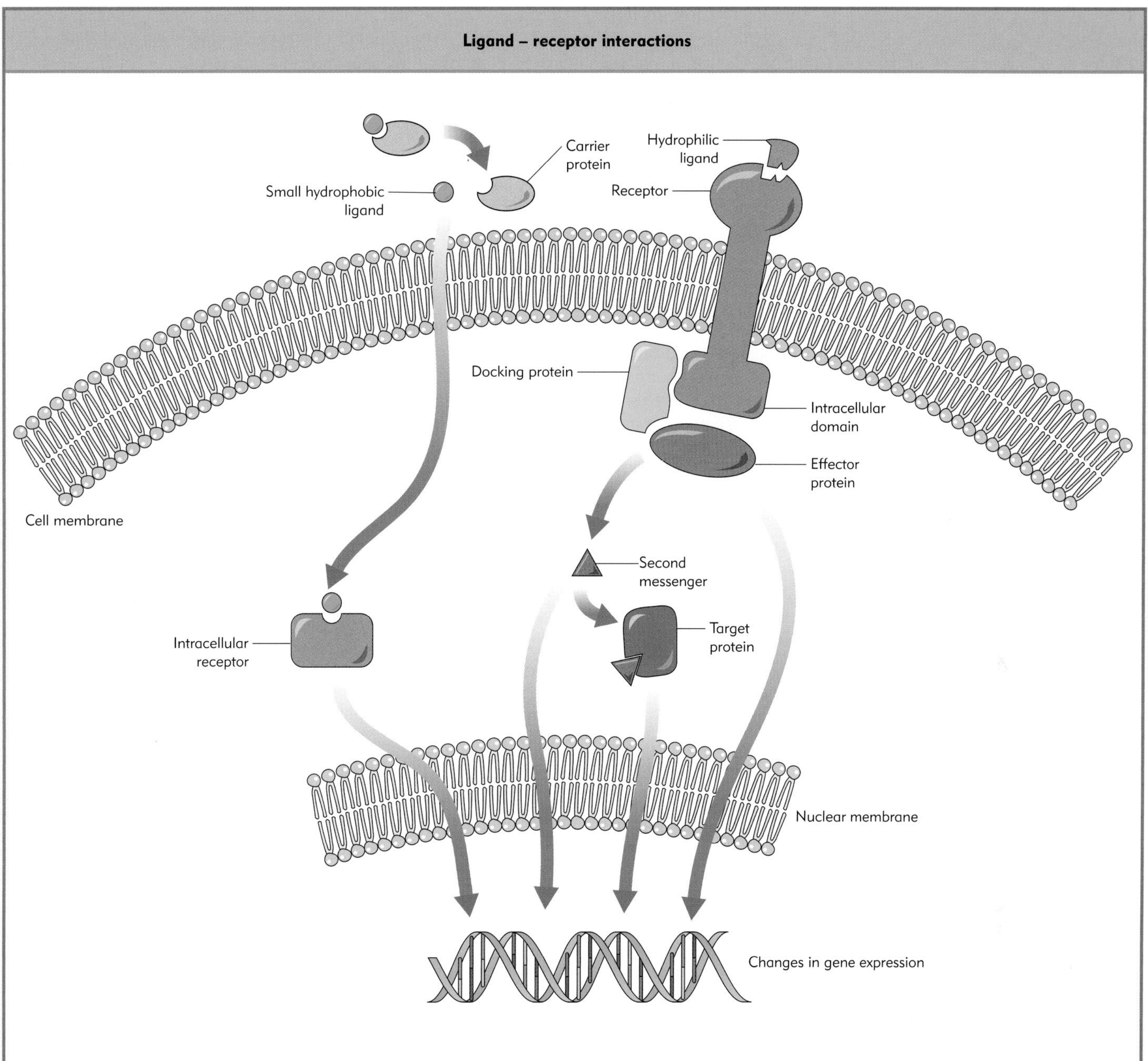

Figure 3.1 Ligand–receptor interactions. Extracellular signals bind to either cell surface receptors or cytoplasmic intracellular receptors. Most signaling molecules are hydrophilic and therefore unable to cross the plasma membrane; they bind to cell surface receptors, which in turn generate one or more intracellular signals (second messengers) inside the target cell or change the activity of effector proteins (e.g. G proteins, protein kinases, ion channels), through their intracellular effector domains. Receptor activation can result in direct changes in the activity of intrinsic enzymatic activities of the receptor intracellular domain, or indirectly via association of the receptor with intracellular mediators, which in turn regulate the activity of effector proteins. Some effectors translocate to the nucleus to control gene expression (e.g. transcription factors) or to other subcellular compartments. Some small signaling molecules, by contrast, diffuse across the plasma membrane and bind to receptors inside the target cell, either in the cytosol (as shown) or in the nucleus. Many of these small signaling molecules are hydrophobic and nearly insoluble in aqueous solutions; they are therefore transported in the bloodstream and other extracellular fluids bound to carrier proteins, from which they dissociate before entering the target cell. (Adapted from Lodish H et al., Molecular Cell Biology, 3rd edition. pp. 853-924; WH Freeman and Co, New York: 1995.)

Additional specificity is imparted by the existence of distinct receptors coupled to different intracellular signaling pathways that respond to the same extracellular signal. Thus a single extracellular signal can elicit different effects on different target cells, depending on the receptor subtype and the signaling mechanisms present. A good example is the neurotransmitter acetylcholine, which stimulates the contraction of skeletal muscle but the relaxation of some smooth muscles. Differences in the intracellular signaling mechanisms also allow the same receptor to produce different responses in different target cells.

The cytoplasmic intracellular receptors are all structurally related and act by directly regulating the transcription of specific genes. In contrast, there are three major classes of cell surface receptor, defined by their signal transduction mechanisms: G protein-coupled receptors, ligand-gated ion channels, and receptor-linked enzymes (Table 3.1). These cell surface receptor proteins act as signal transducers by binding the extracellular signal molecule and converting this information into an intracellular signal that alters target cell function. *G protein-coupled receptors* (GPCRs) interact with specific G proteins in the plasma membrane, which in turn activate or inhibit an enzyme or ion channel. GPCRs constitute the largest family of cell surface receptors, and they mediate the cellular responses to diverse extracellular signals, including hormones, neurotransmitters, and local mediators. There is also a remarkable diversity in the number of GPCRs for the same ligand receptor subtypes. Examples include the multiple receptors for epinephrine, dopamine, serotonin and the opioids. *Ligand-gated ion channels* (ionotropic receptors) are involved primarily in fast synaptic transmission between excitable cells (e.g. the nicotinic acetylcholine receptor at the neuromuscular junction). Neurotransmitter binding to these receptors transiently opens the associated ion channel to alter the ion permeability of the plasma membrane and thereby the membrane potential. The *enzyme-linked cell surface receptors* are a heterogeneous group of receptors that contain intracellular catalytic domains or are closely associated with intracellular enzymes. This receptor class includes the receptor tyrosine kinases, receptor guanylyl cyclases, receptor tyrosine phosphatases, and receptor serine/threonine kinases, in which ligand binding to the receptor activates intrinsic catalytic activity.

The activation of many receptors leads to changes in the concentration of intracellular signaling molecules, termed *second messengers*. These changes are usually transient, which is a result of the tight regulation of the synthesis and degradation (or release and reuptake) of these intracellular signals. Important second messengers include adenosine 3′:5′-monophosphate (cyclic AMP; cAMP), guanosine 3′:5′-monophosphate (cyclic GMP; cGMP), 1,2-diacylglycerol, inositol 1,4,5-trisphosphate (IP_3) and Ca^{2+}. Changes in the concentrations of these molecules following receptor activation are coupled to the modulation of the activities of important regulatory enzymes and effector proteins. The most important second messenger-regulated enzymes are protein kinases and phosphatases, which catalyze the phosphorylation and dephosphorylation, respectively, of key enzymes and proteins in target cells. Reversible phosphorylation alters the function or localization of specific proteins. It is the predominant effector mechanism involved in mediating cellular responses to almost all extracellular signals.

Receptor regulation

The number and function of cell surface receptors are subject to regulation by several mechanisms. Most receptors can be covalently modified by phosphorylation, which can rapidly change their affinity and/or signaling efficiency. For example, β-adrenergic receptors desensitize as a result of phosphorylation of a number of sites in the intracellular carboxy-terminal domain by cAMP-dependent protein kinase, protein kinase C and β-adrenergic receptor kinase (βARK), a G protein-coupled receptor kinase (GRK). The former is activated as a result of receptor stimulation of adenylyl cyclase and results in homologous or heterologous desensitization, whereas the latter is active only on β-receptors occupied by ligand, and therefore results in only homologous desensitization. Phosphorylation by βARK leads to the binding of β-arrestin to the receptor. These processes both serve to uncouple the active ligand–receptor complex from interacting with G_s, creating a negative feedback loop for modulation of β-receptor activity. In other instances, receptor phosphorylation can affect ligand affinity or associated ion channel kinetics rather than G protein coupling. Phosphorylation also often promotes receptor internalization.

Many receptors undergo *receptor desensitization* in response to prolonged exposure to a high concentration of ligand, a process by which the number or function of receptors is reduced, such that the physiological response to the ligand is attenuated (tachyphylaxis). These mechanisms are thought to contribute to the termination of the receptor stimulation, and to prevent overstimulation. Receptor desensitization can occur by several mechanisms, including receptor modification, internalization, downregulation, or modulation. Receptor modification can be a change in conformation that results in spontaneous inactivation, as in the case of some ligand-gated ion channels (e.g. nicotinic acetylcholine receptor, AMPA glutamate receptor) that close in the prolonged presence of the ligand. Receptor internalization by endocytosis is a common mechanism for the desensitization of hormone receptors. The hormone–receptor complex is sequestered by receptor-mediated endocytosis, which results in translocation of the receptor to intracellular compartments (endosomes) that are inaccessible to ligand. This is a relatively slow process that usually terminates the hormone signal. Cessation of agonist stimulation allows the receptor to recycle to the cell surface by exocytosis. In other cases the internalized receptors are degraded and are no longer available for recycling, a process known as receptor downregulation. Receptors must then be replenished by protein synthesis. Receptor downregulation in response to prolonged agonist stimulation can also occur at the level of receptor protein synthesis or mRNA regulation owing to changes in gene transcription and/or mRNA stability. Regulated endocytosis and the delivery of AMPA-type glutamate receptors is also involved in the activity-dependent regulation of synaptic strength by controlling the number of receptors.

CELL SURFACE RECEPTORS: STRUCTURE AND FUNCTION

G protein-coupled receptors

A variety of signals, which include hormones, neurotransmitters, cytokines, pheromones, odorants, and photons, produce their intracellular actions by pathways involving interactions with receptors that activate heterotrimeric guanine nucleotide (GTP)-binding proteins (G proteins). G proteins act as molecular switches to relay information from activated receptors to appropriate intracellular targets. Heterotrimeric G consist of a large α subunit and a smaller βγ subunit dimer. There are various isoforms of each subunit, which have different properties. An agonist-stimulated receptor can activate several hundred G proteins, which in turn activate a variety of downstream effectors, including ion channels and enzymes, to alter the levels of cytosolic second messengers such as Ca^{2+}, cAMP and inositol trisphosphate. G protein-coupled (or linked) receptors (GPCRs) form a large and functionally diverse receptor superfamily; more than 600 (over 2% of total genes) members have been identified so far, making it the largest family of cell surface receptors. These transmembrane receptors cross the membrane seven times, hence they are also known as seven-transmembrane domain, heptahelical, or serpentine receptors. GPCRs transduce a wide variety of extracellular signals, such as light, odorant molecules, biogenic amines, a variety of other small molecules, and peptides. They have an important role in pharmacology – more than two-thirds of all nonantibiotic drugs target GPCRs, and thus they are critical to anesthesiology.

The binding of extracellular signals to their specific cell surface receptors initiates a cycle of reactions to promote guanine nucleotide exchange by G proteins that involves three major steps:

- the signal (ligand) activates the receptor to induce a conformational change;
- the activated receptor turns on a heterotrimeric G protein in the cell membrane by forming a high-affinity ligand-receptor–G protein complex, which promotes guanine nucleotide exchange of GTP for GDP bound by the α subunit of the G protein, followed by dissociation of the α subunit and the $\beta\gamma$ subunit dimer from the receptor and each other;
- the appropriate effector protein(s) is regulated by the dissociated GTP-bound α subunit and/or $\beta\gamma$ subunits, which thereby transduces the signal (Fig. 3.2a).

The dissociation of the G protein from the receptor reduces the affinity of the receptor for the ligand, and the system returns to its basal state as the GTP bound to the α submit is hydrolyzed to GDP by the GTPase activity of the α subunit, and the trimeric G protein complex reassociates to terminate the signal. Several isoforms of G protein α, β and γ subunits exist which mediate the stimulation or inhibition of functionally diverse effector enzymes and ion channels (Table 3.2). Among the effector molecules regulated by G proteins are adenylyl cyclase (Fig. 3.2b), phospholipase C, phospholipase A_2, cGMP phosphodiesterase, and Ca^{2+} and K^+ channels. These effectors then produce changes in the concentrations of a variety of second-messenger molecules or in the membrane potential of the target cell.

Despite the diversity in the extracellular signals that stimulate the various effector pathways activated by GPCRs, these receptors share some global structural similarity, including the seven-transmembrane domain, which is consistent with their common mechanism of action. The GPCRs belong to four different large families that have no sequence homologies between them. The structural domains of GPCRs involved in ligand binding and interactions with G proteins have been analyzed by deletion analysis, in which segments of the receptor are sequentially deleted by site-directed mutagenesis, in which specific single amino acid residues are deleted or mutated, and by constructing chimeric receptor molecules, in which recombinant chimeras are formed by splicing together complementary segments of two related receptors. For example, the agonist isoproterenol binds among the seven transmembrane α helices of the β_2 adrenergic receptor near the extracellular surface of the membrane. The large intracellular loop between α helices 5 and 6 and the C-terminal segments are important for specific G-protein interactions.

Most nonantibiotic drugs in current use target G protein-coupled receptors.

Heterogeneity within GPCR signaling pathways exists at both the level of the receptors and G proteins. A single extracellular signal may have several closely related receptor subtypes. For example, six genes for α-adrenergic receptors, three genes for β-adrenergic receptors and five genes for muscarinic cholinergic receptors have been identified. Likewise, G proteins consist of multiple subtypes. The 16 homologous

Table 3.2 Diversity of G protein-coupled receptor signal transduction pathways. G proteins and their associated receptors and effectors

G Protein[a]	Representative receptors	Effectors	Effect[b]
G_s	β_1, β_2, β_3-adrenergic, D_1, D_5-dopamine	Adenylyl cyclase Ca^{2+} channels	Increased cAMP Increased Ca^{2+} influx
G_i	α_2-adrenergic; D_2-dopamine; m_2, m_4 Muscarinic; μ, δ, κ opioid	Adenylyl cyclase Phospholipase A_2 K^+ channels	Decreased cAMP Eicosanoid release Hyperpolarization
G_q	m_1, m_3 muscarinic; α_1-adrenergic	Phospholipase Cβ	Increased IP_3, DG, Ca^{2+}
G_{olf}	Odorants	Adenylyl cyclase	Increased cAMP (olfaction)
G_t	Photons	cGMP phosphodiesterase	Decreased cGMP (vision)
G_o	?	Phospholipase C Ca^{2+} channels	Increased IP_3, DG, Ca^{2+} Decreased Ca^{2+} influx

[a]G_s, stimulation; G_i, inhibition; G_q, phospholipase C regulation; G_{olf}, olfactory; G_t, transducin; G_o, other.
[b]cAMP, adenosine 3′,5′-monophosphate; cGMP, guanosine 3′,5′-monophosphate; IP_3, inositol 1,4,5-trisphosphate; DG, 1,2,-diacylglycerol.

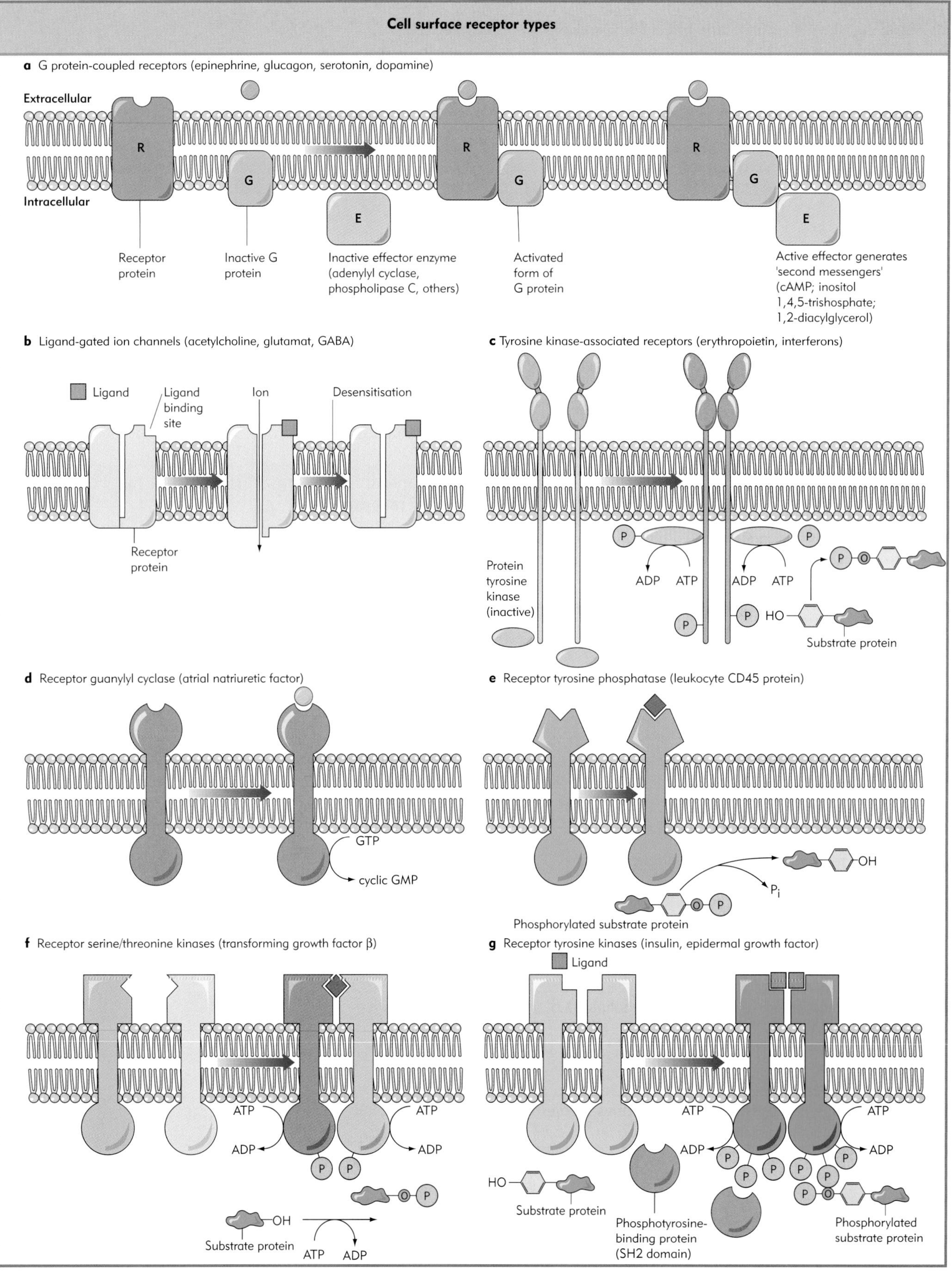

For legend see opposite page.

Figure 3.2, cont'd Cell surface receptor types. Common ligands for each receptor type are shown in parentheses. (a) G protein-coupled receptors. Ligand binding triggers the sactivation of a heterotrimeric G protein, which then binds to and activates an enzyme that catalyzes the synthesis of a specific second messenger or regulates an ion channel. (b) Ligand-gated ion channels. A conformational change triggered by ligand binding opens the channel for ion flow. Continuous occupation of the receptor can result in desensitization of the receptor owing to closure of the ion channel. (c–g) Enzyme-linked cell surface receptors: (c) Tyrosine kinase-associated receptors. Ligand binding causes the formation of a homodimer or heterodimer, triggering the binding and activation of a cytosolic protein tyrosine kinase. The activated kinase phosphorylates tyrosines in the receptor; substrate proteins then bind to these phosphotyrosine residues and are themselves phosphorylated. (d) Activated receptors are monomers with guanylyl cyclase activity that generate the second messenger cGMP. (e) Ligand binding to other receptors activates intrinsic tyrosine phosphatase activity; these receptors can remove phosphate groups from phosphotyrosine residues in substrate proteins, thereby modifying their activity. (f, g) The receptors for many growth factors have intrinsic protein kinase activity. Ligand binding to these receptors causes either identical or nonidentical receptor monomers to dimerize and activates their enzymatic activity. Activated receptors with serine/threonine kinase activity are heterodimers (f), whereas those with tyrosine kinase activity are heterodimers or homodimers (g). In both cases, the activated dimeric receptor phosphorylates several residues in its own intracellular domain. Receptor tyrosine kinases also can phosphorylate certain substrate proteins, thereby altering the activity of these proteins; it is not known whether receptor serine/threonine kinases phosphorylate specific substrate proteins. Specific phosphotyrosine residues in receptor tyrosine kinases function as recognition sites for binding proteins containing SH2 domains. (Adapted from Lodish H et al., Molecular Cell Biology, 3rd edition. pp. 853-924; WH Freeman and Co, New York: 1995.)

α-subunit genes are classified as α_s, α_i, α_o, α_q etc. subtypes based on structural similarities. The different α subunits have distinct functions, coupling with different effector pathways. The different β and γ subunit isoforms may also couple with distinct signaling pathways. Heterogeneity in effector pathways makes divergence possible within GPCR activated pathways. This effector pleiotropy can arise from two distinct mechanisms: a single receptor can activate multiple G protein types, or a single G-protein type can activate more than one effector pathway. Thus, a single type of GPCR can activate several different effector pathways within a given cell, and the predominant pathway may vary between cell types.

The structure and function of the adrenergic receptors for epinephrine and norepinephrine (noradrenaline) and their associated G proteins can be used to illustrate important principles of GPCRs (Fig. 3.3). β-Adrenergic receptors are coupled to the stimulation of adenylyl cyclase, a plasma membrane-associated enzyme that catalyzes the synthesis of cAMP. cAMP was the first second messenger identified, and exists in all prokaryotes and animals. The G protein that couples β-adrenergic receptor stimulation to adenylyl cyclase activation is known as G_s, for stimulatory G protein. Epinephrine-stimulated cAMP synthesis can be reconstituted in phospholipid vesicles using purified β-adrenergic receptors, G_s and adenylyl cyclase, which demonstrates that no other molecules are required for the initial steps of this signal transduction mechanism. In the resting state G_s exists as a heterotrimer consisting of α_s, β, and γ subunits with GDP bound to α_s. Agonist binding to the β-adrenergic receptor alters the conformation of the receptor and exposes a binding site for G_s. The agonist-activated receptor binds the GDP–G_s complex, and thereby reduces the affinity of α_s for GDP, which dissociates, allowing GTP to bind. The α_s subunit bound to GTP then dissociates from the G-protein complex, which exposes a binding site for adenylyl cyclase, to which it binds and activates. The affinity of the receptor for agonist is reduced following dissociation of the complex, leading to agonist dissociation and a return of the receptor to its inactive state. Activation of adenylyl cyclase is rapidly reversed following agonist dissociation from the receptor, as the lifetime of active α_s is limited by the intrinsic GTPase activity of α_s that is stimulated by binding to adenylyl cyclase. The bound GTP is hydrolyzed to GDP, which returns the α subunit to its inactive conformation. The α_s subunit then dissociates from adenylyl cyclase, which renders it inactive, and reassociates with $\beta\gamma$ to reform G_s. Nonhydrolyzable analogues of GTP, such as GTPγS or GMPPNP, prolong agonist-induced adenylyl cyclase activation by preventing the inactivation of active α_s. The mechanism of action of cholera toxin involves selective ADP ribosylation of α_s to inhibit the GTPase activity and prolong $G\alpha_s$ activation. Pertussis toxin promotes ADP-ribosylation of $G\alpha_i$ and prevents its activation by blocking its ability to exchange GDP for GTP.

The activity of adenylyl cyclase can also be negatively regulated by receptors coupled to inhibitory G proteins. An example is the α_2-adrenergic receptor, which is coupled to inhibition of adenylyl cyclase through G_i. Thus the same extracellular signal – epinephrine in this example – can either stimulate or inhibit the formation of the second-messenger cAMP, depending on the particular G protein that couples the receptor to the cyclase. G_i, like G_s, is a heterotrimeric protein consisting of an α_i subunit and β and γ subunits, which can be the same as those in G_s. Activated α_2-adrenergic receptors bind to G_i and lead to GDP dissociation, GTP binding, and complex dissociation, as occurs with G_s. Both the released α_i and the $\beta\gamma$ complex are thought to contribute to adenylyl cyclase inhibition, α_i by direct inhibition, and $\beta\gamma$ by direct inhibition and indirectly, by binding to and inactivating any free α_s subunits. Activated G_i can also open K^+ channels, an example of how a single G protein can regulate several effector molecules.

A hallmark of signal transduction by GPCRs, as well as other receptor/second messenger systems, is their ability to amplify the extracellular signal. *Amplification* is possible because the receptor and the G protein are able to diffuse in the plasma membrane, which allows each agonist-bound receptor complex to interact with many inactive G_s molecules and convert them to their active state. Further amplification occurs when each active $G_{s\alpha}$•GTP complex activates a single adenylyl cyclase molecule, which then catalyzes the formation of many cAMP molecules in the period before the GTP is hydrolyzed, the complex dissociates, and adenylyl cyclase is inactivated.

A number of novel signaling mechanisms have been identified for GPCRs in the last decade. For example, β-arrestin binds to phosphorylated β_2 adrenoceptors to recruit Src-like tyrosine kinases to the membrane and activate MAP kinase and Jun kinase signaling pathways. Thus certain arrestins, which were known to bind to the C-terminal tail of GPCRs phosphorylated by a G protein receptor kinase (GRK) to block G protein receptor interactions and promote receptor recycling via endocytosis, can also initiate other signaling pathways. Direct interaction of the C-terminus of GPCRs with PDZ domains can bypass G proteins to activate intracellular signaling pathways, as in the regulation of the Na^+–H^+ exchanger by β_2 adrenoceptors. These and other *non-G protein mediated effects* indicate that these mechanisms probably represent an important aspect of GPCR signaling. The *regulators of G protein signaling* (RGS) proteins are a recently identified family of signaling molecules that modulate G protein signaling and also act as scaffolding proteins to maintain signaling complexes. Most RGS proteins are GTPase-activating proteins (GAPs), and terminate signaling by activating GTPase activity of Gi and Gq α subunits, in contrast to the receptor, which acts as a guanine nucleotide exchange factor (GEF) to catalyze GDP release from Gα. Other regulators of the G protein cycle include guanine nucleotide dissociation inhibitors (GDIs), which prevent dissociation of GDP from the α subunit and block reassociation of the $\beta\gamma$ subunit, thereby prolonging $\beta\gamma$ signaling, and guanine nucleotide exchange factors (GEFs), which enhance the rate of GTP loading in the presence of activated receptor, thus accelerating the speed of the response. Although GPCRs are classically thought to function as monomers, recent evidence supports the existence of *dimeric or oligomeric complexes*, either between like receptors (homomers) or between different members of the GPCR family (heteromers). Such interactions modulate receptor function and may be required to produce functional native receptors (e.g. $GABA_B$ receptors).

Ligand-gated ion channels

Signals that utilize GPCRs operate with time courses of seconds to minutes, as occurs with slow synaptic transmission or neuromodulation, in which receptor activation is coupled indirectly through a series of steps to a specific change in effector function. Signals that require rapid transduction, such as fast synaptic transmission, utilize ligand-gated ion channels, in which binding of the signal to the receptor directly causes an immediate conformational change in the receptor–ion channel complex to open the associated ion channel (Chapter 6) and selectively change its ion permeability independent of a second messenger. The ligand-binding site and the ion channel are part of the same molecule or multimolecular complex. A common structural pattern for ligand-gated ion channels involves a tetramer or pentamer of subunits surrounding a central ion pore (Fig. 3.4). Ion channel activation is dependent on the continued occupation of receptor by the ligand, and is rapidly reversible upon ligand dissociation. This allows ligand-gated ion channels to mediate rapid onset and rapidly reversible cell signaling.

Ligand-gated ion channels allow the conversion of extracellular chemical signals directly into electrical signals in excitable cells such as neurons and muscle. The ionic selectivity of the ion channel and the membrane potential of the target cell determine whether the ligand-gated ion channel has an excitatory or an inhibitory effect on neuronal excitability or synaptic transmission (Chapter 19). Excitatory neurotransmitters, which include acetylcholine and glutamate, open cation-selective channels that allow Na^+ influx and depolarize the membrane. Inhibitory neurotransmitters, which include γ-aminobutyric acid (GABA) and glycine, open Cl^- selective channels that usually hyperpolarize the membrane or prevent depolarization. In contrast to these neurotransmitter receptors located at the plasma membrane, a subclass of ligand-gated ion channels is located on intracellular endoplasmic reticulum membranes. It includes receptors for intracellular messengers that control Ca^{2+} channels involved in the regulation of intracellular Ca^{2+} concentration (e.g. the ryanodine receptor and IP_3 receptors – see below).

Although their ligand-binding specificities and ion channel selectivities differ, the ligand-gated ion channels that respond to acetylcholine, serotonin, GABA, and glycine consist of structurally homologous subunits and constitute a receptor superfamily. They are heteropentameric membrane-spanning proteins that consist of homologous subunits that interact to form a central transmembrane ion channel. Multiple isoforms of each subunit exist that interact in different combinations to form receptor–ion channel complexes with distinct ligand affinities, sensitivities to drugs, and channel conductance and kinetic properties. Glutamate-gated ion channels (AMPA, kainate, NMDA subtypes) constitute a distinct family of receptors that also consist of multiple subunit isoforms.

Extensive structural and functional information is available for the nicotinic acetylcholine (ACh) receptor, which can be isolated in large quantities from fish electric organs. This receptor contains four subunit types, which exist in the stoichiometry $\alpha_2\beta\gamma\delta$ (Fig. 3.4a). Each subunit of the nicotinic ACh receptor, GABA receptor, and glycine receptor contains four hydrophobic transmembrane domains in its carboxy-terminal region in similar positions within the subunit, with similar deduced membrane topology (Fig. 3.4b). A long intracellular loop is located between the third and fourth transmembrane segments and may mediate interactions with other proteins. The second transmembrane segment is the most hydrophilic of the four, and lines the aqueous ion channel. A large extracellular ligand-binding domain extends over the entire amino-terminal half of the subunit.

Molecular cloning techniques have identified a large number of isoforms of the five different subunit types that constitute the $GABA_A$ receptor (α_1–α_6; β_1–β_4; γ_1–γ_3; ε; δ; and ρ subunits), an important target for general anesthetics, benzodiazepines, and anticonvulsants. Each isoform is homologous and has the general structure shown in Figure 3.4b. Experimental expression of specific subunit isoforms in cultured cells has identified pharmacologic differences produced by various subunit combinations. For example, benzodiazepine sensitivity depends on the specific α or γ subunit isoform present. Alternative splicing of subunit mRNA precursors has also been shown to generate a second isoform of each γ subunit, which may contain an additional phosphorylation site. The many alternative combinations of $GABA_A$ receptors have been shown to have a complex anatomical distribution within the CNS, which may have important functional and pharmacological implications.

Signaling by ligand-gated ion channels is affected by most general anesthetic drugs.

The ligand-gated glutamate receptors are functionally divided into those activated by *N*-methyl-D-aspartate (NMDA) and the non-NMDA receptors, which latter can be distinguished by their sensitivities to α-amino-3-hydroxy-5-methylisoxazole-4-propionic acid (AMPA) and kainate. Expression cloning was used to identify the first non-NMDA receptor subunit structure, from which a family of homologous non-NMDA receptor subunits has been identified (GluR1–GluR7 and KA1–KA2). These subunits have three deduced hydrophobic transmembrane domains with a reentrant P-loop. More than one type of subunit is required to express glutamate-gated cation channel function, which suggests that the functional form of the receptor exists as an oligomer. Alternative splicing results in additional subunit heterogeneity, as seen with the $GABA_A$ receptor. NMDA receptors possess many unique properties among ligand-gated ion channels, which include (in addition to glutamate sensitivity), the requirement of glycine as a co-agonist, slow kinetics, and voltage-dependent blockade by Mg^{2+}. Identification of the structure of an NMDA receptor subunit by expression cloning (NR1) again revealed a topology consisting of three similar transmembrane domains and a reentrant loop. Additional subunits have since been identified (NR2A–NR2C). Although NR1 can produce the above physiological properties in homomeric form, NR2A–NR2C are only functional in a heteromeric form with NR1. The NR2 subunits differ considerably from NR1 in amino acid sequence and subunit lengths owing to variable carboxy-terminal extensions. Although the multiple glutamate receptors overall show considerable sequence diversity, the similarities in their transmembrane sequences justifies their inclusion as a distinct subgroup in one superfamily with the nicotinic ACh receptors.

The structural diversity of ligand-gated ion channels is reflected in a rich pharmacological diversity. Important examples include the actions of neuromuscular blocking drugs on nicotinic ACh receptors at the neuromuscular junction (Chapter 37), of barbiturates and benzodiazepines on $GABA_A$ receptors (Chapter 25), and of phencyclidine derivatives (e.g. ketamine) on NMDA receptors (Chapter 25).

Enzyme-linked cell surface receptors

Enzyme-linked receptors are transmembrane proteins that couple an extracellular ligand-binding domain with an intracellular catalytic domain via a single transmembrane domain. The enzyme activity is either contained within the intracellular domain of the receptor (intrinsic activity) or associated with the intracellular domain of the receptor (associated activity). Although this is a heterogeneous group of receptors, most possess a single transmembrane domain and are associated with the activation of protein kinase activity (Fig. 3.2). The known enzyme-linked receptors are divided into five classes: receptor tyrosine kinases, tyrosine kinase-associated receptors, receptor tyrosine phosphatases, receptor serine/threonine kinases, and receptor guanylyl cyclases.

The best-known receptors in this family are the *receptor tyrosine kinases*, which include the receptors for many peptide/protein growth factors, including epidermal growth factor (EGF), platelet-derived growth factor (PDGF), nerve growth factor (NGF) and related neurotrophins, fibroblast growth factors (FGFs), and insulin and insulin-like growth factor-1 (IGF-1). Signaling through receptor tyrosine kinases is central to many of the cell–cell interactions that regulate embryonic development, tissue maintenance, and repair. Their activity is tightly regulated; perturbation due to mutations results in dysregulated kinase activity and malignant transformation. Ligand binding to the extracellular domain of most receptor tyrosine kinases induces dimerization and activation of the tyrosine kinase intrinsic to the intracellular domain, which catalyzes the phosphorylation of the receptor itself (autophosphorylation) and of specific intracellular proteins, which leads to specific physiological effects and changes in gene expression. Receptor dimerization is important in the activation of the intracellular tyrosine kinase activity, as it allows cross-phosphorylation of the two intracellular domains.

Phosphorylated tyrosines on proteins create high-affinity binding sites for specific intracellular signaling proteins in the target cell, resulting in changes in their localization or activity. These interacting proteins usually contain Src homology-2 domains (SH2 domains), protein interaction modules that recognize phosphorylated tyrosine residues in the receptor. Tyrosine phosphorylation thus acts as a switch to recruit SH2 domain-containing target proteins. Binding of SH2 domain-containing proteins frequently results in their phosphorylation on tyrosine and subsequent activation, or in their interaction with other signaling molecules. Receptor tyrosine autophosphorylation triggers the assembly of a transient intracellular signaling complex that is involved in the signal transduction process (Fig. 3.5). Some proteins in these complexes function only as scaffolding (or adaptor) proteins that bring together other signaling molecules. Other proteins that interact with tyrosine phosphorylated receptors via their SH2 domains are themselves signaling proteins, such as phospholipase Cγ, GTPase activating proteins (GAPs), c-Src-family non-receptor tyrosine kinases, and phosphatidylinositide 3-OH kinase. Activation of phosphatidylinositide 3-OH kinase activates another pleiotropic signaling pathway by phosphorylation of membrane lipids to form phosphatidylinositol-(3,4)-bisphosphate and phosphatdylinositol-(3,4,5)-trisphosphate, which recruits the serine/threonine kinase Akt to the membrane by binding to its PH domain. This allows Akt activation by PDK-1, an Akt kinase, and leads to the phosphorylation of Akt substrates involved in regulating glucose transport, programmed cell death (apoptosis) and cell growth.

An important class of proteins recruited by tyrosine kinase receptors includes regulators of small G proteins. Ras proteins are small G proteins involved in transducing mitogenic signals from the cell surface to the nucleus through a cascade of protein kinases to stimulate cell growth and differentiation (Fig. 3.5). In contrast to the larger heterotrimeric G proteins, small G proteins are monomeric and consist primarily of the GDP/GTP-binding domain. They are involved in many functions, such as regulation of the cell cycle and the cytoskeleton. Ras activation by growth factor receptor tyrosine kinases requires the adapter proteins Grb2, Shc, and Sos, which couple receptor activation to Ras activation. Binding of growth factor to its receptor leads to autophosphorylation. An SH2 domain in Grb2 interacts with a phosphotyrosine residue on the intracellular portion of the activated receptor tyrosine kinase (e.g. EGF receptor) or on the adapter protein Shc. Grb2 then binds and activates Sos through two SH3 domains on Sos, thereby linking the receptor with Sos, a guanine nucleotide exchange factor (GEF) that activates Ras by stimulating the release of GDP and subsequent GTP binding. The active GTP-bound form of Ras then recruits and activates the Raf-1 protein kinase. Activated Raf-1 protein kinase initiates a protein kinase cascade that involves the phosphorylation and activation of MAP-kinase kinase (MEK), which then phosphorylates and activates MAP-kinase (mitogen-activated protein kinase, also called ERK) by phosphorylation of both threonine and tyrosine residues (an unusual dual-specificity kinase). Activated MAP-kinase signals downstream by phosphorylating various effector molecules, such as phospholipase A_2, and transcription factors involved in gene regulation. The *MAP-kinase pathway* is a highly conserved eukaryotic signaling pathway involving a kinase cascade that couples receptor signals to cell proliferation, differentiation, and metabolic regulation. Activated GTP-Ras is slowly converted to the inactive, GDP-bound form by its intrinsic GTPase activity, which can be accelerated by a GAP (GTPase-activating protein).

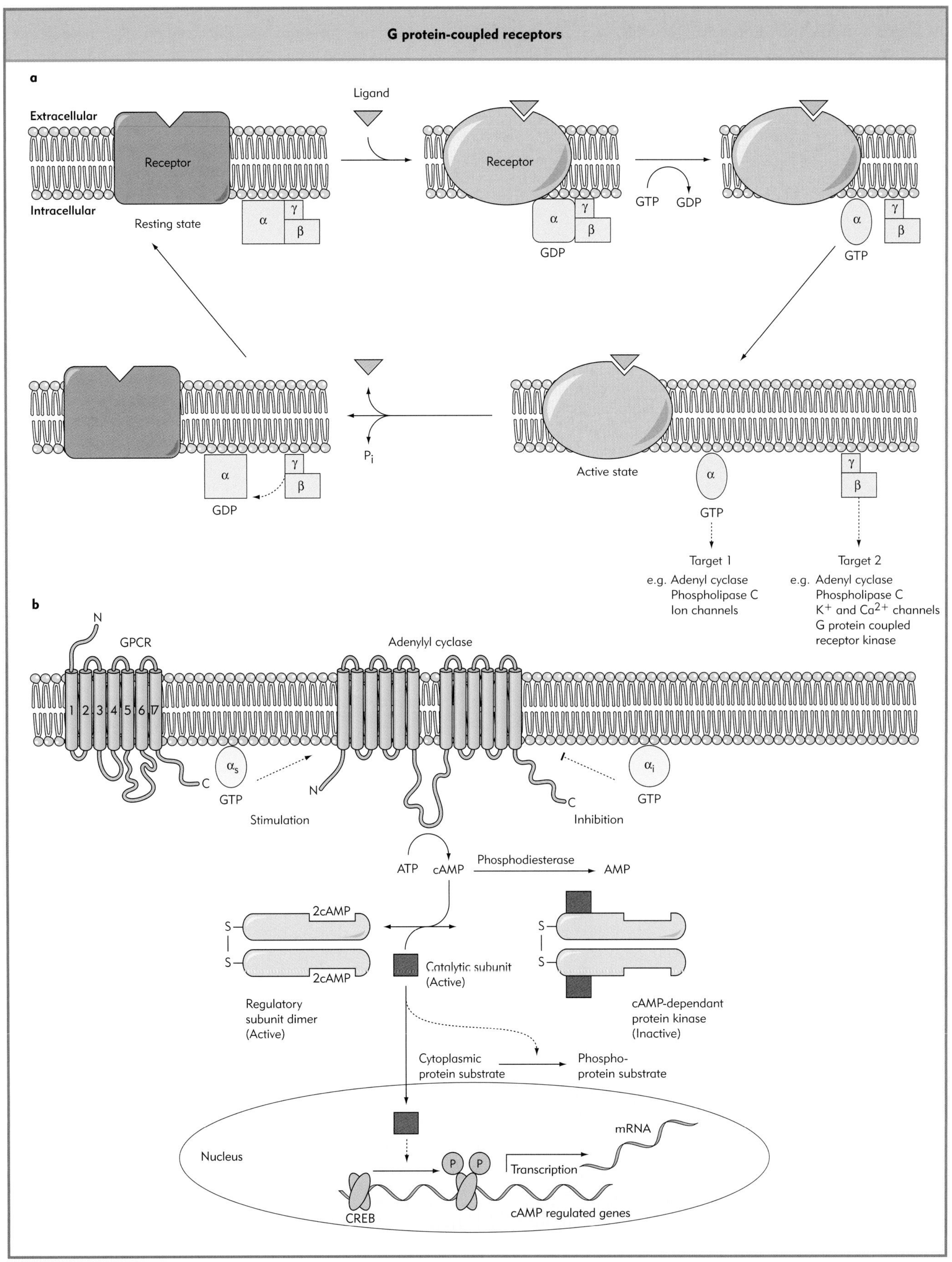

For legend see opposite page.

Figure 3.3, cont'd G protein-coupled receptors. (a) General features. Many receptors belong to this class, including those for neurotransmitters, hormones, odorants, light, and Ca^{2+}. These receptors associate with heterotrimeric G proteins comprised of three subunits, α, β, and γ. G proteins are not transmembrane proteins but are associated with the membrane by covalently bound fatty acid molecules. In the resting state GDP is bound to the α subunit, which in this form interacts with the βγ complex. When the ligand binds to the receptor the conformation of the receptor changes, leading to α subunit and inducing a change in the conformation of the α subunit such that GDP dissociates and GTP binds. The GTP-bound α subunit is no longer capable of interacting with the receptor or βγ. GTP-bound α and βγ interact with specific targets that differ for each isoform of α or βγ subunit. After a short time GTP is hydrolyzed to GDP and α-GDP reassociates with βγ. At about the same time the ligand leaves its receptor, which returns to its resting state. G protein, guanine nucleotide-binding protein; Pi, inorganic phosphate. (b) The adenylyl cyclase/protein kinase A (PKA) pathway. cAMP is formed from ATP by a class of transmembrane enzymes, adenylyl cyclases. A cytosolic form (soluble adenylyl cyclase) has also recently been identified which may function as a bicarbonate sensor. Transmembrane adenylyl cyclases are activated by two related subtypes of G protein α subunit, α_s (stimulatory, which is ubiquitous) and α_{Olf} (olfactory, which is found in olfactory epithelium and a subset of neurons). Adenylyl cyclases are inhibited by α_i (inhibitory). In addition, some adenylyl cyclases can be stimulated or inhibited by βγ, or Ca^{2+} combined with calmodulin. Cyclic AMP is inactivated by hydrolysis into AMP by phosphodiesterases, a family of enzymes which is inhibited by theophylline and related methylxanthines. cAMP has only two known targets in vertebrates: one is a cAMP-gated ion channel which is most prominently found in olfactory neurons; the other is cAMP-dependent protein kinase which is present in all cells. cAMP-dependent protein kinase is a tetramer composed of two catalytic subunits and two regulatory subunit. When cAMP binds to the regulatory subunits (two molecules of cAMP bind to each regulatory subunit), they dissociate from the catalytic subunits. The free active catalytic subunit phosphorylates numerous specific substrates, including ion channels, receptors, and enzymes. In addition, the catalytic subunit can enter the nucleus, where it phosphorylates transcription factors. One well-characterized transcription factor phosphorylated in response to cAMP is CREB (cAMP-responsive element-binding protein). In the basal state, CREB forms a dimer which binds to a specific DNA sequence in the promoter region of cAMP-responsive genes, called CRE (cAMP-responsive element). CREB is unable to promote transcription when it is not phosphorylated, whereas phospho-CREB strongly stimulates transcription. Genes regulated by CREB include immediate-early genes c-Fos and c-Jun. CREB is also activated by a Ca^{2+} calmodulin-dependent protein kinase. (Adapted from Lodish H et al., Molecular Cell Biology, 3rd edition. pp. 853-924; WH Freeman and Co, New York: 1995.)

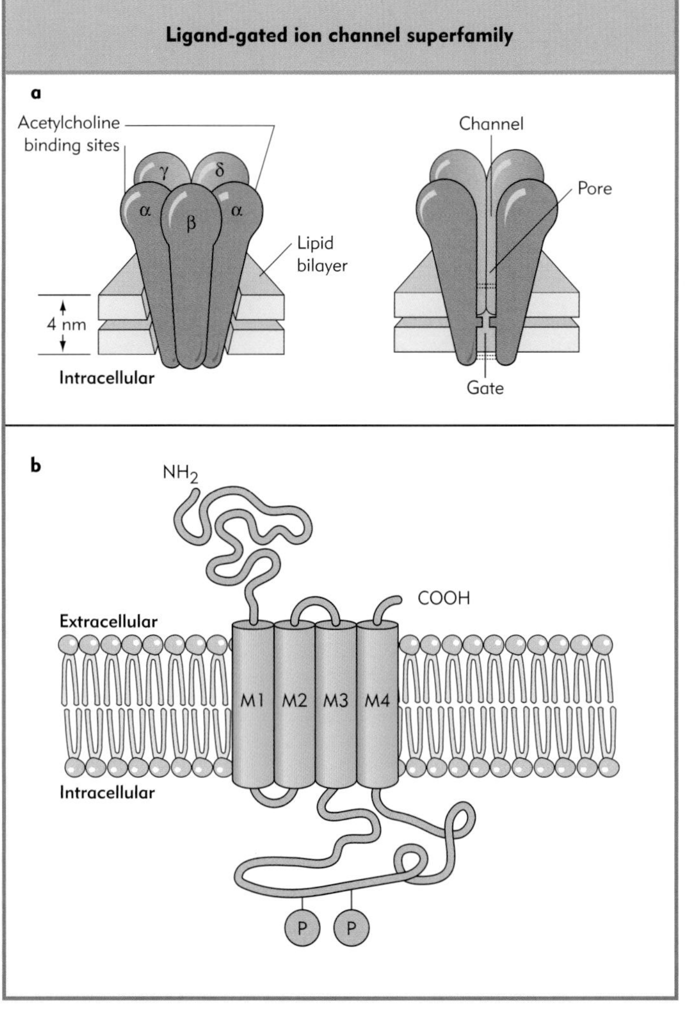

Figure 3.4 Ligand-gated ion channel superfamily. (a) The nicotinic acetylcholine receptor, a representative ligand-gated ion channel. Five homologous subunits (two αs, β, γ, δ) combine to form a transmembrane aqueous pore. The pore is lined by a ring of five transmembrane α helices, one contributed by each subunit. The ring of α helices is probably surrounded by a continuous rim of transmembrane β sheet, made up of the other transmembrane segments of the five subunits. In its closed conformation the pore is thought to be occluded by the hydrophobic side chains of five leucine residues, one from each α helix, which form a gate near the middle of the lipid bilayer. The negatively charged side chains at either end of the pore (dotted lines) ensure that only positively charged ions pass through the channel. Both of the α subunits contain an acetylcholine-binding site; when acetylcholine binds to both sites, the channel undergoes a conformational change that opens the gate, possibly by causing the leucine residues to move outward. (b) Transmembrane topography of each of the four subunit types of the nicotinic acetylcholine receptor. M1–M4 represent the four transmembrane domains of the receptor subunit. A region of the intracellular loop of each subunit is phosphorylated by cAMP-dependent protein kinase, protein kinase C, and a protein–tyrosine kinase. Phosphorylation of the receptor in this region increases its rate of rapid desensitization. (Adapted from Lodish H et al., Molecular Cell Biology, 3rd edition. pp. 853-924; WH Freeman and Co, New York: 1995.)

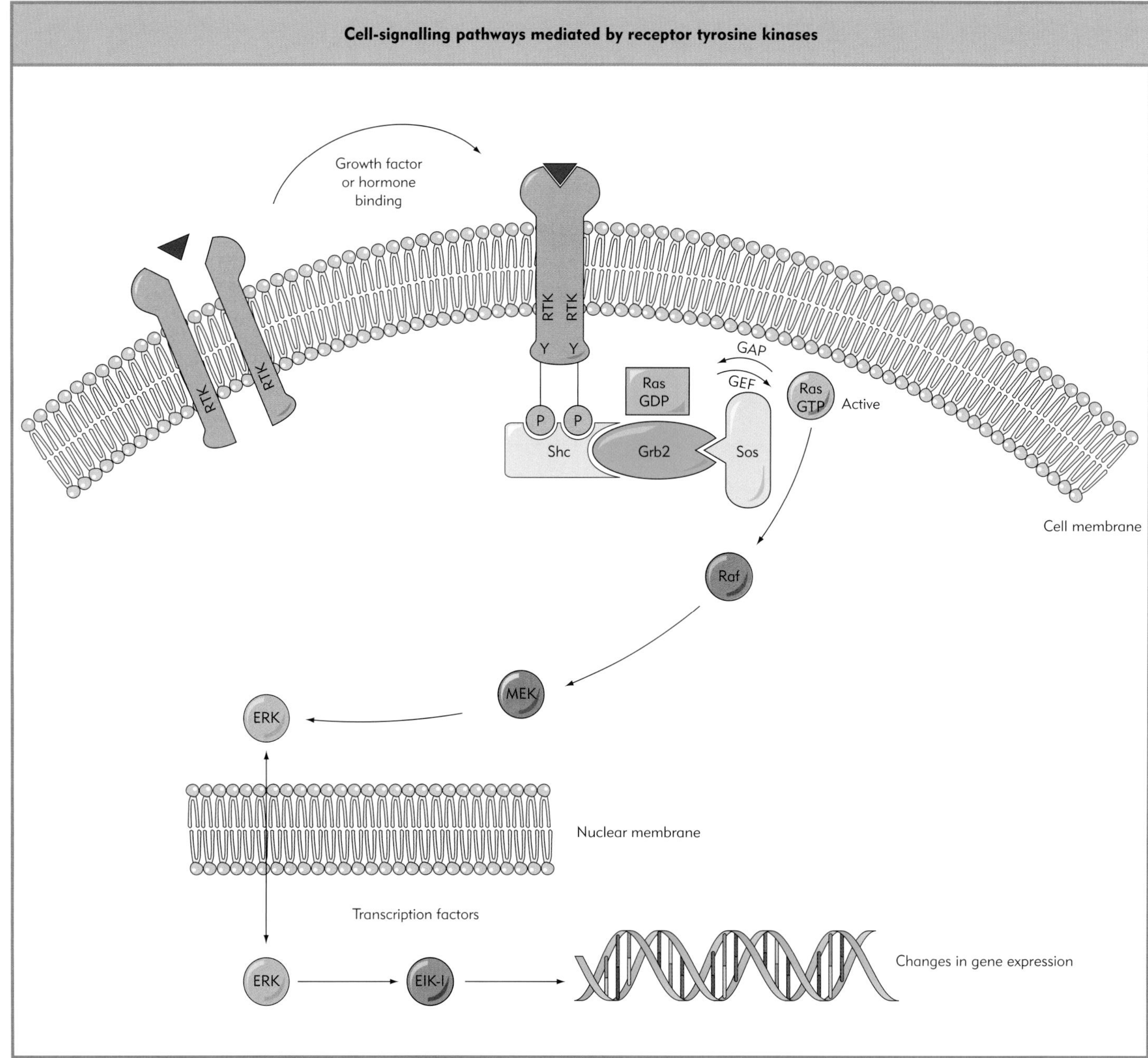

Figure 3.5 Cell-signaling pathways mediated by receptor tyrosine kinases. Binding of a hormone such as insulin leads to dimerization, autophosphorylation, and activation of a receptor tyrosine kinase (RTK). On receptor stimulation, the adaptor protein Shc binds to activated, tyrosine phosphorylated receptors and becomes phosphorylated. Tyrosine-phosphorylated Shc subsequently interacts with the SH2 domain of Grb2, which binds by its SH3 domains to the guanine nucleotide exchange factor (GEF) Sos, which activates the small GTP-binding protein Ras. Sos enhances GDP dissociation from Ras, promoting its activation by rebinding GTP; Ras then slowly hydrolyzes GTP to GDP and becomes inactive. Activated Ras in turn activates Raf-1, a serine/threonine protein kinase. Raf-1 phosphorylates and activates MEK (MAP kinase), a bifunctional protein tyrosine and protein serine/threonine kinase. MEK (extracellular signal-regulated kinase [ERK] kinase) activates ERK (MAP kinase) by phosphorylation on both tyrosine and threonine. ERK itself phosphorylates and activates cytoplasmic proteins such as S6 kinase, which stimulates protein synthesis, insulin-stimulated protein kinase $p90^{rsk}$, and nuclear transcription factors such as Elk-1 and c-Jun. Ras functions as a GDP/GTP-regulated binary switch at the inner surface of the plasma membrane to relay extracellular signals to the cytoplasmic signaling cascades. A linear vectoral pathway exists between the activation of receptor tyrosine kinases, Ras, a serine/threonine kinase cascade (Raf→MEK→ERK) and transcription factors to provide a link between the cell membrane and the nucleus. (Adapted from Lodish H et al., Molecular Cell Biology, 3rd edition. pp. 853-924; WH Freeman and Co, New York: 1995.)

Tyrosine kinase-associated receptors are comparable to the receptor tyrosine kinases, but instead of activating an integral tyrosine kinase activity they work through associated nonreceptor tyrosine kinases. This diverse group of receptors includes those for some hormones (prolactin, growth hormone, leptin), many cytokines, interferons, and growth factors (e.g. erythropoietin). The associated tyrosine kinases belong to the Janus family (e.g. JAK1 and JAK2) of nonreceptor tyrosine kinases. Other nonreceptor tyrosine kinases, such as those of the c-Src family, are involved in transducing signals from membrane receptors, including lymphocyte antigen receptors. Integrins, which are receptors for extracellular matrix proteins, associate with the tyrosine kinase FAK (focal adhesion kinase). These receptors function like the receptor tyrosine kinases, except that the tyrosine kinase domain is a separate entity that interacts with the receptor noncovalently. As with the receptor tyrosine kinases, ligand binding usually induces receptor dimerization, tyrosine kinase activation, and phosphorylation of distinct sets of substrate proteins.

Receptor tyrosine phosphatases are a large and diverse group of membrane-bound enzymes that reverse the action of tyrosine kinases by catalyzing the dephosphorylation of specific phosphotyrosine residues. Receptor tyrosine phosphatases include an extracellular domain of variable length and composition, a single membrane-spanning domain, and one or two intracellular catalytic domains. CD45, the prototype of this family, has a single transmembrane domain and is activated by crosslinking with antibodies to the extracellular domain. The natural ligand for CD45, or for other members of this family, is unknown.

Receptor serine/threonine kinases constitute a family of receptors for the transforming growth factor-β (TGF-β) family of signaling proteins, including activin and inhibin. These receptors consist of a single transmembrane domain with an integral serine/threonine protein kinase domain within the intracellular portion of the receptor.

Another class of receptor is linked to the activation of proteolytic enzyme cascades. Proteolysis can be involved at several levels of receptor function, including maturation and activation by the ligand. Some transmembrane receptors activate a cascade of intracellular proteases that results in cell death. For example, receptors for Fas ligand and tumor necrosis factor (TNF) associate with various intracellular proteins which, among other things, activate aspartate-specific proteases (caspases).

The *receptor guanylyl cyclases* are discussed below.

SECOND MESSENGERS AND PROTEIN PHOSPHORYLATION

Work by Sutherland and his colleagues in the 1950s on the hormonal control of glycogen metabolism in liver showed that epinephrine and glucagon stimulate glycogenolysis by increasing the synthesis of the intracellular second messenger cAMP. Subsequently, Krebs and his colleagues discovered a protein kinase in skeletal muscle that is activated by increases in cAMP, and demonstrated that epinephrine stimulates glycogenolysis through activation of this protein kinase. Since this groundbreaking work, the mechanisms of action of a number of extracellular signals have been shown to involve second messengers and/or regulation of protein phosphorylation. Protein phosphorylation involves either direct activation of a receptor-associated protein kinase or an alteration in the level of a second messenger, which in turn regulates a specific protein kinase or protein phosphatase (Fig. 3.6). The regulation of the state of phosphorylation of specific substrates by a variety of protein kinases represents a final common pathway in the molecular mechanisms through which most hormones, neurotransmitters, and other extracellular signals produce their biological effects.

Protein phosphorylation represents a final common pathway by which most hormones and neurotransmitters produce their cellular effects.

Protein phosphorylation is the covalent modification of key substrate proteins by phosphoryl transfer, which in turn regulates their functional properties. All protein phosphorylation systems have three components in common: a substrate protein (phosphoprotein) that exists in either the dephospo- or the phospho-form, a protein kinase that catalyzes phosphoryl transfer from the terminal (γ) phosphate of ATP to a specific hydroxylated amino acid of the substrate (serine, threonine or tyrosine), and a protein phosphatase that catalyzes dephosphorylation of the phosphorylated substrate (Fig. 3.6). Second messengers involved in the control of protein phosphorylation by extracellular signals include cAMP, cGMP, Ca^{2+} (with calmodulin), and 1,2-diacylglycerol, each of which activates one or more distinct protein kinases.

Protein kinases are divided into two major classes, serine/threonine kinases and tyrosine kinases (already discussed above), and a minor class of dual specificity kinases. The serine/threonine kinases are further divided into those that are regulated by known second messengers and those that are not (the Ca^{2+}- and cyclic nucleotide-dependent protein kinases and the receptor serine/threonine protein kinases). Almost 2% of human genes encode protein kinases (>500 genes), most of which are serine/threonine kinases (395 genes), and there are at least 15 serine/threonine and 56 tyrosine phosphatase genes. Adding phosphate to a protein can change its conformation, thereby activating or inhibiting a catalytic domain, or form part of a binding motif recognized by other proteins that facilitates protein interactions and the formation of multiprotein complexes. Kinases can be rather specific in their substrate specificity, whereas the catalytic subunits of the phosphatases are relatively nonspecific. Additional specificity is conferred by targeting to specific protein complexes and subcellular domains, and by interactions with various regulatory subunits. Protein kinases are emerging as potentially important therapeutic targets with improved specificity over receptor-based targets. In oncology, small molecule inhibitors of the Abl tyrosine kinase (imatinib; Gleevec) and aurora kinases (VX-680) identified by structure-based approaches suppress tumor growth in vivo.

Protein kinases are emerging as potentially important therapeutic targets.

Cyclic AMP

Cyclic AMP, the first intracellular messenger to be identified, operates as a signaling molecule in all eukaryotic and prokaryotic cells. Various hormones and neurotransmitters regulate the levels of cAMP. Transmembrane adenylyl cyclases form a class of membrane-bound enzymes that catalyze the formation of cAMP, usually under the control of receptor-mediated G protein-coupled stimulation (by α_s and α_{Olf}) and inhibition (by α_i). Depending on the isoform, adenylyl cyclases are also sensitive to other regulators, such as β subunits of heterotrimeric G proteins and Ca^{2+}. Soluble adenylyl cyclase is a recently identified nontransmembrane enzyme that is localized to a number of subcellular compartments and produces cAMP in response to bicarbonate. The rapid degradation of cAMP to adenosine 5′-monophosphate by one of several isoforms of cAMP phosphodiesterase provides the potential for rapid reversibility and responsiveness of this signaling mechanism. Most of the actions

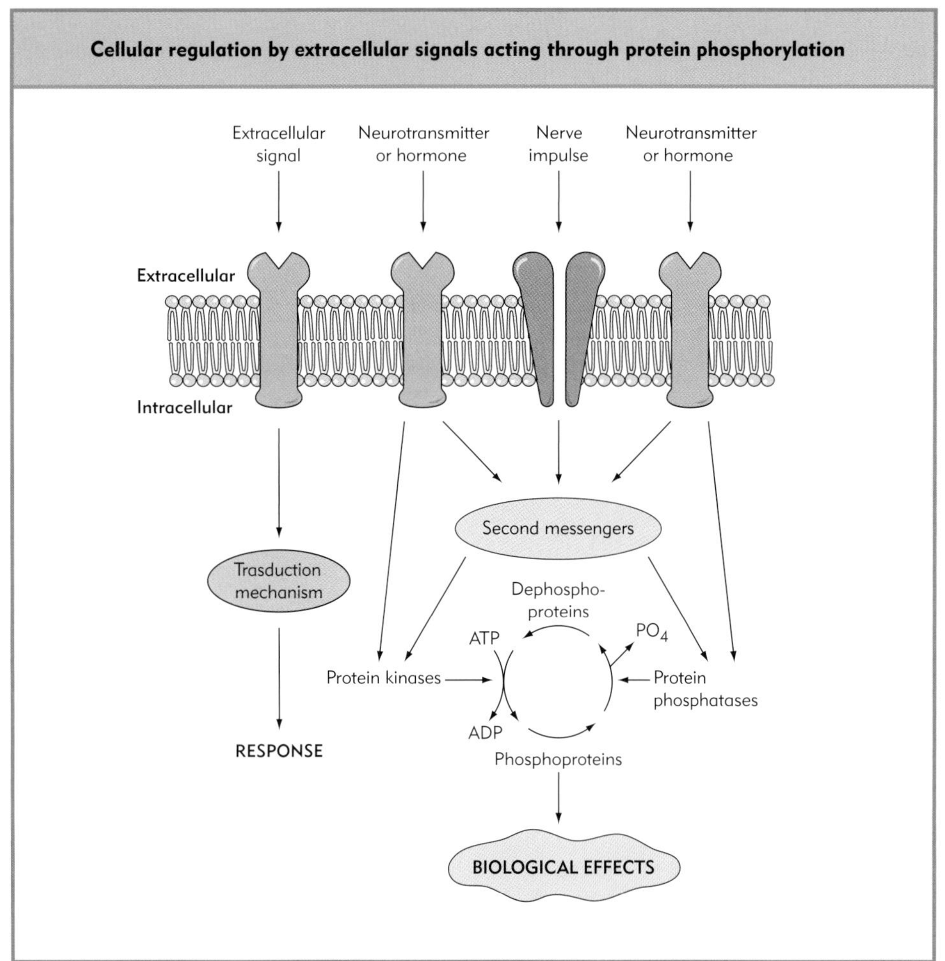

Figure 3.6 Schematic diagram of cellular regulation by extracellular signals acting through protein phosphorylation. A generalized scheme for cell surface receptor-mediated signal transduction is shown on the *left*. Extracellular signals (first messengers), which include various neurotransmitters, hormones, growth factors, and cytokines, produce specific biological effects in target cells via a series of intracellular signals. Cell membrane receptors for many extracellular signals are coupled to the activation of protein kinases, either directly by activating a protein kinase intimately associated with the receptor, or indirectly through changes in the intracellular levels of second messengers (*right*). Protein kinases are enzymes that transfer a phosphoryl group from ATP to serine, threonine or tyrosine residues. Prominent second messengers involved in the regulation of protein kinases include cAMP, cGMP, Ca^{2+}, and 1,2-diacylglycerol. Other protein kinases are themselves regulated by phosphorylation and participate in kinase cascades (Fig. 3.5). The activation of individual protein kinases causes the phosphorylation of specific substrate proteins (phosphoproteins) in target cells. Specificity of the sites phosphorylated is conferred by the surrounding amino acid sequence. In some cases these substrate proteins, or third messengers, are the immediate effectors for the biological response, and in other cases they produce the biological response indirectly, through additional intracellular messengers (e.g. the MAP kinase cascade). Protein phosphatases are also subject to regulation by extracellular signals acting either directly or through second messengers (e.g. Ca^{2+} acting on Ca^{2+}/calmodulin-dependent protein phosphatase-2B), or by the phosphorylation of specific protein phosphatase modulator proteins. Many, if not all, membrane receptors and ion channels are themselves regulated by phosphorylation/dephosphorylation. (Adapted from Lodish H et al., Molecular Cell Biology, 3rd edition. pp. 853-924; WH Freeman and Co, New York: 1995.)

of cAMP are mediated through the activation of cAMP-dependent protein kinase (PKA) and the concomitant phosphorylation of protein effectors on specific serine or threonine residues.

The widespread distribution of PKA throughout the animal kingdom and in all cells led to the hypothesis that the diverse effects of cAMP on cell function are mediated through the activation of this enzyme, which is the principal intracellular receptor for cAMP. Other known receptors for cAMP are the hyperpolarization-activated cyclic nucleotide-gated (HCN) channels. PKA exists as a tetramer composed of two types of dissimilar subunits, the regulatory (R) subunit and the catalytic (C) subunit (Fig. 3.3b). In the absence of cAMP, the inactive holoenzyme tetramer consists of two R subunits joined by disulfide bonds, bound to two C subunits (R_2C_2). The binding of cAMP to the R subunits of the inactive holoenzyme lowers their affinity for the C subunits and leads to the dissociation from the holoenzyme of the two free C subunits expressing phosphotransferase activity. Each R subunit contains two binding sites for cAMP, which activate the kinase synergistically and exhibit positively cooperative cAMP binding.

The phosphorylation of specific substrates by PKA represents the next step in the molecular pathway by which cAMP produces its biological responses. Substrates for PKA are characterized by two or more basic amino acid residues on the amino-terminal side of the phosphorylated residue. The identification and characterization of the specific substrate(s) phosphorylated in response to cAMP is an important goal in the study of agents whose actions are mediated by cAMP. The various substrates for PKA present in different cell types explain the diverse tissue-specific effects of cAMP. They include ion channels, receptors, enzymes, cytoskeletal proteins, and transcription factors (e.g. CREB; cAMP-responsive element binding protein).

Cyclic GMP/nitric oxide

Cyclic GMP is a key intracellular signaling molecule in virtually all animal cells and is involved in signal transduction pathways activated by nitric oxide (NO). Tissues contain multiple forms of guanylyl cyclase and cGMP phosphodiesterase, the enzymes that regulate the intracellular concentration of cGMP. Guanylyl cyclases exist in both soluble and particulate (plasma membrane) forms. Soluble forms of the enzyme are activated by NO formed from L-arginine by the activation of NO synthase. Nitric oxide signaling is important in the control of vascular tone, neurotransmission, and macrophage function. The vasodilators nitroglycerin or nitroprusside produce smooth muscle relaxation via the formation of NO and activation of the guanylyl cyclase system. Soluble guanylyl cyclase contains a heme moiety which binds NO and other oxidants to stimulate enzyme activity. The family of NO synthases includes constitutive neuronal (nNOS) and endothelial (eNOS) forms and an inducible (iNOS) macrophage form. The eNOS and nNOS forms are dependent on Ca^{2+}/calmodulin binding for activation, whereas iNOS is constitutively active owing to tightly bound intrinsic Ca^{2+}/calmodulin and is regulated by protein expression. NOS knockout mice indicate that nNOS is involved in neurotransmission and ischemic neuronal damage, eNOS in blood pressure regulation, and iNOS in immunomodulation. Nitric oxide is thought to be the endogenous regulator of guanylyl cyclase activity that mediates the action of several vasodilators, including acetylcholine, bradykinin, and substance P (Fig. 3.7). These transmitters stimulate the production of a diffusible mediator known as endothelium-derived relaxing factor (EDRF), which has been identified as NO or a closely related molecule. Nitric oxide is a key physiological mediator of Ca^{2+}-mediated signaling pathways such as NMDA receptors and voltage-gated Ca^{2+} channels, which activate Ca^{2+}/calmodulin-dependent forms of NO synthase.

The NO/guanylyl cyclase signaling pathway has received considerable attention as the first example of a signaling system that involves a gaseous signaling molecule. Recent evidence suggests that carbon monoxide (CO) also acts as a gaseous signaling molecule to stimulate guanylyl cyclase. Because it readily

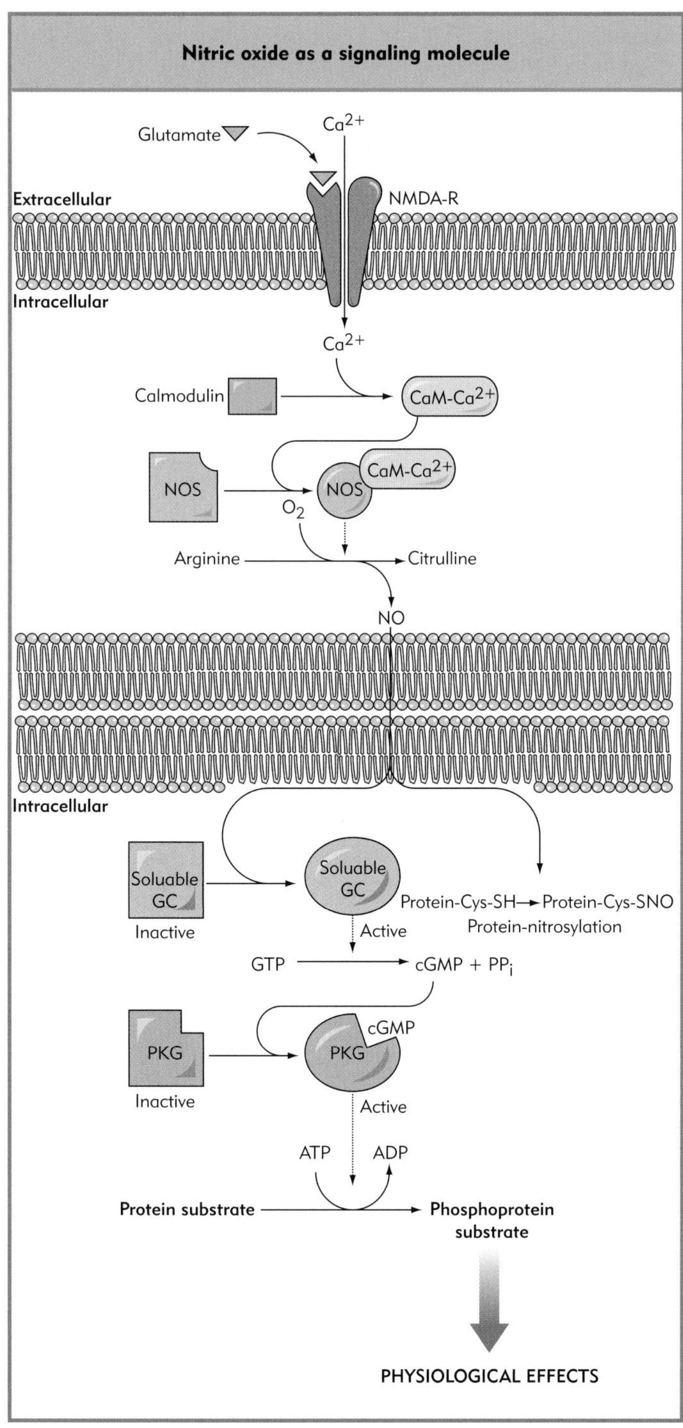

Figure 3.7 Nitric oxide as a signaling molecule. Nitric oxide (NO) is a gas which is highly diffusible and chemically reactive. It is used as a locally active intracellular or intercellular messenger. The enzyme responsible for the formation of NO is NO synthase (NOS). This is activated by Ca^{2+} complexed to calmodulin. In neurons, opening of glutamate receptors of the NMDA subtype is a major source of Ca^{2+} influx, which can lead to the activation of NOS. NOS is a complex enzyme which uses molecular oxygen, O_2, to generate NO by transforming arginine into citrulline. Nitric oxide can cross membranes readily and diffuse to neighboring cells. Thus, the rest of the cascade depicted in the figure can take place in a cell different from that in which NO was generated, as illustrated. A major target of NO is soluble guanylyl cyclase. This enzyme is activated by NO and uses GTP to form cGMP, a second messenger that remains within the cell in which it is produced. Cyclic GMP exerts its effects by activating several enzymes, one of which is cGMP-dependent protein kinase, which is homologous to cAMP-dependent protein kinase. Phosphorylation of specific proteins by cGMP-dependent protein kinase accounts for some of the physiological effects of NO. Nitrosylation of cysteine thiols in certain proteins is dynamically regulated and provides an additional effector mechanism for NO. Cys, cysteine; GC, guanylyl cyclase; NMDA-R, *N*-methyl-D-aspartate subtype of glutamate receptor; PKG, cGMP-dependent protein kinase; CaM, calmodulin. (Adapted from Lodish H et al., Molecular Cell Biology, 3rd edition. pp. 853-924; WH Freeman and Co, New York: 1995.)

diffuses within a restricted volume across cell membranes, NO formed in one cell is able to activate guanylyl cyclase in the same cell as a second messenger (autocrine effect) as well as in neighboring cells as a transmitter (paracrine effect), but as a free radical its diffusion is limited by its high chemical reactivity and short half-life. The chemical reactivity of NO underlies its recently identified signaling roles not involving guanylyl cyclase activation. Higher concentrations of NO can result in nitrosylation of cysteine residues or nitration of tyrosine residues in proteins. Protein nitrosylation and nitration exhibit key properties of physiological transduction mechanisms, including modulation of substrate function, substrate specificity, and reversibility by denitrosylase and denitrase enzymes. Nitric oxide donors (e.g. nitroglycerin, nitroprusside), inhibitors of NO synthase, and NO itself are providing new approaches to the management of a number of diseases, including sepsis, ARDS, pulmonary hypertension, ischemia, and degenerative diseases.

The seven particulate forms of guanylyl cyclase serve as cell surface receptors for a variety of different peptide ligands, including the natriuretic peptides (e.g. atrial natriuretic peptide; ANP). These receptors contain a single transmembrane domain flanked by an extracellular peptide-binding domain and intracellular guanylyl cyclase and protein kinase-like catalytic domains. They are activated by ligand binding and are insensitive to NO. Some forms of particulate guanylyl cyclase are also sensitive to intracellular Ca^{2+}.

The cellular responses to cGMP are mediated in specific tissues by regulation of phosphodiesterases (PDE), cyclic nucleotide-gated ion channels (CNG), and cGMP-dependent protein kinase (PKG). Of the five families of phosphodiesterases, there are cGMP-stimulated, cGMP-inhibited, and cGMP-specific families. Inhibition of the cGMP-specific isoform PDE 5 by the popular drugs sildenafil (Viagra), tadalafil (Cialis), and vardenafil (Levitra) increase cGMP, activate PKG, and result in vasodilation of the penile vessels and erection. The CNG channels are voltage-gated cation channels that modulate membrane potential and are involved in retinal photoreceptor transduction. cGMP-dependent protein kinase is a serine/threonine kinase that exists as a soluble dimer of identical subunits (type I) or a membrane-bound monomer (type II). It is activated by increases in intracellular cGMP, the formation of which is catalyzed by guanylyl cyclase. The primary mechanism of inactivation of PKG is hydrolysis of cGMP by cyclic nucleotide phosphodiesterase. Each subunit of type I PKG contains a cGMP-binding domain and a catalytic domain, which is homologous to cAMP-dependent protein kinase catalytic subunit. Upon binding of cGMP, a conformational change occurs in the enzyme that exposes the active catalytic domain; the mechanism of activation of the type II kinase has not been determined. In contrast to cAMP-dependent protein kinase, which is present in similar concentrations in most mammalian tissues, PKG has an uneven tissue distribution. Relatively high concentrations of the type I enzyme are found in lung, heart, smooth muscle, platelets, cerebellum, and intestine; the type II enzyme is widely distributed in the brain and intestine. *In vitro*, cGMP-dependent and cAMP-dependent protein kinases show similar substrate specificities. Although many physiological substrates for cAMP-dependent protein kinase have been identified, only a few specific physiological substrates for PKG have been found. Many of the phosphorylated targets of the type I enzyme result in smooth muscle relaxation, and are thus part of the eNOS signal transduction pathway.

Calcium and inositol trisphosphate

Along with cAMP, Ca^{2+} controls a wide variety of intracellular processes. Ca^{2+} entry through Ca^{2+} channels or its release from intracellular stores triggers hormone and neurotransmitter secretion, initiates muscle contraction, and activates protein kinases and many other enzymes. The concentration of free Ca^{2+} is normally maintained at very low levels in the cytosol of most cells ($<10^{-6}$ M) compared to the extracellular fluid ($\sim10^{-3}$ M) by a number of homeostatic mechanisms. A Ca^{2+}-ATPase in the plasma membrane pumps Ca^{2+} from the cytosol to the cell exterior at the expense of ATP hydrolysis, a Ca^{2+}-ATPase in the endoplasmic and sarcoplasmic reticulum concentrates Ca^{2+} from the cytosol into intracellular storage organelles, and an Na^+/Ca^{2+} exchanger, which is particularly active in excitable plasma membranes, couples the electrochemical potential of Na^+ influx to the efflux of Ca^{2+}. The Ca^{2+}-ATPase has a higher affinity for Ca^{2+} and a lower capacity than the Na^+/Ca^{2+} exchanger. Although mitochondria have the ability to take up and release Ca^{2+}, they are not widely felt to play a major role in cytosolic Ca^{2+} homeostasis under normal conditions.

Changes in intracellular free Ca^{2+} concentration can be induced directly by depolarization-evoked Ca^{2+} entry down its electrochemical gradient through voltage-gated Ca^{2+} channels (as in neurons and muscle) and by extracellular signals that activate Ca^{2+}-permeable ligand-gated ion channels (e.g. the NMDA receptor), or indirectly by extracellular signals coupled to the formation of IP_3 (Fig. 3.8). IP_3 is formed in response to a number of extracellular signals that interact with GPCRs coupled to the activation of phospholipase C (through G_q, G_{11}). Phospholipase C hydrolyzes phosphatidylinositol-4,5-bisphosphate to IP_3 and diacylglycerol; further degradation of diacylglycerol by phospholipase A_2 can result in the release of arachidonic acid. All three of these receptor-regulated metabolites are important second messengers. IP_3 increases intracellular Ca^{2+} by binding to specific IP_3 receptors on the endoplasmic reticulum which are coupled to a Ca^{2+} channel that allows Ca^{2+} efflux into the cytosol. IP_3 receptors are similar to the Ca^{2+} release channels (ryanodine receptors) of muscle sarcoplasmic reticulum that release Ca^{2+} in response to excitation. Ryanodine receptors are stimulated by elevations of cytosolic free Ca^{2+}, and are responsible for Ca^{2+}-induced Ca^{2+} release, which can lead to Ca^{2+} waves in some cells. Diacylglycerol remains in the plasma membrane where it activates protein kinase C, whereas arachidonic acid, in addition to its metabolism to biologically active prostaglandins and leukotrienes, also activates protein kinase C. The Ca^{2+} signal is terminated by hydrolysis of IP_3 and by the rapid reuptake and extrusion of Ca^{2+}.

Ca^{2+} carries out its second-messenger functions primarily after binding to intracellular Ca^{2+}-binding proteins, of which *calmodulin* is the most important. Calmodulin is a ubiquitous multifunctional Ca^{2+}-binding protein, highly conserved between species, that binds four atoms of Ca^{2+} with high affinity. Ca^{2+} can also bind to C2 domains found in several proteins (e.g. protein kinase C, phospholipase A_2, synaptotagmin). Most calmodulin-regulated enzymes appear to be activated by a similar mechanism. Calmodulin does not usually bind to the enzyme in the absence of Ca^{2+}; however, in the presence of micromolar concentrations of Ca^{2+}, calmodulin undergoes a marked conformational change, exposing hydrophobic binding sites. The exposed hydrophobic domain of the Ca^{2+}–calmodulin complex

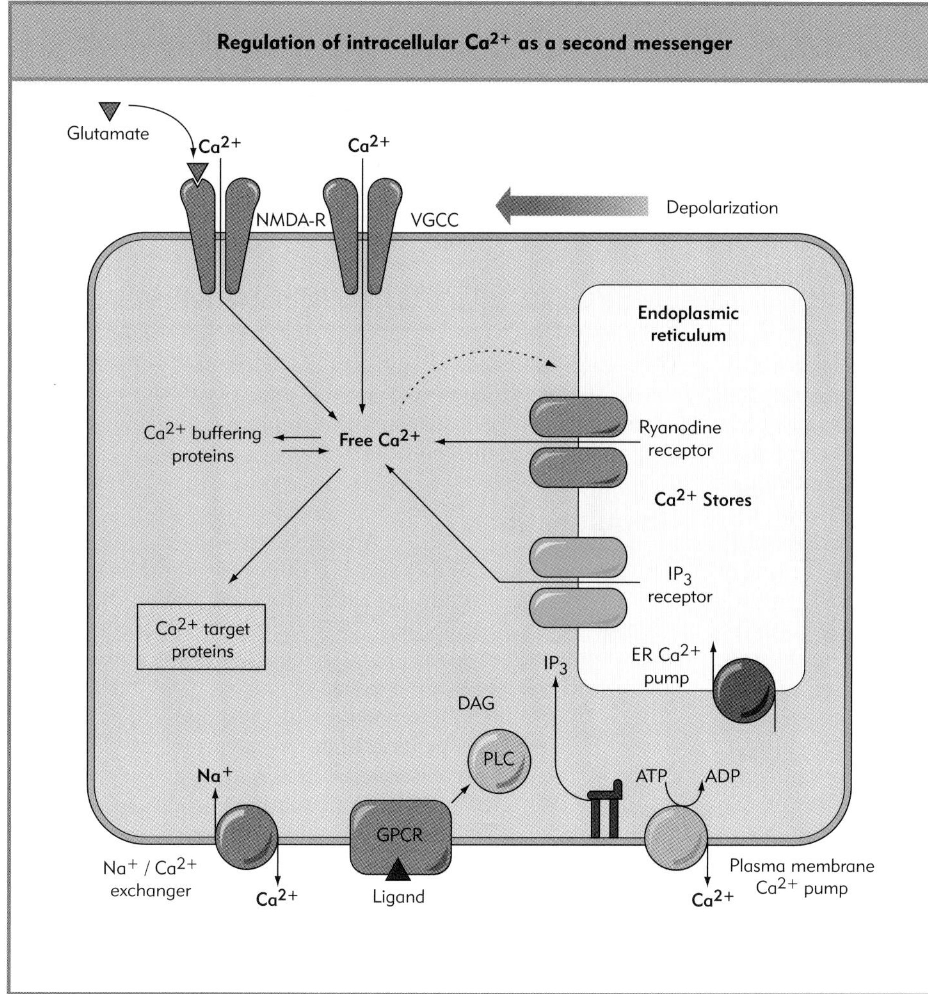

Figure 3.8 Regulation of intracellular Ca^{2+} as a second messenger. Ca^{2+} is a divalent cation whose concentrations are relatively high in the extracellular space (around 1.2 mM) and more than 10 000 times lower within the cytosol (around 100 nM). In resting conditions the plasma membrane is impermeable to Ca^{2+}. In neurons it can penetrate through specific channels, which include voltage-gated Ca^{2+} channels (VGCC) and glutamate receptors of the NMDA subtype (NMDA-R). When these channels are open, in response to depolarization in the case of VGCC or in the presence of glutamate in the case of NMDA receptor, Ca^{2+} flows into the cytosol following both its concentration gradient and the electrical potential. Ca^{2+} can also be released into the cytosol from internal stores (the endoplasmic reticulum). Two types of Ca^{2+} channel are responsible for the release of Ca^{2+} from internal stores. One is the IP_3 receptor, the opening of which is triggered by inositol-1,4,5-trisphosphate (IP_3), a second messenger generated by phospholipase C from phosphatidylinositol 4,5-bisphosphate. The other is the ryanodine receptor, named after ryanodine, a drug that triggers its opening. In the cytosol, Ca^{2+} is mostly bound to specific binding proteins. Some of them function as buffering proteins, preventing excessive rises in cytosolic free Ca^{2+}. Others are the actual targets of Ca^{2+}, which account for the potent biological effects of this cation. Among the best-characterized targets are calmodulin and calmodulin-related proteins, which undergo a conformational change enabling them to interact with, and activate, a number of enzymes. Free Ca^{2+} in the cytosol is maintained at very low levels by several highly active processes, which include Ca^{2+} pumps and Ca^{2+} exchangers. The Ca^{2+} pumps have a high affinity but a low capacity for Ca^{2+} and are used for fine tuning of Ca^{2+} levels. They are located on the plasma membrane and the membrane of the endoplasmic reticulum, and their energy is provided by ATP hydrolysis. Na^+/Ca^{2+} exchangers, whose driving force is provided by the Na^+ gradient, have a large capacity but a low affinity for Ca^{2+}. ER, endoplasmic reticulum; GPCR, G protein-coupled receptor; PLC, phospholipase C; DAG, diacylglycerol. (Adapted from Lodish H et al., Molecular Cell Biology, 3rd edition. pp. 853-924; WH Freeman and Co, New York: 1995.)

interacts with a calmodulin-binding domain present in a variety of effector proteins, including the Ca^{2+}–calmodulin-dependent protein kinases, which along with protein kinase C mediate many of the effects of Ca^{2+} in cells. Ca^{2+}–calmodulin-dependent activation of protein kinases was originally observed for phosphorylase kinase and myosin light-chain kinase (Chapter 38). Subsequently, Ca^{2+}–calmodulin-dependent protein phosphorylation was found to be widespread in various tissues. Ca^{2+}–calmodulin kinases I, II, and IV, myosin light-chain kinase, and phosphorylase kinase appear to be responsible for most Ca^{2+}–calmodulin-dependent protein kinase activity. Ca^{2+}–calmodulin kinase I has a widespread species and tissue distribution, and, like phosphorylase kinase or myosin light-chain kinase, exhibits a restricted substrate specificity. In contrast, the isozymes of Ca^{2+}–calmodulin kinase II exhibit a relatively broad substrate specificity. This kinase is therefore referred to as the multifunctional Ca^{2+}–calmodulin-dependent protein kinase.

Protein kinase C (PKC) is a family of serine/threonine protein kinases that consists of 12 structurally homologous phospholipid-dependent isoforms with conserved catalytic domains, but distinguished by their variable N-terminal regulatory domains and cofactor dependence. PKC is activated by Ca^{2+}, diacylglycerol, and membrane phospholipid. PKC is a intracellular receptor for, and is activated by, the tumor-promoting phorbol esters. The Ca^{2+}-dependent or conventional isoforms of PKC (cPKC) are components of the phospholipase C/diacylglycerol signaling pathway. They are regulated by the lipid second messenger 1,2-diacylglycerol, by phospholipids such as phosphatidylserine, and by Ca^{2+} through specific interactions with the regulatory region. Binding of diacylglycerol to the Cl domain of cPKC isoforms (α, $\beta 1$, $\beta 2$, γ) increases their affinity for Ca^{2+} and phosphatidylserine, facilitates PKC translocation and binding to cell membranes, and increases catalytic activity. The novel PKC isoforms (nPKC; δ, ε, η, θ, μ) are similar to cPKCs, but lack the C2 domain and do not require Ca^{2+}. The atypical isoforms (aPKC; ζ, λ) differ considerably in the regulatory region, and do not require Ca^{2+} or diacylglycerol for activity. The cPKC holoenzyme contains a hydrophobic regulatory domain which interacts with Ca^{2+} and phospholipids (C2), and with diacylglycerol and phorbol esters (C1). A hydrophilic C-terminal catalytic domain can be cleaved from the holoenzyme by proteolysis to yield a fragment that is catalytically active in the absence of Ca^{2+}, diacylglycerol, and phospholipid, illustrating the negative modulatory role of the regulatory domain. PKC has a broad substrate specificity, which differs from those of both cyclic nucleotide-dependent and Ca^{2+}–calmodulin-dependent protein kinases. Additional specificity is provided by specific targeting subunits that localize activated PKC near its important substrates, receptors for activated C-kinase or RACKs.

Protein kinase C is activated by micromolar concentrations of Ca^{2+} and membrane phospholipids, of which phosphatidylserine is the most active. The addition of low concentrations of diacylglycerol increases the affinity of cPKC for Ca^{2+}. cPKC and nPKC isoforms are activated by an increase in the concentration of diacylglycerol produced by receptor-stimulated phosphatidylinositol turnover. The activation of the kinase by diacylglycerol, although dependent on micromolar concentrations of Ca^{2+}, does not appear to be dependent on increases in intracellular Ca^{2+}. Tumor-promoting phorbol esters appear to substitute for diacylglycerol in the activation of PKC. The hydrolysis of phosphatidylinositol 4,5-bisphosphate produces diacylglycerol and IP_3, and the latter compound mobilizes Ca^{2+} in cells. Activation of PKC results from the synergistic actions of increases in the intracellular concentrations of both Ca^{2+} and diacylglycerol. The contributions of each second messenger may vary, however, depending on the cell type or receptor-mediated event. Activation of PKC, which is predominantly cytosolic, leads to its translocation to the plasma membrane, where it undergoes protease-mediated downregulation in the presence of continuous stimulation. Translocation of PKC may be important in targeting the enzyme to specific substrates and cellular compartments.

Protein phosphatases

The phosphorylation of specific sites on proteins is transient and regulated by protein phosphatases, which remove the phosphate groups transferred by protein kinases (Fig. 3.6). Protein phosphatases exhibit distinct substrate specificities and are tightly regulated; regulation of both protein phosphorylation and dephosphorylation increases the complexity and flexibility of this regulatory mechanism. The protein phosphatases involved in the dephosphorylation of most of the known proteins phosphorylated on serine or threonine residues are accounted for by four groups of enzymes: type 1 protein phosphatases (protein phosphatases-1) and type 2 protein phosphatases (protein phosphatases-2A, -2B, and -2C). Protein phosphatases-1, -2A, and -2B share homologous catalytic subunits, and are complexed with one or more regulatory subunits. Protein phosphatase-2C is distinct and relatively minor in most tissues. Protein phosphatases-1, -2A, and -2C all exhibit relatively broad substrate specificities, whereas that of protein phosphatase-2B appears to be more restricted. Multiple forms of both cytosolic and membrane-bound (receptor) phosphotyrosine-protein phosphatases exist which are distinct from the phosphoserine/phosphothreonine-protein phosphatases.

Protein phosphatases, like protein kinases, are under tight physiological regulation. Protein phosphatase-2B (also known as calcineurin), is activated by Ca^{2+} plus calmodulin. Calcineurin is a target for inhibition by cyclosporin A and FK506 used in transplant therapy and autoimmune disorders, and has been implicated as a schizophrenia susceptibility gene. Protein phosphatase-1 is regulated indirectly by cAMP, which stimulates the phosphorylation and activation of two potent and specific inhibitor proteins (DARPP-32 and phosphatase inhibitor-1). This provides a positive feedback mechanism for amplifying the effects of cAMP, and a mechanism for cAMP to modulate the phosphorylation state of substrate proteins for protein kinases other than PKA. Protein phosphatase-1 is also regulated by its interaction with regulatory subunits. A complex of protein phosphatase-1 with phosphatase inhibitor-2 (together known as the Mg^{2+}/ATP-dependent protein phosphatase, or $PP1_I$) is inactive in its basal state, but is activated by phosphorylation. Tissue-specific targeting subunits also localize protein phosphatase-1 to important subcellular sites of action in many tissues.

EMERGING SIGNALING MECHANISMS

The rich diversity of cell signaling mechanisms is apparent in the classic pathways identified in the past 50 years, but fundamentally novel mechanisms with important physiological roles continue to be identified.

Ubiquitination

Post-translational modification of proteins to alter their function, activity, or localization typically involves the addition and removal of small molecules, for example by phosphorylation, methylation, nitrosylation, etc. Conjugation of the conserved 76 amino acid residue protein ubiquitin via its C-terminal glycine residue to specific lysine residues in proteins (ubiquitination) was well recognized for its role in targeting proteins for degradation by the 26S proteasome. Ubiquitination involves a cycle of reactions: after cleavage of the ubiquitin precursor, ubiquitin is adenylated by ATP and linked to an activating enzyme (E1) through a high-energy thioester bond, passed to a conjugating enzyme (E2), and then attached to a substrate protein by a ubiquitin-protein ligase (E3). Polyubiquitination of diverse proteins marks them for degradation by the 26S proteasome, a remarkable protein machine that catalyzes ATP-dependent protein unfolding and proteolysis. The ubiquitin–proteasome system is the principal mechanism for the turnover of short-lived proteins; an example is the periodic degradation of cyclin activators and inhibitors of cyclin-dependent kinases during progression of the cell cycle.

Recent findings indicate that mono-ubiquitination can function as a reversible nonproteolytic modification that controls protein function in endocytic trafficking, retroviral budding, and transcriptional regulation by histone modification. Several ubiquitin-binding domains function to recognize this protein modification to facilitate protein–protein interactions, similar to SH2 domain– phosphotyrosine residue interactions. Mono-ubiquitination is highly regulated, often at the level of the E3 ligase, and reversible by de-ubiquitinating enzymes, hallmarks of physiological signaling pathways. A number of ubiquitin-like modifiers have also been discovered, with mechanistic parallels to the ubiquitin pathway but distinct cellular functions. For example, SUMO (small ubiquitin-related modifier) is reversibly conjugated to specific proteins, including a number of signaling molecules. Sumoylation is involved exclusively in nonproteolytic signaling functions, including the regulation of transcription factors, signaling pathways, and chromosome function.

Proteolytic pathways

Proteases are usually perceived as degradative enzymes that break down proteins for the purposes of elimination. However, proteases can act as exquisite control switches for many pivotal cellular processes, such as embryonic development, immune response, and wound healing. Proteases play important role in a number of signaling cascades, including ubiquitin-targeted protein degradation by the proteasome (above), blood coagulation (Chapter 53), and apoptosis (Chapter 2). Extracellular proteases are involved in the maturation, processing, and degradation of many peptides and proteins. For example, angiotensin-converting enzyme (ACE) is a protease involved in blood pressure regulation that catalyzes the conversion of angiotensin I into angiotensin II and the inactivation of bradykinin, leading to vasoconstriction, a target for the clinically important ACE inhibitors. Recently proteases have been found to activate cell surface receptors, either directly or indirectly, to initiate intracellular signaling cascades. Protease activated receptors (PARs) are G protein-coupled receptors that are activated by protease cleavage of an extracellular domain that unmasks a self-activating ligand that interacts with the receptor. For example, thrombin cleaves PARs on the platelet and the endothelial cell membrane to regulate their responses to coagulation. A distinct protease-mediated signaling event involves regulated intramembrane proteolysis (RIP), in which sequential proteolysis first outside the membrane (by a metalloprotease of the ADAM family) is followed by a second cut inside the membrane (by a γ-secretase) to release a peptide messenger cleaved from the receptor itself. These messengers can act as transcription factors, mRNA-binding proteins, or modulators of other signaling pathways. For example, Notch, a transmembrane receptor critical during development, is activated by two successive proteolytic cuts following interaction with its ligand; the resulting intracellular peptide fragment translocates to the nucleus, where it modulates gene transcription. Similar processing of amyloid precursor protein (APP) can lead to the accumulation of amyloid-β protein and the formation of plaques in Alzheimer's disease.

Acetylation and methylation

Post-translational modification of histones, the main protein component of chromatin, plays a key role in the storage and expression of genetic information encoded in DNA. Histones can be modified in several ways, including the highly reversible mechanisms involving phosphorylation (serine and threonine; see above) and acetylation (lysine), or more stable methylation (lysine and arginine). These modifications can recruit binding/effector molecules to chromatin as described above for phosphorylation signaling. Histone acetylation involves the transfer of an acetyl group from acetyl Co-A to the ε-amino group of lysine side chains by histone acetyltransferase (HAT). The removal of the acetyl groups is catalyzed by histone deacetylases (HDAC). Acetylation can alter DNA binding, protein–protein interaction, or subcellular localization. Histone acetylation is a dynamic process induced by HATs and reversed by HDACs. There is a general correlation between transcriptional repression and histone deacetylation. The involvement of histone acetylation in cell cycle regulation has made histones a promising new target for cancer therapy. Methylation of histone lysine residue ε-amino groups by methyltransferases has been linked to gene transcription and heterochromatin assembly, and demethylases have also been identified recently. There are considerable interactions between histone acetylation, phosphorylation, and methylation in the regulation of histone function.

Key references

Ciechanover A, Heller H, Elias S, Haas AL, Hershko A. A heat-stable polypeptide component of an ATP-dependent proteolytic system from reticulocytes. Biochem Biophys Res Commun. 1978;81:1100–5. (First example of ubiquitin-mediated proteolysis.)

Krebs EG, Fischer EH. The phosphorylase-b to phosphorylase-a converting enzyme of rabbit skeletal muscle. Biochim Biophys Acta 1956;20:150–7. (Discovery of protein phosphorylation as a regulatory mechanism.)

Rall TW, Sutherland EW, Berthet J. The relationship of epinephrine and glucagon to liver phosphorylase. J Biol Chem. 1957;224:463–75. (Idenitification of cyclic AMP as a second messenger.)

Further reading

Berridge MJ, Lipp P, Bootman MD. The versatility and universality of calcium signalling. Nature Rev Mol Cell Biol. 2000;1:11–21.

Blume-Jensen P, Hunter T. Oncogenic kinase signalling. Nature 2001;411:355–65.

Carroll RC, Beattie EC, Von Zastrow M, Malenka RC. Role of AMPA receptor endocytosis in synaptic plasticity. Nature Rev Neurosci. 2001;2:315–24

Cell-to-cell signaling: hormones and receptors. In: Lodish H et al., eds. Molecular cell biology, 5th edn. pp. New York: WH Freeman & Co; 2003:853–924.

Cell communication. In: Alberts B et al., eds. Molecular biology of the cell, 4th edn. New York: Garland Publishing; 2002; 831–906.

Chang L, Karin M. Mammalian MAP kinase signalling cascades. Nature 2001;410:37–40.

Downward J. The ins and outs of signalling. Nature 2001;411:759–62.

Hamm HE, Gilchrist A. Heterotrimeric G proteins. Curr Opin Cell Biol. 1996;8:189–96.

Hanafy KA, Krumenacker JS, Murad F. NO, nitrotyrosine, and cyclic GMP in signal transduction. Med Sci Monit. 2001;7:801–19.

Hicke L. Protein regulation by monoubiquitin. Nature Rev Mol Cell Biol. 2001;2:195–201.

Hunter T. Protein kinases and phosphatases: the yin and yang of protein phosphorylation and signaling. Cell 1995;80:225–36.

Pawson T, Gish GD, Nash P. SH2 domains, interaction modules and cellular wiring. Trends Cell Biol. 2001;11:504–11.

Pawson T, Scott JD. Signaling through scaffold, anchoring and adaptor proteins. Science 1997;278:2075–80.

Schlessinger J. Cell signaling by receptor tyrosine kinases. Cell 2000;103:211–25.

Yamakura T, Bertaccini E, Trudell JR, Harris RA. Anesthetics and ion channels: molecular models and sites of action. Annu Rev Pharmacol Toxicol. 2001;41:23–51.

Chapter 4

Principles and techniques of molecular biology

Kirk Hogan

TOPICS COVERED IN THIS CHAPTER

- **General principles**
- **Classic versus molecular genetics**
- **DNA structure, replication, and repair**
- **RNA structure, transcription, transcriptional regulation, translation, and the genetic code**
- **Gene structure, RNA processing, and genomic and complementary DNA**
- ***In vitro* molecular biology**
    - Chromosome sorting, nucleotide isolation, and cleavage
    - Nucleotide separation
    - Nucleotide visualization
    - Nucleotide probes
    - In vitro hybridization, and Southern, Northern, and Western blotting
    - In situ hybridization
    - Nucleotide propagation: cell-based cloning, nucleotide libraries
    - Nucleotide propagation: cell-free cloning and the polymerase chain reaction
    - DNA sequencing
- **Genome structure, mutation, the human genome project, and bioinformatics**
    - Recombinattion, genetic maps, and genetic linkage
    - Site-directed mutagenesis
    - Expression cloning
    - Gene transfer
    - Transgenic animals
    - Gene knockouts
    - Gene therapy

GENERAL PRINCIPLES

Deoxyribonucleic acid (DNA) and ribonucleic acid (RNA) comprise a cell signaling system that defies the death of an organism, if not the extinction of a species. Not only are the nucleic acids responsible for coordinating the cellular mechanisms that underlie growth, development, disease, and senescence, but also their biochemical morphology enables successful adaptations to be communicated to an organism's progeny. To fulfill these diverse roles, nucleic acids are forever suspended in tension between the demands of error-free replication and those for the continuous variation required to fuel selection. Too much or too little stability in regions of an individual's DNA sequence that are unique, or in those that are shared with other individuals, entails identical lethal consequences.

It is now possible to measure with precision the extent of variation between creatures, from the identity of whole organism clones to that of phylogenetic ancestors long extinct. Moreover, we have the capacity to introduce variation, to enable better understanding of the mysteries of anesthesia, or to ameliorate pain. Described below are the fundamental concepts and tools of nucleic acid investigations (molecular biology). Inevitably, these principles and techniques will improve many areas of anesthetic practice, including presymptomatic diagnosis (malignant hyperthermia, plasma cholinesterase deficiency), anesthetic genotoxicology (compound A), workplace safety (nitrous oxide, viral pathogens), and therapeutic interventions (xenogenic organs, recombinant proteins, gene therapy for pain). As nucleic acids are involved in virtually all cellular processes, the same set of tools can be used to address questions of outwardly unrelated origin. Although the vernacular of molecular biology is huge and daunting, the underlying notions are usually simple and concrete, reflecting the parsimony that unites nucleic acid structure with function.

CLASSIC VERSUS MOLECULAR GENETICS

With the advent of contemporary molecular biology, the definition of a gene has shifted from abstract units of inheritance of specific traits to the correspondence of DNA sequence with expressed proteins and RNA. Nevertheless, an explicit distinction between the genotype and phenotype of an organism has been preserved. The genotype, or genetic constitution, of an organism can be described with extraordinary precision, and differences between species, populations, individuals, and even cells within the same individual can be compared. Conversely, the phenotype, or characteristics that result from the interaction of an organism's genotype and its environment, is much more indefinite. The perceived phenotype is largely a function of how well the investigator is able to observe (e.g. how accurate is the in vitro halothane contracture test used to phenotype malignant hyperthermia susceptibility?) and categorize biologic phenomena (e.g. how is the state of anesthesia defined?). The net result is that mapping phenotypic observations of interest to concrete DNA sequences inevitably risks confusing biochemical with semantic logic.

With the exceptions of sex chromosomes and mitochondrial DNA (which is inherited only from the mother), the human genome is diploid, with each gene present twice at a given chromosomal locus. *Mitosis* is the process of DNA replication in cell division that generates new diploid cells for development and replacement. *Meiosis* is DNA replication in the testis and ovary that results in the creation of haploid sperm and egg cells. The copy at one locus of a matched pair of chromosomes is inherited from the mother, and that of the other from the father. Each copy of a gene at a specific locus is called an *allele*. An organism that carries two unaltered, normal alleles is *wild type*. An altered allele is *mutant*. When a specific allele at a particular genetic locus is both necessary and sufficient for a trait to be expressed, given an otherwise normal genetic and environmental background, the trait (not the gene) is said to be inherited in a mendelian fashion. Authentic mendelian traits are *dominant* if detectable in the heterozygote with a single copy of the allele, and *recessive* if two copies of the allele in the homozygote are needed for detection. Alleles at the level of the genotype (i.e. in reading actual DNA sequence) are codominant, as both may be discerned unambiguously without reference to an expressed trait. In some conditions the heterozygote may have an intermediate phenotype, which is then referred to as semidominant. Pathologic and nonpathologic human mendelian traits are recognized and cataloged, each with a six-digit call number, in Online Mendelian Inheritance in Man (OMIM), with weekly updates on the Internet (http://www3.ncbi.nlm.nih.gov/Omim).

Mendelian single-gene traits are the exception rather than the rule.

Mendelian traits are inherited in patterns (e.g. *autosomal dominant*) that may often reflect more of an informed guess than an actual genetic mechanism. An outwardly identical trait may be caused by mutations in different genes (locus heterogeneity), or by distinct mutations in the same gene (allelic heterogeneity). Furthermore, different mutations in the same gene may give rise to apparently unrelated phenotypes. A basic mendelian pattern may be disguised by pleiotropic alleles (widespread and divergent effects of the genotype), the presence of phenocopies (phenotypes produced by environmental factors and masquerading as genetic traits), incomplete *penetrance* (the probability that an individual who has the genotype manifests the phenotype), and variable *expressivity* (the genotype gives rise to different phenotypes in related individuals). For a trait with high penetrance and variable expressivity, each affected individual manifests the genotype, but in different ways. A trait with reduced penetrance and limited expressivity is identical in all affected individuals, but some who have the genotype may show no sign of the trait. Because the human genome is complex and outbred, and because environmental factors vary enormously between individuals, truly mendelian single-gene traits are the exception rather than the rule. Mutant alleles at several (oligogenic inheritance) or many (polygenic inheritance) loci, with greater or lesser contributions from genetic interactions (epistasis) and environmental factors (multifactorial inheritance), are required to account for most human phenotypes.

DNA STRUCTURE, REPLICATION, AND REPAIR

Although Avery had established DNA as the carrier of genetic information by 1944, its structure was not elucidated until 1952. Ten years elapsed before the molecular mechanisms that underlie DNA self-replication and protein assembly were correlated with its structure. Both DNA and RNA are composed of linked sequences of nucleotides, each consisting of a base, a five-carbon sugar (pentose), and a phosphate group. Two classes of base are used: *pyrimidines* (cytosine (C), thymine (T) in DNA, and uracil (U), which substitutes for T in RNA) and *purines* (adenine (A) and guanine (G)) (Fig. 4.1). The covalent addition of a pentose to N_1 of a pyrimidine or N_9 of a purine creates the *nucleosides* (one base plus one sugar) cytidine, thymidine, uridine, adenosine, and guanosine. The difference between ribose (RNA) and deoxyribose (DNA) is the hydroxyl group at the 2′ position of the sugar (Chapter 1). A phosphate group is added to the 5′ position to form the cytidylic (C), thymidylic (T), uridylic (U), adenylic (A), and guanylic (G) acid *nucleotides* (one nucleoside plus one, two, or three phosphate groups) that constitute the basic repeat units of nucleic acids.

Nucleotides that form the nucleic acid chain are connected by a covalent phosphodiester bond between the 5′ and 3′ positions of adjacent sugar rings. Each nucleic acid chain begins with a free 5′ phosphate, and terminates with a free hydroxy group at the 3′ position. The designations 5′ (upstream) and 3′ (downstream) serve as a shorthand to orient relative position along the DNA and RNA linear sequence. Double-stranded DNA takes the shape of an antiparallel helix of two polynucleotide chains. The phosphate groups confer a net negative charge to the outside of the nucleic acid helix. Like rungs of a ladder, the bases point inward and are joined such that the distance between the two phosphorylated sugar backbones remains constant. This results from the regular pairing of one purine with one pyrimidine, either A with T bound by two hydrogen bonds, or G with C linked by three hydrogen bonds. The capacity of these noncovalent hydrogen bonds to break and reform under physiologic conditions is of crucial importance in nucleic acid function.

The A–T and G–C dyads are referred to as *base pairs* (bp) and represent the basic unit of distance along the nucleic acid molecule (e.g. a kilobase (kb) equals 10^3 bp, a megabase (Mb) equals 10^6 bp]. Because a given purine only binds with a specific pyrimidine, one strand of DNA is complementary to the other, which permits the reproduction of DNA, with one strand serving as a template for synthesis of its companion. Partner strands of the helix are oriented in an antiparallel direction, with the sense strand running from 5′ to 3′ and the complementary antisense strand from 3′ to 5′. Synthesis of new DNA molecules during replication proceeds in the 5′ to 3′ direction. The enzyme helicase first unwinds the double strand, which allows each single strand to serve as a template for the synthesis of an identical daughter strand catalyzed by DNA polymerase.

Each of the daughter DNA duplexes contains one parental strand and one newly synthesized strand. As the two parental strands are antiparallel in orientation only, the leading strand is continuously synthesized 5′ to 3′ from the origin of replication. The second lagging strand is assembled in small 5′ to 3′ fragments,

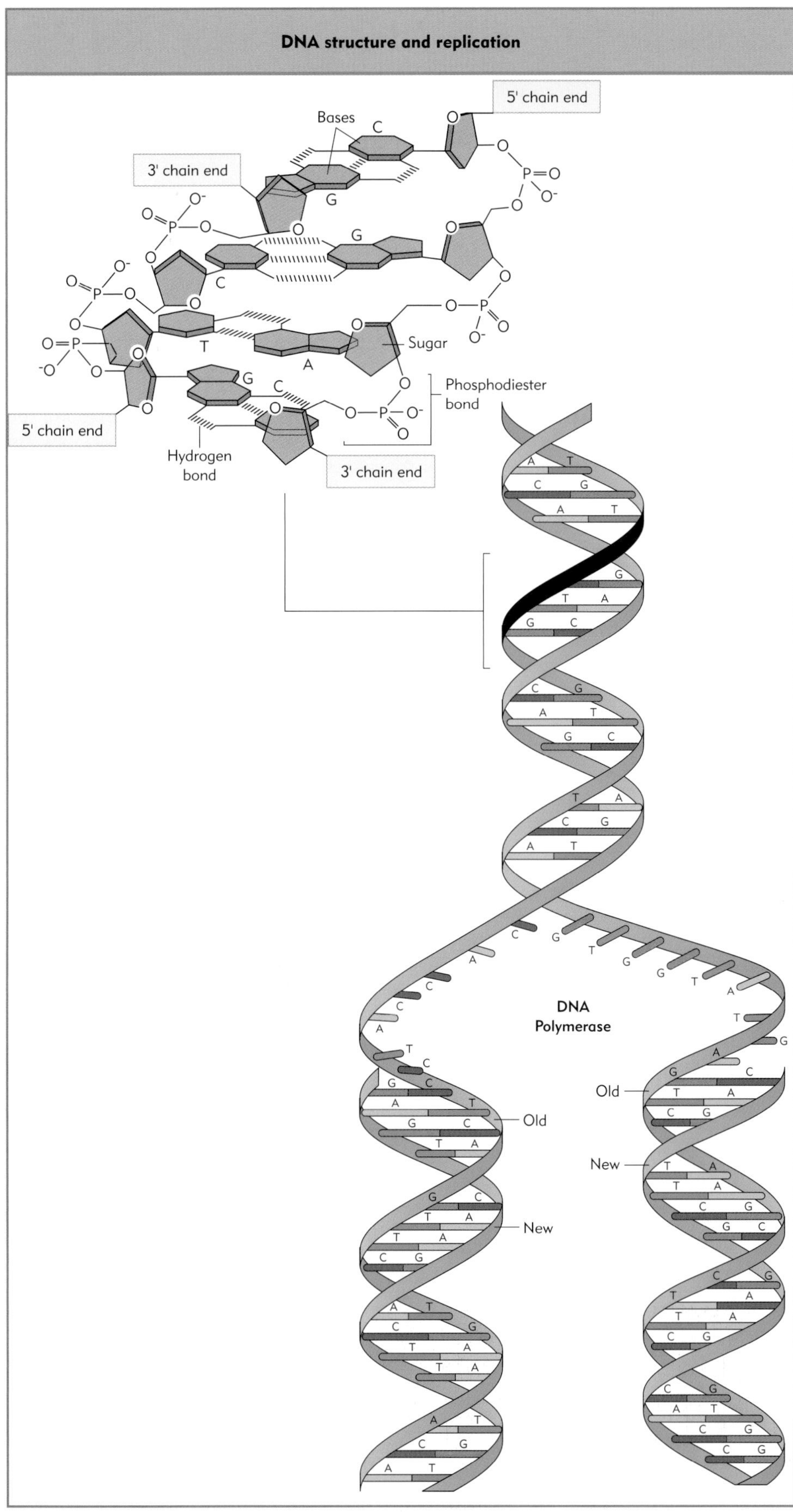

Figure 4.1 DNA structure and replication. The DNA strands in the 'double helix' consist of a deoxyribose sugar backbone held together by phosphodiester bonds. The two chains, which run in opposite (antiparallel) directions, are linked by either two (A–T) or three (G–C) hydrogen bonds between complementary purine and pyrimidine base pairs. During replication the strands unwind and separate, such that each is able to serve as a template for the synthesis of a new complementary, antiparallel daughter strand using DNA polymerase. Each daughter duplex contains one parental and one new DNA strand that is identical in sequence and structure to the parental duplex.

which are covalently joined by DNA ligase. About 8 hours is required for complete DNA replication in cultured human cells. Most errors that occur during DNA replication are corrected by DNA repair enzymes (glycosylase, phosphodiesterase, helicase), which continuously scan the DNA sequence to detect and replace damaged nucleotides. Two major repair pathways, single-base excision and polynucleotide excision (the latter for larger lesions up to 30 bp), recognize and remove most changes in the DNA duplex. Alterations of fewer than 20 bp/year arise in a mammalian germline cell with a genome size over 3000 Mb.

RNA STRUCTURE, TRANSCRIPTION, TRANSCRIPTIONAL REGULATION, TRANSLATION, AND THE GENETIC CODE

The replacement of T with U and ribose for deoxyribose makes RNA chemically less stable than DNA. The single-stranded RNA polynucleotide chain is able to adopt secondary structures of functional significance. Three kinds of RNA, each synthesized by a different RNA polymerase, are present in the cell. The first step by which the genetic information encoded by DNA is converted to protein assembly is transcription, whereby a single strand of messenger RNA (mRNA) is assembled from 5′ to 3′ in the cell nucleus, to be identical in sequence with its sense DNA strand (Fig. 4.2).

In subsequent steps in the cytoplasm, mRNA serves as a template for the synthesis of amino acids into proteins (translation). Most (up to 99%) RNA in the cell is ribosomal (or rRNA), which does not code for proteins. Ribosomes that comprise rRNA and specific protein constituents are the active sites of translation, and contain binding sites for the interacting molecules necessary for initiation, elongation, and termination of peptide chains. Twenty distinct transfer RNA (tRNA) molecules in cloverleaf conformations participate in translation by recognition and aminoacyl-tRNA synthetase-mediated covalent binding of a specific amino acid to an acceptor arm. *Codons* are mRNA triplets, each of which encodes a single amino acid (Fig. 4.3).

Of the 64 possible codons (4^3 combinations of nucleotides), 20 amino acids are designated. Thus, the *genetic code* is degenerate or redundant (i.e. several different codons may designate the same amino acid). A loop within another arm of each tRNA carries an anticodon nucleotide triplet complementary to an mRNA codon, which assures an orderly assembly of the nascent polypeptide chain in procession from the amino terminus to the carboxy terminus of the peptide corresponding to the 5′ to 3′ orientation of the DNA sequence. Successive amino acids are incorporated in the growing chain by peptide bonds created by a condensation reaction between the amino group of the incoming amino acid and the carboxyl group of the preceding amino acid (Chapter 1). Translation is begun at the initiation codon AUG, which encodes the amino acid methionine. Three codons (UAA, UAG, UGA) do not signify an amino acid, but are 'nonsense codons' that terminate translation at the 3′ end of the open reading frame. As a result of the triplet code, each stretch of DNA and the corresponding transcribed RNA contains three potential translation frames. The *open reading frame* is that string of codons flanked on the 5′ end by an initiation codon, and on the 3′ end by a termination codon. It is therefore possible to infer DNA or RNA sequence one from the other, if either is known. Peptide translation products commonly undergo a variety of *post-translational modifications* that involve chemical (e.g. hydroxylation, phosphorylation) and side-chain (e.g. glycosylation) alterations, as well as cleavage of precursors to mature proteins.

For biochemical purposes, a *gene* is defined as a segment of DNA responsible for the production of one or more related polypeptide chains or structural RNA molecules. The gene or, more accurately, the transcription unit is a sequence of DNA that can be transcribed into a single mRNA, tRNA, or rRNA using a specific RNA polymerase. Included in the transcription unit are regions that precede (proximal promoter) and follow (distal terminator) the coding sequence. Upstream promoter sequences (e.g. a TATA box 25 bp 5′ from a transcriptional start site) serve to bind various *transcription factors* (TFs), positioning and activating RNA polymerase to begin transcription. The TFs are referred to as *trans*-acting because they themselves are the products of genes located elsewhere in the genome, and move to their specific *cis*-acting sites of action upstream of a gene about to undergo transcription. Genes with expression regulated by external factors, including hormones or internal signaling molecules (e.g. cyclic adenosine monophosphate (cAMP)), are preceded by response elements capable of binding the signaling factor. Transcription is further stimulated by *cis*-acting elements (enhancers) for sequence-specific regulatory proteins that function independently of orientation and proximity to the coding sequence and are responsible for tissue-specific and developmental regulation of the ~30 000 genes per cell which are differentially expressed along 40 Mb of sequence.

A gene is a segment of DNA that encodes one or more related polypeptide or structural RNA molecules.

The activation of gene expression is complex and involves the state of DNA methylation (which represses transcription), modification of chromatin-associated histone proteins, and the state and stage of the cell in its cycle. The heteronuclear RNA transcript is processed shortly after transcription to mRNA with the addition of a 5′ cap (guanosine), a substrate for methylation that contributes to the efficiency of mRNA transport to the cytoplasm, and splicing to facilitate translation. Most genes have 5′ leader and 3′ trailer untranslated sequences added after the initiation of transcription. At the 3′ terminus, an untranslated poly(A) tail of 150–200 A nucleotides is added after an endonucleic cleavage of about 20 bases 3′ to an AAUAAA RNA sequence. This poly(A) tail may stabilize the mRNA transcript in the cytoplasm, and assist transport and translation.

GENE STRUCTURE, RNA PROCESSING, AND GENOMIC AND COMPLEMENTARY DNA

The majority of mRNA transcripts are interrupted by large segments of intervening sequences, or *introns*, which are eventually edited out to leave only the coding sequences or *exons* linked together. Noncoding intron sequences, which contain defective copies of functional genes (pseudogenes and gene fragments) and repetitive *noncoding DNA*, are highly polymorphic as they are not subject to the same selective pressure as exons. On average, a polymorphic allele is detected once in 10^3 bp of human exon sequence, and intron polymorphisms

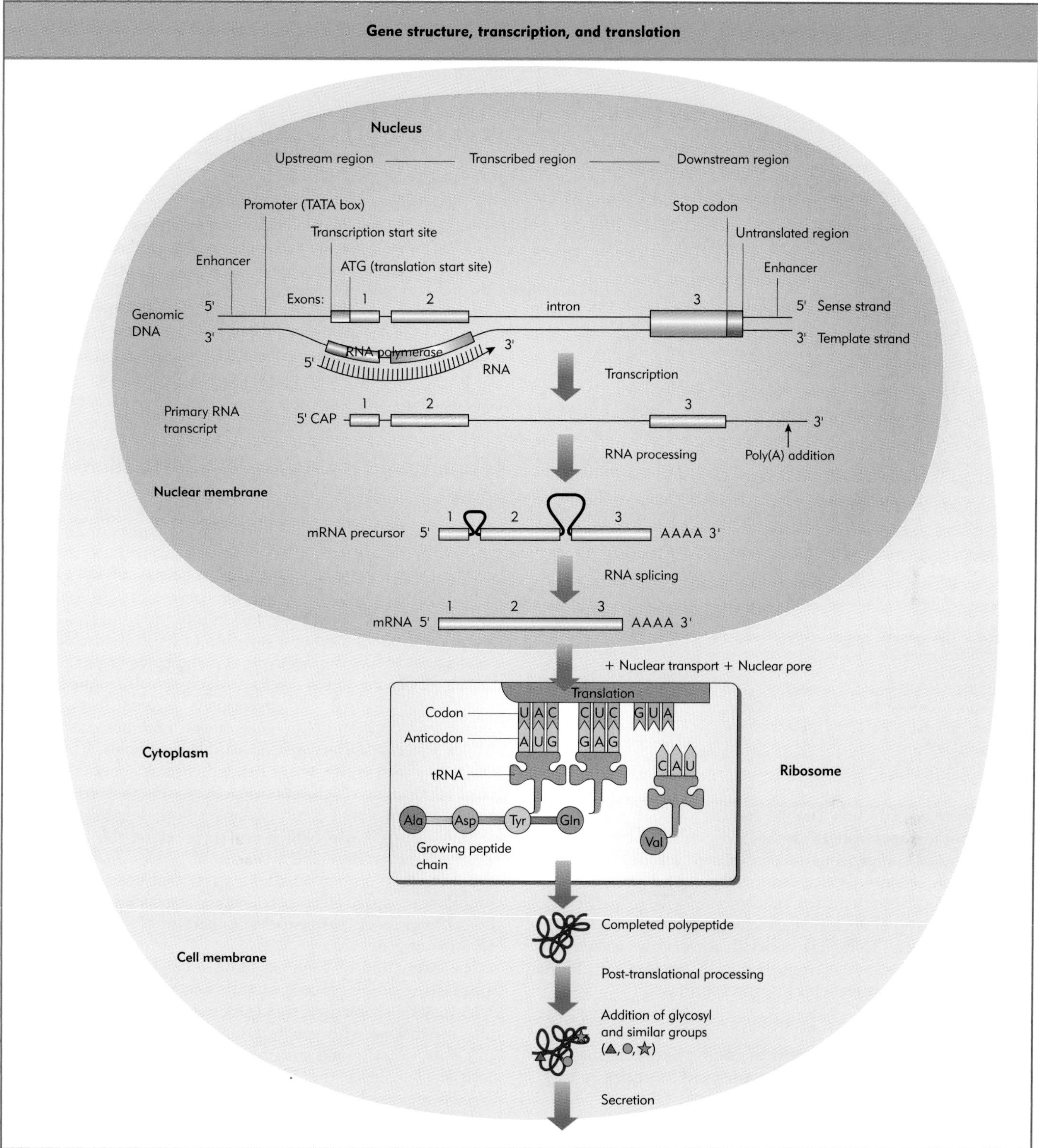

Figure 4.2 Gene structure, transcription, and translation. Information transfer between nucleotide sequence and protein synthesis begins with transcription of DNA into complementary mRNA. This step is catalyzed by RNA polymerase and coordinated by a variety of *cis*-acting enhancers and promoters and *trans*-acting transcription factors (TF). Within the cell nucleus the mRNA transcript is edited to remove noncoding regions and splice exon segments (1–3 above) together. Processing of RNA is completed with 5′-capping and 3′-polyadenylation prior to transport to cytoplasmic ribosomes for translation into peptide chains. The genetic code is deciphered from 5′ to 3′ at the ribosome, which corresponds to the assembly of the protein from the amino to the carboxy terminus, by codon–anticodon recognition between the mRNA transcript and tRNAs specific for each amino acid. Further modifications of the gene product take place after translation, so that the protein can play its enzymatic or structural role in the cell. Ala, alanine; Asp, aspartic acid; Gln, glutamine; Tyr, tyrosine; Val, valine.

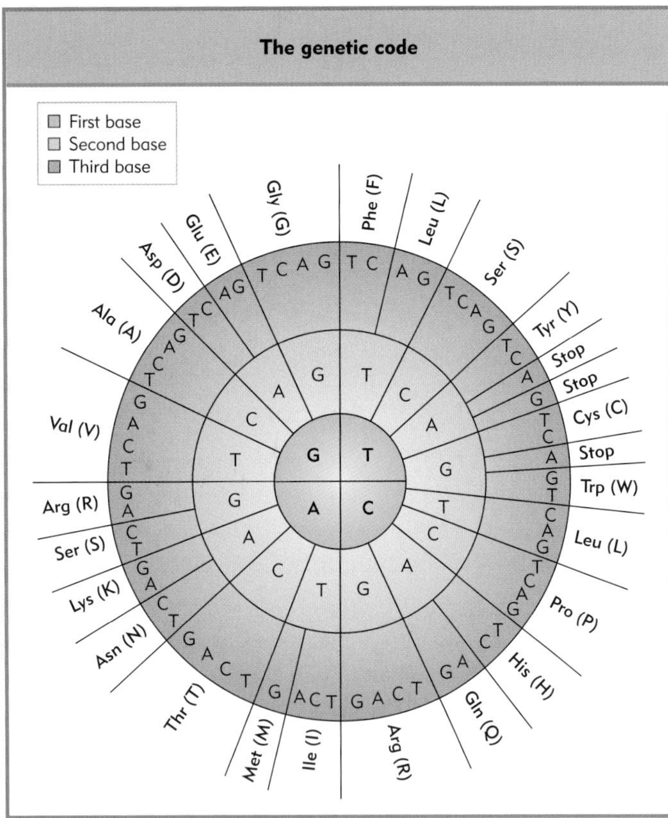

Figure 4.3 The genetic code. Codons composed of three nucleotides are translated into amino acids according to the rules shown, with the first, second, and third positions chosen from the inner to outermost circles, respectively. Arg, arginine; Asn, asparagine; Cys, cysteine; Glu, glutamic acid; Gly, glycine; His, histidine; Ile, isoleucine; Lys, lysine; Met, methionine; Phe, phenylalanine; Pro, proline; Ser, serine; Thr, threonine; Trp, tryptophan.

appear once in 10^2 bp. The functional roles of introns are unclear, but it is speculated that they may act as TF binding sites and regions of spontaneous recombination. *Splicing* occurs at consensus sequences of splice donor and acceptor junctions, and results in the formation of a spliceosome, a large particulate complex made up of nuclear ribonucleoprotein particles (RNPs) and small nuclear RNPs, U1 and U2. Alternative patterns of splicing from the same heteronuclear RNA can lead to mRNAs that encode different proteins by exon shuffling.

Most mRNA transcripts consist of coding exons separated by noncoding introns, which are removed by splicing.

Genomic DNA is isolated from eukaryotic cells and contains both introns and exons. In addition to the elements described above, genomic DNA represents all of the boundaries between introns and exons, together with all of the internal noncoding sequences. *Complementary DNA (cDNA)* is synthesized in vitro from mRNA transcripts isolated from tissues that express the genes of interest. The synthesis of cDNA employs the enzyme reverse transcriptase, which (like other DNA polymerases) uses a template sequence, a primer (usually oligodeoxythymidylic acid (oligo(dT)) annealing to the mRNA poly(A) tail), and the four deoxynucleotide triphosphates (dNTPs). Unlike other DNA polymerases, reverse transcriptase is able to use RNA as a template for synthesis, creating a cDNA molecule that corresponds to the edited open reading frame.

IN VITRO MOLECULAR BIOLOGY

The cellular mechanisms required for nucleotide segregation, lengthwise and end-to-end cleavage, sorting, recognition, editing, and replication have been elucidated by virtue of their conservation in widely divergent organisms, including prokaryotes (bacteria) and eukaryotes (yeast, mammalian cells). To detect variations in DNA sequence directly, and to correlate them with variations between cells, individuals, families, and species, tools were needed to repeat these processes in vitro. A revolution in human biology was heralded by the discovery and availability of restriction endonucleases (1962), DNA ligases (1967), vectors (1973), DNA sequencing (1977), and the polymerase chain reaction (PCR) (1984).

Chromosome sorting, nucleotide isolation, and cleavage

The complement of human chromosomes consists of 22 homologous pairs of autosomes, numbered by convention from the largest (1) to the smallest (22), and one pair of sex chromosomes. Together, the *human genome* consists of 3 000 000 000 base pairs (Fig. 4.4). During the mitotic interphase, chromosomes are decondensed and invisible to light microscopy. The use of agents to halt the cell cycle at metaphase permits the visualization of chromosomes, each of which reveals unique banding patterns when stained with appropriate reagents. Together with the size and position of the centromere, chromosome banding enables accurate differentiation of the autosomes. The representation of the entire set of banded chromosomes is a karyogram. Alterations of chromosomal structure that arise during meiotic crossover may result in duplications, deletions, or translocations up to 4 Mb, which are apparent on the karyogram. These and other large abnormalities of genetic material (aberrations in chromosomal number, e.g. triploidy, or structure, e.g. chromosome rings, inversions), when associated with specific clinical syndromes, may provide important clues to the sublocalization of genes.

The extraction of genomic DNA of high molecular weight from cells is simple. If it is of sufficient molecular weight, the DNA may be spooled on to a glass rod. In fact, the main difficulty in working with genomic DNA from eukaryotic cells in bulk is its viscosity and susceptibility to shearing forces. Much more challenging is the isolation of RNA. Ubiquitous tissue ribonucleases are hardy and can even survive autoclaving.

The human genome consists of 3 000 000 000 base pairs in 46 chromosomes encoding about 30 000 genes.

Endonucleases are enzymes that cleave phosphodiester bonds within a nucleic acid chain. *Restriction enzymes* are a class of endonuclease that recognize short sequences of double-stranded DNA and cleave at or near a recognition sequence (Fig. 4.5). Selection from a catalog of restriction endonucleases, each with known recognition-specific sequences, enables the segregation of

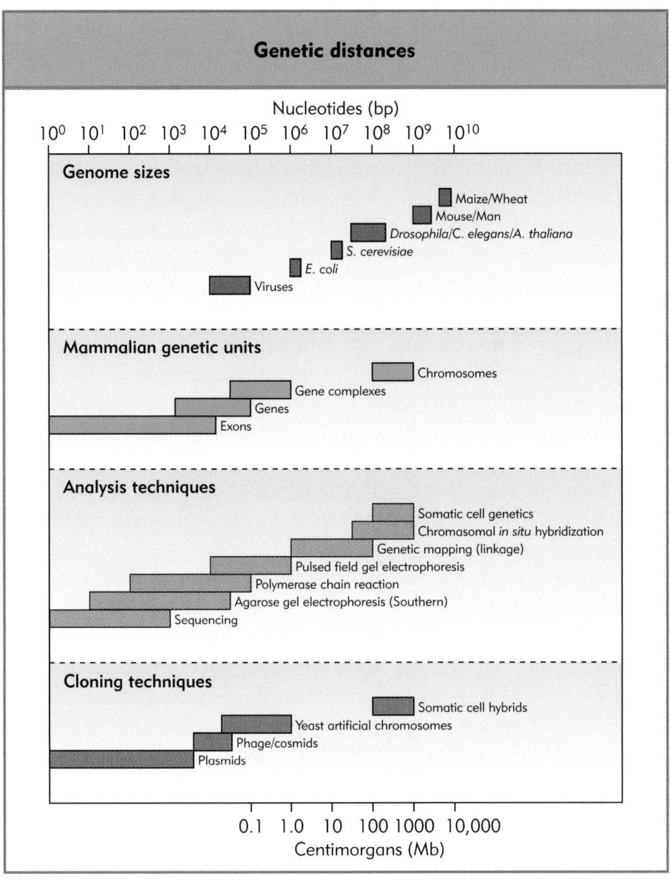

Figure 4.4 Genetic distances. (*E. coli, Escherichia coli; S. cerevisiae, Saccharomyces cerevisiae; C. elegans, Caenorhabditis elegans; A. thaliana, Arabidopsis thaliana.*)

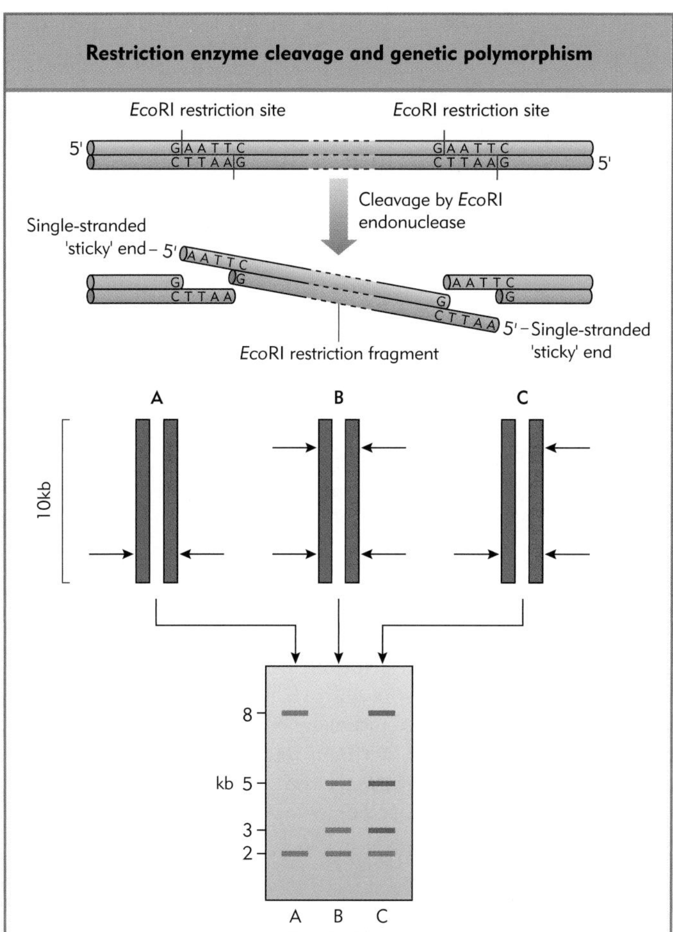

Figure 4.5 Restriction enzyme cleavage and genetic polymorphism. A molecule of DNA contains many short nucleotide sequences recognized by restriction endonucleases that bind and cut the DNA duplex at that site (e.g. the enzyme EcoRI cleaves wherever it encounters the sequence GAATTC, to leave staggered 'sticky' ends). The presence or absence of the recognition site can be inferred by the size of fragments separated by gel electrophoresis after enzymatic digestion. Unambiguous ordering of fragment sizes is used to discriminate chromosomal regions inherited from either parent (i.e. genetic 'markers'). In the example shown, a single digest of a 10 kb fragment is sufficient to detect each homozygote (A and B) from the heterozygote in which all four possible configurations are represented.

DNA fragments by size, based on the estimated frequency of the recognition site. Smaller fragments are generated by digestion with frequent cutters, whereas larger fragments are produced by rare cutters with longer and less frequently encountered recognition sites. The resultant fragments may have either blunt or sticky ends – the overhangs of the latter are especially useful for the ligation of DNA from dissimilar sources. The number and arrangement of restriction sites can be assembled into a restriction map of a particular DNA sequence or even a whole genome.

Detection of *restriction fragment length polymorphisms* (RFLPs) was the first technique developed that used DNA sequence as a marker for the presence of mutant alleles in genes. An RFLP is a specific DNA fragment resulting from restriction endonuclease digestion of DNA, which differs in length between two alleles of the same gene in an individual, or between two individuals. The difference resides in the presence or absence of the specific cleavage site required by the enzyme, which may depend on a single base-pair change. In the presence of the site, two smaller fragments are generated after digestion. In its absence, only a single larger fragment results. The polymorphism is represented by the lengths of the fragments, which are easily measured.

Nucleotide separation

Fragments of DNA that arise from restriction endonuclease digestion are separated according to size on agarose or polyacrylamide gels. As a result of their phosphate groups, DNA fragments are negatively charged and are therefore repelled from the negative electrode toward the positive electrode as they sieve through a porous gel. Smaller fragments move faster. Agarose gel can separate DNA fragments that range in size from 100 bp to 25 kb. Pulse-field gel electrophoresis enables the separation of very large fragments of DNA up to several Mb using alternating current in two different directions.

Nucleotide visualization

Ethidium bromide binds DNA by intercalating between base pairs, which causes the DNA helix to partially unwind. Deoxyribonucleic acid bands in gels stained with ethidium are fluorescent on exposure to ultraviolet light. Silver staining for small fragments in polyacrylamide gels and radiolabeling fragments prior to gel separation are alternative strategies for tracking the presence of a DNA sequence of interest. Although these approaches can indicate the presence of DNA, none can disclose the base-pair composition of the DNA fragment that has been isolated. For this, probe-based tactics are necessary.

Nucleotide probes

A probe is any single-stranded nucleic acid of known composition that can be labeled with a marker and hybridized (bound) to an unknown target nucleic acid on the basis of base complementarity. Labeled nucleic acid probes allow investigators to interrogate genetic material in solution, fixed on a filter, separated in an electrophoretic gel, or on a histologic section. Nucleic acid probes can be used to detect a single nucleotide species from thousands of messages of varying abundance. Such DNA probes may be 15–50 bp oligonucleotides synthesized on the basis of prior knowledge of the DNA target, PCR (see below) products (<15 kb), or full-length genomic or cDNA inserts (0.1–300 kb) cloned from libraries and isolated by cell-based cloning (see below). When no DNA sequence is available but the protein sequence is known, the DNA sequence can be deduced from the genetic code, and an array of degenerate synthetic oligomer nucleotides synthesized to represent all possible codon combinations. A variety of methods (nick translation, kinasing, random primer, RNA transcription) have been devised to incorporate nucleotide precursors with radionuclide (^{32}P, ^{3}H, or ^{35}S) tags. After hybridization to radiolabeled probes and washing, the filter is exposed to a film with autoradiographic emulsion. The resultant autoradiograph reveals the pattern of hybridization. Nonradioactive methods use nonisotopic adducts (biotin-labeled probes incubated with colorimetric streptavidin or fluorescent dyes).

In vitro hybridization, and Southern, Northern, and Western blotting

Sequences of DNA may be specifically identified by binding or molecular hybridization, which is the formation of a duplex between two complementary nucleotide sequences. All nucleotide hybridization tests are based on the fact that two antiparallel single-stranded nucleic acid molecules recognize one another and bind on the basis of hydrogen bonding (e.g. DNA:DNA, DNA:RNA, and RNA:RNA). The probability of hybridization depends on the free energy available for the formation of a particular structure, and is the sum of the individual base-pairing reactions involved. The total number of complementary bases in the two sequences is a major factor in determining the ability to form a stable hybrid, but the base-pair composition also plays a role. Multiple G–C pairings with three hydrogen bonds form a more stable duplex than A–T-rich (with two hydrogen bonds) structures.

The interaction between duplex strands of nucleic acid is strongly temperature dependent. Duplex stability is measured by the melting temperature, defined as the temperature that corresponds to the midpoint in observed transition from the double-stranded to the single-stranded form. The transition is easily assayed by measuring optical density as the mixture is gradually heated. Besides homology indexed by the percentage of mismatches between probe and target, hybrid formation is a function of the mole percentage of G–C pairs in the probe, probe length, salt and nucleic acid concentration, the degree of reannealing of the probe to itself, and the presence of other denaturing agents (e.g. formamide). Manipulation of these variables helps to determine the specificity (stringency) of conditions that favor duplex formation. Duplexes formed when the two strands have a high degree of base homology withstand high stringency conditions (e.g. high temperature, low salt, high formamide) better than duplexes of lesser homology. In certain applications highly stringent conditions may be desired, whereas relaxed conditions, which allow imperfect duplex formation in the presence of mismatched nucleotide pairs, may be useful early on in gene searches (e.g. using a gene sequence from one species as a probe to identify homologs in a genomic DNA library (see below) derived from a second species). In most hybridization experiments the labeled probe is bound to its complementary target, excess probe is washed away, and the specifically bound residual is detected. A common application of hybridization technologies is filter hybridization, in which denatured (single-stranded) DNA or RNA is immobilized on an inert support such that self-annealing is prevented, but the bound sequences are accessible for hybridization with a labeled nucleic acid probe.

In Southern blotting, DNA from any source is extracted, purified, fragmented with restriction endonucleases, and size-separated on an agarose gel (Fig. 4.6). The gel contents are transferred or 'blotted' on to a solid-support nitrocellulose or nylon filter. The flow of buffer by capillary action causes denatured DNA fragments to pass out of the gel on to the filter paper, with preservation of their relative positions. The DNA is hybridized with a complementary labeled single-stranded DNA nucleic acid probe and the nonspecifically bound excess probe is discarded. Thus, a restriction map of a particular DNA sequence is generated by digestion with a panel of restriction enzymes. Deoxyribonucleic acid fingerprinting using multilocus patterns that represent the summed contribution of two alleles at many variable loci throughout the genome enables unequivocal distinction between any two individuals who are not identical twins.

Laser scanning for evidence of hybridization of sample cDNA to oligonucleotide probes representing thousands of genes fixed to glass *chip microarrays* enables simultaneous screening of thousands of alleles. This technology potentially identifies any genotype of interest to perioperative caregivers within several hours. Adaptation of these methods to ascertain patterns of gene expression by organ, cell, subcellular structure, or pathologic process yields insights into the components of complex events.

Probes representing thousands of genes fixed to glass chip microarrays enables simultaneous screening of thousands of alleles.

Northern blotting is the RNA counterpart of Southern blotting, and may be useful for the estimation of the steady-state level of specific mRNA transcription, or expression pattern, at the time of extraction from the tissue. It is also valuable in the detection of transcripts of differing sizes (alternate splice variants), and may indicate the presence of promoters, splice sites, or untranslated segments not apparent on Southern blotting of genomic DNA. Western blotting employs the same matrix and detection formats, but the targets are proteins and the labeled probes are antibodies.

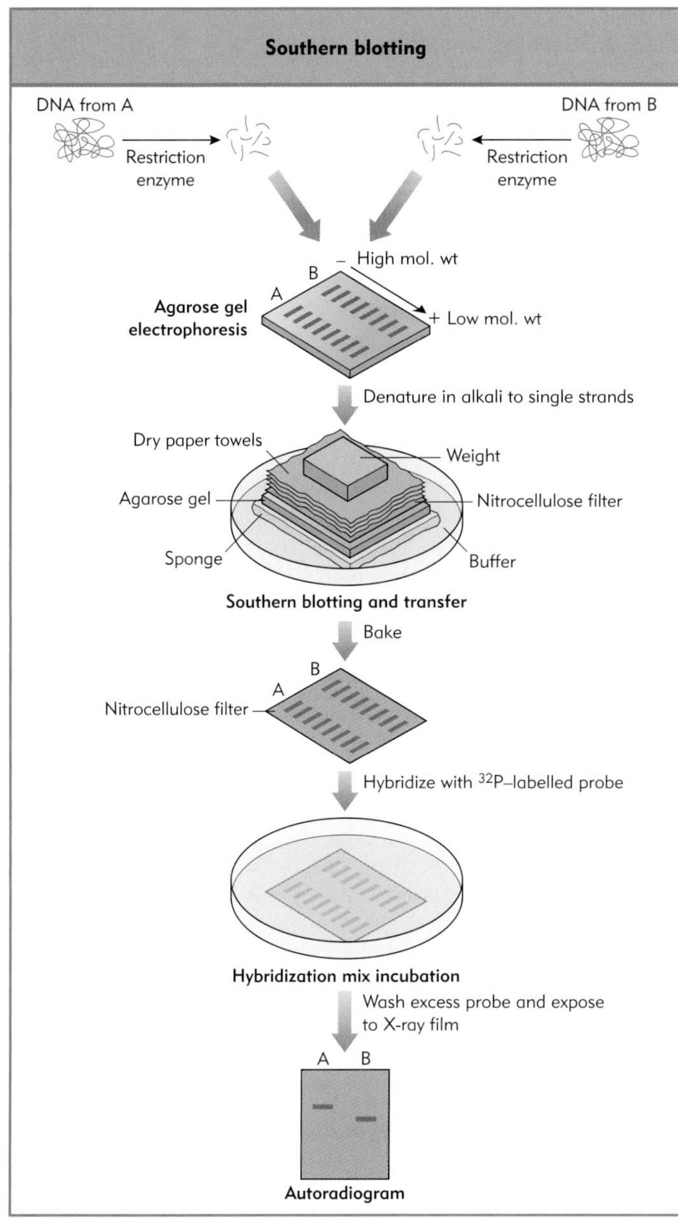

Figure 4.6 Southern blotting. Deoxyribonucleic acid samples are digested by a restriction endonuclease and fractionated by size on agarose gel by electrophoresis. The positions of DNA fragments complementary to the probe are detected as bands on the developed autoradiogram.

In situ hybridization

In situ hybridization, the technique of hybridization applied to cells, reveals the tissue or cellular distribution of nucleic acid sequences. Both the cellular localization of a specific DNA or RNA sequence (tissue in situ hybridization) and the chromosomal assignment (chromosomal in situ hybridization) of a probe can be established. Other than choosing between DNA and RNA targets, differences between in situ hybridization protocols center on maintaining tissue morphology while rendering the tissue permeable to the probe without losing the target. The sensitivity of in situ hybridization relies on the fraction of target in the tissue that is accessible for hybridization, the mass of probe relative to the target (saturation), and the specific activity of the probe. Noise in the hybridization reaction correlates with the extent to which the probe is able to bind nonspecifically to the background. The specificity of hybridization is controlled by the sequence and stringency conditions, and can be measured using other probes (e.g. those that bind to the poly(A) tails of most mRNA species) as controls.

Nucleotide propagation: cell-based cloning, nucleotide libraries

Because a particular fragment of DNA may represent only a small fraction of the DNA in a cell, techniques are required to selectively amplify and purify the sequence of interest before its structure and function can be investigated (i.e. by sequencing or in vitro expression). Cell-based cloning is an in vivo technique in which foreign DNA fragments are attached to DNA sequences capable of independent replication, which are then propagated in suitable host cells. *Recombinant DNA* refers to novel hybrid DNA molecules constructed from DNA sources that cannot occur naturally. *Vectors* are DNA molecules capable of continuing a usual lifecycle after the insertion of foreign DNA. A vector with a foreign recombinant DNA insert capable of replication in bacteria represents a recombinant DNA clone. Cloning of recombinant DNA in bacteria allows the production of large amounts of the inserted fragment. The common property of all vectors is a site at which foreign DNA can be inserted without disrupting function. Plasmid vectors are autonomous circular DNAs capable of self-replication without incorporation into host-cell chromosomes. Most plasmid inserts are limited in size, usually <5 kb (Fig. 4.7). Phages are viruses that infect bacteria and, unlike plasmids, are capable of extracellular existence. Up to 23 kb DNA sequences can be stably packaged in phage particles. Cosmid vectors are plasmids with some phage sequences. Perpetuated in bacteria as plasmids, but retrieved by packaging in vitro into phages, cosmids carry inserts up to 45 kb in length.

The ends of the DNA insert, whether cDNA or genomic DNA fragments, must be engineered to link with the vector at a specific locus. Any DNA fragment can be successfully cloned by generating sequences of the foreign DNA that are complementary to sequences of the vector and then selecting a unique restriction site in the vector to be used as the cloning site. The ends of the insert sequence are ligated to the complementary vector ends with DNA ligase. Often the restriction site is within a marker gene in the vector, so that interruption of the gene by the DNA insert can be used to select appropriate clones. If the interrupted gene confers antibiotic resistance (e.g. to ampicillin), the recombinant clones will be sensitive to the antibiotic. In other systems, inserts interrupt the β-galactosidase gene required to metabolize lactose. Recombinant clones are unable to cleave an artificial substrate (X-gal). Wildtype clones that lack the recombinant DNA inserts produce a blue color, whereas recombinant clones do not.

The recombinant plasmid molecule that consists of foreign DNA and vector-specific sequence is introduced into bacterial host cells, usually a strain of *Escherichia coli*, by the process of transformation. The host bacteria are made competent by pretreatment with calcium chloride, and exposed to heat in the presence of the plasmid. Although only a small percentage of the competent cells take up foreign DNA, they can be selected and

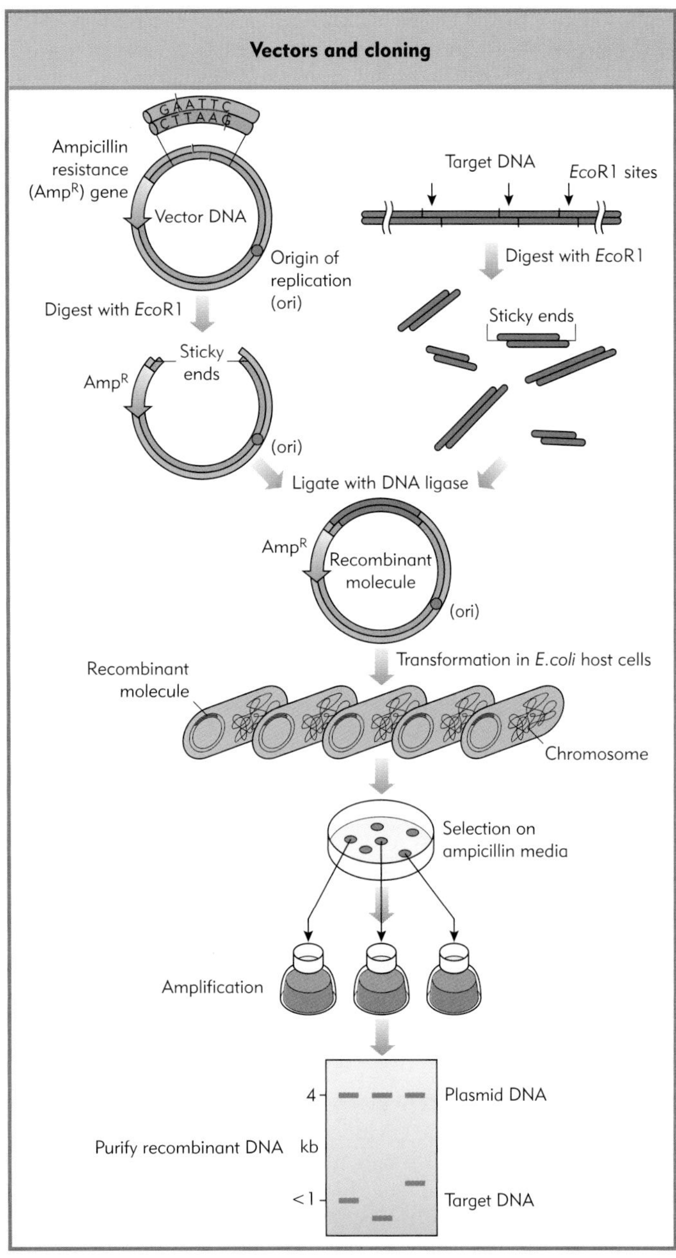

Figure 4.7 Vectors and cell-based cloning. Multiple copies of a DNA fragment of interest can be created by cell-based cloning. To clone DNA, a circular plasmid vector is linearized (cut) with a restriction endonuclease, to leave the vector and insert with compatible ends for ligation. The plasmids, which carry sequences for replication origin (ori) and antibiotic resistance (AmpR), are introduced into *E. coli* host cells by transformation and replicate as drug-resistant elements. Bacterial colonies that contain the vector molecule are selected on antibiotic-containing media and amplified in culture. Bacterial and plasmid-vector DNA are discarded, and target recombinant DNA is purified by electrophoresis.

replicated many times. The transformed bacterial colonies are selected in antibiotic-containing media and undergo secondary expansion to scale up large yields of cell clones, each with the desired insert. When the foreign DNA is ligated into phage DNA the recombinant DNA is first packaged into the phage, which is allowed to infect the bacteria.

Preparation of the DNA insert and host vector with restriction endonucleases not only ensures specific recombination, but permits later isolation and recovery of the cloned insert. To retrieve the cloned DNA the bacteria are lyzed and the plasmid DNA is extracted. Separation of the insert from its cloning vector is accomplished by restriction endonuclease digestion, followed by gel electrophoresis and visualization of the fragments with ethidium bromide staining. The gel band that contains the foreign DNA can be sliced out and eluted, and recombinant DNA molecules subcloned into a different vector molecule for structural or functional assays. Cloning vectors capable of accepting DNA inserts up to 3.0 Mb have been developed. Bacterial artificial chromosomes were created to counteract the instability of large eukaryotic inserts (>300 kb) cloned in bacterial hosts, but usually give only low yields of recombinant DNA. Cloning in yeast cells with the construction of yeast artificial chromosomes (YAC) enables the propagation of exogenous DNA fragments up to 2 Mb in length, and has become essential for physical mapping of genomes. However, YACs are also hampered by relatively low yields of recombinant DNA.

Species-specific genomic DNA and tissue-specific cDNA fragments are available as libraries of clones supplied in plasmids, phages, and cosmids. DNA sequences that are extremely rare in the starting population can be represented in a library of clones created by restriction endonuclease digestion, from which they can be selected and amplified. Hybridization is the most widely used method for screening a library to select individual clones of interest with DNA or RNA probes (Fig. 4.8). In colony hybridization with plasmid vectors or plaque hybridization with recombinant phage vectors, bacterial cells are used to propagate recombinants on an agar surface, which are transferred to a nitrocellulose or nylon membrane, denatured, and hybridized to a labeled probe. The position of positively hybridized probes identifies colonies that contain the cDNA sequence, which may be picked and expanded. Subsequent rounds of cloning and library rescreening (using one end of a newly identified clone to detect an overlapping clone) enables ever larger DNA fragments in the region of interest to be characterized by chromosome walking.

Interspecies somatic cell hybrids are created by radiation fragmentation of human cellular components. During the fusion of rodent and human cells, hybrids that contain human, rodent, and recombinant human–rodent chromosomes are created. Hybrid cells randomly lose chromosomes in subsequent culture, which allows the selection of hybrid panels with one or a few remnant human chromosomes. Matching the presence or absence of a particular nucleic acid probe by hybridization on the panel with the presence or absence of known chromosome fragments leads to unambiguous identification of the chromosome that contains the gene from which the probe was derived.

Nucleotide propagation: cell-free cloning and the polymerase chain reaction

If the sequence of regions that flank both ends of a specific DNA fragment is known, it is possible to selectively amplify picogram (10^{-12} g) quantities of DNA using PCR. Defined as the in vitro enzymatic synthesis and amplification of specific DNA sequences, PCR is a simple and efficient technique to produce over 100 billion copies of a single molecule of DNA within hours (Fig. 4.9). Its advantages are its capacity to use minute samples to produce a high yield of amplified target DNA, the specificity of the reaction, the flexibility of the methods, and the rapidity and simplicity of the automated procedure. Owing to these attributes, PCR has been successfully used to amplify degraded

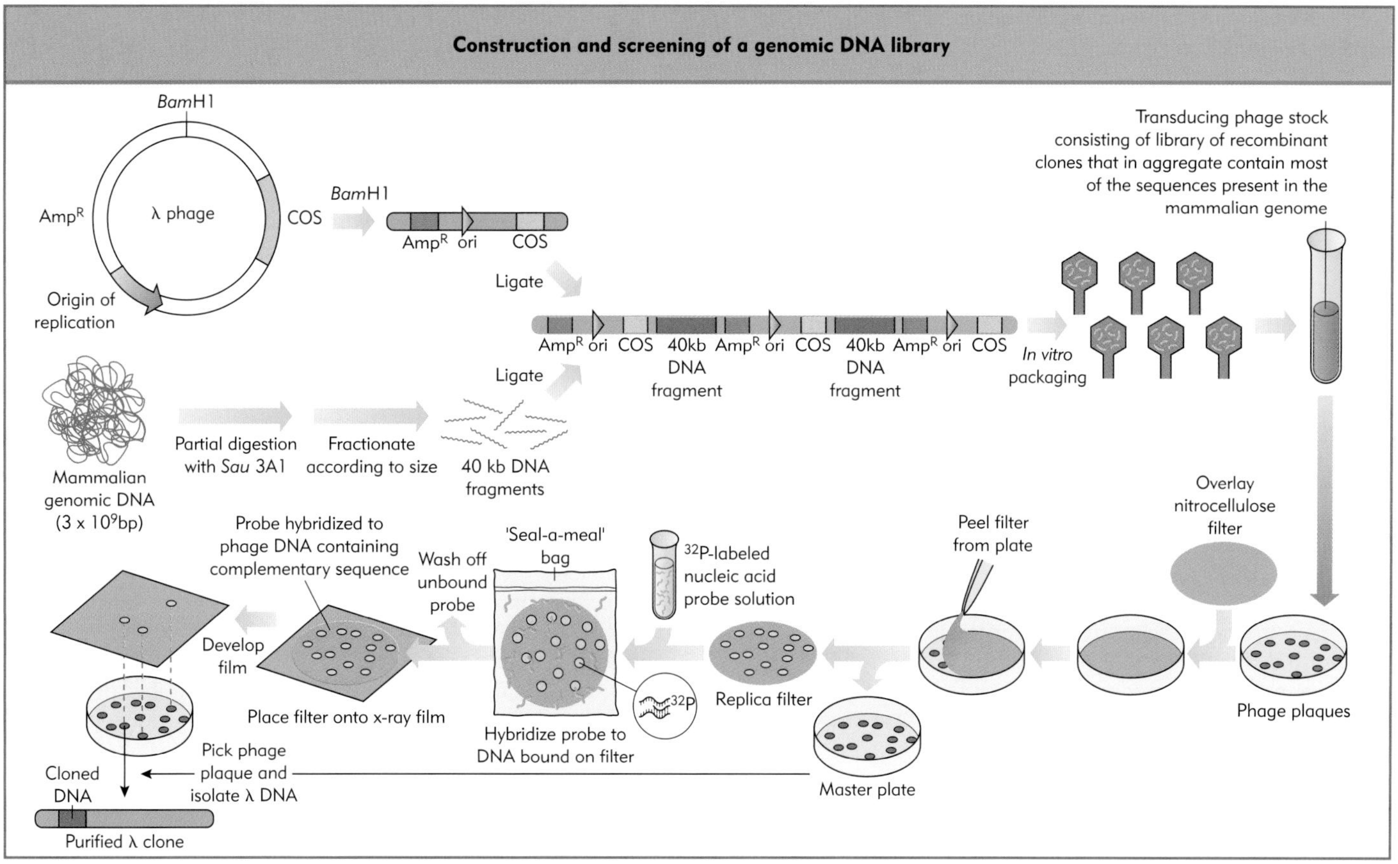

Construction and screening of a genomic DNA library

BamH1
Amp^R
λ phage
COS
Origin of replication
BamH1
Amp^R ori COS
Ligate
Amp^R ori COS 40kb DNA fragment Amp^R ori COS 40kb DNA fragment Amp^R ori COS
Ligate
In vitro packaging
Transducing phage stock consisting of library of recombinant clones that in aggregate contain most of the sequences present in the mammalian genome
Mammalian genomic DNA (3 x 10^9bp)
Partial digestion with *Sau* 3A1
Fractionate according to size
40 kb DNA fragments
Overlay nitrocellulose filter
Peel filter from plate
Phage plaques
^{32}P-labeled nucleic acid probe solution
Replica filter
Master plate
'Seal-a-meal' bag
Hybridize probe to DNA bound on filter
Wash off unbound probe
Probe hybridized to phage DNA containing complementary sequence
Develop film
Place filter onto x-ray film
Pick phage plaque and isolate λ DNA
Cloned DNA
Purified λ clone

Figure 4.8 Construction and screening of a genomic DNA library. To construct a genomic DNA library, easily accessible cells (e.g. leukocytes) are harvested, lyzed, and their DNA extracted. Partial digestion with a restriction endonuclease cleaves the DNA at a small number of available sites (with the pattern differing between molecules), which results in a near-random cleavage in aggregate. The series of overlapping restriction fragments that represents most of the sequences present in the genome is packaged in phage, and bacterial plaques are adsorbed from the master plate to overlying filters. The filters are screened by hybridization to a radiolabeled probe and placed on radiographic film. Plaques that contain the recombinant fragment of interest appear as spots on the film, and can be picked from the master plate for amplification and purification. COS sequences are 12 bp sticky ends at either terminus of linear bacteriophage λ (l) DNA molecules.

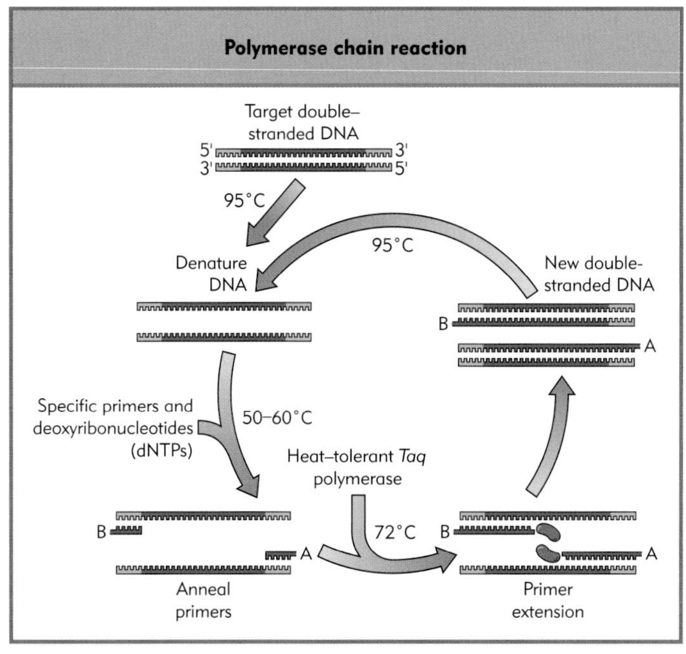

Figure 4.9 The polymerase chain reaction. In the first step of PCR, target double-stranded DNA is denatured at high temperature (e.g. 95°C) for 1–2 minutes to give single-stranded DNA (denaturation step). Next, 20–30 bp oligonucleotide primers specific for the flanking regions on opposite strands are annealed to the denatured DNA (annealing step) at 50–70°C. The primers are designed to be complementary to the opposite strands of DNA and not to one another, and bind at the 5′ ends of the cDNAs in a 5′ to 3′ orientation. Next, a heat-tolerant DNA polymerase uses the oligonucleotides as primers to synthesize cDNA with both strands as templates (primer extension step). Taq DNA polymerase, originally isolated from *Thermus aquaticus* living in the geysers of Yellowstone National Park, is active at temperatures used for extension (70–72°C), and survives subsequent 95°C denaturation steps. The strands are heat denatured, the cycle is begun again, and the template amplified in a geometric expansion over 30-40 cycles. A programmable heating and cooling thermal cycler makes replication of DNA fragments rapid and cost-effective.

DNA from Egyptian mummies, Neanderthal remains, and dyes used in Paleolithic cave art.

Major disadvantages compared with cell-based cloning include template contamination, the need for target-sequence information for primer assembly, limited PCR product sizes (usually <15 kb), and the absence of proofreading mechanisms to correct copying errors. Because PCR may be successful in the presence of several DNA bases in the primer that are not complementary to the template DNA, it is possible to assemble amplified PCR fragments with modified restriction endonuclease recognition sites for use in subcloning, or to introduce site-directed mutations into amplified products of target DNA to investigate functional expression in host cells (see below). Knowledge of the intron–exon structure of a gene expressing pathogenic alleles allows exon-specific amplification by PCR using primers complementary to 5′ and 3′ boundary intron sequences. The resultant PCR products can then be analyzed for mutations by rapid screening methods or by direct sequencing. If primers are assembled to anneal with specific sequences that exhibit the pathogenic allele (allele-specific oligonucleotides) at the 3′ terminus of the primer, the presence of the mutant allele is inferred by the presence of the appropriately sized PCR product. Small deletions and insertions are readily detected by a change in the size of PCR products, or by a failure to produce any fragment if the primer is unable to anneal in the area of deletion.

DNA sequencing

The resolution of the fine structure of DNA by direct sequencing was achieved in 1977. Subsequent refinements of the technique using novel cloning vectors and oligonucleotides led to the Sanger dideoxy sequencing method now in widespread use. The basic principle in sequencing methods is the assembly of a population of synthetic single-stranded DNA molecules in which each base of a specimen is represented by DNA fragments of a length that conforms to the sample sequence that extends to that point, and not beyond (Fig. 4.10). Typically, several hundred base pairs of specimen sequence (up to 400 bp) can be read with high fidelity. Synthesis of new oligonucleotide primers based on homology with this sequence enables ongoing sequencing using the same clone of template DNA. Novel sequencing methods now make it feasible to use double-stranded vectors such as plasmids and λ phage, provided a short sequence of insert or vector is known to construct the priming oligonucleotides.

GENOME STRUCTURE, MUTATION, THE HUMAN GENOME PROJECT, AND BIOINFORMATICS

The human genome is the total DNA content in human cells, including the complex nuclear genome and a simple mitochondrial genome that specifies only a small proportion of mitochondrial functions in its 37 genes. The number of genes in the nuclear genome, estimated by genomic sequencing and random sequencing of partial cDNA clones, known as expressed sequence tags (ESTs), is estimated to be 30 000–40 000, encoded by 3% or less of the 3000 Mb genome. Human genes vary tremendously in size and internal organization. On average, a human gene consists of 10–20 boundaries between intron and exon sequences, 1–2 kb of coding, and 10–30 kb of genomic

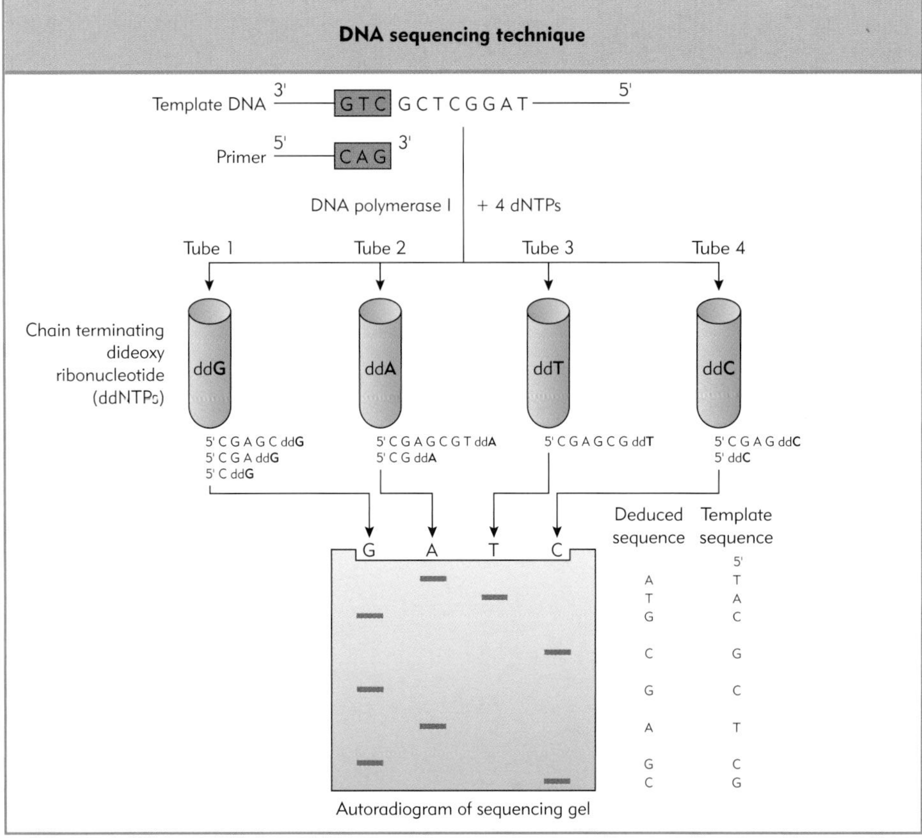

Figure 4.10 Sanger dideoxy DNA sequencing. The DNA to be sequenced is inserted into a polycloning site of the M13 phage vector, which can produce single-stranded DNA as a template. A universal oligonucleotide primer is annealed to the strand of sample DNA, and synthesis of new strands is initiated in vitro by the addition of DNA polymerase I and dNTPs. Deoxyribonucleic acid polymerase I is able to incorporate the dideoxynucleotides (ddNTPs), but cannot add further to the chain to form a new phosphodiester bond with the next incoming nucleotide. Thus, a series of DNA molecules is constructed in each of four reaction tubes; the series differ in length depending on the location of a particular base relative to the 5′ end, as a result of 3′ chain termination by a specific ddNTP. The synthesized strands are labeled by radionuclide or fluorescent markers linked either to the four bases individually, or to the primer itself. The four tubes of reaction products, which consist of DNA fragments of the same sequence that differ in length by one base, are separated into four parallel lanes of a polyacrylamide gel, one for each ddNTP. After autoradiography or laser dye detection, the sequence is read from one band to the next according to the lanes in which the bands appear.

sequence. Genes as small as several hundred base pairs without introns and as large as the dystrophin gene, with 15 kb of coding sequence and 60 introns that span an entire genomic sequence of 2.5 Mb, are well described. Overlapping genes, genes within genes, multiple copy numbers of the same gene, and gene families with homology between members have been identified. Intron sequence is characterized by microsatellite (1–4 bp) and minisatellite (1–20 kb) tandem repeats of high copy number and variable length, but of unknown functional significance.

Mutation, which produces heritable changes in DNA, includes both large changes (loss, duplication, or rearrangement of chromosome segments) and small point modifications (loss, duplication, or alteration of segments of DNA as small as a single base pair). Based on estimates of gene frequency in a population and reproductive failure of a genotype because of natural selection, mutation rates for most organisms are 10^{-5}–10^{-7} per locus per generation. This low level of mutation represents a balance that allows occasional evolutionary novelty at the expense of disease or the death of a proportion of members of a species. Methods available to detect human genes that carry novel mutant alleles are chosen according to the size of the defect. Visible chromosomal rearrangements that give rise to dysmorphic syndromes may represent contiguous gene defects disrupting a monogenic locus of interest. Animal models, traits associated with previously mapped loci, and candidate proteins in plausible pathways may indicate specific genes for direct sequencing. If there are no such shortcuts, investigators may resort to genetic maps of linked markers and positional candidate genes (see below). Once a mutation is identified, to screen individuals at risk is relatively simple using PCR-based approaches. Single base-pair alterations produce mismatches that modify the ability of a PCR product to form heteroduplexes with tagged RNA probes. More commonly, conformational changes in single-strand DNA fragments (single-strand conformation polymorphism, SSCP) that differ at one base pair are discriminated by gel electrophoresis to detect known mutations (Fig. 4.11).

A major goal of the Human Genome Project was achieved in 2001 with completion of a full-length composite sequence. Ultimately, a genomic DNA sequence (physical map) will be assembled so that meaningful variations from normal can be compared with their respective phenotypes, and thereby improve the diagnosis and management of disease. The genomic DNA sequence map will incorporate all the information obtained in the construction of earlier, lower-resolution physical maps (e.g. cytogenetic maps, restriction maps, and cDNA maps; Fig. 4.12).

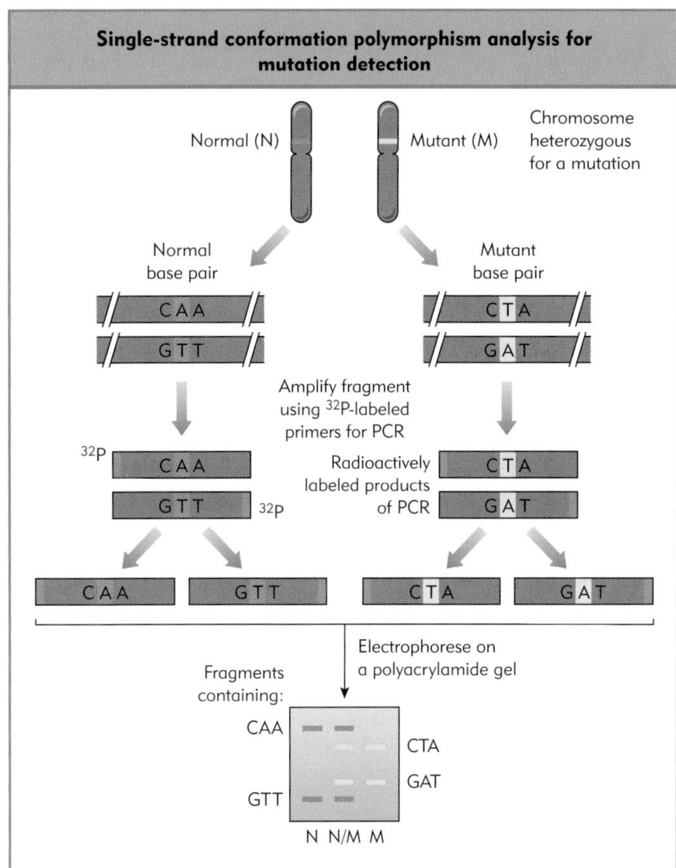

Figure 4.11 Single-strand conformation polymorphism analysis for mutation detection. Single-strand DNA forms complex structures stabilized by weak intermolecular bonds based on DNA composition that can be discriminated by altered electrophoretic mobility. Denatured PCR products tagged with radiolabeled primers are loaded on nondenaturing polyacrylamide gels – samples that differ by a single base pair may be resolved. In the example shown, two bands are apparent from each of the homozygous normal (N) and mutant (M) strands, whereas all four bands are present in DNA from the heterozygote (N/M). Although SSCP is a sensitive technique with which to screen PCR products for mutations, it is limited to fragments of several hundred bp and cannot indicate the exact nature or position of the genetic alteration if this is not already known.

Recombination, genetic maps, and genetic linkage

The basic principle in *genetic mapping* is to order loci using meiotic recombination to index the size of the intervening distance. Any phenotypic or genotypic character that is polymorphic and mendelian can be used as a marker for the presence of a genetic locus. In the simplest case of X-linked conditions, analysis of pedigrees using gender as a marker leads to many gene assignments to the X chromosome. For the remaining 22 autosomes, tremendous genetic variation arises during the first stage of meiosis, from independent assortment of maternal and paternal chromosomes to the gamete to recombination or *crossing-over* (the exchange of chromosomal material between homologous chromosomes during meiosis). Taking advantage of the low probability of reassortment by crossing-over between genetic loci in close linear approximation, linkage analysis allows the detection of regions of the genome that contain genes associated with traits and diseases inherited in a mendelian single-gene manner. The strength of the approach is that no assumptions need be made regarding the nature of the gene or its expressed product. Its weaknesses include the need for pedigrees of substantial size and specific character (e.g. several affected individuals in three generations), a clear-cut phenotypic diagnosis, and assumptions about gene number, mechanisms of inheritance, expressivity, and penetrance that may or may not prevail.

Linkage refers to the co-inheritance of a marker and a region of DNA sequence thought to underlie a specific trait. Ideal markers are highly polymorphic (i.e. at least two or more alleles exist at the locus) and the least common allele has a frequency of at least 1% in the general population. Individuals are most likely to be heterozygous for markers that are highly polymorphic, which makes it possible to track the inheritance of a particular marker-tagged chromosome within a family. In the simplest version of linkage analysis (Fig. 4.13), if a marker is

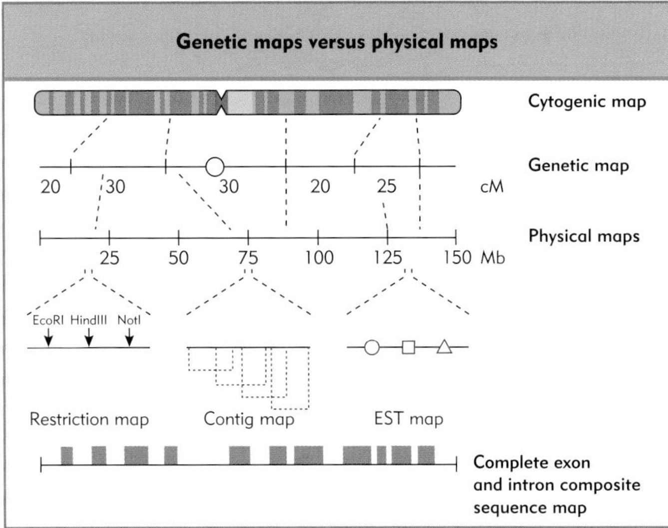

Figure 4.12 Genetic maps versus physical maps. Genetic maps represent the order of loci by the frequency of recombination events between two loci. Genetic loci in close approximation – <1 cM apart – rarely dissociate in meiosis, whereas the greater the interval between loci, the greater the likelihood that they sort independently. The genetic distance of 1 cM corresponds loosely to the physical distance of 1 Mb, but is not constant throughout the genome (see text). When completed, the highest-order human physical map of exon and intron sequence will encompass lower-resolution cytogenetic, restriction, contig (contiguous overlapping DNA clones assembled by chromosome walking), and cDNA physical maps, and will incorporate chromosome-specific genetic maps.

mapped to a specific locus and a marker at a second locus is linked to the first, then the two loci must reside on the same chromosome. The map distance defined as a frequency of recombination between loci of 1% ($\theta = 0.01$) is 1 centiMorgan (cM), which is estimated to represent about 1 Mb, but genetic maps and physical maps are not isologous. Recombination is more frequent at the ends of chromosomes, occurs more often in females than in males, and may be especially common in recombination 'hotspots'. Linkage is observed by simultaneous inheritance through successive generations of identical alleles at the loci in question, with no evidence for recombination between the two. As few families are ideal for linkage analysis, mathematical models that calculate the LOD score (logarithm of the odds ratio) are required to compare the likelihood that an observed association of alleles occurs as a result of varying degrees of linkage rather than by chance alone. A LOD score of 3 or more favors the probability of linkage at 1000:1, and is taken as evidence of true linkage. Once a set of markers (haplotype) in a chromosomal region has been found to be co-inherited (co-segregate) with a trait of interest, fragments of DNA sequence from that region can be searched for causal genes using chromosome walking. As the number of mapped genes in the Human Genome Project has increased, it is now more common to seek candidate genes that have already been mapped to the linked locus (positional candidates) for analysis using intragenic markers and direct mutation searches. Alternatively, association studies aim to identify DNA sequence variations that correlate with the presence or absence of a trait in matched but unrelated population samples. Higher-order statistical models are required for quantitative trait loci (QTL) mapping, in which

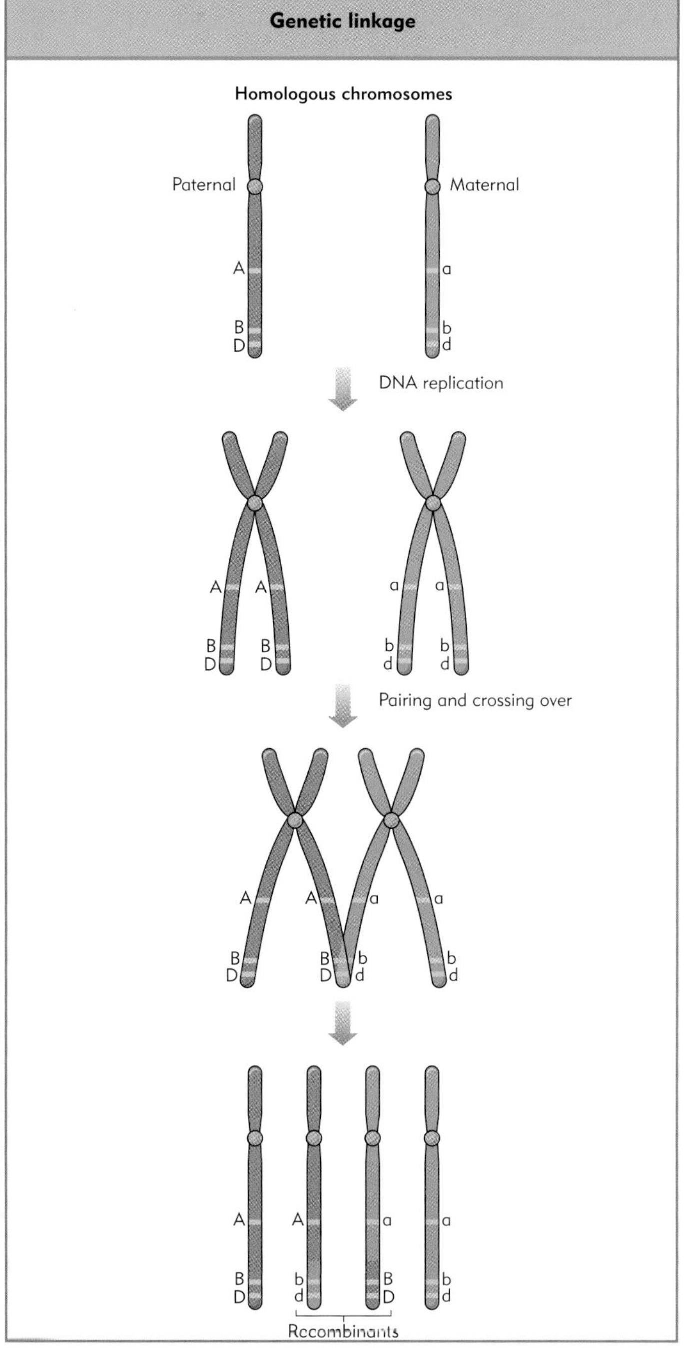

Figure 4.13 Genetic linkage. By isolating a series of polymorphic markers at loci linked to a locus associated with a specific trait or disease, it is possible to track the inheritance of specific chromosomal regions in families without knowledge of the function of the locus in question. If two loci are closely linked (e.g. Bb and Dd), their alleles are transmitted together to the gamete. Exchange of chromosomal material between homologous chromosomes during meiosis is a crossover event. The smaller the distance between two loci, the less probable a crossover event (recombination) between the two becomes, and therefore the likelihood of recombinational events between two loci can be used to define genetic distances.

many genes contribute to the inheritance of the trait, for example predisposition to diabetes or hypertension.

Site-directed mutagenesis

If a gene has been cloned and a suitable assay is available, molecular genetic techniques allow dissection and mapping of the operational elements within the gene and the protein, as well as investigation of the pathophysiologic consequences of disease-causing alleles. The techniques of site-directed mutagenesis precisely alters one or more nucleotides in a DNA clone using either cell-based or cell-free PCR approaches. With PCR, primers are designed to be dissimilar to the target sequence by incorporating novel nucleotides in the PCR product, but not sufficiently different to inhibit amplification. Denatured PCR products of two reactions with partially overlapping sequences that contain the mutation of interest can then be combined to create a larger fragment with the mutation at midpoint in the sequence. In add-on mutagenesis, modified primers introduce a convenient restriction site, labeled group, promoter sequence, or other useful component to the 5′ end of the PCR product. Using the normal gene as a control, the mutant gene product may then be expressed in host cells and functional changes compared with the wild type gene product.

Expression cloning

Most cloning efforts in the past have been aimed at the acquisition and amplification of DNA to investigate its structure and function. More recently, the generation of bulk amounts of a specific protein for therapy (insulin, growth hormone) or for direct studies of peptide function has become feasible, with the design of cloning systems that promote the expression of eukaryotic genes in bacterial cells (expression cloning). An expression vector contains bacterial promoter sequences of DNA required to transcribe the cloned DNA insert and translate its mRNA into protein (i.e. sequences that position the mRNA on the ribosome and an initiation codon). The foreign DNA fragment may be cloned into a site within the coding region of a prokaryotic gene. Expression vectors are most appropriate for cDNA inserts, as bacteria lack the mechanisms for intron splicing. They often include an inducible promoter, which overcomes the detrimental effects of foreign gene expression by switching on the foreign gene after the bacteria have been selected and propagated. The expression of eukaryotic proteins in bacterial cells may be useful in the identification and characterization of novel genes by antibody screening of a cDNA library in bacterial cells that express foreign proteins (phage display library). Clones that react positively for a specific antibody are isolated and used as probes for genomic library screens.

In the absence of many post-translational processing systems in bacterial prokaryotic cells, eukaryotic gene products may be unstable or reveal no biologic activity. Expression of eukaryotic genes in eukaryotic cells allows the detection and quantification of a gene product, which might otherwise be impossible in bacteria. A crucial step in the development of DNA-mediated transfection techniques was the creation of mammalian expression vectors, which allow the transcription and translation of foreign genes in a wide variety of recipient cell types. Mammalian expression vectors contain a eukaryotic transcription unit, in addition to a prokaryotic plasmid region composed of a replication origin (ori) and an antibiotic resistance cistron (e.g. AmpR). To obtain a high level of expression in a broad range of host cell types, the transcription unit derived from a simian virus (SV40) that contains an early promoter is placed upstream (5′) from the insert coding region. The function of the SV40 transcription unit is to direct transcription, the processing and transport of the foreign mRNA to the host cell cytoplasm. An intervening intron sequence improves mRNA stability and transport to the cytoplasm, and a 3′ polyadenylation site prevents 'readthrough' to a prokaryotic plasmid sequence. Other modifications include restriction endonuclease sites for the insertion of DNA sequences, or a eukaryotic DNA replication origin may be added for specific applications. To measure the function of exogenously introduced DNA it is necessary to construct a foreign gene such that its expression can be distinguished from that of the host cell gene. Foreign gene elements are marked by fusion with functional reporter genes expressing easily assayed proteins that are otherwise absent or expressed at low levels in mammalian cells (e.g. chloramphenicol acetyltransferase, *E. coli* β-galactosidase, and firefly luciferase).

Gene transfer

Despite the various mechanisms evolved by host cells to sequester and degrade foreign DNA, many physicochemical and viral techniques have been contrived to surmount obstacles to gene transfer. The major attribute of nonviral vectors is the absence of infectious and neoplastic hazards, whereas their greatest deficit is inefficient transfer. After physicochemical transfer, plasmid transgenes are maintained in the nucleus as episomal DNA, but as they are nonreplicating they may not be useful vectors in regenerating tissue. In the most fundamental method, plasmid DNA is delivered directly into the nucleus using microinjection. Although microinjection bypasses cytoplasmic and lysosomal degradation, only several hundred cells can be modified in a given experiment. Calcium phosphate–DNA co-precipitation to micrometer-size particles is a convenient and versatile technique for endocytosis-mediated gene transfer. It is effective with a wide range of cell types and can be used with both plasmid and high molecular weight genomic DNAs, although the efficiency of transgene expression is below that required for most therapeutic applications. Electroporation, the technique used to create whole animal clones by nuclear transfer, generates pores in the cell membrane for DNA entry in the presence of transient, high-voltage pulses that result in stable transfectants. Upon cessation of the pulse, the pores close and entrap the transgene. Many cells do not survive the electric shock, and even under optimal conditions most do not take up the foreign DNA. Particle bombardment with the 'gene gun' requires minimal manipulation of target cells and is able to deliver controlled dosages of DNA that coat the heavy projectile beads. However, expression is transient, with minimal stable integration of foreign DNA in the nuclei of treated cells. Artificial cationic liposomes that contain small plasmid DNAs are able to fuse to cells in tissue culture and deliver DNA into the mammalian host cell. In the past this technique was confined to low molecular weight DNA fragments, and yields of expression in vivo were low, but recent modifications of liposome composition and DNA packaging promise to make liposome-mediated gene transfer the method of choice, particularly in applications for which it is possible to select stable transfectants.

For long-term expression of introduced DNA, viral transfection vectors are most effective, but carry risks.

For long-term expression of large inserts in vivo, viral transfection vectors are preferred. The gene to be expressed is cloned into a site in the viral genome that replaces essential viral sequences and renders the recombinant host virus defective. The recombinant viral genome is then co-transfected into packaging cells in culture, and DNA from a second, defective helper virus carries functional genes that lack the recombinant viral genome. Cells that take up both the recombinant host virus and the helper virus express proteins required for replication of the introduced DNA. The DNA is packaged into infectious particles that are harvested to transfect cell targets for expression of protein from the cloned gene. Retroviral vectors capable of reverse transcriptase-mediated synthesis of cDNA are able to integrate into chromosomal DNA, accommodate large inserts (up to 7 kb), and are highly efficient, easily manipulated, and propagate through daughter cells after mitosis. Chromosomal integration after viral transfection allows the transgene to be perpetuated by replication following cell division, which provides long-term stable expression at the risk of host cell death or undesired modification. Unfortunately, they do not readily transfect nondividing cells, may cause harmful insertional mutagenesis, and may be prone to rescue of the crippled helper virus by contamination with wild type replication-competent viruses. Adenoviral vectors enable gene delivery into differentiated postmitotic cells, with limited risk of wild type contamination. As adenoviral infection is ubiquitous in mammals, pre-existing immunity may account for unstable and depressed levels of expression. Other viral vectors are under investigation. A shared theme is that the qualities of a vector that promote gene transfer are closely entwined with properties that endanger the host.

Transgenic animals

Using transgenic animals, the consequences of discrete nucleotide alterations may be investigated in genetic backgrounds otherwise identical to those of the unmanipulated organism. Hence, a whole animal expression–cloning system is produced by transfection of exogenous DNA into cultured cells capable of differentiation into the cells of the adult animal. If the exogenous gene is found in only a proportion of cells, the animals are partially transgenic. If the foreign DNA is transferred into fertilized oocytes or embryonic stem (ES) cells that contribute to the development of the whole organism, the animals are fully transgenic and will transmit the modified genome to their offspring. Methods used in the assembly of transgenic animals include pronuclear microinjection of DNA into random chromosomal sites of individual oocytes, retroviral transfer into pre- or postimplantation embryos, and injection of modified ES cells into host blastocysts, using coat color as a proxy to identify chimeras (organisms derived from more than a single zygote) that carry mutations for subsequent backcrossing (Fig. 4.14).

Transfer of foreign DNA into fertilized oocytes or embryonic stem cells is used to create transgenic animals.

Gene knockouts

The introduction of a transgene into a preselected endogenous locus is a form of site-directed in vivo mutagenesis termed *gene targeting*. Gene targeting in ES cells leads to the creation of an animal in which all the nucleated cells carry a mutation at the gene of interest. This is usually accomplished by electroporation of a cloned gene that is closely related in sequence to an endogenous gene of an ES cell. Selected from the treated ES cells are those in which recombination between the introduced gene and its corresponding chromosomal homolog (homologous recombination) has occurred. The modified ES cells are injected into the blastocyst of a foster mother to produce an animal in which all of the nucleated cells have been mutated at the site of interest. If the mutagenesis results in the inactivation of gene expression, the mutation is termed a 'knockout' and the effect of the mutation on development and physiology is measured. Often the knockout mutation is lethal, but viable cells can be harvested for further investigation. On occasion little or no change may be detected in the phenotype of the animal, which indicates that other (redundant) genes are able to fulfill the required functions of the inactivated locus.

Targeted degradation of a specific gene's mRNA transcript is perhaps the greatest technical advance in molecular biology since the advent of the polymerase chain reaction. In *RNA interference* (RNAi) either small fragments of RNA are introduced exogenously, or the cell is engineered for their endogenous production by administration of DNA, which will direct the formation of specific RNA oligonucleotides. Outside the nucleus, the short double-stranded 21–23 bp interfering RNAs (siRNAs) bind to their target mRNA transcript, thereby recruiting RNases to the nucleic acid–protein RNA-induced silencing complex (RISC). siRNA duplexes are unwound by helicases in the RISC, and the resulting single-stranded RNA guides target identification. When single-stranded RNA base-pairs with its target mRNA, the RISC RNase degrades the target mRNA, synthesis of the protein encoded by the targeted mRNA is blocked, and the cell's phenotype is specifically altered (Fig. 4.15). Selective gene silencing mediated by RNAi has rapidly become a powerful tool in defining gene function, and RNAi-based drugs are currently entering trials in experimental models.

RNA interference targets degradation of a specific mRNA.

Gene therapy

In the broadest sense, gene therapy is the genetic modification of a patient's cells to enable the treatment of disease. This definition embraces many potential avenues for intervention, including the transfer of whole or partial genes from identical or foreign genomes, synthetic genes, and antisense oligonucleotides to eliminate damaged cells or protect normal tissues from destruction. Originally envisaged as a method to correct human diseases that arise from single-gene defects, gene therapy currently encompasses a much broader range of applications in acquired disorders, infectious diseases, oncology, degenerative diseases, and symptom management. Owing to profound ethical, legal, and social considerations, for the foreseeable future human gene therapy will be restricted to addressing disorders of somatic rather than germline cells.

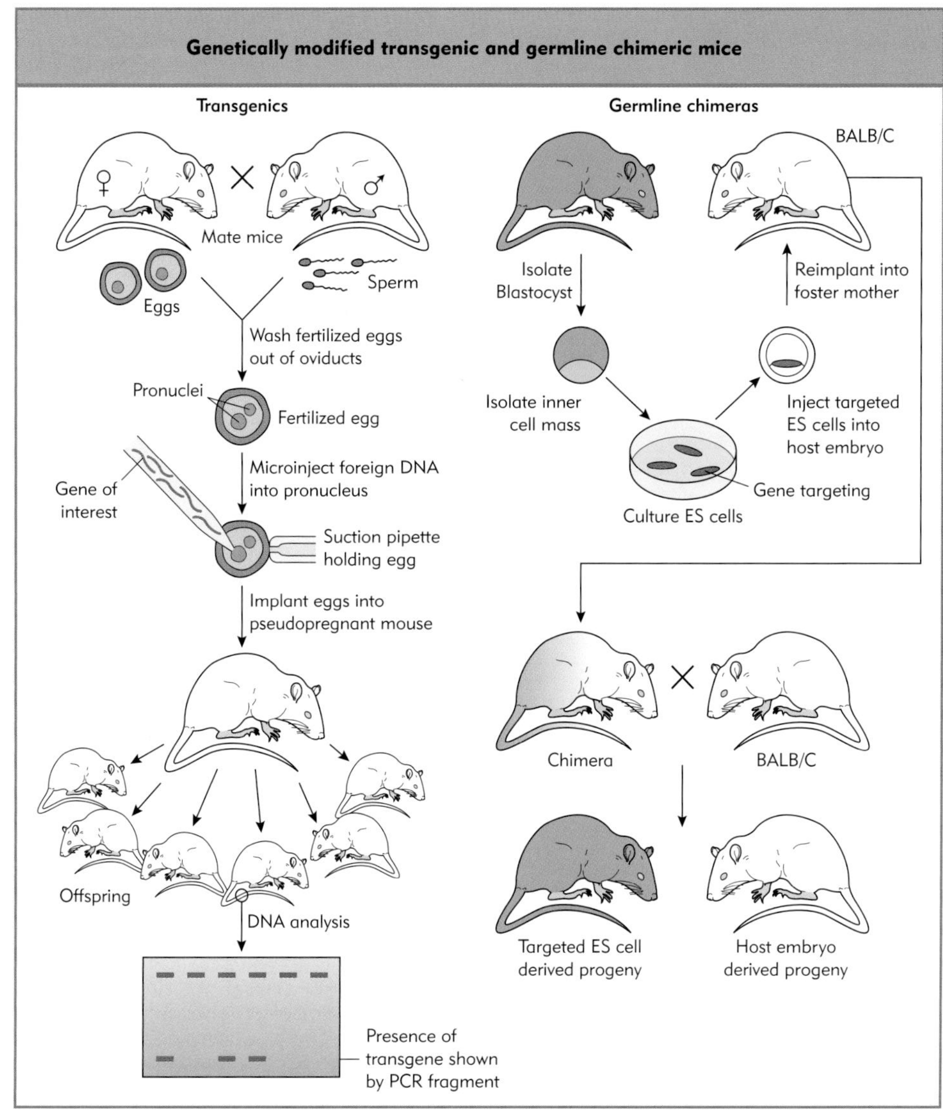

Figure 4.14 Genetically modified transgenic and germline chimeric animals. To create transgenic animals, fertilized eggs are transferred to pseudopregnant foster mothers after microinjection of the gene of interest into one of the pronuclei. Southern blotting of DNA from tail cells is used to screen the offspring for the presence of the transgene. To generate germline chimeras, ES cells isolated from the blastocyst are gene targeted for a mutation by homologous recombination in culture, injected into blastocysts from a different strain, and reimplanted into a pseudopregnant foster mother. Chimeric animals are bred to identify germline chimeras in which a proportion of the progeny arise from ES-derived gametes using coat color as a marker. Backcrossing and interbreeding of chimeras produces animals that are heterozygous or homozygous for the genetic modification. (BALB/C is a host mouse strain.)

Strategies that involve the modification of somatic cells can be classified into in vivo ‘direct’ and ex vivo ‘indirect’ gene therapies (Fig. 4.16). In vivo methods, with transgene vectors directly introduced into the tissue space of a living organism, are limited by poor specificity and stability of gene transfer because of the inability to select and amplify transformed cells, which increases the need for repeated treatments that may engender immunogenicity. Ex vivo methods are based on grafting target cells that are transfected, selected, and expanded in vitro to deliver a required gene product fabricated in the host cell. Selectivity and specificity are expedited by the physical removal and isolation of autogenic or allogenic target cells. To serve as ex vivo platforms for expression of transgenes, the host cells must be harvested, purified, and banked easily and safely. They must be tolerant to genetic manipulation by various means, survive transplantation without immunosuppression, and express the transgene for an appropriate interval with minimal oncogenic, infectious, and immunogenic potential.

Well-characterized genes, and methods to transfer genes into appropriate target cells considered in earlier sections of this chapter, are prerequisites for gene therapy. Identification of conditions with well-defined phenotypes and clear-cut therapeutic end points to monitor efficacy is an additional significant barrier. For the ideal clinical target, the biochemical pathophysiology must be understood, a suitable animal model must be available or created using transgenic technologies, the human and appropriate model animal genes must have been cloned (e.g. genes that encode ligands, receptors, and metabolic enzymes), outcomes must be quantifiable and controlled (i.e. using identical vectors with nontherapeutic reporter genes replacing the gene of interest), and the shortcomings of competing approaches must be balanced by the magnitude of the clinical problem. Many of the conditions faced by anesthesiologists (e.g. cancer pain syndromes) meet these criteria, and knowledge of the fundamental pathophysiology of other disorders (e.g. complex regional pain syndromes) must be expanded before gene therapy will serve a management role.

Methods to regulate the bioactivity of the gene product offer the prospect of temporal specificity to complement the topographic specificity realized by confining cell targets to discrete populations. These methods include control of transcription with the administration of second drugs coupled to promoters

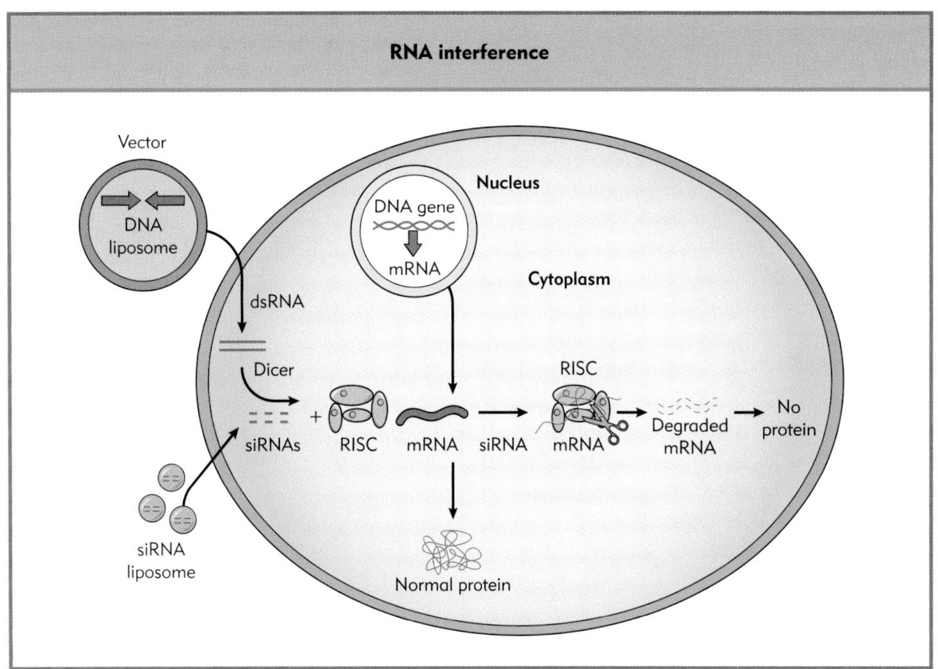

Figure 4.15 RNA interference. Taking advantage of cellular processes aimed at the destruction of viral invaders, mRNA transcripts are cleaved by RNase enzymes that recognize the RNA-induced silencing complex (RISC) formed by the binding of short interfering 21–23 bp RNA oligonucleotides (siRNAs) to their mRNA targets. siRNAs may be packaged for external application to the cell, or they may be internally produced by the cell after transfection with double-stranded DNA with the desired sequence composition, and then processing by an enzyme (Dicer) to the effective length.

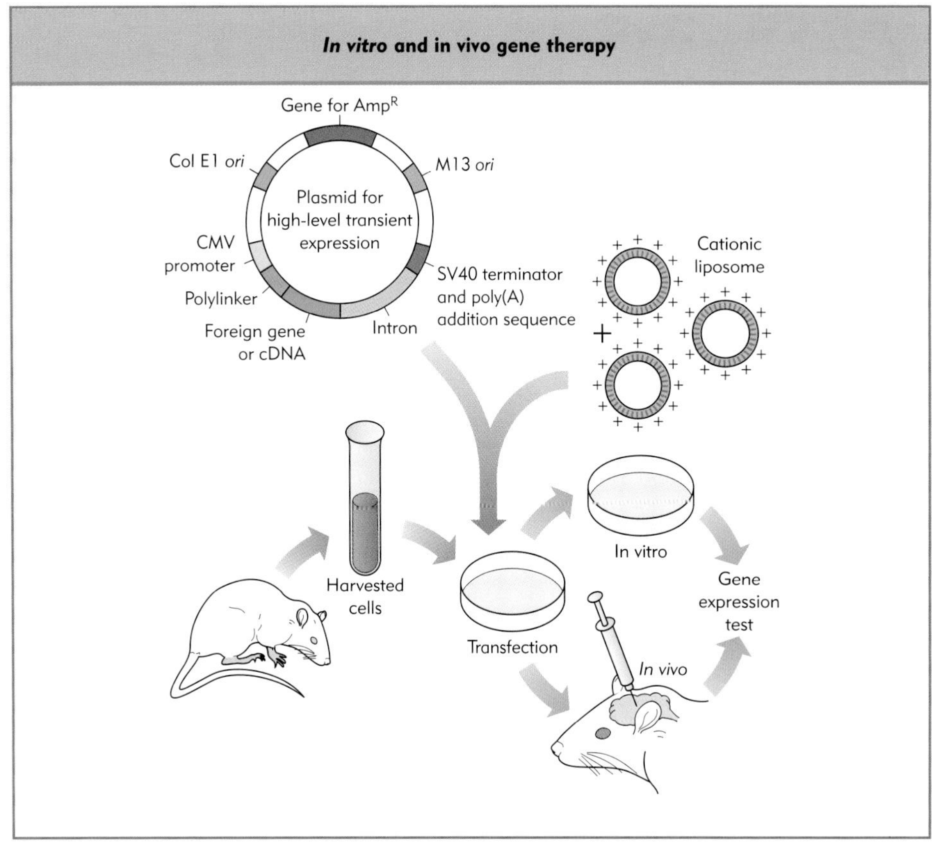

Figure 4.16 Gene therapy. Mammalian expression vectors contain prokaryotic regions required for replication (ori) and antibiotic resistance (AmpR), together with promoter (CMV), polyadenylation, and intervening intron sequences to improve mRNA stability and transport. Ex vivo gene therapy entails modification of harvested primary cells by transfection, in this example with a plasmid DNA–cationic lipid complex, and reimplantation into the organism. Expression of the transgene is monitored in vitro and in situ. In vivo gene therapy refers to direct injection of viral or nonviral vectors into targeted host cells. (Adapted from Morgan E. The aquatic ape hypothesis. London: Souvenir Press; 1982.)

(tetracycline, antiprogestins), or channeling gene products through alternative pathways of RNA splicing, post-translational modification, or pharmacokinetic transport and elimination. In this fashion, alterations engineered at the most fundamental molecular level of the cell may be placed directly under the will of the patient (i.e. patient-controlled gene therapy), while limiting toxicity and tolerance and maintaining bioactivity in reserve as needs dictate.

Antisense oligonucleotides derived from RNA sequences modulate endogenous nucleic acids through complementary hybridization. Specific binding of an oligomeric antisense compound to its target may selectively impair such vital functions as replication, transcription, translocation, translation, splicing, and catalytic RNA activity. The overall effect is altered expression of the targeted gene. Antisense oligonucleotides are widely used as research reagents to elucidate the function of particular genes, or to distinguish between functions of various components of a biological pathway. Clinical applications of therapeutic antisense oligonucleotides are being developed in a number of areas.

Key references

Sambrook J, Russel DW. Molecular cloning: a laboratory manual, 3rd edn. Cold Spring Harbor: Cold Spring Harbor Laboratory Press; 2001.

Vogel F, Motulsky AG. Human genetics: problems and approaches, 3rd edn. Heidelberg: Springer Verlag; 1997.

Watson JD, Gilman M, Witkowski J, Zoller M. Recombinant DNA, 2nd edn. New York: WH Freeman and Co; 1992.

Further reading

Carlson EA. Defining the gene: an evolving concept. Am J Hum Genet. 1991;49:475–87.

Frankel WN, Schork NJ. Who's afraid of epistasis? Nature Genet. 1996;14:371–3.

Hogan K. To fire the train: the second malignant hyperthermia gene. Am J Hum Genet. 1997;60:1303–8.

Joyner AL (ed.). Gene targeting: a practical approach, 2nd edn. Oxford: IRL Press; 2000.

McPherson MJ, Hames BD, Taylor GR. PCR2: a practical approach. Oxford: IRL Press; 1995.

Milhavet O, Gary DS, Mattson MP. RNA interference in biology and medicine. Pharmacol Rev. 2003;55:629–48.

Phillips M1 (ed.). Gene therapy methods. Methods in Enzymology v. 346: 2002.

Phimster B (ed) The chipping forecast. Nature Genet. (Suppl). 1999;21:1–60.

Singer M, Berg P. Genes and genomes. Mill Way: University Science Books; 1991.

Ventner JC et al. The sequence of the human genome. 2001;291:1304–51.

Wolf U. The genetic contribution to the phenotype. Hum Genet. 1995;95:127–48.

Chapter 5 Genomics and proteomics

Marek Brzezinski, Gregory A Michelotti and Debra A Schwinn

TOPICS COVERED IN THIS CHAPTER

- **DNA variability**
  - Genetics – historic background
- **Molecular biology tools**
  - Tools used to incorporate genetic analysis into clinical studies
- **Perioperative risk and outcome**
- **Genomics and proteomics**
  - Microarray analysis
  - Proteomics
  - The 'omic' revolution

Innovations in molecular genetics have changed the face of medicine. In 2003 the Human Genome Project produced the first sequence of the 2.9-gigabase (Gb) human genome. This achievement coincided with the 50th anniversary of the determination of double-helical structure of DNA. The human genome contains approximately 30 000 protein-encoding genes, consistent with other mammalian genomes. In fact, about 85% of human and rodent genes are identical in their coding sequences, and more than 99% of human DNA is identical between individuals. However, variations in the exact DNA sequence do exist between individuals, making each person unique. This genetic variability may have important implications in physiology and medicine.

Although the human genome only contains about 30 000 genes, variation at the protein level is far more extensive, creating possibly more than 1000 000 modified human proteins. Such diversity at the protein level results from extensive post-transcriptional, translational, and post-translational modifications. Whereas genetic variability at the DNA level can be examined using DNA sequencing techniques, analysis of large-scale variability at the RNA and protein levels can be accomplished via microarray and proteomics approaches. This chapter provides basic information on approaches for the analysis of DNA sequence variation, and for high-throughput analysis of RNA and protein alterations resulting from diseases or clinical interventions. This information should facilitate the incorporation of new genetic/genomic tools into clinical research and practice.

DNA VARIABILITY

Genetics – historic background

Today, the Czech monk Mendel is widely considered to be the founding father of modern genetics. His landmark article 'Experiments in plant hybridization', published in 1865, proposed the principles of heredity and introduced the concept of recessive and dominant genes. The term 'genetics' was first coined at the beginning of the 1900s by a British zoologist, William Bateson. In 1902, Garrod described the inheritance of a biochemical disorder in his article 'The incidence of alkaptonuria: a study in chemical individuality'. His book, *Inborn Errors of Metabolism*, written under the influence of Mendel's work, marked the beginning of 20th century biochemical genetics. It was not until 1944, however, that Avery and co-workers demonstrated that DNA was the hereditary material in the living cell. In 1953, Watson and Crick revealed the double-helix structure of the DNA molecule, and in 1966 Crick introduced the concept – now the central dogma of genetics – that every cellular protein is encoded in RNA which is derived from the DNA sequence (Fig. 5.1). Recent milestones include the discovery of recombinant DNA in the mid-1970s, cloning of DNA fragments, development of the polymerase chain reaction, and the development of automated sequencing machines. These remarkable advances led in the mid-1980s to the idea to sequence the human genome. In 1990, supported by a broad international consortium, the Human Genome Project was initiated.

The genome is the active genetic complement of an organism.

The term genome, publicized with the Human Genome Project, derives from the combination of words '*gene*' and 'chromos*ome*,' and is defined as the entire genetic complement of an organism. The term was coined by Winkler in 1920 to describe the haploid set of chromosomes within all genes. Chromosome 22 was the first human chromosome to be completely sequenced by the Human Genome Project, in 1999. Chromosome 21 followed in 2000 and chromosome 20 in 2001. Finally, the first draft of the human genome was published in

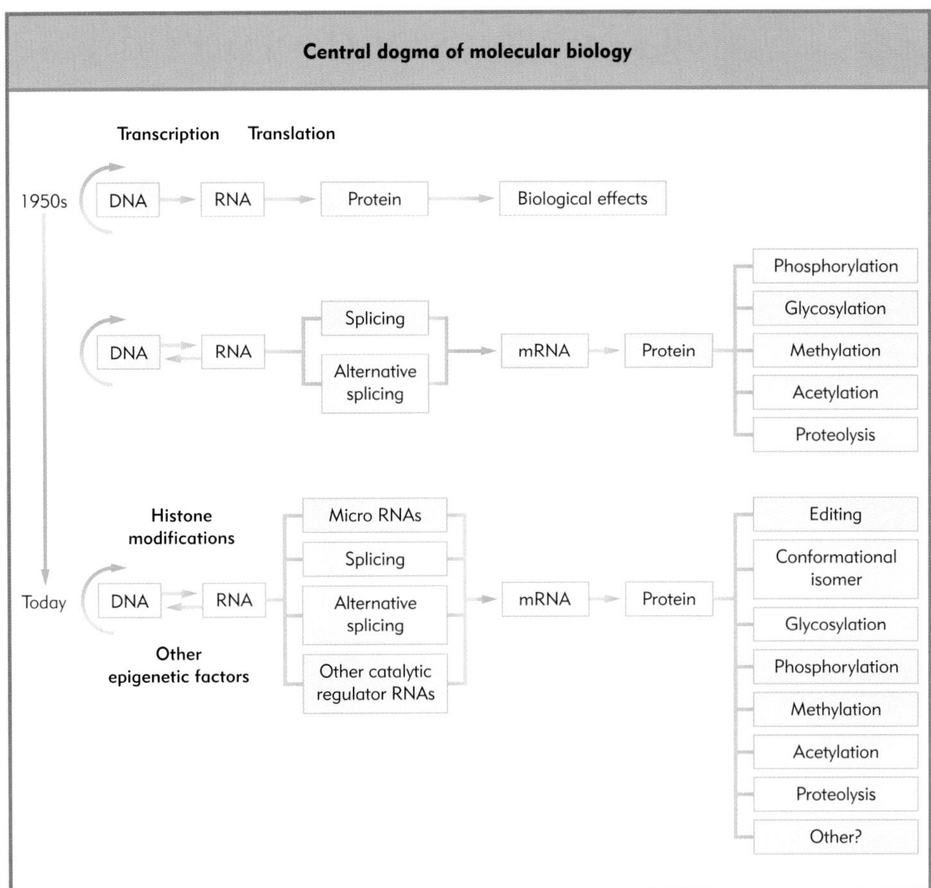

Figure 5.1 Central dogma of molecular biology. Unidirectional gene expression, proposed in the 1950s, has evolved into a more complex model with multiple factors affecting gene expression at the transcriptional, translational and post-translational levels. A single gene can give rise to multiple gene products via alternative splicing and/or editing RNA to mature mRNA, resulting in multiple isoforms, as well as post-translational modifications (see text for description). By influencing protein enzymatic activity, changing half-life, biological stability etc., protein regulation mechanisms have a direct impact on ultimate biological activity.

2001. To fully appreciate the extent of this Herculean task, one must realize that the human genome consists of approximately 3 billion bases. In April 2003 the 'finished' sequence of the human genome was announced.

MOLECULAR BIOLOGY TOOLS

The basic concepts of molecular biology, such as DNA, RNA, proteins, genetic code, and gene structure, are discussed in detail in Chapter 4. A *gene* is considered a coding unit of heredity composed of a specific DNA sequence located at a locus (or site) within a chromosome. Each gene encodes a specific protein(s). The most common DNA sequence for a particular gene is referred to as the *wildtype allele*, and any rarer, less expressed DNA sequence variants are termed *variant alleles*.

Single nucleotide polymorphisms (SNP) are variations in single bases of DNA between organisms, and provide useful genetic markers for clinical phenotypes.

An *allele* is defined as any alternative form of a gene occupying the same chromosomal position as that gene. Such allelic variation may occur secondary to insertion, deletion, translocation, or inversion of a DNA fragment. A variation in the DNA sequence that has an allele frequency of ≥1% is defined as a *polymorphism*. DNA sequence variants with allele frequency of <1% are sometimes defined as *mutations*. DNA polymorphism is quite common; DNA variants occur every few hundred base pairs. The most common allelic variation is the *single-nucleotide polymorphism* (SNP). SNPs can be defined as a variation in single nucleotide bases of DNA between individuals:

...ATGCGATCGATTCTGAATCCCCGA... Individual A
...ATGCGATCGATGCTGAATCCCCGA... Individual B

Genome-wide maps describe the most common SNPs. One of the most commonly used databases is dbSNP, an international database available via the National Institutes of Health (USA) websites (www.ncbi.nlm.nih.gov/SNP).

Two types of SNP exist with regard to clinical effects. The first type leads to changes in a *phenotype* that can be clinically appreciated (e.g. changes in clinical endpoints such as blood pressure, bleeding, or enzyme function). A second type (the majority) are clinically silent; such polymorphisms are called *background SNPs*. Both types of SNP are useful markers for genetic studies of disease association.

A *haplotype* is defined as an arrangement of alleles (i.e. genetic polymorphisms) of closely linked loci within a single chromosome that tend to be inherited together. The ability to categorize human chromosomes by sections, i.e. *haplotypes*, is convenient. Because genetic variability is most often the result of chromosomal crossovers over generations, regions of each chromosome segregate together. The use of haplotypes in clinical medicine can therefore eliminate the need to identify the actual genetic mutation involved/associated with a disease. Clinical outcomes can be predictable simply from the presence of a known genetic marker, as this can predict the presence/absence of a disease-altering genetic variant nearby on the chromosome.

Tools used to incorporate genetic analysis into clinical studies

Genetic linkage studies take advantage of the fact that the genes of a given chromosome tend to be inherited together, by a similar concept to that described for haplotypes. The closer different genes are located to each other on the chromosome, the higher the chance for those 'linked genes' to be inherited together. Genetic linkage studies follow genes using specific genetic variants known as 'markers' that are distributed across all chromosomes. These have been used to identify specific chromosome regions present in specific populations with a given disease.

Linkage disequilibrium studies are based on the assumption that there is a difference between observed and predicted frequencies of haplotypes in a population, i.e. that there is a *linkage disequilibrium* (LD) between alleles (i.e. SNPs). The extent of LD depends on factors such as mutations, natural selection, genetic drift, and population admixture. The degree of LD varies highly from one genomic region to the next, sometimes described as deserts and islands of genetic variability.

Genetic variation influences perioperative outcome and complications.

Genetic association studies are designed to assess whether a genetic variant is 'associated with' a disease. A population is tested to determine whether a particular genetic variant is enriched in individuals with disease characteristics. Association studies have been particularly successful in identifying genes involved in polygenic disorders (diseases where more than one gene is involved). Conducted in a population-based sample of affected and appropriately matched unrelated controls, association studies have greater statistical power to uncover the small clinical effect of multiple genes.

Candidate-gene studies have been developed to enhance the efficiency of genetic studies. In contrast to a generalized approach, using markers spread across the genome without consideration of their function or their distribution in a specific gene, candidate-gene studies concentrate on genes selected according to our current knowledge of disease mechanisms.

PERIOPERATIVE RISK AND OUTCOME

Some genetic variability in humans can be considered 'background,' leading to distinctive personal traits (for example eye color), but with no clinical consequences. Other genetic variants can have important clinical ramifications. Although the majority of classic single-gene diseases are rare, DNA variation can have more subtle effects in complex diseases where multiple genes interact to produce a final outcome, or phenotype. In such situations (e.g. diabetes, hypertension, atherosclerosis), genetic variability can contribute to disease onset, severity, progression, etc. An increasing body of evidence supports the influence of genetic variation on perioperative outcome and complications. Some of these variants important to anesthesiologists are described below.

Several genes predictive of perioperative vascular response have been identified. For instance, a significantly increased vascular sensitivity to α-adrenergic receptor stimulation (phenylephrine) was found in patients with the endothelial nitric oxide synthase G894T gene polymorphism and patients homozygous for the deletion genotype of the angiotensin-converting enzyme insertion/deletion polymorphism of intron 16 (DCP1). Variability in the β_2-adrenoreceptor gene has been associated with increased mean arterial blood pressure response to the stress stimulus of tracheal intubation (Fig. 5.2).

Several genes predictive of a postoperative hypercoagulable state associated with thrombosis have been identified. The factor V Leiden genotype, resulting from a point mutation in factor V (A1691G), is the most common genetic polymorphism associated with primary venous thrombosis. Factor V Leiden has also been linked to an elevated incidence of postoperative venous thromboembolism, stroke, and coronary artery bypass graft (CABG) thrombosis.

Increased attention has been paid to identifying genotypes associated with an increased risk of acute or delayed restenosis after revascularization surgery. The human platelet antigen-1b (HPA-1b or PI A2) polymorphism has been linked to post-CABG thrombotic occlusion, myocardial infarction, and death. Homozygosity for the G allele of myocardial chymase (CMA-1905) has been identified as an independent risk factor for accelerated post-CABG atherosclerosis.

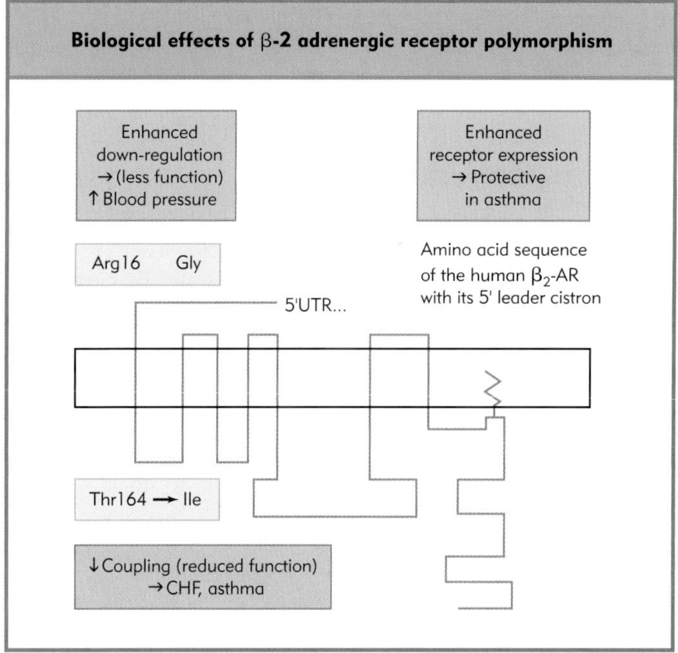

Figure 5.2 Association of genetic polymorphisms with perioperative outcomes. β_2-Adrenergic receptor (AR) genetic polymorphisms are clinically relevant in diseases such as hypertension, asthma, and congestive heart failure. In the β_2AR gene, genetic alterations in the upstream leader sequence (an introductory regulatory sequence occurring immediately upstream from where the protein coding sequence begins) result in enhanced β_2AR expression. Resultant increased airway β_2ARs protect against methylcholine-induced bronchoconstriction. An association exists between the Gly16 polymorphic form of the β_2AR and vascular hyporesponsiveness to agonist in normotensive individuals, resulting in elevated systemic blood pressure compared to individuals with the Arg16 receptor. Finally, the β_2AR variant Ile164 appears to accelerate the clinical course of patients with congestive heart failure (CHF).

The severity and intensity of the postoperative inflammatory reaction (i.e. the modulation of the surgery-induced immune response) may depend on genotype. For example, the IL-6 gene promoter G-572G>C and G-174G>C polymorphisms significantly increase the IL-6 response to the inflammatory stimulus after heart surgery with cardiopulmonary bypass (CPB). The apolipoprotein (APO) ε-4 polymorphism and TNF-α gene polymorphisms may exert a proinflammatory effect in patients undergoing CPB. Interestingly, the TNF-α gene polymorphism influences plasma TNF-α concentration and outcome in patients with severe sepsis. Finally, evidence suggests that genotype influences two important causes of postoperative morbidity: postoperative neurocognitive and renal outcomes.

Gene association studies are not without limitations. Most populations originate from multiple ethnic and racial groups, bringing unique and varied genetic backgrounds. This introduces genetic '*wobble*', which can only be overcome by either properly powering a study for a primary main endpoint, or by carefully screening the population to be as homogeneous as possible. Furthermore, genetic association studies are only as good as the clinical phenotyping used; therefore each clinical endpoint examined should be both quantifiable and reproducible.

GENOMICS AND PROTEOMICS

Following the Human Genome Project, a need for systematic high-throughput method to assign function to genes ushered in modern *genomics*. Today, *genomics* encompasses the comprehensive study of whole sets of genes, gene products, and their interactions – as opposed to studies of single genes or proteins. The genomics approach is anchored in the 'central dogma' of molecular biology: DNA→RNA→Protein (Fig. 5.1).

Microarray analysis

Because only active genes are transcribed, levels of different mRNA sequences in a tissue reflect the functional activity of the entire genome for a particular physiological state. By comparing one clinical state to another (e.g. disease versus no disease), *functional information* about genes and their *control mechanisms* can be uncovered by examining many genes and proteins; such studies are known as 'expression profiling'.

Microarray analysis has emerged as a key method of studying genomics at the RNA level. This approach offers simultaneous analysis of thousands of gene products in a single process (Fig. 5.3). Some call microarray analysis '*the essence of genomics*'. This method embeds thousands of small fragments of complementary DNA (cDNA; Chapter 4), called probes, in a predetermined order on to a solid matrix (e.g. nylon membrane, silicon, or glass). Each of the probes represents a microarray spot. Thousands of such spots fit on to a single matrix. The term 'chip' is often used to describe the solid matrix with these thousands of probes. The selection of exact DNA probes varies widely between chips and depends on the experimental or diagnostic objective. Although genomic DNA with complete introns and exons is particularly useful to study SNPs, only genes that are actively expressed (represented by complementary DNA clones or expressed sequence tags (ESTs)) can be used to analyze gene expression patterns. There are predominantly two competing platforms. One utilizes very high-density glass slides that contain hundreds of thousands of oligonucleotide sequences on a glass chip about 1.5 cm^2 in size. In this platform, each transcript is represented as a probe set, made up of probe pairs comprised of perfect match (PM) and mismatch (MM) probe cells. This probe pairing strategy identifies and minimizes the effects of nonspecific hybridization and background signal. The intensities of each probe pair are used to determine expression levels for each gene and facilitate chip-to-chip comparisons between independent experiments. An example of this platform is the Affymetrix GeneChip®, named after the company that pioneered large-scale microarray production using photolithographic DNA synthesis technology. The second platform utilizes distinct DNA fragments (typically 70-mers, but can also be cDNA fragments) attached as an array of distinct spots on a suitably treated glass slide via a mechanical robotic spotting process. Two distinct samples, typically the reference and the test sample, are given fluorescent red and green labels, respectively, and are combined in solution and applied to the array. The relative amounts of red and green fluorescence at each spot provides a measurement of relative numbers of red- and green-labeled fragments attached at the spot, and thus of the relative numbers of fragments in the reference and test samples. The most commonly used labels are the Cy5 (red) and Cy3 (green) fluorescent dyes. Because they lack internal standards, such studies typically require a larger number of independent confirmations; however, they can be made in a single investigator's laboratory and are much less expensive than competing platforms, making them popular.

Microarray analysis allows simultaneous determinations of the expression of thousands of genes, for use in the molecular characterization and diagnosis of disease states.

Possible applications for DNA microarrays include studying the physiologic consequences of genetic variants, gene identification, and/or screening for mutations and polymorphisms. Genomic profiling already facilitates early disease identification, thereby also potentially facilitating early intervention. Moreover, genomic studies should improve our knowledge of the molecular characterization of disease, help refine diagnostic tests, and ultimately identify novel targets for therapeutic intervention.

Proteomics

Information provided by microarray gene expression analysis regarding levels of mRNA may not accurately reflect expression at a protein level in all cases (Fig. 5.4). Futhermore, post-transcriptional control mechanisms enable transcribed RNA to be spliced in multiple ways to yield different protein forms. Further changes can be introduced following translation from RNA to proteins, such as glycosylation, phosphorylation, lipid attachments, and/or proteolytic processing. In fact, more than 200 known post-translational modifications may produce a variety of protein products from the same single gene, such that the number of human proteins may be between 100 000 and 1000 000, or roughly between four and 50 proteins for every gene. This has led to the emergence of a new field to study protein modifications at the molecular level, called *proteomics*.

Proteomics involves characterizing the total set of proteins in a given cell at a given time. Such studies examine the *dynamic protein products* of the genome – which, it can be argued, are the

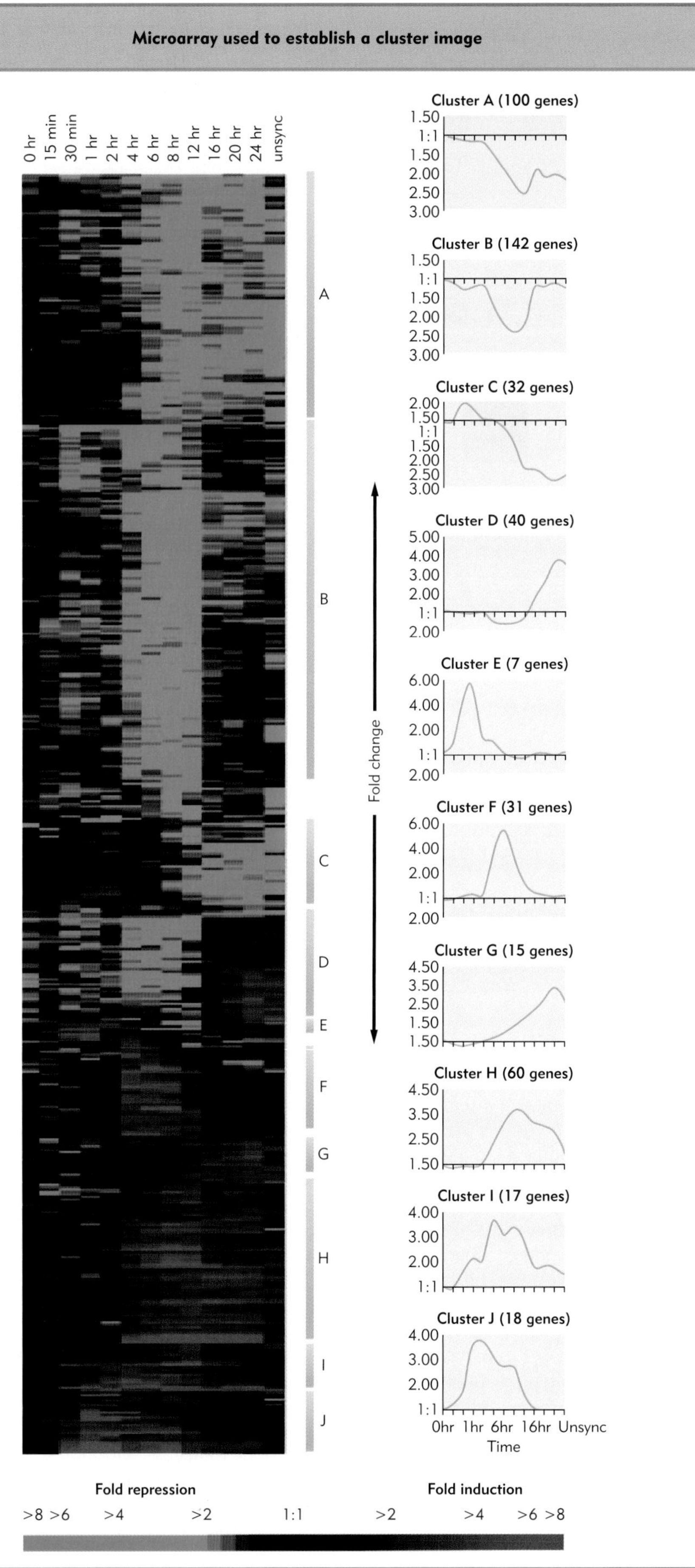

Figure 5.3 Microarray analysis of mRNA expression profiles. Example of microarray use to establish a cluster image of different classes of gene expression profiles. RNA was isolated from human fibroblast cells following a time course of serum stimulation and differentially expressed genes were identified by microarray analysis. There were 517 genes grouped into categories on the basis of their most likely role (indicated by A–J). The expression pattern of each gene is displayed as a horizontal strip. The color scale at the bottom represents the ratio of mRNA levels, i.e. gene activity, at the indicated time after serum stimulation to its level in the serum-deprived (time zero) fibroblasts. The graphs show the average expression profiles for the genes in the corresponding 'cluster'. 'Unsync' denotes exponentially growing cells. Reproduced with permission from: Iyer VR et al. The transcriptional program in the response of human fibroblasts to serum. (Science 1999;283:83–7.)

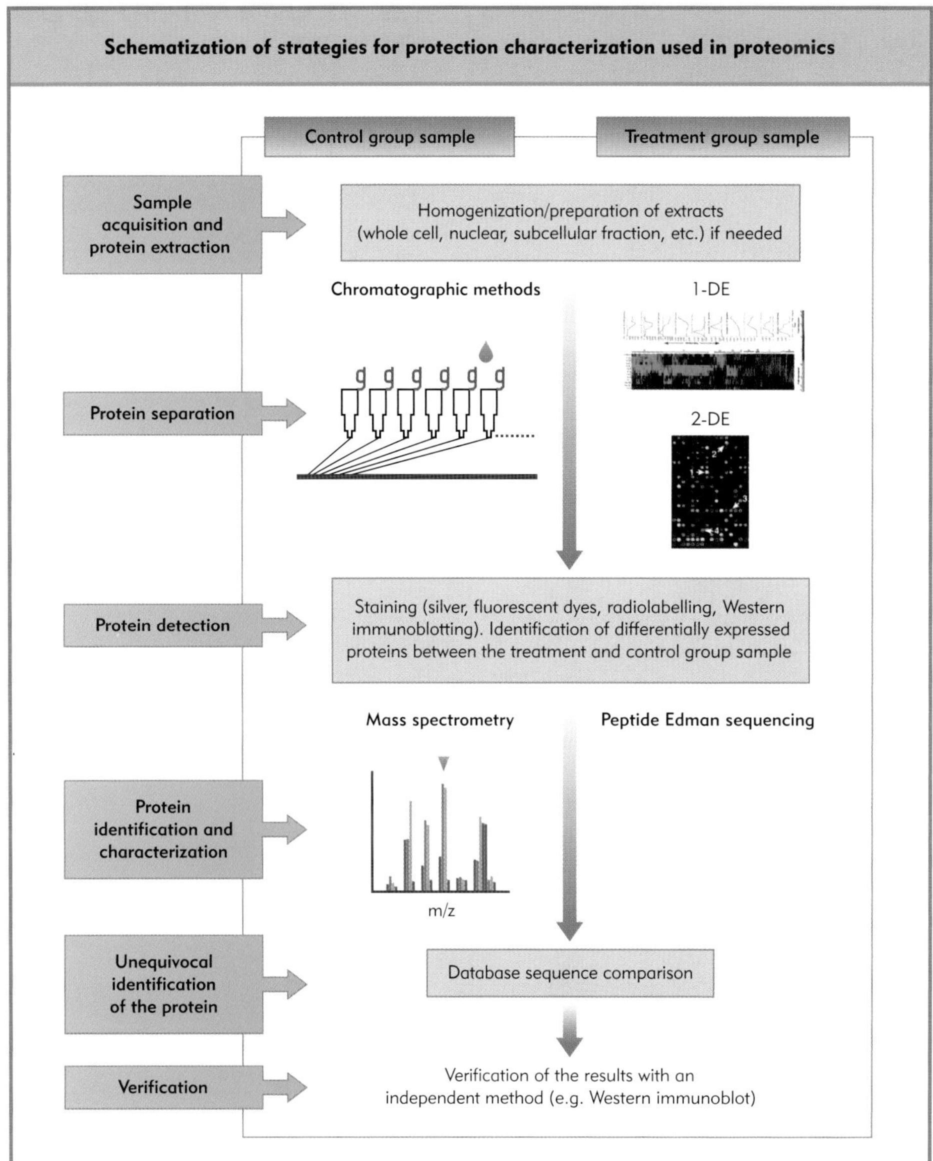

Figure 5.4 Schematization of strategies for protein characterization used in proteomics. Proteomics is an expanding field, with new techniques and methods rapidly developing. Currently there are six basic steps in proteomic analysis: sample acquisition and protein extraction, separation, detection, identification and characterization, final identification and verification. 1-DE, 1-dimensional electrophoresis; 2-DE, 2-dimensional electrophoresis. (Modified with permission from Graves PR, Haystead TA. Molecular biologist's guide to proteomics. Microbiol Mol Biol Rev. 2002;66:39–63.)

most biologically important molecules in a cell – rather than focusing on '*static*' DNA. By studying all proteins expressed in a cell simultaneously, together with their interactions, proteomics offers a more global and integrated view of biology. The aim is to identify proteins that undergo changes in abundance, modification, or localization in response to a particular disease state, treatment, trauma, stress, etc. In this way proteomics complements other functional genomic techniques. In combination with other genome-wide approaches, proteomics enhances the identification of complex genotypes predictive of disease and/or drug responses (Fig. 5.5).

Proteomics is the large-scale study of gene expression at the protein level, which provides insight into the activity level of all proteins.

The most straightforward proteomic approach first separates and isolates proteins using chromatography, single-dimension (1-DE) gel electrophoresis, or two-dimensional (2-DE) gel electrophoresis (Fig. 5.4). In the second step, silver stain or other dyes are used to detect the protein spots. Information for the identification and characterization of proteins is obtained through mass spectrometry or Edman peptide sequencing. In the last step, identified protein sequences are analyzed by comparison with existing databases of amino acid and nucleotide sequences in order to determine the identity of a protein spot.

Recently protein arrays and antibody chips have been developed to improve, simplify, and expedite the analysis of the proteome. In this context, single-stranded oligonucleotides (either DNA or RNA) called aptamers have been used; these molecules can fold into an almost endless array of structures, which then interact directly with proteins. Using a technique called SELEX (systematic evolution of ligands by exponential enrichment), nuclease-resistant DNA or RNA aptamers are selected by their ability to bind protein targets with high affinity and specificity in the same range as antibodies. This process has been used to successfully create aptamers to a variety of targets, including receptors, growth factors, and adhesion molecules implicated in the genesis of some kinds of cancer. The

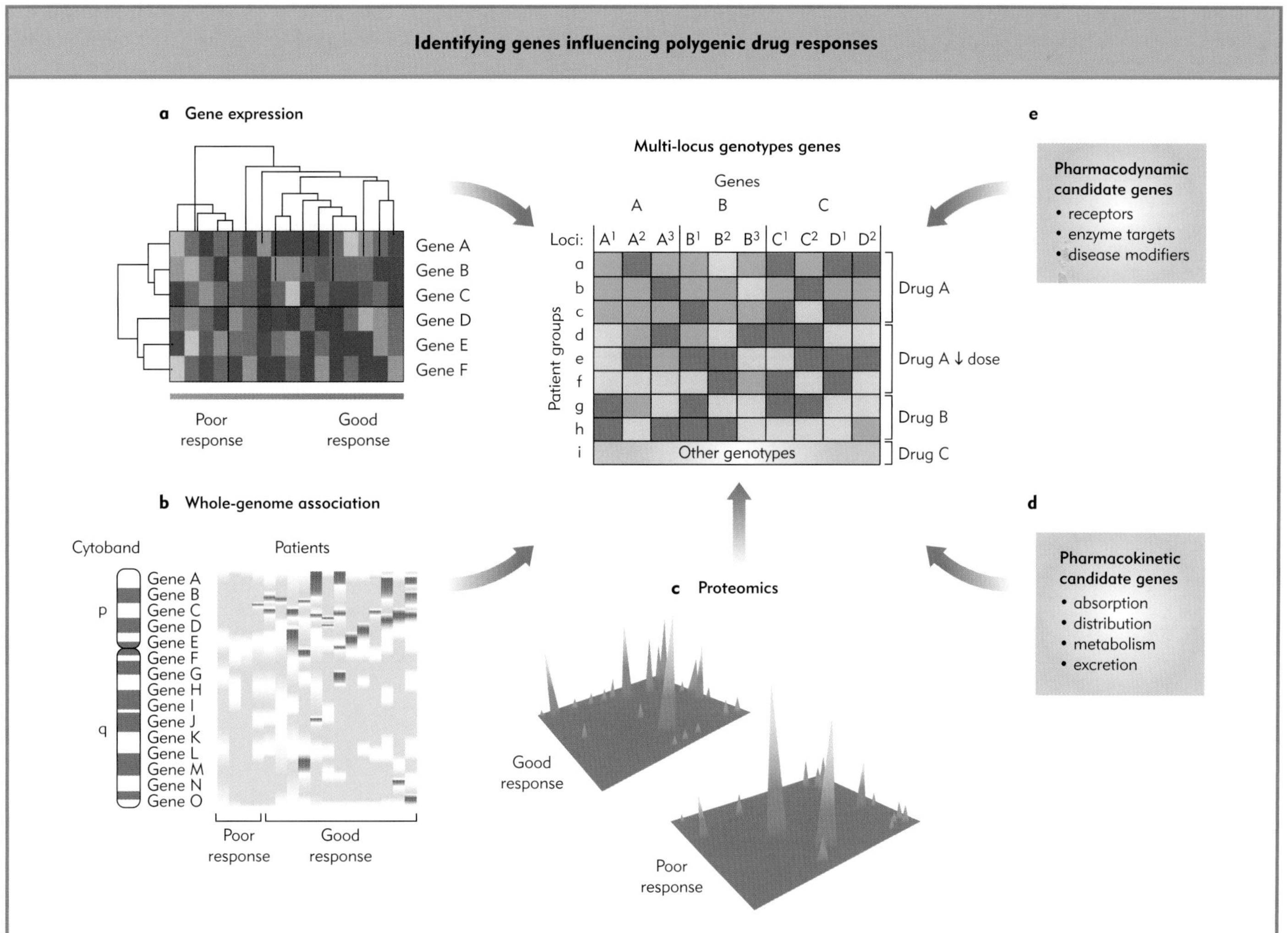

Figure 5.5 Identifying genes influencing polygenic drug responses. Three genome-wide approaches, gene-expression analysis, genome-wide scans, and proteomics, can be used to identify potential candidate genes that influence a specific drug response (e.g. the promotion of antileukemic effects). (a) DNA microarray analysis of cancer cells for six genes (rows) in 16 patients (columns), four with a poor response and 12 with a good response. (b) SNP haplotype map showing 16 gene loci on one chromosome for four patients with a poor response and 13 with a good response. (c) LC-MS (liquid chromatography/mass spectrometry) analysis of plasma or tumor tissue to identify differences in proteins (see yellow peaks) between good and poor responders. (d, e) The conventional 'candidate gene' approach, based on clinical pharmacology studies of proteins (e.g. receptors) and pathways known to be involved in a drug's pharmacokinetic or pharmacodynamic response. The middle panel represents a subset of the final product, a panel of multiple genes and loci that collectively segregate patients into groups that respond best to one of several drugs or doses. (Modified with permission from Evans WE, Relling MV. Moving towards individualized medicine with pharmacogenomics. Nature 2004; 29: 464–8).

automation of the SELEX process could lead to generalized use of this technology for specific protein identification over standard antibody approaches, and increase the feasibility of creating protein chips.

The possibilities of proteomics go far beyond the simple 'uncovering' of the proteome of a particular cell. Proteomics opens the door to study all protein isoforms, protein modifications, protein interactions and functions, and to create a complete three-dimensional map of a cell, indicating where specific proteins are located. Proteomics can help with the identification of functionally crucial post-translational modifications in response to a variety of intracellular and extracellular signals.

The integration of proteomic data together with information gained by genomic approaches should create powerful tools to comprehensively describe and modify cellular interaction mechanisms. In parallel, gene expression profiles help identify cellular pathways and mechanisms leading to changes in the expression of particular proteins. Even without knowing the mechanisms involved, identification of differentially expressed proteins in specific diseases offers a way to identify novel medical targets, and so revolutionizes drug development.

The 'omic' revolution

Recently we have witnessed the emergence of a variety of 'omic' disciplines. The suffix 'omic' describes the ability to analyze components of a living cell in its entirety. In addition to *proteomics*, there are *phenomics*, which studies the complete set of mutational phenotypes; *epigenomics*, which looks at the complete set of methylation and acetylation alterations in the genome; *ligandomics*, which examines the complete set of organic small molecules; and *metabolomics*, which describes small metabolic products present in a cell, to mention just a few. Integrated 'omic' databases might in future provide the key to a final understanding of all products, processes, and interactions in the human cell, from genome to genome product and ultimately to function, specifically identifying changes present with specific diseases.

CONCLUSIONS

Concepts of genetic variability and new genomic approaches have revolutionized medicine. In the future, rather than simply tabulating patient risk factors (e.g. age, race, sex), a detailed genetic history may be taken into account. In the near future, a preoperative 'gene chip' designed to highlight the most notable genetic variants important in bleeding, inflammatory, and neurologic responses to perioperative stress may be developed. Mechanistically, information gleaned by genomic approaches will unveil both new disease mechanisms and targets for therapies and interventions. At that point we will have far more detailed information for use in designing the most appropriate and safest anesthetic plan for a given patient.

Key references

Avery O, MacLeod C, McCarty M. Studies on the chemical nature of the substance inducing transformation of pneumococcal type. J Exp Med. 1944;79:137–58.

Evans GA. Designer science and the 'omic' revolution. Nature Biotechnol. 2000;18:127.

Lander ES et al. Initial sequencing and analysis of the human genome. Nature 2001; 409:860–921.

Nature Insight: Human genomics and medicine. Nature 2004; 429: 439–81.

Tabor HK, Risch NJ, Myers RM. Opinion: Candidate-gene approaches for studying complex genetic traits: practical considerations. Nature Rev Genet. 2002;3:391–7.

Tyers M, Mann M. From genomics to proteomics. Nature 2003;422: 193–7.

Venter JC et al. The sequence of the human genome. Science 2001;291:1304–51.

Waterston RH et al. Initial sequencing and comparative analysis of the mouse genome. Nature 2002;420:520–62.

Watson JD, Crick FH. Molecular structure of nucleic acids; a structure for deoxyribose nucleic acid. Nature 1953;171:737–8.

Further reading

Ansell SM et al. Primer on medical genomics. Part VI: Genomics and molecular genetics in clinical practice. Mayo Clin Proc. 2003;78:307–17.

Cahill D. Protein and antibody arrays and their medical applications. J Immunol Meth. 2001;250:81–91.

Davies KE. The application of DNA recombinant technology to the analysis of the human genome and genetic disease. Hum Genet 1981;58:351–7.

Dennis C, Gallagher R. The human genome. New York: Nature/Palgrave; 2002.

Franco RF, Reitsma PH. Genetic risk factors of venous thrombosis. Hum Genet. 2001;109:369–84.

Henrion D et al. The deletion genotype of the angiotensin I-converting enzyme is associated with an increased vascular reactivity in vivo and in vitro. J Am Coll Cardiol. 1999;34:830–36.

Kim NS et al. The effects of beta2 adrenoceptor gene polymorphisms on pressor response during laryngoscopy and tracheal intubation. Anaesthesia 2002;57:227–32.

Kwok PY et al. Increasing the information content of STS-based genome maps: identifying polymorphisms in mapped STSs. Genomics 1996;31:123–6.

Liggett SB. Beta(2)-Adrenergic receptor pharmacogenetics. Am J Respir Crit Care Med. 2000;161:S197–201.

Lorentz CP et al. Primer on medical genomics part I: History of genetics and sequencing of the human genome. Mayo Clin Proc. 2002;77:773–82.

Philip I et al. G894T polymorphism in the endothelial nitric oxide synthase gene is associated with an enhanced vascular responsiveness to phenylephrine. Circulation 1999;99:3096–8.

Risch N, Merikangas K. The future of genetic studies of complex human diseases. Science 1996;273:1516–17.

Schwinn DA, Booth JV. Genetics infuses new life into human physiology: implications of the human genome project for anesthesiology and perioperative medicine. Anesthesiology 2002;96:261–3.

Tefferi A et al. Primer on medical genomics part II: Background principles and methods in molecular genetics. Mayo Clin Proc. 2002;77:785–808.

Zotz RB et al. Prospective analysis after coronary-artery bypass grafting: platelet GP IIIa polymorphism (HPA-1b/PIA2) is a risk factor for bypass occlusion, myocardial infarction, and death. Thromb Haemost. 2000;83:404–7.

Chapter 6

Molecular physiology

Kevin J Gingrich and Jay Yang

TOPICS COVERED IN THIS CHAPTER

- **Membrane potential**
- **Ion channels**
    - Physiology
    - Molecular structure
- **Carriers, pumps and transporters**
    - Transporters as a current source
    - Transporter reversal
- **Electrophysiological techniques**
    - Two-electrode voltage clamp
    - Patch clamp technique
    - Lipid bilayer technique
    - Extracellular recording
- **Fluorescent techniques for measuring intracellular ions**

Ion channels are specialized membrane-spanning proteins that mediate rapid transmembrane ionic fluxes to produce alterations in membrane potential critical for the initiation and propagation of action potentials, synaptic transmission, and muscle contraction. Carriers, pumps, and transporters form another class of membrane protein that carry ion fluxes essential to cellular homeostasis. In addition, they transport neurotransmitters and large organic molecules involved in metabolism. Electrophysiologic studies have identified the governing physiologic principles and provided functional characterization of these proteins. The techniques of molecular biology have advanced our knowledge of the molecular structures underlying their functions. The importance of ion channels and carrier proteins in normal cell function is self-evident, but some may also serve as targets for anesthetic agents and other therapeutic drugs. This chapter reviews the fundamental electrical principles that govern the behavior of all cells, membrane potential, the properties of ion channels and carrier proteins, and the methods used to study them.

MEMBRANE POTENTIAL

Membrane potential is the voltage difference between the inner and outer surfaces of the cell membrane. Precise control of membrane potential is critical to cell homeostasis and to cell function in electrically excitable tissues. Membrane potential is determined by the membrane electrical properties, the nature of charged particles (ions) separated by the membrane, and the movement of ions through the membrane and embedded ion channels. Electrical properties determine, in part, the movement of ions across cell membranes. Electrical properties derive from fundamental physical laws and include the concepts of *electrical current*, *potential or voltage*, *capacitance*, and *resistance* (Chapter 12). To illustrate these concepts, consider two parallel plates composed of a conducting material that allows the easy passage of ions (Fig. 6.1a). A nonconducting gas between the plates prohibits ion movement and electrically insulates one from the other. Overall, this configuration is a capacitive element which stores charge on parallel plates. Current (I) is defined as the flow of positive charge (Q) per unit time and has units of amperes (A). However, current can also be carried by anions (negatively charged ions), where the direction of actual ion flow is opposite to that of current. Current delivered to the upper plate by the flow of cations leads to a net positive charge that electrostatically repels cations on the lower plate, driving them off and resulting in a net negative charge. Separated positive and negative charges create an electric field between the plates with a magnitude described by a *potential* or *voltage* (V) difference. The electric field exerts a force (F_V) on an ion, with magnitude proportional to the voltage and in a direction towards the unlike charge. Therefore, voltage or potential differences drive positive charges in the form of current from positive to negative polarity.

Capacitance (C) is a measure of the ability of an electrical element to store charge. An electrical circuit equivalent of a capacitive element has two parallel lines representing parallel plates (Fig. 6.1b). Capacitance is expressed in terms of the amount of charge stored for the applied voltage and has units of Farads (F). Application of voltage to a capacitor induces a transient charging current that continues until the applied and capacitive voltages equalize.

Resistance (R) is the opposition to current flow and has units of ohms (Ω). As resistance increases, higher voltages are required to induce the same current through the element. Resistance is defined by the ratio of the applied voltage to the induced current (Fig. 6.1c). *Conductance* (G), the reciprocal of resistance, describes the ease with which ions are passed and has units of mho (the reverse spelling of ohm) or siemens (S).

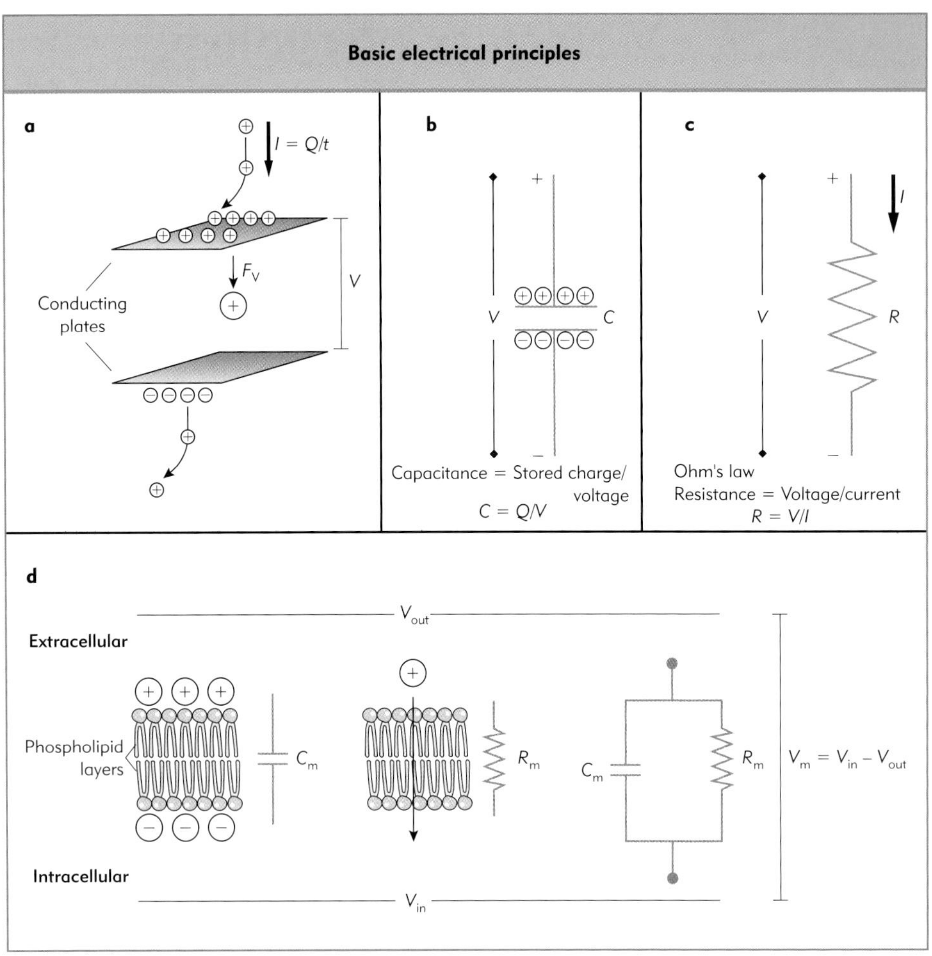

Figure 6.1 Basic electrical principles. (a) Two parallel conducting plates separated by a non-conducting gas constitute a capacitive element. Ions are represented by circles, with – and + signs indicating polarity. Current (*I*) carried by cations is delivered to the upper plate. The voltage or potential difference (*V*) between the plates is indicated. A large cation placed between the plates experiences an electromotive force (F_V) arising from the electric field and the voltage difference. (b) The electrical circuit equivalent of a capacitive element. Charges are shown on each plate. (c) The electrical circuit equivalent for resistance (*R*). (d) The cell membrane is composed of a phospholipid bilayer; each molecule has a polar phosphate group and two nonpolar long-chain hydrocarbons. The cell membrane can store charges, demonstrating its capacitance (C_m). The membrane permits limited passage of cations, constituting a finite resistance (R_m). Alongside is the overall equivalent electrical circuit, which combines capacitive and resistive elements. The voltage difference is the trans-membrane voltage (V_m).

The cell membrane separates the intracellular and extracellular environments (Chapter 2). Molecules energetically prefer surroundings with similar physicochemical properties. The properties of aqueous environments are determined by the polar nature of water molecules. As a result, polar or charged molecules favor the company of water molecules and are called 'water loving' or *hydrophilic*. Long uncharged carbon chains prefer the absence of water molecules and are called 'water fearing' or *hydrophobic*. Because the extracellular and intracellular environs are aqueous they attract the polar hydrophilic phosphate heads of membrane phospholipids while repelling the nonpolar hydrocarbon tails; this favors the formation of a phospholipid bilayer as molecules align in this manner (Fig. 6.1d). This bilayer allows the passage of small nonpolar molecules, but is virtually impermeable to ions and large or polar molecules (e.g. sugars and amino acids), which must enter and exit the cell by means of ion channels and transporters. Because the membrane impedes ion flow it electrically insulates the intracellular and extracellular solutions, which themselves are excellent conductors because of their high ion concentrations. This arrangement results in significant membrane capacitance (C_m). Ions, to a small degree, penetrate the bilayer, resulting in a finite but large membrane resistance (R_m). The electrical properties of the membrane can be represented by an equivalent circuit involving resistance and capacitance elements (Fig. 6.1d, right). The voltage across this circuit is the membrane potential or voltage (V_m). Events that force V_m towards negative potentials are *polarizing* and those that drive V_m towards positive potentials are *depolarizing*. Thus the electrical properties of a cell can be represented by an electrical circuit made up of familiar electrical elements (resistors and capacitors).

Many ions have different intracellular and extracellular concentrations, resulting in transmembrane concentration differences or gradients. These gradients, combined with ion-selective channels, provide for the control of resting membrane potential, which is critical to cell function. In addition, gated channels allow for the modulation of membrane potential (Chapter 19). In the face of a concentration gradient representing a chemical potential, particles move by diffusion to give a net movement from the area of high concentration to that of the lower. As a simplification, the chemical potential gives rise to a diffusional force (F_D) that pushes particles down the concentration gradient. The effects of diffusional forces and ion-selective or semipermeable channels on membrane voltage are shown in Figure 6.2. The permeant cation has a greater concentration inside than outside, similar to K^+ in actual cells. When the gated ion channel opens, F_D pushes the permeant cation through the channel pore to the outside solution. This charge movement constitutes an outward channel current. The permeant cation accumulates on the outer membrane surface because of electrostatic attraction from its partner anion, which itself is drawn to the inner membrane surface. These charges, stored in the membrane capacitance, result in a negative membrane potential. In electrically quiescent cells, the resting membrane voltage is negative. Outward currents cause additional polarization or *hyperpolarization*. Conversely, inward currents drive the mem-

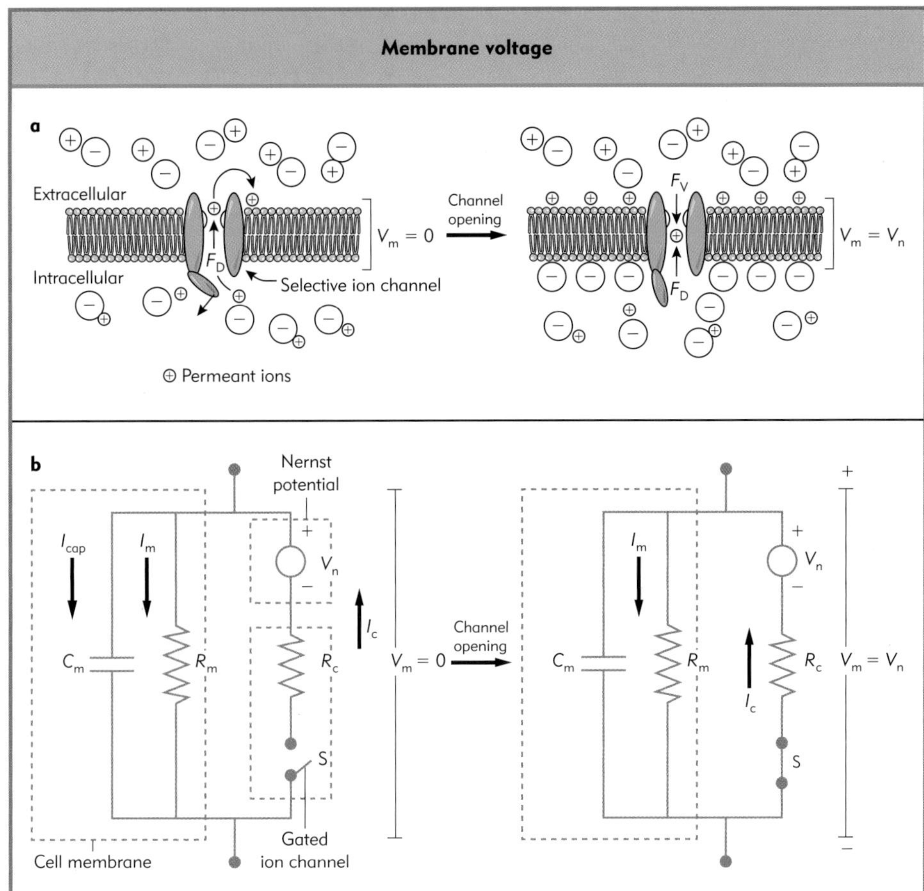

Figure 6.2 Membrane voltage. (a) Larger impermeant cations are at a high concentration outside and permeant cations are inside. Channel opening allows the diffusional force (F_D) to drive permeant cations through the channel, where they collect on the outer surface as a result of electrostatic attraction with partner anions that move to the inner surface. In the new equilibrium condition, the diffusional force (F_D) is equal to the electromotive force (F_V) as a result of V_m. At this equilibrium, V_m is equal to the Nernst potential (V_n) for the permeant ion. (b) The Nernst potential is shown as a source of voltage that can induce an ion channel current. Initially V_m is zero. When the channel opens (closure of switch S) the channel current (I_c) is composed of capacitive charging current (I_{cap}) and transmembrane resistive current (I_m). At the new equilibrium I_c is equal to I_m. The current magnitude is such that the voltage induced in R_m (membrane resistance) is equal to V_n, assuming $R_m >> R_c$. Therefore, V_m equals V_n.

brane voltage to more positive values and cause *depolarization.* The outward current continues until the forces owing to diffusion and the increasing membrane potential equalize. The Nernst equation describes the magnitude of the membrane voltage (*Nernst potential*) that exerts a force (F_V) that matches the diffusional force, thereby stopping ion flow through the channel. The equation for the Nernst potential of ion X is:

■ Equation 6.1

$$V_X = (RT/zF) \times \ln\frac{[X_{out}]}{[X_{in}]}$$

where R is the universal gas constant, T is temperature in Kelvin, F is the Faraday constant, z is the valence of the ion, the brackets indicate concentration, and subscripts *in* and *out* designate inside and outside the cell, respectively. Applying the constants and converting to $\log_{10}$:

■ Equation 6.2

$$V_X = 61 \times \log_{10}\frac{[X_{out}]}{[X_{in}]} \text{ in mV at 37°C}$$

If we assume $[K^+_{out}] = 0.01$ mol/L and $[K^+_{in}] = 0.1$ mol/L, we obtain a Nernst potential for K^+ (V_K) of –61 mV. Thus, when $V_m = -61$ mV, K^+ will stop flowing through the channel. If there are only K^+ channels present, the voltage at which the measured current reaches zero and reverses polarity, the *reversal potential* (V_R), is equal to V_K. At equilibrium, the membrane potential is called the *resting membrane potential* and is equal to the reversal potential.

There are many ion-selective channels in cells, each with its own Nernst potential. The reversal potential will then depend on all permeant ions. The Goldman, Hodgkin, and Katz equation is used to determine the reversal potential for two (X and Y) or more permeant ions:

■ Equation 6.3

$$V_{X,Y} = (RT/zF) \times \ln\frac{(P_X \times [X_{out}]) + (P_Y \times [Y_{out}])}{(P_X \times [X_{in}]) + (P_Y \times [Y_{out}])}$$

where the constants are the same as in Equation 6.1 and P is the permeability for each ion when its channel is open. Permeability represents the ease with which a concentration gradient induces a flow of ions, and here reflects channel conductance summed over all channels present. The reversal potential is the voltage at which the net current through the membrane is zero. For two ions, this means that current carried by ion X is of equal magnitude and opposite polarity to that of Y.

ION CHANNELS

Physiology

Ion channels are ion-selective macromolecular protein pores that traverse the cell membrane and may therefore affect the membrane potential, which is vital to excitable cells. Ions are passed with high efficiency, such that a few picoamperes (10^{-12}A) of current are generated by the ionic flow of a single open channel. This high efficiency means that relatively few channels – of the order of thousands – are needed in a particular cell to support its electrical function. The majority of ion channels fall into two broad categories: *voltage-gated* or *ligand-gated*. Gating is the progression of the channel through various conformational states, including a resting closed state and an open ion-conducting state. A triggering stimulus (membrane depolarization or ligand binding) causes the transition from resting to open through the process of activation. Permeation is the passage of ions through the open channel. In this way, gating regulates ion permeation. Figure 6.3 shows a simple topologic model of a generic voltage-gated cation channel. Permeation occurs via the channel pore, which begins on the extracellular face as the outer vestibule and narrows to a selectivity filter responsible for ion discrimination. The pore then widens to an inner vestibule (in which there are binding sites for local anesthetics in Na^+ channels or antagonists in Ca^{2+} channels; Chapters 32 and 40). An activation gate is shown at the inner channel mouth, which is closed at rest and obstructs the pore. Membrane depolarization triggers activation by exerting force on a charged voltage sensor, leading to the open conformation. Persistent depolarization induces further gating that closes the channel by shutting an inactivation gate. Consequently, voltage-gated ion channels have three primary conformational states: resting and inactivated closed states, and an open conducting state. In contrast, ligand-gated ion channels are activated by ligand (such as a neurotransmitter) binding to an extracellular receptor site. Like voltage-gated channels, they manifest resting and open states. However, a persistent ligand presence induces a closed desensitized state which is the correlate of the inactivated state of voltage-gated channels. Examples of common gated ion channels and their physiologic roles are given in Table 6.1.

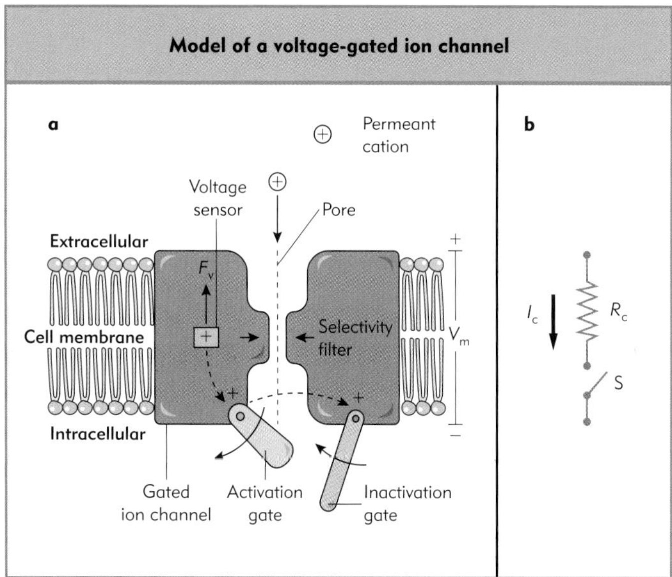

Figure 6.3 Model of a voltage-gated ion channel. (a) A simple general model of a voltage-gated ion channel residing within the cell membrane. A selectivity filter performs ion discrimination. An activation gate is shown at the intracellular mouth, which normally occludes the pore in the resting closed state and prevents permeation. Depolarization of the membrane voltage (V_m) exerts a force (F_V) on a positively charged voltage sensor, which triggers conformational changes leading to activation, gate opening, and ion permeation. Prolonged activation, caused by persistent depolarization, leads to closure of a normally open inactivation gate at the inner mouth. Negative V_m drives the permeant cation into the cell. (b) An electrical circuit can be drawn to describe a gated ion channel where the resistive element (R_c) is resistance to ion flow of the channel pore, I_c is the induced channel current, and the switch (S) represents the regulatory effect of channel gates on pore patency. When all gates are open, S is closed.

Molecular structure

Functional entities that define channel behavior (such as the selectivity filter, voltage sensor etc.) have structural correlates. The molecular structure of an ion channel defines its properties. Channel proteins span the membrane and have a hydrophobic exterior surface compatible with the hydrophobic environment of the lipid bilayer. The channel pore is lined with hydrophilic amino acids, providing a water-like environment for the ion to traverse the membrane. These pores are designed to pass ions of a particular kind, either anions (negatively charged ions) or cations (positively charged ions), as determined by the selectivity filter. Cationic channels are generally more selective than anionic channels. Many ligand-gated ion channels (e.g. the acetylcholine-gated channels that mediate neuromuscular transmission or the glutamate-gated channels that are largely responsible for excitatory synaptic transmission) are permeable to several cations. Numerous ion channels have been cloned and their function directly assayed using oocytes harvested from South African clawed frogs (*Xenopus laevis*). These oocytes are large enough to be injected with messenger RNA (mRNA) from other species and are capable of synthesizing the encoded foreign protein (heterologous protein expression). Messenger RNA is derived from complementary DNA (cDNA) purified or cloned from tissues rich in the channel of interest. Mutant cDNA clones with engineered alterations in the primary structure of the protein can be expressed and the properties of the mutated ion channel can be studied electrophysiologically to determine which regions of the protein are critical for a given channel function.

Most voltage-gated ion channel proteins are composed of multiple subunits or domains, with each containing six α-helical hydrophobic transmembrane regions, S1–S6. Voltage-gated K^+ channels (K_V; the subscript v indicates voltage-gated) are composed of four separate subunits (Fig. 6.4a,b). The subunits are assembled to form the central pore in a manner that also determines the basic properties of gating and permeation of the channel type. The peptide chain (H5 or P loop: permeation loop) between the membrane-spanning segments S5 and S6 projects into and lines the water-filled pore, as do portions of S6. The voltage sensor is composed of charged amino acid residues (lysine and arginine) on S4 that move outward during depolarization to trigger channel opening. Mutated K^+ channels with varying numbers of positively charged amino acids in S4 show distinct voltage-dependent gating, supporting the idea that the S4 segment is a voltage sensor. Inactivation involves the movement of the N-terminus into the inner mouth, thus obstructing the permeation pathway. The inactivation gate of Shaker channels, K^+ channels with a very rapid rate of inactivation, is the peptide forming the N-terminus, which acts like a 'ball on a chain' to plug the inner mouth to prevent further permeation. When the inside of the cell where the N-terminus of the K^+ channel resides is treated with a proteolytic enzyme (digesting away the peptide), inactivation is eliminated. Subsequently, if a

Table 6.1 Common gated ion channels

Voltage-gated channels	Abbreviation	Role
Na	I_N	Rapid rising phase of action potential
K^+ Delayed rectifier Inward rectifier	 I_K I_{KR}	 Termination of action potential Determines resting membrane potential
Ca^{2+} Low voltage activated or transient	LVA or T-type	Automaticity in the heart, Ca^{2+} influx in nerve
High-voltage activated (HVA) Neuron Muscle	HVA HVA N-type HVA L-type	 Synaptic transmission Ca^{2+} influx

Ligand-gated channels	Neurotransmitter	Primary permeable ion(s)	Role
$GABA_A$	GABA	Cl^-	Inhibition in CNS
Glycine	Glycine	Cl^-	Inhibition in spinal cord
Kainate	Glutamate	Na^+, K^+	Excitation in CNS
AMPA	Glutamate	Na^+, K^+	Excitation in CNS
NMDA	Glutamate	Na^+, Ca^{2+}	Excitation in CNS
Nicotinic acetylcholine	Acetylcholine	Na^+, K^+	Excitation in CNS and neuromuscular junction

AMPA, 2-amino-3-hydroxy-5-methylisoxozole-4-propionic acid; GABA, γ-aminobutyric acid; NMDA, *N*-methyl-D-aspartate.

synthetic polypeptide corresponding to the N-terminal amino acids of the ion channel is introduced to the cell, inactivation reappears, clearly supporting the notion that the structural basis for fast inactivation resides in the N terminus. The current understanding of the structure of K_V channels derives from experiments described above, as well as the study of changes in channel function produced by modifications in the primary peptide sequence. X-ray crystallography, which determines the complete structure of the protein in a crystal, has been successfully applied to bacterial channels much smaller than K_V channels. However, results from the small bacterial K^+ channel KcsA are relevant to the structure of K_V, as the primary peptide sequence and function of KcsA are similar to the S5, P-loop, and S6 regions of K_V. Therefore, KcsA can be viewed as a truncated form of K_V, thereby allowing extrapolation of structural conclusions in KcsA to these regions of K_V. Three fundamental structural features proposed for K_V were confirmed by the crystallographic findings in KcsA: 1) KcsA contains two α-helical transmembrane-spanning segments (Fig. 6.5c) in agreement with S5 and S6 of K_V; 2) P-loops contribute to the channel selectivity filter (Fig 6.5c); and 3) four subunit proteins coassemble in a axial fashion to form a functional channel (Fig. 6.5d). The complete structural picture of K_V awaits successful application of X-ray crystallography to this channel protein.

The pore-forming α subunit of Na^+ and Ca^{2+} channels contains four repeats of the six transmembrane-spanning motifs or domains (I–IV). These channels coassemble with accessory subunits that modulate channel gating but do not contribute to the pore. The structure of voltage-gated Na^+ and Ca^{2+} channels is fundamentally similar to that of K^+ channels (Fig. 6.4e).

Most ligand-gated ion channels comprise multiple subunits or groups of subunits; however, in these, each subunit contains four hydrophobic transmembrane regions (Fig. 6.4f,g). The subunits assemble in a pentameric fashion, such that segment M2 from the five subunits forms the central pore and determines permeation characteristics. Channel activation is triggered by ligand binding to site(s) on the extracellular segment of the polypeptide chain. Ligand binding causes a conformational change that opens the channel pore. Molecular cloning has identified numerous isoforms of the subunits of ligand-gated ion channel receptors (Chapter 20). The reason why so many receptor subunit isoforms exist is unclear. The exact subunit composition of the γ-aminobutyric acid (GABA) type A receptor probably has significance for the action of general anesthetics.

CARRIERS, PUMPS AND TRANSPORTERS

The cell membrane preserves the intracellular milieu, thereby excluding the free movement of larger and charged molecules in and out of cells. Substrate molecules required for cell metabolism, such as glucose and amino acids, metabolic end-products, and essentially all charged molecules must be transported. Carriers, pumps, and transporters are proteins that allow movement of these molecules across the cell membrane. Like voltage-gated ion channels, some protein carriers are highly selective

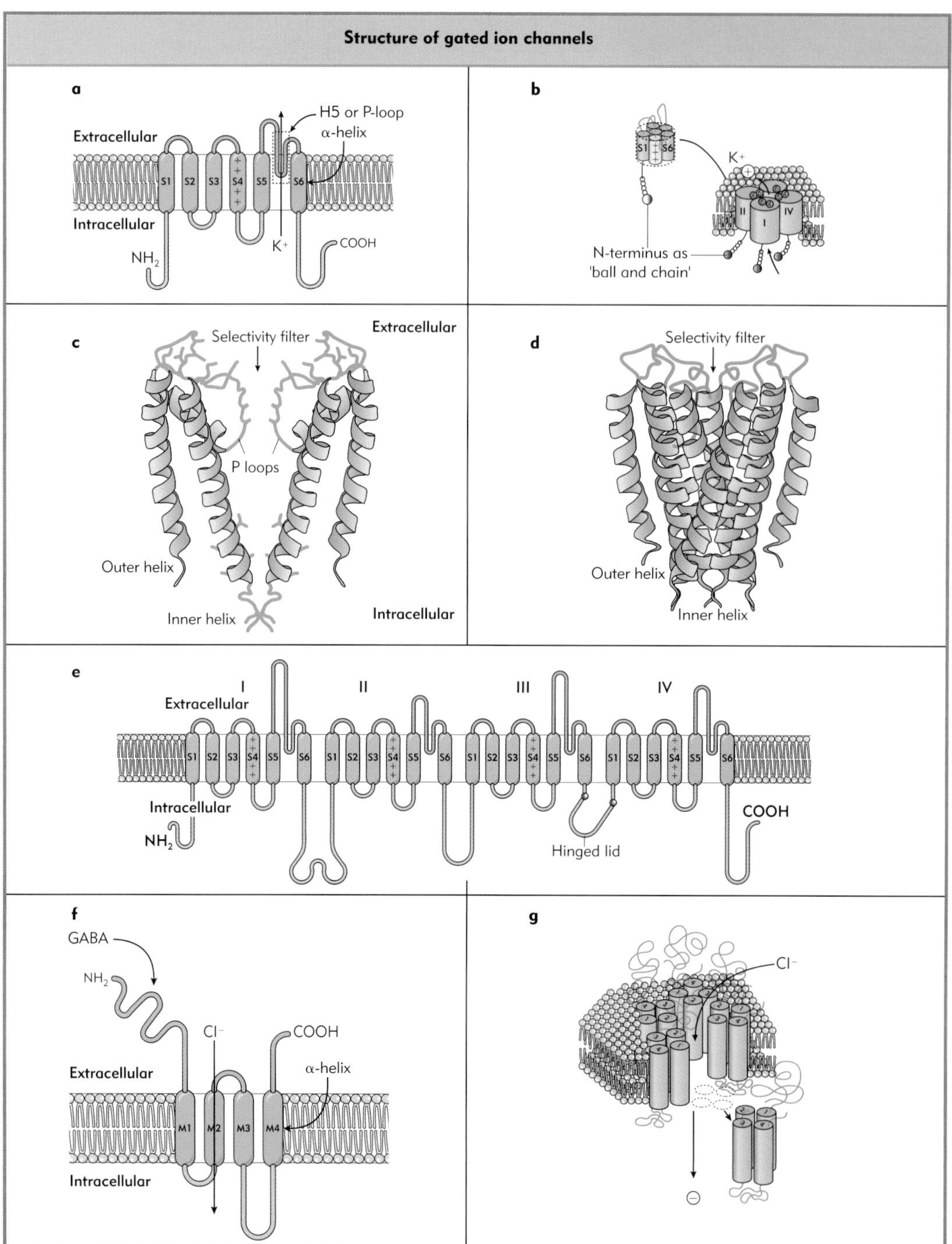

Figure 6.4, cont'd Structure of gated ion channels. (a) Proposed tertiary structures of a typical K^+ channel based on amino acid hydrophobicity deduced from cloned channel mRNA sequences and the X-ray structure of the channel. The voltage-gated K^+ channel consists of four subunits, each containing six membrane-spanning segments (S1–S6). Positively charged residues in S4 act as a voltage sensor. Residues of H5 (P-loop) line the pore and contribute to the selectivity filter, which is located between S5 and S6. S6 residues also contribute to the pore. (b) The four subunits assemble to form a K^+ channel in which the N terminus acts like a 'ball on a chain' to mediate fast (N-type) inactivation by occluding the permeation pathway at the inner mouth. X-ray crystallography of the bacterial KcsA K^+ channel supports fundamental structural features of K_V channels. (c) Two KcsA subunits showing inner and outer transmembrane-spanning segments which are coiled α-helical structures as proposed for similar S5 and S6 regions of K_V channels in panel (a), and the contribution of P-loops to the selectivity filter. Straight lines represent components of individual amino acids. (d) Coassembly of four subunits to form a complete channel (tetramer) with selectivity filter as indicated (see text). KcsA lacks fast inactivation and hence the N-terminus is small and mostly membrane bound. (e) In Na^+ channels, the α-subunit comprises four repeats (domains I–IV) that are strikingly similar to a single K^+ channel subunit. The α-subunit alone forms the channel pore, although other auxillary subunits also exist. Voltage sensors are charged residues of S4 in each domain. All P-loops contribute to the pore, as well as portions of S6 in domain IV. The cytoplasmic loop between domains III and IV underlies fast inactivation and is considered a 'hinged lid'; it closes to occlude the pore. The structure of Ca^{2+} channels (not shown) is similar to that of the Na^+ channels. (f) The ligand-gated $GABA_A$ receptor has subunits containing four membrane-spanning segments (M1–M4). M2 contributes to the pore and a chloride ion is shown traversing it. (g) Five subunits assemble to form a $GABA_A$ channel. This general structure also applies to several other ligand-gated ion channels (e.g. those for glycine, serotonin, nicotinic acetylcholine; see also Chapter 19). (c and d modified with permission from Doyle DA, Cabral JM, Pfuetzner RA et al. The structure of the potassium channel: molecular basis of K^+ conduction and selectivity. Science 1998;280:69–77.)

whereas others resemble neurotransmitter-gated ion channels which move two or more molecules at the same time. Therefore, in many ways carrier proteins functionally resemble ion channels. *Carrier proteins* are classified as active or passive, depending on whether the translocated molecules are moved up or down their electrochemical gradients, respectively. The electrochemical gradient is determined by the concentration difference across the membrane and membrane potential, and determines the direction of passive transmembrane movement of a molecule. Active carrier proteins expend energy through ATP hydrolysis to move molecules against the electrochemical gradient. They are further subdivided into *primary active* or *secondary active*, depending on whether the transporter is directly or indirectly coupled to the energy-supplying process (Fig. 6.5). The best-known primary active transporter is the Na^+/K^+-ATPase, which is present in all eukaryotic cells. This primary active transporter maintains the Na^+ and K^+ ionic gradients by translocating Na^+ outward and K^+ inward against their electrochemical gradients. The Ca^{2+}-ATPase, abundant in Ca^{2+} storage organelles such as skeletal muscle sarcoplasmic reticulum, moves Ca^{2+} against its electrochemical gradient. The ionic gradients established by these primary active transporters provide the potential energy necessary for the rapid membrane electrical events critical to the function of excitable membranes. Secondary active transporters lack endogenous ATPase activity and move molecules against their electrochemical gradient by coupling to an already established potential energy source. In most cases, movement of Na^+ and/or K^+ drives secondary active transport. Examples include the Na^+/K^+-dependent glutamate transporters, Na^+/Cl^--dependent GABA transporter, Na^+–Ca^{2+} exchanger, and the Na^+–glucose cotransporters (SGLTs).

Passive transporters move molecules down their electrochemical gradient, which is sometimes referred to as *facilitated* or *carrier-mediated diffusion*. The carrier has a maximum rate, which indicates the involvement of a specific binding process. As the concentration gradient for the transported molecule is increased, a maximum transport velocity (V_{max}) is reached that depends on the total binding sites available. The Na^+-independent amino acid and glucose transporters are examples of passive transporters. For an uncharged molecule, the electrochemical gradient is the concentration gradient. For charged molecules, transport depends on membrane potential as well. Transporters can translocate a single molecule in one direction (*uniport*), or two or more molecules in the same (*symport*) or opposite (*antiport*) directions (Fig. 6.5).

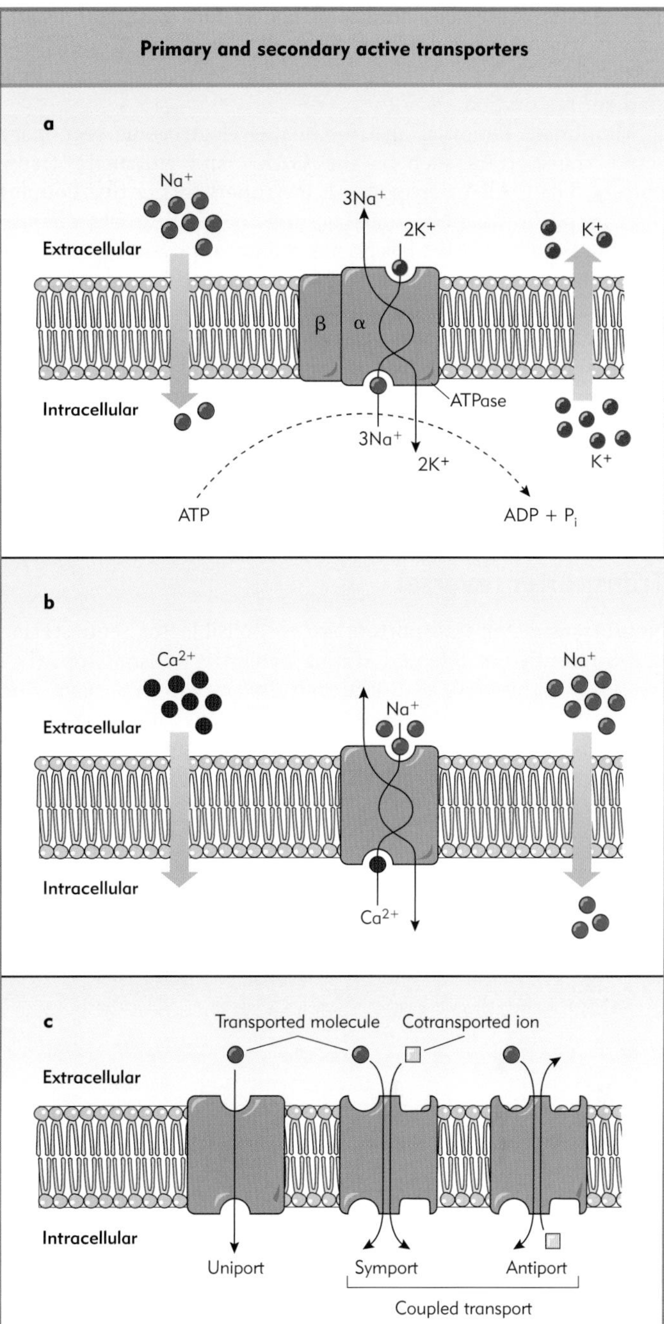

Figure 6.5 Primary and secondary active transporters. (a) The primary active transporter Na^+/K^+-ATPase has two binding sites for K^+ (red) facing the extracellular surface and three binding sites for Na^+ (blue) on the intracellular side. The movement of Na^+ outside and K^+ inside both against their respective concentration gradients (green arrows) is accomplished by energy derived from the hydrolysis of ATP. (b) The secondary active transporter Na^+–Ca^{2+} exchanger binds three Na^+ (blue) on the outside and one Ca^{2+} (black) inside. The translocation of Ca^{2+} against its concentration gradient is driven by the coupled movement of Na^+. This carrier protein has 11 transmembrane domains; it does not hydrolyze ATP. (c) Three types of protein transporter exist, depending on the coupling between the ions or molecules that they transport. Both active and passive transporters can function as uniporter, symporter, or antiporter. (Modified from Guyton 1991 and Alberts et al. 1994, with permission.)

Transporters as a current source

The Na^+/K^+-ATPase couples the translocation of three Na^+ outward and two K^+ inward, both against their electrochemical gradients. Because of the unequal 3:2 coupling, there is a net movement of positive charge out of the cell. In electrical terms, the Na^+/K^+-ATPase is *electrogenic*, as it produces a net outward current. An electrogenic pump has two major implications for cell function. First, its transmembrane current affects membrane potential. For the Na^+/K^+-ATPase, the outward current hyperpolarizes the membrane. Inhibition of this pump by drugs such as digoxin therefore depolarizes the cell membrane by removing this hyperpolarizing effect. Second, electrogenic pumps are influenced by membrane potential. Depolarization of the membrane enhances cation pumping. Therefore, during times of intense membrane depolarization, such as during skeletal muscle activity with exercise, ionic gradients can run down. Under these conditions, Na^+/K^+-ATPase activity is increased, enhancing gradient restoration.

Membrane potential also modulates electrogenic secondary active transporters such as the GABA and glutamate transporters. The GABA transporter is a symport carrier that couples the transport of two Na^+, one Cl^-, and one GABA molecule into the cell. Because GABA has no net charge, at physiologic pH this results in net transport of one positive charge into the cell for each cycle. The glutamate transporter is an antiport carrier that couples the inward translocation of two Na^+ and a glutamate anion, with outward transport of K^+ and OH^-. Glutamate is negatively charged at physiologic pH, resulting in net transport of one positive charge into the cell. Thus both GABA and glutamate transporters are electrogenic, causing a net inward current, and, like the Na^+/K^+-ATPase, they are sensitive to membrane potential.

Transporter reversal

Neurotransmitter transporters are responsible for sequestering neurotransmitters released during synaptic transmission. The rapid sequestration of neurotransmitters away from postsynaptic receptors ensures rapid termination of the signal, which allows for high-speed information transfer. They may also serve as a nonvesicular source of neurotransmitter release during pathophysiologic conditions (e.g. ischemia). Under normal conditions, the GABA transporter removes the inhibitory neurotransmitter GABA from the extracellular space against its concentration gradient. With increased neuron excitability, such as during a hypoxic–ischemic insult to the brain or seizure, the membrane depolarizes and the intracellular Na^+ concentration rises. Both factors oppose the normal inward electrogenic GABA transporter activity. In fact, under these conditions the GABA transporter may reverse, translocating Na^+, Cl^-, and GABA outward. γ-Aminobutyric acid can activate GABA receptors, inducing membrane hyperpolarization and reducing electrical activity (Fig. 6.6a) such that reversal of the GABA transporter serves as a negative feedback mechanism, reducing neuronal excitability at times of greatest need.

In contrast, reversal of the glutamate transporter during ischemia or neuronal hyperexcitability can result in greater glutamate release into the extracellular space, causing increased neuronal damage (Fig. 6.6b). During neuronal hyperexcitability, the increased intracellular Na^+ and extracellular K^+ concentrations and the depolarized membrane potential favor reversal of the glutamate transporter, resulting in the outward translocation of glutamate from the cytoplasmic pool. Released glutamate can activate its receptors, leading to further neuronal excitation and ultimately to neuronal death ('excitotoxicity'). The significance of this positive-feedback self-exacerbating mechanism in vivo may be limited by the effect of extracellular acidosis to block transporter function. Malfunction of the glutamate transporter may be important for the pathophysiology of a variety of neurodegenerative diseases.

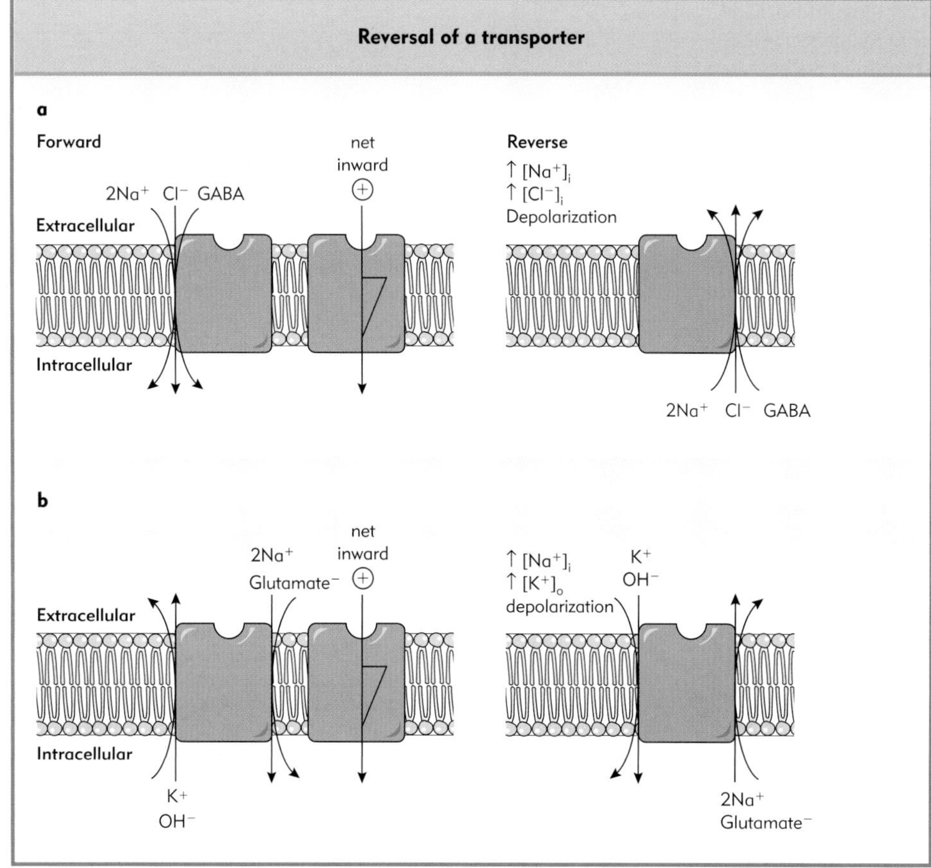

Figure 6.6 Reversal of a transporter. Transport proteins can operate in the forward or reverse direction. (a) The Na^+/Cl^--dependent GABA transporter under physiologic conditions (left) transports GABA along with the cotransported ions from the extracellular to the intracellular space. The net inward current flow is denoted as an inwardly directed current source. Under the conditions indicated (right), the transporter may operate in the reverse direction serving as a nonvesicular source of GABA release, which can act on its receptors to decrease neuronal excitability. (b) Normal forward operation of the Na^+/K^+-dependent glutamate transporter (left) sequesters extracellular glutamate. This transporter is also electrogenic, causing an inwardly directed current. Under the conditions indicated (right), reversal of this transporter releases intracellular glutamate, exacerbating the excitotoxicity of neurons.

ELECTROPHYSIOLOGICAL TECHNIQUES

A dramatic increase in our understanding of ion channels and carrier proteins has resulted largely from combining the powerful techniques of molecular biology (Chapter 4) and electrophysiology. This section provides an overview of selected electrophysiologic techniques that allow precise measurements of transmembrane currents and voltages.

Two-electrode voltage clamp

Channel currents are determined by the nature of channel opening, resistance or conductance of the permeant ion(s), the Nernst potential, and membrane voltage. In order to study ion channel function, the essence of ion channel physiology, channel currents are precisely measured during the delivery of a triggering stimulus (a membrane voltage change for voltage-gated ion channels, or a pulse of agonist for ligand-gated channels).

In the 1950s the two-electrode voltage clamp technique yielded the first observations of currents through voltage-gated ion channels and remains an indispensable tool in ion channel physiology. This technique employs two electrodes to control or 'clamp' membrane voltage (V_m) (Fig. 6.7). The glass microelectrodes contain conducting solutions and communicate electrically with the cell cytosol. A voltage-sensing electrode in combination with a bath electrode provides measurement of the membrane potential (V_m). When the voltage-gated channel opens, the resultant current (I_c) drives V_m away from V_{ref}. This increases the error, causing an increase in I_a (current delivered by the amplifier) that exactly matches I_c to equalize V_m and V_{ref}. As a result, the change in I_a reports I_c under constant V_m. Two-electrode voltage clamp controls the voltage of the entire cell membrane, and therefore reports an average activity of all channels, which is known as *whole-cell* or *macroscopic* current. Two-electrode voltage clamp can only be used in cells large enough to tolerate puncture by two microelectrodes (e.g. cardiac Purkinje cells). As a result single-electrode voltage clamp techniques were developed, but the nature of currents through individual or *single channels* remained a mystery until the 1970s, when Neher and Sakmann developed the patch clamp technique, for which they received a Nobel Prize.

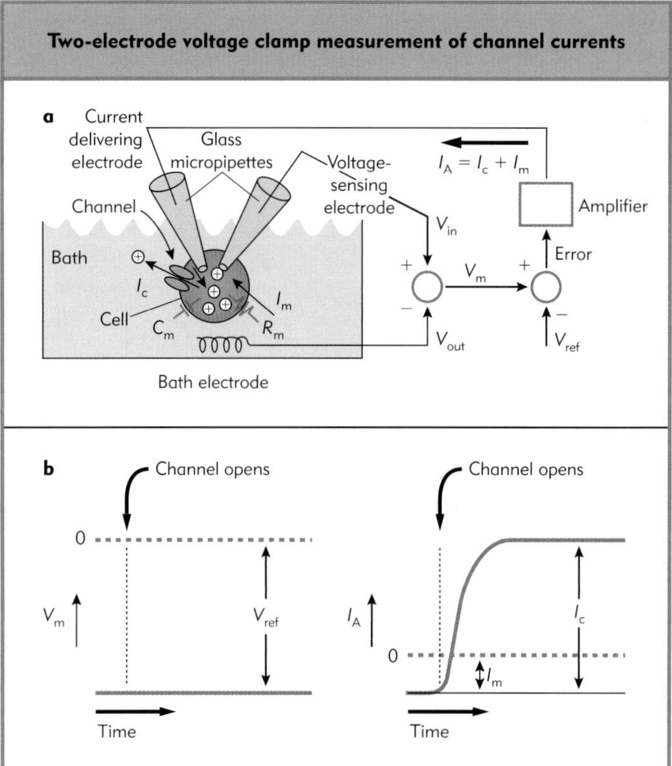

Figure 6.7 Two-electrode voltage clamp measurement of channel currents. (a) The method is illustrated for a single cell with a gated ion channel selective for an intracellular cation (circle with + sign) that is concentrated in the cytosol. Electrical elements representing membrane capacitance (C_m) and resistance (R_m) are superimposed on the membrane. The intracellular voltage (V_{in}) is assayed by a glass micropipette (diameter 10^{-6} m) and voltage-sensing electrode. The transmembrane voltage (V_m) is determined by comparing V_{in} with the bath voltage (V_{out}) detected by the bath electrode (coiled wire); V_m is compared with its desired value (V_{ref}). The difference represents an error signal that is fed to an amplifier; this then generates a proportional current (I_A) that is delivered to the cell via a second electrode (current delivering). (b) Changes in V_m (left) and I_A (right) over time are also shown. Initially, when the gated channel is closed, I_A is equal to the negative resistive current (I_m) necessary to cause the voltage induced in R_m and, therefore, V_m to equal V_{ref} (< 0 mV). Channel opening results in an outward hyperpolarizing current. The setup delivers additional current equal to I_c in order to maintain equality between V_m and V_{ref} (negative feedback control). This technique allows the measurement of ion channel current at constant V_m.

Patch clamp technique

The patch clamp technique provides voltage clamp of a membrane patch (hence the name). A single glass micropipette is pushed on to the cell membrane and negative pressure is carefully applied to form a 'tight seal', characterized by high resistance (giga-Ohm, $>10^{12}\Omega$). In essence, the electrode isolates and captures all ions flowing through the ~2 μm^2 membrane bounded by the micropipette. In this fashion, ionic current passing through a single channel in the membrane patch can be collected and measured. These *single-channel* or *microscopic currents* reflect closed or open conducting states (Fig. 6.8). Open channels conduct *unitary current*, which is determined by channel conductance, ionic conditions, and membrane potential. Single channel activity reports transitions between numerous possible conformational states; the analysis of these data requires probabilistic techniques such as histogram analysis. The patch clamp technique has a number of variations for the measurement of single channel currents, which include cell-attached inside-out, cell-free inside-out and outside-out, as well as whole-cell formations for measuring whole cell currents.

Lipid bilayer technique

The lipid bilayer technique also allows the study of single channel activity. The recording chamber comprises two wells separated by a thin wall containing a 250 μm diameter hole, which is painted with lipid solution to form a lipid bilayer. Channel-containing vesicles are introduced in one well and fuse with the lipid covering the hole, thereby inserting the channel. The voltage across the lipid bilayer is clamped and the channel current studied.

Extracellular recording

Much has been learnt about the fundamental properties of excitable membranes through voltage clamp techniques that

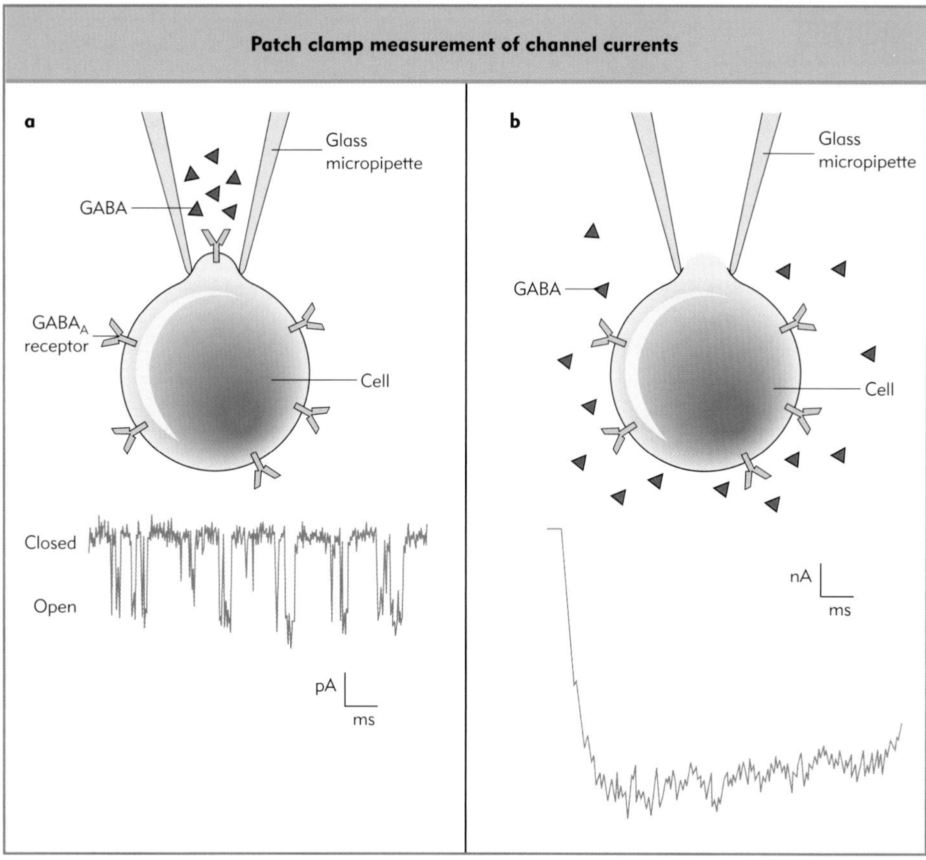

Figure 6.8 Patch clamp measurement of channel currents. In the 'membrane patch' arrangement (a) a glass micropipette is pushed on to the cell membrane and negative pressure is applied to the micropipette lumen to form a high-resistance seal. γ-Aminobutyric acid (GABA) in the pipette triggers the opening of the channel, which is reported as a Cl^- current below. These single-channel records demonstrate that individual channels open in a quantal fashion to conduct a unitary current. The membrane patch can be 'ripped' off the cell to achieve a cell-free inside-out configuration (not shown), which allows the delivery of agents to the cytoplasmic side of the channel and membrane. In the 'whole-cell' configuration (b) transient negative pressure applied to the micropipette lumen disrupts the membrane patch, allowing the pipette lumen to communicate with the cell cytosol electrically. Delivery of GABA to the cell exterior triggers channel opening. The recorded current reflects the averaged activity of numerous channels in the entire membrane.

require intracellular microelectrodes. However, essentially all clinical information is obtained through extracellular recording (e.g. electrocardiogram, electroencephalogram, sensory- and motor-evoked potentials). Extracellular recording of electrical activity is based on two fundamental principles: excited membrane serves as a current generator, and current flowing between any two points on a tissue can be recorded as a resistive voltage difference.

The first principle is easy to understand based on the preceding discussions on gated ion channels. The net current flow across a short segment of axon or a membrane patch changes from zero at rest to net inward current at the peak of an action potential (inward Na^+ channels are fully open) to net outward current during the falling phase of an action potential (outward K^+ channels are fully open), and back to zero. These events sequentially cause the excitable membrane to be a current sink, then a current source, before returning to zero current. The charge flow that feeds the current sink or accepts the current source comes from the extracellular space surrounding the excitable membrane. When many membrane patches act as a time-dependent current generator, a corresponding extracellular current flow occurs. Quantitatively, the transmembrane current (i.e. the net current that flows across the cell membrane via the ion channels) is directly proportional to the first derivative of the extracellular action current. In experimental recording situations, such as extracellular recording from a hippocampal slice preparation, this relationship is utilized and the first derivative of the initial upstroke of the extracellular action current is used as an indirect measure of the transmembrane current indicative of the synaptic strength. In clinical situations when a fairly well defined large amount of excitable tissue undergoes a more or less uniform change in its excitability (such as during the stimulation of a nerve bundle during a nerve conduction test), the total extracellular current flow resulting from these changes is recorded as the compound action potential. When billions of nerve cells all fire in a synchronous manner in the brain, all individually contributing a miniscule amount of extracellular current, the net aggregate extracellular current flow as recorded on the surface of the scalp is the *electroencephalogram* (EEG) (Chapter 14).

The second principle states that the final magnitude of the recording is a product of the actual current flow and the extracellular resistance between the two recording points. For a given amount of current flow, the ohmic voltage drop is proportional to the resistance. Therefore, a low-resistance contact provided by the electrocardiogram pads and the precise placement of the leads becomes essential for obtaining reproducible results (Chapter 13).

FLUORESCENT TECHNIQUES FOR MEASURING INTRACELLULAR IONS

Ion channels and protein carriers maintain vital intracellular ion and substrate concentrations. Direct physicochemical techniques, such as radioisotopic tracer or ion-selective microelectrode methods, allow the measurement of intracellular ion concentrations. Optical methods based on ion-selective indicators are also useful. Their principal advantages are that they are noninvasive and allow high spatial resolution of intracellular ion concentrations at the level of individual cells and organelles.

The physical principles underlying optical measurement of intracellular ions should be familiar to clinical anesthesiologists. The method is based on a concentration-dependent change in the absorbance/emission of light at a given wavelength, analogous to the principles underlying oxygen saturation determination by pulse oximetry. Thus, determination of the functional oxygen saturation of hemoglobin is accomplished by comparing light absorbance at 660 and 940 nm. At 660 nm, reduced hemoglobin (higher extinction coefficient) absorbs light better than oxyhemoglobin (lower extinction coefficient), whereas at 940 nm the converse is true. Modern pulse oximeters take measurements of light absorption at these two wavelengths nearly 500 times a second, and calculate the relative amounts of oxyhemoglobin and reduced hemoglobin and determine the hemoglobin oxygen saturation. Optical methods of determining ion concentrations follow the same principle. Binding of specific ions to their respective indicator molecule results in altered spectral properties. Unlike hemoglobin, many of the newly developed ion-selective indicators are fluorescent molecules. Light at shorter wavelengths (excitation wavelength) is absorbed and lower-energy light at a longer wavelength is given off (emission wavelength). Upon binding of a specific ion to its indicator, the emission and/or the excitation spectrum changes. For example, the commonly used Ca^{2+} indicator Fura-2 has a characteristic emission peak at 510 nm. This molecule shows a Ca^{2+}-dependent increase in fluorescence with excitation at 340 nm and concomitant decreases in fluorescence with excitation at 380 nm. As the availability of free Ca^{2+} increases, the light intensity ratio measured at 510 nm owing to excitation at 340 nm compared to 380 nm increases. Ion-selective indicators for other divalent ions (e.g. Mg^{2+}, Zn^{2+}, Cu^{2+}), for monovalent ions (e.g. Na^+, K^+, Cl^-), and for other inorganic ions are also available.

Key references

Alberts B, Johnson A, Lewis J, Raff M, Roberts K, Walter P. Carrier proteins and active membrane transport. In: Lewis J, Rass M, Roberts K, Watson JD, eds. Molecular biology of the cell, 4th edn. New York: Garland; 2002.

Amara SG, Arriza JL. Neurotransmitter transporters: three distinct gene families. Curr Opin Neurobiol. 1993;3:337–44.

Attwell D, Barbour B, Szatkowski M. Nonvesicular release of neurotransmitter. Neuron 1993;11:401–7.

Catterall WA. Structure and function of voltage-gated ion channels. Annu Rev Biochem. 1995;65:493–531.

Doyle, DA, Cabral JM, Pfuetzner RA et al. The structure of the potassium channel: molecular basis of K^+ conduction and selectivity. Science 1998;280:69–77.

Hamill OP, Marty A, Neher E, Sakmann B, Sigworth FJ. Improved patch-clamp techniques for high-resolution current from cells and cell-free membrane patches. Pfluger Arch. 1981;391:85–100.

Hille B (ed) Ion channels of excitable membranes, 3rd edn. Sunderland, MA: Sinauer; 2001.

Rabow LE, Russek SJ, Farb DH. From ion current to genomic analysis: recent advances in GABA, receptor research. Synapse 1995;21:189–274.

Richerson GB, Gaspary HL. Carrier-mediated GABA release: is there a functional role? Neuroscientist 1997;3:151–7.

Further reading

Kandel ER, Schwartz JH, Jessel TM (eds) Principles of neural science, 4th edn. Norwalk, CT: Appleton & Lange; 2000.

Sakmann B, Neher E (eds) Single-channel recording, 2nd edn. New York: Plenum; 1995.

Chapter 7

Sites of drug action

Brian J Pollard

TOPICS COVERED IN THIS CHAPTER

- **Nature of receptors**
- **Drug–receptor interactions**
  - Structure–activity relationships
  - Drug–receptor interaction
- **Concentration–response relationships**
  - Antagonists
- **Biological responses**

Applied pharmacology is central to the practice of anesthesia. Following intravenous administration of a drug, the desired effects – and the unwanted effects – are rapid and usually immediate. The observed effect is not the direct result of the drug itself, however, but a response by the organism to the presence of the drug. Original beliefs held that this was due to a physical interaction, the drug combining with the cell to induce a physical change, e.g. a change in size, shape, surface tension, or osmotic pressure. The pioneering work of Langley and Ehrlich at the beginning of the 20th century, however, gave rise to the concept of surface groups on cells that could exhibit specific binding properties with external molecules. It was Ehrlich who named these groups 'receptors'. Since then, a vast array of drugs, toxins, transmitters, hormones, etc. have been shown to act by transferring information to cells by interaction with receptors. The activation of a receptor necessitates a direct chemical bonding between the ligand and the receptor, the latter functioning as a specific recognition/binding site for the former.

Studies by Clarke, also in the early part of the 20th century, centered on the quantitative relation between concentration and action. Clarke examined the responses to graded increasing concentrations of acetylcholine and showed that when plotted in the form of a graph a curve resulted which could be expressed mathematically by the equation:

■ Equation 7.1

$$x = k\frac{y}{(100 - y)}$$

where x is the concentration of acetylcholine, y is the effect expressed as a percentage of maximum possible effect, and k is a constant.

The simplest explanation for this relationship was a reversible monomolecular reaction between two entities – the drug and a single binding site on the cell.

NATURE OF RECEPTORS

A receptor is an entity that binds to a drug or a transmitter substance and puts into action a chain of events leading to an effect (or part of an effect, if it is necessary to exceed a threshold). These must be differentiated from certain other sites that bind drugs, e.g. plasma proteins. These latter sites, often called 'acceptors', possess an affinity for the drug but result in no response. The presence and concentration of these inactive acceptor sites may considerably influence the action of a drug, either by removing it from the active biophase, thereby decreasing the expected effect, or by acting as a storage site and potentially prolonging the effect.

Receptors have three notable properties: *sensitivity, selectivity,* and *specificity*. A response results from very low concentrations (sensitivity). A response is only produced by a narrow range of structurally similar chemical entities (selectivity). The response to an agonist that is acting on the same set of receptors is always the same because the cells themselves (specificity) determine it. Although the concept of receptors on the surface of cells was established, they remained a conceptual entity until the 1970s, when the techniques of electron microscopy and biochemistry began to allow their visualization and purification.

Receptors have traditionally been classified according to the target systems to which they relate, and on the basis of effects and the relative potency of selective agonists and antagonists, e.g. cholinergic muscarinic, cholinergic nicotinic, adrenergic. In most systems, detailed studies with more selective agonists and antagonists have revealed many subdivisions, e.g. adrenergic α_1, α_2, β_1, β_2, β_3. An alternative classification results from the anatomical location of the receptors. Here, the tissue supporting the receptors could be used to categorize receptors: for example, most cholinergic muscarinic receptors lie on smooth muscle or glandular tissues, whereas a particular subtype of cholinergic nicotinic receptor lies on striated muscle. One further classification has become available relatively recently following advances in molecular biology. The isolation and study of single receptors has allowed the actual amino acid sequence to be determined. Receptors can now be classified in a very detailed manner, according to the gene sequence encoding the receptor.

Molecular characterization of receptors used to be very difficult because they are present in extremely small concentrations compared with other membrane proteins. Destruction of the membrane using detergents will secure the release of the membrane proteins, including those containing receptors. Those containing the ligand-binding sites can then be isolated and purified. Such purification processes are complex and tedious in view of the very small concentrations of receptors available, and this limited research until relatively recently. Molecular biological techniques have now revolutionized this field. Messenger RNA encoding the receptor being examined is used to create the complementary DNA, which is replicated by insertion into bacteria. The DNA produced, which is capable of encoding a particular receptor, is then harvested from the bacterial cells following cell lysis and used to express the receptor in cells that would not normally contain that receptor. The new receptor can then be examined using routine ligand-binding techniques. Using these techniques it is possible to produce receptors at a very much higher density than in normal cells (overexpression), and further purification and studies are facilitated. More detailed studies to determine the receptor structure are then possible, and purified receptors can be inserted into other artificial lipid membranes to facilitate further studies of receptor function under more physiological conditions.

Cell membranes are made up of a phospholipid bilayer, the hydrophobic parts of which lie within the membrane and the hydrophilic parts of which line the surface (Fig. 7.1). Proteins are an important constituent of the cell membrane and are orientated within the membrane according to their hydrophilic and hydrophobic characteristics. The majority of drug-binding sites are situated on proteins, glycoproteins, or lipoproteins, and the unique three-dimensional structure of these substances permits highly individualized binding sites to be created. In the case of a water-soluble drug, the binding site will lie within the hydrophilic head of the protein on the outer surface of the cell membrane. In the case of a lipophilic drug, the binding site probably lies within the cell membrane itself. The whole structure usually spans the membrane, such that the outer section contains the binding site for the drug or ligand, the transmembrane part is made up of amphiphilic helices of lipophilic amino acids capable of transmitting or functioning as a gate, and the intracellular section is capable of interacting with other intracellular proteins to promote second-messenger systems. The transmembrane proteins cannot move into or out of the membrane, although they are capable of lateral motion, floating in a lipid film in a dynamic fashion. Lateral motion may be very important, allowing the receptor proteins to interact freely (or relatively freely) with adjacent proteins. Many receptors appear to depend on such interactions as a part of their action to trigger the ongoing response. The reverse may be true, however, in that binding of a ligand to one receptor might alter the affinity of the binding of another ligand to an adjacent receptor, thus modulating drug and hormonal actions.

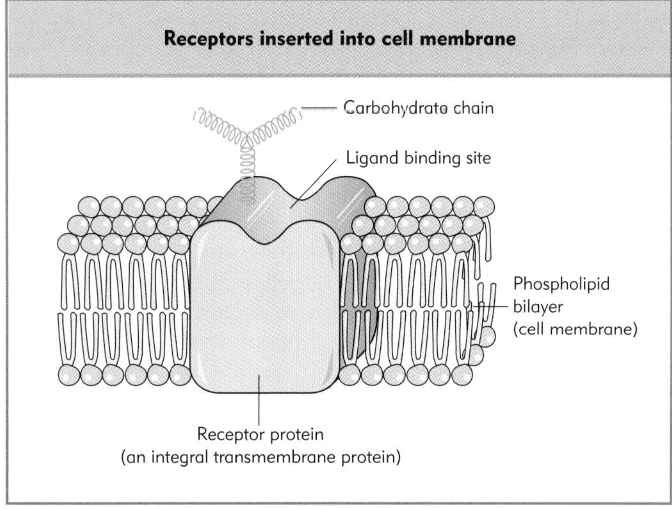

Figure 7.1 Receptor inserted into cell membrane.

DRUG RECEPTOR INTERACTIONS

There are a number of properties common to transmembrane receptors, in particular the recognition of extracellular drugs or ligands and the transmission of information to the intracellular region. Ligands combine directly with receptors. This bonding is usually electrostatic (ionic) in nature. Other forms of electrostatic bonding, e.g. hydrogen bonds and van der Waals forces, act to further stabilize binding. Covalent bonds are not common and are usually irreversible. The formation of ionic charges, and also the hydrophilicity, depends upon the pH of the medium and the pK_a of the molecule. These are extremely important in the context of drug–receptor interactions and can be manipulated externally to change binding properties, prolong or inhibit drug receptor interactions, etc. Hydrogen bonds are very weak and serve principally as reinforcements to other types of ionic bond. The importance of hydrogen bonds in biological systems is considerable: for example, the macromolecular structure of DNA and similar proteins depends upon the presence of large numbers of hydrogen bonds.

Structure–activity relationships

Drugs act at receptors, which are specific groups on the surface of cells. A large number of different receptors exist, each with its own individual family of related drugs. In general, there is little or no crossreactivity between these separate families. For example, tubocurarine has an action at the nicotinic acetylcholine receptor, and diazepam at the benzodiazepine receptor. Neither has any effect on the other receptor. Tubocurarine and diazepam differ considerably in their chemical structure, and it might therefore be expected that the characteristics and shape of the molecule would be relevant to activity. The whole molecule is not necessarily involved, however. Pancuronium and atracurium, for example, all have the same effect as tubocurarine on the nicotinic acetylcholine receptor whereas midazolam, temazepam and lorazepam all affect the benzodiazepine receptor. It would thus appear logical to infer that there must be some component part of each molecule which is common to a series, and which possesses the ability to combine with the receptor. That moiety on benzodiazepines must be different from that on the cholinergic agonists.

The study of structure–activity relationships has enabled us to determine a number of factors with respect to the receptors. Information concerning, for example, the number of binding sites and their spatial configuration, the probable nature of the binding forces, and the requirements for activation may be deduced. Although traditional structure–activity relationships continue to be important in the elucidation of receptor structure, newer methods have been developed. Of particular importance are computational techniques involving advanced graphics. These enable predictions to be made of energies between bonds, and the conformations of the bound versus the unbound states of drug–receptor complexes. Advances in recombinant DNA technology have allowed the primary structures of receptors to be copied. X-ray crystallography and magnetic resonance imaging have also played a vital role.

The simplest model concerning the relationship between drug (or ligand or agonist) concentration and observed response is derived from the Law of Mass Action and assumes that the two entities (agonist and receptor) are combining in a reversible manner to form a third. In its simplest form, this may be expressed by the following equation:

■ Equation 7.2

$$[\text{Drug (D)}] + [\text{Receptor (R)}] \rightarrow [\text{Drug–Receptor complex (DR)}]$$

Unless the drug forms a completely irreversible union with the receptor (an uncommon state of affairs), the drug–receptor complex can dissociate into its two component parts and the equation is bidirectional:

■ Equation 7.3

$$[D] + [R] \underset{k_{21}}{\overset{k_{12}}{\longleftrightarrow}} [DR] \rightarrow \text{Effect}$$

The rate of forward reaction, k_{12} (formation of drug–receptor complex), depends upon the concentration of drug [D] and the concentration of receptors [R]. The rate of dissociation of drug–receptor complex (k_{21}) depends upon its concentration [DR]. Therefore, when steady state is reached,

■ Equation 7.4

$$k_{12}\,[D][R] = k_{21}\,[DR]$$

$$\text{rearranging, } \frac{[D][R]}{[DR]} = \frac{k_{21}}{k_{12}} = K_D$$

The ratio k_{21}/k_{12} is usually replaced by the single term K_D, the dissociation constant. It must be noted that in this scheme it has been assumed that the reaction is totally reversible, that all receptor sites have an equal affinity for the drug, that binding to some receptor sites does not affect the binding to others, and that there are no other nonspecific binding sites present. Clearly, this is an 'ideal' situation and not one that pertains in many clinical circumstances. Fractional receptor occupancy may be expressed as a function of ligand concentration [L] at equilibrium, and the result is a rectangular hyperbola (Fig. 7.2a). The equilibrium dissociation constant K_D is equal to the concentration of ligand at 50% receptor occupancy, and is more easily determined from the semilogarithmic plot of log [L] against [LR] (Fig. 7. 2b). Note the similarity of these ligand-binding graphs to the dose (concentration)–response graphs below.

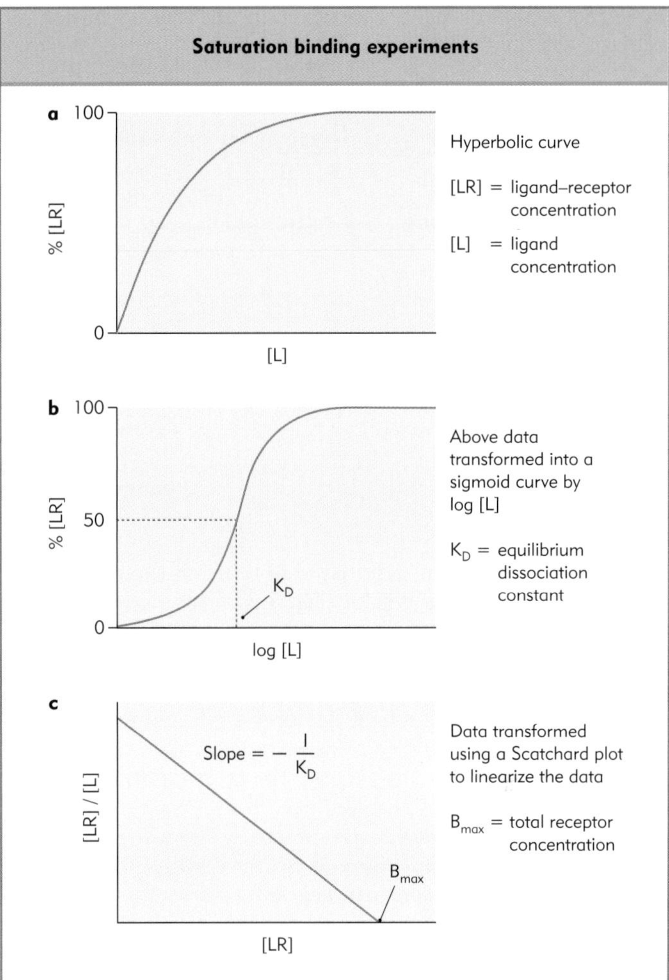

Figure 7.2 Hyperbolic curve of ligand receptor concentration (%LR) against ligand concentration [L]. The same data transformed by taking logarithms of [L]. A sigmoid curve results. K_D, the equilibrium dissociation constant, is equal to [L] at 50% receptor occupancy.

At equilibrium, the sum of the total number of free receptors [R] and the total number of receptors bound to drug [DR] must equal the overall total of existing receptors, which we can denote by the term $[R_{total}]$. Thus, $[R_{total}] = [R] + [DR]$.

Substituting for [R] in Equation 7.2 and rearranging gives the following:

■ Equation 7.5

$$K_D = \frac{[D]\,[R_{total} - DR]}{[DR]}$$

which can be further rearranged as:

■ Equation 7.6

$$\frac{[DR]}{[R_{total}]} = \frac{[D]}{K_D + [D]}$$

When all of the receptors $[R_{total}]$ are occupied by agonist, the maximum effect (E_{max}) will be produced. When no receptors are occupied, there will be no effect. Between these two extremes, the effect (E) will be proportional to the concentration of receptors occupied [DR]. Thus,

■ Equation 7.7

$$\text{therefore}\ \frac{E\ [DR]}{E_{max}\ [R_{total}]} = \frac{[D]}{K_D + [D]}$$

The measured response, r, is equal to E/E_{max}, so:

■ Equation 7.8

$$r = \frac{[D]}{K_D + [D]}$$

and

■ Equation 7.9

$$[D] = K_D \times \frac{r}{1 - r}$$

If drug concentration is displayed in terms of the response, r, a rectangular hyperbola results (Fig. 7.3). This is the standard concentration–response relationship graph and is identical to that derived by Clarke (see above). It is also clear that K_D is the concentration of agonist that will occupy half of the receptors at equilibrium. When K_D is small, the receptors have a high affinity for the agonist (few drug molecules are required to occupy 50% of the receptors), and when K_D is high, the receptor affinity is low.

The rectangular hyperbola describing the relationship between drug concentration and measured effect is particularly difficult to construct and to use. It is therefore common to display the data as the response against the logarithm of the concentration (or dose) of drug, where the response is expressed as a percent of maximum response. This yields a sigmoid-shaped graph (Fig. 7.4). This transformation is particularly useful because the section from approximately 20% to 80% of maximal response is a straight line, allowing a more precise estimate of the EC_{50}. Additional advantages of this semilogarithmic plot are that it is possible to visualize effects over a wide range of drug doses (concentrations), and also to more easily compare the effects of different agonists and antagonists.

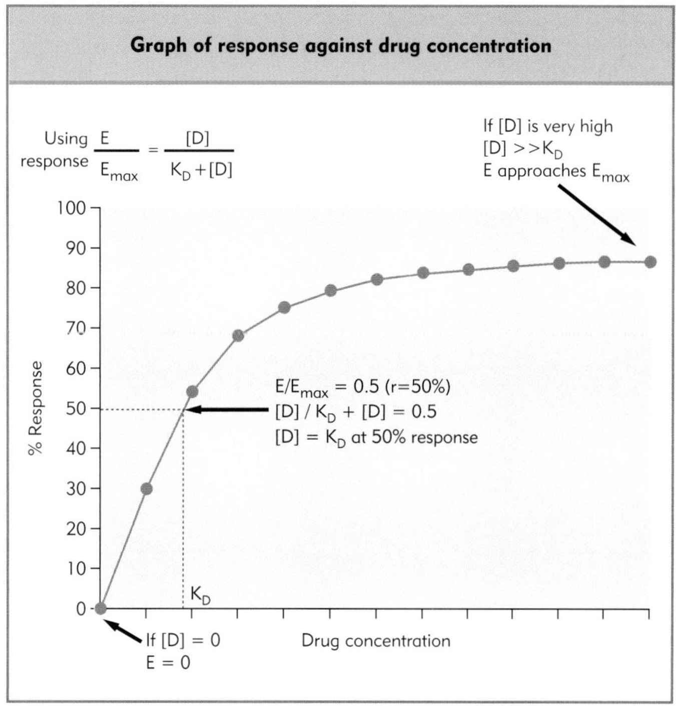

Figure 7.3 Graph of response against drug concentration (a 'dose–response curve') demonstrating the similarity to the ligand-binding graphs (Fig. 7.2). Key points referring to the derived equations have been illustrated.

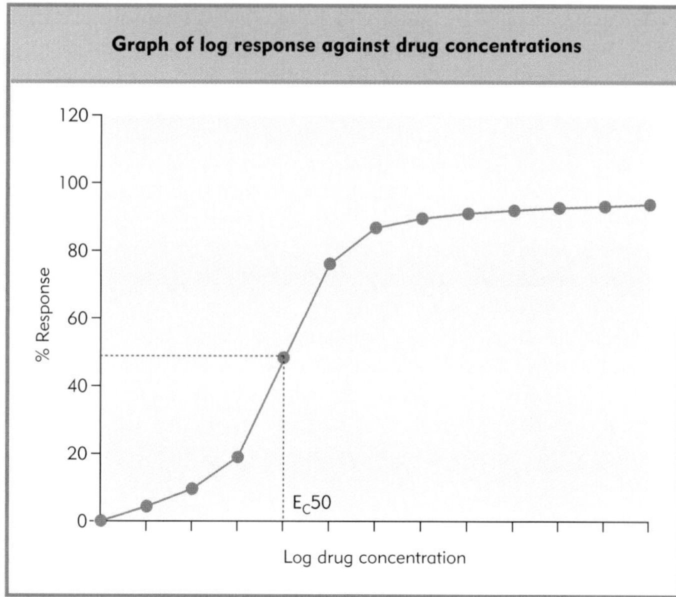

Figure 7.4 Graph of response against log drug concentration (the 'log dose–response curve'). The section from about 20% to 80% is linear, making it easier to use and to determine standards of comparison, e.g. the ED_{50} or EC_{50}.

The log dose–response graph is difficult to use outside the range 20–80% of maximum response because of nonlinearity, and it may not be possible to confine data to the central linear section. A further transformation can be obtained by taking logarithms of both sides of the equation:

■ Equation 7.10

$$\text{Log}[D] = \text{Log}K_D + \text{Log}\left(\frac{r}{1 - r}\right)$$

Thus a graph of log[D] against $\log\left(\frac{r}{1 - r}\right)$ will produce a straight line, the intercept of which gives the value for $\log K_D$ (Fig. 7.5). This relationship is known as the Hill plot (named after A V Hill). If the agonist and receptor combine on a 1:1 basis, then the slope of the line should be unity.

The term 'Log $\left(\frac{r}{1 - r}\right)$' is also referred to as the logit (or logistic) transformation, and this has the effect of extending the ends of the scale of r and is linear between about 2% and 98% of maximum response. It allows points to be reliably plotted out to between approximately 5% and 95% of maximum response.

There is an alternative approach, namely that of probit analysis. This considers the response as being due to a statistical summation of the probabilities that any individual drug entity and receptor entity will combine to initiate an effect. The response axis is replaced by an axis that represents the proportion (or percentage) of positive receptor interactions for that given dose and response. As the concentration of agonist rises, the proportion (or rate) of receptor interactions increases until

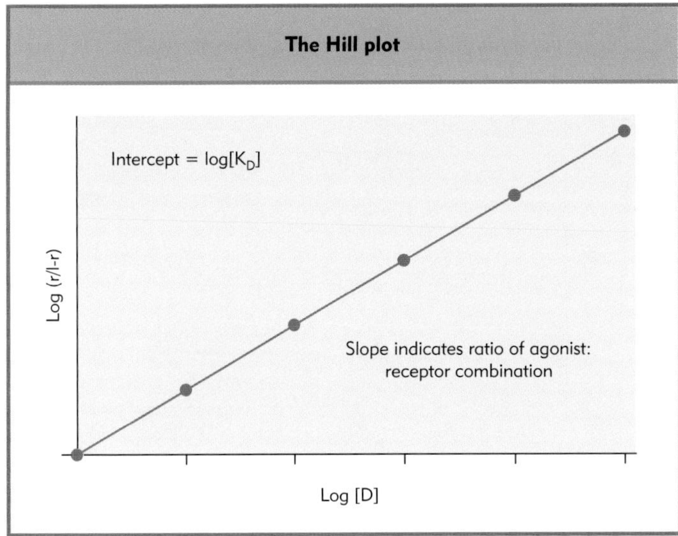

Figure 7.5 The Hill plot.

the 50% response point is reached. The proportional increase for each unit increase in dose then declines with further increases in dose, although the total number of receptors occupied must be increasing. The frequency distribution of quantal responses to many drugs has been shown to be described by such a normal (gaussian) distribution. Conversion of a response to its probit value requires complex mathematics, and it is easier to use either a table of probit values or graph paper marked with a probit scale. The effect of probit analysis is almost identical to that of logit analysis, in that it expands the ends of the scale of response and converts the sigmoid relation between log concentration and response to a straight line between about 2% and 98%.

There is one further technique occasionally applied to biological data, namely arcsine transformation (alternatively known as the angular transformation or inverse sine transformation). The equation $y = \sin^{-1}x$ is applied to the data, where x is the square root of the original variable. As the original variable increases from 0 to 1, y increases from 0° to 90°, and equal changes in x correspond to greater changes in y towards the ends of the scale. The result is therefore again to convert a sigmoid curve (which might be regarded as having the appearance of a section of a sine wave) into a straight line between about 2% and 98%.

Drug–receptor interaction

The two principal theories underlying the interaction between drugs and receptors are the occupation theory and the rate theory, although many others have been postulated.

The occupation theory of drug action is the most logical, and holds that the observed response is a direct function of the number of receptors occupied by drug. The resulting response therefore depends on the receptor density, the dissociation constant K_D, the intrinsic efficacy of the receptors for the drug and the efficiency of the process converting receptor activation to cellular response.

The occupation theory has its origins in the work of Clarke, who showed that there were many situations where the effect of a drug was linearly proportional to receptor occupancy. The occupation theory can readily explain the shape of the dose–response relationships from the equations described above. There are, however, some discrepancies, and a number of assumptions have to be made. In particular, the concentration of drug in the active biophase surrounding the receptor will not change instantaneously, owing to pharmacokinetic factors.

A variant on the occupation theory is the operational model. This originates with the experimental observation that most drug concentration–response curves describe a rectangular hyperbola. Thus the model can be tested by producing a saturation curve. It is simpler than the occupation model in that drug responses can be described in terms of only three parameters: the dissociation constant, the receptor concentration, and the concentration of drug–receptor complex that elicits half-maximal response.

The rate theory of drug action is based on the kinetics of onset and offset of drug binding to the receptors. It recognizes that receptors have to be occupied by drug for the effect to be produced, but holds that the drug is constantly binding with and dissociating from the receptors in a dynamic fashion. The response should then be a function of the rate of interaction between agonist and receptors, and not the actual occupation. This theory can also be mathematically shown to predict the same shapes of graph for the dose–response and log dose–response relationships. The dissociation constant K_D is also equal to the concentration of agonist at half-maximal response. The time curve of a response under the rate theory differs from that predicted by the occupation theory. At zero time, as the drug is administered, [DR] is zero. According to the rate theory, the response should immediately rise to a transient peak and then decrease exponentially very rapidly to a plateau (equilibrium response). It is the equilibrium response that is the measured response. Theoretically, the plateau responses are the same as those predicted by the occupation theory. According to the rate theory, however, peak response may considerably exceed the maximum response that would be possible according to the occupation theory. It is hard to reconcile these theoretical considerations, and the existence of these instantaneous maximum values is almost impossible to test experimentally. The rate theory also supports the observation that agonists act more rapidly than antagonists. It also supports the concept that the probability of an agonist and a receptor combining will depend on their relative concentrations, which has already been supported by using probit analysis as a tool in the analysis of concentration–response relationships.

A third model, the receptor inactivation model, combines elements from both the occupation and the rate theories. This theory proposes first, that an agonist binds to a receptor with an onset rate k_1 and an offset rate k_2. Second, it proposes that the agonist–receptor complex can transform into an inactive state incapable of further activation for a set time, which is governed by a rate constant of k_3. Again this theory fulfils the theoretical criteria but is extremely difficult to test experimentally.

In an attempt to further simplify this field, a recent proposal has suggested that a two-state model is adequate. This theory proposes that a dynamic equilibrium exists between the inactivated and the activated forms of the receptor. The transition from inactivated to activated is rooted in probability theory, such that the probability of a receptor existing in the activated state is high in the presence of agonist and very low in the absence of agonist. The ratio of inactivated to activated is tissue specific and probably receptor specific. In the normal situation, in the unstimulated state there are negligible activated receptors present. In transgenic animals, however, where receptors may be overexpressed more than 1000-fold, there is a greater probability of activated receptors existing in the absence of agonist. According to this theory, agonists bind selectively to stabilize the activated state, and thus the equilibrium is driven towards the right. Antagonists would bind equally to both states, thus promoting the default position of the great majority of receptors being in the inactive state and also preventing an agonist from disturbing this equilibrium. Inverse agonists would bind selectively to the inactive form of the receptor, thus having the opposite effect to an agonist.

CONCENTRATION–RESPONSE RELATIONSHIPS

The binding of a drug to a receptor is necessary for the transmission of the signal. There may be an increase or a decrease in activity of a second-messenger system or a blockade of effect, depending on the substance binding to the receptors. Although consideration has been given to the theoretical interaction between ligands and receptors, such receptor theories may not fully explain the amount of drug that would be required for a given effect. Drugs may fall into a number of different categories with respect to their interactions with receptors.

- **Agonist** An agonist is a ligand or drug that binds to a receptor and causes activation. In an adequate concentration it can cause maximal activation of all receptors (a full agonist). According to the theories above, an agonist alone should completely stabilize the activated form such that in sufficient concentration the reaction would be driven totally to the right and 100% response can be obtained by occupying all receptors (Fig. 7.6).
- **Potency** When considering agonists, the term potency is used to differentiate between different agonists that activate the same receptor and which can all produce the same maximal response, but which do so at different concentrations (Fig. 7.7). The most potent drug of a series has the lowest K_D, and vice versa.

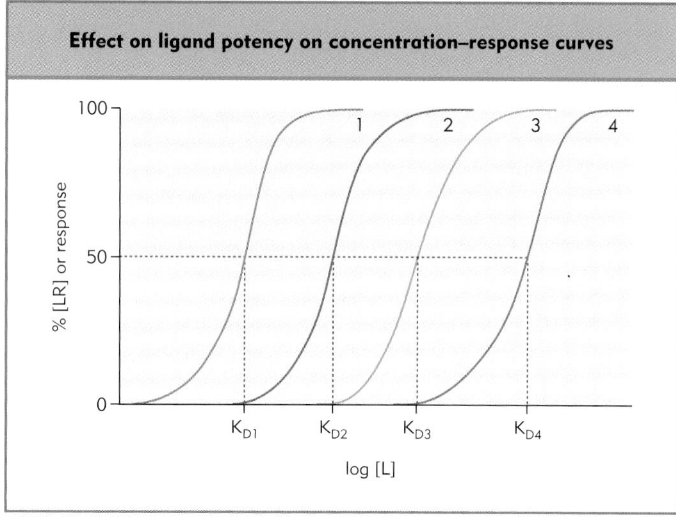

Figure 7.7 Effect of agonist (drug, ligand) potency on concentration–response curves. All are identical, parallel sigmoid curves. They are all capable of producing the same 100% response and differ only in potency. Drug 1 is the most potent and has the smallest K_D, whereas drug 4 is the least potent and has the highest K_D.

- **Affinity** The affinity of a drug is its ability to bind to the receptor. It can be calculated as $1/K_D$.
- **Efficacy** The efficacy of a drug is its ability to produce the appropriate change in the receptor, which leads to stimulation or propagation of the signal. It refers to the maximum possible effect that can be achieved with that drug (Fig. 7.8). The term *intrinsic activity* is often used instead of efficacy, although this more accurately describes the relative maximum effect obtained when comparing compounds in a series. Efficacy may be due to the extent to which an agonist produces the appropriate conformational changes within the receptor/gating molecule.

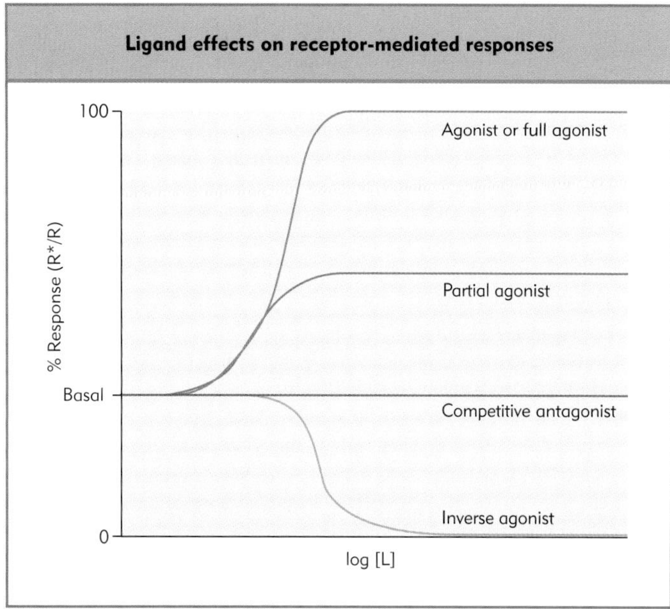

Figure 7.6 Ligand (drug) effects on receptor-mediated responses.

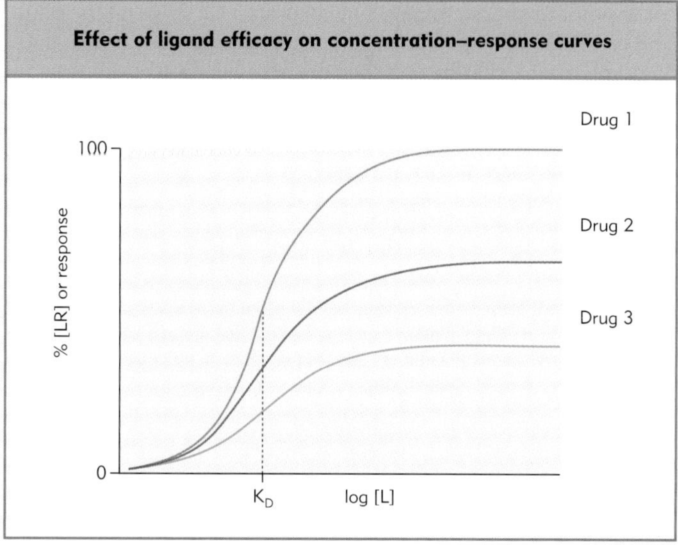

Figure 7.8 Effect of efficacy on concentration–response curves. All three drugs are equipotent, as the curves are not shifted to the left or to the right and they all have the same K_D. Drug 1 is the most efficacious and drug 3 the least.

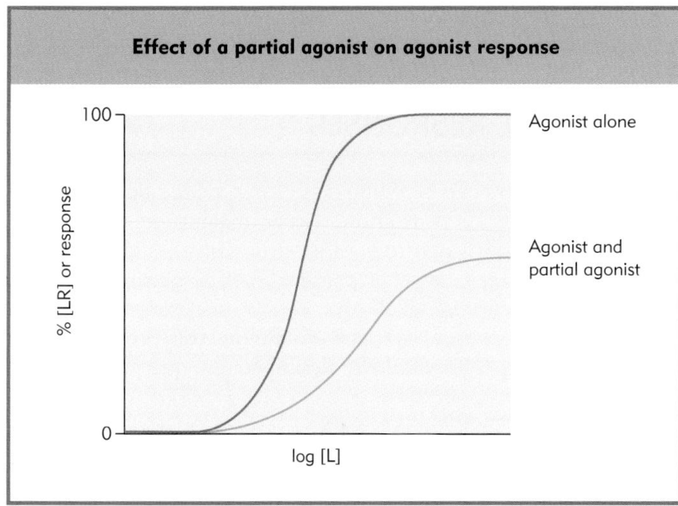

Figure 7.9 Effect of agonist in presence of a partial agonist. A full agonist alone will produce 100% response. The addition of a partial agonist reduces the maximal possible response to the agonist. The responses at lower concentrations of agonist depend on the concentration of partial agonist. In the example illustrated, the concentration of partial agonist is sufficient to produce an effect even in the absence of full agonist.

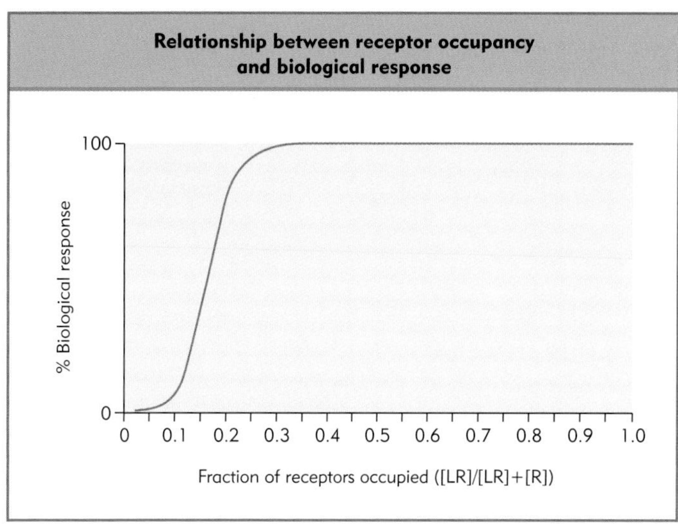

Figure 7.10 The relationship between receptor occupancy and biological response. In this example maximal response can be obtained with only about one-third of the receptors occupied. Further addition of agonist beyond this point will cause more receptors to be occupied, but the response cannot be further increased beyond 100%.

- **Partial agonist** A partial agonist activates a receptor but cannot produce a maximum response (Fig. 7.6). It may also be able to block (at least partially) the effects of a full agonist (Fig. 7.9). It has been postulated that partial agonists possess both agonist and antagonist actions, and the term 'dualist' or 'agonist–antagonist' has been used. A partial agonist has a lower efficacy than a full agonist.
- **Inverse agonist** These substances produce effects opposite to that of an agonist (Fig. 7.6). They appear to bind preferentially to the inactivated receptor to stabilize the system. They may under some circumstances have a theoretical advantage over antagonists in situations where a disease state is partly due to an upregulation of receptor activity, such that there is an increased probability of the activated form of receptor at resting state.
- **Allostery** Proteins are dynamic structures that can alter their structural conformation depending on state of activation, surrounding proteins, etc. This ability is described as allostery. The binding of one ligand or entity may affect the subsequent binding of another, identical or different substance. Recent evidence suggests that this may result from there being several graded states between inactivated and activated, rather than an all-or-none response with just two forms of the receptor.
- **Spare receptor concept** The relationship between the number of receptors stimulated and the response is usually nonlinear. A maximal, or almost maximal, response can often be produced by activation of fewer than all of the receptors present (Fig. 7.10). A good example can be found in the neuromuscular junction. Occupation of over 70% of the receptors by antagonist molecules is necessary before there is a reduction in response, implying that a maximal response is obtained by activation of only 30% of the total number of receptors.
- **Tolerance** Individual variation can result in a situation where an unusually large concentration of drug is required to produce the response. The usual reason for this is chronic exposure to the agonist, and the result is tolerance or tachyphylaxis. The underlying mechanism in many cases may not be clear. Common causes include enzyme induction, depleted neurotransmitter, protein conformational changes, and changes in gene expression.

Antagonists

An antagonist is a substance that inhibits or blocks the action of an agonist. Antagonism may be competitive or noncompetitive, reversible or irreversible. It may or may not take place at the same receptor, and may involve more than one process simultaneously.

Competitive antagonists compete with agonists for a common receptor-binding site. The extent of the competitive antagonism is dependent upon the concentration of agonist and its dissociation constant, and also upon the concentration of antagonist and its dissociation constant. In the presence of the competitive inhibitor, the fractional occupation of receptor by agonist will decrease. Because the nature of the interactions is competitive, increasing the concentration of agonist can still produce the same maximum response as in the absence of the antagonist. A large excess of agonist favors a normal response. A plot of the log dose of agonist against response in the presence of a competitive antagonist also produces a sigmoid curve which is parallel and displaced to the right (Fig. 7.11a). Increasing the concentration of competitive antagonist shifts the curve further to the right.

Noncompetitive antagonists attach to the receptor, or to a nearby group, and prevent the receptor from initiating the response, whether or not it is activated. The antagonist does not necessarily alter the ability of the agonist to combine with the receptor, and agonist can therefore combine with either normal or inactivated receptor. The presence of the antagonist has therefore effectively reduced the number of available receptors, and because the response depends upon the number of receptors activated, the maximum possible response is reduced (Fig. 7.11b). The more noncompetitive antagonist that is present, the greater will be the reduction in possible maximum response. The drug should still be combining with the receptor (whether normal or inactivated) with the same affinity (K_D is the same). The EC_{50}

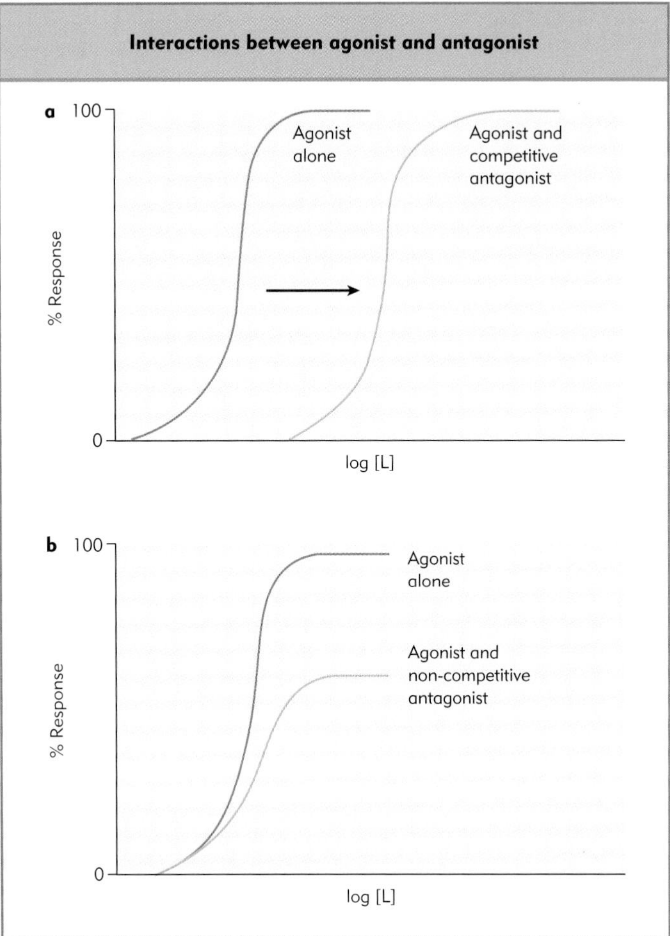

Figure 7.11 Interactions between agonists and antagonists. In the case of a competitive antagonist the curve is shifted to the right in a parallel fashion. The maximum possible response remains the same, but a higher concentration of drug is required in the presence of antagonist. A noncompetitive antagonist will reduce the maximum possible response to the agonist.

remains the same, although it is 50% of a different maximum from the situation pertaining in the absence of antagonist. Increasing the concentration of agonist will have no effect on the maximum response obtainable. Plots of the response against log dose of agonist produce a family of curves similar to those in Figure 7.11b. It can be seen that graphical analysis can be used to discriminate easily between competitive and noncompetitive antagonism.

If the antagonist reacts in an irreversible manner with the receptor the receptors will be permanently removed from the pool. This is irreversible antagonism. Under these circumstances it may be necessary to await the manufacture of new receptors. In the meantime, a normal log dose–response relationship is seen, but the maximum possible response will be less. A family of curves similar to those in Figure 7.11b for a noncompetitive antagonist will result.

It is possible for antagonism to result from a mechanism unrelated to block of drug receptors. Examples might be the inhibition of a second-messenger system which is activated by the receptor, or alteration in cellular excitability by another means. This type of antagonism is sometimes referred to as physiological antagonism. It also must be remembered that it is possible for some antagonists not to act by one mechanism alone, but by several different mechanisms simultaneously.

BIOLOGICAL RESPONSES

Responses to drugs can be defined as either graded or quantal. In a graded response there is an increasing magnitude of response with increasing dose of drug. Most drugs possess this type of action. In some cases, however, there is an all-or-nothing response where, once a certain level of receptor occupancy has been exceeded, the response is triggered. Below the threshold, the response is absent. This would be described as a quantal response.

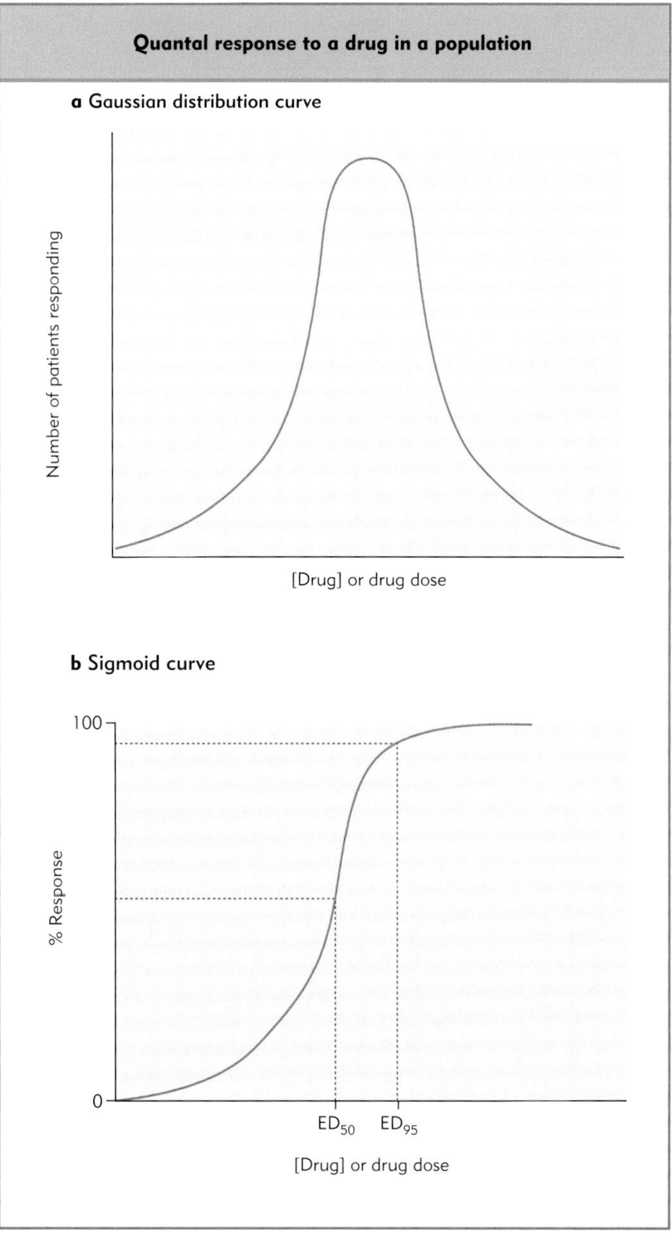

Figure 7.12 Quantal drug responses. (a) Gaussian distribution curve describing a normal quantal dose–response relationship. (b) The result of transforming the data by plotting the cumulative percentage response (number of patients responding) against the dose. The effective dose in 50% of patients (the ED_{50}) can be readily determined.

The nature of the drug interaction with the receptor may itself be described as quantal, as the receptor is either occupied by drug or not. It is the nature of the response of the organism to the presence of drug that is being considered here, though, and if the response increases with increasing receptor occupancy, then it is a graded response, irrespective of the nature if the interaction at molecular level.

Quantal responses are subject to individual variations, whereby different concentrations of a drug will be required to trigger the response in different individuals. The frequency of the response in the population then becomes the important variable in describing quantal effects. When the number of individuals (e.g. patients) who respond is plotted against the concentration (dose) of drug to trigger that response, a population distribution type of graph is produced which might or might not be gaussian in nature (Fig. 7.12a). Such graphs are very difficult to use and to define mathematically, and do not lend themselves to routine use in pharmacology. If the relationship is replotted in the form of cumulative percentage response against dose, however, a sigmoid curve results (Fig. 7.12b) which resembles the log dose–response curve described above. This is much easier to manipulate and is linear between the points of 20% and 80%, allowing ED_{50} etc. to be determined, although in clinical practice this is now the effective dose at which 50% of the patients respond to the drug in the defined manner. If the basic population distribution curve has resulted in a skewed distribution, then it may be necessary to convert the dose axis to its logarithm to produce a sigmoid curve.

Most drug responses are graded in nature, for example the effect of epinephrine on heart rate. As the dose is increased, the heart rate rises. An example of a quantal response might be the dose of induction agent to produce loss of consciousness. Perhaps the classic quantal response is mortality. In animal studies this is regularly used in safety studies of a new drug, where the dose is steadily increased and mortality is the measured outcome, allowing the dose to produce 50% mortality (the LD_{50}) to be determined. If the ED_{50} can also be determined, one of the basic pharmacological standards, the therapeutic index, can be determined, which is the ratio of the ED_{50} to the LD_{50}. The higher the therapeutic index, the safer the drug. In the context of clinical studies, the true therapeutic index related to mortality cannot, of course, be measured, and so the appearance of a predefined unwanted effect (again a quantal response) is used as a surrogate for the lethal dose in place of the actual LD_{50}.

Key references

Clarke AJ. The reaction between acetylcholine and muscle cells. J Physiol. 1926;61:530–46.

Clarke AJ. The reaction between acetylcholine and muscle cells. Part II. J Physiol. 1927;64:123–43.

Clarke AJ. The factors determining tolerance of glucosides of the digitalis series. J Pharmacol Exp Ther. 1913;4:399–424.

Ehrlich P. On immunity with special reference to cell life. Proc Roy Soc Lond B. 1900;66:424–48.

Langley JN. On the contraction of muscle chiefly in relation to the presence of receptive substances. Part 4. The effect of curari and of some other substances on the nicotine response of the sartorius and gastrocnemius muscles of the frog. J Physiol. 1909;39:235–95.

Langley JN. On the physiology of salivary secretion. Part II. On the mutual antagonism of atropin and pilocarpin, having special reference to their relations in the sub-maxillary gland of the cat. J Physiol. 1878;1:339–69.

Langley JN. Croonian Lecture 1906. On nerve endings and on special excitable substances in cells. Proc Roy Soc Lond B. 1906;78:170–94.

Paton WDM. A theory of drug action based on the rate of drug–receptor combination. Proc Roy Soc Lond B. 1961;154:21–69.

Further reading

Ross EM. Pharmacodynamics. In: Hardman JG, Limbird LE, Molinoff PB, Ruddon RW, Gilman AG, eds. The pharmacological basis of therapeutics, 9th edn. New York: McGraw-Hill;1996:24–41.

Chapter 8

Pharmacokinetic principles

Steven L Shafer

TOPICS COVERED IN THIS CHAPER

- **The physiologic basis of pharmacokinetics**
    - Volume of distribution
    - Clearance
    - Protein binding
    - Stereochemistry
- **Mathematical principles of compartmental pharmacokinetics**
    - Zero and first order processes
    - Bolus pharmacokinetics
    - Infusion pharmacokinetics
    - Absorption pharmacokinetics
    - Multicompartment pharmacokinetics
    - Plasma-effect site equilibration
- **Clinical application of pharmacokinetics**
    - Onset of drug effect
    - Maintenance of drug effect
    - Offset of drug effect

Pharmacokinetics is the study of how drugs are distributed in the plasma and tissues, and how they are eliminated from the body. Pharmacodynamics relates drug concentration to drug effect. The fundamental principle of pharmacokinetics is that the time course of drug administration, which includes the dose, rate and route of administration, determines the concentration of drug in the plasma, which then determines the concentration of drug at the site of drug effect, called the 'biophase.' In turn, the time course of drug in the biophase determines the time course of the pharmacodynamic response. This chapter will address pharmacokinetics from three perspectives: the physiological basis of pharmacokinetics, mathematical relationships for the pharmacokinetic models relevant to the intravenous drugs used in clinical anesthesia, and how pharmacokinetic principles and mathematical models can be used clinically to optimize pharmacotherapy in the perioperative period.

THE PHYSIOLOGIC BASIS OF PHARMACOKINETICS

Volume and clearance are the fundamental physiological concepts of pharmacokinetics. Volume represents the dilution of drug as it is progressively distributed among the blood and body tissues. Clearance is the process by which drug is transferred between tissues or removed from the body.

The volume of distribution (Figure 8.1A) is readily envisioned as the dilution of drug into body fluids and tissues. The volume of distribution follows from the definition of concentration:

■ Equation 8.1

$$\text{Concentration} = \frac{\text{amount}}{\text{volume}}$$

By simply measuring the concentration of drug in the body, one can readily calculate the volume of distribution from the dose administered by rearranging Equation 1:

■ Equation 8.2

$$\text{Volume} = \frac{\text{amount (or dose)}}{\text{concentration}}$$

Volume and clearance are fundamental concepts in pharmacokinetics: volume represents the dilution of drug into fluids and tissues, and clearance is the flow of blood or plasma that is completely cleared of drug.

The traditional definition of clearance is the flow of blood or plasma that is completely cleared of drug. This can be envisioned as the flow of drug to an organ that completely removes drug (Figure 8.1B). For a drug like propofol, Figure 8.1B is an accurate representation of clearance, because the liver removes nearly all of the propofol delivered. Thus, propofol clearance is the same as liver blood flow. However, for other drugs the liver only removes a fraction of the drug delivered. For example, the liver removes about half of the fentanyl delivered, such that fentanyl clearance is about half of liver blood flow. The extraction ratio is the amount of drug removed by an organ per unit time, divided by the total amount of drug delivered. The hepatic extraction

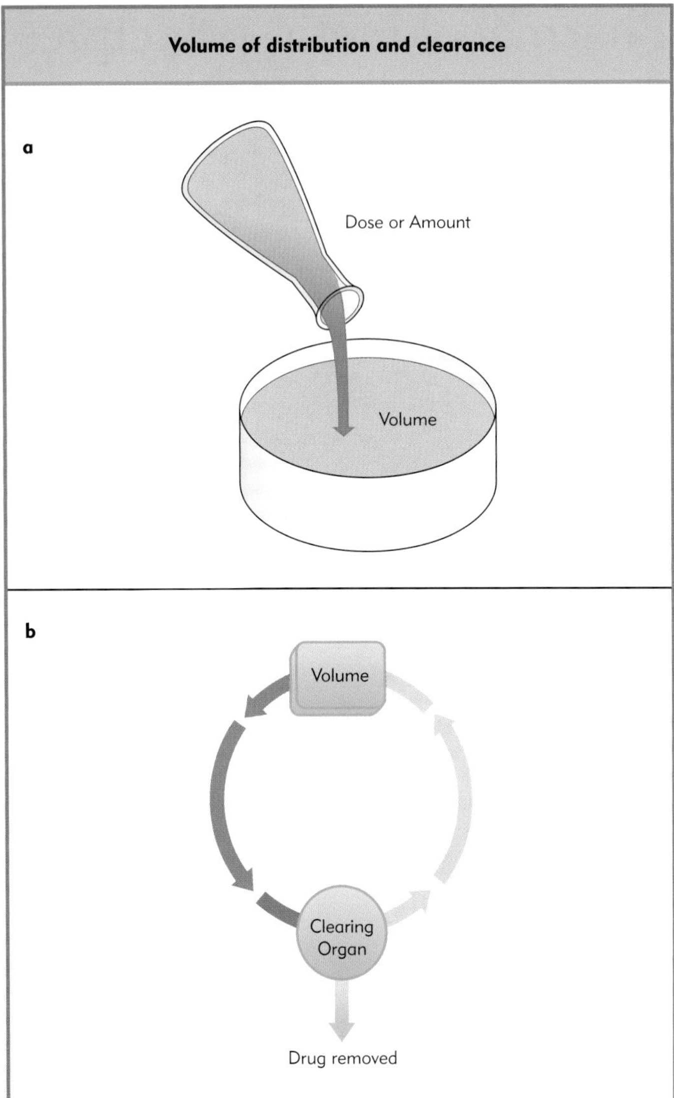

Figure 8.1 Volume of distribution and clearance. A, The volume of distribution is the apparent volume into which the drug has been diluted, based on the initial concentration. **B,** Clearance, represented as the plasma flow to a tissue that completely eliminates the drug. The more general view of clearance is the flow to the clearing organ times the fraction of drug extracted.

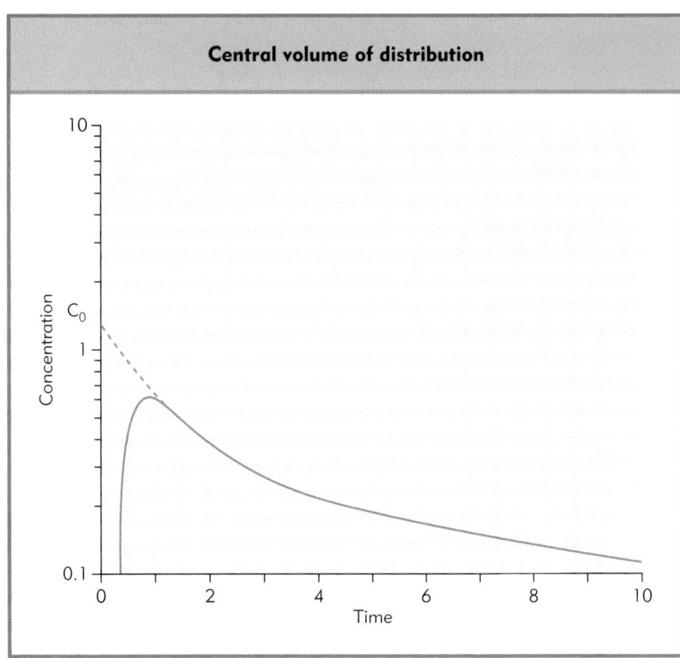

Figure 8.2 The central volume. This is based on the erroneous concept that the highest drug levels following bolus injection occur instantly. The peak at time 0, C_0, is never actually measured, but is the extrapolation (dashed line) of measurements made at subsequent times. The actual concentrations resemble the solid line, and include an initial transport delay.

ratio of propofol is nearly 1, while the hepatic extraction ratio of fentanyl is closer to 0.5.

Volume of distribution

CENTRAL VOLUME OF DISTRIBUTION

The central volume represents the dilution volume at the instant the drug is introduced into the plasma. Returning to Equation 8.2, if concentration is measured right after a bolus injection of drug, then the volume calculated by Equation 8.2 is the central volume of distribution. This would typically represent the blood volume of the upper arm, heart, and great vessels, as well as any uptake into the pulmonary parenchyma prior to the blood reaching the arterial circulation.

The concept of the central volume is based on a notion that the plasma concentration instantaneously peaks at time 0 following a bolus injection, and then continuously declines, as shown in the dotted line in Figure 8.2, where C_0 is the peak at time 0. Of course, the actual concentration in the blood at the instant drug is injected is 0, because it takes time for the drug to travel from the injection site to the sampling site. The solid line in Figure 8.2 shows the true time course of concentration following intravenous injection, where there is a delay between the moment of the injection (at time 0) and when drug appears at the sampling site. To accurately describe the first few minutes after injection requires a model such as that shown in Figure 8.3. The standard compartmental model adequately describes the concentrations from roughly 30 seconds onwards, but fails miserably prior to that. But it is so mathematically simple compared to the recirculatory model shown in Figure 8.3, we will use it for our pharmacokinetic analysis.

Central volume is highly influenced by many factors, including study design, the site of blood sampling (arterial samples yield higher concentrations, and hence smaller volumes, than venous samples) and timing of samples (samples drawn near the arterial peak at 30-45 seconds yield high concentrations, and hence smaller central volumes of distribution). Central compartment volume is also influenced by pulmonary uptake and lipophilicity. Highly lipophilic drugs (e.g. sufentanil) show relatively lower concentrations, and hence larger central volumes, then less lipophilic drugs (e.g. alfentanil).

PERIPHERAL VOLUMES OF DISTRIBUTION

Most anesthetic drugs distribute extensively into peripheral tissues. These appear as peripheral volumes of distribution, linked to the central compartment by 'intercompartmental clearance'. Typically multicompartment models for anesthetic drugs link each peripheral compartment to the central compartment.

The size of the peripheral volumes of distribution reflects the tissue solubility of a drug relative to the solubility in blood or

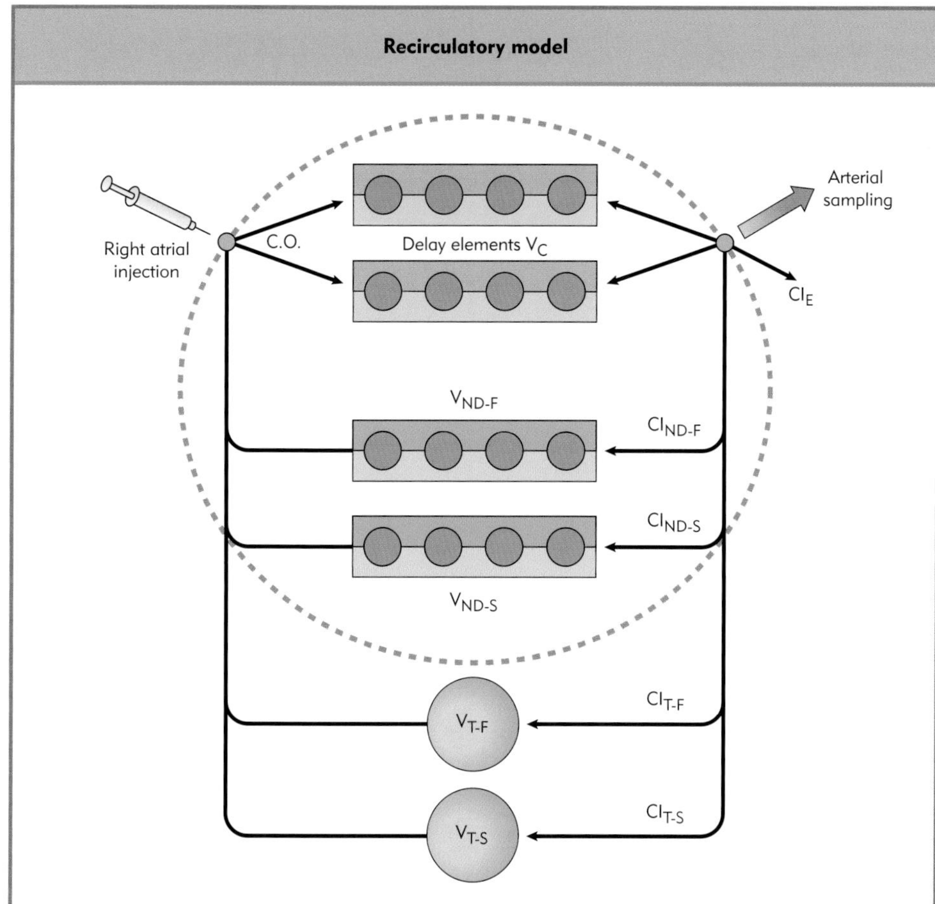

Figure 8.3 A recirculatory model accounting for the transit delays, pulmonary uptake, and initial mixing in the first minute after drug administration. Accurate modeling of the central volume of distribution requires all of the components within the circle. V, volume; Cl, clearance; C.O., cardiac output; E, elimination; ND-F, fast non-distribution; ND-S, slow non-distribution; T-F, fast tissue; T-S, slow tissue. (Adapted from Krejcie et al. J Pharmac Exp Ther 1994; 269:609-616. Copyright © 1994 by American Society for Pharmacology and Experimental Theories.)

plasma. Because we typically do not know the solubility of drugs in peripheral tissues, we assume that the solubility everywhere is the same as in plasma, and that the concentration at steady state in all compartments is the same. While not technically accurate, this simplifying assumption does not compromise our ability to understand or use pharmacokinetics to predict drug behavior. However, it can lead to volumes of distribution that vastly exceed total body volume for drugs that are highly lipid soluble (e.g. propofol's total volume of distribution is thousands of liters). Changes in body habitus and composition influence peripheral volumes of distribution. For example, lipid solubility predicts the volume of distribution for benzodiazepines, which explains the increase in volume of distribution and duration of drug effect in elderly patients.

Volume of distribution at steady state: During an intravenous infusion, the concentration eventually comes to steady state, where the rate of metabolism equals the infusion rate. The concentration of drug in the plasma reflects the dilution of drug into the volume of distribution at steady state (Vd_{ss}) defined as:

■ Equation 8.3

$$Vd_{ss} = \frac{X_{\text{total drug}}}{C_{\text{plasma}}}$$

where $X_{\text{total drug}}$ is the total amount of drug in the body. Vd_{ss} is the mathematical sum of the central volume and the peripheral volumes of distribution, based on the assumption that the concentration in all compartments at steady state is the same.

Clearance

HEPATIC CLEARANCE

Biotransformation of drugs typically reduces the lipophilicity, resulting in metabolites that are more likely to be excreted by the kidney, or discharged into the intestine. Biotransformation reactions occur in nearly all tissues, but the main site is the liver. There are two types of biotransformation reactions: those that expose a linking group, called 'Phase I' reactions, and those that then add a water-soluble moiety to the drug, called 'Phase II' reactions (Fig. 8.4).

The linking groups exposed in a Phase I reaction are typically oxygen or nitrogen. For some drugs this is accomplished by cleaving the molecule to expose the oxygen (O-dealkylation) or nitrogen (N-dealkylation), or altering an existing oxygen to increase reactivity (deamination). Alternatively, this may be accomplished by adding an OH group (aliphatic hydroxylation, aromatic hydroxylation, N-oxidation) or a double bonded oxygen (S-oxidation). The phase I reactions are often catalyzed by cytochrome P 450 ('CYP') enzymes present in the endoplasmic reticulum. Of these, the most important is CYP 3A4, which is responsible for the metabolism of over half of all drugs, including many intravenous drugs used in anesthesia (fentanyl, alfentanil, sufentanil, methadone, midazolam, triazolam, alprazolam, diazepam, droperidol, lidocaine, bupivacaine, ondansetron), and CYP 2D6, which catalyzes the conversion of codeine, a prodrug, into morphine, codeine's active metabolite. CYP 3A4 is induced by rifampin, glucocorticoids, barbiturates, phenytoin, carba-

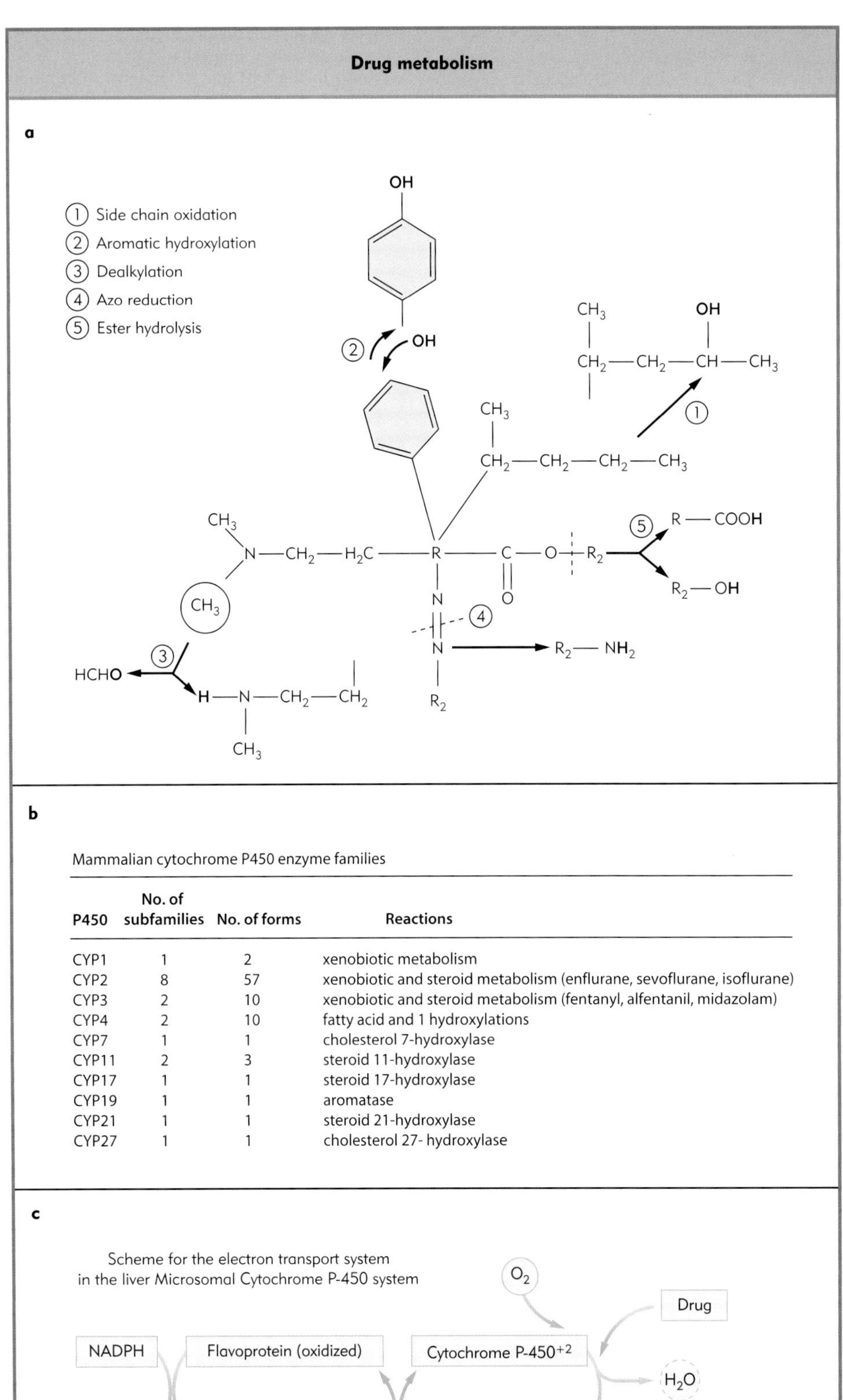

Mammalian cytochrome P450 enzyme families

P450	No. of subfamilies	No. of forms	Reactions
CYP1	1	2	xenobiotic metabolism
CYP2	8	57	xenobiotic and steroid metabolism (enflurane, sevoflurane, isoflurane)
CYP3	2	10	xenobiotic and steroid metabolism (fentanyl, alfentanil, midazolam)
CYP4	2	10	fatty acid and 1 hydroxylations
CYP7	1	1	cholesterol 7-hydroxylase
CYP11	2	3	steroid 11-hydroxylase
CYP17	1	1	steroid 17-hydroxylase
CYP19	1	1	aromatase
CYP21	1	1	steroid 21-hydroxylase
CYP27	1	1	cholesterol 27- hydroxylase

Figure 8.4 Drug metabolism. A, Types of phase 1 biotransformation reactions. **B,** Mammalian cytochrome P450 enzyme families. **C,** Scheme for the electron transport system in the liver microsomal P_{450} system.

d

Localization of phase I and phase II reactions of drug and xenobiotic metabolism in the liver (with examples from anesthetic practice)

Phase I	
Oxidation - mainly in the smooth endoplasmic reticulum	
Aliphatic hydroxylation	Thiopental, methohexital, meperidine, ketamine
Aromatic hydroxylation	Lidocaine, bupivacaine, mepivacaine, fentanyl, propranolol
Epoxidation	Phenytoin
O-dealkylation	Pancuronium
N- dealkylation	Ephedrine, amide local anesthetics, ketamine, fentanyl, morphine, atropine, diazepam
N-oxidation	Morphine, meperidine
S-oxidation	Chlorpromazine
Oxidative deamination	Epinephrine amphetamine
Desulphuration	Thiopental
Dehalogenation	Halothane, enflurane, sevoflurane
Reduction mainly in the cytoplasm	
Nitroreduction	Nitrazepam, dantrolene
Carbonyl reduction	Warfarin
Alcohol dehydrogenase	Chloral hyrate, ethanol
Hydrolysis mainly in the cytoplasm	
Ester linkage breakdown	Procaine, cocaine, succinylcholine, propanidid, pancuronium, atracurium, mivacurium, esmolol, remifentanil
Phase II: in both cytosol and endoplasmic reticulum	
Glucuronidation	
O-glucuronides	Morphine, lorazepam, propofol,
N-glucuronides	diazepam
Sulphation	Morphine, steroid hormones
Acetylation	Procainamide, hydralazine
Methylation	Morphine, norepinephrine
Amino acid conjugation	Salicylic acid (with glycine)
Glutathione conjugation	Acetaminophen

Figure 8.4, cont'd D, Phase 1 and phase 2 reactions.

mazepine, and St. John's Wort, and is inhibited by macrolide antibiotics (e.g. erythromycin, and troleandomycin), and the azole class of antifungals (e.g. ketoconazole). Grapefruit juice inhibits CYP 3A4 in the intestinal mucosa, increasing the bioavailability of CYP 3A4 substrates taken orally, but has no effect on systemic clearance of drugs because it does not affect CYP 3A4 in the liver. Although oxidation and reduction typically are catalyzed by the cytochrome P-450 system, there are notable exceptions, such as aldehyde oxidase, peroxidase, azoreductase, nitroreductase, and alcohol dehydrogenase. Hydrolysis of esters (e.g. etomidate and remifentanil), and amides is a phase I reaction that is typically not catalyzed by a P450 system.

The Phase I step may be followed by a second reaction, called (as expected) the Phase II step. In the Phase II reaction, the drug undergoes conjugation, typically by glucuronic acid, acetate, glutathione, sulfate, or an amino acid. Often this step will mask an existing functional group on the drug. The effect of conjugation is to transform hydrophobic molecules into water soluble molecules through addition of polar groups. Conjugation usually occurs in the cytosol, rather than through the P-450 system, although glucuronidation can involve the P-450 system as well. Some anesthetic drugs are primarily deactivated through conjugation without first undergoing a phase I biotransformation. For example. propofol and morphine are both cleared by glucuronidation.

Hepatic metabolism is responsible for the systemic clearance of nearly all intravenous anesthetic drugs. In general, the rate of hepatic metabolism is proportional to drug concentration, and clearance is constant over the range of concentrations used clinically. Constant clearance is a fundamental assumption of 'linear' pharmacokinetics. Simply stated, linear pharmacokinetics means that if the the dose is doubled, the concentration doubles. This is such an important concept that we will explore clearance in detail, understanding why it is that clearance for anesthetic drugs is constant, and metabolism is proportional to concentration, even though metabolism is intrinsically saturable.

Hepatic metabolism is responsible for the systemic clearance of nearly all intravenous drugs used in anesthesia.

The rate of hepatic metabolism, R, can be calculated as the concentration difference between the drug flowing into and out of the liver the liver, times the rate of blood flow:

■ Equation 8.4

$$\text{Rate of drug metabolism} = R = Q(C_{inflow} - C_{outflow})$$

where Q = hepatic blood flow (about 1.4 L/min in an adult), C_{inflow} is drug concentration in arterial blood perfusing the liver, and $C_{outflow}$ is drug concentration in venous blood draining the liver (Figure 8.5).

The concentration of drug flowing out of the liver can be related to intrinsic hepatic metabolic capacity:

■ Equation 8.5

$$\text{Rate of drug metabolism} = R = Q(C_{inflow} - C_{outflow}) = Vm\frac{C_{outflow}}{Km + C_{outflow}}$$

where Vm is the maximal rate of metabolism and Km is the $C_{outflow}$ that yields metabolism at 50% of the maximum rate (Vm) (Figure 8.6).

Metabolism increases linearly with concentration when the outflow concentration is less than ½ of Km, which is the basis of linear pharmacokinetics. Since at concentrations used clinically $C_{outflow} < ½\, Km$ for all drugs used in anesthesia, anesthetic drugs have linear pharmacokinetics.

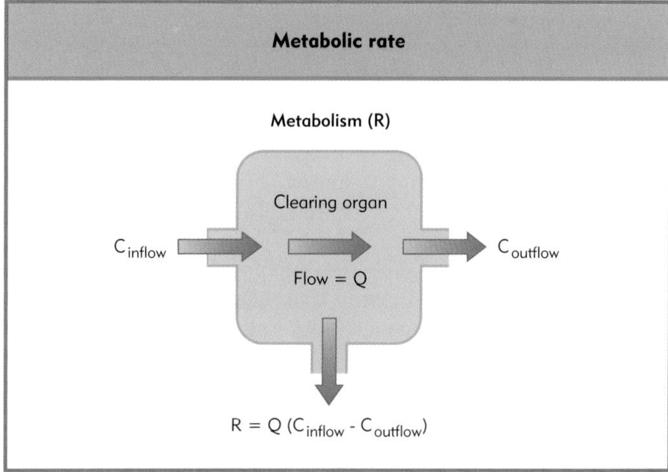

Figure 8.5 The metabolic rate can be calculated as the difference between the inflowing and outflowing concentrations times hepatic drug flow.

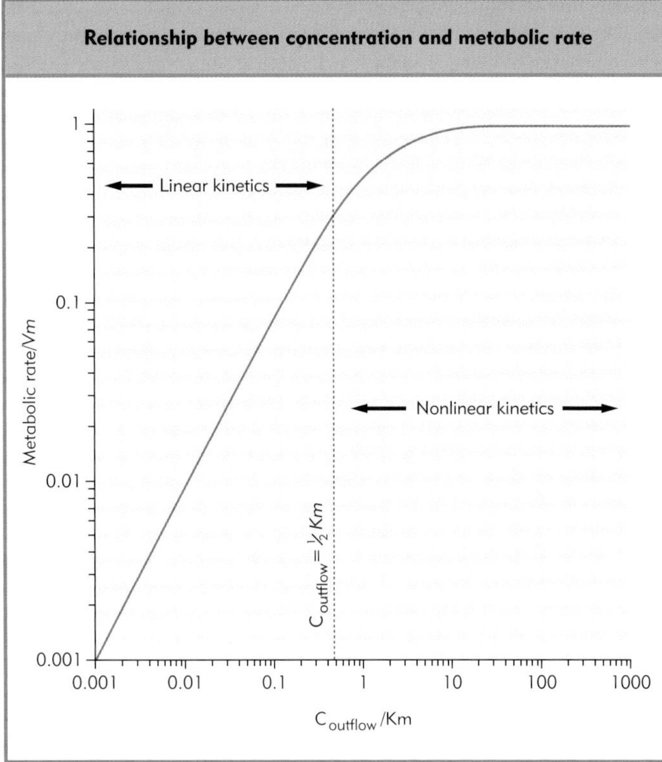

Figure 8.6 The relationship between concentration, in units of *Km*, and the rate of drug metabolism, in units of *Vm*. When the outflow concentration is less than ½ *Km*, a change in concentration is matched by a proportional change in metabolic rate. By normalizing $C_{outflow}$ to *Km* and the metabolic rate to *Vm*, the relationship is true for all values of *Vm* and *Km*. (Adapted from Longnecker DE, Tinker JH, Morgan GE Jr. Principles and Practice of Anesthesiology, 2nd Ed, Copyright © Mosby 1997.)

Hepatic clearance is the flow of blood or plasma that is entirely cleared of drug. Metabolism can be related to clearance by dividing Equation 8.5 by the inflow drug concentration:

■ Equation 8.6

$$\begin{aligned}\text{Clearance} &= \frac{\text{Rate of drug metabolism}}{C_{inflow}}\\ &= Q\,\frac{C_{inflow} - C_{outflow}}{C_{inflow}}\\ &= \frac{VmC_{outflow}}{C_{inflow}(Km + C_{outflow})}\end{aligned}$$

Thus clearance is the ratio of drug metabolism to inflow drug concentration (C_{inflow}), and is a measure of the efficiency of drug metabolism. If the liver is completely efficient, the rate of metabolism equals the rate at which drug flows into the liver, which equals $Q \times C_{inflow}$. Substituting $Q \times C_{inflow}$ for metabolism in Equation 8.6 demonstrates that clearance equals hepatic blood flow, Q, if the liver metabolizes all of the drug it sees.

Clearance is the blood flow times the extraction ratio.

The second relationship of Equation 8.6 introduces the extraction ratio: the fraction of drug flowing into the liver ($Q \times C_{inflow}$) that is extracted by the liver, $Q \times (C_{inflow} - C_{outflow})$. Thus, the extraction ratio is $\frac{C_{inflow} - C_{outflow}}{C_{inflow}}$, and therefore clearance can be expressed as the liver blood flow times the extraction ratio. Equation 8.6 can be rewritten as:

■ Equation 8.7

$$\begin{aligned}\text{Clearance} &= \frac{R}{C_{inflow}}\\ &= Q \times ER\\ &= \frac{VmC_{outflow}}{C_{inflow}(Km + C_{outflow})}\end{aligned}$$

where R is the rate of drug metabolism and ER is the extraction ratio. Solving this equation for the extraction ratio gives:

■ Equation 8.8

$$ER = \frac{Vm - R}{Vm + KmQ - R}$$

In the linear range (which applies to all anesthetic drugs at clinically used doses) R, the rate of metabolism, is much less than Vm, so the extraction ratio can be simplified to:

■ Equation 8.9

$$ER = \frac{Vm}{Vm + KmQ}$$

By definition *Km* is the venous drug concentration at which the metabolic rate is half maximal (i.e., ½ *Vm*). Thus, *Km* times Q is the flow of drug *from the liver,* in amount per unit time, when the liver is operating at half maximal metabolic rate. If *Km* times Q is small relative to *Vm*, then the enzymatic activity of the liver is fully engaged even when the concentration in the venous blood is very low. Put another way, a low *Km* × Q relative to *Vm* means that the liver metabolizes nearly all drug it sees, implying a high extraction ratio close to 1. If *Km* × Q is large relative to *Vm*, the enzymatic activity slows even while the venous blood still has high drug concentrations. Thus, a high *Km* × Q, relative to *Vm*, is associated with a low extraction ratio.

The liver removes nearly all the propofol delivered, resulting in an extraction ratio of nearly 1 (i.e. 100%). For drugs like propofol the metabolic clearance is simply liver blood flow. Consequently, any reduction in liver blood flow reduces clearance for drugs with high extraction ratios and such drugs are said to be 'flow dependent.' The capacity of the liver to metabolize 'flow dependent' drugs is much greater than the flow of drug to the liver at clinically relevant doses. Increases or decreases in hepatic function have little influence on flow-dependent drugs, unless liver blood flow changes as well.

For many drugs (e.g. alfentanil), the extraction ratio is considerably less than 1, and clearance is limited by the capacity of the liver to metabolize the drug ('capacity dependent'). Changes in liver blood flow have little effect on clearance of these drugs, since the liver metabolizes only a fraction of the drug it sees.

Drugs with high hepatic extraction ratios have *flow dependent* clearance, while those with low extraction ratios have *capacity dependent* clearance.

Figure 8.7A relates changes in clearance with changes in liver blood flow. For drugs with an extraction ratio of nearly 1 (e.g. propofol), clearance changes linearly with liver blood flow.

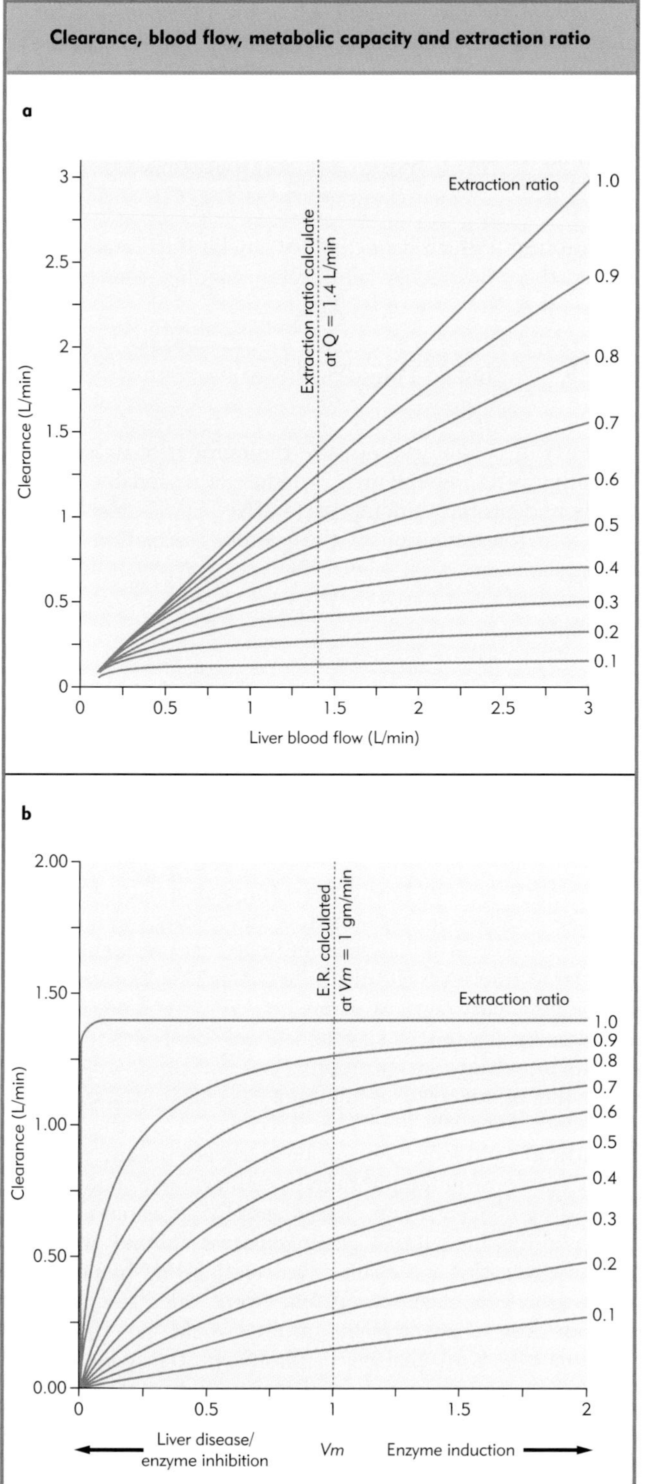

Figure 8.7 Relationships between clearance, blood flow, metabolic capacity and extraction ratio. A, Changes in clearance as a function of changes in liver blood flow for drugs with extraction ratios ranging from 0.1 to 1, calculated at an hepatic blood flow *(Q)* of 1.4 l/min. For drugs with high extraction ratios, clearance approximates liver blood flow, and changes accordingly with changes in liver blood flow. Drugs with low extraction ratios are relatively insensitive to changes in liver blood flow. **B,** Changes in *Vm* have little effect on drugs with a high extraction ratio, but cause a nearly proportional decrease in clearance for drugs with a low extraction ratio. (Adapted from Wilkinson GR, Shand DG. Commentary: a physiological approach to hepatic drug clearance. Clin Pharmacol Ther 18:377-390. Copyright 1975, with permission from the American Society for Clinical Pharmacology and Therapeutics.)

Drugs with a low extraction ratio (e.g. alfentanil) show almost no change in clearance with changes in liver blood flow. Figure 8.7B relates changes in clearance with changes in *Vm* (metabolic capacity). Changes in *Vm*, as might be caused by liver disease (reduced *Vm*) or enzymatic induction (increased *Vm*), have little effect on drugs with a high extraction ratio. However, drugs with a low extraction ratio have a nearly linear change in clearance with a change in intrinsic metabolic capacity *(Vm)*. Returning to Equation 8.7, when $C_{outflow}$ is much smaller than *Km*, clearance can be simplified to:

■ Equation 8.10

$$\text{Clearance} = \frac{C_{outflow}Vm}{C_{inflow}Km}$$

Combining Equations 8.8 and 8.10 we can develop an explicit derivation of clearance in the linear range:

■ Equation 8.11

$$\text{Clearance} = \frac{VmQ}{KmQ + Vm}$$

Because *Vm* and *Km* are often not known, it is useful to replace these by a single term that summarizes the hepatic metabolic capacity, the 'intrinsic clearance'. Consider what happens if hepatic blood flow increases to infinity with no change in hepatic metabolic capacity. Since the finite capacity of the liver could only metabolize an infinitesimal fraction of the drug were hepatic blood flow infinite, $C_{outflow}$ becomes indistinguishable from C_{inflow}. In the setting of infinite hepatic blood flow, clearance becomes $\frac{Vm}{Km + C_{inflow}}$. By definition, if $C_{inflow} = 0$ pharmacokinetics are in the linear range and clearance $= \frac{Vm}{Km}$. This is the intrinsic clearance, Cl_{int}. From this we can calculate (derivation not shown) that intrinsic clearance is directly related to the extraction ratio:

■ Equation 8.12

$$\text{Extraction ratio} = \frac{Cl_{int}}{Q + Cl_{int}}$$

and hepatic clearance:

■ Equation 8.13

$$\text{Hepatic clearance} = \frac{Q\ Cl_{int}}{Q + Cl_{int}}$$

RENAL CLEARANCE

The kidneys use two mechanisms to clear drugs: filtration at the glomerulus, and excretion into the tubules. Renal blood flow is inversely correlated with age, as is creatinine clearance, which can be predicted from age and weight according to the equation of Cockroft and Gault (value for women is 85% of this):

■ Equation 8.14

$$\text{Creatinine clearance (ml/min)} = \frac{(140 - \text{age (yr)}) \times \text{weight (kg)}}{72 \times \text{serum creatinine (mg\%)}}$$

Even with normal serum creatinine concentrations the creatinine clearance is substantially decreased in elderly patients. Nearly all intravenous drugs used in anesthetic practice are cleared by the liver or in the plasma (e.g. esters). The exception is pancuronium, which is about 85% renally excreted, such that its dose must be reduced in elderly patients, *even in the presence of normal serum creatinine.*

Age is an independent predictor of creatinine clearance.

DISTRIBUTION CLEARANCE

Distribution clearance is the transfer of drug between the blood or plasma and peripheral tissues. It reflects tissue blood flow and the permeability of capillaries and tissues to the drug. For a drug which readily crosses into peripheral tissues, such as propofol (a lipophilic anesthetic), the sum of metabolic clearance and distribution clearance approaches cardiac output. For drugs which are metabolized directly in the plasma, such as succinylcholine and remifentanil, the sum of metabolic and distribution clearance can exceed cardiac output. Distribution clearance depends on regional blood flow, which in turn is a function of cardiac output. Decreases in cardiac output decrease distribution clearance and increase plasma concentrations.

The distribution clearance reflects, at least in part, the lipophilicity of a drug. Since drugs need to pass through lipid membranes to reach their site of pharmacological activity, most drugs are at last partly lipophilic. Most anesthetic drugs are highly lipophilic, promoting passage of the drugs across the blood–brain barrier.

Distribution clearance is also affected by specialized transporters. In general, anesthetics move by passive diffusion, rather than transport systems. The exception is morphine, which is actively removed from the CNS by the transporter P-glycoprotein. This accounts for the unusually slow onset of morphine drug effect.

In the case of local anesthetics, the lipophilicity is partly determined by whether the drug is protonated. To provide adequate shelf-life, local anesthetics are typically provided in an acid vehicle with a pH of around 4, where nearly all of the drug is protonated. Since it is the un-ionized form that crosses the cell wall, the transfer of local anesthetics into the nerve, and hence the onset of neural blockade, can be enhanced by first alkalinizing the solution.

Protein binding

Virtually all intravenous anesthetic drugs are reversibly bound to plasma proteins. Generally, acidic drugs (e.g. salicylates, barbiturates) bind to serum albumin, while basic drugs (e.g. fentanyl, diazepam, propranolol) also bind to globulins, lipoproteins and glycoproteins. Basic drugs also bind to acute-phase proteins such as α1-acid glycoprotein. Since the levels of these proteins vary with age and disease, this is a source of pharmacokinetic variation. Only free unbound drug can diffuse across lipid membranes. The relationship between drugs and their binding proteins can be described by the law of mass action:

■ Equation 8.15

$$[D] + [Sites] \underset{k_{off}}{\overset{k_{on}}{\rightleftharpoons}} [Bound\ Drug]$$

where [D] is free drug concentration, [Sites] is the concentration of *available unbound protein binding sites,* [Bound Drug] is the concentration of drug bound to plasma proteins, k_{on} is the rate constant for binding, and k_{off} is the rate constant for dissociation of bound drug. The above formula implies that the rate of formation of bound drug is:

■ Equation 8.16

$$\frac{d[Bound\ Drug]}{dt} = [D][Sites]k_{on} - [Bound\ Drug]k_{off}$$

At equilibrium (which happens very quickly) d[Bound Drug]/dt = 0, and there is no longer net protein binding. This permits us to solve for k, the ratio of k_{on}/k_{off}, as:

■ Equation 8.17

$$k = \frac{k_{on}}{k_{off}} = \frac{[Bound\ Drug]}{[D][Sites]}$$

It is nearly impossible to measure the number of unbound protein binding sites. The plasma protein is a reasonable surrogate for unbound protein binding sites, offset by a scalar that gets folded into the definition of the protein association rate constant, k_a:

■ Equation 8.18

$$k_a = \frac{k_{on}}{k_{off}} = \frac{[Bound\ drug]}{[D][Sites]}$$

We are often interested in the free fraction of drug, *f*:

■ Equation 8.19

$$f = \frac{[D]}{[Bound\ drug] + [D]}$$

For drugs that are not bound (free fraction = 1.0), there is no relationship between free fraction and protein concentration (Figure 8.8). For many anesthetic drugs that are highly protein bound (free fraction <20%), there is a nearly linear change in free fraction with changes in protein concentration. However, there is never greater than a proportional change in free fraction and thus free drug concentration.

Free (i.e. unbound) drug equilibrates between the plasma and the tissues. If protein binding is decreased, then the free drug concentration gradient increases between plasma and peripheral tissues. As a result equilibrium is achieved at a lower total plasma drug concentration. This gives the appearance that the drug has distributed into a larger *apparent* volume of distribution. However, this is a result of calculating Vd_{ss} based on total plasma drug concentration. If Vd_{ss} were calculated based on unbound drug concentrations, there would be virtually no change in Vd_{ss} with changes in plasma protein concentration, because only a trivial amount of the total free drug is in the plasma.

Decreases in protein binding may increase the clearance of drugs with low hepatic extraction ratios by increasing the driving gradient into the liver. However, for drugs with high hepatic extraction ratios, there will be no change since the liver metabolizes all of the drug it sees, regardless of whether it is bound or not.

Decreases in protein binding can increase clearance of drugs with low hepatic extraction ratios, and increase the apparent potency of a drug.

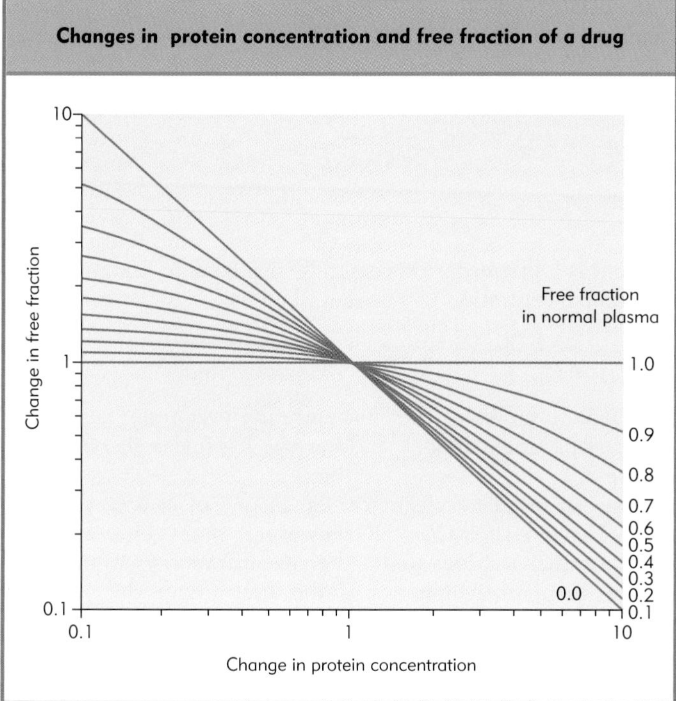

Figure 8.8 The relationship between changes in protein concentration and changes in free fraction of a drug. There is no change in free fraction with changing protein concentration for a drug that is not bound to plasma proteins (free fraction ≈ 1). However, for drugs that are highly protein bound, at typical clinical doses any change in protein causes a nearly inversely proportional change in free fraction.

Decreases in protein binding also increase the apparent potency of a drug. An increase in free fraction increases the driving pressure to the site of drug effect, and thus increases the concentration in the effect site. Thus, decreased protein binding may decrease the dose required to produce a given drug effect even in the absence of other pharmacokinetic changes.

Stereochemistry

Many anesthetic drugs are chiral, and are supplied as racemic mixtures (Chapter 1). Since the body is a chiral environment, enantiomers can have distinct pharmacokinetic and pharmacodynamic properties. For example, see the discussion of ketamine and etomidate in Chapters 24 and 25.

MATHEMATICAL PRINCIPLES OF COMPARTMENTAL PHARMACOKINETICS

Zero and first order processes

Many processes happen at a constant rate. These processes are called zero-order processes, the rate of change (dx/dt) for a zero-order process is constant:

■ Equation 8.20

$$\frac{dx}{dt} = k$$

If x represents an amount of drug, then the units of k are amount/time. The value of x at time t, $x(t)$, is the integral of the equation from 0 to t:

■ Equation 8.21

$$x(t) = x_0 + kt$$

where x_0 is the value of x at time 0. This is, of course, the equation of a straight line with a slope of k and an intercept of x_0.

Other processes occur at a rate proportional to the amount. The rate of change for a first-order process is:

■ Equation 8.22

$$\frac{dx}{dt} = kx$$

Here, the units of k are simply 1/time, since x on the right hand side already includes the units for the amount. The value of x at time t, $x(t)$, is the integral of the equation from 0 to t:

■ Equation 8.23

$$x(t) = x_0 e^{kt}$$

where x_0 is the value of x at time 0. If $k > 0$, $x(t)$ increases exponentially. If $k < 0$, $x(t)$ decreases exponentially. In pharmacokinetics, the exponent is negative, i.e. concentrations decrease over time. It is customary to explicitly express the minus sign:

■ Equation 8.24

$$x(t) = x_0 e^{-kt}$$

Figure 8.9A shows the relationship between x and time, as described by Equation 8.24 (where k is positive, so $-kt$ is < 0). This exponential relationship is typical of drug concentrations after an intravenous bolus. The amount of drug continuously decreases, and the slope continuously increases (i.e. becomes less negative) as the amount of drug falls from x_0 to 0. This relationship can be linearized by taking the natural logarithm (Figure 8.9B) such that:

■ Equation 8.25

$$\begin{aligned}\ln(x(t)) &= \ln(x_0 e{-}kt)\\ &= \ln(x_0) + \ln(e^{-kt})\\ &= \ln(x_0) - kt\end{aligned}$$

The half-life, is $t½$, or the time for x to fall by 50%, can be calculated as the time for x to fall from x_1 to $x_1/2$, based on the slope, $-k$:

■ Equation 8.26

$$k = \frac{\Delta\ln(x_1)}{\Delta t} = \frac{\ln(x_1) - \ln\left(\frac{x_1}{2}\right)}{t½} = \frac{\ln\left(\frac{x_1}{\left(\frac{x_1}{2}\right)}\right)}{t½} = \frac{\ln(2)}{t½} = \frac{\sim 0.693}{t½}$$

Using this relationship, we can compute k from $t½$, or vice versa, depending on what is experimentally measured.

Bolus pharmacokinetics

Returning to Figure 8.1, if we add x units of drug into volume, V, the concentration, C, is x/V. The rate at which drug is removed from the system is $Cl \times C$:

■ Equation 8.27

$$\text{rate of drug elimination} = \frac{dx}{dt} = Cl \times C = Cl\frac{x}{V} = \frac{Cl}{V} = kx$$

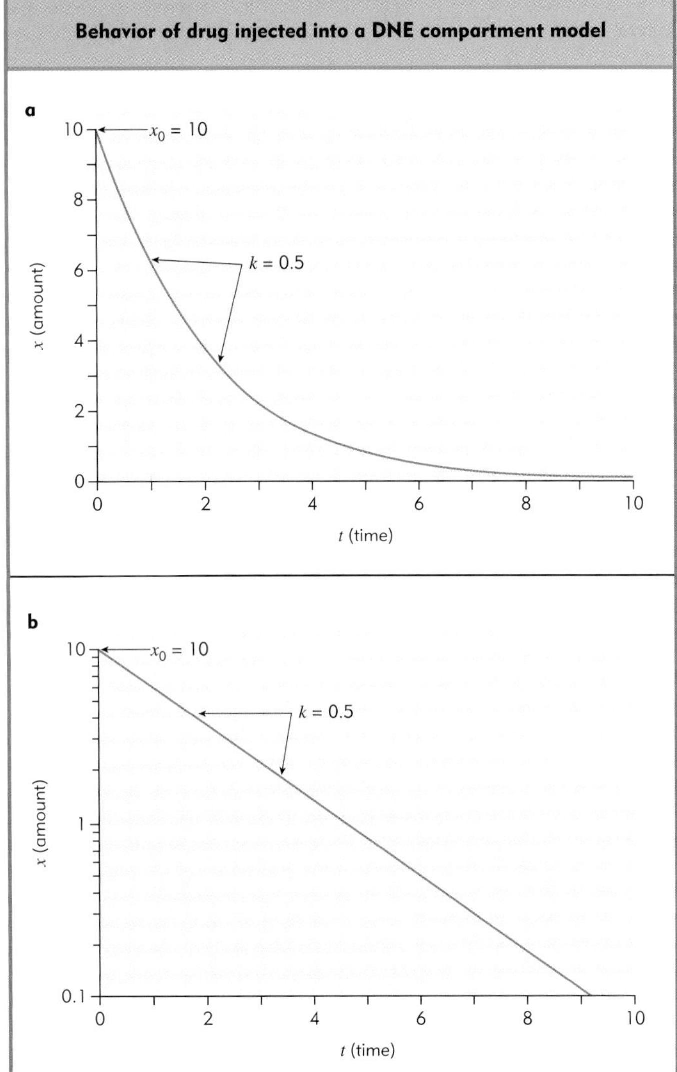

Figure 8.9 Behavior of drug injected into a one compartment model, showing the exponential decay. A, The relationship is $x(t) = x_0\,e^{-kt}$, with $x_0 = 10$ and $k = 0.5$. **B,** The same exponential decay curve, $x(t) = x_0\,e^{-kt}$, but now plotted on a log Y axis.

This is a first-order process, because the rate is proportional to x, and the rate constant, k, equals $\frac{Cl}{V}$. We can rearrange $k = \frac{Cl}{V}$ to derive a fundamental pharmacokinetic relationship:

■ Equation 8.28

$$Cl \text{ (clearance)} = k \text{ (rate constant)} \times V \text{ (volume of distribution)}$$

Equation 8.28 indicates that if we know the volume and clearance, we can calculate k as $\frac{Cl}{V}$. Of course, knowing k we can calculate half-life as $\frac{0.693}{k}$.

Let $C_0 = \frac{x_0}{V}$, where C_0 is the concentration at time 0, x_0 is the dose of drug we added to the volume V. This is the equivalent of an intravenous bolus. To understand the time course of concentration, divide each side of equation 8.27 by V, to turn amounts into concentration:

■ Equation 8.29

$$\frac{dx/V}{dt} = k\frac{x}{V}$$

$$\frac{dC}{dt} = kC$$

Since it is a first order process, referring back to Equation 8.24, plasma concentration will be described by:

■ Equation 8.30

$$C(t) = C_0e^{-kt}$$

This equation defines the 'concentration over time' curve for a one compartment model, and has the log linear shape seen in Figure 8.9.

We can calculate clearance, Cl, in one of two ways. If we know V and k, then $Cl = kV$. However, a more general solution is to consider the area under the concentration vs. time curve, known in pharmacokinetics as the 'area under the curve' or AUC. By definition, the area is the integral of concentrations over time, given by Equation 8.30, the integral of which is:

■ Equation 8.31

$$\begin{aligned} \text{AUC} &= \int_0^\infty C_0e^{-kt}dt \\ &= \int_0^\infty \frac{x_0}{V}\left(e^{\frac{Cl}{V}t}\right)dt \text{ (substituting } C_0 \text{ and } k\text{)} \\ &= \frac{x_0}{V} \times \frac{V}{Cl} \text{ (evaluating the above integral)} \\ &= \frac{x_0}{Cl} \end{aligned}$$

We can rearrange Equation 8.31 for clearance, Cl:

■ Equation 8.32

$$Cl = \frac{x_0}{AUC}$$

Since x_0 is the dose of drug, clearance equals the dose divided by the area under the curve. This is a fundamental property of all linear pharmacokinetic models, and applies to one compartment models, multicompartment models, and to any type of drug dosing (provided the total systemic dose is used as the numerator). It directly follows that AUC is proportional to dose for linear models (i.e. models where Cl is constant).

A fundamental property of all linear pharmacokinetic models is that clearance equals the dose divided by the area under the curve.

Infusion pharmacokinetics

For an infusion at a rate of I (for Input), plasma concentration continues to rise as long as the rate of drug going in the body, I, exceeds the rate at which drug leaves the body, $C \times Cl$. Once $I = C \times Cl$ drug is entering and exiting at the same rate. At equilibrium, we can simply rearrange the definition of steady state, $I = C \times Cl$, to identify the steady state concentration:

■ Equation 8.33

$$C_\infty = \frac{I}{Cl}$$

Thus, the steady state concentration during an infusion is the rate of drug input divided by the clearance. This is similar to the equation describing the concentration following a bolus injection: $C = x_0/v$. Thus volume relates initial concentration to the size of the initial bolus, and clearance relates steady-state concentration to the infusion rate. It follows that the initial concentration following a bolus is independent of the clearance, and the steady state concentration during a continuous infusion is independent of the volume.

The time for the plasma concentration to rise to 50% of the steady state concentration can now be derived. The rate of change in x, the amount of drug in the compartment, is:

■ Equation 8.34

$$\frac{dx}{dt} = I - kx(t)$$

where I is the rate of drug entering, $x(t)$ is the amount of drug present at time t, and $k\,x(t)$ is the rate of drug exiting. We can calculate $x(t)$ as the integral from time 0 to time t, knowing that $x_0=0$ (i.e. we are starting with no drug in the body).

■ Equation 8.35

$$x(t) = \frac{I}{k}(1 - e^{-kt})$$

As $t = \infty$, $e^{-kt} \approx 0$, and Equation 8.35 reduces the steady state amount:

■ Equation 8.36

$$x_\infty = \frac{I}{k}$$

For 50% of that amount, we know that $\frac{x_\infty}{2} = \frac{I}{2k}$. Substituting $\frac{I}{2k}$ for $x(t)$ in Equation 8.35, we get:

■ Equation 8.37

$$\frac{I}{2k} = \frac{I}{k}(1 - e^{-kt})$$

Solving Equation 8.37 for t, we get $\frac{\ln(2)}{k}$. This is, of course, the half-life, $t½$. We can similarly show that we will get to 75% of the steady state concentration following 2 half-lives, 88% following 3 half-lives, 94% following 4 half-lives, and 97% following 5 half-lives. Usually, by 4-5 half-lives, we consider the patient to be at steady state.

Steady state occurs by 4-5 half-lives of the infused drug.

Absorption pharmacokinetics

So far we have focused on intravenous drug delivery, but with minor changes the same mathematics can describe non-intravenous drug delivery. With intravenous dosing, all of the drug reaches the systemic circulation. For other forms of dosing (e.g. oral, intramuscular, epidural, etc.) not all of the drug may reach the systemic circulation. In these cases, the total drug reaching the circulation is not the administered dose, but the administered dose times f, the fraction 'bioavailable:'

■ Equation 8.38

Systemic dose = administered dose $\times f$

When drugs are absorbed, one must also account for the delay in reaching the systemic circulation. Typically the drug is in a depot, from which it is released over time at a rate proportional to the amount of drug in the depot. This is, again, a first order process, and so it is modeled as an exponentially decreasing infusion rate. We can model this exponential decrease in delivered drug as:

■ Equation 8.39

$$A(t) = fD_{oral}k_a e^{-k_a t}$$

where $A(t)$ is the absorption rate at time t, f is the fraction bioavailable, D_{oral} is the dose given orally (or by another non-intravenous route), and k_a is the absorption rate constant. The integral of $k_a\, e^{-k_a t}$ is 1, so that the total amount of drug absorbed is $f \times D_{oral}$. We can use this rate of drug absorption in the differential equation that describes the net flow of drug into the body:

■ Equation 8.40

$$\frac{dx}{dt} = A(t) - kx(t) = D_{oral}fk_a e^{-k_a t} - kx(t)$$

This is the rate of absorption at time t, $A(t)$, minus the rate of exit, $kx(t)$. To solve for the amount of drug, x, in the compartment at time t, we integrate this from 0 to time t, knowing that $x(0) = 0$:

■ Equation 8.41

$$x(t) = \frac{D_{oral}fk_a}{k - k_a}(e^{-k_a t} - e^{-kt})$$

Multicompartment pharmacokinetics

Unfortunately, *none of the drugs used in anesthesia can be accurately characterized by one compartment models.* Distribution of anesthetic drugs into and out of peripheral tissues plays a crucial role in the time course of anesthetic drug effect. Anesthetic drugs are modeled by extending the principles of one-compartment models to account for uptake of drug by peripheral tissues. The plasma concentrations over time following a bolus of an intravenous drug resemble the curve in Figure 8.10. In contrast to Figure 8.9, Figure 8.10 is not a straight line even though it is plotted on a log vertical axis. The concentrations continuously decline, the rate of decline is initially very steep, and the curve continuously becomes less steep (i.e. the slope continuously increases), until it becomes 'log-linear'.

For many drugs, three distinct phases can be distinguished. There is a rapid 'distribution' phase (solid line in Figure 8.10) immediately after the bolus injection. This phase is characterized by very rapid movement of the drug from the plasma to the rapidly equilibrating tissues. The first hydraulic model in Figure 8.10, constructed based on fentanyl pharmacokinetics, permits an intuitive interpretation of this rapid phase. The small tank in the center of the model is the plasma compartment. Initially, drug has three places to go: either of the peripheral tanks, or out the open pipe and down the page. By virtue of having a large concentration gradient against the two tanks and the central metabolism (open pipe), the plasma levels drop quickly.

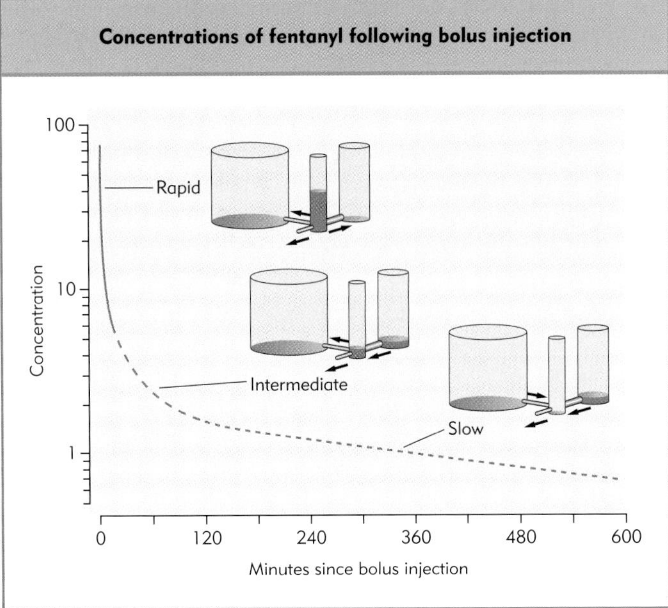

Figure 8.10 The concentrations of fentanyl following a bolus injection, with a superimposed hydraulic representation of a three compartment model. The central tank in the hydraulic model represents the central compartment (plasma). The height of the water in each tank represents the apparent concentration.

The second phase (dashed line in Figure 8.10) is characterized by the plasma levels dropping below those in the rapidly equilibrating tissues, so that the flow to the tank has reversed. The reversed flow between the plasma and the rapidly equilibrating tank slows the decline in plasma concentration.

The terminal phase (dotted line in Figure 8.10) is a straight line when plotted on a semilogarithmic graph. The terminal phase is sometimes called the 'elimination phase' because the primary mechanism for decreasing drug concentration during the terminal phase is drug elimination. This is a misnomer, because the rate of elimination is much slower than during earlier phases, because the plasma drug concentration is less. The distinguishing characteristic of the terminal elimination phase is that the relative proportion of drug in the plasma and peripheral volumes of distribution remains constant. As seen in the tank model, during terminal phase drug is returning from peripheral compartments of distribution into the plasma. Thus, the liver is fighting against the entire body load drug, and the rate of decrease is therefore quite slow.

Curves which continuously decrease over time, with a continuously *increasing* slope (e.g. Figure 8.10), can be described by a sum of exponentials.

■ Equation 8.42

$$C(t) = Ae^{-\alpha t} + Be^{-\beta t} + Ce^{-\gamma t}$$

where t is the time since the bolus, $C(t)$ is the drug concentration following a bolus dose, and A, α, B, β, C, and γ are parameters of a pharmacokinetic model. A, B, and C are called coefficients, while α, β, and γ are called exponents. Following a bolus injection all 6 of the parameters in Equation 8.42 will be greater than 0.

The most important reason to use polyexponential pharmacokinetic models is that **such models describe the data.** Mathematical pharmacokinetics is an empirical science: the models describe the data, not the processes by which the observations came to be. Fortunately, polyexponential functions permit us to use many of the one compartment ideas just developed, with some generalization of the concepts. Additionally, Equation 8.42 can be transformed into a model of volumes and clearances that has an appealing, if not necessarily accurate, physiologic flavor. Figure 8.11 shows one, two, and three compartment models, corresponding to pharmacokinetic models with one, two, and three exponents. Equation 8.42 also has useful mathematical properties. For example, its integral, the AUC, is $A/\alpha + B/\beta + C/\gamma$.

Polyexponential pharmacokinetic models describe the three distinct phases observed for most drugs, and can be transformed into more intuitive compartmental models.

The concentrations over time following bolus injection are the sum of three separate functions, which can be graphed separately or superimposed as shown in Figure 8.12. At time 0 (t = 0), Equation 8.42 reduces to the sum of the coefficients A, B, and C, which equals the concentration immediately following a bolus. Usually, $A > B > C$. Thus, the initial contribution to the decrease in concentration is primarily from the A component, because $Ae^{-\alpha t} >> Be^{-\beta t} >> Ce^{-\gamma t}$ (assuming $\alpha > \beta > \gamma$). The exponents usually differ in size by about an order of magnitude. Each exponent is associated with a half-life. Thus, a drug described by three exponents has three half-lives: two rapid half

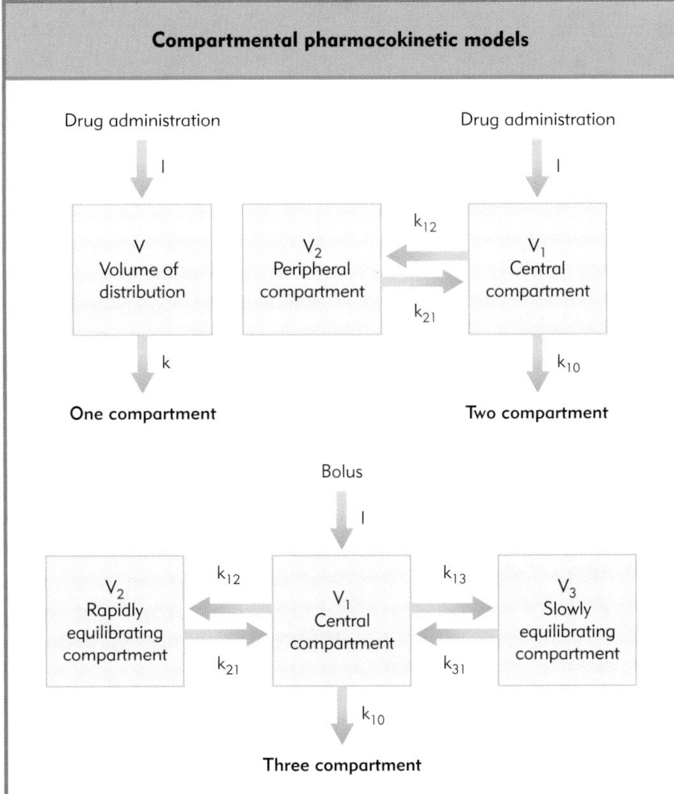

Figure 8.11 One, two, and three compartment pharmacokinetic models. In the two and three compartment pharmacokinetic models, drug is administered into a central compartment, from which it is cleared by metabolism. Drug distributes into peripheral volumes of distribution.

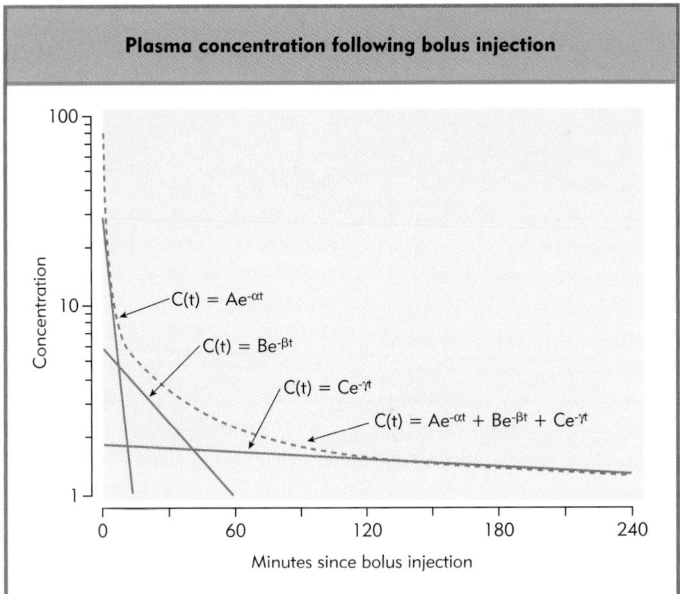

Figure 8.12 The plasma concentration following bolus injection into a three compartment model (dotted line). This can be frequently described as the algebraic sum of three exponential functions. The solid lines represent the individual exponential functions, $A e^{-\alpha t}$, $B e^{-\beta t}$, $C e^{-\gamma t}$.

lives, calculated as $0.693/\alpha$ and $0.693/\beta$, and a terminal half-life (sometimes inappropriately called the 'elimination half-life'), calculated as $0.693/\gamma$.

As seen in Figure 8.12, over time the function approaches the slowest (smallest) exponent. For reasons that mostly reflect pharmacokinetic naivete, the 'half-life' quoted in textbooks and discussed among physicians is usually the slowest (smallest) exponent. The terminal half-life for drugs with more than 1 exponential term is nearly uninterpretable. The terminal half-life may nearly describe, or tremendously overpredict, the time it will take for drug concentrations to decrease by 50% after drug administration. The terminal half-life places an upper limit on the time required for the concentrations to decrease by 50%. Usually, the time for a 50% decrease is much faster than that upper limit.

Polyexponential models can be mathematically transformed from the unintuitive exponential form to an intuitive, if still fanciful, compartmental form, as shown in Figure 8.11. The fundamental parameters of the compartment model are the volumes of distribution and clearances. The central compartment (compartment 1) includes the rapidly mixing portion of the blood and the first-pass pulmonary uptake. The peripheral compartments are composed of those tissues and organs showing a time course and extent of drug accumulation different from that of the central compartment. In the three compartment model, the smaller peripheral compartment may *very roughly* correspond to splanchnic and muscle tissues and the huge compartment may correspond to body fat. If drugs are highly soluble in body tissues (e.g. lipophilic drugs), there will be a large amount of drug in the body, relative to the plasma drug concentration, and the Vd_{ss} may be huge.

Plasma-effect site equilibration

The concept of the effect site is required to understand the clinical application of pharmacokinetic concepts. Figure 8.13 shows the time course of fentanyl and alfentanil concentrations during and after a brief infusion, and the delay in the onset and offset of drug effect relative to the rise and fall of opioid concentration. This delay represents the time required for the drug to transit to the site of drug effect, called the 'effect site' or 'biophase.' The biophase is added to pharmacokinetic models through the addition of an additional compartment (Figure 8.14). By definition, the effect compartment is so small that it receives almost no drug from the central compartment, and thus has no influence on the plasma pharmacokinetics. The rate

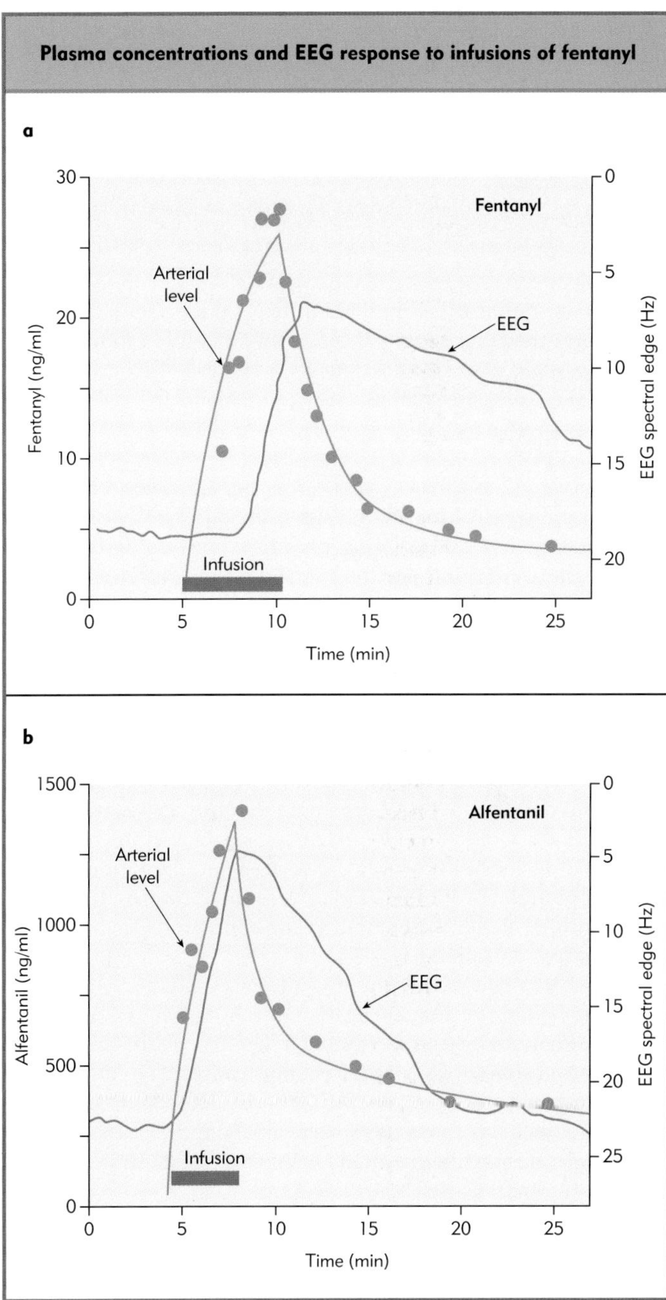

Figure 8.13 The plasma concentrations and electroencephalogram (EEG) response to infusions of fentanyl (top) **and alfentanil** (bottom). The time course of the infusion is shown by the horizontal bar. Arterial concentrations rise quickly during the infusion, and decay quickly when the infusion is terminated. With fentanyl there is a delay of 3–5 minutes between the response in the plasma and the EEG response. The EEG responds much more quickly for alfentanil, reflecting the faster blood–brain equilibrium.

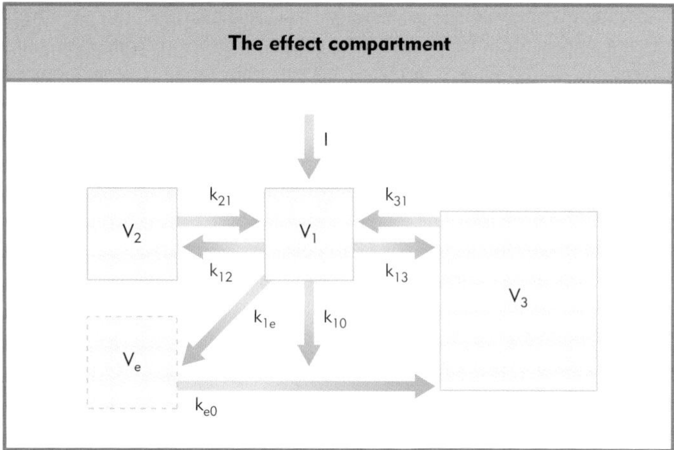

Figure 8.14 The effect compartment. The effect site is a compartment that is added to a conventional pharmacokinetic model to account for the delay between the time course of drug concentration and the pharmacological response. *Ve*, the volume of the effect site, is negligible with respect to V_1.

constant k_{e0} defines the elimination from the effect site, which determines the time course of blood–brain equilibration:

■ Equation 8.43

$$\frac{dCe}{dt} = k_{e0}(Cp - Ce)$$

where *Cp* is the plasma concentration and *Ce* is the effect site concentration. Following a bolus dose, the onset of drug effect is a function of *both* the plasma pharmacokinetics and k_{e0}. For drugs with a very rapid decline in plasma concentration following a bolus (e.g. adenosine, with a half-life of several seconds), the effect site concentration will peak within several seconds of the bolus, regardless of k_{e0}. This happens because the plasma concentrations drop so quickly that after a few seconds there is no longer a driving gradient into the effect site. For drugs with a rapid k_{e0} and a slow decrease in concentration following bolus injection (e.g. pancuronium), the time to peak effect site concentration will be determined more by the k_{e0} than by the plasma pharmacokinetics. k_{e0} has been characterized for many drugs used in anesthesia. Plasma-effect site equilibration is rapid for thiopental, propofol, and alfentanil, intermediate for midazolam, fentanyl, sufentanil, vecuronium and pancuronium, and slow for morphine.

Figure 8.15 shows the plasma and effect site concentrations following boluses of fentanyl, alfentanil, or sufentanil, as a percent of initial plasma concentration. The rapid plasma-effect site equilibration (large k_{e0}) of alfentanil causes the effect site concentration to peak about 90 seconds after bolus injection. Fentanyl effect site concentrations peak about 3–4 minutes after a bolus injection, while sufentanil effect site concentrations peak about 5–6 minutes after bolus injection.

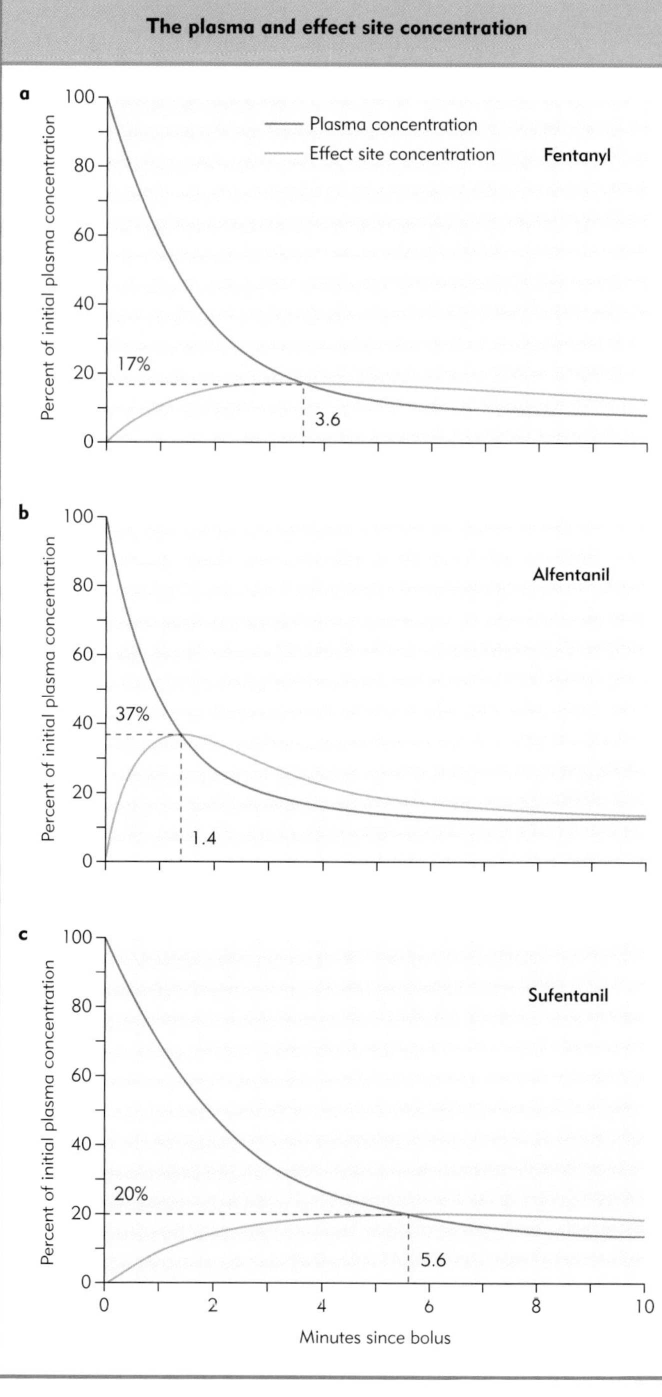

Figure 8.15 The plasma and effect site concentrations, as a percent of initial plasma concentration, following a bolus of fentanyl, alfentanil, or sufentanil. Alfentanil has the most rapid equilibration between brain and effect site, which produces both a more rapid rise in effect site concentration. (Adapted from Shafer SL and Varvel JR, Pharmacokinetics, pharmacodynamics, and rational opioid selection. Anesthesiology. 1991 Jan; 74(1):53-63.

CLINICAL APPLICATION OF PHARMACOKINETICS

Onset of drug effect

Most anesthetics begin with a bolus dose of intravenous drug. Returning to Equation 8.1, we can rearrange the definition of concentration to find the amount of drug required to produce any desired target plasma concentration, C_T, for a known volume:

■ Equation 8.44

$$\text{Bolus} = C_T \times V$$

This simple textbook solution ignores the complexity of anesthetic pharmacokinetics. For all anesthetic drugs there are several volumes: V_1 (central compartment), V_2 and V_3 (the peripheral compartments), and Vd_{ss}, the sum of the individual volumes. V_1 is usually much smaller than Vd_{ss}. The 'textbook' recommendation is to choose something between V_1 and Vd_{ss}. Unfortunately, the range between these is usually so large as to be useless. For example, the fentanyl concentration required to attenuate the hemodynamic response to intubation with propofol is approximately 3 ng/ml. The V_1 and Vd_{ss} for fentanyl are 13 liters and 360 liters, respectively. According to Equation 8.44, the dose of fentanyl required to attenuate the hemodynamic response is between 39 μg (3 ng/ml ÷ 13 liters) and 1080 mg (3 ng/ml ÷ 360 liters).

Since plasma is not the effect site of aneshetic drugs, using plasma concentration to calculate the initial bolus is illogical.

Since plasma is not the site of drug effect, the common teaching of using plasma concentration to calculate the initial bolus is illogical. It is better to consider the time course of drug effect. Once we know the k_{e0} of an intravenous anesthetic, we can design a dosing regimen that yields the desired concentration at the site of drug effect. Figure 8.15 shows the plasma and effect site concentrations following a fentanyl bolus. The plasma concentration decreases continuously, while the effect site peaks several minutes after the bolus. To avoid overdose, we should select the bolus that produces the desired peak concentration in the effect site. This can be calculated based on the volume of distribution at the time of peak effect, $Vd_{\text{peak effect}}$:

■ Equation 8.45

$$Vd_{\text{peak effect}} = \frac{\text{bolus dose}}{C_{\text{peak effect}}\ (\text{plasma})}$$

where $C_{\text{peak effect}}$ (plasma) is the plasma concentration at the time of peak effect. Once we know $Vd_{\text{peak effect}}$, we can calculate the loading dose necessary to produce any desired target concentration, C_T, at the time of peak effect:

■ Equation 8.46

$$\text{Bolus} = C_T \times Vd_{\text{peak effect}}$$

The $Vd_{\text{peak effect}}$ for fentanyl is 75 liters. To produce a peak fentanyl effect site concentration of 3 ng/ml requires 225 μg, which produces a peak effect in 3.6 minutes. This is a clinically reasonable suggestion, particularly compared with the useless suggestion based upon V_1 and Vd_{ss}.

Maintenance of drug effect

The rate at which drug exits the body is the systemic clearance, Cl, times the plasma concentration. To maintain a steady target concentration, C_T, drug must be delivered at the same rate that drug is exiting the body. Thus, the infusion rate to maintain a target concentration, C_T, is often presented as:

■ Equation 8.47

$$\text{Maintenance infusion rate} = C_T \times Cl$$

This equation makes perfect sense for a one compartment model, but fails when applied to drugs described by multicompartment pharmacokinetics (e.g. all intravenous anesthetic drugs). Such drugs distribute into peripheral tissues for many hours during an infusion until steady state is reached. Thus Equation 8.47 is only correct after the peripheral tissues have equilibrated with plasma. At all other times, this maintenance infusion rate will be too slow.

There are several more sophisticated approaches. One approach is to start at higher infusion rates, based on nomograms or other dosing guides, and then turn down the infusion rate by titrating to drug effect. The rigorous pharmacokinetic approach is to compute the amount of drug moving into peripheral compartments, and adjust the dose accordingly. Unfortunately, the equation for the infusion rate so calculated is:

■ Equation 8.48

$$\text{Maintenance infusion rate} = C_T \times V_1(k_{10} + k_{12}e^{-k_{21}t} + k_{13}e^{-k_{31}t})$$

The infusion rate calculated by the above equation is initially rapid, and the rate decreases over time. At equilibrium ($t \to \infty$) the infusion rate decreases to $C_T \times V_1 \times k_{10}$, which is the same as $C_T \times Cl$ (equation 8.47). While few anesthesiologists would choose to mentally solve this equation during administration of an anesthetic, most understand the implications: the rate of drug administration must be continuously titrated downward during anesthesia to avoid overdosing the patient as drug accumulates in peripheral tissues.

TARGET CONTROL INFUSION SYSTEMS

Although Equation 8.48 is not easily applied by the practicing clinician, it is readily solved by computers. In 1968, Kruger-Thiemer described using pharmacokinetics to administer drugs for multicompartment models, exactly as described above. About 10 years later his recommendations were incorporated into an anesthetic dosing system by Schwilden. The result is an infusion device, called a 'Target Controlled Infusion' (or just TCI) that is very analogous in use to a vaporizer, but for intravenous drugs. Using validated pharmacokinetic models, the system will rapidly achieve, and then maintain, a target concentration. Performance is limited by underlying pharmacokinetic variability, but such systems perform quite well; typically measured concentrations are within 20–25% of the targeted concentrations. The only commercially available target controlled infusion system at this time is the Diprifusor for propofol. Several research TCI systems are available over the internet (e.g. STANPUMP, available at http://anesthesia.stanford.edu and RUGLOOP available at http://users.skynet.be/fa491447/).

Offset of drug effect

Although the terminal half-life is typically thought to be important in governing the offset of drug effect, this is almost never the case for anesthetic drugs. The terminal half-life sets an upper limit on how long it will take the plasma concentrations to fall by 50%. However, often the offset of drug effect is far faster for anesthetic drugs because of their polyexponential (i.e. multicompartment) pharmacokinetic profile.

This relationship has been explored in detail for the opioids fentanyl, alfentanil, and sufentanil. Figure 8.16 shows the relationship between a fentanyl infusion that is designed to maintain a constant effect site concentration (i.e. a TCI system with a single target) and the time required for decreases in effect site concentration of various percents after the infusion is terminated. If only modest doses of fentanyl are used, so that the

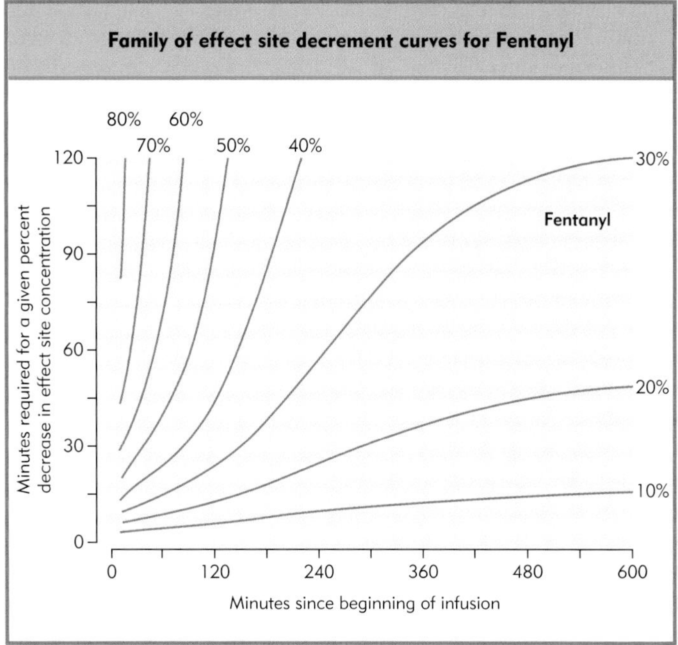

Figure 8.16 The family of effect site decrement curves for fentanyl. The X axis is the duration of an infusion that targets a steady concentration in the effect site (i.e. a TCI infusion targeting the effect site). The Y axis is the time required for a decrease of a given percentage in the effect site concentration after the infusion is terminated. The curves represent the time required for decreases ranging from 10% to 80%. The highly non-linear shape of the curves reflects the multi-compartment nature of anesthetic drugs, and shows how accumulation of drug in peripheral tissues can dramatically lengthen the duration of drug effect, particularly after many hours of anesthesia.

desired offset of drug effect at the end of anesthesia can be accomplished with just a 10% decrease in fentanyl concentration, then the fentanyl can be turned off shortly before the end of the case and patients will awaken quickly. This describes standard clinical use of fentanyl, where the concentrations are maintained quite low and only a modest decrease, if any, is required at the end of anesthesia for adequate ventilation. However, if higher concentrations are maintained, so that the fentanyl concentration the concentration at the end of the case must decrease by 30% for adequate ventilation, then there may be a significant delay in emergence from anesthesia if the case extends longer than 2 hours.

Figure 8.17 explores this relationship for fentanyl, alfentanil, sufentanil, and remifentanil, looking at decreases of 20%, 50%, and 80%. These are called the 20%, 50%, and 80% effect site decrement curves, respectively. There is no accumulation for remifentanil, even though it has a terminal half-life of about 90 minutes. Fentanyl, alfentanil, and sufentanil are indistinguishable in terms of recovery for anesthetics of 30 minutes or less. For anesthetics longer than 30 minutes, sufentanil produces faster recovery than fentanyl or alfentanil for anesthetics less than 3 hours. This also demonstrates the uselessness of half-lives

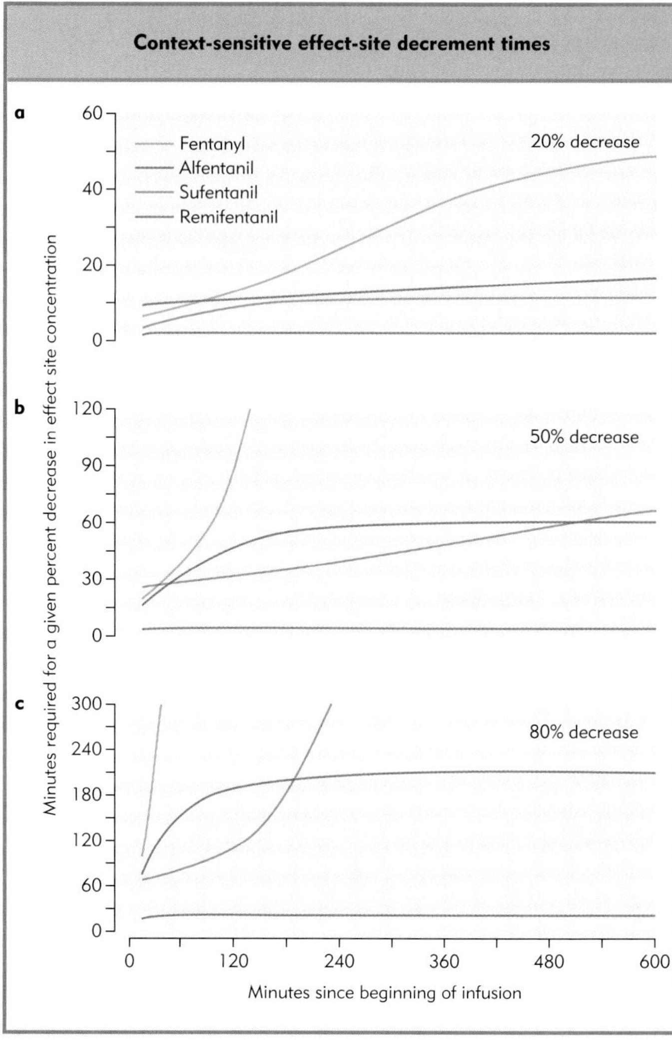

Figure 8.17 The 20%, 50%, and 80% context-sensitive effect-site decrement times for fentanyl, alfentanil, sufentanil, and remifentanil. These curves show the relationship between infusion duration and the time required for decreases in effect site concentration of 20%, 50%, and 80% when the infusion is terminated. The time for the 50% decrease is similar to the "context-sensitive half-time" which describes the time for a 50% decrease is *plasma* drug concentration.

in predicting recovery, because sufentanil has the slowest terminal half-life among these opioids.

Hughes et al simplified this relationship to look at the 50% offset in plasma concentration, which they termed the 'context-sensitive half-time'. The 'context' is the duration of an infusion that maintains a steady drug concentration in the plasma. For anesthetics with relatively rapid plasma-effect site equilibration, the context sensitive half-time and the 50% effect site decrement times are indistinguishable. One cannot predict the shapes of these decrement curves a priori. Computer simulations are required to predict the time course of recovery following administration of drugs described by multicompartment pharmacokinetics.

Key references

Ariens EJ. Stereochemistry, a basis for sophisticated nonsense in pharmacokinetics and clinical pharmacology. Eur J Clin Pharmacol 1984;26:663-668.

Cockcroft DW, Gault MH. Prediction of creatinine clearance from serum creatinine. Nephron 1976;16:31-41.

Greenblatt DJ Arendt RM Abernethy DR Giles HG Sellers EM Shader RI. In vitro quantitation of benzodiazepine lipophilicity: relation to in vivo distribution. Br J Anaesth 1983;55:985-989.

Hughes MA, Glass PSA, Jacobs JR: Context-sensitive half-time in multicompartment pharmacokinetic models for intravenous anesthetic drugs. Anesthesiology 1992;76:334-341.

Kruger-Thiemer E: Continuous intravenous infusion and multicompartment accumulation. Eur J Pharmacol 1968;4:317-324.

Schwilden H. A general method for calculating the dosage scheme in linear pharmacokinetics. Eur J Clin Pharmacol 1981;20:379-386.

Scott JC, Stanski DR. Decreased fentanyl and alfentanil dose requirements with age. A simultaneous pharmacokinetic and pharmacodynamic evaluation. J Pharmacol Exp Ther 1987;240:159-166.

Shafer SL, Varvel JR. Pharmacokinetics, pharmacodynamics, and rational opioid selection. Anesthesiology 1991;74:53-63.

Wilkinson GR, Shand DG. Commentary: a physiological approach to hepatic drug clearance. Clin Pharmacol Ther 1975;18:377-390.

Further reading

Goodman and Gilman, Benet LZ, Kroetz DL, Sheiner LB. Pharmacokinetics: the dynamics of drug absorption, distribution, and elimination. In: Hardman JG, Limbird LI, Molinoff PB, Ruddon RW, Goodman Gilman A, eds. Goodman and Gilman's The Pharmacological Basis of Therapeutics, New York:McGraw-Hill;1996:3-27.

Homer TD, Stanski DR: The effect of increasing age on thiopental disposition and anesthetic requirement. Anesthesiology 1985;62:714-724.

Maitre PO, Vozeh S, Heykants J: Population pharmacokinetics of alfentanil: The average dose-plasma concentration relationship and interindividual variability in patients. Anesthesiology 1987;66:3-12.

Minto CF, Schnider TW, Egan TD et al: The influence of age and gender on the pharmacokinetics and pharmacodynamics of remifentanil. I. Model development. Anesthesiology 1997;86:10-23.

Schnider TW, Minto CF, Gambus PL, Andresen C, Goodale DB, Shafer SL, Youngs EJ. The Influence of Method of Administration and Covariates on the Pharmacokinetics of Propofol in Adult Volunteers. Anesthesiology 1998;88:1170-1182.

Sheiner LB, Stanski DR, Vozeh S et al: Simultaneous modeling of pharmacokinetics and pharmacodynamics: Application to d-tubocurarine. Clin Pharmacol Ther 1979;25:358-371.

Wagner, J.G. 1993. Pharmacokinetics for the Pharmaceutical Scientist, Technomic Publishing Company, Lancaster, PA.

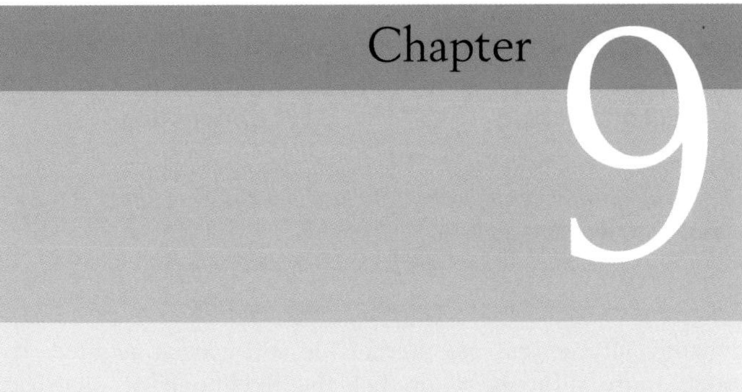

Anesthetic drug interactions

Klaus T Olkkola

TOPICS COVERED IN THIS CHAPTER

- **Types of drug interaction**
- **Mechanisms of drug interaction**
  - Pharmaceutical drug interactions
  - Pharmacokinetic drug interactions
  - Pharmacodynamic drug interactions

When two or more drugs are given together, the pharmacological response may be greater or smaller than the sum of the effects of the drugs given separately. One drug may antagonize or potentiate the effects of the other, and there may be also qualitative differences in response. Although some drug interactions increase toxicity or result in loss of therapeutic effect, others are beneficial. In fact, modern anesthetic techniques depend on the utilization of beneficial drug interactions. A sound combination of drugs can increase the efficacy and safety of drug treatment.

Drug interactions are in some instances an important cause of toxicity. However, the clinical significance of such interactions has occasionally been exaggerated. In many cases our knowledge of adverse drug interactions is based only on case reports.

It is not reasonable to try to list all possible anesthetic drug interactions. It is more important that anesthesiologists understand the principal mechanisms of interactions. Such knowledge will enable drug interactions to be anticipated and, if necessary, avoided. This chapter reviews the mechanisms of drug interactions and presents an overview of possible interactions in anesthesia, intensive care, and pain medicine, with an emphasis on the undesirable consequences of drug interactions.

TYPES OF DRUG INTERACTION

When the effect of two drugs given together is simply the sum of their individual effects, they are said to have an additive interaction. Different types of interaction can be described by isoboles, which are isoeffect curves. These curves show dose combinations that result in equal effects (Fig. 9.1). Isoboles are well suited to describe quantitatively desirable drug interactions, but they cannot be used to describe qualitatively changed responses. Isoboles also illustrate synergistic and antagonistic drug interactions (Table 9.1).

A small drug-induced change in the pharmacokinetics or pharmacodynamics of another drug cannot normally be regarded as clinically significant. A drug interaction is clinically significant only when it results in either unexpected toxicity or loss of efficacy. During a well-monitored intraoperative period or in intensive care this normally requires at least a 50% change in the pharmacokinetic or pharmacodynamic variables describing the response to the drug. Thus, clinically significant adverse drug interactions are not frequently a major problem during the intraoperative phase.

Adverse drug interactions are not a major problem in the intraoperative period.

There is little information on the prevalence of clinically significant adverse drug reactions in the perioperative period, but it has been estimated that in the USA the overall mortality attributed to adverse drug reactions may be as high as 200 000 per year. Owing to the high standards of intraoperative monitoring in developed countries, fatal adverse drug interactions are rare. However, anesthesiologists face the problem of undesirable consequences of drug interactions both in pre- and postoperative periods and in pain medicine. Many patients undergoing surgical operations are taking medication unrelated to surgery. A recent pharmacoepidemiologic study demonstrated that half of the population of adult general surgical patients were taking such medicines. On average, these patients were taking nine different drugs, the number of which increased with age, vascular surgery, and other major procedures. This means that anesthesiologists must be aware of the basic principles of drug interaction to be able to adjust their perioperative strategies according to the patient's condition and concomitant medication. The incidence of adverse drug reactions increases exponentially as the number of drugs prescribed rises, and this is most likely due to drug interactions. The patients with poorest ASA physical status are at the greatest risk of drug interactions.

Isobologram

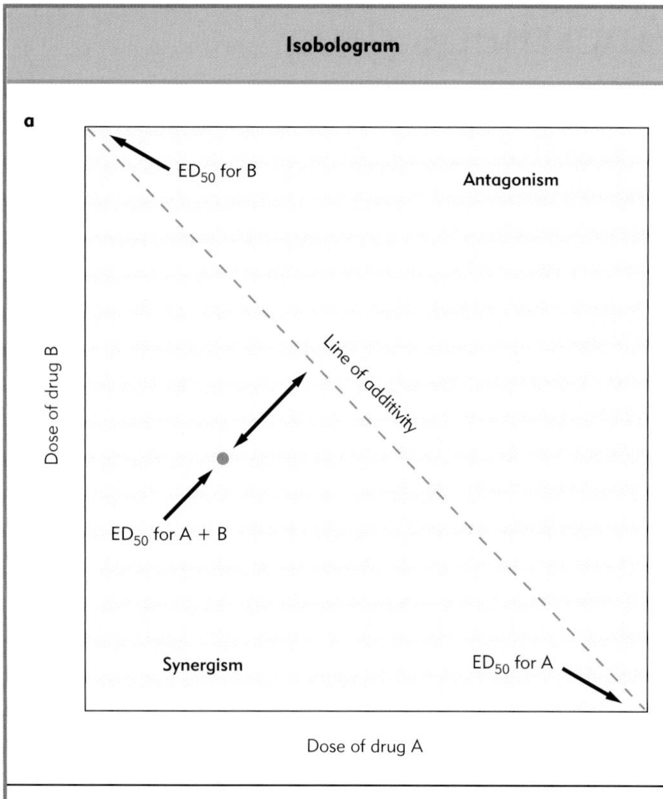

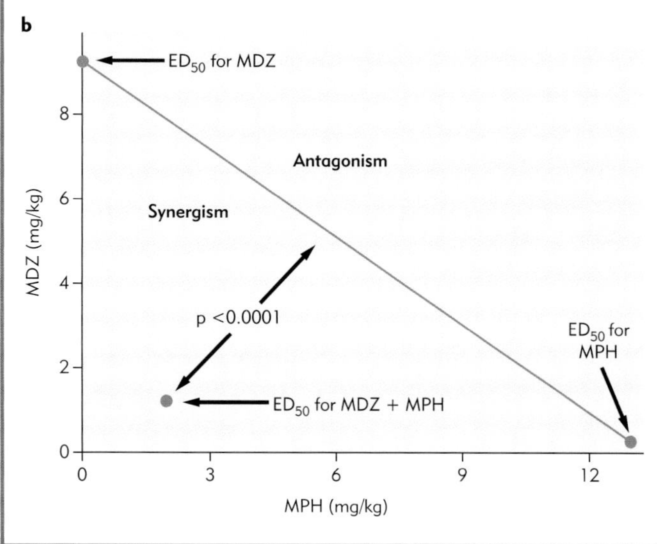

Figure 9.1 Isobologram. (a) The axes are the dose axes of individual drugs A and B. The line of additivity connects isoeffective doses of the two drugs when administered alone. If the isobole (isoeffect curve) bows toward the origin, then the two drugs have a synergistic (supra-additive) interaction. If the isobole bows away from the origin, then the two drugs antagonize each other (infra-additive interaction). (b) Example of an isobologram for the interaction of morphine (MPH) and midazolam (MDZ). Data are for the ED_{50} for loss of righting reflex, which corresponds to loss of consciousness (hypnosis), in rats. (With permission from Kissin et al, 1990).

MECHANISMS OF DRUG INTERACTION

Drugs may interact on a pharmaceutical, pharmacodynamic, or pharmacokinetic basis (Table 9.2). A number of drugs may interact simultaneously at several different sites. Many pharmacodynamic interactions are predictable and can be avoided. It is much more difficult to predict the likelihood of pharmacokinetic interactions despite good prior knowledge of the pharmacokinetics of individual drugs.

Table 9.1 Definition of terminology of drug interactions

Type of interaction	Description
Additive	1 + 1 = 2
Supra-additive (synergism)	1 + 1 >2
Infra-additive (antagonism)	1 + 1 <2

Drugs may interact on a pharmaceutical, pharmacodynamic or pharmacokinetic basis.

Pharmaceutical drug interactions

Pharmaceutical interactions usually occur before the drug is given to the patient. Chemical interactions can occur because of acid–base reactions, oxidation–reduction, salt formation, hydrolysis, or epimerization reactions. For instance, when injecting sodium thiopental with rocuronium through the same intravenous tubing, a precipitate will form instantaneously because of the change in pH. Correspondingly, mixing of calcium salts and $NaHCO_3$ results in the formation of an insoluble salt. There are no difficulties in recognizing such interactions; however, other

Table 9.2 Mechanisms of drug interaction

Mechanisms
Pharmaceutical interactions (i.e. in vitro interactions)
Chemical or physical incompatibility
Pharmacokinetic interactions
Interference with absorption
Change in gastrointestinal pH and motility
Binding and chelation of drugs
Toxic effects on gastrointestinal tract
Change in regional blood flow
Drug distribution (plasma protein-binding displacement)
Drug elimination
Drug metabolism
Stimulation
Inhibition
Changes in hepatic blood flow
Interference with biliary excretion and enterohepatic circulation
Modification of renal excretion
Competition for active renal tubular secretion
Changes in urinary pH
Pharmacodynamic interactions
Competition for same receptors
Action on the same physiological system
Modification of conditions at the site of action

interactions take place without a visible change. For instance, many catecholamines undergo auto-oxidation with light, and epinephrine (adrenaline) loses its efficacy when mixed with alkali.

Physical interactions are due to physical events that may occur during the administration of drugs. Damage to blood because of the use of hyperosmotic solutions and adsorption to plastic infusion sets are common examples of physical pharmaceutical drug interactions. Although most pharmaceutical interactions can be regarded as undesirable, the interaction between protamine and heparin is an example of a beneficial interaction. Acidic heparin loses its pharmacological activity when it forms a stable complex with basic protamine.

As it is impossible to be aware of all possible pharmaceutical interactions, it is important to recognize the most significant ones and to know how they can be avoided or minimized. Some general principles help anesthesiologists to avoid pharmaceutical interactions. It is important that drugs are given as intravenous infusions only when it is really necessary; the oral route should be used whenever possible. The use of multiple drugs in the same infusion fluid should be avoided. NaCl 0.9% and 5% dextrose are regarded as the safest carrier solutions. $NaHCO_3$, dextran, mannitol, blood, and hyperalimentation solutions should not be used because they can react with many drugs to be infused. Bivalent cations also frequently cause problems in infusion solutions. All additions should be marked clearly on the infusion set. The clearness of the solution should always be checked prior to the commencement of infusion. Because numerous incompatibilities have been demonstrated, drugs should never be mixed unless the absence of reaction has been clearly established. Some factors affecting the stability of infusible drugs are shown in Table 9.3.

Pharmaceutical interactions are not limited to drugs administered intravenously. An example of a significant pharmaceutical interaction is the reaction between soda lime and the volatile anesthetics sevoflurane and halothane. The reaction occurs especially with dry soda lime, and may result in diminished anesthetic delivery and delayed onset of anesthesia. However, the use of intraoperative gas monitoring helps to avoid problems associated with the degradation of volatile anesthetics by soda lime.

Pharmacokinetic drug interactions

ABSORPTION

Drugs can influence the absorption of other drugs by changing gastrointestinal pH and motility, intraluminal binding or chelation, changing regional blood flow, inhibition or stimulation of first-pass metabolism, or through toxic gastrointestinal effects. Subcutaneous and intramuscular absorption of drugs can be delayed or decreased following the administration of drugs affecting regional blood flow (vasoactive agents or drugs that affect hemodynamics, such as volatile anesthetics). However, this mechanism has essentially no relevance with regard to anesthesia.

Because the rate of absorption of orally administered drugs is directly proportional to the rate at which drugs pass from stomach to intestine, all drugs that slow the gastric emptying rate delay the gastrointestinal absorption of drugs. Gastric emptying before elective surgery is normal, but premedication with opioids and anticholinergic agents delay it. Figure 9.2 demonstrates the effect of heroin on the oral absorption of acetaminophen (paracetamol). Opioids may significantly delay the onset of action of orally administered drugs, although the bioavailability would not be changed.

Table 9.3 Factors affecting the stability of infusible drugs

pH
Solvent
Buffers
Other drugs
Preservatives
Dilution
Duration of storage
Mixing
Light
Temperature

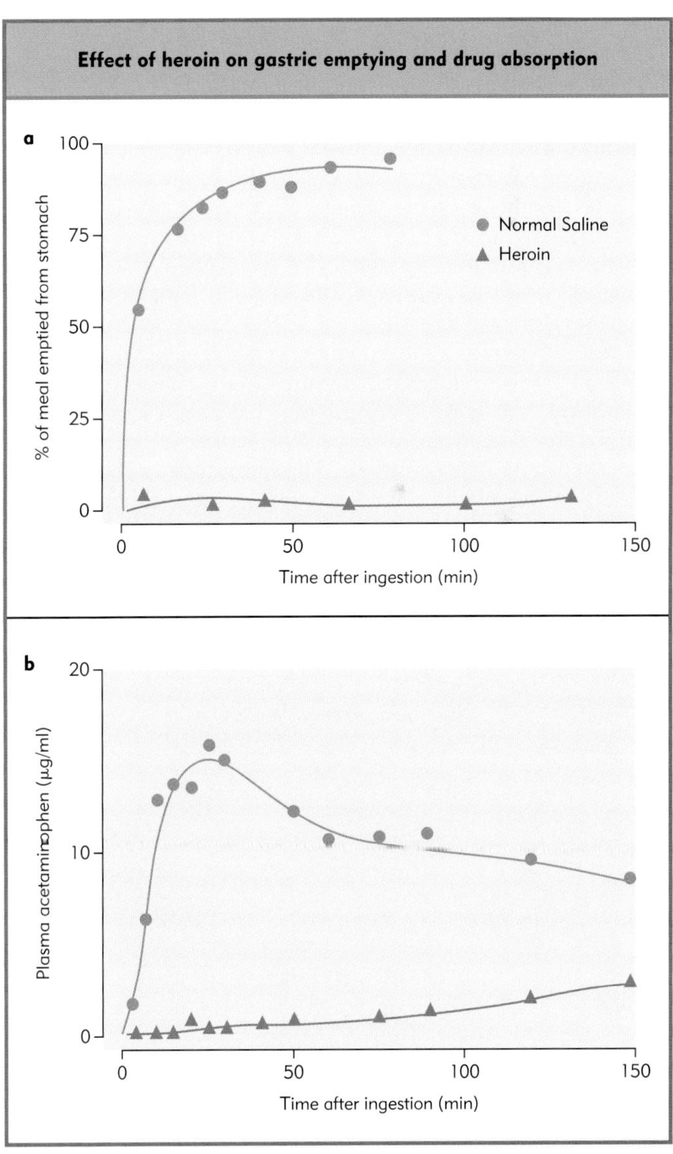

Figure 9.2 Effect of heroin on the rate of gastric emptying. The effect of 10 mg of heroin was measured on gastric emptying (a) and acetaminophen (paracetamol) absorption (b). (With permission from Nimmo et al. 1975.)

Before reaching the systemic circulation, many drugs are subjected to first-pass metabolism in the gut wall and liver (Chapter 8). The biotransformation of drugs during first pass and during elimination from the systemic circulation is usually divided into phase I and phase II reactions. Many drugs are lipophilic and cannot be excreted through the kidneys until they have been transformed into more favorable water-soluble forms. Phase I reactions include oxidation, reduction, and hydrolysis. Phase I reactions alter a functional group of the drug, whereas phase II reactions are conjugation reactions in which the drug or its metabolite is attached to a water-soluble molecule or group, such as glucuronic acid, glutathione, sulfate, acetyl group, methyl group, or glucosamine, making the whole complex more hydrophilic (Fig. 9.3). Oxidation is the most important phase I reaction and is catalyzed by cytochrome P450 enzymes (CYP450).

Inhibition or induction of cytochrome P450 enzymes can enhance or reduce therapeutic effect.

CYP enzymes are divided into families, subfamilies, and specific isozymes, according to the homology of their amino acid sequences. The first Arabic numeral indicates a family (an amino acid sequence homology of 40–55%), the letter thereafter the subfamily (homology more than 55%), and the last number the individual isozyme. CYP1, CYP2 and CYP3 are involved mainly in the metabolism of drugs and other xenobiotics, whereas those belonging to the families CYP4, CYP5, and CYP7 have endogenous functions.

Table 9.4 shows some common substrates, inhibitors, and inducers of cytochrome P450 enzymes. Many substrates are also inhibitors of the same CYP enzyme. Co-administration of an inhibitor and a substrate of any CYP enzyme can increase the plasma substrate concentrations. The magnitude of the increase depends on the inhibitor, its dose, and the interval between the administration of the inhibitor and the substrate. If the substrate has low oral bioavailability, an inhibitor is likely to cause a major increase in substrate concentrations if the substrate is administered orally. For example, ketoconazole can increase the area under the oral triazolam concentration versus time curve (AUC) approximately 30 times, compared to the administration of triazolam with placebo. Correspondingly, the AUC of oral midazolam is increased approximately 16 times. Although the major part of the increases in AUC values is explained by the change in first-pass metabolism of triazolam and midazolam, their concentrations are also increased as a result of the change in elimination clearance.

Inhibition of CYP enzymes is not the only mechanism that can cause clinically significant drug interactions. The concomitant adminstration of CYP enzyme inducers can greatly increase first-pass metabolism and reduce or even eliminate the therapeutic effect. Inhibition or induction of CYP enzymes can cause the AUC values of oral midazolam to vary 400-fold (Fig. 9.4).

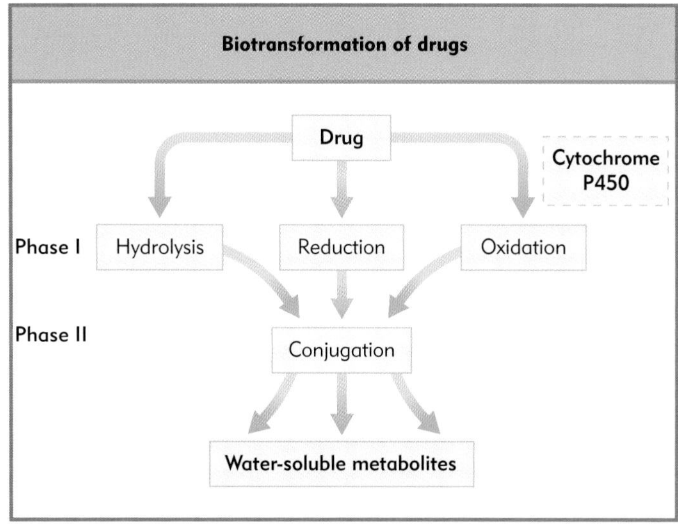

Figure 9.3 Biotransformation of drugs.

DISTRIBUTION

Drug distribution can be affected by numerous factors. Cardiac output and regional variations in perfusion influence the rise of alveolar concentrations of gases and blood concentrations of intravenous anesthetics. Essentially, all drugs are bound to blood components – red blood cells and plasma proteins. Protein-binding interactions have been studied extensively in vitro. Concomitantly administered drugs compete for binding sites on blood and tissue proteins to produce displacement interactions. Because only the unbound (free) fraction of a drug is pharmacologically active, an increase of the free concentration of drug increases its pharmacological effects. The clinical significance of these interactions in anesthesia is often grossly exaggerated (Fig. 9.5).

Protein-binding interactions have been studied extensively, but have limited clinical significance.

In the most common situation the displacer is added to the drug treatment regimen of a patient taking a low extraction-ratio drug. If the displacer has a long elimination half-life relative to the drug, the total plasma drug concentration is decreased when the patient is given the displacer. Because the pharmacokinetics of the displacer is the rate-limiting step in the interaction, the slow accumulation and correspondingly slow elimination of the displacer results in insignificant changes in the unbound drug concentration and hence the therapeutic response. Many anesthetics, including volatile anesthetics, are able to displace drugs from plasma protein binding sites in vitro, but this does not appear to have significant clinical consequences.

ELIMINATION

Metabolic drug interactions can either increase or reduce the metabolism of drugs. Enzyme induction can significantly reduce drug concentrations and effects. Compounds known to enhance drug metabolism include drugs such as rifampicin, barbiturates, phenytoin, and carbamazepine. Smoking and heavy consumption of ethanol also induce hepatic microsomal CYP enzymes. The administration of the inducing drug causes stimulation of not only its own metabolism, but also the metabolism of many unrelated drugs which are substrates for the same microsomal enzymes. Induction usually develops within a period of days or weeks. Table 9.4 shows some common substrates, inhibitors and

Table 9.4 Common substrates, inhibitors, and inducers of cytochrome P450 enzymes

CYP1A2	CYP2C9	CYP2C19	CYP2D6	CYP2E1	CYP3A4
Substrates					
Lidocaine Ropivacaine Amitriptyline Imipramine Clomipramine Theophylline Caffeine	Phenytoin Celecoxib Diclofenac Ibuprofen Valdecoxib S-Warfarin	Diazepam Clomipramine Imipramine Moclobemide Omeprazole Propranolol	Codeine Ethylmorphine Oxycodon Tramadol Amitriptyline Clomipramine Nortriptyline Fluoxetine Venlafaxine Debrisoquine Paroxetine Haloperidol	Desflurane Enflurane Halothane Isoflurane Sevoflurane Acetaminophen	Midazolam Triazolam Alfentanil Buprenorphine Codeine Fentanyl Ethanol Bupivacaine Lidocaine Ropivacaine Valdecoxib Granisetron Ondansetron Venlafaxine Methylprednisone Cortisol Lovastatin Simvastatin Cyclosporin HIV protease inhibitors
Inhibitors					
Cimetidine Ciprofloxacin Fluvoxamine	Miconazole Fluconazole	Fluvoxamine Ketoconazole Omeprazole	Fluoxetine Paroxetine Haloperidol Quinidine Celecoxib Valdecoxib	Disulfiram	Itraconazole Ketoconazole Diltiazem Verapamil Erythromycin Fluvoxamine Grapefruit juice
Inducers					
Smoking	Phenobarbital Rifampicin	Phenobarbital Rifampicin		Ethanol	Carbamazepine Phenobarbital Rifampicin Glucocorticoids

inducers of CYP enzymes; this information allows clinicians to predict drug interactions on the basis of their metabolic pattern.

Recent studies have shown that many dietary supplements and natural products can modify the pharmacokinetics of drugs. For example, the common plant St John's Wort (*Hypericum perforatum*) has gained popularity as an antidepressant. It is a potent inhibitor of CYP3A4 and can have potentially hazardous interactions with substrates of CYP3A4. Grapefruit juice is also an inhibitor of CYP3A4 and greatly increases the concentrations of CYP3A4 substrates such as triazolam, amiodarone, nisoldipin, and felodipin. Other grapefruit-induced interactions are caused by inhibition of intestinal P-glycoprotein. P-glycoproteins are transporters that mediate the transport of various compounds through cell membranes. High levels of P-glycoproteins have been identified in luminal surfaces of the small and large intestine, proximal tubules of the kidneys, and in the luminal surface of biliary tract and hepatocytes. The genes for both P-glycoprotein transporters and CYP3A enzymes are located on the same chromosome, and many inhibitors of CYP3A enzymes are also inhibitors of P-glycoprotein.

Intravenous hypnotics

Because the intravenous hypnotics propofol, thiopental, and etomidate are usually used only for the induction of anesthesia, enzyme induction or inhibition does not have major effects on their pharmacokinetics and effects in humans. Following the induction of anesthesia, the cessation of the effect is mainly due to redistribution and not elimination. Thiopental is a barbiturate that is eliminated mainly by metabolism in the liver. During long-term infusions, enzyme inhibition and induction are likely to change its pharmacokinetics significantly. Propofol has a high extraction ratio and systemic clearance that exceeds hepatic blood flow. From a theoretical point of view, its elimination is dependent on blood flow and not on changes in enzyme activity.

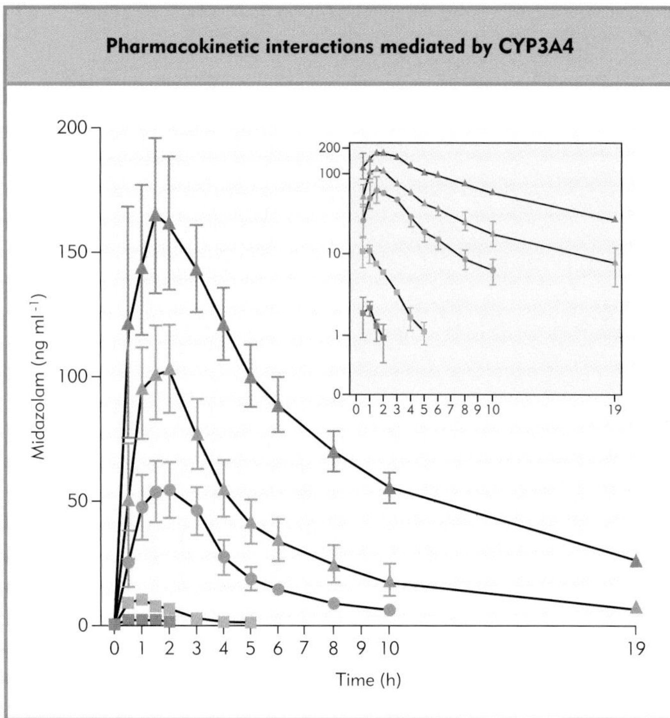

Figure 9.4 Plasma concentrations (mean values ± SEM; *n* = 9) of midazolam after an oral dose of 15 mg without pretreatment, 7.5 mg during and 4 days after pretreatment with the CYP3A4 itraconazole 200 mg daily for 4 days, and 15 mg 1 day and 4 days after pretreatment with the CYP3A4 inducer rifampicin 600 mg daily for 5 days. Plasma concentrations during the itraconazole phases were corrected for a 15-mg dose of midazolam. Orange circles: control, without pretreatment; blue triangles: during itraconazole; orange triangles: 4 days after itraconazole; blue squares: 1 day after rifampicin; green squares: 4 days after rifampicin. (From Backman et al. The area under the plasma…than with rifampicin. Eur J Clin Pharmacol. 1998; 54; 53-58.)

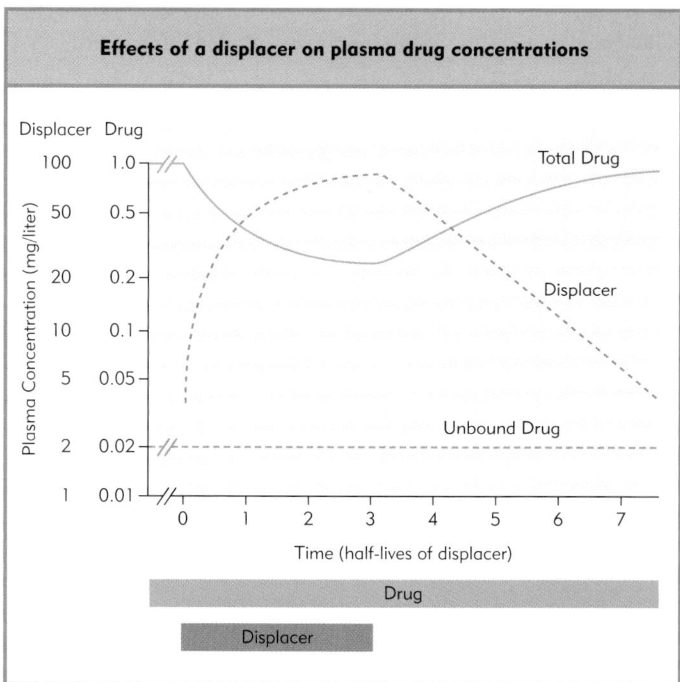

Figure 9.5 Effects of a displacer on plasma drug concentrations. When constantly infused, the unbound (free) concentration of a drug with a low extraction ratio remains virtually unchanged if a displacer with a long half-life, relative to the drug, is either infused or withdrawn. The change in plasma drug concentration reflects the displacement. (From Rowland and Tozer. Clinical Pharmacokinetics: Concepts and Applications. Lea& Febiger 1989 p. 264.)

Although there is evidence that alfentanil can cause a minor increase in propofol plasma concentrations, propofol does not have clinically significant pharmacokinetic drug interactions in humans. Midazolam is a CYP3A4 substrate; its elimination is significantly reduced by strong inhibitors of CYP3A4. Ketamine is cleared almost exclusively by hepatic metabolism. With an extraction ratio of 0.8, its elimination is dependent on liver blood flow. No clinically significant pharmacokinetic drug interactions have been described.

Analgesics

Analgesics are used throughout the perioperative period and also in the long-term treatment of pain. Clinically significant drug interactions are much more likely during the treatment of chronic pain than during the short-lasting and well-monitored intraoperative period.

Clinically significant drug interactions are more likely during chronic pain treatment than in the intraoperative period.

Fentanyl has a high extraction ratio, which makes it unlikely to have clinically significant pharmacokinetic drug interactions during elimination. For example, itraconazole, a potent inhibitor of CYP3A4, does not affect the pharmacokinetics of fentanyl. Interestingly, treatment for 2 days with another CYP3A4 inhibitor, ritonavir, used in the treatment of HIV infections, caused a threefold increase in the concentrations of intravenous fentanyl. Such an increase is of major clinical significance and, if the dose is not reduced, may cause fatal respiratory depression. However, the effect of ritonavir on the metabolism of other drugs is complicated. Longer treatment with oral ritonavir decreased the AUC of oral meperidine (pethidine) by 67%. The AUC of the metabolite normeperidine was increased, suggesting induction of hepatic pethidine metabolism.

Inhibition of CYP3A4 increases the concentration of alfentanil. Although there is little information on the metabolic interactions of morphine, rifampicin and possibly other inducers may reduce the clinical efficacy of morphine by increasing its metabolism. Enzyme induction also increases the metabolism of methadone. Codeine is considered to be a prodrug whose effects are mediated by its minor active metabolite morphine. It is demethylated and glucuronated to yield morphine, codeine-6-glucuronide, and norcodeine, which are then further metabolized. Inhibition or deficiency of CYP2D6 decreases the analgesic efficacy of codeine significantly.

There is little information on the effect of enzyme induction or inhibition on the pharmacokinetics of nonsteroidal anti-inflammatory drugs (NSAIDs). Many commonly used NSAIDs are substrates of CYP enzymes and their metabolism is likely to be changed by enzyme induction and inhibition. However, their large therapeutic index limits the clinical significance of this. Chronic ethanol consumption increases the toxicity of acetaminophen, but otherwise acetaminophen does not appear to have clinically significant pharmacokinetic interactions with other drugs.

Muscle relaxants

The depolarizing muscle relaxant succinylcholine is metabolized by plasma cholinesterase. Drugs that inhibit plasma cholinesterase prolong the time to recovery following succinylcholine. These drugs include the anticholinesterase ecothiopate, the antineoplastic drug cyclophosphamide, and the MAO inhibitor phenelzine.

Modern nondepolarizing neuromuscular blockers are structurally either aminosteroids or benzylisoquinolinium compounds. Enzyme-inducing agents such as glucocorticoids and antiepileptic drugs antagonize the neuromuscular blocking effects of nondepolarizing neuromuscular blockers. The antagonism is more pronounced with the aminosteriods that undergo mainly hepatic metabolism but it occurs also with the benzylisoquinolinium derivatives, which undergo nonenzymatic breakdown (Chapter 37).

Local anesthetics

Local anesthetics can be classified by structure into the aminoesters, which are metabolized by plasma cholinesterase (cocaine, procaine, chloroprocaine, amethocaine, tetracaine), and the aminoamides (lidocaine, prilocaine, mepivacaine, bupivacaine, ropivacaine, etidocaine), which are metabolized by the liver. Ester local anesthetics do not appear to have clinically significant pharmacokinetic interactions.

Amide local anesthetics are metabolized by CYP3A4 and/or CYP1A2. Parenteral lidocaine has not been reported to have clinically significant interactions with inhibitors of CYP enzymes. However, as a drug with a high extraction ratio its elimination clearance is directly proportional to cardiac output. Its elimination is affected by β-blockers which, in addition to decreasing cardiac output, also affect the enzymatic activity in liver.

Bupivacaine has been reported to interact with inhibitors of CYP3A4, but these interactions are not likely to have clinical consequences. Ropivacaine is metabolized mainly by CYP1A2, but also by CYP3A4. Its clearance is reduced by 77% with concomitant administration of the CYP1A2 inhibitor fluvoxamine. Erythromycin, a CYP3A4 inhibitor, alone had only a minor effect on the pharmacokinetics of ropivacaine. However, the combination of fluvoxamine and erythromycin further increased the area under the drug plasma concentration–time curve by 50%. Clinicians should be aware of the possibility of increased toxicity of ropivacaine when used together with inhibitors of CYP1A2. Concomitant use of CYP1A2 and CYP3A4 inhibitors further increases ropivacaine concentration.

Volatile anesthetics

Modern volatile anesthetics are eliminated mainly in unchanged form by exhalation and by CYP-catalyzed biotransformation with varying extents of metabolism: halothane (20%), enflurane (10%), sevoflurane (5%), isoflurane (0.2%), and deslurane (0.02%). The metabolism is mediated mainly in the liver by CYP2E1. Although the metabolism of volatile anesthetics can certainly be modified by compounds affecting CYP2E1, these interactions are of minor clinical importance. Disulfiram, an inhibitor of CYP2E1, can be used to reduce the risk for halothane hepatitis, but because of the limited use of halothane in the adult population and the availability of alternative volatile anesthetics, there is no need to use disulfiram pretreatment prior to general anesthesia.

Volatile anesthetics can affect the pharmacokinetics of other drugs. Halothane reduces the elimination of fentanyl, theophylline, meperidine, and lidocaine in dogs. These changes are due to both decreased liver blood flow and decreased hepatic intrinsic clearance. Halothane has strong hemodynamic effects and can therefore affect the pharmacokinetics of drugs whose elimination is dependent on liver blood flow. This effect is not likely to last longer than the duration of anesthesia. There is little information on the effects of halothane on the pharmacokinetics of co-adminstered drugs in humans, and even less information on the effects of the other volatile anesthetics enflurane, isoflurane, sevoflurane, and desflurane. There is no evidence that volatile anesthetics would have clinically significant pharmacokinetic interactions in humans.

Pharmacodynamic drug interactions

Although pharmacokinetic interactions are of academic interest and may in some cases have clinical significance, pharmacodynamic interactions are far more common and have greater significance in anesthetic practice. In fact, modern 'balanced anesthesia' techniques are based on pharmacodynamic interactions. Many pharmacodynamic interactions are predictable with a good knowledge of pharmacology. In most cases pharmacodynamic drug interactions can be regarded as desirable. A sound combination of drugs having synergistic effects facilitates the use of smaller and less toxic doses of the individual drugs.

Pharmacodynamic drug interactions are of greater clinical significance than pharmacokinetic drug interactions in anesthesia.

Drugs acting at the same receptor can compete at receptor sites. One drug can have a greater affinity than the other for the receptor. If it has no activity, the actions of the second drug are antagonized. Examples of such interactions in anesthetic practice are the interactions between naloxone and opioids, β-blockers and catecholamines at β-adrenergic receptors, flumazenil and benzodiazepines at $GABA_A$ receptors, etc.

The concurrent use of drugs acting at the same site or on the same physiological system can result in either increased or decreased effect. The most typical example is the combined use of several drugs acting on the central nervous system. When used in combination, inhalational anesthetics have an additive interaction. Interactions between intravenous anesthetics may be additive. Examples of such interactions are the ketamine–thiopental and ketamine–midazolam interactions. The lack of synergism is most likely due to the different mechanisms of action of ketamine and the two other anesthetics. Ketamine inhibits excitatory transmission by decreasing depolarization through blockade of NMDA receptors. Thiopental and midazolam exert their effects by allosteric modulation of the $GABA_A$ receptors (Chapter 25).

The interactions between benzodiazepines and opioids are synergistic. The hypnotic effects of propofol, midazolam, alfentanil, and their binary and triple combinations have been studied in humans (Fig. 9.6). The ratios of a single-drug fractional dose (ED_{50} = 1.0) to a combined fractional dose (in fractions of single-drug ED_{50} values), indicating the degree of supra-additivity (synergism), were: 1.4 for propofol–alfentanil, 1.8 for midazolam–propofol, 2.8 for midazolam–alfentanil, and 2.6 for propofol–midazolam–alfentanil. Accordingly, propofol–midazolam–alfentanil interaction produces a profound hypnotic

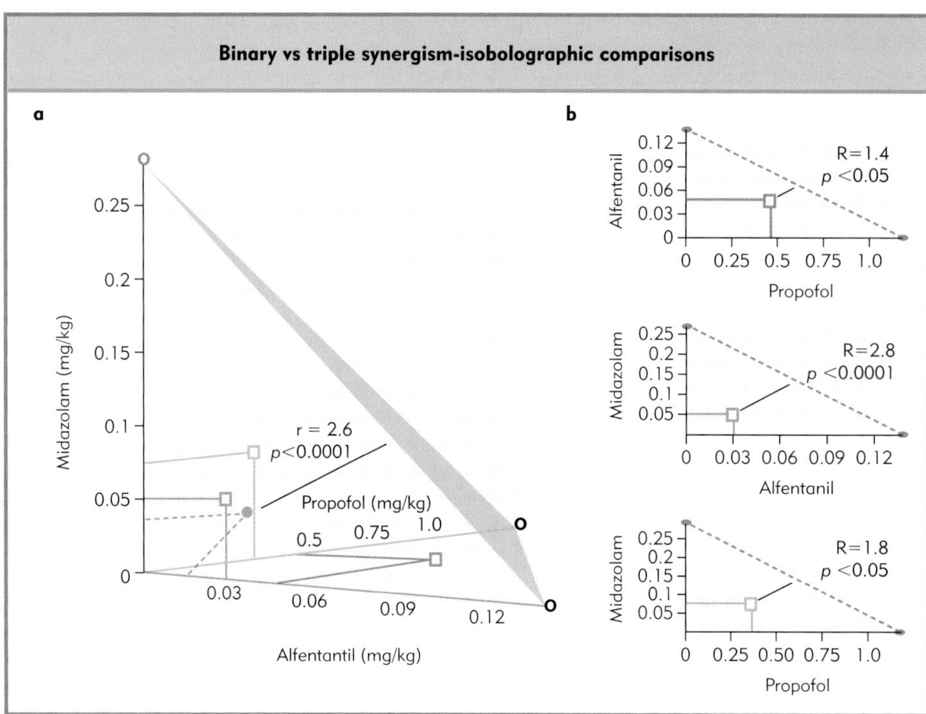

Figure 9.6 Binary versus triple synergism. ED_{50} isobolograms for the hypnotic interactions between midazolam, alfentanil, and propofol. (a) Triple interactions. The purple area shows an additive plane passing through three single-drug ED_{50} points (small open circles, o); the closed circle (●) is an ED_{50} point for the triple combination, and the open squares (□) are ED_{50} points for the binary combinations. The ratio (R) of the single-drug dose (ED_{50} = 1) to combined fractional dose (in fractions of single-drug ED_{50} values) reflects the degree of synergism. The *P* value is the significance of the difference from the additive effect. (b) Binary interactions: the dotted lines are lines of additivity. (From Vinik et al., 1994. REF: Vinik et al. Triple Anesthetic Combination: Propofol-Midazolam-Alfentanil. Anesth Analg 1994: 78: 354-8.)

synergism which is not significantly different from that of the binary midazolam–alfentanil combination.

Volatile anesthetics potentiate the effects of neuromuscular blocking agents in a dose-dependent manner. Although there are quantitative differences in the magnitude of the interaction, depending on the volatile anesthetic and the neuromuscular blocking agent, the interaction can be demonstrated for all volatile anesthetics. Desflurane appears to be able to potentiate the effect more than isoflurane and sevoflurane (Fig. 9.7). The mechanism of potentiation of neuromuscular blockade by inhalational agents is controversial. It may be increased blood flow to the muscle, increased sensitivity of the motor endplate, decreased release of acetylcholine, change in the conductance of the ionic channels of the endplate, and/or induction of relaxation via the central nervous system.

Changes in electrolyte balance may alter the effects of several drugs, especially those that act on neuromuscular transmission. The antiarrhythmic actions of quinidine and lidocaine are antagonized by hypokalemia, and the sudden release of K^+ from muscle following the injection of succinylcholine can cause ventricular arrhythmias in patients on digitalis therapy. Nondepolarizing neuromuscular blocking agents may produce prolonged neuromuscular blockade in the presence of hypokalemia in patients taking thiazide diuretics. Hypokalemia causes hyperpolarization of the motor endplate, and thereby antagonizes the action of acetylcholine for a pharmacodynamic interaction.

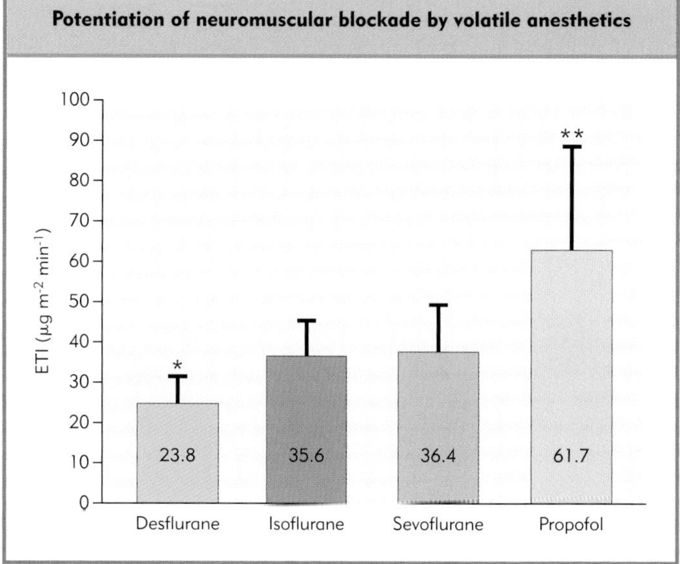

Figure 9.7 Mean effective therapeutic infusion rate (ETI), of cisatracurium (±SD) to maintain neuromuscular blockade constant at 90% during desflurane, isoflurane, sevoflurane, or propofol anesthesia. $^{**}P<0.002$: propofol vs volatile anesthetics; $^{*}P<0.02$: desflurane vs. propofol, sevoflurane, isoflurane. (With permission from Hemmerling et al. 2001).

CONCLUSIONS

Although drug interactions are an important cause of toxicity, their clinical significance has been overemphasized by pharmacologists and some clinicians. Despite all that is written on the subject, the clinical importance of harmful drug interactions is largely unknown. The problem is that the actions of many drugs cannot be measured under clinical conditions, and interactions are unlikely to be recognized unless they cause major adverse effects. During the intraoperative period patients are usually so well monitored that any undesirable drug interactions are unlikely to cause adverse effects. Thus the intraoperative period is less problematic with regard to drug interactions than the pre- and postoperative periods. If anesthesiologists have a sound knowledge of basic pharmacological principles and are aware of the mechanisms of action and pharmacokinetics of the drugs they use, most undesirable drug interactions can be avoided, and desirable interactions can be used for the benefit of the patient.

Anesthesiologists should be especially alert when anesthetizing patients being treated with drugs having a high probability of pharmacokinetic interactions. Such drugs include anticoagulants, cardiac glycosides, antiarrhythmics, antiepileptics, cytotoxic and anti-HIV drugs, and hypoglycemic agents. It is vital that the minority of clinically important interactions are distinguished from the majority, which are only of chance occurrence or academic interest.

Key references

Chyka PA. How many deaths occur annually from adverse drug reactions in the United States? Am J Med. 2000;109:122–30.

Dresser GK, Spence JD, Bailey DG. Pharmacokinetic–pharmacodynamic consequences and clinical relevance of cytochrome P450 3A4 inhibition. Clin Pharmacokinet. 2000;38:41–57.

Fugh-Berman A. Herb–drug interactions. Lancet 2000;355:134–8.

Grandison MK, Boudinot FD. Age-related changes in protein binding of drugs: implications for therapy. Clin Pharmacokinet. 2000;38:271–90.

Levy RH, Thummel KE, Trager EF et al. (eds) Metabolic drug interactions. Philadelphia: Lippincott Williams & Wilkins; 2000: 1–793.

Quinn DI, Day RO. Clinically important drug interactions. In: Speight TM, Holford NHG, eds. Avery's drug treatment. Auckland: Adis; 1997:301–38.

Rowland M, Tozer TN. Clinical pharmacokinetics: concepts and applications, 2nd edn. Philadelphia: Lea & Febiger; 1989.

Wood M. Pharmacokinetic drug interactions in anesthetic practice. Clin Pharmacokinet. 1991;21:285–307.

Further reading

Backman J, Kivistö KT, Olkkola KT, Neuvonen PJ. The area under the plasma concentration–time curve for oral midazolam is 400-fold larger during treatment with itraconazole than with rifampicin. Eur J Clin Pharmacol. 1998;54:53–8.

Desmeules J, Gascon MP, Dayer P, Magistris M. Impact of environmental and genetic factors on codeine analgesia. Eur J Clin Pharmacol. 1991;41:23–6.

Hemmerling TM, Schuettler J, Schwilden H. Desflurane reduces the effective therapeutic infusion rate (ETI) of cisatracurium more than isoflurane, sevoflurane, or propofol. Can J Anesth. 2001;48:532–7.

Jokinen MJ, Ahonen J, Neuvonen PJ, Olkkola KT. The effect of erythromycin, fluvoxamine, and their combination on the pharmacokinetics of ropivacaine. Anesth Analg. 2000; 91:1207–12.

Kennedy JM, van Rij AM, Spears GF et al. Polypharmacy in a general surgical unit and consequences of drug withdrawal. Br J Clin Pharmacol. 2000;49:353–62.

Kharasch ED, Hankins D, Mautz D, Thummel KE. Identification of the enzyme responsible for oxidative halothane metabolism: implications for prevention of halothane hepatitis. Lancet 1996;347:1367–71.

Kissim I, Brown PT, Bradley EL Jr. Sedative and hypnotic midazolam-morphine interactions in rats. Anesth Analg 1990; 71:137–43.

Nimmo WS, Heading RD, Wilson J, Tothill P, Prescott LF. Inhibition of gastric emptying and drug absorption by narcotic analgesics. Br J Clin Pharmacol. 1975;2:509–13.

Olkkola KT, Backman J, Neuvonen PJ. Midazolam should be avoided in patients receiving the systemic antimycotics ketoconazole or itraconazole. Clin Pharmacol Ther. 1994;55:481–5.

Trisel LA. Handbook on injectable drugs, 12th edn. Bethesda: American Society of Hospital Pharmacists; 2003.

Vinik HR, Bradley EL Jr, Kissin I. Triple anesthetic combination: propofol–midazolam–alfentanil. Anesth Analg. 1994;78:354–8.

Vuyk J. TCI: supplementation and drug interactions. Anaesthesia 1998;53:35–41.

Chapter 10

Adverse drug reactions

Philip M Hopkins

TOPICS COVERED IN THIS CHAPTER

- **Drug administration errors**
- **Drug intolerance**
- **Drug idiosyncrasy**
    - Acetylator status
    - Cytochrome P450 variants
- **Plasma cholinesterase variants**
- **Glucose-6-phosphate dehydrogenase deficiency**
- **The porphyrias**
- **Malignant hyperthermia**
- **Allergic drug reactions**

An adverse drug reaction can be considered as any potentially harmful untoward outcome of therapeutic drug administration. The unwanted outcome may be a side effect of the drug, an exaggeration of the therapeutic effect, a failure of the therapeutic effect, or a totally unexpected effect. A classification of adverse drug reactions is given in Table 10.1.

This chapter focuses on the general principles of the mechanisms of adverse drug reactions that can be applied to a wide range of drugs, to idiosyncratic drug reactions relevant to anesthesia, and to allergic reactions to drugs. The mechanisms of direct organ toxicity and secondary effects tend to be specific to individual drugs and will be covered where appropriate in the relevant chapter. Drug interactions are discussed in Chapter 9.

Table 10.1 Classification of adverse drug reactions

Administration errors
Intolerance
Idiosyncrasy
Anaphylaxis/anaphylactoid
Direct organ toxicity
Secondary effects
Drug interaction

DRUG ADMINISTRATION ERRORS

A recent audit at a large UK teaching hospital reported that there were prescribing anomalies in the prescription charts of 60% of patients surveyed. Although some of these errors were minor and probably of little potential consequence, others were more worrying. They included prescription of the wrong drug (substitution of drugs with similar names), the wrong route of administration, the wrong dose, and incorrect dosing intervals. The dosing errors were a mixture of under- and overdosing, and included some doses that were incorrect by three orders of magnitude.

For some drugs, dosing information that forms the knowledge base for prescribers may be inaccurate and thus the cause of erroneous dosing. Several examples exist in anesthetic practice where dosing regimens for a drug developed in a nonanesthetic context have been applied directly to the perioperative situation. This applies to several drugs that were introduced into clinical practice in the days when licensing legislation was not as rigorous as it is now. A classic example of this is morphine. The traditional quoted dose for severe postoperative pain is 0.15 mg/kg given intramuscularly. This was, however, determined as the effective dose for battlefield casualties. It is now appreciated that battlefield casualties are an inappropriate model for postoperative pain, as their pain tolerance is high as a result of the psychological and neurohumoral response to the situation.

Another example is the use of traditional antiemetic drugs for the prevention and treatment of postoperative nausea and vomiting. None of the currently available antiemetics was developed primarily for perioperative use: many were first introduced as treatments for motion sickness or other vestibular disorders, for migraine, or for the treatment of side effects of radiation therapy or cytotoxic chemotherapy. Droperidol, a butyrophenone, was introduced into anesthetic practice as a neuroleptic agent in a dose of approximately 0.1 mg/kg. Although neurolept anesthesia as a technique has diminished in popularity, it did demonstrate the antiemetic efficacy of droperidol. It is interesting that this efficacy was maintained at doses 10 times lower than those used for the neuroleptic effect. It may well be that antiemetic phenothiazines and antihistamines are also being used in inappropriately high doses in the perioperative setting, with an inevitable increase in side effects.

DRUG INTOLERANCE

Even when given the intended correct dose of a drug some patients will exhibit an adverse effect. When this occurs as a result of variation of the individual's drug response within a unimodal population variation in response, the phenomenon is termed drug intolerance. The cause of drug intolerance is invariably multifactorial, with both environmental and genetic factors involved. This is in contrast to idiosyncratic reactions (see below), in which genetic factors determine a bimodal population response to a drug.

The propensity for adverse drug effects is often described in terms of the therapeutic index. In animal testing of new drugs the therapeutic index is calculated from the ratio of the LD_{50} (the dose that causes death in 50% of animals) to the ED_{50} (the dose that produces the desired effect in 50% of animals). The LD_{50} and ED_{50} are calculated from cumulative quantal dose response curves (see Chapter 7). This is illustrated in Figure 10.1a. Figure 10.1b, however, illustrates a limitation of the therapeutic index. This illustrates two drugs, A and B, that have the same ED_{50} value, but because the population variability in response to drug B is greater than that of drug A, the ED_{95} (dose that produces the desired effect in 95% of subjects) is considerably higher for drug B than for drug A. This is of great clinical importance, as we would wish any dosing regimen to have the desired effect in as many individuals as possible, and so the ED_{95}, the ED_{99}, or even the $ED_{99.9}$ would be the best dose to select, provided it does not encroach on doses that produce important unwanted effects. Similarly, the LD_{50} has limited clinical value, as indeed does the dose required to produce any unwanted effect in 50% of individuals, as the clinical pharmacologic requirement is to have as few individuals as possible with an unwanted effect. Figures 10.1c and 10.1d further illustrate this principle for the two drugs described in Figure 10.1b. A more clinically useful concept, therefore, to describe the likelihood of drug intolerance is the *certain safety factor*. This relates the dose to produce a specified unwanted effect in a defined proportion of the population to the dose that will be ineffective in the same proportion of the population. The proportion of the population used in the calculation depends on the severity of the unwanted effect. The most frequently used proportion is 1%, and in this case the certain safety factor is calculated as TD_{01}/ED_{99}, where TD is the toxic dose. If the unwanted effect is especially serious lower proportions may be used, e.g. $TD_{0.1}/ ED_{99.9}$, $TD_{0.01}/ED_{99.99}$, etc. The doses used in the calculation of the certain safety factor also define the limits of the *therapeutic window*.

The certain safety factor is more clinically useful as an indicator of drug tolerance than the therapeutic index.

DRUG IDIOSYNCRASY

Pharmacogenetic variation has been identified in drug metabolism (acetylation, cytochrome P450 variants, plasma cholinesterase variants), inability to compensate for drug effects (glucose 6-phosphate dehydrogenase deficiency, acute porphyrias), and in drug effects themselves (malignant hyperthermia). Each of these examples will be discussed separately.

Acetylator status

Acetylation is one of the nonmicrosomal phase II conjugation reactions. The gene controlling the enzyme involved, *N*-acetyltransferase, exists in one of two forms that determines the acetylator status – slow or fast – of an individual. The prevalence of slow acetylation is 60% in Caucasians and 10–20% in Asians. Drugs subject to *N*-acetylation include isoniazid, hydralazine, procainamide, some sulfonamides, sulfasalazine, nitrazepam, and caffeine. Slow acetylators are at higher risk of side effects of these drugs, such as peripheral neuropathy with isoniazid, lupus syndrome with hydralazine and procainamide, allergic reactions and hemolysis with sulfonamides, and gastrointestinal side effects with sulfasalazine.

Cytochrome P450 variants

The cytochrome P450 group of enzymes are responsible for the great majority of microsomal phase I oxidation reactions. Four classes of cytochrome P450 enzyme (CYP1–4), each with several subgroups, are important in drug metabolism. Polymorphisms in at least four cytochrome P450 enzymes have been found that are associated with reduced or even absent enzyme activity. Most drugs have the potential to be metabolized by more than one subtype of enzyme, but clinically important reductions in metabolism will be seen if there are reductions in the activity of an enzyme that normally predominates in the metabolism of the drug.

CYP2D6

This enzyme is involved in metabolism of approximately 25% of drugs, many of which are relevant to anesthesiologists. The drugs include β-blockers (metoprolol, propranolol), antiarrhythmics (amiodarone, flecainide), antidepressants (nearly all tricyclics and selective serotonin reuptake inhibitors), and neuroleptics (phenothiazines and butyrophenones). It has been estimated that approximately 6% of Caucasians and 1% of Asians have reduced CYP2D6 activity.

CYP2C9

This enzyme is involved in the metabolism of warfarin. Individuals with deficient CYP2C9 activity are prone to hemorrhagic complications of warfarin administered in otherwise standard dosage regimens.

CYP2C19

This enzyme is responsible for the oxidation of diazepam and the proton pump inhibitors, such as omeprazole. Reduced activity of this enzyme is especially prevalent in Asians (20%, versus 3% in Caucasians). Affected individuals require reduced doses of diazepam but have a beneficial therapeutic effect when given proton pump inhibitors in the treatment of *Helicobacter pylori* infection.

CYP3A4–5

The CYP3A enzymes are responsible for 50% of drug oxidation reactions. Polymorphisms leading to reduced activity occur in approximately 6% of Caucasians. Of relevance to anesthesia is that they account for individuals who are slow metabolizers of midazolam, feutanyl and other important anesthetic drugs (Chapter 9).

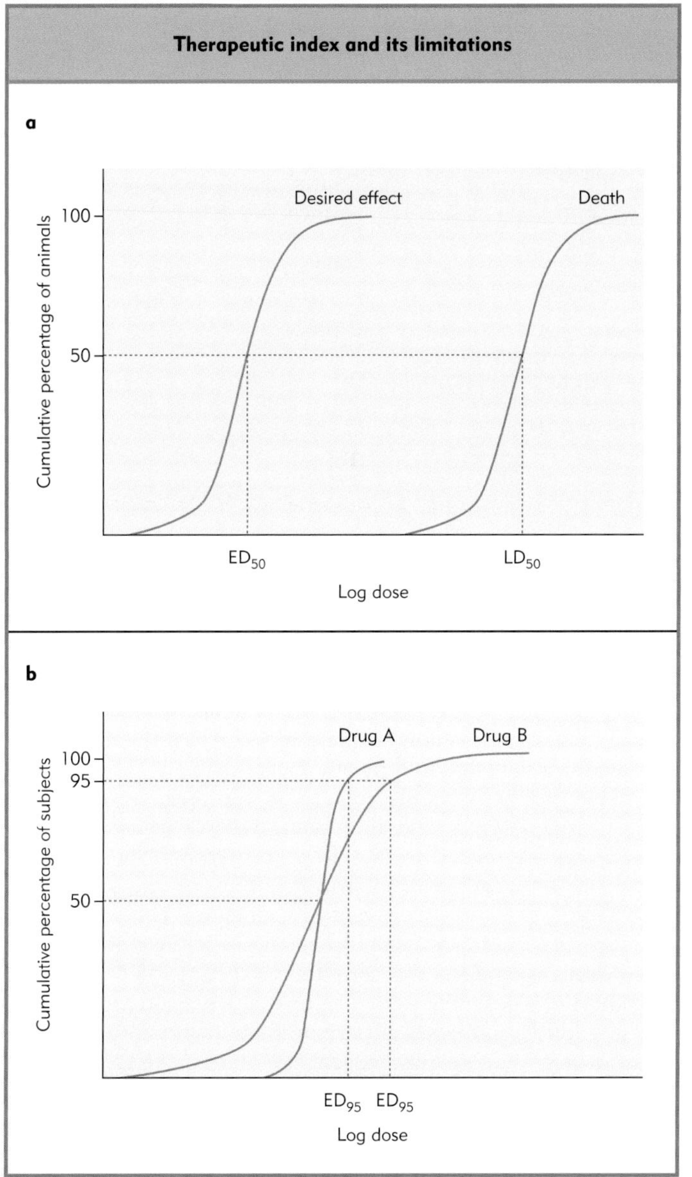

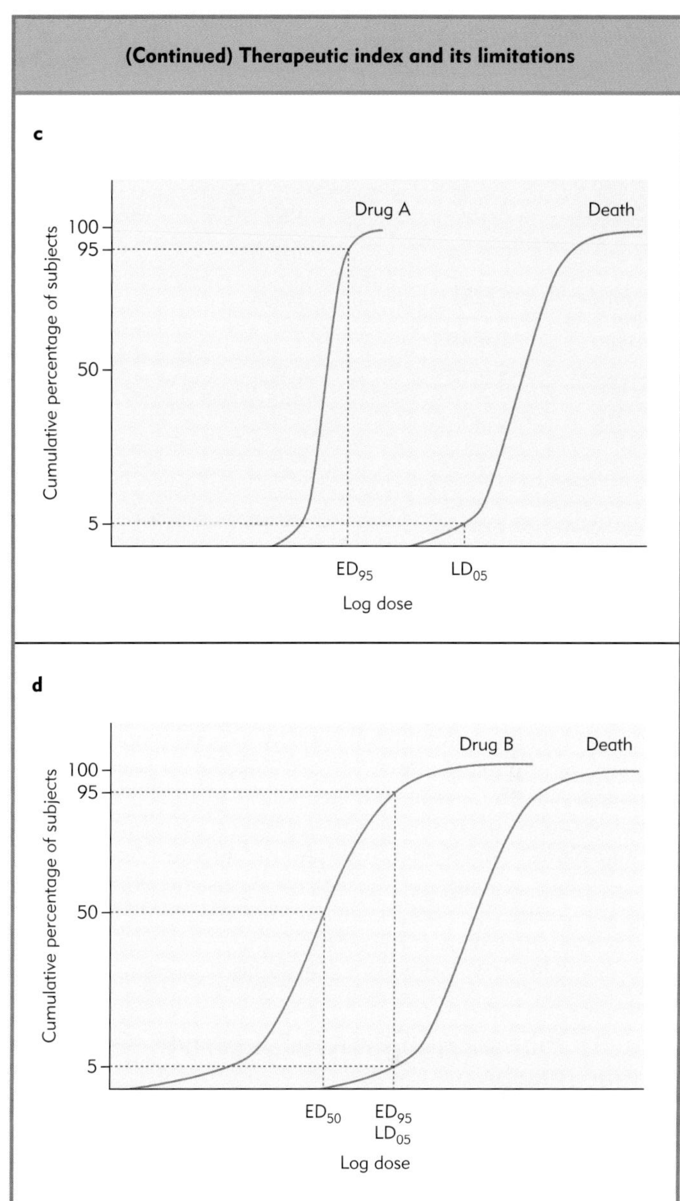

Figure 10.1 The therapeutic index and its limitations. (a) How cumulative quantal dose response curves for the desired drug effect and for death are used to determine ED_{50} and LD_{50} values respectively in animal experiments: these values are necessary to define the therapeutic index of a drug. (b–d) One limitation of using the ED_{50}. The two curves in (b) are the cumulative quantal dose–response curves for two drugs having the same effect. Drugs A and B have identical ED_{50} values but there is greater population variability in the response to drug B than to drug A. (c, d) The cumulative quantal dose–response curves for the desired effect and death for drugs A (c) and B (d). So, although the ED_{50} dose of each drug does not encroach on the dose–response curve for death with either drug (c and d), it can be seen that the ED_{95} value for drug B is identical to the LD_{05} value for the drug (d). This is not the case for drug A (c), which therefore has a greater certain safety factor.

PLASMA CHOLINESTERASE VARIANTS

Plasma cholinesterase (also known as pseudocholinesterase, serum cholinesterase, nonspecific cholinesterase, butyrylcholinesterase, S-type cholinesterase) is responsible for the breakdown of succinylcholine in the plasma. Indeed, it was the recognition of individuals who had prolonged paralysis after the administration of succinylcholine ('scoline apnea') that led to the identification of genetic variants of plasma cholinesterase. Investigation of those affected by scoline apnea revealed the clinical condition to be inherited as an autosomal recessive trait. We now know that the plasma cholinesterase gene lies on the long arm of chromosome 3.

Plasma cholinesterase phenotyping through the measurement of enzyme activity and response to in vitro inhibitors can now be complemented by genotyping (Table 10.2). The first in vitro inhibitor of cholinesterase activity to be used was dibucaine (cinchocaine). In this test the dibucaine number is given by the percentage inhibition of cholinesterase activity of the sera of the patient by dibucaine 10 mM using benzoyl choline as the substrate. Normal individuals have a dibucaine number of 71–85. Patients homozygous for the atypical allele have a dibucaine number of 20, whereas those heterogenous for the atypical allele have an intermediate dibucaine number of 52–65. The use of sodium fluoride 50 mM as an alternative inhibitor to dibucaine enabled the identification of the fluoride-resistant allele. In

Table 10.2 Plasma cholinesterase variants

Name	Base change	Frequency	Enzyme activity (%)	Duration of action of sux
Usual	None	0.98	100	Normal
Atypical	A209T	0.02	30	2 hrs
Silent	G351A	0.0003	Zero	3–4 hrs
Fluoride	C728T	0.003	40	1–2 hrs
H type	G424A	?	10	2–3 hrs
K type	G1615A	0.0013	70	<1 hr
J type	A1490T	?	34	1–2 hrs

The names of the variants were given after their characterization by enzyme activity and inhibitor studies. The variants are due to missense mutations in the plasma cholinesterase gene, which lies on chromosome 3. The normal duration of action of succinylcholine (sux) is 4–6 minutes, depending on the dose administered.

addition to succinylcholine, the nondepolarizing neuromuscular blocking drug mivacurium is metabolized by plasma cholinesterase. The investigation of patients with a prolonged action of either of these drugs can use the traditional phenotyping or a genotyping approach. However, it should be appreciated that a negative mutation screen should be followed by measurement of enzyme activity and inhibitor effect, as there may well be undiscovered mutations in the plasma cholinesterase gene. In addition to succinylcholine and mivacurium, ester local anesthetics, heroin, diamorphine (to 6-acetylmorphine), aspirin and methylprednisolone acetate are metabolized by plasma cholinesterase, at least in part. In contrast, atracurium, remefentanil, esmolol, and 6-acetylmorphine are ester drugs that are not dependent on plasma cholinesterase for their metabolism.

GLUCOSE-6-PHOSPHATE DEHYDROGENASE DEFICIENCY

Erythrocytes are one of the cell types that utilize the pentose phosphate pathway for carbohydrate metabolism. The first step in the pentose phosphate pathway is the conversion of glucose-6-phosphate by glucose-6-phosphate dehydrogenase (G6PD). In this reaction $NADP^+$ is used as a cofactor and is converted to NADPH. NADPH is important in erythrocytes for restoring the levels of reduced glutathione required to combat hydrogen peroxide released within the cell in the presence of oxidants. Individuals with G6PD deficiency are therefore exposed to high levels of hydrogen peroxide in their red cells in the presence of oxidant drugs such as primaquine, chloraquine, chloramphenicol, some sulfonamides, and vitamin K analogs. Administration of these drugs to those with G6PD deficiency results in hemolytic anemia. The prevalence of G6PD deficiency is highest in those areas where falciparum malaria is endemic. This is assumed to reflect a survival advantage of G6PD deficiency to falciparum malaria.

THE PORPHYRIAS

The porphyrias are a group of disorders characterized by the excessive build-up of precursors of heme. These precursors, porphyrinogens, are excreted in the urine, where they are spontaneously converted on exposure to light and air to purple-colored porphyrins. The metabolic pathway of synthesis of heme is shown in Figure 10.2. Under normal circumstances heme synthesis is very tightly regulated by efficient feedback inhibition of heme on δ-aminolevulinic acid (ALA) synthetase. Acute attacks can be precipitated by any factor that places a stress on the heme synthesis pathway, such as bleeding, or metabolic stress (fasting, dehydration, infection, stress). The features of an acute attack are related to the effects of porphyrinogens on the nervous system, which include motor, sensory, and autonomic dysfunction.

Of particular importance to anesthesia is the potential for many drugs to induce the activity of ALA synthetase. These drugs have the potential to induce or exacerbate an acute attack in a susceptible individual. There is some uncertainty and controversy as to the porphyrinogenicity of some drugs. A good example of this is propofol. In animal experiments propofol has been shown to induce ALA synthetase activity, but there are anecdotal reports of its safe use in patients who have acute porphyria. On the other hand, porphyrin levels have been shown to increase after maintenance anesthesia with a propofol infusion in patients with acute porphyrias. Table 10.3 lists drugs of relevance to anesthesia and indicates how safe they are to use in patients with acute porphyria.

MALIGNANT HYPERTHERMIA

Malignant hyperthermia (MH) was first reported in 1960. It is an autosomal dominant condition in which susceptible individuals have a defect in skeletal muscle intracellular calcium regulation. Under most circumstances homeostatic mechanisms compensate for increased calcium turnover, but the potent inhalation anesthetics and succinylcholine cause a massive acceleration of calcium release that overwhelms the compensatory mechanisms. The resulting increased intracellular calcium concentration leads directly to increased muscle contractile activity and metabolic stimulation. Metabolism is further increased indirectly in response to the increased contractile activity and the demand for ATP to fuel sarcoplasmic reticulum and sarcolemmal calcium ATPase pumps. Under these con-

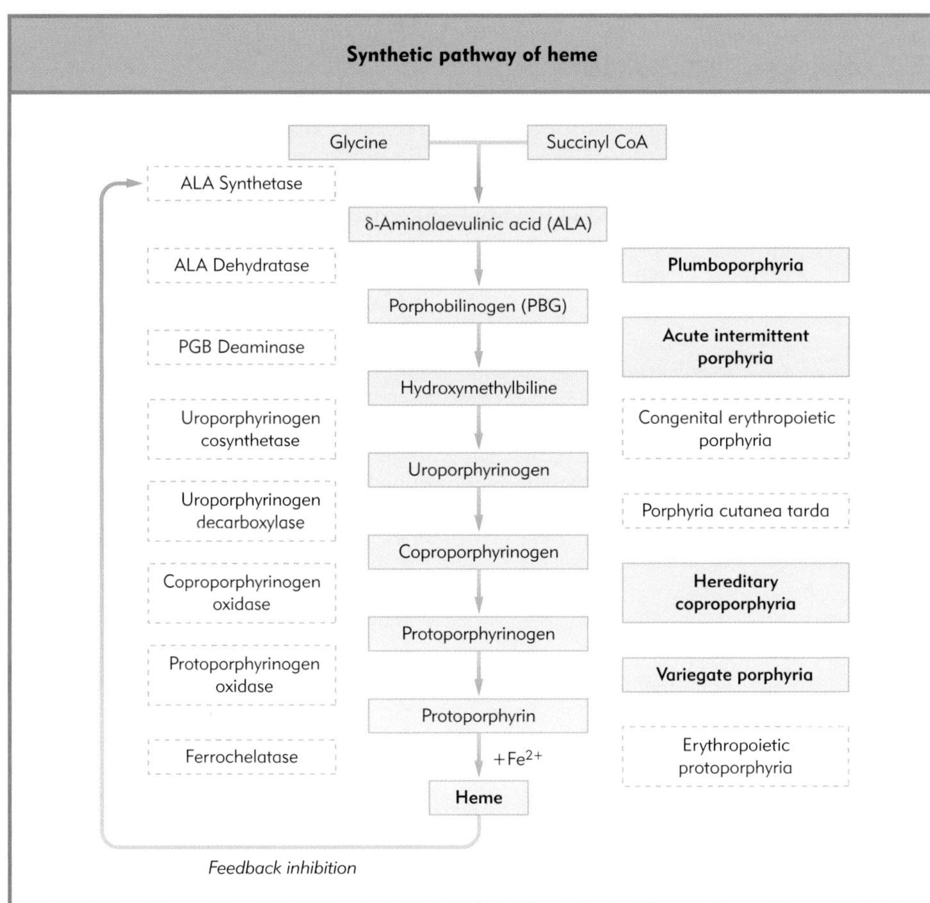

Figure 10.2 The synthetic pathway of heme from glycine and succinyl coenzyme A. The intermediary compounds in the pathway are given in the central column and the enzymes for each step on the left-hand side. The rate-limiting step is that catalyzed by ALA synthetase, which is under feedback control by heme. On the right-hand side the various types of porphyria are listed adjacent to the enzyme deficiency responsible for the condition. The acute porphyrias are shaded. (Adapted from James MF& Hift RJ. Porphyrias. British Journal of Anaesthesia 2000; 85: 143-53, © The Board of Management and Trustees of the British Journal of Anaesthesia. Reproduced by permission of Oxford University Press/British Journal of Anaesthesia.)

ditions oxygen supply cannot match demand, and there is overproduction of carbon dioxide, lactate, and heat. The other primary feature of an MH reaction is rhabdomyolysis. This results from a combination of excessive muscle activity and depletion of ATP, which is required to maintain cell membrane integrity.

The principal gene responsible for determining MH susceptibility is the skeletal muscle ryanodine receptor gene (*RYR1*), which encodes the protein forming the sarcoplasmic reticulum calcium release channel (see Chapter 35). More than 100 mutations or polymorphisms of *RYR1* have been described, and over 20 of these have been demonstrated to lead to functional protein defects consistent with MH susceptibility. Such functional mutations have a potential use in presymptomatic diagnosis of the disorder. The molecular genetics of MH, however, is not always straightforward. Whereas *RYR1* mutations or polymorphisms are likely to be implicated in the great majority of patients, some of these mutations or polymorphisms may need to be present in combination with other *RYR1* variants, or indeed polymorphisms of other genes involved in skeletal muscle calcium regulation, for an individual to be at risk from a clinical reaction.

Other than all the potent inhalation anesthetics (halothane, enflurane, isoflurane, sevoflurane, desflurane) and succinylcholine, no other drugs are implicated as triggers of MH. Some others, such as lidocaine, ketamine, nitrous oxide, phenothiazines, have been implicated in the past as MH triggers, but it is now agreed that these were erroneously implicated as a result of misdiagnosis or poorly designed laboratory experiments.

ALLERGIC DRUG REACTIONS

Allergic reactions to drugs administered intravenously are acute type I hypersensitivity reactions (Chapter 54). By definition, these responses occur on a second or subsequent exposure to an allergen. However, it is recognized that approximately 50% of anaphylactic-like or anaphylactoid reactions that occur in anesthesia do so in patients receiving the drug on the first occasion. True anaphylactic reactions involve mast cell degranulation resulting from the production of allergen-specific IgE. Anaphylactoid reactions can occur through complement activation (classical or alternative pathways) or through a direct drug action on the mast cell itself. There is little rationale in the use of a 'test dose' in the prevention of allergic drug reactions. True anaphylaxis can occur after exposure to the smallest dose of antigen. Direct mast cell degranulation (nonIgE-mediated response) is probably dependent on the mass of drug and its rate of administration. However, in these circumstances there is unlikely to be any response to a test dose, but the full dose will cause the reaction. It is therefore advisable to administer intravenous drugs slowly.

The products of mast cell degranulation that are the mediators of the anaphylactic or anaphylactoid response include principally histamine and other vasoactive amines, but also proteases (such as tryptase) and lipid-derived mediators (such as leukotrienes and prostaglandins). These mediators can affect the skin (flushing and urticaria), the vasculature (vasodilatation and increased capillary permeability), and the respiratory system (bronchoconstriction, inflammation, and increased bronchial secretions). Not all of these features occur in every anaphylactic/anaphylactoid reaction. Some reactions are characterized by the predominance of vasodilatation, whereas in others bronchoconstriction predominates. This probably reflects the presence of two main types of mast cell: mucosal mast cells that are located in the lungs and the gut, and connective tissue mast cells that are ubiquitous. The relationship between individual drugs and the spectrum of clinical features is not consistent between patients suffering reactions, although some drugs (e.g. atracurium, morphine) frequently produce cutaneous reactions without systemic vasodilatation or bronchoconstriction. This suggests that cutaneous connective tissue mast cells are particularly sensitive to these drugs.

Our ability to investigate suspected anaphylactoid reactions is somewhat crude. Histamine release is difficult to measure because the serum half-life of the amine is so short. Its metabolite, methylhistamine, is, however, more stable and can be detected in the urine. Alternatively, mast cell degranulation can be demonstrated by serum mast cell tryptase levels, and complement assays may point to a particular mechanism. The

Table 10.3 Recommendations for the use of drugs during anesthesia in the acute porphyrias

	Drugs	Recommendation
Inhalational agents	Nitrous oxide	Use
	Cyclopropane	Use
	Halothane	Use
	Enflurane	UWC
	Isoflurane	UWC
	Sevoflurane*	UWC
	Desflurane*	UWC
Intravenous induction agents	Propofol	Use
	Ketamine	UWC
	Barbiturates	Avoid
	Etomidate	Avoid
Analgesics	Acetaminophen	Use
	Alfentanil	Use
	Aspirin	Use
	Buprenorphine	Use
	Codeine	Use
	Fentanyl	Use
	Pethidine (meperidine)	Use
	Morphine	Use
	Naloxone	Use
	Sufentanil	Use
	Diclofenac	UWECO
	Ketorolac*	UWECO
	Phenacetin	UWECO
	Tilidine	UWECO
	Pentazocine	Avoid
Neuromuscular blocking drugs	Tubocurarine	Use
	Pancuronium	Use
	Succinylcholine	Use
	Alcuronium	UWC
	Atracurium	UWC
	Rocuronium*	UWC
	Mivacurium*	UWC
	Vecuronium	UWC
Neuromuscular block reversal agents	Atropine	Use
	Glycopyrrolate	Use
	Neostigmine	Use
Local anesthetics	Bupivacaine	Use
	Lidocaine	Use
	Prilocaine	Use
	Procaine	Use
	Tetracaine	Use
	Cocaine	UWC
	Mepivacaine	UWC
	Ropivacaine	ND/avoid
Sedatives and antiemetics	Domperidone	Use
	Droperidol	Use
	Phenothiazines	Use
	Temazepam	Use
	Triazolam	Use
	Benzodiazepines other than listed	UWC
	Cimetidine	UWC
	Diazepam	UWC
	Lorazepam	UWC
	Metoclopramide	UWC
	Midazolam	UWC
	Ondansetron	UWC
	Oxazepam	UWC
	Ranitidine	UWC
	Chlordiazepoxide	UWECO
	Nitrazepam	UWECO
Cardiovascular drugs	Epinephrine	Use
	Magnesium	Use
	Phentolamine	Use
	Procainamide	Use
	α-agonists	Use
	β-blockers	Use
	β-agonists	Use
	Diltiazem	UWC
	Disopyramide	UWC
	Sodium nitroprusside	UWC
	Verapamil	UWC
	Hydralazine	UWECO
	Nifedipine	UWECO
	Phenoxybenzamine	UWECO

* No data, and recommendation is based on drugs of a similar class.
Use, may be used safely; UWC, use with caution, as there is insufficient evidence to indicate complete safety, although they are probably safe; UWECO, use with extreme caution only, as there is insufficient evidence to indicate safety and some rationale for their not being safe; avoid, do not use, as there is good evidence that they could initiate or exacerbate a porphyrinogenic response. (Adapted from James MF& Hift RJ. Porphyrias. British Journal of Anaesthesia 2000; 85: 143-53, © The Board of Management and Trustees of the British Journal of Anaesthesia. Reproduced by permission of Oxford University Press/British Journal of Anaesthesia.)

availability of allergen-specific radioallergosorbent tests (RAST) for anesthetic drugs is limited, although one exists for succinylcholine. There are many enthusiasts for skin-prick testing following suspected anaphylactic reactions. A positive weal and flare reaction following the introduction of an allergen to the skin is produced by an IgE response and, by implication, is said to be indicative of true anaphylaxis. However, protocols for skin-prick testing of potential drug allergens vary widely, as do the interpretation of the results. As with skin-prick testing of, for example, airborne allergens, the specificity of drug allergen testing is low. Furthermore, in some individuals IgE may be absent from the skin but present in serum or bronchial secretions, and in these individuals skin-prick testing will give a false-negative result.

There is little rationale for the use of a 'test dose' to prevent allergic drug reactions.

The greatest controversy with drugs used in anesthesia is the proportion of anaphylactic reactions in which nondepolarizing neuromuscular blocking drugs are implicated. In France, for example, muscle relaxant drugs are implicated in approximately 60% of anesthesia-associated type I hypersensitivity reactions. In Australia and North America, however, reactions to muscle relaxants other than succinylcholine are considered rare. The explanation for this apparent epidemiological anomaly is probably the use of intradermal testing (which has a high false-positive rate) or different degrees of drug dilution in the conduct of skin-prick tests: there is a growing body of evidence that skin-prick tests for nondepolarizing neuromuscular blockers have a high false-positive rate unless the drug is diluted to at least 1:1000. The studies that provide this evidence involve conducting skin-prick tests on subjects who have never received general anesthesia, and in whom any positive response to the skin-prick test should be presumed to be erroneous. An alternative explanation for these findings is that individuals may be immunologically sensitized to neuromuscular blocking drugs by environmental exposure to chemicals used in, for example, perfumes or air fresheners; however, no positive links have so far been established.

These limitations of diagnosis make quantification of the incidence of hypersensitivity reactions difficult. A reasonable consensus would be that they occur in approximately 1:10 000–1:40 000 anesthetics. Drug groups other than muscle relaxants that are most commonly implicated are intravenous anesthetics, antibiotics, and plasma substitutes. Latex sensitivity is becoming an increasing problem and accounts for 20–50% of hypersensitivity reactions during anesthesia. Reactions to latex are characterized by their development after 30–60 minutes of surgery, whereas drug reactions tend to occur within seconds or a few minutes of administration. The use of chlorhexidine as an antibacterial coating to bladder and central venous catheters has also been associated with severe systemic hypersensitivity reactions.

Key references

Barta C, Sasvari-Szekely M, Devai A, Kovacs E, Staub M, Enyedi P. Analysis of mutations in the plasma cholinesterase gene of patients with a history of prolonged neuromuscular block during anesthesia. Mol Genet Metab. 2001;74:484–8.

Dhonneur G, Combes X, Chassard D, Merle JC. Skin sensitivity to rocuronium and vecuronium: a randomized controlled prick-testing study in healthy volunteers. Anesth Analg. 2004;98:986–9.

Mertes PM, Laxenaire MC, Alla F; Groupe d'Etudes des Reactions Anaphylactoides Peranesthesiques. Anaphylactic and anaphylactoid reactions occurring during anesthesia in France in 1999–2000. Anesthesiology 2003;99:536–45.

Robinson RL, Anetseder MJ, Brancadoro V et al. Recent advances in the diagnosis of malignant hyperthermia susceptibility: how confident can we be of genetic testing? Eur J Hum Genet. 2003;11:342–8.

Further reading

James MF, Hift RJ. Porphyrias. Br J Anaesth. 2000;85:143–53.

Halsall PJ, Hopkins PM. Inherited disease and anesthesia. In: Healy TEJ, Cohen PJ, eds. A practice of anesthesia, 7th edn. London: Arnold; 2003: 377–90.

Hopkins PM. Malignant hyperthermia: advances in clinical management and diagnosis. Br J Anaesth. 2000;85:118–28.

Kalow W. Atypical plasma cholinesterase. A personal discovery story: a tale of three cities. Can J Anaesth. 2004;51:206–11.

Chapter 11

Basic physical principles

Paul CW Beatty

TOPICS COVERED IN THIS CHAPTER
- **What is physics?**
- **Mass, force, work, and energy**
- **Pressure and density**
- **States of matter and latent heat**
- **Gas laws**
- **Avogadro's hypothesis**
- **Calorimetry and heat transfer**
  - Thermal or heat capacity
- **Solubility and diffusion**

WHAT IS PHYSICS?

Physics is natural science's attempt to describe the fundamental laws of the world around us. This may seem a rather grandiose way of starting a chapter in a book devoted to explaining the application of the basic sciences in anesthesia, but it is the very nature of physics that often most foxes medical scientists. Physics asks and answers simple fundamental questions. It follows the implications of those questions to their logical and sometimes extraordinarily strange conclusions. The key to understanding it is to do the same. When in doubt, ask simple questions! Physics describes in detail what it finds using the clarity and economy of mathematics. As a result, descriptions in the physical sciences require precision. The starting point for many physical descriptions is a few basic concepts inspired by experimental observation. These concepts lead to basic definitions of quantities defined by number and unit. In the end, however, physics resolves into a single theme: the description of the natural laws that govern energy transfer. All the topics to be covered in this chapter are concerned with energy in one form or another.

MASS, FORCE, WORK, AND ENERGY

The first major problem that was addressed by physics was how and why things move. Intuitively we know that heavy objects require more effort to pick up from ground level. People also noted that, when dropped from a height, objects moved faster and faster until they hit the ground. Initially, it was thought that the heavier the object the faster it would fall, but Galileo proved that this rate of increase in speed (acceleration) was independent of the weight of the object. Therefore, the next question was, what makes objects fall? When objects fall or move in any way, what controls how they move? Does the motion of things on earth say anything about how the planets move in the heavens? One other observation was important. Intuitively, people realized that the same volumes of different materials had different weights. However, Archimedes showed that the weight of an object immersed in water was reduced by the equivalent of the weight of water it displaced. Is there some property of materials that makes the weight of the water and the reduction in weight of the object equivalent?

It was Newton, through his Laws of Motion and Theory of Gravity, who answered all these questions, and by doing so founded physics as we think of it. The definitions and principles he used are shown in Table 11.1.

The ultimate concept derived from Newton's laws is that of energy. Energy can be defined as the capacity to perform work. However, as work is about moving forces and forces are about creating motion, energy can be thought of as the property of an object that creates motion. In the case of gravity, when an object is dropped from a high tower it has a far higher velocity at impact than if dropped only a few meters. Thus, it can create more change in motion in other bodies upon impact. The faster it moves, the more capacity for creating motion it has. This energy that the object has by virtue of its motion is *kinetic energy*.

The capacity to do work was in the object before it fell. The higher the tower from which the object falls, the further the separation of the object from the ground, and the more work is done against gravity. Thus, there is an energy that an object has by virtue of its position in a region over which a natural force acts. This is *potential energy*. Potential energy can be converted into kinetic energy, and vice versa. In a closed system – i.e. one in which energy does not flow out or in – energy is always conserved. The nature of the energy in a system leads to energy being referred to in different ways in different circumstances. For instance, the energy associated with motion may be called mechanical energy, or that with chemical reactions chemical energy, and so on, but all energy ultimately is the same and in the SI system is designated by the unit joule (J).

Table 11.1 Definitions and principles of physics

Newton's laws of motion
I An object remains at rest or continues in motion in a straight line unless acted on by an external force.
II The rate of change of momentum of an object is proportional to the applied force.
III To the action of every force, an equal and opposite opposing force is generated.

Force – that which causes or changes motion (SI unit: Newton, N = kg m/s^2)
Mass – A measure of the amount of matter in a body (SI unit: kilogram, kg)
Velocity – The rate of change of position of an object (speed of motion) in a given direction (SI unit: meter per second, m/s)
Force of gravity – The force that causes objects to fall toward a body and controls the motions of the planets; it is proportional to the product of the masses of the two objects involved and inversely proportional to their distance apart
Momentum – The mass of an object in motion multiplied by its velocity (SI unit: kilogram meter per second, kg m/s)
Acceleration – The rate of change of the velocity of an object in motion. Thus, Newton's second law of motion means that force equals mass multiplied by acceleration
Work – Work is done when the point of application of a force moves; the work done equals the force multiplied by the distance moved by the force's point of application (SI unit: joule, J); the concept of work is fairly intuitive, as is the concept of power
Power – The rate of doing work or the work done per unit time; power equals the work done divided by the time taken to do it (SI unit: watt, W).
Kinetic energy – The energy an object has by virtue of its motion (SI unit: joule, J)
Potential energy – The energy an object has by virtue of its position or state (SI unit: joule, J)
Law of Conservation of Energy – In a closed system for which no energy leaves or enters, the amount of energy in the system is constant
Law of Conservation of Momentum – When two or more objects act upon one another their total momentum does not change unless external force is applied; this is derived from Newton's Third Law of Motion
Pressure – Force per unit area of application (SI unit: Pascal, Pa = N/m^2)
Density – The mass per unit volume of a substance (SI unit: kilogram per cubic meter, kg/m^3)
Absolute pressure measurement – A pressure measurement made with reference to vacuum
Relative or gauge pressure – A pressure measurement made with reference to atmospheric pressure
Latent heat – The latent heat (e.g. vaporization) is the energy required to convert 1 kg of a substance from one phase to another without change in temperature at a given pressure (SI unit: joules per kilogram, J/kg)
Fick's Law – The rate of diffusion is proportional to the gradient of concentration
Graham's Law – The rate of diffusion through a permeable material is inversely proportional to the square root of the molecular weight of the diffusing molecule
Henry's Law – Given an inert gas in contact with a liquid, the mass of gas that dissolves in the liquid is directly proportional to the partial pressure of the gas above the liquid

PRESSURE AND DENSITY

As physical quantities, pressure and density are also related to gravity and Newton's laws. Torricelli, an Italian scientist, performed the classic experiment that revealed this in 1643, and invented the barometer at the same time (Fig. 11.1). He filled a closed glass tube with mercury and placed the open end of the tube in an open dish of mercury. With the tube inclined from the vertical he noted that the mercury filled the tube. However, as the tube was raised to the vertical, when the length of the mercury column above the surface of the mercury in the dish reached a specific length (0.76 m) a space formed at the top of the tube (known as Torricelli's vacuum). His explanation was that atmospheric pressure kept the column of mercury in the tube. He also noted that the upper level of the mercury varied from day to day.

Consider the basic mechanical unit of the mercury, an atom, to be a solid ball. The atoms of mercury in a barometer do not move perceptibly. Therefore, by Newton's Third Law of Motion, they must experience no net force. Consider the forces that act on a mercury atom about halfway up and near to the center of the tube of the barometer. The forces the atom experiences in a horizontal plane from neighboring atoms must be equal, otherwise it would move. Similarly, all the oblique forces it receives from the layers above and below must balance and be equal. The force it experiences from the layer of atoms vertically above it is slightly less than the force it bears down with upon the layer of atoms below, but is still balanced. The difference is the force caused by gravity on its own mass. The force that bears down is the force caused by the weight of all the atoms above this atom. The net force upward, which supports the column of mercury above the layer in which our atom lies, is the sum of all the infinitesimal forces experienced by all the atoms in the layer, which, except at the contact point between the mercury and the tube, must be equal. The size of the atoms and the cross-sectional area of the tube limit the number of atoms that can be packed into one horizontal layer. Thus, the net force upward is proportional to the cross-sectional area of the tube, or (in other words) the force per unit area across the layer is constant. This gives the basic definition of pressure (see Table 11.1).

The actual value of the pressure is determined by the weight of the column of mercury above the point of measurement. In

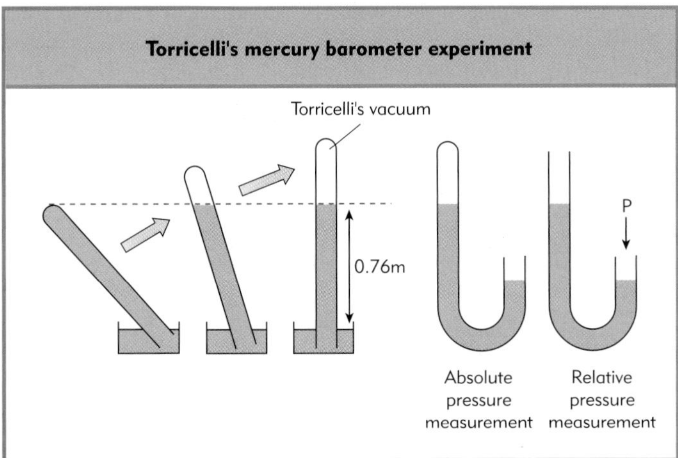

Figure 11.1 Torricelli's mercury barometer experiment.

the barometer, all the infinitesimal forces are resolved and it is the atmospheric pressure at the surface of the mercury in the dish that supports the column of mercury and balances the pressure at the bottom of the barometer tube. The weight of the mercury column is given by the number of atoms in the column, which is determined by the mass of the individual atoms and the number that can be packed into the volume of the column. This is the density (ρ) of the substance.

The pressure P is given by Equation 11.1, in which h is the column height, a the cross-sectional area, and ρ the density of mercury.

■ Equation 11.1

$$P = (hag\rho)/a = hg\rho$$

Equation 11.1 means that, as density and acceleration caused by gravity (g) are constant in the barometer, atmospheric pressure can be measured by reference only to the height of the mercury column above the surface of the mercury in the dish. Hence units of pressure measurement such as millimeters of mercury (mmHg) are used.

Because Torricelli's barometer essentially has a vacuum at one end of its column of mercury, it measures pressure with reference to this vacuum, a true zero pressure, to give an absolute pressure measurement. Torricelli's vacuum is not actually a vacuum, as it contains a saturated vapor of mercury, which exerts a saturated vapor pressure.

Absolute pressure measurements are most often found in hyperbaric medicine or in the measurement of vacuum itself. If a barometer's mercury column and dish are replaced by an open-ended 'U'-tube, one end of which is connected to a pressure source to be measured, then the pressure measurement made is relative to atmospheric pressure (Fig. 11.1).

STATES OF MATTER AND LATENT HEAT

Three states of matter are of interest to anesthesiologists: solid, liquid, and gas. These are three stable states in which molecules exhibit distinctly different bulk physical characteristics. The difference between the states is the degree of intermolecular interaction that exists. In gases the molecules move around freely and are very unstructured, and virtually no intermolecular forces exist. In liquids molecules still move easily, but they display some evidence of wanting to cohere, such as forming droplets under surface tension; slight but significant intermolecular forces exist. Solids are hard and resist deformation. The molecules within them can form regular, ordered patterns called crystal structures; the intermolecular forces are strong.

In all three states, thermal energy is held in the molecules as the kinetic energy associated with the velocity of their random motions. In the gas phase these motions involve collisions, both with the sides of the vessel containing the gas and with other molecules. The more heat there is in the gas, the higher the molecular velocities. In the liquid or solid phases kinetic energy is associated with molecular vibration or limited molecular motion. The more heat, the greater the amplitude of the vibrations and the more kinetic energy present in that form of motion. The amount of thermal energy present is expressed as temperature.

To change from one state of matter to another, for example from liquid to gas, the kinetic energy of the vibrations must be increased until the intermolecular forces can no longer hold the molecules together as liquid and they break free. This can be achieved by heating the liquid. As the liquid heats up, the vibrations increase until the point is reached at which the kinetic energy in the vibrations is equal to the kinetic energy the molecules would have in the gaseous state at the same temperature. However, gas does not form. The intermolecular forces still exist, so a residual potential energy must be supplied to the molecules for the gas to form. This energy is *latent heat*. It does not result in extra vibrations in the molecules and is therefore supplied at the volatilization temperature, or boiling point. The difference between these two is simply the conditions. In boiling, heating is vigorous enough to cause the conditions to be met for gas formation throughout the liquid volume all at once. Thus bubbles of gas form spontaneously in the bulk of the liquid.

The same principles apply to cooling a liquid or gas. If the vibrations are reduced sufficiently, intermolecular forces can establish themselves. So, a practical way of solidifying a liquid is to remove thermal energy (heat) by cooling the liquid. If the temperature change in the liquid is plotted against time, as this process proceeds a point occurs at which the temperature of the liquid ceases to fall but the liquid begins to solidify. At this point the molecular vibrations have been reduced to a level such that the only energy that must be removed for solidification is the latent heat. As cooling proceeds this occurs and solidification takes place at the same temperature, the freezing point. In the opposite direction, it is the melting point.

GAS LAWS

In explaining latent heat, the concept of molecular kinetic energy in gases was introduced. This is the basis of the kinetic theory of a gas, which considers the molecules in a gas as a collection of elastic balls in free, random motion inside a container. They obey Newton's laws of motion and therefore travel in straight lines unless they hit each other or the vessel walls. No energy is lost in any collision, that is, the collisions are perfectly elastic. No intermolecular forces are present, and gravity does not affect the system. These assumptions do not hold for real gases, but they hold well enough to be useful.

Kinetic theory links Newton's laws of motion and the gas laws through a molecular description of the source of pressure in gases. When a molecule strikes the wall of the vessel that contains the gas, it bounces off the wall. Figure 11.2 shows what happens to a molecule (mass m) as it strikes the wall at an angle θ. It is reflected off the wall at the same angle and, because no energy is lost in the collision, it leaves at the same velocity (v) as it had on striking the wall. If we resolve its momentum into a part perpendicular to the wall and a part parallel to the wall before and after the collision, then, as the direction of flight has changed, the change in momentum in the direction of the wall is $2mv\sin\theta$. Because momentum is conserved, Newton's laws show that the result of the collision is the creation of a tiny instantaneous force (f) that acts on the wall of the container. In a real gas container billions of such collisions occur each second. The average force they exert in 1 second over a unit area of one wall of the vessel volume (V) is the average force per unit area, or pressure (P).

To quantify P, we need to know how many collisions occur per second. In a cubic container of side length l, a molecule that collides perpendicularly with one wall will, after recoil, travel back to the opposite wall and there be reflected back, before striking the first wall again. Therefore, the average time between collisions with the original wall is $2l/v\sin\theta$ or $v\sin\theta/2l$ collisions per second. The average change in momentum per second is $m(v\sin\theta)^2/l$ and the average force over that wall is $m(v\sin\theta)^2/l^3$. On average, only one-third of all the molecules (N) in the container have components of velocity in the direction of one wall. Therefore, the equation for one wall (Equation 11.2) applies, where V is the volume of the container. Rearrangement gives Equation 11.3.

■ Equation 11.2

$$P = \frac{[0.33Nm(v\sin\theta)^2]}{l^3} = \frac{[0.33Nm(v\sin\theta)^2]}{V}$$

■ Equation 11.3

$$PV = 0.33Nm(v\sin\theta)^2$$

The motion of the molecules in the gas is clearly governed by statistical considerations. Thus, to derive bulk properties such as the gas laws from kinetic theory, average measures applicable to the whole gas need to be used in the model. For instance, what should the value of the average molecular velocity be? The answer is the root mean square velocity, c, which replaces $v\sin\theta$ in Equations 11.2 and 11.3. The kinetic energy for the whole of the gas, E, in the container is 0.5 Nmc^2, where N is the total number of molecules of mass m, which gives Equation 11.4, in which R is a constant (*the gas constant*) and T is a variable proportional to the average kinetic energy of the molecules, known as temperature.

■ Equation 11.4

$$PV = 0.33\ Nmc^2 = 0.67E = RT$$

Equation 11.4 is the ideal gas equation, which summarizes all the gas laws determined empirically.

Given this development of the concept of temperature, when T = 0 no molecular motion occurs. This is the definition employed in the SI system, in which temperature is measured in degrees Kelvin (°K). The freezing point of water is 0°C or 273.16°K.

Boyle's Law states that at a constant temperature, pressure varies inversely with volume. If temperature T is held constant, it follows from the ideal gas law that the pressure P is inversely proportional to volume V (Equation 11.5).

■ Equation 11.5

$$P \ \alpha \ \frac{1}{V}$$

As the volume of the container is reduced the molecules have less distance to travel between collisions with the walls, and thus the rate of collisions rises and therefore so does pressure.

Charles' Law, or Gay Lussac's Law, states that at a constant pressure the volume of a given mass of gas varies directly with the absolute temperature. In contrast, at constant volume V, the pressure P is directly proportional to absolute temperature T (Equation 11.6).

■ Equation 11.6

$$P \ \alpha \ T$$

As temperature rises the amount of kinetic energy of the gas increases and the average velocity of the molecules increases, so the change in momentum for each collision increases and the pressure rises.

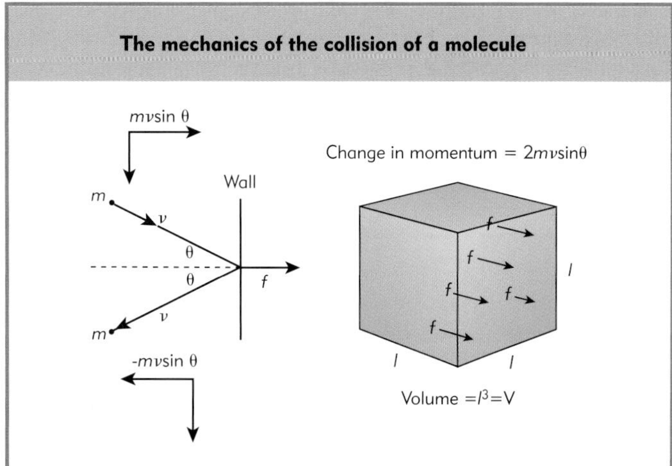

Figure 11.2 The mechanics of the collision of a molecule of an ideal gas with the wall of the container holding the ideal gas.

AVOGADRO'S HYPOTHESIS

Avogadro's Hypothesis states that equal volumes of gas at the same temperature and pressure contain the same numbers of molecules. Avogadro's Hypothesis is implicit in the kinetic theory description of the gas laws. Because temperature is the measure of internal energy, if temperature, volume, and pressure are constant then the number of molecules in the given volume must be the same, irrespective of the mass of the molecules.

In SI units, 1 mole (mol) of a substance is the quantity that has a mass equal to its molecular mass. Molecular mass is the ratio of the mass of a substance's molecule to one-twelfth the mass of an atom of carbon 12 (^{12}C).

The number of molecules in a mole of anything is thus the molecular mass of the substance divided by the mass of one molecule of the substance, which is the molecular mass multiplied by one-twelfth the mass of a carbon-12 atom. This is always a constant, and the number is Avogadro's number, 6.02 ×

10^{23}. Thus 1 mol contains Avogadro's number of molecules. At standard temperature and pressure (STP, i.e. 0°C and 760 mmHg) 1 mol of gas occupies 22.4 L.

If the total mass of the gas is M (= Nm) and the atomic mass of the gas is M_a, then the number of moles of the gas is M/M_a. As 1 mol of gas contains Avogadro's number of molecules, N_a, Equation 11.7 is another form of the ideal gas equation.

■ Equation 11.7

$$PV = \left(\frac{M}{M_a}\right)N_a kT$$

If we define a new constant R [J/(K mol)] as the gas constant ($N_a k$), then the most familiar form of the ideal gas equation is given (Equation 11.8).

■ Equation 11.8

$$PV = \left(\frac{M}{M_a}\right)RT = nRT$$

Dalton's Law of Partial Pressures states that in a mixture of gases the pressure exerted by one gas is the same as it would exert if it occupied the container alone. From kinetic theory, in a mixture of two gases the collisions of the molecules of each gas with the container can be considered separately. So the pressure that results from one gas can be derived from the ideal gas equation and added to the pressure from the other to give the total pressure (Equation 11.9).

■ Equation 11.9

$$P_t = P_a + P_b = \left(\frac{RT}{V}\right)\left[\left(\frac{M}{M_a}\right) + \left(\frac{M}{M_b}\right)\right]$$

CALORIMETRY AND HEAT TRANSFER

Calorimetry is the measurement of the amount of heat evolved, absorbed, or transferred. The techniques used for calorimetry vary with the mechanisms of heat transfer. To understand these mechanisms it is best to start with kinetic theory and gases.

Kinetic theory assumes that the total kinetic energy in a gas is simply the sum of all the molecular kinetic energies. Thus, the higher the temperature, the higher the average velocity of the molecules. Because the number of collisions that a molecule can have increases with its velocity, the higher the temperature of a gas, the higher the number of collisions averaged over time. This energy is transferred in collisions between the molecules and the walls of the vessel. Momentum and energy are conserved in these collisions, but molecules can still change their velocities. In collisions of molecules of the same gas in which one molecule is of higher velocity than the other, on average the velocity of the faster molecule is reduced by the collision and the velocity of the slower molecule is increased. Thus, if a body of gas of a higher temperature mixes with a gas of a lower temperature the collisions tend to heat the cooler gas and cool the hotter gas. In this way, the transfer of molecular kinetic energy from molecule to molecule can pass heat.

In gases it is the collisions between free mobile molecules that transfer the energy, but in liquids and solids the molecules are constrained by intermolecular forces. However, they can still possess kinetic energy, either as a more limited motion similar to that of gas molecules, or as vibrational kinetic energy while still held in place in a solid crystal lattice. This kinetic energy can be coupled from molecule to molecule by intermolecular forces. Coupling of kinetic energy by molecular coupling is the first mode of heat transfer – *conduction*.

The speed at which heat spreads is indicated by the thermal conductivity of the substance. In gases thermal conductivity is closely allied to the process of diffusion (described later). Conduction in solids is much more complex than this simple treatment allows, but can be described by quantum mechanics.

The calorimetry of conduction is concerned with bringing objects of different temperatures together and measuring their common temperature after heat transfer has ceased. This raises the concept of objects having a capacity to hold heat.

Thermal or heat capacity

The thermal capacity of a body is the quantity of heat required to raise its temperature by 1 K (SI unit is the joule, J). The thermal capacity divided by the mass of the object is the specific thermal capacity. The thermal capacity of 1 mol of a substance is the molar thermal capacity.

For the most part, calorimetry is carried out to determine an unknown quantity of heat or the details of heat flow in a specific physical or chemical process. Thus, calorimetry can be used only to measure heat flow within a closed system (i.e. heat does not flow to the outside world). If heat flow cannot be prevented by insulation or placing the calorimeter in a vacuum, corrections for heat flow into or out of the calorimeter have to be made.

If we take two metal objects of thermal capacities C_1 and C_2, heat them to two different temperatures T_1 and T_2, and place them in contact in a well-insulated calorimeter, heat flows between them by conduction and eventually they reach a single temperature, T_A. Because no heat is lost (assuming a perfect calorimeter), the heat balance in the system can be represented by Equation 11.10.

■ Equation 11.10

$$T_1C_1 + T_2C_2 = T_A(C_1 + C_2)$$

Convection is also explained in terms of kinetic theory and the gas laws, but a twist is that in practice it can only occur naturally in bodies of fluids under gravity. In a container of gas under gravity at constant pressure, if part of the gas is heated locally it effectively occupies more volume and is less dense. It thus tends to rise as a body and mix with the cooler gas around it. If it rises and is cooled by coming into a colder part of the container it then sinks, and a circulating current is formed that mechanically mixes the gases and thus transfers heat more rapidly. In calorimetry, convection effects aid heat transfer if fluids are involved. Stirring or otherwise mixing the fluids is even more effective and quicker, and can be thought of as forced convection.

Whereas convection is a bulk effect and conduction is governed by molecular considerations, *radiation*, the final physical heat-transfer process, is exhibited on a submolecular basis. Some of the kinetic energy in a heated molecule is stored as vibrations of the molecular structure itself and of the electrons that surround it. Thus, some of the kinetic energy results in the motion of charged particles, and this movement creates electromagnetic fields that can radiate electromagnetic waves in the infrared range. (Electromagnetic radiation is considered in Chapter 12.) If this infrared radiation intercepts another molecule it can interact with that molecule and increase its internal kinetic energy and hence its temperature. This heat transfer mechanism is the only one that can take place in a vacuum. Because infrared radiation has a relatively short wavelength, like visible light it effectively travels in straight lines. Radiative heat transfer is thus a line-of-sight phenomenon. Again, a detailed description of radiation requires some appreciation of quantum mechanics, and is very complex.

Conduction, convection, and radiation are the three physical methods of heat transfer from one body to another. However, heat is only a specific form of energy. If heat locked up as potential energy in any way is transferred to another place and released as heat again, then heat transfer has, in a very general sense, taken place. In the body, heat generation is biochemical from the chemical potential energy in food and oxygen in respiration. The heat generated is transferred from the body by conduction to the air, convection of air at the skin, losses from chemical binding of energy in exhaled carbon dioxide, and losses from latent heat changes in sweating or humidification of ventilatory gases in the upper respiratory tract (Chapter 64).

Calorimetry of the heat transfer of the body as a whole aims to account for all the sources of energy transfer and measure them. This is carried out in a whole-body calorimeter for metabolic studies.

SOLUBILITY AND DIFFUSION

The process of diffusion can be explained very simply from kinetic theory. If two different gases (or any fluids in any sense) are separated by a physical barrier and that barrier is removed, the kinetic motion of the molecules of the gases mixes them and equalizes their energy until they are perfectly mixed. At this point they are constrained only by the walls of the vessel that contains them.

Of more interest in medicine is how fast this mixing proceeds, which can be expressed in terms of the number of molecules transported through a given area in a given time. This rate of mass transport through another gas or liquid per area per second (M) is proportional to the density gradient ($\partial P/\partial z$). This is Fick's Law (Equation 11.11), in which D is the diffusion coefficient and is proportional to how far molecules travel before collisions. It is thus inversely proportional to gas density and proportional to mean molecular velocity (and hence absolute temperature). Mass transport is one of the fundamental physical principles that underlie gas exchange during respiration throughout the body.

■ Equation 11.11

$$M = D\left(\frac{\delta P}{\delta z}\right)$$

If a membrane permeable to the gas is placed in the way of diffusing molecules, molecular motion is limited by the channels or pores through which the gas can diffuse. In this situation the rate of diffusion becomes dependent on the molecular weight of the gas (Graham's Law).

Another limiting factor to gas transport is the solubility of the gases in blood. Henry's Law governs this when gases are not bonded chemically in the liquid, such as oxygen in hemoglobin. Even in this case, the gas bound by hemoglobin in red cell bodies is exchanged first with plasma and then the cells of tissue or the alveoli, so Henry's Law still plays a part in diffusion limitations to the exchange of oxygen.

The kinetic theory explanation of Henry's Law is the mirror image of the kinetic theory explanation of how saturated vapors are formed. The gas molecules in the liquid have kinetic motion, and some have enough velocity to leave the surface of the liquid. In the gas phase above the liquid, molecules collide with the gases present and some fall back into the liquid. Eventually the rate of loss of molecules from the gas phase equals the rate of emergence of molecules from the liquid, which is a dynamic equilibrium. The partial pressure exerted by the gas at this point is the saturated vapor pressure of the gas.

Henry's Law describes the same equilibrium from the point of view of dissolving the gas. At the equilibrium point the liquid has become saturated with all the gas it can hold. The concept of partial pressure can be applied to its state in the liquid – hence the idea of partial pressures or tensions to measure saturated and other concentrations of gas in a liquid. The pressures involved are temperature dependent, with the amount of gas dissolved decreasing with increased temperature.

Henry's Law is couched in terms of the mass of gas or the partial pressure, but it is possible to express the amount of gas dissolved in terms of the volume of gas in the liquid phase to the gas present in the same volume of the gas phase. This gives a ratio called the partition coefficient or Ostwald solubility coefficient (λ).

The partition coefficient has the advantage that it allows gas exchange to be expressed in terms of volumes directly related to other physiologic volumes, such as tidal volume. It is of particular use in compartmentalized models of gas exchange. Because gases dissolve inertly in many tissues (as if these tissues were liquids), a partition coefficient for a complex tissue can be estimated from the weighted sum of the partition coefficients of the tissues' basic chemical constituents. Thus, the partition coefficient of blood can be estimated by combining the coefficient for olive oil to represent lipids, and saline to represent plasma.

Further reading

Bragg M. On giants' shoulders. London: Hodder & Stoughton; 1998.

Davis PD, Parbrook GD, Kenny GNC. Basic physics and measurement in anaesthesia, 4th edn. Oxford: Butterworth–Heinemann; 1995.

Macintosh R, Mushin W, Epstein HG. Physics for the anesthetist, 3rd edn. Oxford: Blackwell; 1963.

Ohanian HC. Principles of physics. New York: WW Norton; 1994.

Chapter 12

Electromagnetism, light, and radiation

Paul CW Beatty

ELECTRICITY

Electricity is a general term for the phenomena associated with charged particles (usually electrons or protons) at rest or in motion. (The word electron derives from the Greek *elektron* meaning amber.) Electromagnetic theory is the physics of charged particles in electromagnetic fields. It extends beyond simple electrical phenomena and circuit theory to radio transmission, light waves, X-rays, nuclear magnetic resonance (NMR), and other forms of electromagnetic radiation.

CHARGE, POTENTIAL, AND ELECTROMOTIVE FORCE

Charge is the total quantity of electricity in an object, and can be thought of as the number of charged particles in a body (SI unit is the coulomb, C). Charges can have signs, that is, positive or negative. An attractive force exists between opposite charges and a repulsive force between charges of similar sign. As with gravity, work is carried out when charges are moved against electrostatic forces, and bodies having charge can have potential energy because of the electrostatic field.

The electrostatic measure of potential energy is the electric *potential*. It can be positive or negative, depending on the sign of the charge on the body. The earth is assigned a potential of zero, so that the difference in electric potential between two different bodies is simply the sum of the electric potential of the two bodies above the earth, the potential difference (Table 12.1).

When a conductor connects two points of different potential difference, a current flows between them. For this to occur a source of energy is required to make the electrons flow in the conductor; this is called the electromotive force (EMF) and has the same SI unit as potential (V).

The difference between potential difference and EMF can be very important in physiologic measurements, and hence in anesthesia. Electrical energy is dissipated in an electrical circuit by the resistance and impedance of that circuit only when current flows. Bioelectric phenomena, such as those measured using the electrocardiogram (ECG), electroencephalogram (EEG), etc., are generated deep in the body. Inevitably, resistances between the source of these bioelectric potentials and the skin make it harder to measure the signals. Accurate measurement of these requires as little energy dissipation as possible. Thus, we would like to make measurements potentiometrically (when no current flows).

Charge may be transferred from object to object by electrostatic contact without a conductor, but it is most commonly transferred using conduction through metals, which allow electrons to flow from one body to another. When charge moves or flows it is a current, or charge transferred per unit time. When current flows in a wire a magnetic field is created around the wire and deflects a compass needle in a direction depending on the direction of flow of the current. Attractive or repulsive magnetic forces can be established between parallel wires with currents flowing in the appropriate direction, an effect that is used to define the unit of current (ampere).

Returning to electrostatics, the property that relates electric potential to the amount of charge that an object holds is its capacitance, C, given by Equation 12.1.

■ Equation 12.1

$$C = \frac{Q}{V}$$

Table 12.1 Definitions in electromagnetism

Potential difference – The work performed when one positive electric charge is moved from one point to another (SI unit: volt, V)
Electromotive force – The rate at which energy is drawn from a source and dissipated in an electrical circuit when unit current flows (SI unit: volt, V)
Volt – The potential difference between two points on a conducting wire carrying 1 A of current between which 1 W of power is dissipated
Current – Overall movement of electrons through a conductor, or charge flow per unit time
Ampere – The current that produces a force of 2×10^{-7} N/m^{-1} when flowing in two straight infinitely long parallel conductors 1 m apart in a vacuum
Farad – The capacitance of a capacitor across which exists a potential difference of 1 V when storing 1 coulomb of charge
Power – The power dissipated in a resistance is equal to the product of the potential difference across the resistor and the current flowing through the resistor (SI unit: watt, W)
Inductance – That property of an electrical circuit as a result of which an EMF is generated by a change in current flowing in the circuit (self inductance) or by a change in current in a neighboring circuit that is magnetically linked to the first circuit (mutual induction)
Henry – The SI unit of an inductance in a closed electrical circuit, such that a change in current of 1 A produces a change in EMF of 1 V
Becquerel – A radioactive source with a disintegration rate of one disintegration per second is said to have an activity of 1 Bq (1 Curie, Ci = 3.7×10^{10} Bq)
Gray – When a source of radiation transfers 1 J/kg^{-1} of energy to a body then the absorbed dose is 1 Gray (Gy).

It is this property of a system of electrical conductors and insulators that allows the system to store an electrical charge. Capacitance varies with object shape, as the field intensity around an object and hence the work required to place charge on the object against the field varies with its shape. Figure 12.1 shows a parallel plate capacitor with one plate connected to earth and a positive charge placed on the other plate. This induces negative charges to flow from earth to balance this charge. The force that exists between the plates as a result follows the general form of all electrostatic forces (Equation 12.2), in which E is the field strength or force on a unit charge a distance r from a charge Q; ε is the *permittivity* of the space between the charges.

■ Equation 12.2

$$E = \frac{Q}{(4\pi r^2 \varepsilon)}$$

The permitivity of vacuum, or free space, ε_0, is a constant, but other insulators can increase the permittivity if placed between the charges. Thus, placing an insulator between the plates of a parallel-plate capacitor decreases the force between the plates, decreases the work required to move charge onto the plates, decreases the potential difference induced across the capacitor, and therefore increases capacitance.

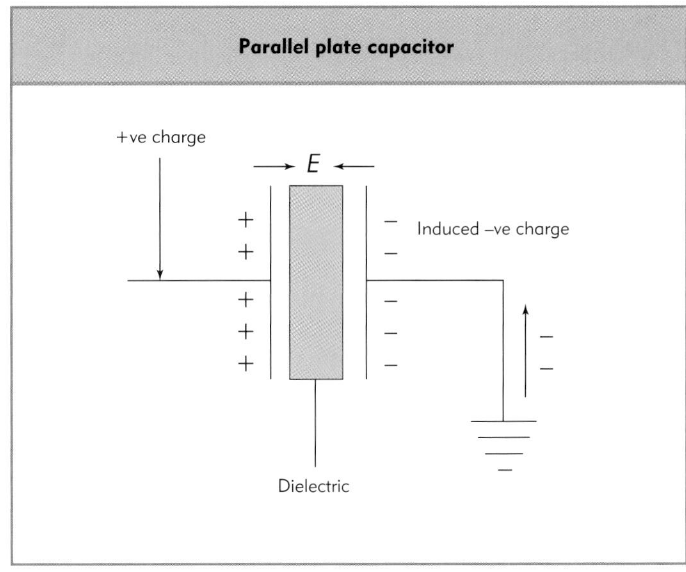

Figure 12.1 The parallel plate capacitor.

The capacitance of a parallel-plate capacitor of which A is the plate area, ε the permittivity of the dielectric in the space between the plates, and d the separation of the plates, is given by Equation 12.3.

■ Equation 12.3

$$C = \frac{A\varepsilon}{d}$$

To increase capacitance, either area or permittivity can be increased or plate separation reduced.

The energy stored in the electric field of a capacitor can be released through a resistor to earth. If this is carried out using a switch, the voltage (V_t) from the capacitor falls exponentially with time to zero from a maximum (V_0) before the switch is thrown (Equation 12.4, in which RC is the time constant of the circuit).

■ Equation 12.4

$$V_t = e^{-t/RC}$$

RESISTANCE, OHM'S LAW, INDUCTANCE, AND IMPEDANCE

How dissipation of energy supplied by a source of EMF occurs depends on whether current flows steadily through conductors in one direction all the time (direct current, DC) or whether it oscillates in direction (alternating current, AC).

Resistance is the simplest process of dissipation. All conductors exhibit resistance, apart from superconductors below specific, extremely low temperatures. Resistance can be thought of simplistically as the result of collisions between the moving electrons that carry the current in a conductor and the molecules or atoms of the main crystal lattice that make up the conductor. The collisions result in transfer of energy that eventually is dissipated as heat within the conductor.

Resistance (SI unit is the ohm, Ω) for a conductor relates current (I) to potential difference (V) across the conductor (Equation 12.5).

■ Equation 12.5

$$R = \frac{V}{I}$$

This is Ohm's Law, given in a more familiar form in Equation 12.6.

■ Equation 12.6

$$V = IR$$

Resistance depends on the shape of the conductor, as current flow is not uniformly distributed even in a uniform conductor. Resistance is proportional to conductor length and inversely proportional to conductor cross-sectional area. Stretching a conductor increases its length, and the resultant increase in resistance is the basis of strain gauges.

Temperature increases can cause conductors to expand, which leads to an increase in resistance by this mechanical effect, as well as affecting electron flow. Resistors used in electronic circuitry are made from metal alloys or films or carbon compounds designed to reduce the effects of changes in ambient temperature.

Different materials have different specific resistances or resistivities. Resistivity (ρ) is the resistance of a unit cube of the conductor at 0°C (SI unit is ohm meters, Ωm), and is generally given by Equation 12.7, where l is conductor length.

■ Equation 12.7

$$\rho = \frac{RA}{l}$$

For resistances in series (Fig. 12.2a), the total potential difference across the resistors is the sum of the potential differences across the individual resistors (Equation 12.8). For resistances in parallel (Fig. 12.2b), Equation 12.9 applies.

■ Equation 12.8

$$V = V_1 + V_2 + V_3 = IR_1 + IR_2 + IR_3$$

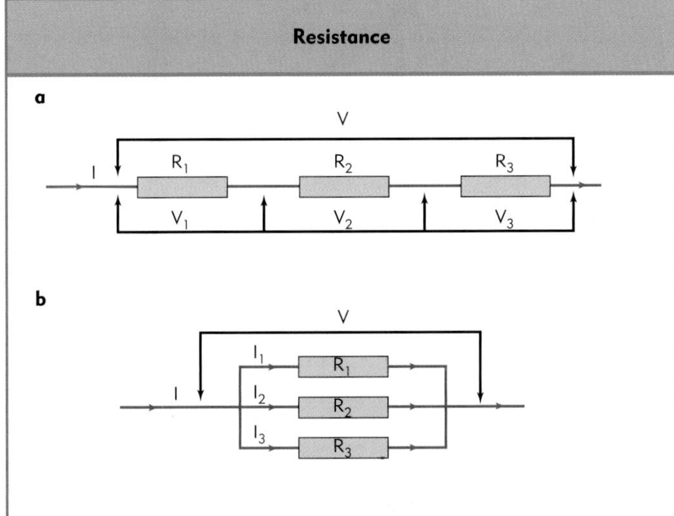

Figure 12.2 Resistance. (a) Resistors in series. (b) Resistors in parallel.

■ Equation 12.9

$$I = I_1 + I_2 + I_3 = \left(\frac{V}{R_1}\right) + \left(\frac{V}{R_2}\right) + \left(\frac{V}{R_3}\right)$$

The way in which resistances dissipate electrical energy is independent of whether the current flow is AC or DC, but this is not true of inductances or capacitances.

In the same way that moving charge into an electrostatic field against electrostatic forces requires work, so moving magnetic poles into a magnetic field requires work. There are no single magnetic poles so, unlike the electrostatic example, moving magnetic poles is more like forcing together two magnetic fields than placing single charges on bodies in the field. Faraday found that if a wire was placed in a permanent magnetic field between the poles of a U-shaped magnet and a current was made to pass along the wire, the wire would kick out of the field. The magnetic field created by the current around the wire opposes the magnetic field of the permanent magnet, which produces a force and hence motion. The direction of motion is given by Fleming's left hand rule (Fig. 12.3).

If a conductor is moved through a magnetic field a current is induced in the conductor (the dynamo effect). If the conductor is placed in a magnetic field that can vary in intensity with time, which is equivalent to moving it in and out of a fixed field, both a time-varying current and an associated magnetic field are induced in the conductor. Time varying (i.e. AC) currents can induce currents in other conductors placed within the influence

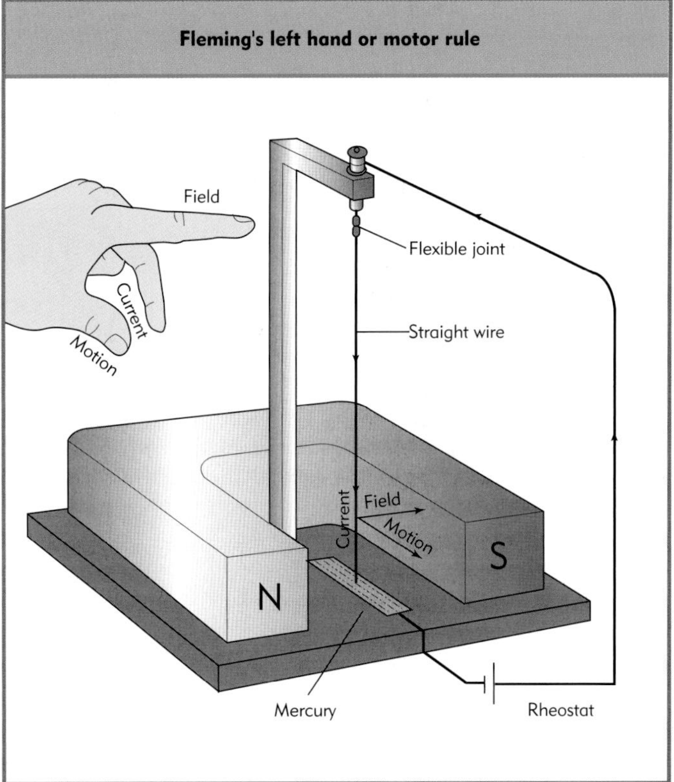

Figure 12.3 Fleming's left hand or motor rule. The first finger, thumb, and second finger of the left hand are held at right-angles to each other; if the direction of the first finger is taken to indicate the direction of a fixed magnetic field and the second finger the direction of current flow in a conductor placed in that field, then the direction of the thumb indicates the direction of force experienced by the conductor in the field.

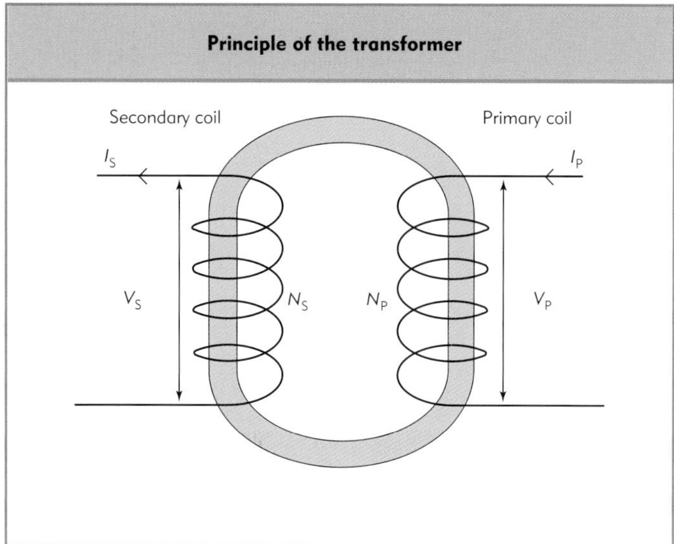

Figure 12.4 The principle of the transformer.

of the magnetic fields created by those currents (*electromagnetic induction*). If two coils or conductors are used, energy is transferred by induction from one coil to the other. This is the principle of the transformer (Fig. 12.4), in which two coils are wound on either side of a circular metal ring composed of a magnetic material such as iron. This core channels the magnetic field produced by the coil that is excited with the AC and transfers it efficiently to the other coil, in which is induced another AC (*mutual induction*).

The coil that is excited in a transformer is termed the *primary*, and the one in which the current is induced is termed the *secondary*. The number of turns in the primary (N_P) and the secondary (N_S) can be different. If this is the case, ignoring losses in the transformer, the EMF (V_S) that the secondary coil can provide is related to the EMF (V_P) used to excite the primary (Equation 12.10).

■ Equation 12.10

$$\frac{V_S}{V_P} = \frac{N_S}{N_P}$$

A conductor has *self-inductance* as well. In a coil, this exists because one turn of the coil sits in the magnetic field of the next turn, and so on. When an AC is applied the changing magnetic fields in one turn produce opposing currents in the neighboring turns, and thus energy is dissipated.

So far we have not discussed the nature of the AC. Any time-varying current causes inductive effects. However, the term AC is conventionally applied to sinusoidal current flows. A sinusoidal waveform is defined by its amplitude and frequency (f). Given a regular waveform such as a sinusoid, is there an AC equivalent for inductors of resistance? The faster the magnetic fields in the inductor reverse, the more energy is dissipated, so any equivalent term must be frequency dependent. The overall dissipation term is called reactance (X_L) and for an inductor of L Henrys is given by Equation 12.11.

■ Equation 12.11

$$X_L = 2\pi fL$$

The effect of dissipation in the inductor does more than reduce the amplitude of the AC that flows through it. It also delays the sinusoidal current, which is termed a phase change.

A similar line of argument applies when a capacitor is excited with a sinusoidal current or voltage. In this case energy is dissipated in continuously reversing the direction of the electric field in the dielectric. This also is dependent on the frequency, and capacitance has reactance too (X_C). Capacitances also induce phase changes in the AC and voltage waveforms (Equation 12.12).

■ Equation 12.12

$$X_C = \frac{1}{2\pi f}$$

Although the concept of reactance is useful for simple electronic calculations, more useful is a quantity that could be used in an AC equivalent of Ohm's law, which relates the amplitude of the current to the voltage across an inductor. This quantity is impedance (Z), which is also frequency dependent. If a resistor, a capacitor, and an inductor are connected in series, the impedance of the three together to AC is given by Equation 12.13.

■ Equation 12.13

$$Z = \{R^2 + [2\pi fL - 1/(2\pi C)]^2\}^{0.5}$$

AMPLIFIERS

The main way that signals and physiologic measurements are processed in medicine is as electrical signals. Even for original signals that are not electrical, transducers or sensors of one form or another are employed to convert them into electrical signals (Chapters 13–15). In any instrument the amplifier is the vital circuit component.

The performance of an amplifier is defined by its gain (A), which is the ratio of the output signal amplitude (v_o) to the input signal amplitude (v_i) (Equation 12.14). A negative gain indicates that the signal is inverted.

■ Equation 12.14

$$A = \frac{v_o}{v_i}$$

Bandwidth is the range of frequencies of signal over which the amplifier amplifies without distortion in frequency (amplifying one frequency more than another) or introducing phase shifts in the signal or components of the signal.

If small signals are to be amplified, the higher the input impedance (Z_i), the more sensitive the amplifier can be. However, input impedance should be resistive, so as not to introduce phase shifts etc. Output impedance (Z_o) should be low, so that the amplifier can provide adequate EMF to drive any form of load or other type of electronic circuit. An amplifier should not produce offset voltages at its own inputs.

The amplifiers used in medical instrumentation are almost invariably operational amplifiers. These are integrated circuits in which the transistors, resistors, and all other components required to construct the amplifier have been manufactured on a single piece of silicon (chip). An operational amplifier (op-amp) has three terminals: inverting input, noninverting input, and output. Voltage signals applied to the inverting input (v_1) with the noninverting terminal (v_2) connected to earth (ground) are amplified and appear at the output inverted, and vice versa for the noninverting input. If signals are applied simultaneously to both, the difference between the signals is amplified and appears at the output. In the latter configuration the amplifier is acting as a differential amplifier.

Operational amplifiers have the following ideal characteristics:

- linear in response both in gain (infinite gain) and phase;
- accurately amplify signals with a very wide range of frequency components (infinite bandwidth);
- stable with temperature;
- very low offset voltages (when $v_1 = v_2$, $v_o = 0$);
- very high (infinite) common mode rejection ratio (CMRR);
- very high (infinite) input impedance; and
- very low (zero) output impedance.

An amplifier with an infinite gain is not very useful. The slightest signal would send it off to infinite gain, which in practice means that the output would immediately saturate at the value of the supply voltage to the device. In practice, the gain and performance of the op-amp is controlled by negative feedback to produce a usable amplifier of known performance that still preserves many of the ideal op-amp characteristics. Negative feedback is applied to the op-amp using two or three external resistors connected to the op-amp terminals.

High CMRR is of particular importance in anesthesia and medical instrumentation. Much of the interference suffered in operating rooms is associated with mains electricity supply and currents flowing in the power supplies of equipment connected to it. The magnetic fields created by these currents induce currents at the mains supply frequency in any conductor within range. These currents are very small but are of the same order as some of the bioelectric potentials, such as the ECG. Because these interfering currents are likely to be the same size in all leads of an ECG or other measuring leads, they should appear as common mode signals at the inputs of any preamplifier used. High CMRR should therefore eliminate these interfering signals. However, even with precision components no pair of resistors can be matched exactly, and if the match is not achieved, CMRR is reduced.

ELECTRICAL HAZARDS AND SAFETY MEASURES

Electricity has three damaging effects on the body and living tissue:

- electrolysis, which causes local chemical breakdown of tissue;
- heating, which causes burns; and
- stimulation of excitable cells (i.e. shock).

Electrolysis

The least well-described hazard is electrolysis. It is a purely local effect and is not life threatening. It can occur wherever a low DC of a few milliamps is applied to the skin for a sufficient time. The skin breakdown that occurs has many of the characteristics of a chemical burn. The effect is proportional to current density, but occurs readily at a few volts. Battery-powered equipment is capable of producing this effect.

Burns

In anesthesia burn injuries to patients are most likely to occur because of faulty or badly applied electrocautery (diathermy) equipment. Surgical electrocautery equipment uses a high-frequency current at about 1 MHz to disrupt or destroy tissue. At these frequencies no neuromuscular effects are produced. Monopolar electrocautery uses a small cutting and/or coagulating electrode in which the current density is high. The cutting effect is proportional to current density, as it is simply the result of dissipating electrical energy in a small volume of tissue. To reduce the current density at exit of the current from the body a large-area electrode is used, usually strapped tightly to the thigh. If this electrode is badly fitted or damaged, local hot spots may develop on the plate or the current may find a lower-impedance return path through ECG electrodes or chance contact between the patient's skin and objects connected to earth (such as the operating table or anesthetic equipment). If these contact areas are small enough and the exit current density high enough, a burn occurs at these sites. Staff can also receive small shocks in these circumstances if they complete the earth return circuit by having contact with the patient. The shock arises because the patient's potential may rise above that of earth until contact is made as the return current tries to find a suitable return path. Bipolar cautery uses two electrodes of similar small size in the form of tweezers. The burning effect takes place between the electrodes and no large earth return electrode is required.

The other indirect burn risk associated with electrical equipment is explosion. When inflammable anesthetic agents were commonly used this was a major hazard. Static electrical discharges and electrical equipment that could cause sparking were potential sources of ignition. Anesthesia is still carried out using gases that readily support combustion (oxygen and nitrous oxide), and there are plenty of paper or cloth drapes and alcohol-based skin preparations to burn. Electrical equipment is still a source of ignition for these fuels. The possibility also exists for ignition from hot components inside anesthetic or monitoring equipment.

Shock

The source of electrical hazard that is most important to anesthetists is shock. The severity of shock is determined by the current involved and the frequency. The maximum neuromuscular effects of electrical currents occur in the frequency range in which cells produce action potentials. This tends to be about 50–60 Hz, the frequency of AC mains supplies.

In terms of life-threatening shock, the heart is the susceptible organ. A sufficient current flow through the heart produces ventricular fibrillation. In *macroshock* an externally applied current produces a sufficient current flow in the thorax to induce fibrillation. However, the other main determinants of shock severity are whether the skin is broken at the point of application of the current, and whether the heart is exposed to direct application of the current (*microshock*). The skin provides a relatively high impedance, which underlying tissues do not. The removal of this protection can reduce the fibrillation threshold by 10 000-fold (Table 12.2).

Limitation of current flow from equipment to patients and staff, under normal operating and fault conditions, is the primary

Table 12.2 Electrical shock

Current	Effect
Macroshock	
1 mA	Threshold of perception
5 mA	Accepted maximum harmless current
10–20 mA	'Let-go' current. Threshold of tetanic contraction of skeletal muscle. The point at which the individual can just let go of a current-carrying conductor
50 mA	Pain, fainting, mechanical injury
100–300 mA	Ventricular fibrillation Respiration center remains intact
6000 mA	Sustained ventricular contraction Defibrillation effect Burns if the current is high enough
Microshock	
10 μA	Recommended safe current limit for directly applied cardiac equipment
50 μA	Maximum fault condition current for cardiac equipment
100 μA	Ventricular fibrillation

method of preventing shock hazard. To do this, both the design of the instrument and the design of the mains supply to that instrument are important (Fig. 12.5).

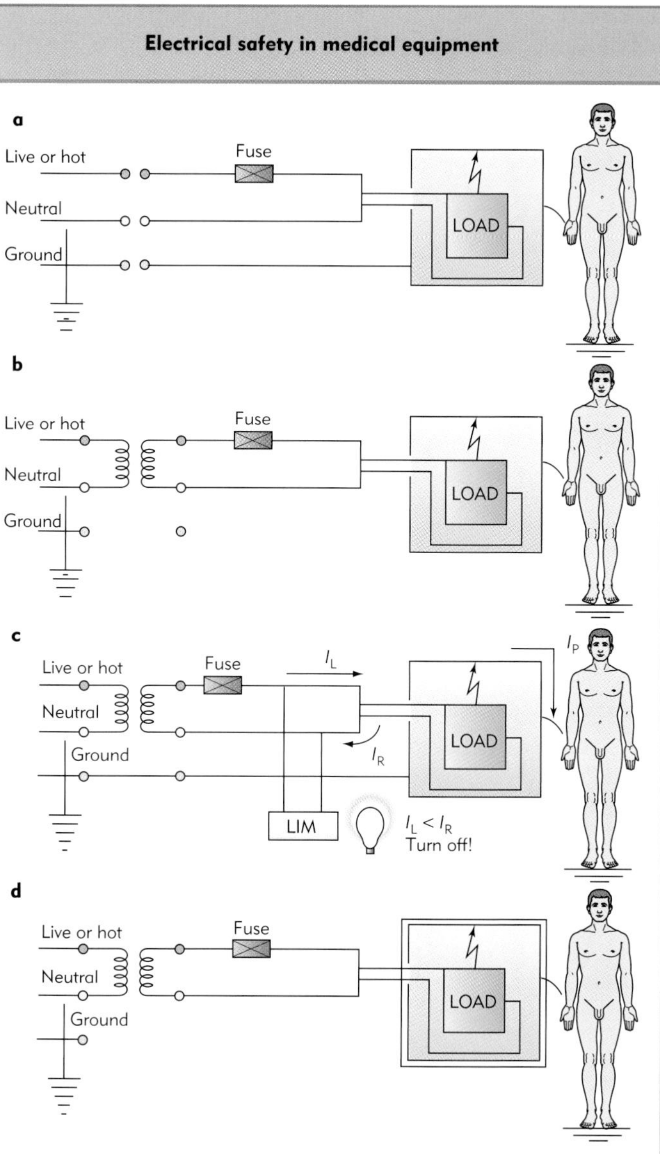

Figure 12.5 Strategies for electrical safety used in medical equipment. (a) Using a simple earth, the earthed case of the instrument conducts the current from the internal instrument fault that shorted the load to the case away from the patient or operator to earth by providing the lowest-impedance conduction path. (b) With an isolation transformer (earth-free system), the transformer eliminates the connection between the earth at the supply and the neutral as far as the instrument is concerned. Under a fault, the patient simply grounds the neutral side of the transformer, but no current flows through the patient. Isolation transformers can be incorporated into the instruments instead of the supply. (c) With an isolation transformer and a line isolation monitor (LIM; residual current detector), the isolation transformer is provided in the supply but an earth connection is maintained. In the event of a fault the LIM detects the difference in current (I_L) between the live (hot) wire and the neutral wire (I_R) created by the current flowing through the patient (I_P). It then cuts the power quickly enough to prevent shock. (d) In double insulation (earth-free system), physically isolating the load twice over from the case makes the instrument safe with the fault.

ELECTROMAGNETIC RADIATION AND LIGHT

Electromagnetic radiation is the collective term for all the electromagnetic fields that propagate across space. The nature of the field follows from considering electrostatic and electromagnetic induction. If an oscillating EMF is applied to a conductor, then associated with the induced current flow is a local electric and magnetic field, both of which vary in time. The laws of induction discussed above are concerned with those fields local or near to the conductor. Also, a field is created at a distance or far from the conductor. This field is a combined electric–magnetic field that propagates away from the conductor at the speed of light. Like the near field, it is capable of inducing currents and EMF in other conductors.

Electromagnetic radiation is a continuous spectrum of waves of different frequencies. These are divided into sections largely related to their interactions with matter, the characteristics of which change with frequency (or wavelength). The common divisions of this spectrum are shown in Table 12.3.

Energy is transmitted in electromagnetic radiation governed by laws given in Equations 12.15 and 12.16, in which λ is the radiation wavelength, f is frequency, c is the speed of light, E is energy, and h is Planck's constant.

- Equation 12.15

$$\lambda f = c$$

- Equation 12.16

$$E = hf$$

This description of electromagnetic radiation views the field as a wave motion. However, when electromagnetic radiation interacts with matter it exhibits particle-like properties as well as wave-like properties. Some effects are best described in terms of wave motion and some by a particle model. The name given to the electromagnetic radiation particle is the *photon*.

Table 12.3 Electromagnetic radiation

Wavelength (m)	Type	Frequency (Hz)
10^{-13}		10^{19}
10^{-12}	γ rays	
10^{-11}		
10^{-10}		10^{16}
10^{-9}	X rays	
10^{-8}	Ultraviolet light (violet)	
10^{-7}		
10^{-6}	Visible light (white)	10^{12}
10^{-5}		
10^{-4}	Infrared light (red)	10^{9}
10^{-3}		
10^{-2}	Microwaves	
10^{-1}		
1	Radio waves UHF	
10	VHF	
10^{2}		
10^{3}		
10^{4}		

Bohr developed a description of the interaction of photons with matter. The idea that electromagnetic radiation carries energy in specific packets or quanta is summarized by Planck's equations above. Einstein explained the photoelectric effect using this idea. He explained why the electrons emitted from metal surfaces when illuminated with light were of a specific energy when the energy from the light reached a specific threshold. Finally, Bohr knew that observation of the details of the spectra of light emitted by elements showed discrete lines of light of specific frequencies.

Bohr combined these facts with Rutherford's view of the structure of the atom (as a small positively charged nucleus with electrons in orbits around it) and suggested that the electrons orbited the nucleus only at specific distances. This meant that the kinetic energy of the electrons in orbit could not take up *any* value but only *permitted* values. Thus, for an electron to be raised to a new orbit of higher energy, the energy supplied must reach the threshold between the two orbits. If the energy is below this threshold the electron stays in the same orbit. This explains the photoelectric effect. If a high-energy electron decays to a lower-energy orbit, a photon of the energy difference is emitted, as energy must be conserved. This explains the discrete nature of the spectral lines.

Bohr's simple atomic model was soon modified by quantum mechanical explanations. However, the basic quantum mechanical nature of photon absorption or emission by electrons in atomic or molecular structures remains a key idea of present-day physics. To atomic properties can be added molecular properties, as we now know that the electrons of constituent atoms in molecules can be shared so they have quantum levels that are a property of molecular structure (Chapter 1).

Absorbance and Beer's Law

Consider a beam of monochromatic light (light of single wavelength and hence photon energy) incident on a sample of substance known to absorb light of this wavelength, termed a *chromophore*, mixed in a nonabsorbing matrix. The amount of absorption of the incident light is the number of photons absorbed, which depends on the probability of a photon interacting with an electron of the correct quantum state. Thus the amount of absorption is proportional to the thickness of the sample, the concentration of the chromophore, and the efficiency of the chromophore at absorbing the light. In such situations slices of equal width through the sample absorb the same proportion of light, which means that the intensity of light falls exponentially with path length through the sample. This is given by Equation 12.17, in which I is the emergent light intensity, I_0 is the incident light intensity, k is a constant, and l is the path length. Taking logarithms of Equation 12.17 and rearranging gives Equation 12.18.

■ Equation 12.17

$$I = I_0 e^{-kl}$$

■ Equation 12.18

$$\log_{10} \frac{(I_0)}{I} = \frac{kl}{2.303}$$

The term $\log_{10} (I_0/I)$ is called variously the absorbance, the extinction coefficient, or the optical density. The expression states that absorbance is proportional to absorbing layer thickness, which is Lambert's Law. Chromophore concentration is implicitly present as part of the constant k. Rewriting Equations 12.17 and 12.18 to show it explicitly gives Equations 12.19 and 12.20, in which ε is the absorption coefficient, c is concentration, and A is absorbance; the latter is Beer's Law.

■ Equation 12.19

$$I = I_0 e^{-k1}$$

■ Equation 12.20

$$\log^{10} \frac{(I_0)}{I} = A = \varepsilon cl$$

Fluorescence

The energy absorbed by the electrons of the chromophore may remain in the chromophore as an excited state. However, one of the following is more likely to result:

- a chain of internal excitations and electron transitions that results in dissipation of the energy as heat to neighboring molecules;
- the excited state may be so energetic that chemical breakdown occurs; or
- after one or two internal transitions the energy is radiated from the molecule as light of a different wavelength or group of wavelengths (*fluorescence*).

If this emitted light is not absorbed by the chromophore its intensity and other properties are measurable. The fluorescent light is emitted in all directions at a lower wavelength than that of the original light. Fluorescence is very useful, as it is specific to the chemistry of the chromophore and may accompany chemical changes. As an alternative measurement to absorbance it has the advantage of greater sensitivity. This arises because, although the light has lost its directionality and is of a lower intensity, it is measured with reference to a true zero light condition.

Lasers

The action of a laser (Light Amplification by Stimulated Emission of Radiation) is in many ways similar to the process of fluorescence. The energy state from which the fluorescent light is emitted is very often a *metastable* electron state. Electrons are temporarily held in this orbit until some process triggers their decay back to an unexcited energy state and a photon associated with the transition is emitted. In the case of fluorescence the delay is small and the metastable state very 'unstable'. However, in laser action the metastable state is relatively 'stable' and the trigger to decay the electron is very specific – the emission of a photon from the metastable state itself.

The original type of laser shown in Figure 12.6 was made from a crystal of ruby. A mirror is placed at one end of the crystal and a half-silvered mirror at the other, all surrounded by a helical flash tube. This tube emits a broad spectrum of visible light, which enters from the sides of the crystal and is reflected up and down the crystal many times by the mirrors. The photons in the blue and green parts of the flash tube spectrum raise unexcited electrons into two ranges of closely packed excited states, called *bands*. However, the electrons rapidly decay from these states to a single metastable state of lower energy. Electrons accumulate in this metastable state as the pumping action continues, until so many electrons are in it that the normal population of electrons between this state and the normal unexcited state becomes inverted. At this point a single decay is enough to start an avalanche of electron decays, as the emission of one photon *stimulates* another electron emission and so on.

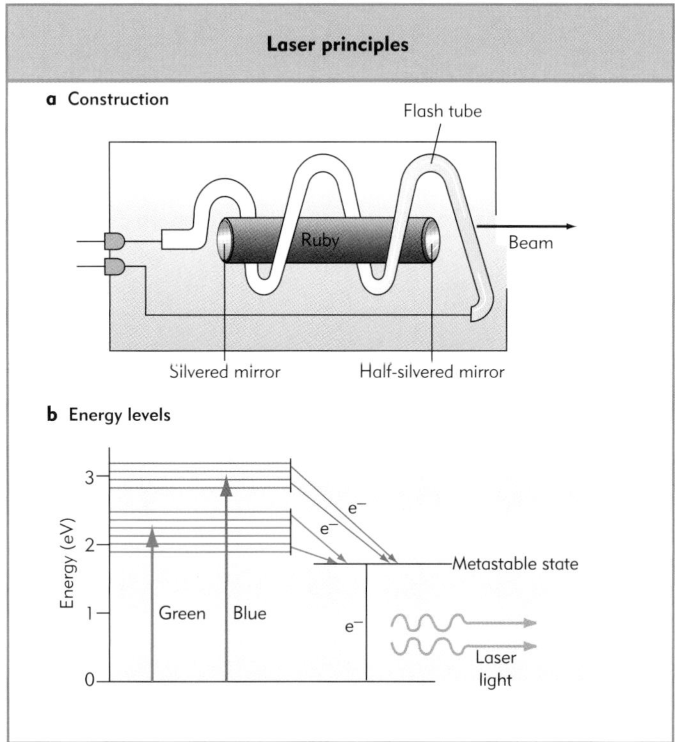

Figure 12.6 The construction of an early ruby laser and the energy levels associated with its action.

What is very particular about the light emitted, however, is that it is not emitted in a random fashion. The stimulation process leads to photons that are in phase, or coherent. The avalanche emission therefore behaves as one wave motion, emerging from the half-silvered end of the crystal as a highly focused, single wavelength and a highly energetic beam.

Laser action has been demonstrated in a wide variety of substances and at a wide range of wavelengths, including microwaves (masers). Gas lasers, such as the helium–neon (which gives red light for plastic surgery), use an electric discharge to pump the electrons in the gas mixture. Considerable power is possible. Laser light interacts with tissue in four ways: thermal heating, photochemically, thermoacoustically, and to produce photoablation. Medical lasers are often very powerful and can be used to cut, weld, or ablate tissues. Medical laser light is often of sufficient intensity to be an ignition risk.

Nuclear magnetic resonance

In the nucleus of an atom each positively charged proton can have a 'spin', a property that can be thought of as if the proton spins on its axis. Associated with this spin is a magnetic field. In the nucleus, protons usually align themselves in pairs of opposite spin to neutralize the overall magnetic field, but in atoms with an odd number of protons this is not possible. This occurs in ^{1}H, ^{13}C, ^{14}N, ^{17}O, ^{23}Na, and ^{31}P, all of which are biochemically important elements common in the body.

Under normal circumstances the orientations of the nuclear fields for individual atoms are random, but when an external magnetic field is applied these orientations align with the field such that the north (N) pole of the particle lines with the south (S) pole of the field. Aligning N–N is also possible, but this state has a higher quantum energy than the N–S orientation and is therefore somewhat like the excited state of an electron in an atom. Nuclei in the magnetic field are not stationary but *precess*, that is wobble, rather like a top or a gyroscope. The frequency at which they precess is fixed by the magnetic field strength. If the nuclei are irradiated with an electromagnetic field at this frequency in the N–S state, they resonate with that field, absorb energy, and can flip to the N–N state. If the electromagnetic radiation is removed, the nuclei decay back to the N–S state in a time that depends on their binding with the atoms around them (effectively the chemistry of the molecules around them). The time constants for these relaxations are quite long (from milliseconds to seconds). The associated electromagnetic radiation can be detected, and if pulses of electromagnetic radiation are used to excite the nuclei, the resultant spin echoes can be gated in time. Because the excitation frequency is atom specific and the echoes have time constants characterized by their interactions, NMR is a very specific analysis tool. It enables the study of one atom type within a sample and it can be carried out in vivo as well as in vitro.

The principle of NMR applies to any spinning, charged atomic particle, including electrons, in which case the equivalent effect is electron spin resonance (ESR). The NMR equipment used to create images of body sections (similar to computed tomography (CT) images) can also be used to examine ESR effects, and is thus given the general name of magnetic resonance imaging (MRI). To reconstruct an image from all the possible echoes in a volume slice of tissue requires sophisticated pulse and gating sequences.

Fiberoptics

In many medical measurement applications it is useful to transmit into or gather light from the body over relatively long path lengths and through small openings or orifices without undue losses. Fiberoptics is a convenient way of achieving this. Fiberoptic cables rely on the principle of total internal reflection of visible light.

A fiberoptic cable is made up of 400–500 individual fibers. These can be made of plastic or glass, and each has a coating that increases its internal reflection. When light is injected into the end it is trapped by the multiple internal reflections and transmitted from one end to the other. The fibers themselves are flexible, and so the whole cable can be bent and shaped as needed. Glass fibers have transmission efficiencies of 60% over 50 cm for wavelengths of 400–1200 nm. Plastic fibers have 70% transmission efficiencies for the same distance, but at a more limited range of wavelengths (500–850 nm).

Fiberoptic cables come in two forms. In *noncoherent* cables (called *light guides*) the fiber diameter is 13–100 nm and no correlation exists between a fiber's spatial position at the entrance to the cable and where it emerges. These are used for transmission of light into the body only. In *coherent* fiber bundles or cables the fibers occupy the same spatial position at entrance and exit, so images can be transmitted faithfully through the bundle. These cables are used for endoscopy.

Fiberoptic cables are relatively more energy efficient at transmitting pulses of information than the equivalent wire conductor, although efficiency is lost in having to create the light pulses initially and to convert them back into electricity at the end of the cable. Fiberoptic cables have the added advantage that the pulses transmitted down the fiber are less distorted by the transmission, which means that the fiber has a greater bandwidth and can transmit more pulses per second than a wire. Fiberoptics is becoming the standard method of transmitting digital information over long distances. In medicine this technology is very attractive as a way of transmitting information from inside the body. Information in this form is immune from electrical interference and the fibers themselves provide electrical isolation from the patient.

RADIOACTIVITY AND RADIATION

Elements are characterized by the number of protons and neutrons in their nuclei. The number of protons is the atomic number, Z, of the element. The atomic number equals the number of electrons in orbit around the nuclei. The number of electrons determines the chemistry of the element. Developing the Bohr model of the atom a little further, more than one electron can exist in each of the orbitals with the same quantum energy. It is found that the greatest chemical stability exists when the outer orbital or *shell* of an atom has an even number of electrons. The shells are given letters to distinguish them, and the maximum number of electrons allowed in each shell rises with the number of shells. The innermost shell, the K-shell has a maximum of two electrons, the L-shell a maximum of eight, the M-shell a maximum of 18, and so on. It is the configuration of the electrons in the outer shell of the element that determines its position in the *periodic table*. Hydrogen, lithium, sodium, rubidium, and francium all have outer shells with one electron. Their ability to lose this electron to form positive ions therefore tends to dominate their chemistry and makes their chemistries similar in many respects.

The number of neutrons in the nucleus of the element does not affect the chemistry of the element, but does affect its mass number, A, which is the total number of neutrons and protons in the nucleus. Elements with the same Z but different A values are *isotopes* of the same element. To distinguish different isotopes in chemical equations, the A value (mass number) is added as a superscript before the chemical symbol and the Z value (atomic number) as a subscript. Thus the three isotopes of hydrogen are given the nomenclature ${}^{1}_{1}H$ (hydrogen), ${}^{2}_{1}H$ (deuterium), and ${}^{3}_{1}H$ (tritium).

The nucleus is held together by strong and weak nuclear forces that are very short range. As with electrons in the shells, protons and neutrons in the nucleus can exist in excited or other states that are described by quantum mechanics. Thus decay of the nucleus is possible, just as ionization of an atom is possible. Spontaneous nuclear breakdown leads to radioactivity.

Most naturally occurring isotopes exist as mixtures of *stable isotopes* that do not exhibit radioactivity. However, some *unstable isotopes* (*radioactive isotopes*) do exist naturally, and others can be created by bombarding stable isotopes with charged subatomic particles.

Types of radioactivity

Disintegration of the nucleus may be accompanied by the emission of particles and/or energy. The three types of radiation associated with nuclear decay are α-, β-, and γ-radiation.

α-RADIATION

α-Radiation consists of heavy, positively charged particles with a mass number 2 and an atomic number 4 (i.e. helium nuclei ${}^{4}_{2}He$). A typical transition that emits α-particles is the breakdown of radium (Ra) into radon (Rn) (Equation 12.21).

■ Equation 12.21

$${}^{226}_{88}Ra \rightarrow {}^{222}_{86}Rn + {}^{4}_{2}\alpha$$

Because α-particles are heavy they do not have a high velocity. They are easily absorbed by passage through a few millimeters of air, tissue, or other material. However, they carry quite a lot of kinetic energy because of their mass, and deposit this effectively in biologic tissues, which results in considerable cellular damage. An α-particle is quite capable of entirely smashing the nucleus of a cell!

β-RADIATION

β-Radiation consists of electrons or positrons, but the majority of isotopes decay by β-particle emission. Isotopes with an excess of neutrons usually decay by this pathway. Loss of a negative charge from the nucleus effectively converts a neutron into a proton, and so the atomic number of the element increases. A typical decay of this type that emits β-particles is the decay of phosphorus-32 into sulfur-32 (Equation 12.22).

■ Equation 12.22

$${}^{32}_{15}P \rightarrow {}^{32}_{16}S + {}^{0}_{-1}\beta$$

Neutron-deficient nuclei can emit a positron (a positively charged electron, the antiparticle of the electron), which reduces atomic number by 1, as with the decay of iron-18 (Equation 12.23).

■ Equation 12.23

$$^{18}_{9}Fe \rightarrow {}^{18}_{8}O + {}^{0}_{1}\beta$$

Because β-particles have low mass they have high velocities and are harder to absorb than α-particles. However, their range in tissue is only a few millimeters. Thus, if a β-active isotope is injected into the body, external detection is not possible. Such isotopes are used for tracer studies in which the radioactivity is measured in samples removed from the body, for example the use of tritiated water (^3H_2O) as a tracer for the measurement of lung water.

Positron decay isotopes are the basis of a relatively new form of functional tissue imaging known as positron emission tomography (PET). In PET, biochemically active isotopes are prepared that decay by positron emission (e.g. glucose). The isotope is injected and taken up by the targeted tissues. Positrons emitted from the isotope are slowed by their interactions with tissue. When a positron encounters an electron, its antiparticle, they annihilate each other and the energy is released as photons, in this case two γ-rays. Because at annihilation neither the electron nor the positron has much momentum, the γ-rays are emitted at 180° from each other. Thus they arrive at two γ-ray detectors on opposite sides of the body at the same time, which can be used to determine where they came from.

As β-particles have low mass they deposit little energy in tissue, and until relatively recently were considered the least dangerous form of radiation. However, it is now recognized that although they do not cause widespread cellular damage, they can break DNA strands in the nuclei of cells and may thus be more dangerous mutagens if ingested than had previously been thought.

γ-RADIATION

γ-Radiation (γ-rays) consists of photons and thus is part of the electromagnetic spectrum. It is given off by radioactive decay as a way of removing excess energy, or as the result of a secondary annihilation (as with the electron–positron example given above). In common with all electromagnetic radiation, γ-rays are very difficult to stop and penetrate many centimeters of tissue (if they do not pass straight through the body). They are highly energetic.

Units of measurement

The amount of radioactivity of a source or its activity is measured in terms of the number of disintegrations per unit time (SI unit is the becquerel, Bq). Of great clinical importance is the absorbed dose of radioactivity, which is measured by the energy transferred to a substance by the radiation (SI unit is the gray, Gy). The absorbed dose needs to be adjusted for the biologic effectiveness of the radiation, which depends on radiation type and target organ. The effective dose is the absorbed dose weighted by terms for radiation type and organ sensitivity (SI unit is the sievert, Sv).

Radioactivity is a probabilistic effect. When an individual atom will decay is not known, but in a given time the number of atoms that decay is a fixed proportion of the number of atoms capable of decaying; this is defined by an exponential decay curve that has the mathematical form of Equation 12.24, in which N is the number of atoms left that can disintegrate, N_0 is the number at the start, k is a constant, and t is time.

■ Equation 12.24

$$N = N_0e^{-kt}$$

The rate at which an exponential curve falls can be defined using two indices: the decay constant (k), and the half-life ($t_{1/2}$). Half-life is the time required for the initial number of atoms to drop to 50% of its initial value (Equation 12.25).

■ Equation 12.25

$$t_{1/2} = \frac{(\ln 0.5)}{-k} = \frac{0.698}{k}$$

Further reading

Ohanian HC. Principles of physics. New York: WW Norton & Company; 1994.

Webster J. Medical instrumentation, 3rd edn. New York: John Wiley & Sons; 1998.

Chapter 13

Electrocardiography

Martin J London

TOPICS COVERED IN THIS CHAPTER

- **Historical perspective**
- **Technical aspects**
  - Power spectrum of the ECG
  - Intrinsic and extrinsic artifacts
  - Technical aspects of electrode placement
  - Clinical sources of artifact
  - Frequency response of ECG monitors: monitoring and diagnostic modes
- **Digital signal processing and computerized ECG**
  - Technical background
- **Lead systems**
  - History and description of the 12-lead sysem
  - Frank leads
- **Detection of myocardial ischemia**
  - Pathophysiology of ST segment responses
  - ECG manifestations of ischemia
  - Clinical lead systems for detecting ischemia
  - Intraoperative lead systems
  - Arrhythmia and pacemaker detection

Interpretation of the electrocardiogram (ECG) is often considered the domain of the cardiologist, but clinicians providing perioperative and critical care also derive important information from it, via the standard 12-lead tracing or as a continuous 'monitoring' modality. With advances in computer technology, the distinction between 'diagnostic' ECG carts and bedside 'monitoring' units is narrowing. Many bedside units are now capable of recording diagnostic-quality 12-lead ECGs for transmission over a hospital network for storage and retrieval. The diagnostic and monitoring capabilities of the ECG for the detection of arrhythmias and myocardial ischemia/infarction continue to develop and expand (Table 13.1). However, there are finite limits defined by the relation between sensitivity and specificity (usually inversely related) for detecting coronary artery disease (CAD) and its consequences. For example, during exercise testing the 12-lead ECG has a mean sensitivity of only 68% and a specificity of 77%. The resting 12-lead ECG is even less sensitive and specific. Thus, other clinical modalities are often required (e.g. transthoracic or transesophageal echocardiography (Chapter 17), pulmonary artery catheterization etc.). Newer, more complex ECG modalities are likely to improve its utility in the future (e.g. continuous vectorcardiography, high-frequency QRS signal averaging etc.). Routine use of digital signal processing techniques greatly facilitates continuous ECG monitoring, both inexpensively and with minimal invasiveness (Table 13.2).

Table 13.1 Clinical information available from electrocardiography. (With permission from London and Kaplan, 1999.)

Anatomy/morphology
Infarction
Ischemia
Hypertrophy
Physiology
Automaticity
Antythmogenicity
Conduction
Ischemia
Autonomic tone
Electrolyte abnormalities
Drug toxicity/effect
Ejection fraction (?)

The practicing anesthesiologist relies on the ECG to make critical decisions at many phases of the perioperative period in patients undergoing cardiac or noncardiac (particularly vascular) surgery. In this chapter, the theory and operating characteristics of ECG hardware used in the perioperative period are presented to facilitate proper utilization and interpretation of monitoring data.

HISTORICAL PERSPECTIVE

Einthoven is universally considered the father of electrocardiography (for which he won the 1924 Nobel Prize). However, Waller actually recorded the first human ECG in 1887, using a glass capillary electrometer. This early device utilized changes in

Table 13.2 Data extraction from electrocardiography to support current and future clinical uses. Data derived with and without ancillary corrective modalities (With permission from London and Kaplan, 1999.)

P wave	**ST-T wave**
Polarity	Slope of ascending/descending limbs
Duration	Area
Mean amplitude	Ratio of area to peak, duration to peak
Area	
Frequency content	
P-R segment	**Power spectrum of variation**
A-H interval	**Arrhythmias**
H-V interval	Morphology
	Coupling interval
QRS complex	
Polarity	
Duration	
Area	
Mean amplitude	
Frequency content	
Late potential-power spectrum	

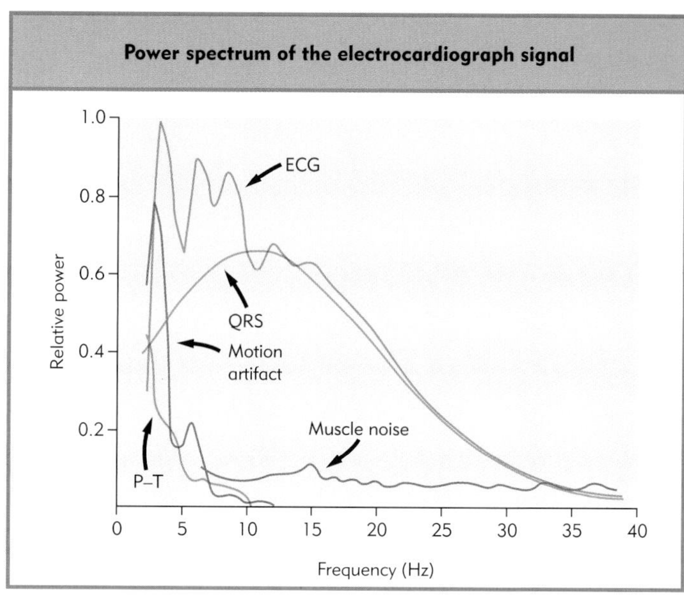

Figure 13.1 Power spectrum of the ECG signal, including its subcomponents and common artifacts (i.e. motion and muscle noise). The power of the P and T waves are low frequency, whereas the QRS complex is concentrated in the midfrequency range. (Reproduced from Thakor NV: From Holter monitors to automatic defibrillators: Developments in ambulatory arrhythmia monitoring. IEEE Trans Biomed Eng BME-31:770, 1984, with permission © 1984, IEEE.)

surface tension between mercury and sulfuric acid in a glass column induced by a varying electric potential. The level of the meniscus was magnified and recorded on moving photographic paper, describing what were initially termed 'A-B-C-D waves'. In 1895, Einthoven published his observations using this crude device. Frustration with its low-frequency resolution led him to develop the string galvanometer, using a silver-coated quartz fiber suspended between the poles of a magnet. Changes induced by the electrical potentials conducted through the quartz string resulted in its movement at right-angles to the magnetic field. The shadow of the string, backlit from a light source, was transmitted through a microscope (the string was only 2.1 mm in diameter) and recorded on a moving photographic plate. Einthoven renamed the signal the P-QRS-T complex (based on standard geometric convention for describing points on curved lines).

Many of the basic clinical abnormalities in electrocardiography were first described using the string galvonometer (i.e. bundle-branch block, δ waves, ST-T changes with angina). This was used until the 1930s, when it was replaced by a system using vacuum tube amplifiers and a cathode ray oscilloscope. A portable direct-writing ECG cart was not introduced until the early 1950s (facilitated at first by transistor technology and subsequently by integrated circuits), which allowed widespread use of the ECG in clinical practice. The first analog-to-digital (A/D) conversion systems for the ECG were introduced in the early 1960s, but their clinical use was restricted until the late 1970s. In the 1980s, microcomputer technology became widely available and is now standard for all diagnostic and monitoring systems.

TECHNICAL ASPECTS

Power spectrum of the ECG

The ECG signal must be considered in terms of its amplitude (or voltage) and its frequency components (generally termed its 'phase'). Voltage considerations differ depending on the signal source. Surface recording involves the amplification of smaller voltages (on the order of 1 mV) than recording sites closer to the heart beneath the electrically resistant layers of the skin (e.g. endocardial, esophageal and intratracheal leads). The 'power spectrum' of the ECG (Fig. 13.1) is derived by Fourier transformation, in which a periodic waveform is mathematically decomposed to its harmonic components (sine waves of varying amplitude and frequency). Spectra representing some of the major sources of artifact must be eliminated during the processing and amplification of the QRS complex. The frequency of each of these components can be equated to the slope of the component signal. The R wave, with its steep slope, is a high-frequency component, whereas P and T waves have lesser slopes and are lower in frequency. The ST segment has the lowest frequency, not much different from the 'underlying' electrical (i.e. isoelectric) baseline of the ECG. Prior to the introduction of digital signal processing (DSP), displaying the ST segment accurately presented significant technical problems, particularly in operating room (OR)/ICU bedside monitoring units (see below). Although the overall frequency spectrum of the QRS complex in Figure 13.1 does not appear to exceed 40 Hz, many components of the QRS complex, particularly the R wave, exceed 100 Hz. Very high-frequency signals of particular clinical significance are pacemaker spikes. Their short duration and high amplitude present technical challenges for proper recognition and rejection to allow accurate determination of the heart rate (HR). The frequencies of greatest importance for optimal ECG processing are presented in Table 13.3.

The ECG is characterized by a power spectrum of harmonic waveform components of varying amplitude and frequency.

Table 13.3 Range of signal frequencies included in different phases of processing in an ECG monitor (With permission from London and Kaplan, 1999)

Processing	Frequency range (Hz)
Display	0.5 (0.05)–40
QRS detection	5–30
Arrhythmia detection	0.05–60
ST segment monitoring	0.05–60
Pacemaker detection	1500–5000

Intrinsic and extrinsic artifacts

Motion artifact and 'baseline wander' result from several causes. Skin impedance has been shown to vary at different skin sites, at different times of the day as well as seasonally (probably related to humidity changes), and may be 50% higher in females. With the application of a silver–silver chloride electrode, impedance decays with a time constant of 6.9 minutes as the conductive gel penetrates the skin. Deformation of the stratum granulosum generates electrical potentials of several millivolts as cells slide over each other or are stretched. Skin potentials up to 64 mV can be measured between two electrodes on the skin surface, varying with the type of electrolyte gel used. Direct current (DC) potentials are actually stored by the electrode itself (termed offset potentials), and vary with the type of electrode used. A striking example of an offset potential is the transient obliteration of the ECG that occurs immediately after electrical defibrillation. Poor electrode contact enhances pickup of alternating current power-line interference (60-Hz signals). The second major physiologic source of artifact is electromyographic (EMG) noise produced by motor activity, either conscious (i.e. during treadmill testing or ambulatory ST segment monitoring) or unconscious (i.e. shivering or parkinsonian tremor). Electromyographic noise is similar in amplitude to the ECG, but is generally of considerably higher frequency. Because it is a random signal, in contrast to the regular repetitive ECG signal, it is amenable to significant attenuation (if not outright elimination) using routine DSP techniques (see below).

ECG artifacts result from skin impedance, electromyographic noise, and electromagnetic interference.

There are also extrinsic or 'non-physiologic' causes of artifact. An important one is termed 'common-mode rejection'. The ECG signal is recorded as the difference in potential between two electrodes and thus is technically a differential signal. Furthermore, the body is not at absolute ground potential, which is why the right leg lead is used as a reference electrode. This higher potential (over that of an absolute ground to earth) is termed common-mode potential, because it is common to both electrode inputs to the differential amplifier used to amplify the ECG signal. Common-mode potential must be rejected or it may alter the ECG signal. The ability of the differential amplifier to reject these potentials (relative to the differential inputs) is termed the common-mode rejection ratio (CMRR). In modern amplifiers, CMRR should be at least 100 000; in newer diagnostic digital ECG units, it is at least 1 million. Adequate CMRR is of great importance in attenuating a variety of environmental factors.

Electrical power-line interference (60 Hz) is a common environmental problem. Power lines and other electrical devices radiate energy, which can enter the monitor via poor electrode contact or cracked or poorly shielded lead cables. Interference can also be induced electromagnetically as these signals radiate through the loop formed by the body, lead cables, and monitor. This type of interference can be reduced by twisting the lead cables together (thereby reducing the loop area) or minimizing the distance between lead cables. In newer diagnostic ECG machines, A/D signal conversion occurs in an acquisition module close to the patient, which effectively reduces the length of the lead cables and the amount of signal induction possible. A line frequency 'notch' filter is often used to remove 60-Hz noise.

Electrocautery (electrosurgery) units generate radiofrequency currents at very high frequencies (800–2000 kHz) and high voltages (1 kV, which is 10^6 greater than the ECG signal). Older units used a modulation frequency of 60 Hz, which spread substantial electrical noise into the QRS frequency range of the ECG signal. Newer units use a modulation frequency of 20 kHz, thereby minimizing this problem. In order to minimize electrocautery artifact, the right leg reference electrode should be placed as close as possible to the grounding pad and the ECG monitor should be plugged into a different power outlet from the electrosurgical unit.

Technical aspects of electrode placement

Monitoring electrodes should preferably be placed directly over bony prominences of the torso (i.e. clavicular heads and iliac prominences) to minimize excursion of the electrode during respiration, which can cause baseline wander. Electrode impedance must be optimized to avoid loss and alteration of the signal. By removing a portion of the stratum corneum (gentle abrasion with a dry gauze pad, resulting in a minor amount of surface erythema, works well), skin impedance can be reduced by a factor of 10–100. Optimal impedance is 5000 Ω or less. The electrode should be covered with a watertight dressing to prevent surgical scrub solutions from undermining electrode contact.

Clinical sources of artifact

Devices with which the patient is in physical contact, particularly via plastic tubing, may at times cause clinically significant ECG artifact. Although the exact mechanism is uncertain, two leading explanations are either a piezoelectric effect due to mechanical deformation of the plastic, or the build-up of static electricity between two dissimilar materials, especially those in motion. This effect has been noted with the use of cardiopulmonary bypass and usually mimics atrial arrhythmias. A grounding lead on the cardiopulmonary bypass machine usually eliminates this. Other clinical devices associated with ECG interference – albeit rarely – include infusion pumps and blood warmers. Isolated power supply line isolation monitors (LIMs) have also been associated with 60-Hz interference. This can be diagnosed by removing the LIM fuses to see if the artifact disappears.

Frequency response of ECG monitors: monitoring and diagnostic modes

Given the importance of the ECG in diagnosing myocardial ischemia, it is important to realize that 'significant' ST segment depression or elevation can occur solely as a result of improper signal filtering in 12-lead ECG machines, and in bedside or ambulatory ST segment monitors. This artifact was a particular problem prior to the introduction of DSP. The American Heart Association (AHA) Committee on Electrocardiography Standardization has addressed specific frequency requirements for monitoring in this setting.

ECG signals must be amplified and filtered before display. To reproduce the component frequencies accurately, each must be amplified equally. Thus, the monitor must have a 'flat amplitude response' over the wide range of frequencies present. Similarly, because the slight delay in a signal as it passes through a filter or amplifier may vary in duration with different frequencies, all frequencies must be delayed equally. This is termed 'linear phase response'. If the response is nonlinear, various components may appear temporally distorted (termed 'phase shift').

ECG signals must be amplified and filtered before display, which can introduce artifact.

Nonlinear frequency response in the low-frequency range (0.5 Hz) can cause artifactual ST depression, whereas phase delay in this range can cause ST segment elevation. Therefore, the AHA recommends a bandwidth from 0.05 to 100 Hz (at 3 dB). Although a completely linear response is desirable, with analog filters it is not generally possible. However, the response at 0.05 Hz should not be reduced by more than 30% (at 3 dB) from the response at 0.14 Hz (Fig. 13.2). Phase response is not well described, but is usually adequate when amplitude response criteria are met. Because greater baseline noise is present when a 0.05 Hz cutoff is used, the 0.5 Hz cutoff is often used to display a more stable signal. This is commonly referred to as 'monitoring mode', whereas the use of a 0.05 Hz low-frequency cutoff is known as 'diagnostic mode'. The difference in ST segment morphology at varying low-frequency cutoffs is illustrated in Figure 13.3. As most newer monitors use signal averaging

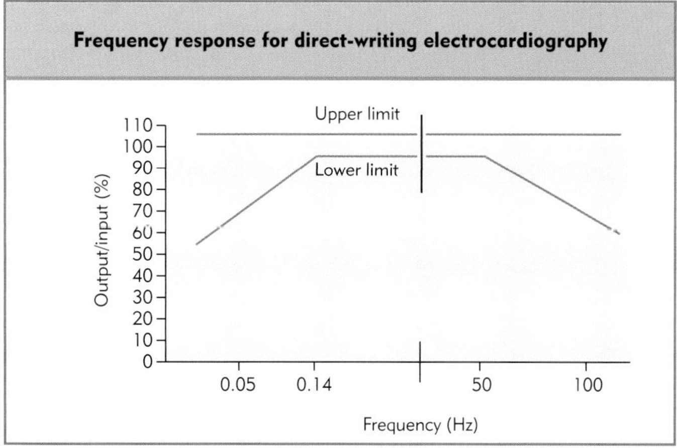

Figure 13.2 Frequency response for direct-writing ECG recommended by the American Heart Association. The bandwidth is demarcated by the upper and lower corner frequencies (in this example 0.05 and 100 Hz). Each of the corner frequencies is located −3 dB (approximately a 30% decrease in voltage) relative to the amplification at a frequency near the middle of the bandwidth (heavy vertical bar). (Reproduced from Pipberger HV, Arzbaecher RC, Berson AS, et al. Recommendations for the standardization of leads and of specifications for instruments in electocardiography and vectorcardiography. Report of the Committee on Electrocardiography, American Heart Association. Circulation 52:11, 1975, with permission; copyright American Heart Association.)

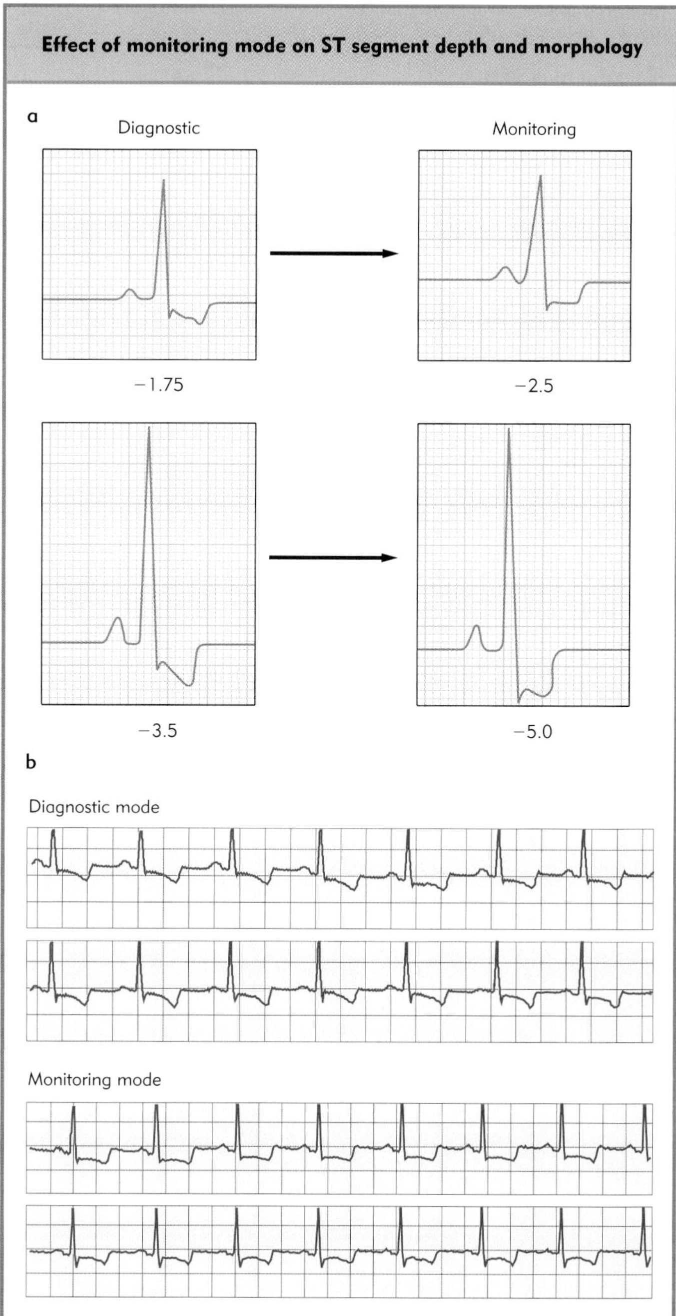

Figure 13.3 The effects of the monitoring mode on ST segment depth and morphology. (a) Effects illustrated using a digital ECG simulator. A SpaceLabs PC2 monitor (Redmond, WA) was switched from monitoring (0.5–40 Hz) to diagnostic mode (0.05–70 Hz). Note the increase in the depth of ST segment depression and the alteration of slope in both leads. (Reproduced from London MJ. Ischemia monitoring: ST segment analysis versus TEE. In: Kaplan JA, ed. Cardiothoracic and vascular anesthesia update. Vol 3, Chap 2, 1993:1–20, with permission). (b) Actual clinical example of monitoring mode exaggerated ST segment depression in a patient with baseline ST segment depression. Notice the subtle wandering of the ECG baseline over several beats that is straightened out in the monitoring mode.

techniques that effectively eliminate most artifact even in the diagnostic mode, the clinician can usually (and should) avoid using the monitoring mode whenever possible.

High-frequency response is of less importance clinically, as the ST segment and T wave reside in the low-frequency spectrum. However, at the commonly used high-frequency cutoff of 40 Hz, the amplitude of the R and S waves may diminish significantly, making it difficult to diagnose ventricular hypertrophy. Significant reduction in QRS amplitude can occur with a major reduction in ventricular function, with obesity, pericardial effusion, and with infiltrative and restrictive cardiac diseases. Newer data document a significant reversible reduction with whole-body fluid accumulation (anasarca).

DIGITAL SIGNAL PROCESSING AND COMPUTERIZED ECG

Technical background

The foundation of DSP is the A/D converter, which samples the incoming 'continuous' analog signal (characterized by variable amplitude or voltage over time) at a very rapid rate and converts the sampled voltage into binary numbers, each of which has a precise time index or sequence. The 'bit size' of the A/D converter controls the number of measurements possible within a given voltage range, according to the formula $2^n - 1$, where n = bit size (i.e. an 8-bit converter divides the input range into 255 intervals). Thus, the larger the bit size, the greater the resolution of the signal. However, greater bit size and higher sampling rates require more powerful microprocessors and more computer memory. Most commercially available units use minimum sampling rates of 256 Hz (resulting in 4-ms increments) with at least 12-bit resolution. The use of lower sampling rates may result in a slight difference in the time at which digitization of each QRS complex begins ('phase shift'), which can distort the signal as noted above. Newer diagnostic ECG units are capable of sampling at 1000 Hz (termed high-resolution or high-RES ECG).

Low-frequency responses, which encompass the ST segment and T wave, are more important clinically than high-frequency responses.

Following A/D conversion, the resultant data bits are inspected by a microprocessor using a mathematical model to determine where reference points ('fiducial points') are located. A common method locates the point of most rapid change in amplitude (located on the downslope of the R wave). This process characterizes the baseline QRS complex (QRS recognition), providing a 'template' on which subsequent beats are overlaid (beat alignment) and averaged (signal averaging). This allows visual display of the QRS complex and quantification of its components, as well as elimination of random electrical noise and wide complex beats that fail to meet criteria established by the fiducial points. Signal averaging is used to reduce noise by the square root of the number of beats averaged (Fig. 13.4). Thus, a 10-fold reduction in noise is accomplished by averaging only 100 beats. Because of the proprietary nature of this technology (the specific algorithms used are patented), methods may vary by manufacturer. Consequently, processed QRS complexes may vary in the 'quality' of representation (i.e. if noise or aberrant beats are averaged into the complex, it will vary from the raw analog complex).

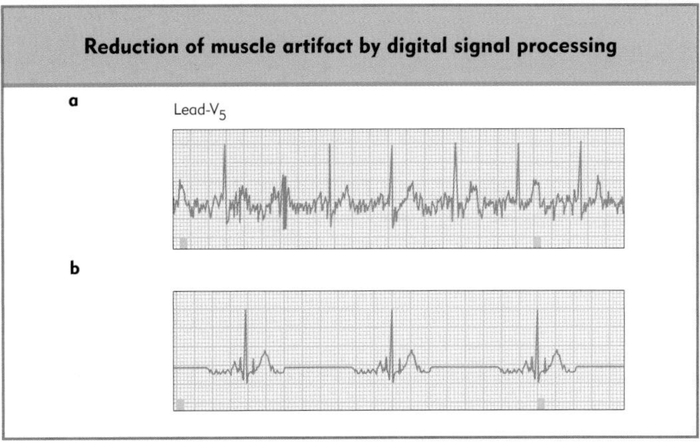

Figure 13.4 Reduction of muscle of muscle artifact (simulated) by digital signal processing using signal averaging (PC2 Bedside Monitor, SpaceLabs, Inc., Redmond, WA). The top tracing contains the initial learned complex ('dominant') on the left followed by real time complexes. The bottom tracing contains median complexes smoothed by signal processing. The degree of noise reduction is proportional to the square root of the number of beats averaged. (From London and Kaplan, 1999, with permission)

The signal averaging process involves comparison of voltages at a particular time point between the incoming complex and a template. The easiest method uses the mean difference between voltages to update the 'template', but the most accurate method uses the median difference (which is less affected by outliers, such as aberrant beats, or other signals that have escaped QRS matching). But median averaging is computationally more complex (i.e. memory intensive) and may have slightly higher baseline noise content. Because median averaging is impractical for continuous data acquisition, 'incremental averaging' is used, a technique that minimizes the influence of outliers. When the incoming value is above the value of the template (by any amount), a small fixed voltage increment is added to the template (generally 10 mV/beat); when it is below the previous beat, the same value is subtracted.

Signal averaging algorithms are used to reduce noise in the ECG.

Most monitors incorporate a visual trend line from which deviations in the position of the ST segment can be rapidly detected to aid online detection of myocardial ischemia. This can be a single summated trend of several 'quasi-orthogonal' leads, or multiple single leads. Nearly all monitors also display on-screen numerical values for the position of the ST segment used for ischemia detection (generally 60–80 ms following the J point). The specific point used is adjustable, which may be helpful with tachycardia (Fig. 13.5). These features enhance the diagnosis of perioperative ischemia, which is difficult to detect without some automated system.

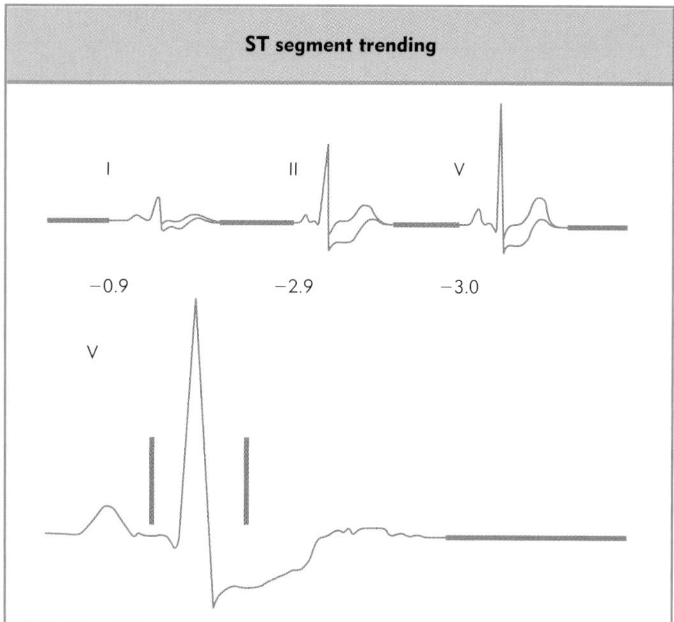

Figure 13.5 The graphic output of the 'ST adjustment' window from a Marquette Electronics (Milwaukee, WI) ST segment analyzer (Series 7010 monitor) demonstrating trending and display of 3 leads (I, II, and a V lead). The initial complex ('learned' when the program was activated) is displayed along with the current complex. The complexes are superimposed to facilitate comparison. ST analysis is performed automatically at 80 msec after the J point, although this point can be manually adjusted by the user. (From London and Kaplan, 1999, with permission.)

LEAD SYSTEMS

Where and how ECG electrodes are placed on the body is a critical determinant of the morphology of the ECG signal. Lead systems have been developed based on theoretical considerations (i.e. the orthogonal arrangement of the Frank XYZ leads) and/or references to anatomic landmarks that facilitate consistency between individuals (i.e. standard 12-lead system). Table 13.4 describes basic mathematical relations between the components of the 12-lead system and the Frank–Lewis orthogonal lead system.

History and description of the 12-lead system

Einthoven established electrocardiography using three extremities as references: the left arm (LA), right arm (RA), and left leg (LL). He recorded the difference in potential between the LA and RA (lead I), LL and RA (lead II), and LL and LA (lead III). Because the signals recorded were differences between two electrodes, these leads were termed 'bipolar'. The RL served only as a reference electrode. As Kirchoff's loop equation states that the sum of the three voltage differential pairs must equal zero, the sum of leads I and III must equal lead II (which is therefore redundant). The positive or negative polarity of each of the limbs was chosen by Einthoven to result in positive deflections of most of the waveforms, and thus has no innate physiologic significance. He postulated that the three limbs defined an imaginary equilateral triangle with the heart at its center. Given the influence of Einthoven's vector analyses of frontal plane forces, others eventually incorporated the other two orthogonal planes (transverse and sagittal).

Wilson refined and clinically introduced the unipolar precordial leads. In order to implement these leads, he postulated a mechanism whereby the absolute level of electrical potential could be measured at the site of the exploring precordial electrode (the positive electrode). A negative pole with zero potential was formed by joining the three limb electrodes in a resistive network in which equally weighted signals cancelled each other out. He termed this the 'central terminal', and in a fashion similar to Einthoven's vector concepts, postulated that it was located at the electrical center of the heart, representing the mean electrical potential of the body throughout the cardiac cycle. He described three additional limb leads (VL, VR, and

Table 13.4 Definitions of electrocardiography leads. (From London and Kaplan, 1999, with permission.)

Lead type	Electrodes used	Definition
Bipolar or limb leads (Einthoven)	LA, RA, LL, RL	I = LA – RA II = LL – RA III = LL – LA
Augmented (Goldberger)	LA, RA, LL, RL	aV_R = RA – 0.5 (LA + LL) aV_L = LA – 0.5 (LL + RA) Av_F = LL– 0.5 (LA + RA)
Unipolar chest leads (Wilson)	$V_1 - V_6$	$V_1 = v_1$ – (LA + RA + LL)/3 $V_2 = v_2$ – (LA + RA + LL)/3 $V_3 = v_3$ – (LA + RA + LL)/3 $V_4 = v_4$ – (LA + RA + LL)/3 $V_5 = v_5$ – (LA + RA + LL)/3 $V_6 = v_6$ – (LA + RA + LL)/3
Orthogonal vector leads (Frank)	I, E, C, A, M, H, F	X = 0.610A + 0.171C – 0.7811 Y = 0.655F + 0.345M – 1.000H Z = 0.133A + 0.736M – 0.2641 – 0.374E – 0.231C

V, precordial voltage (before input to central terminal of Wilson).

VF). These leads measured new vectors of activation, and thus the hexaxial reference system for determination of electrical axis was established. He subsequently introduced the six unipolar precordial V leads in 1935 (Fig. 13.6).

Clinical application of the unipolar limb leads was limited because of their significantly smaller amplitude relative to the bipolar limb leads from which they were derived. They were not clinically applied until 1942, when Goldberger augmented their amplitude (by a factor of 1.5) by severing the connection between the central terminal and the lead extremity being studied (which he termed 'augmented limb leads'). These three lead groups, the bipolar limb leads, the unipolar precordial leads, and the augmented unipolar limb leads, form what was accepted by the AHA as the conventional 12-lead ECG system.

Frank leads

As early as 1920, Mann introduced the concept of vector cardiography (VCG), which measures the time course of the mean instantaneous spatial cardiac vectors. This was represented by a loop in the frontal plane, although it was not until the invention of the cathode ray oscilloscope that it could be directly recorded. Use of the frontal plane bipolar leads has its limitations. Lead I, although oriented horizontally (the x direction), is only an approximation, as current flow in the lead field is not uniform or solely in the x direction (based on the dipole theory). Thus, a number of alternate lead systems allowing more accurate depiction of the vector loop in the three orthogonal axes (transverse x, vertical y, and sagittal z leads) were investigated. The most widely accepted is that of Frank, which uses seven exploring electrodes interconnected by a resistor network to derive approximately uniform vector fields of equal magnitude in the x, y, and z axes. It is properly termed a 'corrected orthogonal lead system', given that it assumes that the body volume conductor is nonuniform, the heart is eccentric as a source, there are a number of dipoles, and there is variation in the vectorial expression of the magnitude of an electrical signal. The Frank lead system allowed standardized recording of the VCG, although it has never been widely accepted owing to its complexity. Nonetheless, the VCG may be superior to the 12-lead ECG in diagnosing myocardial infarction, and in detecting right ventricular hypertrophy or atrial enlargement. Several recent clinical studies report increased sensitivity and earlier detection of perioperative ischemia using continuous computerized vector cardiography, which may facilitate the use of this lead system in the near future.

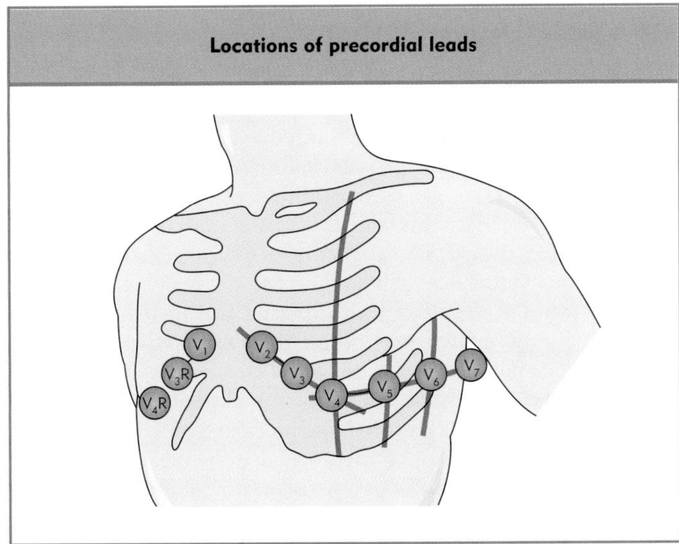

Figure 13.6 The locations of the precordial leads. Heavy vertical lines represent the midclavicular, anterior, axillary, and midaxillary lines, respectively (from left to right). V_1 and V_2 are referenced to the fourth intercostal space and V4 to the fifth space. V_3 lies on a line between V_2 and V_4. V_5 and V_6 lie on a horizontal line from V4. Additional precordial leads can be obtained on the right side (V_3R, V_4R), as well as extending further left from V_6 (V_7). (Reproduced from Friedman HH: Diagnostic Electrocardiography and Vectorcardiography. New York, McGraw-Hill, 1985, p 41, with permission.)

Vector cardiography may be superior to the 12-lead ECG in diagnosing myocardial ischemia.

DETECTION OF MYOCARDIAL ISCHEMIA

Pathophysiology of ST segment responses

The ST segment is the most important portion of the QRS complex for evaluating ischemia. The origin of this segment, at the J point, is easy to locate. Its end, which is generally accepted as the beginning of any change of slope of the T wave, is more difficult to determine. In normal individuals there may be no discernible ST segment, as the T wave starts with a steady slope from the J point, especially at rapid heart rates. The TP segment has been used as the isoelectric baseline from which changes in the ST segment are evaluated, but with tachycardia this segment is eliminated and during exercise testing the P-R segment is used. The P-R segment is used in all ST-segment analyzers as well. Repolarization of the ventricle proceeds from the epicardium to the endocardium, opposite to the vector of depolarization. The ST segment reflects the midportion, or phase 2, of repolarization, during which there is little change in electrical potential. Thus, it is usually isoelectric. Ischemia causes a loss of intracellular potassium, resulting in a *current of injury*. The electrophysiologic mechanism accounting for ST segment shifts (either elevation or depression) remains controversial. The two major theories are based on either a loss of resting potential as current flows from the uninjured to the injured area (*diastolic current*), or a true change in phase 2 potential as current flows from the injured to the uninjured area (*systolic current*). With subendocardial injury, the ST segment is depressed in the surface leads. With epicardial or transmural injury the ST segment is elevated. When a lead is placed directly on the endocardium, opposite patterns are recorded.

ECG manifestations of ischemia

With myocardial ischemia repolarization is affected, causing downsloping or horizontal ST-segment depression. Varying local effects and differences in vectors during repolarization result in different ST morphology recorded by the different leads. It is generally accepted that ST changes in multiple leads are associated with more severe degrees of coronary artery disease (CAD).

The 'classic' criterion for ischemia is 0.1 mV (1 mm) depression measured 60–80 ms after the J point. The slope of the segment must be horizontal or downsloping. Downsloping depression may be associated with a greater number of diseased vessels and a worse prognosis than horizontal depression. Slowly upsloping depression with a slope of 1 mV/s or less is also used, but is considered less sensitive and specific (and difficult to assess clinically). The magnitude of ST segment depression is directly related to the height of the associated R wave. Given that R waves are highest in the lateral precordium and lowest in the inferior regions, some have proposed 'normalizing' ST depression for this variable. However, this is controversial and not practical clinically. Nonspecific ST segment depression can be related to drug use (particularly digoxin). Interpretation on ST segment changes with left ventricular hypertrophy (LVH) is particularly controversial given the tall R-wave baseline, J-point depression, and the steep slope of the ST segment. Although a number of studies have excluded such patients, others (including those using other modalities or epidemiologic studies) note that LVH is a highly significant predictor of adverse cardiac outcome.

Myocardial ischemia induces repolarization abnormalities, reflected in downsloping on horizontal ST segment depression.

The criteria for ischemia with ST-segment elevation (≥ 0.1 mV in two or more contiguous leads), usually due to transmural ischemia but potentially a 'reciprocal change' in a lead oriented opposite to the primary vector with subendocardial ischemia, are used in conjunction with clinical symptoms or elevation of biochemical markers to diagnose acute coronary syndromes. Perioperative studies have also included > 0.2 mV in any single lead, but in fact ST elevation of any kind is rarely reported in this setting (with the exception of cardiac surgery, where it is transiently observed on weaning from cardiopulmonary bypass with relative frequency). ST elevation in a Q-wave lead should not be analyzed for acute ischemia, although it may indicate the presence of a ventricular aneurysm.

Despite the clinical focus on the ST segment for monitoring, the earliest ECG change at the onset of transmural ischemia is the almost immediate onset of a tall, peaked T wave, a so-called 'primary change'. This phase is often transient. A significant increase in R-wave amplitude may also occur at this time. T-wave inversions (symmetrical inversion) commonly accompany transmural ST segment elevation changes, although the vast majority of T-wave inversions and/or flattening observed perioperatively are nonspecific, resulting from transient alterations of repolarization due to changes in electrolytes, sympathetic tone, and other noncardiac factors.

Although repolarization changes are the focus of ischemia detection, computerized ECG analysis using sophisticated signal averaging techniques clearly shows reduced high-frequency components of the QRS complex (150–250 Hz) with ischemia. Such changes are not visible on the standard ECG as they are in the range of 10–20 mV. A recent study using 12-lead analysis documented a higher sensitivity than ST segment analysis. However, this technology is not currently suited for clinical monitoring applications.

Clinical lead systems for detecting ischemia

Early clinical reports of intraoperative monitoring using V_5 in high-risk patients were based on observations during exercise testing in which bipolar configurations of V_5 demonstrated high sensitivity (up to 90%). Subsequent studies using 12-lead monitoring (torso mounted for stability during exercise) confirmed the sensitivity of the lateral precordial leads. However, some studies reported a higher sensitivity of V_4 or V_6 over V_5, followed by the inferior leads (in which most false positive responses were reported). Although the factors responsible for precipitating ischemia during exercise testing and surgical settings may differ (i.e. during exercise testing nearly all ischemia is demand related, whereas in the perioperative period a larger proportion may be due to reduced oxygen supply), the most sensitive leads during exercise testing are clearly useful perioperatively. However, given the relatively low sensitivity and specificity of the ECG (see above), radionuclear or other imaging modalities are now nearly routinely used in addition. Evaluation of other parameters, such as increases in R-wave amplitude and various patterns of heart rate change (e.g. heart rate recovery after exercise, heart rate change related to the slope of the ST segment etc.) have been proposed as more sensitive means to detect ischemia than isolated ST-segment depression, although they are infrequently used.

With the widespread growth in the 1990s of percutaneous coronary intervention (PCI) for acute myocardial infarction and unstable angina, a variety of investigators reported on continuous ECG (3 or 12 leads) monitoring in this setting, extending the classic teaching on localization of sites of occlusion with various coronary lesions. In general, ST segment elevation in leads V_2 and V_3 is most sensitive for occlusion of the left anterior descending artery, lead III most sensitive for the right coronary artery, and circumflex occlusion results in variable responses with primary elevation in the posterior precordial leads (rarely monitored) and reciprocal ST-segment depression in other precordial leads. For transmural ischemia, sensitivity is highest in the anterior rather than the lateral precordial leads. A recent multidisciplinary working group specifically recommended continuous monitoring of leads III, V_3, and V_5 for acute coronary syndrome patients.

Intraoperative lead systems

The detection of perioperative myocardial ischemia has received considerable attention over the last several decades, with the publication of several well-publicized clinical monitoring and therapy (e.g. perioperative β-blockade) studies. Many of these studies demonstrated an association of perioperative ischemia with adverse cardiac outcomes in adults undergoing a variety of cardiac and noncardiac surgical procedures, particularly following major vascular surgery. The ease of use of the new ST segment trending resulted in its routine use in many low-risk surgical patients, which may result in false-positive responses. The clinician must interpret minor ST segment changes in the context of the overall risk profile of the patient to avoid costly diagnostic tests being performed inappropriately. However, recent studies show that transient myocardial ischemia occurs in the absence of significant CAD in unexpected patients, such as parturients, particularly with significant hemodynamic stress and/or hemorrhage.

The recommended leads for intraoperative monitoring, based on several clinical studies, do not differ from those used during exercise testing. The most widely quoted clinical study using continuous computerized 12-lead ECG analysis reported that nearly 90% of responses involved ST segment depression alone (most commonly in V_5 (75%), followed by V_4 (61%)). In approximately 70%, changes were noted in multiple leads. The

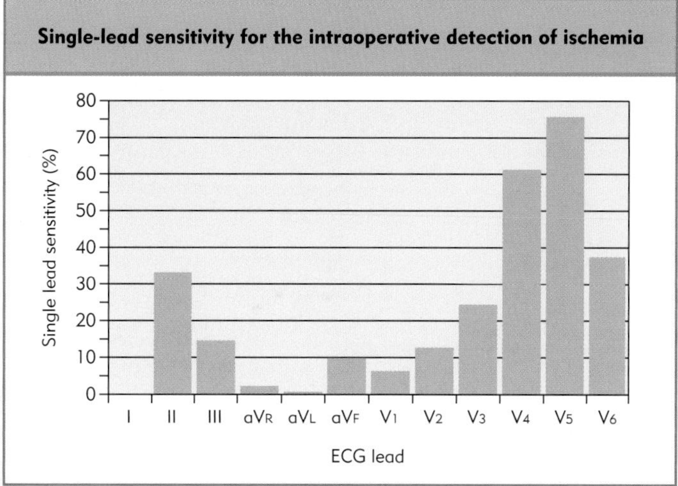

Figure 13.7 Single-lead sensitivity for the intraoperative detection of ischemia based on 51 episodes detected in 25 patients undergoing noncardiac surgery. Sensitivity was calculated by dividing the number of episodes detected in that lead by the total number of episodes. Sensitivity was greatest in lead V_5 and the lateral leads (I, $_aV_L$) were insensitive. (Reproduced from London MJ, Hollenberg M, Wong MG, et al: Intraoperative myocardial ischemia: Localization by continuous 12 lead electrocardiography. Anesthesiology 69:232, 1988, with permission.)

sensitivity of each of the 12 leads is shown in Figure 13.7. When considered in combination (as would be done clinically), the use of both leads V_4 and V_5 increased sensitivity to 90%, whereas the standard clinical combination, II and V_5, was only 80% sensitive. A recent, larger clinical study using a longer period of monitoring (up to 72 hours) extended these observations, reporting that V_3 was most sensitive with ischemia (87%), whereas V_4 was most sensitive in patients with infarction (in this study all were non-Q wave). Analysis of two precordial leads yielded 97–100% of changes. Based on analysis of the resting isoelectric levels of each of the 12 leads, it was recommended that V_4 be monitored, as it was most likely to be isoelectric. No episodes of ST elevation were noted in this study, as opposed to 12% in the earlier study of London et al. Although this literature clearly supports extensive precordial monitoring in patients at risk for subendocardial ischemia, one must be vigilant for the rare patient with acute Q-wave infarction (inferior leads).

Intraoperative monitoring of leads V_4 and V_5 has a sensitivity of 90% for the detection of myocardial ischemia.

Arrhythmia and pacemaker detection

The use of inferior leads allows superior discrimination of P-wave morphology, facilitating the visual diagnosis of arrhythmias and conduction disorders. Although esophageal (and even intracardiac) leads have the greatest sensitivity in detecting P waves, these are rarely used clinically but should be borne in mind for difficult diagnoses. With the increasing use of implantable defibrillators and automatic external defibrillators to treat cardiac arrest from ventricular fibrillation (and pulseless ventricular tachycardia), there is considerable interest in the refinement of arrhythmia detection algorithms and their validation. As expected, accuracy for ventricular rhythms is high and for atrial dysrhythmias lower. In the critical care and ambulatory monitoring setting, a variety of artifacts are common causes of false-positive responses.

The detection of pacemaker spikes may be complicated by very low-amplitude signals and varying amplitude with respiration. Most critical care and ambulatory monitors incorporate pacemaker spike enhancement of small high-frequency signals (typically 5–500 mV with 0.5–2 ms pulse duration) to facilitate recognition. However, this can lead to its own artifact if high-frequency noise enters the signal.

Key references

Chaitman BR. Exercise stress testing. In: Braunwald E, Zipes DP, Libby P, eds. Heart disease, 6th edn. Philadelphia: WB Saunders; 2001:129–55.

Landesberg G, Mosseri M, Wolf Y, Vesselov Y, Weissman C. Perioperative myocardial ischemia and infarction: identification by continuous 12-lead electrocardiogram with online ST-segment monitoring. Anesthesiology 2002;96:264–70.

London MJ, Hollenberg M, Wong MG et al. and the SPI Research Group. Intraoperative myocardial ischemia: localization by continuous 12 lead electrocardiography. Anesthesiology 1988;69:232–41.

London MJ, Kaplan JA. Advances in electrocardiographic monitoring. In: Kaplan JA, Reich DL, Konstadt SN, eds. Cardiac anesthesia, 4th edn. Philadelphia: WB Saunders; 1999:359–400.

Further reading

Balaji S, Ellenby M, McNames J, Goldstein B. Update on intensive care ECG and cardiac event monitoring. Card Electrophysiol Rev. 2002;6:190–5.

London MJ. Multilead precordial ST-segment monitoring: 'the next generation?' Anesthesiology 2002;96:259–61.

Madias JE, Bazaz R, Agarwal H, Win M, Medepalli L. Anasarca-mediated attenuation of the amplitude of electrocardiogram complexes: a description of a heretofore unrecognized phenomenon. J Am Coll Cardiol. 2001;38:756–64.

Marquez MF, Colin L, Guevara M, Iturralde P, Hermosillo AG. Common electrocardiographic artifacts mimicking arrhythmias in ambulatory monitoring. Am Heart J. 2002;144:187–97.

Pipberger HV, Arzbaecher Rc, Berson AS et al. Recommendations for the standardization of leads and of specifications for instruments in electrocardiography and vectorcardiography. Report of the Committee on Electrocardiography, American Heart Association. Circulation 1975; 52: 11–31.

Plonsey R. Electrocardiography. In: Webster JG (ed) Encyclopedia of medical devices and instrumentation. New York: John Wiley; 1988;1017–40.

Stern S. State of the art in stress testing and ischaemia monitoring. Card Electrophysiol Rev. 2002;6:204–8.

Chapter 14

Electrophysiological monitoring

Tod B Sloan

TOPICS COVERED IN THIS CHAPTER

- **Electroencephalography**
- **Evoked potentials**
    - Visual evoked responses
    - Auditory brainstem responses
    - Somatosensory evoked responses
    - Motor evoked responses
- **Electromyography**
- **Sleep, anesthesia, and electrophysiology**

The nervous system functions by electrical activity. This allows diagnostic and monitoring approaches to assess its structural and functional integrity. Although not a replacement for the neurologic examination, the results of electrophysiologic studies can enhance the diagnosis of neurologic dysfunction. In states of altered consciousness or during anesthesia, electrophysiological monitoring can greatly improve our understanding of neurologic functioning and integrity. Electroencephalography (EEG), evoked potential (EP) measurement, and electromyography (EMG), have many aspects in common and will be discussed in this chapter in the context of their intraoperative applications.

ELECTROENCEPHALOGRAPHY

Electroencephalography is based on the spontaneous electrical activity of the cerebral cortex. It represents the summated voltage changes resulting from activity in excitatory and inhibitory synapses in the pyramidal layers II, III, and V of the outer cortex. The activity recorded at an individual scalp electrode represents averaged synaptic electrical activity within 2–2.5 cm of the recording electrode. This local activity may be from intrinsic activity of the local cortex or it may be the result of the influence of other neural regions (most notably the pacemaker-like influence of deeper structures on the background rhythm).

The EEG is recorded by amplifying the electrical activity in a pair of scalp electrodes (referred to as a 'montage'). The signals from these brain regions are amplified through a differential amplifier, and noise is removed by common mode rejection (Chapter 13). In essence, the activity from one electrode is subtracted from the other, eliminating any activity that is present in both electrodes. Filtering out low- and high-frequency activity that is not within the traditional EEG range (0.5–30 Hz) allows further signal improvement. The resulting signal is then displayed visually on a screen or on paper as a plot of amplitude versus time (referred to as time domain) (Fig. 14.1).

Traditional methods of EEG analysis involve visual inspection of the tracings. Frequency content, amplitude, patterns of activity, and the relationship of activity between channels are a few of the factors analyzed. Several rhythms or patterns of activity have been identified in awake patients. These are of limited importance during anesthesia, except for the changes related to anesthesia or physiology (especially ischemia), discussed below, and spike activity associated with seizures. The ability to detect seizure spike activity is unique to monitoring with the EEG and forms the basis of intraoperative monitoring during seizure focus resection.

For intraoperative monitoring, three aspects of the EEG are primarily considered: frequency, amplitude (in microvolts, μV),

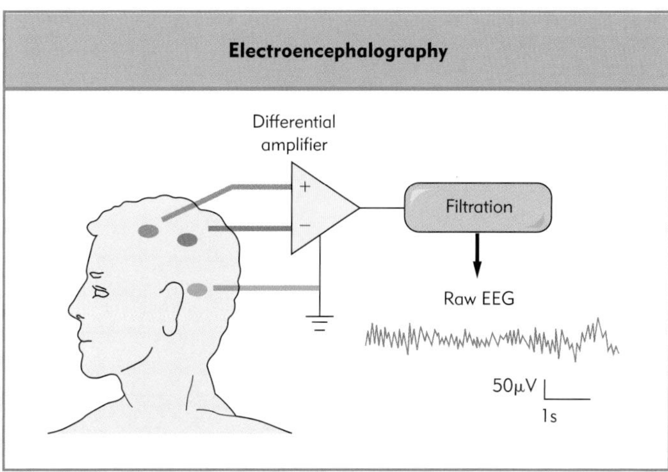

Figure 14.1 Diagram of EEG recording system. The EEG is amplified from two scalp electrodes by a differential amplifier. The activity is filtered to remove unwanted signals such as 60 Hz line frequency and displayed as a plot of amplitude versus time.

and symmetry. Quantitative methods of EEG analysis have also been developed. These focus most commonly on frequency, amplitude, and more complex mathematical analysis.

The frequency content of the EEG is usually described by four frequency bands. Beta (β) frequencies (13–30 Hz) are fast frequencies typical of a normal subject who is awake and alert. The alpha (α) frequencies (8–12 Hz) are typical of a patient who is relaxed with eyes closed. Here the EEG shows an underlying rhythm as if a pacemaker in the thalamus is driving the cortex. Slower EEG frequencies in the theta (θ; 4–7 Hz) or delta (δ; 0–3 Hz) range are seen during sleep, but are usually considered abnormal when awake. In the anesthetized subject, they may result from drug effects (such as with opioids or deep anesthesia) or may be an indication of impending injury (such as ischemia).

Symmetry of activity is an extremely important component of EEG analysis. In general, activity is usually symmetric about the midsagittal line. Any focal increase in activity (such as with a seizure) or focal decrease in activity (such as with local ischemia or stroke) is usually indicative of pathology.

A diagnostic EEG is usually conducted with a large number of electrodes so that recording pairs allow evaluation of the entire cerebral cortex. For intraoperative monitoring, the recording pairs may be limited to the specific regions of interest, as in intracranial aneurysm clipping. For vascular surgery, symmetrically spaced leads allow differentiation between ischemia and deep anesthesia by the evaluation of symmetry. Hence, carotid endarterectomy monitoring might utilize symmetrically placed electrode pairs over the distributions of the right and left anterior, middle, and posterior cerebral arteries.

Symmetrical activity is an important property of the normal EEG.

As with many monitoring techniques, computer processing of the EEG can allow enhancement of the specific variables of interest, although the processed EEG is only as good as the raw data. Early processing methods used simple techniques to determine average amplitude and frequency. Perhaps the most successful was the cerebral function monitor, which determined the amplitude between 2 and 15 Hz (with emphasis around 10 Hz) from a single electrode pair and allowed ready recognition of low-frequency activity.

The most commonly employed technique of computed EEG analysis in current use is based on the mathematical technique of Fourier series analysis. This technique takes a complex wave and determines the amplitudes of a series of sine waves that can mathematically reconstruct the wave. A smoothed *x*–*y* plot results (Fig. 14.2) that depicts the relative amplitude (or power) of each of the component frequencies. These plots give an excellent perspective of both the amplitude and frequency content of the EEG. Spectral edge frequency (SEF) is frequently derived from these data; this is the frequency below which the majority (i.e. 95–99%) of the activity is located. The compressed spectral array (CSA) is a useful variation of this plot in which the effect of time is shown by stacking those *x*–*y* plots in a third dimension (time). The density spectral array (DSA) can reveal some data hidden in the CSA by showing increased amplitude as dark regions (Fig. 14.2).

Several other displays and mathematical signal-processing techniques have been used and have a variety of advantages and disadvantages. Of particular interest is the relationship between sedative drugs and the EEG, allowing the possibility of assessing the depth of sedation during anesthesia. Unfortunately, the profile of EEG changes varies with the drug, so simple measures of the EEG (e.g. amplitude and frequency) are not adequate to sufficiently quantify the EEG for sedation. Hence a variety of methods have been used to find drug-independent measures of sedation. In general, light sedation is characterized by high-fre-

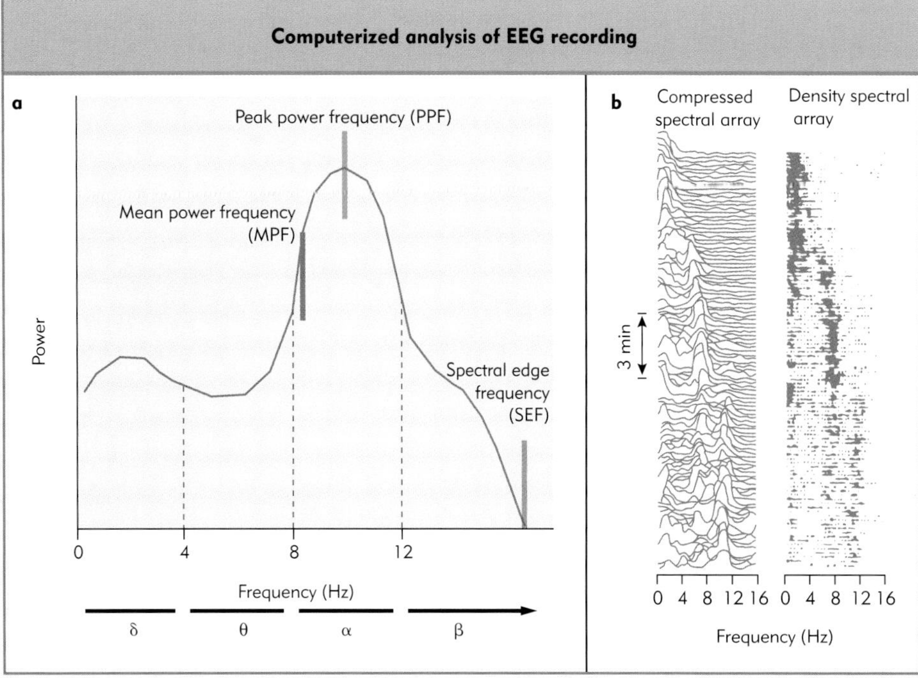

Figure 14.2 Computerized analysis of EEG recording. (a) Frequency amplitude plot after Fourier series analysis. The spectral edge frequency (SEF) is the frequency where 95–99% of the power is contained in lower frequencies. (b) Compressed and density spectral arrays of EEG signals subjected to Fourier series analysis are given for a patient during deepening halothane anesthesia (earlier times in front). Note the progressive loss of high frequency activity. (With permission from Levy et al., 1980.)

quency spatially disorganized activity and a highly variable EEG. Deep sedation is characterized by a shift in activity to the frontal regions, reduced variability, burst suppression (periods of silence between bursts of activity), or a silent EEG. The challenge in this monitoring is assessing between these extremes using drug-independent measures. One approach has been to use many types of mathematical processing to find drug-independent measures. Another method uses a mathematical technique called bispectral analysis, which evaluates the interaction or phase coupling between different EEG frequencies. Other potential monitors of anesthetic depth include semilinear canonized analysis, aperiodic analysis or δ power of the EEG, and measures of the variability of the EEG (referred to as entropy). These techniques convert the processed signal into a number between 0 and 100 for quantifying sedation. Monitoring is usually done using electrodes over the frontal cortex, an area that has been associated with explicit auditory memory. It is of interest that frontal muscle activity (EMG) can also be measured in these frontal electrodes, and the depth of sedation is also inversely related to the EMG activity. Some of these techniques also incorporate the EMG in their analysis. As indicated below, midlatency auditory EP (AEP) and 40 Hz steady-state EPs have also been used for these purposes.

Anesthetic drugs tend to produce either excitation or depression of the EEG (Fig. 14.3). Most agents produce an initial excitatory stage of the EEG characterized by desynchronization (perhaps through loss of inhibitory synaptic function). Amplitude increases as the EEG becomes synchronized, with a predominance of activity in the α range. Increasing dose causes progressive slowing until the EEG achieves burst suppression and finally electrical silence. The volatile anesthetics show these typical effects, although they are not equivalent in the degree of their effects. Isoflurane can produce a flat (isoelectric) EEG at clinically usable concentrations, whereas halothane must be increased to toxic levels (of the order of 10 vol%) to produce a flat EEG.

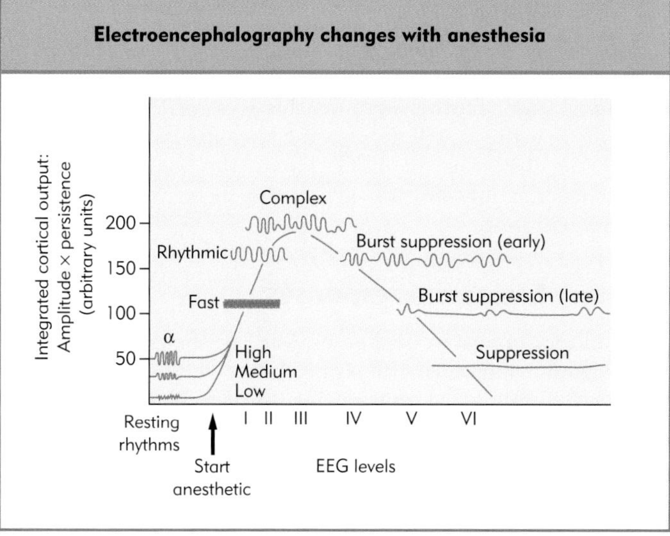

Figure 14.3 Typical changes in the EEG with anesthesia. With increasing depth of anesthesia using an inhalation anesthetic, initial organization into fast frequencies occurs with the formation of rhythmic waves in the α range. Increasing depth of anesthesia causes a reduction in frequency and amplitude until burst suppression and a flat EEG are produced. (From Martin JT, Faulconer A Jr, Bickford RG et al. Electroencephalography in anesthesiology. Anesthesiology. 1959;20:360.)

Some anesthetic agents produce further activation rather than depression of the EEG after the initial excitatory effect, such as spike and seizure activity, but eventually produce EEG depression at higher doses. For example, enflurane at higher doses produces spike activity (especially with hyperventilation). Nitrous oxide also increases activity by producing high-frequency (34 Hz) activity in the frontal area, but does not usually produce spike activity. Nitrous oxide can also reduce the degree of slowing produced by the concomitant administration of a volatile anesthetic agent.

Most general anesthetics produce EEG excitation initially, followed by progressive slowing.

Most intravenous sedative agents also follow this pattern of excitation followed by depression, including the barbiturates, benzodiazepines, propofol, and etomidate. Barbiturates produce a flat EEG at higher doses and have been used to produce a pharmacologic coma, as the decrease in synaptic metabolic rate improves the balance of nutrient and oxygen supply and demand in head injury and cerebral ischema. Low doses of methohexital (methohexitone) (0.5 mg/kg) and etomidate (0.1 mg/kg) can enhance epileptic activity, and propofol can enhance interictal activity in some seizure patients, but electrical silence follows at high doses. The benzodiazepines produce spike-like activity at low doses in some patients, but are frequently used as anticonvulsants.

The opioids do not appear to produce an initial excitement phase but produce a steady decline in EEG frequency, with maintenance of amplitude in the δ range and without producing burst suppression or electrical silence. The effects of ketamine also differ from those of inhalational agents. Ketamine produces high-amplitude θ activity with an accompanying increase in β activity, and has been reported to provoke seizure activity in epileptic but not in normal individuals. Muscle relaxants generally have little effect on the EEG, although succinylcholine (suxamethonium) has an activating effect on the central nervous system during muscle facilitation. Laudanosine, an atracurium metabolite, is a convulsant, but this is not clinically significant with usual doses.

In addition to anesthesia, the EEG is affected by many physiologic variables. Frequency slowing is usually associated with depressed neuronal function. For example, hypoxemia, hypotension, hypocarbia, hypoglycemia, and ischemia cause slowing and flattening of the EEG. Hypercarbia (arterial carbon dioxide tension (P_aCO_2) >90 mmHg) causes high-frequency EEG activity; higher levels are associated with findings similar to those of hypocarbia, and very high levels produce a flat EEG. Hypothermia produces slowing below 35°C, with electrical silence at 7–20°C. Hypothermia is associated with reductions in metabolic rate (both basal and activity dependent) and is protective against cerebral ischemia. The EEG also varies with age, with an adult pattern appearing by 10–15 years of age. Because the effects of many pharmacologic and physiologic factors on the EEG are a reduction in frequency and decreased amplitude, the EEG cannot be used as an isolated monitor but must be interpreted in the context of other information, including anesthetic and physiologic variables.

The EEG is used for intraoperative monitoring during several procedures. Perhaps the most common use is in the detection of ischemia (Fig. 14.4). The response to ischemia is rapid: a flat

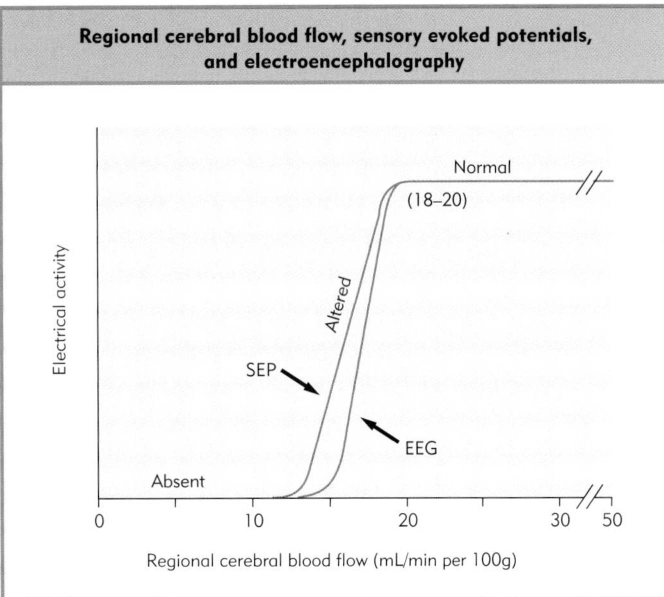

Figure 14.4 Relationship between regional cerebral blood flow, sensory evoked potentials (SEPs), and EEG measurements. As regional cerebral blood flow is reduced below 18–20 mL/min/100 g tissue, the EEG and SEPs become abnormal. Below 12–15 mL/min/100 g the EEG becomes silent; SEPs are lost at slightly lower values because subcortical components of the SEP are more tolerant of ischemia. (From Sloan T. Evoked potentials. In: Albin MA, ed. Textbook of neuroanesthesia with neurosurgical perspectives, Ch.7. New York: McGraw Hill; 1997: 221-76.)

EEG occurs within 20 seconds of complete ischemia. With partial ischemia, the EEG slows at blood flows below 18–20 mL/min/100 g tissue, and becomes flat at 12–15 mL/min/100 g. As cell death does not occur until lower levels of blood flow are reached (<10 mL/min/100 g), the EEG can be used to signal ischemia. The time to infarction is related to the rate of residual blood flow: the more residual flow that is present, the longer the time to infarction. As long as 10–15 minutes may elapse before infarction after graded ischemia produces EEG changes. Hence the EEG may serve to warn of impending stroke and allow attempts to correct the blood flow prior to irreversible injury.

This warning function has made EEG monitoring a component of carotid endarterectomy and intracranial vascular surgery in many centers. Several studies have shown that EEG monitoring can be used to identify patients who may benefit from shunting during carotid endarterectomy and who cannot tolerate temporary clipping of intracranial aneurysms, although the benefits are controversial. Similarly, EEG has been used to monitor patients undergoing cardiopulmonary bypass to determine whether blood flow is adequate, although concomitant hypothermia may reduce the effectiveness of EEG monitoring.

EVOKED POTENTIALS

Whereas the EEG is a measurement of spontaneous electrical activity in the brain (cerebral cortex), EPs are measurements of the electrical potentials produced in response to a stimulus ('evoked') involving specific neuronal tracts. These stimuli may be physiologic in nature (e.g. light flashes to the eyes) or they may be nonphysiologic (e.g. electrical pulses to peripheral nerves). As stimulation focuses testing on a specific neural tract, assessment is also specific.

Evoked potentials are measured using differential amplifiers and filtering, similar to the EEG. Because the amplitude of sensory EPs is very small (<10 μV), a technique known as signal averaging is used to resolve EPs from the much greater EEG (10–1000 μV) and electrocardiogram (ECG) activity. Signal averaging involves repeatedly stimulating the nervous system and measuring the response during the period of stimulated neural activity. The recorded activity is digitized and averaged at each poststimulus time point. After averaging 10^2–10^3 windows (the signal-to-noise ratio increases by the square root of the number of windows averaged), the evoked response becomes apparent, as the desired signal is related to the stimulation but the other activity is not and averages out (Fig. 14.5a).

A typical evoked response output is a plot of voltage versus time (Fig. 14.5b). The electrical response at an active electrode (placed near the neural structure producing the desired electrical activity) is compared with that at a reference electrode. An artifact of stimulation occurs at time zero (coincident with the stimulation), followed by a subsequent series of peaks (both positive and negative) and valleys at later times. The peaks (and valleys) are thought to arise from specific neural generators, and therefore can be used to follow the response at various points along the stimulated tract. The information recorded is usually the amplitude (peak to adjacent trough), the time from the stimulation to the peak (latency), and occasionally the time between peaks (interwave latency, or conduction time).

Visual evoked responses

Visual EPs (VEPs) are produced by light stimulation of the eyes. For diagnostic purposes, stimulation using a checkerboard on which squares alternate between white and black is used; for intraoperative monitoring, light flash stimulation through closed eyes is used. Traditional VEPs are recorded by electrodes over the occiput and are generated by the visual cortex. The retinal response to visual stimulation (electroretinogram; ERG) can also be recorded by electrodes placed near the eyes. By manipulating the color and intensity of the stimulus, the responses of the rods and cones can be separated.

Monitoring of VEPs helps to confirm the structural integrity of the optic tracts, but results may not correlate well with postoperative vision. Furthermore, as this is a cortically generated response, anesthesia will depress the response in a similar manner to the effect on the EEG. Hence the use of depressant agents (such as inhalational agents) may need to be restricted during monitoring.

Auditory brainstem responses

The auditory brainstem response (ABR) or the brainstem auditory evoked response (BAER) is produced when sound activates the cochlea following transmission through the external and middle ear. Vibrations activate the hair cells in the cochlea, which initiates nerve impulses that travel to the brainstem via cranial nerve VIII. The nerve impulse travels via the brainstem acoustic relay nuclei and lemniscal pathways to activate the cortical auditory cortex. The neural pathway of the ABR appears to follow the normal hearing pathway. In the first 10 ms after stimulation three major peaks are usually seen: wave I is generated by the extracranial portion of cranial nerve VIII; wave III is generated by the auditory pathway nuclei in the pons; and wave V is generated by the high pons or midbrain (lateral lemniscus

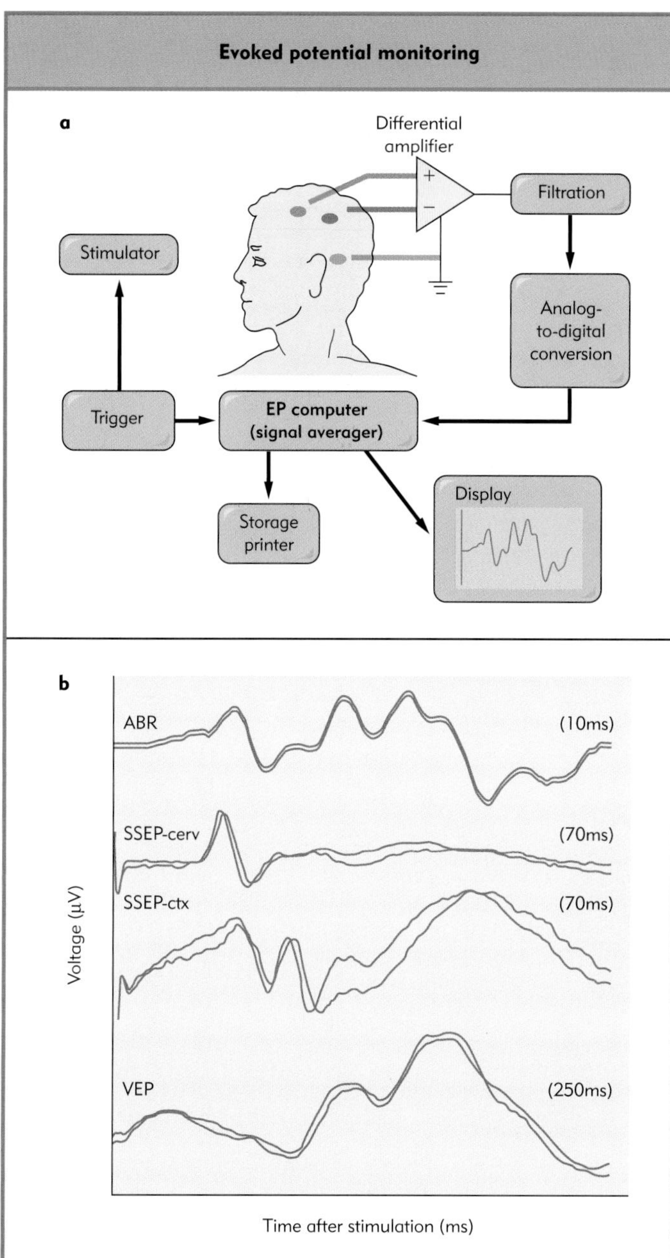

Figure 14.5 Evoked potential (EP) monitoring. (a) EP recording requires a digital computer to conduct signal averaging. A trigger repeatedly causes a stimulus; recording of the voltage change for a set period after each stimulus allows formation of the EP to be demonstrated. (b) Typical sensory evoked responses include the auditory brainstem response (ABR), somatosensory evoked response to median nerve stimulation recorded at cervical (SSEP-cerv) and cortical (SSEP-ctx) locations, and the visual evoked potential (VEP). The timescale for each tracing is shown on the right.

and inferior colliculus). Occasionally a wave II is seen, and wave IV may be resolvable from V (IV and V often blend together). Responses to auditory stimulation can also be recorded over the auditory cortex (cortical AEP) or cortical association areas (response about 300 ms after auditory stimulation; P300). These responses appear to be related to the auditory sensory cortex and cerebral cognitive function areas, respectively.

Testing of ABR is frequently conducted using stimulation with 'clicks' delivered by headphones. Other types of sound have also been used for stimulation, including tone 'pips', which have a more defined frequency content. Usually one ear is stimulated at a time to focus on that neural pathway, with 'white noise' delivered to the other ear to mask stimulatory conditions.

Monitoring of ABR can be used to find the anatomic location of a neural insult and to assist the surgeon during an operation. Procedures in which ABR has been used include surgery on or near the auditory pathways or brainstem (e.g. acoustic neuroma, cerebellopontine angle tumors, posterior fossa procedures). Examination of effects on waves I, III, and V may allow the identification of brainstem injury and determine the general anatomic location based on the specific waves that are altered. Recordings can also be taken from the cochlea and the intracranial portion of cranial nerve VIII.

In general, anesthetic effects on the ABR are not dramatic. Latency increases may be seen as the concentration of potent inhalational agents increases. Nitrous oxide is generally benign unless it causes changes in middle-ear pressure. Some changes can be seen with shifts in body temperature and if cold irrigation fluids are applied into the surgical field. Anesthetic effects on the auditory cortex are much more marked, and these responses have been used to assess the depth of sedation. Both the cortical evoked response (midlatency response) and the steady-state response (40 Hz) have been used.

Somatosensory evoked responses

In the assessment of somatosensory evoked responses a peripheral nerve is stimulated (similar to neuromuscular blockade monitoring) and the neural response is measured. Large mixed motor and sensory nerves (e.g. posterior tibial, common peroneal, ulnar, and median) are usually stimulated, which results in mixed motor and sensory responses. The length of the neural tract involved makes the somatosensory EP (SSEP) potentially one of the most generally applicable monitors because of the many neural structures that can be assessed (peripheral nerve, plexi, spinal cord, brainstem, sensory cortex). It is thought that the incoming volley of neural activity from the upper extremity represents activity primarily in the ipsilateral dorsal column pathway of proprioception and vibration. Stimulation of the peripheral nerve initiates an impulse that ascends the ipsilateral dorsal column, synapses near the nucleatus cuneatus, decussates near the cervicomedullary junction, ascends via the contralateral medial lemniscus, synapses in the ventroposterolateral nucleus of the thalamus, and finally projects to the contralateral parietal sensory cortex (Fig. 14.6). Recordings following stimulation of the lower extremity include additional components in the spinocerebellar pathways; these more anterior pathways may underlie the alterations in the SSEP observed in anterior cord ischemia, which correlate with motor function.

Several alternatives to SSEP monitoring have been developed to overcome some of its limitations. One problem is that the SSEP enters the spinal cord through several roots. Dermatomal EPs (DEPs), produced by stimulation of specified cutaneous dermatomal regions, have been used to evaluate the function of individual nerve roots. Anesthetic effects and poor amplitudes in regions with small cerebral representation (e.g. thoracic dermatomes) limit this technique to some extent. A second problem is that occasionally peripheral nerve stimulation is not sufficient to produce a usable SSEP. One approach to this problem has been to stimulate both extremities simultaneously to increase amplitude, but this response may be less sensitive to

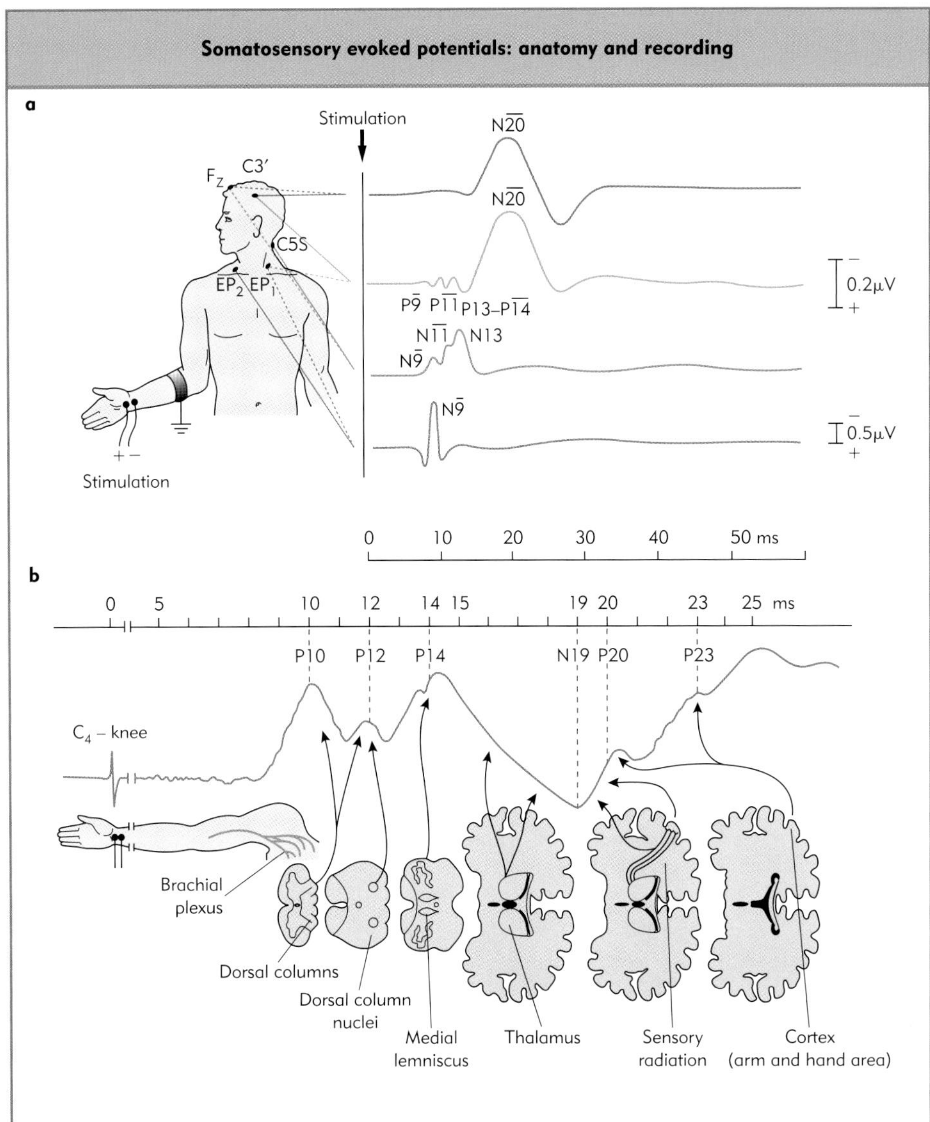

Figure 14.6 Somatosensory evoked potentials: anatomy and recording. (a) Example of evoked potential tracings from various locations for the median nerve SSEP (top). Recordings from Erb's point (EP) over the brachial plexus, cervial spine (C5S), and sensory cortex (C3′, top two tracings) are shown. (With permission from Spehlmann, 1985.) (b) Corresponding anatomy of the nerve and potential peaks. (From Weiderholt WC, Mayer-Harding E, Budnick B, McKeown KL. Stimulating and recording methods used in obtaining short latency somatosensory evoked potentials (SEPs) in patients with central peripheral neurologic disorders. Ann NY Acad Sci. 1982;388:349.)

unilateral insults to the spinal cord. Another approach has been to stimulate the cauda equina via percutaneously placed electrodes. This approach also allows stimulation at spinal levels where no major peripheral nerve is available for stimulation, and produces amplitudes at least twice those of traditional SSEP; however, it may fail to detect unilateral injury. A third problem is that anesthesia can decrease the cortical amplitude. Cortical evoked responses are affected by anesthesia in a fashion similar to the effects on the EEG. Inhalational anesthetic agents (including nitrous oxide) significantly reduce amplitudes and must be used in low concentrations (0.3–0.5 minimum alveolar concentration, MAC), if at all. Anesthesia based on opioids, ketamine, dexmeditomidine, and/or propofol depresses cortical amplitude to a lesser extent. Etomidate and ketamine appear to increase some cortical amplitudes and have been used to facilitate monitoring in very challenging situations. The effect of anesthetic drugs on sensory responses is most pronounced at the cortical level, with decreasing effects on subcortical responses (e.g. ABR).

Inhaled anesthetics significantly depress the amplitude of cortical evoked responses.

Recording locations near the spinal cord have been used as they are less affected by anesthesia. Electrodes can be placed in the spinal bony elements, intraspinous ligament, or subdural or epidural space, either percutaneously or directly by the surgeon. Electrodes can also be used for stimulation, with recording of cortical responses, for peripheral neural or compound muscle action potential (CMAP) responses, or for recording following transcranial motor cortex stimulation. Perispinal stimulation has been used in an attempt to monitor motor tracts. However, like epidural recording, both motor and sensory tracts are stimulated. Despite its limitations, the SSEP and its variations have been used in a wide variety of procedures (Fig. 14.7), notably those in which the spinal cord or cerebral cortex is at risk.

Table 14.1 Intraoperative applications of somatosensory and motor evoked potentials

Peripheral nerve and spinal root procedures	Joint surgery
Neuroma in situ Brachial plexus surgery Spinal root decompression Pedicle screw placement Dorsal rhizotomy for spasticity Cauda equina and prostate procedures	Hip or knee replacement Shoulder arthroscopy Posterior fossa surgery Acoustic neuroma Cerebellopontine angle tumors Retromastoid craniectomy Space-occupying infarcts Microvascular decompression Relief of hemifacial spasm
Spinal procedures	**Sellar or parasellar procedures**
Scoliosis Stabilization and correction of fractures Decompression Tumors AVMs (resection and embolization) Syringomyelia	Transsphenoidal pituitary procedures Supratentorial frontal procedures Repair of basilar skull fracture
Vascular surgery	**Skull base surgery**
Carotid endarterectomy Aortic aneurysm Bronchial artery embolization Spinal angiography and transvascular embolization	Tumors Cavernous sinus
	Stereoencephalotomy
	Parkinson's disease Other movement disorders Intractable pain

AVM, arteriovenous malformation.

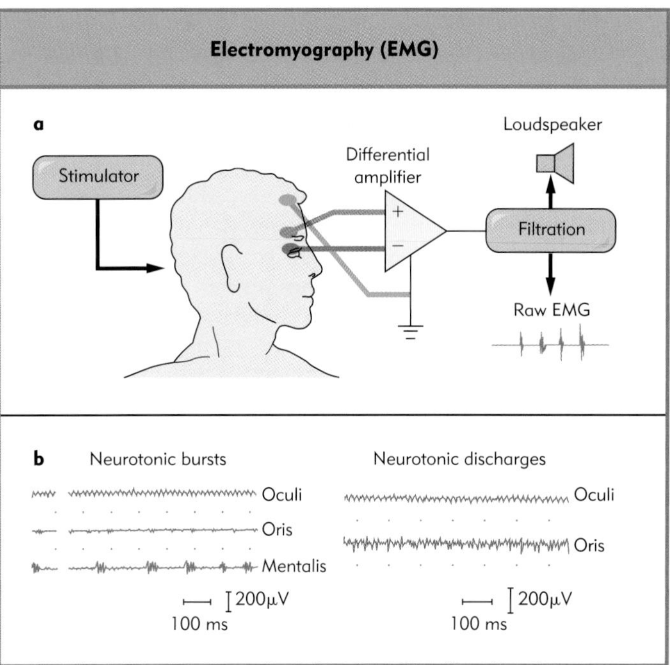

Figure 14.7 Electromyography (EMG). (a) The recording system for orbicularis oculi. (b) Spontaneous EMG activity observed in the operating room is usually one of two types. Neurotonic bursts of activity usually represent mechanical irritation of the nerve (left). Sustained discharge (right) may indicate impending injury as nerve irritation leads to continuous depolarization. (With permission from Cheek, 1993.)

Motor evoked responses

Monitoring of a purely motor tract signal (motor evoked potential, MEP) currently requires stimulation of the motor cortex by electrical impulses applied to the brain or scalp (transcranial electrical motor EP, tcEMEP) or by magnetic stimulation (transcutaneous magnetic motor EP, tcMMEP). The evoked response travels down the lateral corticospinal and ventral corticospinal tracts and is recorded as a peripheral motor nerve response or as CMAP. Contributions of sensory pathways are blocked by synaptic interruptions in the thalamus and brainstem, which prevent transmission down sensory pathways. The major clinical difference between the two cortical stimulation techniques is that the electrical technique is moderately painful, because cutaneous pain receptors are stimulated, whereas the magnetic technique is painless (as long as direct stimulation of the scalp muscles is avoided). These techniques also differ electrophysiologically, as tcEMEP activates the corticospinal neurons directly with additional cortical activation from internuncial activity. In contrast, tcMMEP activates internuncial synapses only at lower stimulation levels.

Responses to transcranial stimulation recorded in the epidural space are preferred by some, because anesthetic effects at the anterior horn cell or neuromuscular junction may reduce or eliminate peripheral responses. The disadvantage of epidural recordings is that they probably represent recording from both lateral pathways; as a result, differentiation of a unilateral injury is difficult. In contrast, muscle recordings can differentiate unilateral changes as well as assess potential injury at several nerve root levels simultaneously. A variety of motor nerves and muscle groups can be monitored by varying the location of the stimulator on the scalp. Some clinical data suggest that recording both epidural and CMAP responses simultaneously may be the most powerful predictor of outcome.

Recording methodology is similar for MEP and SSEP, except that CMAP responses are much larger, requiring fewer signal averages to resolve the signal. Onset latency is measured as the time from stimulation to the beginning of the multipeak response. Amplitude is measured as the peak-to-peak voltage of the response. As with the SSEP, the latency or onset is a measure of average conduction velocity. In addition to latency and amplitude, some researchers refer to threshold, which is the lowest amount of magnetic or electrical stimulation that will still elicit an MEP response.

The use of MEP for spinal cord monitoring has increased because of its utility in the detection of vascular insults. Whereas mechanical stress on the spinal cord may affect both sensory and motor pathways, vascular insults may produce localized injury affecting only motor or sensory tracts. Because motor pathways are supplied by anterior spinal arteries from the aorta via penetrating vessels (notably the artery of Adamkiewicz and radicular arteries), the major concern is a loss of motor function without reflection in the SSEP. This problem is most important in the thoracic spinal cord, which is particularly vulnerable to ischemia because it is not well supplied by collateral vessels and may have only one anterior feeding artery between T4 and L4. Despite the potentials for SSEP to miss anterior spinal cord ischemia, studies suggest that it is not completely insensitive. Motor evoked potentials have been used for many of the same procedures (notably spinal surgery) where the SSEP is used.

The major drawback of the transcranial techniques has been the effects of anesthesia. Because inhalational agents (including nitrous oxide) may obliterate responses at low concentrations through their effects on the cerebral cortex and anterior horn cells, anesthetic techniques based on opioids, ketamine, or etomidate are useful. If muscle responses are to be recorded, neuromuscular blocking agents must be carefully controlled or avoided (see below). For epidural or peripheral nerve responses, neuromuscular blocking drugs may be advantageous in minimizing patient movement during testing and in reducing interference in the recording electrodes from nearby muscle activity. The effects of anesthetic depression are partially overcome by newer multipulse techniques in which magnetic or electrical impulses are delivered to the scalp at 200–500 Hz. Trains of three to five pulses allow the detection of CMAP responses at concentrations of inhalational agents that obliterate responses to single pulses.

ELECTROMYOGRAPHY

Electromyography is the recording of muscle electrical activity by the placement of needles in the muscle. This procedure can detect muscle disorders as well as disorders of the nerves that supply the muscle. It is recognized as an invaluable aid to the neurologic diagnosis of diseases affecting the motor unit. Studies frequently allow localization of a lesion to the muscle, neuromuscular junction, or motor nerves.

The traditional needle electrode examination is conducted by placing a recording electrode within a muscle and examining the electrical activity it produces, using equipment similar to that used in EEG but with much higher frequencies (Fig. 14.8). The activity is displayed on an oscilloscope and played through a loudspeaker, as characteristic sounds assist in diagnosis. Normally, a resting muscle is electrically silent after mild reactivity to the needle insertion. Neuromuscular abnormalities can increase this insertional reactivity and may help to identify hereditary myopathies and axonal loss in the peripheral nerve supplying the muscle. Reduced insertional activity can be seen with muscle diseases associated with fibrosis or fatty replacement of muscle, and in metabolic diseases that reduce the electrical excitability of the muscle.

In a resting muscle, spontaneous activity is not normally seen when the needle electrode is immobile. Irregular spike activity, known as spontaneous fibrillation potentials, is thought to result from recently denervated muscle. Other types of activity are seen with other neuromuscular diseases, including fasciculation potentials (in neuropathies and motor neuron disorders), myokymic discharges (in chronic compressive neuropathies and radiation damage to muscles), and complex repetitive discharges (in chronic neuropathic or myopathic processes).

For nerve conduction velocity measurement, electrical stimulation of a motor nerve elicits a muscle contraction that is measured electrically as a CMAP. By measuring the time from stimulation and the distance from the stimulation site to the muscle, the speed of conduction through the nerve can be determined. By moving the stimulation point along the nerve, the location of a conduction block can be determined. As an example, this technique is used to identify conduction block in the median nerve in carpal tunnel syndrome. A similar method can be used with the SSEP to determine conduction velocities in peripheral nerves, the spinal cord, or central areas (brainstem to sensory cortex: central conduction time).

The CMAP recorded in nerve conduction studies is termed the M response. A later response, termed the H response, can also be recorded at low stimulation intensities. This response is caused by stimulation of sensory fibers in the nerve. These travel centrally to the spinal cord, where a reflex arc activates the motor fibers at the anterior horn cell, resulting in a second CMAP. This is the electrical equivalent of the stretch reflex activity (e.g. the patellar reflex). A second later wave, termed the F wave, is produced because the nerve stimulation causes a wave of depolarization toward the muscle (producing the M wave), and also centrally toward the spinal cord in the motor components of the nerve. The centrally moving motor nerve depolarization is reflected at the spinal cord and results in an outgoing response that produces a second muscle contraction, the F wave, which has limited value in neurologic diagnosis.

Although diagnostic EMG studies have been performed during anesthesia, an anesthesiologist is more likely to encounter EMG as a monitor to assess the integrity of the nerve supplying a monitored muscle. Current methods for EMG in the operating room involve recording electrodes in the muscle of interest, with visible and audible presentation of the electrical activity. These techniques are superior to the older methods of visible or mechanical detection of muscle activity.

This monitoring system usually focuses on two basic types of spontaneous activity (see Fig. 14.8). First are phasic 'bursts'. These neurotonic discharges are brief (<1 s), relatively synchronous motor unit discharges that result from single discharges of multiple axons. The discharge is usually caused by mechanical stimulation of the nerve (nearby dissection, ultrasonic aspiration or drilling, retraction), but can also be caused by thermal (irrigation, lasers, drilling, electrocautery) and chemical or metabolic insults. These short bursts of activity are not usually associated with injurious stimuli, but often indicate that the nerve remains intact and is in the vicinity of the operative field.

More injurious stimuli can cause longer tonic or 'train' activity, which is an episode of continuous, synchronous motor unit discharges. These have audible sounds with a more musical quality and have been likened to the sound of an outboard motor boat engine, swarming bees, popping corn, or an aircraft engine. These trains are often associated with nerve compression, traction, or ischemia, and are usually an indication of enduring nerve injury. The proposed mechanism of the repetitive discharge is a depolarization of the resting membrane potential to near or above the firing threshold.

Electromyography (EMG) can be used as a monitor for nerve injury in any nerve with a motor component; anesthetic effects are limited to muscle relaxants.

Electromyography can be used to monitor any nerve with a motor component. The most common application is for facial nerve monitoring during facial surgery and posterior fossa neurosurgery, where tumors commonly grow to involve the facial nerve, although EMG can be used for other cranial nerves with motor components (Table 14.2). The frequent involvement of the facial nerve with tumors in the cerebellopontine angle and acoustic neuroma (or vestibular schwannoma) has led to the application of facial nerve monitoring during resection of these

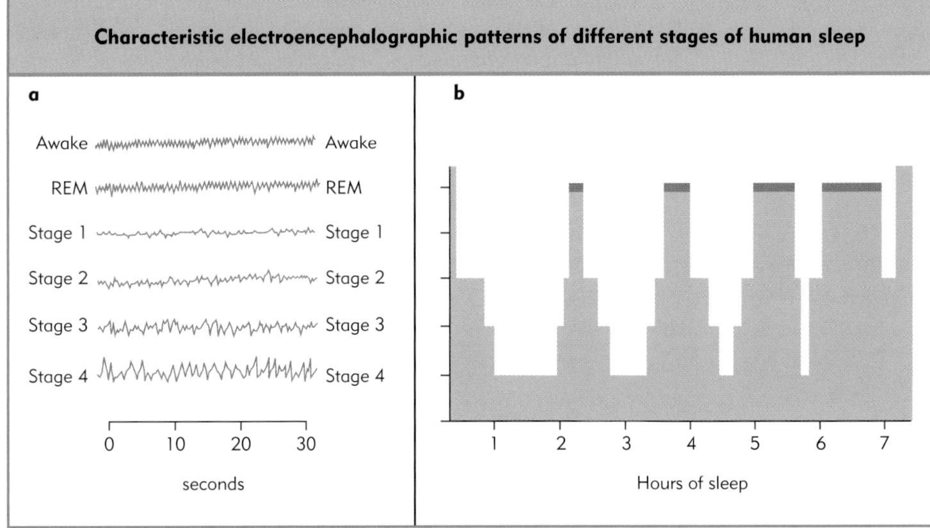

Figure 14.8 Characteristic electroencephalographic patterns of different stages of human sleep. (a) EEG recording during a typical night for a young adult in the waking state and during progressively deeper levels of non-REM sleep. (b) The dark bars represent periods of REM sleep. (With permission from Domino EF. Drugs for sleep disorders. In: Brody TM, Larner J, Minneman K, Neu HC(eds). Human Pharmacology: Molecular to Clinical, 2nd edn. St Louis MO: Mosby; 1994:449-55.)

Table 14.2 Recording locations for cranial nerve monitoring by electromyography

III	Oculomotor	Inferior rectus
IV	Trachlear	Superior oblique
V	Trigeminal	Masseter, temporalis
VI	Abducens	Lateral rectus
VII	Facial	Orbicularis oculi, orbicularis oris
IX	Glossopharyngeal	Posterior soft palate (stylopharyngeus)
X	Vagus	Vocal folds, special endotracheal tubes, cricothyroid muscle
XI	Spinal accessory	Sternocleidomastoid, trapezius

tumors in an attempt to salvage function. Monitoring can warn that the nerve is in the immediate operative field and at risk of injury. Using a handheld stimulator, the surgeon can stimulate the nerve at 1–5 Hz. Repetitive bursts in synchrony with the stimulation verify nerve integrity or confirm that structures for removal are not the nerve. If an injury pattern evolves, stimulation can be used to determine which segment of the nerve is injured.

Monitoring of facial nerve function for resection of acoustic neuroma is accomplished by placing closely spaced bipolar recording electrodes in the orbicularis oris and orbicularis oculi. The value of identifying nerve integrity is that over 60% of patients who have intact nerves will regain at least partial function within a few months of the operation, whereas loss of response is associated with a poor outcome. The excellent outcome data obtained when facial nerve monitoring is used during acoustic neuroma has prompted a National Institutes of Health (NIH) consensus panel to identify facial nerve monitoring as a routine part of acoustic neuroma surgery.

Electromyography has also been used during spinal surgery. For example, monitoring can observe for spontaneous muscle activity as nerve roots are irritated by surgery (e.g. pedicle screws) or as they are activated by specific stimulation. For example, during surgery on the cauda equina, the anal sphincter and various leg muscles can be monitored. Electromyography has also been used during selective dorsal rhizotomy, performed to relieve leg spasticity and thereby improve gait in cerebral palsy. Finally, during pedicle screw surgery low amounts of current applied to the screw hole or pedicle screw can signal a misplaced screw that may pose a threat to the spinal nerve root or spinal cord.

In general, major anesthetic effects on EMG recordings are limited to the use of muscle relaxants. As most EMG monitoring is for detection of nerve integrity, complete neuromuscular blockade eliminates any response and renders the technique useless. As with MEP recording, EMG responses from intentional electrical stimulation can be monitored during partial neuromuscular blockade. However, concern has been raised about partial blockade masking transient responses from mechanical nerve stimulation, and it may be prudent to avoid paralysis during EMG monitoring if these responses are desired.

Because of its ability to evaluate both the structural and the functional integrity of the nervous system, electrophysiologic monitoring has become a valuable tool during surgery in which neural structures are at risk of injury. In some cases, monitoring is indispensable (e.g. seizure focus ablation); in others it is a standard of care (e.g. facial nerve monitoring in acoustic neuroma, and spinal monitoring during scoliosis correction), and in many others it is a valuable adjunct.

SLEEP, ANESTHESIA, AND ELECTROPHYSIOLOGY

Sleep is an essential, readily reversible physiologic state characterized by unconsciousness, reduced muscle tone, analgesia, amnesia, respiratory and autonomic disturbances, and dreaming (Chapter 30). Human sleep is divided into five stages, characterized by different motor, autonomic, and polygraphic (EEG, EMG, eye movement) activities (Fig. 14.8). The major distinction is between rapid eye movement (REM) and non-REM (stage I–IV) sleep. The initial stage of sleep is non-REM, during which the EEG progressively becomes more synchronized and slows, the person becomes more difficult to arouse (most difficult during stage IV), the pupils constrict, and muscle tone, blood pressure, and heart rate decrease. REM sleep occurs about every 90 minutes, lasting longer later in the sleep period, and is interspersed between periods of non-REM sleep to give a total of 6–8 hours of sleep. During REM sleep the EEG is desynchronized in a similar manner to that observed during arousal; there is tonic inhibition of muscle tone, interrupted by phasic motor events (e.g. REM), autonomic instability (e.g. irregular respiration, hypotension, and hypertension), and dreaming. The proportion of time spent in REM sleep and in stages III and IV of non-REM sleep decreases with age.

Natural sleep and anesthesia share many similarities, but they are clearly distinct. Both are characterized by unconsciousness, impaired thermoregulation, analgesia, amnesia, and atonia (in REM sleep). The EEG in sleep is characterized by predictable rhythmic variations generated endogenously. The effects of anesthetics on the EEG are agent specific and dose dependent, but can resemble patterns observed in certain stages of sleep (e.g. the spindles observed with barbiturates). Natural sleep is characterized by autonomic variability, whereas most anesthetics produce autonomic stability even in the face of painful stimuli. Finally, in contrast to anesthesia, natural sleep is characterized by easy arousability and spontaneous movements.

Key references

Cheek JC. Posterior fossa intraoperative monitoring. J Clin Neurophysiol. 1993;10:412.

Levy WJ, Shapiro HM, Maruchak G et al. Automated EEG processing for intraoperative monitoring: a comparison of techniques. Anesthesiology 1980;53:229.

Martin JT, Faulconer A Jr, Bickford RG et al. Electroencephalography in anesthesiology. Anesthesiology. 1959;20:360.

Rampil IJ. A primer for EEG signal processing in anesthesia. Anesthesiology. 1998;89:980–1002

Spehlmann R. Evoked potential primer. Boston, MA: Butterworths; 1985.

Weiderholt WC, Mayer-Harding E, Budnick B, McKeown KL. Stimulating and recording methods used in obtaining short-latency somatosensory evoked potentials (SEPs) in patients with central and peripheral neurologic disorders. Ann NY Acad Sci. 1982;388:349.

Further reading

Adams DC, Heyer EJ, Emerson RG et al. The reliability of quantitative electroencephalography as an indicator of cerebral ischemia. Anesth Analg. 1995:57–76.

Blume WT. Current trends in electroencephalography. Curr Opin Neurol. 2001;14:193–7.

Deletis V, Shils J (eds) Neurophysiology in neurosurgery. New York: Academic Press; 2002.

Holland NR. Intraoperative electromyography. J Clin Neurophysiol. 2002;19:444–53.

Keene DL, Whiting S, Ventureyra EC. Electrocorticography. Epileptic Disord. 2000;2:57–63.

Kumar A, Bhattacharya A, Makhija N. Evoked potential monitoring in anaesthesia and analgesia. Anaesthesia 2000;55:225–41.

Neidermeyer E, Lopes de Silva F (eds) Electroencephalography: basic principles, clinical applications and related fields, 3rd edn. Baltimore, MD: Williams & Wilkins; 1993.

Padberg AM, Bridwell KH. Spinal cord monitoring: current state of the art. Orthop Clin North Am. 1999;30:407–33, viii.

Rampil IJ. Electroencephalogram. In: Albin MA, ed. Textbook of neuroanesthesia with neurosurgical perspectives, Ch. 6. New York: McGraw Hill; 1997:193–219.

Schramm J, Zentner J, Pechstein U. Intraoperative SEP monitoring in aneurysm surgery. Neurol Res. 1994;16:20–2.

Slimp JC. Intraoperative monitoring of nerve repairs. Hand Clin. 2000;16:25–36.

Sloan T. Evoked potentials. In: Albin MA, ed. Textbook of neuroanesthesia with neurosurgical perspectives, Ch. 7. New York: McGraw Hill; 1997:221–76.

Chapter 15

Basic principles and limitations of hemodynamic monitoring

Richard Teplick

Many therapeutic decisions regarding patient management are based on information gathered from monitors, especially invasive pressure monitors and the electrocardiogram (ECG). However, without a full understanding of the principles and limitations of such devices, such data can be inaccurate, imprecise and misleading. This chapter provides a background to help understand how such devices obtain and process data.

PATIENT MONITORING SYSTEMS

Early bedside patient monitors could usually display one ECG channel and several invasively measured pressures. The ECG was displayed after being processed by filters with different user-selectable bandwidths, and several adjustments were often required to sense the heart rate and calibrate the displayed ECG. Pressures were obtained by amplifying the electrical signal from the transducer, a device that converts pressures into electrical signals. These signals were displayed on the monitor screen and also used to deflect a voltmeter. Pressures could be read either from the voltmeter, which was calibrated in pressure rather than volts and swung between systolic and diastolic with each beat, or directly from the display screen. In the latter case, horizontal markings had to be placed on the screen corresponding to the pressures in the range of interest, e.g. 25 mmHg, 50 mmHg, 75 mmHg, and so on, for systemic pressure. The pressure calibration procedure was complex. The pressure amplifiers first had to be adjusted to give the proper deflections on the meter, and then the display amplifiers had to be adjusted to yield the proper deflections on the screen.

Over the past several decades, monitors have become much more complex electronically and much simpler to use. They also can monitor many more parameters, such as oxygen saturation, temperature, cardiac output, and noninvasive blood pressure. The most important change has been the incorporation of digital computer technology to produce the so-called 'smart' monitors. In current-generation monitors all input signals, such as ECG and pressure signals, are converted into digital data by rapid sampling, stored and than analyzed by a microprocessor. The incorporation of microprocessors permits the selection of an enormous number of display options, plus the generation of many derived variables.

Four characteristics are shared by the current generation of monitors. First, they process the electrical signal coming from transducers in ways not clearly specified by the manufacturer. Second, the screens are not as tall as they were on many older monitors. Consequently, reading pressures directly from calibrated screens is difficult or impossible. This shortcoming is especially evident if several waveforms are displayed simultaneously. Third, the monitors emphasize numerical displays, which are derived by processing the data in a variety of ways that are usually unavailable to the user, and without data revealing the accuracy and precision of the processed data. Fourth, relatively simple knobs and buttons have given way to complex software requiring devices such as 'soft keys', trim knobs or touch screens to traverse menus and select options.

The impressive display and computational capabilities can mask major limitations in the ability of a monitor to perform some fundamental tasks. For example, as discussed below, there may be considerable error in the numerical values displayed for central pressures. This can be surmounted to some extent by displaying the pressure waveform on a screen calibrated with horizontal lines at specified pressure increments, so that pressures can be read directly from the display screen. However, usually these calibrations are too coarse to read the pressures accurately. Consequently, often the waveform is frozen, a cursor is manually moved to the portion of the waveform of interest, and the corresponding pressure is displayed numerically. This multistep process correctly implies that the numerical pressure displays are inaccurate. It would seem desirable to be able to measure the desired pressures continuously without the need to interact with the monitor, and that standards should be set for the accuracy of the numerical displays. This is not the case, most probably because the medical community has not clearly defined its needs to the manufacturers. This, in turn, may be because the reasons for monitoring parameters such as central pressures have not been clearly delineated, so that the requisite accuracy and precision of the displays cannot be specified. To understand the use and limitations of bedside monitors and the pros and cons of the evolving technologies, it is necessary to understand the basic principles governing transducers and monitors.

SIGNAL REPRODUCTION

To assess the signal reproduction fidelity of monitoring devices such as ECG recorders or invasive pressure displays, a method is needed to compare quantitatively the actual signal, e.g. intravascular pressures, with those displayed on the monitor. Quantitatively describing and therefore comparing waveform shapes and arterial pressure waveforms, however, is difficult if not impossible. Fortunately, repetitive patterns such as pressure waveforms can be described accurately as the sum of a sequence of sine or cosine waves determined using an analysis called Fourier decomposition. The resulting sequence of sine waves representing a waveform f(t) is called a Fourier series and has the general form:

Equation 15.1

$$f(t) = \frac{A_0}{2} + \sum_{k=1}^{\infty} A_k \mathrm{Sin}\left(\frac{k\pi t}{2} + \alpha_k\right)$$

where t is time, A_k is the amplitude and α_k is the phase of the kth term of the series. The kth term in the summation is termed the kth harmonic. The term $A_0/2$ is the average value of the signal, e.g. the mean pressure. The amplitude, A_k, determines the size of the kth sine wave and the phase, α_k, determines the offset of the sine wave from the usual value of zero at $t = 0$. Many waveforms can be described very precisely with a finite number of terms in the Fourier series. However, this number depends upon the particular waveform and the intended use of the Fourier description. An example of a Fourier series used to describe a square wave is shown in Figure 15.1. The first four sine waves of the series that describe the square wave are shown in Figure 15.2. In this illustration, the values of α_k are such that all of the sine terms always have the value zero at 1.5 s, 3.5 s, and 5.5 s. The amplitude, A_k, and phase, α_k, for the first 21 harmonics are shown in Table 15.1. Notice that these coefficients are nonzero only for odd values of k, except for A_0, which equals the mean value of the square wave. In addition, their values decrease rapidly after the first several harmonics but remain relatively constant thereafter. Consequently, very high-frequency harmonics add relatively little to defining the shape of the square wave, although they are required to define the sharp corners. In fact, for waveforms that have abrupt changes, such as a square wave, the ripple at the corners will remain constant regardless of the number of terms used in the series, because the amplitudes of the higher harmonics remain relatively constant even though they are much smaller than of the lower harmonics and therefore contribute less to the overall shape.

Essentially any periodic waveform can be represented by a Fourier series as a sum of sine waves.

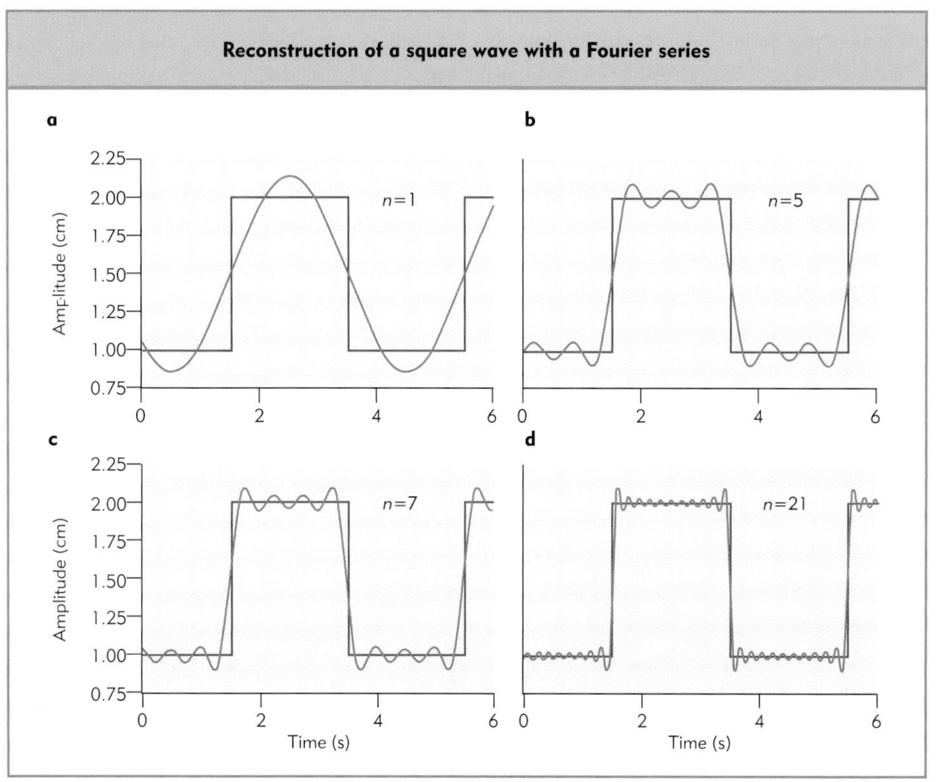

Figure 15.1 Reconstruction of a square wave with a Fourier series. The square wave repeats itself every 4 s and has an average amplitude of 1.5 cm. N is the number of harmonics in the Fourier approximation. Panel a shows a single sine wave that also repeats itself every 4 s and thus has a frequency of 0.25 Hz, which is the fundamental frequency. Notice that the maximum amplitude of this sine is approximately 0.64, so it oscillates between 0.86 and 2.14, providing a relatively poor description of the square wave. As depicted in panels b, c, and d, this approximation improves as more harmonics are added. Nonetheless, even with 21 harmonics (panel d) the sharp corners are not perfectly reproduced. Typically, sharp corners require very high harmonics to be reproduced accurately. However, if the amplitude change occurs very abruptly, as in the square wave in this figure, regardless of the number of terms used in the series, the ripple at the corners will remain constant. This is known as the Gibbs phenomenon.

The first seven harmonics of the Fourier series for a square wave

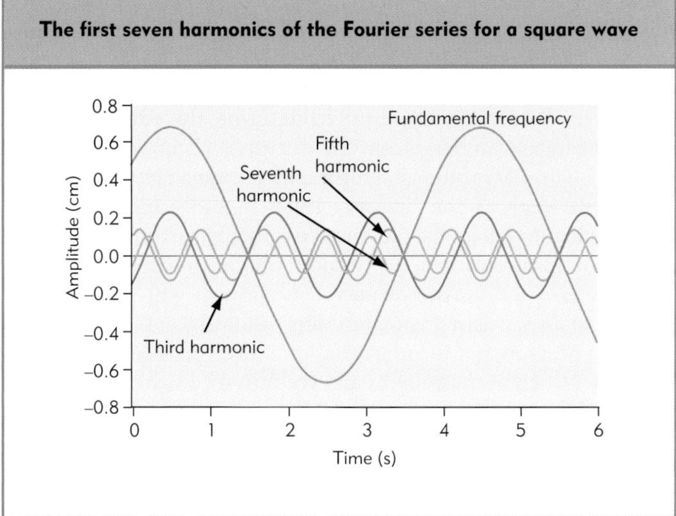

Figure 15.2 The first seven harmonics of the Fourier series for the square wave shown in Figure 15.1. The mean of 1.5 for the square wave is subtracted from each sine wave, so they are shown oscillating around zero. For a square wave all even harmonics are zero. Notice that to reconstruct the square wave, the different harmonics have different heights (amplitudes) and lead or lag each other by differing amounts (phase). Also, the higher harmonics have smaller amplitudes, so that eventually the addition of even higher harmonics would contribute very little to the shape of the square wave. The number of harmonics needed to reconstruct the square wave would depend upon it was being used for, e.g. visualization versus controlling a machine, the latter probably requiring many more harmonics.

Because essentially any periodic waveform can be represented as a Fourier series, knowledge of the magnitude and phase of each harmonic is sufficient to describe the shape of the waveform quantitatively. Ideally, to avoid distortion of a waveform by the monitoring system, the monitor should preserve the relationships between the magnitudes and phases of each term of the Fourier series describing the measured waveform. The range of frequencies that can be transduced without amplitude distortion is termed the bandwidth or frequency response. The transducing system is said to have a flat frequency response over that range. However, because monitoring systems change the amplification of the Fourier terms gradually outside the bandwidth, by convention the bandwidth is defined as the range of frequencies over which the amplification does not vary by more than three decibels (db), which is approximately 30%. A decibel is defined as 20 Log[amplification], so –3 db = 20 Log[0.7079], and so –3 db corresponds to a decrease in amplification of approximately 70%, whereas +3 db corresponds to an increase in amplification of approximately 140%.

Table 15.1 Phases and amplitudes of first 21 harmonics of square wave shown in Figure 15.1

Harmonic	Amplitude	Phase
0	1.5	
1	0.64	0.79
3	0.21	–0.79
5	0.13	0.79
7	0.09	–0.79
9	0.07	0.79
11	0.06	–0.79
13	0.05	0.79
15	0.04	–0.79
17	0.04	0.79
19	0.03	–0.79
21	0.03	0.79

The lowest frequency that needs to be amplified without distortion is usually dictated by the lowest or fundamental frequency of the signal to be monitored. For example, ECG monitors are usually designed to display heart rates that are greater than 30 beats per minute (bpm), corresponding to a fundamental frequency of 0.5 Hz (Hz, or hertz, is the number of cycles – in this case beats per second). Consequently, amplification is relatively constant for frequencies above 0.5 Hz but decreases below this value. A result of the decrease in amplification below 0.5 Hz is that the phase of the Fourier terms of the ECG signal near 0.5 Hz also changes, which produces phase distortion of the reproduced signal. Although phase distortion has little effect on audio signals because the human ear is insensitive to such distortions, it can distort digital signals, and therefore the ECG. To surmount this, the low end of the bandwidth of most ECG system is 0.05 Hz, i.e. amplification is constant above 0.05 Hz, usually until 100 Hz.

PRESSURE MONITORING

Blood pressures are measured invasively using an intravascular cannula and transducing system, a blood pressure cuff via auscultation, or oscillometrically by following cuff volume change. All of these methods are subject to errors that can be readily detected if the principles and limitations are discussed below are understood. Estimation of central pressures using Doppler techniques will not be discussed.

Invasive pressure monitoring

TRANSDUCERS

Pressure transducers convert pressure into an electrical signal by exposing one side of a diaphragm or piezoelectric crystal within the transducer to the pressure to be measured and the other to atmospheric pressure. This pressure difference causes the diaphragm or crystal to flex, and the resultant displacement is converted into an electrical signal either by changing the length or property of a material so that its resistance changes or, for piezoelectric crystals, by generating a small voltage. The pressure-induced displacement causes a change in a voltage, termed the excitation voltage, that is applied to the transducer. The relationship between applied pressure and changes in the excitation voltage defines the sensitivity of the transducer. Most transducers used for hemodynamic monitoring are standardized to produce a change of 50 μV per volt of excitation per cmHg of pressure. That is, their sensitivity is 50 μV/V/cmHg and, unlike older transducers, does not vary appreciably among transducers. Because the diaphragm is stiff (typically, 100 mmHg of pressure causes a volume displacement of 0.001 mm^3), its movement can track even rapidly changing portions of pressure pulses.

TRANSDUCER CALIBRATION

To measure pressures accurately, invasive transducing systems, i.e. the cannula, the associated tubing, transducer and monitor, have to meet three criteria: static calibration, linearity, and dynamic range.

Static calibration

Although newer transducers and monitors have little need for controls to compensate for differences in transducer characteristics, occasionally transducer sensitivity drifts, the cable develops short circuits, or the monitor amplifiers fail, resulting in inaccuracies – pressure measurement errors that may not be apparent to the user but which can be detected easily by performing a static calibration. This requires two steps: zeroing, and then calibration with a known pressure source. Zeroing ensures that a monitor indicates zero pressure in the absence of any applied pressure. To zero a transducer, both sides of the diaphragm are exposed to ambient pressure and the monitor is adjusted to show zero pressure. This usually entails opening the stopcock closest to the transducer to expose the transducer to atmospheric pressure. For older monitors 'zeroing' was accomplished by turning a knob that adjusted part of the electronic bridge used to make the pressure measurement. New monitors do this automatically when requested. Zeroing may also be required to compensate for slight differences in sensitivity due to manufacturing or temperature differences.

Once zeroed, the static gain (sensitivity) of the system can be checked by applying a known pressure to the transducer. If the corresponding pressure is not displayed on the monitor, the cable and then the transducer should be changed in succession. Because the gain of current, monitors usually cannot be adjusted by the user; if the problem remains after the above steps, the monitor must be serviced. Because of improved manufacturing, the static gain usually does not have to be checked.

A transducing system must not only read an applied pressure correctly, it must also be linear. This means that if a multiple of the pressure used for static calibration is applied to the transducer, the monitor should also show the same pressure multiple. Were this not true, the transducer would be nonlinear. However, this is seldom, if ever, a problem with current equipment.

Signal definition and dynamic performance

Successful static calibration does not guarantee accurate reproduction of pressure waveforms. The transducing system must also be able to reproduce accurately the rapid pressure changes that occur in the systemic and pulmonary circulation. To ensure that these pressures are transduced with high fidelity, dynamic performance must be tested.

The shapes of pressure waveforms vary considerably between patients, and even within the same patient at different times and with different interventions. These shapes often do not conform to the expected appearance. For example, arterial pressures may actually have narrow sharp systolic peaks, although this can also be an artifact. Fortunately, pressure-transducing systems can be tested easily to determine whether they are introducing artifacts into displayed waveforms by determining their dynamic response. As described below, using a Fourier series, any repetitive signal, including pressure waveforms, can be described as a sum of sine waves. Each sine wave has a specified amplitude, phase, and frequency. The lowest frequency is determined by the heart rate and is termed the fundamental frequency. All higher frequencies, termed harmonics, are multiples of the fundamental frequency. For example, if the heart rate were 120 bpm, the fundamental frequency would be 120 bpm divided by 60 s/min, which is 2 Hz (two beats per second). The second harmonic would have a frequency of 4 Hz, the third 6 Hz, and so on. The number of harmonics required to describe the pressure waveform accurately depends on the features of interest. As discussed below, reproduction of rapidly changing aspects of a waveform, such as the dicrotic notch in the arterial pressure, requires higher harmonics. If the transducing system distorts the phase, or especially the amplitude relationships between the requisite harmonics, the displayed waveform will be distorted. For accurate visualization and determination of systolic and diastolic pressures of most arterial pressure waveforms, only the first six to eight harmonics are required. Higher harmonics usually have amplitudes that are sufficiently small that they may be neglected without distorting the waveform. However, additional harmonics may be required to accurately depict arterial waveforms having unusual shapes, such as sharp spikes, or to calculate parameters such as the rate of change of pressure with time, dP/dt, which may require harmonics as high as 90. Thus, for a heart rate of 120, the sixth harmonic is 12 Hz, so sine waves with frequencies of 2 Hz, 4 Hz, 6 Hz, 8 Hz, 10 Hz, 12 Hz, and possibly 14 Hz and 16 Hz would be required to depict a usual arterial pressure waveform accurately. Consequently, to display the pressure waveform on the screen without significant shape distortion and determine pressures (other than mean pressure) accurately, the measurement system would have to transduce and process sine waves with frequencies up to at least 12 Hz without changing their relative amplitudes or phases. Higher frequencies need not be amplified at all, but if they are, the amplification must not be greater than that for the lower frequencies.

The transducer and tubing can distort the amplitude and phase relationships of a pressure waveform.

Although most amplifiers can meet this requirement easily, the transducer, and especially the tubing, may distort the amplitude and phase relationships of even the low-frequency Fourier components of a pressure waveform because of the relatively high compliance and low resistance of the tubing and the inertia of the fluid filling the tubing. This distortion may be quantified by modeling the response of the transducer and tubing to intra-arterial pressure, P(t), by the second-order differential equation:

■ Equation 15.2

$$\frac{d^2I(t)}{dt^2} + 2\alpha\omega_o \frac{dI(t)}{dt} + \omega_o^2 I(t) = P(t)$$

where I(t) is the current output from the transducer, α and ω_o are, respectively, the damping coefficient and the resonant frequency of the system. If the transducing system is pressurized and then the pressure source is abruptly disconnected, it will oscillate (resonate) at a frequency close to ω as long as the system is underdamped, i.e. the damping coefficient, α, is less than 1, which is always the case for clinical pressure monitoring systems. The actual oscillation frequency, termed the damped natural frequency (DNF), is affected by the damping coefficient so that:

■ Equation 15.3

$$DNF = \omega_o \cdot \sqrt{1 - \alpha^2}$$

The damping coefficient determines how rapidly the oscillations die out; the closer it is to 1, the more rapidly the oscillations die out.

To understand how ω and α affect the reproduction fidelity of a waveform by the monitoring system, it is useful to determine the frequency response of the system. Mathematically, this is done by setting P(t) = Po cosine(ωt), where Po is a constant, and solving Equation 15.2 to determine the degree of amplification as a function of frequency. The solution to this equation for a given frequency is completely characterized by its resonant frequency and damping coefficient.

Because of the transducing system's tendency to oscillate, depending on the value of α it either amplifies or attenuates the magnitudes of the Fourier harmonics of the pressure waveform near the DNF. An example is shown in Figure 15.3 for a typical transducing system with a resonant frequency, ω, of 20 Hz and a damping coefficient, α, of 0.3. The relative amplitude (amplification) is the ratio of the heights of the output sine wave to the input sine wave, e.g. the ratio of the amplitude of the Fourier component of the waveform processed by the monitor to that of the interarterial pressure waveform at the same frequency. In this example there is no amplification of the mean pressure, so the relative amplitude at zero frequency is 1. Ideally, the amplification should not change with frequency, i.e. should be 1 for all frequencies. Changes in amplification at different frequencies as shown in Figure 15.3 distort the displayed waveform. Notice in Figure 15.3 that amplification of sine waves below approximately 5 Hz is nearly constant, as indicated by the relative amplitude of 1. However, above 5 Hz, as frequencies approach the DNF there is progressive amplification with an amplification of 3 db (an amplification of approximately 1.41) at 12.7 Hz. From Equation 15.2 the DNF can be calculated to be 18 Hz rather than the resonant frequency, ω, of 20 Hz. This simulated system also has a 3 db attenuation in amplification at 29 Hz. Assuming a maximum 3 db change in amplification would be acceptable, the maximum fundamental frequencies that would not distort a pressure waveform using the system in Figure 15.3 would be 2.1 (12.7 / 6) if six harmonics were adequate and 1.6 if eight harmonics were required. The corresponding heart rates would be 127 and 95, respectively.

Distortion of a pressure waveform can manifest as a spurious increase in systolic pressure.

As shown in Figure 15.4, as the damping coefficient increases, progressively less amplification occurs near the DNF, until above 0.7071 there is no amplification but rather a progressive attenuation with increasing frequency. The relationships between the damping coefficient, the DNF and the frequencies at which 3 db changes occur are shown in Table 15.2. This table and Figure 15.4 show that a damping coefficient in the range 0.4–0.7 will yield the flattest frequency response. Unfortunately, the damping coefficient in most transducing systems is seldom

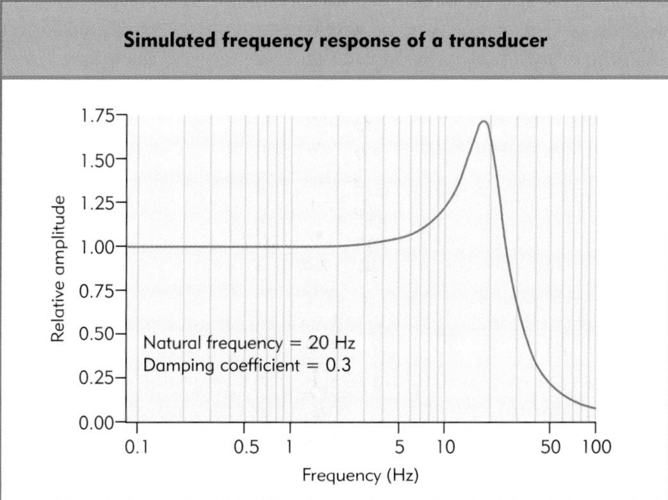

Figure 15.3 Simulated frequency response of a transducer with a resonant frequency of 20 Hz and a damping coefficient of 0.3. The horizontal axis shows the sine wave frequency on a logarithmic scale from 0.1 to 100 Hz. The vertical axis shows the amplitude of a sine wave as a function of frequency relative to the mean, which is normalized to have an amplitude of unity. Note that as the frequency approaches 18 Hz, the damped natural frequency (DNF), there is progressive amplification of sine waves, becoming most pronounced at frequencies near the DNF. This amplification will distort the resultant pressure waveform, but the importance depends on what features are of interest. At frequencies greater than approximately 13 Hz amplification exceeds 3 db (an amplification of 1.41), the conventional definition of bandwidth. Frequencies higher than the DNF are attenuated rapidly decreasing to less than unity above approximately 29 Hz. The width of the resonant peak is determined by the damping coefficient, which does not vary widely among commercial pressure transducers. In this example, if a patient had a heart rate of 120 bpm the arterial pressure waveform probably would not be greatly distorted, because the amplitude of all Fourier coefficients below the sixth harmonic (12 Hz) would undergo less than 3 db amplification. However, certain features, such as sharp peaks or the dicrotic notch, would not be reproduced accurately because they require higher frequencies to reconstruct. Such distortion could be avoided if the damped natural frequency or damping coefficient (see text) were higher.

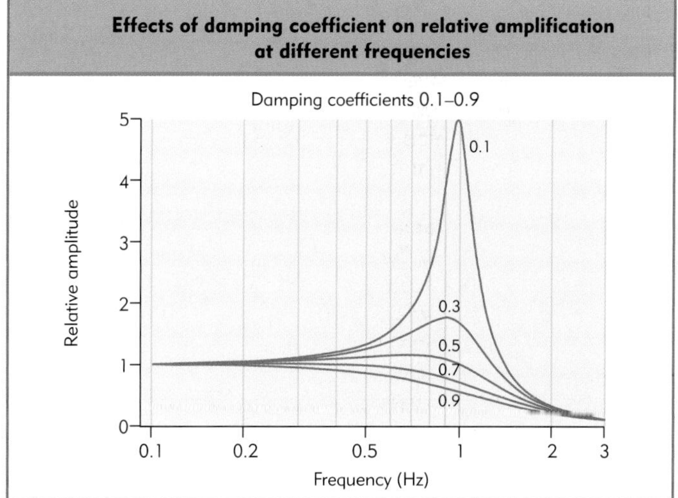

Figure 15.4 Effects of damping coefficient on relative amplification at different frequencies. All of these simulated systems have a resonant frequency of 1.0 Hz. As the damping coefficient decreases, the damped natural frequency also decreases in accordance with Equation 15.2. For a damping coefficient less than approximately 0.3, frequencies greater than approximately 0.55 Hz are markedly amplified. For damping coefficients between approximately 0.4 and 0.7, amplification never reaches 3 db and the bandwidth is relatively flat. The flattest bandwidth is achieved with a damping coefficient of 0.71. Above a damping coefficient of 0.71 3-db attenuation occurs at progressively lower frequencies. From this figure, it appears that transducing systems with damping coefficients in the range 0.4–0.71 can accurately reproduce pressure waveforms with frequency components close to the true resonant frequencies of the system.

Table 15.2 Effects of damping coefficient on damped natural frequency and the frequencies for 3 db changes in amplitude for transducing system simulated as a second-order system with a resonant frequency of 1

Damping coefficient	Damped natural frequency	3 db increase		3 db decrease
0.1	0.99	0.55	1.29	1.54
0.2	0.98	0.57	1.23	1.51
0.3	0.95	0.64	1.11	1.45
0.4	0.92			1.37
0.5	0.87			1.27
0.6	0.80			1.15
0.7	0.71			1.01
0.8	0.60			0.87
0.9	0.44			0.74
1.0	0.00			0.64

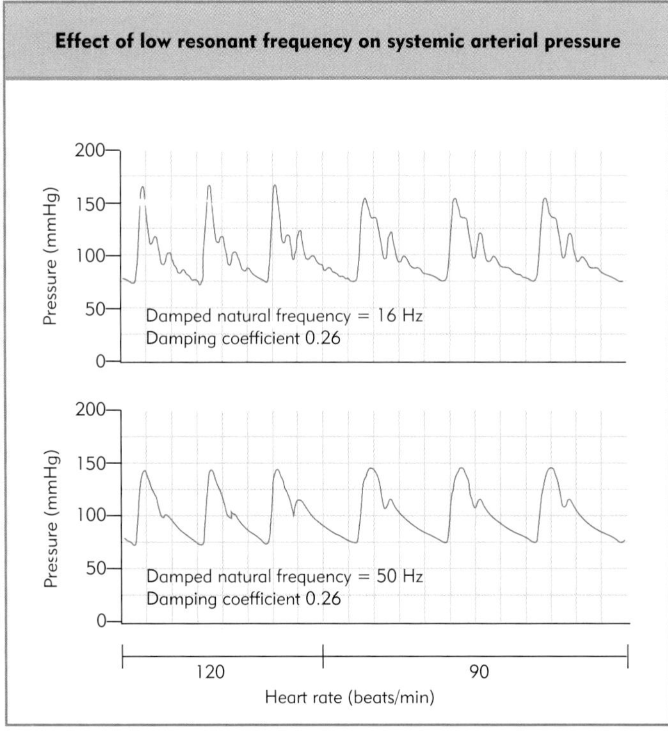

Figure 15.5 Effects of a low resonant frequency of the transducing system on systemic arterial pressure at two different heart rates. The damped natural frequencies (DNF) for the top and bottom pressure waveforms are 16 and 50 Hz, respectively. The damping coefficient is 0.26 for both waveforms. The bottom waveforms serve as standards for comparison. Diastolic pressure and mean pressure (not shown) are virtually unaffected by the frequency response of the transducing system. However, the increase in systolic pressure by almost 25 mmHg at a heart rate of 120 bpm (left half of top trace) and 15 mmHg at a heart rate of 90 bpm is an artifact due to the low DNF. This distortion is accompanied by marked oscillations of the waveform (ringing). The improvement in accuracy at a rate of 90 bpm is due to the lower-frequency response required at lower heart rates.

greater than 0.25, and often less than 0.2, for which 3 db amplification occurs at 55% of the DNF. Therefore, for such systems six to eight times the fundamental frequency should be less than approximately 55% of the DNF. For example, for a heart rate of 60 bpm the eighth harmonic is 8 Hz, so the system should resonate at least at 15 Hz (8/0.55). If, however, the heart rate were 120 bpm the eighth harmonic would be 16 Hz, so the system should resonate at least at 29 Hz. If the damping coefficient were lower, the resonant frequency should be higher.

Distortion of the pressure waveform is generally manifest as a spurious increase in systolic pressure if the higher harmonics of the pressure waveform are close to the resonant frequency. This occurs because the higher harmonics are needed to reproduce abrupt changes in pressures, and these harmonics would be amplified more than lower harmonics, thereby accentuating areas of the waveform where pressure changes abruptly, such as systolic pressure. This is illustrated in Figure 15.5. In contrast, if the frequencies of the first eight harmonics are above the DNF they will be attenuated and therefore fine definition of the waveform would be lost, causing systolic pressure to be underestimated, the waveform to appear sluggish, and abrupt changes such as the dicrotic notch to disappear.

The dynamic performance of the transducer system can easily be determined by measuring the response to an abrupt change in pressure. This 'pop test', shown in Figure 15.6, is performed as follows: 1) the transducer-catheter system is closed both to air and to the patient by turning the stopcock nearest the arterial cannula to a 45° position; 2) the system is pressurized with the flushing solution (usually to 300 mmHg); 3) the occluded stopcock is rapidly opened to air, and oscillations in the subsequent waveform are observed. The damping coefficient and resonant frequency can be determined from the period of the resultant oscillations and the rate at which their amplitudes decrease by solving Equation 15.2 for this change, with the initial conditions that $P(t) = 0$, $P(0) =$ equals the pressure just before opening the stopcock, and that the first derivative of pressure at time zero is zero.

Gardner studied the dynamic performance characteristics required for accurate measurement of blood pressure and described the pop test in detail. He used an analog computer to simulate transducing systems with different natural frequencies and damping coefficients. Two patients' arterial waveforms were applied to this simulated system. He determined a relationship between the natural frequency and the damping coefficient that appeared to reproduce these two waveforms adequately (Fig. 15.7). Note that, as expected, as the resonant frequency decreases the limits on the acceptable damping coefficient become narrower. Below a resonant frequency of approximately 13 Hz, the waveform was distorted regardless of the damping coefficient. Because the heart rate was 118, this corresponds to approximately the sixth harmonic. That is, adequate reproduction of the original waveform could be achieved if the first six harmonics could be transduced without amplitude distortion.

The most common cause of low resonant frequency is air in the tubing, especially near the transducer, because it increases the compliance of the system. This effect is magnified when the tubing between the cannula and the transducer is long, because of the increases in the inertia of the fluid and in tubing resistance and compliance. Current disposable transducer systems resonate above 40 Hz if carefully set up. Tubing length, stopcocks, and flush devices are the major factors decreasing resonant frequency.

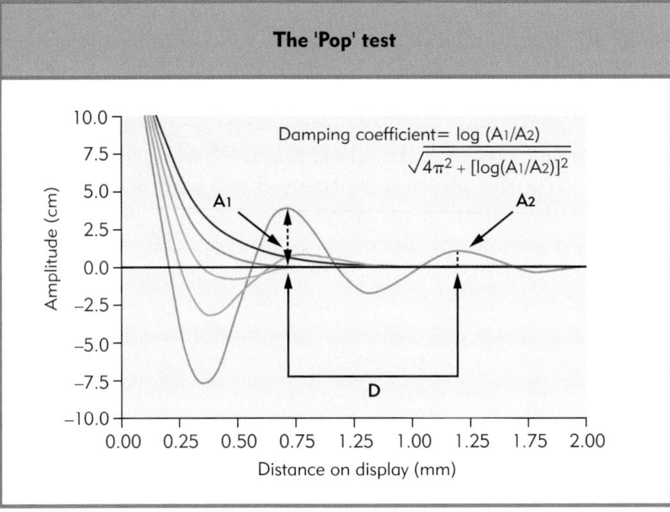

Figure 15.6 'Pop tests' for transducers with the same resonant frequency and five different damping coefficients. As the damping coefficient increases towards 1 the oscillations die out more rapidly and the damped natural frequency decreases. The pop test can be used to determine the damped natural frequency and damping coefficient of a catheter-transducer system. This is illustrated for the pop test yielding the largest oscillations, e.g. the smallest damping coefficient, 0.1. The system is pressurized as described in the text and is then abruptly opened to air. This process, which is equivalent to striking a tuning fork, causes the system to oscillate at its DNF. The DNF can be determined by dividing the rate at which the waveform moves across the screen, the sweep speed, by the distance between peaks. In this example, the distance between peaks, D, is approximately 0.75 mm on the display screen, which has the usual sweep speed of 25 mm/s. Therefore, the damped natural frequency is 25/0.75 = 33 Hz. The damping coefficient, which describes how rapidly the oscillations die out, can be calculated from the ratio of the amplitudes of two successive oscillations, A_1 and A_2, as:

In this example, the ratio of A_1 to A_2 is approximately 4.25, so the damping coefficient is 0.23. If the sixth or eighth harmonic of the pressure waveform is higher than approximately 18 Hz, which is 55% of the DNF, Figure 15.5 and Table 15.2 indicate that inaccuracies in the pressure waveform will become evident. Consequently, the heart rate should be below either135 or 180 bpm to keep the eighth or sixth harmonic, respectively, within this range.

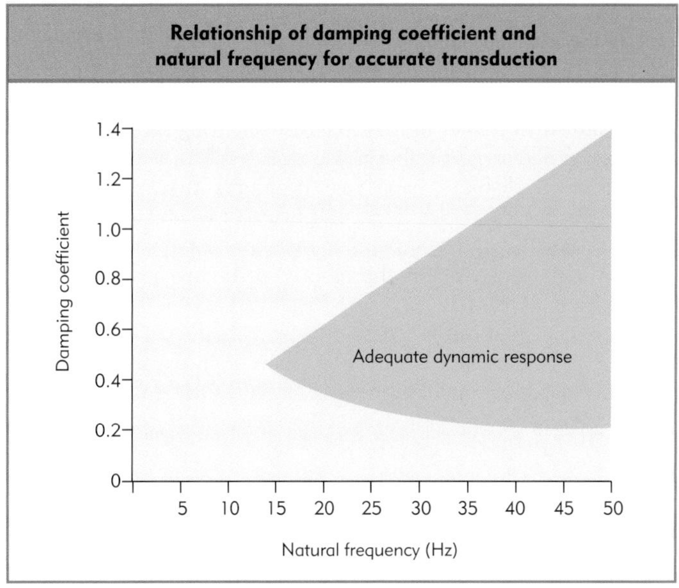

Figure 15.7 Relation between natural frequency and damping coefficient suggested for accurate transduction of waveforms. A computer was used to simulate transducing systems with different natural frequencies and damping coefficients. A measured arterial pressure waveform thought to require the greatest dynamic response of the 37 waveforms examined was used as input to the computer. The effects of varying the damped natural frequency and the damping coefficient on the computer-processed waveform were examined visually. The region labeled 'Adequate Dynamic Response' shows the relation between natural frequency and damping coefficient required for accurate visual reproduction of the input waveform.

Most monitors use filters to try to compensate for the frequency responses of transducing systems. These filters also prevent the spikes often seen on arterial pressure waveforms. Although as discussed above, such spikes can be artifacts, if the frequency response of the system is adequate the spikes are real. Most of these filters prevent amplification of frequencies above approximately 12 Hz, although this can usually be adjusted by the user. It is difficult to understand how such filters could compensate for all systems, as resonant frequencies may vary widely. However, this issue has not been studied carefully, and the effects of such filters on displayed waveforms have not been well defined. The presence of such filters may prevent the use of a pop test because high-frequency oscillations are prevented from being visualized.

NUMERICAL DISPLAYS

Current monitors usually dedicate part of the screen to the numerical display of systolic, diastolic, and mean blood pressures. Because these displayed pressures would be distracting and difficult to read if they were updated with each beat, all monitors display pressures determined by some type of averaging scheme. Older devices used a moving average in which the pressures from each new beat were used to update the average pressures. Specifically:

■ Equation 15.4

$$Pd_i = Pd_{i-1} + \frac{Pm_i - Pd_{i-1}}{K}$$

where Pm_i and Pd_i are the measured and displayed pressures (systolic, diastolic or mean) for beat i, Pd_{i-1} is the pressure displayed for the previous beat (i-1), and K is a constant. For larger values of K the displayed pressure is affected less by beat-to-beat changes in measured pressure, Pm_i. Following a sustained abrupt change in pressure, the change in displayed pressure at beat I would be:

■ Equation 15.5

$$Pd_i = Pm_n - (Pm_n - Pd_0)\cdot\left(\frac{K-1}{K}\right)^i$$

where Pm_n is the new measured pressure and Pd_0 is the original displayed pressure. If K were 1, the displayed pressure would be updated to the new pressure within one beat. As K is increased above 1 the displayed pressure will change more slowly with each beat. For example, if the displayed systolic pressure were 100 mmHg and there was an abrupt change to 120 mmHg, for a K of 5 the first updated pressure would be 100 + (120 – 100)/5 = 104. The next pressure would be 104 + (120 – 104)/5 = 107. After 17 beats the displayed pressure would be 119.5. If K were only 3, the displayed pressure would be 119.5 mmHg after only nine beats. Although it takes longer to display a sustained pressure change with larger values of K, the displayed pressure also will not change much with transient pressure changes. Although usually proprietary, a value of 8 has been recommended for systemic arterial pressures. However, this will generally not display end-expiratory central pressures correctly (see below). To surmount this, an algorithm was developed for which K varies according to how much the mean pressure, MAP, of each new beat differs from the MAP of the preceding beat. For greater differences in MAP, larger weighting factors are used so that the displayed pressures are affected less.

Numerical displays have two problems that render them inaccurate and imprecise. First, because of the averaging system, for pressures that are changing the numbers displayed may differ substantially from the actual pressures at the instant of measurement. For example, the pressure displayed just before the onset of respiration may differ markedly from the actual pressure at this time, because the displayed pressure incorporates pressures from a number of preceding beats. The magnitude of this difference depends on the weighting scheme used, the true change in pressure, and the respiratory rate. Second, the actual weights and schemes for changing them vary between manufacturers. The information about weighting algorithms and their performance specifications are rarely available. Nonetheless, manufacturers should be asked for data describing the performance of their numerical displays. For these reasons, if accurate pressures are desired at a particular instant, such as end-expiration, or the onset of the QRS complex of the ECG, the numerical pressures should be disregarded. Instead, pressures should be determined from calibrated displays or chart recordings.

Numerical displays can be inaccurate due to their systems of signal averaging and weighting.

AUSCULTATED PRESSURES

The standard method for measuring arterial blood pressure was, and still may be, auscultating for Korotkoff sounds. This entails wrapping a blood pressure cuff around the upper arm, inflating it to a pressure above systolic, then slowly deflating it and listening over the brachial artery with a stethoscope for the Korotkoff sounds. These sounds have five phases: I) a clear tapping sound (systolic pressure); II) soft murmurs; III) louder murmurs; IV) muffling; and V) disappearance. The genesis of phase I is controversial. It is thought to reflect either turbulent flow or rapid opening and closing of the artery. Phases II and III reflect the gradual increase in flow as the arterial constriction is relieved. Phase V corresponds most closely to invasively measured diastolic pressure. The auscultatory technique has many potential sources of error. First, because the sounds depend upon flow, if flow is limited or absent, as might occur with severe vasoconstriction or outflow obstruction, the sounds will be difficult or impossible to hear. Second, the pressures obtained depend on the cuff size, how it is applied, and transmission of the cuff pressures to the underlying artery. In general, cuffs that are too narrow for the circumference of the arm lead to spuriously increased pressures, and vice versa. Third, if the cuff is deflated rapidly relative to the heart rate, systolic pressure can be underestimated and diastolic pressure overestimated. For these reasons, this method cannot be considered the gold standard for pressure measurement. In general, auscultated pressures tend to underestimate invasively measured systolic pressures and overestimate diastolic pressures. The importance of such errors depends on the purpose of the measurement: they are probably relatively unimportant in monitoring acute changes, such as might occur during anesthesia or in intensive care units, where the magnitude rather than the precise value of the change is important, and important for chronic measurements such as diagnosing and managing hypertension.

Often auscultated and invasively measured arterial pressures are discordant. This is particularly common when systolic pressure occurs at the top of a sharply peaked narrow spike. Such spikes are often considered 'overshoot' artifacts, especially if the auscultated systolic pressure corresponds to the 'shoulder' of such a waveform. However, if the transducing system is calibrated accurately and the dynamic response is sufficiently high, there is no reason not to accept the invasive rather than the auscultated pressure as the true systolic pressure. Conversely, an inadequate dynamic response can produce a spike that is an artifact by amplifying high-frequency components, as described above. If the spike is real, the lower pressure determined by auscultation probably occurs because the energy or flow associated with the pressure peak is insufficient to cause the requisite turbulence or 'flapping' of the vessel wall to produce the phase I (systolic) Korotkoff sound. The more important question is why is the pressure being measured and the recognition that systolic pressures may vary widely throughout the arterial tree, generally increasing unpredictably with distance from the aortic root (see below).

OSCILLOMETRICALLY DETERMINED PRESSURES

The most common method for determining blood pressure today is probably by automated oscillometry. This technique measures the volume changes in a standard blood pressure cuff resulting from flow-induced pulsations in the underlying vessels as the cuff pressure is decreased. Rather than measuring volume, the changes in cuff pressure resulting from the volume changes are actually measured. As the cuff automatically deflates below systolic pressure, the volume of the cuff and therefore its pressure begins to oscillate with the pulsatile changes in vascular volume. As cuff deflation continues, the magnitude of the volume oscillations increases, reaching a maximum, which usually plateaus and then decreases back to zero. Mean blood pressure, MAP, is usually determined as the lowest cuff pressure during the plateau of maximum oscillations.

Although all automated devices calculate MAP approximately as described above, the method used to determine systolic and diastolic pressures varies between manufacturers, and even with software revisions within the same company. Criteria used to detect systolic and diastolic pressures often are based on the change in shape of the envelope defining the increase and decrease in the initial and final oscillations. Unfortunately, the specific criteria used are seldom available from the manufacturer. Measured pressures are also affected by the methods used to reject artifacts. Consequently, automated devices developed by different companies may yield clinically relevant differences in measured pressures. There have also been many comparisons between auscultated and intra-arterial pressures. Most of these studies show relatively small discrepancies, which, as mentioned, are probably not clinically important in the acute setting. Moreover, although most studies show an oscillometric underestimation of systolic pressure relative to invasively measured arterial pressures, this could be a result of inadequate frequency responses of the invasive measurement system. However, this problem may be accentuated and is of greater clinical relevance in the hypotensive or hypertensive patient and for ambulatory monitoring.

INTERPRETING PRESSURES

Questions about how or when to measure pressures usually can easily be answered once the purpose of making the measurements is clearly defined. Rather than trying to classify hemodynamic measurements into patterns, e.g. hemodynamic profiles, it is more constructive to use the data to assess physiologic or pathophysiologic concerns, or to test hypotheses about the state of the cardiovascular system.

Systemic pressures

The shape of the arterial pulse is determined by the properties of ventricular contraction and the characteristics of the vascular system as the pressure wave travels down the vascular tree (Figure 15.8). These changes, caused by reflected waves within the vascular system, generally reduce the width of the pressure waveform and increase systolic pressure as distance from the aortic root increases. However, the magnitude of these changes varies among patients, and within a patient when conditions such as temperature or sympathetic tone change. These effects become less marked with age as the aorta becomes less compliant, but in children they have been reported to increase systolic pressure between the aortic root and iliac artery by more than 50%. In contrast to systolic pressure, mean and diastolic pressures are usually only slightly lower in peripheral arteries than in the root of the aorta. Changes in the characteristics of either the heart or the vascular system can also produce changes in the features of the arterial pulse, such as the position of the dicrotic notch, which tends to be seen later in the pressure waveform more distally in the circulation.

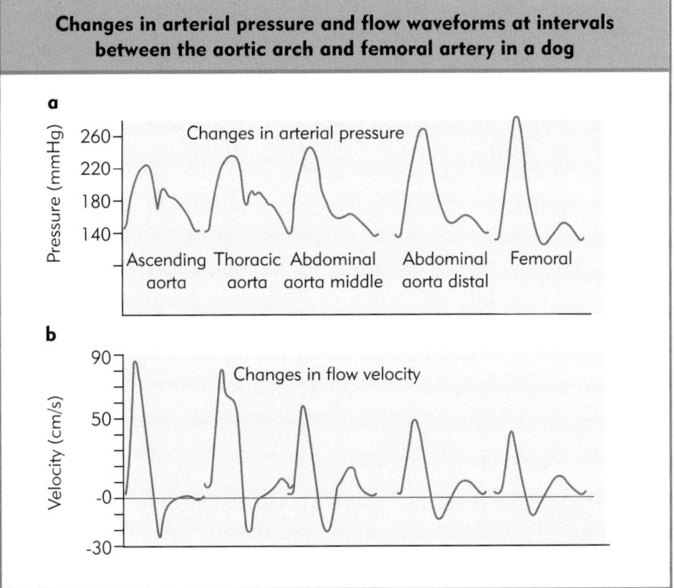

Figure 15. 8 Changes in arterial pressure and flow waveforms at intervals between the aortic arch and the femoral artery in a dog. Systolic pressure increases with distance from the arch, whereas diastolic pressure remains relatively constant. Also, the shape of the waveform changes, with transformation of the dicrotic notch into a dicrotic wave. Because of the compliance of the vasculature, the relationship between pressure and flow at any instant varies with location, such that flow during diastole becomes more pronounced at more distal locations in the circulation. (Adapted from McDonald DA. Blood flow in arteries, 2nd edn. Baltimore: Williams & Wilkins;1974: p. 356, with permission.)

Intravascular systemic arterial pressure tracings may exhibit considerable variation, especially in systolic pressure, during the respiratory cycle. Usually pressures decrease during spontaneous breaths. In contrast, during mechanical breaths, systemic arterial pressure usually increases initially and then decreases (the nadir occurring at about the time that airway pressure has returned to baseline), and gradually rises back to baseline. The length of time required for this last phase varies considerably, ranging from a few beats to 12 beats or more. The exact mechanisms for these variations in pressure are complex and depend on respiratory effects on venous return, pulmonary vascular blood volume, and ventricular load.

Mean arterial blood pressure is the most relevant measurement since perfusion of most organs depends on it.

Mean arterial pressure is probably the most relevant measurement because the perfusion of most organs depends upon it. Moreover, it is the nearly constant throughout the circulation and is directly measured by automated noninvasive and invasive devices, so that measurement at any location approximates the value at any other site. When measured invasively it is determined by integration, not calculation. Systolic pressure is the most difficult to measure accurately and varies unpredictably between the site of measurement and other sites. Fortunately, it also is rarely relevant clinically. Diastolic pressure is also difficult to measure noninvasively, but is relatively constant throughout the arterial system. Its relevance is also uncertain, although it has often been asserted that it is the upstream pressure for the coronary circulation. This cannot be correct, as it occurs during that portion of systole when the inflow to the coronaries has its nadir, and there are no experimental studies validating this concept. The location of the transducer also assumes importance under some conditions, such as the determination of cerebral perfusion pressure, or in strokes. When used for this purpose it should be leveled at the ear, because when leveled at the left atrium in patients who are not supine, the measured pressures are higher than those at the head.

Central pressures

ALTERATIONS DURING RESPIRATION

As with other measurements, the correct method for measuring central vascular pressures (central venous pressure, CVP; right atrial pressure, RAP; pulmonary artery pressure, PAP; pulmonary capillary wedge pressure, PCWP; and left atrial pressure, LAP) depends on the purpose of the measurement. Unlike the respiratory variations in systemic arterial pressures, respiratory changes in central pressures are artifacts. If the purpose of the CVP, RAP, LAP, or PCWP is to estimate the end-diastolic pressure, EDP, of the ventricles, measurements made just before inspiration, i.e. at end-expiration, provide the most accurate and precise estimates. This cannot be done using a monitor's numerical displays because, as described above, they reflect some type of average over a variable number of beats, some of which are unlikely to occur during end-expiration, and are therefore unlikely to be accurate reflections of EDP. However, these pressures can be determined accurately from a waveform displayed on a calibrated screen.

WAVEFORM FEATURES

The presence of atypical or abnormal configurations in central pressure waveforms can also lead to errors in measurement. For example, the typical atrial waveform consists of an A wave, caused by right atrial contraction; a C wave, caused perhaps by bulging and downward movement of the atrioventricular (AV) valves during isovolumic contraction; and a V wave that occurs during atrial filling. Because the AV valves are normally closed from approximately the onset of systole until the peak of the V wave, atrial pressures during this time cannot reflect ventricular EDP. Moreover, because EDV, and hence EDP, increases with atrial contraction, the only time that atrial pressures can reflect EDP is after the A wave and before the onset of systole. Therefore, it is logical to measure atrial pressures at approximately the onset of the QRS complex of the ECG. Because A, C, and V waves usually have amplitudes of only a few mmHg, measurements made at other times during the cardiac cycle generally do not introduce appreciable error. However, the A and V waves can have large amplitudes that would cause error in numerical displays independently of the display's unreliability in displaying end-expiratory pressures. These errors would be apparent and readily avoided if pressures were measured directly from the waveform displayed on a calibrated screen. This is most easily accomplished by superimposing the ECG on the pressure waveform. Unfortunately, this cannot be done on most current generation monitors.

OTHER SOURCES OF CENTRAL PRESSURE MEASUREMENT ERROR

Occasionally, overinflation of the balloon in a pulmonary artery catheter can yield an erroneous PCWP. This error probably results from transient obstruction of the catheter tip by the balloon or the vascular wall, allowing pressure from the pressurized flushing system to build up within the transducer. Because correctly measured PCWP never exceeds pulmonary arterial diastolic pressure, this problem is readily detected by such a discrepancy. Balloon deflation, followed by slow reinflation, usually corrects this problem.

The term catheter whip is commonly used to describe pulmonary and systemic arterial waveforms having unusually sharp peaks (spikes) or oscillations (ringing) of uncertain origin. Catheter whip also implies that such features are caused by mechanical motion of the catheter during the cardiac cycle, or by a low resonant frequency of the transducing system. Because a pulmonary artery catheter passes through the right side of the heart into the pulmonary artery inflow tract, the former explanation seems plausible. Moreover, because of the length and relatively large compliance of the pulmonary catheter lumen, it is difficult to obtain a resonant frequency much above the low teens. This low resonant frequency could produce both spiking and the oscillations described as ringing. Ringing that persists throughout the cardiac cycle suggest that a low resonant frequency may be the cause. Ringing may pose a substantial problem in measuring pulmonary artery diastolic pressure, often used as a surrogate for the wedge pressure because the portion of the diastolic oscillation that should be taken as diastolic pressure is uncertain, and it may produce very large errors in the numerical displays. One solution is to 'eyeball' the most stable point in the oscillations and use this as the diastolic pressure. It is also possible that filtering or increasing the damping coefficient could minimize this problem. Incorrect values should be suspected if the measured pulmonary artery diastolic pressure is lower than the PCWP. This is not usually a problem with the CVP or PCWP because they do not have significant high-frequency harmonics.

Estimation of the LAP from the PCWP theoretically depends on a static column of blood between the catheter tip and left atrium created by balloon occlusion of the branch of the pulmonary artery containing the catheter tip. Because this seems unlikely, as there are many different arterial channels to the veins, even if there is flow generally the venous resistance is low, so that the pressure drop due to continued venous flow is negligible. It has been asserted that if the tip of a pulmonary artery catheter lies in zones 1 or 2 of the lungs described by West et al. (Chapter 47), the PCWP may systematically overestimate LAP. However, it seems improbable that placement of the catheter tip in zones 1 or 2 would be a source of error in estimating LAP. First, placement of the catheter tip in a zone 1 region is unlikely because of the low blood flow in this zone, although changes in ventilation or position theoretically can convert other zones to zone 1 areas. Regardless, although blood flow through alveoli may be absent in zone 1, flow to extra-alveolar (corner) vessels should still exist, thereby providing the requisite continuity between the catheter tip and the left atrium. If such continuity were lost, A, C, and V waves would not be observed on the PCWP trace and the PCWP should reflect alveolar rather than left atrial pressure, and therefore, by the definition of zone 1, be higher than pulmonary artery diastolic pressure. Second, placement of the catheter tip in a zone 2 region should not cause error because there is, by definition, normally flow in these regions, although it may be independent of venous pressure. Therefore, there must be continuity between the catheter tip and the left atrium, even disregarding the extra-alveolar vessels. If inflation of the balloon caused all vascular channels in this zone to collapse, vascular continuity to the left atrium would be lost and the PCWP would reflect alveolar pressure rather than LAP, although this is unlikely because of the multiple arteriovenous pathways. As in a zone 1 region, A, C, and V waves then should not be observed and PCWP should exceed LAP, but this has not been reported. Nonetheless, the literature is confusing on this issue because studies have incorrectly implied that there is no flow and hence no patent arterial–left atrial channel in these regions. The discrepancies between PCWP and LAP attributed to the catheter tip lying in zone 2 could be a result of increased venous resistance caused by the partial collapse of the pulmonary veins in these zones. This would result in a relatively large pressure drop between the catheter tip and the left atrium, owing to continued venous flow after balloon inflation. An additional source of confusion in some studies that found differences related to the zone of the lung is the use of values for PCWP and LAP averaged over respirations. These considerations suggest that having a catheter tip in zones 1 or 2 is unlikely to be the source of spuriously large PCWP–LAP differences. Nonetheless, the possibility of this occurrence highlights the importance of visually examining the PCWP waveform for A, C, and V waves.

MEASUREMENT OF CARDIAC OUTPUT

Cardiac output is usually measured clinically by indicator dilution. The principle involved is the measurement of pulmonary or systemic arterial changes in the concentration of an indicator such as color or cold intravenous solutions injected into venous blood. Room-temperature dextrose or saline are the most common thermal indicators used clinically. Thermodilution depends on measuring changes in blood temperature in the pulmonary artery with a thermistor. Indocyanine green, a dye used less commonly than temperature as an indicator, requires its concentration to be measured at a site in the arterial circulation. Although other noninvasive techniques based on Doppler velocity or changes in impedance are available, the validity of these methods is still controversial. It is important to recognize that achieving a high correlation with a standard method measurement such as thermodilution is not sufficient to validate the method. Correlation only indicates the degree to which the two methods are linearly related, not how well they agree. For example, a correlation of 0.9 means that 81% (0.9^2) of the variation between the two methods is accounted for by a straight line. However, to be accurate, the slope of the line should be 1 and the intercept 0, otherwise the difference between the two methods varies with the cardiac output. For example, if the slope and the intercept of the line relating the two methods were 0.8 and 0.75, respectively, then at low outputs, output using the new method would overestimate that of the standard method, the overestimation decreasing at higher outputs until at an output of 3.75, (0.75/(1.0 – 0.8)) the measured outputs would be equal. Above 3.75 the new method would progressively underestimate the standard measurement.

Dilutional methods

Dilutional methods for calculating cardiac output are based on the Stewart–Hamilton equation, which is an expression of conservation of mass. If an indicator were injected into the venous circulation and none were lost from the circulation or recirculated, the amount recovered at the detection site if all blood flow passed by this site would equal the amount injected. Consequently:

■ Equation 15.6

$$\text{Injected} = \int_0^T q(t)\cdot c(t)\cdot dt$$

where *Injected* is the total quantity of indicator injected, c(t) and q(t) are the instantaneous concentration and blood flow as functions of time, t, at the detection site, and t is the time required for the entire cardiac output to pass by the detection site. If blood flow is constant, this equation may be rewritten as:

■ Equation 15.7

$$\text{Injected} = Q\int_0^\infty c(t)\cdot dt$$

where Q is the cardiac output. Therefore, cardiac output would equal the amount injected divided by the integral of concentration with respect to time, which equals the area under the concentration curve. Even if the total cardiac output did not pass by the sampling site, the change in indicator concentration would be the same in every arterial branch. Consequently, the area under the concentration curve would be the same regardless of where it is measured, and therefore cardiac output can still be estimated using Equation 15.7 by measuring indicator concentration in a branch of the pulmonary artery or of the systemic arterial circulation.

The important assumptions in indicator dilution techniques, then, are as follows:

1. At some point distal to the injection site of the indicator and proximal to the measurement site, all blood passes through a single channel, or at least intermixes. This ensures that the indicator is diluted by the total blood flow.
2. Any changes in flow during the measurement period must occur rapidly, and the average flow must not change during the measurement period. This assumption may be violated by respiration, because it may change output during the measurement period.
3. The indicator must remain in the vascular space, and large shifts of fluid to or from the vascular space cannot occur during the measurement period. If the third assumption were not true, the concentration of the indicator would change independently of blood flow.

DYE DILUTION METHOD

The dye dilution method entails injecting a bolus of a known quantity of dye through a central venous catheter. The change in concentration of the indicator resulting from mixing with blood is detected by withdrawing blood from an arterial catheter at a fixed rate and passing it through a densitometer. This device measures the optical density of the blood to determine the concentration of the indicator. The output from the densitometer is used to generate a curve showing the concentration of the dye over time. Because the dye is not cleared with a single pass through the circulation, some of the indicator recirculates and mixes with some of the initial bolus, causing a second peak in the curve (Fig. 15.9). If this additional peak were included in calcu-

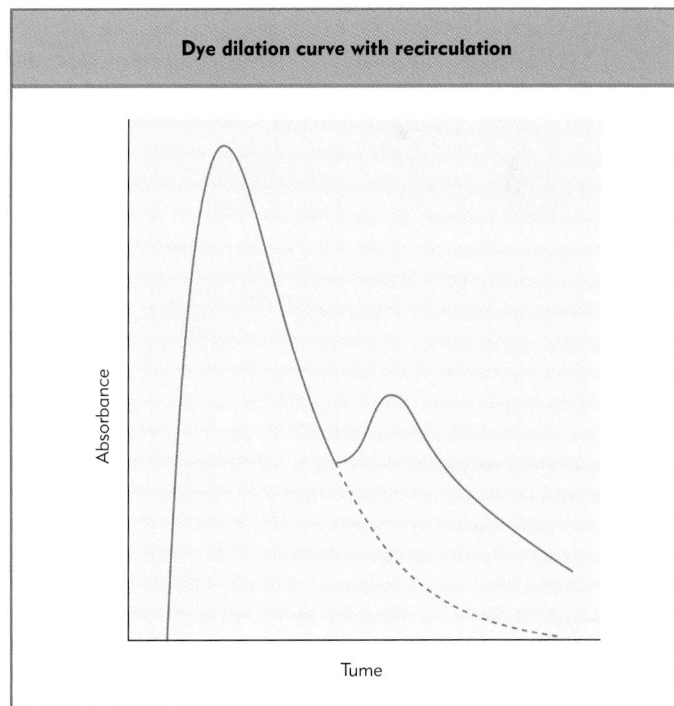

Figure 15.9 Dye dilution curve with recirculation (solid line). The dotted line represents a monoexponential extrapolation from the portion of the solid curve just before recirculation occurs (second peak). The areas under the solid curve before the recirculation peak and below the dotted extrapolation are used to compute cardiac output.

lating the area under the concentration curve the area would be spuriously increased, yielding a falsely low cardiac output. To correct for recirculation of indicator, after the curve has decayed to approximately 25–30% of the peak value, the rest of the curve is calculated by extrapolation, usually assuming a monoexponential decrease in concentration, as shown in Figure 15.9. The validity of this assumption during respiration has not been established. The shape of the dye curve also can yield valuable information about intracardiac shunting. For example, a right-to-left shunt might manifest itself as an early recirculation peak on the curve.

THERMODILUTION TECHNIQUES

Cardiac output

The thermodilution technique entails injecting a known amount of cold fluid at a known temperature below blood temperature (most often room temperature, but occasionally 0°C), into the right atrium. The resulting change in temperature of pulmonary arterial blood is measured by a thermistor on the tip of a pulmonary artery catheter. These data are used to produce a thermodilution curve, which resembles the dye-dilution curve (Fig. 15.9) except that the recirculation peak is usually absent. Cardiac output is then calculated as:

■ Equation 15.8

$$Q = \frac{K\cdot(Tbi - Ti)\cdot 60\cdot Vol}{\int_0^\infty T_b(t)\cdot dt}$$

where T_{bi} and T_i are the initial blood and injectate temperatures, respectively, $T_b(t)$ is the blood temperature as a function of time, Vol is the volume of injectate, and K is a constant, usually 1.08, that depends upon volume, specific gravity, and specific heat of the injectate and the blood, and heat loss within the catheter. The terms in the numerator of this equation, which define the amount of cold injected, are incorporated into the calibration number set on the cardiac output computer.

Recirculation is usually not a problem with thermodilution. However, because the fraction of venous return coming from the superior and inferior venae cavae varies with respiration and there is normally a difference in temperature between these two veins, the pulmonary artery temperature also varies with respiration. Consequently, it is difficult to determine when the temperature curve returns to baseline. To surmount this problem, the area under the temperature difference curve is usually computed by halting the calculation when the washout curve has decayed to approximately 25–30% of the peak value, and a constant corresponding to the area under a monoexponential curve returning from this point to baseline is added to the area of the curve calculated up to this point.

A monoexponential decay is based on the following model. Assume that a bolus of indicator, q, is injected into the right ventricle and instantaneously mixes with the blood to yield a concentration C_1 equal to q / EDV. Given an ejection fraction, EF, the first beat will eject an amount of indicator equal to EDV × EF × C_1. After the ventricle refills to the EDV, the concentration of indicator will equal the original amount, minus the amount ejected divided by the EDV:

■ Equation 15.9

$$\frac{C_1\cdot EDV - C1\cdot EDV\cdot EF}{EDV} = C_1\cdot(1 - EF)$$

On the next beat, the amount of indicator ejected would equal EDV × EF × the ventricular concentration given by Equation 15.9. The concentration of indicator after refilling back to the EDV would then be:

■ Equation 15.10

$$\frac{C_1\cdot(1 - EF)\cdot EDV - C1\cdot(1 - EF)\cdot EDV\cdot EF}{EDV} = C_1\cdot(1 - EF)^2$$

By a similar reasoning, on each beat the concentration would decrease by 1 – EF, so that on the *n*th beat the concentration would be $(1 - EF)^n$, becoming infinitesimal as *n* becomes very large. For thermodilution, q is the amount of cold fluid injected into the right ventricle and C_n is the temperature after the *n*th beat diluted the cold with blood at body temperature, and is also the temperature a thermistor in the pulmonary artery would detect on the next ejection. In fact, this theoretical decrease in temperature by 1 – EF is the basis of the right ventricular ejection fraction thermodilution catheter (see below). The equation $(1 - EF)^n$ can be approximated by a monoexponential increase in temperature, the approximation becoming exact as EF approaches zero and *n* approaches infinity. This formulation does not account for the gradual rather than abrupt temperature decrease following the bolus injection. However, both portions of the curve can be described using a two-compartment kinetic model with pulmonary blood representing the peripheral compartment, or a random walk model, but neither approach has an obvious computational advantage. Surprisingly, experimentally the temperature areas were the same, whether calculated using the computer algorithm which assumed that 22% of the area of the curve occurred after the height of the curve had decreased to 30% of the maximum, or using the entire curve. This lends some credence to the method used by most cardiac output computers of extrapolating area when temperature returns to a certain percent of baseline.

The theoretical problem with thermodilution cardiac output measurement is that the increase in temperature back towards baseline should not be monoexponential if the stroke volume varies slowly over the measurement period, as expected with respiration, for example. This has not been tested experimentally, but it has been shown that thermodilution outputs may vary by as much as 70%, with measured cardiac output ranging from 5.0 to 8.4 L/min when injection is performed at different times during the respiratory cycle, presumably because respiration causes stroke volume to vary slowly during the measurement period. This range was reduced to 6.3–7.1 L/min if injections were made only at end-exhalation. For this reason, clinically significant differences between sets of three measurements could only be detected for differences of 12–15%. Nonetheless, if the average output is desired, it may be more appropriate to average multiple injections randomly distributed throughout the respiratory cycle. As is the case for pressure measurements, changes in output (more specifically stroke volume) are more useful than the absolute number. Therefore, when measuring cardiac output precision is more important than accuracy, and end-expiratory measurement is advisable.

When measuring cardiac output, precision is more important than accuracy.

Thermodilution has often been shown to overestimate low cardiac outputs. Although this has usually been ascribed to excessive cold loss from blood, more recent data indicate that it is a result of an actual increase in cardiac output resulting from the cold bolus, possibly due to increased contractility from reduced temperature in the coronary circulation. Errors in thermodilution cardiac outputs may also occur in the presence of severe tricuspid valve insufficiency (TI). Such errors might occur because of heat loss in the regurgitant volume so that, in effect, less cold is injected, or because the downslope of the curve is not monoexponential, thereby causing errors in the extrapolated portion of the temperature curve area. In the former case cardiac output should be overestimated, whereas in the latter it would probably be underestimated because of a slower than predicted return to baseline. Interestingly, in a dog model outputs were overestimated by thermodilution, whereas in humans they were underestimated. This difference may have arisen because of different standards of comparison: a pulmonary flowmeter in dogs, and indocyanine green or Fick in humans.

Right ventricular ejection fraction

The theoretical increase in blood temperature by an amount proportional to 1 – EF with each beat predicted for bolus thermodilution cardiac output measurement is the basis of thermodilution estimation of right ventricular ejection fraction (RVEF). The RVEF catheter originally depended on a thermistor that could respond to temperature changes rapidly enough to detect the predicted step increase in temperature followed by a plateau with each ejection. As noted, the temperature of each plateau should be related to the preceding plateau by the constant ratio 1 – EF. To measure the plateau temperature measurements were made at the QRS of the ECG sensed using electrodes within the catheter. Eventually, this gave way to using slower thermistors and identifying the points on the exponential portion of the curve where the plateau should occur from the QRS complex. There are, however, several problems with these techniques. First, there is no gold standard for right ventricular volume. Consequently, validation is dependent on the particular standard of comparison for RVEF. Second, although it has been asserted that the accuracy of thermodilution-measured ejection fraction has been validated, this does not seem to be the case. For example, comparisons with biplane angiography yielded an R^2 of only 0.69, with a regression slope and intercept of 0.76 and 15.5, respectively, indicating an overestimation of RVEF that progressively decreased with increasing EF. Both better (R^2 = 0.85) and worse (R^2 = 0.45) relationships have been found in comparison with first-pass radionuclide scanning, but in both studies, as EF increased the underestimation of radionuclide EF by thermodilution also increased. Tricuspid insufficiency, as expected, also interferes with the measurement of right ventricular EF. However, it is unclear whether this is a result of indicator loss as described above, or invalidation of the assumptions of the thermodilution method because of the addition of progressively diluted indicator to the right ventricle with each beat from the regurgitant volume. Collectively, these data and the theory suggest that measurement of right ventricular ejection fraction by thermodilution is unlikely to be accurate or precise. However, it might be useful in distinguishing between high and low EF in situations when stroke volume is low and RAP is elevated, as might occur, for instance, with high transmural pressures or right ventricular dysfunction. In the former case the EF should be high, and in the latter it should be low.

CONTINUOUS CARDIAC OUTPUT

One of the perceived limitations of thermodilution cardiac output measurement is that it is not continuous. To surmount this, the basic principles have been adapted to provide continuous measurement using heat instead of cold as an indicator. The major obstacles to continuous measurement were the excessive heat required and the thermal noise spectrum from intrinsic blood temperature changes, particularly from respiration, and slow baseline temperature changes. These problems were solved by using pseudorandom binary coded temperature pulses which resemble white noise to form cross-correlations with the resultant temperature measurements. The continuous cardiac output pulmonary artery catheter uses a heating coil placed between the right atrium and ventricle to produce these temperature pulses. Each binary code must last longer than the duration of the corresponding bolus thermodilution washout curve. Because of thermal noise, this process must be repeated at least 10 times before a reliable output can be calculated. Consequently, the minimum time to obtain an output is approximately 5 minutes. Numerous clinical studies have compared continuous cardiac output measurements to both bolus thermodilution and indocyanine green measurements, with generally good agreement. The major disadvantage to the continuous system is that it cannot respond rapidly to changes in cardiac output. Response time to display a change of 0.9 L/min following a 1 L/min abrupt change in output is between 10 and 12.5 minutes. Thus, as with all other measurements, the utility of continuous cardiac output measurement depends on what information is being sought. Certainly, it would not be useful in determining the cause of an acute change in hemodynamics, or in acute drug titration, as its response is much too slow.

NONINDICATOR DILUTION METHODS

Pulse contour analysis

Because systemic blood pressure and stroke volume are related by the properties of the vasculature, it would be possible to predict stroke volume from pressure measurements if the relevant vascular properties were known. Methods to determine stroke volume from measured pressure waveforms rely on estimating these vascular properties. Most methods depend on estimates of aortic compliance and assuming that the vasculature can be modeled as a three-element Windkessel. Most commonly, the Windkessel model consists of a proximal resistance or inductance, called the characteristic impedance, and a parallel capacitor and resistor, representing respectively the compliance and the resistance of the arterial vasculature.

A problem with this method, which is common to all estimates of cardiac output based on pressure measurements, is the need to scale the calculated stroke volume to an independent measurement, usually using thermodilution. Performance of these pulse contour methods has been inconsistent, often showing considerable bias and variation relative to thermodilution. This is to be expected, as there are a large number of assumptions that are inherent in all pulse contour methods. For these reasons, and because an independent measurement of cardiac output is required for calibration, these methods should be viewed cautiously.

Impedance cardiography

Thoracic electrical bioimpedance is the characteristic impedance of the tissue and blood in the thorax, which changes with respiration and the cardiac cycle, largely because of the changes in thoracic vascular volume. Thoracic electrical bioimpedance (TEB) or impedance cardiography isolates the change in TEB due to the cardiac cycle from those due to respiration, and converts the measured impedance into stroke volume. It is based on applying a high-frequency low-current signal and measuring the impedance to this current between two pairs of electrodes, one pair usually placed at the base of the neck and the other placed at the xiphoid level. After processing to remove the respiratory component, the change in impedance from the baseline impedance, Z_0, is related to the change in blood volume of the thoracic vessels, particularly the thoracic aorta. A variety of modifications have been made to the original equation in order to incorporate a truncated conic model of the chest, remove the need for precise measurement of electrode distance, and adjust for ideal body weight and specific blood resistance. Regardless of the exact equation used, the accuracy of stroke volume estimation depends on the ability to dissociate impedance changes resulting from volume changes in aortic blood flow from the 'noise' imparted by shifts in tissue fluid volume and respiratory changes in pulmonary and venous blood volumes. Not surprisingly, complicating factors such as pulmonary edema, pleural effusion, profound peripheral edema, sepsis, and morbid obesity diminish the accuracy of cardiac output determination by TEB. Because studies vary so widely in correspondence with other methods of obtaining cardiac output, and because there are both physical and theoretical problems with TEB, as is the case for pulse-contour measurements, it cannot be reliably used for clinical measurement of cardiac output.

Doppler methods

Although a pulmonary artery catheter capable of continuously measuring beat-to-beat stroke volume from Doppler velocity data was found to be at least as accurate as thermodilution, it was relatively complex to use and failed in the marketplace. More recently, stroke volume has been estimated using nasogastric-sized transesophageal Doppler probes to measure flow velocity in the descending aorta, and multiplying this by aortic cross-sectional area predicted from nomograms or by measured using simultaneous M-mode echocardiography. Because this method estimates flow only in the descending aorta, it must be scaled to account for flow to upper portions of the body arising from the aorta proximal to the measurement site. Despite being relatively noninvasive and easy to use, the method has the following limitations. 1) Estimation of aortic area has the same limitations as the pulse contour method. Interestingly, aortic area is estimated from different data sets and nomograms in the commercial Doppler and pulse-contour devices. 2) Placement to obtain the correct Doppler flow can be time-consuming, has a steep learning curve, and may require frequent repositioning if the patient moves. 3) The assumption that the proportion of total blood flow proximal to the measuring site is constant may be incorrect under some circumstances, such as the initiation of epidural anesthesia. Most data indicate that there is considerable disagreement between esophageal Doppler methods and thermodilution, regardless of how aortic area is estimated. Nonetheless, estimation of changes in cardiac output rather than absolute values generally agrees quite closely with thermodilution. Regardless, problems with placement of the probe, displacement with patient motion, and safety in the presence of a nasogastric tube limit its clinical utility.

MIXED VENOUS OXYGEN SATURATION

Cardiac output measurement is useful to assess cardiac performance, especially using calculated or directly measured stroke volume, whether hypotension is due to low cardiac output, decreased vascular resistance, or both, and as an important element of the delivery of oxygen to tissues. A major limitation in directly relating cardiac output to tissue oxygen delivery is that the distribution of flow to different organs varies with the underlying physiology and pathophysiology, but clinical measurements of flow distribution are not yet available. Even if they were, the distribution within an organ, e.g. between the renal medulla and cortex, or the cardiac endocardium and epicardium, is probably of greater importance. Moreover, interventions such as fluid infusions or inotropic drugs that change cardiac output redistribute flow among organs. This is true even in with changes in normal physiology, as illustrated by the more than fourfold increase in cardiac output associated with some forms of aerobic exercise, such as running a marathon, where the increase in cardiac output is mostly directed to muscle and skin whereas visceral organ flow is reduced. To surmount this limitation, mixed venous oxygen partial pressure $P\text{v}O_2$ or saturation, SvO_2, has been proposed as a measure of adequacy of the balance between oxygen supply and demand.

Mixed venous oxygen content, CvO_2, is related to O_2 consumption, VO_2, arterial O_2 content, CaO_2, and cardiac output, Q, by the following equation:

■ Equation 15.11

$$CvO_2 = CaO_2 - \frac{VO_2}{10 \cdot Q}$$

Oxygen delivery, DO_2, which equals $Q \times CaO_2 \times 10$, is the number of milliliters of O_2 leaving the left ventricle per minute. Oxygen extraction is the ratio of oxygen utilization to oxygen delivery, i.e. VO_2 / DO_2, and represents the fraction of available oxygen taken up by tissues. SvO_2 has an approximate inverse relation with O_2 extraction, as shown by dividing both sides of Equation 15.11 by CaO_2 to yield:

■ Equation 15.12

$$\frac{CvO_2}{CaO_2} = 1 - \frac{VO_2}{10 \cdot Q \cdot CaO_2} = 1 - \frac{VO_2}{DO_2}$$

Because O_2 content equals $1.34 \times$ saturation $\times$ hemoglobin concentration $+ 0.0031 \times PO_2$, ignoring the relatively small contribution of dissolved O_2, and assuming that arterial blood is fully saturated, Equation 15.12 can be approximated as:

■ Equation 15.13

$$SvO_2 = 1 - \frac{VO_2}{DO_2}$$

which shows that an increase in oxygen extraction, VO_2/DO_2 is accompanied by a linear decrease in SvO_2, and vice versa.

Mixed venous oxygen saturation is inversely related to average tissue oxygen consumption.

Although a decrease in SvO_2 has often been cited as detrimental, this is not necessarily true. For example, in vigorous aerobic exercise PvO_2 and hence SvO_2 may decrease greatly because of high muscle O_2 extraction, yet muscle blood supply is obviously adequate. Conversely, as indicated by Equation 15.11, increasing cardiac output without concomitant changes in VO_2 or CaO_2 must result in an increase in CvO_2 and therefore SvO_2, reflecting decreased extraction. However, any such increase in cardiac output is unlikely to be distributed uniformly to all tissues, and so the increase in SvO_2 cannot be assumed to reflect better tissue oxygenation. Moreover, the pattern of redistribution will depend on the method used to increase cardiac output and the state of the cardiovascular system prior to the increase.

Further difficulties in interpreting SvO_2 arise from two other sources: 1) tissues can use different mechanisms to increase O_2 extraction, and 2) SvO_2 reflects an average of the venous O_2 content of each organ weighted by the blood flow through that organ. The major mechanisms to increase extraction are to decrease diffusion distances by recruiting more capillaries, and to decrease intracellular PO_2, thereby increasing the driving force for diffusion. Whereas the latter method causes venous PO_2 to decrease, the former method is also usually accompanied by an increase in blood flow, so that the effects on venous O_2 are unpredictable. Because of the enormous heterogeneity of PO_2, oxygen consumption, and blood flow within most organs, interpreting even individual organ venous PO_2 or SO_2 in terms of the adequacy of oxygenation seems physiologically improbable. Moreover, because mixed venous O_2 reflects an average of the venous PO_2 of each organ weighted by its blood flow, both of which vary enormously in different organs: one organ can be ischemic, whereas another is luxuriously perfused without being reflected in the mixed venous O_2. For example, organs having high extraction, such as the heart, have low venous O_2 content. Conversely, the venous PO_2 of the kidney is relatively high (approximately 60 mmHg.). Because the kidneys generally account for at most 20% of cardiac output, changes in renal venous PO_2 would be essentially undetectable, especially if other organ flow increased, as for example in exercise or sepsis. Thus, although SvO_2 is readily measured using pulmonary artery catheters with fiberoptic sensors or direct sampling, both these theoretical considerations, as well as clinical studies, confirm its inadequacy in assessing tissue oxygenation.

Clinical applications

Although low PvO_2 or SvO_2 may be associated with death in critically ill patients, it remains to be shown that increasing these values via therapeutic interventions affects outcome. Nonetheless, the measurement of SvO_2 has become quite popular because it can be obtained online from specially equipped pulmonary artery catheters. The reasons usually cited for measuring SvO_2 are that: 1) SvO_2 is indicative of tissue oxygenation, 2) changes in SvO_2 provide an early warning of patient instability, and 3) changes in SvO_2 reflect changes in cardiac output. The first premise, as noted above, is clearly incorrect. The second premise may be true but has not been verified clinically. Nonetheless, a change in SvO_2 may motivate a further search for causes, in particular occult bleeding or decreases in PaO_2. However, the former should be readily detectable by changes in blood pressure, heart rate, central pressures, and cardiac output, especially with continuous cardiac output measurement, whereas the latter would be detected by pulse oximetry. Disregarding these considerations, it has proved difficult to define either the rate or the magnitude of change in SvO_2 that should trigger an alarm.

The third premise is true only if VO_2 and CaO_2 are constant, an unlikely occurrence in many critically ill patients but which may apply to patients who are stable. In addition, as noted above, not only may changes in cardiac output reflect appropriate autoregulatory adjustments, it also seems likely that any such change should be just a readily detectable using the measures mentioned above.

One useful role for SvO_2 is in situations such as severe tricuspid regurgitation where thermodilution measurement of cardiac output is likely to be inaccurate. If VO_2 is known, cardiac output may be calculated by measuring CaO_2 and CvO_2 and rearranging Equation 14.11 to solve for Q. If VO_2 cannot be measured, the validity of the thermodilution cardiac output measurement may be estimated by noting that the normal difference between arterial and venous O_2 contents is approximately 5 ml/dl. For normal hemoglobin value, SvO_2 should then be approximately 75%. The decrease in SvO_2 that occurs with decreases in hemoglobin concentrations is easily estimated. If the measured cardiac output is very high or low, yet SvO_2 is normal it is likely that there is an error in cardiac output measurement. Unfortunately, because VO_2 is so variable in the critically ill, a more precise estimate is not possible without directly measuring VO_2.

Conclusions

Because the equipment used to monitor the ECG, pressures and cardiac output has many limitations, it is important to understand the principles governing such equipment. However, many of the potential ambiguities can be resolved by asking the proper questions rather than by making multiple measurements on a schedule and calculating hemodynamic profiles. Such questions should be based on an understanding of the physiology and pathophysiology of the cardiovascular system.

Key references

Davis RF. Clinical comparison of automated ausculatory and oscillometric and catheter-transducer measurements of arterial pressure. J Clin Monit. 1985;1:114–19.

Dhainaut J-F BF, Monsallier JF, Villemant D et al. Bedside evaluation of right ventricular performance using a rapid computerized thermodilution method. Crit Care Med. 1987;148–52.

Ellis DM. Interpretation of beat-to-beat blood pressure values in the presence of ventilatory changes. J Clin Monit. 1985;1:65–70.

Gardner RM. Direct blood pressure measurement – dynamic response requirements. Anesthesiology 1981;54:227–36.

Haller M ZC, Briegel J, Forst H. Evaluation of a new continuous thermodilution cardiac output monitor in critically ill patients: a prospective criterion standard study. Crit Care Med. 1995;23:860–6.

Klienman B. Understanding natural frequency and damping and how they relate to the measurement of blood pressure. J Clin Monit. 1989;5:137–47.

Laupland KB BC. Utility of esophageal Doppler as a minimally invasive hemodynamic monitor: a review. Can J Anesth. 2002;49:393–401.

Maran AG. Variables in pulmonary capillary wedge pressure: variation with intrathoracic pressure, graphic and digital recorders. Crit Care Med. 1980;8:102–5.

McDonald DA. Blood flow in arteries, 2nd edn. Baltimore: Williams & Wilkins; 1974:356.

Ramsey M III. Blood pressure monitoring: automated oscillometric devices. J Clin Monit. 1991;7:56–67.

Summers RL SW, Peacock WF, Ander DS, Coleman TG. Bench to bedside: electrophysiologic and clinical principles of noninvasive hemodynamic monitoring using impedance cardiography. Acad Emerg Med. 2003;10:669–80.

van Lieshout JJ WK. Continuous cardiac output by pulse contour analysis? Br J Anaesth. 2001;86:467–9.

Yelderman M. Continuous measurement of cardiac output with the use of stochastic system identification techniques. J Clin Monit. 1990;6:322–32.

Further reading

Balik MPJ, Hendl J. Effect of the degree of tricuspid regurgitation on cardiac output measurements by thermodilution. Intensive Care Med. 2002;28:1117–21.

Bruner JMR, Krenis LJ, Kunsman JM, Sherman AP. Comparison of direct and indirect methods of measuring arterial blood pressure. Med Instrum. 1981;15:11–21.

Haller M, Zöllner C, Briegel J, Forst H. Evaluation of a new continuous thermodilution cardiac output monitor in critically ill patients: a prospective criterion standard study. Crit Care Med. 1995;23:860–6.

Hamilton WF. Measurement of the cardiac output. In: Handbook of physiology: Circulation. Vol. 1, Section 2. Wash-ington, DC: American Physiology Society; 1962:551–84.

Kaufmann MA, Pargger H, Drop LJ. Oscillometric blood pressure measurements by different devices are not interchangeable. Anesth Analg. 1996;82:377–81.

Ladin Z, Trautman E, Teplick R. Contribution of measurement system artifacts to systolic spikes. Med Instrum. 1983;17:110–2.

Posey JA, Geddes LA, Williams H, Moore AG. The meaning of the point of maximum oscillations in cuff pressures in the indirect measurement of blood pressure. Part I. Cardiovasc Res Bull. 1969;8:15–25.

Chapter 16

Monitoring of gas concentrations

Surinder PS Cheema

TOPICS COVERED IN THIS CHAPTER

- **General principles of measurement**
  - Data acquisition and analysis
  - Partial pressure and concentration
  - Analysers
- **Nonspecific methods**
  - Solubility
  - Thermal conductivity
  - Refractive index
- **Specific methods**
  - Magnetic susceptibility
  - Electrochemical analyzers
  - Absorption and emission of radiation
  - Raman spectroscopy
  - Gas chromatography
- **Capnography**
  - Phase I
  - Phase II
  - Phase III
  - Phase IV
- **Blood gas analysis**
  - Oxygen measurement
  - Measurement of carbon dioxide and pH

Current monitoring standards mandate the continuous measurement of O_2 and CO_2 in the respired gas of anesthetized patients. Analysis of O_2 with an audible alarm to detect a low fraction of inspired O_2 (F_IO_2) is particularly relevant in preventing the delivery of a hypoxic gas mixture to a patient. Continuous display of the exhaled CO_2 (capnogram) confirms intubation of the trachea and the adequacy of both ventilation and cardiac output. Agent monitoring, though not a universal standard of care, allows the identification of the inhaled agent, titration of the anesthetic dose, early detection of vapor depletion or of overdose, and provides evidence of elimination during emergence. A sharp rise in the fractional exhaled N_2 could arise from significant venous air embolism. In addition to the analysis of respired gases both O_2 and CO_2 can be measured in body tissues either in vivo or in vitro. Examples of in vivo measurements include pulse oximetry, transcutaneous oximetry, and near infrared spectroscopy. In contrast, arterial and mixed venous blood gas analysis is a common example of in vitro measurement.

Many different devices are available for measuring individual gases or vapors. Each deploys a physical or chemical property that may or may not be specific to the measured gas. Knowledge of the principles involved in the measurement is vital to the interpretation of gas analysis data and to the understanding of the uses and limitations of individual devices.

GENERAL PRINCIPLES OF MEASUREMENT

All devices have an inherent bias and instability that can be characterized and quantified. Consideration of a generalized model illustrates these operational problems. Figure 16.1a shows a generalized electrical measuring device consisting of a sample port, a sensor in the form of a transducer, and a display of the output of the transducer. In some devices there may be no output from the transducer when the substance to be measured is absent. In this instance no zero calibration is required. When an output is present in the absence of the substance to be measured, this output equates to the zero setting on the display. In addition to the zero calibration at least one further point is required to calibrate the device to encompass the expected range of measurements. In Figure16.1b the line A represents a calibration curve in which 0 and 10 units are the standards: it is assumed that the output of the device between these two points is linear. The sensitivity of the device can be increased by increasing the gain, as shown in curve B. After some time in use the output of the transducer may change in the absence of any change in the samples to be measured. This is referred to as drift, and is illustrated by curve C.

When a step change in the measured sample occurs, as in Figure 16.1c, no change is registered for some time. The change is eventually detected, and when a new equilibrium is reached the full extent of the change is displayed. The time taken to register 10% of the new value is referred to as the dead time (interval AB). The time taken to reach 90% of the final value from the initial 10% increase is the rise time (interval BC). The response time is the sum of the dead time and the rise time. The rise time is particularly important when a continuous graphic display of the output is required. The shorter the rise time the

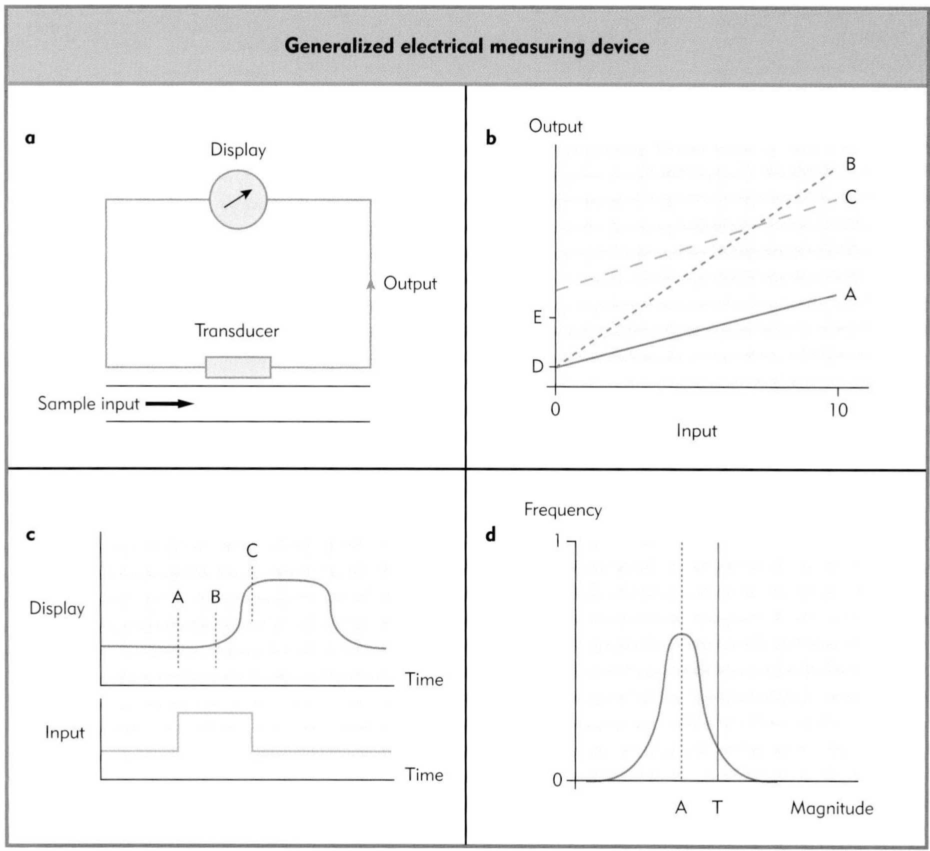

Figure 16.1 (a) Model of a generalized electrical measuring device. (b) On the calibration line A, the outputs D and E represent zero and 10 units, respectively. The device output is assumed to be linear between these points. Increasing the sensitivity increases the device's output for any given sample, as in line B. Continued use may result in drift, as in line C. (c) The inherent delay in displaying a change is shown by introducing a square wave change in the sample being analyzed. The period AB is the dead time and BC the rise time. The total AC is the response time. (d) Measurements on a sample taken with an ideal instrument yield the same correct value T on all occasions. A real instrument yields a spread of values centered on a mean value of A.

less the discrepancy between the displayed and the actual waveforms.

An ideal measuring device should yield the true value every time given the same sample on repeated occasions. This is represented on the frequency distribution by the line with a value of T and a frequency of 1 in Figure 16.1d. In reality a device may consistently under- or overread, as well as failing to produce a single value given the same sample on many occasions. This results in a distribution of measured values for the same sample with a mean and some spread on either side of the mean. The difference between the mean of the measured values (A) and the true value (T) is referred to as the accuracy of the device. The less the difference the greater the accuracy. The ability to reproduce the same measurement given the same sample on many occasions is represented by the spread of values about the mean and is a measure of the precision of the device. The less the spread of values the more reproducible are the measurements for a given sample and the greater the precision of the instrument.

Data acquisition and analysis

Modern gas analyzers function either by analyzing gas at the main breathing circuit (mainstream analyzers) or by extracting a gas sample via a small-bore tube and analyzing it away from the breathing circuit (sidestream analyzer, or diverting system). Currently, mainstream analyzers are used only to detect O_2 in the breathing circuit and CO_2 at the airway connection. Their advantages include the lack of any delay in measurements caused by transport (dead time), no need for a gas sampling line, and relatively easy maintenance. Disadvantages include the added weight at the airway, relative fragility, and the inability to identify other gases in the circuit.

Sidestream analyzers can analyze several gases simultaneously, provide minimum weight at the airway, and are durable. Disadvantages include transport delay time and susceptibility to obstruction of the gas sampling line by water and secretions.

Data can be displayed as concentration (% volumes) or partial pressure (mmHg or kPa: 1 mmHg ≡ 0.133 kPa). If the ambient partial pressure is known, concentration and partial pressures can be derived from measurement of one parameter.

Partial pressure and concentration

Systems that utilize infrared light (infrared spectrometry) or laser emission (Raman spectroscopy) measure the number of molecules of gas present in a mixture. Because pressure is dependent on the number of molecules, these systems identify the absolute partial pressure. When the ambient pressure is known, concentration can be derived as:

■ Equation 16.1
% volume = partial pressure/ambient pressure (mmHg).

If the ambient pressure differs from the value used for calibration of the instrument, the true concentration will be different from the one displayed. The following examples illustrate the importance of proper calibration. If the analyzer at sea level is calibrated to report as a fraction of 760 mmHg (dry gas) rather than at 713 mmHg (water-saturated alveolar gas), the device will overestimate the actual alveolar gas concentration. If the partial pressure of isoflurane is 7.6 mmHg, this would be reported as 1% by a system analyzer calibrated at sea level (ambient pressure of 760 mmHg). If the system is taken to a height of 2000 m above sea level, where the barometric pressure is 598 mmHg, the concentration displayed by this analyzer will still be 1%, although the actual value at this attitude should be 1.3% (7.6 mmHg = 1.3% of 598 mmHg). The system must also correct for the presence of water vapor (partial pressure 47 mmHg at sea level).

Systems that report values as concentration (%) identify components of a gas mixture and determine the percentage contributed by each gas to the total mixture. These systems do not measure partial pressure; using a value for ambient pressure allows calculation of the corresponding partial pressure. Unidentified gases are not recognized, and therefore their presence will artificially elevate the concentration of the remaining components in the mixture. For example, in a patient receiving 1% isoflurane in 100% O_2, the addition of 50% helium, which is not recognized by the system, will artificially elevate the reported concentration of isoflurane to 2%, as the values are read in half the volume of gas. In contrast, a Raman spectroscopy analyzer will provide accurate values by reading the partial pressure of each anesthetic gas.

Analyzers

A wide range of chemical and physical properties is deployed in the measurement of gases and vapors. When the property is nonspecific the instrument quantifies a single agent from a mixture of known composition. In contrast, specific properties allow the agent to be both identified and quantified.

Chemical methods are used primarily for measuring the concentration of O_2 and CO_2 in samples of respiratory gases. The alkalis potassium hydroxide and pyrogallol are used to absorb CO_2 and O_2, respectively, from a sample. Measurement of the reduction in volume allows calculation of the concentration of each gas. With the modified Haldane apparatus accuracies of ± 0.05% (CO_2) and ± 0.1% (O_2) can be achieved.

Physical properties may be unique to a gas or nonspecific. Nonspecific properties are common to all gases and vapors and cannot be used to identify a gas within a mixture. However, when one gas in a mixture has a nonspecific property significantly different from the others, this may be useful in measuring the concentration or partial pressure of that gas. Examples of nonspecific properties used for measurement purposes include solubility, density, viscosity, thermal conductivity, refractive index, and the velocity of sound in a gas.

Specific properties allow the identification of individual components of a mixture as well as quantification. Examples of these properties include the absorption or emission of radiation of a particular wavelength, atomic nuclear properties, susceptibility to a magnetic field, and the conduction of electricity in response to an applied voltage (polarography).

NONSPECIFIC METHODS

Solubility

A quartz crystal contracts slightly when subjected to a potential difference, a phenomenon known as the piezoelectric effect. An alternating voltage of appropriate frequency can make the crystal vibrate at the resonant frequency. In a commercially available device called the 'Emma' a quartz crystal with a thin covering of oil is exposed to the gas to be analyzed. Anesthetic vapor dissolves in the oil layer and changes the resonant frequency of the crystal. The shift in the resonant frequency is related to the amount of vapor dissolved in the oil layer, and in turn to the partial pressure of the vapor through Henry's law. The monitor cannot distinguish different vapors and must be calibrated for a selected agent.

Thermal conductivity

A gas with a high thermal conductivity conducts heat more rapidly than one with a low conductivity. This property is utilized in a katharometer. The device consists of a wire heated by an electrical current and held in a cell through which sample gas is passed at a constant rate. Cooling of the wire by the gas lowers the resistance, which in turn is measured with a Wheatstone bridge. A separate reference chamber containing the gases not being analyzed within the mixture allows the instrument to be zeroed and calibrated. The thermal conductivities of O_2 and N_2 are very similar, and this makes the analysis of one in the presence of the other difficult. Helium and CO_2 have high thermal conductivities, and these can be measured in the presence of either O_2 or N_2 or both. Helium concentrations can be measured to an accuracy of ± 0.01%. Breath-by-breath analysis of CO_2 can also be achieved with appropriate modifications to reduce the rise time. These include a small-volume analysis chamber and a low pressure of gas within the chamber.

Refractive index

The velocity of light in a vacuum is 3×10^8 m/s but falls to 2.3×10^8 m/s in water. The refractive index (a measure of the optical density) of water is 1.3 (3×10^8 m/s ÷ 2.3×10^8 m/s). For gases and vapors the optical density is less than that of water and is dependent on the concentration. The change in the velocity of light on passing through two media of different optical densities can be detected by the pattern of interference using a refractometer. Light from a monochromatic light source is split into two paths. One passes through a cell containing the sample gas, and the other passes through an identical cell containing reference gas. In the Rayleigh refractometer, a laboratory instrument, these cells take the form of two tubes 2 m in length. Light emerging from each cell passes through a small rectangular prism and is then recombined and focused in the eyepiece. If both cells contain the same gas, a series of alternating light and dark bands is seen through the eyepiece as a result of interference, and the optical path length is the same through both limbs of the instrument. However, when the analyzing chamber is filled with sample gas, light emerging from the gas chambers is no longer in phase. The interference pattern is seen to move to the right or the left. Of the two rectangular prisms, one is fixed and the other can be rotated on a Vernier scale. By rotating this prism the optical path length through one limb can be increased or decreased, thereby bringing the two light beams back into phase and restoring the reference pattern of interference. At constant temperature and pressure the rotation of the prism can be calibrated to give the concentration of a particular gas within a known mixture of gases. In the Rayleigh refractometer the reference interference pattern is displayed below the variable pattern so that the two can be matched exactly. This is possible because the original light beam is split into more than two paths. One pair is used for generating the reference pattern, and the other two are used to make the measurement. Refractometers are used principally for the calibration of vaporizers.

SPECIFIC METHODS

Magnetic susceptibility

Most gases, including nitrogen, are repelled by a magnetic field by virtue of their molecular structure, a property referred to as diamagnetism. The two unpaired electrons in the outermost orbital of oxygen result in the molecule being attracted into a magnetic field, and this is referred to as paramagnetism.

Paramagnetic analyzers consist of two identical glass spheres filled with a weakly diamagnetic gas such as N_2 and linked by a short rod. The rod is fixed firmly across a taut wire so that the spheres are free to rotate. The assembly is held inside a cell into which a gas sample can be introduced. The cell in turn lies between the poles of a strong magnet. When O_2 is introduced into the cell it is attracted into the magnetic field, forcing the spheres to rotate from the resting position. In the simplest instrument described by Pauling this rotation is measured by the deflection of a light beam from a small mirror attached to the suspension wire, as shown in Figure 16.2a. The deflected light beam falls upon a translucent scale calibrated from 0 to 100%. The instrument is delicate, and suffers from nonlinearity introduced by nonlinear variations in the strength of the magnetic field and the torque in the suspension wire. These problems are avoided in the Null deflection analyzer (Fig. 16.2b). A small coil through which a current can be passed is attached to the suspension wire, generating a force that counters the rotation of the spheres. The translucent scale is replaced by two photocells and the difference in the output of these is used to generate a current, which precisely counters the rotation of the spheres. The size of the current is proportional to the O_2 concentration. Although null deflection analyzers are accurate to within 0.1% they are prone to interference from water vapor, external vibrations, variations in pressure produced by ventilators, and high flow rates through the analysis chamber. Further improvements in the design have overcome these problems and reduced the response time to 150 ms, as in the Rapid paramagnetic analyzer.

All gases and vapors can be made susceptible to a magnetic field by imposing an electrical charge on the molecules. This is the principle of the mass spectrometer (Fig. 16.3). Molecules of gas in a sample are ionized by bombardment with a stream of electrons. The ionized particles are accelerated through a strong magnetic field towards an electrically charged plate. The magnetic field then deflects the particles on to a row of sensors. The degree of deflection is a function of the mass-to-charge ratio at any given velocity. In practice, the intensity of the magnetic field can be varied by the size of the current that flows through the electromagnets and the velocity of the particles controlled by the voltage on the plate, to which the particles are attracted and accelerated. By carefully adjusting these variables the trajectory of a specific atomic species can be adjusted such that it falls upon a single sensor. The Quadrupole mass spectrometer uses four electromagnets that select out sequentially chosen chemical species and direct them on to a sensor. All gases and vapors can be identified and measured after calibration. However, the mass spectrometer functions as a proportion system and assumes that all gases have been detected; therefore, an unidentified gas in the mixture will artificially elevate the concentration of the detected agents.

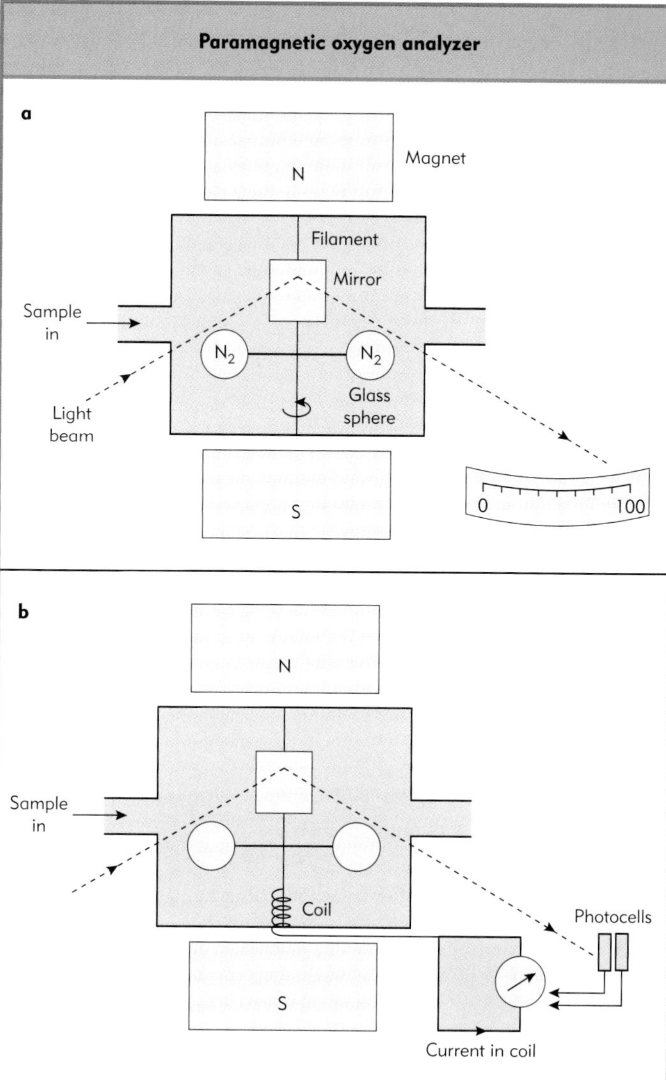

Figure 16.2 (a) Pauling-type paramagnetic oxygen analyzer. (b) Null deflection-type paramagnetic oxygen analyzer.

Electrochemical analyzers

Oxidation is defined as the removal of electrons, and a chemical that accepts electrons is an oxidizing agent. This principle is employed in the polarographic, oxygen or Clarke electrode, and in the fuel cell.

In the polarographic electrode a small voltage of 0.6 V is applied to two electrodes immersed in a buffered potassium chloride electrolyte solution. A current flows, which is proportional to the concentration of O_2 in the electrolyte. Electrons at the platinum cathode react with O_2 and water, generating hydroxyl ions:

■ Equation 16.2

$$O_2 + 4e^- + 2H_2O \rightarrow 4(OH)^-$$

A magnetic sector respiratory mass spectrometer

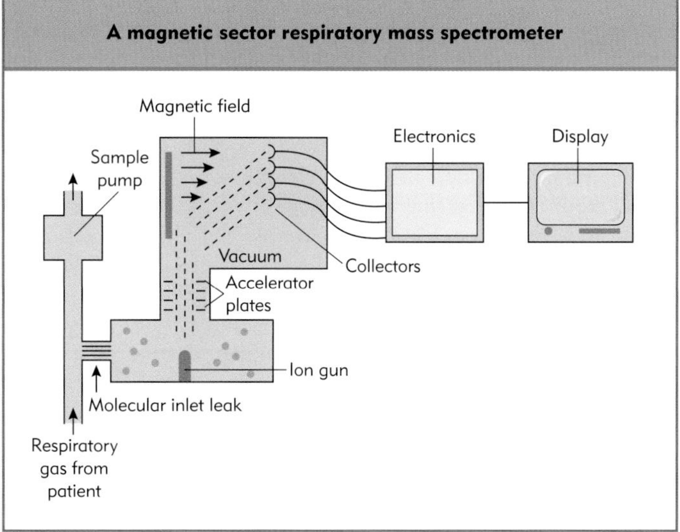

Figure16.3 A magnetic sector respiratory mass spectrometer. Gas molecules enter a vacuum chamber (through the molecular inlet leak) where they are ionized and electrically accelerated. The mass and charge of the ions determine their trajectory in a deflecting magnetic field, and metal dish collectors are placed to detect them. The electrical currents produced by the ions impacting on the collectors are processed and the results are displayed. (With permission from Raemer DB. Monitoring respiratory function. In: Rogers MC, Tinker JH, Covino BG, Longnecker DE, ed. Principles and practice of anesthesiology. St Louis, MO: Mosby; 1992.)

At the silver–silver chloride anode, silver is oxidized to silver chloride:

■ Equation 16.3

$$4Ag \rightarrow 4Ag^+ + 4e^-$$
$$4Ag^+ + 4Cl^- \rightarrow 4AgCl$$

Figure 16.4a shows diagrammatically an oxygen electrode. The output of 7.5×10^{-11}A/$KPaO_2$ is extremely small and depends upon the size of the platinum cathode, the polarizing voltage, the temperature, and the type of membrane used. The membrane, typically polypropylene, protects the electrode from blood and gas samples.

The fuel cell, as the name implies, generates a small potential difference, much like a battery, but differs in that the output is dependent on the concentration of O_2 present and the temperature. The redox reactions that generate this potential difference are illustrated in Figure16.4b. Lead and electrolyte are consumed when O_2 is present, and these are eventually depleted. Nevertheless, most modern fuel cells last 6–12 months. A thermistor is usually incorporated to provide temperature compensation.

Polarographic electrode and fuel cell

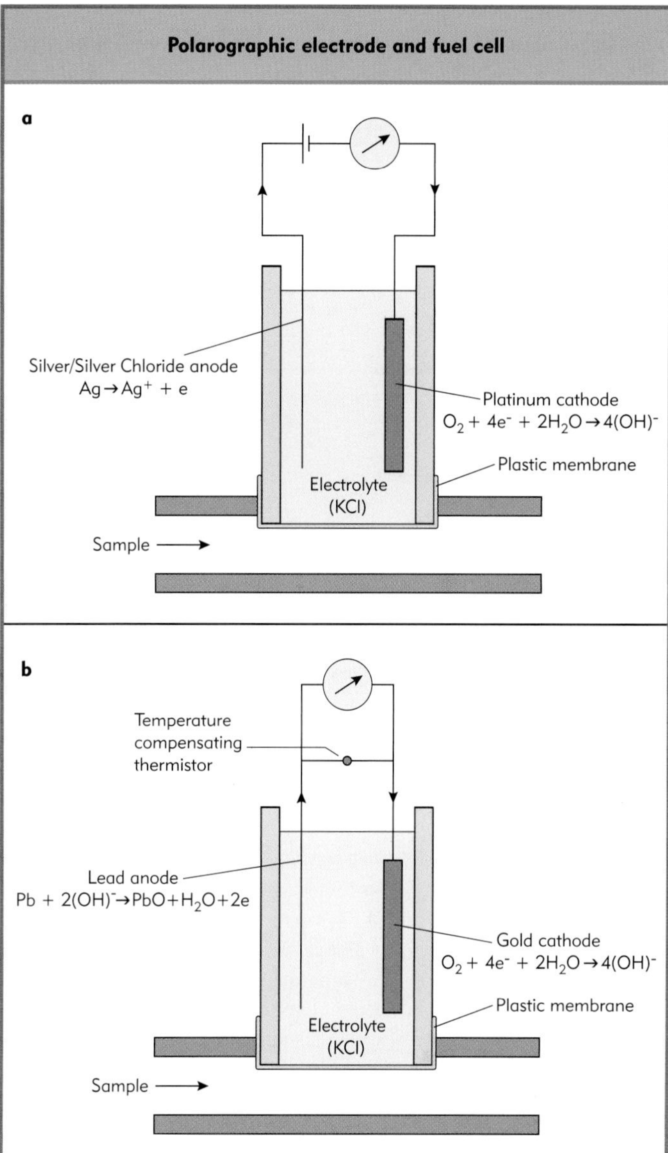

Figure 16.4 (a) A diagrammatic polarographic electrode. (b) A diagrammatic fuel cell.

Absorption and emission of radiation

All gases and vapors, when energized, will emit electromagnetic radiation in the ultraviolet, visible, or infrared parts of the spectrum. These discrete bands of radiation form an emission spectrum characteristic of an individual gas. Conversely, specific wavelengths of radiation are absorbed by an individual gas from a broad spectrum of radiation, forming an absorption spectrum (Fig.16.5).

The N_2 meter is the only example of an emission-based instrument. A sample of gas is drawn by a pump into a glass discharge tube which has an electrode at each end. Gas in the tube is energized by the application of a voltage of up to 2000 V to the electrodes. Electrons in the nitrogen molecules are excited into higher energy levels, from which they return rapidly back to the resting state. The excess energy is emitted as light of specific wavelengths, which is focused on to a photoelectric cell. A filter removes the nonspecific wavelengths before the light intensity is measured. Linearizing circuits are incorporated into the meter, as the measured light intensity is not proportional to the concentration of N_2. Advantages of the instrument include a high specificity and a rapid response time of 20–40 ms.

Absorption of electromagnetic radiation is widely used for the measurement of anesthetic and respiratory gases. Molecules with two or more dissimilar atoms absorb radiation mainly in the infrared (1–15 μm) part of the spectrum. Water, CO_2, N_2O and volatile agents all have significant dipoles and can be detected and measured; O_2 and N_2 are nonpolar and are not detected. These analyzers measure partial pressure, as the absorption

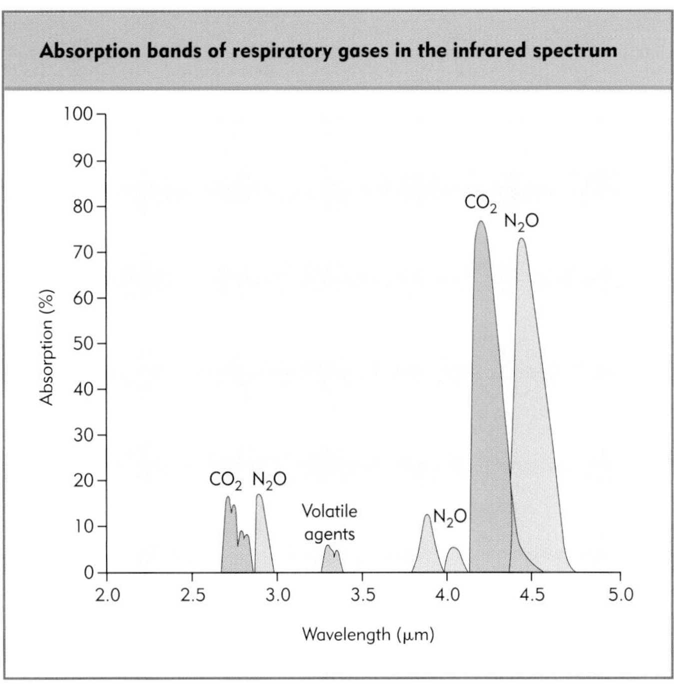

Figure 16.5 Absorption spectra of common anesthetic gases and vapors. (With permission from Raemer, 1992.)

of infrared light depends on the number of molecules. The potential overlap between gases with very similar infrared absorption characteristics (e.g. CO_2 4.3 μm, N_2O 4.4 μm, and most volatile agents) has required analyzers with better resolution of absorption peaks to allow the separation of various compounds. Infrared analyzers may be either dispersive or nondispersive.

In the dispersive type the light is split into a spectrum either with a prism or by diffraction. The light emerging from an analyzing chamber is scanned to detect the wavelengths that have been absorbed, and by applying the Beer–Lambert law the degree of absorption can be related to the concentration of the gas. The infrared spectrophotometer is an example of a dispersive device, and because it produces an absorption spectrum it can be used to measure many different gases. When only one gas in a known mixture is to be measured a nondispersive analyzer is used.

Nondispersive analyzers use a narrow band of infrared light to detect a specific gas. The degree of absorption by the target gas can be quantified by one of several different techniques. In the Luft type analyzer the detector is in the form of a diaphragm, which acts as a pressure transducer. Gas in the analyzing and reference chambers absorbs light to different extents, owing to the difference in the concentration of the gas being measured. Light from the reference and analyzing chambers is of different intensities and falls upon two detector cells separated by a diaphragm. The detector cells are filled with the gas to be analyzed and are hermetically sealed. Absorption of this light results in differential warming and expansion of the gas in the detector cells, resulting in displacement of the diaphragm. In practice the gas in the detector cells is prevented from continuous warming by interruption of the light in the system by a rotating disk with a slit or chopper. Typically light falls upon the detector cells at a frequency of 25–100 Hz, producing a pulsatile output from the detectors. The pulsatile expansion and contraction produced by an intermittent infrared source can also be detected with a microphone, as in photoacoustic spectroscopy (PAS). These devices are designed to measure several gases simultaneously. Each gas is measured by infrared light of a specific wavelength, which is switched on and off by a chopper at a frequency unique to that wavelength. The frequency of the sound from the detecting microphone identifies the gas and the amplitude the concentration. Compared with the detection of light using photoelectric cells, the PAS system has greater zero and gain stability, so that calibration is required at 3-monthly intervals. The response time is also very rapid, with a rise time typically of the order of 300 ms, making possible continuous breath-by-breath measurements.

Overlap of the absorption maxima of different gases leads to errors in measurement. In the case of CO_2, N_2O, and CO these are 4.3, 4.5, and 4.7 μm, respectively. The use of optical filters can narrow down the wavelength band. An alternative method employs a cell filled with the gas producing the interference, placed in the light path to eliminate the effect of that gas. A further source of error is produced by a change in the absorption spectrum of a gas by the physical presence of another. This 'collision or pressure broadening' widens the absorption spectrum of the measured gas, leading to overestimation of the true partial pressure. Calibration with mixtures of gases that are the same as those to be analyzed corrects for pressure broadening.

Raman spectroscopy

Gas molecules in the path of a light beam scatter the photons so that the emergent light intensity is less than that of the incident beam. The photons in the emergent light are identical to those in the incident light, but their direction of travel has been altered by the gas molecules. This is referred to as Rayleigh scattering. Some gas molecules absorb part of the energy of an incident photon and re-emit this as a photon of a different wavelength. This phenomenon, first observed by Raman in 1928, produces scattered light of a wavelength unique to each gas. Raman scattered light has an intensity less than one-millionth of the incident light. Sufficient quantities of Raman scattered light are produced only if the incident light is monochromatic and of very high intensity. This is achieved with an argon laser, making the instrument expensive and a heavy consumer of electrical power.

Gas chromatography

The components of a mixture are more easily identified and quantified once separated into pure samples. The separation and purification is achieved by the technique of chromatography – literally, writing in color. Liquid chromatography allows the separation of dissolved solids and liquids, and gas chromatography separates the components of a mixture of gases. The principles are the same. A gas chromatogram consists of a long tube packed with beads of silica–alumina coated with polyethylene glycol or silicone oil – the stationary phase. Through this, an inert carrier gas, typically nitrogen, argon, or helium, is passed at a constant rate (the mobile phase), thereby moving a sample of gas along the column. Depending on their physical properties, each component of the mixture partitions between the stationary and the mobile phase. Those that dissolve preferentially in the oil of the stationary phase progress along the column slowly, whereas those that are retained in the carrier gas pass along

Table 16.1 Summary of techniques of anesthetic gas and vapor analysis

Techniques	Gases detected				
	O_2	CO_2	N_2O	VA	N_2
IR light spectroscopy		X	X	X	
IR photoacoustic		X	X	X	
Mass spectroscopy	X	X	X	X	X
Raman spectroscopy	X	X	X	X	X
Chromatography	X	X	X	X	X
Polarography	X				
Fuel cell	X				
Paramagnetic	X				
Piezoelectric resonance				X	

VA, volatile anesthetic

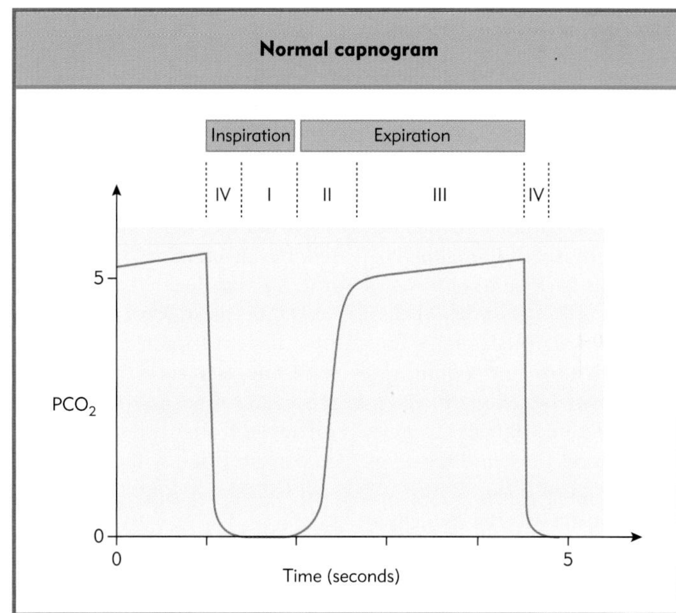

Figure 16.6 Normal capnogram. (Adapted with permission from Raemer DB. Monitoring respiratory function. In: Rogers MC, Tinker JH, Covino BG, Longnecker DE, ed. Principles and practice of anesthesiology. St Louis, MO: Mosby; 1992.)

quickly. The components of a mixture emerge from the chromatogram at different times. The time taken is unique, and identifies the gas or vapor. Calibration of a chromatogram by passing pure samples of each gas to be measured establishes the time to a peak for that gas. The magnitude of each peak is related to the concentration of that component in the original sample, and is measured by one of three techniques: flame ionization, thermal conductivity, or electron capture. Chromatography does not allow continuous measurement, but is very versatile. Many gases, vapors, and drugs in blood samples can be measured even in trace quantities. Table 16.1 summarizes the measurement of common respiratory gases and anesthetic vapors.

CAPNOGRAPHY

A device that measures and displays the numeric value of the inspired ($P_{I}CO_2$) and end-tidal ($P_{ET}CO_2$) carbon dioxide partial pressures is called a capnometer. Current standards of monitoring during anesthesia require a continuous display of the partial pressure of CO_2 in the respired gas against time, i.e. a capnograph. A normal capnograph is divided into two inspiratory phases (IV and I) and two expiratory phases (II and III), as in Figure 16.6. Gas sampled in the inspiratory phase is derived from the breathing system. Phase II gas represents anatomical dead-space gas and phase III alveolar gas. Morphology of the capnograph provides much information concerning the interaction of alveolar ventilation, pulmonary blood flow, and the rate of CO_2 production.

Phase I

Under normal circumstances there is no CO_2 in the inspired air. An elevated phase I implies rebreathing, which may arise from an inadequate fresh gas flow rate or a rise in the respiratory rate when a T-piece breathing system is in use. In the case of a circle system, depletion of the CO_2 absorbant, channeling through the absorber, or sticking of the expiratory valve in the open position results in the same effect.

Phase II

Elimination of anatomical dead-space gas is normally rapid, resulting in an almost vertical upstroke in phase II. Phase II becomes more prolonged if expiration is slowed by an obstruction in the expiratory limb of the breathing system, endotracheal tube, laryngeal mask airway, or intrathoracic airway. Obstruction of the sample line of a sidestream analyzer or a prolonged rise time can have a similar effect.

Phase III

This phase is characterized by a gentle upstroke of the capnogram arising from the normal V/Q mismatch in the lung. The gradient increases if V/Q mismatch worsens. A representative $P_{ET}CO_2$ is obtained only if expiration is not prematurely terminated and alveolar gas is not diluted with breathing system gas. The presence of a normal phase III confirms tracheal intubation and the adequacy of both alveolar ventilation and cardiac output.

Phase IV

The beginning of inspiration is marked by a rapid fall in the PCO_2, as inspired gas is normally free of CO_2. An obstruction to inspiration, a slow sampling rate, or an inadequate fresh gas flow rate in a T-piece breathing system prolongs this phase.

BLOOD GAS ANALYSIS

Respired gases can be measured in vitro in samples of blood taken anaerobically, or in vivo.

Oxygen measurement

Oxygenation can be assessed by measurement of O_2 tension, hemoglobin saturation, or O_2 content; all three are interrelated via the oxygen dissociation curve.

Oxygen tension is measured in vitro with an oxygen (Clark) electrode in a blood gas analyzer. The electrode can be miniaturized and applied to the skin with a contact gel that provides an airtight seal. The skin is heated by an element within the electrode to a temperature of 43°C so that local tissue blood flow increases, oxygen diffusion is more rapid, and measurements are made at a constant temperature. Oxygen in capillary blood diffuses and equilibrates with the electrode, yielding a transcutaneous oxygen partial pressure ($tcPO_2$), an in vivo measurement. Barriers to oxygen diffusion from capillaries, local tissue blood flow, and tissue oxygen consumption will determine the measured value of the $tcPO_2$, which can be expected to be less than the arterial PO_2 (P_aO_2).

Measurement of the oxygen content of blood is referred to as oximetry. The total O_2 content of whole blood is the sum of the dissolved component and that bound to haemoglobin:

■ Equation 16.4

$$CO_2 = (SO_2/100 \times Hb \times Hf) + \alpha\, PO_2$$

where CO_2 is the total content of whole blood, Hb the hemoglobin concentration, $SO_2/100$ the percentage of hemoglobin saturated with O_2, *Hf* is the Hufner factor (1.39 mL/g) and α (0.0031 mL/mmHg at 37°C) is the solubility coefficient of oxygen.

The CO_2 of whole blood can be measured directly with the Lex-O_2-Con apparatus, which employs the fuel cell principle. However, as oxyhemoglobin alone contributes by far the largest proportion of O_2 to the total O_2 content, the measurement of SO_2 has become common in clinical practice. The noninvasive in vivo measurement of hemoglobin saturation is referred to as pulse oximetry (SpO_2). The technique is based on the differences in the absorption spectra of different hemoglobin species (Fig. 16.7). Reduced (Hb) and oxyhemoglobin (HbO_2) have the same absorbance at certain wavelengths known as isobestic points, e.g. 805 nm, but at 625 nm the difference is maximal. Hemoglobin concentration measured at isobestic points measures the total concentration. At a wavelength close to 625 nm the absorbance depends upon the ratio of Hb to HbO_2. Values of the absorbance at two different wavelengths, one of which is at isobestic point, can be used to solve a series of simultaneous equations that give the concentrations of Hb and HbO_2. The percentage saturation is then calculated: $HbO_2/Hb + HbO_2$. In practice, light of the appropriate wavelength is generated by LEDs and a microprocessor rejects the nonpulsatile component of the absorbance so that only the pulsatile values are computed (pulse oximetry) (Fig. 16.8). The reported saturation represents that of arterial blood and is denoted as Sp_aO_2 to indicate the method of measurement. Most pulse oximeters measure to an accuracy of ±2% over the range 70–100%. Laboratory-based oximeters require a sample of whole blood taken anaerobically and make several absorbance measurements at specific wavelengths, depending on the absorption spectra of individual hemoglobin species. Thus the SO_2 and the concentration of other clinically relevant hemoglobin species, such as carboxy- and methemoglobin, can be measured.

Measurement of carbon dioxide and pH

Carbon dioxide dissolved in solution exerts a partial pressure (PCO_2), which can be measured indirectly by measuring the pH, as CO_2 reacts with water to form carbonic acid:

■ Equation 16.5

$$CO_2 + H_2O \Leftrightarrow H_2CO_3 \Leftrightarrow H^+ + HCO_3^-$$

The logarithm of the hydrogen concentration is related to the logarithm of the PCO_2. The change in pH that occurs with a change in the PCO_2 is measured by the Severinghaus CO_2 electrode. An

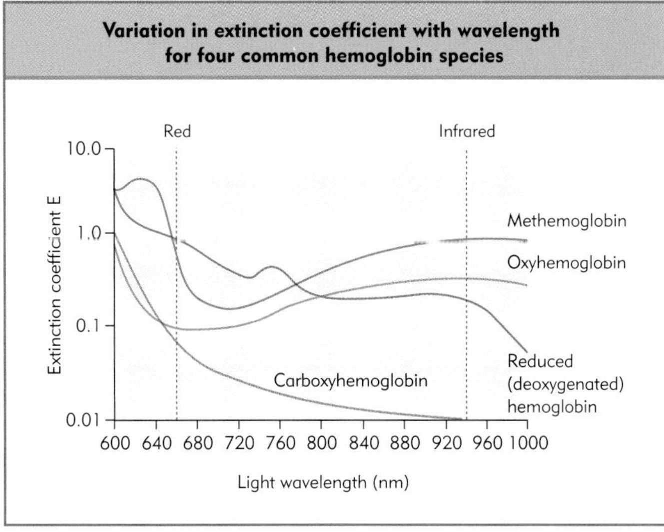

Figure 16.7 Variation in extinction coefficient with wavelength for four common hemoglobin species. The absorbance of carboxyhemoglobin is very similar to that of oxyhemoglobin in the visible red wavelengths. Methemoglobin has a high absorbance over a broad spectrum, giving it a characteristic brown color. (From Tremper KK, Barker SJ. Pulse oximetry: applications and limitations. In: Tremper KK, Barker SJ, eds. International anesthesiology clinics. Advances in oxygen monitoring. Boston, MA: Little, Brown; 1987:155-175.)

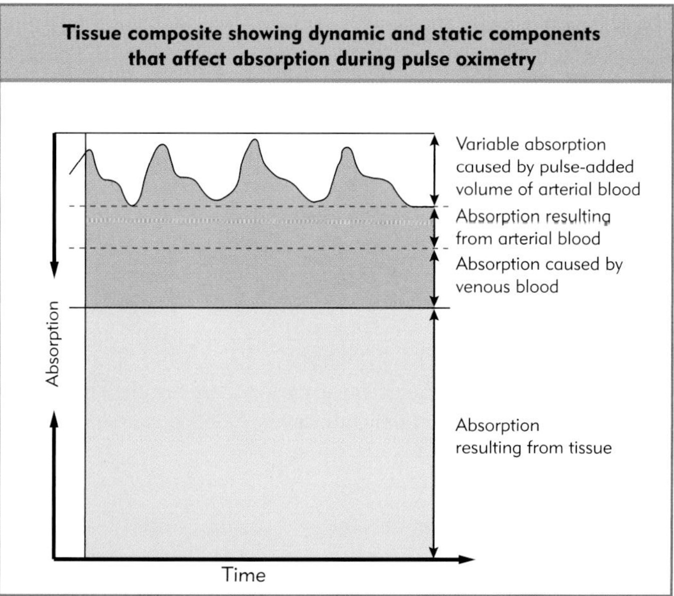

Figure 16.8 Tissue composite showing dynamic and static components that affect light absorption during pulse oximetry. (Adapted from Ohmeda 3700, Pulse oximeter users manual: Copyright© Datex-Ohmeda 1999.)

electrode rests within a blind-ending capillary of pH-sensitive glass. The assembly is immersed in a solution of sodium bicarbonate, which in turn is separated from the sample to be analyzed by a Teflon membrane. Carbon dioxide in the fluid sample diffuses through the Teflon membrane and equilibrates with the solution of bicarbonate. The change in pH sets up a voltage difference between the inside of the glass capillary and the bicarbonate solution outside. At 37°C each 0.1 kPa of CO_2 changes the pH by 0.01. The electrode has to be calibrated with known concentrations of CO_2 and the results expressed as a partial pressure, with appropriate correction for the saturated vapor pressure (SVP) of water at body temperature and for the barometric pressure:

■ Equation 16.6

$$P\text{CO}_2 = (\text{CO}_2 \text{ concentration})/100 \times (\text{barometric pressure} - \text{SVP of water})$$

When 5% CO_2 is used for calibration the instrument should read 4.7 kPa, given that the barometric pressure is 100 kPa and the SVP of water at 37°C is 6.3 kPa.

A miniaturized version of the CO_2 electrode can be used to measure transcutaneous $P\text{CO}_2$. When the arterial $P\text{CO}_2$ is 5.3 kPa the transcutaneous $P\text{CO}_2$ is respectively 2.6 kPa and 3.3 kPa greater in neonates and adults. The relatively slow response time, long set-up time, lack of established physiological norms, and the need to maintain skin temperature up to 44°C has limited the use of this technology.

The pH of a sample of blood is measured against a reference solution of constant pH from which the sample is separated by a glass membrane selectively permeable to hydrogen ions. A difference in pH across the pH-sensitive glass generates a small electromotive force (EMF), which can be measured with a voltmeter of high internal impedance. However, the electrical connections from the voltmeter to the reference and sample solutions also generate small EMFs; this is because whenever a metal makes contact with another dissimilar conductor an EMF is generated across the junction. In the pH electrode the reference solution is connected to one pole of the voltmeter via a silver–silver chloride electrode. The unknown sample is connected to the other pole via a Calomel ($Hg:Hg_2Cl_2$) electrode. The Calomel electrode connects indirectly to the sample through a porous plug filled with a saturated solution of potassium chloride. These electrodes generate a known EMF which, under constant physical conditions, is stable, so that the only variable in the completed circuit is the voltage across the pH-sensitive glass. At 37°C the pH electrode has a sensitivity of 60 mV per unit of pH. The electrode is calibrated with two buffers, one with a pH of 6.841, the same as the reference solution within the electrode. This provides an arbitrary zero. The second has a pH of 7.383, and this establishes a calibration curve. All blood gas analyzers measure at 37°C, but the core temperature of the patient may be different. Both blood gases and pH need to be corrected to the patient's temperature. The effect of changes in temperature on pure solutions of chemicals and gases can be predicted by laws of physics, but body fluids are complex and contain many other organic and inorganic compounds. These cause deviations from the predicted behavior and necessitate empirically derived corrections. An example of an algorithm used to correct pH is that of Rosenthal:

■ Equation 16.7

$$\text{pH}_{(\text{body temp})} = \text{pH}_{(37°\text{C})} - 0.0147(\text{Body temp°C} - 37)$$

Kelman and Nunn have produced algorithms that correct to body temperature, values of $P\text{O}_2$ and $P\text{CO}_2$ measured at 37°C. A detailed account of disturbances of acid–base balance is beyond the scope of this chapter.

Key references

Davis PD, Kenny GNC. Basic physics and measurement in anaesthesia, 5th edn. Edinburgh: Butterworth–Heinemann; 2003.

Gravenstein D, Lampotang S, Huda W, Sultan A. Basic principles of optical radiation and some common applications in anesthesia. J Clin Monit. 1996;12:445–54.

Moyle JTB. Pulse oximetry: principles and practice. London: BMJ Publishing; 1994.

O'Flaherty D. Capnography: principles and practice. London: BMJ Publishing; 1994.

Stock MC. Capnography for adults. Crit Care Clin. 1995;11:219–32.

Sykes MK, Vickers MD, Hull CJ et al. Principles of measurement and monitoring in anaesthesia and intensive care, 3rd edn. Oxford: Blackwell Scientific; 1991.

Further reading

Ganter M, Zollinger A. Continuous intravascular blood gas monitoring: development, current techniques, and clinical use of a commercial device. Br J Anaesth. 2003;91:397–407.

Owen-Reece H, Smith M, Elwell CE, Goldstone JC. Near infrared spectroscopy. Br J Anaesth. 1999;82:418–26

Chapter 17

Ultrasonography

Nikolaos Skubas

TOPICS COVERED IN THIS CHAPTER

- **Sound waves and ultrasound**
- **Interaction of ultrasound with tissue**
- **Pulsed ultrasound and real-time scanning**
- **The ultrasound transducer and beam**
- **Biological effects of ultrasound**
- **Display formats**
- **Imaging artifacts**
- **Doppler echocardiography**
  - Principles
  - Clinical applications
- **Transcranial Doppler**
- **Vessel cannulation**
- **Regional anesthesia**
- **Cardiac function evaluation**

SOUND WAVES AND ULTRASOUND

Sound waves are vibrations comprising alternate compressions (areas with tightly packed molecules) and rarefactions (areas where molecules are spaced apart). Vacuum cannot conduct sound. Sound is depicted as a sine wave with a temporal (duration or period, seconds) and a spatial (wavelength, λ, cm) dimension. Frequency (f, Hz) is the number of sound waves in 1 s, with period $\times f = 1$. Speed (c, m/s) is the velocity of sound through the carrying medium (for the human body, $c \approx 1540$ m/s). As $c = f \times \lambda$, frequency and wavelength are inversely related, so that as the frequency increases the wavelength decreases. This relationship is important in echocardiographic imaging, as greater resolution is produced by smaller wavelengths whereas deeper penetration is accomplished by longer wavelengths. The medium determines the velocity of the sound, so that sounds of different frequencies travel at the same speed in the same medium. The ability to transmit sound is called acoustic impedance (Z) and is related to the density of the tissue (ρ): $Z = \rho \times c$. In general, as the density of a medium increases, the velocity also increases (for example, sound travels faster through bone than through liquids). The amplitude ('strength') of a sound wave is its peak pressure and is measured in dB, where 1 dB = 20 × log (measured sound pressure/reference pressure, where reference pressure = 2×10^{-4} dyn × cm^{-2}). Accordingly, if the measured sound pressure is twice as strong as the reference pressure, its amplitude is 6 dB (20 × log2), and if 100 times stronger its amplitude is 40 dB. Power (in Watts) is the rate of work performed by the sound wave. Power diminishes as sound travels through the body. Intensity (or loudness) is the power of the sound wave in an area (W/cm^2).

Greater resolution requires smaller wavelengths, whereas deeper tissue penetration requires longer wavelengths.

Audible sound has frequencies between 20 and 20 000 Hz, and sound with a frequency higher than 20 kHz is termed ultrasound. Clinical ultrasound has frequencies ranging from 1 to 10 MHz, and because of its very short wavelength is easily manipulated: steered, focused, and directed to a specific target.

INTERACTION OF ULTRASOUND WITH TISSUE

The echocardiographic examination depends on, and is affected by, the interaction of ultrasound with living tissue. These interactions are described by the terms reflection, scattering, refraction, and attenuation.

The basis of diagnostic ultrasound imaging is the reflection of the transmitted ultrasound signal by an interface between media of different acoustic impedances (Fig. 17.1). The amount of reflected ultrasound energy is proportional to the difference in acoustic impedance of the two media (the greater the acoustic mismatch, the greater the amount of sound reflected). Optimal return (maximal reflection) occurs when ultrasound strikes the interface perpendicularly (the angle of incidence is 90°), whereas at any other angle of incidence less energy is reflected. Thus, the amplitude of the recorded (reflected) echo is a function of both the acoustic mismatch and the angle of incidence at the interface. A mechanical aortic prosthesis or a calcified aortic valve creates a brighter echocardiographic image than a native aortic valves because metal and calcium have greater acoustic impedance than normal human tissue (and reflect ultrasound better). Furthermore, an aortic mechanical valve creates a

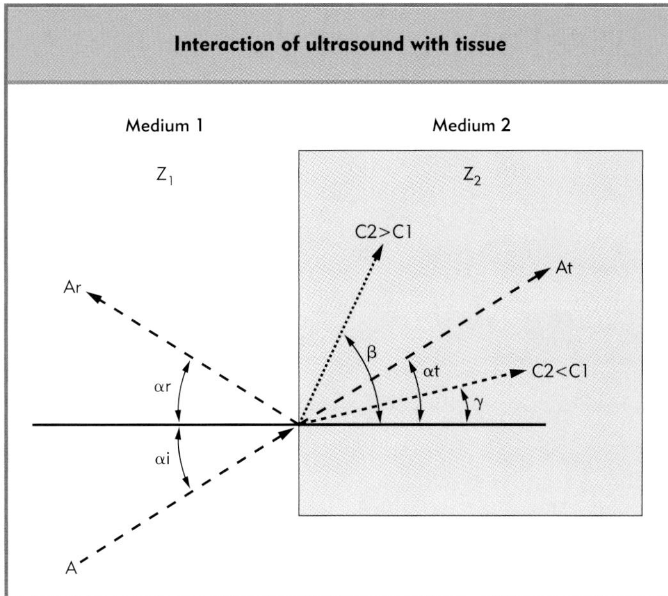

Figure 17.1 Interaction of ultrasound with tissue. A large and smooth interface that separates two media with the same acoustic impedance will let an incident sound wave (A) travel unimpeded (At) through the second medium. However, if the media have different acoustic impedances (Z1≠Z2), the incident ultrasound wave (A) will be reflected (Ar) at an angle αr = αi. The portion of the ultrasound energy of the incident wave A that was not reflected will be transmitted through the second medium at an altered (refracted) direction. If the sound propagation velocity is faster in the second medium (C2>C1), the refraction angle will be larger than the incident angle (β>α). If C1>C2, then γ<α (Snell's law). (Reprinted, with permission, from Skubas N. Principles of echocardiography for the anesthesiologist. The Greek E-Journal of Perioperative Medicine (www.anesthesia.gr/ejournal) 2003;1:26–39.)

'shadow' behind it, as very little ultrasound is transmitted distally. Specular reflections are produced by fairly large (in relation to λ) objects which present a relatively smooth surface to the ultrasound beam. Small structures (width less <λ) or those with an irregular surface produce reflections that are less angle dependent, propagate in all directions, and are less intense (scattered echoes). Although difficult to record (their amplitude is 40–60 dB less than the amplitude of a specular echo), scattered echoes are ever present and are the basis of visualizing objects oriented essentially parallel to the ultrasound beam. The scattered echoes from moving red blood cells are the basis of Doppler echocardiography.

The amplitude of the reflected echo is a function of acoustic mismatch and angle of incidence at the interface.

Refraction is the deflection of the propagated (or transmitted) portion of the ultrasound wave as it strikes, with an oblique angle of incidence, an interface separating media with different acoustic impedances (Fig. 17.1). Refraction cannot occur when ultrasound strikes the interface with a 90° angle of incidence, or when the two media have the same acoustic impedance. Because *c* in human tissue is fairly constant, little refraction occurs while the ultrasound travels inside the body, and the beam path remains straight. The difference between refraction and reflection can be described by using a mirror as the interface surface: watching the approaching cars through a rear-view mirror is refraction, as opposed to watching one's own face (reflection).

Attenuation of ultrasound is the decrease in amplitude, power, and intensity as the ultrasound travels through the body. Attenuation occurs as a result of the absorption and conversion of ultrasound to heat, and scattering at the many small interfaces or elastic discontinuities encountered even in the most homogeneous medium. Changes in acoustic impedance contribute significantly to ultrasound attenuation. Thus ultrasound transducers are constructed so that emitted ultrasound is not significantly attenuated after exiting the transducer, and a water-soluble gel is used to form an airless contact between the transducer and the skin during echocardiographic examination. Generally, for adequate imaging, depth of penetration is limited to approximately 200 × λ, so that lower-frequency (larger wavelength) ultrasound penetrates deeper. In transesophageal echocardiography (TEE) ultrasound travels a short distance and image quality is improved by using higher frequencies, whereas in transthoracic echocardiography (TTE) the structures lie farther away, necessitating the use of ultrasound with larger wavelengths. The attenuation of ultrasound in tissue is approximately 1 dB/cm/MHz; the higher the frequency and the deeper the imaging, the greater the attenuation.

PULSED ULTRASOUND AND REAL-TIME SCANNING

An echocardiography machine that produces a constant sound wave operates in a continuous wave (CW) mode, whereas if it transmits a series of identical pulses, each consisting of only a few cycles, it operates in a pulsed wave (PW) mode. Most echocardiographic imaging systems, either two-dimensional (2D) or Doppler, operate in PW mode. Pulse duration (PD) is the time from the start to the end of that pulse, i.e. the actual time the pulse is 'on', and is determined by the number of cycles and the period of each cycle. In clinical imaging, a pulse consists of 2–4 cycles and lasts 0.5–3 μs. Pulse repetition period (PRP) is the time from the start of one pulse until the start of the next, and includes both the 'on' (transmitting) and the 'off' (listening) time of the pulse. In clinical imaging, PRP ranges from 100 μs to 1 ms. Pulse repetition frequency (PRF) is the number of pulses (resulting in lines of returning data) occurring in 1 second, and ranges from 1000 to 10 000 Hz. PRP and PRF are reciprocals: PRP × PRF = 1 (analogous to period × f = 1). When imaging depth increases, PRP lengthens (with PD constant, the pulse travels farther, and the system dedicates more time for 'listening') and PRF decreases.

In 'real-time' 2D imaging ultrasound data are spatially oriented against time and images are created at a fixed rate. The amount of data collected in a certain period of time is limited by the speed of sound in tissue and the number of images that can be displayed (Table 17.1).

In clinical echocardiography, the quality of imaging (higher line density at a faster sweep rate) is increased by decreasing the depth of examination and/or reducing the size of the scan sector.

THE ULTRASOUND TRANSDUCER AND BEAM

Piezoelectric (PZ, pressure–electric) materials change shape under the influence of an electric field. With the application of an alternating electric current, PZ material alternately contracts

Table 17.1 Variables of real-time imaging

		Imaging situation		
		A	*B*	*C*
	Variable			
1	Imaging depth (cm)	10	15	20
2	Total travel distance (cm)	20	30	40
3	~PRP, or time of flight for one ultrasound pulse (or line) (ms) *	0.13	0.20	0.26
4	PRF (=1 ÷ PRP) (Hz)	7692	5000	3846
5	Sweep (or frame) rate (sweeps/s)	60	45	30
6	Time for each sweep (ms)	17 (1÷60)	22 (1÷45)	33 (1÷30)
7	Lines (or pulses) per sweep	131 (17÷0.13)	110 (22÷0.20)	127 (33÷0.26)
8	Angle of sweep (or scan angle) (°)	60	60	30
9	Line density, or lines (pulses) ÷ degree	2.18	1.8	4.2

*In the total time of flight (PRP) one should add the time required for the transducer to be switched from the receiver to transducer mode – usually 0.02 to 0.01 msec. The PRF would be changed to 7142, 4545 and 3571 Hz, for depth of 10, 15 and 20 cm, respectively.

and expands, generating compressions and rarefactions, i.e. sound waves. Conversely, mechanical stress produced by an ultrasound wave that strikes the PZ material generates an electric charge, with strength (voltage) proportional to the amount of stress applied (the strength of the returning echo). If c in a particular medium is known, the total distance traveled by the ultrasound wave is equal to ($c \times$ time) ÷ 2, and the imaged structure can be appropriately displayed. Such a PZ element is the primary component of an ultrasound transducer, which generates and transmits ultrasound, and receives returning echoes. It consists of the PZ element, electrodes that transmit the current required to excite it and record the voltage produced by the returning echoes, damping material, acoustic insulation, a case, and a face plate to match the acoustic impedance of the tissue and facilitate ideal sound transmission. Basically, the transducer emits a brief burst of ultrasound and then switches to the 'receive' mode to wait for the reflected signals from the acoustic interfaces. This process is repeated both temporally and spatially to generate ultrasound images. The range of frequencies contained in the burst (pulse) of ultrasound is termed frequency bandwidth.

Piezoelectric ultrasound transducers convert electricity to motion, and motion to electricity.

The part of the ultrasound beam in close proximity to the transducer resembles a tube,and is called the near field (Fresnel zone), whereas the diverging, distal conical portion of the beam is called the far field (Frauenhofer zone) (Fig. 17.2). The junction of the near and far fields is the transition zone. The length of the near field is r^2/λ (r = the radius of the transducer 'face'). Although the majority of sound energy produced by a transducer propagates directly away from it to form the main beam, a portion of the energy is transmitted radially, away from the axis of the main beam, creating the side lobes. The intensity of the side lobes decreases as one moves radially, away from the main beam. Side lobes are potential sources of artifact. The focusing of the ultrasound beam, by mechanical or electronic methods, narrows the beam, increases intensity in the near field, and decreases divergence in the far field.

A phased array transducer is comprised of multiple small PZ elements fired individually in a controlled manner in order to steer the ultrasound beam and produce a concentrically curved wave front that can be focused at a given point. The ultrasound beam has three dimensions: axial (parallel to the direction of the ultrasound beam, also called 'linear' or 'longitudinal'), azimuthal (side to side, or lateral), and elevational (perpendicular) (Fig. 17.2). If the phased array elements are circles instead of rectangles, both lateral and elevational dimensions of the ultrasound beam are reduced, and the axial resolution is increased. Image resolution occurs for each of the three dimensions of the beam. Axial resolution (the ability to distinguish two structures that are close to each other, front to back, parallel to the ultrasound beam's main axis) is most precise, and quantitative measurements in 2D and M-mode echocardiography should be made using data derived from a perpendicular alignment between the ultrasound beam and the structure imaged. The smallest resolvable distance between two specular reflectors is 1 λ, so resolution is better with the smaller wavelength (or higher frequency). Lateral resolution (the ability to distinguish two structures that are close to each other, side to side, or perpendicular to the ultrasound beam's main axis) varies with the distance of the specular reflector from the transducer, approaching axial resolution in the focal region. Parallel structures must be separated by more than the width of the ultrasound beam to be 'resolved' as laterally distinct. At greater depths (far field), owing to beam divergence, 'blurring' of the image occurs. Cardiac ultrasound images have a 3–10 mm thickness, resulting in artifacts of elevational resolution (e.g. a linear echo from a calcified atheroma of the aortic wall may appear as a dissection flap). Increasing

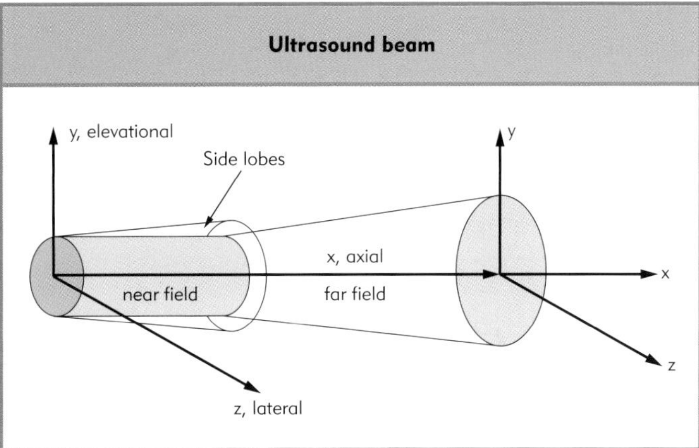

Figure 17.2 Ultrasound beam. The ultrasound beam is three-dimensional, with axial (*x* axis), lateral (*z* axis), and elevational (*y* axis) dimensions. The ultrasound beam is parallel in the near field but takes a conical shape in the far field. Around the near field the ultrasound beam creates side lobes, which may generate imaging artifacts. (Reprinted, with permission, from Skubas N. Principles of echocardiography for the anesthesiologist. The Greek E-Journal of Perioperative Medicine (www.anesthesia.gr/ejournal) 2003;1:26–39.)

transducer frequency improves axial resolution, elongates the near field, and diminishes beam divergence in the far field. However, at the same time, attenuation is increased and the ability of the ultrasound to penetrate deeper cardiac structures is diminished. Penetration is of primary importance because resolution becomes a moot point when ultrasound cannot reach the structures of interest.

BIOLOGICAL EFFECTS OF ULTRASOUND

The biological effects of a sound-emitting system depend on the total acoustic energy (power) produced, the spatial distribution of the energy, and the duration of exposure. Local heating (thermal effect) is directly related to ultrasound intensity, and most likely occurs close to the skin surface (in TTE) or esophageal mucosa (in TEE). The perfusion of tissue by blood has a cooling effect and tends to offset the temperature increase. Cavitation is the formation of gas bubbles by vibration of dissolved O_2 or CO_2, but is not an issue in biological systems because the increased viscosity significantly limits the motion of the bubbles. The mechanical effects of ultrasound, such as radiation forces and radiation torques, probably do not occur in tissue. Duty factor (D) is the fraction of the time the transducer is operating ('on' time) and hence producing biological effects, and is the ratio (%) of PD to PRP. Duty factors for diagnostic ultrasound systems are very low, typically in the range of 0.0005–0.002.

DISPLAY FORMATS

The returning echoes undergo complex manipulation (signal amplification, time-gain compensation, filtering, compression, rectification) to form the final image displayed in 'real time' on the monitor. The basic formats display echocardiographic data along a line that represents the beam axis. In the A-mode format, the amplitude of the recorded echoes is depicted as horizontal deflections (spikes) along a vertical line that represents the depth of their origin. In the B-mode format the returning echoes are depicted as brightness, representing the intensity of the reflectors. The 2D format is a modification of the B-mode: the cross-sectional image is assembled by electronically sweeping the ultrasound beam from one area to another through a fixed plane while continuously transmitting sound pulses and recording the resulting echoes. In the M-mode format (time–motion display) sequential B-mode lines are depicted across the face of the monitor, providing axial information concerning structure and depth, with the time dimension shown on the horizontal axis (Fig. 17.3). M-mode display is valuable for assessing the absolute and relative motion of cardiac structures because it has the highest temporal resolution of any available ultrasound imaging modality. Accurate evaluation of rapid

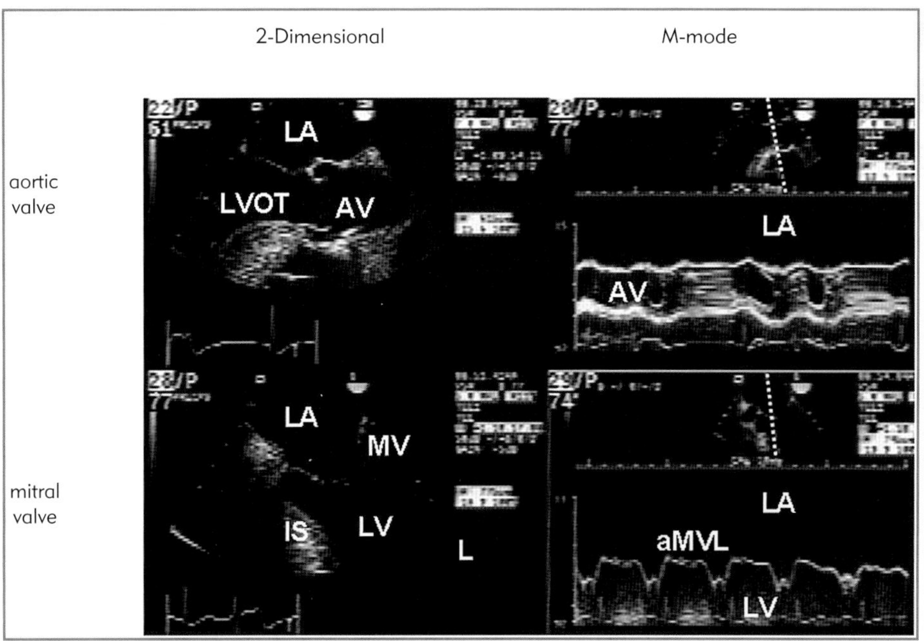

Figure 17.3 Two-dimensional echocardiography display formats. The 2-D display is a cross-sectional image of the heart anatomy (aortic valve on top left, mitral valve on bottom left). M-mode displays the motion of a particular cross-section (represented by the cursor's dotted line) over time (aortic valve on top right, anterior mitral valve leaflet on bottom right). AV, aortic valve; aMVL, anterior mitral valve leaflet; IS, inferoseptal wall; L, lateral wall; LA, left atrium; LV, left ventricle; LVOT, left ventricular outflow tract; MV, mitral valve. (Reprinted, with permission, from Skubas N. Principles of echocardiography for the anesthesiologist. The Greek E-Journal of Perioperative Medicine (www. anesthesia. gr/ejournal) 2003;1:26–39.)

intracardiac motion, such as opening and closing of a valve, high-frequency fluttering of the anterior mitral valve leaflet in aortic insufficiency, oscillations of valvular vegetations, as well as identification of the ventricular endocardial surface, are best viewed in M-mode.

Newer echocardiographic display formats include tissue harmonic imaging and three-dimensional echocardiography. Tissue harmonic imaging is based on the harmonic frequency energy generated as the ultrasound propagates through the tissues. These frequencies result from nonlinear effects of the interaction of ultrasound with tissue. The strength of the harmonic signal increases with depth of propagation, and stronger fundamental frequencies produce stronger harmonics. Harmonic imaging improves endocardial definition and reduces near-field and side-lobe artifacts in patients with poor fundamental frequency imaging. 3D echocardiography is performed by simultaneously transmitting and receiving in a 3D volume, or reconstructing a 3D image by multiple 2D images, to allow the display of images in 3D. The diagnostic accuracy of echocardiography, though limited by the resolution of the instrument, depends on competent interpretation of a skillfully performed comprehensive examination.

IMAGING ARTIFACTS

Imaging artifacts are frequent causes of inadequate or incomplete echocardiographic examination, and knowledge of ultrasound physics helps in their elimination. Suboptimal image quality is due to poor ultrasound penetration, usually because of the interposition of high-impedance structures, such as adipose tissue, lung, or bone. Acoustic shadowing occurs when a structure with a marked difference in acoustic impedance (prosthetic valve, calcium deposit) inhibits transmission of the ultrasound wave beyond that point. The resulting image is devoid of echoes distal to this structure. A different acoustic window is needed to circumvent this problem. Reverberations are multiple linear high-amplitude echo signals originating from two strong specular reflectors, and result in a back-and-forth reflection of the ultrasound signal before it returns to the transducer, limiting evaluation of structures in the far field. Beam width artifacts are due to the 3D structure of the ultrasound beam: images at the edge of the far field or from the side lobes will be displayed in the tomographic section corresponding to the main beam, resulting in imaging of structures that do not belong to that particular location. Range ambiguity results in deep structures appearing closer to the transducer than their actual location when echo signals from an earlier pulse cycle reach the transducer on the next 'listen cycle'. With change of the depth setting or position, this artifact should disappear.

Knowledge of ultrasound physics helps eliminate imaging artifacts.

DOPPLER ECHOCARDIOGRAPHY

Principles

The Doppler phenomenon refers to the change in the frequency of a sound wave reflected by a moving target. The classic Doppler echocardiographic techniques evaluate blood flow velocity with the red blood cells as the moving target. Current ultrasound systems can also apply the Doppler principle to assess velocity within cardiac tissue. The moving myocardium produces higher-amplitude and lower-velocity backscattered echoes than those reflected by red blood cells. This new application is called tissue Doppler (TD).

A moving reflector will backscatter an ultrasound signal (transmitted with frequency f_r) with a frequency (f_s) that is higher or lower than f_r if the target moves respectively towards or away from the transducer. Doppler shifts (the difference $f_s - f_r$ between backscattered and transmitted frequencies) occur only if the target is moving, are audible (0–20 kHz), and can be used to determine the velocity (v) of the moving target, as expressed in the Doppler equation:

■ Equation 17.1

$$v = [c \times (f_s - f_r)] \div [2 \times f_r \times (\cos\theta^\circ)]$$

where c is the speed of sound in blood (1540 m/s), 2 is a factor to correct for the transit time both to and from the target, and ? is the intercept angle between the ultrasound beam and the direction of motion of the moving target. As c and f_r are known, v depends on the Doppler shift and the intercept angle θ (Fig. 17.4). Doppler-derived velocity measurements depend on parallel alignment of the ultrasound beam with the investigated blood flow. The cosine of an angle 0° or 180° is 1, and the angle of intercept can be ignored if the ultrasound beam can be aligned parallel to the direction of motion of the target. With an angle of intercept <20° the cosine is close to 1 (cos20° = 0.94) and the angle can still be ignored. However, with angles of intercept >20°, velocity becomes significantly affected by θ: at 60° the recorded velocity is half of the real one (cos60° = 0.5). The direction of the moving target (blood) can be difficult to ascertain from the 2D image, and one should always bear in mind that the direction in the elevational plane of the ultrasound beam remains unknown.

Doppler echocardiography and 2D or M-mode imaging have quite opposite requirements. 2D imaging is best when the ultrasound beam strikes a large reflective (mirror-like) surface at a perpendicular angle of incidence, whereas Doppler echocardiography will detect no Doppler shift at 90° (cos90° = 0). The best Doppler information is obtained with lower-frequency transducers, a situation the reverse of that for 2D echocardiography. In general, it is difficult to obtain an excellent Doppler examination and an excellent cardiac image simultaneously. Once the reflected signal is received, the multiple frequencies present are analyzed with a process called fast Fourier transform, and the generated display is called spectral analysis (Fig. 17.4b). The amplitude (or strength) of the different frequencies is depicted with gray scale while the velocity is depicted with their distance from the zero baseline. The spectral display contains, at each time point, information regarding the direction of motion, velocity, and signal amplitude.

Continuous-wave Doppler (CWD) echocardiography uses two crystals, one transmitting and one receiving continuously, so that very high-frequency shifts can be measured accurately. The disadvantage of the technique is that all signals along the entire length of the ultrasound beam are recorded simultaneously, and one does not know the location of the individual target, or whether there is more than one moving target (i.e. there is no axial resolution). However, the characteristics of the signal (timing, shape, direction), together with 2D or other modes, helps to determine the depth of origin of the CWD signal. A

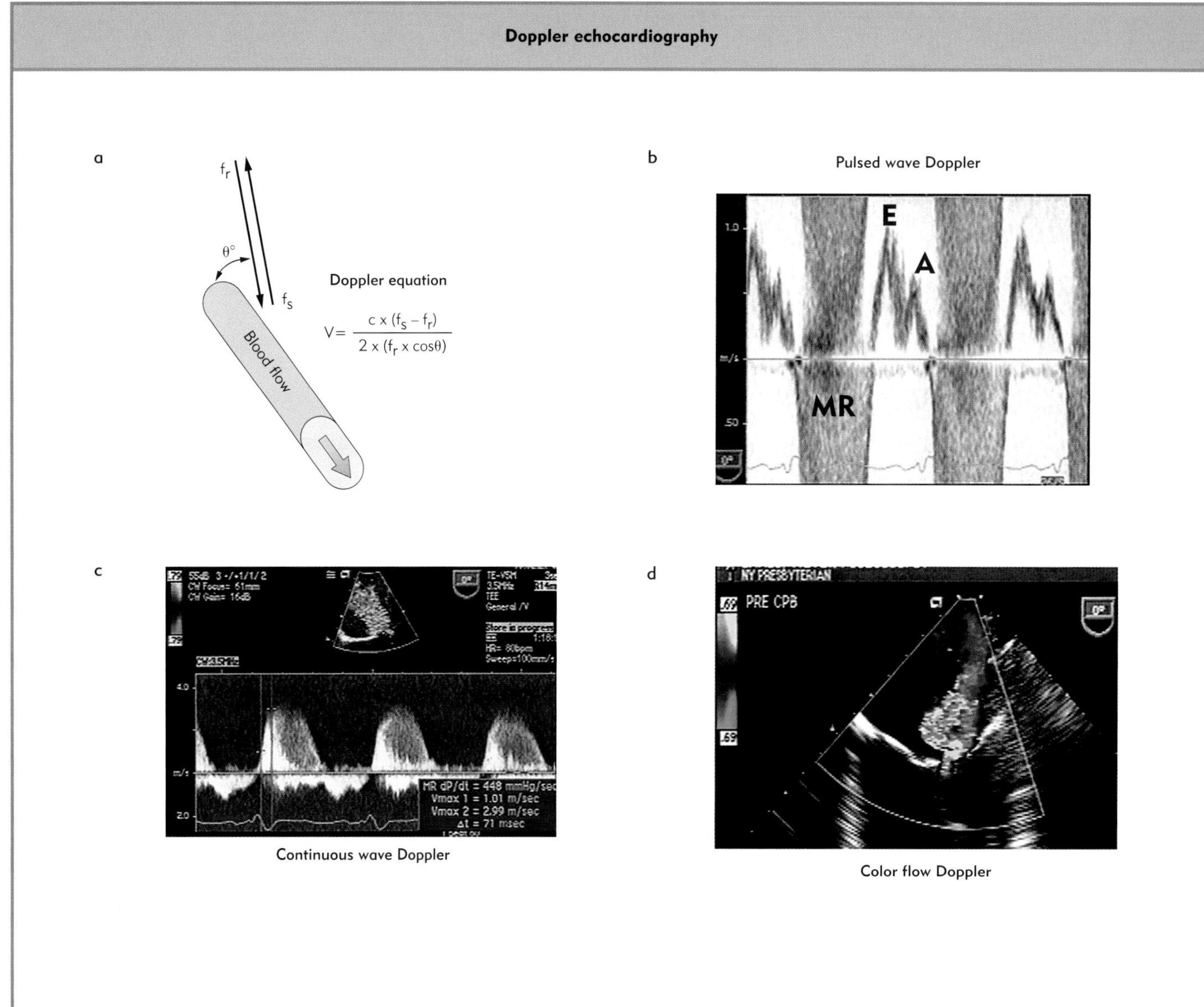

Figure 17.4 Doppler echocardiography. (a) Doppler equation. Doppler interrogation of blood flow through an incompetent mitral valve is displayed. (b) Pulsed wave Doppler displays velocity (*x* axis) over time (*y* axis). The two components of the diastolic transmitral flow are evident (E, early filling; A, atrial contribution). However, the high velocity of the mitral regurgitation can be accurately displayed because of aliasing. The mitral regurgitation signal exceeds the Nyquist limit (75 cm/s), 'wraps around', and reappears on the spectral display. This creates ambiguity, as neither the direction nor the peak velocity of the signal be identified. (c) Continuous-wave Doppler accurately displays the peak velocity and direction of the mitral regurgitation jet. (d) Color flow Doppler displays the turbulence inside the left atrium during mitral regurgitation. (Reprinted, with permission, from Skubas N. Principles of echocardiography for the anesthesiologist. The Greek E-Journal of Perioperative Medicine (www.anesthesia.gr/ ejournal) 2003;1:26–39.)

good-quality Doppler signal has a smooth contour with a well-defined edge, and maximum velocity, onset, and end of flow (Fig. 17.4c).

Pulsed-wave Doppler (PWD) echocardiography allows the sampling of velocities from a specific location by transmitting an ultrasound beam and then sampling the backscattered signal (PWD is a 'time-gated' modification of CWD). Sample volume (usually 5 mm) is the volume of blood or tissue being investigated. PWD is unable to detect high-frequency velocities. A sound wave must be sampled at least twice as fast as its maximum frequency to be characterized correctly. This sampling frequency requirement is the Nyquist limit (or number), and is approximately ½ × PRF. When this is not met, frequency aliasing occurs, which is an ambiguity in the representation of the sound wave. Methods to resolve aliasing include shifting the baseline (an electronic form of 'cut and paste'), using a lower-frequency transducer, increasing the PRF (essentially increasing the Nyquist limit), or using CWD.

Color (flow) Doppler (CFD) echocardiography is a modified Doppler technique: instead of one scanning at a sample volume (PWD), or along the entire axis of the ultrasound beam (CWD), the 2D image is scanned with multiple lines and with multiple sample volumes (usually eight) along each line. The mean (instead of peak, as in PWD and CWD) velocity of laminar blood flow is displayed, and the direction of flow is depicted by using respectively blue color for flow away from and red color for flow towards the transducer (mnemonic, BART: Blue Away, Red Towards). An additional color (green) may be added along the color scale to indicate whether the mean velocity for each of the sample volumes has excessive variability, or turbulence ('variance'). As a pulsed ultrasound technique, CFD is limited by the physics of pulsed waves and is even more limited by aliasing (manifested as color reversal). In addition, the frame rate with CFD is relatively slow because of the electronic manipulations required. To increase the frame rate, one must decrease the sampling size, use lower frequencies, and reduce the scanning angle. In CFD, the change in color may be either due to the blood flow direction relative to the transducer, or secondary to velocity aliasing. Although it is used extensively for evaluation (and quantification) of valvular regurgitation, as an equivalent to the regurgitation of dye during angiography, one should bear in mind that CFD simply records blood velocity, and that the presence of turbulence does not relate to the orifice area. Instrumentation settings and hemodynamic conditions (compliance of the receiving cardiac chamber, afterload, pressure gradient) also affect the recorded velocities. CFD should be used for the investigation or documentation of abnormal flow, and the flow abnormality should be further evaluated by PWD or CWD.

Clinical applications

Flow velocity can be evaluated using all three modes of Doppler echocardiography. CFD allows faster detection of abnormal flows and provides a spatial display of velocities in a 2D view. Quantification of flow is performed with either PWD or CWD or, as for proximal flow convergence in valvular regurgitation, with CFD. PWD is used primarily to assess velocities across normal valves or vessels, to evaluate cardiac function (diastolic and systolic function), or to calculate flow (cardiac output, regurgitant volumes, and intracardiac shunt flow). Based on the simplified Bernoulli equation, the pressure gradient (ΔP) across an orifice is related to the square of the distal (post-orifice) velocity (provided that the pre-orifice velocity is <1.5 m/s): ΔP (mmHg) $= 4 \times v^2$. Intracardiac chamber pressures can also be calculated. Systolic right ventricular or pulmonary artery pressures are equal to the peak velocity of a tricuspid regurgitation jet, if right atrial pressure is known and no pulmonary artery stenosis exists. See Chapter 45 (Valvular heart disease) for applications of Doppler echocardiography in evaluating valvular function.

TRANSCRANIAL DOPPLER

The intracranial arteries can be examined by Doppler ultrasonography (transcranial Doppler, TCD), usually with a 2 MHz probe placed over the temporal window, just above the zygomatic arch, ipsi- or bilaterally to the artery. Middle cerebral artery blood flow velocity is monitored at a depth of ~45–55 mm. The transducer is oriented so that the angle of incidence between the blood flow and the ultrasound beam is minimized. The waveform resembles that of the arterial pulse; systolic, diastolic, and mean velocities and the pulsatility index ([systolic – diastolic] ÷ mean) are recorded. Because the diameter of the vessel is unknown the actual blood flow cannot be quantified, and TCD should be used to display and measure relative changes in blood flow. TCD during carotid endarterectomy is used to manage hemodynamic perturbations (ascertain the adequacy of collateral blood flow, and detect hypoperfusion during cross-clamping) and embolic events. TCD can be used to detect microembolism during tourniquet deflation in knee arthroplasty, and the presence of a patent foramen ovale before neurosurgical procedures in the sitting position. Cerebrovascular reactivity to CO_2 and inhalational anesthetics can be assessed with TCD. TCD can be an auxiliary diagnostic modality in the confirmation of brainstem death (oscillating systolic spikes are found in cerebral circulatory

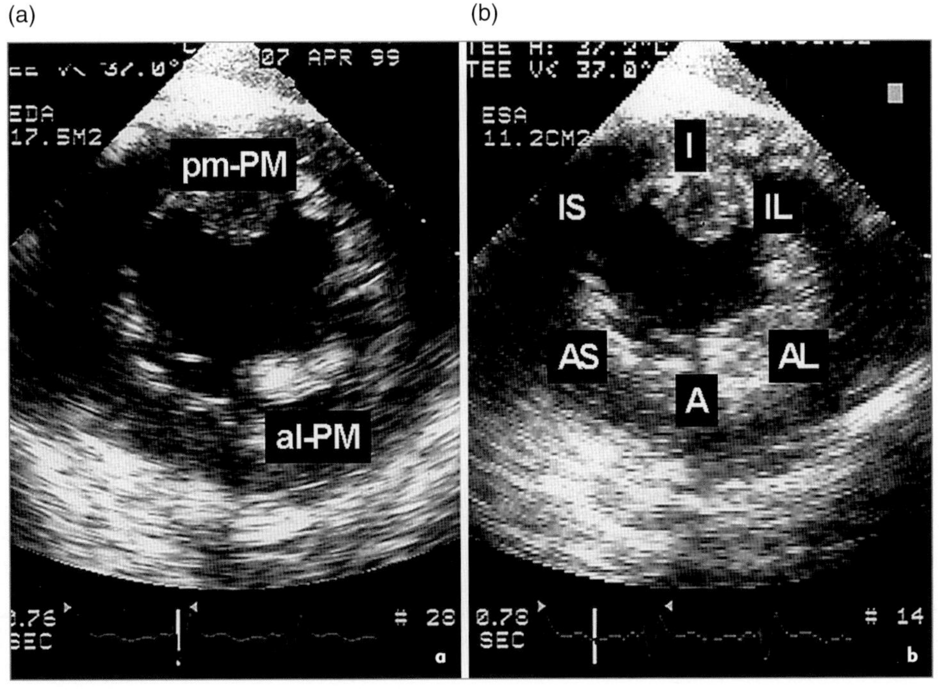

Figure 17.5 Evaluation of systolic function of left ventricle. Midesophageal short axis view of the left ventricle (LV) with transesophageal echocardiography in diastole (a) and systole (b). The systolic function of LV can be evaluated by visual comparison of the end-diastolic (EDA) and end-systolic areas (ESA). Alternatively, the endocardial border can be traced, the areas measured, and the % fraction of area change (FAC) calculated. In the above picture, EDA = 17.5 cm^2, ESA = 11.2 cm^2, % FAC = 36%. (Reprinted, with permission, from Skubas N. Principles of echocardiography for the anesthesiologist. The Greek E-Journal of Perioperative Medicine (www.anesthesia.gr/ejournal) 2003;1:26–39.)

arrest), particularly when sedation precludes the use of electroencephalography.

VESSEL CANNULATION

Real-time ultrasound with or without Doppler guidance is used for vessel location and/or needle guidance during cannulation of the internal jugular or subclavian vein. Compared with the landmark technique, ultrasonography significantly increases the probability of successful catheter placement, reduces complications, and decreases the need for multiple catheter placement attempts. However, the time to successfully place a catheter may be prolonged when using ultrasound guidance.

REGIONAL ANESTHESIA

Using portable devices with linear transducers producing frequencies of 7–15 MHz, normal peripheral nerves appear in transverse scans as round or oval hypoechoic areas encircled by a relative hyperechoic background. Ultrasound has proved helpful for regional anesthesia and interventional pain management techniques by allowing detailed noninvasive assessment of anatomy, aiding in needle positioning and monitoring the spread of the local anesthetic. Ultrasonography results in higher success rates, shorter onset times, and decreased local anesthetic needs and complications compared with the use of nerve stimulators in the performance of regional anesthetic blocks (upper and lower extremity, neuraxial, stellate ganglion, celiac plexus, or lumbar facet).

CARDIAC FUNCTION EVALUATION

The primary role of TEE in cardiac or noncardiac surgery is to confirm anatomy, identify abnormal pathology, assess baseline heart function, monitor and evaluate changes, and guide therapeutic interventions. TEE may be safely performed in most patients, including infants as small as 3 kg. Global systolic and diastolic left and right ventricular function can be evaluated, usually by an 'eyeball' approach, although quantitative TEE measurements of ventricular preload are well validated and are considered more accurate than data derived by pulmonary artery catheter (Fig. 17.5). TEE can detect myocardial ischemia more reliably than electrocardiography or hemodynamic monitoring. The presence and degree of regional systolic dysfunction and its association with coronary blood flow distribution can also be identified and used to guide medical or surgical therapeutic interventions. Valvular pathology and grading of stenotic or regurgitant lesions is also performed by TEE, as well as the assessment of the function of a new valvular prosthesis or repair. The detection of protruding atheromas or aortic intimal thickening >5 mm by TEE dictates alteration of the site or technique of aortic cannulation to decrease the incidence of stroke. The causes of postoperative hypotension or cardiac failure can be investigated using TEE: a hyperdynamic left ventricle with low end-diastolic filling indicates hypovolemia, whereas a dilated and 'sluggish' ventricle is significant for systolic failure. TEE is the test of choice in unstable patients with suspected aortic wall injury or aortic dissection in whom a delay in surgery could prove fatal.

Key references

Fàbregas N, Gomar C. Monitoring in neuroanesthesia: update of clinical usefulness. Eur J Anaesthesiol. 2001;18:423–39.

Feigenbaum H. Instrumentation. In: Feigenbaum H, ed. Echocardiography, 5th edn. Philadelphia: Lea & Febiger; 1994:1–42.

Otto CM. Principles of echocardiographic image acquisition and Doppler analysis. In: Otto CM. Textbook of clinical echocardiography. Philadelphia: WB Saunders; 2000:1–28.

Randolph A, Cook DJ, Calle G, Pribble CG. Ultrasound guidance for placement of central venous catheters: A meta-analysis of the literature. Crit Care Med. 1996;24:2053–8.

Perlas A, Chan VWS, Simons M. Brachial plexus examination and localization using ultrasound and electrical stimulation. Anesthesiology 2003;99:429–35.

Shanewise JS, Cheung AT, Aronson S et al. ASE/SCA guidelines for performing a comprehensive intraoperative multiplane transesophageal echocardiography examination: recommendations of the American Society of Echocardiography Council for intraoperative echocardiography and the Society of Cardiovascular Anesthesiologists Task Force for Certification In Perioperative Tranesophageal Echocardiography. Anesth Analg. 1999;89:870–84.

Weyman AR. Physical principles of ultrasound. In: Weyman AR, ed. Principles and practice of echocardiography, 2nd edn. Philadelphia: Lippincot Williams & Wilkins; 1994:3–28.

Further reading

Boon NA, Bloomfield P. The medical management of valvar heart disease. Heart 2002;87:395–400.

Brickner ME, Hillis L, Lange RA. Congenital heart disease in adults. First of two parts. New Engl J Med. 2000;342:256–63.

Brickner ME, Hillis L, Lange RA. Congenital heart disease in adults. Second of two parts. New Engl J Med. 2000;342:334–42.

Carabello BA. Progress in mitral and aortic regurgitation. Prog Cardiovasc Dis. 2001;43:457–75.

Carabello BA: Aortic stenosis. New Engl J Med. 2002;346:677–82.

Irvine T, Li XK, Kenny A. Assessment of mitral regurgitation. Heart 2002;88(Suppl IV):iv11–iv19.

Rajamannan NM, Gersh B, Bonow RO. Calcific aortic stenosis: from the bench to the bedside-emerging clinical and cellular concepts. Heart 2003;89:801–5.

Reimold SC, Rutherford JD. Valvular heart disease in pregnancy. New Engl J Med. 2003;349:52–9.

Thibault GE. Studying the classics. New Engl J Med. 1995;333:648–52.

Zogbi WA, Enriquez-Sarano M, Foster E et al. Recommendations for evaluation of the severity of native valvular regurgitation with two-dimensional and Doppler echocardiography. J Am Soc Echocardiogr. 2003;16:777–802.

Chapter 18 Statistics

Sue A Hill

TOPICS COVERED IN THIS CHAPTER

INTRODUCTION

The anesthesiologist will meet statistics in many different guises: as summary statistics for audit purposes, when reading and/or reviewing original research papers, when designing research projects, and last – but for some the most important – when preparing for examinations. An understanding of statistics for such diverse reasons requires us to examine underlying principles and appreciate what statistics can or, perhaps more importantly, cannot do. Medical statistics are concerned with collecting data (observations) from a small group of patients (a sample) that is representative of the whole population of similar patients. By analyzing data from this sample, we try and make deductions (inferences) that apply to the population as a whole. Inferential statistics is only useful if the data collected are representative of the population under study and is never precise: the level of accuracy of our deductions and predictions is most commonly described in terms of probabilities and confidence intervals. Thus we use sample *statistics* to estimate true population *parameters*. To ensure that this distinction is retained, different symbols are used for sample compared with population values. Greek lower-case characters are used for the true population parameter and the equivalent lower-case Roman characters for sample statistics. For example, we use m for sample mean and μ for population mean.

There are two underlying principles when dealing with data sets. The first is how to summarize data, and the second is what can be deduced from those data. Unfortunately, mistakes are often made at a preliminary stage of analysis because the nature of the data is misunderstood. Although we have powerful computerized packages for handling complex analyses, the results are meaningless if the methodology does not apply to the type of data collected. So, before we move to a description of how to analyze data, we must ensure we understand the different types of data and whether or not we are able to characterize their distribution(s).

TYPES OF DATA

In general the data we collect fall into two broad groups: things we measure and things we count. The former are continuous data with numerical values that can be given to any number of decimal places, depending on the accuracy of the measuring device; an example is systolic blood pressure. Such data are said to be *continuous quantitative* data. Data that are counted may be divided into interval or categorical types. Interval counts are the number of events that fall into predefined intervals, which themselves are part of a numerically continuous measurement, for example the number of patients admitted to hospital in a day. Here the interval is time, which we know is continuous, but for convenience we use a discrete interval, a day. These type of counted data are *discrete quantitative* data. When we count objects or events that fall into named groups, we also have data that are discrete but which this time are *qualitative* rather than quantitative. If the groups into which such data fall may be ordered in a meaningful way, such as the ASA grading of patients, then we say that the data are *ordinal categorical qualitative* data. For some groups there is no reason to put them in any one particular order, such as ABO blood groups; these data are *nominal categorical qualitative* data. There are a special form of nominal categorical data where only two possible groups exist, such as 'survived' or 'died', which we call *binary categorical* data, or just binary.

DESCRIBING DATA

After collection we need a simple way of summarizing data in order to report our findings. The purpose of summary statistics should not be forgotten: we are using data from a sample to estimate values for the population. Two studies, despite being identically designed, will produce different *statistics* but the population *parameters* remain constant, albeit unknown.

First, it is important to identify the type of data, as the different types are usually summarized in different ways. An initial exploration of the data should involve a graphical method. *Bar charts* and *histograms* are useful to display the frequencies of occurrence of different data values; the former are used for qualitative data and the latter for quantitative. These differ in that only the *heights* of the bars in a bar chart are compared, whereas in histograms the *areas* of the bars are compared. For the examples given above we would use a histogram to display systolic blood pressures and the number of patients admitted per day in a given hospital. A bar chart would be used for the number of patients with each ASA grade or blood group.

A simple bar chart can indicate differences between groups and may identify trends for ordinal data. Histograms can be very useful in identifying the shape of the distribution of our data values. In particular, we often want to know if there is a single 'peak' value, i.e. *unimodal* data, or whether there are two or more peaks, i.e. *multimodal* data. The values of these peaks represent the most frequent observations and are known as the *modes*. Multimodal data suggest that the sample is heterogeneous in some way, so the observations result from the combination of more than one homogeneous group. Nonhomogeneity causes problems when analyzing data, and so whenever a study is planned it is important to be sure that wherever possible each study group is homogeneous.

We also need to know if the data are approximately symmetrical about an average value, or whether there is a tendency for there to be more observations that are higher or lower than the average value. This nonsymmetry is known as *skewness*; a positively skewed distribution of observations has more extreme high values, whereas a negatively skewed distribution has more extreme low values (Fig. 18.1). Skewness is important to identify, as it may make analysis and interpretation more complex.

Some of our data may be *paired*, e.g. two observations on one individual, such as age and height. In this case we use a scatterplot, with each axis representing one of the observations. Such plots are commonly used when considering correlation or regression analysis for associations between two observations.

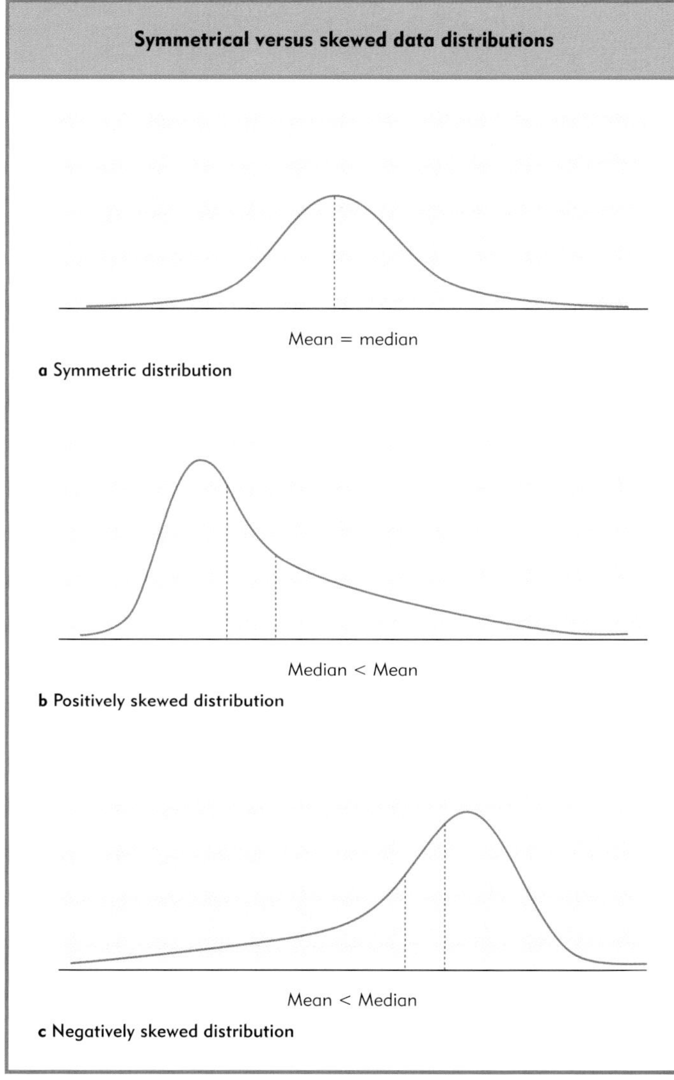

Figure 18.1 Symmetrical versus skewed data distributions. (a) Data that are symmetrically distributed have median = mean. (b) Positively skewed data have median < mean, because the values in the positive 'tail' weight the mean toward a higher value. (c) Negatively skewed data have median > mean, because the values in the negative 'tail' weight the mean toward a lower value.

Central tendency: mean and median

We need a way of describing an 'average' value for each group of data. The mean, m, is obtained by adding all values together and dividing by the total number of observations. This is written mathematically as:

■ Equation 18.1

$$m = \frac{\sum_n x_i}{n}$$

The symbol Σ_n is shorthand for 'add together all n observations', since a single observation is represented by x_i and i takes values 1 to n.

The median is the middle observation when all observations are ranked in order. For an odd number of observations, for example $n = 13$, the median is the value of the seventh observation, because there are six higher and six lower observations. For an even number of observations, for example $n = 12$, there is no single middle observation. Instead, we find the average of the two observations on either side of the middle, the average of the sixth and seventh observations. In both cases we can define the median as the $(n + 1)/2$th observation. For data with a symmetrical distribution the mean and the median population parameters will be the same; for positively skewed data the median is less than the mean, but for negatively skewed data the median is greater than the mean (Fig. 18.1).

We now have a sample *statistic* (mean, m) that estimates the population *parameter* (mean, μ). We can think of this statistic as the 'central tendency of the data'; if we took repeated samples from the same population, then averaged all the sample means we would get an even better estimate of μ. The more samples we take, the closer the average value of the sample means will be to the true population mean. Furthermore, the larger the sample size the better the estimate of the true mean. Means from samples of the same size are distributed approximately normally, with a standard deviation (see below) that becomes smaller as the sample size increases. This is true whatever the underlying distribution of the observations, and is known as the 'central limit theorem'. The standard deviation of the distribution of means from samples of a given size is known as the *standard error of the mean* (SEM). The SEM can be calculated from a single sample using the relationship SEM $= s/\sqrt{n}$, where s is the sample standard deviation and n the sample size.

Spread of data values

In addition to needing a measure of central tendency we also need an estimate of the spread of values about this central value.

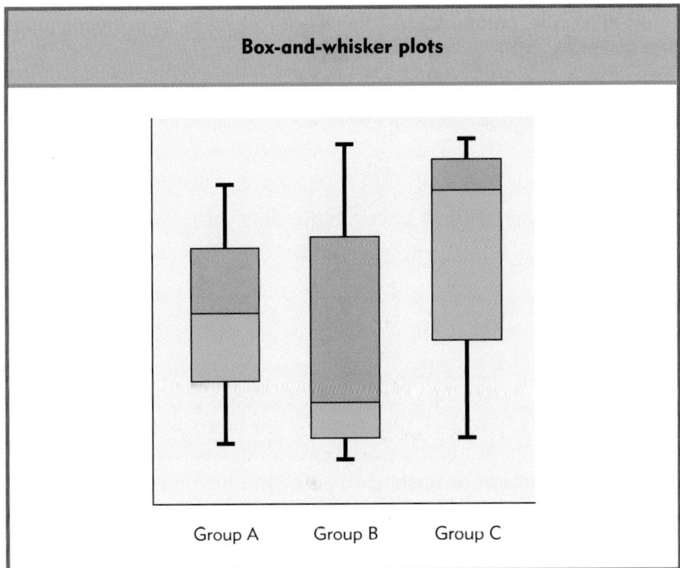

Figure 18.2. Box-and-whisker plots. Box-and-whisker plots can be used to display a summary of data values. The ends of the box represent the upper and lower quartile values, with the line across the box showing the median value. The ends of the whiskers are often the most extreme values. The height of the box therefore shows the interquartile range and the distance between the whiskers shows the range of observed values. Group A is symmetrical data, Group B positively skewed data and Group C negatively skewed data. Note that some computer packages use different criteria for drawing the whiskers to show very extreme observations, known as outliers, so check what your package does.

We could look at the range of values that the observations take, but this is not very helpful as it describes only extremes and not the majority of the observations. A better estimate for spread is the range of values that accounts for the middle 50% of observations when ranked in order – the interquartile range (IQR). To find the IQR for n observations we find the $(n + 1)/4$ and $3(n + 1)/4$th values, interpolating if these do not coincide with actual observations, as we did for the median. Thus for $n = 14$ we need the 3.75th [i.e. (3rd + ¾ (4th – 3rd)] and 10.25th [i.e. (10th + ¼ (11th – 10th)] values to give the lower and upper quartile values, respectively. These values, along with the median and range, can be plotted as a box-and-whisker plot to give an indication of the distribution of the data (Fig. 18.2). Such plots are particularly useful when comparing groups of observations.

Another measure of spread is the *variance* or *standard deviation*. The population variance (σ^2) is the mean square of the difference between the population mean (μ) and all population values: the standard deviation (σ) is the square root of the variance. The sample variance (s^2) for n observations is the sum of the squared differences between the sample mean (m) and observed values divided by $(n - 1)$. Mathematically this is written:

■ Equation 18.2

$$s^2 = \frac{\sum_n (x_i - m)^2}{n - 1}$$

We divide by $(n - 1)$ rather than by n because the sample variance obtained by dividing by n is a biased estimator of the population variance and always underestimates the true variance.

Some texts refer to statistics arising from analysis of the ranking of observations, such as median and IQR, as nonparametric. Such analysis does not require any assumptions to be made as to the distribution of the data, either because the population distribution is not known or because it does not conform to a known mathematically described distribution. On the other hand, statistics calculated using the data values themselves are known as parametric, as they are estimates of the population parameters required to describe the data distribution. There are many mathematically described distributions that data values may take; in the next section we will introduce the three most commonly encountered. These are the normal distribution for continuous numerical data, the Poisson distribution for discrete numerical data, and the binomial distribution used to analyze proportions of observations that fit into just two possible categories, i.e. analysis of binary data.

DATA DISTRIBUTIONS

Parametric distributions can be characterized by the parameter(s) that define the central tendency and spread of the data in a form that can be expressed mathematically. For discrete data each possible count can be associated with a probability that this particular value will occur, and the sum of all probabilities must be 1. For continuous data there is an infinite number of possible values, so the probability associated with any particular value is necessarily very small, but the sum of all these probabilities must also be 1. For continuous distributions we are usually interested in the possibility of a value lying within a particular range, and the probability of this is the area under the curve (AUC) between the two limiting values.

Discrete data

POISSON DISTRIBUTION

A Poisson distribution describes the distribution of the number of *independent* events occurring in a fixed interval; the events occur *randomly* but at a constant mean rate. The data are therefore numerical but discrete. The Poisson distribution is characterized by a single population parameter, μ, which is the mean number of counts during the interval and also the variance. Many naturally occurring events follow such a distribution, such as the number of radioactive particles released in a fixed time period. In medicine the number of admissions to a hospital on a given day of the week, or the number of births in a particular month, may be described by a Poisson distribution.

BINOMIAL DISTRIBUTION

The binomial distribution describes the distribution of the number of 'successes' and 'failures' for binary data on a fixed number of occasions, where the likelihood of success is constant on each occasion. An example is the number of correct responses in an examination of 100 questions (assuming all questions are answered). The binomial distribution is also determined by one parameter, p, where $0 < p < 1$, which is the probability of success. The mean number of successes is np and the variance is $np(1 - p)$. In our example, if we guess the answers then we have a one in two chance of being right, so $p = 0.5$ and the mean number of correct responses for 100 questions is 50, with a variance of 25. To score more we need to work hard and make sure p is greater than 0.5!

Continuous data

We encounter several continuous probability distributions, although the most common is the normal distribution. The families of Student's *t*-distributions, χ^2, and F-distributions encountered in inferential statistics are also continuous probability density functions. The normal and *t*-distributions are both symmetrical, whereas the χ^2 and F-distributions are both highly skewed. Here we will discuss only the normal distribution in detail.

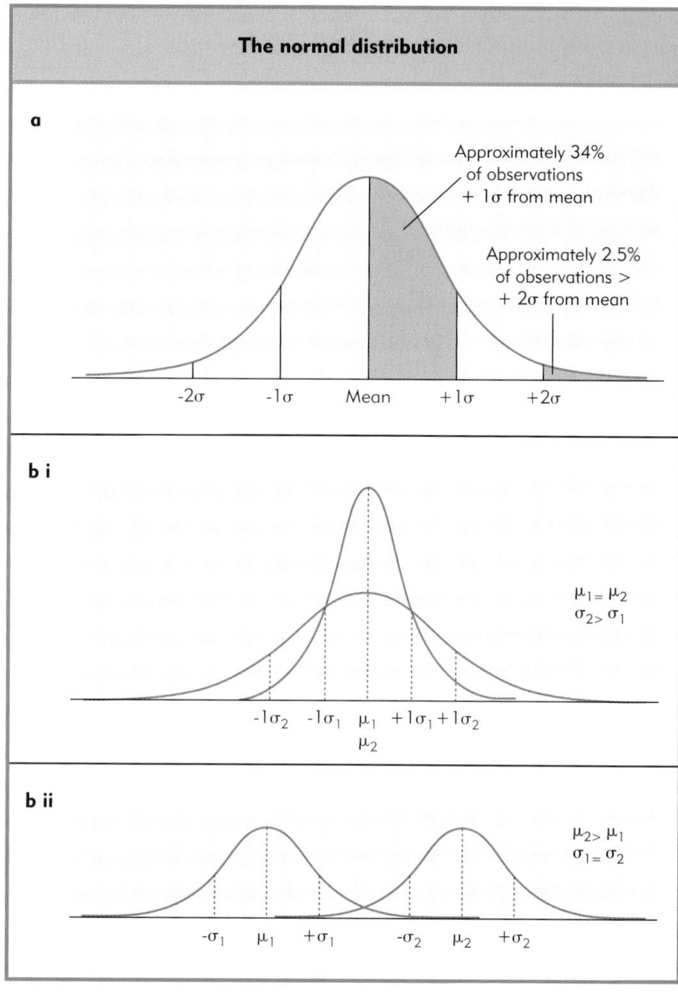

Figure 18.3 The normal distribution is described by two independent parameters, μ, the mean, and σ², the variance. (a) The proportion of observations within one and two standard deviations of the mean. (b) The independence of the two parameters showing two distributors with equal means but different variance (bi) and the same variance but different means (bii).

THE NORMAL DISTRIBUTION

The normal distribution differs from the distributions described above in that it is continuous and the mean and variance of the distribution are *independent* parameters, so both the mean (μ) and the variance (σ^2) are needed to describe it completely. It describes a symmetrical bell-shaped curve where mean = median = mode. Approximately 68% of observations lie within one standard deviation either side of the mean, and approximately 95% of observations lie within two standard deviations either side of the mean (Fig. 18.3a). Because there are two independent parameters describing this distribution, many different normal distributions exist with the same mean but different variance, or with the same variance but different means (Fig. 18.3b). However, all have the same shape and can be transformed into a standard normal curve, which has a mean of 0 and a variance (and also standard deviation) of 1.

The probability that an observation as high as the one we have collected belongs to a given normal distribution must be found from tables. These *Z-tables* are produced for the standard normal distribution. To use such tables it is necessary to transform the observation, x, from our normal distribution with mean μ and standard deviation σ to corresponding values in the standard normal distribution by calculating the *standard normal deviate*, z, where:

■ Equation 18.3

$$z = \frac{(x - \mu)}{\sigma}$$

This effectively converts the observation to a value that is equal to the number of standard deviations from the mean. Thus for a normal distribution described by a mean of 5 and variance of 4, we find z for an observation x = 6 to be $(6 - 5)/2 = 0.5$. From Z-tables we find the probability, p, that an observation as high as this comes from the proposed normal distribution by looking up 0.5 in the table (Fig. 18.4). Because the distribution is symmetrical, Z-tables only show positive z-values, and if the actual z-value is negative then the required probability is $1 - p$, as the total area under the standard normal curve is 1. There are many examples in anesthesia of data taking a normal distribution: mean blood pressure and weight of adult females are just two examples. Sometimes it is important to decide whether or not data conform to a normal distribution. This can be explored

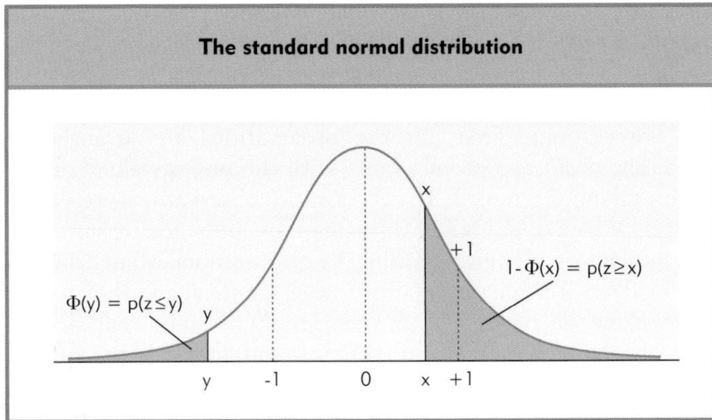

Figure 18.4 The standard normal distribution has a mean of 0 and a standard deviation of 1, with the area under the curve equal to 1. Any observation, n, from a normal distribution can be mapped onto the standard normal by finding the standard normal deviate, z. $z = (n - \mu)/\sigma$, where μ and σ are the mean and standard deviation of the normal distribution from which n is taken. The shaded area on the left of the diagram represents the probability of an observation being fewer than y standard deviations below the mean. This is often written $\Phi(y) = p(z \le y)$, and the values of $\Phi(y)$ are tabulated in Z-tables. The shaded area on the right of the diagram represents the probability of an observation being more than x standard deviations from the mean. As the distribution is symmetrical and we know the area under the curve is 1, this can also be found from tables as $p(z \ge x) = 1 - \Phi(x)$.

graphically using a normal-plot (or z-plot) that plots the observations against their standard normal deviates, which should be linear. If nonlinear, the shape of this plot may suggest a simple transformation that would normalize the data, but may also suggest that the data distribution is complex and so nonparametric analysis may be more appropriate.

CLINICAL STUDIES

Most clinical studies require more of statistical analysis than just a summary of the data. Researchers want to quantify the differences between study groups and draw conclusions from those differences, if present. A full discussion of study design is beyond the scope of this chapter. However, there are several steps involved: (i) formulating a hypothesis, (ii) deciding on the study population, (iii) designing a data collection method that minimizes errors and avoids bias, (iv) estimating sample size for adequate statistical power, (v) and analyzing data and making inferences based on this statistical analysis.

Inferential statistics

Inferential statistics describe the many ways in which statistics derived from observations on samples from study populations can be used to deduce whether or not those populations are truly different. A large number of statistical tests can be used for this purpose; which test is used depends on the type of data being analyzed and the number of groups involved. In medicine generally, and in anesthesia in particular, we are often concerned with drug effects and whether or not a new drug is as effective as a currently available treatment. Studies designed to answer these questions rely on inferential statistics to support or refute the superiority of one treatment over another. First a null hypothesis, H_0, is proposed, which takes the form of a written statement or a mathematical expression. The most commonly proposed null hypothesis is 'no difference(s) exist between the groups, they all come from one population'. Second, an alternative hypothesis, H_1, is proposed that will be accepted if there is good evidence against the null hypothesis. If we are unconcerned about the direction of any difference between groups, H_1 will simply be 'the two populations are different' and we will use a two-tailed test. If we are only interested if the difference is in a particular direction, then we use a one-tailed test. These hypotheses are not probability statements, they relate to the populations represented by the samples, and so have nothing to do with significance probabilities, or p values. The tests all produce a significance probability (p value, or SP) that indicates the likelihood of the observed value of the test statistic belonging to the distribution described by the null hypothesis for the test. A p value of 0.5 suggests that there is a 50% chance that the observation fits the null hypothesis, i.e. a one-in-two chance, whereas a p value of 0.05 suggests that this probability is only 5%, i.e. a 1 in 20 chance. A one-in-two chance is not low enough for us to be sure the null hypothesis is incorrect, whereas a 1 in 20 chance makes it much more likely. At this latter level we might agree that the null hypothesis is incorrect, so a p value of 0.05 is usually taken as the 'cut-off' probability. We say that p values less than 0.05 provide good evidence against the null hypothesis, whereas values greater than this do not. Statistically speaking, we always talk about evidence *against* the null hypothesis, never *for* it; our study is usually designed to reject the null hypothesis, not support it.

Before undertaking an inferential test it is important to understand the type of data being analyzed and whether the data, or transformed data, are normally distributed. If they are, then parametric tests can be used to analyze the data; if not, then nonparametric tests can be used. Nonparametric tests involve the ranks of the observations rather than the observations themselves, so no assumptions need be made as to the actual distribution of data.

PARAMETRIC COMPARISONS OF TWO GROUPS

There are two well-known parametric tests available to compare the mean observations from two groups in order to decide whether or not this *sample* difference is likely to represent a true *population* difference: Student's paired and unpaired t-tests.

Student's paired t-test

Student's paired t-test is used when two groups of the same size are matched exactly in ways other than the experimental intervention. Often this means that the same patients are used for both groups; it is possible to use different patients, but they must be matched very carefully for the test to be valid. The important assumptions of this test are that the variances of the two populations are identical, and that the *differences* between observations from the two populations are normally distributed. There is no need for the two groups of observations to be normally distributed, just their differences. This is not a problem if we know that our groups of observations come from normally distributed data, as the differences between two normally distributed populations with identical variance will also be normally distributed. Our null hypothesis can be stated as H_0: 'there is no difference between the two groups, they come from the same population', or we can write H_0: $\mu_d = 0$, where μ_d is the mean difference between population means. Our alternative hypothesis will then be H_1: $\mu_d \neq 0$, the populations are different because their means are different.

The test statistic is T, the difference between sample means divided by its standard error:

■ Equation 18.4

$$T = m_d/(s/\sqrt{n})$$

Here m_d is the mean difference between the paired observations and s is the standard deviation of those differences. T is distributed according to a t-distribution with $n - 1$ degrees of freedom, where n is the number of pairs of observations. The p value for T will be given by a computer package or can be found from tables. We usually accept that $p < 0.05$ is good evidence against the null hypothesis and we accept the alternative hypothesis.

The t-distributions are symmetrical and describe the distribution of means of samples of a given size taken from a normal distribution where the variance is unknown. The shape of this family of curves is similar to that of a normal distribution, but they are 'tail-heavy' in that there are relatively more observations two standard deviations from the mean. The smaller the sample size the more 'tail-heavy' the t-distribution. As the sample size increases, so the t-distribution more closely approximates a normal distribution. The term 'degrees of freedom' is commonly encountered in statistics and represents the number of observations less the number of parameters that have been estimated from the observations. In the paired t-test we estimate just one parameter, so we have n – 1 degrees of freedom.

Student's unpaired *t*-test

Student's unpaired t-test or two-sample t-test is used to compare observations from two study groups when the groups are not matched. The assumptions of this test are different from those of the paired t-test, so it is important to be clear about which test is appropriate. For the unpaired t-test it is not necessary to have the same number of observations in each group, but this time the observations from both groups must come from normally distributed populations and both populations must have the same variance. It is generally accepted that if the variances of the two groups do not differ by a factor more than 3 then this assumption is met. The test statistic is T:

■ Equation 18.5

$$T = (m_1 - m_2)/(s_p\sqrt{(1/n_1 + 1/n_2)})$$

Here m_1 and m_2 are the mean values from the two samples and s_p is the pooled variance calculated from all observations, $n = n_1 + n_2$ (where these are the number of observations in the two groups). T is distributed according to a t-distribution with $(n - 2)$ degrees of freedom. The p value for T will be given by a computer package, or it can be found from tables.

NONPARAMETRIC COMPARISONS OF TWO GROUPS

There is a nonparametric test available for comparing median values from two independent groups where an assumption of normality is not justified, the Mann–Whitney U-test. The null hypothesis for this test is that there is no difference between the median values for the two groups of observations. As for all nonparametric tests the test statistic is calculated after ranking the observations. First, all the observations are arranged in ascending order and given a rank, with the lowest-valued observation taking the rank 1. If two or more observations are equal, then they are each assigned the same rank, obtained by summing the available ranks and dividing by the number of tied observation. Thus if three observations were identical and they would have taken the ranks 3, 4, 5, they are all assigned rank 4. The sum of ranks for each group is then found, and T is the sum of ranks from the group containing the fewest observations. The test statistic is U:

■ Equation 18.6

$$U = n_1 + n_2 + \tfrac{1}{2} n_1(n_1 + 1) - T$$

Here n_1 and n_2 are the number of observations in the two groups. U/n_1n_2 is actually the estimated probability that an observation from the first population will be less than an observation from the second population, so it is a useful statistic. There is also an interpretation of the T statistic alone, attributed to Wilcoxon. Tables are available for critical values of T for groups of different sizes. For groups with 10 or more observations, T is approximately normally distributed with mean $\mu_T = n_S(n_S + n_L + 1)/2$ and standard deviation $\sigma_T = \sqrt{(n_L\, \mu_T/6)}$, and a z-statistic can be calculated as $(T - \mu_T/\sigma_T)$, which can be referred to Z-tables for the normal distribution described above.

QUANTITATIVE PAIRED DATA: CORRELATION AND REGRESSION

In many circumstances we wish to determine whether or not a relationship exists between two observations made on the same subject. For example, we might want to know if there is a relationship between a baby's head circumference and its age. There are two statistical approaches to analyzing paired data: regression, and correlation. Although superficially similar, the two approaches are aimed at answering different questions. In regression analysis statistics can be used to develop an answer to a question such as 'Can we *predict* what the height of a 4-year-old child will be if we have data for height of children from the ages of 2–7 years?' Here we are not only interested in associations, we also want to be able to use those associations to predict future outcomes. The important feature of the data here is that one of the observations is known with certainty – in this example the age of the child – but the other observation may vary from child to child of the same age. We say that we can identify an *explanatory* or *independent* variable and a *response* or *dependent* variable. For correlation we are only answering the question 'is there an *association* between these paired observations?' There is no distinction between the two variables: they have equal standing.

When analyzing paired data it is essential to identify the types of data involved. If the observations are both discrete, then analysis requires a different test for association than if both observations are continuous. In addition, it is important to decide whether only correlation is being sought or if prediction is required, as the two analyses are associated with different assumptions.

Correlation

There are two distinct types of correlation analysis. The first is a parametric test for a linear relationship between two variables, producing Pearson's correlation coefficient. The second is a nonparametric test for nonlinear association between two variables, producing Spearman's rank correlation coefficient. The first uses the principle of least-squares to fit a straight line to the paired data presented, and the correlation coefficient is a measure of how well the data points fit that straight line. The second approach uses a ranking method whereby the first observation for each pair is ranked, then the second in each pair is ranked, and the relationship between the ranks is then analyzed.

Pearson's correlation coefficient can take a value between −1 and +1, with a zero value indicating that there is no linear correlation between the paired observations. A positive correlation coefficient indicates that an increase in one variable is associated with an increase in the other, whereas a negative value indicates that one variable increases as the other decreases. Spearman's correlation coefficient can also take values between −1 and +1, but in this case a zero value indicates that there is no correlation between the paired observations, whether linear or nonlinear. It is clear that some highly correlated data can have a low Pearson correlation coefficient but a high Spearman correlation coefficient (Fig. 18.5a). It is therefore essential to produce a graphical display of the paired data using a scatterplot before determining how to analyze the data for correlation.

Simple linear regression

Simple linear regression is used to predict the value of the *response* variable from that of the *explanatory* variable. There are some assumptions that must be met before such analysis can be undertaken. First, the response variable (y) should be continuous and normally distributed, and second the variance of the response should be constant across the range of explanatory variable values. If these conditions are not met, then either the response variable must be transformed or a different approach to analysis must be taken. The explanatory variable (x) must be interval or continuous data, but there are no assumptions as to its distribution. It is important to explore the data graphically as a scatterplot before deciding on this method of analysis.

The principle behind simple linear regression is the method of least-squares and a straight line is fitted to the data points (x and y):

■ Equation 18.7

$$y_p = a + bx$$

The slope of this regression line is b, which is an estimate of the true population regression coefficient, β. This models the true relationship between the explanatory and the response variable:

■ Equation 18.8

$$y = \alpha + \beta x + \varepsilon$$

Here α is the intercept on the y-axis and ε the random error term that represents the normal variation of the response, y, about its mean value. The error terms represent the variance of y; ε varies with mean 0 and constant variance.

The null hypothesis is that there is no relationship between the response and the explanatory variables. This is equivalent to saying that the slope of the regression line is zero (H_0: $\beta = 0$). The alternative hypothesis is that the regression slope is not zero. The test statistic used to determine whether or not there is a relationship is T:

■ Equation 18.9

$$T = b/(SEB)$$

Here SEB is the standard error of the estimated slope, b. T is distributed according to a t-distribution with $n - 2$ degrees of freedom (because we estimate both α and β from the data) and a p value will be given. Interpretation of the p value is as before: if $p<0.05$ then there is good evidence against the null hypothesis; it is likely that a predictive relationship does exist between the two variables. The value for SEB and the t-probability are

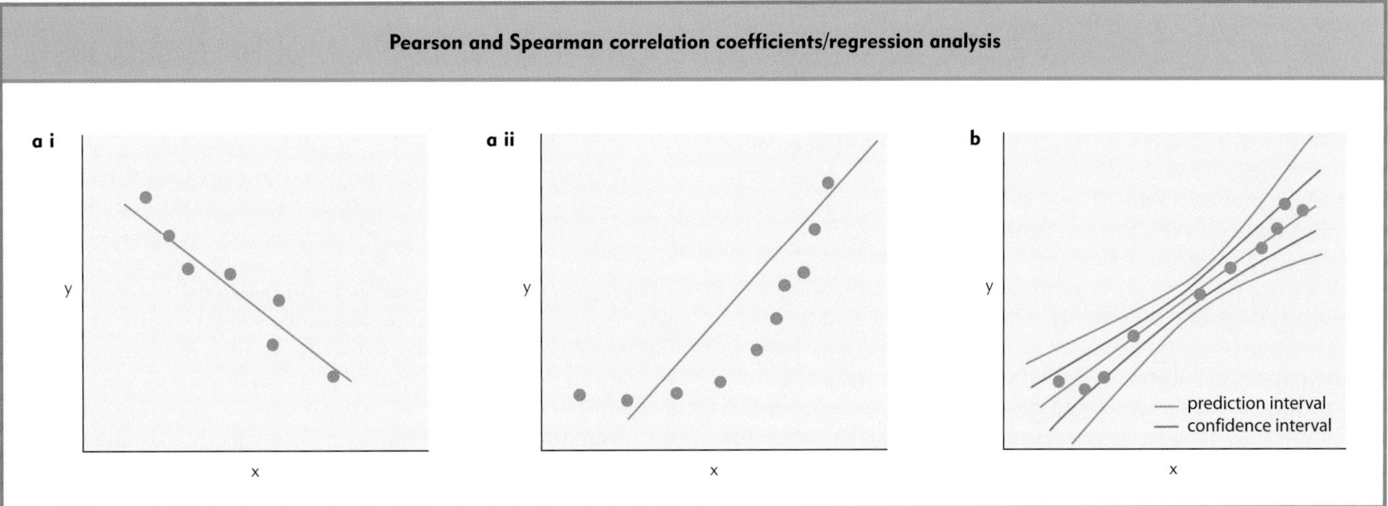

Figure 18.5 Pearson and Spearman correlation coefficients. (a) Pearson's is useful for linear correlation, whereas Spearman's is better at identifying nonlinear correlation. Note that both variables, x and y, are continuous and have equal standing. The correlation coefficients would be exactly the same if the axes were reversed. (b) Regression analysis showing the fitted regression line and 95% confidence and prediction intervals. Note that these intervals are smallest at the point representing the mean values of both variables, and get wider toward extremes. Extrapolating beyond observed values leads to very wide confidence and prediction intervals and is not recommended. The analysis is only valid with the axes as they stand; x and y are not interchangeable (see text for details).

produced by a statistical package. We need to check that the model is a good one by examining the residuals, $(y - y_p)$, where y_p is the predicted value of y as the residuals are estimators for the error terms, ε. This is done within a statistical package and should demonstrate that the residuals are independent, random, and approximately normally distributed about a mean of zero.

Once a regression equation has been developed we can use it to predict a *mean* response for a given value of the explanatory variable, x. The accuracy with which this can be done depends on how well the data points fit the straight line: the closer the fit, the better the estimate. A confidence interval can be calculated for an estimated mean response. If we wish to predict a range of possible values for an individual response we also need to take into account the expected variation in the response, as we know this to be normally distributed. Thus a prediction interval for an individual response will be much wider than the confidence interval for the mean response (Fig.18.5b).

QUALITATIVE DATA: ASSOCIATIONS

We often wish to know whether associations exist between groups of qualitative data. For example, we might wish to determine whether or not patients are more nauseated after neurosurgery on the posterior fossa compared with supratentorial neurosurgery. Here we are dealing with categorical data, and we can tabulate the results of such a study in a table known as a contingency table. The rows could be labeled 'no nausea', 'mild nausea/vomits once or twice', 'severe nausea/vomiting', and the columns labeled 'Posterior fossa surgery' and 'Supratentorial surgery'. This gives a 3 × 2 contingency table with six entries or 'cells', which record the number of patients falling into the six exclusive groups.

The analysis is based on the principle that if the outcome from each of two events is independent, then we can multiply their respective probabilities to obtain the probability of a given outcome in both. In our example, if there is no association we would expect the probability of severe vomiting *and* posterior fossa surgery to be the same as the probability of severe vomiting multiplied by the probability of having posterior fossa surgery. If the two are sufficiently different we can conclude that there is an association between severe vomiting and posterior fossa surgery. The statistical analysis associated with contingency tables produces a test statistic that approximately follows a χ^2 distribution on n degrees of freedom. The number of degrees of freedom is (the number of rows − 1) × (the number of columns − 1), 2 in our example. If the expected value is E and the observed value O, then the test statistic is χ^2:

■ Equation 18.10

$$\chi^2 = \sum \frac{(O - E)^2}{E}$$

The expected values can easily be calculated from the marginal totals and the grand total (Table 18.1). The p value reported can be interpreted as before, with the null hypothesis being that there is no association between the two events in question.

The above analysis can be used for tables of any size, with the proviso that the expected number of observations is always greater than five for any cell. If this is not the case, then rows or columns should be combined to reduce the number of categories. A 2 × 2 contingency table can also be analyzed by a more exact test known as Fisher's exact test, which is more appropriate if the cell counts are small. Alternatively, Yates' correction can be applied, which is a small correction that allows discrete data to be approximated by a continuous distribution. It involves subtracting half from each absolute difference between observed and expected values before producing the square of their difference for calculating the χ^2 statistic.

Table 18.1 Contingency table for association between groups of categorical data. The observed values are shown in (a) and the calculated expected values in (b). To test for association we use the χ^2 test; the χ^2 statistic is calculated from the sum of the squared difference between observed and expected values divided by the expected value. For these data χ^2 is 29.88 on 2 degrees of freedom, giving $p < 0.001$. This gives us strong evidence against the null hypothesis that no association exists. We accept that there is an association between site of surgery and extent of nausa and vomiting.

(a) Observed (O) number of episodes together with marginal totals

	Supratentorial	**Posterior fossa**	**Total**
No N&V	60	18	78
Mild N&V	24	40	64
Severe N&V	6	16	22
Total	90	64	154

(b) Expected (E) value for a cell calculated by multiplying row total and column total for that cell and dividing by the overall total. So for cell 1, no N&V and supratentorial surgery, we find (78 × 90)/154 = 45.6

	Supratentorial	**Posterior fossa**	**Total**
No N&V	45.6	32.4	78
Mild N&V	37.4	26.6	64
Severe N&V	13	9	22
Total	90	64	154

QUANTITATIVE DATA: MULTIPLE GROUPS

Analysis of variance (ANOVA)

Many experimental studies involve the response of more than two groups, and analysis of such data is more complex than just repetitive t-tests or Mann–Whitney U-tests. There is insufficient space to go into detail about the multitude of statistical tests and analysis that can be used for complex data sets. It is important to understand the limitations of t-tests and the implications of p values if multiple tests are carried out. If we assume that a p value of 0.05 is sufficient evidence against the null hypothesis, then if we perform 20 different t-tests on data from the same experiment it is very likely that one of those tests will give a significant result by chance, even if no true difference exists. This is avoided when extending the concept of the unpaired t-test to multiple groups in analysis of variance (ANOVA). Essentially, ANOVA divides variance into between-group and within-group variation. We need to identify true between-group variation. The test statistic calculated in ANOVA is the variance ratio or F statistic, as it follows an F-distribution.

The null hypothesis assumes all data to come from a single normal population, in which case the variance ratio will be 1. If at least one pair of groups differs, then F will be greater than 1. If a significant result is obtained then further analysis, such as Scheffé's test, is needed to decide which pair(s) of groups differ.

There are many forms of ANOVA, depending on how many treatments there are. If there is just one treatment but several groups, then we have one-way ANOVA. If there are two treatments and several groups then we have two-way ANOVA. The important assumptions of ANOVA are that the response variable must be continuous and normally distributed with constant variance across all groups, and there must also be an equal number of comparisons between different pairs of groups. If this is not possible then more complicated multiple regression models may be used instead. The nonparametric equivalent of one-way ANOVA for non-normally distributed data is the Kruskal–Wallis test.

More complex experimental designs can be used to account for variation that occurs independently of treatments but in which we have no interest for the study in question, known as 'blocking'. For example, we would like to know if any of four drug treatments reduces the incidence of vomiting after all kinds of surgery; we are not interested in whether a particular type of surgery is more or less likely to induce vomiting, because we already know this is the case. Here blocking effectively can be used to account for between-surgery variation, which allows treatment groups to be more homogeneous and so enhances the between-treatment effects.

Multiple linear regression

Multiple linear regression is a method of statistical analysis that determines which of many potential explanatory variables are important predictors for a given response variable. As for simple linear regression, the important assumptions are that the response variable is normally distributed with constant variance, and that the error terms are random and independent. This approach can be used to model clinical situations, such as predicting the change in a blood marker for disease when multiple treatments are being administered. The methodology includes ways of determining which variables are important, and may be used to produce a regression model for prediction purposes.

Generalized linear regression model (GLM)

If the response variable is not normally distributed then more complex forms of regression can be used to analyze multiple-treatment data. The response variable can be transformed by a specific function, a link function, which enables a linear regression model to be fitted. In medical research the logistic regression model (LRM) is used to predict a binary outcome (response), such as survival or nonsurvival, given explanatory variables that influence outcome. The link function for the LRM is the logit function, $\log(p/(1 - p))$, where p is the probability of 'success'. The ratio $p/(1 - p)$ is known as the *odds* of success, so by comparing the odds of success after two different interventions we can obtain an *odds ratio*. If an odds ratio is greater than 1 then the outcome from the first treatment is more successful than that from the second. Recovery from an anesthetic can be modeled using LRM, where p is the probability of waking at a given time after discontinuation of drug administration.

ERRORS, POWER, CONFIDENCE, AND BIAS IN CLINICAL STUDIES

The successful design of any clinical study involves careful planning and preparation. Pilot studies are often necessary to estimate the likely differences between groups that can be used to ensure that a larger study has sufficient power to test the hypothesis in question. Those involved in planning must be clear about their aims, and decide *before* the study which intergroup comparisons are central to testing their hypothesis. Failure to do so may result in underpowered studies that are ethically questionable, as they would never have identified a clinically important difference. There must be a clear distinction between clinical and statistical difference: it may be possible to do a large study that identifies a statistically significant difference of 2 mmHg in mean blood pressure, but this small difference is never likely to be of clinical significance.

Errors and power

There are two sources of error inherent in any study that lead to false positive and false negative conclusions. We expect variation to exist, and with normally distributed data about 5% of population values will lie beyond ± 2 SD from the mean, so there is a 1 in 20 chance that an observation will fall into one of these 'tails' but still belong to the population in question. The same is true of test statistics.

A false-positive result arises when the null hypothesis is rejected although it is actually correct. This is also known as a type I or α error, and relates to the significance level chosen by the designer of the study, usually set at 0.05 so that there is a 5% likelihood of obtaining this result by chance even if the null hypothesis is actually correct.

A false-negative result arises when the null hypothesis is accepted when it is actually incorrect. This is also known as a type II or β error, and is usually a result of there being an insufficient number of observations for the result to reach the predetermined significance level. The value $(1 - \beta)$ is known as the *power* of the study and can be determined in advance by calculating the number of observations needed to give a significant result if a minimum clinically relevant difference is identified. Calculating the number of subjects required in a two-group study where the observations are normally distributed may be found using the Altman nomogram (Fig. 18.6). Complicated study designs require the advice of a statistician in calculation group size.

Confidence intervals

Whenever a parameter is estimated by statistical analysis we obtain a point estimate for the population parameter. How can we indicate the certainty we have in this estimate? A confidence interval is a range of values within which we expect to find the true population value. The researcher sets the level of confidence, often 95%, and uses the central limit theorem and standard error to calculate a confidence interval about the point estimate. On 95% of occasions when we repeat the study we would expect the confidence interval to contain the true population parameter. As an example, we can calculate a confidence interval for the mean systolic blood pressure for healthy adults, which is normally distributed data. Let the sample mean (m) be 72 mmHg with $n = 41$ observations having a standard deviation

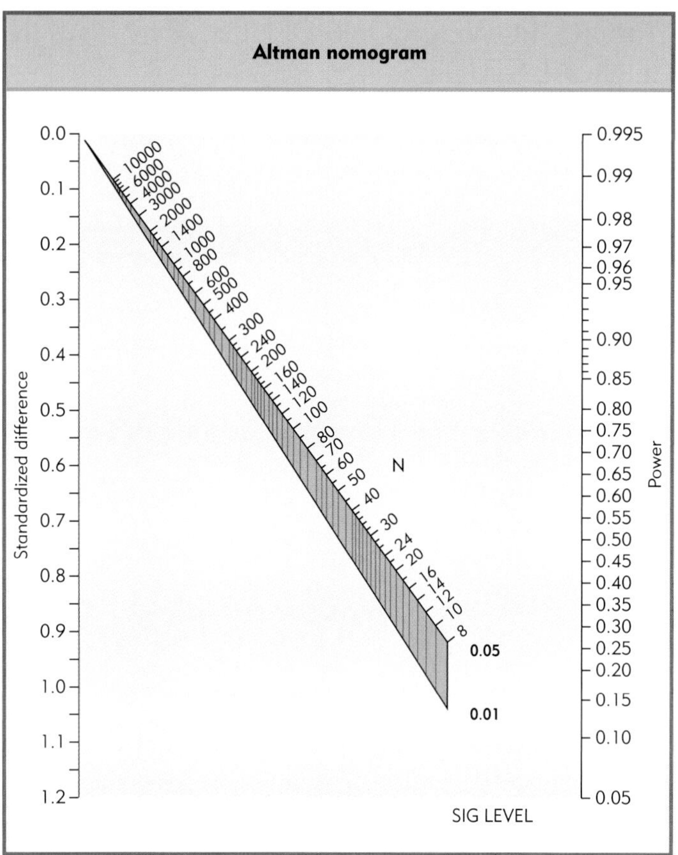

Figure 18.6 Altman nomogram. To estimate the number of observations required for a study involving two groups of equal numbers, first identify the minimum clinically significant difference you would like to demonstrate (d). First, standardize this difference by dividing by the estimated standard deviation (from a pilot study or other source); this gives the standardized difference on the left-hand axis. Second, decide on the power required of the study, usually 0.8 as a minimum; this gives the figure on the right-hand axis. Join these two points with a straight line that intercepts the two given lines. Finally, decide on the significance level for testing the hypothesis, either 0.05 or 0.01. The total number of observations required for the two-group study is the value at the intercept with the line corresponding to the relevant significance level. (Reproduced with permission from Statistics in Practice ed. Gore S and Altman D. How large a sample?, BMJ 1982, Copyright British Medical Association.)

(s) of 6.4 mmHg. The standard error of the mean, SEM, = $s/\sqrt{n}$. A 95% confidence interval (CI) is calculated knowing that we expect 95% of observations in a normal distribution to lie within ± 1.96 standard deviations. Thus the 95% CI for the mean in our example is:

■ Equation 18.11

$$\begin{aligned} 95\%\ \text{CI} &= (m - 1.96 \times \text{SEM},\ m + 1.96 \times \text{SEM}) \\ &= (72 - 1.96 \times 6.4/\sqrt{41},\ 72 + 1.96 \times 6.4/\sqrt{41}) \\ &= (70.04,\ 73.96) \end{aligned}$$

In a similar manner we can calculate confidence intervals for many statistics, such as the difference between two groups when using a two-sample t-test. Confidence intervals are more informative than point estimates with standard deviation, and should always be quoted in research papers.

Bias

Bias occurs when non-random errors are allowed to influence the observations and hence the validity of a statistical analysis. There are two main sources of bias: observer bias and patient bias. Observer bias occurs when the person making the observations knows what result is needed to support the hypothesis, which may either consciously or unconsciously influence the recordings made. Patient bias occurs when patients are aware of the treatment group to which they are allocated, and respond according to what they perceive to be the required result. Blinding the observer and/or the patient to the treatment options may eliminate both types of bias; if both are blinded this is known as 'double blinding'. Errors that may be perceived as bias can also be present when patients are not allocated to study groups in a randomized manner. Thus randomization and double blinding are gold standards for the design of a good clinical study.

SUMMARY

By understanding the type and distribution of data we collect, together with a measure of the clinically important differences, we may design an appropriate clinical study. Such studies will use randomization to avoid bias and be appropriately powered. The gold standard is a randomized double-blind clinical trial. Parametric methods of analysis for normally distributed data may not be valid for highly skewed or non-normal data; equivalent nonparametric tests should be used instead.

Further reading

Altman DG. Practical statistics for medical research. London: Chapman & Hall; 1991.
Castle WM, North PM. Statistics in small doses. Edinburgh: Churchill Livingstone; 1995.
Daly F, Hand DJ, Jones MC, Lunn AD, McConway KJ. Elements of statistics. Harlow: Pearson Education; 1995.
Florey C du V. Sample size for beginners. Br Med J. 1993;306:1181–4.
Gardner MJ, Altman DG (eds). Statistics with confidence. London: British Medical Journal 1989.
Rao PV. Statistical research methods in the life sciences. Pacific Grove, CA: Brooks/Cole; 1998.

APPENDIX

Probability mass and probability density functions for data distributions

All parametric distributions may be expressed mathematically. The mathematical function that describes a discrete distribution is called a *probability mass function* (PMF). The mathematical function that describes continuous data can be drawn as a continuous curve, the *probability density function* (PDF), and the area under this curve must be 1.

Poisson distribution

■ Equation 18.12

$$p(X = y) = (e^{-\mu} \,.\, \mu^{y})/y!$$

where y can take values 0,1,2,.... ($y!$ is y factorial, i.e. $1 \times 2 \times 3 \times \ldots \times y$)

Binomial distribution

■ Equation 18.13

$$p(X = x) = (n!/(x!(n - x)!)).\, p^{x}.\, (1 - p)^{n-x}$$

where x can take values 0, 1, 2,...,n.

Normal distribution

The mathematical expression describing this PDF for the probability of x lying between the values a and b is:

■ Equation 18.14

$$p(a < x < b) = {}_{a}\int^{b} [1/\sqrt{(2\pi\sigma^2)}]\exp[-\tfrac{1}{2}((x - \mu)/\sigma))^2]$$

SECTION 2

Neurosciences

Chapter 19 The structure and function of neurons

Beverley A Orser and Robert E Study

TOPICS COVERED IN THIS CHAPTER

- **Properties of excitable cells**
- **The structure of neurons**
- **Excitatory and inhibitory receptors**
    - Axoplasmic transport
    - Glia
- **Membrane potential**
    - Ion pumps and the generation of the resting potential
- **Electrical properties of neurons**
- **The action potential**
    - Axonal conduction
    - Classification of nerves according to conduction velocity
    - The nature and function of voltage-gated ion channels

PROPERTIES OF EXCITABLE CELLS

General anesthetics target the most complex biological system, the human central nervous system. They are thought to disrupt sophisticated cognitive functions such as perception and memory by altering the balance between excitatory and inhibitory neurotransmission. Not surprisingly, the mechanisms underlying the effects of anesthetics on behavior remain poorly understood. However, new knowledge about the cellular effects of anesthetics is developing hand-in-hand with insights regarding the physiology and pharmacology of neurons. Indeed, anesthetics are important tools in our quest to understand how the brain processes information. Moreover, the rational development of new anesthetic drugs is dependent on identifying their targets clearly and a knowledge of neuronal function.

This chapter focuses on the unique building blocks of the nervous system, neurons and neuroglia (commonly called glia). Neurons are the fundamental units of the nervous system and carry information by conducting electrical impulses. The approximate 10^{12} neurons in the brain are organized into anatomical and functional networks. Glia compose approximately half the volume of the brain and outnumber neurons by at least 10 to 1. Unlike neurons, glia do not generate conducted impulses but provide structural and maintenance support for neuronal tissues. Two-way communication between neurons and glia is essential for axonal conduction, synaptic transmission, and information processing. Here, we describe the salient features of neurons and glia.

THE STRUCTURE OF NEURONS

Neurons have two characteristic structural and functional features: an excitable membrane, and synapses. 'Excitability' means the ability of neurons to generate and propagate stereotypic electrical impulses (*action potentials*). The action potential is the primary means of communication in the nervous system. *Synapses* are specialized points of communication that allow neurons to communicate with each other. Neurons are not 'hard-wired' like electrical circuits, but rather modify synaptic input and store information through changes in protein synthesis and function. Other cells, such as muscle and endocrine cells, also exhibit electrical activity; however, this property is highly developed in neurons. Neurons transmit information using electrical signaling, a property that allows fast communication over long distances. As described in Chapter 20, synapses contain a large number of receptors for chemical neurotransmitters. A single neuron may receive input through hundreds or even thousands of synapses. Conversely, neurons can transmit through hundreds of synapses on to neighboring or distant neurons.

Neurons are characterized by their excitable plasma membrane and synaptic contacts.

The basic architecture of most neurons is fairly consistent, although there is a wide variability of structure (Fig. 19.1). Neurons are organized such that dendrites collect input from other neurons, primarily through synapses, whereas axons transmit output from the cell body or soma to other neurons. The soma contains the nucleus and the protein synthesis machinery for the cell.

Activation of protein receptors for extracellular signals at synapses induces a change in the permeability of the cell to charged particles (ions). The flow of ions generates a current that travels along the dendrite and converges with other dendritic signals at the cell soma. The combined signals, if

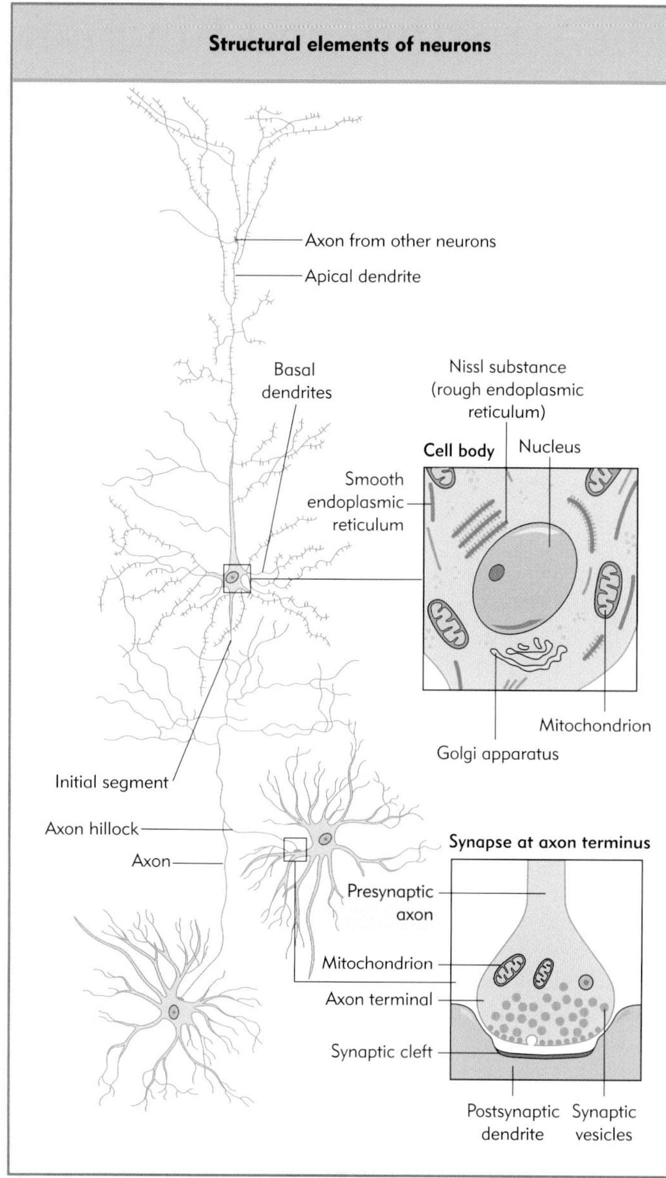

Figure 19.1 The basic structural elements of neurons. A typical CNS neuron exhibiting its major structural attributes, including dendrites (connections of many other neurons to dendrites not shown), a branching axon, and synapses onto other neurons.

sufficiently large, can trigger an action potential. The cell soma exhibits a high degree of excitability, especially at a specialized area at the root of the axon (*axon hillock*). The axon hillock is a trigger site for the generation of action potentials. The action potential propagates away from the soma along the axon, which then contacts other neurons or end organs at distances of a few micrometers to over a meter. Thus, information flows primarily from the dendrite to the axon.

Dendrites tend to have more extensive branching or *arborizations* than axons, with multiple roots in most neurons. By comparison, the axon usually exits as a single fiber, although some may divide extensively along their course. The entire neuron can be electrically excitable, although not uniformly. Dendrites are generally less excitable, transmitting much of the electrical information passively (see below). Although there are many exceptions to this basic dendroaxon model, the above model describes the majority of neurons and provides a foundation for understanding neuronal function.

Synapses can be broadly classified into two groups, excitatory and inhibitory (see Chapter 20). Activation of excitatory synapses increases the membrane conductance to positively charged *cations* (e.g. Na^+, Ca^{2+}) and reduces the membrane potential to more positive values. Conversely, inhibitory synapses are generally permeable to negatively charged *anions* (e.g. Cl^-). Activation of inhibitory synapses causes membrane hyperpolarization and a decrease in the membrane potential away from the potential that generates an action potential (*threshold potential*). Increased inhibitory conductance also depresses neuronal excitability by setting the membrane potential close to the Cl^- or K^+ equilibrium potential, thereby shunting excitatory input (see below).

EXCITATORY AND INHIBITORY RECEPTORS

The principal excitatory and inhibitory neurotransmitters are respectively glutamate and γ-aminobutyric acid (GABA). These chemicals are released from presynaptic terminals and diffuse across the synaptic cleft to activate transmitter-gated ion channels and G protein-coupled receptors (GPCRs) located in the postsynaptic membrane. Generally, transmitter-gated ion channels mediate fast synaptic transmission on a very rapid timescale (µs–ms time range), whereas GPCRs regulate slow synaptic transmission on a slower timescale (generally seconds to minutes). Glutamate activates a family of cation-selective ion channels, whereas GABA activates anion-permeable ion channels. Both glutamate and GABA activate metabotropic GPCRS.

The effect of anesthetics on GABA receptors has been the focus of much research. GABA activates two types of transmitter-gated ion channel ($GABA_A$ and $GABA_C$ receptors) and a type of GPCR ($GABA_B$ receptors). $GABA_A$ receptors have been identified as sensitive targets for many commonly used intravenous and inhaled anesthetics. $GABA_A$ receptors are ubiquitous in the nervous system and regulate inhibition in most neurons. Activation of postsynaptic $GABA_A$ receptors typically generates fast, transient inhibitory postsynaptic currents (IPSCs). Most anesthetics enhance IPSCs by prolonging their duration and increasing the influx of anions. Enhancement of IPSCs is thought to be a major factor that contributes to the neurodepressive effects of general anesthetics.

Most anesthetics enhance inhibitory postsynaptic currents by prolonging their duration.

$GABA_A$ receptors are also expressed in regions of neurons located outside the synapses (Fig. 19.2). These *extrasynaptic* $GABA_A$ receptors are thought to be activated by the low ambient concentrations of GABA present in the extracellular space. The GABA in the extracellular space is released by GABA transport proteins, or spills over from synapses. Extrasynaptic $GABA_A$ receptors generate a persistent tonic inhibitory conductance. There are important differences in the structural and pharmacological properties of extrasynaptic and synaptic $GABA_A$ receptors. Notably, extrasynaptic $GABA_A$ receptors are highly sensitive to low concentrations of intravenous and volatile anesthetics. Studies using genetically modified mice that lack certain populations of extrasynaptic $GABA_A$ receptors indicate that these receptors contribute to the neurodepressive effects of these drugs. Indeed, increasing evidence suggests that extrasynaptic $GABA_A$ receptors are important anesthetic targets.

Axoplasmic transport

A key characteristic of neurons is their length; some cells may extend for a long distance, often more than a meter. However, the machinery for synthesizing proteins and the critical organelles such as mitochondria exists primarily in the cell body, synaptic terminals, and some dendrites. To supply the axon with essential components over such long distances, neurons have developed three transport systems: orthograde axoplasmic transport (away from the soma), retrograde axoplasmic transport (toward the soma), and axoplasmic flow. The first two are quite fast, moving organelles at a rate of up to 40 cm/day. The third involves slow orthograde transport, moving proteins and bulk cytoplasm at a rate of 1–10 mm/day.

Orthograde and retrograde axoplasmic transport both involve adenosine triphosphate (ATP)-driven molecular motors that transport molecules along a rail of microtubules extending the length of the axon. They involve different proteins, some of which are specific for transport in each direction. The principal proteins involved in orthograde and retrograde transport are, respectively, kinesin and dynein. These proteins form links between transported organelles and the microtubule structures along which they move. Kinesin and dynein have properties similar to muscle myosin, and presumably move using a similar ratchet-like mechanism, hydrolyzing ATP in the process. Also, like muscle fibers, axons are rich in actin, but its function in these fast transport processes is not as well understood as its role in muscle. Interestingly, transport in both directions can occur simultaneously along a single microtubule. Slow axoplasmic transport (or flow) transports many soluble proteins and other cytoplasmic components, such as microtubules, along the axon. This supplies the axon and terminals with the wide range of substances required for basic metabolic functions.

The importance of transport away from the axon to the synapse or neuromuscular junction is obvious, but retrograde transport is more obscure. Two known functions of retrograde transport include the movement of synaptic vesicles back to the cell body, presumably for recycling. The second involves endocytosis at the nerve terminal, where vesicles are trafficked back to the cell body. This phenomenon appears to be a form of communication, where information in the form of chemical signals, such as the presence of growth factors in the environment of the nerve terminal, is transported back to the soma. It is particularly important in development and repair of neurons, where connections may be established or eliminated based on such retrograde chemical signaling.

Glia

Glia are nonneuronal cells that are also referred to as glial cells or neuroglia. Glia represent special connective tissue in the central nervous system. Glial function is regulated by neuronal activity. Further, glia signal not only to each other but also back to neurons. Glia are classified into two main groups, astrocytes and oligodendrocytes. Astrocytes are the largest of glial cells, with an average diameter of 40–50 μm. Each contains numerous podia (or foot-like extensions) that make intimate contact with both blood vessels and neurons. Astrocytes play a critical role in regulating the extracellular concentration of ions, neurotransmitters, and metabolites, neuronal development, and supporting synaptic function. Oligodendrocytes are located predominantly in the white matter, where they provide electrical insulation in the form of myelin around the axons. In peripheral nerves, glial cells that form myelin are called Schwann cells (Fig. 19.3). Microglia are small mobile cells that resemble macrophages. Microglia probably arise from the blood and play an immunological role, scavenging debris and generating inflammatory responses via cytokine production.

Glia lack chemical synapses and do not generate action potentials. They connect to each other by low-resistance conduits (or *gap junctions*) that allow the direct exchange of ions and small molecules. Glia are closely associated with neurons, but are separated by fluid-filled spaces that prevent the propagation of action potentials from one nerve cell to neighboring neurons. Two-way communication between neurons and glia is essential for normal functioning of the nervous system. Signaling molecules that are exchanged between neurons and glia include ions, neurotransmitters, gases, cell adhesion molecules, and signaling

Synaptic and extrasynaptic receptors

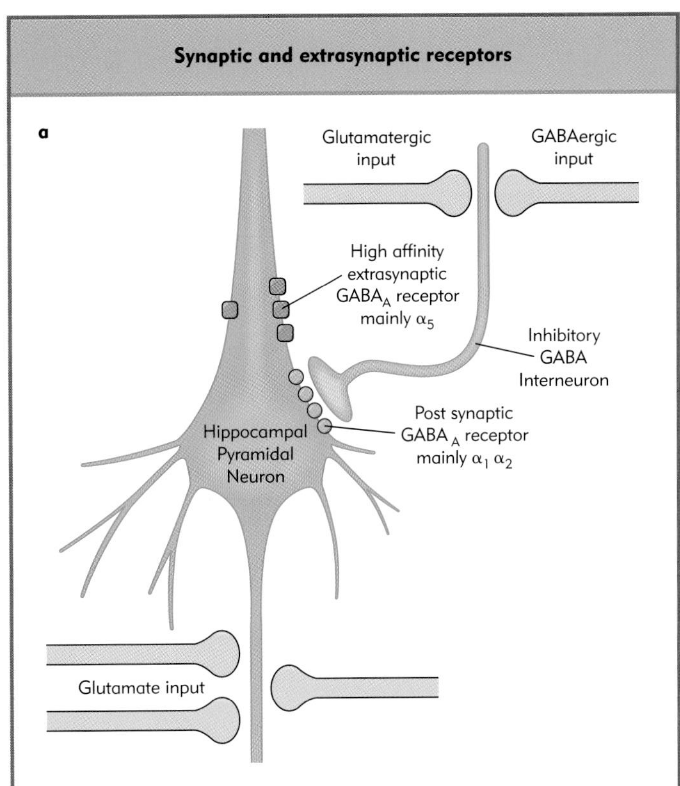

Figure 19.2 Synaptic and extrasynaptic receptors. (a) Synaptic and extrasynaptic inhibitory input to a pyramidal neuron in the hippocampus. Axon terminals that synapse are either excitatory glutamatergic (pink) or inhibitory GABAergic (blue). Pyramidal neurons express both synaptic (blue) and extrasynaptic (pink) $GABA_A$ receptors that are composed of different subunit types. Synaptic receptors detect GABA that is released from the presynaptic terminal and generate fast, transient currents. In contrast, extrasynaptic $GABA_A$ receptors detect GABA that is present in the extracellular space and generate a tonic inhibitory conductance. Extrasynaptic receptors are highly sensitive to many commonly used general anesthetics. (From Bai et al. Distinct functional and pharmacological properties of tonic and quantal inhibitory postsynaptic currents mediated by γ-aminobutyric acid $GABA_A$ receptors in hippocampal neurons. Mol Pharmacol. 2001;59:814–24. Copyright © 2001 The American Society for Pharmacology and Experimental Therapeutics.)

Continued

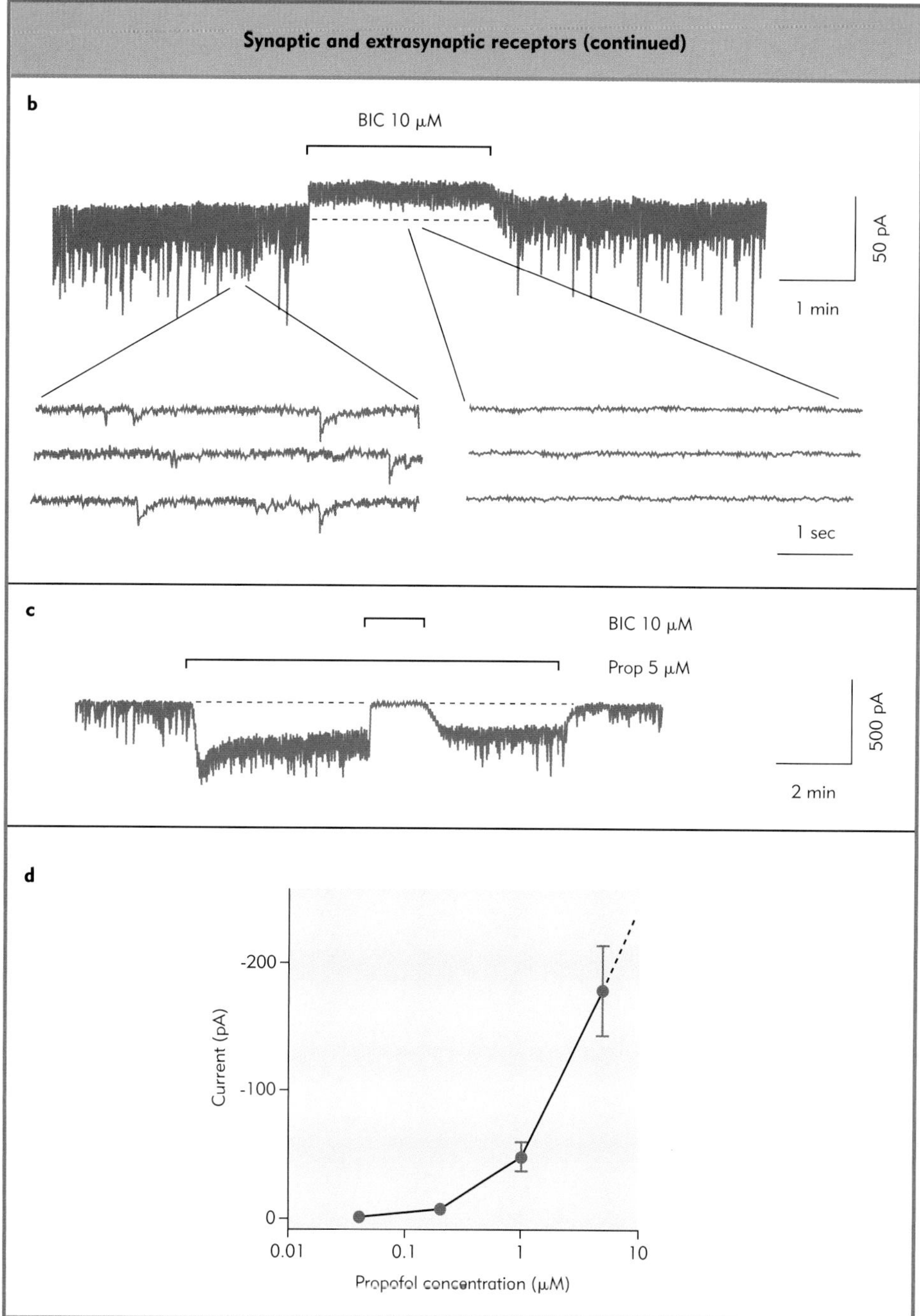

Figure 19.2 cont'd (b) Tonic and postsynaptic currents recorded from hippocampal pyramidal neurons using electrophysiological methods. The tonic current is revealed by an application of the $GABA_A$ receptor antagonist, bicuculline (BIC 10 μM). Bicuculline inhibits a persistent inward current, as shown by the outward shift in the baseline. Bicuculline also blocks postsynaptic currents that are represented by the transient downward deflections. (c) Propofol (Prop 5 μM) increases the tonic current, as shown by an inward shift in the baseline. The effects of propofol are inhibited by bicuculline, indicating that propofol acts on $GABA_A$ receptors. (d) Clinically relevant concentrations of propofol increase the tonic current. The concentration–response plot is shown. Propofol concentrations greater than 10 μM cause a further increase in the tonic current.

proteins. Glial cells communicate with each other through intracellular waves of Ca^{2+} and intercellular diffusion of chemical messengers, rather than the propagation of action potentials. Glia both release and take up neurotransmitters and other extracellular signaling molecules, and thereby play a critical role in coordinating the activity of neurons across networks.

Upon activation, neurons release K^+, transmitters, and metabolites that can accumulate in the extracellular space, and hamper further conduction (see below). Glia are permeable to K^+ and contain protein transporters that pump molecules out of the extracellular space, preventing pathological increases. Glia play an important role in regulating the extracellular concentrations of transmitters, including GABA. Glia and neurons directly exchange a variety of biochemical signals, including proteins. For example, Schwann cells produce proteins that are important for neuronal differentiation and survival, and neurons produce growth factors that can induce the proliferation of Schwann cells.

Additional noteworthy functions of glia occur following neuronal injury. Microglia perform phagocytosis in response to immunological stimuli to clear away cellular debris. Glia also help guide and support the regrowth of axons back to their targets after injury. The appendages of astrocytes are linked by tight junctions that form barriers around capillaries (the so-called blood–brain barrier). This barrier critically limits the diffusion of large molecules, including drugs and proteins, into the nervous system, but can be compromised under pathological conditions.

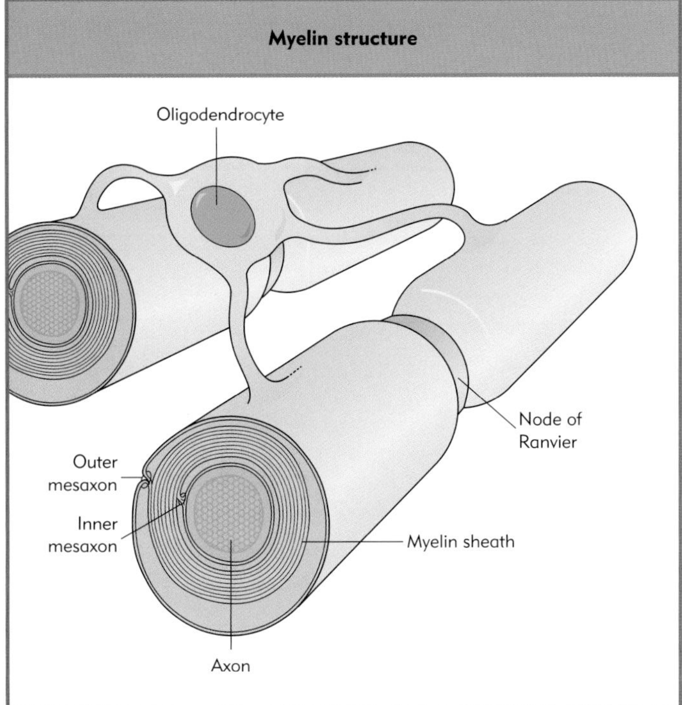

Figure 19.3 Myelin structure. Cross-section of a myelinated axon of the CNS, showing the oligodendroglia cell forming the myelin sheath. The spiral wrapping of the glial cell membrane is shown in cross-section. Myelin is interrupted at regular intervals by a short unmyelinated segment called the node of Ranvier, where the axonal membrane is exposed to the extracellular environment and the current responsible for action potentials crosses.

Tight junctions between astrocytes form a barrier around capillaries, the blood–brain barrier, which limits diffusion into the nervous system.

Instead of action potentials, glia generate 'Ca^{2+} waves', which are caused by the opening and closing of Ca^{2+} channels. These channels allow Ca^{2+} to enter the cytoplasm, and Ca^{2+} subsequently activates the outward flow of K^+. This response is propagated along and between cells, owing to electrically conductive gap junctions that connect the glia. These waves, which are over an order of magnitude slower than action potentials, may have an important role in information processing.

MEMBRANE POTENTIAL

The membrane potential is a fundamental and essential property of all cells. Loss of membrane potential leads to loss of cell viability, as it is required for communication both within and between cells. The membrane potential is an electrical gradient that results from differences in the concentrations of charged organic and inorganic ions across the cell membrane (Chapter 6). Two key elements establish and maintain the membrane potential: protein channels, which are selectively permeable to charged particles, and protein pumps, which actively transport charged particles against electrochemical gradients. Rapid changes in the permeability of the cell membrane (resulting from the opening and closing of ion channels) allows a change in potential that is propagated along the membrane. The change in membrane potential can be integrated over time and space (see below). Regulation of membrane potential is therefore the essence of neuronal function.

Regulation of membrane potential is the essence of neuronal function.

The relationship of ion distributions to membrane potential is a fundamental concept in neuroscience. For most mammalian cells the 'resting' membrane potential inside the cell is negative relative to the outside, usually about −60 to −70 mV. The predominant ions involved are K^+ and organic anions (e.g. proteins and amino acids) on the inside, and Na^+ and Cl^- on the outside (Table 19.1). The membrane potential is established by electrochemical gradients that are generated by energy-dependent ion pumps. These ion pumps actively transport ions across membranes using the energy of ATP hydrolysis. The actual differences in the concentrations of ions across the membrane are determined by the selective permeability of the membrane to specific ions. This selective permeability is imparted primarily by ion channels. Ion channels are proteins that allow certain ions to cross the membrane while excluding others. Some ion channels are nongated or 'leak' channels, indicating that they are usually open. This is in contrast to ion channels that are gated, meaning that they open or close in response to a signal, usually a neurotransmitter or change in membrane potential. Gated channels are critical to rapidly changing the membrane potential for the purposes of information processing, but are usually closed in the resting membrane.

The movement of ions across a semipermeable cell membrane is based on two forces: the relative concentrations of the ions on each side (the concentration gradient) and the relative

Table 19.1 Ionic composition of neuronal intra- and extracellular fluid in the brain. Extracellular fluid (cerebrospinal fluid (CSF) in this case) is high in Na^+ and low in K^+ compared to intracellular fluid. Note that the positive and negative charges balance on each side of the membrane; the negative inside potential present at rest represents an extremely small surplus of negative ions at the inside face of the membrane. Free Ca^{2+} in cytoplasm is very low (~10^{-7} mol/L); it is higher in organelles that store Ca^{2+}.

		Extracellular (CSF) (mmol/L)	Intracellular (mmol/L)
Cations	Na^+	138	10
	K^+	3	120
	Ca^{2+}	1.5	10^{-4}
	Mg^{2+}	2	6.5
	Others	3.5	6.5
	Total positive charge	144.5	136.5
Anions	Cl^-	122	2
	HCO_3^-	25	12
	Organic anions	0.7	94
	Others	0.3	35
	Total negative charge	148	143

charge on either side (the voltage gradient). Charged particles in solution are randomly moving and will tend to diffuse from areas where they are more concentrated to those where they are less concentrated; they will also move toward an opposite charge. The distribution of an ion across the membrane will reach an equilibrium when the concentration forces exactly equal the electrical forces for that ion. The relationship of these electrical and chemical forces was first described in 1888 by Nernst:

■ Equation 19.1

$$E = \left(\frac{RT}{zF}\right)\ln\left(\frac{[\mathrm{Ion_{out}}]}{[\mathrm{Ion_{in}}]}\right)$$

where R is the universal gas constant, T is temperature (Kelvin), z is the valency of the ion, F is the Faraday constant, and E is the equilibrium potential (Nernst potential).

The Nernst equation gives the potential (in volts) across the membrane if the concentrations of the permeable species are known or, conversely, the concentrations of the species if the potential is known at equilibrium. As neuronal membranes are permeable to many ions, the formulation of the Nernst equation must include all permeable ions factored in according to their relative permeabilities. This more complete equation is referred to as the constant-field equation, or the Goldman–Hodgkin–Katz equation, after the investigators who developed it in the 1940s. An illustration of how these equations describe the relationship between membrane potential and ionic concentrations can be clearly demonstrated with glial cells, which are almost exclusively permeable to K^+. Consequently, only this ion needs to be considered. Other ions exist on both sides to nearly balance charge, but the membrane is not permeable to these ions and therefore do not enter into the equation. Most of the other values in the equation are constants under biologic conditions, so if one knows the concentration of K^+ on each side of the membrane the membrane potential of the glial cell can be calculated using Equation 19.1. At normal temperature and pressure, with a monovalent cation:

■ Equation 19.2

$$E = 61\log\left(\frac{[\mathrm{K^+}_{\mathrm{out}}]}{[\mathrm{K^+}_{\mathrm{in}}]}\right)$$

Changes in membrane potential produced by changes in ion permeability are the basis of the action potential and hence communication between neurons.

If $[K^+_{out}]$ is 4 mmol/L and $[K^+_{in}]$ is 120 mmol/L, then E is −90 mV.

As the concentration of K^+ outside the cell changes, the resting potential of the cell changes accordingly, as described by this equation; higher K^+ in the external solution results in a less negative potential (Fig. 19.4). This is also true of neurons, but to a lesser extent because their resting membrane potential is determined by their relative permeabilities to several ions in addition to K^+. Ions with low membrane permeability, such as Na^+, are not necessarily at equilibrium and do not contribute significantly to the resting potential. Although Na^+ is far from equilibrium at resting potential, the cell can rapidly increase permeability to Na^+ in response to a stimulus, causing these ions to flow across the membrane. This changes the membrane potential toward a value determined by the Nernst equation (or, more properly, the Goldman–Hodgkin–Katz equation) using the values resulting from this greater permeability. Such changes in potential produced by changes in ion permeability are the basis of the action potential as well as for much of the electrical communication and integration among neurons.

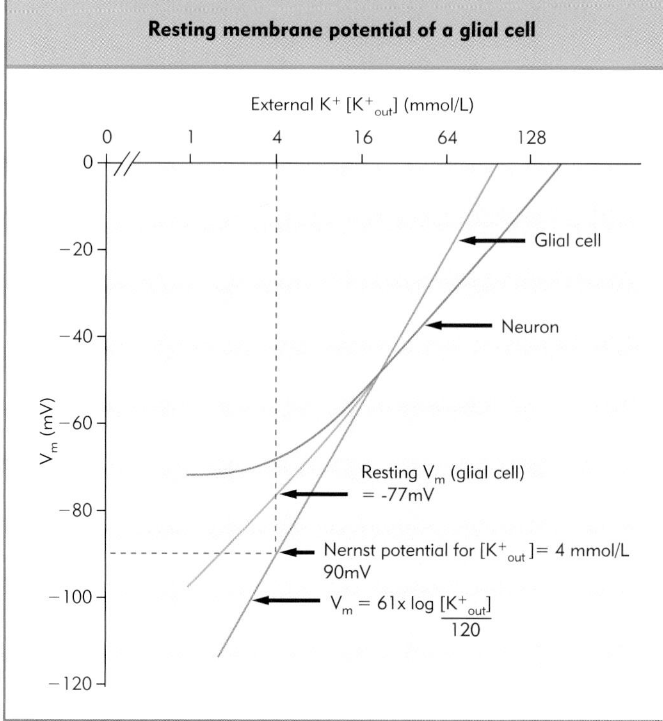

Figure 19.4 The resting membrane potential of a glial cell is dependent on K^+ concentration. Because the resting glial membrane is primarily permeable to K^+, manipulating the external concentration of K^+ alters the resting potential in a manner very close to that predicted by the Nernst equation, as seen by the close correspondence of its resting potential to the line that corresponds to the equation. Neurons, however, have additional ion channels contributing to permeability both at resting and at depolarized potentials, so these cells deviate more from this simple model.

Ion pumps and the generation of the resting potential

The Nernst and Goldman–Hodgkin–Katz equations describe the distribution of permeable ions at equilibrium at a given potential across the membrane, but they do not tell us how that potential was generated. In the example of a glial cell, a membrane permeable only to K^+ is at about −90 mV at 'rest'. However, in most cells the membrane is not perfectly impermeable to all other ions which tend to cross the membrane down their electrochemical gradients, reducing the membrane potential toward zero. To counteract this tendency, neurons and other cells have ion pumps, proteins that utilize the energy of ATP hydrolysis to transport ions across membranes against their electrochemical gradients, thereby maintaining the membrane potential (Chapter 6). The most important ion pump in maintaining neuronal membrane potential is the Na^+/K^+-ATPase or Na^+ pump. This transmembrane protein has the remarkable ability to move three Na^+ ions out of the cell and simultaneously move two K^+ ions into the cell powered by ATP hydrolysis. By moving more positive charges out than in, it causes a net separation of charge across the membrane and is therefore called an *electrogenic ion pump*. Many neurons have a resting potential that is just slightly greater (more negative) than that predicted by the Goldman–Hodgkin–Katz equation because of the active contribution of these electrogenic pumps. Not surprisingly, this pump is highly regulated by the metabolic needs of the cell through second-messenger cascades. The resting potential of most neurons is a dynamic balance between the active pumping of ions and the flow of ions back through ion channels down their electrochemical gradients, which tends to dissipate the potential.

ELECTRICAL PROPERTIES OF NEURONS

The electrical properties of neurons are the foundation for communication. The electrical properties of axons include passive properties that result from ion pumps and nongated channels, and active properties that are attributed to gated channels, particularly those that open or close in response to changes in membrane potential.

Electrical communication requires that the membrane potential changes over time, and that these changes are propagated along the membrane. The changes can be described using the same terminology and mathematics used to describe electrical circuits. In fact, the cell membrane is a capacitor, with the lipid tails of the phospholipid bilayer acting as a dielectric (insulator) and the charged phosphate heads acting as a storage site for positive charges from the intra- and extracellular environments. Nongated channels in the membrane form a conduit for current flow in parallel with the capacitance, and the ion pumps provide the potential energy (voltage) for the flow of current. This situation can be represented schematically as an electrical circuit, as shown in Figure 19.5. The membrane can be considered to act as a resistance–capacitance (RC) circuit. Both the active and the passive behavior of the membrane can be described using this model. When current flows across the membrane, following the opening of a channel or under experimental conditions with the injection of current from an electrode, it may flow almost instantly. However, membrane potential changes as an inverse exponential with time, as it would in an RC circuit. This occurs because much of the initial current (ion) flow charges the capacitance before it changes the potential on the other side of the membrane (Fig. 19.5). Therefore, very fast current flow produces a slower, attenuated change in membrane voltage. An important phenomenon that results from this property is *temporal summation*, in which a series of brief currents across the membrane of a neuron can be additive even though they are asynchronous, because the changes are spread out in time as a result of the membrane capacitance (Fig. 19.5). A phenomenon analogous to this occurs across space in propagation of voltage changes along the membrane. Potential changes are propagated passively along the membrane, as electrical charge will travel to areas where there is less charge of that polarity. If the amount of charge is large enough, it can trigger an action potential at a distant point on the membrane surface. One can best understand this propagation by considering the case of a cylinder such as an axon or dendrite (Fig. 19.6). The circuit model still applies, but here there are many equivalent circuits linked in parallel, with a low resistance to current flow along the cylinder in the extracellular fluid and the cytoplasm, and a higher resistance

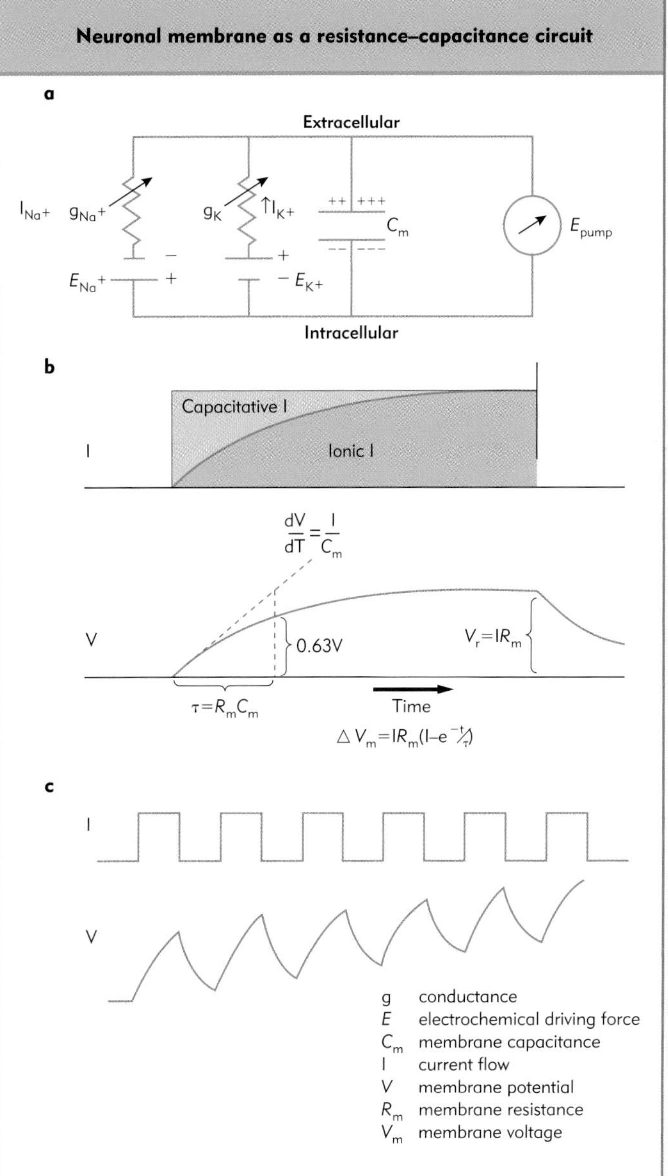

Figure 19.5 The neuronal membrane as a resistance–capacitance circuit. (a) Equivalent circuit representing the cell membrane with only gated ion channels in resting state: the electrochemical driving force (*E*) for ion flux across the membrane is shown for Na^+, K^+, and the electrogenic Na^+/K^+ pump that creates the resting membrane potential. At rest, the conductances for Na^+ and K^+, represented by variable resistors, are nearly closed, so that the resting membrane potential depends mostly on the pump and on a small K^+ conductance. These Na^+ and K^+ conductances do not change in the resting membrane but are altered during the action potential (see Fig. 19.7). (b) The membrane potential changes with ion flow across a membrane, as described by the simple circuit in (a). The initial flow of charge is taken up by the membrane capacitance, so that the voltage across the membrane (the membrane potential) changes more slowly, according to an inverse first-order exponential relationship equivalent to that describing the potential across the capacitor in (a). The initial rate of change in potential is dependent upon the capacitance of the membrane; the final voltage change (V_r) is dependent upon the resistance. The neuronal membrane has a time constant t, equal to the resistance across the membrane (R_m) multiplied by the capacitance (C_m), when the voltage has reached 63% of its value at the end of a long pulse of current. (c) This delay in voltage change across the cell membrane results in short pulses of current flow causing summating changes in membrane potential. This mechanism is found in neurons, where many short current fluxes from dendrites arriving apart may be partially additive.

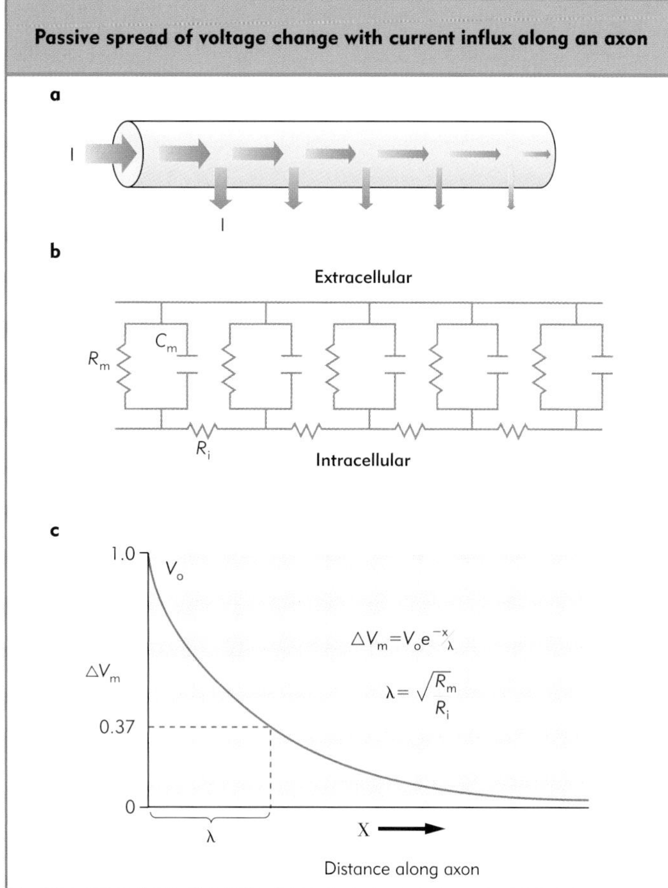

Figure 19.6 Passive spread of voltage change with current influx along an axon. (a) Current flow along an axon, showing the flow across the membrane and within the cytoplasm gradually dissipating (arrow width is proportional to current flow). (b) In an equivalent circuit model of an axon, the resistance and capacitance of the membrane is shown as a series of resistances (R_m) and capacitances (C_m) in parallel. Extracellular fluid resistance is not shown, as it is negligible compared to intracellular resistance (R_i). (c) Voltage change along the axon declines with distance as an inverse first-order exponential. The effective distance that the potential change travels is described by λ, the length constant (or space constant), which is the distance where the decrement is 1/e, or 37% of the initial voltage change. The length constant is dependent on the ratio of the resistance of the axonal membrane to the longitudinal resistance of the cytoplasm.

across the membrane. If current enters at one end of the cylinder there will be a change in membrane potential at that site (with the delay described above), representing a change in the distribution of charge across the membrane. The local change in charge across the membrane also means that there is a difference in charge between this site and adjacent sites on the same side of the membrane, such that current will flow along the membrane. As a result, the potential change will be propagated along the membrane as well. However, the change in potential will decrease with distance along the membrane, because the cell membrane is not perfectly impermeable and will dissipate the charge difference. Consequently, the rate of voltage decrement is dependent not only on the capacitance of the membrane, which determines how much of the charge goes to the capacitor, but also on the relative resistance of the membrane, the cytoplasm, and extracellular fluid. This passive, or electrotonic, conduction is described by λ, the length constant (also called the space constant), which is the distance at which the potential charge has decreased to 1/e (or 37%) of its original value, because it declines as an inverse first-order exponential.

The membrane can be considered to act as a resistance–capacitance (RC) circuit.

The capacitative properties of the cell membrane and the resistive properties of the cytoplasm and the extracellular fluid are quite constant in nearly all neurons. However, the resting resistance of the cell membrane may be quite variable from cell to cell. Length constants of over 100 times the cell body diameter, or more than the length of some very long dendrites, have been measured. This suggests that much of the electrical communication within a neuron can take place with only the passive electrical properties of neurons taking part. Active properties are needed primarily for communication over longer distances.

THE ACTION POTENTIAL

All animal cells have a resting potential, ion pumps, and a membrane that acts like an RC circuit. What distinguishes neurons (and to a lesser extent muscle and endocrine cells) from other cells is their excitability. Excitability is the ability of a cell to generate and propagate a large, rapid potential change in response to a relatively small trigger stimulus. The central phenomenon of excitability is the action potential. In contrast to passive conduction, the action potential conducts without decrement, traveling the entire length of an axon – up to meters – unchanging, regenerating itself constantly along its path. The action potential is a very rapid, stereotyped event: a coordinated sequence of several processes that lead to a specific, rapid depolarization (loss of negative intracellular potential), usually continuing to positive intracellular potentials and then rapidly repolarizing back to negative potentials, all within a few milliseconds. It is a regenerative, all-or-none event set in motion when the membrane potential depolarizes to a threshold level where adequate inward current begins a positive-feedback loop of depolarization (Fig. 19.7).

An understanding of the action potential requires only consideration of voltage-gated Na^+ and K^+ channels.

The action potential depends on the presence of voltage-gated ion channels that respond to changes in membrane potential by opening or closing. This is in contrast to nongated channels, which contribute to the resting membrane potential and are always open. There are many voltage-gated channels involved in neuronal excitability, but an understanding of the action potential requires only consideration of two: Na^+ and K^+ channels. When current (by convention, positive charge) flows into the cell, the cell is depolarized (made less negative inside). Regardless of the source of this current (neurotransmitter-gated channel, propagation of a nearby depolarization, current injection by an experimental electrode), the change in membrane potential is sensed by voltage-dependent Na^+ channels in the membrane. These channels are closed at the resting potential, but if the change in potential is sufficiently large (to above their

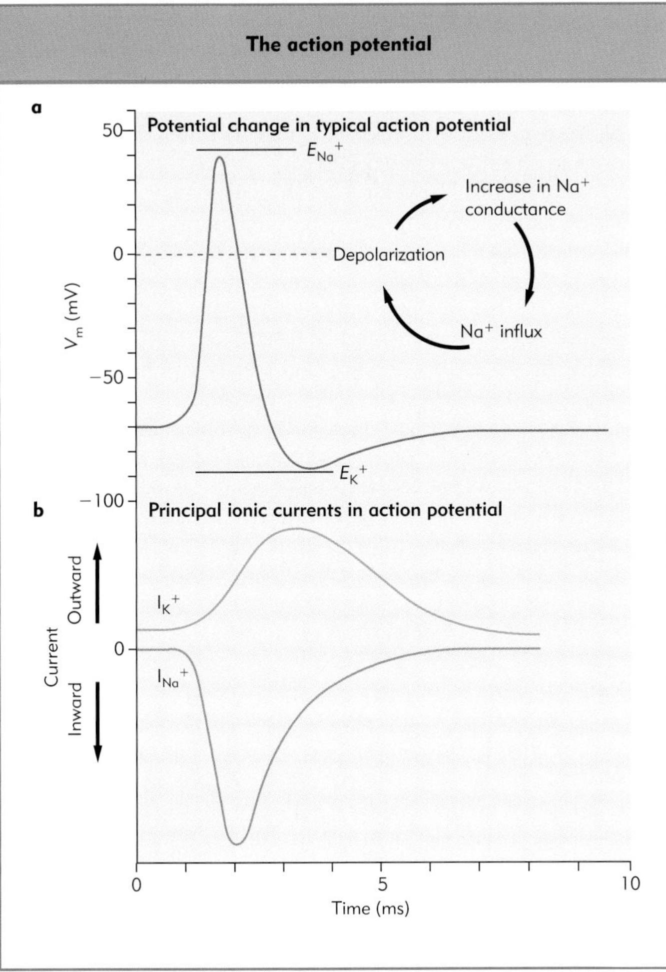

Figure 19.7 The action potential. (a) The potential change of a typical action potential rises from a resting potential of −70 mV, reaching a maximum near the Nernst potential for Na^+ (ENa^+), then declining with a negative undershoot near the Nernst potential for K^+ (EK^+). The action potential is triggered by a positive-feedback loop in which the initial depolarizing stimulus leads to opening of Na^+ channels, which leads to more depolarization. (b) Two principal ionic currents give rise to the action potential. Note that the outward K^+ current is slower and delayed in onset compared to the Na^+ current.

threshold potential), they open rapidly. This allows Na^+ to flow through into the cell, because at the resting potential Na^+ is not at equilibrium across the membrane; in fact, it is far from it. The cell membrane at rest is quite impermeable to Na^+, and the electrogenic ion pumps make the intracellular concentration small relative to that outside the cell. As the resting potential is about −70 mV, there is also a substantial electrical gradient for Na^+ flow into the cell. The equilibrium potential (Nernst potential) for Na^+ is about 50 mV, resulting in a net electrochemical gradient of 120 mV. The initial ion flow through voltage-gated Na^+ channels with depolarization leads to more depolarization and then more channel opening, starting a positive-feedback loop until all the channels that can be opened are open and the membrane potential has approached the Nernst potential for Na^+. The membrane potential can go from a value of −50 mV to as high as +40 mV in less than a millisecond once this process is initiated.

Once the action potential is initiated, the process must be turned off for the membrane to return to its resting potential. The Na^+ channels, once open, close spontaneously after a few milliseconds by a process called inactivation. Another type of voltage-gated channel, permeable to K^+, also opens in response to the depolarization produced by the action potential, but with a small delay compared with Na^+ channels. As discussed above, the Nernst potential for K^+ is near the resting potential. When these K^+ channels open during an action potential the membrane potential is positive, so there is a very strong gradient for K^+ to travel out of the cell, causing an outward current that tends to bring the membrane potential back to its resting state. In fact, there is a small overshoot to most action potentials, during which the membrane potential is more negative than the resting potential for several milliseconds; this is caused by the action of these K^+ channels. The opening of K^+ channels occurs more slowly than that of Na^+ channels; consequently, they do not oppose the action of Na^+ channels until after the action potential has been initiated, assisting primarily in resetting the potential back to the resting level. Because of this, they are referred to as delayed rectifier K^+ channels. The result of these two currents acting in this highly coordinated manner is a potential change (Fig. 19.7). There are several other K^+ channels (not discussed here) that are involved in the regulation rather than in the production of the action potential in various types of neuron.

The action potential has several characteristics that are important for its information-carrying function: threshold, all-or-none behavior, and the refractory period.

The depolarization of the membrane must be of sufficient amplitude and speed to activate an adequate number of Na^+ channels. These Na^+ channels initiate a positive-feedback mechanism that will cause the activation of channels to become regenerative. Otherwise, a small number of channels will be activated, but not enough to depolarize the membrane further to start the positive-feedback loop. The voltage at which the process becomes regenerative and self-sustaining is the action potential *threshold*. This is not a static value, but a dynamic phenomenon dependent on the initial resting potential, the rate of depolarization, the history of recent action potentials, and metabolic modulations.

The second important characteristic of the action potential is its *all-or-none behavior*. This is particularly important in conduction, where an action potential propagates unchanged as long as there are enough voltage-gated Na^+ channels to support it. The two related phenomena of threshold and all-or-none behavior are key to information processing by the nervous system. One of the principal ways of processing information in neurons is the combination of graded excitatory (depolarizing) and inhibitory (hyperpolarizing) influences from synaptic and metabolic sources, which determine whether an action potential will be initiated. This is essentially a calculation at the level of the membrane; once the threshold is reached, it is encoded as an on/off signal that is propagated unchanged as an action potential to the end of the axon.

The third important characteristic of the action potential is the *refractory period*. Once channels have opened to create an action potential, they cannot reopen immediately but require from a few milliseconds to several seconds to return to a fully activatable state. This has several consequences. First, it limits the rate at which action potentials can fire. Second, it allows conduction in only one direction along a segment of axon. The consequence is that if two converging action potentials collide, because the membrane behind each action potential is refractory, conduction will terminate.

Axonal conduction

Propagation of action potentials involves the same process described above acting over space. The inward current caused by Na^+ influx depolarizes the membrane; this depolarization is easily propagated along the membrane toward areas with less charge by electrotonic conduction. As the depolarization spreads to other areas of the membrane, voltage-gated Na^+ channels nearby are opened and the action potential is propagated. The conduction of a typical electrical impulse along a wire decays with distance; however, action potentials maintain their size and shape and will conduct unchanged along a nerve for a theoretically infinite distance. The velocity of this conduction varies tremendously between nerves; depending on their physiologic function, the velocity ranges from several centimeters per second to as much as 10 m/s (Table 19.2, see also Table 22.1). In some pathologic states, such as multiple sclerosis and demyelinating diseases, nerve conduction is drastically affected so that it is slowed and may fail. The factors affecting conduction velocity can be derived from a mathematical analysis of the equivalent electrical circuit model of the membrane and knowledge of the nature of the action potential.

Bigger axons conduct faster. An increase in diameter increases the capacitance of a given length of axon linearly, which tends to slow conduction, but it decreases the resistance of the cytoplasm in proportion to the square of the radius, as this resistance is proportional to the cross-sectional area of cytoplasm. The result is an increase in conduction velocity proportional to the square root of the radius.

Channels that open faster change the membrane potential faster and tend to open nearby Na^+ channels sooner, resulting in faster conduction. This also occurs with increased channel density. For example, the axons of neurons that conduct information about touch and movement have Na^+ channels that open faster than those of neurons that transmit some pain information or control autonomic function, which do not require fast information transmission.

Temperature has complex effects of neuronal excitability. Generally, cooling a nerve will slow conduction by slowing the rate at which Na^+ channels open and close, as well as the rate at which Na^+ traverses the channels. Substantial cooling can actually block conduction. Warming speeds conduction up to a point, but warming over about 40°C causes the channels to close too soon, reducing current flow and hence conduction velocity.

Axonal conduction velocity is increased by wrapping the axon in an insulating layer of myelin over intermittent segments. This can increase conduction velocity up to 10 times more than that achieved in an unmyelinated nerve.

Invertebrates lack myelin. Consequently, they are limited to increasing axonal diameter to speed conduction for signals that must be conducted very fast, such as the signals for flight from danger. The squid, for instance, escapes quickly with signals that travel about 20 m/s along a huge axon that is over 1 mm in diameter. (A preparation of this giant axon was used to great advantage by Hodgkin, Huxley, and others to characterize the electrophysiology of the axon.) This approach, however, is inefficient in terms of space and metabolic requirements, as conduction velocity increases only as the square root of the radius. Myelination allows vertebrates to conduct signals along axons that are only a few micrometers in diameter at rates exceeding that achieved in the squid.

Myelin is a tight, spiral, multilayered wrapping of glial cell membranes around an axon (see Fig. 19.3). Because cell membranes are electrical insulators, they increase the effective resistance of the axon to current flow across its membrane. In addition, the myelin sheath, which is much thicker than the axonal membrane, increases the distance between the charges inside the cell and those in the extracellular fluid, which reduces the effective capacitance of the axon. In an ideal system, an action potential could then be conducted through the axoplasm of a myelinated nerve all the way to its end, where the current would escape into the extracellular fluid and complete the circuit in a similar manner to conductance through an insulated copper wire. However, axoplasm and extracellular fluid are not perfect conductors and myelin is not a perfect insulator, so signals need to be regenerated at regular intervals along the axon. To do this, myelin is interrupted, usually every 1–2 mm along the axon, for a very short distance (a few micrometers), and the axon membrane is exposed to the extracellular fluid. Essentially all the Na^+ channels in the axon are bunched in these zones, called nodes of Ranvier. Current traveling electrotonically in the axon from the nearby node causes a depolarization that is sufficient to trigger the opening of Na^+ channels in the next node, producing a full action potential that is then conducted to the

Table 19.2 Relationship of diameter, conduction velocity, and function in afferent nerve axons. Groups I-IV refers to the classification of muscle afferents. The fiber types Aβ, Aδ, and C refer to cutaneous afferents, although the latter classification, including Aα fibers, is often used when the classification is by conduction velocity alone

	Fiber type	Fiber diameter (μm)	Conduction velocity (m/s)	Function
Myelinated	Aα (group I)	12–20	75–120	Muscle stretch receptors, tendon afferents
	Aβ (group II)	5–12	30–75	Muscle stretch receptors, light touch
	Aδ (group III)	1–5	5–30	Fast pain (immediate, sharp)
Unmyelinated	C (group IV)	0.2–1.5	0.3–1.5	Slow pain (burning, ache)

next node. This node-to-node jump is called *saltatory conduction*. The ability of myelin to allow conduction through the axon with little need to charge the membrane capacitance along the way results in very high conduction velocity within relatively small axons. It is also energy efficient, because ions flow across the membrane only at the nodes. Myelinated axons also show improved gain from an increase in diameter: velocity increases directly with the axon diameter in myelinated axons, versus the square root of diameter in unmyelinated fibers.

Essentially all axonal Na^+ channels are located in the nodes of Ranvier, between which action potentials jump by saltatory conduction.

Classification of nerves according to conduction velocity

Conduction velocity has been used to classify sensory axons because different biologic functions necessitate different conduction velocities (Fig. 19.8). This classification illustrates the relation between action potential conduction velocity and the two strategies used by the nervous system to alter it: axon diameter and myelination. The conduction velocity is also used clinically to diagnosis peripheral neuropathies. Most sensory nerves contain a mixture of fiber types. When such a nerve is stimulated and the action potentials produced are recorded at some distance away, the record contains several impulse peaks (classically four) representing action potentials from hundreds to thousands of axons (compound action potential) arriving at different times according to their conduction velocities. The first peak to reach the recording electrode is that carried by the large-diameter myelinated fibers, the fastest of which are the Aα axons (also called group I afferents), which exist only in nerves innervating muscle (see Fig. 14.6). They are the sensory axons of the muscle spindle reflex arc. The next peak is from the small myelinated fibers, designated Aβ or group II axons, which carry sensory information about mechanical stimuli such as touch. The third peak is the Aδ or group III axons, which carry both mechanosensory information and also some types of pain information, typically that perceived as sharp or lancinating pain. These are even smaller myelinated fibers. The slowest fibers, often conducting at less than 1 m/s, are small-diameter unmyelinated sensory axons. They primarily carry information about temperature and pain, particularly pain that is perceived as burning or aching (Chapters 22 and 23).

The nature and function of voltage-gated ion channels

Specific ion-conducting pores across membranes were demonstrated in the landmark reports of Hodgkin and Huxley in the 1950s that described the action potential in terms of ion currents. Since then we have gained detailed knowledge of the voltage-gated channels involved in excitability, advancing from theoretic concepts to increasingly well-understood molecular entities. This has been made possible by two experimental advances: the patch-clamp recording technique and the application of molecular biology to clone ion channels. In the mid 1970s, Neher and Sakmann succeeded in electrically isolating a single ion channel by sealing a tiny glass electrode around it on

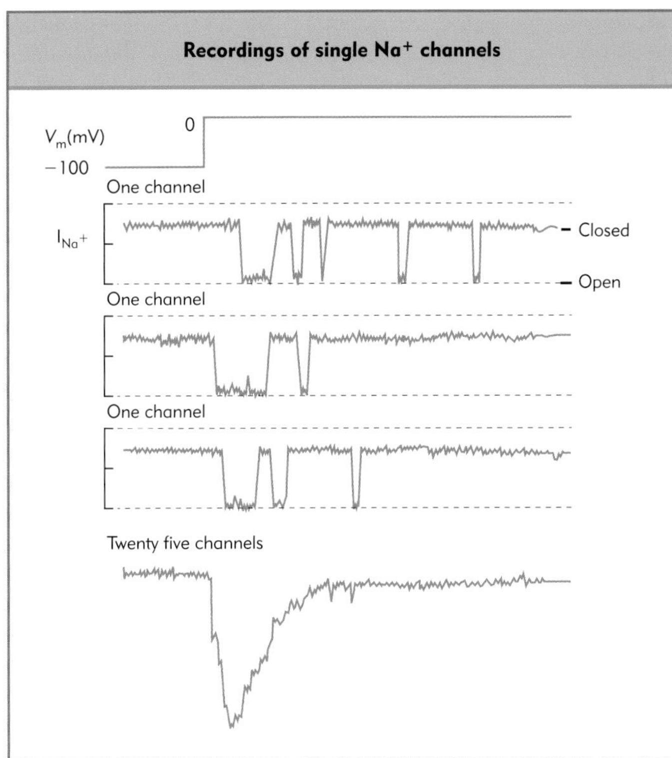

Figure 19.8 Recordings of single Na^+ channels. Schematic of patch clamp recordings of individual Na^+ channels activated by depolarization from a potential of −100 to 0 mV. Note that channels open quickly to a uniform conductance with a more variable time course. Channels open with the initial depolarization, then open less as the membrane is held at 0 mV, representing channel inactivation. When many records of single channels are summed, the resulting trace reconstructs that seen with a whole cell recording (lowest trace).

the surface of a muscle. These studies eventually led to a detailed knowledge of the function of the individual channels that make up the action potential, as well as of many other channels. An example of single-channel recordings is shown in Figure 19.8.

Once ion channels were cloned and expressed in cells lacking such channels, both the molecular structure and the channel activity of these entities could be determined. For example, it was found that several types of voltage-gated Na^+ channel are involved in action potential generation, with different properties depending on the tissue of origin (e.g. brain, peripheral neurons). This has become a recurrent theme with ion channels. As a result, there are more channels identified for each ion than could have been predicted with classic physiologic and pharmacologic approaches, leading to a tremendous opportunity for specific pharmacologic intervention. These ion channels can be grouped into families based on their amino acid sequences.

Voltage-gated channels for Na^+, K^+, and Ca^{2+} are all very similar in structure. They all have a pore-forming subunit with a domain structure of six transmembrane segments. The Na^+ and Ca^{2+} channels each have four domains of this type, whereas K^+ channels have a subunit with only one domain, which functions as a tetramer. The structure of the pore-forming α subunit of a typical Na^+ channel is shown in Figure 33.2. From knowledge of the amino acid sequence of these channels and studies of the effects of known mutations on channel function, certain inferences can be made about their structure. For example, mutants of voltage-gated K^+ channels show that the fourth transmembrane segment of a subunit (the S4 region) is probably responsible for the voltage-sensing properties of the channel. This same region probably confers voltage-sensitive opening of Ca^{2+} and Na^{+} channels as well. A highly hydrophobic region, called the P segment, appears to be the pore- or channel-forming area of the protein, and cytoplasmic segments are involved in closing an open channel. They have positively charged amino acids at the ends of cytoplasmic segments. Following depolarization and channel opening, these amino acids may move and occlude the open channel like a drain plug on a chain. This conformational change may be the molecular mechanism underlying channel inactivation. Such molecular descriptions of ion channel function are just beginning and may lead both to an understanding of the structure–function relationships of channels and to the design of drugs that act on specific functions to alter neuronal excitability (Chapters 6 and 33).

Key references

Caterall WA. Structure and function of voltage-gated ion channels. Annu Rev Biochem. 1995;64:493–531.

Dani JW, Chenjavsky A, Smith SJ. Neuronal activity triggers calcium waves in hippocampal astrocyte networks. Neuron 1992;8:429–40.

Hansson E, Ronnback L. Glial neuronal signaling in the central nervous system. FASEB J. 2003;17:341–8.

Hodgkin AL, Huxley AF. A quantitative description of membrane current and its application to conduction and excitation in nerve. J Physiol. 1952;117:500–44.

Hodgkin AL, Huxley AF. Currents carried by sodium and potassium ions through the membrane of the giant axon of Loligo. J Physiol. 1952;116:449–72.

Peters A, Palay SL, Webster HDF. The fine structure of the nervous system: the neurons and supporting cells. Philadelphia, PA: WB Saunders; 1976.

Further reading

Hille B. Ion channels of excitable membranes, 3rd edn. Sunderland, MA: Sinauer Associates Inc.; 2001.

Kandel ER, Schwartz JH, Jessell T. Principles of neural science, 4th edn. McGraw-Hill/Appleton & Lange; 2000.

Levitan IB, Kaczmarek, LK. The neuron: cell and molecular biology, 3rd edn. New York: Oxford University Press; 2001.

Nicholls JG, Wallace BG, Fusch PA, Martin AR. From neuron to brain, 4th edn. Sunderland, MA: Sinauer Associates Inc.; 2001.

Chapter 20

The synapse

Ken Mackie

TOPICS COVERED IN THIS CHAPTER
- **Presynaptic terminals**
- **Fast and slow synaptic transmission**
- **Excitatory and inhibitory neurotransmitters**
- **Peptide neurotransmitters**
- **Neurotransmitter receptors**
- **Neurotransmitter synthesis and metabolism**
- **Synaptic transmission**
- **Modulation of excitability and synaptic transmission**
- **Neural plasticity**

Synapses are the primary point of communication between neurons. Synapses are highly specialized neuronal structures at which most neurotransmitter release takes place. Their number in the human brain is immense: conservative estimates are that there are about 10^{11} neurons and $>10^{14}$ synapses. The large number of synapses and the ability of neurons to modulate the efficacy or the strength of particular synaptic connections create the complexity and flexibility of the human brain. In addition, the central role played by synapses in the functioning of the nervous system makes synaptic transmission an important target for many anesthetic and other drugs acting on the nervous system.

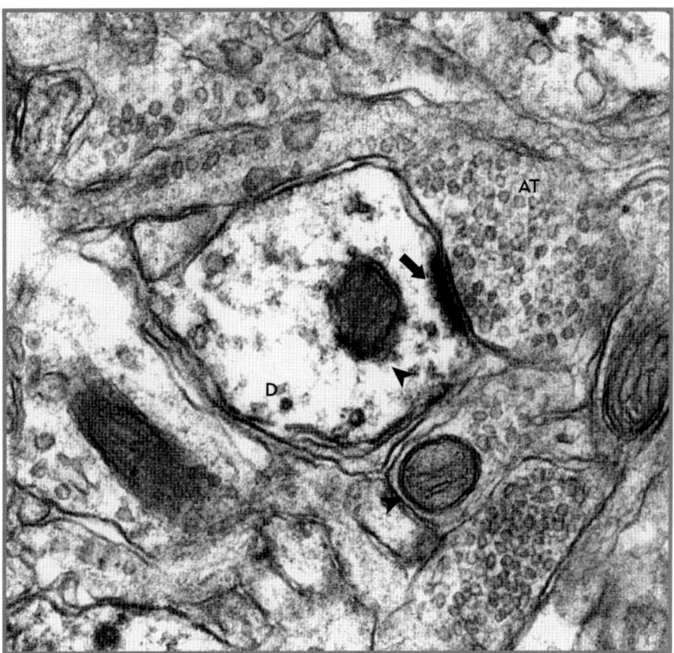

Figure 20.1 Ultrastructure of an excitatory synapse. Electron micrograph of an asymmetric synapse between an axon terminal (AT) and the dendrite (D) of a nonpyramidal cell in rat dorsal cortex. The terminal is packed with small vesicles that contain neurotransmitters. At the synaptic junction (arrow) the presynaptic and postsynaptic membranes are separated by a cleft (synapse), which contains extracellular matrix. The postsynaptic membrane has a prominent coat of dense material (PSD) on its cytoplasmic face. Note the mitochondria in the dendrite and an adjacent terminal (arrowhead). (Micrograph courtesy of Ruth Westenbroek.)

PRESYNAPTIC TERMINALS

Synaptic terminals may take many forms. These include the classic axodendritic (axon terminal to dendrite) type, but also dendrodendritic, dendroaxonal, axoaxonal, etc. Although some of the more specialized synaptic structures occur in specific neuronal structures, it is useful to consider the classic axodendritic synapses as an example. As shown in Figure 20.1, the presynaptic terminal contains synaptic vesicles, mitochondria, and neurofilaments, and is a highly ordered structure.

Specialized structures opposite to presynaptic terminals are present in postsynaptic neurons (Fig. 20.1). In excitatory postsynaptic terminals, a band of electron-dense material is present (the postsynaptic density, PSD). In addition, postsynaptic terminals contain receptors that bind released neurotransmitters, as well as enzymes and ion channels that transduce the signal carried by the neurotransmitter into a physiologic response in the postsynaptic cell.

FAST AND SLOW SYNAPTIC TRANSMISSION

Neurotransmission can be conveniently, if simplistically, divided into two broad types, fast and slow (Fig. 20.2). Fast neurotransmission can be thought of as the point-to-point communication system in the brain. Slow neurotransmission can be

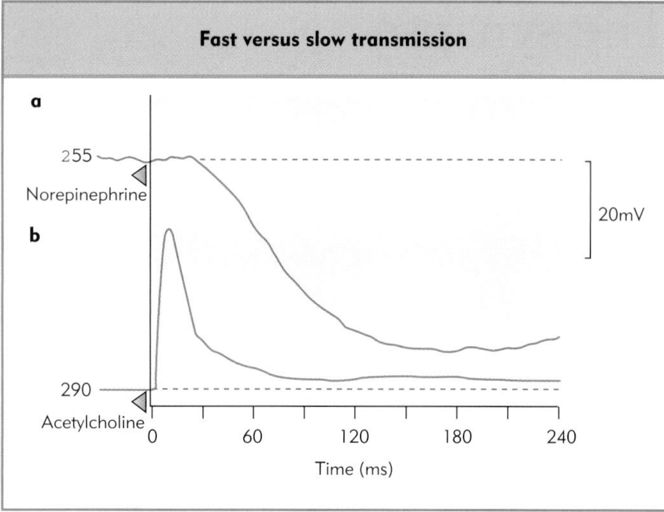

Figure 20.2 Fast versus slow neurotransmission in a guinea-pig submucous plexus neuron. (a) Norepinephrine-induced hyperpolarization of membrane potential mediated by α_2-adrenergic receptors has a latency of approximately 30 ms and reaches its maximum after approximately 180 ms. (b) Acetylcholine (ACh)-induced depolarization mediated by the nicotinic ACh receptor in the same neuron has a very short latency and quickly reaches its peak and inactivates. In both cases a supramaximal amount of drug was applied for 0.5 ms. (From North RA. Drug receptors and the inhibition of nerve cells. Br J Pharmacol. 1989;98:13–28.)

Table 20.1 Fast neurotransmitter systems

Neurotransmitter	Receptor	Significant permeant ions
Excitatory		
Glutamate	NMDA AMPA Kainate	Na^+, K^+, (Ca^{2+}) Na^+, K^+ Na^+, K^+
ACh	Nicotinic	Na^+, $K^+ > Ca^{2+}$
Serotonin (5-hydroxytryptamine)	5-HT_3	Na^+, K^+, Ca^{2+}
ATP, ADP, UTP	P_{2x}	Na^+, K^+, $\pm Ca^{2+}$
Vanillanoids, temperature	VR-I	$Ca^{2+} > Na^+$
Inhibitory		
GABA	GABA	Cl^-, HCO_3^-
Glycine	Glycine	Cl^-

The receptors for these neurotransmitters belong to the superfamily of multimeric ligand-gated ion channels
ADP, adenosine diphosphate; UTP, uridine triphosphate.

thought of as setting the background tone for a collection of neurons and their synapses. A familiar example of fast neurotransmission is the release of acetylcholine (ACh) at the neuromuscular junction (Chapter 36). Cation influx through the nicotinic ACh receptor (a ligand-gated ion channel) results in depolarization of the muscle cell membrane, which leads to Ca^{2+} release from the sarcoplasmic reticulum and muscle contraction. The action of ACh is terminated by its hydrolysis in the synaptic cleft by acetylcholinesterase. Fast neurotransmission in the CNS is mediated by postsynaptic ligand-gated ion channels. Examples include glutamate (*N*-methyl-D-aspartate (NMDA), α-amino-3-hydroxy-5-methylisoxazole-4-propionic acid (AMPA), and kainate (KA) type receptors), γ-aminobutyric acid (GABA; $GABA_A$ receptors), glycine (glycine receptors), ACh (nicotinic ACh receptors), adenosine triphosphate (ATP; purinergic type 2X (P_{2X}) receptors), and serotonin (5-hydroxytryptamine (5-HT_3) receptors) (Table 20.1).

Fast neurotransmission mediates point-to-point communication; slow neurotransmission sets the background tone.

The other major class of neurotransmitter are the 'slow' neurotransmitters, often referred to as neuromodulators (Table 20.2). Their slowness is imparted by their target receptors, often G protein-coupled receptors (GPCRs). After the neuromodulator binds to its GPCR the receptor undergoes a conformational change, activating G proteins (Chapter 3). The activated G proteins dissociate and the α subunit and/or βγ subunits modulate the properties of specific enzymes and ion channels (effectors), setting in motion diverse cellular responses. Often a given neurotransmitter has both 'fast' and 'slow' effects. An example familiar to anesthesiologists is ACh, for which the fast effects (e.g. neurotransmission at the neuromuscular junction) are mediated by nicotinic ACh receptors and the slow effects (bronchoconstriction, salivation, gastrointestinal motility) by muscarinic ACh receptors. Other examples of neurotransmitters that have both fast and slow actions are GABA, serotonin, ATP, and glutamate. Many other neurotransmitters have only slow effects, and include the endogenous opioids, dopamine (DA), catecholamines, eicosanoids, etc. Many of these systems are influenced by anesthetic drugs.

Another class of neuromodulator is the free-radical messengers, including nitric oxide and carbon monoxide. Rather than being stored in vesicles and released, as the classic neurotransmitters mentioned above usually are, they are synthesized 'on demand'. Often functioning as retrograde messengers, they play important roles in neuronal signaling and neural plasticity.

EXCITATORY AND INHIBITORY NEUROTRANSMITTERS

Another classification of neurotransmission is based on the effect of a neurotransmitter on neuronal membrane properties, termed excitatory or inhibitory. For fast neurotransmitters this distinction is fairly clear. Excitatory fast neurotransmitters open ligand-gated ion channels that are preferentially permeable to Na^+, and often to Ca^{2+}. As these ions move down their electrochemical gradients the membrane potential is displaced in a positive direction (depolarizes), making the cell more excitable (that is, more likely to fire an action potential). Conversely, inhibitory fast neurotransmitters open ion channels that are more permeable to Cl^-, which keeps the membrane potential negative and makes the cell less excitable. Excitatory fast neurotransmitters include ACh, glutamate, ATP, and serotonin, whereas the inhibitory fast neurotransmitters in the mammalian CNS are GABA and glycine.

Table 20.2 Slow neurotransmitter systems

Neurotransmitter	Receptor	Ion channels	Second messenger
Glutamate	Metabotropic	↓Ca^{2+}, ↑K^+	↑IP_3/DAG
GABA	$GABA_B$	↑K^+, ↓Ca^{2+}	↓cAMP ↑(IP_3/DAG) – minor
ACh	Muscarinic M_1, M_3, M_5 M_2, M_4	↓Ca^{2+}, ↓K^+ (M-current) ↓Ca^{2+}, ↑K^+	↑IP_3/DAG ↓cAMP
Norepinephrine	α_1 α_2 β_1 β_2 β_3	 ↑K^+, ↓Ca^{2+} ↑Ca^{2+}	↑IP_3/DAG ↑IP_3/DAG ↑cAMP ↑cAMP
Dopamine	D_1, D_5		↑cAMP
Serotonin (5-hydroxytryptamine)	$5\text{-}HT_1$ $5\text{-}HT_2$ $5\text{-}HT_4$ $5\text{-}HT_5$ $5\text{-}HT_6$ $5\text{-}HT_7$	↑K^+, ↓Ca^{2+}	↓cAMP ↑IP_3/DAG ↑cAMP ↓cAMP ↑cAMP ↑cAMP
Substance P	NK_1	↓Ca^{2+}	↑IP_3/DAG
Histamine	H_1 H_2 H_3		↑IP_3/DAG ↑cAMP ↓cAMP, ?
ATP, ADP, UTP	P_{2Y}	↓Ca^{2+}, ↑K^+	↑IP_3/DAG
Adenosine	A_1 A_{2A} A_{2B} A_3		↓cAMP ↑cAMP ↑cAMP ↓cAMP ↑IP_3/DAG
Opioids	μ δ κ	↓Ca^{2+}, ↑K^+ ↓Ca^{2+}, ↑K^+ ↓Ca^{2+}, ↑K^+	↓cAMP ↓cAMP ↓cAMP

The receptors for these neurotransmitters all belong to the superfamily of G protein-coupled receptors containing a predicted seven transmembrane domain structure. Different effects are seen with different subtypes. Not all effects are seen in all cells; the net effect (e.g. on excitability) may be a complex balance of opposing effects. IP_3, inositol trisphosphate; DAG, diacylglycerol; cAMP, cyclic adenosine monophosphate.

Excitatory neurotransmitters make the cell more likely to fire an action potential; inhibitory neurotransmitters suppress firing.

The major excitatory fast neurotransmitter is glutamate, which plays a central role in neuronal function and plasticity. Activation of nonNMDA glutamate receptors (AMPA/kainate receptors) is responsible for most fast glutamatergic neurotransmission. The NMDA receptors only become fully activated by glutamate when their Mg^{2+} block has been relieved by partial depolarization of the neuron; also, NMDA receptor kinetics are much slower. Their activation results in a large Ca^{2+} influx, which has been linked to long-term metabolic, transcriptional, and structural changes, including synaptic plasticity (see below).

These functional differences are reflected in their distinct subunit structures. *N*-methyl-D-aspartate receptors are heteromeric complexes (composed of four or five subunits) of NR1 and NR2 (subtypes A–D) subunits, whereas nonNMDA receptors are composed of GluR (1–7) and KA (1–2) subunits. The major inhibitory fast transmitter is GABA, which is important in regulating neuronal excitability. Activation of pentameric $GABA_A$ receptors is responsible for fast GABAergic neurotransmission; these receptors are thought to be major targets for anesthetic effects (Chapters 24–26). γ-Aminobutyric $acid_A$ receptors are made up from at least 17 different subunits, classified as α (1–6), β (1–4), γ (1–3), δ, ε, and ρ (1–2), with additional diversity from alternative messenger ribonucleic acid (mRNA) splicing. The most common combination in the CNS is two α, two β, and one γ subunit.

Slow neurotransmitters can be classified similarly, although often the distinctions are blurred as a single neuron may express multiple distinct receptors. This occurs because, although the receptors bind the same agonist, they couple to a different spectrum of G proteins that activate different effector systems and produce opposite effects on excitability (a good example of this is the muscarinic ACh receptor family). A related complicating factor in the interpretation of neurotransmitter action is that the same subtype of receptor can couple to different effectors in different cells. Thus, the examples given below are generalities only – specific exceptions exist. Prominent examples of excitatory slow neurotransmitter receptors include substance P, α_1-receptors, bradykinin, group I metabotropic glutamate (mGluR1 and mGluR5), and the odd-numbered (M_1, M_3, and M_5) muscarinic receptors. As one of their actions, many of the excitatory slow neurotransmitter receptors activate phospholipase C (PLC). Specific polyphosphatide-containing membrane lipids (for example, PIP_2 is cleaved by PLC to release inositol trisphosphate (IP_3) and diacylglycerol (DAG)). The release of Ca^{2+} from internal stores (endoplasmic reticulum) is mediated by IP_3, activating several cellular processes that tend to increase excitability. The DAG, in concert with IP_3-released Ca^{2+}, activates protein kinase C (PKC, see Chapter 3), which can also increase excitability. Membrane depolarization by inhibition of a K^+ channel (the 'M-current') is another action of many of these receptors. These actions tend to increase neuronal excitability.

Examples of inhibitory slow neurotransmitter receptors include opioid, even-numbered muscarinic (M_2 and M_4), and α_2-adrenergic receptors. Inhibitory slow neurotransmitters often inhibit adenylyl cyclase, activate K^+ channels (particularly inwardly rectifying K^+ channels), and inhibit N- and P/Q-type voltage-gated Ca^{2+} channels, which are the Ca^{2+} channel isoforms in presynaptic terminals through which Ca^{2+} enters to cause synaptic vesicle fusion and neurotransmitter release (see below). These actions tend to decrease neuronal excitability.

PEPTIDE NEUROTRANSMITTERS

The neuropeptides form an important family of neurotransmitters. Although the number of peptide neurotransmitters continues to expand, a list of the best-studied ones is given in Table 20.3. Those most relevant to the practice of anesthesiology include the endogenous opioids (enkephalins, CGRP, endorphins, dynorphin, and their precursors and metabolites; Chapter 31), substance P, and bradykinin.

Table 20.3 Peptide neurotransmitters

Atrial naturetic factor	Galanin
β-endorphin	Neuropeptide Y
Bradykinin	Neurotensin
Calcitonin gene-related peptide	Oxytocin
Cholecystokinin	Somatostatin
Dynorphin	Substance P
Met-enkephalin	Vasopressin
Leu-enkephalin	Vasoactive intestinal peptide

Peptides are slow neurotransmitters and typically exert their actions by binding to GPCRs (Chapter 3). Whereas classic neurotransmitters, such as glutamate, ACh, GABA, etc., are released from small (40 nm diameter) clear vesicles by the mechanisms outlined below, peptides are often released from large (100 nm diameter) vesicles by less well understood pathway(s). Typically, these large vesicles are distant from active zones. One theory is that these large vesicles only fuse with the membrane and release their contents during strong and prolonged increases in presynaptic Ca^{2+} concentration, as seen during repetitive depolarizations (peptide release is thus frequency dependent). A key difference between peptides and other neurotransmitters is that peptides are synthesized in the cell body and transported to the nerve terminal. Their actions are terminated by proteolysis; thus, replenishment of peptide-containing synaptic vesicles is much slower than that of other neurotransmitter-containing vesicles.

Neuropeptides often coexist with classic transmitters in the same neurons.

A once-prevalent concept in neuropharmacology held that each neuron contained only a single transmitter. However, this concept has recently given way to the idea that neuropeptides coexist in many central and most, if not all, peripheral neurons with classic amino acid or monoamine transmitters. Peptides are thus positioned to increase the information transferred at a given synapse by regulating the amount of transmitter released with a given stimulus or modulating the response of a common target cell.

NEUROTRANSMITTER RECEPTORS

Neurotransmitter receptors can be conveniently divided into two classes. The first are the ligand-gated ion channels, which both bind the neurotransmitter and, when open, allow specific ions to pass through. These are the receptors that underlie fast neurotransmission discussed above (Table 20.1). They consist of a large protein (an assembly of several smaller subunits, e.g. the nicotinic ACh receptor, often composed of two α subunits and β, γ, δ, and/or ε subunits) that both binds the neurotransmitter (usually with two binding sites per channel) and forms the ion pore. In addition, auxiliary subunits are often associated with the pore-forming and ligand-binding subunit. These subunits may convey specific pharmacologic properties (e.g. γ subunits of the $GABA_A$ channel contain the benzodiazepine-binding site).

The second class of neurotransmitter receptor are those that underlie slow neurotransmission (Table 20.2). A classic example of a slow neurotransmitter receptor is a GPCR; other examples include soluble guanylyl cyclase (the receptor for nitric oxide) and receptor tyrosine kinases (see Chapter 3). The effects of many neuromodulators are transduced by GPCRs, as briefly outlined above. Guanylyl cyclase is a 'receptor' for and activated by nitric oxide and related free-radical messengers. Receptor tyrosine kinases bind small peptides (e.g. cytokines and growth factors) in their extracellular domain, which leads to activation of the intracellular tyrosine kinase domain that phosphorylates specific target molecules in the cell. Although these receptors have long been known to play a key role in regulating neuronal growth, differentiation, and survival, it is now clear that they also play an important role in regulating neuronal excitability through their effects on specific ion channels and G protein signaling pathways.

NEUROTRANSMITTER SYNTHESIS AND METABOLISM

The synthesis and metabolism of the small neurotransmitters (ACh, norepinephrine (noradrenaline), DA, epinephrine (adrenaline), glutamate, GABA, glycine, etc.) have been studied extensively. In addition to de novo synthesis, reuptake of released neurotransmitter from the synaptic cleft is an important mechanism used by neurons to recover released neurotransmitter or their metabolites.

Many neurotransmitters are synthesized de novo from amino acids or metabolic intermediates. Figure 20.3 shows the metabolic pathways for the synthesis of ACh, GABA, and the catecholamines (DA, norepinephrine, and epinephrine). Neurotransmitter synthesis and uptake are tightly regulated, enabling the nerve terminal to adjust rapidly to changing demands. This allows the nerve terminal to release larger amounts of neurotransmitter during periods of intense activity, and to slow metabolically costly synthesis during periods of relative inactivity. The best-studied example of regulated neurotransmitter synthesis is that of catecholamines. The rate-limiting step in catecholamine synthesis is the hydroxylation of tyrosine, a process catalyzed by the soluble enzyme tyrosine hydroxylase. Tyrosine hydroxylase activity is inhibited by norepinephrine through competition between it and the necessary cofactor, *tetrahydropteridine*. Thus, as the concentration of norepinephrine increases, enzyme activity declines. However, tyrosine hydroxylase activity increases during periods of nerve stimulation to compensate for the increased neurotransmitter release. This is probably a consequence of its phosphorylation by cAMP-dependent protein kinase, Ca^{2+}/calmodulin-dependent protein kinase II (CaMKII), and PKC. The activity of all three kinases is increased by repetitive depolarization, which results in increased phosphorylation and activation of tyrosine hydroxylase during periods of rapid synaptic transmission.

The synthesis of peptide neurotransmitters is quite different from that of small neurotransmitters. Whereas the latter are synthesized in nerve terminals, peptide neurotransmitters are synthesized in the cell body and transported to the nerve terminal. Like other secreted proteins, peptide neurotransmitters are synthesized and modified in the rough endoplasmic reticulum and transported to the *cis*-Golgi, where they undergo further post-translational modifications (e.g. glycosylation) and are sorted according to their eventual destination. Neurotransmitter-containing vesicles bud off the Golgi stacks and are transported down to the nerve terminal by specific transport proteins.

Most peptide neurotransmitters are synthesized as large prohormones that are processed proteolytically into smaller, biologically active peptides (Fig. 20.4). A typical example is the prohormone pro-opiomelanocortin (POMC), which is cleaved in a tissue-specific fashion to γ-melanocyte-stimulating hormone ((γ-MSH), adrenocorticotropic hormone (or α-MSH and corticotropin-like intermediate lobe peptide), γ-lipotropin (γ-LPH), and β-endorphin. The other opioid peptides – enkephalins and dynorphins – are processed in a similar fashion (Chapter 31).

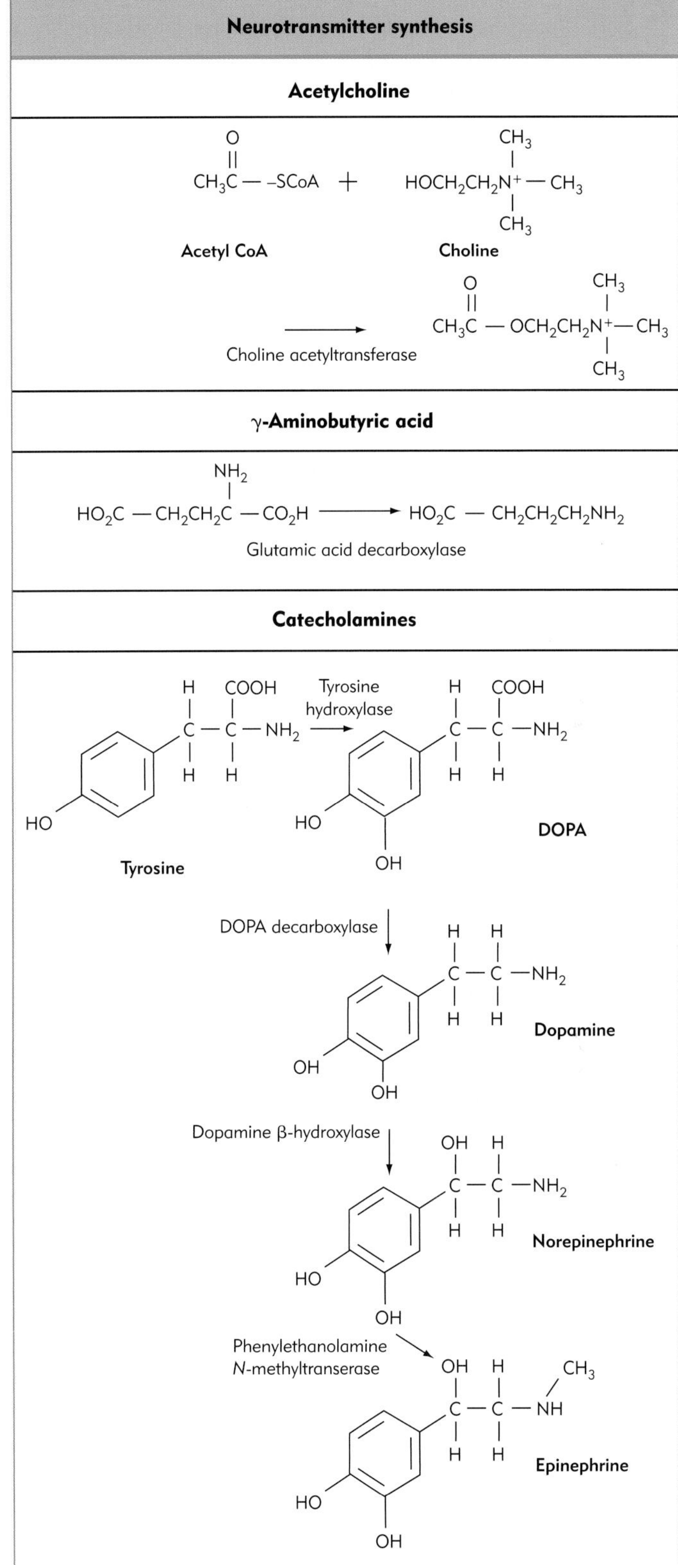

Figure 20.3 Synthetic pathways for small neurotransmitters. Small neurotransmitters, such as ACh, GABA, and the catecholamines, are synthesized in the nerve terminal. The activity of their synthetic enzymes is tightly regulated (see text).

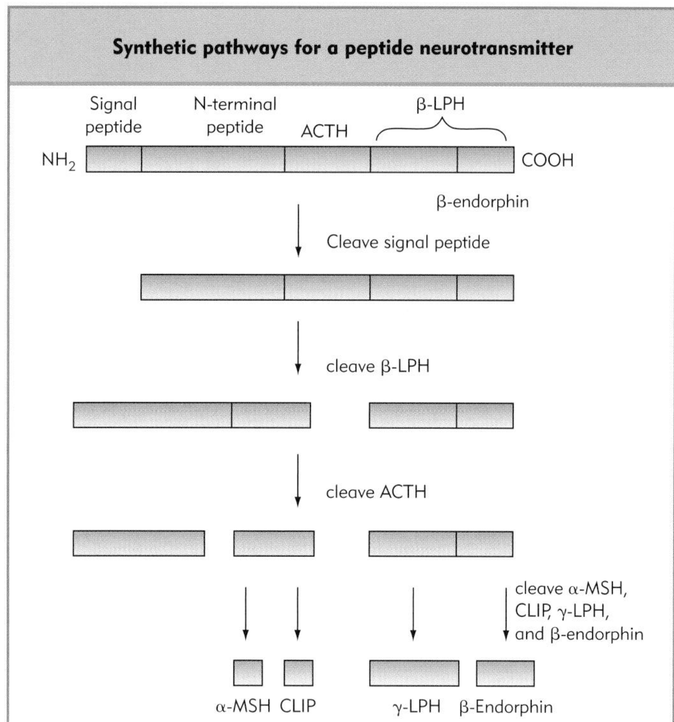

Figure 20.4 Synthetic pathways for a peptide neurotransmitter. Peptide neurotransmitters are often synthesized as a large precursor, cleaved into several biologically active fragments in the soma, packaged into vesicles, and transported to nerve terminals. Processing of the β-endorphin precursor POMC is shown here. (ACTH, adrenocorticotropic hormone; LPH, lipotropin.)

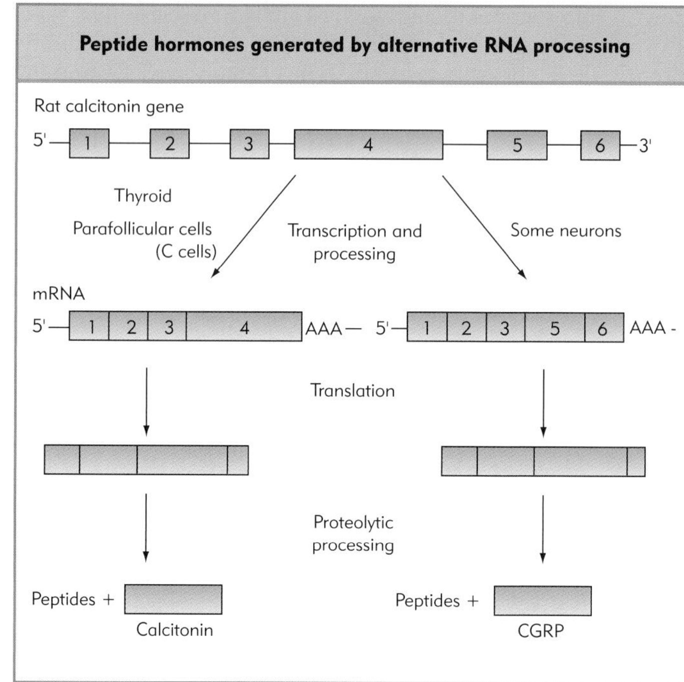

Figure 20.5 Distinct peptide hormones can be generated from a single DNA sequence by alternative RNA processing. Processing of the calcitonin gene to calcitonin and CGRP. Exons in the rat calcitonin gene are numbered 1–6. Exon 4 contains the sequence for calcitonin and exon 5 the sequence for CGRP. In the parafollicular cells of the thyroid the mature RNA transcript contains exons 1–4. In CGRP-expressing neurons the mature transcript contains exons 1–3, 5, and 6. Following translation and proteolytic cleavage, the final peptide products are produced.

Peptide diversity is increased at the level of transcription by alternative RNA processing (Fig. 20.5). The first example of mRNA processing described was for calcitonin and the calcitonin gene-related peptide (CGRP). Here a single gene gives rise to two distinct mRNAs (and proteins) through alternative splicing. These mRNAs are translated into two distinct prohormones that are processed to give calcitonin and CGRP.

Another class of neuromodulator are those derived from fatty acids, examples of which include the prostaglandins, platelet-activating factor, the endogenous sleep factor oleamide, and the endogenous cannabinoids anandamide and 2-arachidonyl glycerol. These compounds are derived from membrane lipids. Their synthesis or cleavage from preformed precursors is driven by specific enzymes (e.g. phospholipase A_2, phospholipase C, and phospholipase D). Often these enzymes are activated by increases in nerve terminal cAMP or Ca^{2+}.

The activities of the small neurotransmitters are terminated by varying combinations of metabolism, reuptake, or diffusion away from the postsynaptic terminal. The relative importance of each of these processes varies between particular synapses and with the type and amount of neurotransmitter released (Fig. 20.6). Examples of metabolism include hydrolysis of ACh to acetate and choline by acetylcholinesterase (Chapter 36), transamination of GABA by GABA-glutamate transaminase to succinic semialdehyde, and modification of catecholamines by monoamine oxidase (in mitochondria) and by catecholamine-O-methyltransferase (in many tissues) to give rise to a number of metabolites that are ultimately excreted in the urine (and often measured as an assay of sympathetic nervous system activity). Examples of reuptake (by both neurons and glia) include the monoamines DA, norepinephrine, epinephrine, and serotonin, as well as glutamate, GABA, glycine, and choline. Here, specific transporters for each neurotransmitter on the presynaptic terminal take up their cognate neurotransmitter into the cell, where it is either metabolized or transported into synaptic vesicles for re-release.

The activity of classic transmitters is terminated by metabolism, reuptake, or diffusion.

In contrast to pumps (e.g. Na^+/K^+-ATPase), which directly couple ion transport to ATP hydrolysis, neurotransmitter transporters concentrate solutes against a concentration gradient by a co-transport (with Na^+ or Cl^-) or antiport (with H^+ or K^+) mechanism that couples transport to the energy stored in transmembrane electrochemical potentials. Two plasma membrane neurotransmitter transporter families have been identified: Na^+/Cl^- dependent (DA, norepinephrine, serotonin, GABA, glycine, and choline) and Na^+/K^+ dependent (glutamate). A distinct H^+-dependent vesicular transporter family (monoamine, GABA and glycine, glutamate, ACh) mediates neurotransmitter transport from the cytoplasm into synaptic vesicles.

Important drugs that affect neurotransmitter transporters include antidepressants, amphetamines, and cocaine, which block the reuptake of norepinephrine, serotonin, and DA. Pharmaco-

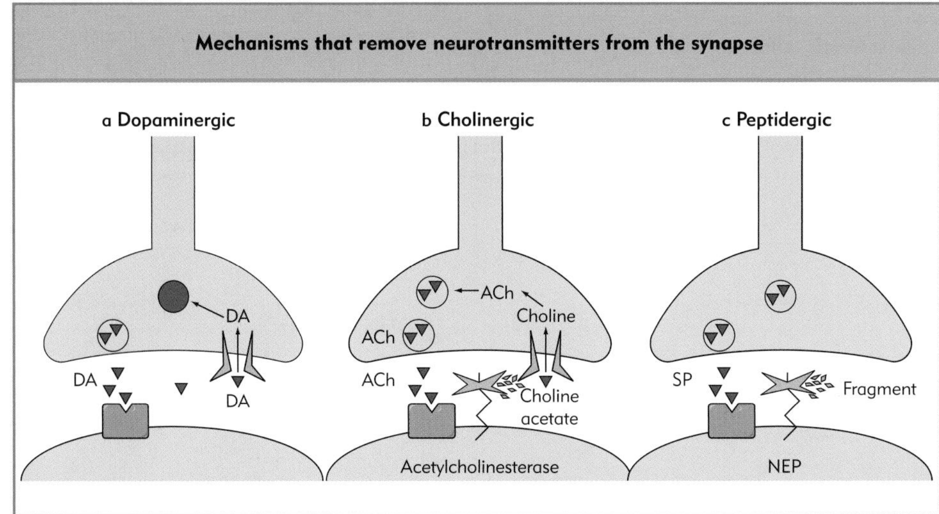

Figure 20.6 Mechanisms that remove neurotransmitters from the synapse. (a) Monoamines and modified amino acids, exemplified by DA, are removed by high-affinity transporters expressed by neurons and glial cells. (b) Acetylcholinesterase rapidly degrades ACh to inactive acetate and choline. Choline is taken up by a choline transporter to be reused for synthesis of ACh. (c) Neuropeptides, exemplified by substance P (SP), are degraded by ectoenzymes, such as neutral endopeptidase (NEP), to fragments that are usually devoid of biologic activity. (Adapted with permission from Böhm SK, Grady EF, Bunnett NW. Regulatory mechanisms that modulate signalling by G-protein-coupled receptors. Biochem J. 1997;322:1–18.)

logical evidence indicates the importance of reuptake for terminating synaptic transmission by most monoamines; for example, noradrenergic transmission is potentiated by inhibitors of norepinephrine reuptake, but not by inhibitors of its metabolism. General anesthetic effects on neurotransmitter transporters have been reported, but their role in the clinical effects of anesthetics is unclear. It is important to note that transporters can operate bidirectionally. Under certain conditions (e.g. anoxia), neurotransmitters can be transported out of the presynaptic terminal (or glia) by these transporters, a nonvesicular form of neurotransmitter release.

Examples of termination of neurotransmitter action by diffusion away from the synaptic cleft include the peptide neurotransmitters and, in some cases, glutamate. Peptides are metabolized by proteolysis. Often the initial products retain biologic activity. Whereas some types of proteolysis occur by nonspecific proteases, others occur by specific neuropeptide-cleaving enzymes (e.g. enkephalinase).

SYNAPTIC TRANSMISSION

The primary function of CNS synapses is deceptively simple: following depolarization of the presynaptic terminal, neurotransmitter is released in a controlled and adjustable fashion, after which the synaptic vesicles are recycled and refilled, allowing the process to be repeated. The molecular details of these steps are slowly emerging. The tight packing in the brain makes it difficult to study individual synapses. However, recent years have seen a remarkable increase in our understanding of the processes involved in synaptic functioning, chiefly neurotransmitter release, as a consequence of a convergence of several fields of research.

- In comparison with CNS synapses, the synapse at the neuromuscular junction is accessible and well understood as a result of work by Katz, Eccles, and others (Chapter 36). Mechanisms found to operate at this synapse form the basis for hypotheses that can be tested in experiments with CNS synapses.
- Our knowledge of the processes involved in vesicular transport between intracellular organelles (e.g. endoplasmic reticulum to Golgi to the cell surface) is well developed. Many of these processes are similar to the events involved in synaptic vesicle translocation to the plasma membrane and recycling (Chapter 2).
- Secretory pathways in yeast have been extensively studied (because of its easy genetic manipulation). Many of the proteins involved in these processes have homologs in the mammalian CNS that are involved in the trafficking of synaptic vesicles, which provides testable hypotheses.
- Simple organisms, such as squid and *Aplysia*, often have specialized large synapses that are amenable to biophysical measurements (e.g. electrophysiologic recording and dye-imaging of Ca^{2+} concentration). Recently, the large size of specialized mammalian synapses, such as the Calyx of Held in the median trapezoid body in the auditory system, have been exploited to explore the presynaptic function in the mammalian CNS.
- When appropriately cultured for several weeks, CNS neurons form functional synapses. The dispersed nature of these synapses makes them accessible to experimental manipulations that are not possible in intact brain, or even brain slices.
- The use of transgenic techniques allows the role of specific proteins in synaptic transmission to be determined.

Although the limitations of each of these approaches must be borne in mind, collectively they have greatly increased our understanding of synaptic function.

Before considering the details of fast synaptic transmission, it is necessary to consider the steps involved in the process (Fig. 20.7). When a synaptic vesicle is loaded with neurotransmitter it is brought to the active zone in a process called docking. The active zone can be defined both morphologically and functionally. Morphologically, it corresponds to a thin band of electron-dense material just below the synaptic membrane, usually opposite the postsynaptic terminal (Fig. 20.1). Functionally, vesicles docked at the active zone are those that are immediately ready to fuse with the membrane and discharge their contents. There are currently two main, competing, hypotheses for vesicle fusion (Fig. 20.7).

Recent research has focused on the complex and highly regulated mechanisms involved in synaptic vesicle release, because of the central role this process plays in neurotransmission. The

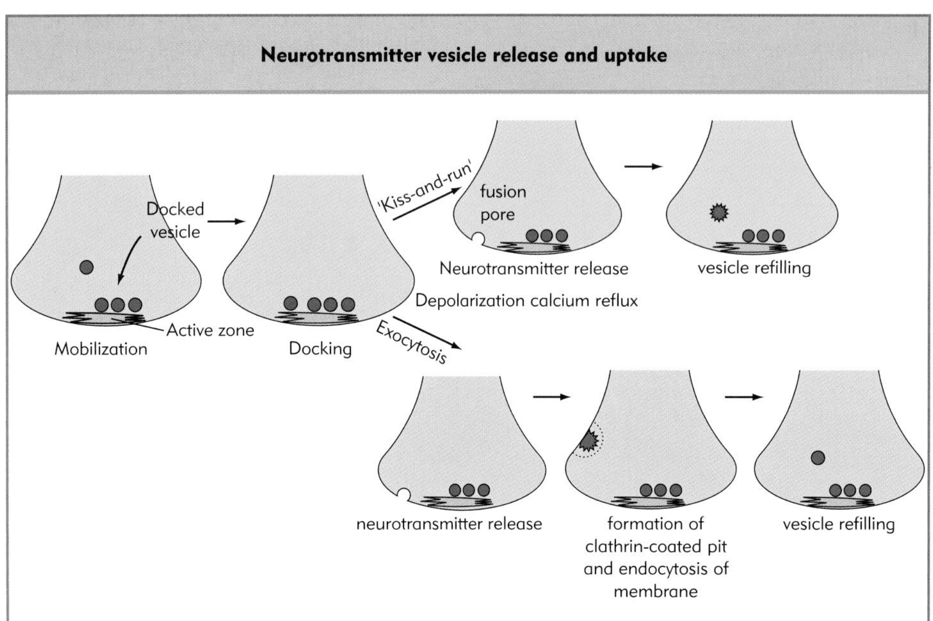

Figure 20.7 Two theories of neurotransmitter vesicle release and reuptake. The upper pathway, termed 'kiss-and-run', involves the transient formation of a fusion pore. This pore opens only briefly, to allow discharge of its contents, closes again, and the vesicle returns to the interior of the synaptic terminal, where it is refilled with neurotransmitter. In the lower pathway, the entire vesicle fuses with and is incorporated into the membrane of the synaptic terminal, discharging its contents in the process. The residual synaptic vesicle membrane is directed to clathrin-coated pits, from which it is retrieved as an intact vesicle by endocytosis and refilled with neurotransmitter.

polar nature of the vesicle and plasma membranes leads to mutual repulsion, which creates a considerable energy barrier that must be overcome to allow fusion and exocytosis. The current hypothesis with the most experimental support holds that specific proteins on discrete sites of vesicles interact with complementary proteins on the synaptic membrane (the SNARE hypothesis), and this interaction is modulated by a third set of proteins. These interactions are strengthened by conditions that promote neurotransmitter release (i.e. elevation in intracellular Ca^{2+}). The energy (ATP)-dependent formation and breakdown of a fusion-core complex regulates vesicle fusion and exocytosis, as illustrated in Figure 20.8.

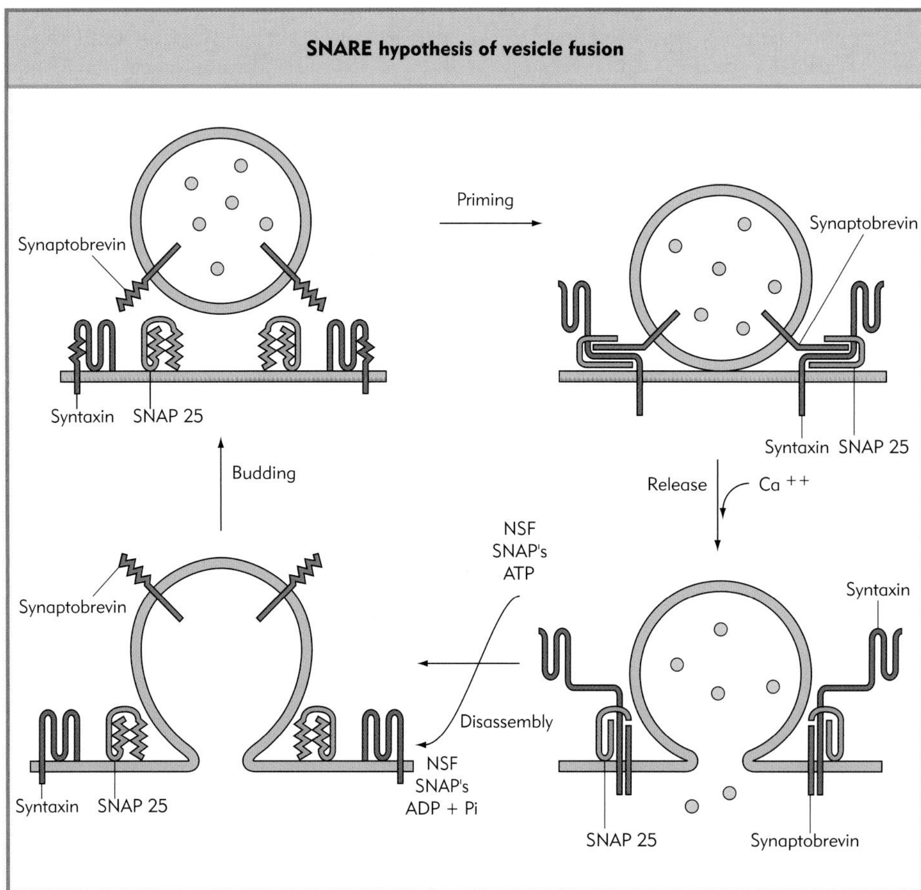

Figure 20.8 The SNARE hypothesis of vesicle fusion, in simplified form. The cytoplasmic domains of synaptobrevin (v-SNARE) interact with syntaxin and SNAP25 (t-SNAREs) to form the 'core complex'. Formation of this complex is a necessary step for vesicle fusion. An increase in intracellular calcium promotes vesicle fusion and transmitter release. After fusion, in an ATP-dependent process requiring NSF and SNAPs, the core complex disassembles and the vesicle membrane is recovered back into the cytoplasm, where it is refilled with neurotransmitter and another round of release occurs.

The term 'SNARE' has its origins in experiments that investigated the shuttling of vesicles from the endoplasmic reticulum to the Golgi, and presumably also underlies the transport of vesicles to target membranes. The proteins and mechanisms involved in vesicular transport, whether between organelles or for exocytosis, are remarkably similar. The vesicle-fusion process was disrupted by alkylation of a protein (*N*-ethylmaleimide (NEM)-sensitive factor, NSF) by NEM. A family of proteins crucial in the process interacted with NSF and were designated SNAPs (soluble NSF attachment proteins). It was found that NSF and SNAPs interact with proteins of both the vesicle being transported, designated v-SNAREs (vesicle SNAP receptors), and the membrane to which it was targeted, designated t-SNAREs (target SNAP receptors). Our current understanding suggests that in the nerve terminal there is one major v-SNARE (synaptobrevin/VAMP) and two major t-SNAREs (syntaxin 1 and SNAP-25: synaptosome-associated protein of 25 kDa, not to be confused with SNAP). These three proteins spontaneously form a tight complex in a 1:1:1 stoichiometry. It is thought that they serve to anchor the synaptic vesicle close to the membrane (the active zone) in a position to fuse with the membrane and discharge its contents. It is likely that interactions between other synaptic vesicles and terminal proteins play a major role. For example, SNAP-25 binds directly to synaptotagmin (see below). The SNARE proteins are cleaved by clostridial and tetanus toxin metalloprotease activity, disrupting neurotransmitter release and producing the pathological, and therapeutic with injection of botulinus toxin, effects of these bacterial toxins.

Synaptic vesicle fusion and exocytosis is a complex unidirectional process mediated by SNARE family proteins.

Although synaptobrevin, syntaxin, and SNAP-25 play major roles in neurotransmitter release, other proteins have critical functions, two of which are briefly discussed here. Small guanosine triphosphate (GTP)-binding proteins are important in providing directionality to a number of vesicular pathways. A similar situation seems to hold in the neuron, for which small G proteins, particularly rab3a, through its interaction with rabphilin and other proteins, provide specificity in the targeting of synaptic vesicles. Also important is synaptotagmin 1. This abundant synaptic vesicle-associated protein binds Ca^{2+}, and thus has been proposed as the Ca^{2+} sensor that drives exocytosis after increases in presynaptic Ca^{2+}. Experimental results to support this hypothesis are the observations that moderate (about 2.2 mmol/L) Ca^{2+} levels increase the binding of synaptotagmin to both membrane phospholipids and the presynaptic membrane protein syntaxin 1, and that targeted deletion of synaptotagmin in *Drosophila* and mice eliminates fast Ca^{2+}-dependent exocytosis.

MODULATION OF EXCITABILITY AND SYNAPTIC TRANSMISSION

Neuronal excitability and synaptic transmission are controlled by many factors, such as the dendritic integration of small synaptic potentials (miniature postsynaptic potentials) that arise from each synaptic contact, events at the cell soma (most notably resting membrane potential), and factors that affect neurotransmitter release. Here the focus is on the factors that affect neurotransmitter release.

In most terminals neurotransmitter release is supported by the entry of Ca^{2+} through two main families of voltage-gated Ca^{2+} channels, designated N-type and P/Q-type, based on their sensitivity to peptide toxins. N- and P/Q-type Ca^{2+} channels are enriched in presynaptic terminals, whereas other Ca^{2+} channels (L-type, R-type, and T-type) are either absent or found at low levels. In addition to their localization in presynaptic terminals, evidence is emerging that the channels tend to cluster in the region of synaptic vesicles as a consequence of their interaction with the t-SNAREs syntaxin 1 and SNAP-25. These interactions position Ca^{2+} channels in a domain close to the putative Ca^{2+} sensors for vesicular release, thereby increasing efficiency. Disruption of the interaction between Ca^{2+} channels and t-SNAREs leads to decreases in evoked (Ca^{2+} channel-dependent), but not asynchronous (Ca^{2+} channel-independent), neurotransmitter release.

Inhibition of Ca^{2+} influx into the presynaptic terminal after its depolarization by an action potential reduces neurotransmitter release and is termed presynaptic inhibition. Both N- and P/Q-type Ca^{2+} channels are inhibited by a wide range of neuromodulators acting via GPCRs. Most of these neuromodulators utilize a membrane-delimited G-protein pathway sensitive to pertussis toxin. These include adenosine, GABA ($GABA_B$), and opioids. For this pathway it appears that a direct interaction of G-protein $\beta\gamma$-subunit dimers with the pore-forming Ca^{2+} channel α_1 subunit makes the channel less likely to open for a given degree of depolarization (voltage-dependent inhibition; Fig. 20.9). Because the probability of vesicle fusion and neurotransmitter release increases as a power function of nerve terminal Ca^{2+} concentration (i.e. the probability of release is proportional to $(Ca^{2+})^n$, $n = 2$–4), even small changes in Ca^{2+}

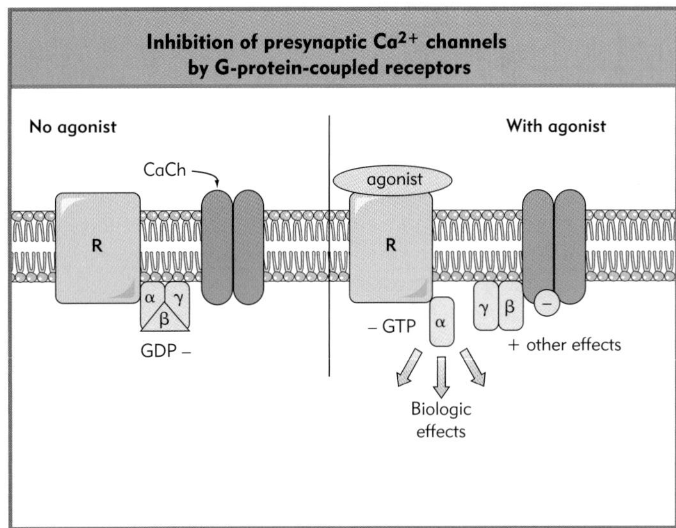

Figure 20.9 Inhibition of presynaptic Ca^{2+} channels by G protein-coupled receptors. In the absence of agonist, voltage-gated Ca^{2+} channels (CaCh) open as the nerve terminal depolarizes. The Ca^{2+} that enters through these channels enables synaptic vesicles to fuse with the presynaptic membrane and release their contents. Following binding of agonist to receptor, G proteins are activated and dissociate into α and $\beta\gamma$ subunits. The $\beta\gamma$ complex binds to the Ca^{2+} channels, which decreases their probability of opening for a given degree of depolarization. This results in less Ca^{2+} influx into the terminal, and thus fewer vesicles fuse and less neurotransmitter is released. In addition to inhibition of the Ca^{2+} channel, the activated G-protein subunits also modulate other processes in the terminal.(GDP, guanosine diphosphate; GTP, guanosine triphosphate.)

influx can profoundly affect neurotransmitter release. The membrane-delimited pathway has its strongest influence in neurons that fire at slow rates (<5 Hz). Presumably, during faster firing more than enough Ca^{2+} for vesicle fusion enters, and even decreases in Ca^{2+} influx of about 50% have little effect on the total number of vesicles released. In addition to the membrane-delimited pathway of Ca^{2+} channel inhibition, another pathway (less well understood) is used by a number of neurotransmitter receptors coupled to PLC, which increases intracellular Ca^{2+} and phosphatidylinositol turnover. Although signaling through this pathway can decrease currents through Ca^{2+} channels, the net effect on neurotransmitter release is more difficult to predict as these receptors often activate PKC (which tends to increase flux through Ca^{2+} channels) and inhibit K^+ currents (which tends to make the neuron more excitable).

Transmitter release is exponentially dependent on nerve terminal Ca^{2+} concentration.

It is likely that GPCRs operating through the membrane-delimited pathway inhibit neurotransmitter release by additional mechanisms. This hypothesis is supported by the observation that, even in the absence of nerve terminal depolarization, spontaneous vesicle fusion and neurotransmitter release occurs. This release is Ca^{2+} independent, yet can be inhibited by activation of the membrane-delimited pathway in a pertussis toxin-sensitive fashion. One explanation for this observation is that activated G proteins or downstream effectors may interact directly with and inhibit some aspect(s) of the release machinery, for example syntaxin I.

In addition to presynaptic inhibition, other mechanisms serve to modulate neurotransmitter release. One well-known example is protein phosphorylation. Here, synapsin I phosphorylation by cAMP-dependent protein kinase and CaMKII during periods of intense neurotransmission facilitates transport of synaptic vesicles to the active zone. Synapsin I is highly enriched in presynaptic terminals, and serves as a link between cytoskeleton and synaptic vesicles, binding to both in its dephosphorylated form. Following its phosphorylation by cAMP-dependent protein kinase or CaMKII, its affinity for vesicles is reduced. This decrease in affinity of the vesicles for the cytoskeleton may allow them to dock at the active zone, from which they are readily released. In addition to the well-defined role of synapsin I phosphorylation in neurotransmission, many of the other proteins involved in synaptic vesicle docking and fusion are also substrates for protein kinases (Chapter 3). However, the functional role of phosphorylation of these proteins remains unclear.

General anesthetics affect excitatory and inhibitory synaptic transmission both presynaptically, by altering neurotransmitter release, and postsynaptically, by altering the responses of neurons to neurotransmitters. Electrophysiologic studies in the CNS indicate that clinically relevant concentrations of general anesthetics affect synaptic transmission rather than axonal conduction or neuronal excitability, by enhancing inhibitory (GABA-mediated) and depressing excitatory (glutamate-mediated) transmission. Many volatile and intravenous general anesthetics potentiate postsynaptic $GABA_A$ receptors and inhibit Na^+ and Ca^{2+} channels (Chapters 24–26). Inhibition of presynaptic Na^+ and/or Ca^{2+} channels may contribute to the anesthetic inhibition of neurotransmitter release.

NEURAL PLASTICITY

Neural plasticity refers to the ability of neurons and particular neuronal networks to change the number and efficacy of their connections. It is commonly believed that plasticity underlies the process of learning, as well as the development of several states of chronic pain after tissue injury (Chapter 23). The facilitation or inhibition of neurotransmitter release by transient increases or decreases, respectively, of presynaptic Ca^{2+} concentration is a simple form of neuronal plasticity. Other forms of plasticity last for some time and persist long after the removal of the triggering event. Many of the early neural plasticity studies relied on invertebrates with simple nervous systems and relatively large neurons that facilitated experimental design and execution. These studies, notably with *Aplysia californica*, show that the brief stimulation of one neuron can strengthen or weaken the communication between two other neurons, and that this effect can last for days. Typically, if the change is to be long-lasting it requires new protein synthesis, protein phosphorylation, and often changes in gene transcription.

In the mammalian CNS, the neural structure that has been the most extensively studied in terms of neural plasticity is the hippocampus. The study of defined neuronal circuits in the hippocampus is facilitated as the pathways between groups of neurons are preserved in the thin sections (brain slices) used for in vitro studies. In addition, the hippocampus plays a role in several learning states, increasing the significance of findings from this structure. The phenomenon most often studied is long-term potentiation (LTP), the strengthening of synaptic connection(s) following an experimental maneuver. The phenomenon of LTP was first observed by Bliss and Lomo, who found that brief high-frequency stimulation of any of the three afferent pathways in the rabbit hippocampus (see below) increased the response to subsequent low-frequency stimulation in the postsynaptic cell. Interestingly, this enhancement of neurotransmission persisted for weeks after a single, brief stimulation. Several of the paradigms used to elicit LTP in the hippocampus mirror the patterns of neuronal firing seen in animals during the learning of a task. A counterpart of LTP is long-term depression (LTD), which has been well studied in the hippocampus and cerebellum. As its name suggests, LTD is a long-lasting inhibition of neurotransmission, and may also contribute to neural plasticity by providing a mechanism to decrease the strength of 'unwanted' synaptic connections.

The circuitry of the hippocampal formation (Fig. 20.10) consists primarily of three excitatory synapses that use glutamate as the neurotransmitter. In the first, the perforant path (projecting from the subiculum and entorhinal cortex) enters the dentate gyrus, synapsing on to the granule cells. The axons of the dentate granule cells project to the CA3 region of the hippocampus and synapse on the dendrites of the pyramidal cells. These large, distinctive terminals are termed mossy fibers. The axons of the CA3 pyramidal cells project to the dendrites of the CA1 pyramidal cells as the Schaffer collateral pathway. Finally, the axons of the CA1 pyramidal cells project out of the hippocampus back to the subiculum. The hippocampus plays a key role in the consolidation of short-term memories (particularly of objects and people) into long-term memories, a process that appears to take some weeks to accomplish (Chapter 29). The central role of the hippocampus in this process has been established using both lesion studies in primates and case studies

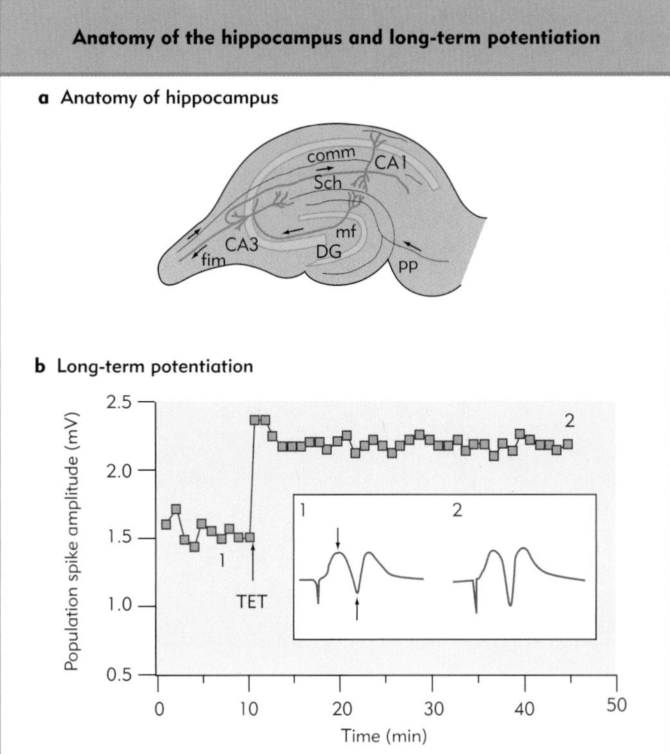

Figure 20.10 Anatomy of the hippocampus and demonstration of the phenomenon of LTP. (a) A thin slice of rat hippocampus illustrates the three sets of excitatory synaptic connections (perforant path, mossy fibers, and Schaffer collaterals). (DG, dentate gyrus; pp, perforant path from the entorhinal cortex to the dentate granule cells; mf, mossy fiber projection from the granule cells to the CA3 pyramidal cells; Sch, Schaffer collaterals, the projection of CA3 pyramidal cells to ipsilateral CA1 pyramidal cells; comm, the commissural pathway, the projection of contralateral CA3 pyramidal cells to CA1 pyramidal cells through the fimbria (fim)). (Modified with permission from Nature 361:31–9.) (b) A typical example of LTP in the perforant path recorded extracellularly from a guinea-pig hippocampal slice. The population spike increases approximately 40% following tetanus stimulation (TET). The inset shows representative population spikes before (1) and after (2) tetanic stimulation. Amplitude was measured as the voltage between the arrows. (Courtesy of Greg Terman, MD, PhD.)

in humans. Ischemia of Ammon's horn (CA fields) results in severe anterograde amnesia, despite intact recall of distant events and unchanged cognitive abilities.

Whereas the phenomenon of LTP has been studied most extensively in the hippocampus, similar processes occur in many other regions of the brain. Of particular relevance to anesthesiologists is neural plasticity and the increased strength of synaptic connections in the dorsal horn of the spinal cord. Increasingly, evidence suggests that this plasticity may underlie the deleterious affects of prolonged painful stimulation and the genesis of certain chronic pain states. This is an area of active basic-science research that may have profound implications in the clinical practice of anesthesia.

Two forms of LTP occur in the hippocampus, associative and nonassociative. Associative LTP is observed at the perforant path and dentate granule cell synapse and the CA3–CA1 pyramidal cell synapse. Nonassociative LTP is found at the mossy fiber–CA3 pyramidal cell synapse. Both forms are produced by high-frequency stimulation of the appropriate afferent path. However, in associative LTP concomitant depolarization of the postsynaptic neuron is required. Interestingly, associative LTP offers a cellular mechanism to encode coincidence between two different events. That is, a synaptic connection is strengthened only if two events, binding of glutamate to AMPA receptors on the postsynaptic cell and depolarization of the postsynaptic cell, occur simultaneously. This is a feature of a 'Hebbian' synapse, an important building block in several theories of neural networks.

Neural plasticity in the spinal cord may underlie the genesis of some forms of chronic pain.

The mechanisms that underlie associative LTP have been extensively studied, and although some aspects remain unclear, the following outline is emerging. The central feature of associative LTP, that concurrent depolarization of the postsynaptic cell is required, is provided by the NMDA-type of glutamate receptor (Fig. 20.11). This receptor is found on dendritic spines and opens after binding of the excitatory amino acid glutamate. Under resting physiologic conditions ions cannot pass through the NMDA receptor, even if glutamate is bound, because its pore is blocked by physiologic concentrations of external Mg^{2+}. However, if the postsynaptic cell is depolarized simultaneously with glutamate binding, Mg^{2+} is displaced from the mouth of the NMDA receptor, allowing the passage of Na^+, K^+, and, most importantly, Ca^{2+} through the channel pore.

The necessity for Ca^{2+} entry through NMDA receptors in the establishment or induction of associative LTP is firmly established, but its mechanisms of action are less clear. The role of protein phosphorylation in the expression of LTP is highlighted by the observation that the introduction of inhibitors of Ca^{2+}/CaMKII or PKC into the postsynaptic cell blocks the induction of LTP. It has been proposed that one or both of these kinases might phosphorylate AMPA receptors, increasing their conductance and strengthening synaptic transmission. In addition, associative LTP may also involve presynaptic events (e.g. increased neurotransmitter release). To link the well-established role of postsynaptic NMDA receptors to presynaptic responses it has been proposed that a retrograde messenger is produced postsynaptically that diffuses to the presynaptic terminal. Experimental support exists that both nitric oxide (or related molecules) and arachidonic acid metabolites may be retrograde messengers. There are several ways in which nitric oxide might act. Stimulation of guanylyl cyclase by nitric oxide would increase presynaptic cyclic guanosine monophosphate (cGMP) levels, which might stimulate cGMP-dependent protein kinase or activate cGMP-gated cation channels. Alternatively, nitric oxide might increase the level of ADP ribosylation of certain presynaptic proteins, thereby enhancing neurotransmitter release.

Because most LTP found in the CNS is associative, this is the type most extensively studied, but we also have a partial understanding of the mechanism of nonassociative LTP. Nonassociative LTP appears to be mediated primarily presynaptically, and NMDA receptors are not involved. Rather, it seems that increased presynaptic CaMKII, which arises during the induction of nonassociative LTP, mediates this process. In addition, this form of LTP is blocked by inhibitors of cAMP-dependent protein kinase, which suggests a role of protein phosphorylation by this kinase. Both Ca^{2+} and cAMP signaling pathways converge at the level of type I adenylyl cyclase (type I AC). Interestingly, mossy fiber LTP is deficient in mice with a targeted disruption of the type I AC gene, which suggests that activation of this isoform of adenylyl cyclase is necessary for nonassociative LTP.

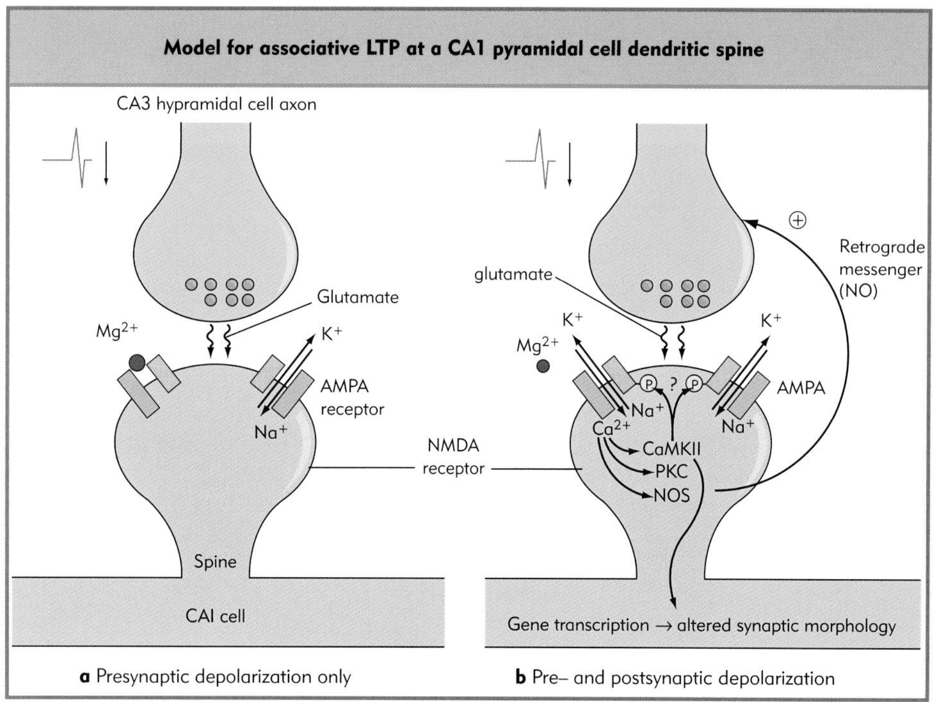

Figure 20.11 Model for associative LTP at a CA1 pyramidal cell dendritic spine. (a) During periods of slow stimulation, glutamate released from the presynaptic terminal only activates AMPA receptors because of the block of NMDA receptors by Mg^{2+}. (b) During periods of intense activity (e.g. synchronous activation of many excitatory synapses on the same dendrite) spine depolarization displaces Mg^{2+}, which allows influx of Na^+ and Ca^{2+} through the NMDA receptor channels. Increased intracellular Ca^{2+} sets in motion several biochemical cascades, resulting in the activation of effectors such as PKC, CaMKII, and nitric oxide synthase (NOS). These and other enzymes act to enhance postsynaptic functions (e.g. to increase the conductance of AMPA receptors). Presynaptic effects, possibly mediated by nitric oxide, are also present, leading to increased neurotransmitter release LTP, long term potentiation.

Key references

Bredt DS, Nicoll RA. AMPA recorder trafficking at excitatory synapses. Neuron 2003;40:361–79.

Deisseroth K, Mermelsteinm PG, Xia J, Tsien RW. Signaling from synapse to nucleus: the logic behind the mechanisms. Curr Opin Neurobiol. 2003;13:354–65.

Malenka RC. The longterm potential of LTP. Nature Rev Neurosci. 2003;4:923–6.

Trachtenberg JT, Chen BE, Knott GW et al. Long term in vivo imaging of experience-dependent synaptic plasticity in adult cortex. Nature 2002; 420:788–94.

Further reading

Boehning D, Snyder SH. Novel neuromodulators. Annu Rev Neurosci. 2003;26:105–31.

Newman EA. New roles for astrocytes: regulation of neurotransmission. Trends Neurosci. 2003;26:536–42..

Freund TF, Katona I, Piomelli D. Role of endogenous cannabinoids in synaptic signaling. Physiol Rev. 2003; 83:1017–66.

Li I, Chin LS. The molecular machinery of synaptic vesicle exocytosis. Cell Mol Life Sci. 2003;60:942–60.

Murthy VN, De Camilli P. Cell biology of the presynaptic terminal. Annu Rev Neurosci. 2003;26:701–28.

Rizo J, Südhof TC. SNAREs and MUNC18 in synaptic vesicle fusion. Nature Rev Neurosci. 2002;3:641–53.

Stevens CF. Neurotransmitter release at central synapses. Neuron 2003;40:381–8.

Chapter 21

Neurophysiology

Patricia Fogarty-Mack and William L Young

TOPICS COVERED IN THIS CHAPTER

- **Cerebral circulation**
- **Cerebrospinal fluid dynamics**
  - Pharmacologic effects on cerebrospinal fluid dynamics
  - Metabolism – cerebral metabolic rate for oxygen
  - Cerebral blood flow and autoregulation
  - Effects of anesthetics on cerebral metabolic rate for oxygen and cerebral blood flow
- **Cerebral edema**
- **Intracranial pressure**
- **Seizures and anticonvulsants**
- **Cerebral ischemia and stroke**
- **Neurotoxicity**
- **Jugular venous oxygen saturation**
  - The neurovascular unit – neurovascular mechanisms of brain function and disease

CEREBRAL CIRCULATION

The primary arterial supply to the brain consists of the anterior circulation, which comprises the paired carotid arteries and their branches, and the posterior circulation, which comprises the paired vertebral arteries and the basilar artery and their branches (Fig. 21.1). Collateral arterial inflow channels are integral for compensatory cerebral blood flow (CBF) changes during ischemia. The circle of Willis, a ring of vessels that encircles the pituitary gland in the subarachnoid space, forms the cornerstone of collateral circulation, although it is incomplete in many patients. The anterior communicating artery connects the carotid circulations, and two posterior communicating arteries join the carotid and vertebral circulations. If the arterial supply is compromised and collateral flow via the circle of Willis is inadequate, other potential collateral pathways may be recruited. These include leptomeningeal communications that bridge 'watershed' areas (i.e. surface connections between the anterior and middle cerebral arteries), pathways from the external to internal carotid (i.e. via facial arteries to the ophthalmic artery), and (rarely) meningeal collaterals.

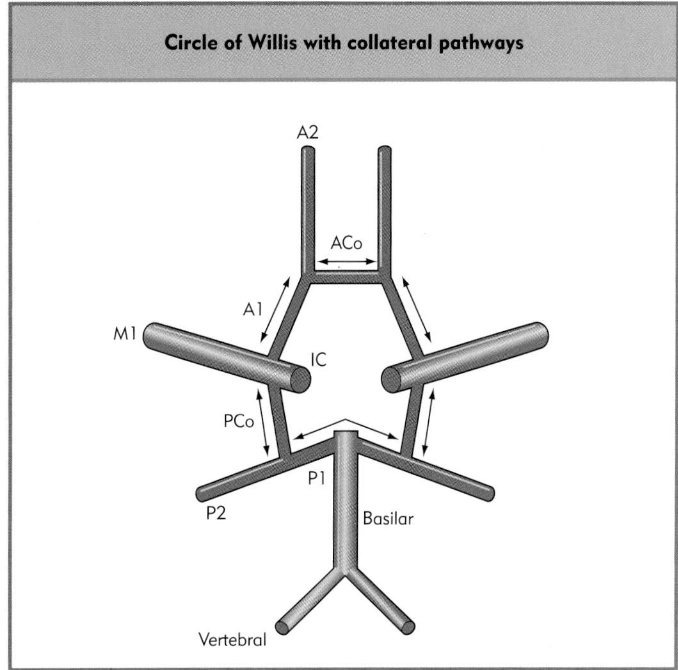

Figure 21.1 Circle of Willis with collateral pathways. The principal pathways for collateral flow are marked by arrows. Not shown are potential pathways from the extracranial circulation. ACo, anterior communicating artery; PCo, posterior communicating artery; A1, A2, M1, P1, P2, anterior, middle and posterior branches; IC, internal carotid artery.

Venous drainage of the brain is complex and variable. Intracerebral veins are thin walled and valveless. They terminate in thick-walled venous sinuses, which are noncompliant and noncollapsible because of their bony connections. The confluence of larger venous sinuses results in significant admixture of blood. Often venous drainage is predominantly unilateral, which may be evident on angiograms.

CEREBROSPINAL FLUID DYNAMICS

Cerebrospinal fluid (CSF) is contained in the two lateral ventricles, the third (cerebral) ventricle, the aqueduct of Sylvius, the fourth (cerebellar) ventricle, the spinal cord central canal, and the subarachnoid space. The total volume of these spaces is approximately 50 mL in infants, 80 mL in small children, 100 mL in large children, and 150 mL in adults. Ventricular volume comprises approximately 17% of this volume in adults. Total volume of extracellular fluid (ECF; interstitial fluid plus CSF) in the brain is 350 mL in adults.

Production of CSF is by the choroid plexus and the ependymal lining of the ventricles, and by cerebral capillary endothelium. At the level of cerebral capillaries little exchange occurs between CSF and ECF because of the impermeability of the blood–brain barrier (BBB). The BBB comprises tight junctions (zonae occludens) that join cells of the capillary endothelium and restrict the movement of molecules with a diameter greater than 20 Å (Fig. 21.2). In addition, capillaries throughout the brain, with the exception of the choroid plexus and several small regions, are surrounded by astrocyte foot processes.

Compared to plasma, CSF has higher concentrations of Na^+, Cl^-, and Mg^{2+}, and lower concentrations of glucose, proteins, amino acids, uric acid, K^+, bicarbonate, and phosphate, though they are isotonic (Table 21.1). The normal concentration of protein in CSF is extremely low (pH = 7.3), and the partial pressure of carbon dioxide ($P\text{CO}_2$) is about 50 mmHg (6.7 kPa).

Comparisons with plasma indicate that active secretion occurs in CSF formation. Regional differences in CSF composition (i.e. higher protein and lower K^+ content in lumbar versus intracerebral CSF) support the hypothesis that sites other than the choroid plexus are involved in the transport of solutes into the CSF. CSF forms at a rate of 0.35–0.40 mL/min (500–600 mL/day); the total CSF volume is replaced three to four times per day. Between 40 and 70% of CSF is produced by the choroid plexus, whereas 30–60% is produced by the ependyma and pia.

Table 21.1 Composition of cerebrospinal fluid and plasma in humans (Reprinted with permission from Cottrell JE, Smith DS. Anesthesia and neurosurgery. St Louis: Mosby-Yearbook; 2001.)

	Mean cerebrospinal fluid value	Mean plasma value
Specific gravity (g/mL)	1.007	1.025
Osmolality (mmol/kg H_2O)	289	289
pH	7.31	7.41
Partial pressure of carbon dioxide (mmHg)	50.5	41.1
Sodium (mEq/L)	141	140
Potassium (mEq/L)	2.9	4.6
Calcium (mEq/L)	2.5	5.0
Magnesium (mEq/L)	2.4	1.7
Chloride (mEq/L)	124	101
Bicarbonate (mEq/L)	21	23
Glucose (mg/dL)	61	92
Protein (mg/dL)	28	7000
Albumin	23	4430
Globulin	5	2270
Fibrinogen	0	300

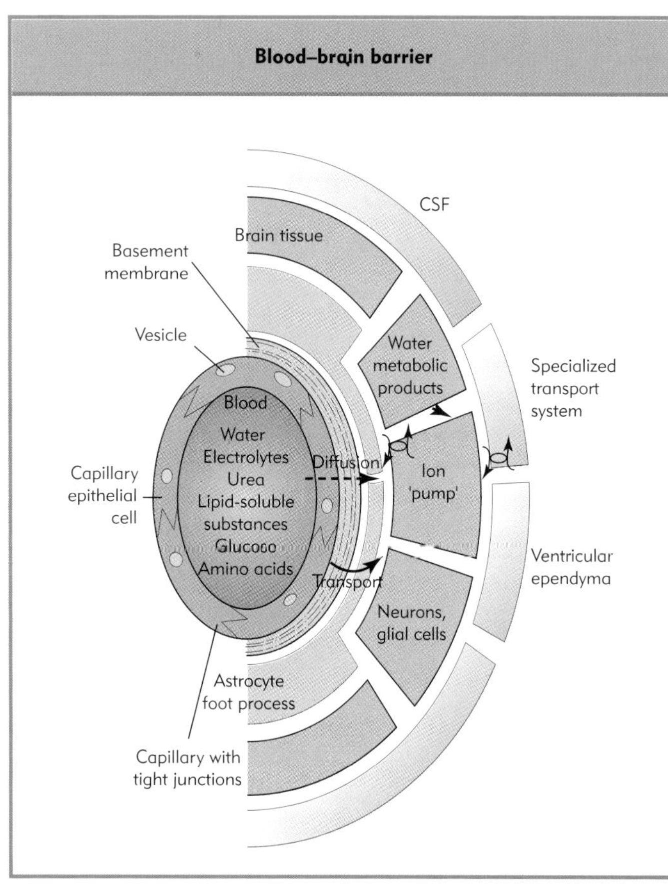

Figure 21.2 Blood–brain barrier. The BBB consists of capillary endothelial cells with tight junctions, a basement membrane, and astrocyte foot processes. Water and constituents of plasma cross the BBB into brain ECF by diffusion or active transport. Water and other cellular metabolites are added to the ECF from neurons and glial cells. (Redrawn with permission from Cottrell JE, Smith DS. Anesthesia and neurosurgery. St Louis: Mosby-Yearbook; 2001.)

The capillary endothelium of the choroid plexus is fenestrated and lacks tight junctions (Fig. 21.3). Thus, blood entering these capillaries is filtered and forms a protein-rich fluid, similar in composition to interstitial fluid elsewhere in the body, within the stroma of the choroid plexus. The choroid plexus interstitium is separated from the macroscopic CSF spaces by epithelial cells that contain apical tight junctions, which restrict passive solute exchange. First, Na^+ is moved from the interstitial fluid into the epithelial cell, and from there into the CSF. Whether this occurs via diffusion or via membrane pumps dependent on ATP is unclear. Water follows the resultant osmotic gradient, both into the epithelial cell and out to the CSF. From epithelial cells, Cl^- is coupled to Na^+ transport and enters the CSF passively, as does bicarbonate, along an electrochemical gradient. Water, Ca^{2+}, and Mg^{2+} may also enter the CSF via 'leaky' epithelial tight junctions. Extrachoroidal CSF formation results from water produced by the oxidative metabolism of glucose (60%) and through ultrafiltration from cerebral capillaries (40%).

Glucose concentration in CSF is 60% that of blood (when blood glucose is <270 mg/dL). Glucose enters the CSF by facilitated transport; at normal blood-glucose levels diffusion of

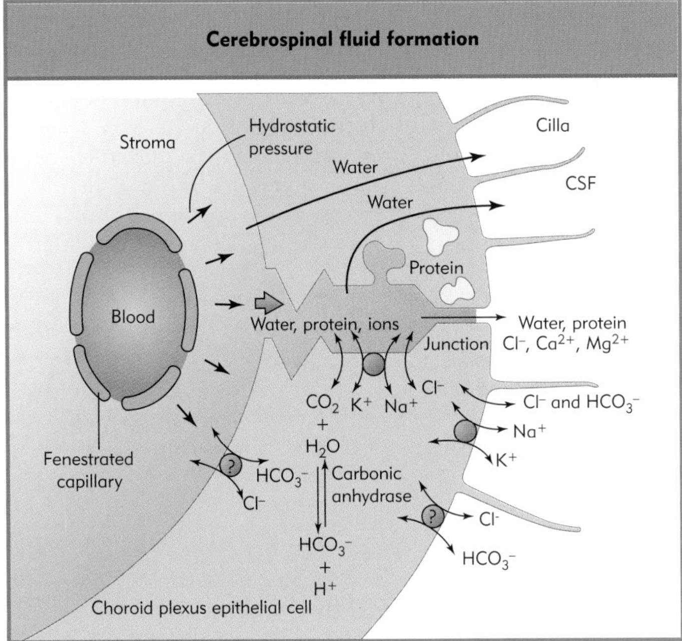

Figure 21.3 Cerebrospinal fluid formation. The ATP-dependent membrane pumps transport Na^+ across the abluminal surface into the choroid plexus cell and across the secretory surface, into the macroscopic CSF space, in exchange for K^+ and H^+. Water moves from the stroma to the CSF as it follows the concentration gradient produced by the ion pumps. (Redrawn with permission from Cucchiara RF, Michenfelder JD, eds. Clinical neuroanesthesia. New York: Churchill Livingstone; 1990.)

glucose into the CSF is insignificant. Glucose is removed from the CSF into the blood via several mechanisms – ouabain-sensitive and -insensitive fluxes, diffusion, and metabolism by periventricular tissue.

The protein concentration of CSF is usually 0.5% that of serum because of the inability of protein to cross the BBB. Of CSF protein, 60% enters at the choroid plexus, where the epithelial apical tight junctions are less restrictive than those in other cerebrovascular sites. Vesicular transport across the choroid plexus endothelium may also play a role.

A decrease in cerebral perfusion pressure (CPP) reduces CSF formation, especially if the decrease results from a combination of arterial hypotension and increased intracranial pressure (ICP). If CPP remains above 70 mmHg (9.3 kPa), an increase in ICP to 20 mmHg (2.7 kPa) does not reduce CSF formation. Reduced CSF production because of arterial hypotension is caused by both a reduction in choroid plexus blood flow, which is further diminished by increased ICP, and a decrease in hydrostatic pressure in the choroid plexus vasculature.

Various routes are taken by the CSF from areas of production to areas of reabsorption. From the lateral ventricles, CSF moves through the foramina of Monro to the third ventricle, and then through the aqueduct of Sylvius into the fourth ventricle. From the fourth ventricle it may pass through the foramina of Luschka into the cerebellopontine angle and prepontine cisterns, or through the foramen of Magendie to the cisterna magna. After leaving the cisterna magna, CSF passes into the subarachnoid space that surrounds the cerebellum, or flows inferiorly along the dorsal surface of the spinal cord to return along the ventral surface of the cord to the basilar cisterns. CSF flow is determined by:

- hydrostatic pressure of 15 cmH_2O (1.5 kPa) at the site of CSF formation;
- cilia on ependymal cells directing flow toward the fourth ventricle and its foramina; and
- respiratory variations and vascular pulsations.

Reabsorption of CSF occurs via arachnoid villi and arachnoid granulations, which consist of arachnoid cells protruding into the subarachnoid space through the wall of an adjacent venous sinus, and are located in dural walls that border the superior sagittal sinus and venous lacunae intracranially (85–90% of reabsorption) and that border the spinal dural sinusoids on dorsal nerve roots (10–15%). The endothelium of the villus acts as a barrier that limits the rate of passage of CSF and solute into venous blood. Flow through the subarachnoid villi is determined by the transvillus hydrostatic pressure gradient (6 cmH_2O (0.6 kPa)), which is equal to CSF pressure (15 cmH_2O (1.5 kPa)) minus venous sinus pressure (9 cmH_2O (0.9 kPa)).

Pharmacologic effects on cerebrospinal fluid dynamics

Anesthetics and other drugs affect CSF dynamics by changing the rate of formation or the rate of reabsorption of CSF. The mechanisms by which anesthetics alter CSF dynamics are unclear. Enflurane may increase choroid plexus metabolism and so increase CSF formation, and halothane may reduce its formation secondary to stimulation of vasopressin receptors. Hypocapnia may also affect CSF dynamics. The effects of volatile anesthetics and intravenous agents on CSF dynamics are summarized in Table 21.2. The clinical implication of these effects is probably minimal for all but the most prolonged anesthetic times.

Anesthetic effects on CSF dynamics are clinically insignificant except for very long exposures.

Diuretics usually reduce the formation of CSF. Acetazolamide, a carbonic anhydrase inhibitor, decreases the number of hydrogen ions available for exchange with Na^+ on the abluminal side. It may also decrease formation by an effect on bicarbonate, and may constrict the choroid plexus, which results in decreased blood flow. Furosemide (frusemide) reduces formation by reducing the transport of Na^+ and Cl^-. Mannitol reduces both choroid plexus output and ECF flow from cerebral tissue to the CSF compartment. Corticosteroids may affect both rate of formation and resistance to absorption (RA). In situations where RA is increased, such as meningitis and pseudotumor cerebri, methylprednisolone and prednisone return RA toward normal values. Dexamethasone decreases formation by up to 50% by inhibiting the Na^+,K^+-ATPase pump at the choroid plexus epithelial membrane.

Metabolism – cerebral metabolic rate for oxygen

Neuronal function is usually completely dependent on the oxidative metabolism of glucose to provide ATP, except in certain states such as chronic starvation, in which the brain can utilize ketone bodies. The brain accounts for 20% of total resting oxygen consumption; a lack of energy substrate storage and high metabolic rate account for its sensitivity to oxygen deprivation.

Table 21.2 Effects of anesthetics on cerebrospinal fluid dynamics (Reproduced with permission from Albin MS, ed. Textbook of neuroanesthesia with neurosurgical and neuroscience perspectives. New York: McGraw Hill; 1997.)

Inhaled anesthetics	**VF**	**RA**
Desflurane	0,+#	0
Enflurane		
Low concentration	0	+
High concentration	+	0
Halothane	–	+
Isoflurane		
Low concentration	0	0, +#
High concentration	0	-
Nitrous oxide	0	0
Sevoflurane	–	+
Sedative-hypnotic and related intravenous drugs		
Etomidate		
Low dose	0	0
High dose	–	0, –*
Flumenazil		
Low dose	0	0
High dose	0	–
Midazolam		
Low dose	0	+, 0*
High dose	–	0, +*
Pentobarbital (phenobarbitone)	0	0
Propofol	0	0
Thiopental (thiopentone)		
Low dose	0	+, 0*
High dose	–	0, –*
Opioids and other intravenous drugs		
Alfentanil		
Low dose	0	–
High dose	0	0
Fentanyl		
Low dose	0	–
High dose	–	0, +*
Sufentanil		
Low dose	0	–
High dose	0	+, 0*
Ketamine	0	+
Lidocaine (lignocaine)	–*	0

+, increase; 0, no change; –, decrease; *, effect dependent on dose; #, effect occurs only during hypocapnia; V_F, volume of formation; R_A, resistance to absorption.

Brain metabolism can be divided into basal and activation metabolism. Basal metabolism involves basic cellular functions, protein and neurotransmitter synthesis, and primarily maintenance of transmembrane ionic gradients. Activation metabolism is that which is necessary for neuronal activity and synaptic transmission. Metabolic rates differ between different brain regions and is four times higher in gray matter than in white. Positron emission tomography (PET) studies suggest that neuronal activation also may involve nonoxidative metabolism, but this remains controversial.

The coupling of CBF to brain metabolism is preserved under physiologic conditions as well as under general anesthesia (Fig. 21.4). Increases in metabolic demand are met instantaneously by local increases in CBF. Thus, regional CBF increases in contralateral motor areas following hand movement and posterior cerebral artery blood flow velocity increases during visual stimulation.

Cerebral blood flow is coupled to brain metabolism; thus reductions in metabolism due to reduced temperature lead to a decrease in blood flow, volume, and intracranial pressure.

The cerebral metabolic rate for oxygen ($CMRO_2$) is normally 35–55 mL/100 g tissue per minute, but it is higher in children. Regional differences occur throughout the brain, with cortical regions having the highest $CMRO_2$. Brain metabolism decreases with decreasing temperature. For each 1°C decrease in body temperature $CMRO_2$ decreases by about 7%. The metabolic temperature, Q_{10}, is defined as the ratio of $CMRO_2$ at a given temperature (T) divided by the $CMRO_2$ at temperature T – 10°C. The cerebral Q_{10} from 37 to 27°C is between 2.0 and 3.0. Below 27°C Q_{10} increases to 4.5. Between 37 and 27°C most of the effect is thought to result from slowing of biochemical processes, whereas the larger Q_{10} below 27°C is thought to be

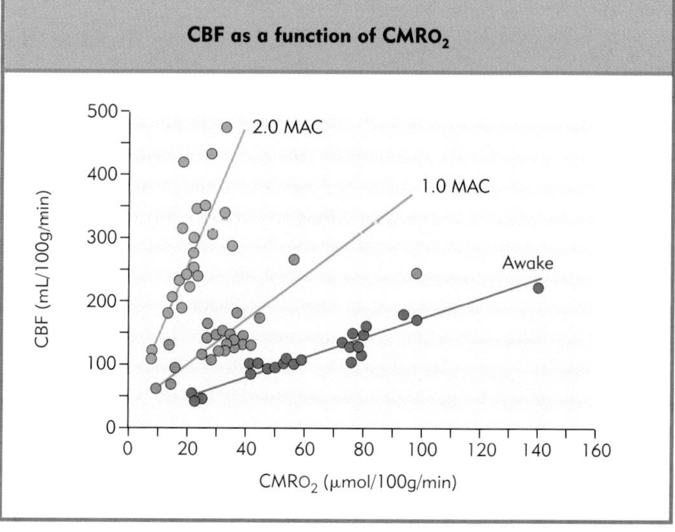

Figure 21.4 Cerebral blood flow as a function of cerebral metabolic rate for oxygen in different brain regions of the rat during isoflurane anesthesia. The volatile anesthetic does not uncouple flow and metabolism: rather, it is 'reset' along a different line. (Redrawn with permission from Cottrell JE, Smith DS. Anesthesia and neurosurgery. St Louis: Mosby-Yearbook; 2001.)

caused by reduced cellular function. As CBF is coupled to metabolism, a reduction in temperature leads to a decrease in CBF; this effect is most prominent in the cerebral and cerebellar cortices, less apparent in the thalamus, and insignificant in the hypothalamus and brainstem.

Cerebral blood flow and autoregulation

Autoregulation is the hemodynamic response of blood flow to changes in perfusion pressure without regard to flow–metabolism coupling. Active vasomotion in response to changes in perfusion pressure and flow–metabolism coupling may or may not be mechanistically related. The prevailing influences in this coupling are thought to be local metabolic factors. Specific factors involved include H^+, K^+, adenosine, glycolytic intermediates, phospholipid metabolites, and endothelium-derived factors (e.g. nitric oxide, NO). The myogenic response of vascular smooth muscle to changes in perfusion pressure (the Bayliss effect) may consist of two mechanisms, one sensitive to mean pressure and the other sensitive to pulsatile pressure. In addition, there is evidence that, irrespective of pressure, flow may affect vascular resistance.

Cerebral vessels have sympathetic and parasympathetic innervation, which is more dense in the anterior than in the posterior circulation, as well as nonadrenergic noncholinergic innervation. Norepinephrine (noradrenaline), acetylcholine, neuropeptide Y, vasoactive intestinal peptide (VIP), calcitonin gene-related peptide (CGRP), and substance P are some of the amines and peptides that may serve as neurotransmitters. The function of the perivascular innervation of the cerebral vasculature remains obscure. Although not essential for hemodynamic autoregulation, it may modify – or in some cases initiate – regulatory responses.

Nitric oxide influences basal arterial tone, including the endothelium-dependent response to acetylcholine in cerebral arteries and vasogenic dilatation because of stimulation of nonadrenergic, noncholinergic nerves. A direct role for NO in CO_2-mediated vasodilatation is not likely, but it may play a permissive role. Although NO does not appear to be important in hypoxia-induced vasodilatation, it may play a role in the cerebral vasodilatory effects of halothane and isoflurane, and is also involved in neuronal transmission.

Cerebral vascular resistance (CVR) is regulated primarily in smaller arteries and arterioles (muscular), not in larger conductance (elastic) vessels, although the contribution of larger conductance arteries, capillaries, and venules is unclear. Ohm's Law is applied as a model to describe the cerebral circulation (Equation 21.1); CPP is given by Equation 21.2, in which MAP is the mean arterial pressure and CVP is central venous pressure.

■ Equation 21.1

$$CBF = \frac{CPP}{CVR}$$

■ Equation 21.2

$$CPP = MAP - \text{outflow pressure (the greater of CVP or ICP)}$$

Cerebrovascular resistance (CVR) can be modeled, though not entirely accurately, by the Hagen–Poiseuille model (Equation 21.3).

■ Equation 21.3

$$CVR = \frac{(8 \times \text{length of conduit})(\text{viscosity})}{\pi(\text{radius})^4}$$

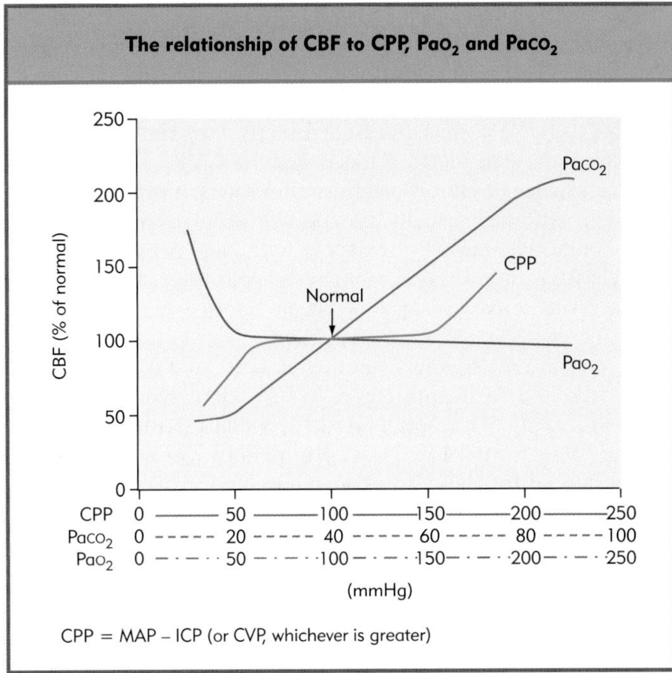

Figure 21.5 The relationship of cerebral blood flow to cerebral perfusion pressure, and to the arterial partial pressures of oxygen and carbon dioxide. (Redrawn with permission from Michenfelder JD. Anesthesia and the brain: clinical, functional, metabolic, and vascular correlations. New York: Churchill Livingstone; 1988.)

In normal individuals CBF is constant (autoregulation) when CPP is roughly 50–150 mmHg (6.7–20 kPa; Fig. 21.5). At the extremes, CBF passively follows changes in CPP, although resistance may not stay fixed and vessel collapse and passive dilatation may potentiate the predicted decline or increase in CBF. The lower limit of autoregulation may be higher in patients who have hypertension, and is probably >50 mmHg (6.7 kPa) even in normal individuals (e.g. 60–70 mmHg (8.0–9.3 kPa)).

Increases in CBF by arteriolar vasodilation lead to increases in cerebral blood volume (CBV). However, at a constant CBF an increase in CPP results in a decrease in CBV as CVR increases to maintain CBF. The physiology of CBV is less well understood than that of CBF. The role of the venous system in autoregulation is unclear. Although the venous system is largely a passive recipient of arterial inflow a slight change in vessel diameter might have a profound effect on CBV, as most CBV is contained within the venous system.

Cerebral blood flow passively follows cerebral perfusion pressure beyond the limits of autoregulation.

Blood viscosity has a major influence on CVR, and hematocrit is the major determinant of blood viscosity. At the microcirculatory level, the Hagen–Poiseuille model does not accurately describe the behavior of flow, because red blood cells that flow near vessel walls create shearing forces, which increase resistance. Therefore, the blood flow is faster in the center of the vessel than in the periphery. In small vessels, cells move faster than the plasma (Fahraeus effect), which reduces microvascular hematocrit (Chapter 43).

Carbon dioxide is a powerful modulator of CVR. Rapid diffusion across the BBB allows CO_2 to modulate arteriolar resistance by its effects on extracellular pH. Systemic pH changes in the presence of an intact BBB do not affect cerebral arteriolar resistance, but H^+ ions released directly into the CSF or the ECF secondary to lactic acidosis reduce CVR. The CSF, via active exchange of HCO_3^-, buffers alterations in pH due to CO_2 diffusion. Although usually assumed to occur over a period of 6–10 hours, this may vary widely in individual patients. Sudden normalization in arterial $P\text{CO}_2$ ($P\text{aCO}_2$) following chronic hypocapnia or hypercapnia may result in relative cerebral hyperperfusion or hypoperfusion, respectively.

At normotension, the response of CBF to $P\text{aCO}_2$ is almost linear from 20 to 80 mmHg (2.7–10.5 kPa). Doubling $P\text{aCO}_2$ from 40 (2.7) to 80 mmHg (10.5 kPa) roughly doubles CBF, and halving $P\text{aCO}_2$ from 40 (5.3) to 20 mmHg (2.7 kPa) halves CBF. Values quoted for the percentage change in CBF secondary to a change in $P\text{aCO}_2$ depend on the method of CBF measurement, but generally range from 3 to 5% change in CBF per mmHg CO_2, with interindividual variations.

The response of CBF to CO_2 is limited by maximal vasodilatation at extreme hypercapnia or maximal vasoconstriction at extreme hypocapnia, similar to blood pressure autoregulation. Hypocapnia may adversely affect cellular metabolism and shift the oxyhemoglobin dissociation curve to the left (Chapter 48). Thus, extreme hypocapnia leads to anaerobic metabolism and lactate production, such that $P\text{aCO}_2$ values <25 mmHg (3.3 kPa) are best avoided.

Arteriolar tone, determined by mean arterial blood pressure, modulates the effect of $P\text{aCO}_2$ on CBF. Moderate hypotension blunts the ability of the cerebral circulation to respond to changes in $P\text{aCO}_2$, and severe hypotension abolishes it (Fig. 21.6).

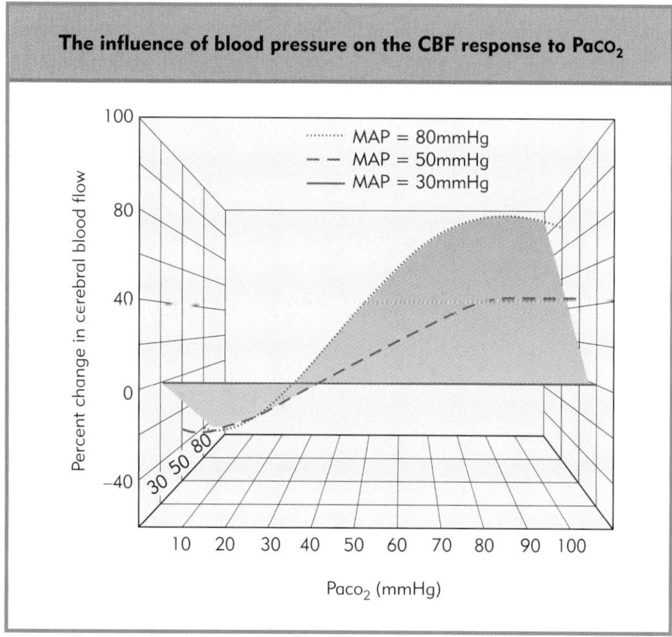

Figure 21.6 The influence of blood pressure on the cerebral blood flow response to arterial partial pressure of carbon dioxide. The effects of alteration of $P\text{aCO}_2$ on cortical blood flow in dogs with normotenson (MAP 80 mmHg, 10.6 kPa), moderate hypotension (MAP 50 mmHg, 6.7 kPa), and severe hypotension (MAP 30 mmHg, 4.0 kPa). (Redrawn with permission from Cottrell JE, Smith DS. Anesthesia and neurosurgery. St Louis: Mosby-Yearbook; 2001.)

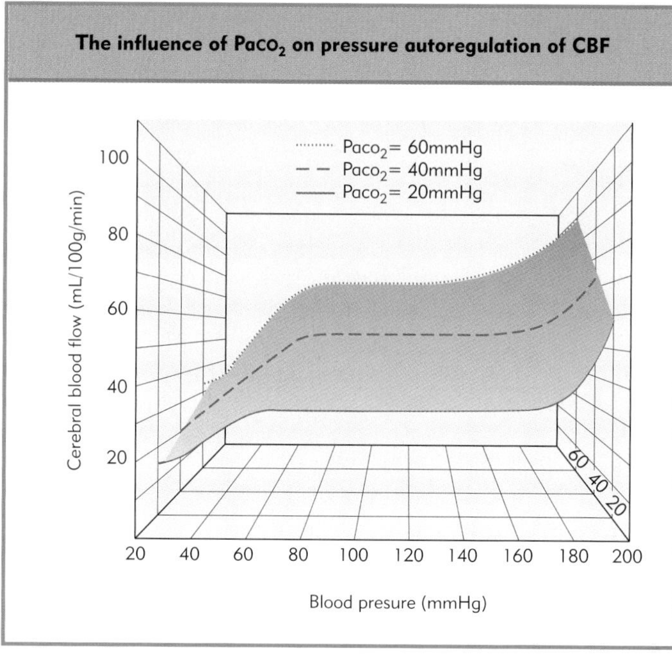

Figure 21.7 The influence of partial pressure of carbon dioxide on pressure autoregulation of cerebral blood flow. The effects of an alteration of blood pressure on CBF at hypocapnia ($P\text{aCO}_2$ 20 mmHg, 2.7 kPa), normocapnia ($P\text{aCO}_2$ 40 mmHg, 5.3 kPa), and hypercapnia ($P\text{aCO}_2$ 60 mmHg). Note the reduction in the autoregulatory plateau with increasing $P\text{aCO}_2$. (Redrawn with permission from Cottrell JE, Smith DS. Anesthesia and neurosurgery. St Louis: Mosby-Yearbook: 2001.)

Conversely, $P\text{aCO}_2$ modifies pressure autoregulation, with hypocapnia widening the autoregulatory plateau and hypercapnia narrowing it (Fig. 21.7). Carbon dioxide responsiveness varies by region according to unknown mechanisms.

Within physiologic ranges, $P\text{aO}_2$ does not affect CBF. However, at $P\text{aO}_2$<50 mmHg (6.7 kPa) CBF begins to increase, and at $P\text{aO}_2$ = 30 mmHg (4.0 kPa) it doubles. Hyperoxia decreases CBF by 10–15% at 1 atmosphere (100 kPa), and hyperbaric oxygenation may reduce CBF further.

Autoregulation and CO_2 reactivity are preserved at moderate hypothermia during cardiopulmonary bypass. Autoregulation may become impaired under pH-stat blood gas management, in which exogenous CO_2 is added to the bypass circuit to maintain 'normal' pH at the patient's actual temperature.

Effects of anesthetics on cerebral metabolic rate for oxygen and cerebral blood flow

Most general anesthetics reduce $CMRO_2$; however, some anesthetics (i.e. enflurane) increase metabolic rate in certain brain structures, with coupling of CBF maintained. With most volatile anesthetics, CBF increases whereas $CMRO_2$ decreases. There is a positive correlation between multiples of minimal alveolar concentration (MAC) and the CBF:$CMRO_2$ ratio, which indicates that the ratio is reset as anesthetic depth increases (see Fig. 21.4).

Halothane causes a dose-dependent reduction in $CMRO_2$ (up to 50%). At low doses (<0.5_vol %), this response predominates and CBF is diminished. At higher concentrations, halothane has a vasodilatory effect and increases CBF if MAP is maintained.

The vasodilatation in cerebral tissue that surrounds brain tumors is more pronounced with halothane than with equipotent doses of enflurane or isoflurane.

Enflurane causes a dose-dependent increase in $CMRO_2$. At high concentrations (3.5_vol %) it produces frequent spiking on the electroencephalogram (EEG) and increases CBF and CMR for glucose (CMR_{glu}) in intercortical and corticothalamic pathways.

In animal studies, isoflurane increases CBF to a lesser extent than does halothane. Also, $CMRO_2$ decreases with increasing concentrations of isoflurane up to 2 MAC, after which no further decrease occurs. In humans who receive nitrous oxide, no change in CBF was noted with isoflurane, whereas $CMRO_2$ decreased (associated with EEG burst suppression). Desflurane and sevoflurane effects on $CMRO_2$ and CBF are similar to those of isoflurane. With desflurane at 1 MAC and hypocapnia, CBF was lower, but at 1.5 MAC, CBF was not different from that with isoflurane. Cerebral pressure autoregulation may be better maintained with sevoflurane than with other volatile anesthetic agents.

The effects of nitrous oxide on $CMRO_2$ and CBF vary widely between species. In dogs, both CBF and $CMRO_2$ increase with a substantial elevation in CBF. In rodents, no change in CBF or $CMRO_2$ occurs. The interaction between nitrous oxide and volatile or intravenous agents is complex. In humans, the addition of nitrous oxide to volatile anesthetics appears to produce an increase in CBF with no or only a slight increase in $CMRO_2$. In humans, the addition of nitrous oxide to intravenous agents does not alter CBF and causes a slight decrease in $CMRO_2$, although baseline vascular tone, other anesthetic agents, and body temperature may affect these results.

Intravenous anesthetics reduce $CMRO_2$, which leads to a decrease in CBF because of flow–metabolism coupling. Thiopental reduces $CMRO_2$ by 55–60% at the point of EEG isoelectricity, after which no further decrease occurs. In isolated cerebral arteries thiopental is a cerebral vasodilator. Barbiturates also attenuate the cerebral vasodilatation produced by ketamine and nitrous oxide. Etomidate also decreases $CMRO_2$ and CBF (by 30–50%). The CBF decrease occurs prior to a reduction in $CMRO_2$, which suggests a component of direct vasoconstriction. As with thiopental, no further decrease in $CMRO_2$ or CBF occurs beyond EEG silence. Propofol decreases CBF and $CMRO_2$ in a dose-dependent manner and, like barbiturates, it dilates isolated cerebral arteries. Ketamine increases CBF and $CMRO_2$ as the result of a direct metabolic stimulating effect, a direct vasodilating effect, and perhaps a cholinergic effect (ketamine-induced CBF increases can be blocked by scopolamine). In humans, ketamine (3 mg/kg) increases CBF by 60%, without a significant change in $CMRO_2$.

In humans, midazolam decreases CBF and $CMRO_2$ by about 30%, an effect reversed by flumazenil.

The effects of opioids on CBF and $CMRO_2$ are influenced by the background anesthetic. In unanesthetized humans and animals up to 1 mg/kg of morphine or 4.4 μg/kg of fentanyl has no effect on $CMRO_2$ or CBF. Combined with nitrous oxide, opioids decrease CBF and $CMRO_2$. At very high doses synthetic opioids may induce seizures, in which case $CMRO_2$ and CBF increase.

Lidocaine (lignocaine), often used during anesthesia to attenuate the sympathetic response to intubation or to avoid coughing, produces a dose-related decrease (up to 30%) in CBF and $CMRO_2$. However, at high doses seizures may be induced and result in increases in $CMRO_2$ and CBF.

CEREBRAL EDEMA

Cerebral edema is defined as an increase in brain intracellular fluid (ICF) and/or extracellular fluid (ECF) volume, which is usually associated with an increase in brain tissue volume and ICP. Several types of edema lead to cerebral edema – vasogenic, ischemic, osmotic, hydrocephalic (interstitial), cytotoxic, edema caused by metabolic storage diseases, and edema caused by increased CBV.

Vasogenic edema is the most frequent type of cerebral edema, and is characterized by increased ECF volume (by up to 50%) secondary to increased permeability of the BBB. Dysfunction of the BBB, whether from tumor, infection, inflammation, or traumatic injury, results in extravasation of a protein-rich fluid under the force of systemic pressure, which accumulates mainly in the white matter. Dysfunction of the BBB appears to be related to opening of tight junctions, increased pinocytosis, and disruption of cells, but can be seen even in cells that appear structurally normal.

Vasogenic cerebral edema due to dysfunction of the blood–brain barrier is the most common form of edema.

Ischemic edema (cytotoxic) occurs following failure of the Na^+, K^+-ATPase pump because of the lack of energy substrate following a prolonged decrease in CBF below the ischemic threshold (Fig. 21.8). Na^+, Cl^-, and H_2O move into the intracellular space. In contrast to vasogenic edema, ischemic edema is more pronounced in gray matter.

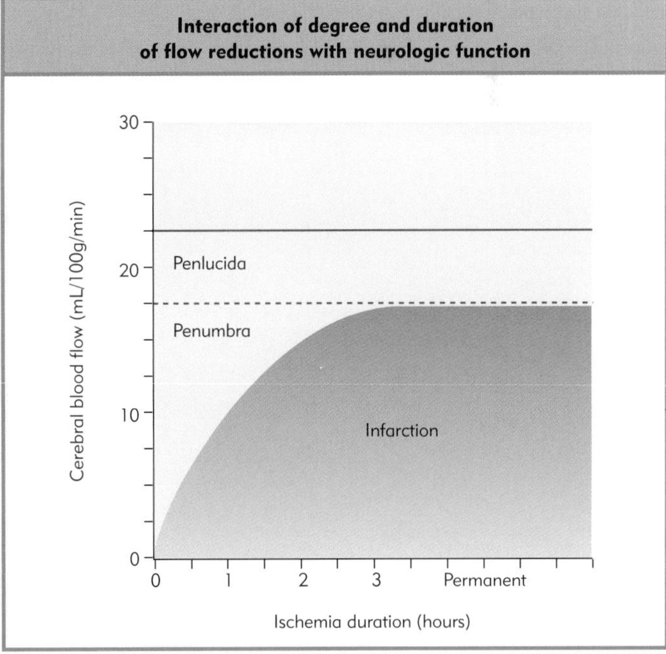

Figure 21.8 Interaction of degree and duration of flow reductions with neurologic function. Tissue that receives blood flow of 18–23 mL/100 g per minute is functionally inactive, but function can be restored at any time with reinstitution of increased perfusion (penlucida). For tissue perfused at lower blood pressures the development of infarction is a function of time. If tissue is restored to adequate perfusion before the time limit of infarction it will recover function (penumbra).

Hydrocephalic edema is similar to lymphedema in other tissues, in which the tissue proximal to an obstruction accumulates fluid in the ECF space. In acute hydrocephalus this occurs in periventricular tissue. Astrocytes are particularly susceptible to this form of edema and undergo cell swelling and eventually cell death.

INTRACRANIAL PRESSURE

The intracranial space contains three components: brain tissue (80–85%), CSF (7–10%), and CBV (5–8%). The pressure caused by the total volume within the nondistensible intracranial space is the ICP. The Monro–Kellie hypothesis states that for ICP to remain normal, an increase in any one of the volumes must be matched by a decrease in another. Brain tissue volume comprises mainly ECF and ICF; CSF volume is determined by the ratio of production to absorption; and CBV is the sum of arterial and venous blood volumes. The presence of an intracranial mass lesion, be it tumor or hematoma, may increase ICP because of a volume effect and/or the position of the lesion (it may obstruct CSF outflow pathways).

Cerebral or intracranial elastance is the change in ICP (ΔP) divided by the change in intracranial volume (ΔV), and intracranial compliance is given by $\Delta V/\Delta P$ (Fig. 21.9). The pressure–volume response (PVR) is defined as the change in ICP after the injection or withdrawal of 1 mL of CSF over 1 second. A normal PVR is less than 2 mmHg/mL, whereas a PVR >5 mmHg/mL signifies reduced intracranial compliance. Although PVR is a sensitive indicator of elastance, it has not been shown to predict outcome in patients who have intracranial hypertension.

The effects of anesthetics on ICP via changes in CSF dynamics are small compared to their effects on CBV. The change in CBV is determined mainly by vasodilatation, but may also be affected by changes in $Pa\text{CO}_2$ and MAP if autoregulation is not intact. Patient positioning, increased CVP and intrathoracic pressure, positive end-expiratory pressure, and coughing may all affect ICP as well. Acute changes in CVP are blunted by venous valves at the thoracic inlet.

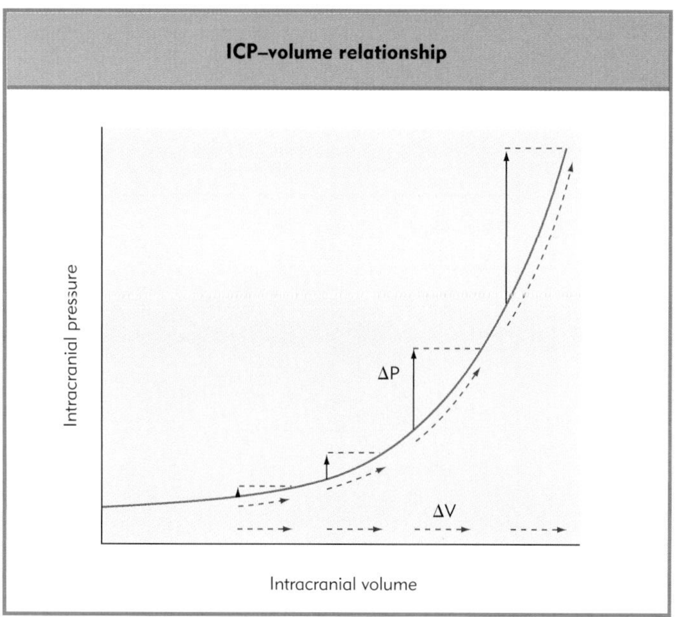

Figure 21.9 The intracranial pressure–volume relationship. The dotted lines and arrows indicate the point to which the volume additions shift the system along the pressure–volume curve. Although for each individual the curve undergoes minor changes in response to therapeutic measures or physiologic changes, the general exponential nature of the curve is retained. (Reprinted with permission from Cottrell JE, Smith DS. Anesthesia and neurosurgery. St Louis: Mosby-Yearbook; 2001.)

Halothane appears to be the most potent of the volatile anesthetics in increasing ICP. This increase can be avoided if hypocapnia is induced prior to the administration of halothane. With enflurane, increases in ICP are minimal in subjects who have normal ICP, but are severe in patients who have space-occupying lesions. In animals, isoflurane alone minimally increases ICP, but increases ICP at high inspired concentrations or in conjunction with nitrous oxide. The increase in ICP with isoflurane lasts only 30 minutes, compared to increases with halothane or enflurane, which last approximately 3 hours. The increase in ICP is attenuated or blocked completely by the institution of hypocapnia (even after the introduction of isoflurane) or thiopental. With space-occupying lesions, ICP may increase when isoflurane concentration is above 1.5 vol%. In animals, sevoflurane produces a minimal increase in ICP and desflurane has no significant effect. Desflurane increases lumbar CSF pressure at 1 MAC, whereas isoflurane does not, but 0.5 MAC desflurane does not affect lumbar CSF pressure in patients who have supratentorial mass lesions. Desflurane has no effect on CSF pressure in patients without mass lesions. Studies of the effect of nitrous oxide on ICP have produced conflicting results. In patients who have decreased intracranial compliance, nitrous oxide may increase ICP.

Volatile anesthetics cause dose-dependent increases in intracranial pressure due to vasodilation, which is antagonized by hypocapnia.

As a result of reductions in CBF and CBV, ICP is reduced by barbiturates. Etomidate decreases ICP without decreasing CPP. Propofol either decreases or does not change ICP; however, CPP may also decrease because of a decrease in MAP. Ketamine causes a substantial increase in ICP. Benzodiazepines produce either no change or a decrease in ICP, which can be reversed by flumazenil. Although opioids produce no effect or small increases in ICP (<10 mmHg, <1.3 kPa), with decreased intracranial compliance opioids may increase ICP secondary to a vasodilatory response to a decrease in MAP. Vasodilation may occur in patients who are not on mechanical ventilation because of an increase in $Pa\text{CO}_2$ that results from opioid-induced respiratory depression.

Succinylcholine increases ICP in lightly anesthetized humans. This effect, which is diminished by pretreatment with intravenous lidocaine (lignocaine) or nondepolarizing muscle relaxants, may result from increased muscle spindle afferent activity, which leads to increased CBF, as well as fasciculation of neck muscles causing stasis in the jugular veins. In neurologically injured patients, succinylcholine causes no change in ICP.

SEIZURES AND ANTICONVULSANTS

A seizure is the manifestation of the excessive discharge of an aggregate of neurons that depolarize synchronously. Seizures are commonly categorized as partial (focal), in which a focal area of neuronal hyperexcitability is surrounded by neurons that remain polarized and unexcited, or generalized, in which depolarization spreads throughout the brain, with EEG involvement of both cerebral hemispheres. A simple partial seizure produces no alteration in consciousness, whereas complex partial seizures involve automatism with variable degrees of responsiveness. A seizure may be partial in onset with generalization, in which a focal electrical disturbance spreads to involve much of the brain and brainstem in producing convulsive seizures. Generalized seizures may be inhibitory (absence or atonic) or excitatory (myotonic, tonic, and clonic). A partial (focal) seizure can cause a postictal focal neurologic deficit (Todd's paralysis). An extensive scheme based on epileptic syndromes, rather than type of seizure, has been developed by the International League Against Epilepsy.

Seizure disorder (chronic) affects 0.5–1.0% of the population, and 2–5% of people experience at least one nonfebrile seizure during their lifetime. Epidemiologic studies suggest a genetic link, with a 2.5-fold increased risk of epilepsy among first-degree relatives, and a multifactorial mode of inheritance involving a number of genes. Common causes of seizures include structural brain lesions and drugs; however, many causative factors exist. The EEG is the most important test in making a diagnosis (Chapter 14). Magnetic resonance imaging is useful in detecting focal areas of atrophy that may be associated with seizure disorder. Examination of the CSF may be useful if infection is contributory.

The many theories regarding the molecular and cellular causes of epilepsy all address the disruption of the delicate balance between cellular depression and excitation. Theories of macrocircuit dysfunction involve the substantia nigra and hippocampus. The substantia nigra is thought to act as a gate, modulating excitation in other brain structures via γ-aminobutyric acid (GABA)-ergic efferents. Hippocampal (medial temporal) sclerosis is often associated with epilepsy, and resection of this area can reduce seizures. Damage to the hippocampus from an initial seizure may predispose to further seizures, which creates a vicious cycle. Microcircuit theories address the excitation– inhibition imbalance on a cellular level. The dormant basket cell hypothesis purports that temporal lobe seizures cause loss of excitatory hippocampal neurons that excite GABAergic interneurons (basket cells), which in turn modulate the effects of the excitatory afferent and other cells in the hippocampus. The mossy fiber sprouting hypothesis involves increased dentate granule cell excitability as a result of loss of mossy cells secondary to damage from seizures, which forces granule cells to synapse on themselves and so increases their response to excitatory stimuli.

Enhanced excitatory amino acid receptor function and diminished number and function of GABA receptors have been reported as molecular mechanisms of epilepsy. Increased levels of extracellular K^+ have been linked to excitatory events in several ways:

- shifting membrane potential closer to spike threshold by partial depolarization;
- increasing the risk of repetitive firing by decreasing postburst hyperpolarization;
- reducing K^+ efflux from cells, thus reducing the $GABA_A$ and $GABA_B$ components of the inhibitory postsynaptic potential; and
- enhanced *N*-methyl-D-aspartate (NMDA) receptor activation.

Genetic polymorphisms in excitatory voltage-gated Na^+ or Ca^{2+} channels can also predispose to epilepsy by affecting their activation/inactivation properties.

Kindling is a phenomenon in which subconvulsive stimuli lead to progressive increases in seizure activity until a generalized convulsion occurs. This process results in increased sensitivity to stimuli despite long stimulus-free periods. Kindling is used extensively as an experimental model of epilepsy in animals.

Treatment of idiopathic seizure disorder is primarily via antiepileptic drugs (AEDs). Mechanisms of action of AEDs include:

- inhibition of repetitive firing by blockade of Na^+ channels (carbamazepine, phenytoin, valproate, lamotrigine, and possibly felbamate (felbate));
- blockade of slow T-type Ca^{2+} channels (valproate, ethosuximide);
- prolonging $GABA_A$ Cl^- channel opening (phenobarbital, clonazepam);
- inhibition of glutamate and aspartate release (lamotrigine);
- blockade of the glycine co-agonist site on NMDA receptors (felbamate); and
- increasing GABA concentration (gabapentin, vigabatrin).

Felbamate, valproate, topiramate, and zonisamide appear to act via several mechanisms. Treatment with AEDs is often monitored by drug levels, although clinical response is more important.

Anesthetic management is affected by AEDs in several ways. Most are metabolized by the liver and induce the cytochrome P450 system, altering the metabolism of other drugs and thus increasing the possibility of pharmacokinetic drug interactions. Increased requirements for fentanyl and nondepolarizing neuromuscular blocking agents in patients chronically treated with phenytoin, carbamazepine, or phenobarbital are secondary to hepatic CYP enzyme induction. Phenytoin-induced increase in the hepatic oxidative and reductive metabolism of halothane may be linked to post-halothane hepatitis. Conversely, sedating AEDs, such as phenobarbital, clonazepam, and gabapentin, may potentiate general anesthetics, so reducing the dosages required. This interaction is consistent with the facilitatory actions of most volatile (Chapter 26) and intravenous (Chapter 25) general anesthetics at the $GABA_A$ receptor.

Enhanced metabolism of fentanyl and neuromuscular blockers is common in patients treated with certain antiepileptic drugs, owing to hepatic CYP enzyme induction.

The effects of AEDs on other organ systems are varied. The immune system may be affected adversely by carbamazepine- and phenytoin-induced leukopenia. Lymphadenopathy, systemic lupus erythematosus, and vasculitis have been noted in patients on AEDs. Valproate affects the hematologic system by an intrinsic system coagulopathy and a dose-related thrombocytopenia. Abnormal hemostasis may be present despite a normal platelet count, prothrombin time, and partial thromboplastin time. Thrombocytopenia is also associated with felbamate, as is aplastic anemia. Anemia may occur with lamotrigine. Liver function tests are usually elevated by 25–75%, usually without clinical significance, although liver failure has been reported with felbamate. Valproate can cause pancreatitis, especially in young patients, in combination with other AEDs. Corticosteroid, thyroxine (T_4), and vitamin D_3 metabolism and function may be altered by phenytoin, carbamazepine, and barbiturates. Protein binding of T_4 and sex hormones may be changed, and the release of calcitonin, insulin, and clotting factors dependent on vitamin K may be impaired. Most patients appear euthyroid because of reduced binding of T_4 to plasma proteins secondary to the extensive protein binding of AEDs.

Carbamazepine metabolism (by CYP3A4) is inhibited by erythromycin and cimetidine, both of which may be used preoperatively. Increased blood levels may lead to toxicity and heart block. Blood levels of AEDs may fluctuate for as long as 1 week after general anesthesia and surgery; therefore, it may be useful to check levels postoperatively.

Certain drugs lower the seizure threshold or activate epileptogenic foci and thus should be avoided in patients with seizure disorders. Methohexital can activate seizure foci and has been used in mapping for surgical resection. Ketamine and propofol have been reported to elicit seizures in patients who have seizure disorder, but their epileptogenic potential is unclear. Although propofol can successfully treat status epilepticus, both seizures and opisthotonos can occur in patients with and without previously diagnosed seizure disorder. Propofol is an effective anticonvulsant for bupivacaine-, picrotoxin-, and pentylenetetrazol-induced seizures in animals, and in seizures produced by GABAergic inhibition; however, seizures produced by a glutamatergic mechanism are augmented by propofol. Antagonism of glycine in subcortical structures has been proposed as a mechanism to explain the seizure-like activity associated with propofol. Inhalational anesthetics exhibit both anticonvulsant and proconvulsant properties in both humans and animals. Isoflurane and desflurane have the least proconvulsant activity. Generally, clinical use of potent agents is anticonvulsant, and isoflurane has been used to treat status epilepticus.

CEREBRAL ISCHEMIA AND STROKE

The assessment of specific anesthetics as cerebral protectants is complicated by several factors. In most studies the anesthetic is added to a standard background anesthetic, such that few studies employ a control group that is not anesthetized. In addition, many models of ischemia are used in different species – global versus focal models and, within focal models, permanent versus temporary ischemia, with variable durations and magnitudes of temporary ischemia. In general, no single anesthetic agent is unequivocally and uniquely cerebroprotective in all settings.

Barbiturates reduce $CMRO_2$, theoretically via enhanced $GABA_A$-receptor activity that leads to increased Cl^- flux. The $CMRO_2$–CBF linkage is preserved, such that CBF is decreased. There is no additional benefit to barbiturate administration beyond that required for EEG silence. The reduction in $CMRO_2$ is not unequivocally cerebroprotective, however. Other possible mechanisms of cerebroprotection by barbiturates include decreased production of free fatty acids during ischemia, and reduced excitatory amino acid release and/or receptor activation following ischemia. A reduction in brain temperature by reducing heat delivery (decreased CBF) might also play a role. Although one primate study found thiopental to be protective after global ischemia the results could not be repeated, and a randomized trial of thiopental loading in comatose survivors of cardiac arrest showed no benefit. In focal ischemia, barbiturates are more effective cerebroprotectants in temporary than in permanent vascular occlusion in animal models. Results from clinical studies that involve middle cerebral artery occlusion, acute stroke, and carotid endarterectomy are conflicting.

Ketamine, which noncompetitively antagonizes the glutamate activation of NMDA receptors (Chapter 25), has been studied in models of focal ischemia. No consistent neuroprotective effect was observed, but lack of temperature control may have affected the results. In a recent study of rat axonal transection (*S*)(+)-ketamine was comparable with the NMDA receptor antagonist MK-801 in producing neuroprotection. Racemic ketamine was somewhat effective, but (*S*)(−)-ketamine was ineffective, indicating stereospecificity.

Both intravenous and volatile anesthetics have neuroprotective properties under certain conditions involving multiple potential mechanisms.

Etomidate reduces $CMRO_2$ and CBF while maintaining systemic blood pressure. In a dog model of global incomplete ischemia (residual EEG activity), etomidate preserved cerebral high-energy phosphates (ATP and phosphocreatinine) and reduced lactic acid accumulation. In doses that achieved EEG silence, etomidate was equally neuroprotective with thiopental in severe forebrain ischemia in rats. Recent studies, however, suggest that etomidate may potentiate ischemic neuronal injury. In addition, in patients undergoing aneurysm clipping cerebral tissue Po_2 decreased after a dose of etomidate causing burst suppression.

The α_2-adrenoreceptor agonists, such as clonidine and dexmedetomidine, may be protective via decreased norepinephrine release following cerebral ischemia. In animal models of focal and global ischemia they protect against immediate and delayed neuronal death.

Volatile anesthetics have been evaluated as potential cerebroprotectants in both global and focal models of ischemia. The mechanism of protection is not known, but may involve cerebral vasodilatation. Most volatile agents produce a sustained increase in CBF in primates. There is a decrease in $CMRO_2$ (linked to EEG activity) and CMR_{glu} with preserved high-energy (e.g. ATP) phosphate metabolism. The mechanism of vasodilatation by volatile anesthetics may be related to NO, because NO synthase (NOS) inhibition blocks increases in CBF secondary to inhaled agents. The role of NO in brain injury is controversial and may be dependent on which NOS isoform (neuronal versus endothelial versus inducible) is inhibited. Therefore, volatile anesthetics may exert a cerebroprotective effect via the NO pathway. Vasodilatation as a result of volatile agents may also be mediated via a prostanoid pathway, as isoflurane-induced vasodilatation is attenuated by indomethacin.

Another potential mechanism for neuroprotection by volatile anesthetics is inhibition of glutamate binding at the NMDA receptor. Isoflurane reduces NMDA receptor and L-glutamate-mediated Ca^{2+} fluxes. However, neither halothane nor isoflurane reduces the amount of glutamate or glycine released following global ischemia. Blockade of Na^+ channels and reduced Na^+ influx may contribute to neuroprotection by volatile and local anesthetics.

In primates subjected to severe temporary focal ischemia, isoflurane provided the same degree of neuroprotection as thiopental. Data from retrospective uncontrolled studies suggest that the EEG threshold for minimal CBF is lower in patients anesthetized with isoflurane (10 mL/100 mg per minute) and sevoflurane (11.5 mL/100 g per minute) compared to enflurane (15 mL/100 g per minute) or halothane (20 mL/100 g per minute) for carotid endarterectomy. However, well-controlled animal studies suggest that cerebroprotection is similar between halothane, enflurane, isoflurane, and sevoflurane.

The effect of nitrous oxide on cerebral ischemia has not been directly evaluated. Studies of the use of nitrous oxide as a sole anesthetic agent would be associated with increases in systemic catecholamines, which may themselves worsen outcome following an ischemic insult. In a rat model, nitrous oxide diminished isoflurane-induced neuroprotection; however, the protective effects of barbiturates were not attenuated. Recent evidence suggests that xenon exhibits significant neuroprotective effects in experimental models.

Other pharmacologic agents under investigation as neuroprotectants include Mg^{2+}, lamotrigine, and dextromethorphan. Mg^{2+}competes with Ca^{2+} for entry into neuronal cells, and blocks NMDA receptors. Lamotrigine, an Na^+ channel blocker, inhibits glutamate release during transient global ischemia in rabbits. Dextromethorphan, an antitussive opioid with no respiratory depression and no addiction potential, is a functional NMDA receptor antagonist.

A confounding factor in studies on the neuroprotective effects of anesthetics is the lack of controlled temperature. In fact, deliberate mild hypothermia – a reduction of 2–3°C – which provides more protection than the volatile agents, has been employed by neuroanesthesiologists for neuronal protection. These small decreases in temperature have relatively minimal effect on $CMRO_2$. Hypothermia may provide protection in part via a decrease in the release of excitatory neurotransmitters following ischemia. In patients who have closed head trauma, deliberate hypothermia appears to improve outcome. In numerous animal models hypothermia has been shown to be neuroprotective; however, in two large clinical trials involving patients with head trauma and subarachnoid hemorrhage, improved neurologic outcome has not been demonstrated in the hypothermic groups.

NEUROTOXICITY

An association between anesthetic agents and neurotoxicity is complicated, with many studies demonstrating conflicting results. Sufentanil, alfentanil, and morphine have been studied in a dog model with chronic intrathecal or epidural catheters and intermittent daily injections over 15–28 days. No morphologic or histopathologic evidence of neurotoxicity was found compared to vehicle controls over a range of doses and concentrations, which were greater than would be used clinically.

NMDA antagonists, which includes nitrous oxide and ketamine, are potentially neurotoxic. The preservative in ketamine, chlorobutanol, induced severe spinal cord lesions in a rabbit model. No evidence of neurotoxicity has been reported for propofol, barbiturates, or volatile anesthetics. In an animal model, anesthetic agents frequently used in pediatric anesthesia (midazolam, isoflurane, nitrous oxide) had neurotoxic effects in immature animals, a finding of potential concern that demands further study (Chapter 25).

Although nondepolarizing neuromuscular blocking agents are highly ionized and do not normally cross the BBB, these agents and their metabolites have been found in the CSF of patients who have neurologic disease, or who are critically ill and in whom the BBB may not be intact. In rat brain cortical slices, pancuronium and vecuronium increased intracellular Ca^{2+} via prolonged activation (rather than inhibition) of nicotinic acetylcholine receptors; atracurium and laudanosine did not have this effect. The clinical relevance of this finding has yet to be established.

JUGULAR VENOUS OXYGEN SATURATION

The CMR for oxygen can be expressed as in Equation 21.4, otherwise as in Equation 21.5, in which $Cao_2 - Cjvo_2$ is the difference in oxygen content in simultaneous arterial and jugular bulb venous blood samples.

■ Equation 21.4

$$CMRO_2 = CBF \times (Cao_2 - Cjvo_2)$$

■ Equation 21.5

$$Cao_2 - Cjvo_2 = \frac{CMRO_2}{CBF}$$

The arterial–jugular bulb oxygen content difference is constant (7–8 mL oxygen/100 mL blood) as long as flow–metabolism coupling is intact. Hypothermia, hyperthermia, and general anesthesia may change baseline values. In head trauma, which disrupts flow–metabolism coupling, $Cao_2 - Cjvo_2$ reflects the adequacy of oxygen delivery for metabolic demand; levels of 4 mL oxygen/100 mL blood indicate increased supply (decreased extraction) relative to demand, whereas levels >9 mL oxygen/100 mL blood indicate global ischemia (increased extraction). Further decreases in oxygen delivery at this point exceed the brain's ability to compensate for hypoperfusion, and infarction may occur. After ischemia and/or infarction, $Cao_2 - Cjvo_2$ decreases, as infarcted tissue does not extract oxygen.

The oxygen content of blood (Co_2 in mL/dL) depends primarily on hemoglobin concentration (Hb), the amount of oxygen dissolved in plasma (to a much lesser extent), and the oxygen saturation of hemoglobin (So_2; Chapter 48):

■ Equation 21.6

$$Co_2 = (Hb \times 1.34 \times So_2) + [0.003 \times Po_2\ (mmHg)]$$

If the hemoglobin concentration and the amount of dissolved oxygen remain constant, $Cao_2 - Cjvo_2$ is primarily dependent on the oxygen saturation of the jugular venous blood:

■ Equation 21.7

$$Cao_2 - Cjvo_2 \propto (1 - Sjvo_2) \text{ and } Sjvo_2 \propto CBF/CMRO_2$$

Fiberoptic intravascular catheters are available which allow the continuous measurement of $Sjvo_2$. Normal $Sjvo_2$ is 66–70%; a saturation >75% indicates either cerebral hyperemia (oxygen supply exceeding demand) or global cerebral infarction. Conversely, decreases in $Sjvo_2$ to <54% indicate 'compensated cerebral hypoperfusion' but not ischemia, whereas a value <40% indicates global cerebral ischemia. If there are fluctuations in the arterial oxygen saturation, cerebral oxygen extraction ratio (OER) may be calculated as:

■ Equation 21.8

$$OER = Sao_2 - \frac{Sjvo_2}{Sao_2}$$

Although $Cao_2 - Cjvo_2$ or $Sjvo_2$ may be useful in identifying patients who have impending cerebral ischemia in spite of adequate CPP, and aid in maximizing therapy in those who have intracranial hypertension, $SjvO_2$ monitoring reflects global cerebral oxygenation and may falsely reassure in the setting of focal ischemia.

The neurovascular unit – neurovascular mechanisms of brain function and disease

Future research in the area of neuroprotection will focus on improving our understanding of the dynamic interactions of the neurovascular unit (NVU). The NVU is a construct defined as brain microvascular endothelium, glia, neurons, and extracellular matrix that maintains spatial relations. Research on the NVU seeks to better define how endothelial injury affects parenchymal damage via multiple cascades of injury. Such cascades include oxidative stress combined with cellular interactions, with activated endothelium leading to inflammatory or metalloprotease damage to the blood–brain barrier. In addition, factors such as tissue plasminogen activator (tPA) may interact with NMDA receptors to increase cell death. Work in this area should provide insight into how to protect the brain from ischemic and hemorrhagic injury.

Key references

Artru AA. Cerebrospinal fluid. In: Cottrell JE, Smith DS, eds. Anesthesia and neurosurgery. St Louis: Mosby-Yearbook; 2001: 83–100.

Brian JE Jr. Carbon dioxide and the cerebral circulation. Anesthesiology 1998;88:1365–86.

Cheng MA, Theard MA, Tempelhoff R. Intravenous agents and intraoperative neuroprotection: beyond barbiturates. Crit Care Clin. 1997;13:185–99.

Cucchaiara RF, Michenfelder JD. Clinical neuroanesthesia. New York: Churchill Livingstone; 1990.

Iadecola C. Bright and dark sides of nitric oxide in ischemic brain injury. Trends Neurosci. 1997;20:132–9.

Joshi S, Ornstein E, Young WL. Cerebral and spinal cord blood flow. In: Cottrell JE, Smith DS, eds. Anesthesia and neurosurgery. St Louis: Mosby-Yearbook; 2001:19–68.

Kofke WA, Templehoff R, Dasheiff RM. Anesthetic implications of epilepsy, status epilepticus and epilepsy surgery. J Neurosurg Anesth. 1997;9:349–72.

Lo EH, Broderick JP, Moskowitz MA. TPA and proteolysis in the neurovascular unit. Stroke 2004; 35: 354-356.

Neuwelt EA. Mechanisms of disease: The blood–brain barrier. Neurosurgery 2004; 54: 131–42.

Sakabe T, Nakatumura K. Effects of anesthetic agents and other drugs on cerebral blood flow, metabolism and intracranial pressure. In: Cottrell ME, Smith DS, eds. Anesthesia and neurosurgery. St Louis: Mosby-Yearbook; 2001: 129–43.

Further reading

Brian JE Jr, Faraci FM, Heistad DD. Recent insights into the regulation of cerebral circulation. Clin Exp Pharmacol Physiol. 1996;23:449–57.

Hansen TD, Warner DS, Todd MM et al. The role of cerebral metabolism in determining the local cerebral blood flow effects of volatile anesthetics: evidence for persistent flow–metabolism coupling. J Cerebr Blood Flow Metab. 1989;9:323–8.

Illievich UM, Zornow MH, Choi KT, Strnat MA, Scheller MS. Effects of hypothermia or anesthetics on hippocampus glutamate and glycine concentrations after repeated transient global cerebral ischemia. Anesthesiology 1994;80:177–86.

Karibe H, Zarow GJ, Graham SH, Weinstein PR. Mild intraischemic hypothermia reduces post-ischemic hyperperfusion, delayed hypoperfusion, blood–brain barrier disruption, brain edema, and neuronal damage after temporary focal cerebral ischemia in rats. J Cerebr Blood Flow Metab. 1994;14:620–7.

Siesjo BK. Pathophysiology and treatment of focal cerebral ischemia. Part I: Pathophysiology. J Neurosurg. 1992; 77:169–84.

Siesjo BK. Pathophysiology and treatment of focal cerebral ischemia: Part II. Mechanisms of damage and treatment. J Neurosurg. 1992;77:337–54.

Chapter 22

Sensory systems

Timothy J Ness and Timothy J Brennan

TOPICS COVERED IN THIS CHAPTER

- **Sensory reception and transduction**
- **Nociceptors and nociceptive afferent neurons**
  - Cutaneous nociceptors
  - Muscle and joint nociceptors
  - Visceral nociceptors
- **Molecular basis of sensory transduction**
- **Spinal pathways and sensory transmission**
  - Anatomy of second-order neurons
  - Intraspinal pathways
  - Anterolateral white matter
  - Dorsal column pathways
  - Functional characterization of the dorsal horn
  - Spinal reflex responses
  - Sites of higher-order sensory processing
- **Dorsal horn neurochemistry**
  - Excitatory neurotransmitters
  - Inhibitory neurotransmitters

Information about the relationship of an organism to its environment is required for homeostasis. The sensory system utilizes specialized transduction mechanisms such as hearing, taste, vision, smell, somatic sensation, visceral sensation and proprioception. Sensory perception and pain modulation are fundamental to the practice of anesthesia as a result of the desire to suppress or abolish the perception of pain and the responses to injury during surgical procedures, childbirth, and acute and chronic pain states. This chapter reviews somatosensory transduction and transmission from the periphery into the central nervous system (CNS), including sensory pathways, neurotransmitter systems, and their modulation. This information is fundamental to understanding the actions of anesthetics and analgesic treatments.

SENSORY RECEPTION AND TRANSDUCTION

The cell bodies of sensory fibers are contained in the dorsal root ganglia (DRG; Fig. 22.1). These unipolar neurons send a single axon to the organ they innervate. Branching of sensory fibers to innervate more than one organ is very rare, indicating that the basis for referred pain from deeper structures such as viscera and muscle to skin is probably convergent inputs at the CNS. Somatic sensory afferents from skin, muscle, and joints and efferent motor fibers are mixed in major nerves and separate into dorsal (sensory) and ventral (motor) roots just before entering or exiting the spinal cord respectively. Visceral afferent fibers are present in major nerves and traverse the sympathetic chain or the pelvic plexus with autonomic efferent fibers. Visceral afferents enter the dorsal root with somatic sensory fibers to synapse in the dorsal horn (Fig. 22.2). Fibers responding to noxious visceral stimuli are also contained in the vagus nerve and transmit sensory information to the brainstem.

Afferent sensory and efferent motor fibers are mixed in major nerves, but separate into dorsal (sensory) and ventral (motor) roots at the spinal cord.

The sensory systems provide information on the modality, location, and intensity of stimuli. Sensory receptors originate from skin, muscle, bone, joints, and visceral structures, and are specialized for particular organs and their unique sensory functions. Specialized sensory receptors transduce stimuli into electrical activity that is conducted by a variety of afferent fibers whose cell bodies are present in dorsal root ganglia for sensory transmission into the spinal cord. The face, head, and parts of the mouth are innervated by the ophthalmic, mandibular, and maxillary divisions of the trigeminal nerve that conduct sensory information to the brainstem (Fig. 22.1). The afferent fibers transmitting sensory information are categorized according to their conduction velocity and the organ of innervation. The conduction velocity of each fiber is dependent on its diameter, which is largely a result of the degree of myelination (Table 22.1).

Sensory fibers from the skin are classified as A and C-fibers, and those from muscle, joint, and tendon as type I, II, III, and IV afferents. The A-fibers are further subdivided into Aβ, and Aδ myelinated afferents. C-fibers are thin, unmyelinated, slowly conducting afferents. Most but not all Aβ-fibers transmit innocuous stimuli. Aδ- and C-fibers transmit a variety of stimuli, but are typically associated with pain transmission.

Skin is classified as glabrous or hairy; both types contain Aβ-, Aδ-, and C-fibers. Glabrous skin exists on the palms and soles of

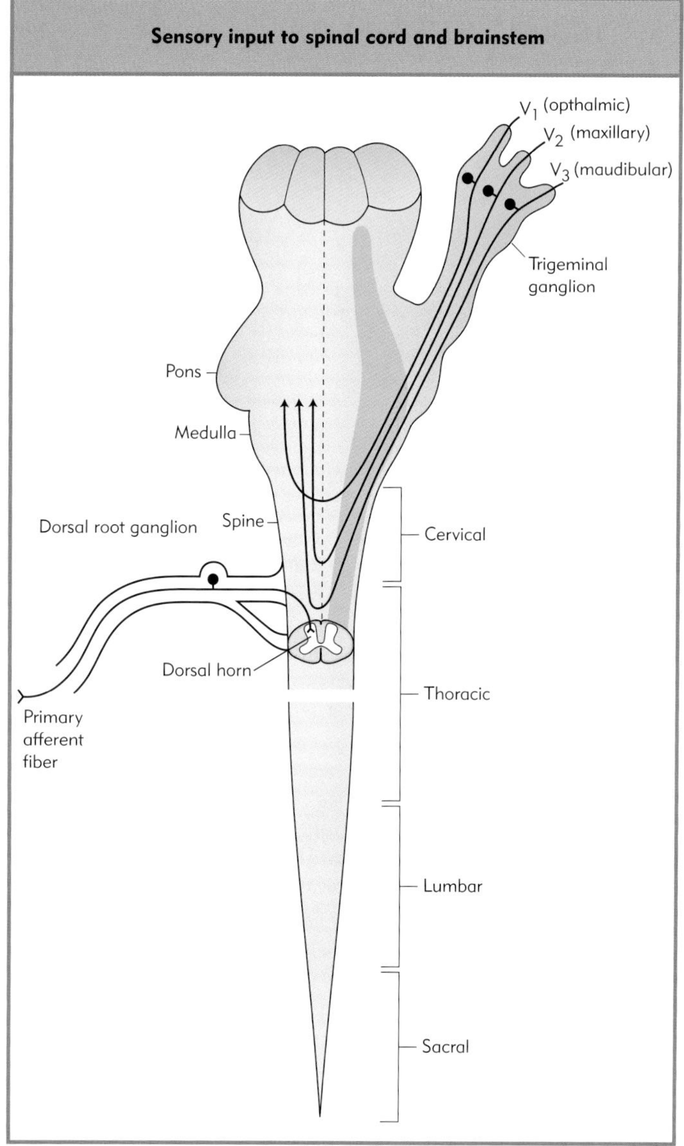

Figure 22.1 Sensory input to the spinal cord and brainstem. The dorsal aspect of the spinal cord and brainstem shows primary afferent input via dorsal root ganglia entering the spinal cord, and trigeminal ganglia into brainstem. Afferents may synapse directly or indirectly on to projecting neurons that ascend to supraspinal centers.

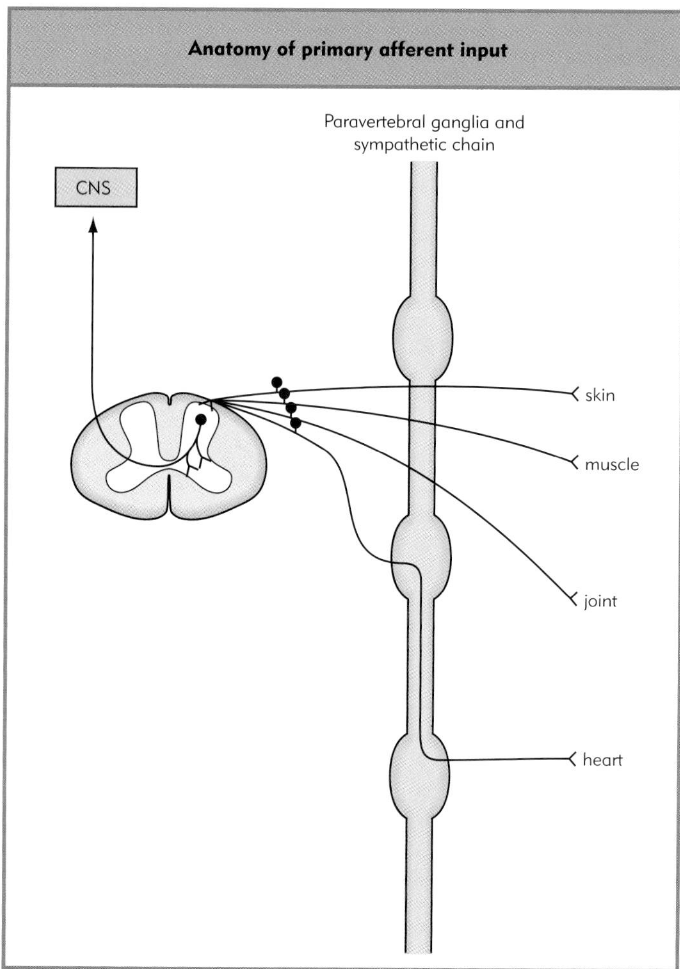

Figure 22.2 Anatomy of primary afferent input to the spinal cord from skin, muscle, joint, and viscera. Somatic afferents from skin, muscle, and joint innervate their respective tissues and enter via the somatic nerve into the dorsal root ganglia, which contain the cell bodies of the afferent fibers. These afferents then enter the dorsal horn of the spinal cord, where they synapse on dorsal horn neurons, some of which ascend to the central nervous system (CNS). Visceral afferents, like those from the heart, course through the sympathetic chain, enter the white ramus with preganglionic sympathetic efferents, and converge with the somatic afferent fibers and enter the dorsal root. The cell body of the visceral afferent nociceptor is also in the dorsal root ganglion. These visceral afferent fibers converge upon dorsal horn neurons that also receive somatic input, which is the basis for referred pain from the viscera to somatic structures.

the feet as well as the face, whereas hairy skin exists in all other areas. Receptors for the skin and tissues just deep to the skin include mechanoreceptors, thermoreceptors, nociceptors, and chemoreceptors. Although the glabrous skin is a small part of the total surface area of the body, mechanoreceptors from this area have been studied extensively. Glabrous skin mechanoreceptors are of two types, rapidly adapting (RA) and slowly adapting (SA). RA mechanoreceptors respond best to the initiation and termination of a mechanical stimulus, but fail to sustain a response during a maintained mechanical stimulus. Meissner corpuscles are specialized receptors that transmit rapidly adapting responses in glabrous skin. Merkel disks are SA type I mechanoreceptors. Merkel disks and Meissner corpuscles have low mechanical thresholds; both are contacted by Aβ-fibers, rapidly conducting sensory fibers. Deep or subcutaneous mechanoreceptors are divided into two classes. Pacinian corpuscles are RA receptors that are also sensitive to vibration. Ruffini corpuscles are SA receptors with sustained responses to stretch.

Hairy skin is well innervated by mechanoreceptors contacted by Aβ-fibers. Lanceolate endings and pilo-Ruffini receptors, as well as Merkel disks and Meissner corpuscles, innervate hair. Lanceolate endings are RA receptors that transduce the velocity of a stimulus, and pilo-Ruffini receptors are SA receptors that respond to mechanical stimulation of the hairs. Other hair receptors have also been described. Some C-fibers present in skin are C-mechanoreceptors, which respond to a variety of innocuous mechanical stimuli.

Sensory fibers from muscle, joint, and tendon are classified as type I, II, III, and IV. Types I, II, and III are myelinated and type IV are thin and unmyelinated. Proprioception, direction, and rate of limb movement are transmitted by receptors originating from muscles, tendons, and joints. Muscle spindles are long

Table 22.1 Afferent fiber types

Group	Myelinated	Organ innervated	Conduction velocity (m/s)
Aβ	Large myelinated	Skin, viscera	30–71
Aδ	Small myelinated	Skin, viscera	4–30
C	Unmyelinated	Skin, viscera	<2
I	Large myelinated	Muscle, tendon, joint	72–120
II	Large myelinated	Muscle, tendon, joint	24–71
III	Small myelinated	Muscle, tendon, joint	6–23
IV	Unmyelinated	Muscle, tendon, joint	<2

encapsulated endings that include both a type I primary sensory axon and a thinner type II sensory axon. Muscle spindles respond to both the onset and the maintenance of muscle stretch. The 1A primary afferent from the muscle spindle is most sensitive to the dynamic component of muscle stretch, whereas the group II muscle spindle afferent is sensitive to the sustained component produced by stretching or contraction. Golgi tendon organs innervate muscle tendons, and have a sustained response to tendon stretch and signal muscle stretch, tension, and contraction. Golgi tendon organs inhibit muscle contraction during extensive stretch. Joint receptors include Ruffini-type joint afferents and Pacinian-like corpuscles. Joint capsule receptors prevent extreme movements in either extension or flexion.

Sensory fibers from the viscera are classified as Aβ-, Aδ- and C-fibers. There are a variety of viscerosensory neurons, including the intrinsic sensory neurons. These afferents reside within the particular organ, for example the intrinsic enteric sensory system. The Aβ visceral mechanoreceptors are few; some may innervate areas around blood vessels. Aδ- and C-fibers transmit noxious stimuli from the viscera.

Thermoreceptors respond to warmth or cold with optimal afferent responses in nonnoxious temperature ranges. Warm receptors are unmyelinated, slowly conducting C-fibers that respond with a temperature range of 30–50°C and a maximum response at approximately 40°C. Cold receptors are lightly myelinated Aδ-fibers that respond maximally at approximately 20°C. Detection of skin temperature is a result of the integrated input from warm and cold receptors, as both discharge in the range of normal skin temperature, approximately 30–35°C. Cooler temperatures inhibit warm receptors and increase the activity of cool receptors, whereas warmer temperatures inhibit the activity of cool receptors and increase the activity of warm receptors.

NOCICEPTORS AND NOCICEPTIVE AFFERENT NEURONS

Nociceptors are contained within viscera, joints, muscles, skin, cornea, and the oropharyngeal cavity. Nociceptive afferent neurons transduce and transmit noxious (tissue-damaging or potentially tissue-damaging) stimuli to the CNS. Nociceptors innervate somatic structures such as skin, muscle, and joints, and also innervate viscera such as the heart, urinary bladder, and stomach. Somatovisceral nociceptors are the free, unencapsulated nerve endings of small myelinated Aδ- and unmyelinated C-fibers. Classification of nociceptors utilizes the organ of innervation, the degree of myelination, and the responses to a variety of stimuli. Activation of nociceptive pathways produces not only pain perception but also autonomic responses, such as sweating, tachycardia, and hypertension. Motor reflexes such as withdrawal or splinting also occur as a result of nociceptive pathway activation.

Cutaneous nociceptors

The most extensively characterized group of nociceptors are those that innervate the skin. Nociceptors in the skin are almost exclusively Aδ- or C-fibers, and are further categorized based on responses to temperature, mechanical or chemical stimuli. In general, cutaneous Aδ- fibers transmit sharp, well localized, fast pain sensations. Aδ mechanical heat (AMH) nociceptors respond to both tissue-damaging mechanical stimuli and heat. AMH nociceptors are divided into those having a high (AMH type I) or a low (AMH type II) threshold response to heat. The distribution of AMH type I and type II nociceptors depends on the type of skin: AMH type I is prominent in hairy skin and AMH type II is present in both hairy and glabrous skin. Aδ-fiber nociceptors also respond to extreme noxious cold temperatures.

Somatovisceral nociceptors are free, unencapsulated nerve endings of Aδ- and C-fibers.

In contrast to the sharp pain signals of Aδ-fibers, C-fibers transmit delayed, dull, poorly localized aching pain. Most C-fibers in the skin are polymodal nociceptors that respond to noxious mechanical stimuli and heat, and have been designated as C mechanoheat (CMH) nociceptors. The threshold for heat activation of CMH fibers is approximately 43°C; these fibers code the threshold and intensity of painful heat. CMH fibers are also chemosensitive, responding to capsaicin, the pungent ingredient in chili peppers, and low pH solutions, and thus are truly polymodal. There are C-mechanonociceptors that do not respond to heat but only to noxious mechanical stimuli. In addition, there are C-fibers that respond to noxious cold. These are a different population of fibers from those that signal cooling.

A unique group of fibers has been discovered and called mechanically insensitive afferents (MIAs). These may be either Aδ- or C-fibers. If they respond at all to a mechanical stimulus, it is only to a high-intensity stimulus. MIA fibers may or may not respond to noxious cold, heat, or chemicals, and may signal the intensity of strong noxious mechanical stimuli better than mechanically sensitive afferents such as AMH and CMH fibers. Following injury, there is some evidence that MIAs may signal mechanical hyperalgesia.

Muscle and joint nociceptors

Muscle nociceptors are less well studied than cutaneous nociceptors despite their clinical importance. Stimulation of muscle nociceptors produces the sensation of deep aching pain. Nociceptive muscle afferent fibers are critical for the generation and transmission of acute pain after muscle injuries such as surgery and trauma, as well as chronic myofascial pain. Muscle nociceptor fibers are designated type III and type IV, small myelinated and unmyelinated afferents, respectively. Stretch and muscle contraction elicit responses in muscle nociceptors. In addition to mechanosensation, both type III and type IV afferents respond to heat and chemical stimuli. Muscle pain may be referred to the overlying skin because of the convergence of both groups of afferents on to common dorsal horn neurons in the spinal cord.

Muscle and joint pain may be referred to overlying skin and visceral pain may be referred to somatic structures because of the convergence of afferent fibers on to dorsal horn neurons.

Joint nociceptors are also designated type III and type IV afferent fibers. Joint receptors respond to both low- and high-threshold mechanical stimuli. MIAs or silent nociceptors (not responding to any stimulus) were discovered in joints and later identified in other organs. Joint MIAs respond poorly even to noxious stimuli, but appear capable of coding painful responses after injury or inflammation, as in trauma and rheumatoid arthritis, respectively.

Visceral nociceptors

Visceral pain is usually characterized by a deep dull aching pain, and is usually referred to somatic structures. Visceral nociceptors signal input from organs such as the heart, esophagus, stomach, biliary tree, and the urogenital system. Activation of visceral nociceptors signals the pain of a myocardial infraction, the burning sensation of reflux esophagitis, and the pain associated with gastritis, kidney stones, or a full urinary bladder. The classification of visceral afferent fibers depends on the organ innervated, the degree of myelination, responses to stimuli, and the location of the nerve terminal. For example, afferent fibers innervating the mucosal surface of the urinary bladder signal stretch, and fibers innervating smooth muscle fibers signal tension. Other visceral afferent fibers innervate the serosal surface of an organ. In general, nociceptors from visceral organs are low-threshold mechanoreceptors which signal intensity-dependent mechanical stimuli. High-threshold mechanically sensitive afferents, which signal the intensity of responses in the noxious range, have also been identified. In addition, silent or mechanically insensitive nociceptors that respond to noxious chemical stimuli have been characterized in several organs. Many nociceptors in the viscera are also sensitive to temperature, in particular heat.

MOLECULAR BASIS OF SENSORY TRANSDUCTION

The responses of sensory neurons to particular stimuli depend on the expression of unique receptors at the terminals of the primary afferent fibers. Considerable efforts have been directed at discovering the molecular basis of sensory transduction. Because nerve terminals are difficult to study owing to their small size, many discoveries have been made using intact, whole cells from sensory ganglia.

Transducers for temperature have been discovered by cloning genes homologous to transient receptor potential (TRP) channels from dorsal root ganglion neurons. The vanilloid receptor-1 (VR1) or TRPV1 responds with inward, depolarizing currents to heat (Fig. 22.3). The threshold for the heat response is approximately 43°C; graded, the response increases with greater temperature. VR1 also responds to capsaicin, a pungent ingredient in peppers that elicits burning pain. VR1 is also sensitive to pH; a reduction in pH to approximately 6.0 depolarizes VR1-expressing cells. This suggests that neurons expressing VR1 receptors may respond to the acidic environment produced by inflammation. Thus, VR1 is one of the heat-transducing molecules that is present on small primary afferent fibers and shares response properties that are characteristic of polymodal CMH and AMH type II nociceptors. VR1 knockout mice are resistant to capsaicin-induced pain and tolerate strong heat better than do wildtype animals, but appear otherwise normal.

After the discovery of the capsaicin receptor, a second TRP channel was isolated and characterized in dorsal root ganglia.

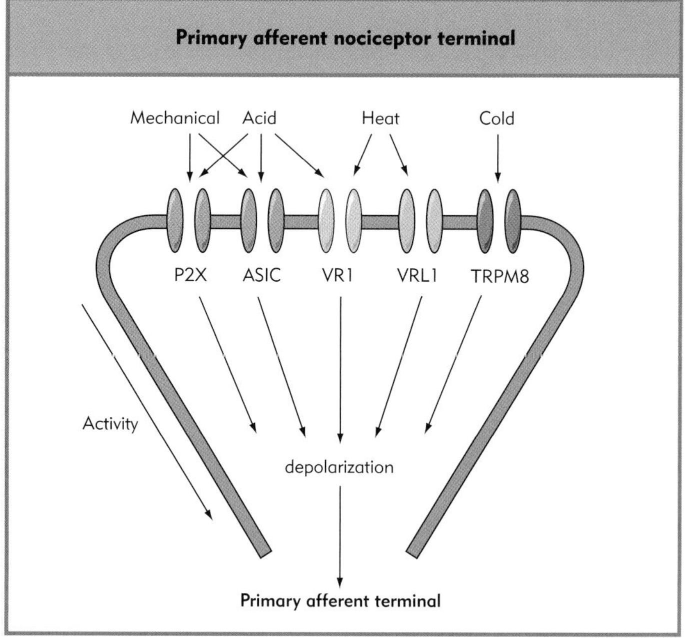

Figure 22.3 Primary afferent nociceptor terminal. Nociceptors are equipped to detect a variety of noxious stimuli, which are transduced into electrical activity at peripheral terminals of unmyelinated C-fibers and thinly myelinated Aδ-fibers. Ionotropic purinergic (P2X) receptors are excited by stretch and modulated by low pH. Acid-sensing ion channels (ASIC) are excited by mechanical stimuli as well as low pH. Both vanilloid receptor 1 (VR1) and vanilloid receptor-like 1 (VRL1) are excited by heat, but only VR1 is activated by low pH. TRPM8 is excited by low temperatures.

This TRP receptor, TRPV2, also known as vanilloid receptor-like 1 (VRL1), does not respond to capsaicin but is activated by high-intensity noxious heat. Because the threshold is approximately 52°C, VRL1 might contribute to the responses of tissue-damaging heat, a characteristic of AMH type I nociceptors.

A third heat-responding TRP channel known as TRPV3 or VRL3 was characterized recently. VRL3 has a lower heat threshold than VR1 or VRL1. VRL3 responds to warm temperatures, but may also contribute responses to heat in the noxious range. A fourth temperature-sensitive TRP channel, TRPM8, responds to cooling temperatures from 15° to 25°C. TRPM8 is also activated by menthol, which produces a cool sensation. VRL3 and TRPM8 probably contribute to temperature-sensitive sensory afferents responding to warm and cool, respectively.

The vanilloid receptors are involved in temperature sensation, but are also sensitive to low pH and specific chemicals.

Because of the limitations in applying mechanical stimuli to cells in culture, transducers for sharp mechanical pain, tension, and stretch have been more difficult to discover. However, some advances have been made in identifying molecules contributing to mechanosensation. P2X receptors are ionotropic purinerigic receptors that are activated by ATP. Mice deficient in one of the P2X receptors, P2X3, demonstrate behaviors indicating difficulty in emptying the urinary bladder. Similarly, P2X receptors contribute to sensory fiber excitation during colon distension. The excitation of P2X2 and P2X3 receptors by ATP is enhanced by acid.

Evidence from other species indicates that the acid-sensing ion channels (ASICs) respond to low pH, but may also be involved in mechanosensation. Three ASIC channels, ASIC1, 2, and 3, are expressed in dorsal root ganglia. Studies using mice deficient in ASIC2 and ASIC3 contribute to the evidence that these channels have a role in mechanosensation. ASIC2 knockout mice showed deficits in RA mechanoreceptors, whereas deletion of the ASIC3 gene caused an increase in the sensitivity of RA mechanoreceptors and a decrease in the sensitivity of high-threshold responses in A-fiber nociceptors. Loss of the ASIC3 receptor also decreased the response of nociceptors to low pH.

SPINAL PATHWAYS AND SENSORY TRANSMISSION

Anatomy of second-order neurons

The site of sensory afferent fiber synapses in the CNS is the dorsal horn of the spinal cord and the trigeminal nucleus. The morphology of neurons in the gray matter of the spinal cord and trigeminal nucleus differs depending on location. Using Rexed's classification system, there are at least 10 different laminae or layers of neurons, the first six of which (I–VI) are termed the dorsal horn in the spinal cord. These laminae, plus the area around the central canal (lamina X), receive the bulk of primary afferent inputs, although information from stretch receptors may also extend to deeper laminae. Spinal dorsal horn neurons receiving excitatory inputs from nociceptive afferents are present throughout the dorsal horn, but are concentrated in laminae I, II, V, VI, and X. Laminar assignment is based on the central location of the neuronal soma. However, dendrites of these neurons may extend throughout multiple laminae, such that the demonstration of primary afferent fiber terminations in specific laminae does not limit connectivity to just neurons of those laminae. Mapping of individual C-fiber primary afferents encoding for cutaneous nociception have demonstrated sites of connectivity that are highly localized into tight 'baskets' typically located in superficial laminae of a single spinal segment. In contrast, single primary C-fiber afferents from deep visceral structures travel via Lissauer's tract to reach multiple spinal segments and multiple laminae (I, II, V, X, and even contralateral sites).

Spinal dorsal horn neurons receiving excitatory inputs from primary afferents encoding nociceptive information frequently have axonal extensions projecting to rostral (and caudal) sites (Fig. 22.4). These sites include other segments of the spinal cord and supraspinal structures such as the thalamus, hypothalamus, midbrain, pons, and medulla. These axons travel within the white matter of the spinal cord, primarily in the anterolateral quadrants and the dorsal midline. Decussation of fibers to the contralateral anterolateral white matter occurs for axons projecting to the thalamus and most other brainstem sites. Many axons with sites of termination in 'reticular' structures remain in the ipsilateral anterolateral white matter. Dorsal column pathways terminate in the gracile and cuneate nuclei of the medulla. Intraspinal pathways exist, as well as extensive collateralization of axons with multiple sites of termination. Novel pathways for ascending nociceptive information may also include dorsolateral spinothalamic pathways related to lamina I neurons.

Intraspinal pathways

Multiple interconnections occur between spinal neurons. On a segmental level this is referred to as interneuron connectivity. When connections are more distant, the pathways of connection

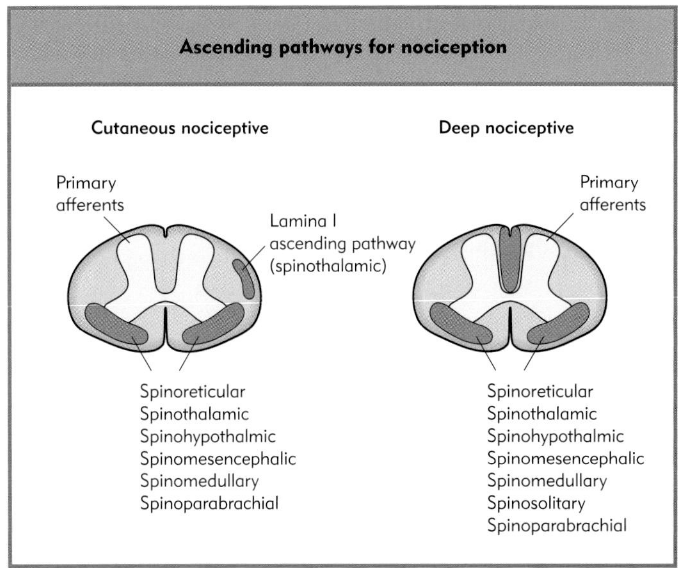

Figure 22.4 Ascending pathways for nociception. White matter pathways from spinal dorsal horn to supraspinal sites are indicated for cutaneous noxious information (left) and deep tissue noxious information (right). The key difference between these sites for the differing modalities is the inclusion of dorsal column pathways for deep tissue information. Other differences may relate to incomplete information on specific pathways for a specific modality.

are termed propriospinal, based on the initial demonstration of a coordinating connectivity between the cervical and lumbar enlargements in quadripeds that allow for coordinated motion. Intraspinal connectivity is particularly evident in neurons receiving visceral afferent input from pelvic structures. With afferent pathways traveling via the pelvic nerve and in association with sympathetic nerve pathways, the site of entry of afferent information for pelvic organs is split between the lower thoracic–upper lumbar and lower lumbar–sacral segments. Cordotomy at the midlumbar spinal cord abolishes the excitatory responses of sacral dorsal horn units to thoracolumbar inputs and thoracolumbar dorsal horn units to their respective pelvic nerve inputs. A more subtle white matter localization of the axonal extensions of propriospinal neurons is presumed to follow the paths of other propriospinal neurons, which include dorsally located white matter paths and some within-gray matter extensions. Collateral intraspinal extensions of ascending axons located within the ventrolateral white matter also exist. Spinocervicothalamic pathways with relay sites in the lateral cervical spinal cord have been demonstrated, but their role in nociception appears limited.

Anterolateral white matter

The traditional pain pathways are the spinothalamic and spinoreticular tracts located within the anterolateral white matter of the spinal cord. Both ipsilateral and contralateral pathways project to supraspinal sites, with the predominant path for afferents to the ventrobasal thalamus residing on the contralateral side. Lesions of the anterolateral spinal white matter reduce ventrobasal thalamic neuron responses to noxious cutaneous stimuli, but not to visceral stimulation. However, ventrolateral medullary neuronal responses and cardiovascular and visceromotor reflex responses to deep tissue stimuli are abolished with ventrolateral white matter lesions. Neurons with projections to other supraspinal sites, such as the hypothalamus, parabrachial nucleus, mesencephalon, pons, and other medullary sites, are excited by deep tissue stimulation. The axonal projections of this specific subset of neurons must follow the same spinal white matter pathways as those of other neurons with similar sites of projection.

The spinothalamic and spinoreticular tracts are traditional pain pathways located within the anterolateral white matter of the spinal cord.

Dorsal column pathways

A spinal pathway in the midline of the dorsal column exists for the rostral transmission of deep tissue nociception. Discrete neurosurgical lesions of this portion of the spinal cord relieve cancer-related pain in patients with pelvic visceral and deep muscle pathology. Parallel animal studies demonstrate that in this area of spinal white matter there are axons of postsynaptic dorsal horn neurons that receive noxious excitatory input from the colon, bladder, and/or uterus. Excitatory responses of neurons located in the ventrobasal thalamus to noxious deep tissue stimuli are attenuated/abolished with lesions of the dorsal midline region of the spinal cord, but are only minimally affected by lesions of the traditional spinothalamic pathways (anterolateral quadrant).

Functional characterization of the dorsal horn

Second-order neurons have also been characterized electrophysiologically according to their responsiveness to cutaneous and deep tissue stimuli. A distinction is made between excitatory responses that are produced by noxious (potentially tissue-damaging) stimuli such as high-intensity mechanical or thermal stimuli and those produced by innocuous stimuli such as hair movement or vibration. Using these criteria, the simplest nomenclature defines neurons as class 1 if excited only by innocuous stimuli, class 2 if excited by both innocuous and noxious stimuli, and class 3 if excited only by noxious stimuli. These classes are further defined by additional properties, e.g. low-threshold class 1 neurons, wide-dynamic-range/convergent class 2 neurons, and high-threshold/nociceptive-specific class 3 neurons. There appears to be a spectrum of responses to all afferent input modalities, with varying overlap.

Nocifensive reflexes evoked by noxious stimuli serve to protect the organism from injury.

Spinal reflex responses

Nocifensive reflexes are those reflexes evoked by noxious stimuli that serve to protect the body from injury. Most motor responses to noxious cutaneous stimuli, such as the flexion–withdrawal response to a pinprick of the foot, are clearly nocifensive. The limb is reflexively pulled away from the damaging stimulus, the threat to the body is removed, and pain generation is minimized. For deep tissue systems, similar reflexes are not always as obvious. Reflexes such as micturition are enhanced by local inflammation, and so can expel toxic urinary contents and thereby serve a protective function, but they may also increase pain owing to increased intravesical pressure. A direct link between tissue damage, protective behaviors, and pain is not always evident. Many responses to deep tissue stimulation in nonhumans correlate with nociception in humans, and in this way are similar to nocifensive reflexes. These include biting/scratching behaviors, and changes in heart rate, blood pressure, respiration, and abdominal muscular tone. These behaviors/reflexes are collectively called pseudoaffective responses by Sherrington, in that they appear to be reflex correlates of emotional responses to painful stimuli. The case for their correlation with accepted nocifensive reflexes is supported when they are inhibited by pharmacological manipulations known to be analgesic (i.e. morphine).

Sites of higher-order sensory processing

Second-order neurons have connectivity to numerous supraspinal sites thought to be important to nociceptive processing (Fig. 22.5). The thalamus is the major relay center between most second-order sensory neurons and the cerebral cortex. Separated into at least two major divisions, the ventrobasal group of the lateral thalamus has direct connections to sites in the somatosensory cortex that are somatotopically organized, and thus are thought to be involved in sensory–discriminative aspects of pain sensation. In contrast, the nuclei of the medial thalamus project diffusely to many different limbic structures and cortical sites, such as insula or cingulate cortex, and thus are thought to be

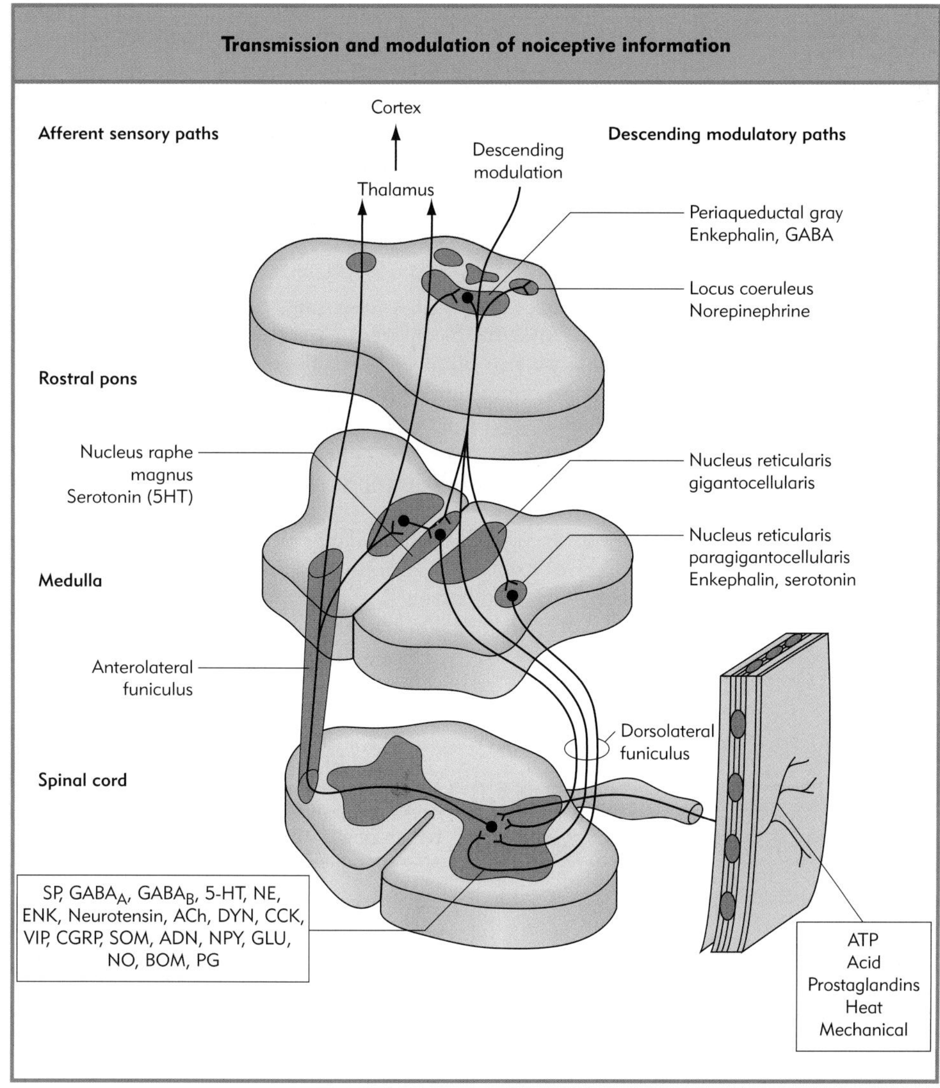

Figure 22.5 Pathways involved in transmission and modulation of nociceptive information. Stimulation of cutaneous nociceptors leads to action potential generation in the primary afferent and concomitant peripheral release of neurogenic inflammatory mediators. Information is relayed to and from a number of brainstem sites (see text). Neurotransmitters are released by afferent fibers, descending terminations, or local interneurons in the dorsal horn, and modulate peripheral nociceptive input. SP, substance P; GABA; 5-HT serotonin; NE, norepinephrine; ENK, enkephalin; ACh, acetylcholine; DYN, dynorphin; CCK, cholecystokinin; VIP, vasoactive intestinal peptide; CGRP, calcitonin gene-related peptide; SOM, somatostatin; ADN, adenosine; NPY, neuropeptide Y; GLU, glutamate; NO, nitric oxide; BOM, bombesin; PG, prostaglandin E. (With permission from Siddall PJ, Cousins MJ. Introduction to pain mechanisms. In: Cousins MJ, Bridenbaugh PO, eds. Neural Blockade in clinical anesthesia and management of pain. Copyright © Lippincott, Williams & Wilkins; Philadelphia 1998:675-713.)

related to the autonomic and affective–motivational aspects of pain sensation. Other sensory pathways, such as hearing, taste, and smell, also relay through the thalamus.

More recently, functional imaging studies using either positron emission tomography (PET) or functional magnetic resonance imaging (fMRI) technologies have identified alterations in regional cerebral blood flow (rCBF) following sensory stimulation. Increased rCBF, which indicates increased neuronal activity, occurs in the somatosensory cortices and in the anterior cingulate cortex. In chronic pain conditions, decreases in baseline bloodflow have been reported in subcortical structures such as portions of the thalamus and the basal ganglia.

The thalamus is the major relay center between sensory input and the cerebral cortex.

Brainstem sites that are activated by noxious peripheral stimuli are part of the 'reticular' system of the CNS. Highly interconnected locally and distally, the reticular activating system (RAS) is a diffuse and diverse network of nuclei activated by events that produce arousal, and is quiescent during sleep or with general anesthesia. Subnuclei of the RAS project to the spinal cord and are the major sources of the monoamines serotonin and norepinephrine in the dorsal horn. Electrical or chemical activation of RAS systems can inhibit or augment nociceptive processing, depending on the site examined.

A characteristic of spinal nociceptive systems is that they are under tonic descending inhibition, such that a common effect of injury to spinal pathways is a release from this inhibition (Fig. 22.5). Hyperreflexive states with secondary spasticity and autonomic lability (autonomic hyperreflexia) can occur following cutaneous and visceral stimuli (e.g. bladder distension). The precise sources of this descending inhibition are not established, but known inhibitory neurotransmitters that arise from supraspinal sites such as the nucleus raphe magnus (NRM) and the locus coeruleus include serotonin and norepinephrine. Electrical stimulation of the periaqueductal gray of the mesecephalon can produce surgical levels of analgesia in rodents via relays in other brainstem sites, such as the NRM.

Spinal nociceptive systems are under tonic descending inhibition involving serotoninergic and noradrenergic pathways.

DORSAL HORN NEUROCHEMISTRY

Excitatory neurotransmitters

The bulk of excitatory neurotransmission in the CNS involves the release of excitatory amino acids (EAAs) such as glutamate and aspartate (Fig. 22.6). Various peptide neurotransmitters lead to neuromodulatory effects via G protein-coupled receptor (GPCR) activation of second-messenger systems and thereby lead to excitatory responses; the most notable of these are calcitonin gene-related polypeptide (CGRP), substance P, and neurokinin A. EAAs act on ligand-gated ion channels to produce immediate excitatory postsynaptic potentials (EPSPs), and also at metabotropic receptors via GPCRs to alter intracellular second-messenger systems in a fashion similar to neuropeptides. Three different EAA-activated ion channels have been characterized, which differ from each other in their regulation by baseline membrane potentials, other agonists, and specific ions. Activation of α-amino-3-hydroxy-5-methyl-4isoxazoleproprionic acid (AMPA) receptors regulates selective Na^+ flow through a ligand-gated ion channel and is responsible for a majority of the fast excitatory transmission in nociceptive systems. AMPA receptors are unaffected by the resting membrane potential of the second-order neuron. In contrast, *N*-methyl-D-aspartate (NMDA) receptors are both voltage and ligand gated, and are permeable to both Na^+ and Ca^{2+}. Activation of the NMDA receptor–channel complex results in sustained depolarization and increased intracellular second-messenger functions of Ca^{2+} following either high-intensity or prolonged stimulation sufficient to remove the intracellular Mg^{2+} gate that holds the channel in an inactive state. The phenomena of 'wind-up' (increasing responses to repeated stimuli of equal intensity) and 'central sensitization' (decreased thresholds for response and/or increased vigor of responses) are blocked by NMDA antagonists and by hyperpolarizing stimuli. As a consequence, activation of inhibitory systems or antagonism of other excitatory systems (i.e. AMPA receptors) can also blunt or block these 'hyperalgesic' phenomena. Selective inhibition of AMPA receptors at a spinal level can lead to an analgesic effect, whereas selective antagonism of NMDA receptors may have minimal effects in the absence of excitatory drive. NMDA receptor antagonists such as ketamine or dextromethorphan produce prolonged analgesic effects when co-administered with opioids. The roles in nociceptive systems of the third excitatory ligand-gated ion channel, the kainate receptor (KA), and of the EAA metabotropic receptors, which act via G-protein mechanisms, are not well understood.

Substance P is a neuropeptide involved in pain processing. Substance P acts by binding to the NK-1 receptor, a G protein-

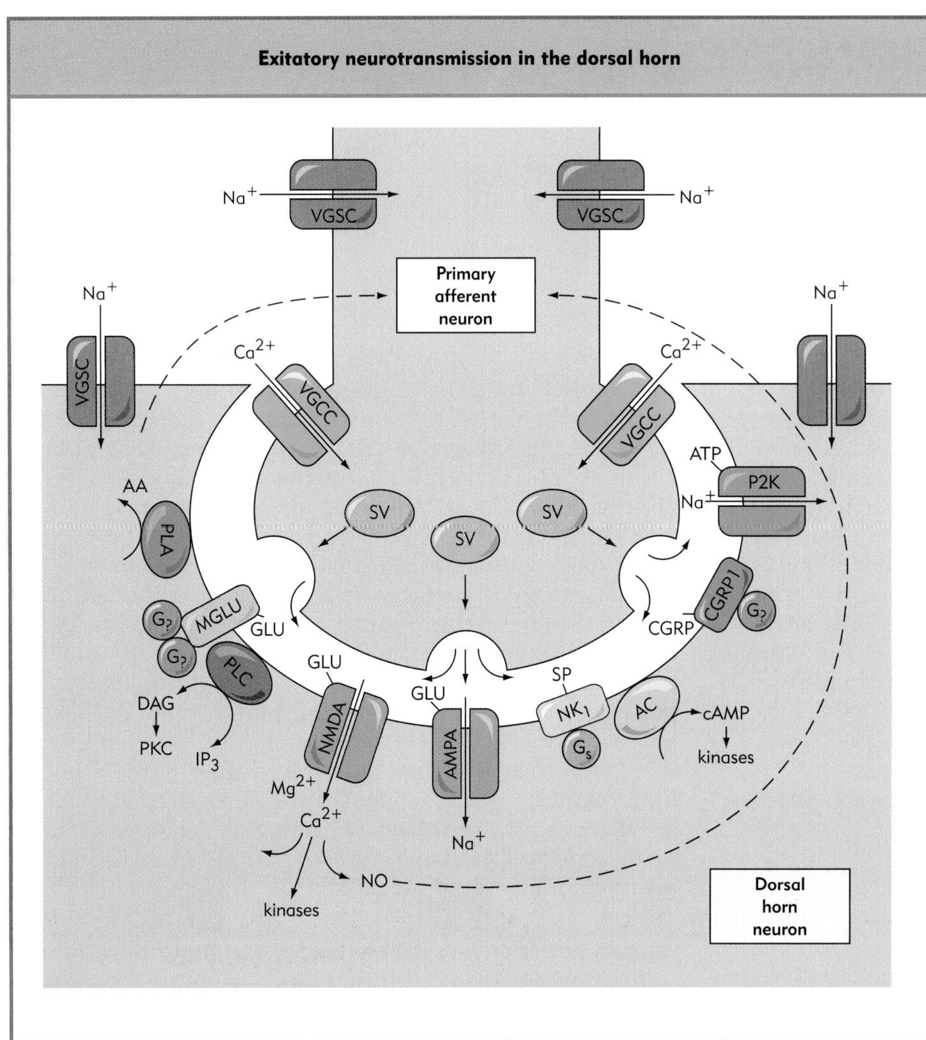

Figure 22.6 Excitatory neurotransmission in the dorsal horn. Action potentials due to voltage-gated Na^+ channels (VGSC) depolarize the nerve terminal of the primary afferent neuron, leading to the opening of voltage-gated Ca^{2+} channels (VGCC). The influx of Ca^{2+} results in synaptic vesicles (SV) fusing with the outer membrane and releasing neurotransmitters, including glutamate (GLU), substance P (SP), calcitonin-gene-related polypeptide (CGRP), and adenosine triphosphate (ATP). GLU opens ligand-gated cation channels: the fast AMPA (α-amino-3-hydroxy-5-methyl-4-isoxazolepropionate) channel and the Mg^{2+} gated NMDA (*N*-methyl-D-aspartate) channel. ATP opens P2X cation channels. Altered intracellular Ca^{2+} and the activation of G protein-coupled receptors (GLU via metabotropic glutamate receptors (mGLU); SP via NK1 receptors; CGRP via CGRP1 receptors) regulate intracellular second messengers and downstream protein kinase activation/expression, with subsequent phosphorylation of multiple receptors, channels, and other substrates involved in mediating their effects. Excitatory postsynaptic potentials due to cation flow may lead to sufficient depolarization to result in activation of voltage-gated Na^+ channels, with subsequent generation of an action potential. Antagonism/blockade of any of the noted receptors–channels will result in reduced neuronal excitation. AC, adenylyl cyclase; PLC, phospholipase C; PLA, phospholipase A; DAG, diacylglycerol; PKC, protein kinase C; IP_3, inositol trisphosphate; AA, arachidonic acid.

coupled receptor in second-order neurons. Typically co-released with glutamate, it promotes membrane depolarization, thereby modifying the gain of nociceptive transmission. It is important in conditions of inflammation, particularly neurogenic inflammation, where it is released from peripheral axons and produces local effects. Substance P appears to not be necessary for acute nociceptive transmission, as pharmacological or genetic knockout of the NK-1 receptor has minimal effects on acute responses. CGRP, a neuropeptide often present in afferent systems, has a yet-to-be-defined role in nociceptive processing.

Inhibitory neurotransmitters

γ-Aminobutyric acid (GABA) and glycine are the two main inhibitory amino acid transmitters of the CNS (Fig. 22.7). GABAergic systems are predominant at supraspinal sites and glycine at spinal sites, but both are present throughout the CNS. GABA mediates fast inhibitory transmission through a ligand-gated ion channel that allows Cl^- flow to produce hyperpolarization. Termed the $GABA_A$ receptor, it is also sensitive to benzodiazepines, barbiturates, propofol, and volatile anesthetics (Chapters 24–26). The slow metabotopic receptor for GABA, the $GABA_B$ receptor, is a G protein-coupled receptor that is coupled to K^+ channel activation and Ca^{2+} channel inhibition. Via actions on motor neurons, $GABA_B$ receptor activation by agonists such as GABA or baclofen leads to decreased spasticity and muscle tone. At brainstem levels, in association with cranial nerve function, $GABA_B$ receptor activation may be analgesic and so is a target in the treatment of various cranial neuralgias.

Glycine acts through both strychnine-sensitive and strychnine-insensitive receptors. The former, a ligand-gated anion channel very similar to the $GABA_A$ receptor, is diffusely located but has prominent actions in the ventral horn of the spinal cord. Also present in spinal sensory systems, the antagonism of glycine effects with strychnine in animal models leads to motor and

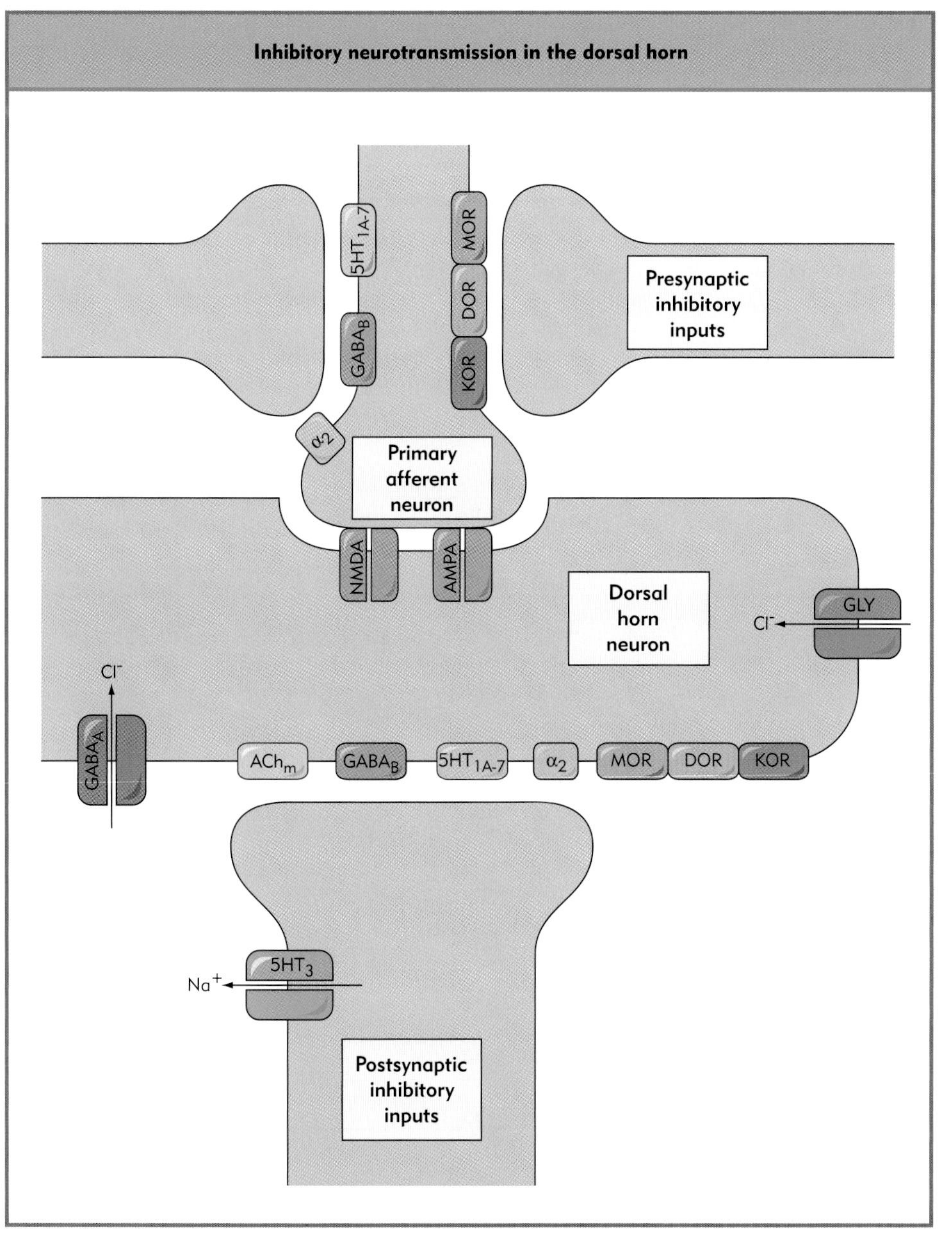

Figure 22.7 Inhibitory neurotransmission in the dorsal horn. Neurotransmission can occur pre- or postsynaptically. Ligand-gated anion channels, such as those for γ-aminobutyric acid (GABA) and glycine (GLY), form the primary ionotropic inhibitory mechanisms. Activation of serotonergic 5HT-3 cation channels activates interneurons that subsequently inhibit dorsal horn neurons. Second messenger-linked systems associated with pre- and postsynaptic inhibitory mechanisms include the μ, δ, and κ opioid receptors (MOR, DOR, and KOR, respectively), multiple families of serotonin receptors (5HT-1A to 5HT-7), α_2-adrenoceptors (α_2), and muscarinic cholinergic receptors (ACh_m).

autonomic hyperreflexia. Paradoxically, glycine can also have excitatory effects when it binds to a separate site at the NMDA receptor complex as a co-agonist. Because of their multiple nonspecific effects, anti- or proglycinergic drugs have not been employed clinically.

Endogenous opioids are the most prominent family of inhibitory neuropeptides in the dorsal horn. Arising from intrinsic spinal interneurons, enkephalins, dynorphin, and endorphins activate G protein-coupled opioid receptors that fall into three major classes (Chapter 31): μ opioid receptors (MOR), κ opioid receptors (KOR), and δ opioid receptors (DOR). Exogenously administered MOR agonists are the mainstay of analgesic therapy for severe pain today, with actions at both spinal and supraspinal sites. Spinal effects arise from the supraspinal administration of MOR agonists acting via descending serotoninergic and noradrenergic mechanisms. MOR agonists administered to spinal sites act both presynaptically on primary afferents to inhibit release of excitatory neurotransmitters and postsynaptically to directly inhibit second-order neurons. KOR agonists, the archetype being endogenous dynorphins, are neurotoxic when administered in high concentrations. Peripherally, these same agents produce analgesia, particularly mediated by deep tissue afferents. DOR agonists hold great promise, having many of the favorable characteristics of MOR agonists. However, selective nontoxic DOR agonists are not available. Cholinergic mechanisms have recently been recognized as important to nociceptive processing, and involve both nicotinic and muscarinic receptors. Cholinergic interneurons may act as intermediary steps for other analgesic treatments, such as descending norepinephrine-related inhibitory systems. These pathways are being targeted for the development of novel analgesic drugs.

Summary, sensory afferent information enters the CNS at the dorsal horn of the spinal cord and the trigeminal nucleus. At this first level of integration, a balance of excitatory and inhibitory influences is translated into coded information that leads to the activation of multiple CNS sites and reflexes. Because of this, either an increase in excitatory inputs or a decrease in inhibitory inputs can have the same sensory consequences. Excitation or inhibition can originate from primary afferent pathways or from segmental (interneurons), propriospinal (nonsegmental intraspinal), and supraspinal sources. The consequences of sensory integration in the CNS determine the sensory experience, which can be modulated by anesthetic and analgesic treatments.

Key references

Hendry FHC, Hsiao SS, Bushnell MC. Somatic sensation. In: Vigmond MJ, Bloom FE, Langus SC et al., eds. Fundamental neuroscience. London: Academic Press; 1999:761–89.

Raja SN, Meyer RA, Rainkamp M, Campbell JN. Peripheral mechanisms of nociception. In: Wall PD, Melvakck R, eds. Textbook of pain. London: Churchill Livingstone; 1999:11–57.

Sanes DH, Reh TA, Harris WA (eds) Development of the nervous system. New York: Academic Press; 2000.

Sawynok J, Cowan A (eds) Novel aspects of pain management: opioids and beyond. New York; Wiley-Liss: 1999.

Willis WD, Coggeshall RE. Peripheral nerves and sensory receptors. In: Willis WD, Coggeshall RE. Sensory mechanisms of the spinal cord, 2nd edn. New York: Plenum Press; 1991:13–45.

Further reading

Caterina MJ, Leffler A, Malmberg AB et al. Impaired nociception and pain sensation in mice lacking the capsaicin receptor. Science 2000;288:306–14.

Hirshberg RM, Al-Chaer ED, Lawand NB, Westlund KN, Willis WD. Is there a pathway in the posterior funiculus that signals visceral pain? Pain 1996;67:291–305.

Julius D, Basbaum AI. Molecular mechanisms of nociception. Nature 2001;413:203–10.

McMahon SB, Morrison JFB. Two groups of spinal interneurones that respond to stimulation of the abdominal visceral of the cat. J Physiol. 1982;322:21–34.

Nauta HJ, Soukup VM, Fabian RH et al. Punctate midline myelotomy for the relief of visceral cancer pain. J Neurosurg. 2000;92(Suppl2):125–30.

Patapoutian A, Peira AM, Story DM et al. Thermo-TRP channels and beyond: Mechanisms of temperature sensation. Nature Rev Neurosci. 2003;4:529–39.

Sugiura Y, Terui N, Hosoya Y, Tonosaki Y, Nishiyama K, Honda T. Quantitative analysis of central terminal projections of visceral and somatic unmyelinated (C) primary afferent fibers in the guinea pig. J Comp Neurol. 1993;15:315–25.

Welsh MJ, Price MP, Xie J. Biochemical basis of touch perception: mechanosensory function of degenerin/epithelial sodium channels. J Biol Chem. 2002;277:2369–72.

Woodworth RS, Sherrington CS. A pseudaffective reflex and its spinal path. J. Physiol (Lond) 1904;31:234–43.

Chapter 23

Physiology of pain

Michael J Hudspith, Philip J Siddall, and Rajesh Munglani

TOPICS COVERED IN THIS CHAPTER

A detailed understanding of sensory perception and the experience of pain is fundamental to the practice of anesthesia. The discipline developed from a need to suppress or abolish the processing of noxious sensory input and the perception of pain during surgical procedures. Anesthesia has flourished and evolved to encompass the management of pain itself in many settings, from acute postoperative pain to chronic pain states.

In the past, pain was often regarded as a simple response by the brain to a noxious stimulus in the periphery; this nociceptive information was then transmitted along well-defined 'pain' pathways. The biologic processes involved in pain perception are, however, no longer viewed as a simple 'hard-wired' system with a pure 'stimulus–response' relationship. The International Association for the Study of Pain has defined pain as '…an unpleasant sensory and emotional experience associated with actual or potential tissue damage, or described in terms of such damage'. In consequence, the perception of pain and its threshold are the result of complex interactions between sensory, emotional, and behavioral factors. Inflammation and nerve injury can reduce pain thresholds and increase sensitivity to sensory stimuli. Conversely, 'battlefield analgesia', in which soldiers receive severe injuries with little immediate awareness of pain is a situation in which thresholds can increase. This chapter emphasizes the dynamic nature of sensory perception, with specific reference to pain and analgesia. Such changes of gain in pain perception can occur over a wide range of timescales: from milliseconds determined by a balance of ion-channel and receptor-operated channel function, through longer-term processes initiated by tropic factors over minutes to hours, leading ultimately to altered gene expression and altered neuronal phenotype and synaptic architecture within the CNS (i.e. synaptic plasticity).

What is the purpose or function of pain? A withdrawal reflex response to an acute noxious stimulus is an understandable and necessary reaction that has an obvious protective function even in the absence of conscious perception. More importantly, the *experience* of pain may lead to the avoidance of potentially harmful situations and possible injury. Immobility and withdrawal due to pain may serve to provide an environment in which healing and restoration of function can occur. The severe deformities developed by individuals with a rare congenital insensitivity to pain illustrate the useful protective function provided by the sensation of pain.

However, chronic pain such as that following nerve injury, the pain associated with migraine, or where pain persists after healing of injury appears to serve no protective or restorative purpose; indeed, the pain itself becomes a disease process. Such chronic pain states are most difficult to treat. This appears to be related to the pathophysiologic processes that occur following inflammation and nerve injury, which are quite different from those seen following acute 'physiologic' pain. Current research efforts are directed toward understanding the pathophysiologic processes associated with chronic pain conditions, which are relevant to our understanding and management of pain in the clinical setting.

Psychologic factors, which include emotional and behavioral responses, are fundamental components in the perception and expression of pain, and the person in pain should always be considered in the context of the interactions between biologic and psychosocial processes. Attempts to manage pain that fail to take these interactions into account will inevitably lead to frustration and failure. Nevertheless, this chapter focuses on the neurobiologic (as opposed to the neuropsychologic) processes in the peripheral nervous system, spinal cord, and higher centers, initiated by a variety of noxious insults that are key to appropriate pharmacologic pain management. A concise overview of the anatomy and physiology of sensory pathways will provide a background for more detailed discussion of central and peripheral adaptive processes pertinent to pain transduction.

PERIPHERAL PAIN MECHANISMS

Primary afferent nociceptors

Stimuli that have the potential to cause damage (e.g. thermal, mechanical, or chemical stimuli) produce cutaneous pain by acting on primary afferent nociceptors; these are generally the initial structures involved in nociceptive processes. Nociceptors are widespread in skin, muscle, connective tissues, blood vessels, and viscera.

Primary afferent nociceptors are pseudounipolar neurons with the cell body located in the dorsal root ganglion (DRG). The peripheral processes of these neurons ramify profusely and innervate a wide variety of tissues, where they lose their perineural sheath. Their central process projects to the spinal cord dorsal horn (Fig. 23.1). Whereas large-diameter myelinated afferents serving low-intensity mechanical stimulus transduction may develop specialized terminal structures (e.g. pacinian corpuscles), nociceptive afferents lack specialized terminal structures and are morphologically 'free' nerve endings. The peripheral axon terminal is not only a transducer of mechanical, thermal, or chemical energy into series of action potentials relayed to the spinal cord, it also releases peptides in response to injury (such as substance P, calcitonin gene-related peptide (CGRP), and neurokinin A) that contribute to peripheral inflammatory processes (Fig. 23.1).

There are two main categories of cutaneous receptor associated with noxious stimulation (Chapter 22). The majority of nociceptors are C-fiber polymodal nociceptors and respond to different modes of stimuli, including noxious thermal (generally above approximately 45°C), noxious mechanical, and noxious chemical stimuli. C fibers (<2 μm diameter) are unmyelinated, with a conduction velocity of less than 2 m/s. However, not all unmyelinated fibers are nociceptors: some respond to heat in the nonnoxious range, and some are activated by nonnoxious mechanical stimuli. The other major group of nociceptors are thinly myelinated Aδ fibers, which have a diameter of 2–5 μm and a conduction velocity of 6–30 m/s. The ratio of myelinated to unmyelinated fibers in cutaneous nerves is about 1:4. Most small-diameter primary afferents are mechanically sensitive, although some are sensitive to thermal stimuli. Approximately 10% of cutaneous myelinated fibers and 90% of unmyelinated fibers are nociceptive.

Brief cutaneous stimuli can result in separate and distinct sensations, which are sometimes referred to as 'fast' and 'slow' pains. Fast pain is thought to be caused by activation of faster-conducting cutaneous Aδ fibers and is perceived as a short-lasting, pricking type of pain. Slow pain is believed to be caused by the activation of slower-conducting cutaneous C fibers, and is perceived as a dull, poorly localized, burning type of pain.

Visceral afferents

Information from nociceptors is transmitted by visceral afferents from visceral organs to the spinal cord and then in the spinothalamic tracts to the brain (Fig. 23.2). The cell bodies are located

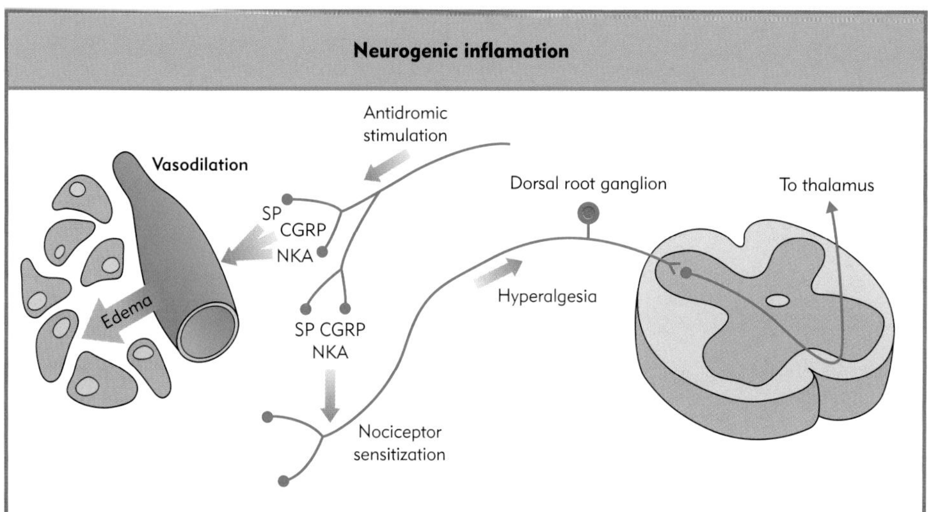

Figure 23.1 Neurogenic inflammation. Antidromic stimulation of nociceptive primary afferents results in the release of neuropeptides from primary afferent peripheral terminals; these neuropeptides bind to peripheral tachykinin receptors to produce vasodilatation, edema, and hyperalgesia (triple response of Lewis). SP, substance P; CGRP, calcitonin gene-related peptide; NKA, neurokinin A.

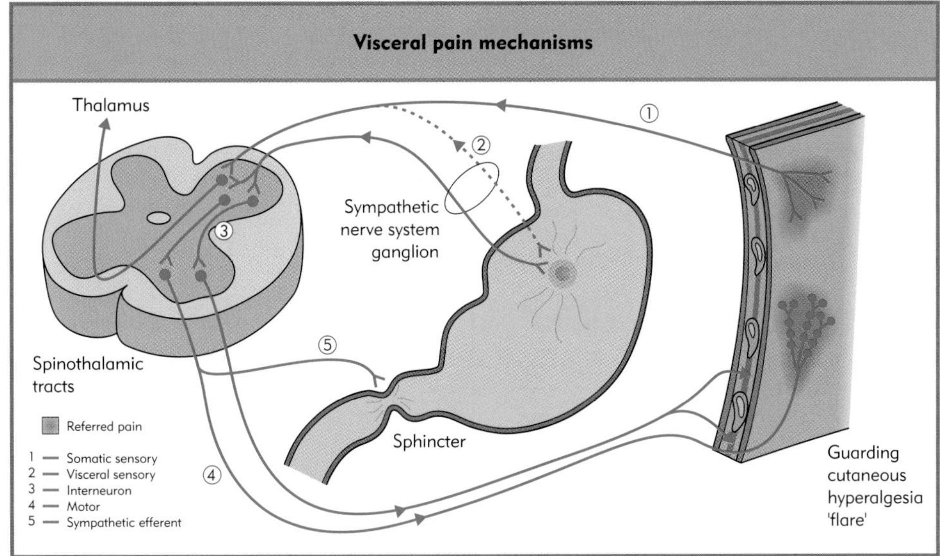

Figure 23.2 Visceral pain mechanisms: convergence of visceral and somatic nociceptive afferents on the same dorsal horn neuron. A small number of somatic nociceptive afferents may dually innervate both visceral and somatic structures. Reflex somatic motor activity results in muscle spasm and 'guarding'. Reflex sympathetic activity may result in altered visceral motility, sphincter spasm, and visceral ischemia, further exacerbating pain.

in the dorsal root ganglia, and fibers travel with sympathetic and parasympathetic axons. Stimuli that are usually painful when applied to the skin, such as thermal and mechanical stimuli, are not usually painful when applied to the viscera. For example, the brain or bowel can be cut without any sensation of pain. Visceral pain arising from hollow organs commonly results from distension or prolonged contraction of smooth muscle wall of the structure.

In contrast to cutaneous pain, which is frequently sharp and well localized to the area of stimulation, visceral pain is diffuse, dull, and poorly localized. It is frequently associated with accentuated visceral autonomic reflexes, manifest as nausea and sweating. The poor localization of visceral pain may be a consequence of the low number of afferent fibers compared with the size of the surface that is innervated; these fibers converge on dorsal horn neurons over a wide number of segments. Visceral afferents converge on second-order dorsal horn cells that also receive cutaneous spinal segmental input. This may give rise to the phenomenon of *referred pain* in dermatomal segments corresponding to their cutaneous innervation, and may result in allodynia and hyperalgesia in this skin area. Cutaneous referral may also be a consequence of considerable branching of peripheral visceral afferents, such that a single DRG cell may have axonal branches supplying both deep and superficial structures.

Sympathetic nervous system

Although visceral nociceptive afferents colocalize with sympathetic efferent nerves and are clearly involved in pelvic, abdominal, and thoracic visceral nociception described above, the sympathetic nervous system (SNS) is best considered as an efferent neuroeffector system modulating cardiovascular, bronchial, visceral, metabolic, and sudomotor function. The role of efferent sympathetic neurons in pain and nociception is considerably more complex. It is well established that the SNS plays a critical role in global behavioral responses to noxious input such as confrontational defense or flight. Within the central nervous system hypothalamic and suprahypothalamic networks of noradrenergic neurons associated with the locus ceruleus (see below) mediate such responses, and their role in arousal, fear, and emotion will modulate the perception of nociceptive input to thalamic and cortical centers.

Much emphasis has been placed on the potential role of peripheral SNS dysfunction in the generation of diffuse burning pain and hyperalgesia following injury. Formerly classified as *reflex sympathetic dystrophy* and *causalgia*, depending on the absence or presence of macroscopic nerve injury, the current terminology is complex regional pain syndromes (CRPS) I and II, respectively. Simplistically, these pain syndromes have been ascribed to the development of sensitivity of peripheral nociceptive afferents to norepinephrine (noradrenaline) or other products of the efferent SNS (hence sympathetically maintained pain). Basic science studies have demonstrated a number of complex and incompletely understood changes involving the SNS that may be responsible for the development of these features (Fig. 23.3). These include the expression of adrenoceptors on nociceptive afferents and the sprouting of sympathetic nerves into the DRG following nerve injury, which may provide in part an anatomic basis for sympathetically maintained pain syndromes.

The clinical features of CRPS reflect neuropathic pain in the presence of autonomic dysfunction. Vasomotor and sudomotor changes, abnormalities of hair and nail growth, and osteoporosis are accompanied by sensory symptoms of spontaneous burning pain, hyperalgesia, and allodynia. There is frequently an associated disturbance of motor function, including weakness, dystonia, or tremor.

Peripheral sensitization/inflammation

Thermal, mechanical, and chemical stimuli activate high-threshold nociceptors that signal information to the first relay in the spinal cord. Signal transduction mechanisms include the vanilloid receptor VR1 (now TRPV1), a nonselective cation channel activated by both noxious heat, and capsaicin, the active constituent of chili peppers; acid-sensing receptors (ASIC) respond to the low pH associated with ischemia and inflammation with increased Na^+ conductance; similar but as yet uncharacterized receptors are proposed to transduce noxious mechanical stimuli.

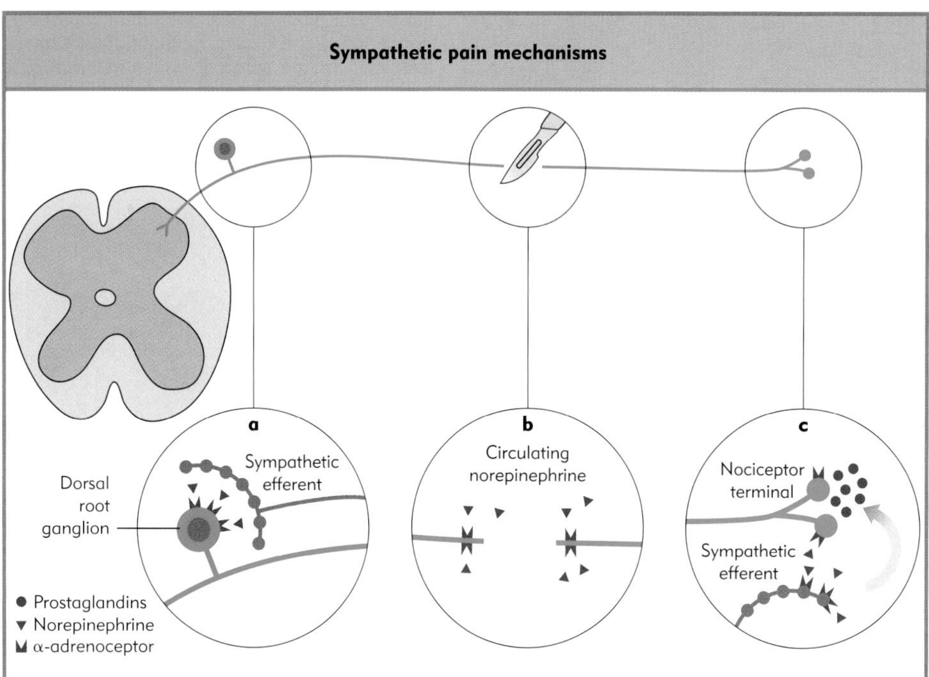

Figure 23.3 Sympathetic pain mechanisms. Injury may result in sympathetic activation of nociceptive afferents at multiple sites. (a) Altered tropic factor availability stimulates sympathetic neurons to form basket-like outgrowths around dorsal root ganglion cells that may drive ganglion activity. (b) Expression of functional α-adrenoceptors at the site of nerve injury results in activation of nociceptive afferents via circulating catecholamines. (c) Peripheral nociceptor afferents may also express α-adrenoceptors and be activated by locally released or circulating catecholamines. Peripheral inflammation results in α-adrenergic-mediated release of prostaglandins from sympathetic terminals, with resultant sensitization.

Pain arising from direct activation or sensitization of primary afferent neurons, especially C fiber polymodal nociceptors is a dynamic process. Nociceptor activation sets in train processes that modify responses to further stimuli; for example, a relatively benign noxious stimulus such as a scratch to the skin initiates peripheral inflammation that reduces the threshold for response of the nociceptor to subsequent sensory stimuli (Fig. 23.4). It is essential to appreciate that surgical or traumatic noxious stimuli are usually prolonged and associated with tissue damage of variable degrees. Clinical pain is therefore almost universally associated with peripheral sensitization.

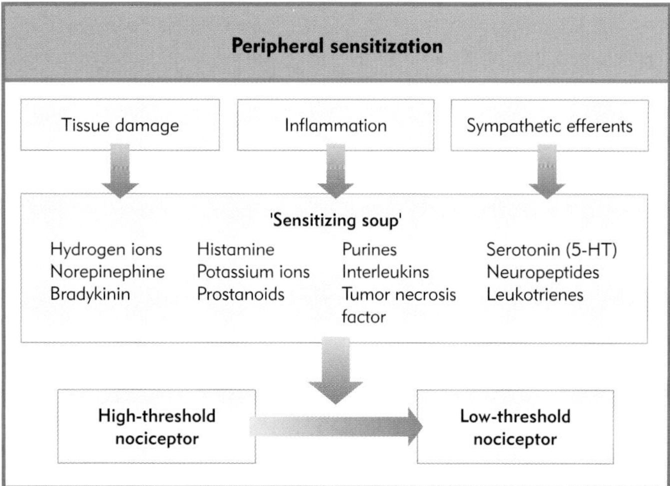

Figure 23.4 Peripheral sensitization. The gain of high-threshold nociceptors can be modified in the periphery by a combination of chemical mediators. Tissue damage and inflammatory cell mediator release is supplemented by neuropeptide and catecholamine release from peripheral nociceptive afferent and sympathetic efferent terminals. (Adapted from Woolf CJ, Chong MS. Pre-emptive analgesia: treating postoperative pain by preventing the establishment of central sensitization. Anesth Analg. 1993;77:362-79.)

Part of the inflammatory response is the release of intracellular contents from damaged cells and inflammatory cells such as macrophages, lymphocytes, and mast cells. Nociceptive stimulation also results in a neurogenic inflammatory response, with the release of compounds such as substance P, neurokinin A, and CGRP from the peripheral terminals of nociceptive afferent fibers. These peptides modify the excitability of sensory and sympathetic nerve fibers, induce vasodilatation and extravasation of plasma proteins, and promote the release of further chemical mediators by inflammatory cells (see Fig. 23.1). These interactions result in a 'soup' of inflammatory mediators, including K^+ and H^+, serotonin, bradykinin, substance P, histamine, cytokines, nitric oxide, and products from the cyclo-oxygenase and lipoxygenase pathways of arachidonic acid metabolism (see Fig. 23.4). These chemicals then act to sensitize high-threshold nociceptors and produce the phenomenon of *peripheral sensitization*. Following sensitization, low-intensity mechanical stimuli that would not normally cause pain are now perceived as painful. There is also an increased responsiveness to thermal stimuli at the site of injury. This zone of 'primary hyperalgesia' surrounding the site of injury is a consequence of peripheral changes and is commonly observed following surgery and other forms of trauma.

Peripheral sensitization may include the SNS, and there is evidence that sympathetic nerve terminals may themselves release prostanoids and products of arachidonic acid metabolism after peripheral injury. This provides a potential link between the peripheral sympathetic efferent and the peripheral nociceptor in CRPS, where pain complaints may vary with sympathetic efferent activity.

Role of nerve growth factor in peripheral sensitization

There is a central role for nerve growth factor (NGF) in the etiology of inflammatory pain. Nerve growth factor belongs to the family of neurotropic peptides, including brain-derived neurotropic factor (BDNF), and neurotropins 3, 4/5, and 6, which specify the phenotypic development of central and peripheral neurons. Neurotropins interact with a low affinity p75 receptor, which may modulate the expression and function of specific high-affinity tyrosine kinase (Trk) receptors for each neurotropin. The biologic effects of NGF are mediated via the TrkA receptor.

Inflammation produces a mixture of mediators that act to sensitize high-threshold nociceptors, thereby producing peripheral sensitization.

The TrkA receptor is expressed on small unmyelinated nociceptive afferents that coexpress the peptide CGRP and innervate a wide variety of peripheral tissues. Within these tissues there is constitutive expression of NGF at low levels by cell types such as fibroblasts, keratinocytes, immune cells, and Schwann cells. This constitutive production of NGF may determine nociceptor phenotype: the 'neurotropic hypothesis'. Inflammation via the cytokines IL-1β and TNF-α is associated with increased NGF expression and has been demonstrated in both animal models of inflammation and human disease, including arthritis and cystitis (Fig. 23.5). The rapid onset of hyperalgesia following experimental subcutaneous administration of NGF strongly suggests a direct peripheral action mediating peripheral sensitization. Tyrosine kinase A receptors are not restricted to nociceptive afferents but are expressed by both mast cells and postganglionic efferents. Nerve growth factor plays a central role in peripheral sensitization mediated by both direct and indirect actions of inflammatory mediators on nociceptive afferents. Furthermore, growth factors may mediate upregulation of various types of Na^+ channel that are more likely to fire spontaneously (akin to pacemaker cells in the myocardium), but also are more sensitive to Na^+ channel blockers such as lidocaine. The development of such Na^+ channels may contribute to the features of spontaneous pain and extreme mechanosensitivity seen in many pain states. Axonal transport of NGF taken up by nerve terminals has tropic effects within the spinal cord dorsal horn, contributing to central sensitization (see below).

Silent nociceptors

Silent or 'sleeping' nociceptors are inactive under most circumstances but become active following inflammation and sensitization by NGF. They have been identified in joint capsules and the walls of viscera. Following sensitization they become responsive and discharge vigorously, even during ordinary movement or visceral distension within the physiological range; they also display changes in receptive fields. This class of nociceptor may contribute to the mechanical allodynia and hyperalgesia associated with peripheral inflammation in arthritis and visceral pain states, such as cystitis or inflammatory bowel disease.

Peripheral nerve injury

Peripheral nerve injury results in a number of biochemical, physiologic, and morphologic changes at the peripheral and spinal level that reflect altered afferent sensory input and which may themselves act as a generator of pain (Fig. 23.6). Nerve damage results in an inflammatory response around the site of injury, with increased production of compounds, including NGF and other tropic factors that normally modulate neuronal growth. Normal sensory processing and primary afferent phenotype are critically dependent on a balance of both retrograde and anterograde axonal transport of tropic factors typified by NGF. For example, following nerve injury there is a loss of the primary afferent peptide transmitters substance P and CGRP, and corresponding upregulation of neuropeptide Y and galanin within the DRG and dorsal horn of the spinal cord. This complex pattern of neuropeptide changes reflects altered tropic factor availability, and the exogenous application of NGF after

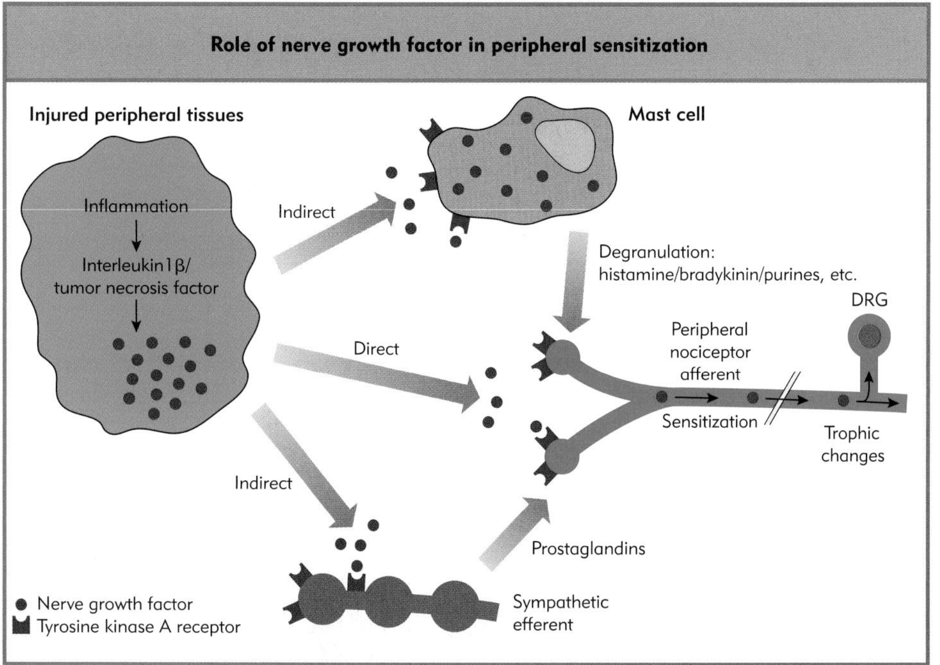

Figure 23.5 Role of nerve growth factor in peripheral sensitization. Nerve growth factor acts both directly and indirectly.

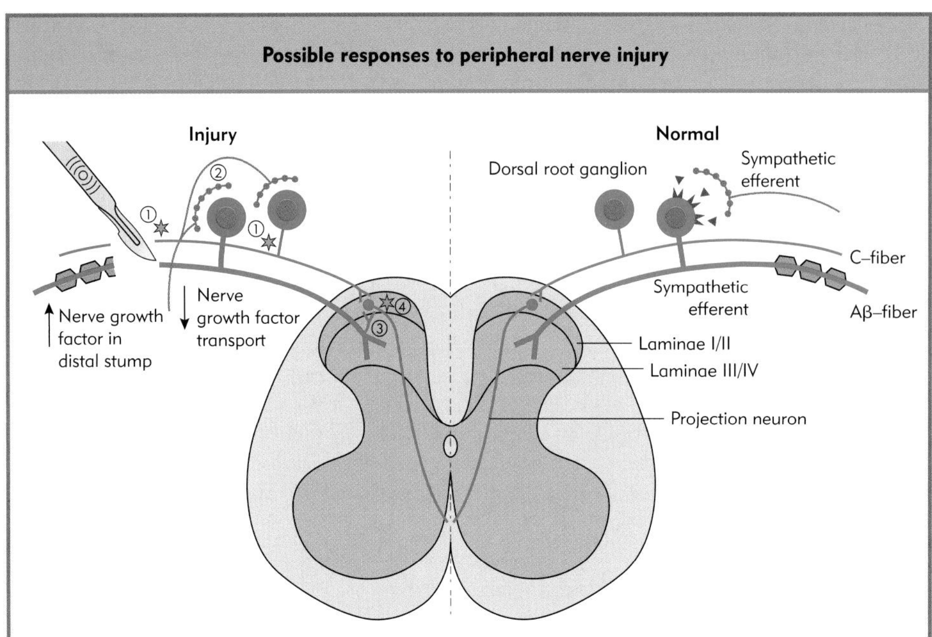

Figure 23.6 Possible responses to peripheral nerve injury. Transverse section of spinal cord and afferent input. 1) Peripheral nerve transection interrupts retrograde axonal transport of growth factors. Sprouting of proximal neuronal stumps produces neuromata expressing altered Na^+ channel isoforms; similar changes occur in the DRG. 2) Sympathetic innervation and activation of DRG neurons (see Fig. 23.3). 3) Aβ fibers within laminae III and IV of the dorsal horn sprout and potentially form synaptic contact with nociceptive projection neurons of lamina II. Nonnociceptive (Aβ) afferent input may therefore activate nociceptive pathways, resulting in allodynia. 4) Altered neuropeptide expression and loss of GABAergic inhibition within the dorsal horn may result in spontaneous activity of dorsal horn projection neurons.

experimental nerve injury can partially reverse such phenotypic changes. Although altered neuronal phenotype within the DRG and dorsal horn may contribute to the development of pathologic pain states, certain changes, such as the upregulation of neuropeptide Y, may also represent adaptive analgesic responses to injury.

Peripheral nerve injury may initiate both excitotoxic and apoptotic death of neurons within the spinal cord dorsal horn. GABAergic interneurons are significantly depleted after peripheral nerve injury. GABA is the major inhibitory transmitter in the spinal cord, and a reduction in the population of GABAergic neurons in the spinal cord may contribute to the hyperalgesia and allodynia seen in chronic pain. The vulnerability of the nervous system through loss of inhibitory control may be accentuated by the increased input from the periphery, as described above, as well as by increased activation of sympathetic nerves, which may 'fire up' the somatosensory system.

Nerve injury involving loss of axonal integrity typically results in trophic factor-mediated sprouting of the peripheral end of the damaged fibers, which may result in neuroma formation. Neuromata express heterogeneous populations of spontaneously and repetitively active Na^+ channels, which may contribute to spontaneous action potential generation after nerve injury. Furthermore, neuromata are typically mechanosensitive and may be sensitive to norepinephrine and sympathetic nerve activity. Damage to the vasa nervorum causes a reduction in the blood supply to myelinated fibers, with resultant demyelination and the production of ectopic impulses.

Reduced inhibitory transmission in the spinal cord may contribute to the hyperalgesia and allodynia seen in chronic pain.

Similar changes occur within the DRG. Partial ligation of a peripheral nerve results in spontaneous firing of these cells, at least in part as a consequence of altered synthesis and expression of Na^+ channels, as described above. Peripheral nerve injury also induces the formation of abnormal basket-like terminations of sympathetic neurons around primary afferent cell bodies in the DRG that may contribute to SNS-mediated pain. Together, changes at the site of nerve injury and in the DRG may give rise to the perception of sharp, shooting, or burning pain in conditions such as diabetic neuropathy, postherpetic neuralgia, and peripheral nerve trauma. Contributing to this state of excitability is the feature of cross-excitation, in which DRG neuron ephaptic discharges may excite otherwise inactive neurons, further contributing to the hyperalgesic and allodynic state.

Clinical implications for peripheral analgesic action

NONSTEROIDAL ANTI-INFLAMMATORY DRUGS

Nonsteroidal anti-inflammatory drugs (NSAIDs) are commonly used for 'peripheral' analgesia and have as one of their actions a reduction in the peripheral inflammatory response. Agents such as aspirin and other NSAIDs provide their anti-inflammatory action by blocking the cyclo-oxygenase pathway (Chapter 32), and it is now apparent that cyclo-oxygenase exists in several isoforms. Most notably COX-1 and COX-2 have been sequenced, but a COX-3 isoform that is a splice variant of COX-1 has recently been described. Whereas COX-1 is constitutively expressed in tissues, including the gastric mucosa, and plays a homeostatic 'housekeeping' role, COX-2 is predominantly induced by inflammation. This has presented an opportunity for the development of agents that have a selective anti-inflammatory effect without gastric side effects. The coxib drugs do indeed demonstrate effective analgesic action with reduced gastrointestinal toxicity, although inhibition of constitutive COX-2 activity in renal and vascular endothelium may produce cardiovascular and renal side effects. Acetaminophen (paracetamol) has minimal effects on peripheral COX-1 or COX-2 in vitro, but may exert central analgesic actions through inhibition of COX-3. As well as the peripheral action of NSAIDs, there is increasing evidence that they exert their analgesic effect through central mechanisms involved in the development and maintenance of spinal cord sensitization. This observation has led to the successful use of intrathecal and epidural NSAIDs in experimental animal pain models.

OPIOIDS

Although opioids traditionally have been considered centrally acting drugs (Chapter 31), there is evidence for the action of opioids on peripheral nociceptor terminals after tissue damage (Fig. 23.7). Opioid receptors are synthesized in the cell body (DRG) and transported toward the central terminal in the dorsal horn and toward the periphery. Peripheral receptors become active within hours of local tissue damage. This occurs with unmasking of opioid receptors and the arrival of immunocompetent cells that possess opioid receptors and have the ability to synthesize opioid peptides. This finding has led to an interest in the peripheral administration of opioids for postoperative analgesia, both at the site of surgery and as supplements to local anesthetics in nerve and plexus blocks. Systematic review of these techniques demonstrates that intra-articular administration of opioids following knee surgery or arthroscopy may be efficacious. Opioids with physicochemical properties that favor peripheral action are under development and may be useful for regional application.

LOCAL ANESTHETICS

Systemic administration of local anesthetic agents such as lidocaine can result in a marked reduction in pain following peripheral nerve injury, and is a useful diagnostic tool in determining the etiology of pain syndromes. Relatively low concentrations of local anesthetic can reduce ectopic activity in specific populations of Na^+ channels in damaged nerves at concentrations below those required to produce conduction block at classic 'tetrodotoxin-sensitive' voltage-dependent Na^+ channels. Although intravenous or subcutaneous lidocaine may be used as an analgesic adjunct in neuropathic malignant pain, oral congeners of local anesthetics such as mexiletine or flecainide and the anticonvulsant lamotrigine are more commonly used for long-term analgesia in neuropathic pain of nonmalignant origin.

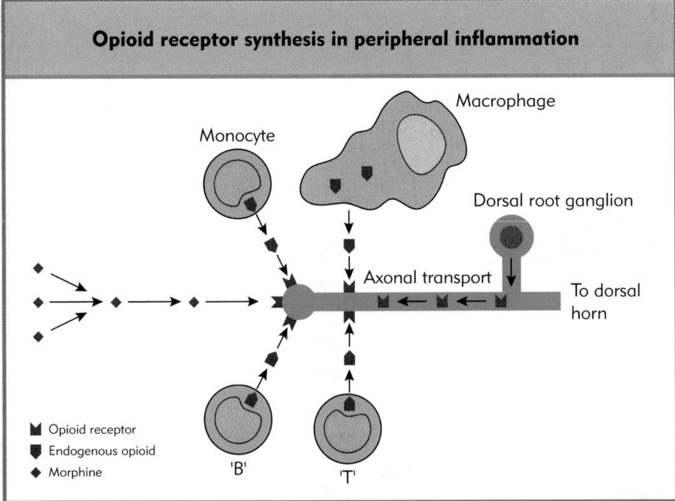

Figure 23.7 Opioid receptor synthesis in peripheral inflammation. Synthesis occurs within the dorsal root ganglia and receptors are transported to the periphery. Peripheral opioid receptors are activated by the release of endogenous opioid peptides from inflammatory cells at the site of injury. Local application of exogenous opioids therefore attenuates firing of sensitized nociceptors. (Adapted from Stein, 1995. © Elsevier, Ltd.)

SYMPATHETIC BLOCKADE

Complex regional pain syndromes have been divided into those that are sympathetically maintained and those that are sympathetically independent. Pain problems that are sympathetically maintained may respond to sympathetic blockade by agents administered systemically, regionally, or around the sympathetic ganglion. Analgesia provided by sympathetic blocks may permit the mobilization and physiotherapy essential to the treatment of the condition. However, there is considerable dispute over the long-term efficacy of repeated sympathetic blocks, whether performed with local anesthetic, neurolytic solutions, or by radiofrequency thermocoagulation.

DORSAL HORN MECHANISMS

Termination sites of primary afferents

The dorsal horns of the medulla and spinal cord are the major sites of termination of nearly all sensory afferents, irrespective of peripheral origin. Small myelinated and unmyelinated fibers tend to aggregate in the lateral aspect of the dorsal root and enter the dorsal horn laterally; larger fibers tend to travel medially. Whereas the principal route of entry for primary afferents is through the dorsal root, a significant number of primarily unmyelinated afferent neurons enter via the ventral root.

In transverse section, the spinal cord gray matter is divided into 10 laminae according to Rexed's classification of their light microscopic morphology. The most superficial of these is lamina I, and the dorsal horn extends to lamina VI. The ventral horn comprises laminae VII–IX, with lamina X being the region surrounding the central canal. The architecture of these laminae is of considerable significance when considering differing modalities of afferent sensory input to the spinal cord.

Unmyelinated C fiber nociceptors terminate principally in lamina II (the substantia gelatinosa). Some unmyelinated fibers also ascend and descend several segments in Lissauer's tract before terminating on neurons that project to higher centers. Small myelinated Aδ nociceptors terminate principally in the superficial dorsal horn (lamina I) and deeper in lamina V. Nociceptors from joints terminate in lamina I as well as more deeply in laminae VI and VII. Large-fiber low-threshold mechanoceptors, which transmit nonnoxious information regarding fine touch, proprioception, and vibration, terminate mainly in lamina III and IV, or more rostrally in the dorsal column nuclei of the medulla oblongata.

The terminations of primary afferent nociceptors transmit information to the first relay of neurons in the dorsal horn, sometimes known as second-order neurons. These are often divided into two main classes: 'nociceptive specific' or 'high threshold', and 'wide dynamic range' or 'convergent' neurons that have different response properties to afferent input and differential distributions in regions of the dorsal horn. Nociceptive-specific neurons are located predominantly within the superficial laminae of the dorsal horn and respond exclusively to noxious input from C and Aδ fibers. Neurons with wide dynamic range represent the majority of nociceptive second-order neurons located in deeper laminae (IV–VI), and approximately 20% of nociceptive neurons in laminae I–II of the dorsal horn. WDR neurons respond to both noxious and nonnoxious inputs, including those from Aβ fibers, but normally do not signal pain in response to a tactile stimulus at a nonnoxious level. However, if they become sensitized and hyperresponsive, they may discharge at a high rate following a tactile stimulus. If the activity of the neuron exceeds a threshold level following this stimulus, then the nonnoxious tactile stimulus will be perceived as painful and give rise to the phenomenon of allodynia.

Outputs from primary afferents

There is a polysynaptic, intraspinal pathway that connects primary afferents to motor neurons. This is a basic pathway that underlies the withdrawal reflex and can occur even in the absence of pain perception, such as under anesthesia or following spinal cord injury. It is heavily modified by local and descending inhibitory influences, and when descending controls are lost (as happens following complete spinal cord injury), the pathway can be activated by nonnociceptive afferents such that even innocuous stimuli will result in a flexor withdrawal response.

An acute noxious stimulus also results in autonomic responses, such as a rise or fall in blood pressure and a change in respiration. Responses appear to be related to the structures involved: nociceptive stimuli from viscera frequently result in a fall in blood pressure, whereas cutaneous stimuli usually lead to an increase in blood pressure. These changes occur as a result of spinal and supraspinal activation of regions involved in autonomic regulation following nociceptor stimulation.

The sensation and interpretation of pain requires activation of those brain regions associated with spatial discriminative and affective components of pain perception. This is clearly a potential (but not inevitable) consequence of activity of the primary afferent nociceptor, and involves integration of the polysynaptic output from the primary afferent through multiple ascending pathways. The exact location of specific supraspinal regions associated with pain perception is complex and incompletely understood, and will be discussed further below. Current research has focused on spinal mechanisms of pain transduction, and these will be reviewed.

Neurotransmitters and neuromodulators

The dorsal horn contains a host of peptide and amino acid neurotransmitters, neuromodulators, and their respective receptors (Chapter 22). Neurotransmission within the dorsal horn encompasses:

- excitatory transmitters released from the central terminals of primary afferent nociceptors;
- excitatory transmission between neurons of the spinal cord;
- inhibitory transmitters released by interneurons within the spinal cord;
- inhibitory transmitters released from supraspinal sources.

The concept of a single neuron releasing a single transmitter within the synaptic cleft clearly does not apply to the dorsal horn. Although exocytotic release of individual peptide or amino acid transmitters may occur, experimental data suggest that this rarely happens under physiologic conditions, and two or more compounds are commonly released at the same time. Differing ratios of cotransmitter release may occur, depending on the intensity of the stimulus. Neurotransmitters may be released in close proximity to pre- or postsynaptic receptors in the dorsal horn; however, it is clear that 'volume transmission' also occurs within the dorsal horn, where spatially distant receptors may be activated by transmitters outside a classic synapse.

Excitatory nociceptor transmission

EXCITATORY AMINO ACIDS

Glutamate is the main CNS neurotransmitter and plays a major role in nociceptive transmission in the dorsal horn. Glutamate acts at α-amino-3-hydroxy-5-methyl-4-isoxazolepropionic acid (AMPA) receptors, *N*-methyl-D-aspartate (NMDA) receptors, kainate (KA), and metabotropic glutamate receptors (Chapters 20, 22).

AMPA receptors are ligand-operated ion channels; the channel is not voltage dependent and permits the selective entry of Na^+ under physiologic conditions. The result is a short-latency excitatory postsynaptic potential (EPSP), and AMPA receptors are responsible for 'fast' transmission of impulses in nociceptive and nonnociceptive pathways (Fig. 23.8). Such information may encode the onset, offset, and intensity of a noxious stimulus. AMPA receptors are not selectively localized to regions of the nervous system involved in nociception, and antagonists at the AMPA receptor may therefore have limited use as analgesics because of their widespread presence and function in the CNS. AMPA receptors may mediate responses in the 'physiologic' processing of sensory information. However, prolonged release of glutamate or concurrent activation of neurokinin receptors results in sustained activation of AMPA and/or neurokinin receptors. This appears to be crucial in the development of abnormal responses to further sensory stimuli by priming the NMDA receptor so that it reaches a state ready for activation.

The NMDA receptor complex is a multimeric channel permeable to Na^+ and Ca^{2+} that is both voltage and ligand gated. At a normal resting potential (–70 mV), Mg^{2+} blocks the ionophore of the NMDA receptor, and binding of glutamate in the presence of its coagonist glycine does not result in channel opening. Priming of the NMDA receptor occurs with depolarization of the membrane to –30 mV, which enables Mg^{2+} to leave the channel (Fig 23.8). This degree of depolarization occurs when glutamate and peptides are co-released after intense afferent activation and act on AMPA and neurokinin receptors in the dorsal horn. Activation of the NMDA receptor causes large and prolonged depolarization associated with Ca^{2+} mobilization in neurons that are already partly depolarized. Activation of NMDA receptors at pre- and postsynaptic loci initiates processes that contribute to the medium- or long-term changes observed in chronic pain states, including central sensitization, changes in peripheral receptive fields, induction of gene transcription, and long-term potentiation (LTP). This last refers to the changes in synaptic efficacy identified as a synaptic correlate of memory in the hippocampus and cerebral cortex, and may play a role in the development of a cellular 'memory' for pain or enhanced responsiveness to noxious inputs.

Release of tachykinins is required to produce intense pain, making this system promising as a drug target.

Metabotropic glutamate receptors comprise three groups (I–III) and at least eight subtypes, mGluR1–mGluR8. Group I are coupled to G_q proteins linked to phosphoinositide hydrolysis and protein kinase C activation, whereas groups II and III couple

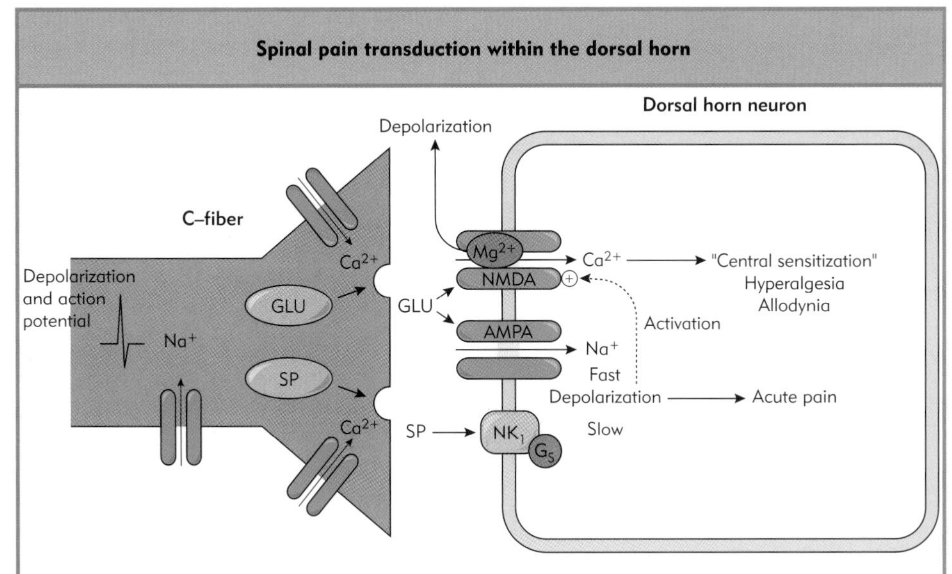

Figure 23.8 The pharmacology of spinal pain transduction within the dorsal horn. Acute pain causes brief postsynaptic depolarization of dorsal horn neurons and activation of central pain pathways. More prolonged afferent input via Aδ and C fibers causes NMDA receptor activation. NMDA, *N*-methyl-D-aspartate; Glu, glutamate; NK_1, neurokinin 1; SP, substance P; AMPA, α-amino-3-hydroxy-5-methyl-4-isoxazolepropionate; G_s, G_s protein. (Adapted from Hudspith MJ. Glutamate: a role in normal brain function, anesthesia, analgesia and CNS injury. Br J Anaesth. 1997;78:731-747. © The Board of Management and Trustees of the British Journal of Anaesthesia. Reproduced by permission of Oxford University Press/British Journal of Anaesthesia.)

negatively to adenylyl cyclase and cAMP signaling pathways through G_i/G_o proteins (Chapters 3, 20). Their role in nociception is currently incompletely defined and they do not appear to be involved in acute 'physiologic' pain. However, there is now compelling evidence that spinal group I mGluRs play a modulatory role in nociceptive processing, central sensitization, and pain behavior. The role of group II and III mGluR is less clear.

Peptides

Small-diameter nociceptive primary afferent fibers are characterized by a variety of peptide transmitters, including substance P, neurokinin A, and CGRP. The release of substance P, which coexists in primary afferents with glutamate, occurs following cutaneous thermal, mechanical, or chemical noxious stimuli and is potentiated by peripheral inflammation. Although historically substance P was considered the major neurotransmitter involved in spinal mechanisms of nociception, experimental data from animals lacking the substance P receptor (NK-1 receptor 'knockout' mice) demonstrate that acute nociception persists in animals lacking substance P-mediated neurotransmission. Rather, substance P plays a modulatory role in nociception, modifying the gain in afferent transmission. Animal data demonstrate that substance P may play an important role in the transmission of prolonged or highly noxious stimuli. The actions of substance P may be potentiated by neurokinin A and CGRP within the dorsal horn, although the role of these peptides is less well understood. Disruption of the preprotachykinin A gene, which encodes for substance P and neurokinin A, significantly reduces the response to moderate-to-intense pain and abolishes neurogenic inflammation without affecting responses to mild pain. The release of these tachykinins from primary afferent nociceptors is therefore required to produce intense pain. Neurokinin A or substance P antagonists are promising targets for the development of new drugs to treat pain.

Intracellular events

NMDA receptor activation and Ca^{2+} mobilization set in train a cascade of secondary events in the neuron that has been activated by prolonged and intense afferent input (Fig. 23.9). Subsequent changes in the neuron increase its responsiveness to further afferent input and lead to some or all of the phenomena described above.

Influx of Ca^{2+} into the neuron activates a number of pathways involving second messengers, including inositol trisphosphate (IP_3), cGMP, eicosanoid, nitric oxide, and protein kinase C (Chapter 3). The exact role of NO in nociceptive processing is unclear, and it does not appear to be important in acute nociception. However, production of NO is implicated in the induction and maintenance of chronic pain states. NO may act as a positive feedback mechanism, acting in conjunction with presynaptic NMDA receptors to upregulate afferent input further, and thereby potentiate nociceptive input. Inhibition of NO synthesis results in a decrease in the behavioral correlates of pain in animal models of neuropathic pain.

Immediate early gene induction and altered protein synthesis are key steps that follow Ca^{2+} mobilization within the dorsal horn, and manifest as longer-term changes in neuronal excitability and ultimately in altered pain behavior. Uncontrolled release of glutamate (as may occur after major nerve or CNS injury) may induce cell death within the CNS. This may be immediate (excitotoxicity); however, more significantly, neuronal and glial death may occur by programmed mechanisms involving protein synthesis (apoptosis) for periods long after the initial injury. Small GABAergic inhibitory interneurons appear to be particularly susceptible, with a net loss of inhibitory tone within the dorsal horn after nerve injury.

SPINAL MECHANISMS FOLLOWING NERVE INJURY AND INFLAMMATION

Central sensitization and synaptic plasticity

NMDA-mediated mechanisms underlying *central sensitization* may occur at both pre- and postsynaptic sites in the dorsal horn. Presynaptic sensitization, in conjunction with retrograde transmission by NO, may further enhance glutamate release from the primary afferent. At the postsynaptic site, NMDA receptor

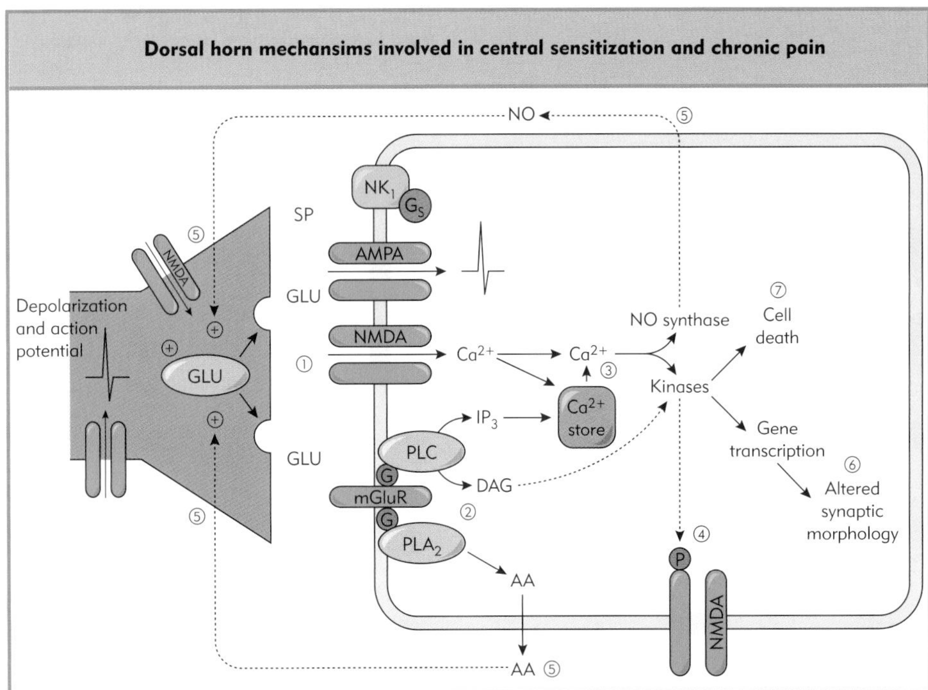

Figure 23.9 Dorsal horn mechanisms involved in central sensitization and chronic pain. There are at least seven places at which changes causing central pain can occur:

1. Enhanced Ca^{2+} entry into the postsynaptic neuron follows GLU release and NMDA receptor activation. Presynaptic NMDA receptors may mediate similar enhancement of Ca^{2+} availability and potentiate glutamate release.
2. The Ca^{2+} signal may be supplemented by Ca^{2+} release from IP_3-gated stores as a consequence of coactivation of mGlu receptors.
3. The rise in Ca^{2+} concentration in the postsynaptic cell initiates a chain of events secondary to the activation of numerous Ca^{2+}-dependent enzymes.
4. Postsynaptic hyperexcitability follows phosphorylation of NMDA receptors, which alters their voltage-gating characteristics.
5. Postsynaptic hyperexcitability may be augmented by release of retrograde transmitter(s) (NO and arachidonic acid?), causing the presynaptic nerve terminal to enhance its release of GLU and SP. Enhanced transmission occurs at the affected synapses.
6. Within the postsynaptic cell, protein kinase activation may lead to gene transcription, altered neuronal phenotype, and changes in synaptic morphology.
7. Within the postsynaptic cell, protein kinase activation may lead to neuronal death, which may be immediate or delayed.

GLU, glutamate; NMDA, *N*-methyl-D-aspartate; AMPA, α-amino-3-hydroxy-5-methyl-4-isoxazolepropionate; mGluR, metabotropic glutamate receptor; PIP, phosphatidylinositol 4,5-bisphosphate; NO, nitric oxide; PLC, phospholipase C; IP_3, inositol 1,4,5-trisphosphate; IP_3R, IP_3 receptor; PLA_2, phospholipase A_2; G, GTP-binding protein; P, phosphorylation site; DAG, diacylglycerol; SP, substance P; NK1, neurokinin 1 receptor. (Adapted from Hudspith MJ. Glutamate: a role in normal brain function, anesthesia, analgesia and CNS injury. Br J Anaesth. 1997;78:731-747. © The Board of Management and Trustees of the British Journal of Anaesthesia. Reproduced by permission of Oxford University Press/British Journal of Anaesthesia.)

activation in second-order neurons results in phosphorylation of the NMDA receptor, such that the voltage gating of the receptor for subsequent stimuli is removed (see Fig. 23.9). Functionally this is manifest as increased gain of transmission for a given afferent input, and the earliest stages in this process are demonstrable electrophysiologically within the dorsal horn as 'wind-up'. Wind-up is a progressive increase in the frequency of firing of second-order spinal neurons elicited by a peripheral stimulus sufficient to excite C fibers at a frequency above 0.5 Hz. A key observation is that low doses of conventional analgesics such as μ opioids administered prior to such stimulation prevent wind-up but do not reverse the established sensitized state. This has had a major impact on the current view of pain and has led to a surge of interest in approaches such as pre-emptive analgesia.

The rationale behind pre-emptive analgesia is to prevent central sensitization by blocking the acute pain stimulus, and thereby to inhibit the supposed progression to 'subacute' or chronic pain. Attempts to demonstrate pre-emptive analgesia in a clinical setting have met with only limited success, which in part reflects methodologic difficulties. More significantly, post-operative and post-traumatic pain has a complex etiology involving both inflammatory and neuropathic components, and will result in prolonged afferent input to the spinal cord. Although 'wind-up' and central sensitization demonstrate that the response of cells in the dorsal horn can outlast the stimulus, they are relatively short-lived (minutes) phenomena, and ongoing afferent input hours or days after the initial injury probably has a key role in clinical pain mechanisms.

Chronic pain necessitates pathophysiologic modulations of synaptic efficacy that persist for days or weeks, an example of which is long-term potentiation (LTP), a form of strengthening of the efficacy of synaptic transmission that occurs following activity across that synapse. LTP has been demonstrated to occur in the spinal cord, and shares many of the physiologic and biochemical features implicated above in the development of chronic pain. Indeed, we may now talk of 'memory traces' within the spinal cord. Such long-term functional changes may coexist with physical changes in synaptic architecture, exemplified by sprouting within the dorsal horn.

Sensory and physiologic changes

Changes that occur in the periphery following trauma lead to peripheral sensitization and primary hyperalgesia. However, the altered processing of sensory input associated with trauma, inflammation, or nerve injury can only be partly explained by peripheral changes.

Following injury, there is increased responsiveness to normally innocuous mechanical stimuli (allodynia) in a zone of 'secondary hyperalgesia' in uninjured tissue surrounding the site of injury. In contrast to the zone of primary hyperalgesia, there is no change in the threshold to thermal stimuli, and these changes are the behavioral manifestation of central sensitization involving WDR neurons. WDR neurons have receptive fields with a central area that has a lower stimulus threshold than its periphery, and central sensitization is associated with an expansion in receptive field size and a reduction in threshold, such that it responds to stimuli outside the region of cutaneous innervation that responds to nociceptive stimuli in the nonsensitized state. Furthermore, there is an increase in the magnitude and duration of the response to stimuli that are above threshold in strength.

Consequently, stimuli that are nonnoxious may activate neural pathways that normally signal nociceptive information, i.e. Aβ afferent input may result in WDR firing at a higher impulse frequency. These changes underlie the enhancement of postoperative pain by movement and coughing, and the perception of pain in dermatomes distant from the incision site; if unresolved, they will result in the development of chronic pain.

Sprouting

Peripheral nerve injury induces morphologic changes in the superficial laminae of the dorsal horn (see Fig. 23.6). Axotomy or chemically induced C-fiber degeneration results in atrophy of laminae I–II nociceptor innervation This has been shown to be associated with the sprouting of central terminals of myelinated Aβ afferents from lamina IV into lamina II. The resultant reorganization of the normal synaptic architecture, possibly as a result of altered NGF availability, creates the potential for functional contact between Aδ fiber terminals (which normally transmit nonnoxious information) and second-order neurons of superficial laminae that normally receive nociceptive input. This mechanism, which develops (at least in animal models) over a period of weeks following nerve injury and persists beyond the period of peripheral nerve regeneration, would provide a mechanism for the pain and hypersensitivity to light touch (allodynia).

However, the time course of dorsal horn sprouting does not follow that of the development of allodynia, which may manifest immediately after nerve injury. Furthermore, drugs that have antiallodynic effects on animal behaviour may have little effect on Aδ fiber-evoked response in electrophysiological studies. Therefore, although sprouting may contribute to the persistence of allodynia under certain circumstances, it seems not to be critical to its initiation.

MODULATION AT A SPINAL LEVEL

The gate theory

The transmission of nociceptive information is subject to modulation at all levels of the neuraxis, from the dorsal horn rostrally. Afferent impulses arriving in the dorsal horn initiate inhibitory mechanisms that limit the effect of subsequent impulses. Inhibition occurs through local inhibitory interneurons and descending pathways from the brain. A model of how this interaction occurs in relation to pain processing was proposed by Melzack and Wall in 1965, and has been termed the 'gate theory' (Fig. 23.10).

Gate theory proposes that transmission or T cells located in the dorsal horn project to the brain; that the output from these cells depends on information entering the dorsal horn in different types of primary afferent; and that such cells could be activated by noxious input from small-diameter primary afferents and by nonnoxious information in large-diameter primary afferents. The output from transmission cells is regulated or modulated by inhibitory cells in the substantia gelatinosa, which also receive information from the primary afferents, but the effect on the inhibitory cell is dependent on whether it is nonnoxious information in large-diameter afferents or noxious information in small-diameter afferents. Nonnoxious input along

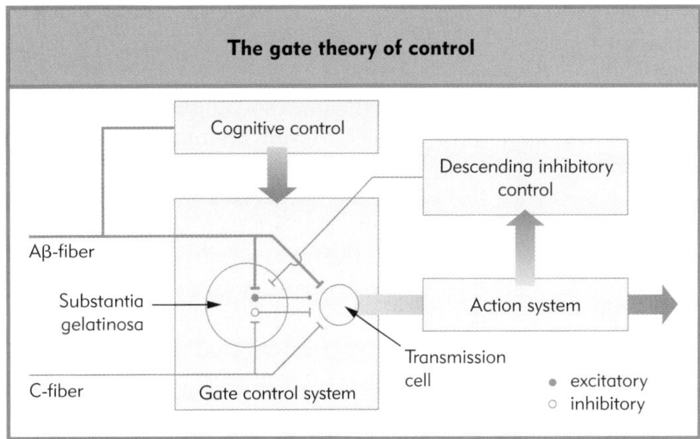

Figure 23.10 The gate theory of control. The activity of transmission cells is modulated by both excitatory and inhibitory links from the substantia gelatinosa and by descending inhibitory controls from the brainstem. The inhibitory link may involve both pre- and postsynaptic inhibition. All other connections are excitatory. (Adapted from Melzack R. Psychological aspects of pain. In: Cousins MJ, Bridenbaugh PO, eds. Neural blockade in clinical anesthesia and management of pain. Philadelphia 1998:781-91. Copyright © Lippincott Williams and Wilkins.)

large-diameter afferents primarily activates inhibitory cells, and therefore reduces output from transmission neurons. Noxious input along small-diameter afferents primarily inhibits the inhibitory cells, and therefore increases the output from transmission cells. Thus, the output from transmission cells to the brain is determined by the relative balance of activity in small- and large-diameter fiber afferents arriving at the dorsal horn. A further level of modulation in the gate theory is that descending pathways from the brain can also act to inhibit transmission of information by transmission cells.

The gate theory has had a significant impact on concepts of pain and has helped to explain why pain may occur in some conditions and why some treatments (such as transcutaneous nerve stimulation and dorsal column stimulation) may be effective. However, it has been difficult experimentally to demonstrate some of the specific circuitry suggested in the original proposal. Although descending inhibitory controls have been demonstrated, most cells in the spinal cord respond to noxious and nonnoxious stimuli and do not fit the proposed characteristics of transmission cells. Clinically, selective large-fiber loss often results in contradiction to that predicted by the gate theory. The theory also fails to explain why some people have pain after complete loss of afferent input, as occurs, for example, following complete spinal cord transection. Although it is an important and helpful advance in our understanding of pain, the gate theory does not completely resolve the specific mechanisms responsible for pain processing.

Gate theory proposes that pain transmission is modulated by inhibitory spinal mechanisms via a balance between modulatory afferents and descending pathways.

γ-aminobutyric acid and glycine

Both GABAergic and glycinergic interneurons are involved in tonic inhibition of nociceptive input; downregulation or loss of these neurons can result in features of neuropathic pain, such as allodynia. Although both $GABA_A$ and $GABA_B$ receptors have been implicated at both pre- and postsynaptic sites, $GABA_A$ receptor-mediated inhibition occurs through largely postsynaptic mechanisms. In contrast, $GABA_B$ mechanisms may be preferentially involved in presynaptic inhibition by suppressing excitatory amino acid release from primary afferent terminals. This finding may help to explain the disparity between laboratory findings, which demonstrate that $GABA_B$ receptor agonists such as baclofen have an antinociceptive action, and clinical experience, which has found that intrathecal baclofen is of limited use in the management of chronic pain. Particularly in neuropathic pain, where there is increased excitability of second-order neurons with no direct relationship to the amount of excitatory amino acids released by primary afferents, intrathecal administration of $GABA_A$ agonists may be more effective.

Clinical implications for modulation of spinal sensitization

REDUCTION OF EXCITORY AMINO ACID RELEASE

The initiation and, under some circumstances, maintenance of central sensitization is dependent on NMDA receptor activation by endogenous glutamate. Riluzole (currently licensed for use in motor neuron disease) and the anticonvulsant lamotrigine attenuate glutamate release and have analgesic properties in experimental pain models. A number of clinical studies suggest that lamotrigine may be useful for the management of refractory neuropathic pain, such as trigeminal neuralgia and central post-stroke pain.

NMDA ANTAGONISTS

The NMDA receptor complex provides many potential targets for modulation of the initial stages of central sensitization, including open channel blockers, competitive NMDA antagonists, and glycine and polyamine site allosteric modulators. The dissociative anesthetic ketamine, the antiparkinsonian drug memantine, the antitussive dextromethorphan, and the antiviral amantidine all bind to the open channel site and have analgesic efficacy in neuropathic pain. Recent evidence suggests that methadone also produces NMDA antagonist-mediated analgesia in addition to μ-opioid actions. Therapeutic manipulation of Mg^{2+} concentration may influence NMDA receptor function, and Mg^{2+} infusions reduce postoperative pain. Psychotomimetic side effects limit the usage of ketamine and other experimental NMDA antagonists, even if administered epidurally or intrathecally. Concerns have also been raised about potential neurotoxicity, particularly with intrathecal administration of potent NMDA antagonists. There remains the potential for the development of NMDA receptor antagonists with a more acceptable side-effect profile, and several agents are being investigated, either for analgesia or for neuroprotection.

NONSTEROIDAL ANTI-INFLAMMATORY AGENTS

The production of arachidonic acid metabolites is part of the cascade that follows NMDA receptor activation. Although the peripheral effects of NSAIDs have been emphasized previously (see Chapter 32), there is considerable evidence for spinal cord targets for NSAID action. Spinally, NSAIDs inhibit cyclooxygenase-mediated processes involved in the maintenance of central sensitization, and may also interact at the strychnine-insensitive glycine site of the NMDA receptor complex. Concerns regarding potential neurotoxicity preclude intrathecal or epidural administration of currently available NSAIDs. The report that COX-3 is abundantly expressed in human brain and spinal cord provides a putative central analgesic and antipyretic action of acetaminophen (paracetamol).

MOLECULAR APPROACHES

Traditional approaches to analgesia have focused on classic ligand–receptor blockade or enzyme inhibition as a means to reduce nociceptive input. The rapid progress in our understanding of the molecular and genetic mechanisms involved in nociception provides the potential for a new and powerful approach to pain management. Although currently in its infancy, the use of agents that modify tropic factor function, or antisense and siRNA strategies to limit gene expression, may make the selective targeting of factors involved in the transmission of nociceptive and neuropathic messages a potentially powerful analgesic tool.

ASCENDING SPINAL TRACTS

Target structures

Fibers associated with the transmission of noxious information may ascend one or two segments from their point of origin before crossing in the dorsal commissure (see Fig. 23.5). Primary afferent nociceptors relay to projection neurons in the dorsal horn, which ascend in the anterolateral funiculus to terminate in the thalamus. En route, collaterals of the projection neurons activate multiple higher centers, including the nucleus reticularis gigantocellularis. Neurons project from here to the thalamus, and also activate the nucleus raphe magnus and periaqueductal gray (PAG) of the midbrain. Descending fibers from the PAG project also to the nucleus raphe magnus and adjacent reticular formation. These neurons activate descending inhibitory neurons that are located in these regions and travel via the dorsolateral funiculus to terminate in the dorsal horn of the spinal cord. Descending projections also arise from a number of brainstem sites, including the locus ceruleus. Several other sites within what is often referred to as the limbic system receive projections from the spinal cord, such as the amygdaloid and septal nuclei. These projections to supraspinal sites are contained within the anterolateral funiculus in the contralateral quadrant of the spinal cord, comprising the spinothalamic, spinoreticular, spinomesencephalic, and spinolimbic tracts. The spinocervicothalamic tracts and the postsynaptic dorsal column pathway provide additional pathways for nociceptive input.

SPINOTHALAMIC TRACT

The spinothalamic tract is regarded as having a central role in pain perception and transmits information regarding pain, cold, warmth, and touch. The cells of origin of the spinothalamic tract are located predominantly within laminae I and IV–VI of the dorsal horn, with some in lamina X and the ventral horn. These cells project mainly to the contralateral thalamus, with some projecting ipsilaterally. The nuclei in the thalamus that receive these projections are located either laterally (ventral posterior lateral and ventral posterior inferior nuclei and medial posterior complex) or medially in the central lateral nucleus and other intralaminar nuclei.

There appears to be a somatotopic organization within the spinothalamic tract, and spinothalamic projection neurons have restricted receptive fields. Fibers arising from more caudal segments tend to be located laterally, and those entering from more rostral segments tend to be located in the more medial and ventral part of the tract. They respond well to noxious mechanical and thermal stimuli, but many also respond to nonnoxious mechanical stimuli.

SPINORETICULAR TRACT

The cells of origin of the spinoreticular tract are located in the deep layers of the dorsal horn and in laminae VII and VIII of the ventral horn. These cells send projections to several nuclei within the reticular formation of the brainstem, including the lateral reticular nucleus, nucleus gigantocellularis, nucleus paragigantocellularis lateralis in the medulla, the pontine nuclei oralis and caudalis, and the parabrachial region. Many spinoreticular neurons are activated preferentially by noxious input, but there is no clear somatotopic organization of the spinoreticular tracts. These projections terminate in close apposition to regions that are involved in blood pressure and motor control and the descending inhibition of pain. Therefore, it appears that this pathway is involved in the basic autonomic, motor, and endogenous analgesic responses to nociceptive input. Central processing of this information may contribute to the negative emotional arousal and behavior associated with anxiety or threat.

SPINOMESENCEPHALIC TRACT

The cells of origin of the spinomesencephalic tract are located predominantly in laminae I and IV–VI of the dorsal horn, with some found in lamina X and the ventral horn. These cells project to several nuclei in the midbrain, including the PAG, cuneiform nucleus, red nucleus, superior colliculus, pretectal nuclei, and Edinger–Westphal nucleus. In contrast to the spinoreticular tract, the spinomesencephalic tract appears to be somatotopically organized, with projections from caudal body regions terminating in the caudal midbrain and projections from rostral body regions terminating in more rostral regions of the midbrain. In contrast to the spinothalamic tract, cells in this tract have large and complex receptive fields. The sites of termination of this tract suggest that some of its components are involved in a range of more organized and integrated motor, autonomic, and antinociceptive responses to noxious input, such as orienting, quiescence, defense, and confrontation.

SPINOLIMBIC PATHWAY

Ascending projections from the brainstem relay information from the spinoreticular tract to the medial thalamus, hypothalamus, and other structures in the limbic system. As well as this multisynaptic pathway, there are direct projections from the spinal cord to the hypothalamus, nucleus accumbens, septal nuclei, and amygdala. Projections to the hypothalamus arise chiefly from cells in the deep dorsal horn and lateral spinal nucleus, as well as from cells in laminae I, VII, and X. Projections to the amygdala arise from cells in the deep dorsal horn and lamina X. These projections may be responsible for the motivational or affective responses associated with pain perception.

SPINOCERVICOTHALAMIC PATHWAY

The spinocervicothalamic pathway comprises neurons that have their cells of origin in lamina IV of the spinal dorsal horn and fibers that ascend in the dorsal part of the lateral funiculus. The fibers terminate in the lateral cervical nucleus at the level of C1 and C2 before crossing and ascending with the medial lemniscus to terminate in the contralateral ventral posterior lateral nucleus and medial part of the posterior complex of the thalamus. Most cells in this tract respond to light touch and do not appear to have a primary role in nociception. However, some do respond to nociceptive stimuli, and therefore it may serve as a potential pathway for the transmission of nociceptive information.

POSTSYNAPTIC DORSAL COLUMN PATHWAY

The dorsal columns and nuclei (gracile and cuneate nuclei) are generally considered to be the pathway for information regarding the nonnoxious sensations of fine touch, proprioception, and vibration. Stimulation of the dorsal columns is normally reported to produce a sensation of vibration rather than pain, although there are reports that mechanical stimulation of the medial aspect of the nucleus gracilis may result in pain. However, recent evidence points to a role of the dorsal column pathway in visceral nociception, and cells in the gracile nucleus respond to noxious stimulation of the viscera. The pathway that supplies this information is referred to as the postsynaptic dorsal column pathway, and has cells of origin in lamina III of the dorsal horn as well as just lateral to lamina X.

Further evidence for a role for the dorsal column nuclei in pain perception comes from the demonstration that a phenotypic change occurs in neurons projecting through the dorsal column following nerve injury. Damage to large myelinated fibers results in the de novo synthesis of substance P within these neurons and may be part of the mechanism responsible for the hypersensitivity to light touch that occurs following peripheral nerve injury.

Clinical implications

Many surgical and percutaneous procedures have been employed to disrupt specific tracts in the spinal cord. These include cordotomy, extralemniscal myelotomy, and commissural myelotomy. The distribution of fibers associated with pain transmission within the anterolateral quadrant would suggest that section of these tracts using an anterolateral cordotomy should be a useful procedure in abolishing or relieving pain. This concept is based on the cartesian or 'private line' model of pain perception, and results are variable and often transient. Sometimes excellent relief can be obtained in the short term, but long-term results are usually disappointing and complications include the return of pain, motor weakness, and loss of bladder and bowel function. Consequently, these procedures are usually limited to the treatment of cancer pain.

Electrical stimulation of the fibers of the dorsal columns (*dorsal column stimulation*, DCS) may activate the proposed gating mechanisms of the dorsal horn and inhibit the nociceptive input associated with neuropathic pain states. The mechanism involves enhanced release of endogenous GABA and attenuation of the release of excitatory amino acids. A direct inhibitory effect on the postsynaptic dorsal column pathway may also contribute to analgesia, although visceral pain is rarely considered an indication for DCS.

SUPRASPINAL STRUCTURES

Thalamus

Axons within the spinothalamic pathway are divided into two main groups, depending on their terminations. One group travels in the anterolateral funiculus and, together with projections from the medulla, pons, and midbrain, terminates more laterally in the ventroposterior nuclei and posterior complex of the thalamus. These axons are believed to be involved in the sensory discriminative component of pain (Fig. 23.11). Another group terminates more medially in the intralaminar nuclei, including the centrolateral, ventroposterolateral, and submedian nuclei, which project to the somatosensory cortex. The centromedian nuclei project more diffusely, including projections to the limbic system, and are believed to be involved in the affective–motivational aspects of pain. The medial thalamus also receives projections from the spinoreticular and spinomesencephalic tracts. Projections from the spinocervical and postsynaptic dorsal column pathways terminate in the ventral posterior lateral nucleus and posterior complex.

Animal studies indicate that there is a spinothalamic projection with terminations in the ventroposterior thalamic nucleus. Neurons in this region have restricted receptive fields and respond to noxious stimuli. These findings suggest that nuclei in this region have a role in the discriminative aspects of pain processing. However, it is interesting that stimulation of the ventrocaudal nucleus (analogous to the ventroposterior nucleus in animals, and supposedly part of the 'pain' pathway) in awake humans rarely results in pain, except in those who have central deafferentation pain. In contrast to cells in the lateral thalamus, cells in the medial thalamus have large, often bilateral, receptive fields, suggesting a minor role in discriminative aspects of pain perception. It has been reported that a nucleus within the medial thalamus is specific for pain and temperature sensation.

Positron emission tomography (PET) studies have identified a number of subcortical structures that are presumed to be involved in nociceptive transmission and pain perception. These include the thalamus, putamen, caudate nucleus, hypothalamus, amygdala, PAG, hippocampus, and cerebellum. Although previous physiologic and anatomic experiments have suggested that some of these structures are responsible for pain transmission, the role of others is unclear. The activation of these subcortical structures may vary with differing pain complaints: studies indicate that whereas an acute experimental painful stimulus results in increased activity in the thalamus, chronic pain caused by cancer and chronic neuropathic pain are associated with a decrease in activity in the thalamus.

Cortical structures

The effect of cortical stimulation and lesions on pain perception is confusing and intriguing. Patients who have had a complete hemispherectomy can have almost normal pain sensation. In the awake human, stimulation of the primary somatosensory cortex typically evokes nonpainful sensations. Neurosurgical lesions of cortical regions produce varying effects, depending on the region ablated. Lesions of the frontal lobe and cingulate cortex result in a condition in which pain perception remains. However, the suffering component of pain appears to be reduced, the person only reports pain when queried, and spontaneous requests for analgesia are reduced. These effects contrast with those seen following lesions of the medial thalamus and hypothalamus, in which there is pain relief but no demonstrable analgesia.

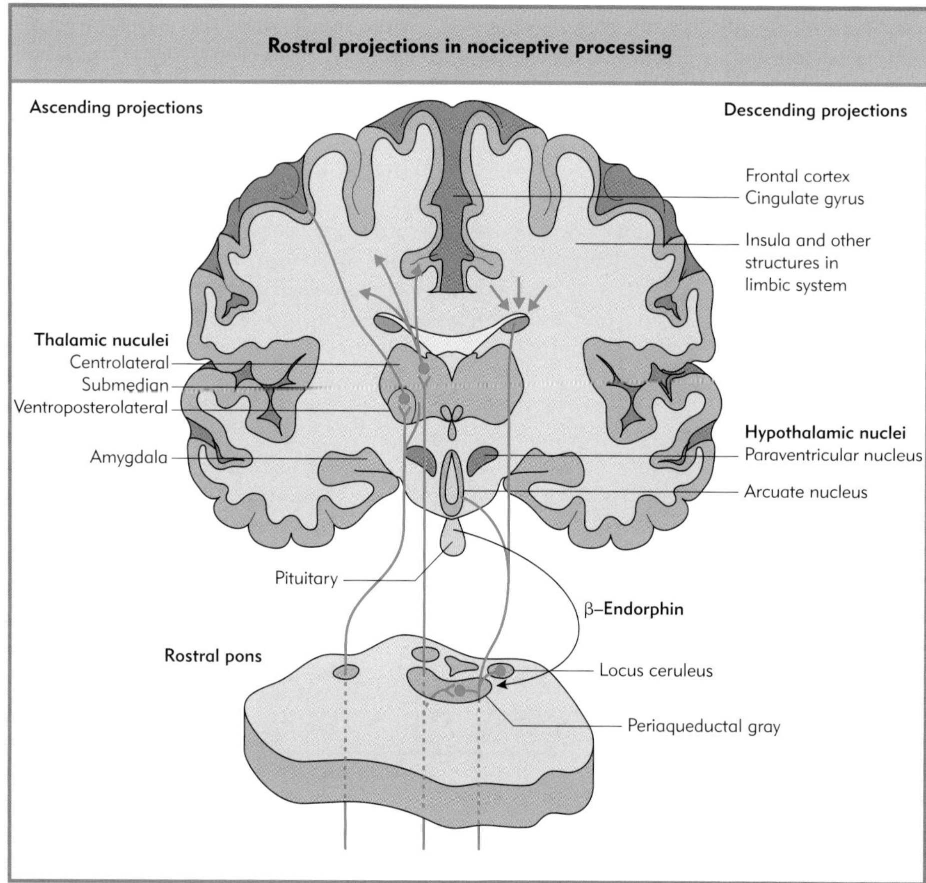

Figure 23.11 Rostral projections of nociceptive progression. Ascending projections terminate in the thalamic nuclear complex. The descending fibers inhibit the transmission of nociceptive information between primary afferents and projection neurons in the dorsal horn. In addition to direct neural connections, endorphins are released into the cerebrospinal fluid and blood, where they can exert an inhibitory effects at multiple centers. (With permission from Siddall PJ, Cousins MJ. Introduction to pain mechanisms. In: Cousins MJ, Bridenbaugh PO, eds. Neural blockade in clinical anesthesia and management of pain. Philadelphia 1998: 675-713. Copyright © Lippincott Williams and Wilkins.)

Both PET and functional magnetic resonance imaging (fMRI) have been helpful in elucidating the cortical regions involved in pain processing, and although there is some inconsistency in the results (perhaps because of the differing stimuli used in various studies) it is clear that no specific 'pain center' or homunculus can be identified where nociceptive signals ultimately reach conscious perception. Painful stimuli result in activation of somatosensory, motor, premotor, parietal, frontal, occipital, insular, and anterior cingulate regions of the cortex, in concert with activation of subcortical structures mentioned above. Although it is by no means clear, it has been suggested on the basis of PET findings that the parietal regions of the cortex are responsible for evaluation of the temporal and spatial features of pain, and the frontal cortex, including the anterior cingulate, is responsible for the emotional response to pain.

Current neurophysiological constructs of consciousness propose massively parallel processing of sensory input by neural networks involving thalamocortical and thalamolimbic loops (Chapter 29). The multiple destinations of nociceptive projections from the spinal cord to thalamic, limbic, and cortical targets indicate that pain 'emerges' from the coordinated processing of this information in areas involved in sensation, emotion, and cognition, and is therefore an inherently complex perception with affective emotional as well as spatial discriminative facets.

Descending modulation

There are powerful inhibitory influences arising from the brain that descend in the spinal cord to modulate spinal reflexes. Interest from those studying pain strengthened with the demonstration in the late 1960s that electrical stimulation of the PAG of the midbrain enabled abdominal surgery to be performed on animals with little evidence of discomfort. It is now known that there are powerful inhibitory (as well as facilitatory) influences on nociceptive transmission acting at many levels of the neuraxis. The PAG receives projections from a number of brain regions, including the amygdala, frontal and insular cortex, and hypothalamus, and acts in concert with the rostral ventromedial medulla (RVM) to provide a descending pain modulatory system. In addition to direct neural connections, endorphins synthesized in the pituitary are released into the cerebrospinal fluid and blood, where they can exert an inhibitory effect at several centers, including the PAG. Descending inhibition may be activated by external factors such as stress (stress-induced analgesia) and noxious input (diffuse noxious inhibitory controls), or can be induced by peripheral or central nervous stimulation.

Although the role of descending systems has been emphasized, there is also evidence for ascending modulation of 'higher' structures. For example, stimulation in the PAG can produce inhibition of the responses of neurons in the medial thalamus. Although it is possible that this inhibition may occur through the activation of descending pathways, it indicates that there are multiple interactions at many levels of the nervous system.

Brain structures involved in descending inhibition

Descending inhibitory influences arise from a number of supraspinal structures, including the hypothalamus, PAG, locus ceruleus, and RVM nuclei, including nucleus raphe magnus and nucleus paragigantocellularis lateralis. Electrical stimulation and microinjection of excitatory amino acids into these regions inhibits nociceptive responses. Descending inhibition does not require 'turning on'. Even though descending inhibition is activated by external stimuli, it is also tonically active and maintains a resting level of inhibitory function. This is demonstrated by reversible spinal cord block, which results in an increased responsiveness of spinal cord neurons.

The midbrain PAG appears to have a major role in descending inhibition. Stimulation in this region results in antinociception; although the PAG does not project directly to the spinal cord, descending fibers from the PAG relay in several structures that are also implicated in descending inhibition. These include the nucleus raphe magnus of the RVM and the paragigantocellular nucleus situated lateral to it. The PAG also appears to be highly organized. It has been demonstrated that analgesia obtained from the lateral PAG is nonopioid in nature, whereas opioid analgesia is obtained from stimulation of the medial PAG.

The midbrain periaqueductal gray matter is important in descending inhibition of spinal nociceptive input.

As with the PAG, electrical or chemical stimulation of the midline nucleus raphe magnus or ventrolateral (paragigantocellular nucleus) medulla results in antinociception. In the RVM, two types of neuron, on-cells and off-cells, have been identified as pain modulatory. On-cells exhibit a sudden increase in firing, whereas off-cells cease firing immediately prior to initiation of a nociceptive response. Fibers descend directly from these regions to the dorsal horn of the spinal cord and may exert a bidirectional control over nociception. Tracts from these structures descend mainly in the dorsolateral funiculus of the spinal cord and terminate in laminae I, II, and V. Stimulation of the locus ceruleus also results in inhibition of nociceptive-evoked dorsal horn activity. This nucleus receives inputs from a number of brain structures and provides descending inputs to the spinal dorsal horn. These descending fibers travel ipsilaterally in the ventrolateral funiculus.

Terminations of descending pathways interact with several different neural elements in the dorsal horn. These include projection neurons that transmit information from the spinal cord to the brain, local interneurons within the spinal cord, and primary afferent terminals. Inhibition may occur presynaptically by modulation of transmitter release, or postsynaptically by either excitation of local inhibitory interneurons or direct inhibition of second-order projection neurons. The bulk of evidence suggests that descending inhibition is exerted via postsynaptic mechanisms.

Neurotransmitter mechanisms

OPIOIDS

Opioid receptors modulate nociceptive input at many sites in the CNS, although functionally these can be divided into supraspinal and spinal sites of analgesia (Chapter 31).

Supraspinally, there is a high density of opioid receptors in the PAG, nucleus raphe magnus, and locus ceruleus. The profound analgesia produced by electrical stimulation of these regions is reversed by the opioid antagonist naloxone, which confirms the importance of endogenous opioid agonists in nociceptive behavior. However, microinjection of opioid agonists into these regions results in complex alterations in pain behavior, reflecting both inhibition and disinhibition (the inhibition of an inhibitory interneuron) of pathways involved in nociception. Subregional differences, dose dependence, and action at specific opioid receptor subtypes further increase the complexity of supraspinal analgesia. For example, high doses of morphine in the clinical setting have occasionally been reported to result in hyperalgesia rather than analgesia.

Opioids act at a spinal level in the dorsal horn by activating presynaptic opioid receptors, which inhibit glutamate and neurokinin release from primary afferent terminals, and postsynaptic receptors, which inhibit second-order neuron depolarization. Particularly within the spinal cord dorsal horn, opioid receptor density and distribution are dynamic: inflammation may enhance and nerve injury markedly reduce opioid-mediated spinal analgesia. Changes in presynaptic opioid receptor number and function, at least in part, underlie these effects.

Opioid analgesic mechanisms are themselves modulated by the release of cholecystokinin (CCK) acting on CCK1 and CCK2 receptors in the dorsal horn and at supraspinal sites such as the RVM. Microinjection of CCK into the RVM of experimental animals produces behavioural signs of neuropathic pain, and pathologic upregulation of this system has been proposed as a mechanism contributing to opioid-resistant chronic pain states in humans.

SEROTONIN

Serotonin has long been suggested to be a major neurotransmitter in descending controls. Serotonin is contained in a high proportion of nucleus raphe magnus cells, and in terminals of descending fibers in the dorsal horn. Electrical stimulation of the nucleus raphe magnus increases the release of serotonin in the spinal cord. Agents that block serotonin synthesis attenuate stimulation-produced analgesia, and the application of some serotonin agonists in the spinal cord inhibits cells responsive to nociceptive stimuli.

Although these findings appear highly suggestive of a role for serotonin in descending inhibition, several other findings indicate that it is not conclusive. Antinociception produced by stimulation of descending pathways cannot always be blocked by serotonin antagonists. Under certain circumstances intrathecal serotonin can facilitate behavioral nociceptive responses, and serotonin agonists can have an excitatory effect on cells in the superficial dorsal horn. These conflicting results may result from motor effects associated with some behavioral responses, differing effects associated with different serotonin receptor subtypes, and observation of effects on inhibitory neurons.

NOREPINEPHRINE

Norepinephrine is also an important neurotransmitter for descending inhibitory controls, and most central noradrenergic neurons originate within the locus ceruleus (LC). Descending projections from the LC give rise to the majority of noradrenergic fibers in the spinal cord. The noradrenergic stress response hypothesis proposes that stimuli that threaten the physical or psychological integrity of the individual generate a central noradrenergic response mediated by the LC: the associated hypervigilance and defensive response is associated with enhanced antinociception. Direct stimulation of noradrenergic cell groups in the brainstem, notably the locus ceruleus, produces antinociception, and norepinephrine-containing terminals are found in the superficial laminae of the spinal dorsal horn. Iontophoretic application of norepinephrine inhibits the activation of dorsal horn neurons by noxious stimuli, and intrathecal norepinephrine results in inhibition of nociceptive responses. Conversely α_2-adrenoceptor antagonists and compounds that reduce the amount of norepinephrine in the spinal cord increase nociceptive responses.

OTHER NEUROTRANSMITTERS

Other transmitters that appear to be important in descending inhibition are acetylcholine, GABA, thyrotropin-releasing hormone, and somatostatin.

Clinical implications

ANTIDEPRESSANTS

Tricyclic antidepressants, typified by amitriptyline, produce spinally and supraspinally mediated analgesia in chronic pain states by mechanisms distinct from those that enhance mood. Tricyclic antidepressants have actions that include the inhibition of uptake of both norepinephrine and serotonin, in conjunction with muscarinic anticholinergic effects (Chapter 28). The selective serotonin-reuptake inhibitors (SSRI) have weaker analgesic actions than traditional tricyclic antidepressants, suggesting that noradrenergic mechanisms are a more significant mode of tricyclic analgesia than the potentiation of serotonergic mechanisms. However, amitriptyline and similar tricyclic antidepressants are moderately potent Na^+ channel blockers and also bind to NMDA receptors with an affinity similar to that of ketamine. The analgesic action of tricyclic antidepressants is therefore likely to involve multiple mechanisms, and they remain a mainstay of pharmacological pain management.

OPIOIDS

Opioids remain the primary analgesics for the management of acute, severe nociceptive pain. Respiratory depression and sedation are supraspinally mediated and limit maximally tolerated systemic doses. Selective targeting of opioid receptors in the dorsal horn via epidural or intrathecal administration is therefore a logical means to achieve analgesia and reduce supraspinally mediated side effects.

Opioid tolerance results in a requirement for increasing doses to achieve a given degree of analgesia for a constant nociceptive stimulus. The mechanisms include opioid-mediated enhancement of cAMP levels, protein phosphorylation, and subsequent upregulation of NMDA receptor mechanisms within the dorsal horn and supraspinal sites. In addition, the accumulation of the morphine metabolite morphine 3-glucuronide, which may antagonize the analgesic action normally produced by opioid receptor activation, may play a supplementary role. Tolerance is rarely of clinical significance in acute pain management, and although frequently described in the context of chronic pain, it is not an inevitable consequence of long-term opioid administration. Neuropathic pain states with pre-existing NMDA receptor activation may predispose to the development of opioid tolerance or insensitivity. Animal studies indicate that the administration of an NMDA antagonist can prevent both the development of tolerance to morphine and the withdrawal syndrome in morphine-dependent rats. Therefore, co-administration of NMDA antagonists such as dextromethorphan or ketamine with opioids may attenuate the development of opioid tolerance and potentiate opioid analgesic mechanisms. The observation that methadone enantiomers are analgesic as a result of NMDA receptor antagonism in addition to μ-opioid receptor activation provides a logical basis for its long-term administration.

NITROUS OXIDE

Nitrous oxide produces analgesia via complex mechanisms involving supraspinal opioid-mediated activation of descending noradrenergic pathways and direct activation of spinal α_2-adrenoceptors. In addition, recent evidence suggests that nitrous oxide inhibits NMDA receptor function.

CLONIDINE

The α_2-adrenergic agonists clonidine and dexmedetomidine exert potent analgesic actions at a spinal level when administered by epidural or intrathecal routes. The activation of pre- and postsynaptic α_2-adrenoceptors inhibits primary afferent transmitter release and second-order neuronal depolarization. Clonidine potentiates spinal opioid analgesia, and combination therapy may be efficacious in neuropathic pain. Epidural and intrathecal clonidine have been demonstrated to provide analgesia in CRPS states that are opioid insensitive.

STIMULATION-PRODUCED ANALGESIA

The demonstration that powerful inhibition of nociceptive responses can be obtained by activation of descending pathways led to a resurgence of interest in techniques such as acupuncture and transcutaneous electrical nerve stimulation. It also led to the development and investigation of new techniques, such as dorsal column stimulation and deep brain stimulation. Although not widely used, deep brain stimulation involves the insertion of fine electrodes into brain regions where inhibition can be obtained. Initial studies focused on the PAG and periventricular gray matter, but other sites, such as the thalamus, are also used and provide significant analgesia in selected patients.

CLINICAL SIGNIFICANCE OF INFLAMMATION AND NERVE INJURY

Peripheral and central sensitization resulting from inflammation or nerve injury is a common consequence of surgical or traumatic injury. In most individuals acute postoperative pain is amenable to 'conventional' therapy with combinations of opioids, NSAIDs, and local anesthetics, and is self-limiting. The resolution of the injury is generally associated with resolution of pain, indicating that, at least at the behavioral level, the manifestations of central sensitization are reversible. Experimental evidence indicating that phenotypic changes outlast behavioral changes in pain models suggests that adaptive analgesic mechanisms usually compensate within the spinal cord.

Pre-emptive analgesia

There is evidence that severe postoperative pain may be a significant predictor of long-term pain, and that steps that reduce or abolish noxious input to the spinal cord during a painful event such as surgery may reduce or minimize spinal cord changes and thereby lead to a reduction of postoperative, and possibly chronic, pain. However, the duration or degree of noxious input that is required before these long-term changes occur remains unclear. Furthermore, it is uncertain how much these long-term changes depend on the afferent barrage during surgery, and how much they depend on continuing inputs from the wound after surgery. At both stages there will be sustained noxious input and, therefore, the potential to produce central sensitization; however, it would be expected that interventions that pre-empt central sensitization and seek to prevent it, rather than attempts to treat it after it has occurred, should be more successful.

The pre-emptive effects of local anesthetics, opioids, and NSAIDs (alone or in combination) administered locally, epidurally, intrathecally, or systemically at a variety of time points before, during, or after surgery have been studied. A number of trials have shown that pre-emptive analgesia results in reduced pain, decreased analgesic requirements, improved morbidity, and decreased hospital stay. However, these are balanced by a similar number that have failed to show benefit. The variability in agent, timing, and method of administration, as well as differences in the type of surgery and anesthetic procedure, have made it difficult to compare many studies of pre-emptive analgesia. Furthermore, many studies have been flawed methodologically. As examples, nitrous oxide and volatile agents may influence central sensitization, and the increased anesthetic requirement in patients not receiving pre- or intraoperative analgesia may influence outcome. Similarly, basic science studies suggest that NSAIDs are equally effective at attenuating sensitization, whether administered pre or post stimulus: postoperative administration of NSAID may mask or minimize opioid pre-emptive effects. Therefore, despite the logical appeal of pre-emptive analgesia and its ready clinical application, further trials are necessary before a definitive statement can be made regarding its benefits and advantages.

Much of the focus of pre-emptive analgesia has been on reducing acute pain in the early postoperative period. Pre-emptive analgesia may also be important in reducing chronic pain, but this has not been systematically evaluated. The finding that preoperative epidural blockade of patients undergoing lower limb amputation resulted in a lower incidence of phantom limb pain at 6 and 12 months after surgery than that seen in a control group having intraoperative block alone generated much interest. Although there are inadequacies in the study design and not all subsequent studies have confirmed their findings, it demonstrates that pre-emptive analgesia may have the potential to prevent the development of chronic pain states. Further studies are required to address this important question.

Chronic pain

ONGOING NOCICEPTIVE INPUT

Perhaps the simplest explanation of chronic pain is that of pure ongoing peripheral nocigenic input. This is typified by chronic inflammatory degenerative conditions (e.g. rheumatoid arthritis or degenerative osteoarthritis). Ongoing activation of peripheral nociceptors with or without the presence of inflammatory mediators results in ongoing peripheral sensitization. However, this is commonly supplemented by central sensitization. Clinical manifestations include ongoing peripheral mechanothermal hyperalgesia, and allodynia. Peripheral nociceptor sensitization may respond to NSAIDs, whereas opioids will attenuate primary afferent transmitter release in the dorsal horn. Conditions of pure peripheral nociceptor activation should respond to conventional analgesics. Opioid resistance suggests the involvement of central sensitization mechanisms.

PERIPHERAL MAINTENANCE OF CENTRAL SENSITIZATION

Central sensitization, once established, can clearly be maintained by ongoing peripheral activation of nociceptive afferents where a peripheral inflammatory or nocigenic stimulus persists. Following nerve injury, spontaneously discharging neuromata and spontaneously active DRG cells provide an alternative mechanism for the maintenance of central sensitization. Sympathetic efferent activity may play a similar role in CRPS pain states, where sprouting of sympathetic neurons results in activation of primary afferent cell bodies within the DRG. Furthermore, sensitized dorsal horn neurons with enlarged receptive fields can be activated by nonnoxious input; an effect that may be potentiated by sprouting of Aβ fibers. Nonnoxious mechanical and proprioceptive afferent input may thereby maintain central sensitization after resolution of the initial injury. These mechanisms underlie zygapophysial facet joint-generated spinal pain, and possibly myofascial pain. Specific blockade of the neuronal mechanisms that maintain sensitization (e.g. local anesthetic blockade of neuroma, facet joint, or efferent SNS innervation) may markedly attenuate spontaneous pain, allodynia, and hyperalgesia and provide insight into the etiology of the pain complaint.

ONGOING CENTRAL SENSITIZATION

Pain perception requires activity only in cortical and associated supraspinal regions many synapses distant from the peripheral nociceptor. Therefore, ongoing afferent input into the spinal cord is not a prerequisite for ongoing pain. If the normal spinal inhibitory mechanisms are overwhelmed by the magnitude of the initial stimulus (e.g. massive loss of inhibitory interneurons), and there is a failure in adaptive analgesic mechanisms that might oppose otherwise uncontrolled excitation in pain pathways, then a self-maintaining state of central sensitization may be established: this may involve abnormal upregulation of endogenous CCK and dynorphin pathways at both spinal and supraspinal sites. The determinants leading to the 'centralization' of pain are imprecisely understood, but the severity and chronicity of noxious stimulus in individuals with genetically determined 'vulnerable neurochemistry' are proposed as key factors.

The concept of a balance between excitation and inhibition is of prime importance in the pathophysiology of pain; for example, cerebrovascular accident, head injury, and spinal cord injury are frequently associated with 'central' pain syndromes (e.g. 'thalamic pain') that reflect aberrant excitatory activity in central neurons involved in pain transduction, resulting in spontaneous pain. Furthermore, a spontaneous loss of spinal and/or supraspinal inhibitory tone and consequent disinhibition of projection neurons should result in spontaneous pain, hyperalgesia, and allodynia. Fibromyalgia and similar diffuse pain syndromes that are not clearly linked to an initial nocigenic event could, at least in part, be explained by such mechanisms.

Centrally mediated and maintained pain will be 'referred' to dermatomes representative of pathologically activated central neurons. Peripheral neural blockade of afferent input from these dermatomes will not abolish spontaneous pain sensation, although hyperalgesia and allodynia may be relieved and the quality of pain altered. Such 'central' pain states rarely respond to conventional analgesic strategies. They are associated with downregulation of opioid receptor number and function, and pain is likely to be independent of primary afferent excitatory amino acid transmitter release, which is a primary target of opioid analgesia. Potentiation of spinal and supraspinal noradrenergic and GABAergic systems, together with suppression of ectopic Na^+ channel activation, may provide significant analgesia, necessitating combination therapy with tricyclic antidepressants, anticonvulsants, and Na^+ channel antagonists.

Peripheral nerve blockade in chronic pain

Peripheral nerve blockade is often used as a diagnostic procedure to predict outcome for nerve section or neuroablative procedures. However, isolated uncontrolled nerve blocks have little diagnostic or predictive value in the assessment of sciatic pain caused by lumbosacral disease. The recent evidence for physiologic and morphologic changes within the spinal cord following sustained peripheral input suggests that there are pitfalls in diagnostic neural blockade. First, chronic pain caused by peripheral nerve damage may no longer be dependent on peripheral input, and there is no evidence that treatments aimed at the periphery modify established central sensitization. For example, a longstanding intercostal neuralgia will not be expected to respond to intercostal neurectomy; indeed, the pain may increase as the processes of central sensitization may be enhanced. Second, diagnostic nerve blocks seek to identify a 'pain' source and can isolate the person from the disease process thought to be responsible for the pain. Using diagnostic nerve blocks in this way can mean that there is little recognition of the complex psychologic issues that can underlie the chronic pain presentation. It may even mean that a psychologic 'diagnosis' is made on the basis of the person's response to a diagnostic procedure. Therefore, diagnostic procedures must be performed in the context of a multidisciplinary assessment, with an understanding of the complex biopsychosocial components of chronic pain and placebo response to interventions.

Transitions from acute to chronic pain

The development of chronic pain represents a cascade of molecular events that are initiated at the time of peripheral stimulation or injury (Fig. 23.12). Many of the changes are common to both acute and chronic pain stages (e.g. the activation of the NMDA receptor, increase in intracellular Ca^{2+}, involvement and upregulation of neuronal nitric oxide synthase, and increase in *c*-fos expression). These changes in ion channel function, second messengers, immediate early genes, and neuropeptides are followed by more permanent changes in the nervous system and may include changes in the synaptic efficacy of pre-existing synapses, nerve sprouting, and the formation of novel synapses via growth factors. These latter changes may be the basis of pain memories in the spinal cord and brain. Particular changes may be prominent in certain conditions (e.g. changes in α_1- and α_2-adrenoreceptor function may contribute to sympathetically maintained pain). It is an attractive concept that inhibiting the earlier events may delay and perhaps prevent some of the later events, and thereby prevent the occurrence of long-term changes associated with persistent pain.

The persistence of pain may be a result of plastic changes in the nervous system, both in the periphery and centrally within the spinal cord, with or without persistence of the original stimulus. Yet it is clear that a group of individuals who have identical injuries will not all develop chronic pain symptoms. Genetic variations between individuals may account for such varying outcomes. Failure to increase the levels of analgesic peptides such as neuropeptide Y, marked declines in GABAergic function, or even accentuated sympathetic responses may predispose to chronic pain in some individuals. The translation of this increased understanding of chronic pain mechanisms to the introduction of novel therapies and elucidating the genetic basis of the predisposition to chronic pain are the challenges for the early 21st century.

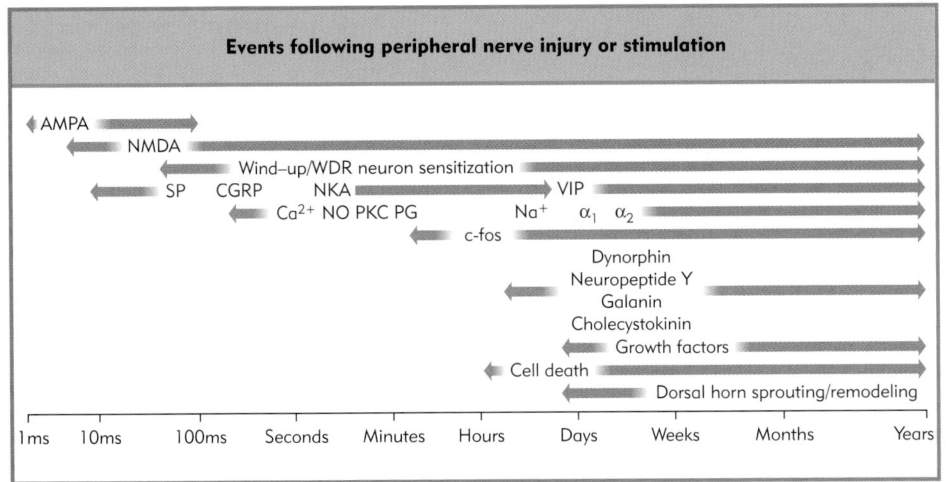

Figure 23.12 The cascade of molecular events that may occur in the spinal cord following peripheral nerve injury or stimulation. Many of the changes are common to both acute and chronic pain stages, but may then be followed by more permanent changes in the nervous system, which may be the basis of pain memories (see text). Inhibiting the earlier events may delay and perhaps prevent some of the later events. AMPA, α-amino-3-hydroxy-5-methyl-4-isoxazolepropionate; NMDA, *N*-methyl-D-aspartate; SP, substance P; CGRP, calcitonin gene-related peptide; NKA, neurokinin A; NO, nitric oxide; PKC, protein kinase C; PG, prostaglandins; VIP, vasoactive intestinal polypeptide. (From Munglani, 1998. © Elsevier, Ltd)

Key references

Bach S, Noreng MF, Tjellden NU. Phantom pain in amputees during the first 12 months following limb amputation. Pain. 1988;33:297–301.

Al-Chaer ED, Traub RJ. Biological basis of visceral pain: recent developments. Pain 2002;96:221–5.

Cao YQ, Mantyh PW, Carlson EJ et al. Primary afferent tachykinins are required to experience moderate to intense pain. Nature 1998;392:390–4.

Hudspith MJ. Glutamate: a role in normal brain function, anesthesia, analgesia and CNS injury. Br J Anaesth. 1997;78:731–47.

Melzack R. Psychological aspects of pain. In: Cousins MJ, Bridenbaugh PO, eds. Neural blockade in clinical anesthesia and management of pain. Philadelphia: Lippincott-Raven; 1998:781–91.

Ren K and Dubner R. Descending modulation in persistent pain: an update. Pain 2002;100:1–6

Rowbotham DJ ed. Advances in pain. Br J Anaesth. 2001;87:1–152.

Schwab JM et al. COX-3: just another COX or the solitary elusive target of paracetamol? Lancet 2003;361:981–2.

Siddall PJ, Cousins MJ. Introduction to pain mechanisms. In: Cousins MJ, Bridenbaugh PO, eds. Neural blockade in clinical anesthesia and management of pain. Philadelphia: Lippincott-Raven; 1998:675–713.

Vanderah TW, Ossipov MH et al. Mechanisms of opioid-induced pain and antinociceptive tolerance: descending facilitation and spinal dynorphin. Pain 2001;92:5–9.

Woolf CJ, Salter MW. Neuronal plasticity: increasing the gain in pain. Science 2000;288:1765–8.

Woolf CJ, Shortland P, Coggeshall RE. Peripheral nerve injury triggers central sprouting of myelinated afferents. Nature 1992;355:75–8.

Further reading

Brodal P. The central nervous system: structure and function, 2nd edn. Oxford: Oxford University Press; 1998.

Dickenson A, Besson JM. The pharmacology of pain. Handbook of experimental pharmacology. Berlin: Springer Verlag; 1997.

Hansson PT, Fields HL et al. (eds) Neuropathic pain: pathophysiology and treatment. Progress in pain research and management, Vol 21. Seattle: IASP Press; 2001.

Munglani R. Advances in chronic pain therapy with special reference to low back pain. In: Kaufman L, Ginsburg R, eds. Anaesthetic review, Vol. 14. Edinburgh: Churchill Livingstone; 1998:153–74.

Munglani R, Hunt SP, Jones GJ. Spinal cord and chronic pain. In: Kaufman L, Ginsburg R, eds. Anaesthetic review, Vol. 12. Edinburgh: Churchill Livingstone; 1996:53–76.

Willis WD Jr, Coggeshall RE. Sensory mechanisms of the spinal cord, 2nd edn. London: Plenum Press; 1991.

Chapter 24

General anesthetics: mechanisms of action

Neil L Harrison

TOPICS COVERED IN THIS CHAPTER

- **Pharmacological criteria for general anesthetic target sites**
  - What is the 'clinically relevant concentration' for a general anesthetic?
  - Anatomical location
  - Stereoselectivity
- **The synaptic effects of general anesthetics**
- **Molecular targets of general anesthetic action**
- **Experimental approaches to studying general anesthetic actions**
- **Targets of the inhaled general anesthetics**
- **The ether anesthetics – isoflurane**
- **The alkane anesthetics**
  - Xenon and nitrous oxide
- **Targets for the intravenous anesthetic agents**
  - Propofol and etomidate
- **Steroidal anesthetics**
- **Barbiturates**
- **Ketamine**
- **Future directions**

Since their introduction into clinical practice nearly 150 years ago, general anesthetics have become some of the most widely used and important therapeutic agents. However, despite over a century of research, the molecular mechanisms of action of general anesthetics in the central nervous system (CNS) have remained elusive. During the 1980s and 1990s, ion channels emerged as promising molecular targets to mediate the CNS effects of this class of drug. $GABA_A$ and NMDA receptors remain promising general anesthetic targets, owing partly to their ubiquitous distribution and essential physiological roles in the CNS. Indeed, for the intravenous agents these may represent the most significant targets.

Recent evidence supports a potential role for a variety of other ion channels in anesthesia, especially in the actions of the volatile anesthetics. These include the 'leak' K^+ channels as well as the HCN family of channels that give rise to 'pacemaker' currents, and some voltage-gated Na^+ channels, especially those at critical presynaptic sites. Most of these targets have widespread distribution in the CNS. Given the uncertainty concerning the exact circuitry that is disrupted to produce the constellation of behavioral effects seen during general anesthesia, it is conceivable that target molecules with more limited distribution (e.g. specific ion channel isoforms) may have a role as molecular mediators of specific components of the general anesthetic state.

It was recognized many years ago that general anesthetics may act on specific targets. For example, from the 1940s onwards Eccles and colleagues studied spinal reflexes in animals under pentobarbital anesthesia, and raised the possibility of anesthetic actions at neurotransmitter receptors important in synaptic transmission. This chapter reviews the actions of general anesthetics on potential target molecules and synaptic circuits within the CNS. All of the targets discussed are involved in the control of neuronal excitability on a subsecond timescale. This makes sense, because general anesthetics act extremely rapidly once they reach their site of action.

PHARMACOLOGICAL CRITERIA FOR GENERAL ANESTHETIC TARGET SITES

Before discussing the actions of specific agents, it is worth reviewing some specific pharmacological criteria that a target molecule (receptor protein or otherwise) must fulfill in order to qualify as a candidate in mediating the behavioral actions of the general anesthetics.

1. The general anesthetic must alter the function of the receptor at behaviorally relevant concentrations.
2. The receptor must be expressed in the appropriate anatomical locations to mediate the specific behavioral effects of the anesthetic.
3. If an anesthetic shows stereoselective effects in vivo, these should be mirrored by anesthetic actions at the receptor in vitro.

What is the 'clinically relevant concentration' for a general anesthetic?

For the potent inhaled anesthetics, the clinically relevant concentrations were first established in the classic studies of Eger and colleagues, in which they defined the 'minimum alveolar concentration' (MAC) necessary to inhibit movement (i.e. produce immobility) in 50% of a human population in response to a skin incision. More recent work defined the lower concentrations of anesthetic associated with hypnosis ('MAC awake') and other cognitive endpoints. Determination of MAC in terms of partial pressures is therefore relatively straightforward owing to the pharmacokinetic properties of these inhaled agents (Chapter 27). A series of aqueous 'MAC equivalent' concentrations has been determined based on the aqueous solubilities.

The issue of clinically relevant concentrations for the intravenous anesthetics in humans is complicated by pharmacokinetic aspects (absorption/distribution/metabolism/elimination) of these drugs, and the consequent difficulty of ascertaining steady-state concentrations in the brain and spinal cord. In some cases (e.g. for propofol and the barbiturates), detailed studies have addressed these issues and reasonable estimates of free anesthetic concentrations in brain have been obtained. In other cases (e.g. ketamine and the steroid anesthetic alphaxalone), only total anesthetic concentrations in blood are known, thus invariably overestimating brain concentrations and therefore underestimating the potency of this class of anesthetics, often by as much as one to two orders of magnitude.

Anatomical location

The idea of specific anatomical locations for anesthetic action was for many years neglected, as it was inconsistent with the prevailing dogma that general anesthetics lacked specificity of action, influencing the membranes of all cells in an indiscriminate manner. The rejection of 'unitary' theories of anesthesia and advances in basic neuroscience have led to renewed interest in anatomical aspects of general anesthetic action, and to a renaissance of rational approaches to these questions. Even today, however, there remains considerable debate about precisely which synaptic circuits are responsible for the various reflexes and behaviors that are perturbed by general anesthetics.

Important pharmacological criteria for general anesthetic target sites are: effects at clinical concentrations, appropriate anatomical location, and appropriate stereoselectivity.

Perhaps not surprisingly, the immobility produced by general anesthetics appears to involve the depression of spinal reflex pathways. Immobilization can be demonstrated independently of drug actions in the brain under certain defined experimental circumstances. What is less clear is whether supraspinal targets can influence these reflex pathways under more typical conditions of anesthetic application. The anatomical location of circuits responsible for the amnestic effects of general anesthetics are presumed to include the hippocampus, the amygdala, and the entorhinal and perirhinal cortices, all of which are implicated in learning and memory in humans. Certainly, synaptic transmission in these areas is altered by a variety of general anesthetics.

The nature of the circuitry underlying the hypnotic effects of anesthetics is less clear; the thalamus, cortex, and parts of the brainstem have all been proposed to be critical for the control of arousal and 'consciousness'. More recently, specific nuclei in the hypothalamus have also been implicated in the regulation of sleep and in the hypnotic actions of general anesthetics.

Stereoselectivity

This represents one of the most powerful tests for the relevance of a putative anesthetic target. A number of general anesthetic molecules possess a chiral carbon atom, and some pairs of stereoisomers have different anesthetic potencies in vivo. Stereoselectivity for producing immobility has been documented for the isomers of etomidate, the barbiturates, ketamine, and steroid anesthetics. The clinical formulation of these anesthetics is usually based on the racemic mixture, with the exception of etomidate, which is prepared by a chiral synthesis. General anesthetic stereoselectivity demolished the traditional 'lipid theories' of anesthetic action. Stereoselectivity has been used to support the plausibility of the $GABA_A$ receptor as a target in mediating the actions of etomidate (Fig. 24.1), pentobarbital (pentobarbitone), and the steroid anesthetics, as in vivo potency and activity at the $GABA_A$ receptor display identical trends. The in vivo stereoselectivity of ketamine isomers is paralleled by the inhibitory action of the stereoisomers at the NMDA receptor.

THE SYNAPTIC EFFECTS OF GENERAL ANESTHETICS

The effects of general anesthetics on synaptic transmission have been studied for over a century, and there is now broad agreement that general anesthetics have effects at both pre- and postsynaptic sites. At inhibitory synapses mediated by GABA, the predominant effect of many anesthetics seems to be an increase in the postsynaptic effect of the neurotransmitter at lower, clinically relevant anesthetic concentrations, at which there may also be an increase in the frequency of spontaneous release of GABA. At higher concentrations, both pre- and postsynaptic function may be depressed. At excitatory synapses mediated by glutamate, the predominant effect of many anesthetics seems to be a decrease in the postsynaptic effect of the neurotransmitter that is observed at higher anesthetic concentrations and, with a few exceptions, this seems to be due to a combination of direct hyperpolarization of the postsynaptic neurons, and/or a decrease in the spontaneous and evoked release of glutamate. The presynaptic effects of general anesthetics have been observed over many years, but the molecular targets of these actions remain mysterious. Potential candidates include the voltage-gated Na^+ and Ca^{2+} channels, and various aspects of the release apparatus, such as the SNARE proteins that mediate synaptic vesicle fusion with the plasma membrane.

Anesthetics have important effects at both presynaptic and postsynaptic sites.

MOLECULAR TARGETS OF GENERAL ANESTHETIC ACTION

A number of excellent reviews over the last decade have summarized work on the molecular and cellular actions of general anesthetics. Much of this has focused on the ligand-gated ion channels (LGIC). Clearly, LGICs are not the only possible molecular targets for general anesthetics: other neuronal proteins, such as voltage-gated ion channels and G protein-coupled receptors, might also play a role in the overall spectrum of

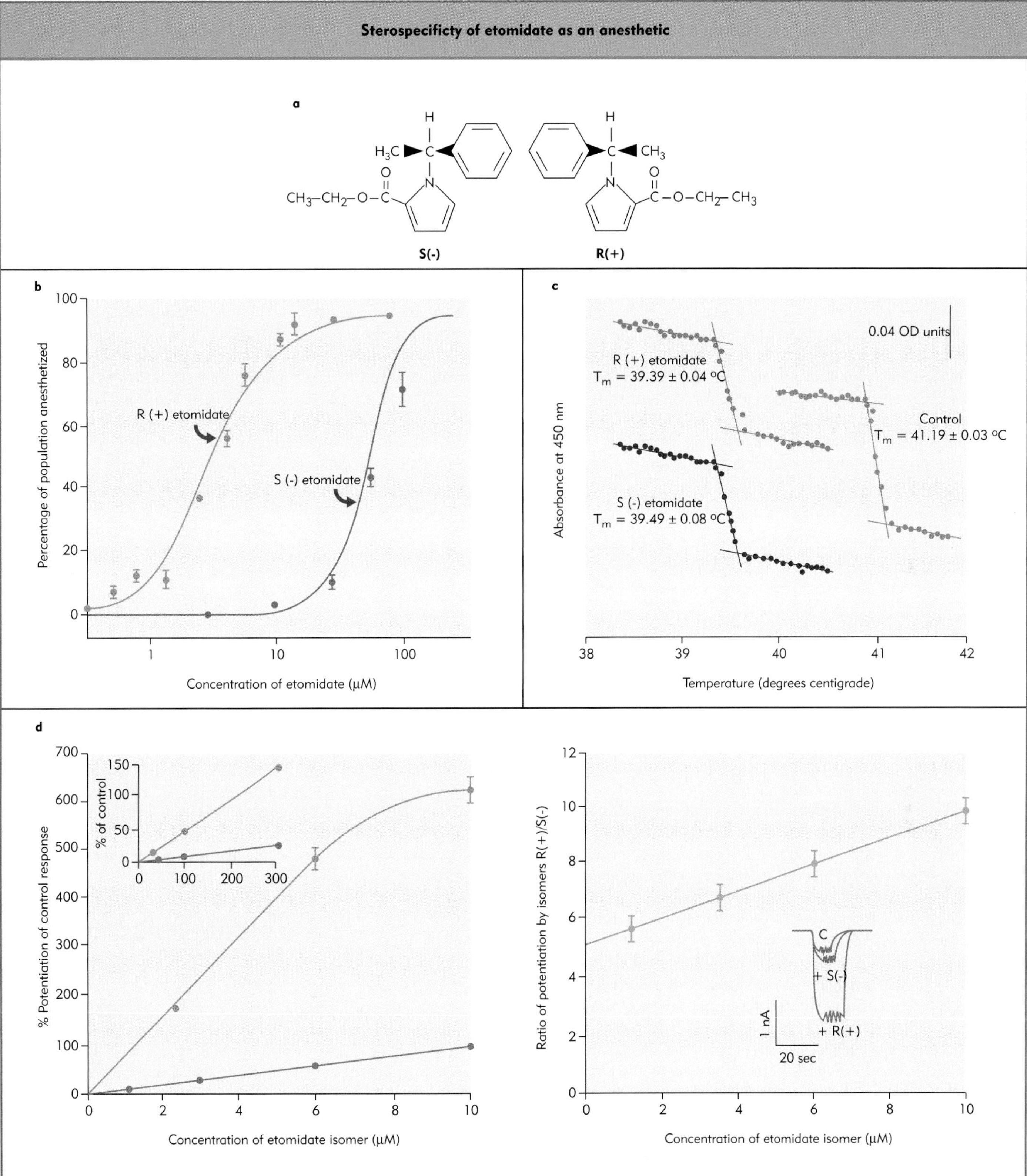

Figure 24.1 Stereospecificity of etomidate action as an anesthetic. (a) The optical isomers of etomidate. The R(+) isomer is used clinically. (b) Potency difference between the optical isomers in producing loss of righting reflex in tadpoles. (c) The etomidate optical isomers show identical potency in altering physical properties of lipid bilayers. (d) The R(+) isomer is >10 times more potent than the S(–) isomers in enhancing neuronal responses to GABA. (Adapted from Tomlin SL, Jenkins A, Lieb WR, Franks NP(1998) Stereoselective effects of etomidate optical isomers on gamma-aminobutyric acid type A receptors and animals. Anesthesiology 88:708-717.)

behavioral actions of some general anesthetics. In the 1980s it was suggested that the majority of voltage-gated ion channels are insensitive to clinically relevant concentrations of general anesthetics. In the last decade, however, it has become obvious that certain Na^+ channels, along with the HCN channels and the voltage-independent 'leak' K^+ channels, may be important and significant exceptions to this proposal.

Detailed studies of general anesthetic actions on G protein-coupled receptors are scarce, and it can be difficult to distinguish effects on the receptor per se from general anesthetic perturbations of second messengers or effector molecules, such as protein kinases and phospholipases. In most cases, the studies reveal that these targets are insensitive to clinically relevant concentrations of anesthetic. Neurotransmitter receptors of the LGIC family are currently strong candidates as molecular mediators of the CNS effects of general anesthetics. These include the $GABA_A$ and glycine receptors, along with the NMDA subtype of iontotropic glutamate receptors. $GABA_A$, glycine, serotonin (5-HT3), and nicotinic acetylcholine receptors (nAChR) form part of an evolutionarily related ligand-gated ion channel gene superfamily. The ionotropic glutamate receptors (AMPA, NMDA receptors) belong to a different ion channel class with a distinct molecular structure (Chapter 20).

EXPERIMENTAL APPROACHES TO STUDYING GENERAL ANESTHETIC ACTIONS

General anesthetic actions at target molecules have been studied using a variety of methods, including protein chemistry, radioligand binding, site-directed mutagenesis, and electrophysiology. Specific binding of radiolabeled general anesthetics has proved exceedingly difficult to demonstrate, owing to the low affinity of the interactions and the high degree of nonspecific binding to neuronal membranes. Some progress has been made in developing anesthetic congeners useful for photoaffinity labeling or other covalent modification of receptors. These limitations contrast with the studies of other classes of agent at LGICs. For instance, the high-affinity benzodiazepine-binding site on the $GABA_A$ receptor has been mapped in some detail thanks to the ability to perform both specific radioligand binding and photoaffinity labeling, which powerfully complements the extensive body of literature from site-directed mutagenesis and heterologous expression and electrophysiological analysis in *Xenopus* oocytes or mammalian cells.

The advent of cloning and recombinant expression techniques greatly accelerated and facilitated attempts to study the molecular sites of action of general anesthetics. Molecular biology techniques are now being used to determine which regions of ion channels are critical for anesthetic modulation. Sensitivity to general anesthetics varies considerably, sometimes even among closely related channels, and this forms the basis for the use of 'chimeric' channels to identify specific regions of a molecule essential to anesthetic modulation. Chimeric receptors are created by joining together, at the cDNA level, complementary fragments of channel subunits, in which the parental subunits exhibit markedly different responses to anesthetic. The analysis of chimeric channels has been used to delimit a region of a receptor essential for general anesthetic modulation, after which site-directed mutagenesis can be used to further identify key residues. Despite potential pitfalls, the use of chimeric receptors has already helped to define putative sites of general anesthetic action on a variety of ion channels. Another useful tool are targeted gene manipulations in mice, in which a variety of manipulations are possible (Chapter 4), including introducing a gene not normally present (transgenic mice), inactivating an endogenous gene ('knockout mice'), or replacing an endogenous gene with an altered copy ('knock-in mice'). Gene targeting in mice has already been very valuable for elucidating the mechanism of action for some anesthetic drugs.

TARGETS OF THE INHALED GENERAL ANESTHETICS

In the 1980s there was really no solid evidence for any molecular target of inhaled anesthetic action at clinically relevant concentrations. This situation changed as research focused increasingly on ion channels that are responsible for the control of neuronal excitability and synaptic transmission within the CNS. Knowledge has advanced rapidly since then, and the spectrum of potentially important targets for the inhaled anesthetics now includes ligand-gated channels, such as the $GABA_A$, glycine and NMDA receptors, and a variety of other channels that can loosely be described as members of the voltage-gated ion channel family. These include some of the 'leak' K^+ channels, certain voltage-gated Na^+ channels, and the HCN family of channels.

The effects of inhaled anesthetics have been best studied so far in the LGICs. A number of volatile general anesthetics act as either *positive* or *negative allosteric modulators* of agonist actions at ligand-gated ion channels. Among the ligand-gated ion channels, there is no known case in which the anesthetic competes for the same binding site as the endogenous neurotransmitter. The most extensively examined LGIC target for general anesthetics has been the $GABA_A$ receptor. A majority of inhaled anesthetics tested enhance the function of the $GABA_A$ receptor at clinically relevant concentrations. This includes all of the anesthetic ethers that have been tested to date, and some of the alkanes as well. Among contemporary inhaled agents, the list includes isoflurane, sevoflurane, desflurane, and halothane. The exceptions known so far are xenon, nitrous oxide, and cyclopropane.

A number of ion channels, both ligand-gated and voltage-gated, are affected by general anesthetics.

THE ETHER ANESTHETICS – ISOFLURANE

The prototypical ether anesthetic in use today is isoflurane, and this has been the most studied of these agents in recent years. The available evidence suggests that the molecular pharmacology of isoflurane is representative of that of the other halogenated ethers. Isoflurane interacts with $GABA_A$ and glycine receptors, but also appears to activate some of the 'leak' two-pore domain K^+ channels, inhibit the function of certain subtypes of nicotinic acetylcholine receptor, NMDA receptors, HCN 'pacemaker' channels, and voltage-gated Na^+ channels.

Isoflurane and enflurane were first shown to interact with $GABA_A$ receptor function by Narahashi and colleagues in 1989. The effects are evident in single-cell electrophysiological experiments as the potentiation of a submaximal GABA response

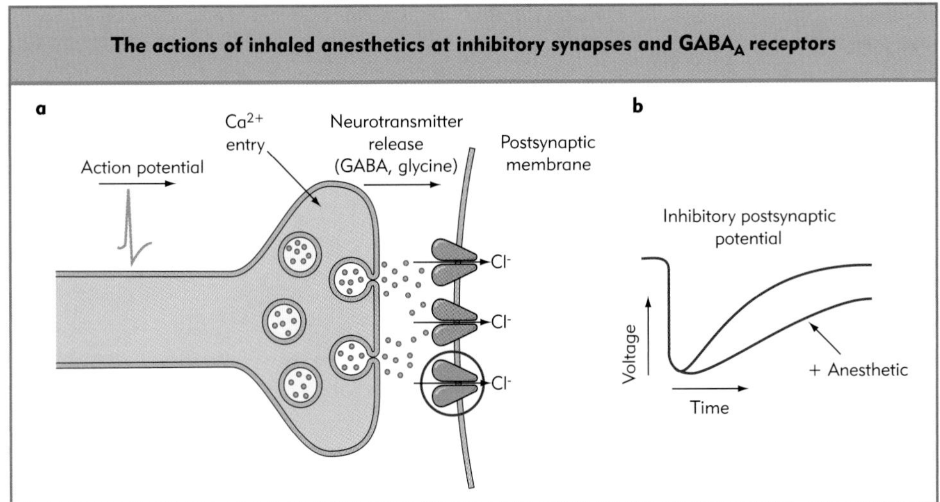

Figure 24.2 The actions of inhaled anesthetics at inhibitory synapses and GABA$_A$ receptors. a, GABA$_A$ receptors bind the neurotransmitters that are released at inhibitory chemical synapses, and open to allow chloride ions to diffuse across the postsynaptic membrane. b, the main effect of volatile anesthetics is to prolong channel opening and, hence, to increase postsynaptic inhibition (From Franks NP, Leib WR. Inhibitory synapses. Anaesthetics set their sites on ion channels. Nature 1997;389:334-335.)

(whether in neurons or in expression systems) or, at the synaptic level, as prolongation of inhibitory postsynaptic potentials or currents (Fig. 24.2). The effects of isoflurane may also be manifest as enhancement of nonsynaptic 'tonic' inhibition. Isoflurane also acts an allosteric modulator of GABA$_A$ and glycine receptors, an observation that led to the identification of critical domains of these receptors, and to the subsequent suggestion that isoflurane interacts with a binding cavity between the transmembrane segments of the α subunits of these receptors (Fig. 24.3). The structure recently derived for the nAChR of *Torpedo* and proposed for the rest of the LGIC family includes such a cavity between adjacent transmembrane helices. The actions at GABA$_A$ and glycine receptors of the other ethers such as enflurane, sevoflurane, and desflurane are essentially the same as for isoflurane.

Isoflurane can activate 'leak' K^+ channels, an effect first identified in the snail *Lymnaea*, and subsequently observed in mammalian species. Activation of these channels hyperpolarizes neurons and decreases spontaneous firing and responsiveness to excitatory synaptic input (Fig. 24.4). Recently, isoflurane has also been shown to inhibit the activity of pacemaker channels, thereby reducing the rate of rise of 'pacemaker' potentials and reducing the bursting frequency of neurons showing autoryhthmicity. Although in general action potentials are unaffected by clinical concentrations of isoflurane, it was shown some time ago that conduction in certain unmyelinated axons was inhibited by inhaled anesthetics. Neurotransmitter release studies also support an action of isoflurane on presynaptic voltage-gated Na^+ channels. More recently, studies of recombinant voltage-gated Na^+ channels are revealing inhibitory effects of isoflurane on specific subtypes of mammalian channels.

Although the GABA$_A$ and glycine receptors have been studied extensively, there are other neurotransmitter receptors that are sensitive to isoflurane, including some of the brain-type nicotinic acetylcholine receptors, and NMDA receptors, in which effects may have been overlooked initially because they appear to be use dependent, that is, block is promoted by receptor activation.

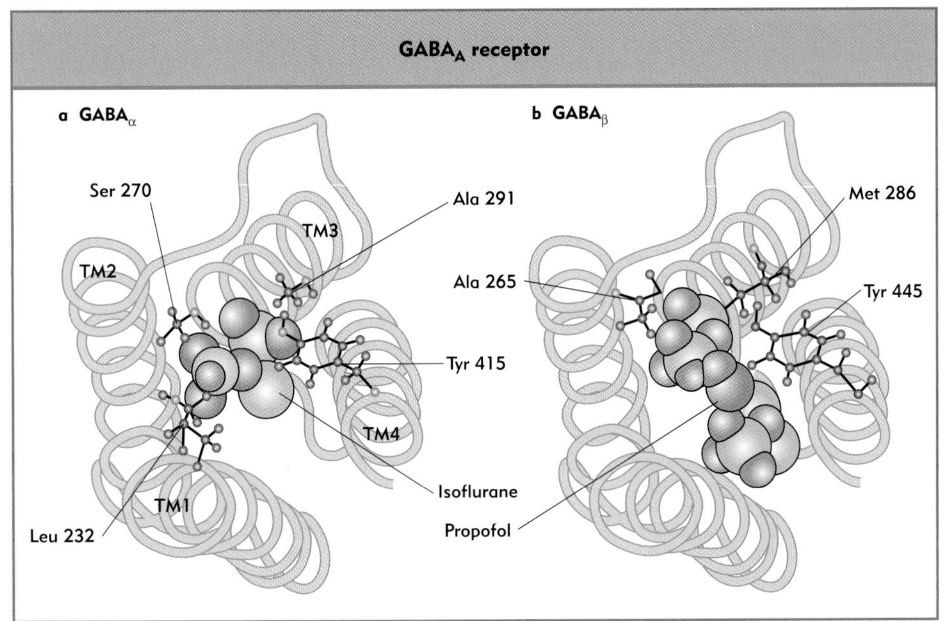

Figure 24.3 Isoflurane and propofol may interact with critical sites in the GABA$_A$ receptor. (a) Model of GABA$_A$ α_1-receptor subunit molecular structure with Leu 232, Ser 270, Ala 291, and Tyr 415 residues rendered in ball-and-stick format. A molecule of isoflurane is shown rendered with a space-filling surface. The transmembrane (TM) α helices are numbered 1–4. (b) Model of GABA$_A$ β_2 subunit with Asn 265, Met 286, and Tyr 445 residues rendered in ball-and-stick format. A molecule of propofol is shown rendered with a space-filling surface with the TM α helices as in (a). (Original figure courtesy of Jim Trudell.)

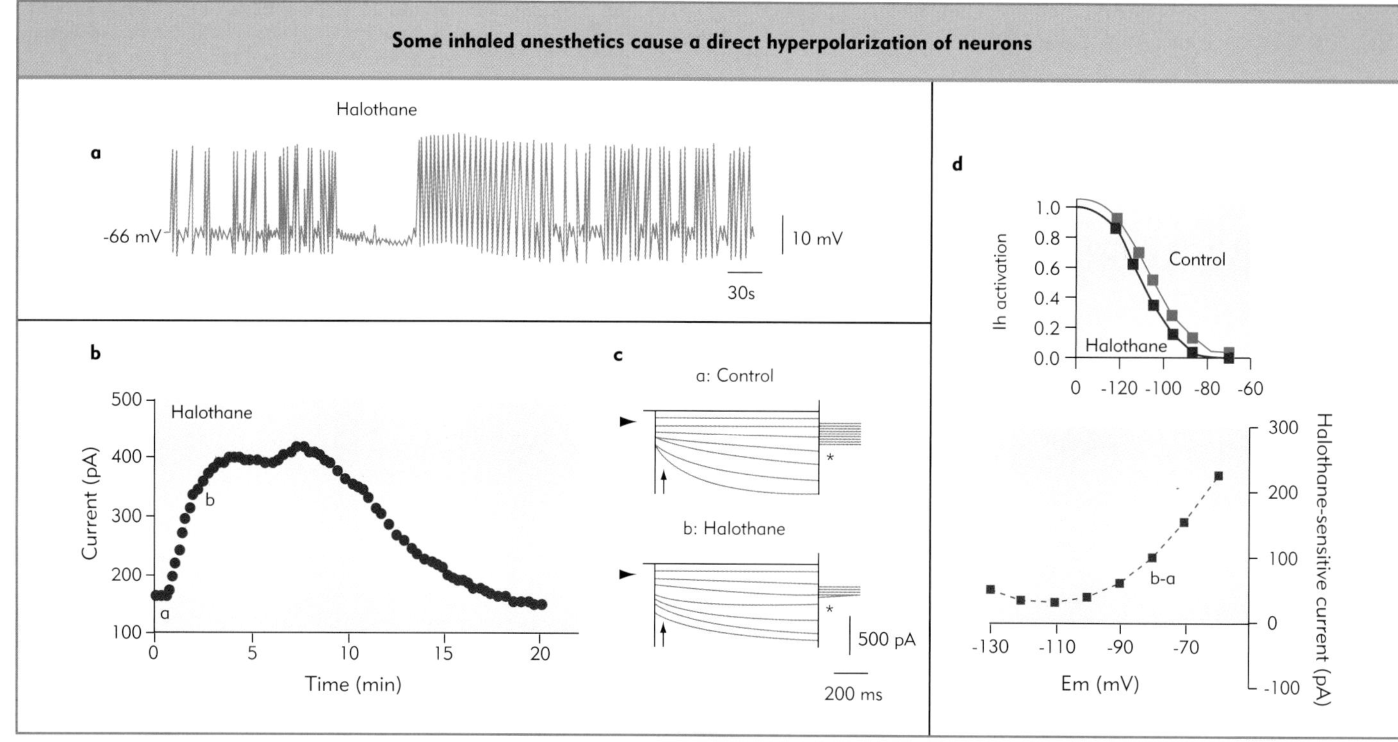

Figure 24.4 Some inhaled anesthetics cause a direct hyperpolarization of neurons. a, effect of halothane (0.35 mM) on a hypoglossal motoneuron recorded under current clamp conditions. Halothane caused a membrane hyperpolarization. b, time series illustrating the outward shift of holding current (at –60 mV) induced by halothane. c, current traces obtained at the times indicated in b in response to the hyperpolarizing voltage steps from –60mV under control conditions (a) and in the presence of halothane (b). d, the halothane-sensitive current was obtained by subtracting control currents (a) from those obtained in the presence of halothane (b). Inset, normalized tail currents from control and halothane were fitted with a Boltzmann function; halothane caused a hyperpolarizing shift in the voltage dependence of I_h activation. (From Sirois et al. The TASK-1 two-pore domain K+ channel is a molecular substrate for neuronal effects of inhalation anesthetics. J Neurosci 2000; 20:6347-6354.)

THE ALKANE ANESTHETICS

Halothane has actions at the $GABA_A$ and glycine receptors that are very similar to those of isoflurane, despite its smaller molecular volume. It also appears to interact with some of the targets mentioned above, such as the twin-pore K^+ channels, although it has received less study than isoflurane. Halothane also has important presynaptic effects that may be mediated via its inhibitory effect on voltage-gated Na^+ channels. Cyclopropane has no activity at $GABA_A$ and glycine receptors but is a good inhibitor of NMDA receptor and nicotinic acetylcholine receptor function.

Xenon and nitrous oxide

Xenon also has no activity at $GABA_A$ receptors but is a good inhibitor of NMDA receptor function. Nitrous oxide also inhibits NMDA receptors, although reports differ regarding its effects on $GABA_A$ receptors.

TARGETS FOR THE INTRAVENOUS ANESTHETIC AGENTS

Propofol and etomidate

Propofol and etomidate both appear to be relatively selective modulators of $GABA_A$ receptors, enhancing $GABA_A$ receptor function at low GABA concentrations, apparently by promoting the gating of the channel, rather than by enhancing agonist binding. Some of the intravenous anesthetic agents, especially propofol and etomidate, open the $GABA_A$ receptor chloride channel in the absence of agonist. This 'direct activation' by general anesthetics usually occurs at high clinical concentrations (e.g. propofol), suggesting a potential contribution to their clinical effects.

$GABA_A$ receptors fulfill all three criteria for a plausible target underlying the anesthetic actions of these compounds. For example, $GABA_A$ receptors are located in all of the regions implicated in the hypnotic, sedative, amnestic, and even immobilizing actions of both propofol and etomidate. Neither of the agents has yet been shown to modulate other ion channels at clinically relevant concentrations, but this possibility has received relatively little attention and so remains open.

Specific amino acid residues within the β subunit of the $GABA_A$ receptor have been identified that are essential for potentiation of $GABA_A$ receptor function by etomidate, consistent with previous studies suggesting that the β subunit of the $GABA_A$ receptor was likely to contain binding sites for these compounds. More recent work using site-directed mutagenesis, protection experiments, and a variety of propofol analogs of different size all appears to support the idea that Met 286 within TM3 of the β subunit is part of a binding site for propofol (see Fig. 24.3). An impressive set of behavioral and pharmacologic studies has now been performed with genetically engineered β_3 and β_2 knock-in mice bearing the mutation β(N265S) which appear to confirm the $GABA_A$ receptor as a primary molecular target of etomidate and propofol.

STEROIDAL ANESTHETICS

Many steroid anesthetics, such as alphaxalone, which are in veterinary but not clinical use, are also relatively selective for the $GABA_A$ receptor. Again, certain steroids have potent actions on other ligand-gated ion channels. For the steroid anesthetics, structure–activity studies comparing in vivo and in vitro potencies support a role for $GABA_A$ receptors in the actions of these compounds. Critical regions of the $GABA_A$ receptor for modulation by steroid anesthetics have yet to be identified.

BARBITURATES

Unlike propofol, etomidate, and the steroid anesthetics, the barbiturates appear much less selective in their action. In addition to their actions at $GABA_A$ receptors, which were first described in the 1970s, barbiturates also potently inhibit AMPA, kainate, and neuronal nicotinic ACh receptors. The optical isomers of pentobarbital display the same order of potency for modulatory actions at the $GABA_A$ receptor as for their in vivo anesthetic actions. A residue within TM1 of the β subunit of the $GABA_A$ receptor has been identified that is apparently necessary for GABA potentiation by pentobarbital. GABA potentiation by barbiturates is not abolished by the specific TM2 and TM3 mutations in $GABA_A$ receptors that abolish potentiation by the volatile anesthetics etomidate or propofol, suggesting that their sites of action may be distinct.

KETAMINE

Compared to the other intravenous anesthetic agents discussed above, the 'dissociative anesthetic' ketamine has a very different in vivo and in vitro profile of action. Ketamine and related arylcycloalkylamines such as phencyclidine produce an atypical anesthesia characterized by a state of sedation, immobility, amnesia, marked analgesia, and a feeling of dissociation from the environment, without true unconsciousness. These compounds can also produce intense hallucinations, especially in adults, which limits their clinical usefulness. In contrast to most other general anesthetics, ketamine does not potentiate $GABA_A$ receptor function at clinically relevant concentrations. Instead, ketamine appears to produce anesthesia by inhibition of NMDA receptors. The blockade of NMDA receptors occurs at clinically relevant concentrations, and is especially effective in interrupting thalamocortical excitatory transmission. The NMDA receptor is blocked in a voltage- and use-dependent manner by ketamine.

FUTURE DIRECTIONS

Recent advances in molecular biology, pharmacology, and gene targeting have provided tremendous opportunities for understanding the actions of general anesthetics on these receptors. The availability of cDNAs encoding the receptor subunits, combined with methods for the introduction of specific mutations into mice, has enabled a series of rapid advances toward the definition of molecular sites of anesthetic action in the brain. The knock-in mouse experiments provide an elegant bridge between in vitro experiments and whole-animal behavior. An elegant series of experiments with benzodiazepines first illustrated the tremendous potential of this approach, which has now been applied to etomidate and propofol. We can expect to see many more such experiments. A potential complication of gene targeting experiments is the existence of multiple targets of general anesthetic action (e.g. for the inhaled anesthetics) and a significant amount of genetic redundancy among the ion channels. This means that targeting of multiple genes may be required to obtain large alterations in anesthetic sensitivity in certain cases.

There is now ample evidence that clinical concentrations of several intravenous general anesthetics influence the function of $GABA_A$ receptors and other important ion channels, and we are on the verge of a molecular understanding of the sites of action of these drugs on $GABA_A$ receptors. However, there is still little information, or at least agreement, about the consequences of actions of these agents on these channels. This problem reflects our basic ignorance of how the brain works, especially at the systems level. We have only a primitive idea how small changes in channel function will influence behavior. We can be optimistic that the construction of mice with mutant molecules that lack the property of regulation by anesthetics will indeed help to address the fundamental question of how modulation of specific receptors influences specific behaviors. It is likely that rapid advances in systems neurobiology will help to fill in some of the gaps in our knowledge between the level of the synapse and the level of cognitive and motor functions in the organism.

Key references

Heurteaux C, Guy N, Laigle C, Blondeau N, Duprat F, Mazzuca M, Lang-Lazdunski L, Widmann C, Zanzouri M, Romey G, Lazdunski M. TREK-1, a K^+ channel involved in neuroprotection and general anesthesia. EMBO J 2004;23:2684-95.

Jurd R, Arras M, Lambert S et al. General anesthetic actions in vivo strongly attenuated by a point mutation in the GABA(A) receptor beta3 subunit. FASEB J 2002;17:250–2.

Krasowski MD, Koltchine VV, Rick CE, Ye Q, Finn SE, Harrison NL. Propofol and other intravenous anesthetics have sites of action on the γ-aminobutyric $acid_A$ receptor distinct from that for isoflurane. Mol Pharmacol. 1998;53:530–8.

Nelson LE, Guo TZ, Lu J, Saper CB, Franks NP, Maze M. The sedative component of anesthesia is mediated by GABA(A) receptors in an endogenous sleep pathway. Nature Neurosci. 2002;5:979–84.

Orser BA, Pennefather PS, MacDonald JF. Multiple mechanisms of ketamine blockade of *N*-methyl-D-aspartate receptors. Anesthesiology 1997;86:903–17.

Sirois JE, Lei Q, Talley EM, Lynch C III, Bayliss DA. The TASK-1 two-pore domain K^+ channel is a molecular substrate for neuronal effects of inhalation anesthetics. J Neurosci. 2000;20:6347–54.

Tomlin SL, Jenkins A, Lieb WR, Franks NP. Stereoselective effects of etomidate optical isomers on gamma-aminobutyric acid type A receptors and animals. Anesthesiology 1998;88:708–17.

Further reading

Campagna JA, Miller KW, Forman SA. Mechanisms of actions of inhaled anesthetics. New Engl J Med. 2003;348:2110–24.

Eger EI 2nd. A brief history of the origin of minimum alveolar concentration (MAC). Anesthesiology 2002;96:238–9.

Franks NP, Leib WR. Inhibitory synapses. Anaesthetics set their sites on ion channels. Nature 1997;389:334–5.

Rudolf U, Antkowiak B. Molecular and neuronal substrates for general anaesthetics. Nature Rev Neurosci. 2004;5:709–20.

Sonner JM, Antognini JF, Dutton RC et al. Inhaled anesthetics and immobility: mechanisms, mysteries, and minimum alveolar anesthetic concentration. Anesth Analg. 2003;97:718–40.

Chapter 25

Intravenous anesthetic agents

Misha A Perouansky and Hugh C Hemmings Jr

TOPICS COVERED IN THIS CHAPTER

- **Cellular targets**
- **Propofol**
  - Chemistry and formulation
  - Pharmacokinetics
  - Mechanism of action
  - Clinical effects
  - Cardiovascular and respiratory effects
  - Other effects
- **Barbiturates**
  - Chemistry and formulation
  - Pharmacokinetics
  - Mechanism of action
  - Clinical effects
  - Cardiovascular and respiratory effects
  - Other effects
- **Etomidate**
  - Chemistry and formulation
  - Pharmacokinetics
  - Mechanism of action
  - Clinical effects
  - Cardiovascular and respiratory effects
  - Other effects
- **Neurosteroids**
- **Benzodiazepines**
  - Chemistry and formulation
  - Pharmacokinetics
  - Mechanism of action
  - Clinical effects
  - Cardiovascular and respiratory effects
  - Other effects
- **Nonbenzodiazepine hypnotics**
- **Ketamine**
  - Chemistry and formulation
  - Pharmacokinetics
  - Mechanism of action
  - Clinical effects
  - Cardiovascular and respiratory effects
  - Other effects
- **Anesthetic neurotoxicity**

The induction of general anesthesia is usually achieved by the administration of intravenous agents, regardless of the technique used for maintenance of anesthesia; they can be combined with inhalation, opioid, balanced, or total intravenous anesthesia (TIVA). The ideal intravenous anesthetic agent would be water soluble, stable, nonirritating, rapid in onset, short-acting with inactive and nontoxic metabolites, and lacking excitatory effects, cardiac or respiratory depression, histamine release, neuromuscular blocking effects, or hypersensitivity reactions. However, there is no ideal intravenous anesthetic agent. A variety of injectable anesthetic drugs of diverse molecular structure are available, with differing pharmacologic profiles and side effects. Appropriate drugs are selected based on the anesthetic goals for each individual, which are dictated by the procedure to be performed and the pathophysiologic state of the patient. This chapter covers the intravenous anesthetic agents that are used primarily for the induction of general anesthesia. Other uses of intravenous anesthetics include the maintenance of general anesthesia, conscious sedation (defined as a minimally depressed level of consciousness with continuous retention of spontaneous airway control and verbal responsiveness), various levels of sedation in the intensive care setting, and brain protection.

The appropriate use of intravenous anesthetics requires an understanding of their pharmacokinetic (Chapter 8) and pharmacodynamic properties. Elimination half-time ($t_{1/2}$), a useful clinical parameter, is directly proportional to the volume of distribution (V_d) and inversely proportional to the clearance (Cl) of the drug; it is approximated by $0.693V_d/\text{Cl}$. Many intravenous anesthetics have very large apparent volumes of distribution at steady state ($V_{dss}>100$ L) because of high tissue:plasma partition coefficients and/or protein binding, which are reflected in a large apparent compartment volume.

The potency of intravenous anesthetics has been defined as the plasma concentration required to prevent a response in 50% of subjects (Cp_{50}) to a specific stimulus, analogous to the use of the minimum alveolar concentration (MAC) to prevent a response in 50% of subjects for volatile anesthetics (Chapter 26). Computer-controlled drug infusion systems are available based on derived pharmacokinetic models (Chapter 8) to allow more effective targeting of blood concentration based on the Cp_{50} (target controlled infusion; TCI).

CELLULAR TARGETS

The primary targets of intravenous anesthetic agents are relatively well defined – these drugs interact with receptors for endogenous neurotransmitters (Chapter 20). Neurotransmitter receptors can be broadly classified as either ionotropic (linked to an ion channel) or metabotropic (linked to a G protein). Most neurotransmitters in the CNS have the potential to activate both classes of receptor. The ionotropic receptors for γ-aminobutyric acid (GABA) and glutamate and the metabotropic α_2-adrenergic receptor for catecholamines are the principal targets for most intravenous anesthetics (Chapter 24).

The *$GABA_A$ receptor* (Fig. 25.1) is a member of the cys-cys loop receptor family that includes the nicotinic acetylcholine, glycine, and $5HT_3$ serotonin receptors. It is the primary target leading to the anesthetic effects (sedation, anxiolysis, hypnosis, amnesia) of all intravenous anesthetics and sedatives except ketamine and the α_2-adrenergic agonists. Advances in molecular biology and genetic engineering have in recent years allowed the identification of the structural requirements and receptor subunit specificities for the actions of several intravenous anesthetic drugs (discussed below).

Glutamate receptors are classified as either NMDA or non-NMDA types. The NMDA-type glutamate receptor plays an important physiologic role in learning and memory and, under pathologic conditions, mediates excitotoxic neuronal damage. It is the primary target for the dissociative anesthetic ketamine and some drugs of abuse (phencyclidine). The nonNMDA receptors are frequently co-localized at synapses with the NMDA receptors and enable their activation by glutamate.

The *α_2-adrenergic receptor* is the only metabotropic receptor that is a main effector of anesthetic–sedative drug action. Its physiologic agonist is noradrenaline. Activation of α_2-receptors produces inhibition of adenylyl cyclase (as opposed to activation of β_1-adrenergic receptors, which stimulates the cyclase). The drugs in anesthetic practice that target this receptor (discussed in Chapter 28) are clonidine, dexmedetomidine, and xylazine (the latter used in veterinary medicine).

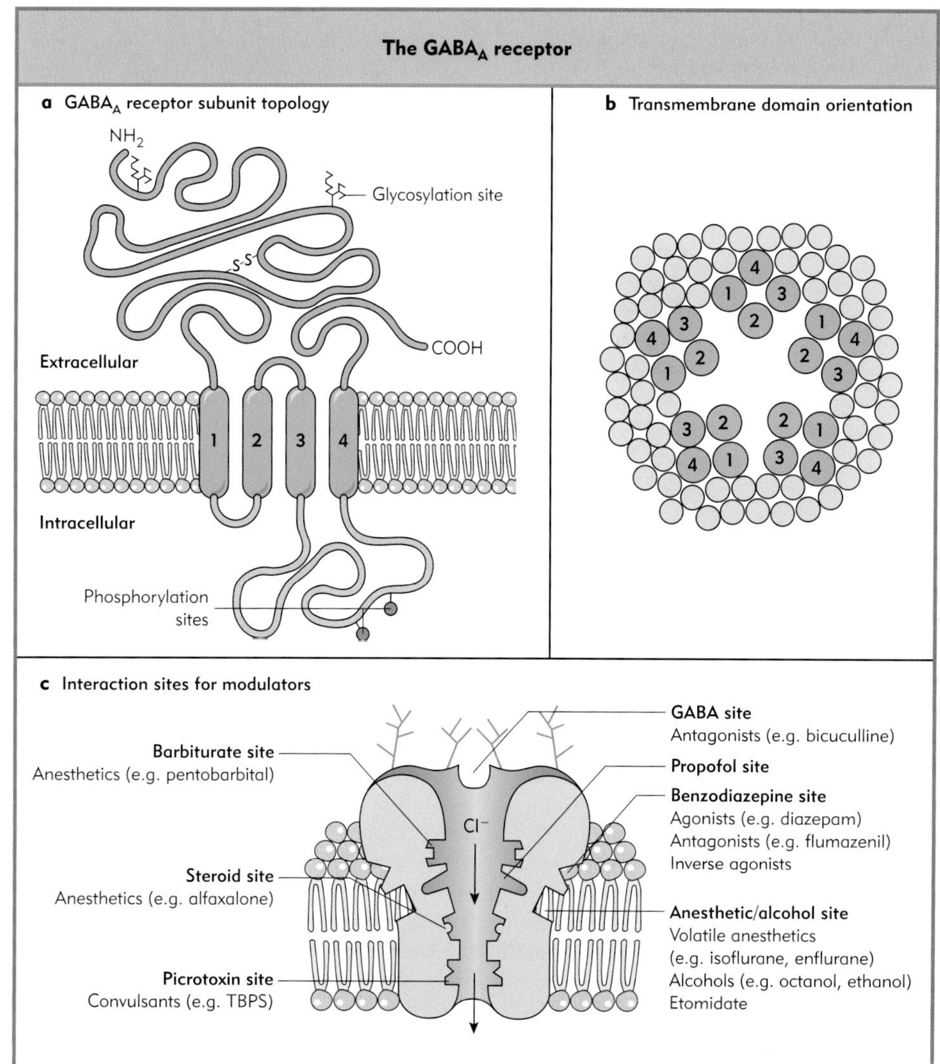

Figure 25.1 The GABA$_A$ receptor is a member of the extensive cys–cys (after the conserved cystine bridge in the N-terminal domain) receptor family that also includes the nicotinic acetylcholine, the glycine, and the serotonin 5HT$_3$ receptors. (a) The generic GABA$_A$ receptor subunit has four hydrophobic transmembrane segments that are thought to form amphipathic α-helices. The N-terminal domain contains *N*-glycosylation sites and forms the agonist-binding site. The large intracellular loop undergoes phosphorylation in several isoforms and mediates interactions with cytoskeletal and signaling molecules. (b) Plane view of the transmembrane hydrophobic segments showing interactions to form a central ion-conducting pore lined by the second transmembrane (TM2) domains. The hetero-oligomeric structure consists of five subunits, with each subunit contributing to the ion channel pore. (c) The GABA$_A$ receptor gates an anion channel permeable to Cl^- and HCO_3^-. The effects of general anesthetics differ from the those of the benzodiazepines (which allosterically modulate GABA binding to potentiate GABA responses) by separate binding sites and their ability to activate/gate the GABA$_A$ receptor channel directly. A separate site at the interface between the second and third transmembrane segments appears to interact with volatile anesthetics, alcohols, and etomidate, as demonstrated by site-directed mutagenesis studies.

PROPOFOL

Chemistry and formulation

Propofol (2,6-di-isopropylphenol) is an achiral, lipophilic, sterically hindered alkylated phenol (Fig. 25.2). It is a very weak acid ($pK_a = 11$) that is unionized at physiologic pH. It exists as an oil at room temperature and is very insoluble in water. Because of its poor water solubility, propofol is formulated at 1% in an oil/water emulsion containing 10% soybean oil, 1.2% egg lecithin, and 2.25% glycerol (as an osmotic agent) with a pH of 6–8.5. A previous formulation, in Cremophor EL, was withdrawn owing to anaphylactic reactions. The oil/water emulsion is an excellent medium for microbial growth, and care must be taken to avoid contamination and to minimize the time between withdrawal from the ampoule and administration (no longer than 6 hours). Recent formulations include the metal chelator ethylenediamine tetra-acetic acid (EDTA) or sodium metabisulfite to impede microbial growth.

The clearance of propofol is greater than hepatic blood flow, consistent with extrahepatic metabolism.

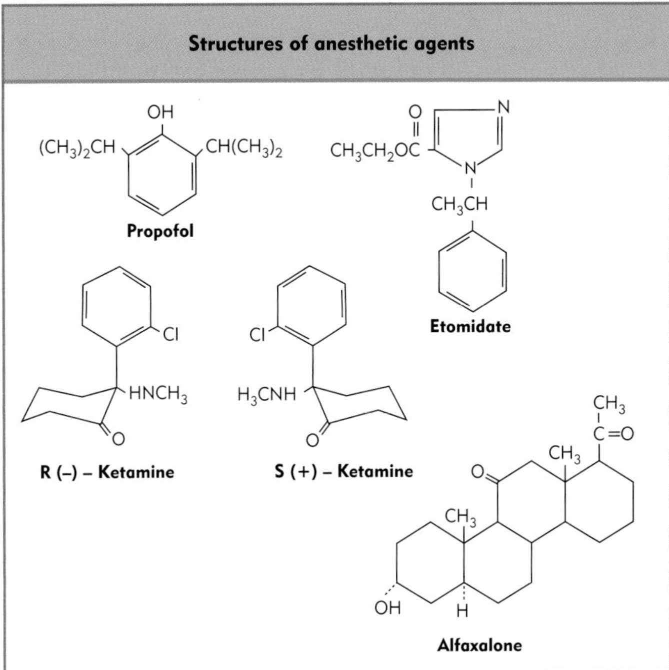

Figure 25.2 Chemical structures of propofol, etomidate, ketamine, and alfaxalone.

Pharmacokinetics

Propofol is a rapidly acting anesthetic that induces anesthesia within one arm–brain circulation time following intravenous injection. Following bolus intravenous injection, plasma concentration decreases rapidly owing to the combined effects of redistribution and elimination. When plasma concentrations are fitted to a three-compartment pharmacokinetic model, the initial and terminal half-lives are less than those of thiopental (Table 25.1). The V_{dss} of propofol is extremely large compared to that of thiopental. However, in contrast to thiopental, the clearance of propofol is also extremely high and exceeds hepatic blood flow, consistent with its extrahepatic metabolism (e.g. in the lungs, kidneys). Propofol is rapidly and completely metabolized by the liver to inactive compounds that are eliminated by the kidney. Despite its hepatic metabolism, the clearance of propofol is not impaired in patients who have cirrhosis. Clearance is also unaffected by renal failure. Although the terminal half-time is long, recovery is rapid as the terminal half-time, which is influenced primarily by the slow mobilization

Table 25.1 Pharmacokinetic properties of intravenous anesthetic agents. Data obtained after a single intravenous dose were analyzed using a three-compartment model for all but ketamine, which was analyzed using a two-compartment model (Modified with permission from Hull CJ. Pharmokinetics and pharmacodynamics, with particular reference to intravenous anesthetic agents. In: Nunn JF, Utting JE, Brown Jr BR, eds. General Anesthesia, 5th edn. London 1989; Butterworths: 96-114 .)

		Propofol	Thiopental	Methohexital (methohexitone)	Etomidate	Ketamine
Water solubility		No	Yes (sodium salt)	Yes (sodium salt)	No	Yes
pK_a		11	7.6	7.9	4.2	7.5
Half-time (t½) Initial (min)		2	8.5	5.6	1	16
Intermediate (min)		50	62	58	12	–
Terminal (h)		4.8	12	3.9	5.4	3.0
Volume of distribution (L/kg)		4.6	2.4	2.4	5.4	3.0
Clearance (mL/min/kg)		25	3.4	11	18–24	19
Protein binding (%)		98	80	85	75	12
Induction dose (mg/kg IV)	adult	1.5–2.5	2.5–4.5	1–1.5 (30 PR)	0.2–0.4 (6–7 PR)	0.5–2.0 (4–6 IM)
	children	2–3	5–6	1–2		
	infants	3–4.5	7–8	2–3		
Active metabolites		No	No	No	No	Yes (minimal)

from lipophilic tissue compartments (e.g. fat), does not reflect its rapid clearance from the central compartment (i.e. propofol has a short context-sensitive half-time). The high lipophilicity of propofol contributes to its rapid uptake into the brain; redistribution and a very high clearance result in a short duration of action. Children have an increased central compartment volume and clearance rate, and require a larger induction dose (about 1.5 times) and maintenance infusion rate, respectively. Propofol is extensively (98%) bound to plasma albumin.

Mechanism of action

As is the case with a number of other general anesthetics, propofol facilitates inhibitory synaptic transmission by potentiating and directly gating $GABA_A$ receptors at inhibitory synapses throughout the CNS (see Fig. 25.1). Targeted mutation of a single residue of the β_3 subunit (N265 to M) in mice by the knock-in technique strongly reduces their sensitivity to propofol and etomidate, but not to the neurosteroid alfaxalone, for the hypnotic and immobilizing actions of these drugs. Propofol can also block voltage-gated Na^+ and Ca^{2+} channels and potentiate glycine receptors, which may also contribute to its CNS effects. Inhibition of $5HT_3$ receptors may underlie its antiemetic properties. In contrast to other anesthetics, propofol appears to have marked subcortical effects, which may be involved in some of its atypical actions (see below). A recent study showed that microinjection of propofol directly into the tuberomammillary nucleus of the hypothalamus, a nucleus involved in specific sleep pathways, induced sedation that was reversed by a $GABA_A$ receptor antagonist. This finding suggests that the sedative effects of propofol may be quite specific and anatomically localized, rather than a generalized global depression of synaptic activity.

Clinical effects

Rapid redistribution and elimination, which result in a rapid return to consciousness with minimal residual effects, and a low incidence of nausea and vomiting make propofol particularly useful for short procedures and ambulatory surgery. The rapid clearance and short context-sensitive half-time of propofol make it useful for maintenance of anesthesia by continuous infusion without significant cumulative effects; plasma concentrations decrease rapidly when the infusion is terminated. Infusion of propofol can be combined with infusions of other short-acting drugs (e.g. remifentanil, alfentanil, sufentanil, mivacurium) for total intravenous anesthesia. Propofol is widely used as a sedative agent and as an adjunct to regional anesthesia.

Propofol possesses a number of unique characteristics, including antiemetic and antipruritic properties, that may result from its effects at subcortical sites. Its marked anxiolytic and euphorogenic properties are useful in sedation. Subhypnotic doses of propofol do not cause an increased sensitivity to somatic pain and may even provide analgesia, in contrast to thiopental, which can be antalgesic. Propofol also acts as an anticonvulsant and can be used for treating refractory epilepsy, though dystonic movements are sometimes confused with seizure activity. The rapid titratability of propofol is very useful for neurosurgical procedures, including awake craniotomy, stereotactic biopsy, and neuroradiology. Propofol exhibits pharmacodynamic synergism with benzodiazepines and opioids in anesthesia induction (hypnotic effect), allowing a reduction in its induction dose.

Cardiovascular and respiratory effects

An intravenous injection of propofol (2 mg/kg) in healthy patients decreases arterial blood pressure by 15–40%; reductions in blood pressure are generally greater with propofol than with comparable doses of thiopental (Table 25.2). Propofol produces significant reductions in systemic vascular resistance and cardiac filling, with little or no direct effect on myocardial contractility. The effect of propofol on heart rate is variable, but in general it produces less tachycardia than thiopental and may produce bradycardia. Propofol resets baroreceptor reflex control of heart rate, resulting in an unchanged heart rate despite lower levels of blood pressure compared with baseline. This mechanism may explain the greater hypotensive effect of propofol compared to thiopental. The hemodynamic effects of propofol may be magnified in hypovolemic or elderly patients, and in those who have impaired left ventricular function. These patients benefit from a reduced dose of propofol in conjunction with slow

Table 25.2 Cardiovascular, respiratory, and CNS effects of intravenous induction agents

Function	Propofol	Thiopental	Etomidate	Ketamine
Heart rate	–/↓	↑	–	↑↑
Systemic vascular resistance	↓↓	–/↓	–	–/↑
Cardiac contractility	↓	–/↓	–	↑
Histamine release	–/↑	↑	–	–
Mean arterial pressure	↓↓	↓	–	↑
Respiration	↓↓	↓↓	–/↓	–/↓
Cerebral blood flow	↓	↓	↓	↑
Cerebral metabolic rate of O_2 consumption ($CMRO_2$)	↓	↓	↓	↑
Intracranial pressure (ICP)	↓	↓	↓	↑/–
CNS excitation	+	–/+	++	++

administration and an intravenous opioid or benzodiazepine to reduce the propofol requirement and minimize cardiovascular effects. Patients should be adequately hydrated before induction to minimize hypotension. The pressor response to tracheal intubation is less marked and intubating conditions are better, owing to better intrinsic muscle relaxation with propofol than with the barbiturates. Propofol produces a minimal increase in plasma histamine levels. Propofol is not arrhythmogenic and does not sensitize the heart to catecholamines. Propofol is a potent respiratory depressant and often produces an apneic period of 30–60 seconds following a normal induction dose. Hiccough, cough, and laryngospasm are less common than with barbiturates, possibly because of greater depression of laryngeal reflexes. Propofol also causes some bronchodilatation, in contrast to thiopental or etomidate, which makes it a useful agent for asthmatic patients.

Other effects

Pain on injection is a significant problem with intravenous propofol. This may be minimized by using larger veins with a rapid carrier infusion rate, by injecting lidocaine (lignocaine) before or with the propofol emulsion, or by injecting a synthetic opioid before the propofol emulsion. The incidence of venous thrombosis and phlebitis following propofol injection is low. Propofol does not have adverse gastrointestinal or hepatic effects; even high doses produce no significant changes in hepatic transaminases, alkaline phosphatase, or bilirubin. Coagulation and fibrinolytic activities are also unaffected. Propofol has significant antiemetic activity, even at subanesthetic doses (10 mg IV). Propofol is also an effective antipruritic and can be used to relieve the pruritus associated with neuraxial opioids. Propofol is more effective in reducing intraocular pressure than thiopental or etomidate. Propofol has no significant direct effects on renal function and does not interfere with cortisol secretion. If used as a prolonged infusion (days), it can lead to hypertriglyceridemia. As with other intravenous anesthetics, propofol does not trigger malignant hyperthermia. Propofol does increase γ-aminolevulinic acid reductase activity in vitro and is therefore potentially porphyrinogenic, but its use has been described in patients who have acute intermittent porphyria without producing a porphyric attack. Propofol has no direct effect on neuromuscular transmission, nor are there significant interactions between propofol and neuromuscular blocking agents. Propofol has been used successfully in pregnancy and obstetrics, but may cause neonatal depression after prolonged infusion.

Excitatory phenomena can occur with induction or emergence from propofol or etomidate anesthesia.

Excitatory phenomena such as tremor, hypertonus, opisthotonos, and spontaneous or dystonic movements can occur with induction or on emergence from anesthesia induced by propofol. Most dystonic reactions have been reported in young female patients in the day-surgery setting; benzotropin 2 mg IV has been recommended for treatment of severe cases. Propofol induces dose-related changes in the electroencephalogram (EEG), from increased β activity with sedation to increased δ activity with unconsciousness, and burst suppression at higher doses. Although propofol can produce EEG burst suppression, it has not been demonstrated to be neuroprotective in clinical practice. Propofol is not likely to induce EEG seizure activity in normal patients, but can be epileptogenic in patients who have seizure disorders. The majority of apparent propofol-induced ‘seizures’ are likely to be caused by spontaneous excitatory movements secondary to selective disinhibition of subcortical centers, which may be avoidable by using adequate doses. Seizure-like phenomena have been reported without pre-existing neurologic or psychiatric disorders; most of these were consistent with convulsions, and the others resembled dystonic movements. Propofol may have anticonvulsant properties similar to thiopental in animal models, but is not recommended for use in epileptic patients by drug safety advisory committees in the UK and Australia. Propofol can shorten the duration of convulsions following electroconvulsive therapy, which may be a therapeutic disadvantage. Propofol depresses somatosensory and motor evoked potentials, but does not appear to affect brainstem auditory evoked potentials (Chapter 14).

Cerebral blood flow (more than cerebral metabolic rate for oxygen, $CMRO_2$), $CMRO_2$, and intracranial pressure (normal or elevated) are reduced by propofol. In contrast, propofol causes direct cerebral arterial and venous dilatation in vitro. Cerebrovascular reactivity to carbon dioxide and autoregulation are preserved. Its marked potential for reducing mean arterial pressure often results in greater reductions in cerebral perfusion pressure than with other agents.

As propofol gained acceptance as a sedative drugs in intensive care units, reports of adverse reactions, some of them fatal, appeared. The constellation of symptoms (metabolic acidosis, lipemic plasma, myocardial failure, hepatomegaly, rhabdomyolysis) was characteristic enough to be summarized as propofol infusion syndrome (PIS). Initially, the reports were limited to children sedated for prolonged periods, but more recently PIS has been reported in adults. The underlying pathophysiology is not understood.

BARBITURATES

Chemistry and formulation

The barbiturates are weak acids and are poorly soluble in water. The most commonly used anesthetic barbiturates, which include thiopental (thiopentone), thiamylal (thioseconal), and methohexital (methohexitone) (Fig. 25.3), are formulated as racemic mixtures of their water-soluble sodium salts. Sodium carbonate is included to maintain an alkaline pH of 10–11, which prevents precipitation of the free acids through acidification by atmospheric carbon dioxide. The alkalinity of these solutions can result in severe tissue damage from extravascular or intra-arterial injections. They will also induce precipitation of drugs that are weak bases, such as pancuronium, vecuronium, rocuronium (e.g. during rapid-sequence induction: complete obstruction of the intravenous catheter can occur), lidocaine, and morphine sulfate. The barbiturates are broadly classified as thiobarbiturates (sulfur at C2: thiopental, thiamylal) and oxybarbiturates (oxygen at C2: methohexital). Substitution of sulfur for oxygen at C2 increases lipophilicity, which results in increased potency, more rapid onset, and shorter duration of action (compare pentobarbital (pentobarbitone) with thiopental, its thio analog). Alkylation of N1 also increases lipophilicity and thereby speeds onset, but it also increases excitatory side effects, such as spontaneous involuntary movements (e.g. as seen with methohexital,

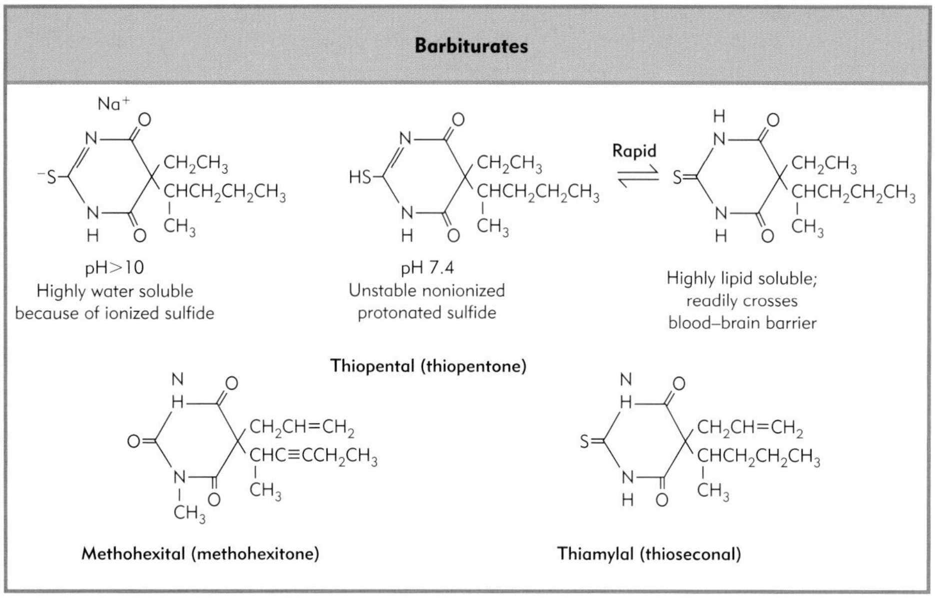

Barbiturates

pH>10
Highly water soluble because of ionized sulfide

pH 7.4
Unstable nonionized protonated sulfide

Rapid

Highly lipid soluble; readily crosses blood–brain barrier

Thiopental (thiopentone)

Methohexital (methohexitone)

Thiamylal (thioseconal)

Figure 25.3 Chemical structures of intravenous barbiturates. The water-soluble sodium salts are formed by association of Na^+ with an unstable structural isomer (tautomer) in alkaline solution, as illustrated for thiopental. At physiologic pH (7.4) the sulfide is protonated, forming an unstable unionized structure that rapidly isomerizes to form a highly lipid-soluble tautomer that readily crosses the blood–brain barrier. Analogous tautomerism occurs for thiamylal and methohexital.

a methylated oxybarbiturate). The L-isomers of thiopental and thiamylal are more than twice as potent as the D-isomers as anesthetics. Both drugs, however, are used as racemic mixtures. Methohexital has two asymmetric carbons, yielding four enantiomers, and is marketed as a racemic mixture of the two α-enantiomers. The β-enantiomers are proconvulsant.

Pharmacokinetics

The short duration of action of thiopental, thiamylal, and methohexital can be explained by their pharmacokinetic properties. Following rapid bolus intravenous administration, these agents distribute rapidly within the intravascular space and to the highly perfused (vessel-rich) tissues, including the brain (Fig. 25.4), resulting in loss of consciousness within one arm–brain circulation time, or about 20 seconds, depending on the cardiac output. Maximal anesthetic depth is achieved within four to five arm–brain circulation times. Subsequently, thiopental is redistributed to muscle, and to a lesser extent to fat. Throughout this period, small but substantial amounts of thiopental are removed by the liver and metabolized. Unlike removal by redistribution to other tissues, liver uptake and metabolism are terminal. Data for thiopental and methohexital (Table 25.1) indicate that the central V_d values (equivalent to the central compartment) exceed the intravascular volume, consistent with their rapid distribution to brain and other highly perfused tissues. The action of a single bolus injection is terminated primarily by redistribution to the much larger apparent V_{dss}, which includes lean vessel-rich tissues such as muscle. Therefore, the appropriate induction dose should be calculated based on lean body mass. This phenomenon may underlie the apparent increased sensitivity to barbiturates of women and the elderly. The high fat:plasma partition coefficient of the lipophilic barbiturates has little effect on their initial distribution because of the poor perfusion of adipose tissue, but it provides a large reservoir for delayed drug uptake with prolonged administration. Because they are acidic lipophilic compounds, most barbiturates bind to plasma albumin.

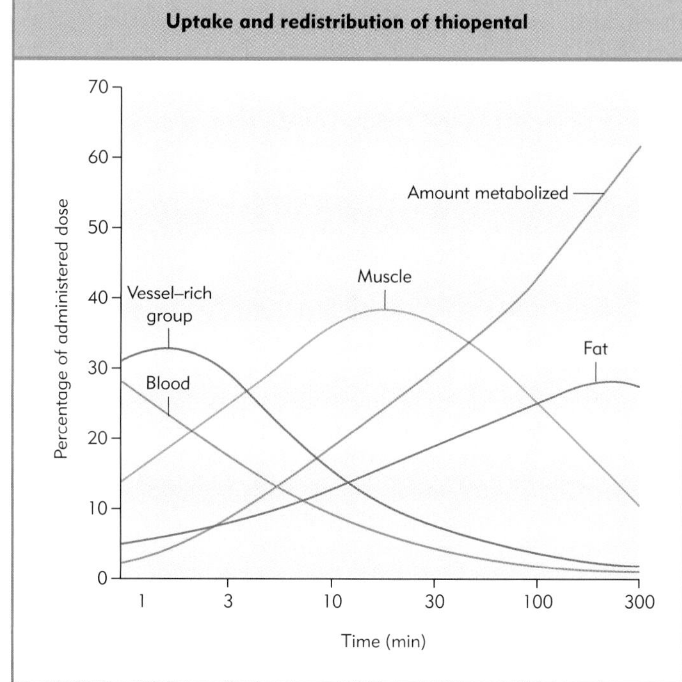

Figure 25.4 Uptake and redistribution of an intravenous bolus of thiopental. The amount of thiopental in the blood rapidly decreases as drug moves from blood to body tissues. The time to peak tissue levels is a direct function of the tissue capacity for barbiturate uptake relative to blood flow. Redistribution between tissues and metabolism results in removal of tissue contents. (Modified from Saidman LJ. Uptake, distribution and elimination of barbiturates. In: Eger EJ, ed. Anesthetic uptake and action. Baltimore, MD: Williams and Williams; 1974:264-284.)

The action of a single bolus dose of thiopental is terminated primarily by redistribution.

The pharmacokinetic properties of the barbiturates also explain the mechanism of delayed recovery observed after large or repeated doses, or after prolonged infusions. The short duration of action depends on a redistribution mechanism, which is limited by the mass of lean tissue and is easily overwhelmed by a large cumulative dose that saturates this reservoir. At this point, the duration of action is no longer related to the initial redistribution half-time, but to the terminal (elimination) half-time, which is relatively slow given its high V_{dss} and low clearance (see Table 25.1). Under these conditions of zero-order elimination (rate is constant and independent of plasma concentration), methohexital is eliminated more quickly than thiopental because of its higher clearance (despite a similar V_{dss}). Recovery is also hastened by the lack of active methohexital metabolites. The ultimate elimination of barbiturates, which is very slow relative to drug uptake by lean tissue and makes little contribution to terminating their effects acutely, is primarily through hepatic extraction and metabolism. The marked prolongation of recovery time with increasing duration of thiopental infusion is reflected in its context-sensitive half-time (Fig. 25.5). The use of barbiturates administered by continuous infusion for maintenance of anesthesia has been largely supplanted by propofol, which allows for more rapid recovery due to its more favorable kinetics. If a barbiturate is used, methohexital is the more suitable owing to its shorter terminal elimination half-time of about 4 hours (compared to 12 hours for thiopental). Thiopental is occasionally administered via continuous infusion to treat intracranial hypertension in the intensive care unit.

Mechanism of action

The principal mechanism of action of the ultrashort-acting anesthetic barbiturates, as suggested by several lines of evidence, is through facilitation of inhibitory synaptic transmission (by both enhancing and mimicking γ-aminobutyric acid (GABA)-mediated Cl^- influx at the $GABA_A$ receptor (see Fig. 25.1). Electrophysiologic evidence suggests that barbiturates also inhibit excitatory synaptic transmission, possibly by blocking postsynaptic nonNMDA subtype glutamate receptors. Remarkably, the ability of pentobarbital to block is critically dependent on a single amino acid in one of the subunits forming the receptor. Barbiturates also block voltage-gated Na^+ and Ca^{2+} channels and can scavenge free radicals, effects that may contribute to their neuroprotective actions. Effects have also been reported at K^+ channels and nicotinic acetylcholine receptors. The barbiturates thus appear to be more promiscuous than propofol or etomidate in affecting multiple targets in addition to $GABA_A$ receptors.

Clinical effects

Considerable information is available concerning the clinical effects of barbiturates, given their early introduction in the 1940s and widespread use thereafter. Until the 1990s, barbiturates were the most popular anesthetic induction agents, but have been superseded by propofol, especially for ambulatory anesthesia. Following intravenous injection, thiopental, thiamylal, and methohexital induce anesthesia in a manner similar to propofol, with a duration of 4–8 minutes. Dose requirements are reduced by pharmacodynamic interactions (opioid or benzodiazepine premedication, acute ethanol intoxication), and by pharmacokinetic effects (anemia, malnutrition, uremia, shock,

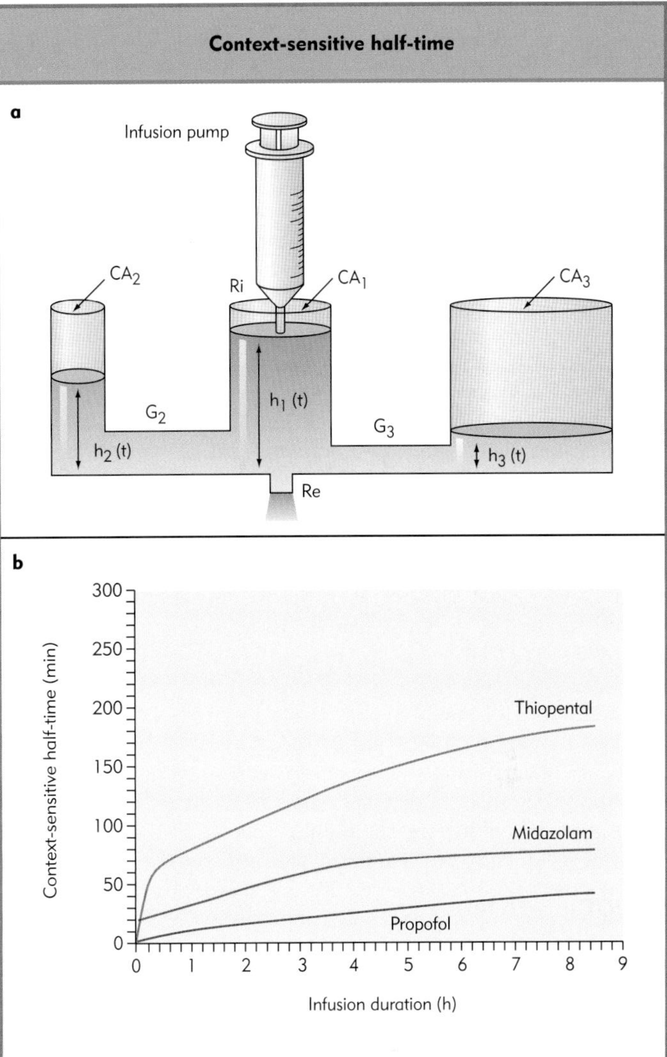

Figure 25.5 (a) Hydraulic model analogy to three-compartment pharmacokinetic model of context-sensitive half-time. The three buckets represent a central (CA_1, blood) and two peripheral (CA_2, muscle; CA_3, fat) compartments into which a lipophilic drug distributes during intravenous administration at a constant rate R_i (symbolized by the infusion pump). Each compartment has a certain capacity to take up the drug (represented by the surface areas CA). The peripheral compartments have different rates of equilibration with the central compartment that are determined by the specific conductances G (analogous to tissue blood flow) and the drug concentration gradients (represented by the height *h* of the fluid columns). The rate at which the drug concentration in the central compartment decreases after discontinuation of the drug infusion depends not only on the rate of elimination (R_e) but is strongly influenced by the amount of drug stored in the peripheral compartments, which in turn is dependent on the length of time the drug has been administered (context sensitivity). Note that the parameter of clinical interest is the half-time (the time for a given drug concentration in the central compartment to decrease by 50%), not the half-life. **(b) Context-sensitive half-times as a function of infusion duration for various drugs used in anesthesia.** Context-sensitive half-time is the time required for the central compartment drug concentration to decrease by 50% at the end of infusion as predicted by agent-specific multicompartment pharmacokinetic models, where context refers to the duration of the infusion. This index is more useful in predicting the time course of recovery of many agents than is elimination half-life. Note the early steep increase in context-sensitive half-time for thiopental compared with propofol. (Modified with permission from Hughes MA, Glass PSA, Jacobs JR. Context-sensitive half-time in multicompartment models for anesthetic drugs. Anesthesiology 1992; 76:334-341.)

or severe systemic disease). Reduced cardiac output prolongs induction and allows higher peak blood drug levels to develop, which decreases the dose requirement. Methohexital is about 2.7 times more potent than thiopental, which is slightly less potent than thiamylal.

With burst suppression of the EEG, thiopental reduces cerebral metabolism and blood flow by ~55%.

Barbiturates are also used by anesthesiologists as anticonvulsants in acute situations; for brain protection during neurosurgery, cardiac valvular surgery or circulatory arrest; and to reduce intracranial pressure in patients who have intracranial hypertension. The cerebroprotective effect of barbiturates has been attributed to a reduction in cerebral metabolism as a result of a dose-related reduction in neuronal activity. However, recent studies indicate that equivalent reductions in cerebral metabolism by hypothermia are more effective for neuroprotection. Reduced neuronal activity is reflected in a dose-dependent depression of the EEG (Chapter 14 and Fig. 25.6a), which progresses from an awake pattern of α activity through high-amplitude and low-frequency δ and θ activity to burst suppression and subsequently electrical silence (5–10 mg/kg body weight followed by 10–20 mg/kg/hour for 90% burst suppression). With burst suppression, there is a maximal decrease of ~55% in $CMRO_2$. EEG changes correlate with serum thiopental concentrations. However, the biphasic nature of the relationship of EEG frequency to thiopental serum concentration makes EEG alone inadequate for monitoring the depth of barbiturate anesthesia (Fig. 25.6b).

Although thiopental is a vasodilator in vitro, dose-dependent reductions in intracranial pressure in vivo preserve cerebral perfusion pressure despite reductions in mean arterial pressure. Cerebral blood flow decreases with anesthetic depth (up to approximately 50% reduction) until the EEG becomes isoelectric, after which there is no further decrease, indicating the relation with $CMRO_2$. The normal coupling between cerebral blood flow and $CMRO_2$ (autoregulation) and arterial partial pressure of carbon dioxide ($PaCO_2$) is not affected. By reducing cerebral blood volume, barbiturates can reduce intracranial pressure, although this action may be lost with severe brain injury. Thiopental can reduce intracranial pressure refractory to mannitol and/or hyperventilation. These properties make the barbiturates particularly useful in neurosurgical patients.

Barbiturates may be useful in reducing the sequelae of temporary *focal* or regional cerebral ischemia by suppressing oxygen consumption in ischemic zones, scavenging oxygen radicals, and increasing perfusion to ischemic zones as a result of vasoconstriction in normal zones (secondary to decreased $CMRO_2$ – 'inverse steal'). Thiopental is the only agent to have shown evidence of long-term cerebral protection in focal ischemia. However, thiopental was ineffective in cerebral resuscitation after *global* ischemia (cardiac arrest) when administered 10–50 minutes after restoration of spontaneous circulation.

Baroreceptor reflex-mediated tachycardia partially compensates for the systemic vasodilation produced by barbiturates, mitigating the reduction in blood pressure.

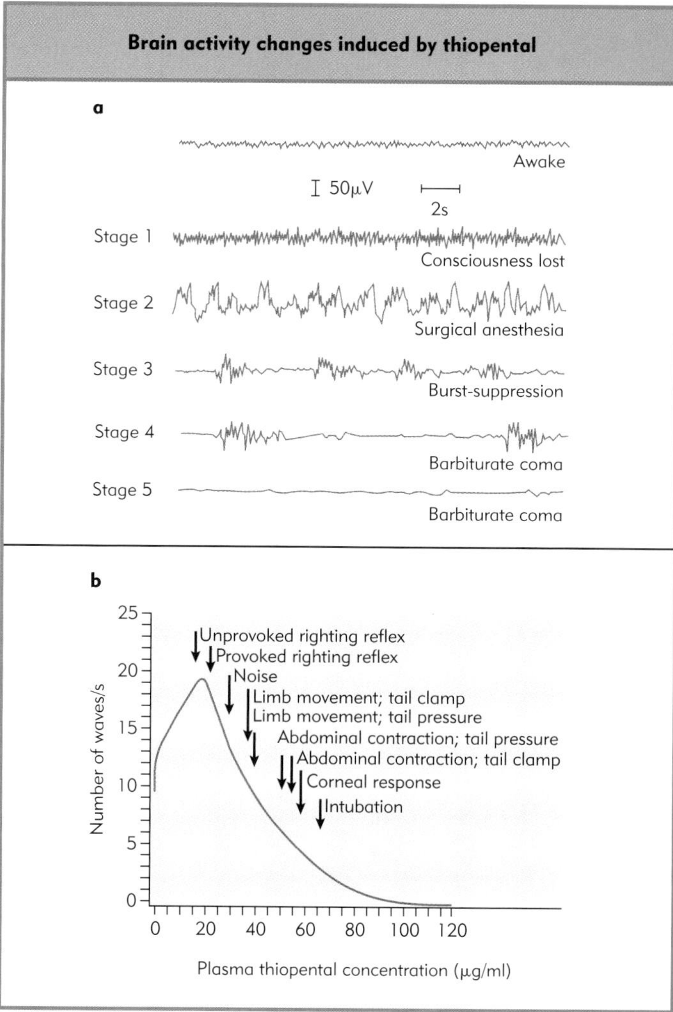

Figure 25.6 Brain activity changes induced by thiopental. (a) EEG shows the changes induced by thiopental. As consciousness is lost in stage 1 there is an increase in frequency and amplitude. Amplitude increases further and frequency is markedly reduced in stage 2, whereas stage 3 is characterized by bursts of electrical activity interspersed between isoelectric periods (burst suppression). Progressive prolongation of isoelectric periods ensues through stage 4 until a continuously isoelectric EEG is obtained in stage 5. (Adapted from Kiersey DK, Bickford RG, Faulconer A Jr. Electroencephalographic patterns produced by thiopental sodium during surgical operations: description and classification. Br J Anaesth 1951; 23:141-152., © The Board of Management and Trustees of the British Journal of Anaesthesia.) (b) EEG effect versus pseudosteady-state plasma thiopental concentration in rats. Modeled values required to suppress response to various stimuli are also shown. Note that the EEG returns to baseline frequency at 40 μg/mL. The biphasic response has also been shown in humans and confounds efforts to relate clinical effect measures to the EEG. (Modified with permission from Gustafsson LL et al. Quantitation of depth of thiopental anesthesia in the rat. Anesthesiology. 1996;84:415-427.)

Cardiovascular and respiratory effects

The principal hemodynamic effects of barbiturates administered by bolus intravenous injection for the induction of anesthesia in healthy, normovolemic patients are a transient reduction in systemic arterial pressure and cardiac output, an increase in heart rate, and no change or an increase in systemic vascular resistance (see Table 25.2). Hypotension results from marked venodilatation, with peripheral pooling of blood and decreased cardiac filling pressure that reduces cardiac output and arterial pressure. The usual doses of thiopental produce minimal myocardial depression, although higher doses reduce contractility. The increased heart rate, which is more marked with methohexital than with thiopental, results from baroreceptor reflex-mediated sympathetic stimulation of the heart, and may partially mask the vasodilation and negative inotropic effects. Thiopental and thiamylal, but not methohexital, can induce histamine release, which exacerbates their cardiovascular effects. The hypotensive effects of barbiturates are more pronounced in patients who have treated or untreated hypertension and under conditions where compensatory mechanisms are impaired, such as hypovolemia, valvular or ischemic heart disease, or shock. The hemodynamic effects of barbiturates can be particularly deleterious in conditions that are worsened by reduced preload or tachycardia, such as myocardial ischemia, congestive heart failure, pericardial tamponade, and valvular heart disease. Barbiturates are not arrhythmogenic but can sensitize the heart to catecholamines (in dogs).

Anesthetic barbiturates are potent central respiratory depressants. They produce dose-dependent decreases in both minute volume and tidal volume. The respiratory rate may increase slightly at lower doses but is reduced by higher doses, which lead ultimately to apnea. The medullary center ventilatory responses to both hypercapnia and hypoxia are depressed. Usual induction doses of barbiturates do not depress laryngeal and tracheal reflexes. Therefore, laryngospasm and, rarely, bronchospasm can occur on induction of anesthesia, especially with upper airway stimulation by secretions, artificial airways, or laryngoscopy. Cough and hiccough are not uncommon, especially with methohexital.

Other effects

Pain on intravenous injection is rare with thiopental but is more common with methohexital. Venous thrombosis and phlebitis may occur up to several days after administration. Intra-arterial or subcutaneous injection can cause tissue irritation or necrosis, depending on the amount and the site of injection. Barbiturates do not acutely affect gastrointestinal or hepatic function. There is a low incidence of postoperative nausea and vomiting. Chronic administration can lead to hepatic enzyme induction, resulting in accelerated metabolism of barbiturates and other drugs. Stimulation of the mitochondrial enzyme δ-aminolevulinic acid reductase, the rate-limiting enzyme in porphyrin biosynthesis, can exacerbate acute intermittent porphyria in susceptible patients; therefore barbiturates are contraindicated in porphyria. Barbiturates can contribute to intraoperative oliguria by reducing renal blood flow and glomerular filtration, an effect that is effectively managed by treating hypotension and providing adequate intravenous fluid. In contrast to etomidate, barbiturates do not suppress adrenocortical stimulation. Thiopental can be safely used for anesthetic induction for cesarean section; however, doses greater than 8 mg/kg may cause neonatal depression as a result of its placental transfer. This effect can be minimized by delivering the baby within 10 minutes of induction. Thiopental has little effect on uterine contractions. Undesirable CNS effects observed with barbiturates include paradoxical excitement with small doses (possibly owing to central disinhibition or an antalgesic effect, especially in the presence of pain) and involuntary skeletal muscle movements (myoclonus, a central excitatory effect). Methohexital (40–50 mg) can trigger seizure foci in susceptible patients, an effect which can be used to advantage in epilepsy surgery and when providing anesthesia for electroconvulsive therapy. Prolonged neurobehavioral effects can be observed for several hours after induction with large or repeated doses. Significant effects on neuromuscular transmission or skeletal muscle function do not occur with barbiturates. Barbiturates have minimal effects on somatosensory or motor evoked potentials, but cause dose-dependent reductions in brainstem auditory evoked potentials.

ETOMIDATE

Chemistry and formulation

Etomidate is a carboxylated imidazole derivative that is chemically unrelated to other general anesthetics (see Fig. 25.2). It is a weak base (pK_a = 4.2) that is poorly water soluble and is currently formulated as a hyperosmotic solution in 35% propylene glycol. (*R*)(+)-Etomidate is synthesized and used as the pharmacologically active stereoisomer.

Pharmacokinetics

The onset of unconsciousness following intravenous injection of etomidate is rapid, occurring in one arm–brain circulation time, as a result of its high lipophilicity, which facilitates penetration of the blood–brain barrier. Duration is dose dependent, but is usually 3–5 minutes with an average dose (0.3 mg/kg). Awakening after a single injection of etomidate is rapid because of extensive redistribution to peripheral tissues, which is reflected in a large but variable V_{dss} (see Table 25.1). Pharmacokinetic investigations of plasma etomidate concentrations after bolus intravenous injection reveal its rapid distribution (half-time 1 minute) and slower elimination (half-time 5.4 hours). Etomidate is rapidly and essentially completely metabolized in plasma and liver by ester hydrolysis to the inactive carboxylic acid derivative. Etomidate clearance is relatively high (18–24 mL/min/kg), similar to that of propofol. The longer terminal half-time of etomidate compared with propofol results primarily from the larger V_{dss} of etomidate. Although etomidate has been used by continuous infusion without evidence of accumulation, large doses will result in cumulative effects. Limited pharmacokinetic data suggest that in hepatic cirrhosis V_{dss} and terminal half-time are approximately twice normal. Etomidate is about 75% bound to both albumin and α_1-acidic glycoprotein in plasma.

Mechanism of action

The general anesthetic properties of etomidate result from the facilitation of inhibitory synaptic transmission at GABAergic synapses through potentiation of $GABA_A$ receptor function. Etomidate preferentially affects $GABA_A$ receptors containing β_2 or β_3 subunits (see Fig. 25.1). The pivotal role of the $GABA_A$ receptor in the mechanism of action of etomidate is supported by the fact that (*R*)(+)-etomidate is much more potent as an anesthetic than (*S*)(–)-etomidate in vivo, and is also a more potent modulator of $GABA_A$ receptors in vitro (enantioselectivity). A single amino acid residue change in the second transmembrane domain of the β_2 (N265) or β_3 subunit (N289) can eliminate the potentiating allosteric effect of etomidate. Targeted mutation of N265 of the β_2 subunit to S265 results in mice that are resistant to the sedative effects of etomidate but still exhibit anesthesia and burst suppression, whereas mutation of N265 of the β_3 subunit to M265 results in mice that are resistant to the anesthetic effects of etomidate. These findings indicate that $GABA_A$ receptors containing the β_2 subunit mediate the sedative properties of etomidate, whereas those containing the β_3 subunit mediate loss of consciousness. This elegant demonstration of subunit-selective actions of an intravenous anesthetic suggests that $GABA_A$ β_3 subunit-selective agents could be used to produce anesthesia with improved recovery as a result of less sedation.

Clinical effects

Despite its rapid onset and short duration of action a number of troublesome side effects and its cost have limited the widespread use of etomidate as an intravenous induction agent. Etomidate has found a niche as an induction agent with fewer cardiovascular and respiratory depressant actions than thiopental. It is particularly useful in the induction of anesthesia in patients who have impaired ventricular function, with cardiac tamponade, or in hypovolemic patients who require emergency surgery in the absence of adequate fluid resuscitation. A short duration of action makes it useful as a sole anesthetic agent in short, painless procedures such as electroconvulsive therapy or cardioversion in patients who have ventricular dysfunction or hypovolemia. Etomidate has effects on the CNS similar to those of barbiturate anesthetics. Dose-dependent changes occur in the EEG, from an awake α pattern to δ and θ activity, and changes culminate in burst suppression at doses greater than 0.3 mg/kg; in contrast to thiopental, β activity is not seen initially. Etomidate also decreases $CMRO_2$ (by about 45%) and cerebral blood flow (by about 35%), and reduces elevated intracranial pressure without reducing arterial blood pressure or cerebral perfusion pressure, thereby producing an increase in the cerebral oxygen supply/demand ratio. This results from direct vasoconstriction and coupled reductions in $CMRO_2$ and cerebral blood volume. Carbon dioxide reactivity is preserved. These properties make it attractive for use in neurosurgical procedures, where its short duration is advantageous. Although etomidate has been used to control status epilepticus, it can also activate seizure foci, a property that can be used to facilitate intraoperative localization. Etomidate can precipitate generalized seizure activity in epileptic patients, and it does not inhibit evoked seizures in patients undergoing electroconvulsive therapy.

Cardiovascular and respiratory effects

Etomidate is remarkable for its relative lack of cardiovascular effects (Table 25.2). In normal patients, or in patients who have mild cardiovascular disease, etomidate (0.15–0.3 mg/kg) has minimal effects on heart rate, stroke volume, cardiac output, and ventricular filling pressures. Arterial blood pressure is also minimally affected, although decreases of up to 20% can occur in patients who have valvular heart disease. Hemodynamic stability results from reduced effects on the sympathetic nervous system and baroreceptor reflex responses. Etomidate produces a smaller change in the balance of myocardial oxygen supply and demand than thiopental or ketamine, and has a twofold lower negative inotropic effect than equianesthetic doses of thiopental. Studies in vitro suggest that the negative inotropic effect of etomidate results from the propylene glycol vehicle and not from etomidate itself. Etomidate does not evoke histamine release and has a low incidence of hypersensitivity reactions.

Etomidate has minimal cardiovascular effects owing to reduced actions on sympathetic and baroreceptor reflex responses and causes less respiratory depression than other anesthetics.

Etomidate causes less respiratory depression than barbiturates, which makes it a useful induction agent for patients when maintenance of spontaneous ventilation is desirable. In most patients minute ventilation and tidal volume are decreased, whereas respiratory rate is increased. Transient apnea may occur, especially in geriatric patients, an effect that may be reduced by premedication. Etomidate does depress the sensitivity of the medullary respiratory center to carbon dioxide, but ventilation is usually greater at a given $PaCO_2$ than with barbiturates.

Other effects

Pain on injection and myoclonus are the most frequent undesirable effects of etomidate. Pain on injection occurs in up to 80% of patients, but its incidence varies with the size and location of the vein used, the vehicle, the speed of injection, and premedication. The use of large veins, a rapid carrier infusion, or opioid premedication decreases the incidence. Induction of anesthesia with etomidate is accompanied by a high incidence of excitatory phenomena (up to 87% of unpremedicated patients), including spontaneous muscle movement, hypertonus, and myoclonus. Although these effects may resemble seizure activity, they are associated with epileptiform EEG activity in only ~20% of patients. As with propofol, excitatory phenomena probably result from disinhibition of subcortical extrapyramidal pathways. The incidence of myoclonus associated with etomidate is reduced by prior administration of opioids or benzodiazepines.

Etomidate causes less depression of evoked potentials than thiopental or propofol. Brainstem auditory evoked responses are unaffected, whereas somatosensory evoked potentials show minimally increased latency and increased amplitude, which can improve poor signals in procedures that employ this monitor (Chapter 14). Etomidate administered by single injection or by continuous infusion directly suppresses adrenal cortical function. Although the clinical significance of this effect following a single injection is unclear, increased mortality has been observed in critically ill patients receiving long-term etomidate infusions. Etomidate reversibly inhibits the activity of steroid 11β-hydroxylase, a key enzyme in steroid biosynthesis. This effect persists for 6–8 hours after an induction dose and is unresponsive to adrenocorticotropic hormone (ACTH). Etomidate has no significant effects on hepatic and renal function. In contrast to other intravenous anesthetics and volatile anesthetics, there is no reduction in renal blood flow. Nausea and vomiting are more common following induction of anesthesia with etomidate (approx. 30%) than with other induction agents. Etomidate is potentially porphyrinogenic and should be avoided in patients with porphyria. There are insufficient data to support the use of etomidate in pregnancy and obstetrics. Etomidate is an inhibitor of plasma cholinesterase and may prolong the action of succinylcholine (suxamethonium) in patients who have plasma cholinesterase deficiency; it may also potentiate the action of nondepolarizing neuromuscular blockers.

NEUROSTEROIDS

A number of other compounds with general anesthetic properties have been used as induction agents but are not currently available for clinical use. Of these, the neurosteroid anesthetics are of particular interest. Neuroactive steroids are a group of compounds which, in addition to their genomic effects, also interact with a host of neurotransmitter receptors and have a variety of neuropharmacologic effects, including – but not limited to – anesthesia, sedation, and hypnosis. Althesin, a proprietary mixture of alfaxalone (the active anesthetic) and alfadolone, is poorly soluble in water (see Fig. 25.2). A formulation in Cremophor EL was withdrawn from the market because of a high incidence of hypersensitivity reactions. In addition to enhancing the effect of GABA, alfaxalone activates $GABA_A$ receptors directly. Minaxolone and 2-aminosteroids have been developed as water-soluble steroid anesthetics but are associated with a high incidence of excitatory phenomena. 5β-Pregnenolone (Eltanolone) was under development as an intravenous induction agent. It is a water-insoluble enantiomeric pair and is formulated in a lipid emulsion. Advantages of this agent include minimal hemodynamic side effects, reduced respiratory depression, a short duration of action, and a low incidence of venous irritation. However, involuntary excitatory movements and urticaria are problems. The mechanism of action of all steroid anesthetics appears to be through facilitation of $GABA_A$ receptors, although they display variable subunit preferences in vitro (see Fig. 25.1).

BENZODIAZEPINES

Chemistry and formulation

The three most commonly used benzodiazepine receptor agonists in anesthesia are midazolam, lorazepam, and diazepam (Fig. 25.7). They are all weak bases with a high degree of protein binding (96–98%). Midazolam, the most lipid-soluble of the three in vivo, is unique in that it undergoes a pH-dependent isomerization that results in ring closure and a large increase in lipid solubility. At pH values less than 4.0 it exists in an open-ring water-soluble configuration, but above pH 4 the ring closes, producing the active lipid-soluble form of the drug. Midazolam is formulated in aqueous solution buffered to pH~3.5. Its imidazole ring confers stability in solution and rapid metabolism. The injectable form of diazepam (pH 6.2–6.8), which is insoluble in water, contains 0.4 mL of propylene glycol, 0.1 mL of ethanol per mL of solution, as well as benzyl alcohol and benzoic acid, and is therefore extremely irritating when given intravenously (less irritating, emulsified formulations are available in some countries). Lorazepam is also formulated in a vehicle of polyethylene glycol, propylene glycol, and benzyl alcohol to increase its solubility.

Midazolam is unique in its formulation as a water-soluble prodrug that undergoes pH-dependent ring closure to form the active lipid-soluble form.

Pharmacokinetics

Protein binding and volume of distribution are similar for the three drugs that are classified as short-, intermediate and long-lasting, but the clearance differs widely, ranging from

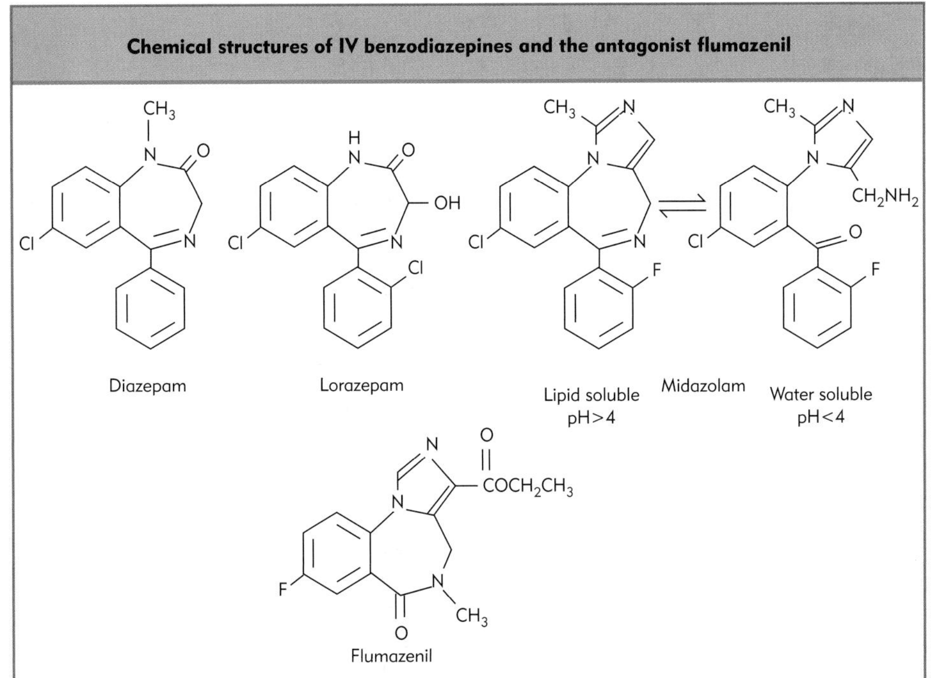

Figure 25.7 Chemical structures of intravenous benzodiazepines and the antagonist flumazenil. The reversible pH-dependent ring opening of midazolam is shown.

Table 25.3 Pharmacokinetic properties of benzodiazepines. As these drugs are frequently referred to by their trade names, some of these are also included. If pharmacodynamic equivalency data are available (e.g. electroencephalography (EEG) effects), relative potency is indicated with reference to midazolam

Drug	Terminal half-time (h)	Equivalent IV/IM dose or total daily PO dose	Potency relative to midazolam (MDZ:drug)
Diazepam (Valium)	25–40	0.3 mg/kg, 4–40 mg/day	1:7
Lorazepam (Ativan)	10–20	0.05 mg/kg, 2–6 mg/day	1:0.5
Midazolam (Versed (USA); Hypnoval (UK))	2–6(15–26)	0.15 mg/kg	–
Chlordiazepoxide (Librium (USA); Librium, Tropium (UK))	5–30	15–100 mg/day	–
Alprazolam (Xanax)	10–15	0.75–4.0 mg/day	1:1
Clonazepam (Klonopin (USA); Rivotril (UK))	18–50	0.5–4.0 mg/day	–
Triazolam (Halcion)	2.5	0.125–0.25 mg/day	–
Temapzepam (Restoril)	10–40	15–30 mg/day	–
Oxazepam (Serax)	5–20	30–120 mg/day	–
Clorazepate (Tranxene)	50–100 (metabolite)	15–60 mg/day	–

6–11 mL/kg/min for midazolam to 0.2–0.5 mL/kg/min for diazepam (Table 25.3). Diazepam is metabolized to active metabolites with slow elimination, whereas midazolam metabolites are cleared rapidly. These properties account for the shorter context-sensitive half-time of midazolam. The recovery profile from a single intravenous dose of the two drugs is, by contrast, similar, as it is determined not by elimination but by redistribution. Lorazepam is metabolized primarily by glucuronide conjugation, a pathway that is less affected by age (slowed elimination), enzyme inhibition/induction, liver dysfunction, and genetic polymorphism than the elimination of the former two drugs.

Mechanism of action

Benzodiazepines bind to a specific site on $GABA_A$ receptors containing the γ subunit. Binding of an agonist to the benzodiazepine-binding site on the $GABA_A$ receptor increases the affinity of the receptor to GABA. Benzodiazepine-insensitive $GABA_A$ receptors are rare (usually containing the α_4 or the α_6 subunit). Recently, the different clinical effects of benzodiazepines have been traced to interactions with $GABA_A$ receptors containing specific γ subunits using site-directed mutagenesis in mice. Sedation, amnesia, ataxia, and some seizure protection are mediated by receptors containing the α_1 subunit, as the α_1H101R mutation eliminates these actions, whereas α_2 subunit-containing receptors mediate anxiolysis and myorelaxation. These insights should allow the design of more specific drugs targeted to very selective effects with minimal side effects.

Clinical effects

Until the introduction of propofol, benzodiazepines were the most commonly used drugs to produce sedation and amnesia in the perioperative, interventional, and intensive care settings. They make excellent sedatives, given their profile of hypnotic, amnestic, anticonvulsant, and myorelaxant properties. The choice of benzodiazepine is guided primarily by pharmacokinetic parameters and cost. Midazolam is the drug of choice when intravenous administration (almost immediate onset) and fast elimination are desirable (e.g. ambulatory surgical setting). Typically, intravenous midazolam is titrated to the desired effect (adequate sedation or dysarthria). Administration via the oral or the rectal route (in the pediatric population) requires that the dose be determined empirically (0.3–0.7 mg/kg); the time to effect is approximately 20 min. Nasal administration of midazolam is also possible. Benzodiazepines can also be used for the induction of general anesthesia and maintenance of hypnosis and amnesia. Tolerance and dependence occur with chronic administration.

Cardiovascular and respiratory effects

Benzodiazepines have minimal cardiovascular and respiratory effects. They do cause respiratory depression, however, particularly in patients with chronic obstructive pulmonary disease. They have marked synergistic interactions with other respiratory depressants (volatile anesthetics, opioids). Induction doses of benzodiazepines have modest hemodynamic effects that are attributable to a decrease of systemic vascular resistance. However, as the stress of endotracheal intubation and surgery is not significantly mitigated by benzodiazepines, adjuvant anesthetics are frequently co-administered. Combination with opioids has supra-additive hemodynamic effects.

Benzodiazepines alone cause minimal respiratory depression, but they have marked synergistic interactions with other respiratory depressants, such as volatile anesthetics and opioids.

Other effects

Benzodiazepines reduce the $CMRO_2$ and cerebral blood flow, and suppress rapid eye movement (REM) sleep. The sleep-like state induced by benzodiazepines differs in its EEG characteristics from nonREM sleep. Overall, benzodiazepines are remarkably safe drugs with a high margin of safety (compared to barbiturates, for example). They are also free of allergenic effects and do not suppress the adrenal gland. Undesirable effects of acutely administered benzodiazepines (respiratory depression, prolonged amnesia) can be reversed with the selective competitive antagonist flumazenil. Flumazenil produces withdrawal (seizures, confusion, agitation) in the presence of physical dependence, and should also be avoided in patients with seizure disorders. Benzodiazepines with a faster recovery profile than midazolam are undergoing clinical trials.

NONBENZODIAZEPINE HYPNOTICS

Zolpidem is an imidazopyridine agonist of the benzodiazepine-binding site of the $GABA_A$ receptor. Other nonbenzodiazepine agonists of benzodiazepine receptors are zolpicone and zaleplon. Zolpidem has a preferential sedative hypnotic effect. It displays high selectivity for receptors containing the α_1 subunit and, unlike benzodiazepines, has little effect on the stages of sleep in normal human subjects and induces markedly less tolerance.

Over the years numerous drugs with general CNS depressant properties have been developed that can induce profound hypnosis. The mechanism of action of most of them involves the $GABA_A$ receptor. Their use has decreased markedly with the advent of the drugs discussed in the preceding sections. Chloral hydrate was widely used in the past to induce sedation in children undergoing uncomfortable procedures. After oral administration chloral hydrate is rapidly metabolized to trichloroethanol, the active compound which acts on $GABA_A$ receptors. Other drugs in this category include paraldehyde, meprobamate, and ethchlorvynol, which are now rarely used.

KETAMINE

Chemistry and formulation

Ketamine, a weak base, is a partially water-soluble arylcyclohexylamine derivative with a pK_a of 7.5 (see Fig. 25.2). It is currently formulated as a racemic mixture of two enantiomers in aqueous solution with sodium chloride and benzethonium chloride. The (*S*)(+)-enantiomer is about three times more potent than the (*R*)(–)-enantiomer in producing anesthesia, and is associated with fewer psychoactive side effects. It therefore has a higher therapeutic index, and is available for use in some countries. There are no apparent differences between the enantiomers in their cardiovascular effects in humans, although some differences have been detected in vitro.

Pharmacokinetics

Following an intravenous injection of ketamine, its plasma concentration shows rapid distribution (half-time 16 minutes) and elimination (half-time 3 hours; see Table 25.2). Ketamine is extremely lipophilic (5–10 times more lipid soluble than thiopental), which leads to a high V_{dss}. As a result of its lipophilicity and its pK_a near physiologic pH, it is rapidly taken up into the brain and has a fast onset of action. The rapid elimination of ketamine is a result of its high clearance, which approximates hepatic blood flow. Ketamine is metabolized by hepatic microsomal enzymes by *N*-demethylation (to norketamine) and hydroxylation to derivatives that are glucuronidated and excreted in the urine. Norketamine has significantly less pharmacologic activity than the parent compound, but may nevertheless be a clinically significant metabolite. The (*S*)(+)-enantiomer of ketamine is cleared more rapidly than the (*R*)(–)-enantiomer, leading to a shorter duration of action for the same dose. Redistribution from highly perfused tissues to lean tissue is responsible for its short duration of action, which is unaffected by hepatic or renal dysfunction following a single dose. Cumulative drug effects can occur with repeated doses or continuous infusion, as ketamine is ultimately dependent on hepatic metabolism for clearance. Chronic administration of ketamine can induce the hepatic enzymes involved in its metabolism, which may lead to tolerance on repeated exposures; pharmacodynamic tolerance may also occur. Ketamine is not extensively bound to plasma proteins.

Mechanism of action

The general anesthetic effects of ketamine result from inhibition of excitatory synaptic transmission by noncompetitive antagonism of the *N*-methyl-D-aspartate (NMDA) receptor, an excitatory ionotropic glutamate receptor subtype (Fig. 25.8; see Chapter 20). Ketamine is relatively selective for inhibition of NMDA receptors, although it also interacts with opioid receptors, muscarinic and nicotinic cholinergic receptors, monoaminergic receptors, and voltage-gated Ca^{2+} and Na^+ channels. Its stereoselectivity in producing anesthesia is also observed in its effects at NMDA receptors and at μ and κ opioid receptors. *N*-methyl-D-aspartate receptor inhibition would be of theoretic benefit in treating glutamate-mediated neurotoxicity. However, ketamine and other noncompetitive NMDA receptor antagonists have neurotoxic effects in several limbic structures when given continuously for several days to rats.

Ketamine is unusual among intravenous anesthetics in not producing its effects primarily through interactions with the $GABA_A$ receptor. The anesthetic effects of ketamine also differ from other agents clinically, and have been described as 'dissociative anesthesia' because of electroencephalographic evidence of dissociation between the thalamocortical and limbic systems. Electroencephalographic activity in the thalamus and cortex exhibit marked synchronous δ-wave bursts, whereas the ventral hippocampus and amygdala exhibit θ waves characteristic of

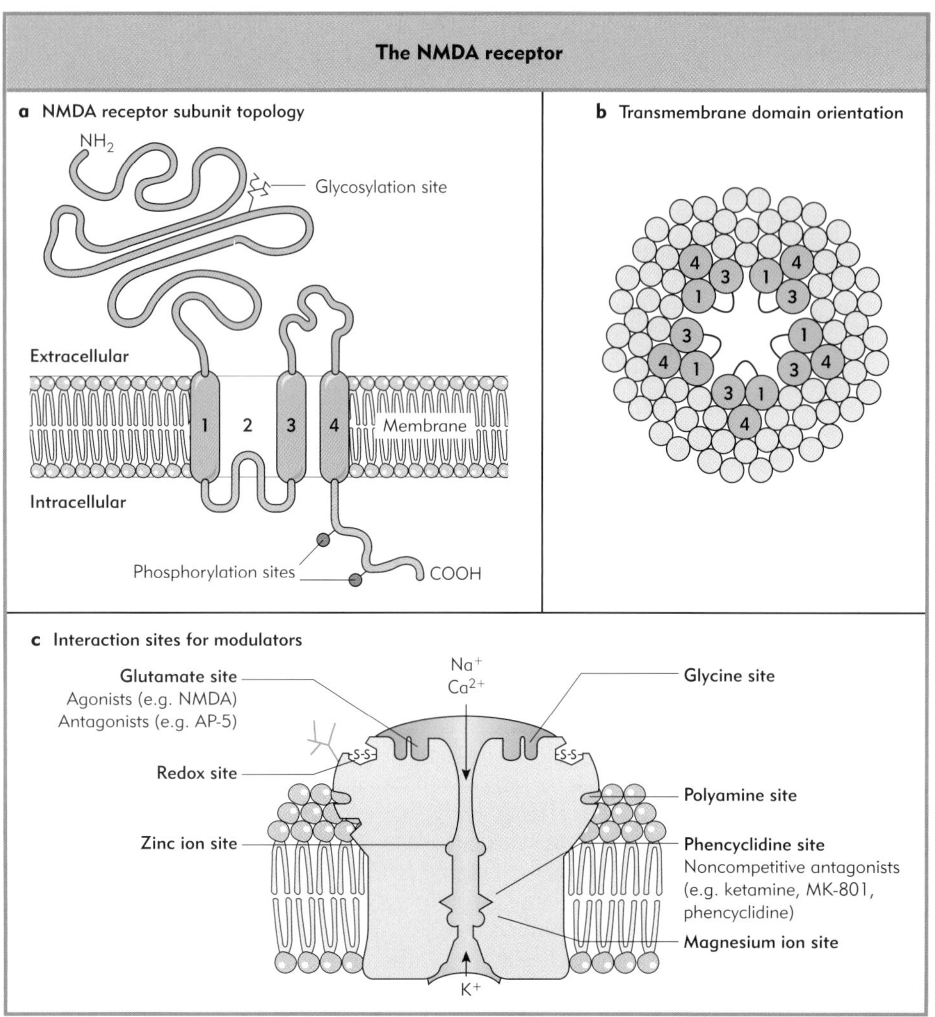

Figure 25.8 The glutamate receptor family. (a) The glutamate receptor family comprises three distinct subgroups: the AMPA receptors (hetero-oligomers of GluR1 to GluR4), the kainate receptors (homo- or hetero-oligomers of GluR5-GluR7, KA1 and KA2) and the NMDA receptors (hetero-oligomers containing both the NR1 and the NR2 (NR2A-D) subunits). AMPA and kainate receptors are frequently grouped together as nonNMDA receptors but have distinct physiologic functions. A typical glutamate receptor subunit has three transmembrane segments and a fourth hydrophobic segment (designated 2) that loops into the membrane without traversing it. Mutation studies of GluR1 to GluR7 and of the NR subunits suggest that this loop is the putative channel-lining segment that defines the ionic permeability of the channels. Blockade of the NMDA-type of glutamate receptors by dizocilpine (MK-801), phencyclidine, and ketamine occurs through binding to a site that overlaps the Mg^{2+} site in the pore. The C-terminal domain undergoes phosphorylation, which regulates channel activity and mediates interactions with intracellular anchoring proteins. (b) Transmembrane hydrophobic segments interact to form a central ion-conducting pore lined by the second hydrophobic segments. The stoichiometry of the hetero-oligomeric glutamate receptors is not known, but may be four or five (as shown), by analogy with the homologous nicotinic cholinergic receptor. (c) The NMDA receptor gates a cation channel that is permeable to Na^+, Ca^{2+}, and K^+ and is gated by Mg^{2+} in a voltage-dependent fashion. Agonists (glutamate, NMDA) and the co-agonist glycine, required for full activation, bind to the extracellular domain. The typical nonNMDA receptor also gates a cation channel that in the presence of the GluR2 subunit has a low permeability for Ca^{2+} and is not affected by Mg^{2+}.

arousal. Dissociative anesthesia is characterized by intense analgesia, amnesia, and a cataleptic-like state of unresponsiveness with occasional purposeful movements. The analgesic effects of ketamine, which occur at subanesthetic doses, result from inhibition of excitatory glutamatergic transmission at both spinal and supraspinal sites. Ketamine possesses only modest affinity for opioid receptors ($\mu > \delta$ and κ), and its central analgesic effects are not antagonized by naloxone.

Despite its undesirable psychotomimetic effects, ketamine has clinically useful characteristics including analgesia, bronchodilation, and reduced cardiac and respiratory depression.

Clinical effects

Ketamine possesses a number of properties that limit its routine clinical use, although some can be advantageous in specific situations. The psychedelic effects of ketamine, which is structurally similar to phencyclidine (PCP, angel dust), are therapeutically undesirable and a source for potential abuse. Emergence reactions, including excitement, confusion, euphoria, fear, vivid dreaming, and hallucinations, occur most frequently during the first hour of emergence. The incidence of emergence reactions (10–30% in adult patients) is lower in children and elderly patients and with use of the (S)(+)-enantiomer, and can be reduced by co-administration of benzodiazepines with a lower dose of ketamine.

The sympathomimetic properties of ketamine give it an important role in the induction of anesthesia under specific conditions. Ketamine is useful in the rapid induction of anesthesia in hemodynamically unstable patients who have acute hypovolemia, hypotension, cardiomyopathy, constrictive pericarditis, or cardiac tamponade, and in patients who have congenital heart disease (with the potential for right-to-left shunting) or bronchospastic disease. Ketamine may be the agent of choice for rapid induction of anesthesia in patients who have acute asthma or cardiac tamponade. Ketamine is also effective by intramuscular injection and can be used for the induction of anesthesia in children and uncooperative patients without necessitating intravenous access. A unique advantage of ketamine is the versatility of administration routes: intravenous, intramuscular, oral, or rectal. The efficacy of epidural or intrathecal ketamine is controversial. Subanesthetic doses of ketamine by intermittent bolus (0.1–0.5 mg/kg IV) or by continuous infusion (10–20 μg/min/kg body weight) can be used to provide intravenous sedation and intense analgesia. These properties are beneficial in short painful procedures (e.g. debridement, dressing changes, skin grafting, closed reduction of bone fractures, biopsies, etc.) and as a supplement to regional anesthesia, both during placement of painful blocks and for inadequate or resolving blocks. It is also gaining acceptance as an adjuvant for the treatment of refractory cancer-related pain. Ketamine combined with a benzodiazepine is also useful for the sedation of pediatric patients for procedures outside the operating room (e.g. cardiac catheterization, dressing changes, radiation therapy, diagnostic radiology etc.). Ketamine has been used in clinical situations requiring high inspired oxygen concentrations (e.g. one-lung anesthesia), and in combination with propofol by infusion with minimal cardiorespiratory depression or psychedelic effects. Despite its disturbing psychoactive properties, ketamine possesses several clinically useful characteristics that promote its use, including analgesia, bronchodilation, and reduced cardiopulmonary depression.

Cardiovascular and respiratory effects

The cardiovascular effects of ketamine result primarily from stimulation of the sympathetic nervous system by a direct effect on the CNS, resulting in tachycardia and hypertension (see Table 25.2). Ketamine increases atrioventricular conduction time and has a direct myocardial depressant effect; these effects are usually masked by the sympathomimetic effect. In patients who have depleted catecholamine stores or exhausted sympathetic nervous system compensatory mechanisms (i.e. critically ill patients, or patients in shock), ketamine may have significant hypotensive effects. Ketamine inhibits catecholamine reuptake by both neuronal and extraneuronal sites and potentiates norepinephrine (noradrenaline) release from sympathetic ganglia, which may contribute to stimulation of the sympathetic nervous system. Both enantiomers of ketamine are potent M1 muscarinic receptor antagonists, which may contribute to its tachycardic effects. The stimulatory cardiovascular effects of ketamine include increases in systemic and pulmonary arterial vascular resistance and pressure, heart rate, cardiac output, myocardial oxygen consumption (MVO_2), coronary blood flow, and cardiac work. These effects are in contrast to the effects of other anesthetic drugs, which produce either no change or hypotension and myocardial depression. The hemodynamic effects of ketamine are not related to dose, and are usually less pronounced following a second dose. The cardiac stimulation produced by ketamine can be blocked by a number of pharmacologic methods, including α- and β-adrenoceptor antagonists, clonidine, benzodiazepines, and volatile anesthetics. Ketamine is relatively contraindicated in patients who have coronary artery disease (it increases myocardial work and MVO_2) or pulmonary hypertension (it increases pulmonary vascular resistance). Equianesthetic doses of the (*S*)(+)-enantiomer may allow for decreased cardiovascular side effects as well as a quicker recovery (because of the reduced dose and more rapid metabolism).

Ketamine does not appreciably depress the ventilatory response to carbon dioxide. Respiratory rate may decrease transiently immediately following induction of anesthesia; apnea rarely occurs following rapid administration. Upper airway reflexes and muscle tone are maintained, which is beneficial during deep sedation. However, ketamine stimulates salivary and tracheobronchial secretions, which can lead to cough and laryngospasm. For this reason, an antisialagogue is recommended in conjunction with ketamine; glycopyrrolate (glycopyrronium) is preferred to atropine or scopolamine (hyoscine) because of its lack of CNS effects. The bronchodilatory effect of ketamine makes it extremely useful in patients who have reactive airway disease or active bronchospasm. The mechanism of this effect is uncertain, but may involve inhibition of catecholamine uptake, anticholinergic effects (muscarinic and/or nicotinic), and/or direct smooth muscle relaxation. Ketamine may be unique in its ability to maintain the functional residual capacity (FRC) upon induction of anesthesia, possibly owing to the maintenance of skeletal muscle tone. Ketamine can stimulate uterine contractions in the first trimester of pregnancy, but has variable effects in the third trimester.

Other effects

Ketamine is a potent cerebral vasodilator that increases cerebral blood flow (more than $CMRO_2$), $CMRO_2$, and intracranial pressure in spontaneously breathing patients, which has made it relatively contraindicated in neurosurgical procedures. However, recent studies indicate that the increase in intracranial pressure can be attenuated by controlled ventilation, hypocapnia, or prior administration of diazepam, thiopental, or propofol. The cerebrovascular effects appear to be direct. Ketamine also produces mydriasis, nystagmus, and excitatory CNS effects, evident in the development of slow-wave θ activity on EEG. However, ketamine does not appear to decrease the seizure threshold in patients who have seizure disorders, and has anticonvulsant efficacy in animals. Ketamine in low doses may control neurogenic pain and reverse the 'wind-up' phenomenon (Chapter 23). Ketamine enhances the amplitude of somatosensory evoked potentials but suppresses the amplitudes of auditory and visual evoked potentials. Ketamine does not impair hepatic or renal function, and its elimination is not significantly altered by hepatic or renal dysfunction. It does not evoke histamine release and allergic reactions are rare, although a transient erythematous rash is not uncommon. Ketamine enhances the action of nondepolarizing neuromuscular blockers, possibly by blocking nicotinic receptors. In contrast to phencyclidine, it does not significantly prolong the action of succinylcholine by inhibition of plasma cholinesterase. Ketamine can increase muscle tone but does not trigger malignant hyperthermia.

ANESTHETIC NEUROTOXICITY

Anesthetic-induced unconsciousness has been traditionally regarded as a fully reversible drug-induced condition without any intrinsic ill effects on the central nervous system. Recent laboratory reports have begun to challenge this complacent assumption. Based on the observation that drugs that increase $GABA_A$-ergic inhibition and/or inhibit NMDA receptors (e.g. ethanol) induce widespread apoptosis in the developing rodent brain, recent studies report widespread neurodegeneration and persistent learning deficits in rats exposed in the early postnatal period to anesthetic doses of midazolam, nitrous oxide, and isoflurane. The most severe effects were induced by co-administration of all three drugs. The importance of these findings for clinical practice is unclear at present.

Key references

Hughes MA, Glass PSA, Jacobs JR. Context-sensitive half-time in multicompartment models for anesthetic drugs. Anesthesiology 1992;76:334–41.

Jurd R, Arras M, Lambert S et al. General anesthetic actions in vivo strongly attenuated by a point mutation in the GABA(A) receptor $beta_3$ subunit. FASEB J, 2003;17:250–2.

Kiersey DK, Bickford RG, Faulconer A Jr. Electroencephalographic patterns produced by thiopental sodium during surgical operations: description and classification. Br J Anaesth. 1951;23:141–52.

Reynolds DS, Rosahl TW, Cirone J et al. Sedation and anesthesia mediated by distinct $GABA_A$ receptor isoforms. J Neurosci. 2003;23:8608–17.

Saidman LJ. Uptake, distribution and elimination of barbiturates. In: Eger EJ, ed. Anesthetic uptake and action. Baltimore, MD: Williams &Wilkins; 1974:264–84.

Further reading

Brain Resuscitation Clinical Trial Study Group. Randomized clinical study of thiopental loading in comatose survivors of cardiac arrest. N Engl J Med. 1986;314:397–403.

Bray RJ. The propofol infusion syndrome in infants and children: can we predict the risk? Curr Opin Anesthesiol. 2002;15:339–42.

Hirota K, Lambert DG. Ketamine: its mechanism(s) of action and unusual clinical uses. Br J Anaesth. 1996;77:441–4.

Jevtovic-Todorovic V et al. Early exposure to common anesthetic agents causes widespread neurodegeneration in the developing rat brain and persistent learning deficits. J Neurosci. 2003;23:876–82.

Mohler H, Fritschy JM, Rudolph U. A new benzodiazepine pharmacology. J Pharmacol Exp Ther. 2002;300:2–8.

Olsen RW. Barbiturates. Int Anesth Clin. 1988;26:254–61.

Smith I, White PF, Nathanson M, Gouldson R. Propofol. An update on its clinical use. Anesthesiology 1994;81:1005–43.

White PF, Schütter J, Shafer A et al. Comparative pharmacology of the ketamine isomers. Br J Anaesth. 1985;57:197–203.

White PF, Way WL, Trevor AJ. Ketamine: its pharmacology and therapeutic uses. Anesthesiology 1982;56:119–36.

Chapter 26

Inhalational anesthetic agents

Ian Smith

The birth of modern anesthesia dates back to the public use of ether by William Morton in Boston on Friday 16 October 1846, and its earlier use by Crawford Long in 1842. Meanwhile, Horace Wells successfully used nitrous oxide in dental anesthesia in 1844. Most of the modern volatile anesthetics are direct descendants of ether, and nitrous oxide remains in use. Despite the increased popularity of intravenous anesthesia in the early 1990s, inhaled anesthetics are currently used in the majority of cases.

PHYSICAL PROPERTIES

Inhalational anesthetics are administered in gaseous form. The five currently in use volatile anesthetics are liquids at room temperature, but readily evaporate. Nitrous oxide and xenon are gases at room temperature. The physical properties of these agents are shown in Table 26.1.

Solubility in blood

The solubility of inhalational anesthetics in blood, as indicated by their blood:gas partition coefficient, determines their speed of onset and, to a significant degree, the rate of recovery. Relatively insoluble agents act more rapidly, as a smaller quantity

Table 26.1 Physical properties of the inhalational anesthetics considered in this chapter

	Halothane	Enflurane	Isoflurane	Desflurane	Sevoflurane	Nitrous oxide	Xenon
Boiling point (°C)	50.2	56.5	48.5	22.8	58.5	−88.5	−108.1
Vapor pressure @ 20°C (mmHg)	243	175	238	669	120	–	–
Molecular weight (Da)	197.4	184.5	184.5	168	200	44	131
Specific gravity (g/mL)	1.87	1.52	1.50	1.47	1.50	–	–
Blood:gas partition coefficient	2.4	1.9	1.4	0.42	0.66	0.47	0.115
Oil:gas partition coefficient	224	98.5	90.8	18.7	53.4	1.4	1.9
MAC (vol%)	0.75	1.7	1.15	7	2.05	104	71
Metabolism (%, approx.)	20	2	0.2	0.02	5	0	0

is removed by dissolving in blood, leaving a higher alveolar concentration to facilitate induction. A more intuitive way of thinking of this is to regard solubility in blood as the inhalational equivalent of volume of distribution. The effect of solubility is considered further in Chapter 27.

The blood:gas partition coefficient of inhalational anesthetics determines their speed of onset and, to a significant degree, the rate of recovery.

Lipid solubility

The solubility of inhalational anesthetics in lipids, as indicated by their oil:gas partition coefficient, correlates reasonably well with their anesthetic potency, according to the Meyer–Overton relationship (Fig. 26.1). This association has been used to suggest that inhalational anesthetics act on a hydrophobic target. However, the use of logarithmic scales makes the correlation appear stronger than it actually is, and alternative mechanisms of action have subsequently been postulated (see Chapter 24).

The oil:gas partition coefficient of inhalational anesthetics correlates with their anesthetic potency.

Structure

The structures of the five volatile anesthetics are shown in Figure 26.2. Halothane is a halogenated alkane and therefore has somewhat different properties (see below) from the other agents, which are all halogenated methyl ethers. Enflurane and isoflurane are structural isomers of each other (they have the same chemical formula and atomic weight), whereas desflurane has just a single atom substitution. All of the volatile anesthetics, except sevoflurane, have an asymmetrical carbon atom and so can exist as stereo- (optical) isomers, with the commercial preparations being racemic mixtures. The individual stereoisomers of some volatile anesthetics differ in potency for some, but not all, of their effects, providing further insight into the possible mechanisms of anesthetic action (Chapter 24). However, these differences are not sufficient to justify the commercial development of pure isomers at present.

Vapor pressure

Volatile anesthetics are liquid at room temperature, but are administered as a gas. The saturated vapor pressure at room temperature for most of the agents is about one-third of an atmosphere, well above the clinically useful dose. An appropriate dose is delivered by diluting a quantity of saturated vapor with a larger volume of carrier gas in a variable-bypass vaporizer. This is achieved by splitting the carrier gas into a fraction that

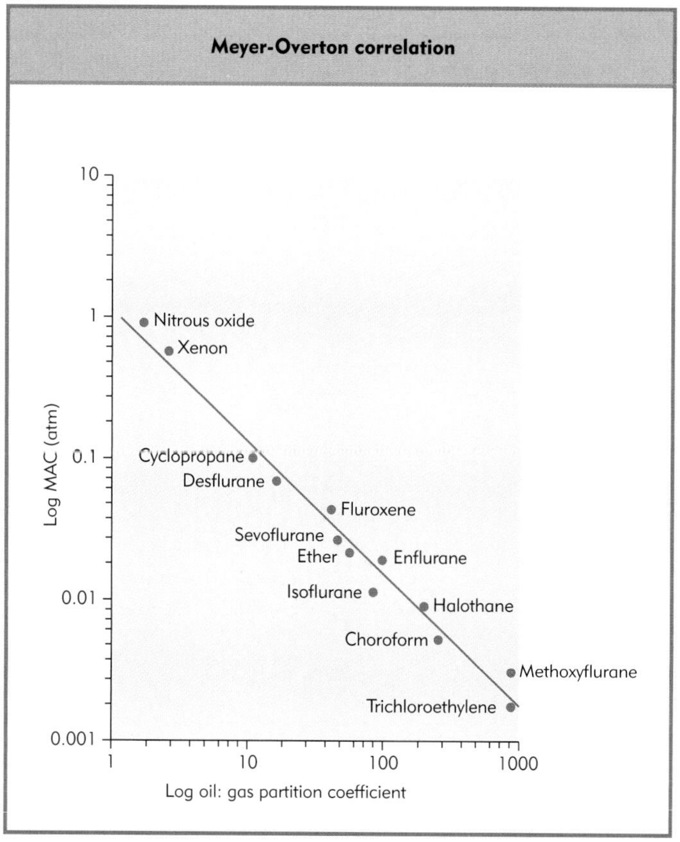

Meyer-Overton correlation

Log MAC (atm): 10, 1, 0.1, 0.01, 0.001

Nitrous oxide
Xenon
Cyclopropane
Desflurane
Fluroxene
Sevoflurane
Ether
Enflurane
Isoflurane
Halothane
Choroform
Methoxyflurane
Trichloroethylene

Log oil: gas partition coefficient: 1, 10, 100, 1000

Figure 26.1 The Meyer–Overton correlation between anesthetic potency and oil:gas partition coefficient for inhaled anesthetics that have been used in humans. Note the logarithmic scales.

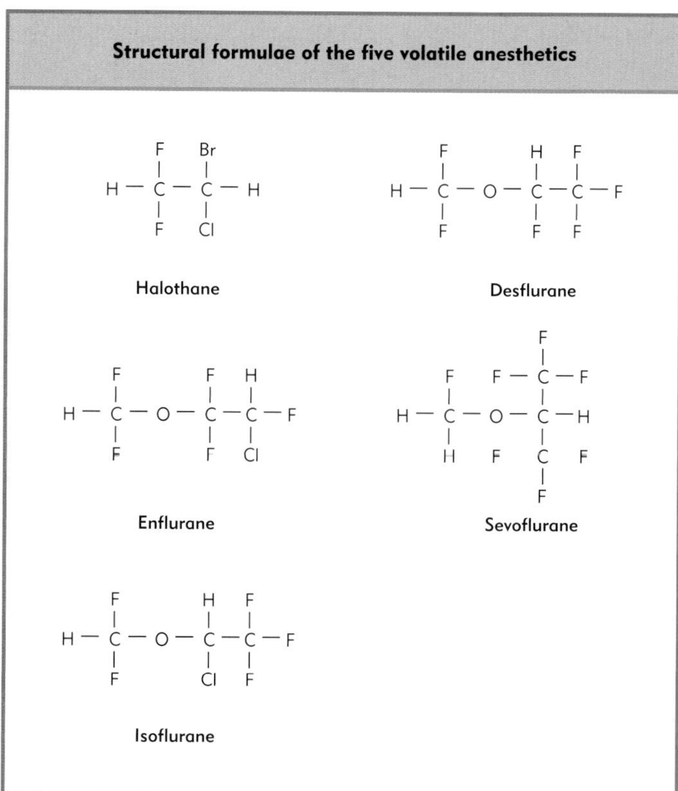

Figure 26.2 The structural formulae of the five volatile anesthetics. Halothane is an alkane, whereas the others are methyl ethers. Enflurane and isoflurane are structural isomers, desflurane differs from isoflurane by a F substituted for a Cl, and sevoflurane has a CF_3 substituted for a Cl and a H substituted for a F.

passes over the liquid anesthetic, thereby becoming saturated with vapor, and a larger portion that bypasses the liquid and subsequently dilutes the vapor. Altering the splitting ratio (varying the bypass fraction) changes the dose or delivered concentration. The vaporizer is also temperature compensated to maintain a constant vapor concentration, with changes in vapor pressure occurring due to variation in ambient temperature and due to the cooling which occurs secondary to vaporization. Modern vaporizers also have a large surface area (produced by a wick) to ensure that the vapor remains saturated in the evaporation chamber.

Because the final delivered concentration depends on the vapor pressure of the anesthetic, vaporizers are agent specific. Filling the vaporizer with the wrong agent could result in under- or overdosage. An overdose will also occur with mixtures, as all agents present will be vaporized. Keyed filling systems and infrared agent analyzers both guard against these eventualities.

Desflurane has a much higher vapor pressure because its boiling point is close to room temperature. A conventional vaporizer would not be able to cope with the large changes in vapor pressure resulting from small variations in ambient temperature, and would also be unable to supply sufficient latent heat for the evaporation of an adequate amount of desflurane. The desflurane vaporizer (TEC 6) is therefore radically different and uses an electrical current to evaporate the drug, which is then metered as a gas. A pressure transducer compensates for changes in temperature and fresh gas flow, with back-up systems for safety. Functionally, this device is used like a conventional vaporizer, although it does require a mains electrical connection and a brief period to warm up before use. Unlike all other vaporizers, it has a low-agent alarm and can be refilled while it is in use.

POTENCY

The determination of anesthetic potency has been complicated by the fact that the vaporizer dial setting does not necessarily reflect the concentration in the breathing circuit, alveoli, blood, or site of anesthetic action (Chapter 27). This is less problematic now that agent analyzers give a reliable approximation of blood concentration, although this may still differ from the effect site concentration, except at equilibrium. The concept of minimum alveolar concentration (MAC) was developed in the 1960s as a measure of the 50% effective dose (ED_{50}) for a given endpoint under conditions designed to ensure reasonable equilibration between the inspired concentration and that in various compartments, including the brain. Thus MAC determinations require a constant concentration to be delivered for at least 15 minutes, and the endpoint used is 'gross purposeful movement' in response to a surgical stimulus. A number of factors can alter MAC (Table 26.2) and these need to be controlled for in MAC determinations and allowed for when deciding on an appropriate anesthetic administration for an individual.

Limitations of MAC

Although MAC is useful in defining relative potency, it has significant limitations. It may be difficult to decide whether a given subject responded sufficiently for this to be termed 'gross purposeful movement'. Given that MAC is usually determined in small numbers of subjects, a difference in the response of just one individual may alter the result. Clinically, it must be remembered that, at MAC, half of all subjects will respond; ensuring that 90–95% of subjects do not respond requires about 1.25–1.3 times MAC. Furthermore, the measured end-expired anesthetic concentration will not equate to MAC at times of changes in drug delivery, where effect site delay prevents proper equilibration.

MAC measures somatic response and not lack of awareness. It is thought that MAC assesses the effect of inhaled anesthetics on spinally mediated reflexes, as destroying the higher centers in animals does not alter its value. MAC is therefore more representative of the 'analgesic' component of anesthesia. A guide to the anesthetic requirement for preventing consciousness (the hypnotic component) is given by MAC-awake. This is determined by allowing the anesthetic concentration to gradually decline and noting the level at which a response first occurs. MAC-awake is typically about half the value of MAC. This may explain why awareness is relatively uncommon in patients who are not 'paralyzed' and who are therefore able to move if anesthesia becomes too 'light'.

Table 26.2 Factors that alter the value of minimal alveolar concentration (MAC)

Factors that decrease MAC	Factors that increase MAC
Drugs α_2 Agonists Barbiturates Benzodiazepines Opioid analgesia Other anesthetics **Other factors** Increasing age Hypothermia Hypoxia Hypotension Pregnancy	**Drugs** Alcohol (chronic) **Other factors** Young age Hyperthermia

MAC-awake is typically about half the value of MAC.

ADVANTAGES AND DISADVANTAGES OF INHALATIONAL ANESTHETICS

Inhalational anesthetics have remained popular because of their relative ease of use and our considerable familiarity with them. Their results are predictable, as there is little metabolism or accumulation, even after prolonged administration. The widespread availability of end-tidal agent analyzers provides further monitoring of drug concentration, in particular leading to more efficient administration at low fresh gas flows and guarding against failures in drug delivery (e.g. disconnection, empty vaporizer). Significant tolerance to the effects of inhalational anesthetics is rare and they do not cause anaphylaxis. In addition to causing unconsciousness, these drugs provide a useful degree of muscle relaxation and somewhat attenuate the responses to noxious stimuli. They can be used in most clinical situations, and specific advantages are discussed under the individual agents.

Inhaled anesthetics can all trigger malignant hyperthermia (see Chapter 10) in susceptible individuals, and this is really the only absolute contraindication to their use. They all appear to contribute to postoperative nausea and vomiting (PONV), and this effect appears to be dose-dependent. However, PONV is a multifactorial entity, and can often be reduced to acceptable levels by a variety of measures.

Inhalational anesthetics do require specialized equipment for their delivery and for waste gas scavenging, although this is widely provided. Significant training is required to use these agents, which have a far smaller margin between safe and lethal doses (therapeutic index) than that of most other modern drugs. The most obvious toxicity is from cardiorespiratory depression. The various anesthetics differ in the patterns of response produced, and these are discussed under the individual agents. Most other forms of toxicity are related to metabolism or interaction with carbon dioxide adsorbents.

METABOLISM

Inhaled anesthetics are metabolized to a far lesser degree than most other drugs, including other anesthetics, and metabolism has no significant impact on their pharmacokinetics. Halothane undergoes the most metabolism and desflurane the least (see Table 26.1). Although metabolism is not necessarily harmful, volatile anesthetic metabolism may lead to toxicity.

Halothane hepatitis

About 20% of administered halothane is metabolized to trifluoroacetic acid, chloride, and bromide. Usually this is harmless, although subclinical and self-limiting hepatic dysfunction, as indicated by abnormal liver enzymes, is not uncommon. The condition is not unique to halothane and may be the result of reactive metabolites, exacerbated by reductions in hepatic blood flow. Rarely fulminant hepatic necrosis occurs, with an incidence of 1:10 000–1:35 000.

Fulminant hepatic necrosis can occur as a result of halothane metabolites, with an incidence of 1:10 000–1:35 000.

This halothane hepatitis appears more common in middle-aged obese women, and is also associated with multiple halothane exposures. It carries a high mortality. It is now thought that trifluoroacetyl–halide compounds can react with liver proteins to form a hapten–protein conjugate, to which a few susceptible individuals form antibodies capable of damaging hepatocytes. Such antibodies have been detected in up to 70% of cases of halothane hepatitis.

The substantial metabolism of halothane means that immune sensitization (and subsequent damage) is more likely than with other inhaled anesthetics. However, enflurane, isoflurane, and desflurane (but not sevoflurane) all form metabolites which are identical to, or immunologically cross-reactive with, those of halothane (Fig. 26.3). Once the patient is sensitized to halothane, hepatitis can occur (and has been reported) after each of these other anesthetics, with an incidence that appears to be correlated with their degree of metabolism.

Fluoride toxicity

Methoxyflurane, which is significantly biotransformed to produce inorganic fluoride ions, was nephrotoxic, although toxicity did not occur if the serum fluoride concentration remained below about 50 μmol/L. This value has subsequently come to be believed to represent a 'threshold' for nephrotoxicity. Enflurane is also metabolized to fluoride, but the fluoride concentration usually remains well below this threshold, lending further support to the theory. Although enflurane has often been said to be contraindicated in patients with pre-existing renal failure or for prolonged use, there are few confirmed reports of nephrotoxicity. In contrast, serum fluoride concentrations exceed 50 μmol/L in about 7% of patients following sevoflurane anesthesia, yet clinically significant nephrotoxicity has never been reported with this agent, despite its use in more than 45 million patients. It now appears that the mechanism of methoxyflurane nephrotoxicity was more complex than a simple increase in serum fluoride; indeed, other forms of fluoride poisoning do not produce the same clinical picture, despite far higher serum fluoride concentrations. Intrarenal fluoride production or the actions of some other metabolic product are possible causes, and the 'threshold' hypothesis of fluoride toxicity has largely been discounted.

INTERACTION WITH SODA LIME

Carbon monoxide

In the presence of extremely dry soda lime, desflurane, enflurane, and isoflurane are degraded to produce carbon monoxide. The amount produced is dose dependent (and so proportional to MAC) and can result in carboxyhemoglobin levels reaching more than 30%. As sufficient drying is only really produced by leaving fresh gas flowing through an out-of-use circle-absorber system for several hours, the problem is largely solved by turning the anesthetic machine off when not in use. Halothane and sevoflurane produce little, if any, carbon monoxide.

In the presence of extremely dry soda lime, desflurane, enflurane, and isoflurane are degraded to produce carbon monoxide.

Compound A

Under clinical conditions, soda lime degrades sevoflurane into compound A (Fig. 26.4). The quantities produced are proportional to sevoflurane concentration and absorbent temperature and inversely related to fresh gas flow. Compound A is nephrotoxic in rats at about 50 parts per million (ppm), concentrations similar to those produced under some clinical circumstances.

Although some workers have detected what they considered to be subtle markers of renal toxicity (enzymuria, proteinuria, glycosuria) following prolonged high-dose low-flow sevoflurane exposure in volunteers, others have been unable to reproduce their findings. In addition, similar markers have been detected after anesthesia with isoflurane, which is not degraded to compound A. As isoflurane has an excellent safety record, these chemical markers presumably have little clinical relevance. Despite its extensive study, including under conditions of pro-

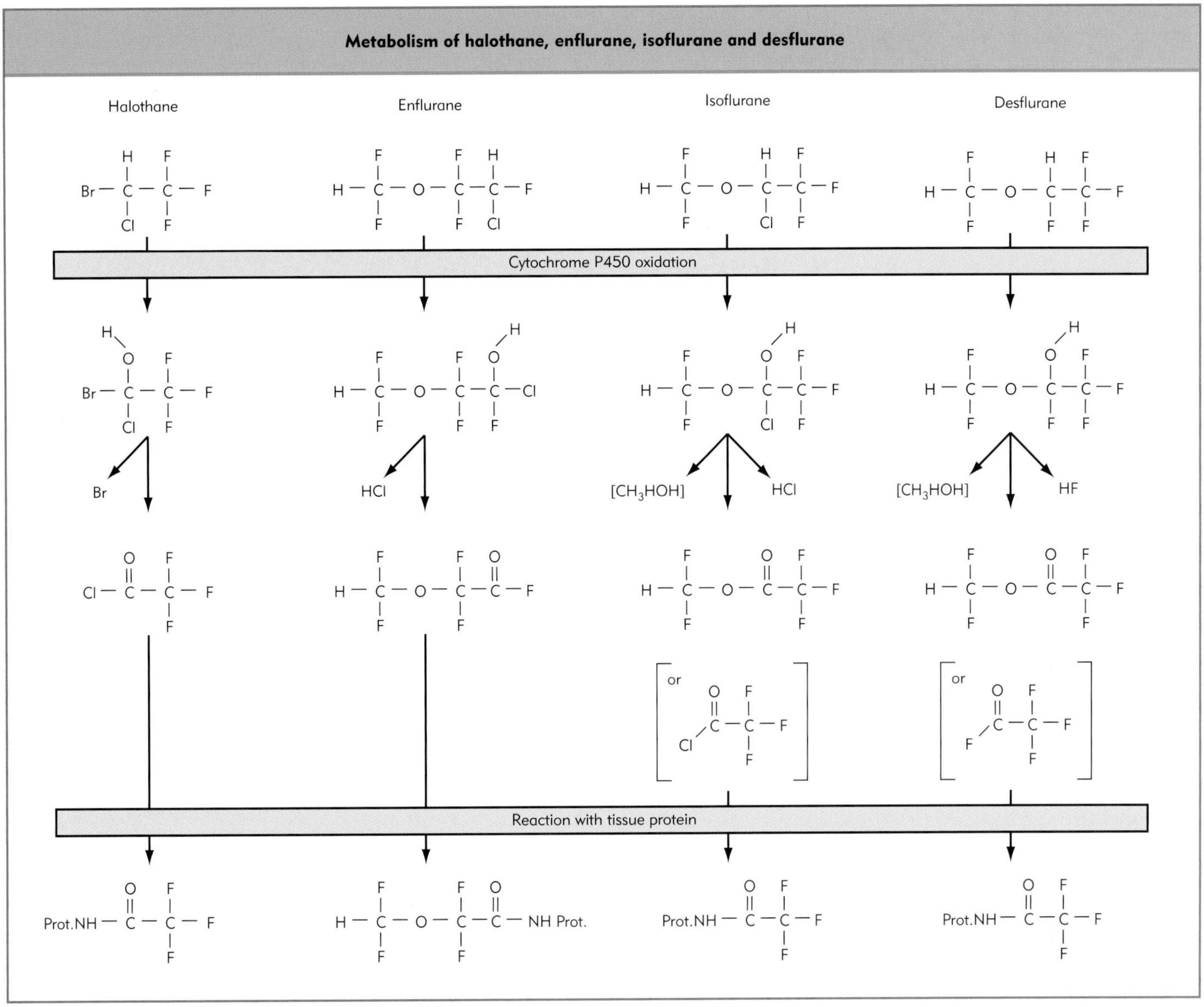

Metabolism of halothane, enflurane, isoflurane and desflurane

Halothane
Enflurane
Isoflurane
Desflurane

Cytochrome P450 oxidation

Br
HCl
[CH_3OH]
HCl
[CH_3OH]
HF

Reaction with tissue protein

Prot.NH
NH Prot.

Figure 26.3 The metabolism of halothane, enflurane, isoflurane and desflurane. Interaction with cytochrome P450 produces oxidative metabolites, which may then interact with tissue proteins to produce molecules that may trigger a cross-reacting immunological response. (Elliott RH, Strunin L. Hepatotoxicity of volatile anaesthetics. British Journal of Anaesthesia 1993;70:339–348. Copyright © The Board of Management and Trustees of the British Journal of Anaesthesia. Reproduced by permission of Oxford University Press/British Journal of Anaesthesia.)

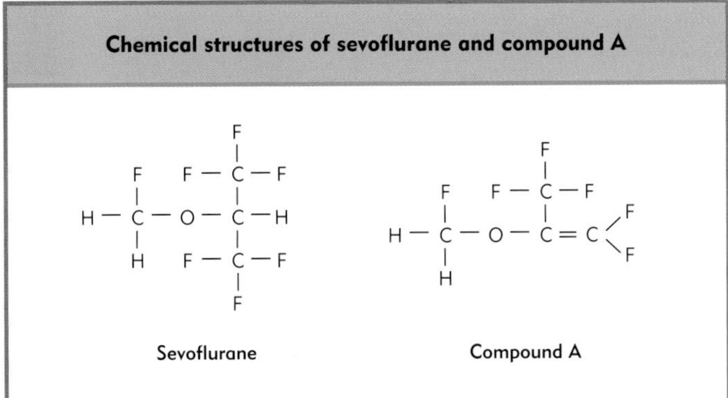

Figure 26.4 Chemical structures of sevoflurane and compound A.

longed and extreme low fresh gas flow, even in patients with established renal failure or receiving other nephrotoxic drugs, clinically significant nephrotoxicity has never been reported following sevoflurane anesthesia.

Other interactions

There have been occasional reports of sevoflurane degradation occurring during inhalational induction, resulting in delayed loss of consciousness and/or irritation caused by toxic products such as formic acid and formaldehyde. As with carbon monoxide production from other anesthetics, this breakdown only occurs in the presence of extremely dry soda lime. With the absorbent in the usual place in the expiratory limb of the circle, moisture from the patient, as well as that produced from the reaction with carbon dioxide, provides sufficient hydration to prevent degradation. The reported cases have all involved equipment where the soda lime was installed on the inspiratory limb.

Although all of the above interactions are either avoidable or do not appear to produce clinical harm, modifying the composition of the soda lime by removing sodium and potassium hydroxide also seems to prevent all of them. One such product (Amsorb) is commercially available.

SPECIFIC INHALATIONAL ANESTHETICS

Halothane

Halothane was once the 'gold standard' against which all other anesthetics were judged, a role which has now been assumed by isoflurane. The demise of halothane is as much due to its slow recovery and adverse cardiovascular effects as to the risk of halothane hepatitis.

CARDIOVASCULAR SYSTEM

Halothane causes a dose-dependent reduction in cardiac contractility, leading to a reduction in cardiac output (Table 26.3). As systemic vascular resistance changes very little, arterial blood pressure also decreases. Regional blood flow shows some variation, with an increase in cerebral blood flow and a reduction in splanchnic and hepatic blood flow. A reduction in sympathetic activity and inhibition of transmembrane calcium flux in the sinoatrial node and conducting system lead to a reduction in heart rate. Reduced automaticity often results in nodal rhythm, but of greater concern is that slow conduction predisposes to re-entry arrhythmias, such as premature ventricular contractions. More dangerous rhythms (e.g. ventricular tachycardia or fibrillation) can also occur, especially with high levels of endogenous catecholamines (e.g. anxiety, light anesthesia, hypercarbia) or when exogenous catecholamines are administered. These effects are not seen with the ether-derivative anesthetics.

RESPIRATORY SYSTEM

Like other volatile anesthetics, halothane is a respiratory depressant. Tidal volume is decreased with an increase in respiratory rate. The respiratory responses to hypoxia and hypercarbia are also depressed (as with other agents). Halothane is relatively nonirritant to the airway. This means that inhalational induction is well tolerated (although somewhat slow, owing to its solubility). This benefit, combined with excellent bronchodilation, has ensured the continued use of halothane, especially in children, although it is rapidly being displaced by sevoflurane.

Halothane also depresses mucociliary transport. Although all volatile anesthetics appear to do this, the greater solubility of halothane, and hence its delayed recovery, may tend to exacerbate the effect.

MISCELLANEOUS EFFECTS

Like other volatile anesthetics, halothane is a generalized central nervous system depressant. Cerebral vasodilatation and impaired autoregulation lead to increases in cerebrospinal fluid pressure. As other agents do this to a lesser degree, halothane is relatively contraindicated in head injuries and with raised intracranial pressure.

Halothane relaxes skeletal muscle and potentiates neuromuscular blocking drugs, although to a lesser extent than the anesthetic ethers. It is a potent uterine relaxant, probably more so than the ethers. Halothane is also a more potent trigger to malignant hyperthermia than ether anesthetics.

Halothane is a relatively unstable molecule and is stabilized by the presence of 0.01% thymol. Regular drainage of vaporizers is required to prevent the accumulation of this stabilizer, which is not evaporated. Halothane is corrosive to metal, plastic, and rubber. The presence of bromine as well as chlorine means that it can have adverse effects on the ozone layer in the upper atmosphere.

Enflurane

As a halogenated ether, enflurane has many properties in common with isoflurane (see below). It is stable without preservatives and noncorrosive. Its relatively high solubility and low potency (relative to maximum vaporizer output) make it difficult to achieve an adequate depth of anesthesia rapidly. It depresses myocardial contractility to a significant degree (Table 26.3), with moderate vasodilatation, a decrease in systemic blood pressure, and a reflex tachycardia. It is also a potent respiratory depressant. Enflurane produces a degree of central nervous system stimulation and a convulsive EEG pattern may be seen, making its use unwise in the presence of epilepsy.

Table 26.3 Cardiovascular effects of the various inhalational anesthetics compared. Arrows indicate an increase, decrease, or no change in the parameter. The number of arrows signifies the approximate magnitude of the effect

	Cardiac output	Systemic vascular resistance	Mean arterial pressure	Heart rate
Halothane	↓	↔	↓	↓↓
Enflurane	↓↓	↓	↓↓	↑
Isoflurane	↓	↓	↓	↑
Desflurane	↔	↓	↓	↑
Sevoflurane	↔	↓	↓	↔
Nitrous oxide	↓	↑	↔	↑
Xenon	↔	↔	↔	↓

Concerns over fluoride production (see above) also limit its use in prolonged anesthesia and in the presence of renal failure.

Enflurane has a number of disadvantages compared to isoflurane and no real benefits. Lack of competition has even resulted in a higher cost than isoflurane, and it is likely that enflurane will soon be withdrawn.

Isoflurane

Isoflurane is now the reference anesthetic and is suitable in most circumstances. Loss of patent protection and competition have made it very inexpensive. The molecule is stable, noncorrosive, and undergoes minimal metabolism. Halogenated with chlorine and fluorine, it causes less environmental damage than halothane (but more than desflurane and sevoflurane).

CARDIOVASCULAR SYSTEM

Isoflurane causes only a modest reduction in myocardial contractility (Table 26.3). The decrease in arterial pressure is largely the result of peripheral vasodilatation and is accompanied by a centrally mediated compensatory tachycardia. Heart rhythm is unaffected and isoflurane, like other substituted ethers, does not sensitize the myocardium to catecholamines.

As systemic arterial pressure is decreased, coronary blood flow should also decrease, although this is compensated for by coronary artery dilatation. In the presence of coronary stenosis, redistributed blood flow might lead to distal ischemia, known as 'coronary steal'. Although isoflurane has long been associated with this phenomenon, the subject is still controversial and outcome studies do not appear to show any detriment from isoflurane anesthesia in patients with coronary artery disease.

RESPIRATORY SYSTEM

Isoflurane is a respiratory depressant, decreasing tidal volume, increasing respiratory rate, and depressing responses to hypoxemia and hypercarbia. Isoflurane is quite irritant to the airway. Although inhalational inductions have been performed, isoflurane is not a good choice for this purpose. Respiratory irritation can also induce transient increases in heart rate and blood pressure if the inspired concentration is rapidly increased. Coughing may also occur in the absence of neuromuscular block.

MISCELLANEOUS EFFECTS

Although isoflurane does cause cerebral vasodilatation, this is not marked at low concentrations and isoflurane has been used extensively in neuroanesthesia. It does not produce any convulsive activity.

Isoflurane relaxes skeletal muscle and potentiates neuromuscular blocking drugs to a greater extent than halothane. It can trigger malignant hyperthermia in susceptible individuals. All these properties are similar to those of other halogenated ethers. Uterine relaxation is noted at relatively high concentrations, but is less marked at clinically relevant concentrations.

Desflurane

Desflurane is notable for its low blood gas solubility and virtual lack of metabolism. Although the latter is a theoretical benefit, it appears to convey no great advantage in practice. In theory, the low solubility should facilitate rapid induction of anesthesia, but desflurane is highly irritant and inhalational induction is not recommended, especially in children. Desflurane is, however, usually well tolerated during the maintenance phase, even in patients breathing spontaneously. Its low solubility does increase the speed of response to changes in delivered concentration, although the irritation can again transiently increase heart rate and blood pressure. Nevertheless, low solubility and rapid response make desflurane an easy agent to use with low-flow anesthesia.

Recovery after desflurane anesthesia is also rapid, due to the low blood gas solubility. After procedures of moderate duration (for example most day-case operations) any improvement in recovery compared to isoflurane is minimal in magnitude and unlikely to be of clinical benefit. However, for anesthesia lasting 2 or more hours differences in recovery become more marked (prolonged anesthesia delays recovery from desflurane less than for other agents), and it is for prolonged anesthesia that desflurane probably has the greatest clinical indication.

Low blood gas solubility and rapid response make desflurane an easy agent to use with low-flow anesthesia.

Other than the properties outlined above, the cardiac (Table 26.3), respiratory, and musculoskeletal effects of desflurane are virtually identical to those of isoflurane. Being halogenated only with fluorine, desflurane appears benign to the upper atmosphere.

Sevoflurane

Sevoflurane differs most notably from isoflurane in its low solubility and minimal airway irritation. However, reference to Figure 26.2 shows that its structure is rather unlike that of the other ether anesthetics, and a number of its properties also show differences.

CARDIOVASCULAR SYSTEM

Sevoflurane causes a moderate reduction in systemic vascular resistance, producing a small decrease in arterial pressure (Table 26.3). However, arterial pressure does not appear to continue to decrease much with deepening levels of anesthesia. Myocardial contractility is virtually unchanged and there is no significant tachycardia or bradycardia. Coronary blood flow also changes little. These properties should result in a greater therapeutic index and reduced cardiovascular toxicity, although no beneficial outcome compared with isoflurane has so far been demonstrated.

RESPIRATORY SYSTEM

Although it is still a respiratory depressant, sevoflurane is the most effective bronchodilator and the least irritant of the inhaled anesthetics. This means that rapid increases in delivered concentration (up to the maximum vaporizer output) and inhalation induction are both well tolerated.

Sevoflurane is the most effective bronchodilator and the least irritant of the inhaled anesthetics.

INHALATIONAL INDUCTION

Sevoflurane rapidly established a place for inhalational induction in children, but has also led to a resurgence of this technique in some adult patients. Advantages include reduced hypotension, maintenance of spontaneous ventilation, and earlier awakening after brief procedures compared to propofol. Various induction techniques have been described, but those where the patient is exposed to 8 vol% sevoflurane from the outset are associated with the most rapid induction and the fewest complications.

Controversy still exists over whether sevoflurane or halothane is preferable for induction in the presence of severe airway compromise. As regular experience with halothane declines, sevoflurane is likely to become the agent of choice by default.

MISCELLANEOUS EFFECTS

Like desflurane, sevoflurane is readily controllable at low fresh gas flows. Equilibration occurs rapidly after an inhaled induction, and in this circumstance it is more efficient to continue with sevoflurane administration than to change to an alternative. This concept has become known as volatile induction and maintenance of anesthesia (VIMA).

Recovery from sevoflurane is acceptably rapid, especially after VIMA for short procedures. However, as with desflurane, no earlier discharge of day-case patients has been observed. Unlike with desflurane, however, recovery after more prolonged exposure is not much improved compared to isoflurane.

Like other ethers, sevoflurane relaxes muscles and attenuates the response to noxious stimuli. The ability to tolerate high delivered concentrations without significant cardiovascular depression or delayed recovery may allow these properties to be exploited to a somewhat greater degree, thereby allowing neuromuscular blocking drugs and opioid analgesics to be avoided in association with a VIMA technique. Avoiding opioids may reduce the incidence of postoperative nausea and vomiting, which may otherwise be more prevalent with this technique.

Sevoflurane has been associated with epileptiform EEG activity, although there is little clear evidence of clinically significant effects. Sevoflurane appears to cause less cerebral vasodilatation than isoflurane, and maintains dynamic cerebral autoregulation to a better degree. These properties may make sevoflurane the agent of choice for neuroanesthesia.

The development of sevoflurane was prolonged because of concerns over its potential for toxicity (see above). This does not seem to be a major problem in practice, although the margin of safety is unknown. The sevoflurane molecule is less stable than that of other ether anesthetics, and is currently stabilized by a minute amount of water (approximately one drop per bottle). However, this is probably more related to attempts to prolong patent protection than to clinically significant instability. Like desflurane, sevoflurane has no significant effect on the ozone layer and is not a 'greenhouse gas'.

Nitrous oxide

Despite being the first agent to demonstrate practical anesthesia, nitrous oxide (N_2O) remains in use, although its popularity is beginning to decline. Nitrous oxide is delivered as a gas, through calibrated flow meters, from pressurized cylinders, either on the anesthetic machine or via a hospital supply line. As the critical temperature of nitrous oxide is above room temperature, it is a liquid when compressed in a cylinder. One consequence of this is that the reading on the pressure gauge (750 psi; 51.7 bar at 20°C) does not alter until all the liquid has evaporated and the cylinder contains only gas. At this point, the pressure declines rapidly as the cylinder quickly empties. This is of relatively less importance now that most nitrous oxide is supplied from pipelines, with large banks of cylinders and back-up systems. In addition, nitrous oxide is used mainly as a supplement, rather than as the sole anesthetic agent, so its temporary unavailability, if recognized, is not disastrous.

The low potency of nitrous oxide means that it cannot be used as a sole anesthetic except in the most frail of individuals. Instead, it is used to provide background analgesia and to reduce the amounts of other anesthetics that are required. The latter may be desirable because of the rapidity with which nitrous oxide may be delivered and eliminated. In addition, nitrous oxide may be less depressant than 'deep' anesthesia with alternative agents. These benefits may be less obvious with desflurane and sevoflurane, which are rapidly acting and minimally depressant. However, nitrous oxide is relatively inexpensive, especially compared to the newer volatile anesthetics that are still covered by patent protection. There may therefore still be a financial benefit to supplementing desflurane or sevoflurane with nitrous oxide.

CARDIOVASCULAR SYSTEM

Nitrous oxide causes mild depression of cardiac output, but this is often compensated for by a degree of sympathetic stimulation, which causes increased vascular resistance and a stable blood pressure (Table 26.3). These depressant effects are modest in comparison to those of some of the inhaled agents, which might be used in higher doses in the absence of nitrous oxide, although this is probably less so for desflurane and sevoflurane. Furthermore, nitrous oxide may be more depressant in the presence of pre-existing cardiac dysfunction. Under some circumstances it can raise pulmonary vascular resistance, and may reverse shunt direction in pediatric patients with congenital cardiac malformations.

RESPIRATORY SYSTEM

Nitrous oxide is less of a respiratory depressant than the volatile anesthetics. It does depress the response to hypoxemia, but has less effect on that to hypercarbia. Tidal volume is slightly reduced, with respiratory rate increasing to maintain minute volume. Airway reflexes are depressed (similar to volatile agents) and there is no significant irritation or odor, making it useful during induction.

Nitrous oxide is thought to facilitate inhalational induction through the second gas effect. In practice, there is little evidence for any clinically significant improvement in the speed or quality of induction, at least with sevoflurane. Postoperative diffusion hypoxia, caused by dilution of inspired air by dissolved nitrous oxide being excreted by the lungs, was once a cause of great concern. Saturation monitoring reveals any effect to be transient, significant hypoxemia in the past more likely being due to the respiratory depressant effects of soluble anesthetics, inadequate reversal of neuromuscular block, and/or excessive opioid analgesia.

CENTRAL EFFECTS

Although the MAC of nitrous oxide is greater than 1 atm, it may still produce amnesia and unconsciousness at safe concentrations in some individuals. However, reliance on nitrous oxide alone, as was once common in obstetric anesthesia, results in a high incidence of awareness and is no longer justified. Nitrous oxide appears to be mechanistically different from the volatile anesthetics. It may produce unconsciousness with virtually no change in bispectral index (Chapter 14), making titration to bispectral index more difficult when nitrous oxide forms a substantial part of the anesthetic. Nitrous oxide is a potent analgesic and much of its action probably results from changes in endogenous opioids. This may be mediated through the inhibition of *N*-methyl-D-aspartate (NMDA) receptors.

MISCELLANEOUS EFFECTS

Nitrous oxide has no significant effect on muscular tone or neuromuscular blocking drugs. Uterine tone is unaffected, and there is no apparent change in renal or hepatic function. Nitrous oxide is nonflammable but, unlike the volatile anesthetics, it does support combustion.

Nitrous oxide has significant deleterious environmental consequences, as it depletes the ozone layer and is also a 'greenhouse gas'. It is far more harmful in this respect than other anesthetic agents, but the vast majority of the nitrous oxide that currently reaches the atmosphere comes from sources other than anesthetic use. Ultimately, this balance may change as other uses are restricted, and environmental concerns will probably eventually force the withdrawal of nitrous oxide from anesthetic practice.

Nitrous oxide is potentially hazardous, predominantly owing to its ability to diffuse into closed spaces and its chronic toxicity.

DIFFUSION INTO CLOSED SPACES

The gut lumen, sinuses, and middle ear all contain air under normal circumstances, and pneumothoraces, pneumoperitoneum, air emboli, various forms of emphysema, and air within the skull or eye cavities may exist in certain individuals. These air-filled spaces all contain oxygen and nitrogen in equilibrium with room air, but when a nitrous oxide–oxygen mixture is breathed, nitrous oxide diffuses into the spaces about 25 times as fast as nitrogen can escape, because of its far greater solubility in blood. As a result, the space will expand and/or become pressurized. Eventually, if time permits, equilibration is achieved and the pressure in the space normalizes until nitrogen is again breathed, at which time contraction and/or subatmospheric pressure may occur.

The effects of nitrous oxide on bowel distension are controversial. Much of the luminal gas is not air, and the system is potentially open-ended. Some workers have reported adverse surgical conditions when nitrous oxide is used (in comparison to its avoidance), but others have not. The effects may be greater in the case of bowel obstruction, although even here opinion is divided. Nitrous oxide causes a modest increase in postoperative nausea and vomiting, and an effect on bowel function may be a contributory factor.

Diffusion of nitrous oxide is undoubtedly hazardous in the presence of a noncompliant air-filled space.

Diffusion of nitrous oxide is undoubtedly hazardous in the presence of a noncompliant air-filled space. The volume of a pneumothorax can double in 10 minutes and bullae may rupture. Eardrum rupture, tympanic graft displacement, hearing loss, and other damage may result from changes in middle ear pressure, especially in the presence of inflammation blocking the eustachian tubes. Pain from blocked sinus cavities may also occur under these circumstances. Intracranial air was once used as a contrast medium. Although this is no longer the case, trauma may result in intracranial air, which may expand with disastrous consequences if nitrous oxide is administered.

A bubble of air (60%) and sulphur hexafluoride is often injected into the eye to provide long-lasting tamponade after retinal detachment surgery. Anesthesia using nitrous oxide 2 days after such surgery has resulted in permanent blindness due to an increase in intraocular pressure.

TOXICITY OF NITROUS OXIDE

Nitrous oxide undergoes virtually no metabolism with the exception of that caused by microbial breakdown in the gut lumen, which is harmless. Nitrous oxide inhibits vitamin B_{12}, which in turn inactivates the enzyme methionine synthetase, thereby inhibiting folate metabolism. This has a number of potential consequences, including megaloblastic anemia, agranulocytosis, and polyneuropathy. Although some changes may be observed after modest exposure, significant toxicity requires a duration of exposure of about 24 hours or more. Consequently, nitrous oxide is not used for intensive care sedation or for very long cases.

A fatality has also been reported in a child with an undiagnosed inborn error of methionine synthesis. It is thought that nitrous oxide further depressed methionine levels, which were already low but survivable.

Nitrous oxide appears to be a mild teratogen in the rat, but does not seem to be mutagenic or carcinogenic in humans. Epidemiological studies have not shown increased fetal abnormalities when nitrous oxide is used during pregnancy. Concerns remain about chronic exposure to low concentrations of nitrous oxide in operating room personnel, who may be at increased risk of bone marrow suppression and, possibly, fetal abnormalities. The majority of evidence shows a lack of adverse effects, and efficient scavenging helps to minimize exposure.

Xenon

Xenon is a noble gas that is present in minute quantities in the atmosphere, hence its name, which is Greek for 'stranger'. Xenon has been known since 1951 to possess anesthetic properties. It has a MAC value of 71% (although recent work suggests this may be closer to 60%) and is very insoluble, with a blood:gas partition coefficient of 0.115. Induction with xenon is very rapid, although limited by the inability to deliver significant overpressure owing to the high MAC value. Recovery is also rapid, faster than that which can be achieved with isoflurane or sevoflurane. Like desflurane but more so, recovery is largely independent of anesthetic duration.

Xenon is a monatomic gas at room temperature. Being virtually inert, it does not bond with other molecules. However, the large outer electron shell can become polarized, allowing interactions with proteins and lipids. Xenon is a potent inhibitor of NMDA receptors (similar to nitrous oxide), but has little effect on GABA receptors or voltage-gated ion channels.

Xenon has undergone considerable investigation in recent years, but has also been used in fairly routine practice in countries such as Russia, which have routinely collected it as a byproduct of air liquefaction.

CARDIOVASCULAR SYSTEM

Xenon produces minimal changes in myocardial contractility, vascular resistance, or blood pressure (Table 26.3). Heart rate may decrease slightly, with increased variability, but to a clinically unimportant degree. It does not sensitize the myocardium to the effects of catecholamines. This remarkable cardiovascular stability is maintained under conditions of a compromised myocardium and in subjects with limited cardiovascular reserve.

RESPIRATORY SYSTEM

Xenon produces relatively benign respiratory effects. It is a mild respiratory depressant, but unlike the volatile anesthetics it reduces the respiratory rate with an accompanying increase in the tidal volume. Inspiratory resistance is slightly increased, owing to its high density and viscosity (respectively 3 and 1.5 times those of nitrous oxide). Although diffusion hypoxia may occur, this is less marked than with nitrous oxide, which is in any case of minimal significance (see above). Xenon is odorless, tasteless, and nonirritant, which would facilitate inhalational induction.

Xenon anesthesia is associated with remarkable cardiovascular stability, which is maintained under conditions of a compromised myocardium and in subjects with limited cardiovascular reserve.

MISCELLANEOUS EFFECTS

Xenon appears to be quite effective at protecting experimental animals against chemical- or hypoxia-induced neuronal damage. This neuroprotection occurs at subanesthetic doses, and has also been observed in animals subjected to cardiopulmonary bypass. Despite this apparent benefit, xenon increases cerebral blood flow, at least transiently, and may raise intracranial pressure following head injury. However, the effects seem to be highly variable, and reactivity to carbon dioxide is maintained. Although it is considered safe when used to enhance cranial CT scans, xenon cannot currently be considered safe for neuroanesthesia.

Xenon is a more potent analgesic than nitrous oxide and is three times more effective at blunting the cardiovascular response to skin incision than equi-MAC concentrations of sevoflurane. Its effects do not correlate well with bispectral index (BIS), with responsiveness occurring at BIS levels usually associated with adequate hypnosis. Auditory evoked potentials may measure the xenon anesthetic state somewhat better.

Xenon seems to have relatively little effect on other organ systems. It does not trigger malignant hyperthermia in appropriate animal models. It is nonflammable and does not support combustion. There is no evidence of mutagenicity, teratogenicity, carcinogenicity, or allergic reactions. Like nitrous oxide, xenon can diffuse into air-filled spaces, but being less soluble, the effect is likely to be less. Xenon diffuses freely through rubber, which may permit significant losses from a breathing circuit.

As a constituent of the atmosphere xenon has no adverse environmental consequences (other than the significant energy expenditure required for its purification).

LIMITATIONS OF XENON

The greatest limitation of xenon is its rarity and hence its cost. Unlike other anesthetics, where the purchase price largely reflects the cost of research and development rather than manufacture, xenon is expensive to produce. It is recovered from the liquefaction of air and purification by way of its increased density, but xenon constitutes only about 0.087 ppm of atmospheric air. Consequently, xenon costs many times more than nitrous oxide, currently around $15 (£10) per liter. The supply is ultimately limited and xenon is already recovered for other uses, including medical imaging, lasers, high-intensity lamps, and space applications. It is therefore unlikely that the price will decrease dramatically.

Because of its extremely low solubility, xenon is ideally suited to closed-circuit anesthesia and its cost would really not permit any other form of delivery. Even so, priming the circuit and the initial wash-in will require a substantial volume of gas, making xenon relatively more efficient for long cases. A 4-hour case has been estimated to cost about US$350, but developments to reduce priming and allow the recycling of xenon after use may make it more affordable. However, such specialized equipment is itself likely to be expensive, and xenon will probably remain limited in its use. The most obvious indication for xenon would be cardiac surgery in seriously compromised individuals, where cardiovascular stability, neuroprotection, and rapid recovery would all be highly beneficial.

SUMMARY

Inhalational anesthetics have a long and well-established track record and remain useful to this day. The usage of both halothane and enflurane has declined considerably, and it is likely that both agents will ultimately be withdrawn as they become commercially unviable. This will leave isoflurane as the 'standard' inhaled anesthetic. Desflurane and sevoflurane have a number of advantages over isoflurane and are probably closer to the ideal agent. It is likely that their use will increase considerably when patent protection ends and their price comes down through competition.

Nitrous oxide remains a popular supplement, although a number of anesthetists have now abandoned it for some, or all, of their cases. Although it may be a desirable supplement, it cannot really be called essential and it is likely that environmental concerns will ultimately cause its withdrawal.

Xenon may soon find a place in the anesthetic armamentarium, but this is likely to be severely limited owing to its high cost and the need for complex equipment for its efficient use. Other than this interesting agent, there seems little prospect of any other new inhalational anesthetics for the foreseeable future.

Further reading

Dingley J, Ivanova-Stoilova TM, Grundler S, Wall T. Xenon: Recent developments. Anaesthesia 1999;54:335–46.

Ebert TJ, Kharasch ED, Rooke GA, Shroff A, Muzi M. Myocardial ischemia and adverse cardiac outcomes in cardiac patients undergoing noncardiac surgery with sevoflurane and isoflurane. Sevoflurane Ischemia Study Group. Anesth Analg. 1997;85:993–9.

Eger EI, II, Saidman LF, Brandstater B. Minimum alveolar anesthetic concentration. A standard of anesthetic potency. Anesthesiology 1965;26:756–763.

Eger EI II. Desflurane: A compendium and reference. Rutherford NJ: Anaquest. Healthpress Publishing; 1993.

Eger EI II. Nitrous oxide, N_2O. New York: Elsevier; 1985.

Elliott RH Strunin L. Hepatotoxicity of volatile anaesthetics.Br J Anaesth. 1993;70:339–48.

Ghatge S, Lee J, Smith I. Sevoflurane: an ideal agent for adult day-case anesthesia? Acta Anaesthesiol Scand. 2003;47:917–31.

Juvin P, Servin F, Giraud O, Desmonts J-M. Emergence of elderly patients from prolonged desflurane, isoflurane, or propofol anesthesia. Anesth Analg. 1997;85:647–51.

Sanders RD, Franks NP, Maze M. Xenon: No stranger to anaesthesia. Br J Anaesth. 2003;91:709–17.

Smith I, Nathanson M, White PF. Sevoflurane – a long-awaited volatile anaesthetic. Br J Anaesth. 1996;76:435–45.

Stenqvist O, Husum B, Dale O. Nitrous oxide: An aging gentleman (Editorial). Acta Anaesthesiol Scand. 2001;45:135–7.

Chapter 27

Pharmacokinetics of inhalation anesthetics

Jerrold Lerman

TOPICS COVERED IN THIS CHAPTER

- **Drug delivery systems**
  - Circuits
  - Vaporizers
- **Pharmacology**
  - Xenon
- **Pharmacokinetics**
  - General principles
  - Determinants of wash-in
  - Ventilation
  - Functional residual capacity
  - Inspired concentration
  - Uptake of anesthetic from the lungs
  - Solubility
  - Cardiac output
  - Alveolar-to-venous partial pressure gradient
- **Specific conditions**
  - Ventilation
  - Hyperventilation
  - Modes of ventilation
  - The concentration effect
  - Second gas effect
  - Overpressure technique
  - Vital capacity inductions
  - Cardiac output
  - Shunts
  - Temperature
- **Tissue uptake**
- **Pharmacokinetics in children**
  - Ratio of alveolar ventilation to functional residual capacity
  - Solubility in blood
  - Solubility in tissues
  - Cardiac output
- **Elimination**
  - General principles
  - Metabolism
  - Methoxyflurane
  - Halothane
  - Sevoflurane
  - Enflurane
  - Isoflurane
  - Desflurane
  - Infants and children

DRUG DELIVERY SYSTEMS

Circuits

The anesthetic circuit serves several purposes, including the delivery of anesthetic, oxygen, heat, and humidity to the patient, and the removal of anesthetics and carbon dioxide from the patient. The circuit also facilitates ventilation, either spontaneous or mechanical. Anesthetic circuits can be simply classified as:

- circuits that include a carbon dioxide absorber (e.g. circle systems);
- rebreathing circuits, where inspired and exhaled gases can mix (e.g. Ayre's T-piece, or the Bain circuit); or
- nonrebreathing circuits, in which a one-way valve separates the inspired and exhaled gases (e.g. the resuscitation self-inflating bag).

Circle systems have a fresh gas hose from the anesthesia machine, a canister (which contains a carbon dioxide absorbent such as soda lime or barium hydroxide lime), a reservoir bag for spontaneous or manual ventilation, two unidirectional valves (one on each of the inspiratory and expiratory limbs), inspiratory and expiratory hoses, and a Y-piece to connect the hoses to the mask or tracheal tube. They may be used with either spontaneous or controlled ventilation, at any fresh gas flow (the lowest flow being 4–7 mL/min/kg body weight oxygen flow, depending on age), for prolonged periods. The absorbent removes CO_2 from the exhaled gas in an exothermic reaction that produces an alkaline medium, heat, and water (Fig. 27.1). When the absorbent is expended, an indicator changes color. Either within or upon exiting the canister, the exhaled gas mixes with fresh gas in the inspiratory limb of the circuit. These circuits are efficient, inexpensive, and environmentally friendly. However, they suffer from several disadvantages, including a slow wash-in and washout of anesthetic (see below), bulky and heavy tubing, and, if high-compliance hoses are used with positive-pressure ventilation, wasted ventilation. Furthermore, unidirectional valves can fail and cause unanticipated rebreathing of exhaled gases, or the inability to ventilate with positive pressure. Finally, concerns exist regarding the degradation of inhaled anesthetics in the presence of absorbents.

All volatile anesthetics are absorbed, degraded and/or adsorbed to varying degrees in the presence of carbon dioxide absorbents. At high temperatures halothane is degraded to 2-bromochloro-

Reactions involved in the chemical absorption of carbon dioxide

Reaction of carbon dioxide with barium hydroxide lime

$Ba(OH)_2 + 8H_2O + CO_2 \rightleftharpoons BaCO_3 + 9H_2O + \text{heat}$

$9(H_2O) + 9CO_2 \rightleftharpoons 9H_2CO_3$

Then by direct reactions and by KOH and NaOH

$9H_2CO_3 + 9Ba(OH)_2 \rightleftharpoons 9BaCO_3 + 18H_2O + \text{heat}$

Reaction of carbon dioxide with soda lime

$CO_2 + H_2O \rightleftharpoons H_2CO_3$

$H_2CO_3 + 2NaOH(KOH) \rightleftharpoons Na_2CO_3(K_2CO_3) + 2H_2O + \text{heat}$

$Na_2CO_3(K_2CO_3) + Ca(OH)_2 \rightleftharpoons CaCO_3 + 2NaOH(KOH)$

Figure 27.1 Reactions involved in the chemical absorption of carbon dioxide. The reaction with barium hydroxide lime involves a direct reaction of barium hydroxide and carbon dioxide and liberates more water than the reaction with soda lime.

ethylene, although the concentration of this product is less than 3% of its lethal concentration. Isoflurane, enflurane, and desflurane are absorbed and degraded to small extents in the presence of soda lime. Sevoflurane undergoes alkaline hydrolysis in the presence of soda lime and barium hydroxide lime (baralyme), producing five compounds, of which compound A, a halogenated alkene, is the most abundant (Fig. 27.2). Several factors increase the rate of degradation of sevoflurane and thus increase the production of compound A, including high concentrations of sevoflurane, low fresh gas flows (i.e. closed circuits), high absorber temperature, prolonged exposure, and dessicated absorbent. The degradation is greater with barium hydroxide lime than with soda lime, and in adults than in infants. Concern regarding the production of compound A stems from the histologic and biochemical changes that have been reported in rat kidney, although similar changes have not been demonstrated in primates or humans. A minimum fresh gas flow of 1 L/min is recommended with sevoflurane for a maximum of 2 MAC-hours in the presence of a carbon dioxide absorbent. Studies have demonstrated that the degradation of sevoflurane may be eliminated if both KOH and NaOH (accelerators within the absorbent) are excluded from the absorbent. Two new absorbents, Amsorb and lithium hydroxide, are free of KOH and NaOH and do not degrade sevoflurane.

All volatile anesthetics are absorbed, degraded and/or adsorbed to varying degrees in the presence of carbon dioxide absorbents.

Carbon monoxide (CO) is a potentially fatal product of the degradation of inhaled anesthetics in the presence of CO_2 absorbents. Carbon monoxide can be formed when inhaled anesthetics interact with dessicated absorbent. The amount of carbon monoxide formed depends in part on the particular inhaled anesthetic (desflurane > enflurane > isoflurane >>> halothane = sevoflurane). Factors that increase the degradation include low moisture content, high temperature, and the use of barium hydroxide lime rather than soda lime. To avoid absorbent desiccation, the fresh gas flow should be disconnected from the anesthesia machine when not in service and the machine turned

Decomposition of sevoflurane by soda lime

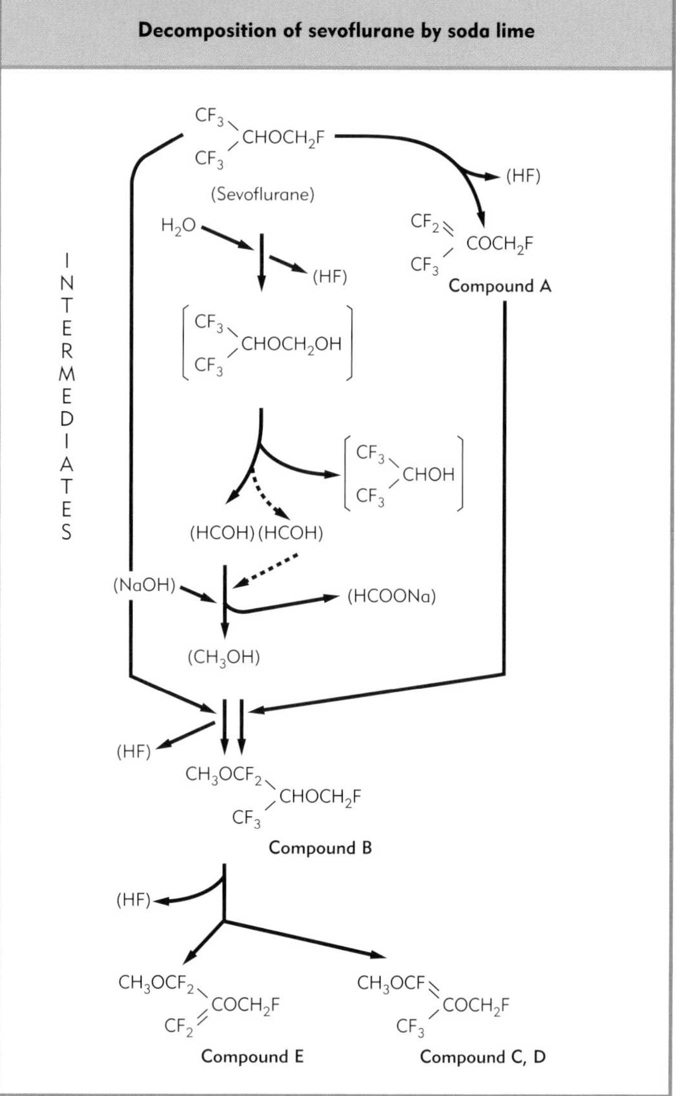

Figure 27.2 Possible mechanism for the decomposition of sevoflurane by soda lime.

off before long periods of disuse. Inhalational anesthetics are not degraded to carbon monoxide when dessicated Amsorb or lithium hydroxide is used.

Recent reports of extreme heat produced within absorbent canisters, leading to canister fire/explosion, have been associated with the use of sevoflurane and dessicated Baralyme. Putative combustible degradation products such as methane may be formed within the canister and then ignited, which can be prevented if dessication of the absorbent is avoided.

Rebreathing circuits have been classified by Mapleson according to their design and function during spontaneous respiration (designated A–F). The most common rebreathing systems in use belong to the Mapleson E or F category. Examples are the Jackson–Rees modification of the Ayre's T-piece, and the Bain circuit, which is a valved coaxial version. Rebreathing is always possible with these circuits, depending on the minute ventilation and fresh gas flow. These circuits deliver rapid wash-in and washout of anesthetic (see below). In the past, large fresh gas flows were used to prevent rebreathing of CO_2. With the widespread availability of capnography, much lower fresh gas flows can be used to maintain end-tidal P_{CO_2} within normal limits. Disadvantages of rebreathing circuits include high cost (due to large fresh gas flows used in the past), environmental concerns (due to wasted large fresh gas flow, including nitrous oxide), minimal heat conservation, and negligible gas humidification.

Vaporizers

Vaporizers are devices that deliver the desired concentration of anesthetic vapor to the breathing circuit. They are situated on the anesthetic machine, upstream from the fresh gas outlet. As reservoirs, vaporizers store a volume of liquid anesthetic. As controllers, they add a calibrated volume of anesthetic vapor to the fresh gas to yield the desired inspired concentration of anesthetic. Most modern vaporizers are temperature-compensated concentration-calibrated variable bypass devices designed for use with a specific anesthetic (Fig. 27.3). The desflurane vaporizer is not a variable bypass device and depends on electricity to maintain high temperature and pressure within the vaporizer, as described below.

The delivery of a known concentration of anesthetic vapor is achieved using a variable bypass system. Fresh gas is split into two streams: a smaller stream that passes through the vaporizer, and a larger stream that bypasses it. The concentration-calibrated controller directs a fraction of fresh gas into the vaporizer, where it becomes saturated with anesthetic vapor. Upon exiting the vaporizer, this smaller stream mixes with the larger bypass stream to yield the inspired concentration set on the controlling dial. The low boiling point of desflurane precludes delivery by a variable bypass system. Instead, desflurane is delivered via an electrically heated (398°C) and pressurized (1500 mmHg) vaporizer that injects a known volume of desflurane vapor into the fresh gas flow to yield the dialed inspired concentration.

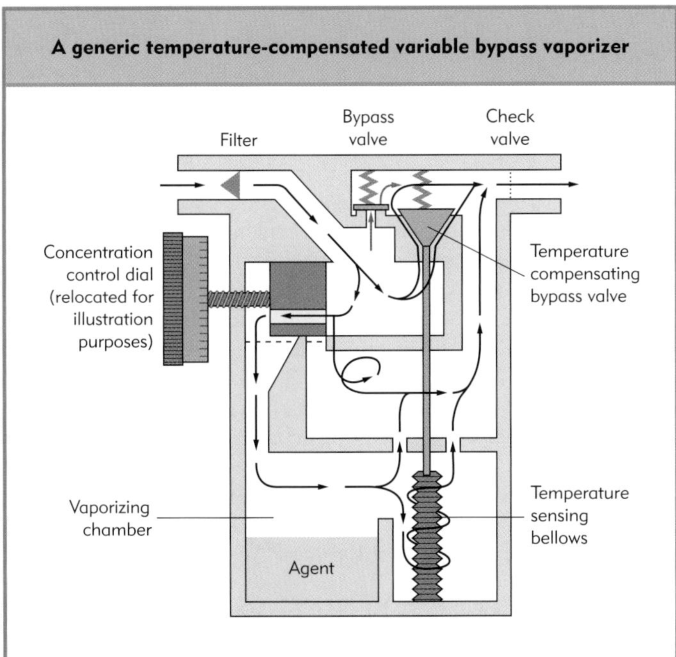

Figure 27.3 A generic temperature-compensated variable bypass vaporizer. Temperature compensation is achieved by a gas-filled temperature-sensing bellows that controls a temperature-compensating bypass valve. Other vaporizers use a bimetallic strip incorporated into a flap valve in the bypass gas flow. (With permission from Eisenkraft JB. Anesthesia vaporizers. In: Ehrenwerth J, Eisenkraft JB, eds. Anesthesia equipment: principles and applications. St Louis, MO: Mosby; 1993:57-88.)

Several techniques are used to control vaporizer output during changes in vaporizer temperature, including expandable bellows and bimetallic strips (composed of nickel and brass). As vaporizer temperature increases, the bellows expand or the strip bends to increase bypass flow. This increase compensates for the increase in anesthetic concentration (vapor pressure) in the effluent that results from the increase in temperature. Because the relationship between temperature and vapor pressure of volatile anesthetics is nonlinear, vaporizers are calibrated within a narrow operating temperature range.

The volume of liquid anesthetic vaporized per hour is approximately 3 × dialed vol% × fresh gas flow.

Each vaporizer is calibrated for use with one inhaled anesthetic. If a vaporizer is filled with an anesthetic for which it was not intended, output may be greater, less, or no different from the 'dialed' concentration, depending on the characteristics of both the vaporizer and the anesthetic. The volume of liquid anesthetic vaporized per hour may be estimated by the simple expression 3 × dialed vol% × fresh gas flow (L/min), where 3 is a factor that corrects for time and volume units. Thus, 1 vol% halothane at a gas flow of 6 L/min vaporizes 18 mL of liquid halothane per hour.

Modern vaporizers are well-engineered devices capable of delivering the dialed inspired concentration from 0.2 to 15 L/min for most anesthetics and concentrations. However, the dial indicator may overestimate the delivered concentration at higher dial settings when fresh gas flow exceeds 5 L/min. Vaporizer performance can be affected by factors other than fresh gas flow rate, including carrier gas composition (nitrous oxide dissolves in the liquid anesthetic and decreases vaporizer output during the early period of administration), atmospheric pressure (at high altitude, vaporizer output increases substantially in terms of volume percentage, but much less in terms of potency), filling the vaporizer with an anesthetic for which it is not calibrated, and back-pressure in the fresh gas circuit (although most vaporizers and anesthesia machines have back-pressure compensation valves). The maximum inspired concentration that a vaporizer can deliver is determined by a number of characteristics of the anesthetic, including the concentration at which it is flammable, its potency, its wash-in profile, and its lethal concentration.

PHARMACOLOGY

This subject is covered in more detail in Chapters 24 and 26. The potent inhalational (volatile) anesthetics are polyhalogenated alkanes (halothane) or ether derivatives (methylethyl ethers – methoxyflurane, enflurane, isoflurane, desflurane – or methylisopropyl ether – sevoflurane). They share physicochemical properties, including reduced flammability, boiling point at approximately 50°C (with the exception of methoxyflurane (104°C) and desflurane (23°C)) and stability in the liquid and vapor phases (Table 27.1).

The potency of inhalational anesthetics is measured by the minimum alveolar concentration (MAC), which is the concentration

Table 27.1 Properties of the inhalation anesthetics. The data regarding the percentages of compounds metabolized in vivo are from studies in both humans and animals

Physical properties	Halothane	Enflurane	Isoflurane	Sevoflurane	Desflurane
Chemical structure	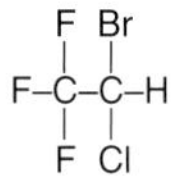 F Br F–C–C–H F Cl	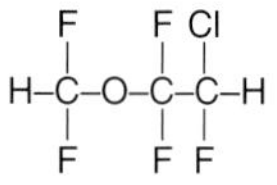 F F Cl H–C–O–C–C–H F F F	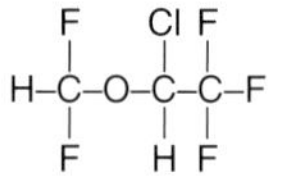 F Cl F H–C–O–C–C–F F H F	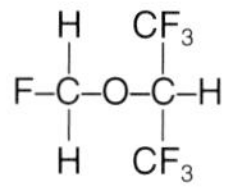 H CF_3 F–C–O–C–H H CF_3	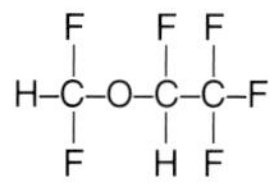 F F F H–C–O–C–C–F F H F
Molecular weight	197.4	184.5	184.5	200.1	168
Boiling point (°C)	50.2	56.5	48.5	58.5	22.8
Vapor pressure (mmHg)	243	175	238	120	669
Percent metabolized in vivo	15–20	2.4	0.2	5.0	0.02
Solubility					
Blood:gas ratio in adults	2.4	1.9	1.4	0.66	0.42
Blood:gas ratio in neonates	2.1	1.8	1.19	0.66	–
Fat:blood ratio in adults	51	–	45	48	27
Minimum alveolar concentration (MAC)					
MAC in adults	0.75	1.7	1.2	2.05	7.0
MAC in neonates	0.87	–	1.6	3.2	9.2

that prevents movement in response to a standardized skin incision in 50% of subjects (Chapter 26). The MAC values for volatile anesthetics in neonates and adults are shown in Table 27.1. Minimum alveolar concentration decreases with increasing age; it is maximal in infancy, and decreases thereafter and with decreasing gestational age to 24 weeks (Fig. 27.4). For sevoflurane, MAC appears to vary less with age; the MAC in neonates and infants (1–6 months of age) is 3.2% and that in older infants and children up to 12 years of age is 2.5%. Minimum alveolar concentration is lowered by a number of factors in addition to age, including co-administration of other agents (e.g. nitrous oxide, opioids, α_2-agonists, etc.), lower temperature, and pregnancy.

Effect of age on the minimum alveolar concentration

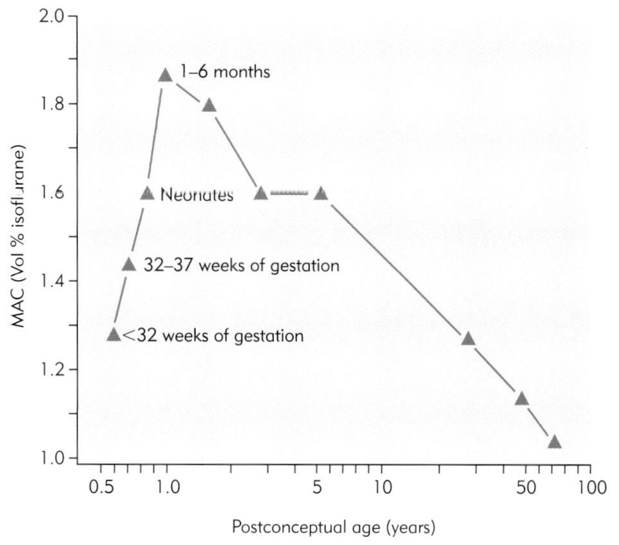

Figure 27.4 Relationship between age and the minimum alveolar concentration (MAC) for isoflurane. MAC increases throughout gestation, reaching a maximum in infants 1–6 months of age. Thereafter, MAC decreases with increasing age.

Xenon

Xenon, a naturally occurring noble gas that is present as 8×10^{-6}% of the atmosphere, or approximately 0.05 ppm, has been under investigation as an anesthetic for more than five decades. It is produced by fractional distillation of air. As a noble gas, it is chemically inert and does not undergo metabolism.

Unlike nitrous oxide and the polyhalogenated hydrocarbons, xenon neither pollutes the environment nor depletes the ozone layer. Xenon is nonteratogenic, confers low toxicity, does not trigger MH reactions, facilitates rapid induction and recovery from anesthesia (blood:gas partition coefficient of 0.15) and has a high MAC (63%). It also confers analgesic properties. Its lack of negative inotropy and vasodilation makes it suitable for patients with limited cardiovascular reserve. It may also confer neuroprotective effects, protecting neuronal cells against ischemic injury. Recently, the first randomized trial in which xenon and isoflurane were compared in healthy patients demonstrated that xenon was a safe anesthetic. It induced anesthesia rapidly, maintained hemodynamic stability, and resulted in rapid and complete recovery.

Xenon has been limited in its clinical use because of high costs, attributable to the costs of production and delivery systems. Xenon is currently under development as a substitute anesthetic for nitrous oxide, with the advantages of providing cardiostability, particularly in those with limited cardiovascular reserve, rapid onset and offset of action, analgesia, and neuroprotection. Because of its expense and high MAC value, xenon is best suited for closed-circuit anesthesia where very low flows may make it cost-effective.

PHARMACOKINETICS

General principles

The increase in the ratio of inhaled anesthetic fraction or partial pressure in the alveoli (F_A) to that in inspired fresh gas (F_I) with time is known as wash-in. The relationship between F_A/F_I and time during this wash-in period is described by the differential equation:

■ Equation 27.1

$$\frac{dF_A}{dF_I} = -t/\tau$$

where t is time and τ is the time constant. The units of t are time, and thus the ratio dF_A/dF_I is dimensionless. The time constant for wash-in of inhaled anesthetics is defined as the ratio of the capacity of the reservoir (V) into which the anesthetic is delivered to the flow rate of anesthetic (Q) into the reservoir:

■ Equation 27.2

$$\tau = \frac{V}{Q}$$

To solve Equation 27.1, the ratio F_A/F_I, must be defined at the extremes of time: at $t = 0$, when F_A/F_I is zero, and at $t = \infty$, when F_A/F_I approaches 1.0. Equation 27.1 is then integrated to yield:

■ Equation 27.3

$$\frac{F_A}{F_I} = 1 - e^{-t/\tau}$$

Using Equations 27.2 and 27.3, we can estimate the time to equilibration of F_A and F_I in the lungs, assuming uptake of anesthetic from the lungs is negligible. For adults, the functional residual capacity (FRC) is 2 L and alveolar ventilation is 4 L/min. Hence, τ is 2/4 or 0.5 minutes. When t equals 1τ, $F_A/F_I = 1 - e^{-1}$ or 0.63. Thus, the alveolar fraction is 63% of the inspired fraction. The values for F_A/F_I for larger multiples of 2, 3, and 4τ are 84, 92, and 96%, respectively. Based on these values, it takes four half-lives, or approximately 2 minutes in this example, to reach 96% equilibration of F_A with F_I in the adult.

Determinants of wash-in

The rate of increase in F_A/F_I (wash-in) depends on a balance of the rate of anesthetic delivery to and removal (or uptake) from the lungs. If delivery to the lungs is unopposed (negligible uptake), then the increase in F_A/F_I progresses unopposed and rapidly towards equilibration (i.e. unity), as for the wash-in of nitrous oxide and desflurane (and of other inhalation anesthetics in the first 2 minutes of wash-in). This interval represents unopposed wash-in of anesthetic into the lungs and has implications for the maximum deliverable inspired concentration by a vaporizer (see below). However, if delivery to the lungs is opposed by rapid removal (as in the case of a more soluble anesthetic such as halothane), then F_A/F_I increases more slowly (Fig. 27.5a). The wash-in of inhalational anesthetics depends on six factors. The first three determine the rate of anesthetic delivery to the lungs: ventilation, FRC, and inspired concentration. The second three determine its rate of removal from the lungs: solubility, cardiac output, and alveolar-to-venous partial pressure gradient.

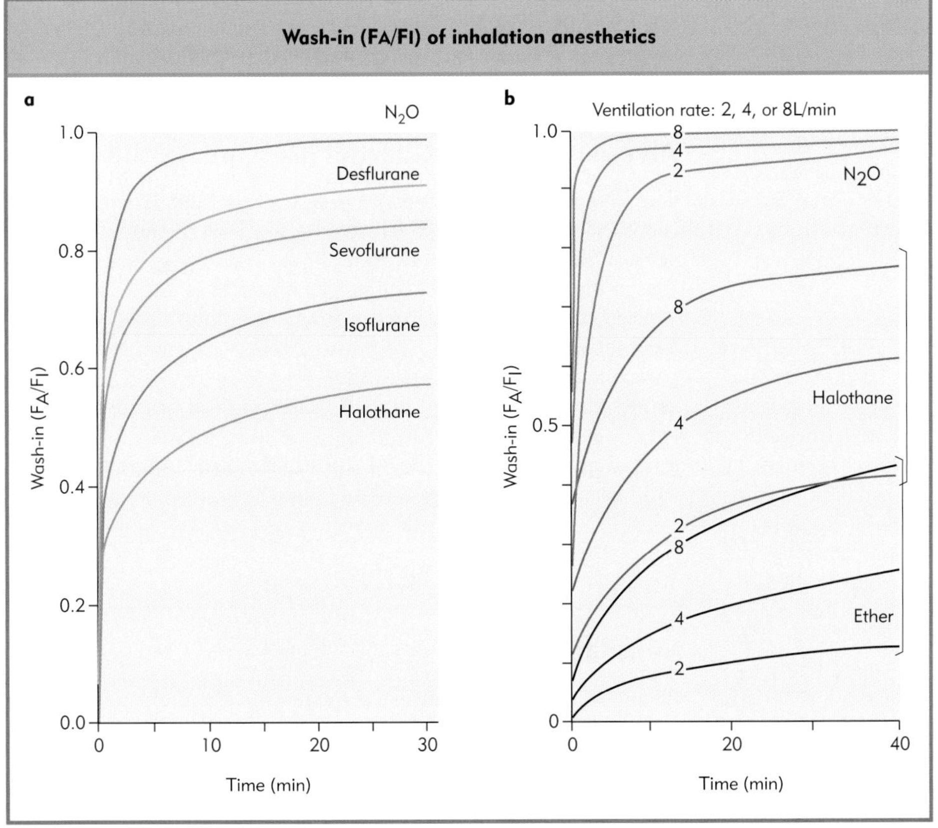

Figure 27.5 Wash-in (F_A/F_I) of inhalation anesthetics. (a) The wash-in of anesthetics increases as their solubility in blood decreases. (b) Increasing alveolar ventilation at a fixed cardiac output increases wash-in. The effect of ventilation on wash-in increases with increasing anesthetic solubility in blood.

Ventilation

With regard to anesthetic wash-in, ventilation refers exclusively to alveolar ventilation (Chapter 47), which is the fraction of minute ventilation that directly affects wash-in. Changes in alveolar ventilation result in parallel changes in the rate of increase in F_A/F_I (Fig. 27.5b).

> **Wash-in of inhaled anesthetics depends on lung delivery (ventilation, FRC, and inspired concentration) and removal (solubility, cardiac output, and alveolar–venous partial pressure difference).**

Functional residual capacity

The value of τ depends on the ratio of the volume of the reservoir into which the gas flows, the FRC (V), to the alveolar ventilation (Q), as in Equation 27.2. Changes in FRC lead to parallel changes in τ during wash-in, provided alveolar ventilation remains constant. In clinical situations such as obesity and restrictive lung defects, in which FRC is reduced, wash-in is more rapid.

Inspired concentration

The inspired concentration of an inhalational anesthetic is the physical force that drives anesthetic into the lungs, blood, and tissues. The greater the inspired concentration, the greater the driving force and the more rapid the increase in the ratio F_A/F_I. This factor significantly affects only oxygen, nitrous oxide, and xenon, because they are given in concentrations greater than 50%.

Uptake of anesthetic from the lungs

Uptake of anesthetic from the lungs is the product of three factors: cardiac output, solubility or the blood/gas partition coefficient (λ), and the alveolar-to-venous partial pressure gradient. If any of these factors decreases, uptake decreases in parallel. As a consequence, the partial pressure of anesthetic remaining in the lungs increases more rapidly until it equilibrates with the F_I.

Solubility

Inhalational anesthetics partition from the gas phase into two physiologic compartments, an aqueous phase and a protein/lipid phase. This is analogous to the distribution of oxygen and carbon dioxide in blood between the aqueous phase and hemoglobin. The *partial pressure* of the anesthetic determines the amount that is dissolved in the aqueous phase (Table 27.1). The remainder of anesthetic is bound to proteins and lipids in liquids and tissues. The solubility of inhalational anesthetics is defined as the ratio of the concentrations of anesthetic in two phases when the partial pressure of the anesthetic in the two phases has equilibrated (partition coefficient).

The rate of increase of wash-in is inversely related to anesthetic solubility in blood: anesthetics that are less soluble wash in more rapidly than those that are more soluble. This is because the diminished uptake of less soluble anesthetics from the lungs results in the accumulation of more anesthetic in the lungs, and its partial pressure increases more rapidly than for the more soluble anesthetics (Fig. 27.5). Thus, the alveolar partial pressure of less soluble anesthetics equilibrates more rapidly with inspired partial pressure than does the alveolar pressure of the more soluble anesthetics. The same holds true for the tissue partial pressure of anesthetics.

> **The equilibration of alveolar partial pressure with inspired partial pressure (wash-in) is more rapid for less soluble inhaled anesthetics.**

Cardiac output

Uptake of inhalational anesthetic from the lung involves movement of anesthetic across the alveolar capillary membranes and removal of anesthetic by blood traversing the pulmonary capillaries. Lipid membranes offer negligible resistance to anesthetic movement. Removal of anesthetic from the lungs depends on two remaining factors: pulmonary blood flow (or cardiac output), and the alveolar-to-venous partial pressure gradient. The greater the pulmonary blood flow, the greater the uptake of anesthetic by blood, which in turn increases the quantity of anesthetic delivered to tissues. However, the greater uptake of anesthetic from the lungs actually slows the rate of wash-in. Because the difference in anesthetic partial pressures (not concentrations) between the lungs or blood and tissues is the driving force along which anesthetics move from lung into blood and from blood into tissues, the slower rate of increase of alveolar partial pressure slows the accumulation of anesthetic in fluids and tissues. Thus, an increase in cardiac output actually slows the rate of increase of both wash-in and the partial pressure of anesthetic in tissues (Fig. 27.6). Conversely, as cardiac output decreases, so too does the uptake of anesthetic from the lungs. This speeds the equilibration of F_A and F_I. When blood flow to brain and heart is preserved in states of low cardiac output, the rapid increase in alveolar and blood anesthetic partial pressures rapidly depresses vital organ function.

Alveolar-to-venous partial pressure gradient

The alveolar-to-venous partial pressure gradient is the physical force that drives inhalational anesthetics from the alveolus to the venous blood. As anesthetic partial pressure in tissues approaches that in blood, so too does the partial pressure of anesthetic in the venous blood returning to the lungs approach alveolar values. The net effect is a decrease in the alveolar-to-venous anesthetic partial pressure gradient and, therefore, a decrease in the uptake of anesthetic from the lungs. As this gradient approaches zero (i.e. the partial pressures of anesthetic in tissues, blood, and lungs equilibrate), uptake of anesthetic also approaches zero. This occurs faster for less soluble anesthetics.

SPECIFIC CONDITIONS

Ventilation

Changes in ventilation affect the rate of wash-in of more soluble inhalational anesthetics to a greater extent (Fig. 27.5b). The rate of uptake of more soluble anesthetics from the alveoli is greater than that of less soluble anesthetics by a factor of their relative solubilities. Hence, more soluble anesthetics depend on their

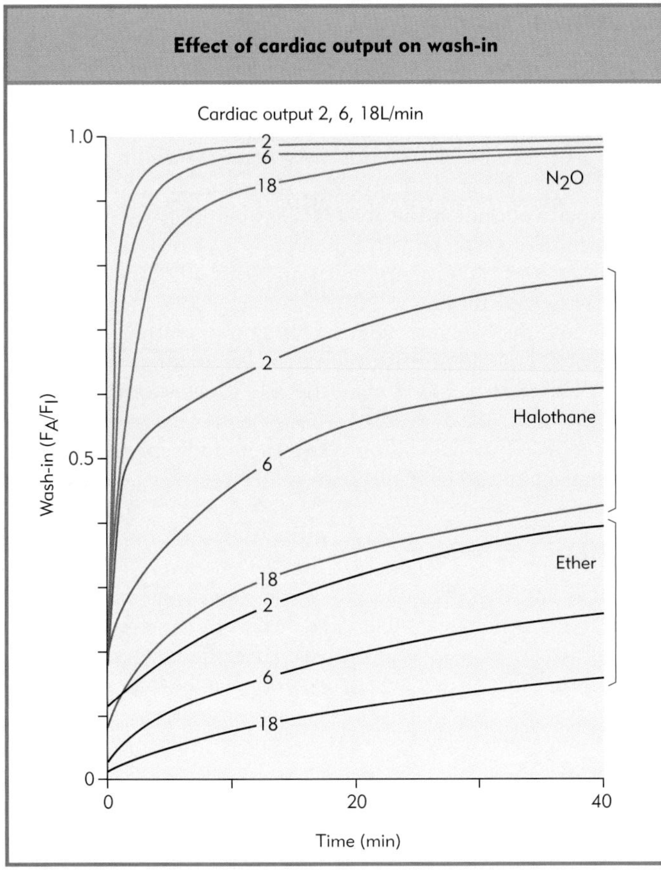

Figure 27.6 Effect of cardiac output on wash-in. Increasing cardiac output at a fixed alveolar ventilation decreases wash-in. The effect of cardiac output increases with increasing anesthetic solubility in blood.

rates of delivery (i.e. alveolar ventilation) to compensate in part for the greater uptake. Wash-in of less-soluble anesthetics is rapid because there is little uptake of anesthetic from the lungs, and F_A/F_I equilibrates rapidly. The slower wash-in of more soluble anesthetics is attributed to the rapid removal of anesthetics from the alveoli because of their high solubilities in blood and tissues.

Wash-in of insoluble anesthetics is rapid because there is little uptake of anesthetic from the lungs.

Hyperventilation

Increases in ventilation (or hyperventilation) should speed the rate of alveolar-to-blood-to-tissue anesthetic movement, and thus reduce the time for equilibration. However, increases in alveolar ventilation may also affect tissue blood flow. For example, hyperventilation decreases arterial CO_2 tension, which in turn decreases cerebral blood flow. Because the delivery of anesthetic to the brain depends on its blood flow, hyperventilation may actually increase the value of τ for anesthetic partial pressure equilibration within the brain. The net effect of hyperventilation is a balance of an increase in delivery of anesthetic to the alveoli and a decrease in delivery of anesthetic to brain.

The effect of hyperventilation on the rate of increase of anesthetic partial pressure in the brain depends to a large extent on the blood solubility of the anesthetic. In the case of a soluble anesthetic, hyperventilation increases the delivery of anesthetic to the blood while decreasing cerebral blood flow. The net effect is to speed the rate of increase of anesthetic partial pressure in the brain. In contrast, hyperventilation with a less soluble anesthetic minimally increases the delivery of anesthetic to the blood but decreases cerebral blood flow. The net effect is a slowing of the equilibration of anesthetic partial pressures within brain. After the initial period, hyperventilation speeds the rate of equilibration of anesthetic partial pressures within the brain. For anesthetics of intermediate solubility such as halothane, these opposing effects of hyperventilation are offsetting during the initial period of anesthesia (Fig. 27.7). After this initial period, however, the rate of increase of anesthetic partial pressure within the brain exceeds that during normocapnic ventilation.

Modes of ventilation

Two feedback mechanisms function in response to inhalational anesthesia: respiratory and cardiovascular. The respiratory feedback mechanism is a negative feedback loop in which *spontaneous ventilation* decreases as the depth of anesthesia increases (respiratory depression). This limits the depth of anesthesia by attenuating the delivery of anesthetic to the lungs. Although the delivery of anesthetic to the lungs subsides, anesthetic present in tissues redistributes from organs in which it is present at a high partial pressure (such as the brain) to others in which it is present at a low partial pressure (such as muscle). When the

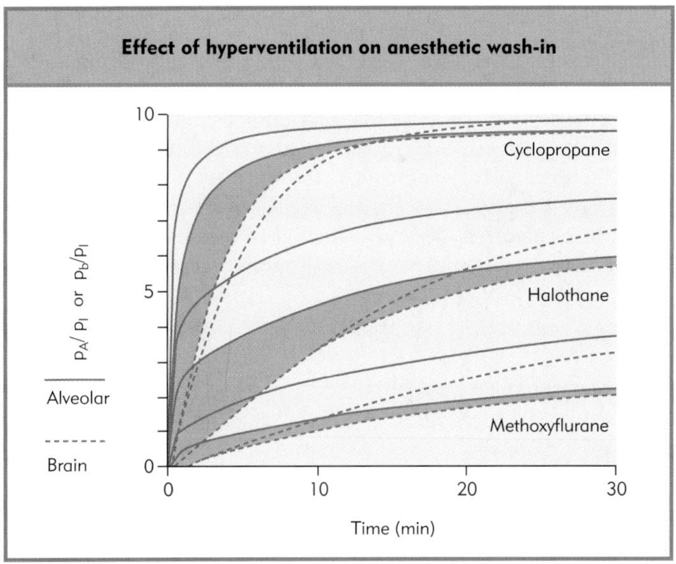

Figure 27.7 The effect of hyperventilation on the wash-in of three inhalation anesthetics of different solubilities: cyclopropane (less soluble), methoxyflurane (very soluble), and halothane (intermediate solubility). Two conditions are delineated: normocapnia (denoted by the curves joined by the purple shading) and hypocapnia induced by hyperventilation (other curves). Compared with the normocapnic state, hyperventilation speeds the rise of alveolar anesthetic partial pressure for all three anesthetics, although the effect is greatest with the most soluble and least with the least soluble anesthetic. In contrast, hyperventilation delays the rise of brain anesthetic partial pressure most with the least soluble and least with the most soluble anesthetic. The effect on halothane is intermediate. P_A, alveolar partial pressure; P_b, brain partial pressure; P_I, inspired partial pressure of anesthetic. (Adapted with permission from Munson ES, Bowers DL. The effects of hyperventilation on the rate of cerebral anesthetic equilibration. Anesthesiology 1967;28:377–81.)

partial pressure of anesthetic in the brain has decreased to a threshold level, respiration increases. This is a protective mechanism that prevents anesthetic overdose with spontaneous ventilation by limiting the delivery of anesthetic to vital organs.

The cardiovascular feedback mechanism is a positive feedback loop in which cardiac output decreases as the depth of anesthesia increases. As cardiac output decreases the uptake of anesthetic from the lungs decreases, and thus the rate of increase of alveolar-to-inspired anesthetic partial pressure increases further. This is reflected in an increase in the partial pressure of anesthetic in blood and a greater driving force for anesthetic delivery to tissues. The increase in anesthetic partial pressure in tissues further depresses organ function such as cardiac output, with a further increase in anesthetic partial pressure in alveoli, blood, and tissues.

Anesthetic uptake is regulated by a negative respiratory feedback mechanism and a positive cardiovascular feedback mechanism.

The significance of these feedback loops to the pharmacokinetics of volatile anesthetics has been demonstrated in adult dogs, which were allowed to breathe *spontaneously* while anesthetized with halothane at between 0.3 and 4 vol%. F_A/F_I increased to approximately 0.65 after 15 minutes, where it remained for up to 50 minutes. All of the dogs survived. In a second experiment, dogs were ventilated *mechanically* while anesthetized with halothane at similar inspired concentrations. The F_A/F_I plateaued only in those dogs given an inspired concentration of 1.5% or less. The F_A/F_I increased relentlessly to approximately 1.0 in those dogs that were anesthetized with 4% and 6% halothane; within 1 hour most of those dogs experienced circulatory collapse (Fig. 27.8). Thus, spontaneous ventilation remains an effective negative feedback mechanism for preventing an overdose of a volatile anesthetic. In contrast, *controlled ventilation* exposes patients to a positive feedback mechanism that may result in a relentless downward spiral of circulatory depression and cardiac arrest unless anesthetic partial pressure is reduced.

The concentration effect

The concentration effect results from two factors: a concentrating effect and an augmentation in effective ventilation. When an inhalational anesthetic is administered in a low concentration (1 vol%), uptake of half of this anesthetic results in a concentration of approximately 0.5 vol%. The net effect of the uptake of this small volume on the alveolar gas volume is small; ventilation is minimally affected. If, however, the anesthetic is administered in an 80 vol% concentration, uptake of half of the anesthetic contracts the residual gas volume. The net concentration is not 50 vol% of the original concentration but rather 66 vol%, because of the concentrating effect on the smaller residual gas volume. This effect, along with the additional ventilation that follows the contracted alveolar volume, leads to a concentration that exceeds 70 vol%. The only anesthetic administered today that is subject to the concentration effect is nitrous oxide.

Second gas effect

When two anesthetics are administered one in a large concentration and another in a small concentration, the concentration effect of the first anesthetic may increase the concentration of the second. This effect, which is produced by the same two mechanisms that explain the concentration effect above, has been demonstrated in dogs, but its clinical relevance has been questioned.

Overpressure technique

In order to establish rapidly the desired partial pressure of anesthetic in the alveoli or brain, its inspired partial pressure may be adjusted to a value that is several times greater than the desired alveolar partial pressure (overpressure technique). For example, if the target alveolar (or brain) partial pressure of an anesthetic is 1.0 vol%, then the inspired partial pressure could be adjusted to a value of 3 vol%. During the early period of anesthesia F_A/F_I increases rapidly, reaching a ratio of 0.3 (Fig. 27.5a) and thus achieving the target alveolar or brain partial pressure of 1 vol% more quickly than when starting at 1 vol%.

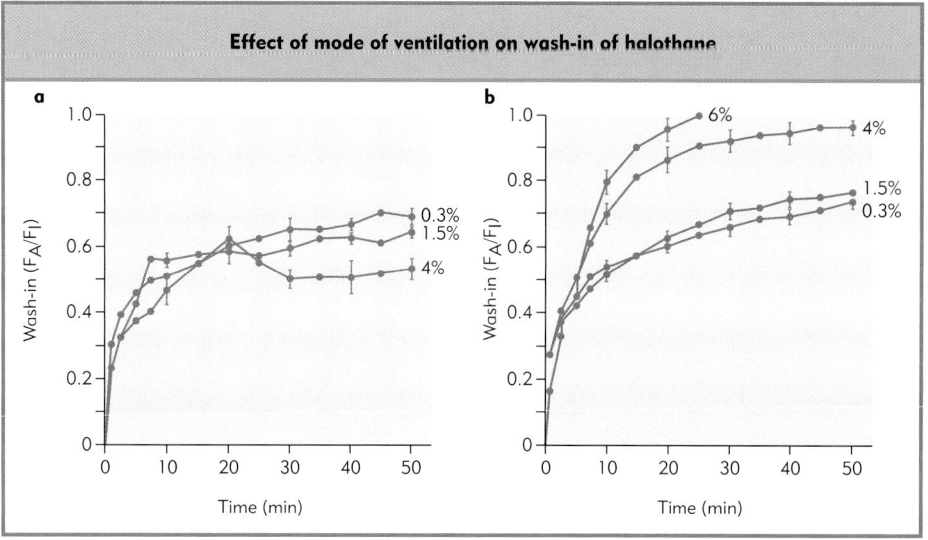

Figure 27.8 Effect of mode of ventilation on wash-in of halothane. Wash-in (the rate of rise of the ratio of alveolar (F_A) to inspired (F_I) anesthetic partial pressure) is shown for (a) spontaneous and (b) controlled ventilation. The negative feedback effect of spontaneous ventilation limits the rate of rise of F_A/F_I. All dogs survived. The positive feedback effect of decreased cardiac output during controlled ventilation resulted in death in those dogs anesthetized with 4% or 6% halothane.

Vital capacity inductions

The traditional technique used for induction of anesthesia by inhalation is a stepwise increase in inspired concentration every few breaths. With the introduction of sevoflurane, single-breath vital capacity inductions have become popular. The stepwise technique was conceived out of concerns that laryngospasm and breathholding might occur if high concentrations of halothane were administered too rapidly. These concerns have not been supported with recent evidence. To perform a single-breath induction, the anesthetic circuit is first primed with the maximum deliverable concentration of anesthetic and the patient then performs one or more vital capacity inhalations. These inductions are more rapid than graded stepwise inductions.

Cardiac output

Changes in cardiac output affect the rate of increase in alveolar-to-inspired anesthetic partial pressure of soluble anesthetics to a greater extent than with less soluble anesthetics. Soluble anesthetics are removed from the alveoli in greater quantities, and therefore in the presence of an increased cardiac output, the rate of rise of alveolar-to-inspired partial pressures of soluble anesthetics is slower than that of less soluble anesthetics. This is reflected in parallel changes in the partial pressure of more soluble anesthetics in tissues, as the anesthetic partial pressure in the blood equilibrates with that in the alveoli.

Shunts

Left-to-right shunts (where blood is recirculated through the lungs) do not usually affect the wash-in of inhalational anesthetics provided cardiac output and its distribution remain unchanged. In contrast, right-to-left shunts (where venous blood bypasses the lungs and mixes with arterial blood) exert a significant effect on wash-in of inhalational anesthetics. The magnitude of this effect depends on the solubility of the anesthetic: right-to-left shunts affect less soluble anesthetics (i.e. nitrous oxide, desflurane, and sevoflurane) to a much greater extent than the more soluble anesthetics (i.e. halothane and methoxyflurane). In the model shown in Figure 27.9, each lung is represented by one alveolus and is perfused by one pulmonary artery. When the tracheal tube is positioned at the midtracheal level (i.e. no shunt), ventilation is divided equally between both lungs, yielding equal anesthetic partial pressures in both pulmonary veins. However, when the tip of the tube is advanced into one bronchus (right-to-left shunt), all of the ventilation is delivered to one lung; ventilation to the intubated lung is doubled, whereas ventilation to the second lung is zero. Under these conditions, normocapnia is maintained. In the case of a more soluble anesthetic, the partial pressure of anesthetic in the combined pulmonary venous drainage of the lungs is approximately the same as under normal conditions in the trachea, as the increased ventilation to the intubated lung speeds the rise of alveolar-to-inspired anesthetic partial pressure such that it compensates for the presence of the shunt (Fig 27.9b). However, when a less soluble anesthetic is administered in the presence of a right-to-left shunt, the increased ventilation to the intubated lung minimally affects the rate of rise of alveolar-to-inspired anesthetic partial pressures in that lung, because changes in ventilation do not appreciably affect the wash-in of less soluble anesthetics (Fig 27.9c). In this case, the anesthetic partial pressure in the combined pulmonary venous drainage lags behind that which would occur in the absence of a right-to-left shunt.

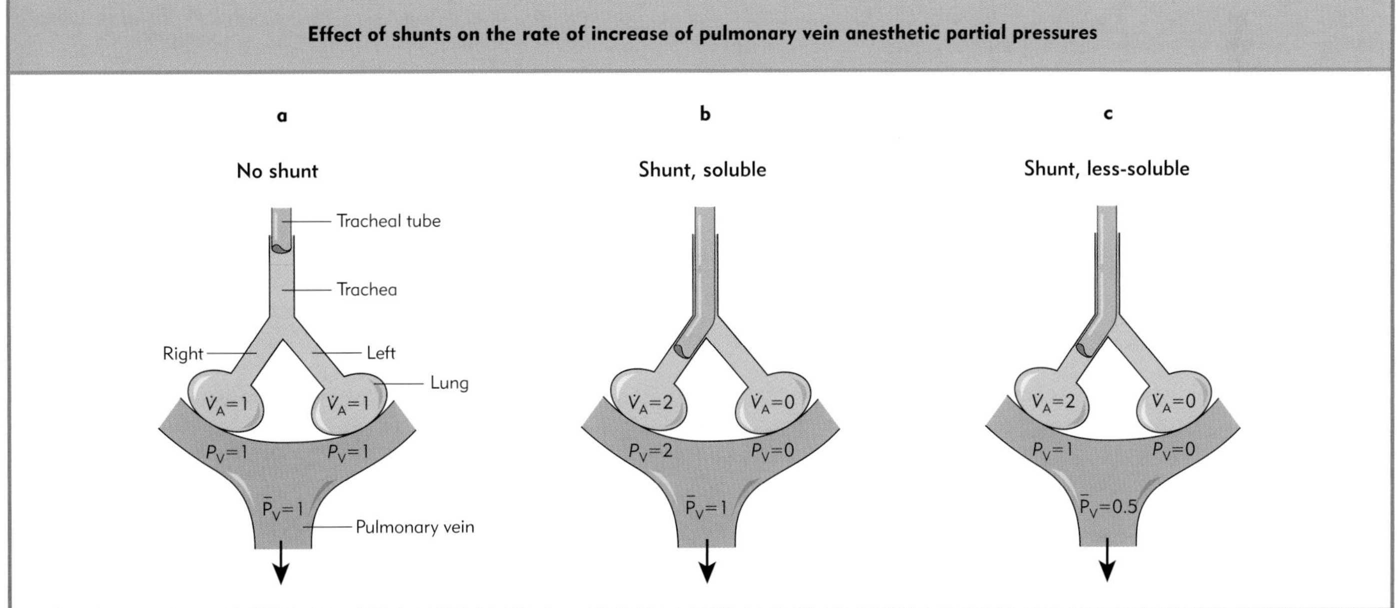

Figure 27.9 The effect of shunts on the rate of increase of pulmonary vein anesthetic pressures varies with the solubility of the anesthetic. If a soluble anesthetic is administered in the presence of a right-to-left shunt (b), normocapnia is maintained and hypoxic pulmonary vasoconstriction is negligible. Here, the increase in ventilation to the intubated lung offsets the effect of the shunt. However, a right-to-left shunt in the presence of a less-soluble anesthetic (c) limits the increase in anesthetic partial pressure in the pulmonary vein (P_V). Because an increase in alveolar ventilation does not substantially affect the wash-in of a less soluble anesthetic, the shunted blood slows the rate of rise of P_V. Arrows indicate the direction of blood flow.

Right-to-left shunts significantly affect the wash-in of less soluble inhaled anesthetics.

Temperature

The solubility of inhalational anesthetics in blood and tissues is inversely related to temperature: as the temperature decreases, the solubility increases. Solubility increases 4–5% for every 1°C reduction in temperature. As temperature decreases and solubility increases, the rate of rise of alveolar-to-inspired anesthetic concentration slows. This effect is most prominent during cardiopulmonary bypass, when temperatures as low as 10–18°C are used.

TISSUE UPTAKE

The uptake of anesthetic by the body is the sum of uptake by all tissues. Initially, uptake of anesthetic by tissues is great and the partial pressure of anesthetic in the venous blood returning to the lungs is low. As the partial pressure of anesthetic in tissues approaches that within the alveoli, the partial pressure of anesthetic in venous blood also increases. This diminishes the alveolar-to-venous partial pressure gradient, one of the determinants of anesthetic uptake from the lungs, and anesthetic uptake diminishes.

Anesthetic uptake can be estimated by grouping tissues according to the time to anesthetic partial pressure equilibration within the tissues; this is related to the relative solubility of the inhalational anesthetics in and perfusion to the tissues. Tissues have been divided into four groups: vessel-rich group (VRG), muscle group (MG), fat group (FG), and vessel-poor group (VPG). The VRG comprises five organs: brain, heart, kidney, splanchnic (liver), and endocrine glands. The VPG includes bone and connective tissues.

The time constant for equilibration of anesthetic partial pressure in a tissue is defined as the ratio of the capacity of the organ and the blood flow to the organ. The capacity of the tissue reservoir for anesthetic is the product of the volume of the tissue and the solubility of the anesthetic in that tissue (tissue:blood partition coefficient). The time constant for organs is thus defined as:

■ Equation 27.4

$$\tau = \frac{V\lambda_{t/b}}{Q}$$

where $\lambda_{t/b}$ is the tissue:blood partition coefficient, V is tissue volume and Q is tissue blood flow. Because the volume of most tissues and their blood flow is constant, changes in the value of τ are determined by the partition coefficient. For example, the time to equilibration of anesthetic partial pressures in tissues such as the brain may be expressed in terms of τ as:

■ Equation 27.5

$$\tau = \frac{\text{Volume of the brain (mL)} \times \text{brain/blood solubility}}{\text{Brain blood flow (mL/min)}}$$

The rate of rise of anesthetic partial pressure in tissues follows a pattern determined by the delivery of anesthetic to these tissues. That is, tissues perfused with a greater fraction of the cardiac output equilibrate more rapidly: VRG > MG > VPG > FG.

Uptake of anesthetic by the VRG is denoted by the initial flattening of the wash-in curve for inhalational anesthetics. Without uptake by the VRG, wash-in would continue to increase as rapidly as it did during the first minutes of wash-in. The effect of uptake of anesthetic by the VRG is to slow the rate of rise of alveolar-to-inspired partial pressure.

Wash-in of inhalational anesthetics into the VRG is usually complete within the first 15–20 minutes of anesthesia. In adults, these tissues comprise 8% of body weight but receive 75% of cardiac output. Accordingly, τ for the VRG is small and anesthetic partial pressures equilibrate rapidly in these organs. For example, the time to 1τ, or 63% equilibration of halothane partial pressure in the VRG, is 3 minutes and the time to 4τ or 96% is 12 minutes. The wide range of values of τ for different tissues is attributable to tissue:blood solubility (the greater the solubility, the greater the value of τ) and blood flow.

After equilibration of anesthetic partial pressure in the VRG, wash-in should increase rapidly. However, the rate of increase of wash-in is slower than expected because of the uptake of anesthetic by the MG. Uptake by this group becomes prominent approximately 20 minutes after induction of anesthesia and continues for approximately 200 minutes. The value of τ for anesthetic in the MG is greater than that in the VRG by 10–30-fold. This may be attributed to a relatively lower cardiac output per unit muscle mass and a greater solubility of anesthetics in muscle. The time to equilibration of anesthetic partial pressure in muscle is 2–6 hours, depending on the anesthetic.

After equilibration of anesthetic partial pressure in the MG, uptake continues by the VPG and FG, as reflected by their large τ values. Fat represents 20% of body weight but receives only 6% of cardiac output in the healthy adult. Although perfusion of fat per unit volume is only 10–20% less than that of muscle, the solubility of anesthetics in fat is 10–30 times greater than that in muscle. On the basis of Equation 27.4, the value of τ for fat is 10–30 times that in muscle, or 1.5–40 hours depending on the anesthetic, such that uptake of anesthetic by fat usually contributes minimally to the total tissue uptake.

PHARMACOKINETICS IN CHILDREN

The rate of rise of alveolar-to-inspired partial pressures of inhalational anesthetics is more rapid in neonates and infants than in adults. This observation has been attributed to four differences between infants and adults. The order of these four factors reflects their relative contributions to this effect. The net effect of these differences between neonates and adults is to speed the equilibration of anesthetic partial pressures in alveoli and tissues, and thereby speed the rate of rise of wash-in in infants and children compared to adults.

Ratio of alveolar ventilation to functional residual capacity

The greater the ratio of alveolar ventilation to FRC, the more rapid the wash-in of anesthetic (see Fig. 27.5). In neonates this ratio is approximately 5:1, compared to only 1.5:1 in adults. The greater ratio in neonates is attributable to the threefold greater metabolic rate and concomitant oxygen consumption in neonates compared to adults (Table 27.1).

Wash-in of inhaled anesthetics is more rapid in infants owing to greater alveolar ventilation: FRC ratio; lower anesthetic solubilities in blood and tissues; and greater cardiac index.

Solubility in blood

The solubility of inhalational anesthetics in blood varies with age. The blood solubilities of halothane, isoflurane, enflurane, and methoxyflurane are 18% less in neonates and the elderly than in young adults. These differences may be attributed to differences in blood constituents: the blood:gas partition coefficients of isoflurane and enflurane correlate directly with serum albumin and triglyceride concentrations; that of halothane correlates directly with serum cholesterol, albumin, triglyceride, and globulin concentrations; and that of methoxyflurane correlates directly with serum cholesterol, albumin, and globulin concentrations.

Solubility in tissues

The solubilities of halothane, isoflurane, enflurane, and methoxyflurane in tissues of the VRG in neonates are approximately 50% of those in adults. The decreased tissue solubilities are attributable to greater water content and decreased protein and lipid concentrations in neonates. The solubilities of volatile anesthetics in muscle increase with age. The reduced solubility of anesthetics in the muscle of neonates may be attributed to the low protein content of muscle in the first few months of life, whereas the increased solubility in the elderly reflects the increased protein and fat content of muscle in this age group. The reduced solubility in the muscle of neonates speeds the equilibration of anesthetic partial pressure in muscle during the interval when uptake by muscle is greatest, that is, between 20 and 200 minutes.

Cardiac output

The greater cardiac index in neonates compared with adults speeds the equilibration of alveolar and inspired anesthetic partial pressures. This may be explained by the preferential distribution of cardiac output to the VRG in neonates. This is because the VRG receives a greater proportion of cardiac output in neonates because it comprises 18% of the body weight compared to only 8% in adults.

ELIMINATION

General principles

The washout of inhalational anesthetics follows an exponential decay (the inverse of wash-in) and varies inversely with blood:gas solubility; that is, the lower the solubility, the more rapid the wash-out (Table 27.1). However, elimination of inhalational anesthetics depends on other factors as well, including duration of anesthetic exposure and, to a lesser extent, metabolism. Recovery from anesthesia parallels the washout of inhalational anesthetics.

Washout of inhalational anesthetics differs from wash-in in two respects. First, during wash-in, the inspired concentration of anesthetic can be increased to compensate for the rapid uptake of anesthetic from the lungs. However, during washout the minimum partial pressure of the anesthetic cannot be less than zero. Therefore, the inspired concentration of anesthetic cannot increase the rate of washout of inhalational anesthetics. Second, during washout anesthetic exits tissues in sequence (VRG, MG, VPG, and FG) but may also redistribute to tissue groups, particularly with the more soluble anesthetics.

The effect of the duration of anesthesia on the rate of washout depends in part on the solubility of the anesthetic. For anesthetics with low solubilities, washout is rapid and the duration of anesthesia has an attenuated effect. For anesthetics that are very soluble, the rate of washout varies inversely with the duration of anesthesia.

Percutaneous loss of inhalational anesthetics is small compared to expired and metabolic losses. These losses depend on the blood solubility of the anesthetic. Quantitatively, percutaneous losses of inhalational anesthetics do not affect their pharmacokinetics.

Metabolism

The metabolism of inhalational anesthetics depends primarily on cytochrome P450 enzyme systems located in the endoplasmic reticulum of hepatocytes. The two major pathways for metabolism are the oxidative and reductive pathways. Of the oxidative pathways, dehalogenation and O-dealkylation are involved. Dehalogenation is the result of hydroxylation of the halogenated carbon, which decomposes to a carboxylic acid and inorganic halogens. The presence of two halogens on the terminal carbon provides optimal conditions for dehalogenation, whereas the presence of three halogens dramatically reduces the probability of dehalogenation. O-Dealkylation is the result of hydroxylation of an alkyl group adjacent to the oxygen of the ether bond. The intermediate compound rapidly decomposes to an alcohol and an aldehyde. The aldehyde may be oxidized by aldehyde oxidase to carboxylic acid, or reduced by alcohol dehydrogenase to an alcohol. The reductive pathway has only been demonstrated for halothane.

The extent of in vivo metabolism of inhalational anesthetics ranges from 50% for methoxyflurane to 0.02% for desflurane (Table 27.1). With the exception of halothane and methoxyflurane, metabolism of inhalational anesthetics accounts for the elimination of 5% or less of the anesthetic administered; consequently, the contribution of metabolism to their pharmacokinetics is small.

Methoxyflurane

Methoxyflurane is an ether anesthetic that is oxygenated either at the methyl carbon or at the dichloroethyl carbon, with the release of large quantities of inorganic fluoride, dichloroacetic acid, and, possibly, methoxydifluoroacetic acid. Defluorination of methoxyflurane occurs in the presence of cytochrome P450, glutathione *S*-transferase, and possibly also by a nonenzymatic pathway that requires vitamin B_{12} and glutathione. Plasma inorganic fluoride concentrations in excess of 95 μg/dL (50 μmol/L) have been associated with high-output renal insufficiency, although recent evidence suggests that renal insufficiency depends on the local renal production of inorganic fluoride by the metabolism of methoxyflurane by renal cytochrome P450 CYP 2E1 isozyme. Metabolism of methoxyflurane is increased after pretreatment with phenobarbital, diphenylhydantoin, ethanol, diazepam, and isoniazid.

Metabolism accounts for the elimination of <5% of inhaled anesthetics, except for halothane and methoxyflurane.

Halothane

Halothane is extensively metabolized via the cytochrome P450 system. The products of oxidative metabolism are inorganic bromide, chloride, and trifluoroacetic acid; the products of reductive metabolism are inorganic bromide and fluoride. An alternate reductive pathway requires an electron donor (usually cytochrome P450 enzyme system) and an anaerobic milieu. This pathway results in several volatile halogenated compounds (1,1-difluoro-2-chloroethylene, 1,1,1-trifluoro-2-chloroethane, and 1,1-difluoro-2-bromo-2-chloroethylene). Inorganic fluoride is also released with the first metabolite. Peak plasma inorganic fluoride concentrations are low (<28 μg/dL (<15 μmol/L)) even after 19.5 MAC.h halothane in adults. Metabolism of halothane is increased after administration of phenobarbital or isoniazid, and after prolonged exposure to subanesthetic concentrations of halothane.

Sevoflurane

Sevoflurane is metabolized by CYP 2E1 via oxidation of the α-carbon. The profile of plasma inorganic fluoride production after sevoflurane anesthesia in adults without hepatic enzyme induction is similar to that of enflurane. Maximum fluoride concentrations reach 66 μg/dL (25–35 μmol/L) within 1 or 2 hours of discontinuation of the anesthetic, but decrease to less than 9.5 μg/dL (5 μmol/L) within several hours. The rapid decrease in serum inorganic fluoride after discontinuation of the anesthetic is attributed to the rapid washout and minimal metabolism of sevoflurane. Plasma inorganic fluoride concentrations are approximately 20% greater after prolonged exposure (>13 hours) to sevoflurane and in mildly obese patients compared to concentrations after brief exposures in nonobese adults. Metabolism of inhalational anesthetics within the kidney may explain why some anesthetics that release inorganic fluoride cause high-output renal insufficiency (i.e. methoxyflurane) and others (sevoflurane) do not. The reduced affinity of renal CYP 2E1 for sevoflurane compared to that for methoxyflurane results in a subtoxic intrarenal concentration of inorganic fluoride and hence less damage to renal tubular cells. Defluorination of sevoflurane is increased after pretreatment with phenobarbital, diphenylhydantoin, ethanol, and isoniazid.

Enflurane

Enflurane is metabolized to only a small extent via oxidative dehalogenation at the chlorofluoromethyl carbon by CYP 2E1. The resultant inorganic fluoride yields serum concentrations that are considered subtoxic.

Isoflurane

Isoflurane is metabolized to a small extent via oxidation of the α-carbon, yielding trifluoroacetic acid, inorganic fluoride, and several intermediate compounds. The maximum serum concentration of fluoride after isoflurane is <9.5 μg/dL (5 μmol/L), although plasma fluoride concentrations in excess of 95 μg/dL (50 μmol/L) have been reported after prolonged administration (19.2 MAC.h). Enzyme induction increases the metabolism of isoflurane, although metabolism does not contribute significantly to its elimination.

Desflurane

Of the inhalational anesthetics, desflurane is the least metabolized in vivo. The reduced metabolism is attributed to the substitution of fluoride for chlorine on the α-carbon, thereby decreasing the affinity of this substrate for cytochrome P450 enzymes. Inorganic fluoride levels after desflurane anesthesia are less than 5.7 μg/dL (3 μmol/L) even after prolonged exposure.

Infants and children

The metabolism of inhalational anesthetics in neonates and infants is less than in adults. This has been attributed to reduced activity of hepatic microsomal enzymes, reduced fat stores, and more rapid exhalation of the anesthetics. After 131 MAC.h isoflurane, plasma inorganic fluoride levels are not elevated.

Key references

Eger EI II. Anesthetic uptake and action. In: Baltimore: Williams & Wilkins; 1974.

Eisenkraft JB. Anesthesia vaporizers. In: Ehrenwerth J, Eisenkraft JB, eds. Anesthesia equipment: principles and applications. St Louis: Mosby; 1974:57–88.

Ledez KM, Lerman J. The minimum alveolar concentration (MAC) of isoflurane in preterm neonates. Anesthesiology 1987;67:301–7.

Munson ES, Bowers DL. The effects of hyperventilation on the rate of cerebral anesthetic equilibration. Anesthesiology 1967;28:377–81.

Smith TC. Anesthesia breathing systems. In: Ehrenwerth J, Eisenkraft JB, eds. Anesthesia equipment: principles and applications. St Louis: Mosby; 1993:89–113.

Yasuda N, Lockhart SH, Eger EI II et al. Comparison of kinetics of sevoflurane and isoflurane in humans. Anesth Analg. 1991;72:316–24.

Further reading

Kobayashi S, Bito H, Obara Y et al. Compound A concentration in the circle absorber system during low-flow sevoflurane anesthesia: comparison of Dragersorb Free, Amsorb and Sodasorb III. J Clin Anesth. 2003;15:33–7.

Rossaint R, Reyle-Hahn M, Schulte Am Esch J et al. Multicenter randomized comparison of the efficacy and safety of xenon and isoflurane in patients undergoing elective surgery. Anesthesiology 2003;98:6–13.

Sanders RD, Franks NP, Maze M. Xenon: no stranger to anaesthesia. Br J Anaesth. 2003;91:709–17.

Struys MM, Bouche MP, Relly G et al. Production of compound A and carbon monoxide in circle systems: an in vitro comparison of two carbon dioxide absorbents. Anaesthesia 2004;59:584–9.

Versichlen LF, Bouche MP, Rolly G et al. Only carbon dioxide absorbents free of both NaOH and KOH do not generate compound A during in vitro closed-system sevoflurane: evaluation of five absorbents. Anesthesiology 2001;95:750–5.

Chapter 28

Anesthetic adjuvants and other CNS drugs

Francis Bonnet, Emmanuel Marret and Robert A Veselis

Anesthetic adjuvants are drugs active within the CNS that strengthen the effects of anesthetic agents. Anesthetic adjuvants are used because of their anesthetic-sparing properties, to prolong the anesthetic effect, and to avoid implicit or explicit memory during anesthesia, which is one of the main uses for benzodiazepines. Modern techniques of monitoring the depth of anesthesia facilitate the prevention of 'awakening' and 'recall'. New anesthetic agents aid a rapid return to consciousness, and so anesthesiologists are less interested in prolonging the duration of anesthesia in the postoperative period. The use of benzodiazepines has consequently declined, to the benefit of other adjuvants. The prevention of postoperative pain by drugs that act synergistically with opioids is now facilitated by agents such as α_2-adrenergic agonists and NMDA (*N*-methyl-D-aspartate) glutamate receptor blockers. This chapter reviews the roles of these drugs as anesthetic adjuvants, and then discusses the pharmacology of other CNS-active drugs relevant to anesthesiology.

α_2-ADRENERGIC AGONISTS

Pharmacology

α_2-adrenergic agonists belong to three main chemical classes: phenylethylates (e.g. methyldopa, guanabenz), imidazolines (e.g. clonidine, dexmedetomidine, mivazerol, azepexole) (Fig. 28.1), and oxaloazepines (e.g. rilmelidine).

Clonidine is the prototypal α_2-adrenergic agonist, having a 200-fold selectivity for α_2 over α_1 adrenoceptors. Clonidine is moderately lipid soluble and has a large volume of distribution (approximately 2 L/kg) and a relatively long terminal elimination half-life (12–24 hours). Clonidine is almost completely absorbed after oral administration, with a peak effect between 60 and 90 minutes. The analgesic effect of clonidine is more closely related to its CSF than its plasma concentration.

Dexmedetomidine, also an imidazoline compound, is eight times more selective for α_2 adrenoreceptors than clonidine. The distribution half-time ($t_{1/2\alpha}$) of dexmedetomidine is about 6 minutes, and the estimate of the terminal elimination half-time ($t_{1/2\beta}$) is 2 hours, both considerably shorter than those of clonidine. Dexmedetomidine undergoes extensive liver transformation into methyl and glucuronide conjugates.

Role of α_2-adrenergic receptors

α_2-adrenergic receptors are G protein-coupled receptors, coupled via pertussis toxin-sensitive G_i proteins to pathways that produce hyperpolarization. Three distinct human α_2-adrenoreceptor subtype genes have been cloned, identified pharmacologically as α_{2A}, α_{2B} and α_{2C}. The dorsal horn of the spinal cord contains α_{2A} subtype receptors, whereas both α_{2A} and α_{2C} receptors are found in primary sensory neurons. Binding of agonist to the receptor results in a conformational change in structure, facilitating interaction with the G_i protein (Fig. 28.2; see also Chapter 3). The affinity of the α subunit of G_i for GDP is decreased, it is replaced by GTP, and the G protein consequently dissociates and couples to the effector. The affinity of the agonist decreases and the agonist leaves its binding site. The intrinsic GTPase in the dissociated α subunit is activated and it hydrolyzes bound GTP into GDP. At the level of the dorsal horn of the spinal cord, activation of G_i-gated K^+ channels results in neuronal membrane hyperpolarization, causing a decrease in excitability.

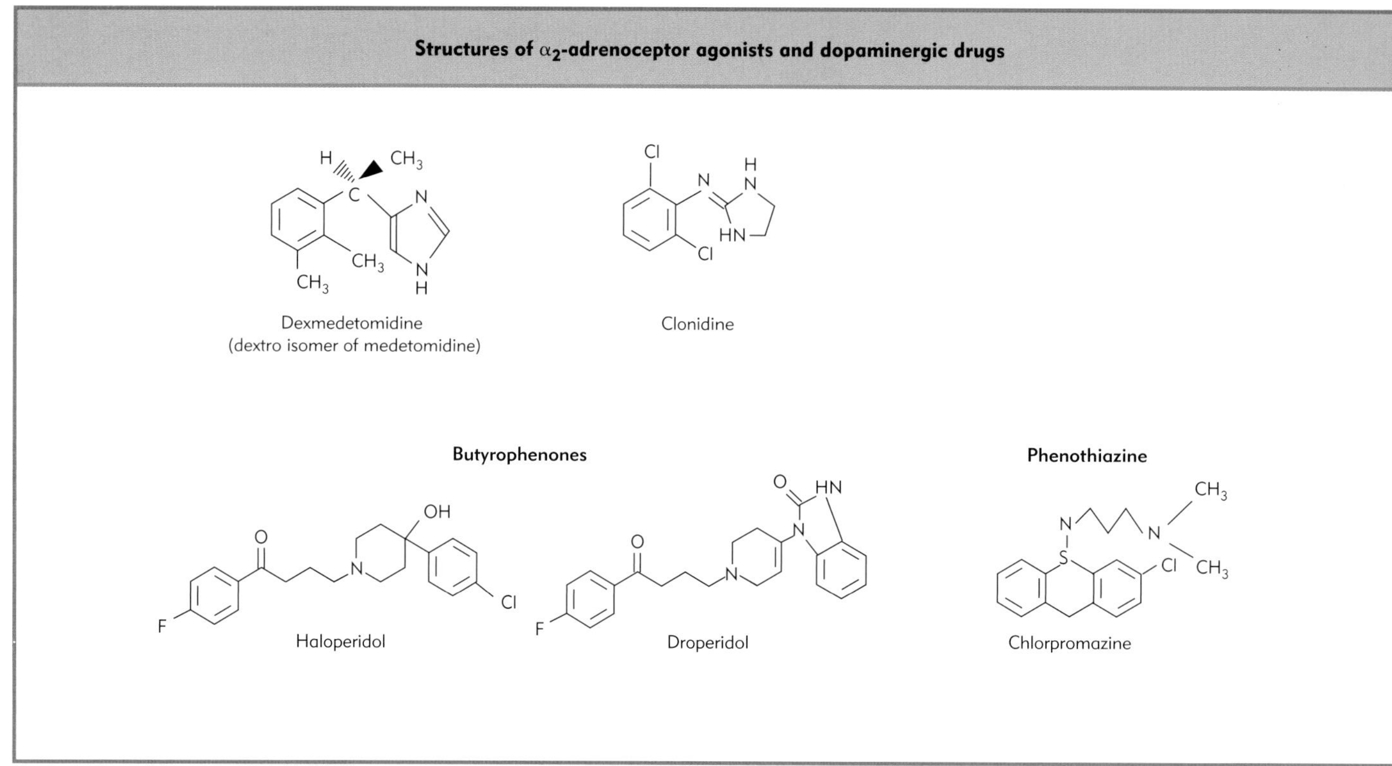

Figure 28.1 Structures of α_2-adrenoceptor agonists and dopaminergic drugs.

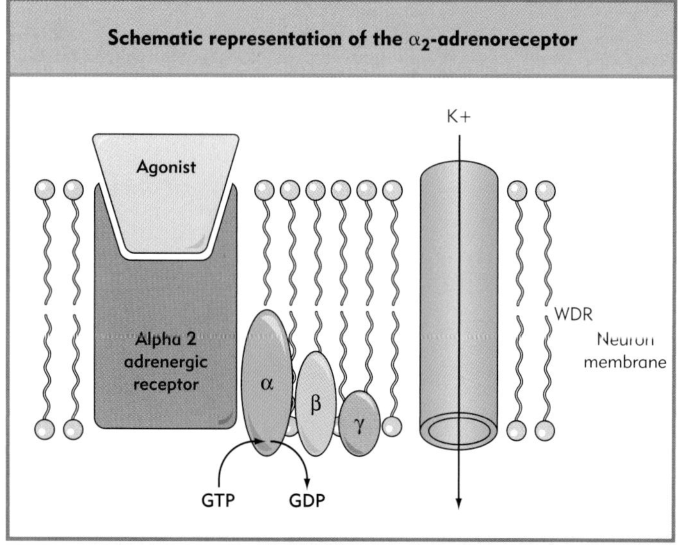

Figure 28.2 Schematic representation of the α_2-adrenoreceptor and its relation to a G_i protein. Binding of the agonist (norepinephrine–clonidine–dexmedetomidine) to the α_2-adrenergic receptor facilitates contact with a pertussis toxin-sensitive G_i protein and promotes the dissociation of GDP from the α subunit. GTP binding activates the G protein; the α subunit interacts with a K^+ channel and facilitates opening, resulting in K^+ inflow that hyperpolarizes the plasma membrane of the wide dynamic range (WDR) neurons of the dorsal horn of the spinal cord. The effecter of the G protein depends on the site and receptor subtype.

Effects of α_2-adrenergic agonists on the central nervous system (Table 28.1)

α_2-adrenergic agonists induce *sedation*. Sedation is due to the depression of the locus ceruleus, a brainstem nucleus that has been implicated in the sleep–wake cycle. Sedation is related to stimulation of α_2-adrenergic receptors, and is antagonized by α_1-adrenergic agonists. This explains why less selective agents, such as clonidine, that also stimulate α_1-adrenergic receptors, do not achieve complete anesthesia. The locus ceruleus is implicated in the anesthetic-sparing effect of α_2-adrenergic agonists, and in their preventive and/or therapeutic effect in withdrawal syndrome after opioid or cocaine administration.

α_2-Adrenoceptor agonists such as clonidine and dexmedetomidine reduce requirements for both intravenous and volatile general anesthetics.

Because of their sedative properties α_2-adrenergic agents have an *anesthetic-sparing effect*. Anesthetic sparing is best documented during the induction period, but it may also be demonstrated for the maintenance phase of anesthesia. Clonidine premedication results in a 30–35% decrease in propofol and thiopental requirements for anesthesia induction. Clonidine and dexmedetomidine also decrease the requirements for isoflurane and sevoflurane. Whereas the sparing effect of clonidine 'plateaus'

Table 28.1 Spectrum of action of α_2-adrenergic agonists

Effects on the central nervous system	Clinical effect
Depression of the activity of WDR neurons	Analgesia
Depression of the locus ceruleus	Sedation; anesthetic-sparing effect; treatment of opioid and alcohol withdrawal
Depression of sympathetic autonomic nervous system	Hypotension; bradycardia; prevention of hypertension; improvement in perioperative glucose control; prevention of myocardial ischemia and perioperative cardiac complications; prevention of perioperative renal ischemia
Depression of hypothalamic thermoregulatory mechanism	Inhibition of shivering; decrease thermal threshold for shivering
Peripheral effects	
Inhibition of nerve fiber action potential	Strengthening of local anesthetic block; prolongation of duration of analgesia
Inhibition of peripheral norepinephrine release (?)	Intra-articular analgesia
Depression of neurons of the spinal cord anterior horn	Increase in local anesthetic-induced motor block
Stimulation of subendothelial α_1- and α_2-adrenoceptors	Transient hypertension after intravenous bolus administration
Stimulation of α_2-adrenergic gut receptors	Inhibition of duration of postoperative ileus

WDR, wide dynamic range.

between 25% and 40%, anesthetic sparing following the more selective dexmedetomidine may be up to 90%. Moreover, dexmedetomidine acts synergistically with opioids (fentanyl) to reduce the requirements for enflurane. Finally, clonidine reduces the end-tidal concentration of isoflurane when patients first respond by opening their eyes to verbal command at the end of anesthesia (MAC-awake).

α_2-adrenergic agonists produce *analgesia* through stimulation of α_2-adrenergic receptors located on the dorsal horn of the spinal cord. They mimic the effect of the endogenous neurotransmitter norepinephrine, which is released through the activation of descending inhibitory pathways originating from the periaqueductal gray, the locus ceruleus, and the dorsal raphe nucleus. Norepinephrine and α_2-adrenergicagonists depress the activity of wide dynamic range neurons in the superficial dorsal horn evoked by stimulation of Aδ and C peripheral nociceptive fibers. Clonidine and related compounds also stimulate intermediate spontaneously active neurons located in the deeper layers of the dorsal horn of the spinal cord, which are thought to release acetylcholine and/or enkephalins, whereby they inhibit wide dynamic range neuronal activity. Norepinephrine, clonidine, dexmedetomidine, and related compounds produce analgesia in many behavioral paradigms in different animal species. Although the precise site for this effect is not known, neuraxially administered clonidine may induce nitric oxide release, thereby providing a possible explanation for its analgesic effect, although others have implicated a peripheral site for the analgesic mechanism. In animal behavioral studies, α_2-adrenergic agonists interact synergistically with both opioid and cholinergic agonists (or cholinesterase inhibitors such as neostigmine). Finally, there are nonspinal analgesic mechanisms; for example, clonidine strengthens the depression by local anesthetic agents of nerve fiber action potentials, and intra-articularly administered clonidine has a local analgesic action.

The use of α_2-adrenergic agents in clinical practice is commonly limited by the occurrence of *hypotension and bradycardia*, which are mediated via central mechanisms. α_2-adrenergic agonists depress both spontaneous and evoked sympathetic activity through a decrease in the firing of the adrenergic cardiovascular neurons located in the vasomotor center of the brainstem. Activation of α_2-adrenergic receptors located in neurons of the nucleus tractus solitarius enhances the inhibitory action of this nucleus on the sympathetic neurons of the medulla. α_2-adrenergic agonists also inhibit presynapic sympathetic neuronal activity in the lateral horn of the thoracic spinal cord; this effect is reversed by local administration of the cholinesterase inhibitor neostigmine. Besides central effects, α_2-adrenergic agents produce peripheral vasoconstriction that only partly compensates for central depression of sympathetic nervous tone. Abrupt discontinuation of α_2-adrenergic agonists following chronic administration may induce a withdrawal syndrome, including rebound hypertension and myocardial ischemia.

Hypotension and bradycardia are prominent effects of α_2-adrenergic agonists.

α_2-adrenergic agonists alter thermoregulatory control and produce a decrease in the threshold for vasoconstriction and shivering during hypothermia. The antishivering effects result from central hypothalamic thermoregulatory inhibition rather than peripheral action on thermogenic muscular activity.

Although α_2-adrenergic agonists have no significant effects on respiratory rate or tidal volume during resting ventilation, ventilatory drive is modestly attenuated.

Recent evidence indicates that dexmedetomidine may be useful as a neuroprotective agent in conditions associated with cerebral ischemia.

Practical aspects of drug administration

α_2-adrenergic agonists may be used as premedication, providing sedation, amnesia, and anxiolysis. The dose of clonidine must be decreased in older patients to avoid hypotension on anesthetic induction. Young ASA 1–2 patients may receive 2–4 μg/kg, but 1–2 μg/kg is more appropriate for elderly patients. Bradycardia may occur in relatively young, unstimulated patients receiving dexmedetomidine. In children, clonidine premedication is well accepted and improves facemask tolerance on anesthetic induction. Premedication with α_2-adrenergic agonists allows a significant reduction in anesthetic requirement for induction. Premedicant use of α_2-adrenergic agonists blunts sympathetic activation and the resulting hypertension and tachycardia due to orotracheal intubation. α_2-adrenergic agonists also prevent tachycardia and hypertension on emergence from anesthesia. Recovery from anesthesia is delayed only when anesthetic protocols do not appropriately reduce the amount of hypnotic agent given concomitantly.

Although the occurrence of hypotension and bradycardia may prevent the use of α_2 agonists in all patients, there are some clinical conditions in which the benefits outweigh these concerns:

- In drug addicts and alcoholics sympathetic hyperactivity is well controlled by α_2-adrenergic agonists, which may also reduce the risk of withdrawal.
- Patients suffering from chronic cancer or noncancer pain often have considerably elevated opioid requirements in the perioperative period that may be significantly reduced by α_2-adrenergic agonists.
- Hypertensive patients are particularly vulnerable to marked swings in blood pressure perioperatively, which are reduced by premedication with α_2-adrenergic agonists.
- Clonidine premedication provides mild to moderate hypotension for ear or orthopedic surgery without using excessive amounts of anesthetic agents.
- Premedication with clonidine or dexmedetomidine lowers intraocular pressure (IOP) and is the preferred premedicant in patients with elevated IOP.
- Improved hemodynamic control may prevent perioperative myocardial ischemia when using α_2-adrenergic agonists during cardiac or vascular surgery, with a reduction in cardiac morbidity and mortality.
- Premedication with clonidine enhances the duration of spinal blockade and the quality of analgesia after intrathecal local anesthesia. However, there is an increased risk of hypotension and bradycardia in patients undergoing spinal anesthesia who receive doses of clonidine in excess of 150 μg.
- Clonidine increases the threshold of toxic plasma concentrations of bupivacaine and reverses its intracardiac conduction disturbances.
- The combined intrathecal administration of clonidine and a local anesthetic improves the quality and duration of the block and prevents shivering; however, there is more associated hypotension. Consequently, when used in combination with local anesthetics the maximum dose of intrathecal clonidine should not exceed 1 μg/kg.

Analgesia

Bolus administration of epidural clonidine provides analgesia in a dose-dependent fashion. Compared to morphine, clonidine has a lower efficacy and shorter duration. Pain relief is improved when clonidine is administered by continuous infusion; for complete pain relief doses as high as 100–150 μg/h are required, in which setting hypotension, bradycardia, and sedation are prominent. Consequently, the use of epidural clonidine for postoperative analgesia is preferable in combination with other analgesic drugs (e.g. opioids) with which there is enhanced analgesia. Nevertheless, once the dose of clonidine (in combination) exceeds 150 μg bolus or 20 μg/h by continuous infusion, hypotension is a frequent occurrence. This probably explains why epidural clonidine has not superseded the standard combination of epidurally administered local anesthetic and opioid agents.

α_2-adrenergic receptor agonists enhance both central and peripheral neural blockade by local anesthetics.

Epidural clonidine has been used as an adjuvant to enhance the analgesic effect of local anesthetics in women in labor. In a range of 30–150 μg, epidural clonidine prolongs the analgesic effect of epidural bupivacaine. Epidural clonidine inhibits shivering in parturients, but this is obtained at the expense of systemic effects, including sedation, hypotension, and bradycardia. Because clonidine crosses the placenta, epidural clonidine also reduces the heart rate of the fetus, although no deleterious effect has been reported in newborns. The epidural clonidine dose must therefore be limited to less than 1 μg/kg in parturients.

NMDA RECEPTOR BLOCKERS

Agents that block *N*-methyl-D-aspartate (NMDA)-type glutamate receptors have gained interest for anesthesiologists in recent years. Because of its capability to block NMDA receptors, ketamine acts synergistically with opioids and can prevent acute tolerance to opioid administration. Consequently, low-dose ketamine administration protocols have been designed to improve postoperative analgesia and reduce opioid side effects.

Ketamine

The pharmacology of ketamine as an anesthetic is discussed in Chapter 25. Ketamine is commonly used as a racemic mixture of two optical enantiomers, R(−) and S(+). S(+) ketamine has an approximately fourfold greater affinity for the NMDA receptor than the R(−) enantiomer. Ketamine preparations commonly contain a preservative, benzothenium chloride, which is neurotoxic. Consequently a preservative-free solution of ketamine should be administered spinally or epidurally.

Ketamine induces dose-dependent depression of the CNS that leads to a dissociative state characterized by amnesia and analgesia but a variable degree of loss of consciousness. Ketamine has other properties that make it different from other anesthetic agents: it stimulates the sympathetic nervous system and induces catecholamine release, increasing or maintaining arterial blood pressure while its own direct in vitro effect is to depress myocardial contractility; it induces bronchial dilatation; and finally, it only weakly depresses respiratory drive. Unlike most anesthetic agents, ketamine does not interact with $GABA_A$ receptors, but mainly with NMDA receptors, and probably also with opioid, monoaminergic, and cholinergic receptors. In addition, ketamine has local anesthetic properties, explaining why it produces an anesthetic block after spinal administration. The role of NMDA receptors in excitatory synaptic transmission, plasticity, and neurodegeneration in the CNS has redefined the role of ketamine as an adjuvant to other anesthetic and analgesic agents used perioperatively.

Role of NMDA receptors (Fig. 28.3)

Glutamate, the most abundant excitatory neurotransmitter in the central nervous system, activates three families of ionotropic receptor: NMDA, AMPA, and kainate receptors (Chapter 20). Simultaneous binding of glutamate and glycine is required to activate NMDA receptors, which are normally blocked at resting membrane potential by extracellular Mg^{2+}. Activation of NMDA receptor permits Ca^{2+} entry. NMDA receptors consist of a heteromeric combination of one NR1 subunit and at least one of four NR2 subunit subtypes (NR2A, B, C, D). Glycine- and glutamate-binding sites occur on homologous regions of the NR1 and NR2 subunits, respectively. Affinity for agonists and antagonists depends on the NR2 subunit. Ketamine selectively blocks NMDA receptors by two distinct mechanisms: it decreases the frequency of channel opening by an allosteric mechanism, and it blocks the open channel by binding at the phencyclidine site, thereby reducing channel open time. Ketamine inhibits NR1/NR2A and NR1/NR2B glutamate receptors, independently of the effect of Mg^{2+}, but in a superadditive manner. In addition, ketamine potentiates the effects of volatile anesthetics on NMDA receptors.

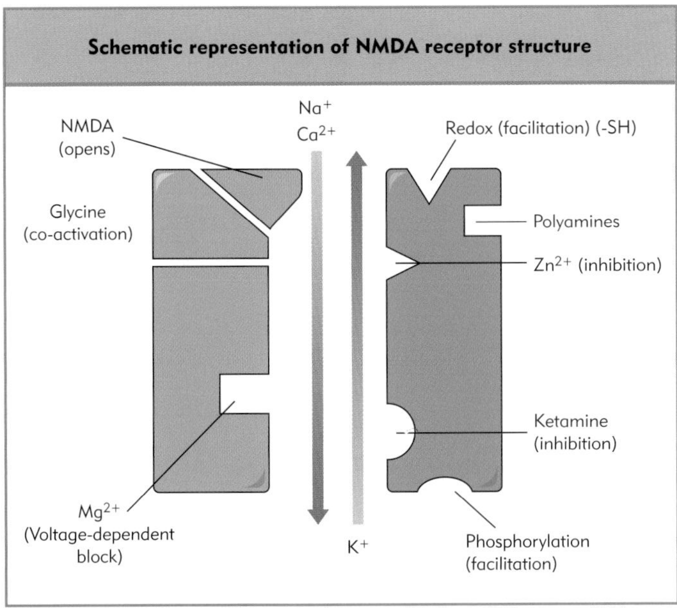

Figure 28.3 Schematic representation of NMDA receptor structure. The ion channel is permeable to Ca^{2+}, K^+, and Na^+. The binding site of *N*-methyl-D-aspartate is indicated with the obligatory coagonist glycine site. Ketamine interacts with the phencyclidine site inside the receptor to block receptor function noncompetitively. The site is distinct from those of other inhibitors (Mg^{2+}, Zn^{2+}) or facilitators (polyamines, phosphorylation) of the receptor.

NMDA receptors are important for learning and conditioning. The hippocampus plays an important, although not unique, role in learning and memory. Hippocampal activation is essential to establish new memory. The occurrence of long-term potentiation (LTP) in hippocampal postsynaptic cells, secondary to activation of NMDA receptors, is thought to induce synaptic plasticity, which is considered a key mechanism of implicit memory. NMDA antagonists prevent LTP. Thus low doses of ketamine in healthy volunteers produce a dose-dependent impairment to working, episodic, and procedural memory.

At the level of the dorsal horn of the spinal cord, NMDA receptors do not participate in normal synaptic transmission because of their voltage-dependent block by Mg^{2+}. Following postsynaptic depolarization by a constant drive of noxious afferent input, Mg^{2+} block is removed, allowing Ca^{2+} entry, which causes activation of downstream protein kinases and results in phosphorylation of NMDA receptors. Magnesium block at resting potential is consequently decreased and Ca^{2+} channel open time is prolonged. This phenomenon participates in *central sensitization* (Chapter 23). NMDA receptors have been identified in unmyelinated and myelinated axons in peripheral somatic tissues. Local administration of glutamate results in nociceptive responses that are attenuated by peripheral administration of NMDA antagonists. Similarly, hyperalgesia and inflammation induced by the administration of an irritant substance are inhibited by local application of an NMDA antagonist. Thus, peripheral administration of ketamine enhances the local anesthetic and analgesic effect of bupivacaine and inhibits the development of primary and secondary hyperalgesia after an experimental burn injury in humans.

Glutamate release induced by hypoxia can cause ischemic neuronal damage (excitotoxicity). Blockade of NMDA receptors has a neuroprotective effect on lesions induced by cerebral hypoxia in laboratory animals.

Practical aspects of drug administration

COMBINATION WITH OPIOID

Ketamine enhances the analgesic effect of opioids in healthy volunteers. Pre-, intra-, and/or postoperative administration of intravenous ketamine decreases postoperative visual analog scale (VAS) pain scores and reduces patient-controlled morphine administration. Ketamine is given as a bolus or a continuous infusion that is occasionally administered during the postoperative period. Bolus doses (0.15–2 mg/kg) are lower than anesthetic doses (2–5 mg/kg). Ketamine has also been combined with morphine for patient-controlled administration in a ratio of 1:1. Preoperative administration is no more effective than postoperative administration in terms of VAS scores for pain intensity or opioid consumption in most studies, which raises questions as to its action as a pre-emptive analgesic.

COMBINATION WITH LOCAL ANESTHETICS

The combination of intravenous or epidural ketamine with local anesthetics results in a significant strengthening and prolongation of the duration of analgesia. Epidural administration seems to be more effective than intravenous administration. Small intravenous doses (0.25 mg/kg) of S(+) ketamine also improve postoperative analgesia produced by epidural ropivacaine. Ketamine can more than double the duration of analgesia of caudal blocks, comparable to clonidine. The optimal dose of 0.5 mg/kg results in more than 20 hours of effective analgesia without side effects.

COMBINATION WITH GENERAL ANESTHETICS

Intravenous bolus or a continuous infusion of ketamine can be administered before induction or during anesthesia to prevent recall from anesthesia or the development of hyperalgesia, especially in patients receiving remifentanil. Patients receiving a 0.15 mg/kg bolus followed by a 2 μg/kg continuous intravenous infusion required less remifentanil during the operative procedure and had lower pain intensity scores and morphine demand postoperatively. This result is supported by experimental studies showing that concomitant ketamine administration with opioids prevents rebound hyperalgesia. Ketamine has a propofol-sparing effect during anesthetic induction.

BENZODIAZEPINES

Benzodiazepines are hypnotic, anticonvulsant, and sedative agents that produce amnesia and muscle relaxation; they are used as adjuvants to anesthetic agents or as sedatives. The CNS effects of benzodiazepines are rapidly reversed by flumazenil, a selective antagonist. Benzodiazepines differ from anesthetic agents by their pharmacokinetics and by their mechanism of action on $GABA_A$ receptors.

Pharmacology

Benzodiazepines are anxiolytic/hypnotic agents with a chemical structure that includes a benzene ring fused to a seven-membered ring with a phenyl radical (Fig. 28.4). Examples include diazepam (1963), flunitrazepam (1973), and midazolam (1986), the first benzodiazepine produced primarily for use in anesthesia, which results from the addition of an imidazole ring. Benzodiazepines are very lipid soluble, explaining a large volume of distribution and accumulation after continuous or prolonged administration. The imidazole ring in the structure of midazolam accounts for its stability in aqueous solutions and its more rapid metabolism. Pharmaceutical preparations of midazolam are buffered to a pH of 3.5 because the midazolam ring remains open at pH values less than 4, maintaining the water solubility of the drug. Following oral administration of benzodiazepines, bioavailability depends on hepatic first-pass metabolism, which is 80% for diazepam and flunitrazepam, and 50% for midazolam. Benzodiazepines are extensively bound to plasma protein; owing to their lipid solubility they achieve a rapid distribution in a large volume of distribution. The volume of distribution of benzodiazepines is increased in obese patients. Benzodiazepines undergo microsomal oxidation in the liver by cytochrome P450 enzymes, demethylation, and glucuronidation. Substitution of a hydroxyl group leads to a new series of compounds (lorazepam, oxazepam, temazepam) that undergo hepatic hydroxylation. Most of the metabolites are inactive, but diazepam and midazolam can produce active compounds (desmethyldiazepam, and 1-,4-hydroxymidazolam, respectively), that can accumulate in renal failure. Compared to general anesthetic agents, benzodiazepines have very long elimination half-lives (Table 28.2). This is responsible for a prolonged duration of action after repeated or continuous administration, whereas the duration of

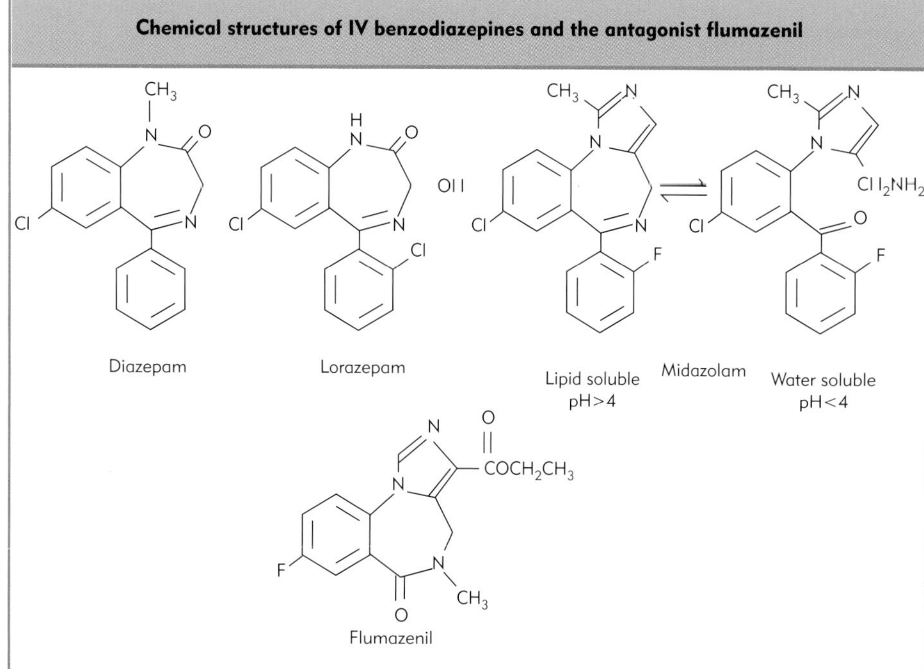

Figure 28.4 Chemical structures of intravenous benzodiazepines and the antagonist flumazenil. The reversible pH-dependent ring opening of midazolam is shown.

Table 28.2 Physicochemical and pharmacokinetic characteristics of benzodiazepines

	Diazepam	Flunitrazepam	Midazolam
Molecular weight (Da)	284	313	362
p*Ka*	3.4	1.8	6.2
Water soluble	No	No	Yes
Lipid soluble	Yes	Yes	Yes
Volume of distribution (L/kg)	1–1.5	0.5–2	1–1.5
Clearance (mL/kg/min)	0.2–0.5		6–8
Elimination half-life (h)	30–40	15–30	1–4

action is determined by the distribution phase after a single administration. Elimination half-life is prolonged in aged patients and those with hepatic failure.

Benzodiazepines induce amnesia, decrease anxiety, produce sedation, prevent and treat seizures, and relax muscle, but have no analgesic properties. Midazolam is especially rapidly acting and more potent than other benzodiazepines. Premedication with benzodiazepines results in an anesthetic-sparing effect for either intravenous or volatile anesthetic agents. The sedative effects of midazolam with alfentanil or fentanyl are synergistic. Benzodiazepines, especially midazolam, enhance the respiratory depressant effect of opioids, as those inexperienced with their use have too often learned.

Benzodiazepines produce vasodilatation that can lead to arterial hypotension and low cardiac output in hypovolemic patients. Prolonged administration in critical care patients can lead to withdrawal symptoms (nausea, tachycardia, hypertension, agitation).

Role of the $GABA_A$ receptor

The $GABA_A$ receptor (Chapter 20) is the main target of benzodiazepines. Binding occurs at a site distinct from the GABA binding site, thereby increasing Cl^- current by modulating GABA binding. The acute sedative and amnestic effects of benzodiazepines is mediated by the α_1 subunit of $GABA_A$ receptors, as demonstrated by a point mutation of histamine 101 to arginine, which renders the receptor insensitive to these effects of diazepam. An analogous mutation in the α_2 subunit eliminates the anxiolytic and myorelaxant effects.

The sedative/amnestic and anxiolytic/myorelaxant actions of benzodiazepines have been assigned to distinct receptor subtypes using genetic techniques.

Benzodiazepines increase the opening frequency of $GABA_A$ chloride channels in response to GABA, leading to enhanced inhibitory postsynaptic currents. A specific site has been identified for benzodiazepine binding. $GABA_A$ receptors are extensively distributed in the CNS. Midazolam acts on $GABA_A$ receptors of the hippocampus, explaining the effect of benzodiazepines on memory. More generally, benzodiazepine-binding sites are distributed in the frontal and occipital cortex and the limbic system.

Practical aspects of drug administration

Benzodiazepines are used as premedication and as sedative agents. They are especially appropriate as oral premedicants because of their sedative and amnesic effects. Anesthetic requirements are reduced in a dose-related manner by midazolam, but awakening following general anesthesia is delayed. In children, midazolam can also be administered by oral, rectal, or nasal routes. The shorter elimination half-life of midazolam gives it an advantage as a sedative over other benzodiazepines. Midazolam is an alternative to propofol for intravenous sedation during invasive diagnostic or surgical procedures. Because midazolam can induce respiratory depression, sedation requires adequate monitoring. Compared to propofol, midazolam administration results in a more delayed recovery of cognitive function, making it less appropriate for short-term sedation, especially during ambulatory procedures. For these patients, midazolam-induced amnesia is more a problem than an advantage. Finally, midazolam is used for sedation in critical care patients. In these patients, not all problems related to sedation are resolved by midazolam: a paradoxical reaction (i.e. agitation, confusion) may be observed on induction of sedation, delayed sedation over several days can result from long-term administration especially in cases of hepatic or renal failure, and withdrawal symptoms can be observed several days after cessation of infusion.

The action of benzodiazepines on the $GABA_A$ receptor can be blocked by flumazenil, a specific antagonist. Flumazenil has a shorter duration of action (elimination half-time 20–25 minutes) than the agonists. It is consequently used more as a diagnostic tool to identify the mechanism of alteration in consciousness in patients suspected of drug intoxication than as a therapeutic agent in the same setting.

DOPAMINERGIC AGENTS

The dopamine system plays a key role in motor and reward activities. There are two main CNS dopaminergic pathways. One originates in the substantia nigra and projects to the caudate putamen (striatum) and is related to movement control, particularly in planning or organization of movement sequences. Loss of dopamine in the substantia nigra results in Parkinson's disease, and blockade of dopamine receptors by major tranquilizers can exacerbate Parkinson's disease symptoms or result in tardive dyskinesia.

The other pathway originates in the ventral tegmental area of the mesencephalon and projects to areas in the limbic system (amygdala, septal area, nucleus accumbens) and the prefrontal cortex. Projections to the prefrontal cortex may modulate executive behaviors. Damage to, or dopamine deficiency in, this area of the cortex produces increased perseveration (inappropriate repetition of a previously rewarded response) and abnormalities in working memory, behavioral inhibition, affect, attention, planning, drive, and social interactions. This mesolimbic system rewards the organism for behavior that responds to cues that signal the availability of incentives or reinforcers. Exogenous stimulation of this system by various drugs (marijuana, cocaine, alcohol, etc.) can result in addictive behaviors.

Dopamine receptors have been classified pharmacologically and biochemically into two classes: D_1 (D_1 and D_5 subtypes) and D_2 (D_2, D_3, and D_4 subtypes), which have distinct cellular locations and intracellular signaling mechanisms. Dopamine D_1 receptors may be particularly important in the reinforcing effects of addictive drugs.

Haloperidol is a D_2 dopamine receptor antagonist used as an antipsychotic and major tranquilizer that is the drug of choice for treatment of severe agitation in the postoperative period. There is also a large body of literature on the use of haloperidol in the intensive care unit setting. It has been administered in a doubling dose fashion, as a continuous intravenous infusion, and in large doses if necessary. Initially 1–2 mg are administered, and if agitation is severe the dose is doubled until the agitation is controlled. Patients requiring doses of 300–1200 mg/day have been reported. Once the initial agitation is controlled, a maintenance dose is given every 6 hours, or an infusion of 1–20 mg/h can be used. Serious complications are rare. Tardive dyskinesia can occur but is infrequent with acute intravenous administration. The QT_C interval of the ECG should be monitored, as *torsades de pointes* has been reported. When combined with a benzodiazepine, smaller doses of haloperidol are effective to treat severe agitation. Consequently, a combination of agents is preferred to treat major delirium, or in prophylaxis of acute drug withdrawal.

The signs and symptoms of neuroleptic malignant syndrome resulting from antipsychotic and other CNS drugs resemble those of malignant hyperthermia, but their etiologies are distinct.

One complication of large and prolonged doses of haloperidol is the neuroleptic malignant syndrome (NMS). This is more common with oral than with acute intravenous administration. This syndrome results from the central effects of chronic administration of haloperidol and other psychoactive drugs (e.g. other butyrophenones, phenothiazines, monoamine oxidase (MAO) inhibitors, lithium, or combinations thereof). Patients usually develop impaired motor function, with generalized rigidity, akinesia, and/or extrapyramidal disturbances. Deterioration in mental status occurs, with coma, stupor, and/or delirium. Most notably, hyperthermia develops, with diaphoresis, blood pressure and heart rate fluctuations, and tachypnea. The syndrome may be quite similar to that of acute malignant hyperthermia, but their etiologies are distinct and the onset of NMS generally requires several days to several weeks. Treatment involves discontinuation of the inciting drugs and symptomatic control of temperature, acid–base balance, intravenous fluid balance, and muscle tone. Recovery is slow because the drug effects dissipate very slowly. Dantrolene can aid in therapy of NMS by lowering muscle heat production and thereby reducing body temperature.

ADDICTIVE DRUGS

The reasons for addiction with certain drugs are a current area of much research, with huge socioeconomic implications. Compared with drug enforcement, research in this area is vastly underfunded. Although 20–50% of trauma patients that present to large city emergency rooms in the USA have positive blood/urine tests for cocaine or its metabolites, there is almost no research or literature regarding the administration of anesthesia in these circumstances.

Cocaine

Cocaine is an inhibitor of catecholamine (principally norepinephrine) reuptake at nerve terminals. The resultant synaptic catecholamine excess results in central stimulant effects and peripheral vasoconstrictive effects. The addictive properties of cocaine are related to its dopaminergic effects. Cocaine, as well as amphetamines, binds to the dopamine transporter, which clears dopamine from the synaptic cleft. A key site for addictive drug action is the nucleus accumbens, the projection site of the mesolimbic dopaminergic pathway.

Acute intoxication with cocaine can result in seizures, focal neurologic symptoms or signs, headache, transient loss of consciousness, hyperthermia, and hyperglycemia. Other signs of peripheral catecholamine release include diaphoresis and pupillary dilatation. Psychiatric disturbances include agitation, anxiety or depression, psychosis and paranoia, and suicidal ideation. The agitation can be severe and responds poorly to normal doses of sedatives. Hemodynamic instability is common. Arrhythmias frequently occur and are the presumed cause of sudden death from cocaine. The combination of ethanol with cocaine is particularly toxic.

Depending on the time course of drug administration and the chronic patterns of stimulant use, a variety of hemodynamic responses can be seen during anesthesia. These range from severe hypertension, tachycardia, and profound vasoconstriction to hypotension unresponsive to indirect sympathomimetics (e.g. ephedrine). Vasoconstriction can result in cerebral aneurysm rupture or acute myocardial infarction, and can be so severe that peripheral pulses are not palpable. This has led to the erroneous administration of vasopressors. The vasoconstriction persists past the acute hemodynamic effects of cocaine administration. In fact, coronary vasoconstriction can occur for up to 6 weeks after the last use of cocaine, resulting in anginal symptoms or electrocardiogram changes. The hemodynamic response depends on whether cocaine is acutely preventing catecholamine reuptake or whether these stores are already depleted. For instance, there are reports indicating either no response or a severe hypertensive response to ephedrine.

Chronic use of cocaine impairs cognitive function, even when no drug is present. It can also lead to thrombocytopenia. Pulmonary changes occur in chronic users, especially with inhalation. These patients are particularly vulnerable to pulmonary edema, pulmonary hemorrhage, pneumothorax, and bronchospasm, and can develop interstitial fibrosis.

Ethanol

Ethanol is a sedative agent, and acute ingestion decreases anesthetic requirements. In fact, ethanol has been used as a standardized control for the sedative effects of various anesthetic drugs. Acute intoxication results in delayed gastric emptying. It also depresses left ventricular function with autonomic compensation, resulting in tachycardia and a reduced ejection fraction. Preload should be maintained at higher levels to maintain normal cardiac function.

Chronic alcohol abuse may have varying effects on anesthetic requirements; most evidence indicates that higher doses are needed. The larger required doses may just reflect altered pharmacokinetic parameters, with no change in CNS sensitivity. Consequently, the anesthetic requirements in alcohol abusers are variable and depend on the degree of chronic consumption, any acute ingestion (which the patient may not reveal), and various physiologic changes accompanying chronic alcohol abuse. Careful titration of anesthetic drugs is required in this situation. A difficult problem occurs postoperatively, when patients can develop withdrawal symptoms.

Withdrawal

Acute withdrawal from various addictive substances, particularly that precipitated by the administration of an antagonist, can be lethal, with pulmonary edema, seizures, arrhythmias, or myocardial infarction. A common component of withdrawal is the stress response, marked by the release of corticotropin-releasing factor, particularly in the amygdala. A major problem is how to manage patients requiring surgery who chronically abuse addictive substances. The intraoperative course may be stormy, but the use of general anesthetics masks many withdrawal symptoms, and indeed can be used as a means to allow rapid detoxification. The more difficult management problem occurs in the postoperative acute care unit where the usual sedation regimens may be ineffective. Various regimens have been suggested that involve the administration of benzodiazepines, major tranquilizers, or the substance itself (e.g. intravenous ethanol), which seem to be equally effective. The administration of sympatholytic agents (β-blockers, central α_2 agonists) may be effective in ameliorating some of the peripheral (hypertension, tachycardia) symptoms but not the central (craving, hallucinations) withdrawal symptoms. The use of β-blockers may exacerbate coronary vasospasm, which can occur with acute cocaine use.

ANTIDEPRESSANTS

Depression is an underreported and undertreated disease. With the advent of newer, more effective, and better tolerated agents, greater use is being made of antidepressants in the general population. A plethora of such drugs is now available, and anesthesiologists frequently encounter patients receiving these medications (Fig. 28.5).

The most important interactions of antidepressants with anesthetics in the perioperative period occur with monoamine oxidase (MAO) inhibitors. There are numerous case reports of severe hemodynamic alterations under general anesthesia in patients treated with MAO inhibitors. Unfortunately, MAO inhibitors are used when other therapies fail, and discontinuation of these drugs before surgery is not without risk. Other antidepressant drugs seem to have few interactions with anesthesia, but most are relatively new. Even though tricyclic antidepressants and MAO inhibitors have been in use for decades, only recently have blunted responses to catecholamines been reported in patients taking chronic therapy with these agents.

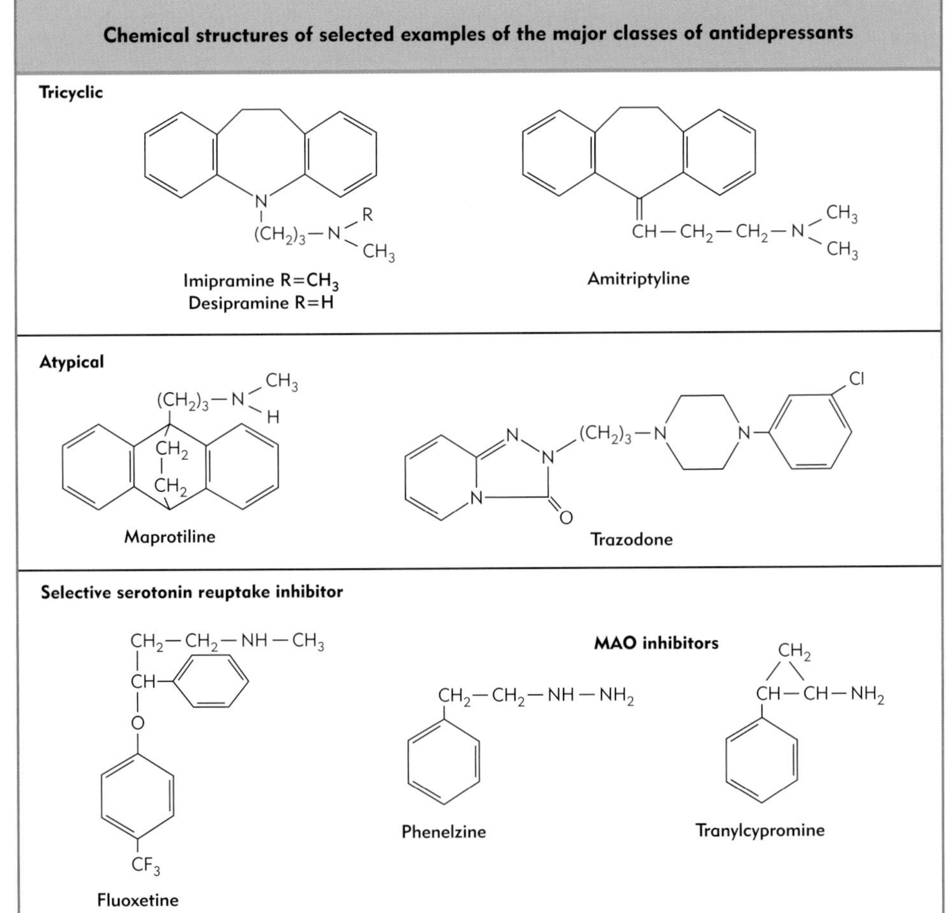

Figure 28.5 Structures of selected antidepressants.

In addition to the older and tricyclic and tetracyclic antidepressants, serotonin (5-HT) reuptake inhibitors (fluoxetine, sertaline, and paroxetine) and antidepressants with atypical mechanisms of action (bupropion, trazodone, venlafaxine, and nefazodone) are now available. Antagonism of monoamine transport is the primary cellular action of many antidepressant medications. However, an increased synaptic concentration of monoamines, which occurs minutes after administration, does not explain the antidepressant response, which is often delayed by a matter of weeks. Furthermore, antidepressants have widely different effects on norepinephrine and serotonin reuptake, but all have comparable efficacy. Other drugs that increase norepinephrine at the synapse (e.g. levodopa and amphetamine) have no clinical effect in depression. A common effect is that chronic administration of any of the antidepressants increases the efficiency of serotonergic transmission, albeit by different mechanisms. Serotonergic pathways are broadly distributed in the CNS, including the limbic forebrain, which is implicated in affective illness.

Most newer antidepressants are associated with a risk of clinically significant drug interactions. A rapidly growing body of literature provides evidence for a distinct profile of cytochrome P450 inhibition and drug interaction risks with individual antidepressants. The most commonly used agents, tricyclic antidepressants, were originally synthesized from the phenothiazines. In common with phenothiazines, side effects include sedation, anticholinergic and sympatholytic effects, cardiotoxicity (orthostatic hypotension, flattened T waves, prolonged PR and QRS intervals), and increased sensitivity to catecholamines. Long-term treatment with these substances can lead to intraoperative blood pressure fluctuations, tachycardia, and arrhythmias. Acute administration of tricyclic antidepressants may exaggerate the blood pressure response to catecholamines; long-term therapy may result in downregulation of receptors, depletion of endogenous stores, and a decrease in the response to catecholamines.

Monoamine oxidase inhibitors are used as treatment for depression not responsive to initial drug therapy. In contrast to the irreversible blockade produced by many MAO inhibitors, moclobemide produces a reversible blockade and this results in fewer side effects. MAO inhibitors are the antidepressants associated with the highest incidence of adverse interactions with anesthesia, though it is likely that moclobemide will have fewer such interactions than earlier MAO inhibitors.

Meperidine (pethidine) in particular has been associated with severe interactions with MAO inhibitors. A syndrome of coma, hyperpyrexia, and hypertension can occur. A similar interaction with other opioids does not occur, or is very rare. The mechanism appears to be an inhibition of neuronal serotonin uptake by meperidine, which results in toxic central serotonergic effects. Monoamine oxidase inhibitors may modify the response to catecholamines, with potentiation of catecholamine effects or hypertensive reactions. Anesthetic interactions with MAO inhibitors seem to be idiosyncratic, as meperidine, ketamine, and various catecholamines have been administered without incident to patients receiving MAO inhibitors. Treatment for this idiosyncratic reaction is supportive. For patients taking long-term MAO inhibitor therapy, it takes some time for normal adrenergic responsiveness to return following discontinuation of the drug. Refractory hypotension may occur in this situation, possibly as a result of receptor downregulation.

MAO inhibitors are associated with a high incidence of adverse interactions with anesthesia.

Selective serotonin reuptake inhibitors (SSRIs) apparently have very few side effects, and no significant adverse interactions with anesthetics have been reported. Drugs of this class differ substantially in their pharmacokinetics and effects on P450 enzymes. Most have a half-life of approximately 1 day. Fluoxetine, however, has a half-life of 2–4 days, and its active metabolite, norfluoxetine, has an extended half-life of 7–15 days. A discontinuation syndrome can occur with cessation of therapy, and is most evident with drugs having short half-lives (paroxetine, venlafaxine, and fluvoxamine). The syndrome includes nausea, lethargy, insomnia, and headache; it also occurs with abrupt discontinuation of tricyclic antidepressants. Consequently, discontinuation of SSRIs before anesthesia is not recommended. Selective serotonin reuptake inhibitors are associated with hyponatremia from the syndrome of inappropriate antidiuretic hormone release (SIADH), especially in elderly patients.

Lithium was the first effective drug used to treat psychiatric disorders. Since the end of the 1990s it has had a major role in the treatment of bipolar affective disorder, with particular efficacy in the manic phase. It also has a role in treating recurrent depression. The major toxicity is renal, which is rare if therapeutic levels are adequately monitored. Lithium may potentiate the action of neuromuscular blocking drugs and may theoretically decrease anesthetic requirements. It can affect the T waves of the ECG.

ANTICONVULSANTS

Enhanced excitatory amino acid receptor function and diminished number and function of GABA receptors have been reported as molecular mechanisms of epilepsy. Increased levels of extracellular K^+ have been linked to excitatory events in several ways: by shifting membrane potential closer to spike threshold by partial depolarization; by increasing the risk of repetitive firing by decreasing post-burst hyperpolarization; by reducing K^+ efflux from cells, thus reducing the $GABA_A$ and $GABA_B$ components of the inhibitory postsynaptic potential; and by enhanced *N*-methyl-D-aspartate (NMDA) receptor activation. Kindling is a phenomenon in which subconvulsive stimuli lead to progressive increases in seizure activity until a generalized convulsion occurs. This process results in increased sensitivity to stimuli despite long stimulus-free periods. Kindling is used extensively as an experimental model of epilepsy in animals.

Treatment of idiopathic seizure disorder is primarily via antiepileptic drugs (AED); see also Chapter 21. Mechanisms of action of AEDs include:

- Inhibition of repetitive firing by blockade of Na^+ channels (carbamazepine, phenytoin, valproate, lamotrigine, and possibly felbamate);
- Blockade of Ca^{2+} channels (valproate, ethosuximide);
- Prolonging $GABA_A$ Cl^- channel opening (phenobarbital, clonazepam);
- Inhibition of glutamate and aspartate release (lamotrigine);
- Blockade of the glycine coagonist site on NMDA receptors (felbamate);
- Increasing GABA concentration (gabapentin, vigabatrin).

Treatment with AEDs is often monitored by drug levels, although clinical response is more important.

Anesthetic management is affected by AEDs in several ways. Most are metabolized by the liver and induce the cytochrome P450 system, altering the metabolism of other drugs. Increased requirements for fentanyl and nondepolarizing neuromuscular blocking agents in patients chronically treated with phenytoin, carbamazepine, or phenobarbital are secondary to hepatic enzyme induction. A phenytoin-induced increase in hepatic oxidative and reductive metabolism of halothane may be linked to post-halothane hepatitis. Conversely, sedating AEDs, such as phenobarbital, clonazepam, and gabapentin, may potentiate general anesthetics, so reducing the dosages required. This interaction is consistent with the facilitatory actions of most volatile (Chapter 26) and intravenous (Chapter 25) general anesthetics at the $GABA_A$ receptor. The effects of AEDs on other organ systems are varied. The immune system may be affected adversely by carbamazepine- and phenytoin-induced leukopenia. Lymphadenopathy, systemic lupus erythematosus, and vasculitis have been noted in patients on AEDs. Valproate affects the hematologic system by an intrinsic system coagulopathy and a dose-related thrombocytopenia. Because abnormal hemostasis may be present despite a normal platelet count, prothrombin time, and partial thromboplastin time, a bleeding time test is recommended prior to surgery. Thrombocytopenia is also associated with felbamate, as is aplastic anemia, and anemia may occur with lamotrigine. Liver function tests are usually elevated by 25–75%, usually without clinical significance, although liver failure has been reported with felbamate. Valproate can cause pancreatitis, especially in young patients, in combination with other AEDs. Corticosteroid, thyroxine (T_4), and vitamin D_3 metabolism and function may be altered by phenytoin, carbamazepine, and barbiturates. Protein binding of T_4, and sex hormones may be changed, and the release of calcitonin, insulin, and clotting factors dependent on vitamin K may be impaired. Most patients appear euthyroid because of reduced binding of T_4 to plasma proteins secondary to the extensive protein binding of AEDs.

Carbamazepine metabolism (by CYP3A4) is inhibited by erythromycin and cimetidine, both of which may be used preoperatively. Increased blood levels may lead to toxicity and heart block. Blood levels of AEDs may fluctuate for as long as 1 week after general anesthesia and surgery; therefore, it may be useful to check levels postoperatively.

Certain drugs can lower the seizure threshold or activate epileptogenic foci, and thus should be avoided in patients who have a seizure disorder. For example, methohexital can activate seizure foci and has been used in mapping for surgical resection. Ketamine and propofol have been reported to elicit seizures in patients who have seizure disorder, but their epileptogenic potential is unclear. Although propofol can successfully treat status epilepticus, both seizures and opisthotonos have been reported in patients with and without previously diagnosed seizure disorder. Propofol is an effective anticonvulsant for bupivacaine-, picrotoxin-, and pentylenetetrazol-induced seizures in animals and in seizures produced by GABAergic inhibition; however, seizures produced by a glutamatergic mechanism have been augmented by propofol. Antagonism of glycine in subcortical structures has been proposed as a mechanism to explain the seizure-like activity associated with propofol. Inhalational anesthetics exhibit both anticonvulsant and proconvulsant properties in various studies in both humans and animals, with isoflurane and desflurane having the least proconvulsant activity. Generally, clinical use of volatile agents is anticonvulsant. In fact, isoflurane has been used to treat status epilepticus.

Key references

Eisenach J, Detweiler D, Hood D. Hemodynamic and analgesic actions of epidurally administered clonidine. Anesthesiology 1993;78:277–87.

Hirota K, Lambert DG. Ketamine: its mechanism(s) of action and unusual clinical uses. Br J Anaesth. 1996;77:441–4.

Kalibayashi T, Maze M. Clinical uses of α_2-adrenergic agonists. Anesthesiology 2000;93:1345–9.

Khan ZP, Ferguson CN, Jones RM. Alpha-2 and imidazoline receptor agonists. Their pharmacology and therapeutic role. Anaesthesia 1999;54:146–65.

Kohrs R, Durieux ME. Ketamine: Teaching an old drug new tricks. Anesth Analg. 1998;87:1186–93.

Maze M, Fujinaga M. α_2-Adrenoreceptors in pain modulation. Which subtype should be targeted to produce analgesia? Anesthesiology 2000;92:934–6.

Petrenko AB, Yamakura T, Baba H, Shimoji K. The role of *N*-methyl-D-aspartate (NMDA) receptors in pain: a review. Anesth Analg. 2003;297:1108–16.

Whitwam JG. Flumazenil and midazolam in anaesthesia. Acta Anaesth Scand. 1995;108:15–22.

Further reading

Armand S, Langlade A, Boutros A et al. Meta-analysis of the efficacy of extradural clonidine to relieve postoperative pain: an impossible task. Br J Anaesth. 1998;81:126–34.

Bruce DL. Alcoholism and anesthesia. Anesth Analg. 1983;62:84–96.

Hudspith MJ. Glutamate: a role in normal brain function, anaesthesia, analgesia and CNS injury. Br J Anaesth. 1997;78:731–47.

Kofke WA, Templehoff R, Dasheiff RM. Anesthetic implications of epilepsy, status epilepsies and epilepsy surgery. J Neurosurg Anesth. 1997;9:349–72.

McFarlane HJ. Anaesthesia and the new generation monoamine oxidase inhibitors. Anaesthesia 1994;49:597–9.

Rudolph U, Mohler H. Analysis of $GABA_A$ receptor function and dissection of the pharmacology of benzodiazepines and general anesthetics through mouse genetics. Annu Rev Pharmacol Toxicol. 2004;44:475–98.

Schmid RL, Sandler AN, Katz J. Use and efficacy of low-dose ketamine in the management of acute postoperative pain: a review of current techniques and outcomes. Pain 1999;82:111–25.

Chapter 29

Consciousness and cognition

Kane O Pryor and Robert A Veselis

TOPICS COVERED IN THIS CHAPTER

- **Consciousness**
  - Defining consciousness
  - Biological theories of consciousness
  - Unconscious states
  - Anesthesia – pharmacological unconsciousness
  - Pathological unconsciousness
- **Cognition**
  - Memory
  - Anatomy of memory
  - Cellular mechanisms of memory
  - Anesthesia and memory

CONSCIOUSNESS

René Descartes' 1637 dictum '*Cogito, ergo sum*' marks the origin of an intellectual dialog on consciousness. Since that time, consciousness and free thought have been regarded as existential components of what it is to be human. In this context, anesthetic agents possess the remarkable property of being able to predictably and reversibly remove consciousness and cognition, and yet permit most other organ functions to continue relatively unperturbed. Retrospectively, it is surprising that the introduction of anesthesia did not harbinger the development of a new science of consciousness. However, in the mid-nineteenth century the possibility that consciousness might have a physical explanation was itself a novel, if not heretical, idea. It was only in the late twentieth century that neural science came to regard a physical explanation for consciousness as a legitimate and serious academic pursuit. By that time, academic anesthesiology had concentrated most of its attention on other physiological and pharmacological questions.

The last two decades have seen a renaissance in the scientific investigation of consciousness and cognition, with the development of positron emission tomography (PET) and functional magnetic resonance imaging (fMRI) standing as revolutionary advances in the ability to study the functioning brain. The development of these modalities has also greatly facilitated the study of how brain function is affected by anesthetic drugs. Studies using anesthetic drugs enable direct comparison of brain function during pharmacologically altered states of consciousness with that during normal consciousness. The attractiveness of these studies is the ability to correlate regional changes in brain activity with changes in behavioral performance on carefully focused neuropsychological tests, theoretically providing insight into which neural structures may perform particular behavioral functions. This chapter introduces fundamental concepts involved in the study of consciousness and cognition that are related to anesthesia.

Defining consciousness

There is no consensus on how to approach the question of a scientific explanation for consciousness. Much of current research is devoted to establishing the *physical nature* of the neural correlate of consciousness (NCC) – the required neuronal events that bring an aspect of consciousness into existence – without necessarily addressing the question of exactly how the NCC creates a unified, subjective, and qualitative consciousness.

Consciousness challenges scientific methodology, largely because of its inability to be objectively observed. Science can only directly observe the *correlates* and *mechanisms* that mediate consciousness; consciousness as experienced is absolutely subjective and cannot be separated from the sole observer. Thus, the foundation task of the science is to establish a lexicon of definitions that characterize those properties of consciousness that are universal. In this regard, the question of consciousness may be one of the last to be legitimately shared by both science and philosophy.

The irreducible features of consciousness are its *qualitativeness*, its *subjectivity*, and its *unity*. Most scientific research is focused on the unity of consciousness – the integration of innumerable discrete elements of a percept into a singular, unified, conscious experience. Secondarily, this unified consciousness is *continuous*, traveling as an unbroken stream that integrates immediate perception and thought with previous contextual information and memory. It is also *selective*, or at least *non-deterministic*, in that there is a degree of 'free will' in the inclusion or exclusion of stimuli from the attention of the perceptual foreground. This selectivity can move freely over an essentially infinite number of potential conscious elements, yet consciousness is remarkably *stable* in time intervals associated with working processes (milliseconds to seconds).

Conscious experience requires the existence of the conscious state – the presence of the ability to perceive the internal (and usually the external) environment. The distinction between the *state* and the *content* of consciousness is of neurobiological importance, as clearly the conditional processes that *enable* consciousness are quite distinct from those that form subjective conscious experience. The development of the electroencephalogram (EEG) created an objective, nonbehavioral measurement of the state of consciousness, enabling neuroscience to progress in understanding the mechanisms that support the conscious state, even when the question of conscious experience remained enigmatic.

Until relatively recently, definitions of consciousness inherited Descartes' concept of *cartesian dualism*, the belief that mind and brain are not reducible forms of a common nature. In classic dualistic thinking, the perception of the external world by physical processes in the brain is integrated and observed in the *cartesian theater* of the mind, which is nonphysical. As reductionism came to dominate scientific methodology, classic dualism was renamed the *cartesian error*. However, it is by no means universally accepted that reductionism will provide the answer to consciousness and the nature of mind.

Biological theories of consciousness

The *state* of consciousness is dependent on a system of neuronal pathways originating in the upper brainstem, hypothalamus, and basal forebrain, termed the *ascending reticular activating system*, or the *ascending arousal system*. The ascending arousal system has two major branches. One branch travels through the thalamus to modulate the rhythmicity and synchronicity of thalamic relay and other neuronal signaling to diffuse thalamocortical projections. The other branch travels though the lateral hypothalamus, integrating projections from hypothalamic and cholinergic basal forebrain nuclei before projecting diffusely to cortical structures (Fig. 29.1). Bilateral lesions of either branch result in permanent loss of consciousness.

Consciousness depends on patterns of coherent neuronal activity in the thalamus, which in turn are modulated by the ascending arousal system.

Consciousness is dependent upon patterns of coherent neuronal activity in the thalamus, which in turn are dependent upon modulatory input from the ascending arousal system. In the waking state, the resting membrane potential of the thalamic relay neurons is maintained close to the threshold potential by neuroexcitatory projections from the rostral pons and basal forebrain. In this state, termed the *transmission* or *spike mode*, thalamic relay neurons accurately transmit excitatory sensory input onward to thalamocortical projections through a single 'spike' firing potential. At the level of the outer cortex, this nonrhythmic complexity of thalamocortical firing patterns results in fast, low-voltage desynchronized wave activity, and is the source of the β waves of the electroencephalogram. Conversely, in the *burst mode* the thalamic relay neurons are in a hyperpolarized state, supported by projections from inhibitory GABAergic interneurons in the reticular nucleus of the thalamus. In the hyperpolarized state the relay neurons are unable to reach the firing threshold in response to sensory inputs. Instead, the neurons exhibit a slow, rhythmic bursting pattern that is mediated by changes in voltage-gated Ca^{2+} channels and Ca^{2+}-activated potassium channels. A feedback loop is created through reciprocal projections from thalamic relay neurons to the reticular nucleus, resulting in a slow, global, rhythmic thalamocortical firing pattern, which appears as high-amplitude, synchronized slow-wave activity at the level of the

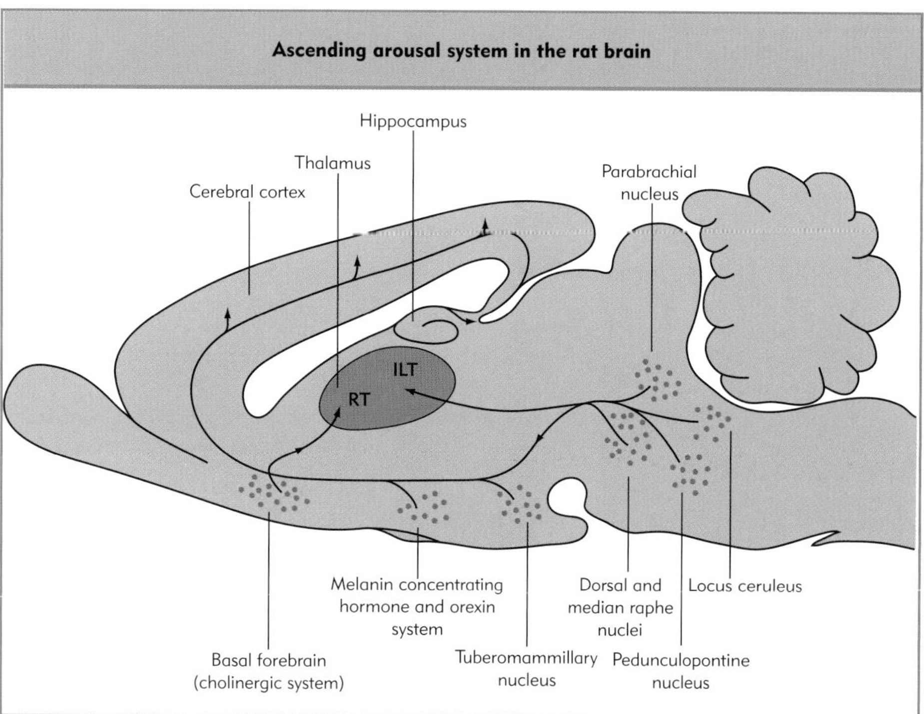

Figure 29.1 The ascending arousal system consists of the axons from nuclei in the upper brain stem, hypothalamus, and basal forebrain. These pathways diffusely innervate the thalamus and cerebral cortex and keep them in a state in which they can transmit and respond appropriately to incoming sensory information. Damage to either the main pathway in the brainstem or its branches in the thalamus or hypothalamus can cause loss of consciousness. RT, reticular nucleus of the thalamus; ILT, intralaminar thalamic nuclei. (From Saper CB. Brain stem modulation of sensation, movement, and consciousness. In: Kaplan ER, Schwartz JH, Jessell TM, eds. Principles of Neural Science. New York: McGraw-Hill, 2000; 889-909; Fig. 45.10).

cortex, and is the source of delta (δ) and theta (θ) activity on the EEG.

Several lines of research suggest that the subsequent element necessary for the presence of consciousness involves coherent oscillation through re-entrant pathways in corticothalamocortical loops that connect critical neuronal groupings. The neuronal components of corticothalamocortical circuits involve deep-layer corticothalamic neurons, thalamocortical neurons, thalamic reticular neurons, and GABAergic thalamic interneurons (Fig. 29.2). There is also an excitatory glutamatergic circuit between neocortical and thalamocortical neurons, and an inhibitory circuit between thalamocortical neurons and GABAergic thalamic reticular neurons. The initiation and perpetuation of coherent oscillatory activity requires thalamic relay neurons to be in the transmission mode, which is contingent upon tonic excitatory input from cholinergic, noradrenergic, and histaminergic projections from the brainstem and hypothalamus. The anatomical structure of a resonant loop does not appear to be fixed, but does appear to be highly dependent on the oscillatory frequency: resonance in the gamma (γ; 30–50 Hz) range may occupy only a single cortical column, whereas slow-wave resonant loops may cross hemispheres to become a global cortical process. Thus, corticothalamocortical loops can be thought of as a dynamic functional structure.

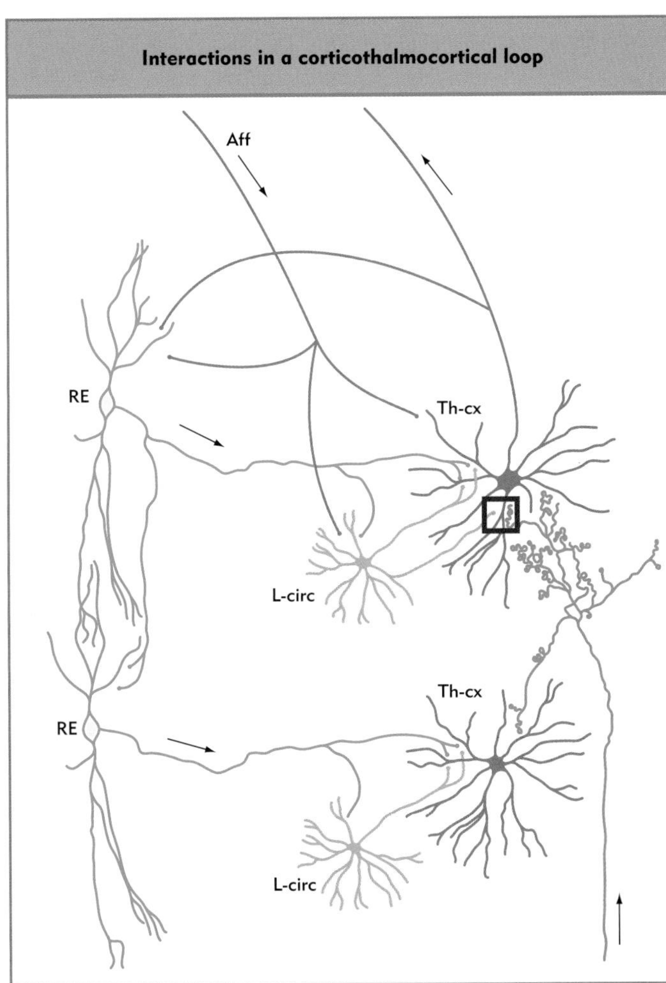

Figure 29.2 Interactions between GABAergic thalamic reticular (RE) neurons, local-circuit (L-circ) neurons, and thalamocortical (Th-cx) neurons in a corticothalamocortical loop. Afferent input (Aff) predominantly excites the *top* Th-cx neuron. RE neurons modulate the activity through actions on Th-cx and L-circ neurons. The circuit receiving the predominant afferent input (the *top* Th-cx neuron) will be amplified, whereas the adjacent weakly excited loops (the *bottom* Th-cx neuron) will be inhibited. The system is thus capable of a dynamic response to complex afferent input. (From Steriade M. Impact of network activities on neuronal properties in corticothalamic systems. J Neurophysiol. 2001;86:1–39.)

According to several theories, the individual perceptual elements of consciousness are probably supported within the substrate of these corticothalamocortical resonant columns. The afferent content entering the loop can derive from a projection of sensory modality input, thus mediating conscious perception of the external world, or from intrinsic processes, existing entirely within a 'closed' brain system. The thalamus receives greater input from widespread cortical structures than from the external sensory system, suggesting that the intrinsic processes are predominant. It is possible that these 'closed loop' intrinsic systems support what is perceived as thought and imagination, and that dreaming in REM sleep involves a hyperattentiveness to intrinsic processes, accompanied by isolation from external sensory input.

Synchronized oscillations in the high-frequency (γ) band, especially around 40 Hz, are associated with conscious activity. In the waking state, the presentation of a stimulus is able to reset and synchronize coherent 40 Hz activity over wide regions of the brain with a high degree of spatial organization. In REM sleep this coherent 40 Hz activity exists but is not reset by external stimuli. It is not seen at all in δ sleep (Fig. 29.3). Corticothalamocortical loop complexes support 40 Hz oscillations, probably

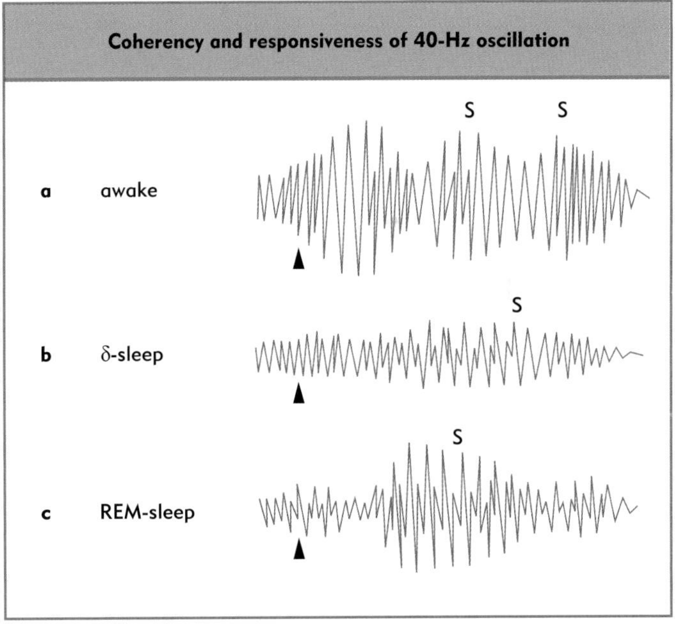

Figure 29.3 Coherency and responsiveness of 40-Hz oscillation during wakefulness, REM sleep, and δ sleep. Shown is a single epoch of 40-Hz oscillations following the presentation of a single auditory stimulus (arrow), recorded using a 37-channel magnetoencephalogram in a healthy subject. When awake (a) the stimulus is followed by a reset of 40-Hz activity, and then by two further spontaneous oscillations (S). With sleep (b and c) the stimulus produced no resetting of the rhythm. However, spontaneous 40-Hz oscillations (S) are seen in REM sleep independent of the stimulus. 40-Hz oscillations responsive to stimuli characterize the awake conscious state, whereas oscillations which are not responsive to external stimuli are seen in the dreaming state. (After: Llinas R, Ribary U. Consciousness and the brain. The thalamocortical dialogue in health and disease. Ann N Y Acad Sci 2001; 929: 166-75. Originally after: Llinas R, Ribary U. Coherent 40-Hz oscillation characterizes dream state in humans. Proc Nat Acad Sci USA 1993; 90: 2078-81. Copyright © 1993 National Academy of Sciences, USA)

through inherent properties of thalamic nuclei in connection with a series of feedforward and feedback mechanisms in the circuit. Although the theory that coherent 40 Hz oscillations represent the neural correlate of consciousness has fallen out of favor, they may still be highly significant in the mechanism of consciousness, possibly through 'amplifying' critical neuronal networks above random activity, without actually increasing the firing rate.

Like other theories of 'elemental reductionism', re-entrant loop theories are crucial to understanding the neural correlates and functional mechanisms that underlie the processing of individual perceptual elements. There has been substantial progress in describing neural correlates for elements of visual perception, language, hearing, recognition, and other discrete perceptual functions. However, *understanding the perceptual fragments does not explain how all the elements come to be perceived as a unitary and continuous stream of qualitative consciousness*. This is what physicist Christoph von der Malsburg termed the *binding problem*: what structure or function *binds* the elements of perception to form the unified oneness of conscious experience?

There is little prospect that a generally accepted answer to this problem lies in the near future, but several – albeit incomplete – neurobiological theories of consciousness have been developed. The quest for a unified theory of consciousness remains one of the most difficult and elusive goals in all science.

Unconscious states

The transition from consciousness to unconsciousness occurs when thalamic relay neurons become sufficiently hyperpolarized to switch to the burst mode, thus interrupting afferent input into corticothalamocortical loops. Hypothetically, this 'state change' can occur as a result of a decrease in the excitatory tonic input, an increase in inhibitory GABAergic neurotransmission, and/or direct hyperpolarization at nodes in the loop. Loss of consciousness is also associated with a decrease in γ band activity and an uncoupling of synchronous activity across brain regions, but these may represent secondary effects of corticothalamocortical loop disruption.

Anesthesia – pharmacological unconsciousness

Although at high doses anesthetic agents cause depression of global brain function, it is clear that the initial transition into unconsciousness is due to critical regional and functional effects. Quantitative EEG studies demonstrate that the loss of consciousness associated with anesthesia is invariantly associated with four changes: 1) a significant drop in γ band activity; 2) an increase in slow-wave activity; 3) an increase in power and coupling in anterior regions; and 4) an uncoupling of inter- and intrahemispheric interactions. These changes imply a loss of cooperative processes between neuronal populations. Variable-resolution electromagnetic tomography (VARETA), which localizes the corresponding structures in three-dimensional space, suggests that the critical structures include the thalamus, basal ganglia, superior frontal gyrus, anterior cingulate gyri, and precentral, paracentral, and certain prefrontal gyri. PET studies demonstrated that the loss of consciousness due to propofol anesthesia is associated with reduced cerebral blood flow in the thalamus and similar frontal and prefrontal structures (Fig. 29.4). *Thus, one prominent hypothesis is that the critical common event in anesthesia-induced unconsciousness is the disruption of corticothalamocortical re-entrant activity, most likely resulting from hyperpolarization of thalamocortical neurons*. Thalamocortical hyperpolarization may itself follow inhibition of the mesencephalic reticular formation and disinhibition of the nucleus reticularis of the thalamus. It is likely that GABAergic anesthetics, such as volatile anesthetics, barbiturates, benzodiazepenes, and propofol, at a minimum facilitate hyperpolarization through pre- and postsynaptic actions at GABAergic interneurons in the reticular nucleus of the thalamus. As it is likely that consciousness and unconsciousness are the result of quantal states of re-entrant activity (either supra- or subthreshold), the unconsciousness induced by anesthetics may not be the endpoint of a gradual descent, but instead a fairly sudden state change – the *thalamocortical switch*. However, the hypothesis that GABAergic anesthesia-induced thalamocortical hyperpolarization is *always* the result of direct action at the thalamus has recently been challenged: recent PET studies with thiopental *do not* show a prominent reduction in cerebral blood flow in the thalamus during the transition to unconsciousness, even though the EEG is consistent with thalamocortical depression. Thus, thiopental may induce thalamocortical hyperpolarization through downstream, indirect effects. The actions of anesthetic agents acting at NMDA receptors are more complex, and may involve 'unbinding' of coherent processes without necessarily terminating corticothalamocortical loop activity.

Loss of consciousness with anesthesia is due to critical regional and functional effects evident on EEG.

Pathological unconsciousness

Consciousness is impaired when any of the processes described above are disrupted. Pathological loss of consciousness can result from three forms of dysfunction: 1) impairment of the ascending arousal system, which prevents the thalamus from entering transmission mode; 2) dysfunction of the forebrain (diencephalon and telencephalon), which leads to direct corruption of thalamocortical processes; or 3) a combination of these. Impairment of the ascending arousal system and the diencephalon commonly results from a structural injury, usually following trauma or cerebrovascular insult, whereas loss of consciousness due to impairment of the telencephalon is more often due to a global process causing encephalopathy, with pyramidal neurons in laminae III and V being the most vulnerable to injury.

Lesions of either branch of the ascending arousal system may result in *coma*, a state of profound unrousability. There is a degradation of excitatory tonic input to thalamic relay neurons, which are then dominated by inhibitory input from the reticular nucleus of the thalamus. Characteristically, the EEG is profoundly slowed and synchronized, as thalamic relay neurons enter an exaggerated state of burst mode firing. Direct injury to the thalamus may result in complete loss of the EEG if thalamic relay neurons are unable to initiate thalamocortical firing; in less severe injury some thalamocortical activity may be present, but it is sufficiently disrupted to prevent the establishment of a conscious field.

Unconsciousness that results from dysfunction of the cerebral hemispheres represents a loss of the content of consciousness, even when the conditions that support the state of consciousness remain intact. Irreversible injury may result in a *persistent vegetative state*. Because brain functions below the level of the

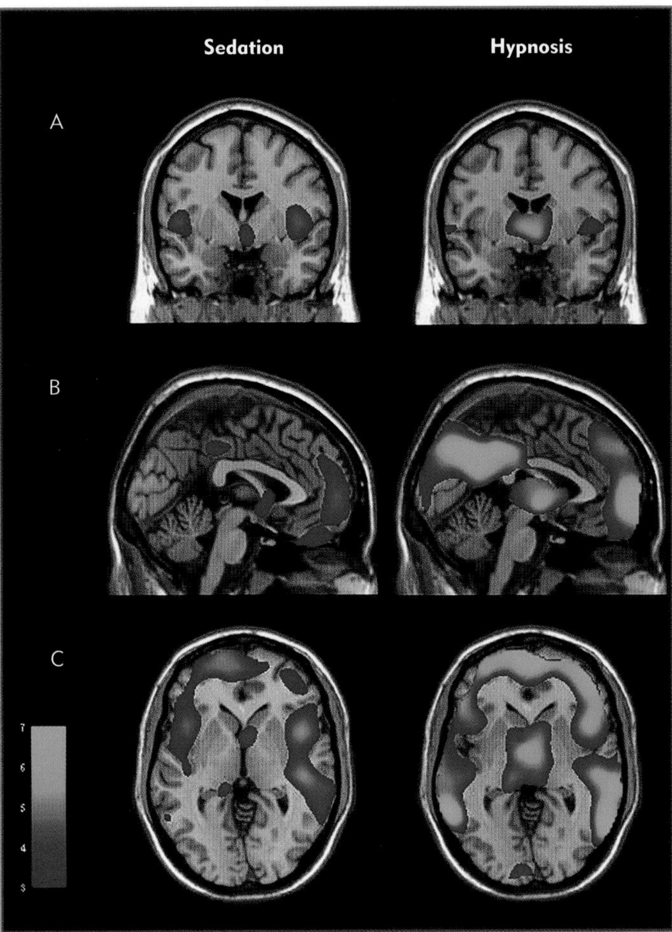

Figure 29.4 Reductions in regional cerebral blood flow (rCBF) associated with different concentrations of propofol. Data were obtained using ^{15}O PET imaging, and analyzed by statistical parametric mapping from four subjects (A, B, and C represent the coronal, sagittal, and horizontal planes, respectively). The transition from blue to green indicates a *reduction* in rCBF compared to baseline. Areas without coloration did not have a reduction in rCBF greater than the threshold ($p < 0.05$). At sedative concentrations rCBF is maximally reduced in prefrontal and parietal association areas, prominently involved in working memory and organizational processes. At hypnotic concentrations, in addition to these areas, thalamic activity is specifically reduced. This suggests that the initial transition to unconsciousness is not due to diffuse reduction in cortical activity, but rather to a discrete state change – the thalamocortical switch.

telencephalon may remain intact, patients in this state may exhibit actions that give the illusion of consciousness, such as a sleep–wake cycle, facial expressions, and visual fixation on objects; however, these actions are performed without the existence of any cognitive content. This is distinct from *brain death*, in which all lower brain functions cease, and only reflexive actions mediated by the spinal cord remain.

COGNITION

The cognitive faculties of the brain are the processing systems that ultimately create the substrate for the content of consciousness. Thought, learning, memory, perception, language, and planning of movement emerge from the complex associative interactions of cortical regions that perform discrete simple processing functions. Simple processing elements are integrated in a progressive hierarchy that involves areas of *association cortex*. For example, modalities of a visual input – such as color, motion, orientation, depth, and contour – are initially processed in discrete regions of primary visual cortex in the occipital lobe. A unified visual modality is formed via hierarchical integration within the surrounding *unimodal* visual association area in the occipitotemporal region, and is then connected to other modalities such as audition and language via projections to the large *multimodal* posterior association area in the parietotemporal region.

Memory

The cognitive function of greatest interest to anesthesiologists is memory. The ability to directly manipulate memory mechanisms such that profound, reversible memory impairment occurs is an elemental component of anesthetic practice. Consequently, one of the goals of anesthesiology research is to understand how anesthetic drugs cause memory impairment. At the same time, anesthetic drugs are a powerful tool to elucidate the underlying mechanisms involved in memory. *Working memory* (often called 'short-term memory') is the transient storage and manipulation of information that is part of other cognitive functions, such as speech or vision. It integrates immediate perceptual experience and can hold information for only short periods (seconds), but is capable of circularly rehearsing information to perpetuate its existence in the foreground of attention (such as when rehearsing a telephone number). The content of working memory is given context and meaning through parallel access to long-term memory systems that subserve knowledge, experience, or skills. Working memory comprises two slave systems: a *visuospatial sketchpad* for temporary storage of visual images, and a *phonological loop* for articulatory rehearsal of verbal material. A third system, the *central executive*, directs the foreground of attention across the components of working memory.

The ability to reversibly impair memory is an essential element of anesthesia.

Information beyond the transience of working memory enters into *long-term memory*. This singular description is somewhat misleading, as long-term memory can clearly be divided into several distinct modalities. *Explicit* (declarative) memory is memory as we usually think of it – the information that is recalled into consciousness, usually involving the complex association of multiple contextual elements of information about an object or concept. Explicit memory can be further divided into two forms. *Episodic* (autobiographical) memory is the memory of personal experience that is temporally based, with information about time and place embedded in the memory. *Semantic* (factual) memory is the complex knowledge of facts, language, and other concepts that remain long after the extinction of the episodic memory for how the knowledge was acquired.

Explicit memory is the result of four distinct functional processes. *Encoding* is the immediate processing of a stimulus that initiates a memory trace, and is dependent on attentional mechanisms. *Consolidation* is the process by which the initially unstable memory trace is transformed to a more stable state. *Storage* processes create a long-term and stable retention of a memory, and *retrieval* is the final process in which disparate elements of stored information are reconstituted into a unified memory percept. Studies of memory and neuroplasticity suggest that working memory and the different stages of long-term memory may not be sequential, but are independent processes acting in parallel.

Implicit (nondeclarative) memory refers to processes which are learned and which alter behavior, but which do not involve conscious processes. The development of motor skills is the archetype of implicit memory. Others include procedural skills, associative learning such as fear conditioning, nonassociative learning such as habituation, and priming behavior, which is that most often used in experiments to evaluate implicit memory formation under anesthesia. Priming occurs when a prior event, for which there is no explicit memory, influences subsequent performance when the subject is allowed to choose a response or free-associate. A classic – and now illegal – use of priming is in subliminal advertising, whereas classic pavlovian conditioning exemplifies associative learning. Figure 29.5 depicts a simple taxonomic schema for memory systems, including the neuroanatomical structures prominently involved in long-term memory behaviors.

Anatomy of memory

The current concept of memory is one in which there are multiple memory *systems* that involve a group of structures in several regions of the brain. A given structure may be dynamically involved in several memory systems, with each system responsive to others that function as *modulators* of activity. For example, the basolateral amygdala complex (BLAC) is critically involved in interpreting the emotional context of a memory, in modulating memory consolidation processes in the hippocampus and other regions, and in forming fear-conditioned implicit memory. The BLAC represents a common node at which multiple neural networks converge and interact, but the systems themselves are quite distinct. Several structures are known to be critical in performing particular memory behaviors (Fig. 29.6).

HIPPOCAMPUS

The hippocampus, within the medial temporal lobe (MTL), was once thought to be the exclusive locus of several memory functions, but is now understood to be one component of systems that subserve these behaviors. It is important in the initial consolidation and stabilization of early long-term memory, but does not appear to be involved in the long-term storage of explicit memory. The surrounding cortical masses, which include the entorhinal and perirhinal cortices, are critical for the transfer of initial stabilized memory trace to long-term memory, which is probably spread diffusely throughout the neocortex, and which probably occurs over a period of days to weeks. The left hippocampus may modulate the integration and binding of elements of a retrieved memory, especially those involving contextual information, whereas the right hippocampus is important in the development of spatial representation.

BASAL GANGLIA

The caudate nucleus and putamen are critically involved in a memory system that is independent of the hippocampal system and which operates in parallel, sometimes with competitive interference between the two systems. Where the hippocampal

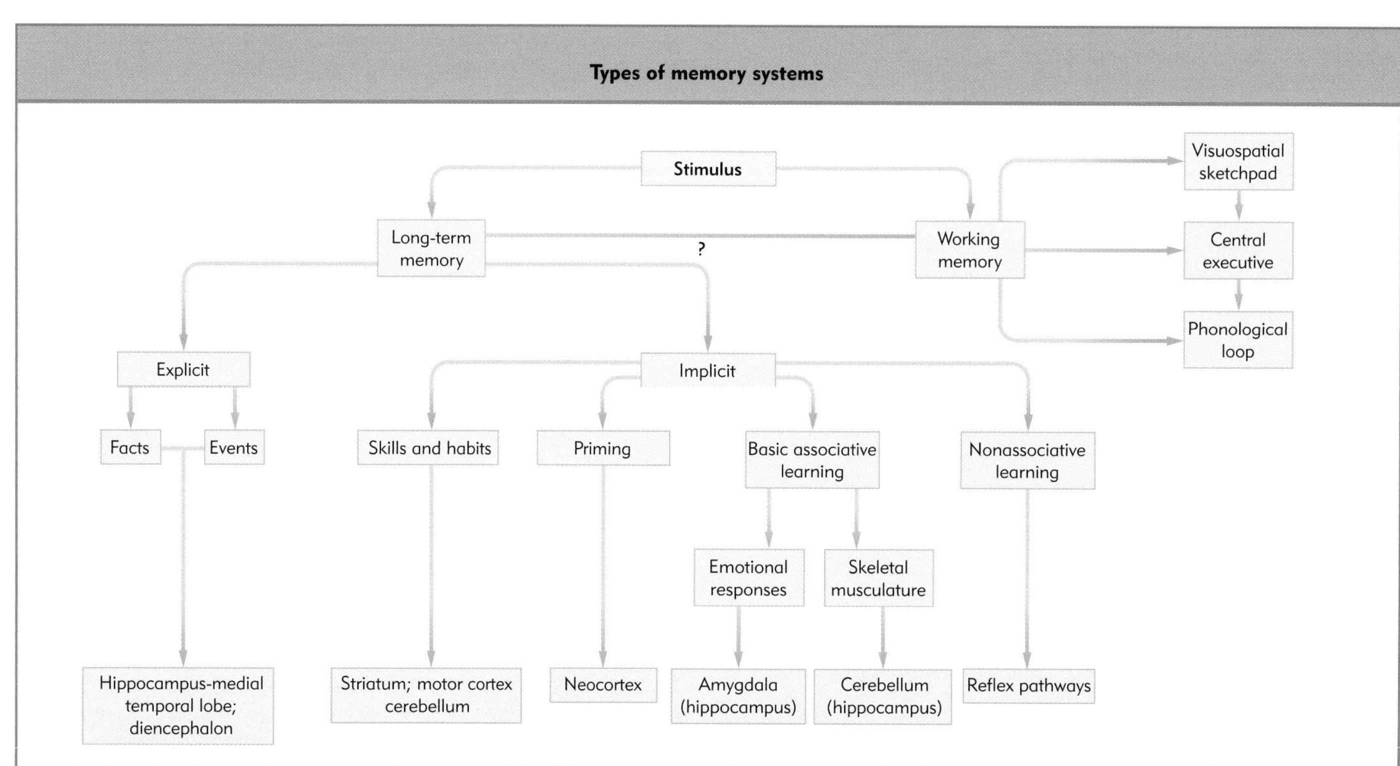

Figure 29.5 Types of memory systems. A simple taxonomic schema for different forms of memory and critical structures for explicit and implicit memory are shown. Working memory appears to involve diffuse areas of the neocortex, although prefrontal areas are particularly important for organizational and executive functions. (Adapted with permission from Squire LR, Zola-Morgan S. The medial temporary lobe memory system. Science 1991; 253:1380-6. Copyright © 1991 AAAS.)

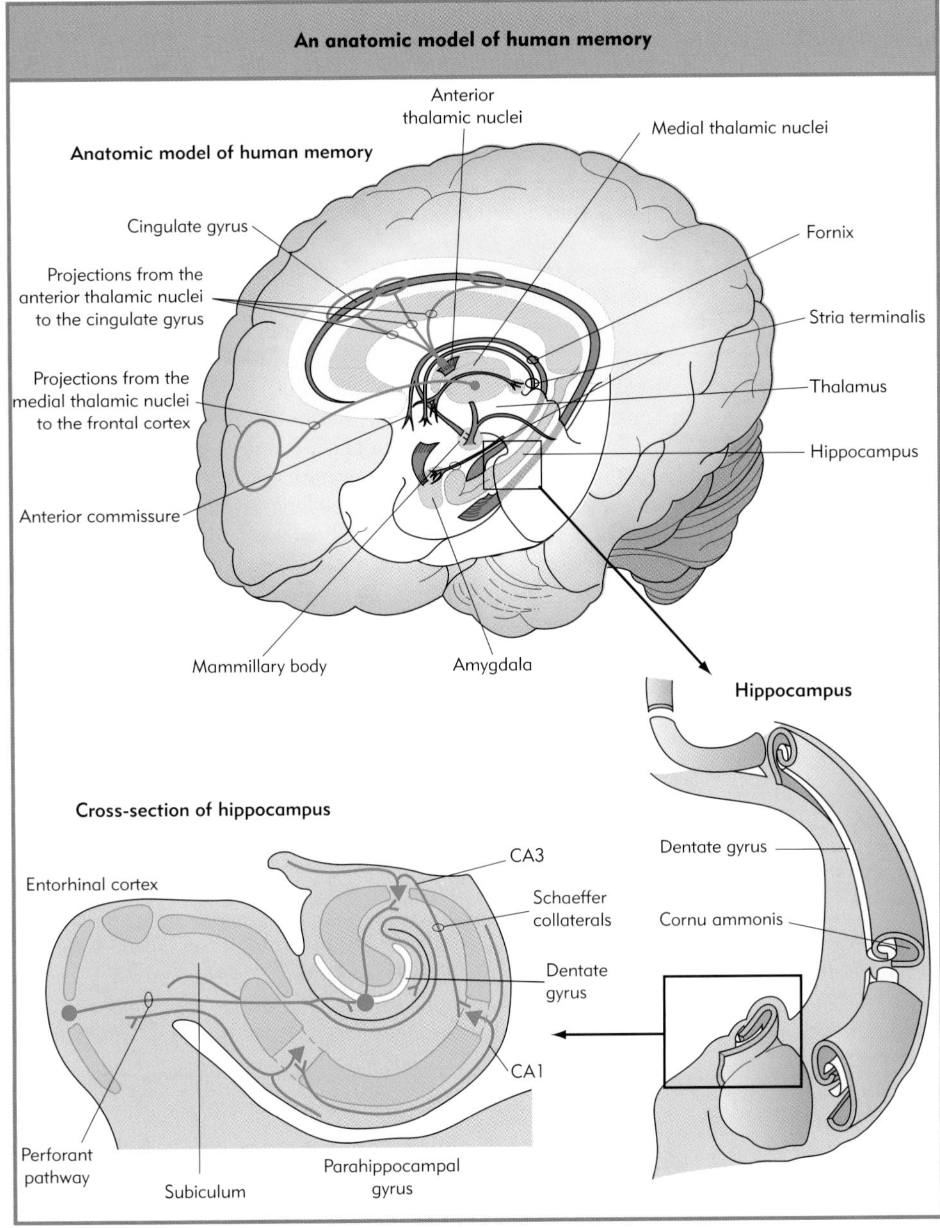

Figure 29.6 An anatomic model of human memory. The various components of memory are widely distributed, but key structures are involved in certain steps. The microscopic diagram (bottom left) shows the flow of information from the entorhinal cortex and subicular region to the dentate gyrus via perforant fibers to synapse on to granule cells in the hippocampus. The axons from these form a bundle, the mossy fiber pathway, that runs to the pyramidal cells in the CA3 region. These cells send excitatory input to the CA1 region via Schaffer collaterals. The efferents from the hippocampus travel through the fornix to the septal nuclei, the hypothalamus, the mammillary bodies, and the anterior nuclei of the thalamus, which in turn project to the cingulate gyrus. Some of these structures (e.g. the cingulate gyrus and the septal nuclei) also provide afferents to the hippocampus. In this way, the arrangement of neurons in the hippocampus and tracts to and from the hippocampus form a recurrent network. This system has been extensively studied as a model of synaptic plasticity – the modification of synaptic interactions that have the ability to store information. For example, CA1 and CA3 fields exhibit long-term potentiation to form spatial memories.

system mediates cognitive, spatial, or declarative memory, the caudate–putamen system appears to mediate stimulus-response 'habit' formation, taxon, and complex procedural memory.

AMYGDALA

A small structure in the MTL, the amygdala complex is an important modulator of memory encoding, storage, and consolidation processes occurring in other brain regions. Functional neuroimaging studies clearly demonstrate that the amygdala is prominently involved in modulating memory processes during states of negative emotional arousal – an explanation for the common experience that strong negative memories tend to be better remembered. Amygdala activity modulates processes occurring in the hippocampus, possibly through long-term potentiation, and also the caudate nucleus, possibly through modulation of stimulus-response processes – which is consistent with the pattern of predominantly glutamatergic neuronal projections from amygdala nuclei. The modulatory role of the amygdala is probably enabled via the release and action of stress hormones such as epinephrine and cortisol, and is enhanced or attenuated by the actions of centrally acting β-adrenergic agonists and antagonists, respectively.

PREFRONTAL CORTEX

The prefrontal cortex performs functions of cognitive control, and is prominently – though not exclusively – involved in working memory organization via central executive processes. It is involved in the organization of material prior to encoding, as well as the verification, monitoring, and evaluation of representations that have been retrieved from long-term memory. Subjects with damage to prefrontal regions demonstrate disorganization, and have severe problems when irrelevant information must be ignored, or when required to shift strategies; confabulation is common, which is probably due to an impairment of cognitive control processes that regulate retrieval task parameters and the verification and monitoring of recollected information.

CEREBELLUM

The cerebellum is critical in motor learning and in associative forms of implicit memory, such as the formation of a conditioned response. The cerebellum is also involved in some cognitive, linguistic, and emotional functions through cross-projections to the limbic system and prefrontal cortex.

Cellular mechanisms of memory

The sea slug *Aplysia californica* has provided a simple system for the detailed study of elementary forms of implicit learning, and several vertebrate models have been used to study potential mechanisms for explicit memory, especially involving the hippocampus. How any of these findings relate to human memory is unclear.

In *Aplysia*, the simplest forms of short-term learning – habituation and sensitization – occur through presynaptic modulation of synaptic *plasticity*. *Habituation* results in a decrease in the presynaptic release of glutamate from sensory neurons. *Sensitization* results from facilitation of presynaptic transmission at sensory neurons induced by the activity of modulatory interneurons. For example, after a single stimulus interneurons release serotonin, which binds to 5-HT receptors on the presynaptic sensory neuron. A G-protein–cyclic AMP–protein kinase A (PKA) cascade follows, which together with protein kinase C enhances neurotransmitter release from the sensory neuron's terminal for a few minutes. In *classic conditioning* a similar presynaptic mechanism, also involving Ca^{2+}/calmodulin activation, is accompanied by a postsynaptic component, which is probably a form of NMDA-receptor-dependent long-term potentiation (see below).

When a stimulus is repeated, such that long-term sensitization or classic conditioning is induced, a different molecular process occurs which involves new protein synthesis. In *long-term sensitization*, persistent activation of PKA recruits mitogen-activated protein kinase (MAPK), and the two kinases translocate to the nucleus, where they activate a transcription factor called CREB-1 (cAMP response element-binding protein) and suppress the inhibitory actions of CREB-2. A cascade of gene activation follows which results in the growth of new synaptic connections. *Long-term classic conditioning* involves a similar CREB-dependent process.

In the vertebrate hippocampus, transmission along each of the three major pathways is modulated by what has occurred previously in a process called *long-term potentiation* (LTP). Stimulus along any of the pathways increases the amplitude of subsequent excitatory postsynaptic potentials. LTP has an early and a late phase. The early phase is cooperative and associative, and involves NMDA receptors, Ca^{2+}/calmodulin-dependent kinase II (CaMKII), the formation of postsynaptic nonNMDA receptors, and possibly nitric oxide. The late phase involves new mRNA and protein synthesis, and recruits the cAMP–PKA–MAPK–CREB pathway. LTP may be involved in the formation of a long-term explicit memory trace. In the cerebellum and other regions, a different process called *long-term depression* (LTD) appears to mediate synaptic plasticity. LTD reduces synaptic transmission from granule cells to Purkinje cells in a reorganization that is 'error-driven'.

Anesthesia and memory

Sufficient general anesthesia completely ablates contextually rich explicit memory. However, explicit awareness during anesthesia can and does occur at a rate of around 0.2%. It is unlikely that the occurrence of 'anesthesia awareness' represents a patient-specific idiosyncratic resistance to the normal memory impairment caused by anesthetic drugs. Anesthesia awareness is most reasonably explained by an insufficient administration of anesthesia *relative* to the level of neuroexcitation induced by surgical stimulation and the patient's basal state. Awareness is most likely in patients who are physiologically unable to tolerate appropriate doses of anesthetic drugs, and who are in a physiologically hyperstimulated and stressed state that activates the ascending arousal system and higher structures. Thus, trauma and obstetric emergency patients, who possess both risk factors, have the highest incidence of awareness. Many studies suggest that some implicit memory processes can continue in the presence of clinically relevant concentrations of anesthetic drugs, even when no explicit memory is evident.

ANESTHESIA AND EXPLICIT MEMORY

Theoretically, explicit memory could be impaired at any of four stages – encoding, consolidation, storage, or retrieval. Functional neuroimaging (FNI) studies show that GABAergic anesthetic drugs at high concentrations cause a widely distributed reduction in cerebral metabolism and blood flow, suggesting that the memory impairment effects at these levels are due to nonspecific disruption of memory processes. However, memory impairment is also evident at drug concentrations substantially lower than those required for global cerebral depression. In this case, FNI and electrophysiological studies suggest that anesthetic drugs cause loss of explicit memory through *very specific mechanisms* that critically disrupt a distinct component of memory function. The intravenous GABAergic drugs, especially midazolam, propofol, and thiopental, have been the most extensively studied in this regard.

Awareness under general anesthesia is most likely due to insufficient dosing relative to the level of basal and surgically induced neuroexcitation.

Deep anesthesia (hypnosis) of any kind causes memory impairment through the removal of normal attention mechanisms. Unattended stimuli do not enter either working or explicit memory systems, and in the extreme unresponsive state of general anesthesia no encoding takes place. There is no single electrophysiological marker for attention or sedation, but anesthesia-induced unconsciousness has a profound effect on the components of the event-related potential (ERP) that are associated with initial encoding, such as the P3. As drug concentration increases, FNI shows global cerebral depression, but this is preceded by a series of critical events leading to unconsciousness, the most important of which is depression of thalamic neurons via GABAergic mechanisms, leading to hyperpolarization, a disconnection of the anterior and posterior brain, and a disruption of corticothalamocortical re-entrant activity (see above).

Memory impairment at lower levels of anesthesia, where the subject is not profoundly unconscious, is more intriguing. The loss of attention mechanisms remains important, and drugs are able to impair encoding through a nonspecific sedative effect. However, for some drugs there is also a discrete amnesic effect on specific memory processes. This is apparent clinically in patients given a small dose of midazolam or propofol who are capable of conversing (demonstrating intact working memory and early long-term memory processes), but who repeat themselves minutes later with no memory of the previous conversation (demonstrating that memory consolidation/storage was interrupted). Thus, midazolam and propofol have a strong amnesic effect *independent* of their sedative effect on attention. The specific amnesic effect of propofol involves information that has *successfully been acquired and encoded* into early long-term memory but subsequently lost, presumably though disruption of consolidation and storage. Benzodiazepines have a similar memory effect. Thiopental has a weak amnesic effect, whereas fentanyl has none. Dexmedetomidine also exerts its memory impairment predominantly through sedation, via α_{2A}-adrenoreceptor binding at the locus ceruleus, an important modulator of vigilance and a principal source of noradrenergic innervation to the forebrain. Anticholinergic drugs such as scopolamine have a similar effect on memory to the benzodiazepines.

Current knowledge of memory mechanisms suggests disruption of hippocampal processes, in particular long-term potentiation (LTP), as a mechanism for these specific amnesic effects. The hippocampal-complex structures are rich in GABA and NMDA receptors, and animal studies have shown specific LTP processes to be altered by propofol and isoflurane. The point in the memory process at which the amnesic effects are evident is consistent with our current understanding of the role of the hippocampus in consolidation and early storage. However, it is far from clear that LTP and the hippocampus is the site of propofol's amnesic effects.

EEG MONITORING AND EXPLICIT MEMORY

A number of quantitative EEG analysis algorithms have been designed to measure the depth of anesthesia. The *bispectral index (BIS)* algorithm incorporates a Fourier analysis of EEG data and a bispectral analysis of phase shift at critical EEG frequencies. A multivariate regression model derived from four common anesthetic combinations establishes a single score between 0 (no electrical activity in the brain) and 100 (completely awake). The *patient state index (PSI)*, which uses two anterior, a midline central, and a midline posterior electrode also incorporates a Fourier analysis, and then calculates variance in a number of 'critical features', such as the absolute δ power at the vertex, and the posterior relative power on the slow δ band. A multivariate model, which includes some 'self-normalization' components, generates a score from 0 to 100. The *Narcotrend* monitor (currently used in Europe) uses discriminant analysis to yield probabilities for the degree of similarity between the measured EEG epoch and prevalidated EEG epochs, divided into 14 substages of anesthesia and then converted to a number between 0 and 100. Finally, the *auditory evoked potential (AEP) monitor* calculates an index (ARX AEP index; AAI), based upon changes in amplitude and latencies of the middle latency auditory evoked potentials (MLEAPs).

The BIS is the most extensively studied of these monitors and has been used as an indicator of adequate anesthesia and complete memory impairment. Early studies of the other monitoring systems suggest that they may have a similar ability to the BIS in predicting depth of anesthesia. The existence of EEG-derived monitors has been well publicized in the lay press, usually in the context of discussion about intraoperative awareness. However, it is important to appreciate that no EEG-based device has been shown to measure depth of anesthesia across all possible anesthetic combinations and pathological brain states, and the American Society of Anesthesiologists has not adopted any EEG-derived monitor of anesthesia depth as a standard.

Severe impairment of explicit memory usually occurs even at relative high BIS values (85–90), in the absence of a marked neurohormonal stress response which is able to modulate memory formation. Some weak, contextually poor explicit memory may be formed at values above 60, although it is difficult to distinguish this from implicit memory behavior. Most studies show no memory at BIS levels of 40–60. One notable study with trauma patients suggested that some implicit memory formation can occur at these lower values, but it is not clear how fluctuations in hypnotic state or the modulatory actions of the hormonal stress response may have contributed to that finding. The role of EEG monitoring in reliably predicting implicit memory has not been defined.

MEMORY FORMATION DURING ANESTHESIA (MFDA)

Some form of unconscious memory formation can – but does not necessarily – occur during adequate general anesthesia. There are a number of difficulties in characterizing MFDA, primarily the uncertainty of what exact form of memory is involved. One possibility is that MFDA is a weak (i.e. contextually poor) form of explicit memory. Another is that it represents a preservation of some of the implicit memory mechanisms seen in the normal waking state. Inherently, many studies make this assumption by using experimental paradigms based on validated models for studying implicit memory in awake subjects. The most common experimental design involves priming for an auditory word list played during anesthesia. There is an inherent danger in making the assumption that MFDA *equals* classic priming, and that a failure to demonstrate classic priming indicates the absence of MFDA. There is a third, compelling possibility: that MFDA is a novel form of memory.

It is likely that some form of unconscious memory can occur during adequate general anesthesia.

There is ample evidence from both natural sleep and drug studies that cortical processing of stimuli is possible during unconsciousness. Electrophysiologic responses are well documented during sleep, including the P3 and K-complex, and similar responses have been demonstrated during drug-induced unresponsiveness. PET studies of rCBF demonstrate a continued localization of response to auditory stimuli during unresponsiveness. During sedation, this localized response appears to involve an increased area of activation relative to baseline, involving the sensory association areas surrounding the primary sensory cortex. Normally, memory formation involves widely distributed association areas, but there is evidence that perisensory cortical areas are able to adopt some rudimentary memory function when extended cortical networks are not activated. This is supported by molecular studies, which have demonstrated protein induction and LTP in perisensory areas. Thus, one theoretically possible explanation for MFDA is that neuronal activation still present in primary sensory regions may be able to sustain higher orders of cognitive activity, sufficient to allow the

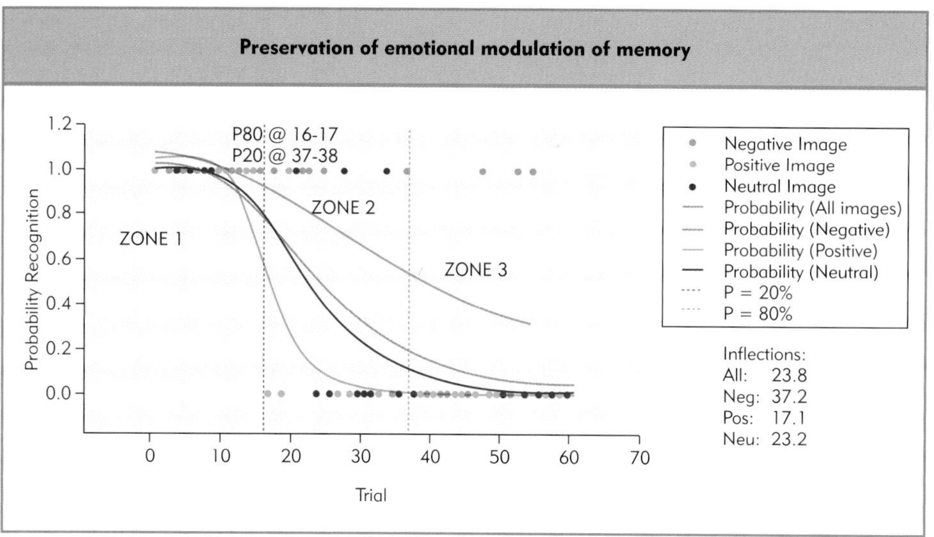

Figure 29.7 The preservation of emotional modulation of memory during subanesthetic doses of GABAergic drugs. Subjects are shown a random sequence of negative (red), positive (green), and neutral (blue) pictures, with an interval of 10 seconds (shown on the *x*-axis). During this sequence, drug concentration at the effect site (brain) is increasing. As the sequence progresses, subjects have reduced memory for all pictures as the drugs reach concentrations sufficient to cause amnesia. However, memory impairment for the negative images is substantially less than that for the positive images.

formation of a weak memory trace, which is relatively advantaged as there is little or no cognitive competition at the time.

Another attractive hypothesis is that the amygdala may be centrally involved in MFDA. The amygdala complex is an important modulator of memory encoding, storage, and consolidation processes, and its modulatory role is enabled via the action of stress hormones such as epinephrine and cortisol released in response to surgery. FNI studies suggest that the amygdala, like other MTL structures, is relatively resistant to the effects of GABAergic drugs compared to other neocortical regions. This might be explained by the fact that limbic structures in humans have a unique distribution of $GABA_A$ receptor subtypes, most notably a concentration of the α_5 subunit. At the same time, animal studies suggest that the basolateral amygdala complex (BLAC) may be involved in mediating the amnesic effects of GABAergic drugs: removal of the BLAC completely blocks the amnesic effects of propofol and diazepam.

The amygdala is critical in implicit memory behaviors involving emotional, and in particular fear, conditioning. These amygdala functions are robust: amnesiacs demonstrate intact emotive modulation despite profound explicit memory deficits, and some form of memory processing may occur in the amygdala even during normal REM sleep. Emotional modulation of memory – a key behavioral marker of amygdala activity – continues during subanesthetic concentrations of GABAergic drugs, even when explicit memory is considerably attenuated (Fig. 29.7). An amygdala-based theory for MFDA suggests that in the setting of the stress response to surgery the amygdala continues to exert modulatory effects on memory mechanisms, but with a poorly defined or absent cognitive associate. Several poorly understood perianesthetic phenomena – postanesthesia nightmares, dysphoria, depression, anxiety, perianesthesia disinhibition, emotional lability, and aggression – can be hypothesized to follow from disturbances in the implicit and explicit functions of the amygdala and limbic structures.

β-adrenergic blockers have been repeatedly shown to attenuate the modulatory effects of emotive information on explicit and implicit memory behavior, and FNI studies suggest that this is mediated via attenuation of amygdala activity at the time of encoding. The α_2-adrenergic agonist dexmedetomidine may also exert similar effects on emotional memory and fear conditioning. A reduction in noradrenergic output from the locus ceruleus would be expected to attenuate amygdala-mediated modulation of memory. If β-blockers or α_2-adrenoreceptor agonists modulate MFDA, they may one day have a place in the prevention of postanesthesia psychological and visceral sequelae.

Key references

Alkire MT, Haier RJ, Fallon JH. Toward a unified theory of narcosis: Brain imaging evidence for a thalamocortical switch as the neurophysiologic basis of anesthetic-induced unconsciousness. Consciousness Cognition 2000;9:370–86.

Erk S, Kiefer M, Grothe J, Wunderlich AP, Spitzer M, Walter H. Emotional context modulates subsequent memory effect. Neuroimage 2003;18:439–47.

Ghoniem MM. Awareness during anesthesia. Anesthesiology 2000;92:597–602.

Kim JJ, Lee HJ, Han J-S, Packard MG. Amygdala is critical for stress-induced modulation of hippocampal long-term potentiation and learning. J Neurosci. 2001;21:5222–8.

Lubke G, Kerssens C, Phaf H, Sebel PS. Dependence of explicit and implicit memory on hypnotic state in trauma patients. Anesthesiology 1999;90:670–80.

Nelson LE, Lu J, Tianzhi G, Saper CB, Franks NP, Maze M. The alpha2-adrenoceptor agonist dexmedetomidine converges on an endogenous sleep-promoting pathway to exert its sedative effects. Anesthesiology 2003;98:428–36.

Steriade M. Corticothalamic resonance, states of vigilance and mentation. Neuroscience 2000;101:243–76.

Veselis RA, Reinsel RA, Feshchenko V. Drug-induced amnesia is a separate phenomenon from sedation: electrophysiologic evidence. Anesthesiology 2001;95:896–907.

Veselis RA, Reinsel RA, Feshchenko V, Dnistrian AM. A neuroanatomical construct for the amnesic effects of propofol. Anesthesiology 2002;97:329–37

Further reading

John ER. A field theory of consciousness. Consciousness Cognition 2001;10:184–213.

Llinas R, Ribary U. Consciousness and the brain. The thalamocortical dialogue in health and disease. Ann NY Acad Sci. 2001;929:166–75.

McGaugh JL. Memory – a century of consolidation. Science 2000;287:248–51.

Roberts AC, Glanzman DL. Learning in *Aplysia*: looking at synaptic plasticity from both sides. Trends Neurosci. 2003;26:662–70.

Simons JS, Spiers HJ. Prefrontal and medial temporal lobe interactions in long-term memory. Nature Rev Neurosci. 2003;4:637–48.

Zeman A. Consciousness. Brain 2001;24:1263–89.

Chapter 30

Sleep and anesthesia

Ralph Lydic and Helen A Baghdoyan

TOPICS COVERED IN THIS CHAPTER

- **Sleep as a public health concern**
- **Sleep deprivation and restriction**
- **Neurobiology of sleep and anesthesia**
  - Pontine reticular formation and REM sleep
  - Pontine reticular formation and state-dependent alterations in breathing
  - Modulation of cortical excitability by muscarinic cholinergic receptors

States of anesthesia and sleep are overtly similar functions of the nervous system, yet there is only a rudimentary dialog between sleep research and anesthesia research. Before 1998, anesthesia textbooks contained no detailed consideration of natural sleep. This chapter addresses the need for a dialog between these fields by reviewing the relevance of sleep for anesthesiology. Sleep neurobiology and sleep disorders medicine are recent developments. The chapter begins with a brief historical perspective on the awareness of sleep as a public health concern, followed by consideration of the negative impact of sleep deprivation and restriction. Substantial data support our working hypothesis that brain regions generating sleep are preferentially involved in regulating anesthetic states. Therefore, the chapter concludes with evidence that advances in sleep neurobiology may help elucidate the mechanisms of anesthetic action.

SLEEP AS A PUBLIC HEALTH CONCERN

The United States National Commission on Sleep Disorders Research found in 1990 that 40 million Americans had sleep disorders, that sleep deprivation was a significant health problem, that the cardiovascular consequences of obstructive sleep apnea accounted for approximately 38 000 deaths per year, and that the direct costs of sleep disorders and sleep deprivation were as high as $15.9 billion. Despite these statistics, sleep education in medical schools was almost nonexistent, and few young physicians and scientists were aspiring to careers in sleep disorders medicine or sleep research. In 1993, the Commission published its findings and identified three major problems. Subsequent sections of this chapter review data showing how each of these problem areas is especially relevant for anesthesiology.

The first problem addressed by the Commission was the large number of patients with undiagnosed and untreated sleep disorders. By 2010, sleep difficulty was estimated to affect 79 million Americans, and 40 million would suffer from debilitating excessive daytime sleepiness. For a more complete history of sleep disorders medicine see Dement's chapter in *Principles and practice of sleep medicine.*

Many patients have undiagnosed and untreated sleep disorders.

For the anesthesiologist, these patients present a special set of medical management problems. Anesthesia patients with obstructive sleep apnea (OSA) require special management of the upper airway, yet most such patients present for anesthesia with their OSA undiagnosed and untreated. The second major problem was that sleep deprivation is a pervasive societal problem. Data now make it clear that sleep deprivation is a risk factor for tasks that require vigilance. The final problem identified was inadequate sleep education and research.

In addition to the upper airway management issues associated with sleep apnea, another factor promoting an interest in sleep by anesthesiologists is the increasing use of sedation analgesia. During conscious sedation patients commonly exhibit traits characteristic of wakefulness, such as the ability to follow verbal commands, combined with traits characteristic of sleep. These sleep-like traits include diminished sensory processing, impaired judgment, gaps in recall, and significant alterations in autonomic control. The complex and dissociated states characteristic of conscious sedation differ from states of general anesthesia. Successful monitoring of patients undergoing conscious sedation could be facilitated by an understanding of sleep-like states.

SLEEP DEPRIVATION AND RESTRICTION

Workloads and call schedules make sleep restriction and sleep deprivation of interest to anesthesiologists. These concerns were reinforced with the 1999 publication by the US Institute of

Medicine which attributed as many as 98 000 deaths per year to medical errors. Recent research by Howard et al. shows that decrements in cognitive and psychomotor performance associated with prolonged intervals of work are relevant for anesthesiology, and convincing data demonstrate the negative effects of sleep loss. Chronically restricting sleep to 6 hours or less per night for 14 days causes progressive decrements in psychomotor vigilance, working memory, and cognitive performance equivalent to deficits in performance caused by two nights of total sleep deprivation. Subjects were not aware of their cognitive deficits. An important point to emerge from these data is a lack of support for the view that humans adapt to chronic sleep restriction.

Sleep restriction causes progressive decrements in psychomotor vigilance, working memory, and cognitive performance equivalent to ethanol intoxication.

The safe and effective delivery of anesthesia is more complex than operating a motor vehicle, and many lines of evidence emphasize the relationship between fatigue and motor vehicle accidents. The National Highway Traffic Safety Administration estimates that 100 000 police-reported crashes each year are the direct result of driver fatigue. The loss of even 1 hour of sleep associated with the shift to daylight saving time increases the number of traffic accidents. Post night-call residents and staff have an increased probability of falling asleep while driving. Sleep deprivation causes intervals of sleep that invade ongoing wakefulness, and these micro-sleeps can occur without the awareness of the sleep-deprived person. Bonnet's data show that one must be asleep for at least 2 minutes in order to know that one has slept. A study by Marcus and Loughlin found that 17% of 58 anesthesia residents had motor vehicle accidents, and 72% had near-miss accidents; this problem reflects lack of sleep, and is not unique to anesthesiology. The US Accreditation Council for Graduate Medical Education (ACGME), which functions to accredit the nearly 8000 postgraduate training programs, has begun to address the problem of fatigue-related accidents by issuing recommendations and regulations regarding resident work hours. Residents are now limited to an 80-hour maximum working week, must have at least one 24-hour period off per week, and must work no more than every third night on call. In contrast to the hours-of-service plan used by the Federal Motor Carrier Safety Administration, the ACGME guide does not incorporate circadian data documenting performance decrements that peak at predictable times in each 24-hour day.

For a discipline devoted to the precept of 'do no harm' it is relevant that the risk of driving when sleepy endangers others. This danger is illustrated by the 2001 Selby road/rail accident in the UK. This accident was caused by a car driver who fell asleep, lost control of his vehicle, and caused a passenger train accident. Ten people died and more than 70 required hospital treatment. The car driver survived and was sentenced to 5 years in prison. The sentence was upheld by a 2003 appeal ruling that the Selby crash victims were 'unlawfully killed'. Compensation claims against the driver amounted to more than £20 million.

In the US as well, the societal and medicolegal perspective on driving while sleepy are changing. In 2003 the New Jersey State Senate passed into law a bill that included 'fatigued driving' as part of the vehicular homicide statute. Fatigue is operationally defined as being without sleep for a period in excess of 24 consecutive hours. Hospital administrators and residency program directors will want to know their level of risk and responsibility for fatigue management. Sleep loss similar to that experienced by medical residents and on-call staff causes performance decrements equivalent to decrements associated with blood ethanol levels that indicate intoxication. Risk assessment should incorporate the psychophysical data showing similarities between neurobehavioral impairments caused by ethanol and impairment caused by sleep deprivation.

NEUROBIOLOGY OF SLEEP AND ANESTHESIA

Sleep is not merely the loss of wakefulness. Sleep is actively generated by the CNS and involves two interacting processes. The first is mediated by the suprachiasmatic nuclei (SCN). The SCN are bilateral hypothalamic structures that regulate the timing of sleep to occur at a specific phase during the 24-hour day. All physiological and behavioral variables exhibit significant circadian (24-hour) rhythms. The disruption of sleep referred to as 'jet lag' provides an example of the circadian control of sleep. Individuals with jet lag experience an inability to sleep at their habitual clock time and a profound sleepiness at clock times when they would normally feel alert. The second process regulating sleep occurs at the level of the brainstem, and is manifest as the periodic oscillation between the rapid eye movement (REM) phase and the nonREM (NREM) phases of sleep. An activated electroencephalogram (EEG), somatic motor atonia (EMG), rapid eye movements, autonomic dysregulation, and the human experience of dreaming are features of REM sleep. Nomenclature is not uniform and REM sleep is synonymous with paradoxical sleep or active sleep. During a sleep interval there is a periodic oscillation between the REM and NREM phases. The NREM/REM cycle occurs as an ultradian (<24-hour) rhythm. The periodicity of the NREM/REM cycle is species specific, and in humans averages about 90 minutes. These hypothalamic (circadian) and brainstem (ultradian) sleep-generating systems interact in a poorly understood manner. Electrophysiological recordings of SCN neurons demonstrate enhanced cell firing during the REM phase of sleep and diminished SCN discharge during the NREM stage. In humans, the interaction between circadian and ultradian sleep rhythms, together with environmental task load, accounts for variations in normal sleep requirement. Sleep need is highly variable, but normal sleep requirements are about 8 hours (see Kryger et al. for an excellent review).

Efforts to elucidate the cellular and molecular mechanisms regulating sleep are directly analogous to the search for mechanisms of anesthetic action. Table 30.1 outlines some of the similarities and differences between states of sleep and anesthesia.

Few studies have characterized the effects of anesthesia on sleep. The ability to establish a direct, causal link between anesthetic drugs and alterations in sleep is complicated by potentially confounding variables. Pain is a complex psychophysiological experience and there is a high variability in nociceptive stimulation associated with different surgical procedures. Potential confounds also include coexisting disease or trauma, and the polypharmacy associated with anesthesia care. Research into the effect of anesthesia on sleep also must incorporate the fact that

Table 30.1 Comparison of anesthesia and sleep onset, maintenance, and offset (From Lydic, R. Pain: A bridge linking anesthesiology and sleep research. Sleep 24: 10-12, 2001.)

	Anesthesia	Sleep
Onset	Drug-induced Not significantly altered by previous sleep or circadian history Failure to initiate is nonexistent Not significantly altered by environmental factors, such as caffeine intake, environmental temperature, noise, and light	Endogenously generated Significantly influenced by circadian phase and duration of prior wakefulness Failure to initiate is a recognized pathology Environmental factors significantly modulate sleep onset
Maintenance	Duration is dependent on agent dose and independent of previous wakefulness Without surgical stimulation, depth of anesthesia can be held constant for long periods of time Failure to maintain is nonexistent Environmental factors (noise, light, temperature) do not alter anesthetic maintenance; sensory input blocked	Duration is a function of prior wakefulness and circadian factors Rhythmically oscillates between stages 1, 2, 3, 4, and REM sleep Failure to maintain is a recognized pathology Environmental cues easily disrupt sleep maintenance; sensory input blunted and/or enhanced
Offset	Resumption of normal wakefulness is slow (hours to days) Duration of anesthesia and elimination of agent or active metabolites determines timing of wakefulness Reanesthetizing patient easily achieved immediately following offset Offset accompanied by agent side effects (nausea, vomiting, emergence delirium)	Resumption of normal wakefulness is rapid (minutes) Timing of waking is modulated by sleep duration and circadian rhythm Immediate initiation of second sleep interval difficult following offset of normal night of sleep Offset normally associated with reports of feeling rested and refreshed

anesthesia is a state that can be produced by different classes of molecules (Chapter 24). Finally, few anesthesiology studies have used objective measures of sleep in relation to sedative and anesthetic drugs.

An objective measure of sleepiness is the multiple sleep latency test (MSLT). Individuals undergoing an MSLT are given four to six nap opportunities throughout the day and instructed to allow themselves to sleep. During the test objective measures of EEG and behavior are recorded. The drive to sleep, or sleepiness, is evaluated relative to normative data indicating that the average sleep latency for a healthy, non sleep-deprived adult in the United States is about 11 minutes. Lichtor and colleagues used the MSLT to evaluate sleep tendency as a measure of recovery after drugs used for ambulatory surgery, and found that sleepiness as measured with the MSLT persisted for up to 8 hours after sedation. Efforts to understand the effects on sleep of drugs used in anesthesia also must elucidate how different molecules alter the specific stages of sleep. Preclinical and clinical data concur that opioids obtund wakefulness but inhibit the REM phase of sleep, whereas γ-aminobutyric acid ($GABA_A$) agonists promote NREM sleep but suppress REM sleep. Studies using systemic drug delivery have the advantage of emulating clinical practice, but the disadvantage of nonspecific agonist actions throughout the nervous system. Therefore, studies seeking to elucidate the cellular and molecular basis for sleep and anesthesia focus on specific brain regions. For example, the hypothalamic tuberomammillary nucleus (TMN), thought to promote wakefulness, plays a role in the sedative response to $GABA_A$ agonists. Administration of a $GABA_A$ antagonist into the TMN decreased the sedative response to propofol and pentobarbital. The remainder of this chapter highlights animal models and regions of the pontine brainstem that show particular promise for identifying mechanisms that generate states of sleep and anesthesia.

Depressed breathing and decreased cortical excitability are characteristic of both NREM sleep and general anesthesia.

Brain mechanisms that generate anesthesia-induced physiological traits also generate traits characteristic of natural sleep (e.g. depressed breathing and decreased cortical excitability). Advances in mouse genetics and the availability of a draft sequence of the mouse genome have encouraged the National Heart, Lung, and Blood Institute to develop a major program to support the phenotyping of sleep using mice (http://nhlbi.nih.gov/resources/pga/index.htm). The mouse may be a particularly good animal model for studies aiming to identify mechanisms regulating states of sleep and anesthesia, and state-dependent alterations in autonomic control. Koblin and colleagues pioneered the selective breeding of mice for anesthetic resistance and susceptibility. The mouse genome has a 99% homology with the human genome, therefore these preclinical studies suggest that different responses to anesthesia by patients result, in part, from genetic differences in the central nervous system. This concept is the basis for pharmacogenetics and has enormous potential for advancing anesthesiology (Chapter 5). Continuation of this line of research has provided support for the feasibility of identifying the multiple genes and alleles that contribute to the variability in anesthetic potency and perioperative outcome. Available evidence from mice suggests that sleep may be modulated by relatively few genes. Genetic regulation of the complex trait of sleep is likely to involve alterations in pathways contributing to central cholinergic neurotransmission. Acetylcholine (ACh) modulates behavioral and EEG arousal. The data reviewed below provide an essential first step using mice to characterize the cholinergic regulation of sleep and anesthesia. The results support the view that ACh is a lower-level phenotype regulating arousal.

Pontine reticular formation and REM sleep

Human data since the 1970s consistently show that the onset of REM sleep is significantly delayed by intramuscular injection of scopolamine, and significantly enhanced by intravenous administration of cholinergic agonists or acetylcholinesterase inhibitors. Microinjection of cholinomimetics into a region of the pontine reticular formation causes a REM sleep-like state that is site dependent, concentration dependent, and blocked by atropine. Microdialysis data reveal that ACh release in this same region of the pontine reticular formation is significantly increased during REM sleep and during the REM sleep-like state caused by pontine microinjection of cholinomimetics. These data encouraged efforts to determine whether the cholinergic model of REM sleep could be successfully developed in mice.

The states of sleep and wakefulness recorded in B6 mice reveal excellent homology with sleep recorded in humans. This homology is consistent with convergent evolutionary perspectives and with the genetic homology between human and mouse. Enhancing cholinergic neurotransmission increases human REM sleep, and microinjection of neostigmine into the pontine reticular formation of B6 mice causes a REM sleep-like state (Fig. 30.1). Because neostigmine prevents the degradation of ACh, these data support the interpretation that ACh in the pontine

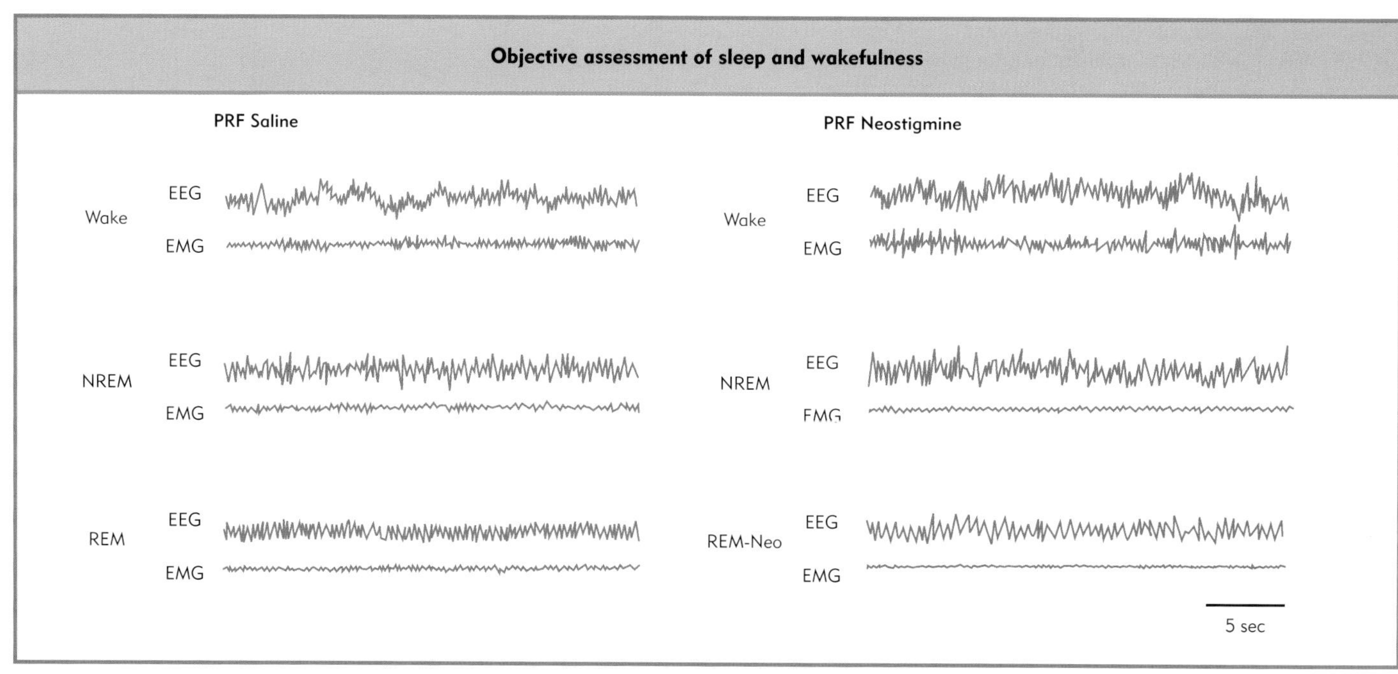

Figure 30.1 Objective assessment of sleep and wakefulness in C57BL/6J (B6) mice. Electroencephalogram (EEG) and electromyogram (EMG) recordings from a mouse with implanted electrodes used to objectively score states of wakefulness (Wake), nonrapid eye movement (NREM) sleep, and rapid eye movement (REM) sleep. During wakefulness, the EEG is characterized by a low-amplitude mixed-frequency pattern. Following microinjection of saline into the pontine reticular formation (PRF) the EMG recordings during wakefulness show a normally high amplitude, indicating motor tone and movement. During NREM sleep, EEG amplitude is high and EEG frequency is slow, relative to wakefulness. EMG activity is markedly decreased, indicating the absence of movement. The REM phase of sleep is characterized by a low-amplitude rhythmic EEG signal and a low-amplitude EMG signal. These patterns of EEG and EMG activity are similar to those recorded in humans. The frame on the right shows similar recordings from the same mouse after microinjecting neostigmine into the PRF. Drug delivery causes a REM sleep-like state. These data are consistent with the view that endogenous ACh in the PRF is involved in REM sleep generation. (Coleman, C.G., R. Lydic, H.A. Baghdoyan. M2 muscarinic receptors in pontine reticular formation of C57BL/6J mouse contribute to REM sleep generation. Neuroscience 2004;126(4):821-30.)

reticular formation has a causal role in REM sleep generation. Additional data show that the REM sleep-like state caused by pontine microinjection of neostigmine is concentration dependent and blocked by atropine. These pharmacologic data are consistent with the conclusion that the REM sleep-like state in B6 mice is mediated by muscarinic cholinergic receptors. This conclusion is further supported by the finding that the cholinergic agonist carbachol causes a concentration-dependent atropine-sensitive activation of guanine nucleotide-binding proteins (G proteins) in the pontine reticular formation of B6 mice (Fig. 30.2). G proteins were significantly activated in the same regions of the pontine reticular formation where microinjection of neostigmine causes a REM sleep-like state.

Acetylcholine in the pontine reticular formation plays a causal role in REM sleep generation.

Pontine reticular formation and state-dependent alterations in breathing

The depression of breathing asssociated with sleep and anesthesia is clinically relevant for both anesthesiology and sleep disorders medicine. The mechanisms causing state-dependent respiratory depression remain poorly understood. This gap in our knowledge encourages the development of nonhuman animal models that can help elucidate the mechanisms by which sleep and anesthesia depress breathing. Breathing during the cholinergically induced REM sleep-like state is characterized by decreased rate, prolonged periods of apnea, and periodic patterns (Figs 30.3 and 30.4). The brain has no pain receptors, and one can make microinjections into specific brain regions of intact unanesthetized mice (Fig. 30.3a) and quantify the effect on sleep and breathing. For studies of breathing, mice are placed in a whole-body plethysmograph after drugs have been delivered to the pons. Typical recordings of breathing after pontine injection of saline (Fig. 30.3b) can be contrasted with altered breathing caused by pontine injection of neostigmine (Fig. 30.3b,c). Periodic breathing is a characteristic of both obstructive and central sleep apnea, and is thought to reflect instability of the central respiratory generating network. The observations of respiratory pauses (Fig. 30.3d) and periodic breathing (Fig. 30.3e) during neostigmine-induced REM sleep demonstrate causal modulation by pontine cholinergic neurotransmission. These changes in breathing (Fig. 30.4) are evoked from a region of the pons that contains no major clusters of respiratory neurons. This means that pontine neurons regulating arousal can significantly alter networks devoted to respiratory rhythm generation.

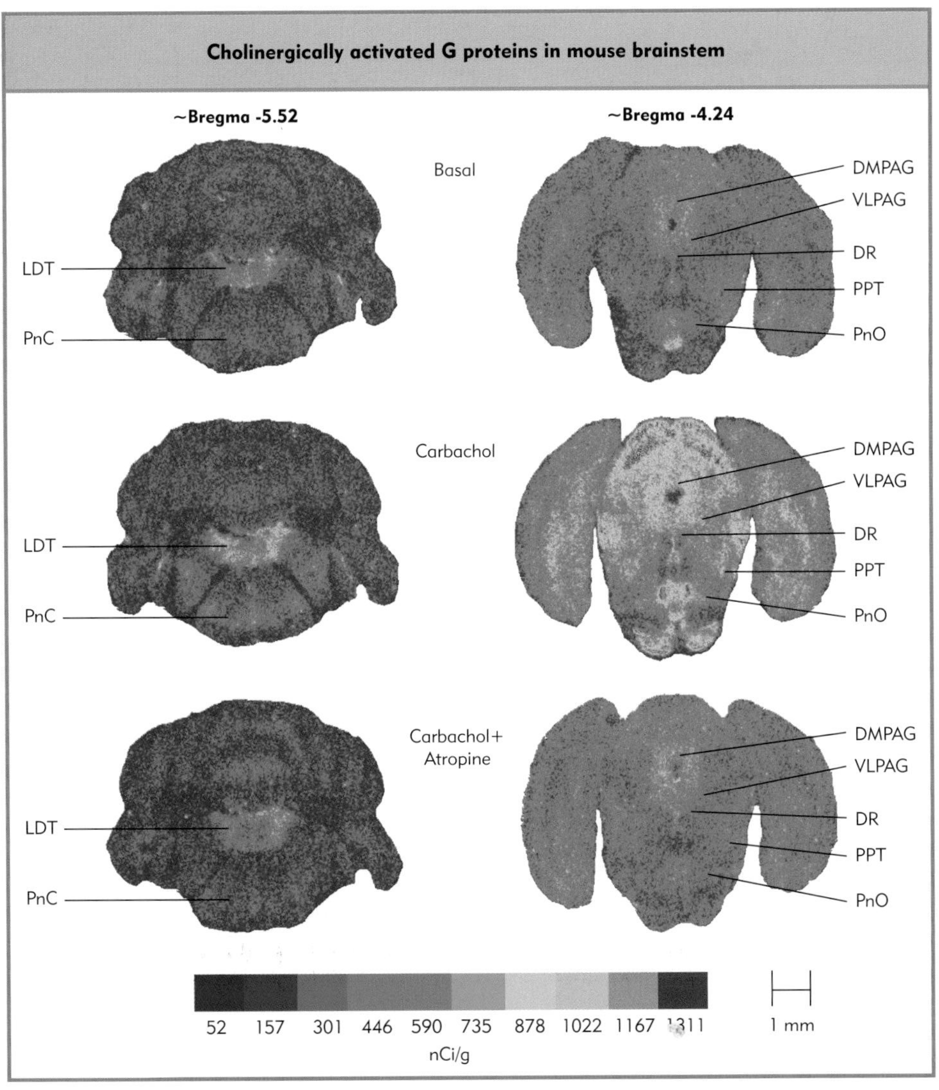

Figure 30.2 Cholinergically activated G proteins in mouse brainstem. In vitro [^{35}S]guanylyl-5′-*O*-(γ-thio)-triphosphate ([^{35}S]GTPγS) autoradiography permits visualization and quantification of G proteins that have been activated as a result of an agonist binding to its receptor. These coronal images from mouse brainstem show total [^{35}S]GTPγS binding for two brainstem levels (columns) and three in vitro treatment conditions (rows). Treatments included basal (no agonist) to provide control levels of G-protein activation (top), the cholinergic agonist carbachol (1 mM) to show activated G proteins (middle), and carbachol (1 mM) plus the muscarinic receptor antagonist atropine (0.1 mM) to block carbachol-induced G-protein activation (bottom). Note that the sections treated simultaneously with carbachol and atropine showed levels of G-protein activation similar to basal, indicating that the carbachol-stimulated increases in [^{35}S]GTPγS binding resulted from the activation of muscarinic cholinergic receptors. Nuclei known to play functional roles in arousal and/or nociception are labeled as follows: DMPAG, dorsomedial periaqueductal gray; DR, dorsal raphe nucleus; LDT, laterodorsal tegmental nucleus; PnC, pontine reticular nucleus, caudal part; PnO, pontine reticular nucleus, oral part; PPT, pedunculopontine tegmental nucleus; VLPAG, ventrolateral periaqueductal gray. (Reprinted with permission from DeMarco GJ, Baghdoyan HA, Lydic R. J Comp Neurol 2003;457:175-184. Copyright © 2003 Wiley-Liss, Inc., a subsidiary of John Wiley & Sons, Inc.)

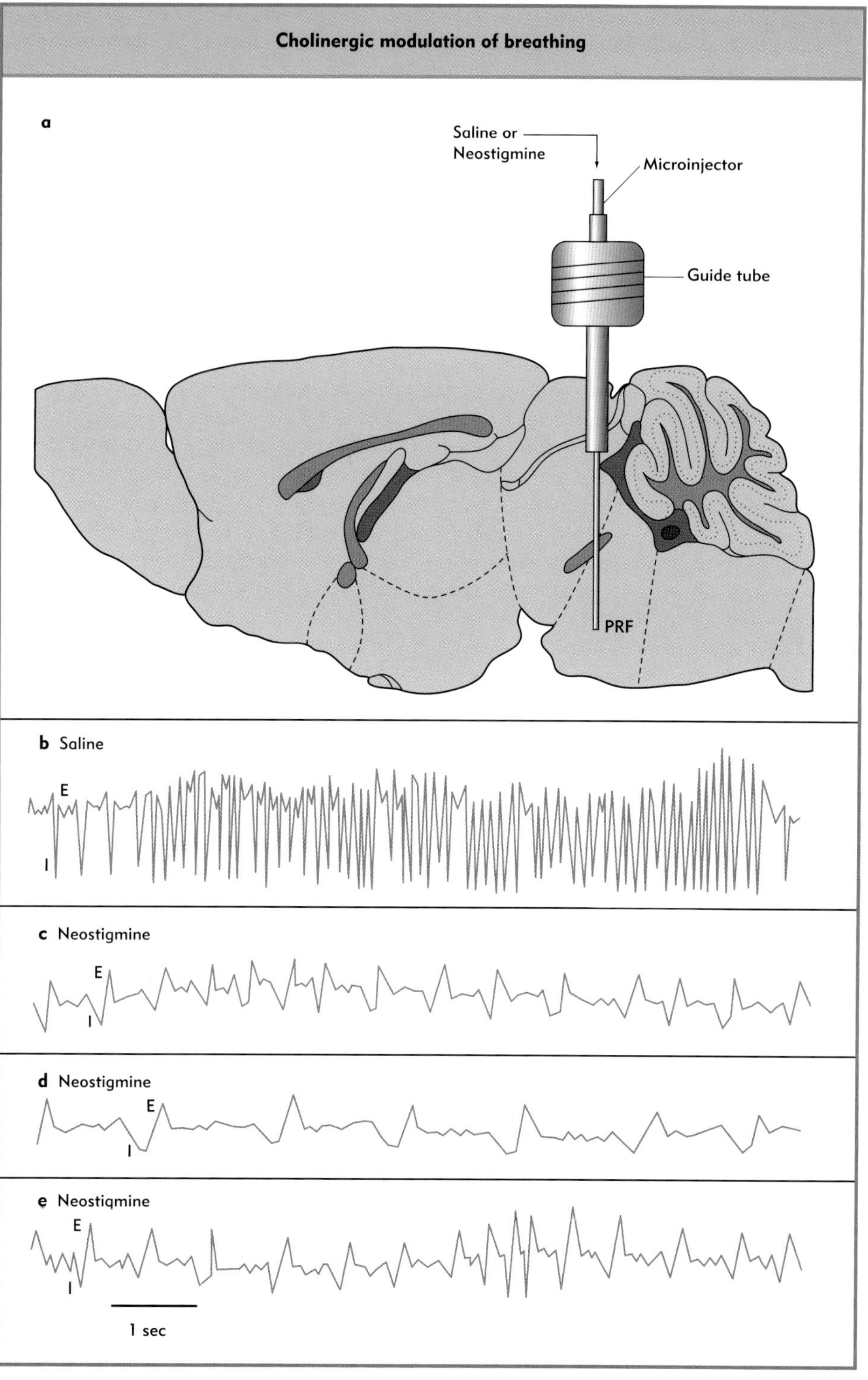

Figure 30.3 Drug delivery by intracerebral microinjection and plethysmographic measures of breathing recorded from C57BL/6J mice. (a) Sagittal view of mouse brain illustrating stereotaxic placement of a guide tube for microinjection into the pontine reticular formation (PRF). After drug delivery to the PRF, the mouse is placed in a whole-body plethysmograph for quantitative studies of breathing. (b–e) Each of the four frames shows a 10-second recording of breathing. Respiratory traces are labeled to indicate inspiration (I) and expiration (E). (b) The normally rapid rate of breathing during quiet wakefulness is shown following a control microinjection of saline (50 nL) into the PRF. (c–e) The reduction in respiratory rate and irregular pattern of breathing during the REM sleep-like state produced by microinjecting neostigmine (0.133 μg/50 nL, 8.8 mM) into the PRF. Tracings b–e were recorded within a 5-minute period. Note the neostigmine-induced decreased rate of breathing (c), periods of apnea (d), and periodic breathing (e). (Reprinted with permission from Lydic R, Douglas CL, Baghdoyan HA. Microinjection of neostigmine into the pontine reticular formation of C57BL/6J mice enhances rapid eye movement sleep and depresses breathing. Sleep 2002;25:835–41.)

Pontine neurons regulating arousal modulate respiratory rhythm-generating networks.

Of greater concern for the anesthesiologist is airway management during induction and extubation. Data from cats and rats show that microinjection of cholinomimetics into the pontine reticular formation also causes significant hypotonia of upper airway muscles. Owing to the technical limitations associated with the small size of mice (20–25 g), changes in mouse upper airway muscles as a function of sleep and anesthesia have not yet been measured. Breathing and the ventilatory response to hypercapnia are genetically determined phenotypes. Thus, mouse models show great promise for ongoing and future efforts to understand the mechanisms that cause breathing to be depressed during states of sleep and anesthesia.

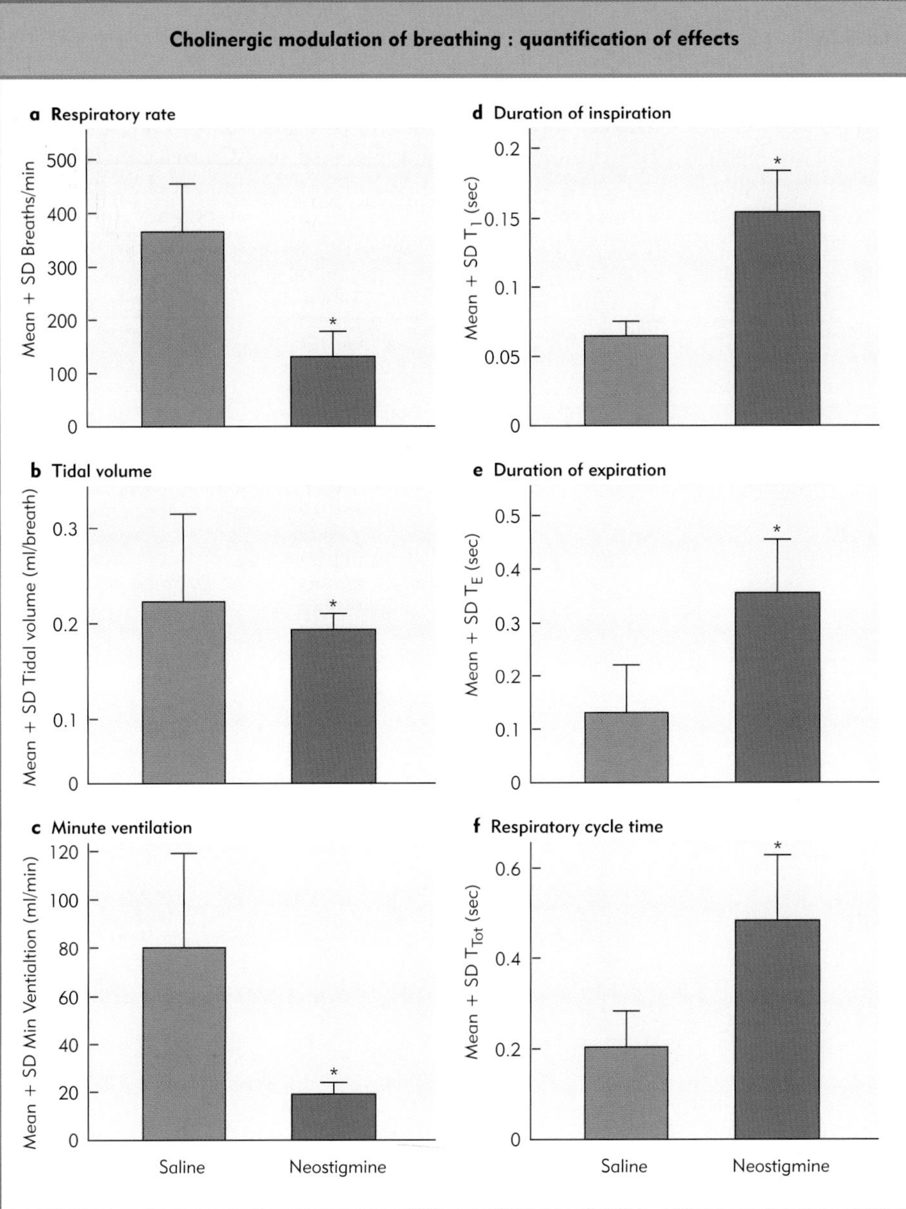

Figure 30.4 Quantification of breathing after pontine reticular formation microinjection of saline or neostigmine. A, respiratory rate; B, tidal volume; C, minute ventilation; D, duration of inspiration (Ti); E, expiration (Te); and F, total respiratory cycle time (Ttot). The neostigmine-induced REM sleep-like state provides a model of respiratory depression characterized by a significantly decreased rate of breathing (A), decreased minute ventilation (C), and increased respiratory cycle (F) time due to increased inspiratory (D) and expiratory (E) time. *$p<0.05$. (Reprinted with permission from Lydic R, Douglas CL, Baghdoyan HA. Microinjection of neostigmine into the pontine reticular formation of C57BL/6J mice enhances rapid eye movement sleep and depresses breathing. Sleep 2002;25:835–41.)

Modulation of cortical excitability by muscarinic cholinergic receptors

EEG recordings from mice (see Fig. 30.1) are homologous to human EEG recordings during sleep and wakefulness. States of wakefulness and REM sleep are characterized by low-amplitude fast waves referred to as an activated EEG. In contrast, during states of light anesthesia and NREM sleep the EEG has a slower frequency and larger amplitude. When combined with behavioral and autonomic monitoring, the EEG provides a tool for diagnosing seizure disorders, for hypnotic/sedative drug development, and for objectively quantifying states of sleep and levels of light anesthesia.

EEG characteristics of NREM sleep include increased activity in the 0.5–4 Hz range called δ waves, and 7–14 Hz waves referred to as sleep spindles. Responsiveness to external stimulation decreases as EEG δ power increases. The EEG correlates of sleep are actively generated by the brain. Synaptic hyperpolarization of thalamocortical neurons generates EEG spindles and effectively disconnects the cortex from afferent input, thus helping to maintain states of sleep or anesthesia. Cortical levels of ACh are positively correlated with an activated EEG. These data fit well with the concept that cortical activation is caused by ascending projections from the pontine reticular formation. The direct relevance of these concepts for efforts to understand sleep and anesthesia were emphasized by the findings that volatile anesthetics diminish behavioral arousal and deactivate the cortical EEG, that ACh excites cortical neurons, and that brainstem cholinergic input to the thalamus blocks EEG spindle generation.

The EEG correlates of sleep are actively generated.

Recent studies provide insight into the pre- and postsynaptic muscarinic cholinergic receptors through which ACh causes cortical activation. Such studies must confront the complexity of five different muscarinic receptor subtypes (M1–M5). Neuropharmacological studies of the relationship between ACh and the EEG are also limited by a lack of ligands that are highly selective for any single muscarinic receptor subtype. The studies described below focus on cholinergic regulation of the prefrontal cortex, because prefrontal cortex is especially vulnerable to anesthesia and to sleep deprivation. Functions of the prefrontal cortex that are particularly relevant for sleep and anesthesia include autonomic control, regulation of attention and arousal, and consolidation of working memory. Evidence reviewed below supports muscarinic receptor regulation of cortical excitability.

Acetylcholine release in the prefrontal cortex is modulated by muscarinic autoreceptors of the M2 subtype. Microdialysis delivery of scopolamine to the prefrontal cortex causes a concentration-dependent increase in ACh release, suggesting that prefrontal cortical ACh release is modulated by muscarinic autoreceptors (Fig. 30.5). The order of potency to cause an increase in ACh release by different muscarinic receptor antagonists was scopolamine = AF – DX 116>pirenzepine. Based on the differential relative selectivities of these antagonists for the five muscarinic receptor subtypes, the results support the con-

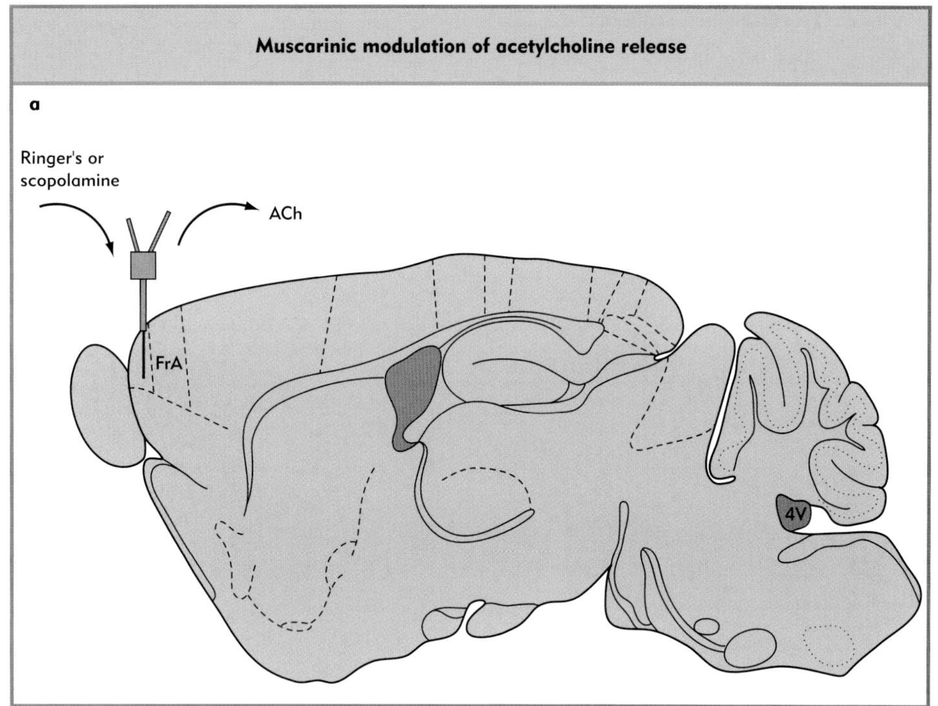

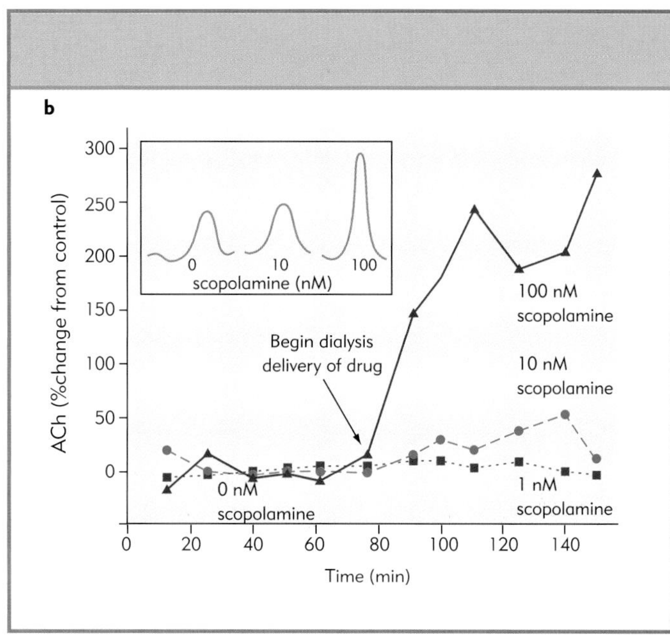

Figure 30.5 Release of acetylcholine (ACh) in the prefrontal cortex of C57BL/6J mice is modulated by muscarinic autoreceptors. (a) Sagittal schematic view of mouse brain showing a microdialysis probe in the prefrontal cortex (FrA). The probe is dialyzed with Ringer's solution (control) followed by Ringer's containing drug (scopolamine) and endogenous ACh is measured. (b) Plot of ACh release in prefrontal cortex measured as a function of time (abscissa) during dialysis delivery of scopolamine. The inset shows chromatographic peaks corresponding to ACh. The left peak represents control levels of ACh measured during dialysis with Ringer's (0 nM scopolamine). The middle peak represents ACh during dialysis delivery of 10 nM scopolamine, and the right ACh peak during dialysis with 100 nM scopolamine. Thus, scopolamine caused a concentration-dependent increase in ACh release, indicating modulation by muscarinic autoreceptors. (Reprinted with permission from Douglas CL, Baghdoyan HA, Lydic R. M2 muscarinic autoreceptors modulate acetylcholine release in prefrontal cortex of C57BL/6J mouse. J Pharmacol Exp Ther. 2001;299:960–6.)

clusion that ACh release in the prefrontal cortex is modulated by muscarinic autoreceptors of the M2 subtype.

Acetylcholine acting at postsynaptic M1 muscarinic receptors causes EEG activation. Microdialysis drug delivery can be combined with quantitative evaluation of cortical EEG and measures of ACh release to identify the postsynaptic muscarinic receptor subtype that modulates EEG activation (Fig. 30.6). Dialysis delivery of the muscarinic antagonist AF-DX 116 to the prefrontal cortex increased ACh release ipsilateral to the probe and decreased the number of halothane-induced EEG spindles contralateral to the probe. These findings from anesthetized B6 mice are relevant to sleep and anesthesia because the EEG spindles caused by halothane anesthesia are indistinguishable from those characteristic of NREM sleep. A functional consequence of increased ACh release on one side of the cortex is activation of the EEG in the contralateral cortex (Fig. 30.6). These preclinical data fit well with clinical studies showing that physostigmine reverses propofol-induced unconsciousness.

The finding of a decrease in the number of EEG spindles caused by increased ACh release stimulated efforts to identify the subtype of postsynaptic muscarinic receptor mediating the cholinergically induced EEG activation.

Acetylcholine acting at cortical postsynaptic muscarinic receptors causes EEG activation.

Comparing the potencies of different antagonists for increasing ACh release while blocking spindles (i.e. activating the EEG) revealed that the subtype of postsynaptic muscarinic receptor mediating EEG activation is M1. These conclusions are summarized by Figure 30.7, which illustrates several key points. First, cholinergic neurons in the substantia innominata region of the basal forebrain provide most of the ACh-releasing terminals to the prefrontal cortex. Second, cholinergic activation of cortical neurons on one side of cortex can activate the EEG by decreasing

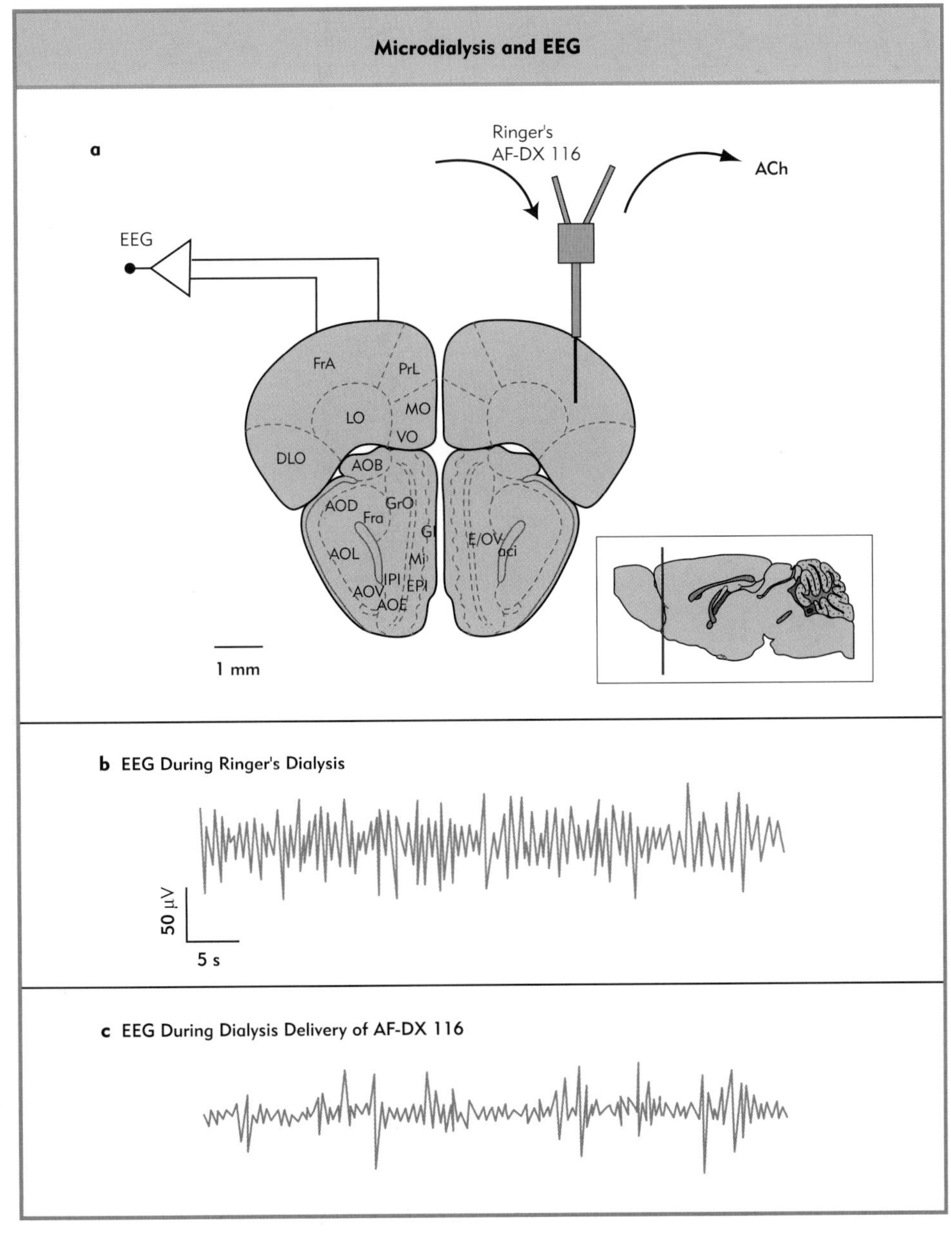

Figure 30.6 Microdialysis and EEG recorded from prefrontal cortex of C57BL/6J mouse. (a) Drawing of a coronal section from the mouse brain atlas, placement of a microdialysis probe in the prefrontal cortex (also called frontal association cortex, or FrA), and recording of the EEG from the contralateral FrA. Insert at lower right gives a midsagittal perspective of the mouse brain. The vertical line denotes the level of the coronal section along the rostral (left) to caudal (right) axis. (b) The cortical EEG recorded during halothane anesthesia is characterized by 7–14-Hz bursts, or spindles, under control conditions (dialysis with Ringer's). Halothane-induced EEG spindles are similar to those that occur spontaneously during the NREM phase of sleep in all mammals, including humans. (c) Dialysis delivery of the muscarinic receptor antagonist AF-DX 116 activates the contralateral EEG by decreasing the number of EEG spindles. (Reprinted with permission from Douglas CL, Baghdoyan HA, Lydic R. Prefrontal cortex acetylcholine release, EEG slow waves, and spindles are modulated by M2 autoreceptors in C57BL/6J mouse. J Neurophysiol. 2002;87:2817–22.)

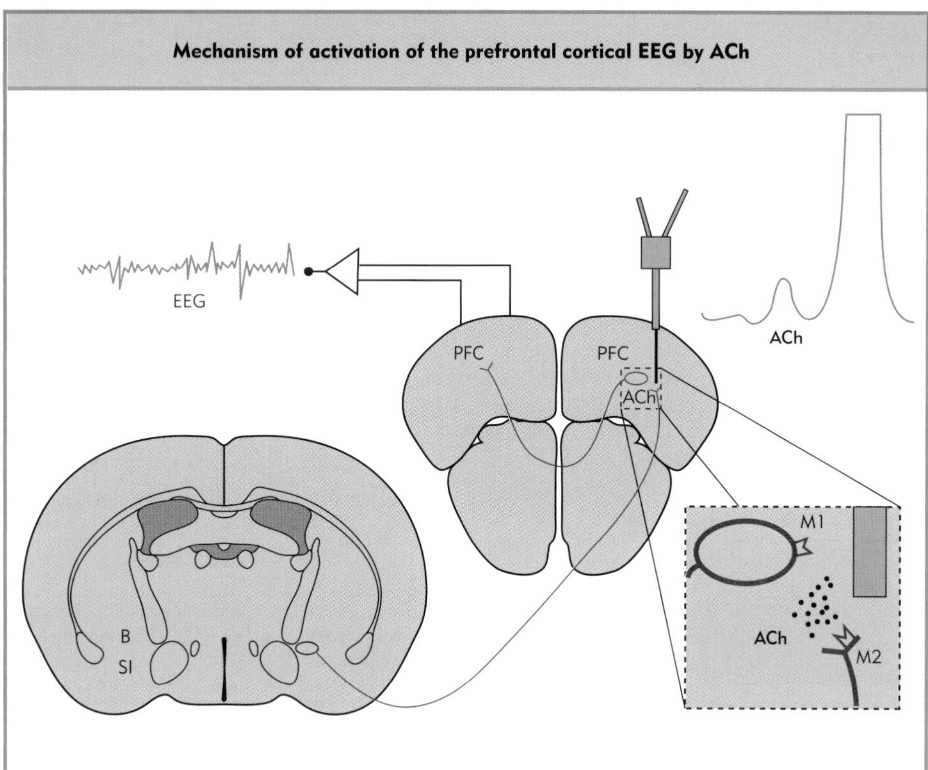

Figure 30.7 Mechanism for activation of the prefrontal cortical EEG by ACh. Cortically projecting neurons of the substantia innominata (SI) and basal nucleus of Meynert (B) are the main source of ACh released in the cortex. Release of ACh in the prefrontal cortex is modulated by M2 autoreceptors (inset) residing on terminals originating from the substantia innominata and the basal nucleus of Meynert. Increased ACh in one prefrontal cortex (PFC) causes EEG activation in the contralateral PFC. Thus one functional consequence of increasing ipsilateral ACh release in the PFC is activation of the contralateral EEG via postsynaptic M1 receptors (inset). (Reprinted with permission from Douglas CL, Baghdoyan HA, Lydic R. Postsynaptic muscarinic M1 receptors activate prefrontal cortical EEG of C57BL/6J mouse. J Neurophysiol. 2002;88:3003–9.)

EEG spindles recorded from the contralateral cortex. Third, the inset of Figure 30.7 illustrates presynaptic localization of M2 muscarinic receptors and postsynaptic localization of M1 muscarinic receptors. Blocking presynaptic M2 autoreceptors increases ACh release, which in turn activates postsynaptic M1 receptors of cortical neurons projecting to the contralateral cortex. The result of ACh binding to postsynaptic M1 receptors is activation of the contralateral EEG, as indicated by a diminished number of spindles. This is one mechanism by which ACh can increase cortical excitability and promote brain arousal.

CONCLUSIONS

The brain is the end organ for both sleep and anesthesia, yet the interaction between research in sleep and that in anesthesia remains minimal. Neuronal systems that evolved to generate states of sleep are preferentially involved in generating states of anesthesia. Thus, sleep neurobiology can enrich efforts to elucidate the mechanisms of anesthetic action. Greater interaction between anesthesiology and sleep neurobiology can be expected to benefit both disciplines and contribute positively to clinical care.

Acknowledgments

Supported by National Institutes of Health Grants HL40881, MH45361, HL57120, HL65272, and the Department of Anesthesiology. We thank M.A. Norat for editorial assistance.

Key references

Baghdoyan HA, Lydic R. Neurotransmitters and neuromodulators regulating sleep. In: Bazil CW, Malow B, Sammaritano M, eds. Sleep and epilepsy: the clinical spectrum. New York: Elsevier Science; 2002:17–44.

Deboer T, Vansteensel MJ, Détári L, Meijer J. Sleep states alter activity of suprachiasmatic nucleus neurons. Nature Neurosci. 2003;6:1086–90.

Dement WC. History of sleep physiology and medicine. In: Kryger MH, Roth T, Dement WC, eds. Principles and practice of sleep medicine, 3rd edn. Philadelphia: WB Saunders; 2000:1–14.

Howard SK, Rosekind MR, Katz JD, Berry AJ. Fatigue in anesthesia: implications and strategies for patient and provider safety. Anesthesiology 2002;97:1281–94.

Kryger MH, Roth T, Dement WC, eds. Principles and practice of sleep medicine, 3rd edn. Philadelphia: WB Saunders; 2000.

Lancel M. Role of $GABA_A$ receptors in the regulation of sleep: Initial sleep responses to peripherally administered modulators and agonists. Sleep 1999;22:33–42.

Lichtor JL, Alessi R, Lane BS. Sleep tendency as a measure of recovery after drugs used for ambulatory surgery. Anesthesiology 2002;96:878–83.

Lydic R, Baghdoyan HA. Neurochemical evidence for the cholinergic modulation of sleep and breathing. In: Carley D, Radulovacki M, eds. Sleep-related breathing disorders: experimental models and therapeutic potential.New York: Marcel Dekker; 2003: 57–91.

Lydic R, Baghdoyan HA. Cholinergic contributions to the control of consciousness. In: Yaksh T, Lynch C, Zapol WM, Maze M, Biebuyck JF, Saidman LJ, eds. Anesthesia: biologic foundations. Philadelphia: Lippincott Raven; 1998:433–50.

Nelson LE, Guo TZ, Lu J, Saper CB, Franks NP, Maze M. The sedative component of anesthesia is mediated by GABA(A) receptors in an endogenous sleep pathway. Nature Neurosci. 2002;5:979–84.

Tafti M, Franken P. Genetic dissection of sleep. J Appl Physiol. 2002;92:1339–47.

Steriade M, Timofeev I. Neuronal plasticity in thalamocortical networks during sleep and waking oscillations. Neuron 2003;37:563–76.

Further reading

Koblin DD, Dong DE, Deady J, Eger EI. Selective breeding alters murine resistance to nitrous oxide without alteration in synaptic membrane lipid composition. Anesthesiology 1980;52:401–7.

Kohn LT, Corrigan J, Donaldson MS, Richardson WC, eds. To err is human: building a safer health system. Washington, DC: National Academies Press; 2000.

Marcus CL, Louglin GM. Effect of sleep deprivation on driving safety in housestaff. Sleep 1996;19:763–6.

Meuret P, Backman SB, Bonhomme V, Plourde G, Fiset P. Physostigmine reverses propofol-induced unconsciousness and attenuation of the auditory steady state response in bispectral index in human volunteers. Anesthesiology 2000;93:708–17.

Roehrs T, Burduvali E, Bonahoom A, Drake C, Roth T. Ethanol and sleep loss: A dose comparison of impairing effects. Sleep 2003;26:981–5.

Sonner JM, Gong D, Eger EI. Naturally occurring variability in anesthetic potency among inbred mouse strains. Anesth Analg. 2000;91:720–6.

Tagaito Y, Polotsky VY, Campen MJ et al. A model of sleep-disordered breathing in the C57BL/6J mouse. J Appl Physiol. 2001;91:2758–66.

van Dongen HP, Maislin G, Mullington JM, Dinges DF. The cumulative cost of additional wakefulness: dose–response effects on neurobehavioral functions and sleep physiology from chronic sleep restriction and total sleep deprivation. Sleep 2003;26:117–26.

Chapter 31

Opioids

Gavril W Pasternak

TOPICS COVERED IN THIS CHAPTER

- **Endogenous pain-modulatory systems**
- **Opioid drugs**
    - Morphine-related compounds
    - Phenylpiperidines
    - Methadone and propoxyphene (dextropropoxyphene)
    - Mixed agonist/antagonists
- **Pharmacokinetics**
- **Opioid receptors**
    - The μ receptors
    - The δ receptors
    - The κ receptors
    - Opioid receptor transduction mechanisms
- **Opioid analgesia**
    - Tolerance and dependence
    - Opioid rotation
    - Anti-opioid systems
- **Other opioid actions**
    - Respiratory depression
    - Gastrointestinal transit
    - Other effects
- **Clinical pharmacology**

Opioids have long been used in the relief of pain. The search for nonaddicting agents and for analgesics that avoid the many side effects encountered with current drugs has led to the synthesis of thousands of analogs. Although this search has not yielded such agents, it has provided important pharmacological tools in our understanding of opioid actions. We now know that the opioids act through a complex system of receptors and opioid peptides, components of the endogenous opioid systems.

Opioids have unique actions in the relief of pain. Unlike local anesthetics, which interfere with all sensation, opioids act upon pain without interfering with objective sensations such as touch and temperature. Pain is made up of two components, fast and slow pain (Chapter 23). Fast pain is carried through neospinothalamic pathways and conducts well-localized 'objective' aspects of painful sensations. Neurons in the dorsal horn of the spinal cord receive input from sensory nerves, cross the midline, and then ascend to the contralateral thalamus. Thalamic neurons then project directly to the sensory cortex. Damage to the sensory cortex, as seen in stroke, leads to the loss of these sensations. Slow pain is transmitted rostrally more slowly because of extensive synaptic interactions in the brainstem and limbic structures. Unlike fast pain, slow pain is poorly localized and is responsible for the 'hurt', or suffering, component of pain. Opioids specifically target 'slow pain', relieving the 'hurt'. Indeed, patients often comment after receiving an opioid that the pain is still there but does not hurt.

Opioids specifically target 'slow pain', relieving the hurt of pain without eliminating pain itself, by activating an endogenous pain-modulatory system.

ENDOGENOUS PAIN-MODULATORY SYSTEMS

Pain is an essential, although unpleasant, sensation that protects the individual by warning of potential injury or damage. Yet it is easy to think of situations in which pain must be suppressed. A wounded combatant, for example, must still defend himself. Thus the sensory nervous system is able to filter nociceptive stimuli, modulating the perception of pain. The first clinical study implying such a system came from studies comparing the morphine needs of wounded soldiers in World War II to those of civilians undergoing elective surgery. Despite far more serious wounds, soldiers required fewer analgesics than did civilians. Experimental evidence emerged from studies of direct brain stimulation. Stimulation of specific brain regions induced potent analgesic action in experimental animals and humans. Only certain brain regions were capable of producing these actions, and the analgesic activity could be prevented by naloxone, a specific opioid antagonist. This provided the first evidence for an endogenous pain-modulatory system that could be activated by opioids.

The endogenous opioid system comprises a family of peptides and their receptors. Pharmacologically, opioid peptides share many characteristics, including the ability to produce analgesia. However, their mechanisms of action are very different. The enkephalins were the first opioid peptides identified, followed soon after by the dynorphins and β-endorphin. Structurally, all opioid peptides have striking similarities. Met^5-enkephalin and Leu^5-enkephalin are highly related pentapeptides that differ only in their C-terminal amino acid (Table 31.1). Enkephalins are endogenous ligands for the δ-class of opioid receptors. Peptides within the dynorphin family are longer than the enkephalins. Dynorphin A, the most intensely studied member of this family, contains 17 amino acid residues and is the endogenous ligand for the κ_1-opioid receptor. Like other members of this opioid peptide family, dynorphin A contains the sequence of Leu^5-enkephalin at its N-terminus. Less is known about other members of this family, such as dynorphin B or α-neoendorphin. β-endorphin is the third member of the opioid peptide family. It is larger than the other opioid peptides, containing 31 amino acid residues. Its precursor, pro-opiomelanocortin (POMC), encodes only one opioid peptide, but also generates several other physiologically important peptides, including adrenocorticotropic hormone (ACTH), which is co-released from the pituitary with β-endorphin (Chapter 66).

The presence of an enkephalin sequence within the dynorphin series and in β-endorphin suggested that the enkephalins might be breakdown products of these larger peptides. However, this is clearly not the case; each of the three major families of opioid peptides is encoded by separate genes (Fig. 31.1). The opioid peptides are derived from larger precursors through extensive proteolytic processing. Although prepro-opiomelanocortin contains only β-endorphin, the other precursor peptides contain multiple copies of opioid peptides. The isolation and cloning of all three precursors unequivocally established that each generates distinct neurotransmitters.

Regional differences exist in the distribution of the various opioid peptides within the CNS. The enkephalins are widely distributed, implying a wide range of actions beyond simple analgesia. In contrast, β-endorphin is limited to the pituitary and the arcuate region of the hypothalamus, although these areas have extensive projections.

Table 31.1 Opioids and related peptides

	Structure
Leu^5-enkephalin	Tyr-Gly-Gly-Phe-Leu
Met^5-enkaphalin	Tyr-Gly-Gly-Phe-Met
Dynorphin A	Tyr-Gly-Gly-Phe-Leu-Arg-Arg-Ile-Arg-Pro-Lys-Leu-Lys-Trp-Asp-Asn-Gln
Dynorphin B	Tyr-Gly-Gly-Phe-Leu-Arg-Arg-Gln-Phe-Lys-Val-Val-Thr
α-neoendorphin	Tyr-Gly-Gly-Phe-Leu-Arg-Lys-Tyr-Pro-Lys
β-neoendorphin	Tyr-Gly-Gly-Phe-Leu-Arg-Lys-Tyr-Pro
β-endorphin	Tyr-Gly-Gly-Phe-Met-Thr-Ser-Glu-Lys-Ser-Gln-Thr-Pro-Leu-Val-Thr-Leu-Phe-Lys-Asn-Ala-Ile-Ile-Lys-Asn-Ala-Tyr-Lys-Lys-Gly-Glu
Endomorphin-1	Tyr-Pro-Trp-Phe-NH_2
Endomorphin-2	Tyr-Pro-Phe-Phe-NH_2
Orphanin FQ/ nociceptin	Phe-Gly-Gly-Phe-Thr-Gly-Ala-Arg-Lys-Ser-Ala-Arg-Lys-Ala-Asp-Glu

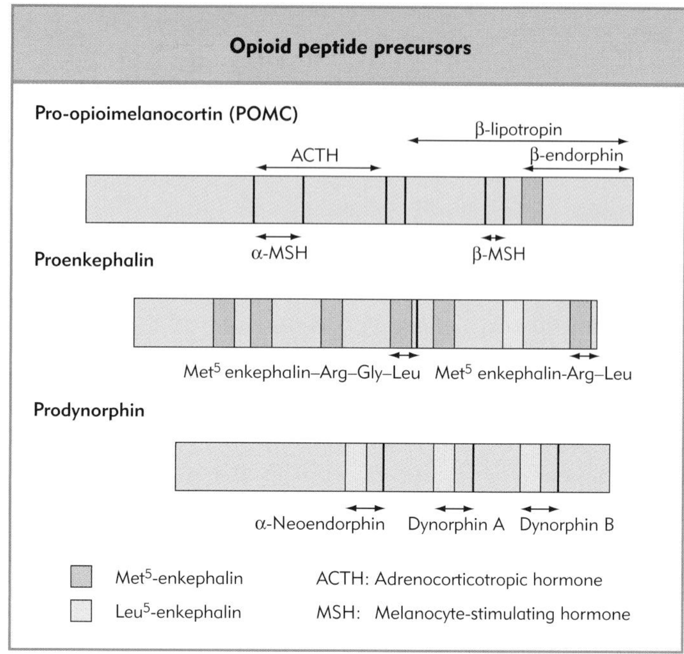

Figure 31.1 The opioid peptide precursors.

A major difficulty faced in early studies of the enkephalins was their instability because of rapid enzymatic degradation in vivo. The development of metabolically stable derivatives has greatly facilitated the evaluation of these compounds. In addition to enhancing their stability, variations in structure have led to extraordinary differences in selectivity for the various opioid receptors. For example, the synthetic opioid D-Ala^2–$MePhe^4$–$Gly(ol)^5$-enkephalin (DAMGO) is a very selective morphine-like drug with properties quite different from those of the natural enkephalins. These synthetic opioid peptides provide highly selective agonists and antagonists for most opioid receptors, which have become important investigational tools.

Another pair of opioid peptides, the endomorphins, has been isolated recently. Endomorphin-1 and endomorphin-2 are tetrapeptides that are structurally distinct from other members of the opioid peptide family. The major difference between the endomorphins and other opioid peptides is their high selectivity for μ-receptors, which suggests that they may represent endogenous ligands for these receptors. Our knowledge of the endomorphins is quite limited, but it is likely to open new areas in drug development and provide insights into the μ-opioid system.

Opioid peptides are derived from larger precursors through extensive proteolytic processing.

The recent cloning of the opioid receptors has identified a receptor within the opioid family that has poor affinity for traditional opioids. Although this receptor is related to the opioid κ_3 receptor, they are not identical. The endogenous ligand for this receptor is orphanin FQ, or nociceptin, a heptadecapeptide with some similarities to dynorphin A (Table 31.1). The pharmacology of this peptide is complex. For example, it was originally proposed to be hyperalgesic. More recent studies have demonstrated that it can functionally reverse the analgesic actions of a number of opioids, but it can elicit analgesia in other paradigms.

OPIOID DRUGS

Morphine-related compounds

Morphine and codeine were first isolated from opium, an extract of *Papaver somniferum* which contains a mixture of alkaloids (Fig. 31.2). Structurally, they differ only in the presence of a methyl group at the 3-position. Codeine must be metabolized to morphine by 3-O-demethylation for full analgesic effect. This reaction is catalyzed by the genetically polymorphic P450 isozyme CYP2D6, which is absent in about 8% of the British population, and which is inhibited by tricyclic antidepressants, selective serotonin reuptake inhibitors, neuroleptics, quinidine, etc. Because codeine acts through its metabolism to morphine and these individuals are unable to convert codeine to morphine, they do not respond to codeine. Morphine 6-glucuronide (M6G) is a potent morphine metabolite with pharmacologic properties that are distinct from those of morphine. Heroin (diacetylmorphine, diamorphine) is not used for therapeutic purposes in the USA but is used in the UK, and remains the major opioid of abuse. It is synthesized from morphine by acetylation at both the 3- and the 6-positions. When administered, the 3-acetyl group is rapidly removed enzymatically in vivo to form 6-acetylmorphine, the active component of heroin. Nalorphine (Fig. 31.3) was the first opioid antagonist identified and reverses the actions of morphine. It differs structurally from morphine only in the replacement of the *N*-methyl group with an *N*-allyl moiety. It is not used clinically, as it also has activity at κ receptors and produces severe dysphorias and psychotomimetic actions.

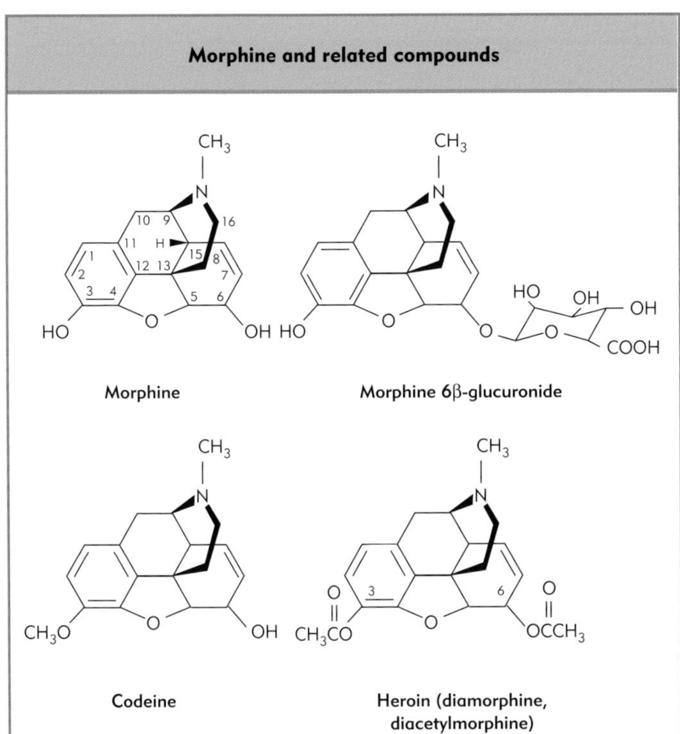

Figure 31.2 Structures of morphine and related compounds.

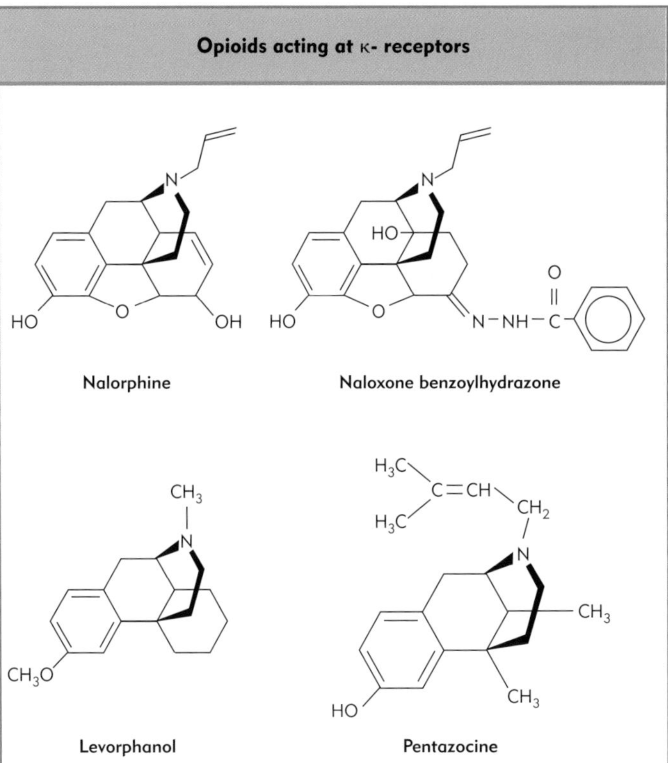

Figure 31.3 Structures of opioids acting at κ receptors.

Metabolism has important consequences for the action of morphine and its relatives codeine and heroin.

Opium also contains thebaine, which has been used to make a number of additional opioid compounds, many of which are important clinically (Fig. 31.4). Hydromorphone is a potent analgesic, as is oxymorphone. Oxycodone is widely used in combination with acetominophen (paracetamol) or aspirin. Naloxone and naltrexone (Fig. 31.5) are both pure opioid antagonists and are used clinically. It is interesting that the simple replacement of the *N*-methyl group of oxymorphone with an *N*-allyl moiety converts this potent analgesic to the pure antagonist naloxone.

A number of these agents are now available in slow-release formulations, including morphine and oxycodone. The ability to increase the dosing interval to up to 12 hours has been a major advantage clinically, although care must be taken with dose titration, as it may take several days to reach steady-state levels of the drug.

Phenylpiperidines

The first phenylpiperidine used was meperidine (pethidine) (Fig. 31.4), one of the most widely used opioids for many years. Loperamide is a structurally similar compound which is a peripherally acting μ-opioid agonist. Fentanyl and its analogs are highly potent opioids that act predominantly through μ receptors (Fig. 31.6). However, they differ pharmacologically from morphine in a number of ways, as discussed below. Their short half-lives and rapid onset and offset have led to their extensive use in anesthesiology. Fentanyl is now also available as

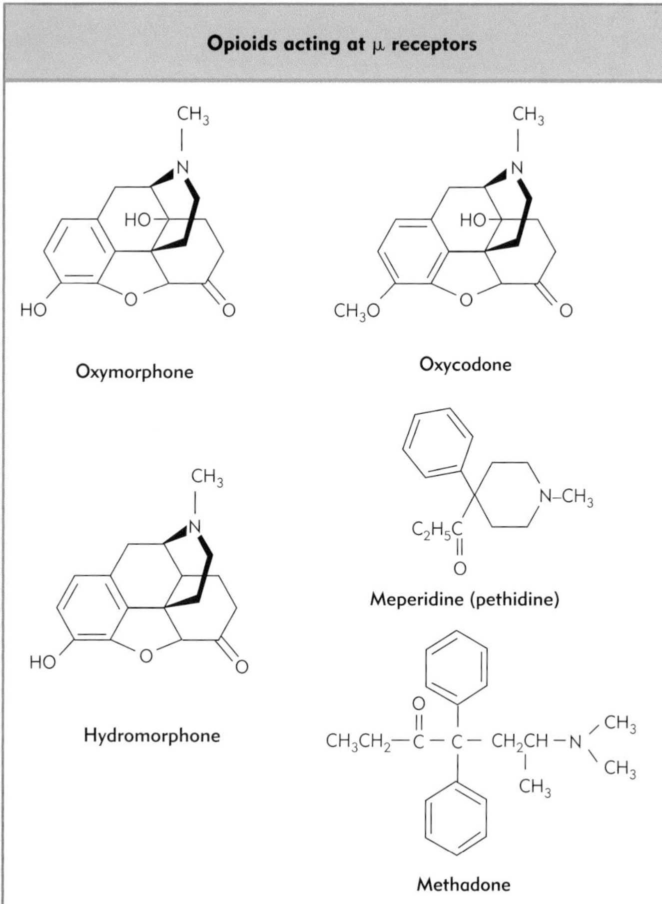

Figure 31.4 Structures of opioids acting at μ receptors.

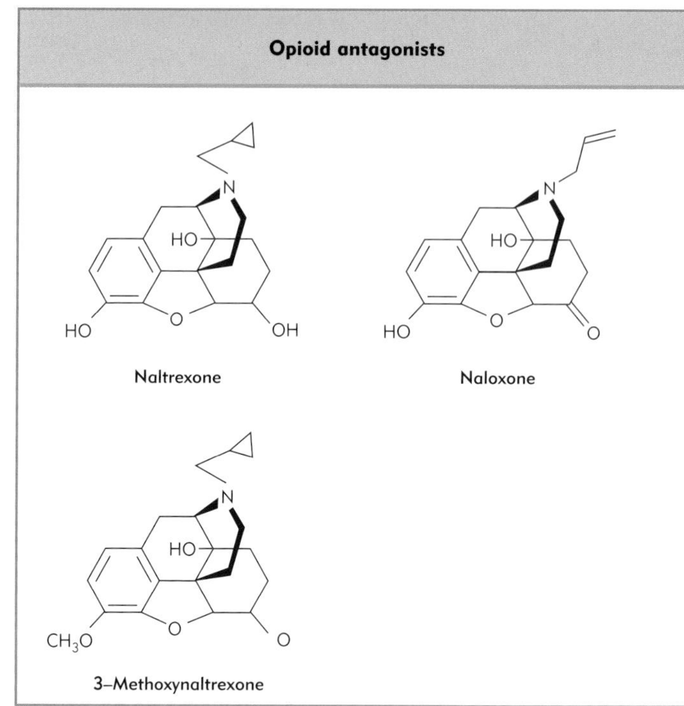

Figure 31.5 Structures of opioid antagonists.

a transdermal patch, which has advantages particularly for patients who cannot take medications orally.

Methadone and propoxyphene (dextropropoxyphene)

Methadone (Fig. 31.4) is a μ-opioid with actions similar to those of morphine. One of the first synthetic opioids, methadone is used extensively in the management of opiate abuse, but it is also a valuable analgesic. It has a long half-life, permitting less frequent dosing. Propoxyphene (dextropropoxyphene), which is structurally related to methadone, is a weak opioid widely used in conjuction with either acetominophen or aspirin.

Mixed agonist/antagonists

Pentazocine (Fig. 31.3) is the most widely used drug with mixed agonist/antagonist properties (partial agonists). It has analgesic actions mediated primarily through κ_1 receptors, but also has antagonist activity at μ receptors which can precipitate withdrawal in highly dependent patients. Thus, the use of pentazocine should be limited to opioid-naive patients. Nalbuphine and butorphanol are also mixed agonist/antagonists. Their analgesic actions also are mediated through κ receptors, and they are partial agonists at μ receptors; like pentazocine, they show antagonist activity toward full μ agonists. Buprenorphine has a similar profile, but dissociates slowly from μ receptors and is poorly antagonized by naloxone. Tramadol, which is structurally distinct from other opioids, is a partial μ agonist with minimal κ affinity. Its antinociceptive effects are not fully antagonized by naloxone, and may also involve inhibition of norepinephrine and serotonin reuptake.

PHARMACOKINETICS

In addition to their widely varying receptor selectivities, opioid analgesics also can be differentiated by their durations of action (Table 31.2). In general, the duration of analgesia corresponds to the elimination half-time of the drug, but some need to be given more frequently than anticipated to maintain analgesic activity. Half-times vary depending on the route of administration and mechanism of clearance. This is particularly an issue with the antagonist naloxone. Its duration of action is typically far less than that of the agonists it is used against. Thus, it is often necessary to give multiple doses or infusion of naloxone to ensure the continued reversal of the agonist effect.

The duration of opioid effect is determined primarily by elimination half-time, with important contributions from lipid solubility and p*K*a.

Some physicochemical and pharmacokinetic properties of the fentanyl family of opioids are summarized in Table 31.3 and Figure 31.7. Simple comparison of their elimination half-times does not predict the rates of decrease in effect-site concentration detected by pharmacokinetic studies. An intravenous bolus of fentanyl undergoes rapid distribution to highly perfused tissues. Peak concentrations occur in brain in 2–3 minutes, with peak analgesia about 2 minutes later. Brain levels rapidly decline

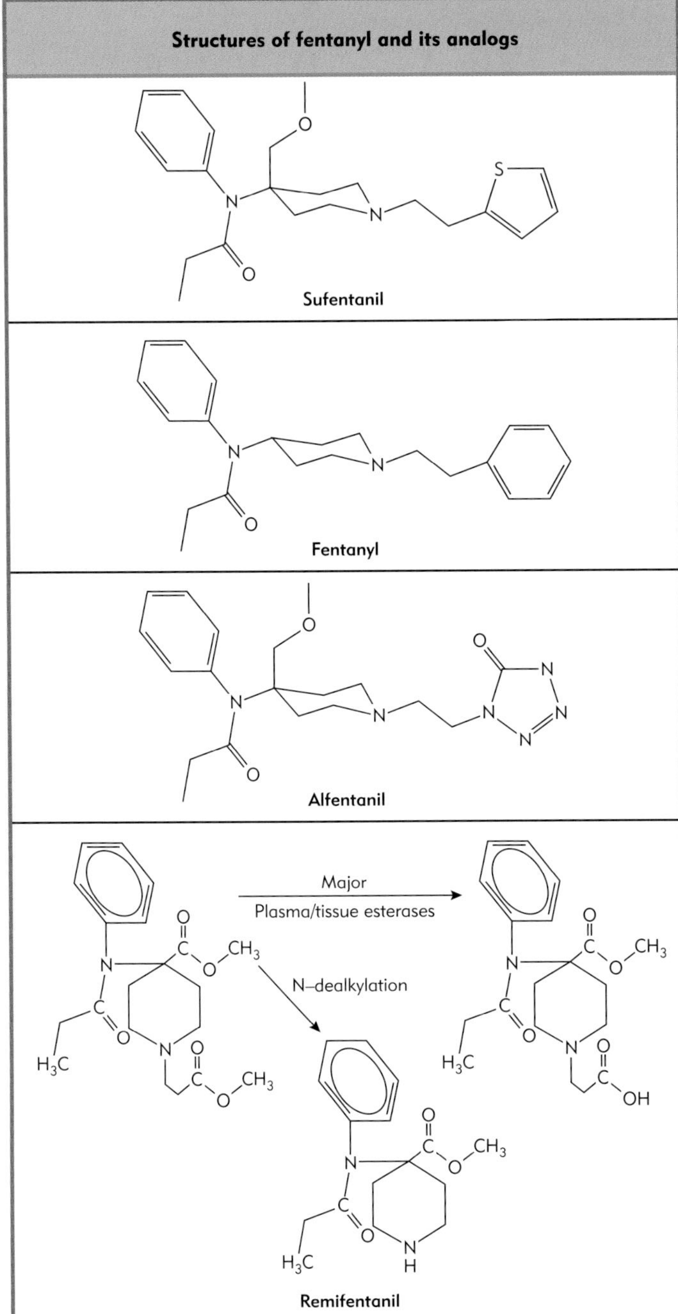

Figure 31.6 Structures of fentanyl and its analogs. The metabolic pathway of remifentanil is also shown. Its major metabolite is <0.001% as potent as remifentanil.

through redistribution into the high volume of distribution (V_d), followed by a slower elimination through hepatic metabolism (by *N*-dealkylation) as the drug re-enters the central compartment. This slow elimination phase can result in prolonged and cumulative effects with repeated or large doses, as reflected in the steep increase in the context-sensitive half-time (the time to a 50% decrease in effect-site concentration after termination of an infusion, which depends on the rates of distribution and elimination ($t_{1/2b}$) *and* on the duration of infusion) (Fig. 31.7). Alfentanil exhibits similar pharmacokinetics, but its reduced lipophilicity results in less protein and lipid binding, a lower

Table 31.2 Elimination half-times of opioids

Drug	Approximate half-time
Remifentanil	10 min
Naloxone	75 min[a]
Alfentanil	90 min
Morphine	120 min
Hydromorphone	150 min
Oxymorphone	150 min
Nalbuphine	150 min
Sufentanil	150 min
Butorphanol	180 min
Codeine	180 min
Meperidine (pethidine)	200 min
Fentanyl	220 min
Propoxyphene (dextropropoxyphene)	8 h
Levorphanol	15 h
Methadone	24 h

[a]Note that the half-time of the μ-receptor antagonist naloxone is far shorter than that of most clinically used opioids.

V_d, and more rapid clearance by cytochrome P450 CYP3A4. Consequently, alfentanil is much less likely to produce cumulative effects (Fig. 31.7). Despite its lower lipid solubility, the onset of alfentanil action is much faster than that of fentanyl. The initial plasma concentration is higher because of its lower central V_d, and its more acidic pK_a means that it is 90% nonionized at blood pH and is, therefore, diffusible across the blood–brain barrier. Sufentanil has the highest lipid solubility, with a large V_d and high clearance by hepatic *N*- and O-dealkylation compared to alfentanil. Its context-sensitive half-time demonstrates its utility in short procedures compared to alfentanil and fentanyl (Table 31.3). Remifentanil, a 4-anilidopiperidine, has a unique metabolic and pharmacokinetic profile. It undergoes rapid methyl ester hydrolysis by tissue and plasma esterases (not plasma cholinesterase) to relatively inactive metabolites; as a result, its effect is terminated by rapid metabolic clearance rather than redistribution (Fig. 31.7). This results in rapid reduction in plasma concentration after bolus or prolonged infusion independent of age, weight, sex, or hepatic and renal function. It is a potent, fast-acting μ opioid with a rapid recovery, which is useful for infusions or short, painful procedures. Its short-duration analgesic effect requires pre-emptive use of longer-acting analgesics at discontinuation of infusion to prevent postoperative pain.

OPIOID RECEPTORS

Opioid receptors are members of the family of G protein-coupled receptors (Chapter 3). Despite major advances in our understanding of these receptors, many questions remain. There are three major classes of opioid receptor: μ, δ, and κ; although they share the ability to elicit analgesia, their pharmacologic

Table 31.3 Physicochemical and pharmacokinetic properties of the fentanyl family of opioids

Parameter	Remifentanil	Alfentanil	Fentanyl	Sufentanil
Lipid solubility (octanol: water solubility coefficient)	17.9	129	816	1727
pK_a	7.1	6.5	8.4	8.0
Nonionized fraction at blood pH	67	89	8.5	20
Volume of distribution (L/kg)	0.47	0.75	4.0	2.9
Elimination half-time (min)	9-11	94	219	164
Clearance (L/h/kg)	2.48	0.48	0.78	0.76
Relative potency	1	0.014	1	9

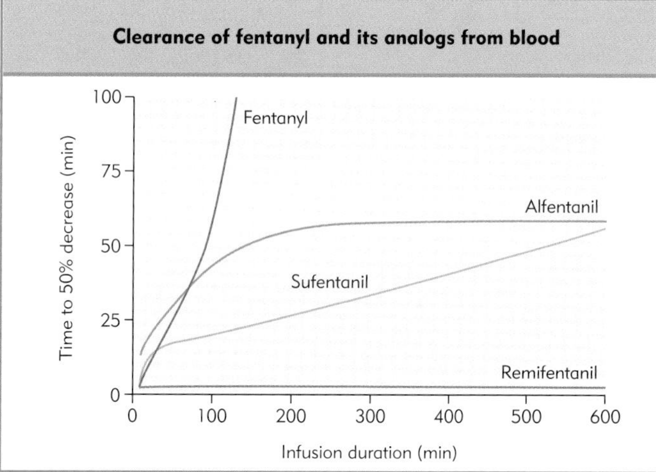

Figure 31.7 Clearance of fentanyl and its analogs from blood. A simulation of the time necessary to achieve a 50% decrease in drug concentration in the blood (or plasma) after variable times of intravenous infusions of remifentanil, fentanyl, alfentanil, and sufentanil. Note that alfentanil has a longer context-sensitive half-time than sufentanil, despite having a shorter elimination half-time. (From Egan TD, Lemmens HJM, Fiset P, et al. The pharmacokinetics of the new short-acting opioid remifentanil (G187184B) in healthy adult male volunteers. Anesthesiology. 1993;79:881–92.)

properties differ. Highly selective agonists and antagonists demonstrate their distinct mechanisms of action in animal models. They display no cross-tolerance and selective antagonists can reverse the actions of one class without blocking others. This makes each opioid receptor class a potential therapeutic target. However, the vast majority of clinically used drugs are μ agonists, despite their undesirable respiratory depressant and constipating actions. Subtypes of these families have been proposed from both traditional pharmacological approaches and molecular cloning studies, although the relationships between the subtypes defined pharmacologically and those identified at the molecular level are not entirely clear. Four genes encoding opioid receptors have been identified, encoding μ (*MOR-1*), δ (*DOR*-1), κ_1 (*KOR-1*), and a related orphan opioid clone (*KOR-3/ORL1*) that binds the novel peptide orphanin FQ/nociceptin.

Opioid receptors belong to three major classes defined pharmacologically, each a potential therapeutic target.

The μ receptors

Morphine and related alkaloids act primarily through μ receptors to produce their classic actions, foremost among which is analgesia (Table 31.4). Most clinically used analgesics act at μ receptors, including morphine, oxymorphone, methadone, and the fentanyl series. Many opioid side effects are also produced through μ receptors, such as constipation and respiratory depression. The μ receptors are antagonized by a number of drugs. Some are highly selective and only block μ receptors (β-funaltrexamine), but these are not available clinically. Others reverse the actions of a variety of opioids and show only slight selectivity for μ receptors (e.g. naloxone, which is used extensively clinically).

Pharmacologic evidence suggests three functionally defined subtypes of μ receptor. The initial characterization of μ-receptor subtypes was based on the opioid antagonist naloxonazine, with naloxonazine-sensitive opioid actions defined as μ_1 and naloxonazine-insensitive actions as μ_2 (Table 31.4). Both types elicit analgesia but at different sites within the CNS. The μ_1 sites are important for supraspinal and peripheral analgesia, whereas μ_2 sites mediate morphine analgesia at the spinal level. The respiratory depressant actions of morphine and many of the signs of dependence are mediated through μ_2 receptors, raising the possibility of producing μ_1-selective agonists analgesics lacking gastrointestinal or respiratory depressant activity. Conversely, a μ_2 antagonist might prove useful to reverse the respiratory and gastrointestinal actions of morphine and related compounds.

The third functionally defined member of the μ-receptor family is perhaps the most intriguing. It mediates the actions of morphine-6β-glucuronide (M6G), a very potent morphine metabolite. When administered directly into the CNS to bypass the blood–brain barrier, M6G is over 100 times more potent than morphine. The importance of the M6G receptor is due to its distinct mechanisms of action and the ability of a number of other μ-receptor opioids to act through them, including heroin. However, the actions of M6G are sensitive to naloxonazine, implying that this class of receptor is most appropriately considered a subdivision of μ_1 receptor. Evidence for this third

Table 31.4 Opioid receptor classification and localization of analgesic actions

Receptor	Clone	Analgesia	Other actions
μ Receptors	MOR-1		
μ_1	–	Supraspinal, peripheral	Prolactin release, acetylcholine release in the hippocampus, feeding
μ_2	–	Spinal	Respiratory depression, gastrointestinal transit, dopamine release by nigrostriatal neurons, guinea pig ileum bioassay, feeding
	M6G	Spinal and supraspinal	–
κ receptors			
κ_1	KOR-1	Spinal and supraspinal	Psychotomimetic, sedation
κ_2	–	Unknown	Diuresis, feeding
κ_3	KOR-3/ORLI(?)	Supraspinal	Unknown
δ receptors		Mouse vas deferens bioassay,	dopamine turnover in the striatum, feeding
δ_1	–	Supraspinal	–
δ_2	DOR-1	Spinal and supraspinal	–

Some of the actions attributed to a general family of receptor have not yet been associated with a specific subtype. The correlations in this table are based on animal studies, which can show species differences.

μ-receptor subtype comes from a variety of sources. A new antagonist, 3-methoxynaltrexone, unlike the other μ antagonists, is selective for the M6G site and blocks both M6G and heroin analgesia at doses that are inactive against morphine. Genetic evidence also supports the existence of this receptor class. The CXBK strain of mouse is insensitive to morphine. Yet M6G and heroin retain their analgesic activity. Other μ-receptor drugs, including methadone, also retain analgesic activity in these animals, providing indications for an even greater complexity of μ-receptor actions.

The μ opioid receptor, termed MOR-1, it is a typical G protein-coupled receptor with seven transmembrane domains arranged to form a doughnut-like structure spanning the membrane, with the binding pocket for the drug located in the center. Morphine and other μ-acting drugs bind to this site with high affinity, confirming that it represents a μ receptor. The *MOR-1* gene contains four exons, and splice variants have been identified in all species that have been examined, included humans. The most prominent variants involve 3′-splicing, which changes only the amino acids at the tip of the intracellular C-terminus (Fig. 31.8). Since the binding pocket of the receptor is defined by exons 1, 2 and 3, it is not surprising that they all maintain high selectivity for morphine and related compounds, consistent with their designation as μ receptors. However, the C terminus is important in transduction mechanisms, and differences among the variants can be shown for a variety of μ opioids. The variants also differ in cellular and subcellular localization. They are often expressed in different regions of the CNS, and even when seen in the same region they may be expressed in different cells. Furthermore, ultrastructural studies indicate different subcellular localizations within neurons as well.

The presence of these variants supports earlier suggestions of μ-receptor subtypes. However, specific splice variants have yet to be correlated with the pharmacologically defined μ-receptor subtypes. Additional molecular approaches also indicate pharmacological differences between the μ opioids. Antisense mapping studies provide a method of decreasing mRNA levels for a specific protein with a specificity far greater than that of any of the available antagonists. In antisense mapping, probes are designed to examine different mRNA sequences corresponding to various exons, which provides the opportunity to attribute functional activity to specific splice variants. Antisense mapping analysis of the four exons of *MOR-1* reveals dramatic differences between the actions of morphine and those of M6G. Probes targeting exon 1 effectively block morphine analgesia without interfering with M6G analgesia. Conversely, probes targeting exon 2 are inactive against morphine but block M6G analgesia. These studies imply that both morphine and M6G act through receptors related to *MOR-1* but which represent distinct transcripts from each other.

Knockout mice provide yet another assessment of the functional significance of the cloned receptors (see Chapter 4). Disruption of MOR-1 in a number of models eliminates morphine actions. Similarly, in one knockout mouse in which the first exon of the *MOR-1* is deleted, morphine is inactive. However, these same mice respond to M6G and heroin, further supporting differences between morphine and the other two drugs at a genetic level. Other MOR-1 splice variants are still expressed in the exon-1 knockout mouse, implying that one of these variants is responsible for M6G and heroin analgesia. In knockout mice in which exon 2 is inactivated, both morphine and M6G are completely inactive. Thus, M6G acts through a receptor that is a product of the *MOR-1* gene distinct from receptors responsible for morphine analgesia.

MOR-1 exon-1 knockout mice have also proved valuable in assessing other opioid analgesics. For example, fentanyl has been

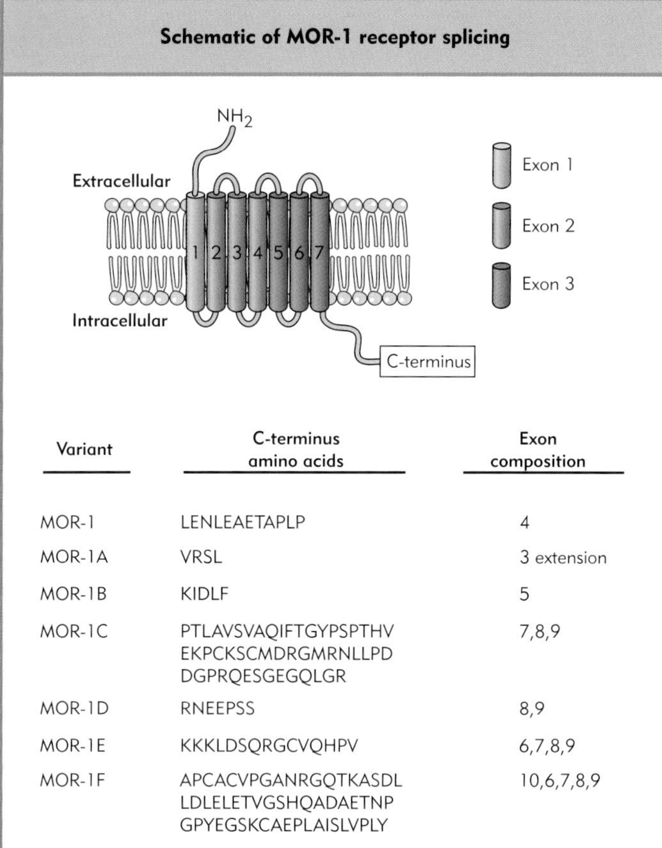

Variant	C-terminus amino acids	Exon composition
MOR-1	LENLEAETAPLP	4
MOR-1A	VRSL	3 extension
MOR-1B	KIDLF	5
MOR-1C	PTLAVSVAQIFTGYPSPTHV EKPCKSCMDRGMRNLLPD DGPRQESGEGQLGR	7,8,9
MOR-1D	RNEEPSS	8,9
MOR-1E	KKKLDSQRGCVQHPV	6,7,8,9
MOR-1F	APCACVPGANRGQTKASDL LDLELETVGSHQADAETNP GPYEGSKCAEPLAISLVPLY	10,6,7,8,9

Figure 31.8 Schematic of MOR-1 receptor splicing. The schematic illustrates a series of 3′ splice variants of MOR-1 in mouse. Similar types of splicing have been observed in other species, including humans. The transmembrane domains are defined by exons 1, 2, and 3, and make up the binding pocket of the receptor for opioids. Additional exons comprise the C terminus. The intracellular loops and C terminus are important in the transduction systems responsible for the actions of opioids.

classified as a drug acting upon μ receptors based on extensive pharmacologic testing. Yet fentanyl also is active in the *MOR-1* exon 1 knockout mouse, implying that it can act through M6G mechanisms distinct from those of morphine, and therefore has pharmacological properties distinct from those of morphine. The availability of these genetic models will provide new insights into the pharmacology of many analgesics, both newly developed and those already widely used.

The δ receptors

The δ receptors are highly selective for enkephalins. They were first identified in mouse vas deferens bioassays, and subsequently in brain by receptor-binding studies. Like μ receptors, δ receptors produce analgesia both spinally and supraspinally. A δ receptor encoded by *DOR-1* has been cloned and demonstrates the anticipated selectivity for enkephalins and related compounds. Two δ receptors have been proposed pharmacologically, δ_1 and δ_2, which can be differentiated by both agonists and antagonists. Spinal δ_2 receptors mediate analgesia, and both δ subtypes are active supraspinally. The cloned δ receptor appears to correspond to the δ_2 subtype. Although δ receptors remain a viable therapeutic target, no agents acting at δ receptors are yet available clinically.

The κ receptors

The κ receptors were identified initially based on the pharmacology of opioid analogs such as ketocyclazocine. Their existence was firmly established with the discovery of dynorphin A, the endogenous ligand for the κ_1 receptor, and the development of highly selective agonists such as U50,488 and U69,593, and the antagonist norbinaltorphimine. Many of the mixed agonist/antagonist opioids act at the κ_1 receptor, including pentazocine. Although several of the highly selective κ_1 agonists were analgesic in clinical trials, unpleasant side effects prevented further development. In addition to a significant diuretic action, these drugs produce psychotomimetic effects and dysphoria. The suggestion of subtypes within the κ_1-receptor group has raised the possibility of more selective analgesic agents lacking these side effects.

The κ_2 receptor was identified in binding studies. By using nonselective agents that label most opioid receptors, binding to established receptors could be displaced, leaving binding to the κ_2 site. Although easily demonstrated biochemically, the pharmacology of these sites remains unclear, primarily because of the absence of selective drugs. The approach used in the binding studies is not applicable to in vivo pharmacology. There is evidence that this receptor is produced by dimerization of κ and δ receptors.

The κ_3 receptor was first proposed based on the binding and pharmacologic actions of naloxone benzoylhydrazone (Fig. 31.3). Subsequent studies suggest that the κ_3 receptor corresponds to the nalorphine receptor. A number of clinical analgesics act in part through κ_3 receptors, including levorphanol and nalbuphine.

With the isolation of cDNAs encoding the traditional opioid receptors, an additional member of the family was cloned from mouse (*KOR-3*), rat, and human (*ORL1*). Several lines of evidence associate this gene with the κ_3 receptor, although they are clearly not identical. First, a monoclonal antibody that selectively labeled the κ_3 receptor recognized the new receptor. Second, antisense probes designed from this clone blocked κ_3-mediated analgesia. Despite this close association, this receptor differed from the κ_3 receptor. Although κ_3 receptors bind many traditional opioids with high affinity, the new receptor does not. Furthermore, an endogenous ligand for the new clone, orphanin FQ/nociceptin, does not compete for κ_3-receptor binding. The relationship between the two receptors is still not established; they could represent splice variants of a single gene, or totally distinct entities. A number of splice variants have been identified and several have unique pharmacologic profiles.

Opioid receptor transduction mechanisms

In general, the opioid receptors are inhibitory, acting primarily through the $G_i\alpha$ and $G_o\alpha$ classes of G protein. They inhibit adenylyl cyclase (μ, δ, and κ), and can also stimulate K^+ channel activity (μ and δ) and inhibit Ca^{2+} channel activity (κ) (Fig. 31.9). Chronic opioid exposure can lead to molecular adaptations, including upregulation of the cAMP pathway, with increased expression of specific subtypes of adenylyl cyclase and cAMP-dependent protein kinase (PKA) involving the CREB transcription factor. Drug-induced regulation of this and other transcription factors may represent molecular mechanisms underlying persistent alterations of neuronal function characteristic of addiction and tolerance.

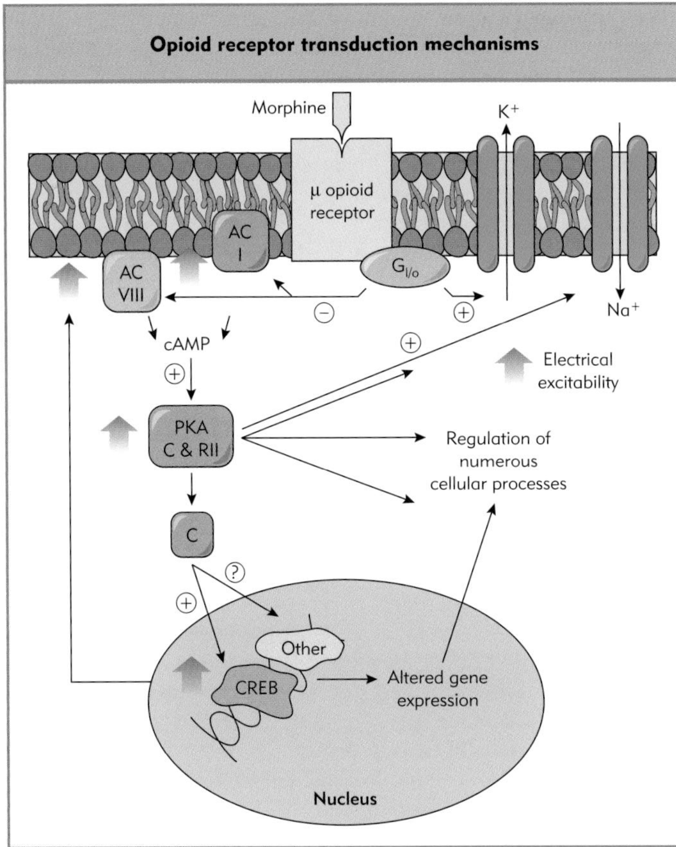

Figure 31.9 Opioid receptor transduction mechanisms. Opioids acutely inhibit neurons by increasing the conductance of an inwardly rectifying K^+ channel through coupling with $G_{i/o}$, as well as by decreasing a Na^+ current through coupling with $G_{i/o}$ and the consequent inhibition of adenylyl cyclase. Reduced concentrations of cAMP decrease PKA activity and the phosphorylation of the responsible channel or pump. Inhibition of the cAMP pathway also decreases phosphorylation of numerous other proteins, and thereby affects many additional processes. It reduces the phosphorylation state of CREB, which may initiate some of the longer-term changes. Upward bold arrows summarize the effects of chronic morphine administration in the locus ceruleus, the major noradrenergic nucleus in the brain, which is involved in opioid withdrawal. Chronic morphine increases concentrations of adenylyl cyclase types I and VIII (AC I and VIII), PKA catalytic (C) and regulatory type II (RII) subunits, and several phosphoproteins, including CREB. These changes contribute to the altered phenotype of the drug-addicted state. The intrinsic excitability of locus ceruleus neurons is increased by enhanced activity of the cAMP pathway and Na^+-dependent inward current, which contributes to the tolerance, dependence, and withdrawal exhibited by these neurons. (From Nestler EJ, Aghajanian GK. Molecular and cellular basis of addiction. Science. 1997;278:58–63. Copyright © 1999 AAAS.)

OPIOID ANALGESIA

Opioid pharmacology is quite complex, and extends far beyond the use of opioids as analgesics. Opioids suppress the hurt, or subjective, component of pain, with each opioid receptor class acting through distinct receptor mechanisms in different locations within the CNS. The complexity of the system is markedly increased by extensive synergistic interactions between various regions, the development of tolerance and dependence, and the existence of anti-opioid systems. Finally, there are wide ranges in genetic sensitivity to different classes of opioid. This is attributed to a number of factors, including opioid receptors themselves and the activity of anti-opioid systems.

Opioids exert both central and peripheral analgesic actions. Morphine analgesia has been most widely studied. Despite extensive information regarding the clinical pharmacology of morphine, our understanding of the receptor systems rests predominantly on animal models. Systemic morphine analgesia is mediated primarily through supraspinal μ systems, with some involvement of peripheral and spinal mechanisms. A number of brainstem regions mediate morphine analgesia, including the periaqueductal gray, the nucleus raphe magnus, and the locus ceruleus. At the spinal level, μ receptors in the dorsal horn are responsible for morphine analgesia. Morphine also acts peripherally on sensory neurons through a μ-receptor mechanism. This is illustrated by the antihyperalgesic effect of loperamide, a μ agonist that does not cross the blood–brain barrier and is locally active, and by the actions of topical opioids.

Although all the locations are active alone, they are more effective in combination, displaying profound synergistic interactions. Synergy was first demonstrated between spinal and supraspinal systems. Although morphine is active when given either supraspinally or spinally, its potency is markedly increased by giving divided doses into both regions. Synergy is not limited to spinal/supraspinal interactions. Within the brainstem, synergy has been demonstrated between the periaqueductal gray and the locus ceruleus, and between the periaqueductal gray and the nucleus raphe magnus. Peripheral mechanisms also synergize with central ones. These interactions are most pronounced between peripheral and spinal systems, although peripheral/supraspinal interactions also occur. The importance of these interactions cannot be overstated. Small spinal doses of morphine, for example, can reduce the ED_{50} (median effective dose) for systemic morphine in mice by as much as 100-fold. This may help explain the utility of epidural morphine. When given epidurally, morphine concentrations at the spinal level are very high. However, there also is significant systemic absorption, leading to blood concentrations similar to those seen with intramuscular injections. Although spinal morphine alone is active, it is likely that the overall efficacy of this approach is enhanced by spinal/systemic synergy. These interactions also suggest that the utility of epidural drugs can be enhanced by the concomitant administration of systemic drugs.

Opioids differ in their ability to relieve pain, and patient responses can vary. The mixed agonist/antagonists are easily distinguished from morphine. Differences also exist among μ-receptor drugs, as illustrated above by the distinct activities of morphine, M6G, fentanyl, and heroin. Unfortunately, it is not yet possible to predict which agent will be most effective for a particular patient or a particular type of pain, and clinicians are encouraged to switch medications empirically. Also, opioids are not completely cross-tolerant. Patients tolerant to one agent may not be as tolerant to another, which must be considered when changing agents.

Tolerance and dependence

Tolerance is the progressive decline in the activity of a drug with prolonged use. Although it is frequently encountered with opioids, tolerance can usually be overcome by increasing the dose, by switching to a different drug, or both. Opioid tolerance can be quite profound, resulting in a requirement for doses 100 times higher than those used in naive patients. Tolerance is not usually a problem unless dose-limiting side effects prevent further escalation of the dose. Importantly, the need to escalate opioid doses may result from other factors, such as progressive disease in cancer patients.

Tolerance involves a number of mechanisms. Early studies focused on receptor transduction mechanisms, which are affected by chronic exposure to opioids. The most intriguing system associated with tolerance involves the *N*-methyl-D-aspartate (NMDA)–nitric oxide cascade (Chapters 20 and 22). Blockade of NMDA glutamate receptors has no effect on the analgesic activity of opioids such as morphine, yet NMDA antagonists can effectively block the progressive tolerance seen with opioids in animal models, which demonstrates that the mechanisms responsible for analgesia and tolerance can be dissociated. Blockade of nitric oxide synthesis has similar effects. This system may offer important targets in the treatment of pain.

Dependence invariably develops with continued opioid use. However, the presence of dependence should not interfere with their appropriate use. Dependence is a physiologic response and does not imply addiction, which involves drug-seeking behavior. All patients chronically on opioids become dependent, yet very few given opioids for pain management ever become addicted, although those with a prior history of drug abuse are a greater concern.

Dependence invariably develops with continued opioid use, but addiction, characterized by drug-seeking behavior, is rare in pain management.

Dependence raises several important clinical issues. First, patients taking opioids long term should not be given mixed agonist/antagonists, which can precipitate withdrawal. Withdrawal is also a concern when stopping opioids abruptly, although patients who are drug dependent can be easily tapered off opioids without evidence of withdrawal. Withdrawal signs and symptoms include nausea, diarrhea, yawning, rhinorhea, piloerection, sweating, increases in temperature and blood pressure, coughing, and insomnia. Their severity may vary depending on the degree of dependence and the rate of elimination of the drug. Agents such as methadone that are long lasting may have a milder, but protracted, withdrawal period. The dose can usually be decreased by 50% every 2 days without manifestations of withdrawal.

Opioid rotation

Although μ opioids show cross-tolerance, this is often not complete. This is important, particularly when switching drugs in highly tolerant patients. The equianalgesic tables often used to compare doses among opioids were obtained primarily from naïve patients and fall short when used in tolerant patients. Incomplete cross-tolerance is used clinically, an approach termed opioid rotation. When switching a tolerant patient to a new opioid, it is common practice to calculate the appropriate dose based on the tables and then reduce it by 50% or more. This often enables the restoration of analgesic activity with fewer side effects.

Anti-opioid systems

There is extraordinary variability in individual response to nociceptive stimuli and to analgesics. Although cultural factors play a role, genetic factors also may prove important. Marked differences in sensitivity to opioid analgesics exist between various strains of mice. Sensitivities of the various opioid receptor subtypes vary independently of each other. Some strains respond well to morphine and related μ-receptor drugs, but not to κ-receptor agents. Others display a reduced sensitivity to all opioid classes. These differences in analgesic sensitivity can correspond to levels of receptors, but in most situations do not.

Pain and the analgesic efficacy of endogenous opioid systems are modulated by recently identified anti-opioid transmitter systems. These systems include cholecystokinin, neuropeptide FF, orphanin FQ/nociceptin, and the σ system. The σ receptors were first identified based on the pharmacology of benzomorphan opioids, but it has become obvious that σ receptors do not belong in the opioid receptor family. Unlike the opioid receptors, which belong to the G protein-coupled family, σ receptors do not have the same distinguishing structures, such as seven transmembrane-spanning domains. Structurally, σ receptors have little similarity to any known membrane receptor and their functions remain to be elucidated.

Despite our limited understanding of σ-receptor functions at the biochemical level, many σ receptors and antagonists have been identified. (+)-Pentazocine is a potent agonist at σ_1 receptors. Unlike its optical isomer, (−)-pentazocine, which is a potent opioid analgesic, (+)-pentazocine has little affinity for opioid receptors. One of the most useful σ antagonists is haloperidol, which binds σ receptors as potently as dopamine receptors. (+)-Pentazocine blocks opioid analgesia regardless of which opioid receptor system is involved, whereas (−)-pentazocine is a clinically useful analgesic. Blockade of σ receptors with haloperidol reverses the actions of (+)-pentazocine. Opioid systems typically show little tonic activity, as demonstrated by the inactivity of naloxone in measures of pain sensitivity. In contrast, σ systems appear to have important tonic activities, which may explain the varying analgesic sensitivities of some mouse strains, particularly for the κ systems. Haloperidol shifts the dose response for morphine almost twofold in a number of strains of mice. Similarly, it enhances the analgesic actions of δ- and κ-acting drugs. However, in a mouse strain that is not very sensitive to κ drugs, haloperidol increased the κ-receptor sensitivity over 10-fold, indicating tonic activity of the σ system. This and other anti-opioid systems may prove important in our future understanding of the sensitivity of patients to opioids and nociceptive input.

OTHER OPIOID ACTIONS

Opioids have a number of actions other than analgesia. Some, such as nausea, are mediated through unknown mechanisms. However, a number of undesirable side effects are mediated by opioid receptors. The two most problematic effects are respiratory depression and constipation.

Respiratory depression

Respiratory depression is common with μ opioids. It is rarely a problem in the outpatient setting in the absence of underlying pulmonary disease, but problems may be more common in the perioperative setting. Morphine and related opioids reduce respiratory drive by shifting the ventilation–arterial carbon dioxide partial pressure (P_aCO_2) response curve down and to the right. Therefore, patients who retain carbon dioxide are most sensitive to the respiratory depressant actions of opioids. Respiratory depression is mediated through μ receptors and can be readily reversed by naloxone. The difficulty with current antagonists is that they also reverse analgesia and, in patients who are opioid dependent, can precipitate withdrawal. Although lower doses can be used to titrate respiratory depression without completely antagonizing analgesia, κ-acting drugs have less respiratory depressant activity and their use should be considered in patients with respiratory compromise. However, most of the κ-acting agents currently available also have antagonist activity at μ receptors and can precipitate withdrawal in patients who are opioid dependent.

Gastrointestinal transit

Morphine and other μ-acting opioids act both centrally and through receptors located in the myenteric plexus to impede gastrointestinal transit, which can lead to constipation. As with respiratory depression, the subpopulation of μ receptors responsible for the constipating action of opioids can be differentiated from that mediating analgesia. Theoretically, oral opioids should present a greater problem than parenteral ones, but constipation remains a frequent issue even in patients on parenteral drugs, and should be addressed early in all patients chronically taking opioids. One future approach towards avoiding constipation is through the use of an oral antagonist, alvimopam, which has no significant systemic absorption.

Other effects

Opioids also have a number of additional actions, including bradycardia, hypothermia, and miosis. All are naloxone sensitive, implying a role for opioid receptors. In addition, the fentanyl series of agents has been associated with rigidity, but the receptor mechanisms associated with this action are incompletely understood. Opioids can also alter the function of the immune system by suppressing cytokine production and perhaps by inducing apoptosis in lymphocytes, although the immunological consequences of opioid action are not well defined.

CLINICAL PHARMACOLOGY

Owing to the widely varying nature of pain and the genetic sensitivities of the patient, the treatment of pain depends on individualization. Assessing pain intensity can be difficult, and successful treatment requires an understanding of each patient. Nociceptive stimuli are not perceived equally by everyone, owing to both genetic and situational factors. For example, an acute episode of excruciating back pain in a patient with a remote history of cancer may subside dramatically if the patient is assured that it does not imply tumor recurrence. Pain has meaning, and understanding its meaning to the patient is essential in assessing its severity. In any event, the only accurate measure of pain is the patient's report. Acute pain is often associated with well-recognized autonomic signs. However, these signs are typically lost in chronic pain syndromes, despite the persistence of pain.

Treatment of pain should focus on the simplest regimen with the fewest side effects. Treating pain requires an understanding of the type of pain involved and the utility of various drugs for specific types of pain. Somatic pain is well treated by opioids, whereas other types, such as neuropathic pain, are far less responsive. For many neuropathic pain syndromes other classes of drug are useful, including antidepressants such as amitriptyline and anticonvulsants such as carbamazepine and gabapentin (Chapter 28). Pain should be treated aggressively with the goal of keeping the patient pain free. Patients should not wait until pain returns before taking their next analgesic dose. It is easier to prevent pain than to take it away, and patients on round-the-clock dosing typically require less opioid over 24 hours than those taking opioids on an as-needed basis.

Key references

Lord JAH, Waterfield AA, Hughes J, Kosterlitz HW. Endogenous opioid peptides: multiple agonists and receptors. Nature 1977;267:495–9.

Pasternak GW. Pharmacological mechanisms of opioid analgesics. Clin Neuropharmacol. 1993;16:1–18.

Reisine T, Bell GI. Molecular biology of opioid receptors. Trend Neurosci. 1993;16:506–10.

Shafer SL, Varvel JR. Pharmacokinetics, pharmacodynamics, and rational opioid selection. Anesthesiology 1991;74:53–63.

Yeung JC, Rudy TA. Multiplicative interaction between narcotic agonists expressed at spinal and supraspinal sites of antinociceptive action as revealed by concurrent intrathecal and intracerebroventricular injections of morphine. J Pharmacol Exp Ther. 1980;215:633–42.

Further reading

Burkle H, Dunbar S, van Aken H. Remifentanil: a novel, short-acting μ opioid. Anesth Analg. 1996;83:646–51.

Nestler EJ, Aghajanian GK. Molecular and cellular basis of addiction. Science 1997;278:58–63.

Pasternak GW, Standifer KM. Mapping of opioid receptors using antisense oligodeoxynucleotides: correlating their molecular biology and pharmacology. Trends Pharmacol Sci. 1995;16:344–50.

Payne R, Pasternak GW. Pain. In: Johnston MV, Macdonald RL, Young AB, eds. Principles of drug therapy in neurology. Philadelphia: Davis; 1992:268–301.

Pleuvry BJ. Opioid receptors and their relevance to anaesthesia. Br J Anaesth. 1993;71:119–26.

Reisine T, Pasternak GW. Opioid analgesics and antagonists. In: Hardman JG, Limbird LE, eds. Goodman and Gilman's pharmacological basis of therapeutics, 9th edn. New York: McGraw-Hill; 1995:521–55.

Rosow C. Alfentanil. Semin Anesth. 1988;VII:107–12.

Standifer KM, Pasternak GW. G proteins and opioid receptor-mediated signalling. Cell Signal. 1997;9:237–48.

Chapter 32

Nonopioid analgesic and anti-inflammatory drugs

Ian Power

TOPICS COVERED IN THIS CHAPTER

- **Nonopioid analgesic and anti-inflammatory drugs and pain pathophysiology**
  - Acetaminophen (paracetamol)
- **Nonsteroidal anti-inflammatory drugs (NSAIDs)**
  - Cyclo-oxygenase isoenzymes (COX-1 and COX-2)
  - Efficacy
  - Adverse effects
  - Cyclo-oxygenase-2 selective inhibitors (COX-2 inhibitors)
- **Other nonopioid drugs used in pain management**
  - NMDA antagonists
  - α_2 adrenoceptor agonists
  - Tramadol
  - Anticonvulsants
  - Tricyclic antidepressants
  - Lidocaine
  - Steroids

Although opioids remain the basis for the treatment of postoperative pain, they have a number of important deficiencies that justify the use of alternative analgesics. Moreover, with the increasing emphasis on ambulatory surgery, with patients being discharged from hospital care so soon after surgery, it is impossible to rely on opioids alone for postoperative pain relief. Modern medical practice necessitates the use of alternative nonopioid analgesic and anti-inflammatory drugs to complement and sometimes replace opioids to improve analgesia, minimize side effects and facilitate acute rehabilitation. Our current understanding of the pathophysiology of pain is that multiple and diverse processes are involved at the site of tissue damage in the periphery, in the peripheral nerves, in the spinal cord, and in the brain, with powerful descending efferent modulating pathways being activated. Control of this complicated pathophysiological process requires the use of a range of pharmacological modalities, as in the use of balanced, or multimodal, analgesia. Analyses of the evidence for the safety and efficacy of drugs used to provide analgesia also support the use of approaches combining the use of nonopioids and opioids.

NONOPIOID ANALGESIC AND ANTI-INFLAMMATORY DRUGS AND PAIN PATHOPHYSIOLOGY

Pain is a multifactorial phenomenon that cannot be controlled with simple analgesic monotherapy, as neuronal pathways are not hard wired but are plastic and involve processes that signal and temporarily increase pain sensation after tissue damage. Unlike many sensations, pain does not accommodate with repetitive stimulation, but increases by the processes of peripheral and central sensitization (Chapter 23). Single-drug therapy is unlikely to be successful in modulating the nervous system response to tissue damage, as so many chemical and neuronal factors are involved. This becomes obvious upon consideration of the changes that occur after tissue damage at the periphery, in the primary nerve afferents, in the dorsal horn of the spinal cord, the important central pain pathways, and the descending modulating influences.

The nerve endings of Aδ mechanothermal and C polymodal nerve fibers are the receptors for painful stimuli, or nociceptors, and they normally have a high threshold for activation. Pain is produced by direct stimulation of these nerve endings, but the inflammatory response after tissue damage enhances their sensitivity to further stimuli and reduces their threshold for activation. Tissue damage releases many chemical factors, including bradykinin, histamine, substance P, prostaglandins, leukotrienes, purines, cytokines, 5-HT, neuropeptides, norepinephrine, nitric oxide, hydrogen ions, and potassium ions, forming an inflammatory soup that affects the nerve endings, converting them from 'high-threshold' to 'low-threshold' nociceptors. The inflammatory soup produces 'peripheral sensitization', where sensitivity is enhanced in the area of tissue damage so that now even low-intensity mechanical stimuli are sensed as pain. The afferent nerve axons are not simply electrical conductors of nociceptive information, but instead may contribute to the pain process. Nerve damage results in increased production of peptides, including nerve growth factor, which affect the response of other nerves to painful stimuli. The ends of damaged nerves also form sprouts, fire spontaneously, and become sensitive to norepinephrine.

A zone of secondary hyperalgesia develops in uninjured tissue after damage around the area of local primary sensitization. This is evidence of 'central sensitization', produced by changes in the dorsal horn of the spinal cord, the site of termination of the primary afferents. A painful stimulus not only activates dorsal horn neurons, but the neuronal response increases during the stimulus, with 'wind-up' of activity in the spinal cord neurons. The phenomenon of wind-up is dependent on activation of postsynaptic *N*-methyl-D-aspartate (NMDA) receptors, stimulated by the excitatory amino acid transmitter glutamate and antagonized by the nonopioid analgesic ketamine. Central sensitization produces an expansion of the receptive field of the dorsal horn neurons, a reduction in their threshold, and an increase in the intensity and duration of their response to stimuli.

This brief description of pain pathophysiology depending on changes at the receptor, the afferent nerve, and the dorsal horn of the spinal cord is presented to confirm that effective pain relief is unlikely to result simply from the administration of opioids alone. Instead, multimodal analgesia, utilizing other nonopioid agents that affect peripheral inflammation (anti-inflammatories), block afferent nerve activity (local anesthetics), and modulate central pain processes (NMDA antagonists, α_2 agonists, tricyclic antidepressants, and anticonvulsants) is needed. Moreover, 'neuropathic pain' (burning, stinging pain, perhaps with allodynia and dysesthesia, that responds poorly to usual doses of opioids) can present soon after tissue damage, requiring the use of specific, nonopioid analgesics. The remainder of this chapter describes the pharmacology of specific nonopioid analgesic and anti-inflammatory drugs.

Acetaminophen (paracetamol)

Acetaminophen is the active metabolite of the earlier, more toxic, drugs acetanilide and phenacetin. It can be given orally, rectally, or parenterally, has little anti-inflammatory activity, and is an effective analgesic and antipyretic (Fig. 32.1).

Acetaminophen is absorbed rapidly from the small intestine after oral administration, can be given rectally, and recently parenteral preparations have been introduced into clinical practice. Acetaminophen has lower protein binding (hence fewer potential drug interactions than nonsteroidal anti-inflammatory drugs, NSAIDs) and a higher volume of distribution than NSAIDs. The recommended dose in adults is 0.5–1 g orally or rectally every 3–6 hours when necessary, and a maximum of 6 g a day in divided doses for acute use and 4 g a day for chronic use.

The mechanism of action of acetaminophen is not well understood, but it may inhibit prostaglandin synthesis in the central nervous system, with few peripheral nervous system effects. Unlike morphine acetaminophen has no apparent binding sites, and unlike NSAIDs it does not inhibit peripheral cyclo-oxygenase activity. There is growing evidence of a central antinociceptive effect of acetaminophen. Postulated mechanisms include central COX-2 inhibition, inhibition of a central cyclo-oxygenase, COX-3, that is selectively susceptible to acetaminophen, and modulation of descending serotoninergic pathways that suppress spinal cord nociceptive transmission. Acetaminophen may also inhibit prostaglandin production at the cellular transcriptional level, independent of cyclo-oxygenase activity. Nitroacetaminophen is new potent nitric oxide-releasing version with anti-inflammatory and analgesic properties, with a described mechanism of action in the spinal cord that differs from that of acetaminophen.

EFFICACY

The efficacy of acetaminophen for the relief of severe pain after surgery has been confirmed by many studies. McQuay and Moore have enabled comparison of the efficacy of acetaminophen with other types of analgesic for acute pain relief after surgery by developing the concept of number needed to treat (NNT), using meta-analyses of well designed studies of postoperative analgesia (*www.jr2.ox.ac.uk/bandolier/booth/painpag/*). From such work, the NNT of acetaminophen is 3.8 (3.4–4.4); morphine 10 mg intramuscularly is 2.9; ibuprofen 400 mg 2.4; and codeine 60 mg 16.7. The combination of acetaminophen 1000 mg plus codeine 60 mg has a NNT of 2.2. Acetaminophen is therefore an effective analgesic, with potency somewhat less than a standard dose of morphine, or of the nonsteroidal anti-inflammatory drugs.

Acetaminophen is an effective adjunct to opioid analgesia, and regular administration can reduce opioid requirements by 20–30%. The addition of an NSAID to acetaminophen also improves efficacy. Therefore, acetaminophen is an integral component of multimodal analgesia in combination with NSAIDs and opioids. Intravenous acetaminophen has been shown to be an effective analgesic after surgery, although there is some evidence of a ceiling effect.

Acetaminophen is an effective adjunct to opioid analgesia, and regular administration can reduce opioid requirements by 20–30%

ADVERSE EFFECTS

Acetaminophen has fewer side effects than the NSAIDs and can be used when the latter are contraindicated (asthma, peptic ulcers, bleeding diathesis). However, acetaminophen overdose can produce severe liver damage. A small amount of acetaminophen undergoes cytochrome P450-mediated hydroxylation, producing a toxic metabolite that is normally rendered harmless by liver glutathione conjugation. With excessive doses the rate of reactive metabolite formation exceeds that of glutathione conjugation, and the result is centrilobular hepatocellular necrosis. Doses of more than 150 mg/kg taken within 24 hours may result in severe liver damage, hypoglycemia, and acute tubular necrosis. Individuals taking enzyme-inducing agents are more susceptible. Early signs include nausea and vomiting, with right subcostal pain and tenderness. Damage is maximal 3–4 days after ingestion, and may lead to death. Treatment includes gastric emptying and the administration of methionine or acetylcysteine. Plasma acetaminophen concentration versus time from ingestion indicates the risk of liver damage after overdose (acetylcysteine is given if the plasma acetaminophen concentration is greater than 200 mg/L at 4 hours and 6.25 mg/L at 24 hours after ingestion). In children the dose changes with age (6–12 years 250–500 mg 6-hourly), necessitating care to avoid inadvertent overdose. The new nitroxyacetaminophen may have less hepatic toxicity than the parent drug.

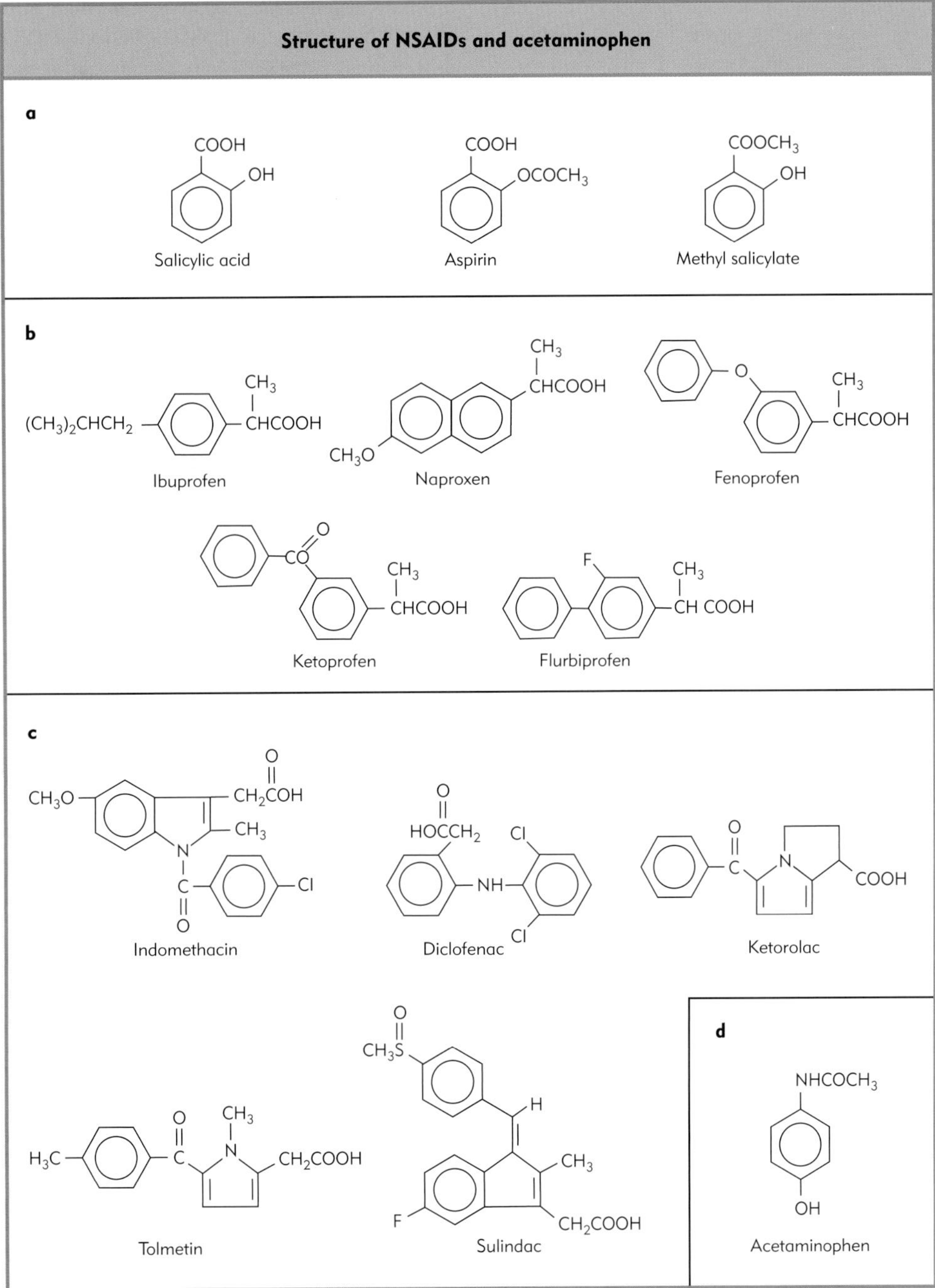

Figure 32.1 Chemical structures of NSAIDS and acetaminophen. a. Salicylates, b. arylpropionic acids, c. acetic acids, d. acetaminophen.

NONSTEROIDAL ANTI-INFLAMMATORY DRUGS (NSAIDs)

The introduction of injectable preparations of the 'aspirin-like' NSAIDs ketorolac, diclofenac, ketoprofen, and tenoxicam promised perioperative analgesia free from the opioid disadvantages of respiratory depression, sedation, nausea and vomiting, gastrointestinal stasis, or abuse potential. Extensive clinical investigation and the use of NSAIDs have confirmed that they are effective postoperative analgesics, but that they have significant contraindications and serious adverse effects. NSAIDs have a spectrum of analgesic, anti-inflammatory, and antipyretic effects.

NSAIDs are effective postoperative analgesics but have significant contraindications and serious adverse effects.

NSAID absorption is rapid by all routes of administration, whether enteral or by injection. The drugs are highly protein bound, have low volumes of distribution of the order of 0.1 L/kg, and the unbound fraction is active. Consequently, NSAIDs can potentiate the effects of other highly protein-bound drugs by displacing them from protein-binding sites (oral anticoagulants, oral hypoglycemics, sulphonamides, and anticonvulsants).

NSAIDs can potentiate the effects of other highly protein-bound drugs by displacing them from protein-binding sites.

Many of the effects of NSAIDs and aspirin are mediated by inhibition of prostaglandin synthesis in peripheral tissues, nerves, and the central nervous system. Aspirin acetylates and irreversibly inhibits cyclo-oxygenase, whereas NSAIDs act by competitive inhibition. However, the NSAIDs and aspirin may have other mechanisms of action independent of any effect on prostaglandins, including effects on basic cellular and neuronal processes.

Prostaglandins were initially described as locally active substances from the prostate gland that produced smooth muscle contraction. Many are now recognized, based on a 20-carbon chain molecule, being one family of the 'eicosanoids' ('eicosa' = Greek for '20'), oxygenated metabolites of arachidonic acid and other polyunsaturated fatty acids that include leukotrienes. The rate of prostaglandin synthesis is normally low, being regulated by tissue stimuli or trauma that activates phospholipases to free arachidonic acid, from which prostaglandins are produced by prostaglandin endoperoxide (PGH) synthase, which has both cyclo-oxygenase and hydroperoxidase enzymatic sites. Prostaglandins have many physiological functions, including gastric mucosal protection, maintenance of renal tubular function and renal vasodilatation, and bronchodilation; endothelial prostacyclin produces vasodilatation and prevents platelet adhesion, and platelet thromboxane produces aggregation and vessel spasm (Fig. 32.2).

Two subtypes of cyclo-oxygenase enzyme ('constitutional' COX-1, and 'inducible' COX-2) have been identified. NSAIDs, like aspirin, are 'nonselective' cyclo-oxygenase inhibitors that inhibit both COX-1 and COX-2. New 'COX-2 inhibitors' have been developed, and these inhibit selectively the inducible form.

Nonselective COX-1 and COX-2 inhibition confers both the analgesic and the adverse (peptic ulceration, renal impairment, bleeding and aspirin induced asthma) effect profile of NSAIDs.

Cyclo-oxygenase isoenzymes (COX-1 and COX-2)

The COX enzyme was first isolated in 1976, but more recently isoenzymes have been isolated. The two isolated COX isoenzymes have 75% amino acid homology with complete preservation of the catalytic sites for cyclo-oxygenase and peroxidase activity, with almost identical enzyme kinetics.

COX-1 is a membrane-bound hemoglycoprotein with a molecular weight of 71 kilodaltons (kDa) found in the endo-

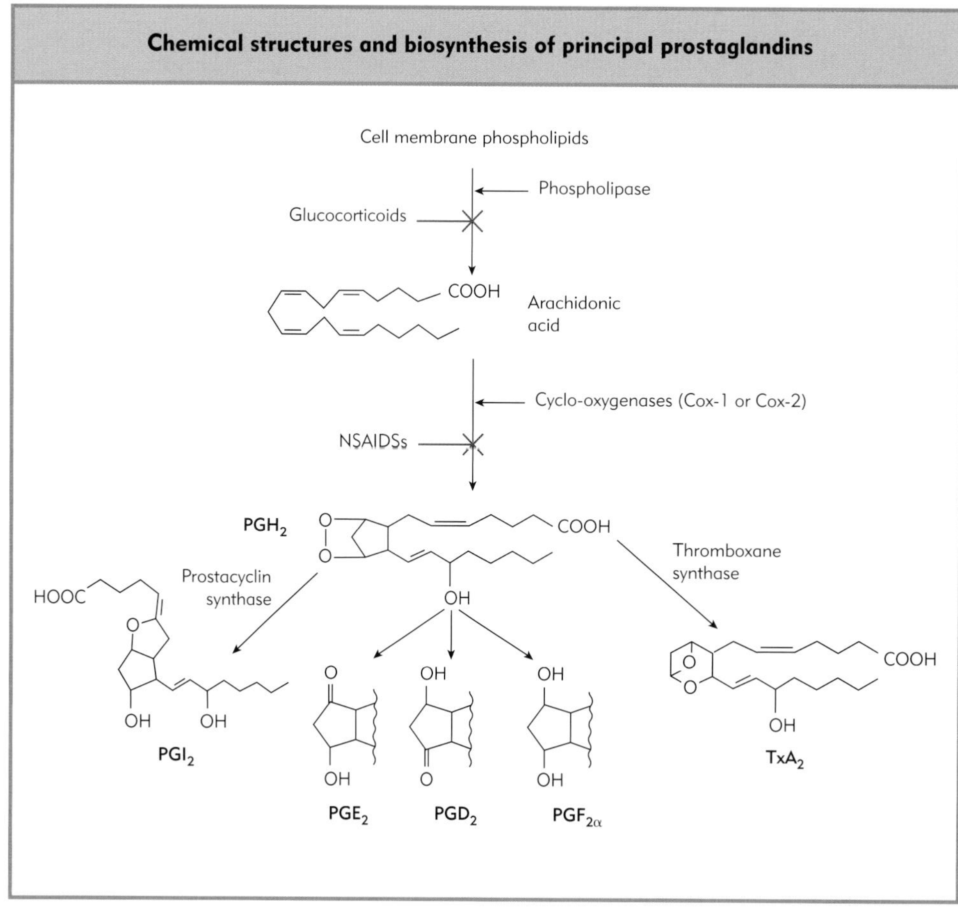

Figure 32.2 Chemical structures and biosynthesis of principal prostaglandins. Endoperoxide PGH_2 differs from PGI_2 (prostacyclin), PGE_2, PGD_2, and $PGF_{2\alpha}$. (TX, thromboxane).

plasmic reticulum of prostaglandin-producing cells. The enzyme cyclizes arachidonic acid and then adds a 15-hydroperoxy group to form the endoperoxide PGG_2, which is then reduced to the hydroxy form of PGH_2 by a peroxidase in the same COX enzyme protein. The COX–1 isoenzyme integrates into only a single leaflet of the lipid bilayer, and this is described as a 'monotopic' arrangement. The enzyme has three independent folding units: an epidermal growth factor-like domain, a membrane-binding domain, and an enzymatic domain. The α-helices of the membrane-binding domains form a channel entrance to the active site, are inserted into the membrane, and thereby allow arachidonic acid to gain access to the interior of the lipid bilayer. The sites for cyclo-oxygenase and peroxidase activity are spatially distinct but adjacent to each other. The COX active site is a long hydrophobic channel with tyrosine 385 and serine 530 at the apex. NSAIDs block COX-1 halfway down the channel by hydrogen bonding to the polar arginine at position 120 (reversible). Aspirin acetylates serine 530, irreversibly preventing access for arachidonic acid.

COX-2 has a molecular weight of 70 kDa with similar sites to COX-1 for the attachment of arachidonic acid, and a similar three-dimensional structure to COX-1. However, its active site has a greater volume, because it has a larger central channel with a wider entrance and a secondary internal pocket. Therefore, COX-2 can accommodate larger drugs than COX-1. A single amino acid difference at position 523 is critical for COX-1 and COX-2 selectivity of the NSAID. In COX-2 a valine molecule replaces the isoleucine molecule present at position 523 in COX-1. This valine molecule is smaller (by one methyl group) and produces a gap in the wall of the channel, giving access to a side pocket, which is the binding site of the COX-2-selective inhibitors. The larger isoleucine at position 523 in COX-1 blocks access of drug molecules to the side pocket.

The genes for the two isoenzymes are found on different chromosomes: chromosome 9 for COX-1 and chromosome 1 for COX-2. Under physiological conditions COX-1 activity predominates to produce prostaglandins that regulate rapid physiological responses such as vascular homeostasis, gastric function, platelet activity, and renal function. The concentration of the COX-1 isoenzyme is low, but this may increase two- to fourfold in response to stimulation by hormones or growth factors. Low concentrations of COX-2 can normally be detected in the brain, the kidney, and the gravid uterus. COX-2 mRNA expression by monocytes, synovial cells, and fibroblasts may be increased 10–80-fold when stimulated by growth factors, cytokines, bacterial lipopolysaccharides, or phorbol esters. These factors increase COX-2 production and tissue PGE_2 concentrations, resulting in pain and inflammation.

Efficacy

The efficacy of single-dose NSAIDs as postoperative analgesics has been examined and confirmed by many studies. The NNT of ketorolac 10 mg is 2.6, that of diclofenac 50 mg 2.3, and ibuprofen 400 mg 2.4. For comparison the NNT of morphine 10 mg intramuscularly is 2.9, and codeine 60 mg 16.7. Individual studies have confirmed that NSAIDs are effective postoperative analgesics and, when given in combination with opioids, produce better analgesia and reduce opioid consumption by 25–50%. NSAIDs are insufficient for sole use to relieve very severe pain immediately after major surgery, although they are very useful analgesic adjuncts, improving pain relief while reducing opioid requirements. They are of considerable value in day-case surgery, where they can be given by injection at the time of surgery and then continued by mouth after discharge from hospital.

NSAIDs are effective postoperative analgesics, and when given in combination with opioids produce better analgesia and reduce opioid consumption by 25–50%.

Adverse effects

Prostaglandins are local tissue hormones that regulate function, and interference with their synthesis can produce problems. With acute use the main concerns are the potential to produce peptic ulceration, interference with platelets, renal impairment and bronchospasm in individuals who have 'aspirin-induced asthma'. In general, the risk and severity of NSAID-associated side effects increases with age.

The main adverse effects of NSAIDs are the potential to cause peptic ulceration, interference with platelets, renal impairment, and bronchospasm in individuals who have 'aspirin-induced asthma'.

The gastric and duodenal epithelia have protective mechanisms against acid and enzyme attack involving prostaglandin production, and chronic NSAID use is associated with peptic ulceration and bleeding. One meta-analysis has estimated the risk of perforations, ulcers, and bleeds associated with NSAID use, finding that the pooled relative risk from nine cohort studies comprising over 750 000 person-years of exposure was 2.7 (95% CI: 2.1, 3.5). Unfortunately, acute gastroduodenal damage and bleeding can occur with short-term NSAID use. Concerning ketorolac, a postmarketing surveillance study concluded that the risk of gastrointestinal hemorrhage was small but increased with the use of higher doses, in older subjects, and with use for more than 5 days.

Platelet cyclo-oxygenase is essential for the production of the cyclic endoperoxides and thromboxane A_2 that mediate vasoconstriction and platelet aggregation, the primary hemostatic response to vessel injury. Aspirin acetylates cyclo-oxygenase irreversibly, but NSAIDs inhibit platelet cyclo-oxygenase in a reversible fashion. Single doses of NSAIDs such as ketorolac and diclofenac inhibit platelet function (prolong skin bleeding time and inhibit platelet function in vitro), but do not tend to increase surgical blood loss in normal patients. However, the presence of a subclinical bleeding diathesis, or the administration of anticoagulants, may increase the risk of significant surgical blood loss when NSAIDs are given.

Renal prostaglandins have important physiological roles, including the maintenance of blood flow and glomerular filtration, regulation of tubular electrolyte handling, and modulation of the actions of renal hormones. The adverse renal effects of chronic NSAID use are well recognized. In certain clinical settings where there are high plasma concentrations of the vasoconstrictors renin, angiotensin, norepinephrine, and vasopressin, intrarenal vasodilators, including prostacyclin, are produced and renal function can then be impaired by NSAID administration. The co-administration of other potential nephrotoxins, such as gentamicin, may increase the renal effect of NSAIDs. Nevertheless, with careful patient selection and monitoring the incidence of NSAID-induced renal impairment in the perioperative period is low.

Precipitation of bronchospasm is a recognized phenomenon in individuals with asthma, chronic rhinitis, and nasal polyps. Such 'aspirin-induced asthma' affects 10–15% of asthmatics, can be severe, and features cross-sensitivity with NSAIDs. A history of aspirin-induced asthma is a contraindication to NSAID use after surgery, although there is no reason to avoid NSAIDs in other asthmatics. The mechanism is unclear, but the reaction increases with cyclo-oxygenase inhibitor potency. Cyclo-oxygenase inhibition may increase the availability of arachidonic acid for the production of inflammatory leukotrienes by lipo-oxygenase pathways. Aspirin-induced asthma is less common in children, and the susceptibility may be established in adult life by viral illness.

There is some suggestion that bone healing can be affected by NSAIDs. Prostaglandin production is involved in animal models of bone healing, but there is little research evidence that this putative inhibitory effect of NSAIDs is important clinically.

Cyclo-oxygenase-2 selective inhibitors (COX-2 inhibitors)

New drugs have been developed that selectively inhibit the inducible cyclo-oxygenase enzyme COX-2, and spare the constitutive enzyme COX-1 (see above). The COX-2 inhibitors currently available include meloxicam, nimesulide, celecoxib, valdecoxib, and parecoxib, the injectable valdecoxib precursor (Fig. 32.3). Rofecoxib has recently been withdrawn by the manufacturer. By sparing physiological tissue prostaglandin production while inhibiting inflammatory prostaglandin release, COX-2 inhibitors offer the potential of effective analgesia with fewer side effects than the NSAIDs.

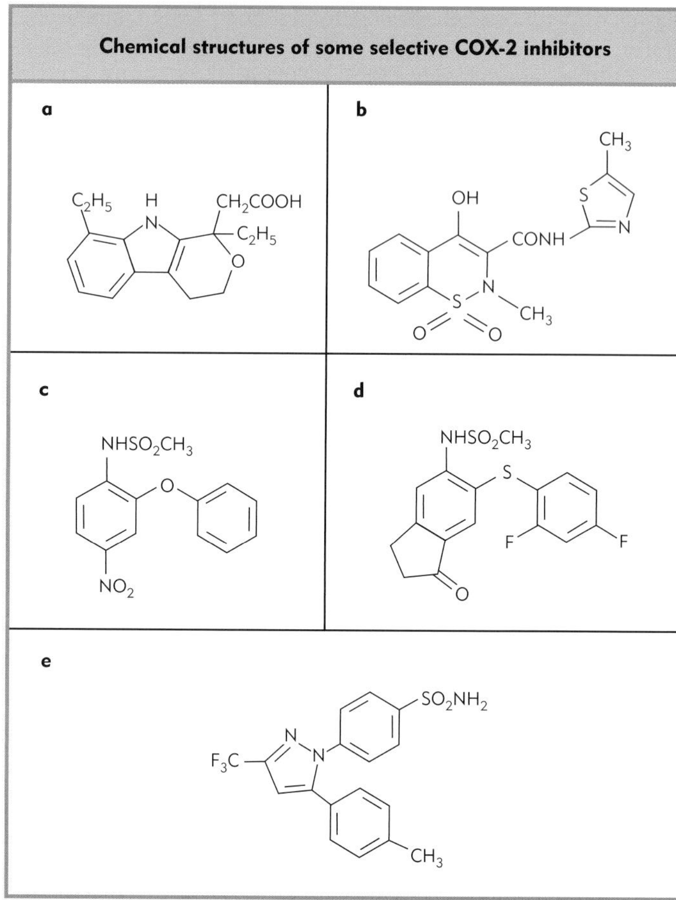

Figure 32.3 Chemical structures of some selective COX-2 inhibitors. a. Etodolac, b. meloxicam, c. nimesulide, d. L-745,337, and e. celecoxib.

EFFICACY

Extensive clinical studies have confirmed that COX-2 inhibitors can produce effective analgesia for moderate to severe acute pain, as after surgery, similar to that of NSAIDs. Quoted NNTs are comparable to those for conventional NSAIDs: celecoxib 200 mg 4.5; rofecoxib 50 mg 2.3; parecoxib 20 mg IV 3.0; parecoxib 40 mg IV 2.2; valdecoxib 20 mg 1.7.

ADVERSE EFFECTS

Large outcome studies have demonstrated that COX-2 inhibitors produce less clinically significant peptic ulceration than NSAIDs. It has been estimated that the number of patients needed to treat with COX-2 inhibitors in preference to NSAIDs to avert one clinical event in one year is 40–100. However, peptic ulceration remains a significant adverse effect of the COX-2 inhibitors, and there is continuing debate on their role in patients who have other risk factors for complicated ulcer disease: the elderly, those taking aspirin or corticosteroids, those with a previous ulcer, or those with *Helicobacter pylori* infection.

Platelets do not produce COX-2 but only COX-1, and so COX-2-selective inhibitors do not impair platelet function. Clinical studies have confirmed the lack of an antiplatelet effect of COX-2 inhibitors, and a reduction in surgical blood loss in comparison to NSAIDs. The question has been raised whether COX-2 inhibitors can produce a tendency to thrombosis, because they inhibit endothelial prostacyclin production while sparing platelet function. Indeed, some outcome studies of peptic ulceration have demonstrated a lower incidence of thrombotic episodes in patients given naproxen rather than a COX-2 inhibitor, and this is the reason for the withdrawal of rofecoxib.

COX-2 is resident, or constitutive, in some tissues, including the kidneys, and current opinion holds that COX-2 inhibitors have similar adverse effects on renal function to conventional NSAIDs.

Recent work in patients known to suffer from aspirin-induced asthma has provided encouraging evidence that COX-2 inhibitors do not produce bronchospasm in such individuals when administered at analgesic doses.

At present the effect of COX-2 on bone healing, as with NSAIDs, remains a potential effect demonstrated under specific laboratory conditions, but with little evidence as yet of clinical importance.

OTHER NONOPIOID DRUGS USED IN PAIN MANAGEMENT

NMDA antagonists

The activation by excitatory amino acids (glutamate) of spinal cord dorsal horn *N*-methyl-D-aspartate (NMDA) receptors is essential for the development of central sensitization after tissue damage. The anesthetic agent ketamine is a potent NMDA receptor antagonist, and relatively low-dose ketamine given by subcutaneous or intravenous continuous infusion (5–15 mg/h) produces significant pain relief. When combined with opioids, ketamine improves analgesia and reduces side effects. Unfortunately, the side effects of ketamine, including hallucinations, limit its use. A notable advantage of ketamine is that it is effective for both nociceptive and neuropathic pain, which presents as burning stinging pain with allodynia and dysesthesias. Ketamine can be of particular benefit in clinical situations where the pain may be of a mixed nociceptive and neuropathic nature (e.g. severe burns, or cancer pain with nerve involvement). Dextromethorphan, a component of cough mixtures, is an alternative, although less potent, NMDA receptor antagonist that has been shown to reduce opioid requirements following oral or abdominal surgery.

α_2 adrenoceptor agonists

The α_2 adrenoceptor agonists clonidine and dexmedetomidine have been shown to provide effective analgesia after a variety of surgical procedures. Their use has concentrated on the spinal or epidural administration of clonidine to take advantage of the known attenuating effect of stimulating spinal α_2-receptors on pain perception. In general, α_2 agonists are useful only as adjuncts to conventional opioid analgesics because of the side effects of sedation, hypotension, and bradycardia, which can be marked. Epidural administration has been shown to be more effective than the systemic route, supporting the theory that clonidine acts via spinal α_2-receptors. Indeed, high-dose epidural clonidine (8 μg/kg bolus and then 2 μg/kg/h) has been successfully used as a sole analgesic following major abdominal surgery, but with a significant incidence of sedation and hypotension. There is some evidence that systemic clonidine administration may have some analgesic effect. Clonidine, when given orally as a premedication (5 μg/kg), reduces both the requirements for postoperative morphine and the incidence of nausea and vomiting. Clonidine is useful in the treatment of neuropathic pain, and can also be used to modify opioid withdrawal states. In addition, spinal infusions of clonidine with opioids and local anesthetic agents may be of considerable benefit in the treatment of complex regional pain syndromes (CRPS).

Tramadol

Tramadol is a centrally acting analgesic with a unique, dual mechanism of action – it exerts agonistic properties at opioid receptors and interferes with neurotransmitter reuptake. Tramadol inhibits the reuptake of the natural neurotransmitters norepinephrine (noradrenaline) and serotonin, and also binds weakly to μ-opioid receptors, blocking the transmission of pain signals to the brain. Tramadol's only active metabolite, O-demethyltramadol has greater affinity for μ-opioid receptors than does tramadol. The μ-opioid receptor antagonist naloxone only partially blocks the effect of tramadol on nociceptive activity.

Anticonvulsants

Anticonvulsants are useful for the alleviation of neuropathic pain. Drugs used include carbamazepine, phenytoin, sodium valproate, and the newer agents gabapentin, lamotrigine, and vigabatrin. Suggested mechanisms of action include frequency-dependent block of sodium channels, calcium channel blockade, and potentiation of GABA inhibition of spinal nociceptive pathways via increased release or reduced breakdown. Meta-analyses of clinical studies have demonstrated that anticonvulsants are effective for neuropathic pain, but with frequent adverse effects. For example, the NNT for carbamazepine for trigeminal neuralgia is 2.6, whereas the number needed to harm (NNH) is only 3.4 patients. Therefore, the effectiveness of anticonvulsants for neuropathic pain must be balanced against their adverse effects, which may be serious. Common side effects include sedation, rashes, nausea, anorexia, dizziness, confusion, and ataxia. Serious side effects are blood dyscrasias, subacute hepatic impairment, renal failure, and Stevens–Johnson syndrome. Newer agents such as gabapentin offer the potential of similar efficacy with an improved safety profile, but gabapentin does produce the significant adverse effects of pancreatitis, altered liver function tests and Stevens–Johnson syndrome.

Tricyclic antidepressants

The tricyclic antidepressants used to relieve neuropathic pain all potentiate noradrenergic activity by inhibiting norepinephrine reuptake at nerve endings, probably in descending modulatory inhibitory pain pathways. The antidepressants have similar NNT and NNH to the anticonvulsants and are again effective for the relief of neuropathic pain, but with the cost of common side effects, many related to a vagolytic effect. Some tricyclic side effects are transitory, such as dry mouth and sedation, but others are serious, including postural hypotension, urinary retention, narrow angle glaucoma, paralytic ileus, and cardiac arrhythmias. The elderly are particularly susceptible to side effects when given tricyclic antidepressants. Unfortunately, newer antidepressants with a better side effect profile have not been shown to be as effective for the treatment of neuropathic pain.

Lidocaine

The amide local anesthetic lidocaine can be a very useful diagnostic test and treatment for neuropathic pain. The dose is 0.5–1.5 mg/kg/h by subcutaneous or intravenous infusion, and may be continued for a number of days to control neuropathic pain quickly before long-term oral therapy is instituted if required.

Steroids

The role of corticosteroids as analgesics is limited to short-term relief of neuropathic pain where nerve compression is a feature.

SUMMARY

There is good evidence that patients suffering acute pain benefit from the use of multimodal or balanced analgesia whereby opioids, local anesthetics, and other nonopioid analgesics are combined to improve pain relief and minimize side effects. In this way acetaminophen, NSAIDs or COX-2 inhibitors are used in clinical practice in combination with opioids and local anesthetic agents for neuronal blockade to provide the best evidenced-based approach to the relief of acute pain. In certain circumstances the nonopioids ketamine and clonidine may also confer specific advantages in managing acute pain. For chronic pain, anticonvulsants and antidepressants are used in combination with opioids for many pain states, and NSAIDs and COX-2 inhibitors with due consideration of its cardiovascular side-effects are in common use for chronic joint pain. Acute neuropathic pain, as after surgery or trauma, is now being recognized early, and may be controlled with ketamine or lidocaine by infusion before long-term anticonvulsant or tricyclic antidepressant therapy is commenced.

Key references

Bonnefont J, Courade JP et al. Mechanism of the antinociceptive effect of paracetamol. Drugs 2003;63:1–4.

Cousins MJ, Power I. Acute and postoperative pain. Handbook of Pain Management. Melzack R and Wall PD, Churchill Livingstone: 2003;13,30.

Hawkey CJ, Skelly MM. Gastrointestinal safety of selective COX-2 inhibitors. Current Pharmaceutical Design 8(12): 2002;1077–89.

Jaquenod M, Ronnedh C et al. Factors influencing ketorolac-associated perioperative renal dysfunction. Anesthesia Analgesia 1998;86:1090–7.

Kam PCA, Power I. New Selective Cox-2 Inhibitors. Pain Reviews 2000;7(1):3–13.

Keeble JE and Moore PK. Pharmacology and potential therapeutic applications of nitric oxide-releasing non-steroidal anti-inflammatory and related nitric oxide-donating drugs. British Journal of Pharmacology 2002;137(3):295–310.

Lee ACM, Craig JC, Knight JF, Keneally JP. Effects of nonsteroidal anti-inflammatory drugs on post-operative renal function in normal adults (Cochrane Review). In: The Cochrane Library. Chichester, UK: John Wiley & Sons, Ltd(1); 2004.

NHMRC. Acute pain management: scientific evidence. Canberra, Australia., National Health and Medical Research Council; 1999.

Ofman JJ, MacLean CH et al. A metaanalysis of severe upper gastrointestinal complications of nonsteroidal antiinflammatory drugs. Journal of Rheumatology 2002;29(4):804–12.

Strom BL, Berlin JA et al. Parenteral ketorolac and risk of gastrointestinal and operative site bleeding, a postmarketing surveillance study. Journal of the American Medical Association 1996;275(5):376–82.

Szczeklik A, Stevenson DD. Aspirin-induced asthma: Advances in pathogenesis, diagnosis, and management. Journal of Allergy and Clinical immunology 2003;111(5):913–21.

Warner TD, Mitchell JA. Cyclooxygenase-3 (COX-3): Filling in the gaps toward a COX continuum? Proceedings of the National Academy of Sciences of the United States of America 2002;99(21):13371–3.

Chapter 33

Pharmacology of local anesthetics

Thomas S McDowell and Marcel E Durieux

TOPICS COVERED IN THIS CHAPTER

- **Chemistry of local anesthetics**
  - Structures of local anesthetics
  - Physicochemical properties
- **Mechanisms of action**
  - Blockade of neuronal voltage-gated Na^+ channels
  - Differential block
  - Interactions with G protein-coupled receptor systems
  - Molecular mechanisms of local anesthetic-GPCR interactions
- **Local anesthetic pharmacokinetics**
  - Effect site concentration
  - Absorption and metabolism
- **Local anesthetic toxicity**
  - Anaphylaxis
  - Systemic toxicity
  - Neurotoxicity
  - Methemoglobinemia

This chapter covers the pharmacology of the local anesthetics, including their mechanisms of action, metabolism and excretion, and toxicities. The 'classic' action of these versatile compounds, namely blockade of axonal conduction, is mediated by actions on voltage-gated Na^+ channels, and this mechanism will be described in detail. It has become increasingly clear that these compounds affect other signaling systems as well. Interactions with G protein-coupled receptors in particular may be responsible for a number of beneficial effects of the compounds.

CHEMISTRY OF LOCAL ANESTHETICS

Structures of local anesthetics

All local anesthetics used clinically contain three major structural features (Table 33.1). These are a hydrophobic end containing an aromatic ring; an aliphatic end, which usually contains a tertiary amine (exceptions include prilocaine, which contains a secondary amine, and benzocaine, containing no amine groups); and either an ester or an amide linkage between the two ends. The type of linkage determines the route of metabolism. As a memory aid, local anesthetics with amide linkages are spelled with two 'i's, whereas those with ester linkages are spelled with only one 'i'.

Cocaine was the first local anesthetic to be used clinically. In the late 1800s it was employed for topical anesthesia and later for neuraxial and peripheral nerve blocks, despite its side effects and toxicity. Procaine was synthesized in the early 1900s and for almost 50 years was the most widely used local anesthetic, until the introduction in 1948 of lidocaine, the first amide local anesthetic. Lidocaine is still the most versatile and the most widely used of these compounds. It is used intravenously as an antiarrhythmic drug and as a supplement to general anesthesia, injected for regional anesthesia in the form of peripheral and neuraxial blocks, and as a topical anesthetic on both mucosal surfaces and keratinized skin, applied as either a solution, gel, ointment, or patch. Bupivacaine, introduced in 1963, is valued for its longer duration of action than lidocaine and its propensity to preferentially block sensory fibers while sparing motor fibers, particularly at low concentrations. Unfortunately, bupivacaine is highly cardiotoxic, which limits its use. Ropivacaine, formulated as a pure S(–) enantiomer, and the S(–) enantiomer of bupivacaine, levobupivacaine, retain the favorable properties of bupivacaine with less cardiac toxicity.

Local anesthetic lipid solubility correlates with potency and duration of action.

A number of other compounds have the ability to block Na^+ channels, and therefore act as local anesthetics. Some of these are of potential clinical interest, as they may allow other modes of administration or have a prolonged duration of action. Mexilitine is an orally available local anesthetic and is used in chronic pain therapy. Tricyclic antidepressant drugs, such as amitriptyline, are potent neuronal Na^+ channel blockers with half-times measured in hours, compared to minutes for lidocaine. They are being studied as long-acting local anesthetics to provide nerve blockade of much longer duration (up to days). Concerns about neuronal toxicity have been raised, however, and it is not clear whether these compounds will ultimately be useful for this application. Derivatives (such as *N*-phenylethyl-amitriptyline and *N*-methyl-amitriptyline) are also under investigation.

Table 33.1 Structures and properties of local anesthetics

	Structure	pKa	Partition Coefficient	Potency (procaine=1)	Speed of onset	Duration of action
Esters						
Cocaine		-	-	2	Fast	Medium
Procaine	$H_2N-C_6H_4-C(=O)-OCH_2CH_2-N(C_2H_5)_2$	9.1	1.7	1	Slow	Short
Tetracaine	$H_9C_4(H)N-C_6H_4-C(=O)-OCH_2CH_2-N(CH_3)_2$	8.6	221	8	Slow	Long
Benzocaine	$H_2N-C_6H_4-C(=O)-OC_2H_5$	-	-	-	Fast	Short
2-Chloroprocaine	$H_2N-C_6H_3(Cl)-C(=O)-O-CH_2-CH_2-N(C_2H_5)_2$	9.3	9.0	1	Fast	Short
Amides						
Lidocaine	$(CH_3)_2C_6H_3-NH-C(=O)-CH_2-N(C_2H_5)_2$	8.2	43	2	Fast	Medium
Mepivacaine		7.9	21	2	Fast	Medium
Bupivacaine		8.2	346	8	Medium	Long
Ropivacaine		8.2	115	6	Medium	Long
Prilocaine	$CH_3C_6H_4-NH-C(=O)-CH(CH_3)-NH-C_3H_7$	8.0	25	2	Fast	Long
Etidocaine	$(CH_3)_2C_6H_3-NH-C(=O)-CH(C_2H_5)-N(C_2H_5)(C_3H_7)$	8.1	115	6	Medium	Long

Adapted from Strichartz GR et al. Fundamental properties of local anesthetics. II. Measured octanol:buffer partition coefficients and pKa values of clinically used drugs. Anesth Anal. 1990 Aug;71(2):158-70.

Physicochemical properties

All local anesthetics are lipophilic, owing to the presence of an aromatic ring in their structures. Lipid solubility, assessed quantitatively by the relative solubility in octanol compared with solubility in an aqueous solution, varies widely among different local anesthetics, however. The degree of lipid solubility correlates with the potency of a local anesthetic as well as the duration of clinical action. The increased potency may be explained by the fact that more lipid-soluble local anesthetics are better able to pass through hydrophobic barriers such as the myelin sheath and the cell membrane to reach their sites of action (see below). Increased duration of action may be due to increased storage in local tissues, such as fat and muscle, at the site of injection, thus leading to less absorption and uptake into the bloodstream and removal from the site of action.

Tertiary amine groups make local anesthetics weak bases, with pK_a values ranging from around 8 to 9. This means that at physiological pH (~7.4) most local anesthetic molecules are protonated, and therefore have a net positive charge. Because local anesthetics must be able to pass through hydrophobic environments to reach their site of action (see below), compounds with a lower pK_a (and thus with a greater fraction of molecules in the more lipid-soluble uncharged form at a given pH) gain access to the cell more easily. Once inside the cell, the molecules are probably reprotonated. The charged form of most local anesthetics is more potent at blocking the Na^+ channel (see below).

Commercial preparations of local anesthetics are usually formulated as the hydrochloride (HCl) salts to improve the aqueous solubility and stability of the drug. These solutions are quite acidic, with pH ranging from 3 to 7. Sodium bicarbonate is often added to local anesthetic solutions prior to use to raise their pH, thereby increasing the fraction of uncharged local anesthetic molecules and theoretically improving the speed of onset or the duration of the block. The addition of bicarbonate may also reduce the pain felt during injection of the local anesthetic, which is due in part to the acidity of the solution. Conversely, local anesthetics are less effective when injected into inflamed tissues, which may be due in part to the acidity of the extracellular fluid in this setting (pH ~6.5–7.0) causing more of the drug molecules to be protonated. Inflamed tissues also have increased local blood flow, which may decrease local anesthetic tissue concentrations by increasing absorption into the blood.

MECHANISMS OF ACTION

Blockade of neuronal voltage-gated Na^+ channels

Local anesthetics are used primarily to block conduction in peripheral nerve axons and their terminals. Blockade of sensory fibers produces localized analgesia and anesthesia, whereas blockade of motor fibers produces localized immobility, and blockade of sympathetic fibers produces a localized sympathectomy with vasodilation, anhidrosis, and other sympatholytic effects. Local anesthetics prevent nerve conduction in axons primarily by blocking voltage-gated Na^+ channels, ion channels that cause rapid depolarization during the first phase of the action potential in excitable cells (see Chapter 19). Local anesthetics also block voltage-gated Ca^{2+} channels and various types of K^+ channels, which may modulate Na^+ channel block or otherwise alter neuronal excitability.

Na^+ channels are normally closed at the resting membrane potential (–60 to –80 mV). When activated by a small depolarization, they open rapidly to cause the upstroke of the action potential. The channels then rapidly inactivate, limiting the depolarization and giving the action potential its characteristic brief time course (along with K^+ channel activation). Subsequent depolarizations cannot open the channel from its inactivated state; it must undergo a conformational change to return to the closed state from the inactivated state before it is reprimed to open again. Repriming only occurs at negative membrane potentials.

Local anesthetics block nerve conduction by inhibiting voltage-gated Na^+ channels at an intracellular site, probably within the pore of the channel.

Early insights into the molecular mechanisms of Na^+ channel block by local anesthetics came from experiments performed by Strichartz over 30 years ago. He showed that two quaternary ammonium derivatives of lidocaine, QX-314 and QX-222, which unlike lidocaine each carry a permanent positive charge, did not inhibit Na^+ channel currents in nerve axons when applied to the bath, but produced a profound block when applied to the axoplasm. This indicates that local anesthetics act at an intracellular site that the charged molecules cannot access when applied outside the nerve axon. He also showed that these lidocaine analogs showed little inhibition on the first test depolarization used to open the Na^+ channels, but that inhibition increased cumulatively with subsequent depolarizations (Fig. 33.1). Because

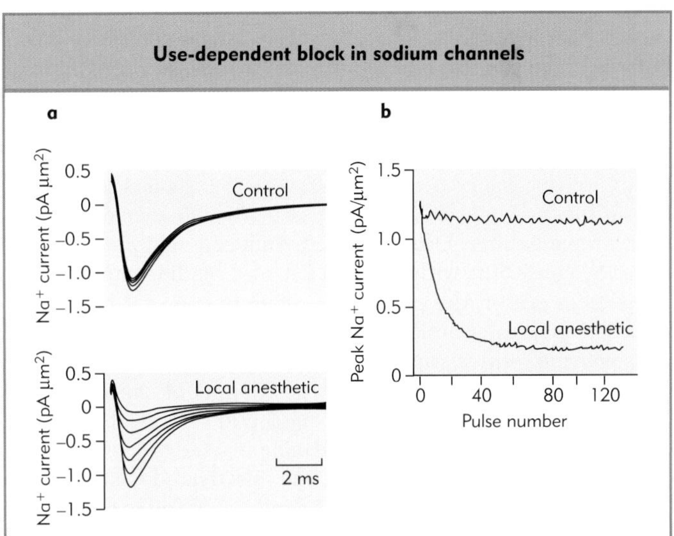

Figure 33.1 Phasic block of voltage-gated Na^+ currents by local anesthetics. Na^+ currents (I_{Na}) were measured in isolated canine cardiac Purkinje cells by the patch clamp technique during a train of voltage steps from –150 mV to 0 mV at a frequency of 10 Hz. Panel A shows current traces at various times during the pulse train in control conditions (top) and during intracellular perfusion of a permanently charged lidocaine analog (QX222). In the presence of QX222, I_{Na} decreased progressively during the pulse train. In panel B, peak current amplitudes are plotted against pulse number in the train. (Reproduced from The Journal of General Physiology, 1994, 103, 19–43. By permission of The Rockefeller University Press.)

the magnitude of inhibition was small at rest but increased when the Na^+ channel was opened, the binding site for the lidocaine analogs was theorized to be within the pore of the channel, and therefore not accessible when the channel was in the closed state. This type of inhibition became known as 'use-dependent' or phasic block, whereas inhibition after holding the channel closed for long periods was termed tonic block. Subsequently, the terms 'guarded receptor hypothesis' or 'modulated receptor hypothesis' have been suggested. These theories maintain that local anesthetics bind preferentially to channels that are either open or inactivated, either because they are hindered from accessing their site when the channel is closed (the site is 'guarded'), or because they may bind to the closed state of the channel with lower affinity (the site is 'modulated' by the channel conformation). Local anesthetics, once bound to the channel, stabilize and prolong the duration of the inactivated state, thus preventing Na^+ channel opening during further depolarizations.

As more is learned about the molecular structure of the voltage-gated Na^+ channel, the local anesthetic binding site has been explored in greater detail. The Na^+ channel is a heteromer composed of a large pore-forming α subunit and smaller auxiliary β subunits. The α subunit is composed of nearly 2000 amino acids arranged in four homologous domains (I–IV), each consisting of six membrane-spanning α-helical segments (S1–S6) that coalesce to form the pore of the channel (Fig. 33.2). The S6 segments of each domain are thought to line the channel pore. Short segments of the protein linking the S5 and S6 segments at the extracellular surface in all four domains line the outer rim of the pore and form the selectivity filter that keeps the channel from conducting ions other than Na^+ when it is opened. The S4 segments in all four domains, which contain a large number of positively charged amino acids, are probably the sensor by which the channel detects changes in transmembrane voltage. These voltage sensors move in response to changes in the membrane electric field which induces conformational changes in the protein that initiate channel gating. The short cytoplasmic linker between domains III and IV is important for fast inactivation of the channel.

Selective site-directed mutation of individual amino acid residues in Na^+ channel α subunits has revealed information about how local anesthetics interact with the channel to produce phasic block. Mutations of residues in the S6 segments of all four domains alter local anesthetic-induced inhibition of the channel, consistent with the concept of a binding site for local anesthetics within the pore. In α subunits from rat brain (Na_v 1.2 channels), three amino acids in the S6 segment of domain IV, an isoleucine residue at position 1760, a phenylalanine residue at position 1764, and a tyrosine at position 1771, appear to be particularly important for local anesthetic effects (Fig. 33.2). Mutating phenylalanine 1764 to alanine markedly decreased the affinity of local anesthetics for the inactivated state of the channel. This mutation, as well as similar mutations at residues 1760 and 1771, also decreased the ability of local anesthetics to induce phasic block. The isoleucine at position 1760, which is at the extracellular end of the putative local anesthetic binding site, appears to act like a stopper within the pore, preventing local anesthetics from accessing their binding site from the extracellular side of the channel. Changing the isoleucine at this position to an alanine increased the rate of local anesthetic washout from the site, and also allowed the permanently charged QX-314 molecule to block the channel when applied extracellularly. These and other mutations of the S6 segments, however, also have significant effects on channel gating even in the absence of a local anesthetic, making definitive conclusions about the local anesthetic binding site impossible.

Differential block

After peripheral nerve or neuraxial blocks, motor function is often resistant to local anesthetics or returns to normal sooner than sensory function. In addition, low concentrations of epidural local anesthetics are frequently used in the postoperative period to selectively reduce pain sensations but preserve motor function. Based on clinical observations like these, as well as some early experiments in animals and isolated nerves, it has been suggested that local anesthetics produce a differential block of nerve axons based on size, with small, slowly conducting sensory nerve axons (Aδ myelinated and C unmyelinated fibers) being more susceptible than large, fast-conducting motor axons (Aα myelinated fibers). More careful analysis reveals that this 'size principle' only appears to be true for myelinated axons. Unmyelinated C-fibers, particularly those with the slowest conduction velocities, are actually among the fibers most resistant to local anesthetic block in experimental animals and in vitro (Fig. 33.3). In addition, the anatomic distribution of axons within a peripheral nerve bundle may affect the susceptibility and speed of onset of block, with axons near the surface and closer to the site of application of local anesthetic being exposed to higher concentrations than those buried deeper in the nerve.

Sensory function is more sensitive to local anesthetic block than motor function, possibly related to greater sensitivity of small diameter myelinated fibers.

It is not entirely clear why unmyelinated C fibers are relatively resistant to local anesthetic block. One reason could be the difference in Na^+ channel isoforms expressed by these neurons. A number of different types of Na^+ channel are found in peripheral nerves, including Na_v 1.6, which is clustered at the nodes of Ranvier in myelinated nerves, as well as Na_v 1.2 and Na_v 1.7. Two isoforms found primarily in peripheral nerves with C-fiber axons, termed Na_v 1.8 and Na_v 1.9, are interesting in that they are resistant to block by the classic pufferfish Na^+ channel toxin tetrodotoxin (TTX). These TTX-resistant channels are also less susceptible to block by local anesthetics, which may explain in part the resistance of unmyelinated fibers to local anesthetics (Fig. 33.4).

Interactions with G protein-coupled receptor systems

In addition to blockade of Na^+ channels, local anesthetics affect the function of a number of other systems, such as voltage-gated K^+ and Ca^{2+} channels, nicotinic acetylcholine receptors, and various types of G protein-coupled receptors. Interactions with other ion channel types tend to require greater concentrations of local anesthetics than those required for Na^+ channel blockade. For example, in anterior pituitary cells lidocaine inhibits Na^+ currents at 170 μM, K^+ currents at 1.9 mM, and Ca^{2+} currents at 2.6 mM. Whether disregarding these interactions because of these concentration requirements is appropriate remains an open question.

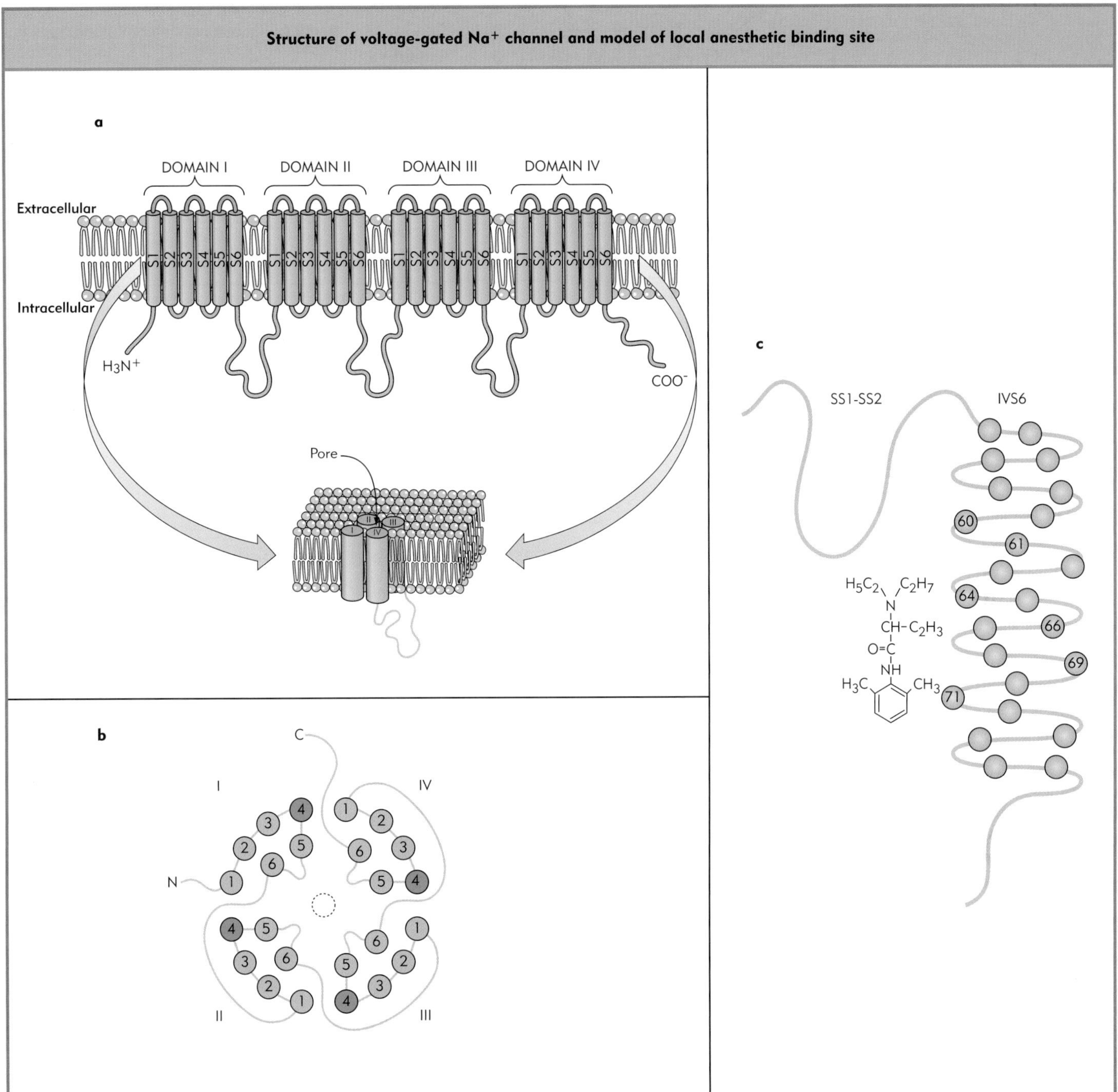

Figure 33.2 Structure of the voltage-gated Na⁺ channel and a model of the local anesthetic binding site. Panel A shows a linearized representation of the voltage-gated Na⁺ channel consisting of four homologous domains (I–IV), each containing 6 α-helical membrane spanning segments (S1–S6) predicted by maps of amino acid hydrophobicity. The four similar domains come together to form a channel with a central conducting pore. The predicted structure of the channel as seen from outside the cell (panel B) comprises a pore formed by the amino acid loop between S5 and S6 (P). Segment 4, indicated by the positive charge symbols, may be the voltage sensor that opens the channel in response to depolarization. Panel C is a detailed schematic of the S6 segment from domain IV, showing how a molecule of lidocaine may interact with residues 1760 (isoleucine), 1764 (phenylalanine), and 1771 (tyrosine) in the pore of the channel. Copyright © 1999 AAS. (From Ragsdale DS, McPhee JC, Scheuer T, Catterall WA. Molecular determinants of state-dependent block of Na⁺ channels by local anesthetics. Science 1994;265:1724–8. Copyright © 1999 AAAS.)

Recently, Ca^{2+}-signaling G protein-coupled receptors (GPCRs) – that is, GPCRs linked to release of Ca^{2+} from intracellular stores – have been identified as a target for local anesthetics. A number of well-described clinical actions of local anesthetics that are difficult to explain by Na^+ channel block can be accounted for by inhibition of GPCR signaling. In particular, the inflammatory modulating actions of local anesthetics might result from interactions with GPCR-mediated inflammatory signaling. Inhibition of several GPCRs can occur at local anesthetic concentrations that are easily attained systemically during clinical use. Some receptor systems are exquisitely sensitive to local anesthetics, and are inhibited at nanomolar concentrations.

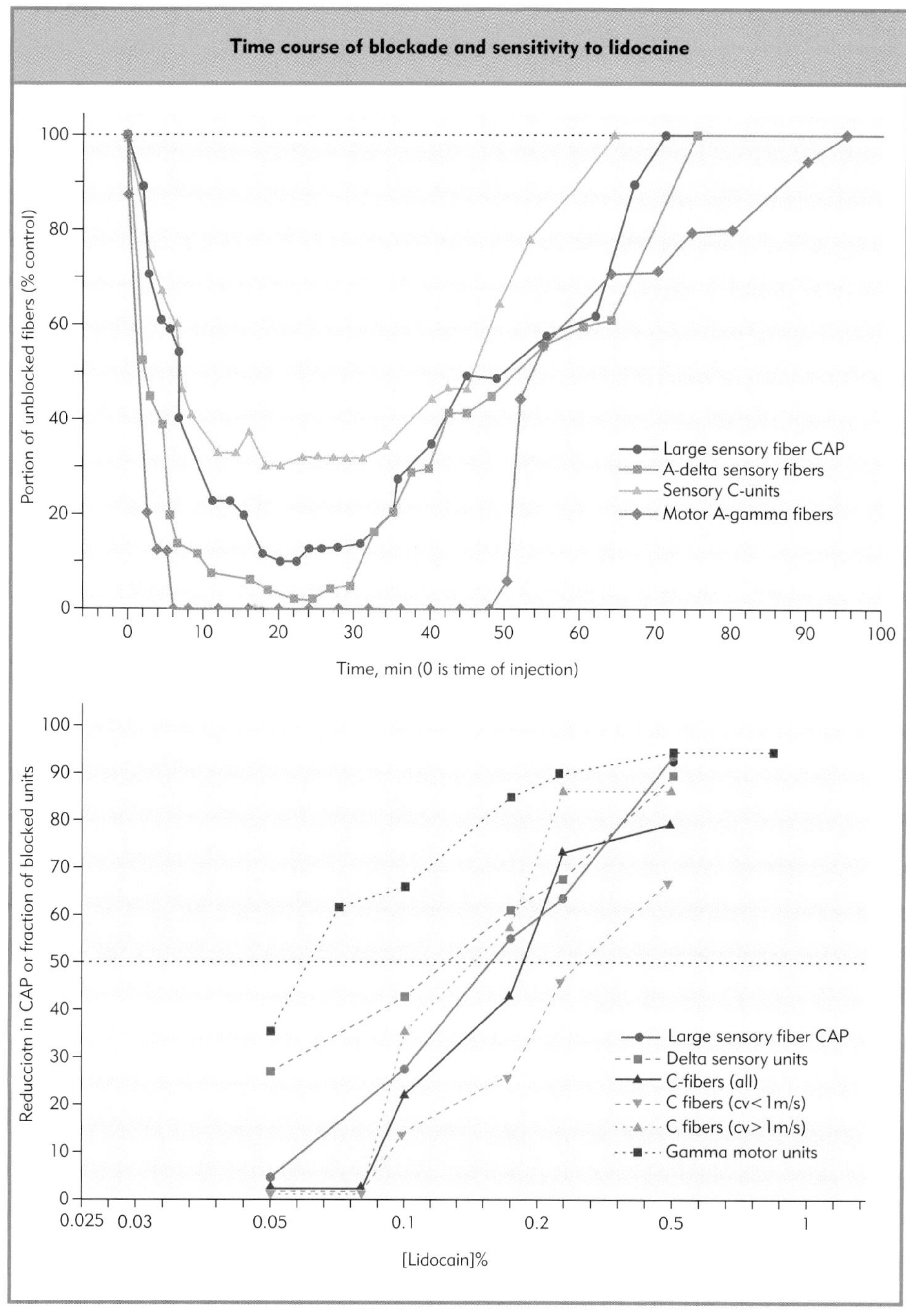

Figure 33.3 Time course of blockade and sensitivity to lidocaine of different fiber types in a peripheral nerve. Nerve activity was recorded in dorsal and ventral spinal roots in response to stimulation of the distal sciatic nerve after injection of lidocaine at the sciatic notch. Panel A shows the averaged responses of 15–33 fibers after injection of 0.1 mL of 0.5% lidocaine. Transmission of action potentials was reduced in all fiber types, but the degree and duration of block were less for C-fibers than for other sensory fibers. Panel B shows concentration–response relations for lidocaine effects on different fiber types. C-fibers with conduction velocities (cv) <1 m/s were the least sensitive to block by lidocaine. CAP, compound action potential. (From Gokin AP, Philip B, Strichartz GR. Preferential block of small myelinated sensory and motor fibers by lidocaine. Anesthesiology 2001; 95:1441–54.)

Prolonged exposure (hours) greatly enhances the sensitivity of GPCR signaling to local anesthetics. Local anesthetic interactions with GPCR signaling provide a potential explanation for part of the efficacy of these drugs in inflammatory and chronic pain.

Molecular mechanisms of local anesthetic–GPCR interactions

The mechanisms of action of local anesthetics on GPCR signaling have been elucidated largely by studies in recombinant systems. When expressed in *Xenopus* oocytes, Ca^{2+}-signaling GPCRs activate one of several G proteins (G_q, G_{11}, G_{14}, or G_o), which in turn activate phospholipase C (PLC; see Chapter 3). Activated PLC cleaves membrane phosphatidylinositol bisphosphate (PIP_2) into inositol trisphosphate (IP_3) and diacylglycerol (DAG). IP_3 induces intracellular Ca^{2+} release by activating a receptor channel on intracellular stores. This increase in intracellular Ca^{2+} can be measured and used as an index of GPCR function.

Initial findings demonstrated a wide range of sensitivities of various GPCRs to local anesthetics, even when studied in identical settings. Thus the M1 muscarinic acetylcholine receptor is remarkably sensitive: the IC_{50} for lidocaine was 18 nM. At the other end of the spectrum, the AT_{1A} angiotensin receptor is completely insensitive to local anesthetics. Other receptor systems, such as those for the inflammatory mediator thromboxane A_2 (TX) and the putative inflammatory signaling molecule lysophosphatidate (LPA), show intermediate sensitivities. In

Variable lidocaine sensitivities of Na^+ channels

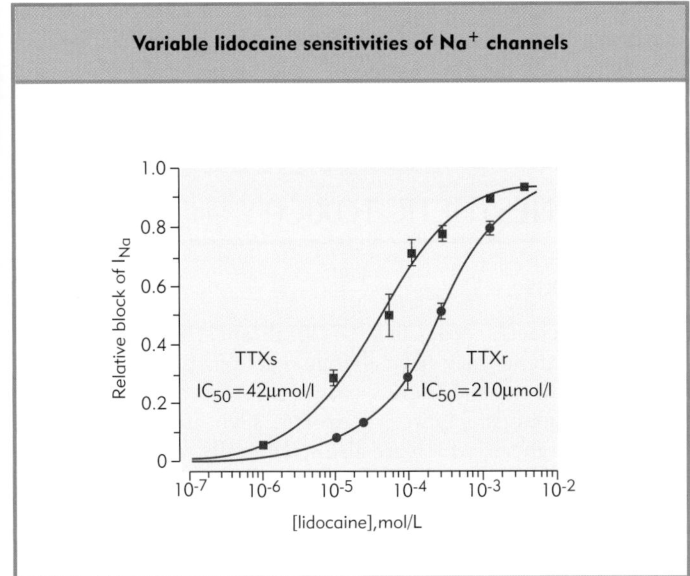

Figure 33.4 Concentration–response relations for block of tetrodotoxin-sensitive (TTXs) and TTX-resistant (TTXr) Na^+ channels by lidocaine. Na^+ currents (I_{Na}) were recorded from isolated rat dorsal root ganglion neurons using the patch clamp technique. TTXs currents were blocked by <200 nM TTX, whereas TTXr currents were recorded in the presence of 300 nM TTX. TTXr Na^+ channels were almost five times less sensitive to lidocaine than TTXs Na^+ channels. (From Scholz A, Kuboyama N, Hempelmann G, Vogel W. Complex blockade of TTX-resistant Na^+ currents by lidocaine and bupivacaine reduce firing frequency in DRG neurons. J Neurophysiol. 1998; 79:1746–54.)

Local anesthetic block of G protein-coupled receptor

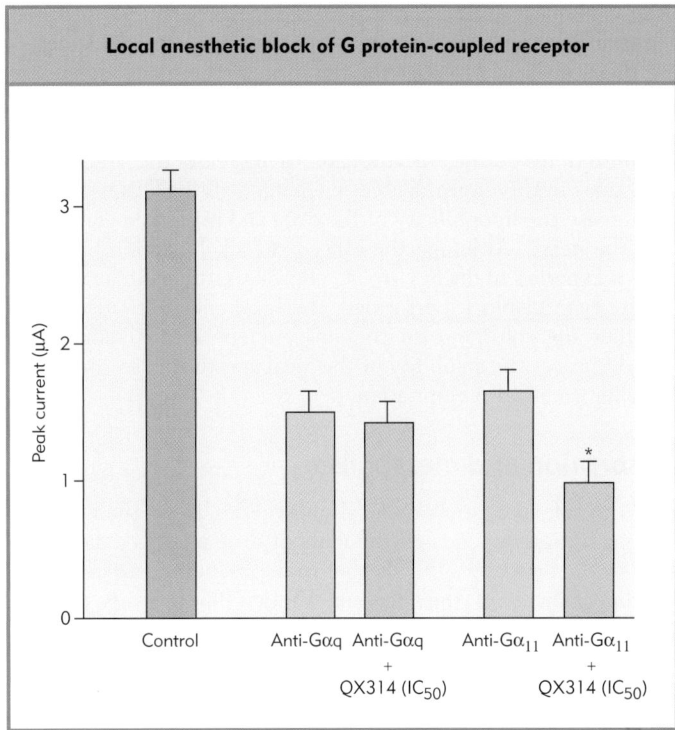

Figure 33.5 Local anesthetic block of G protein-coupled receptor signaling is dependent on $G_{\alpha q}$ protein. M1 muscarinic acetylcholine receptors were expressed recombinantly in *Xenopus* oocytes, and Ca^{2+}-activated Cl^- currents induced by methylcholine were measured (purple bar). Injection of antisense oligonucleotides directed against $G_{\alpha q}$ or $G_{\alpha 11}$ reduced signaling (green bars), indicating that this receptor couples to these G proteins. The local anesthetic QX314, applied intracellularly at half-maximal inhibitory concentration (IC_{50}, orange bars) no longer affected receptor signaling in the absence of $G_{\alpha q}$, indicating that this protein is essential for the inhibitory effect of the local anesthetic on this G protein-coupled receptor-signaling pathway. (From Hollman MW et al. Local anesthetic inhibition of G protein-coupled receptor signaling by interference with Galphaq protein function. Mol Pharmacol 2001; 59: 294-301. Copyright © 2001 The American Society for Pharmacology and Experimental Therapeutics.)

contrast, sensitivity to intracellular local anesthetic (such as the nonpermeable lidocaine analog QX314) is similar among the receptor systems. As the molecular structures of these receptors are quite different, this finding suggests that intracellular QX314 may interact instead with a molecule within the downstream signaling pathway. However, the IP_3 channel and its downstream signaling pathway do not appear to be a target, as Ca^{2+} release induced by direct injection of IP_3 into oocytes was not sensitive to local anesthetics.

The similar potencies for intracellular local anesthetics on various receptors, and the lack of effect on the downstream signaling pathway, suggest an effect on G protein coupling to receptors. These findings have been confirmed by direct knockdown of various G protein α subunits using antisense oligonucleotides. In each case, the effect of local anesthetic was eliminated if, and only if, the G_q protein was removed (Fig. 33.5). Knockdown of any of the other G-protein α subunits was without effect. Therefore, the intracellular effects of local anesthetics on Ca^{2+}-signaling GPCRs are probably explained by an inhibitory action on the G_q α subunit.

LOCAL ANESTHETIC PHARMACOKINETICS

Effect site concentration

Local anesthetics are generally directed to the site of their desired effect either topically, to block conduction in peripheral nerve endings, or by injection near nerves, nerve roots, or plexuses to provide regional anesthesia. Mucosal surfaces are readily anesthetized by the topical application of benzocaine and lidocaine solutions, gels, aerosols, or lozenges. Tetracaine solutions are commonly used to anesthetize cornea and conjunctiva. Keratinized skin is an effective barrier against most local anesthetics, but specialized preparations such as the lidocaine patch (5%) and the EMLA patch and cream can provide very superficial anesthesia of the skin if given enough time. EMLA (eutectic mixture of local anesthetics) is a combination of 2.5% lidocaine and 2.5% prilocaine in an emulsion. The term 'eutectic' refers to a combination of drugs (lidocaine and prilocaine) which has a lower melting point than either drug alone. Thus these agents are liquids in the emulsion at room temperature, which facilitates their absorption.

To ensure successful conduction block when administering local anesthetics by injection, an adequate volume and concentration of the drug must be administered close to the target nerves. Even then, to reach the axoplasm where they act, local anesthetic molecules must traverse several layers of connective tissue surrounding the nerve axons without being taken up by muscle, fat, and blood. Only a few percent of the total mass of local anesthetic injected peripherally actually enters the nerve. Two methods are used to improve drug penetration into the nerve. Vasoconstrictors such as epinephrine (adrenaline) are often added to the injectate to reduce absorption into and removal by the blood. This increases the amount of drug entering the nerve and prolongs the duration of the block, as well as decreasing blood levels of local anesthetics and reducing systemic toxicity. Second, local anesthetic solutions are frequently alkalinized by adding bicarbonate to increase the fraction of molecules in the unprotonated, uncharged state. This is thought to increase the lipophilicity of the drug and improve penetration into the nerve. Although the efficacy of alkalinization has been shown experimentally in vitro, its clinical usefulness may depend on the type of block performed, the local anesthetic used, and whether the solution also contains epinephrine. Alkalinization also decreases the solubility of the local anesthetic, so care must be taken to avoid precipitation.

Absorption and metabolism

The rate of absorption of local anesthetics from their site of administration depends on the mass of drug injected, the blood flow to the injection site, whether vasoconstrictors are used, and the lipophilicity of the local anesthetic. Blood levels of local anesthetics after an intercostal block, where blood flow is high, are greater than after peripheral blocks and subcutaneous injections. As indicated above, systemic effects may be quite relevant for a number of the clinical actions of local anesthetics, in which case blood concentrations become very important. Epidural administration of local anesthetics leads to significant but nontoxic blood concentrations between 1 and 5 μM, which are likely to contribute to their clinical effects. Intravenous administration of local anesthetics to attain such levels can be performed safely with a relatively simple dosing scheme, such as 3 mg/min for body weight >70 kg and 2 mg/min for body weight <70 kg in adults. This will attain blood levels that have clinically relevant actions on the heart and inflammatory system, yet do not lead to toxic levels. In patients with liver failure or in the very elderly, a dose reduction is indicated.

Most local anesthetics are highly protein bound to albumin and α_1-acidic glycoprotein.

Most local anesthetics are highly protein bound in the blood; albumin and α_1-acidic glycoprotein are the primary binding proteins. Changes in the levels of these circulating proteins lead to changes in the free (active) fraction of local anesthetics in plasma. For example, decreases in albumin levels during pregnancy and chronic disease increase free plasma levels of local anesthetics. Levels of albumin and α_1-acid glycoprotein are low in newborns, which also makes them susceptible to systemic toxicity. On the other hand, levels of α_1-acid glycoprotein are increased (and the extent of local anesthetic binding increases) with trauma, surgery, myocardial infarction, uremia, and smoking.

Local anesthetics are removed from the bloodstream primarily by metabolism, followed by urinary excretion of the metabolites. For ester-linked local anesthetics, metabolism occurs primarily by ester hydrolysis catalyzed by plasma esterase to produce an amine and either *p*-aminobenzoic acid (PABA) or a PABA derivative. The PABA metabolites of ester-linked local anesthetics may produce anaphylactic reactions in susceptible individuals (see section on Toxicity). Amide-linked local anesthetics are metabolized in the liver by the cytochrome P450 enzymes CYP1A2 and CYP3A4 by *N*-dealkylation, amide bond hydrolysis, and hydroxylation. Impairment of hepatic function and decreases in hepatic blood flow (e.g. associated with heart failure) prolong the elimination of amide-type local anesthetics. A metabolite of prilocaine, *o*-toluidine, can cause significant methemoglobinemia (see section on Toxicity).

LOCAL ANESTHETIC TOXICITY

Anaphylaxis

True anaphylactic reactions to local anesthetics are rare. However, patients may have allergic reactions to metabolites of ester-linked local anesthetics, namely PABA and structurally similar compounds. Hydroxybenzoates such as methylparaben and other parabens, which are also structurally related to PABA, may be included in both ester- and amide-linked local anesthetic-containing solutions as bacteriostatic preservatives, and these agents may also cause allergic reactions. Adverse reactions experienced by patients receiving local anesthetics and reported as allergic reactions may in some cases reflect systemic toxicity due to high blood levels of local anesthetics, either from absorption or accidental intravascular injection, or due to an adverse response to an additive, such as epinephrine.

Systemic toxicity of local anesthetics is concentration dependent, with CNS toxicity occurring at lower concentrations than cardiac toxicity.

Systemic toxicity

Low blood levels of local anesthetics, achieved either by slow absorption from an injection site or by intravenous administration, can have beneficial effects on the central nervous system, the cardiac conduction system, and the immune system, as noted above. Above these therapeutic levels local anesthetics can produce toxic effects, primarily via actions in the central nervous system and the heart. Toxic blood levels of local anesthetics can be caused by the administration of excessive amounts of drug, by rapid absorption, and/or by impaired metabolism. Perhaps more commonly, toxicity is seen after accidental intravascular injection of local anesthetic, leading to rapidly developing but short-lived toxic reactions. For lidocaine, in which toxicity has been well documented, symptoms vary according to the blood concentration. At therapeutic concentrations below about 5 μg/mL (21 μM) lidocaine produces sedation and has antiarrhythmic effects. Slightly higher concentrations produce excitatory effects in the central nervous system, presumably reflecting the blockade of Na^+ channels in inhibitory neurons. Symptoms include tinnitus and altered sound perception, lightheadedness, and circumoral numbness or paresthesias. Higher blood levels produce severe excitatory reactions, including agitation and confusion, muscle twitching or tremors, and seizures. As concentrations increase to 15 μg/mL and above, central nervous system inhibition predominates, producing unconsciousness and central cardiorespiratory depression. At concentrations above 20–25 μg/mL, cardiac conduction and contractility are also depressed, leading to cardiac arrest.

More potent local anesthetics, such as bupivacaine and ropivacaine, also produce systemic toxicity, although at lower blood levels. Bupivacaine is unusual in that it has extremely high potency at cardiac Na^+ channels, such that toxicity related to its cardiac effects is observed before CNS toxicity is apparent. Interestingly, the R(+) enantiomers of local anesthetics with a chiral carbon, such as bupivacaine, have higher affinity at the cardiac Na^+ channel than the S(−) isomer. This enabled the development of the less cardiotoxic drugs levobupivacaine, the S(−) isomer of bupivacaine, and ropivacaine, which is structurally and clinically similar to bupivacaine, except that it is formulated as a pure S(−) isomer.

Neurotoxicity

Local anesthetics rarely have neurotoxic effects when used for peripheral nerve blocks. Spinal nerve roots, however, seem to be more susceptible to injury by local anesthetics. This may be due in part to the lack of a connective tissue sheath surrounding and protecting the nerve from high concentrations of local anesthetics. Intrathecal lidocaine in particular has been implicated as a cause of cauda equina syndrome (primarily its use with intrathecal microcatheters, which were subsequently removed from the market) and a more recently described condition, transient neurologic syndrome (TNS), sometimes referred to as transient radicular irritation (TRI). Symptoms of TNS occur hours after resolution of the initial spinal block, and include pain and paresthesias in the lower back, buttock, and lower extremities. These symptoms are short lived, usually disappearing in less than 1 week.

The mechanism of TNS is unknown. The symptoms are not associated with any positive neurological finding, and are transient. It occurs more commonly in outpatients and when the lithotomy position is used intraoperatively. It has been reported after spinal anesthesia with most local anesthetics, but is much more commonly associated with the use of lidocaine. The incidence is not altered by changes in the baricity of the solution, or by changes in the dose or concentration of lidocaine, even down to 0.5%. The risk of TNS associated with intrathecal lidocaine has made its continued use controversial, despite its long safety record.

Methemoglobinemia

Benzocaine and a metabolite of prilocaine (*o*-toluidine) can cause clinically significant methemoglobinemia, a condition in which the ferrous iron atom (Fe^{2+}) in hemoglobin is oxidized to the ferric form (Fe^{3+}), which does not bind O_2. Cytochrome b5, which is regenerated by the enzyme methemoglobin reductase, usually keeps the iron in its reduced state, but it has a limited capacity if there is too much oxidizing agent, or multiple agents working in combination. Nitrates such as nitroglycerin, sulfonamides, antimalarials, and perhaps acetaminophen can also produce methemoglobin. Individuals with hereditary alterations in the reducing enzymes are also more susceptible. Treatment of methemoglobinemia with methylene blue (1–2 mg/kg IV) accelerates the reduction of methemoglobin by an alternative pathway for hemoglobin reduction.

Because both benzocaine and prilocaine (when used in EMLA) are commonly used topically, this may invite the misconception that these agents are completely safe. To prevent methemoglobinemia, follow the maximum dosing guidelines listed for the benzocaine-containing product (e.g. a 1-second spray of aerosolized benzocaine), and follow the recommended guidelines for EMLA application, particularly in small children.

Key references

Butterworth JF, Strichartz GR. Molecular mechanisms of local anesthesia: a review. Anesthesiology 1990;72:711–734.

Catterall WA. From ionic currents to molecular mechanisms: The structure and function of voltage-gated sodium channels. Neuron 2000;26:13–25.

Hollmann MW, Wieczorek KS, Berger A, Durieux ME. Local anesthetic inhibition of G protein-coupled receptor signaling by interference with Galpha(q) protein function. Mol Pharmacol. 2001;59: 294–301.

Ragsdale DS, McPhee JC, Scheuer T et al. Molecular determinants of state-dependent block of Na^+ channels by local anesthetics. Science 1994;265:1724–8.

Strichartz GR. The inhibition of sodium currents in myelinated nerve by quaternary derivatives of lidocaine. J Gen Physiol. 1973;62:37–57.

Strichartz GR, Sanchez V, Arthur GR et al. Fundamental properties of local anesthetics. II. Measuring octanol:buffer partition coefficients and pK_a values of clinically used drugs. Anesth Analg. 1990;71:158–70.

Further reading

Hanck DA, Makielski JC, Sheets MF. Kinetic effects of quaternary lidocaine block of cardiac sodium channels: a gating current study. J Gen Physiol. 1994;103:19–43.

Hollmann MW, Durieux ME. Local anesthetics and the inflammatory response: a new therapeutic indication? Anesthesiology 2000;93:858–75.

Hollmann MW, Gross A, Jelacin N, Durieux ME. Local anesthetic effects on priming and activation of human neutrophils. Anesthesiology 2001;95:113–22.

Lambert LA, Lambert DH, Strichartz GR. Irreversible conduction block in isolated nerve by high concentrations of local anesthetics. Anesthesiology 1994;80:1082–93.

Pollock JE. Transient neurologic symptoms: Etiology, risk factors, and management. Reg Anesth Pain Med. 2002;27:581–6.

Rowlingson JC. Toxicity of local anesthetic additivies. Reg Anesth. 1993;18:453–60.

Scholz A. Mechnisms of (local) anaesthetics on voltage-gated sodium and other ion channels. Br J Anaesth. 2002;89:52–61.

Strümper D, Durieux ME. Antidepressants as long-acting local anesthetics. Reg Anesth Pain Med. 2004;29:277–85.

Yu FH, Catterall WA. Overview of the voltage-gated sodium channel family. Genome Biol. 2003;4:207.

Zaric D, Christiansen C, Pace NL et al. Transient neurologic symptoms (TNS) following spinal anaesthesia with lidocaine versus other local anaesthetics (Cochrane Review). In: The Cochrane Library, Issue 1, Chichester, UK: John Wiley & Sons; 2004.

Chapter 34

Autonomic nervous system

Christofer D Barth and Thomas J Ebert

TOPICS COVERED IN THIS CHAPTER

- **Central organization**
- **Anatomy of the peripheral sympathetic nervous system**
- **The baroreflex and other neural reflexes**
- **Anesthetics and the sympathetic nervous system**
- **Autonomic pharmacology**
  - Parasympathetic nervous system
  - Parasympathetic agonists
  - Parasympathetic antagonists
  - Sympathetic nervous system
  - The α-adrenoceptors
  - The β-adrenoceptors
  - Endogenous catecholamines
  - Dopamine
  - Norepinephrine
  - Epinephrine
  - Synthetic β agonists
  - β_2 agonists
  - β antagonists (blockers)
  - α_1 agonists
  - α_2 agonists
  - α antagonists

The autonomic nervous system (ANS) controls the visceral motor neuronal network. ANS connections maintain body homeostasis by integrating signals from somatic and visceral sensors to modulate organ perfusion and function. The efferent components of the ANS are the sympathetic and parasympathetic nervous systems (SNS and PNS). Their tonic activity maintains cardiac activity and visceral and vascular smooth muscle in a state of intermediate function (Fig. 34.1) from which rapid increases or decreases in autonomic outflow can adjust blood flow and organ activity in response to the environment. There is generally no voluntary control of the ANS, although conscious modulation can occur transiently (biofeedback or mental stress). The SNS exits the spinal cord at thoracolumbar sections and has been called the 'fight or flight' division. Its activation under stress (e.g. blood loss, temperature change, or exercise) increases sympathetic neural activity to the heart and other viscera, peripheral vasculature, sweat glands, ocular muscles, and piloerector muscles. Activation can affect sympathetic output in a highly differentiated manner; however, generalized activation leads to increases in cardiac output, blood glucose, pupillary dilation, and body temperature. In contrast, the PNS exits from the craniosacral portions of the central nervous system; it is responsible for 'rest and digest'. Activation of the PNS slows heart rate and respiration, and increases glandular epithelium secretion and digestion (Fig. 34.1).

Autonomic nervous system dysfunction can lead to severe hypotension during anesthesia.

Anesthesiologists should have a thorough understanding of the ANS and its function. First intravenous and inhaled anesthetics may cause hypotension directly through vascular smooth muscle dilation and cardiac depression. The ANS counteracts this effect; therefore, ANS dysfunction can lead to severe hypotension during anesthesia. Second, both general and neuraxial anesthesia alter autonomic tone and reflexes. Third, in pathologic states such as shock or hypertensive crisis, the ability of the ANS to maintain homeostasis is limited. Many drugs and therapeutic maneuvers used to restore physiologic equilibrium directly target ANS effector sites. Fourth, acute and chronic pain disorders often involve altered ANS functions. Finally, the general goals of anesthesia can be considered to be unconsciousness, amnesia, immobility, analgesia, and blockade of autonomic responses to noxious stimuli. In fact, most anesthetics are titrated to blunt the neuroendocrine response to stress, and the autonomic responses (heart rate and blood pressure) are used to gauge the stress response.

CENTRAL ORGANIZATION

The basal 'tone' of the ANS is determined by input to the lower brainstem. The primary relay or integration region is the medullary vasomotor center, which integrates neural information from the central autonomic network (CAN) and peripheral sensors. The CAN consists of four primary areas: the cerebral cortex, amygdala, hypothalamus, and medulla. The CAN receives input from peripheral visceral and somatic receptors. Humoral

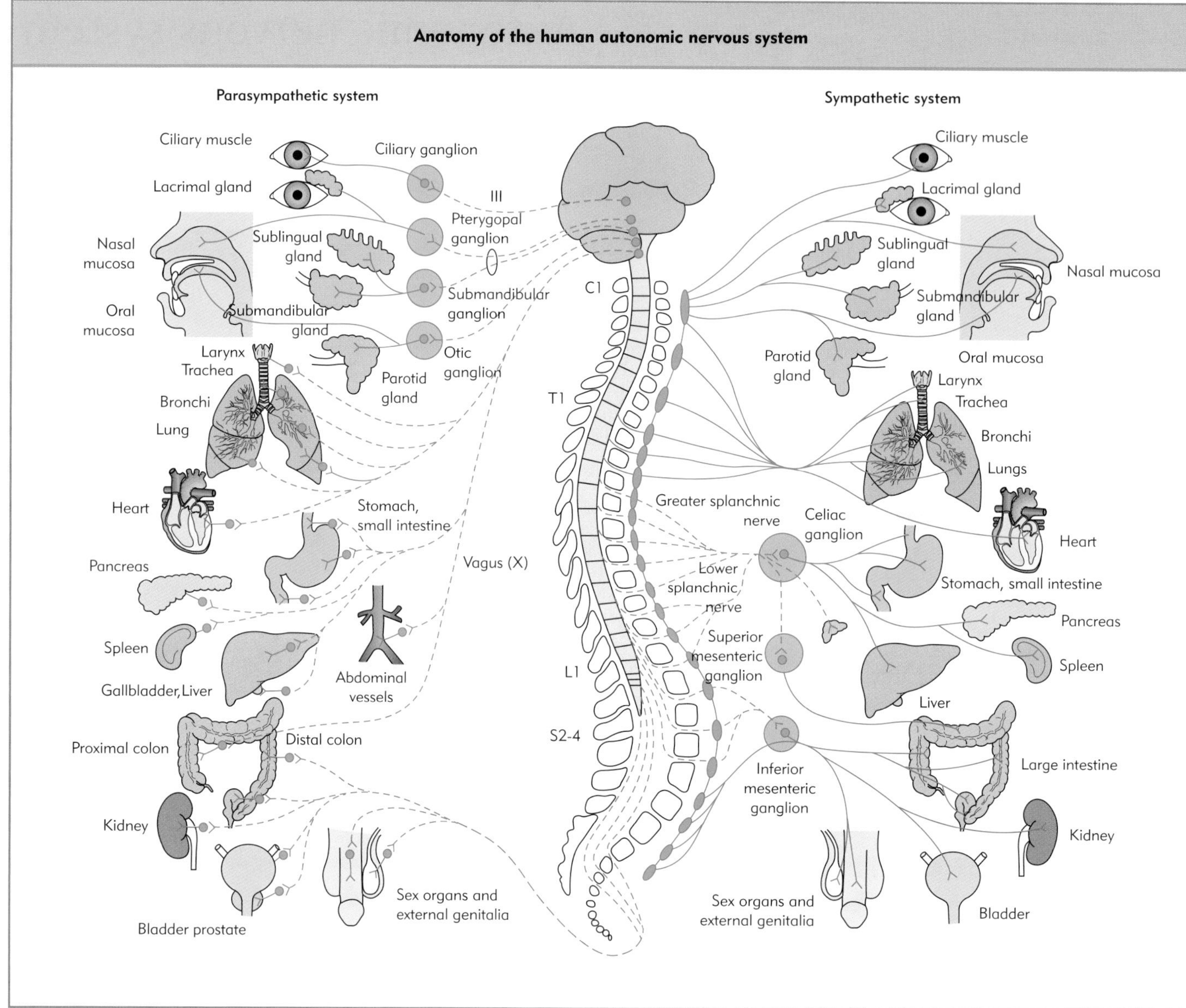

Figure 34.1 Anatomy of the human autonomic nervous system. Preganglionic and postganglionic fibers are indicated by broken and solid lines, respectively.

substances also modulate the CAN via the circumventricular organs where the blood–brain barrier is absent. Angiotensin, arginine-vasopressin, and various cytokines appear to cross into the central nervous system (CNS) at the subfornical organ, in the lamina terminalis of the anterior wall of the third ventricle, and at the area postrema in the fourth ventricle. These circulating substances modify various 'visceral' reflexes initiated from peripheral receptors in blood vessels and tissues. The CAN is not completely automatic or autonomous; rather, it can be transiently influenced by both environmental and somatic sensors. In biofeedback, conscious relaxation methods can reduce blood pressure and heart rate, and the simple act of thinking about exercise increases heart rate and metabolic waste products from muscular activity trigger ascending neural signals that modify the ANS.

The medullary vasomotor center is the first relay for afferent input from peripheral sensors, including the baro- and chemoreceptors and gastrointestinal receptors. Ascending signals synapse in the nucleus tractus solitarius (NTS), located bilaterally in the dorsal medulla. The NTS relays information to higher centers of the CAN, such as the amygdala and hypothalamus, and also has connections with the ventrolateral medulla (VLM). From the rostral VLM, efferent sympathetic outflow projects to the intermediolateral column of the thoracolumbar spinal cord and increases sympathetic discharge. Neurons in the rostral VLM discharge with a rhythm linked to heart rate, and are suppressed during high-pressure baroreceptor discharge at peak pulse pressure. The caudal VLM interconnects with the rostral VLM and contains neurons that can suppress preganglionic sympathetic outflow.

The SNS consists of preganglionic fibers that arise from the intermediolateral column and exit the spinal cord between the first thoracic (T1) and the third lumbar (L3) level (Figs 34.1 and 34.2). Most of these fibers make synaptic connections in the 22 pairs of ganglia termed the bilateral sympathetic chain. The preganglionic fibers are so named because they are presynaptic

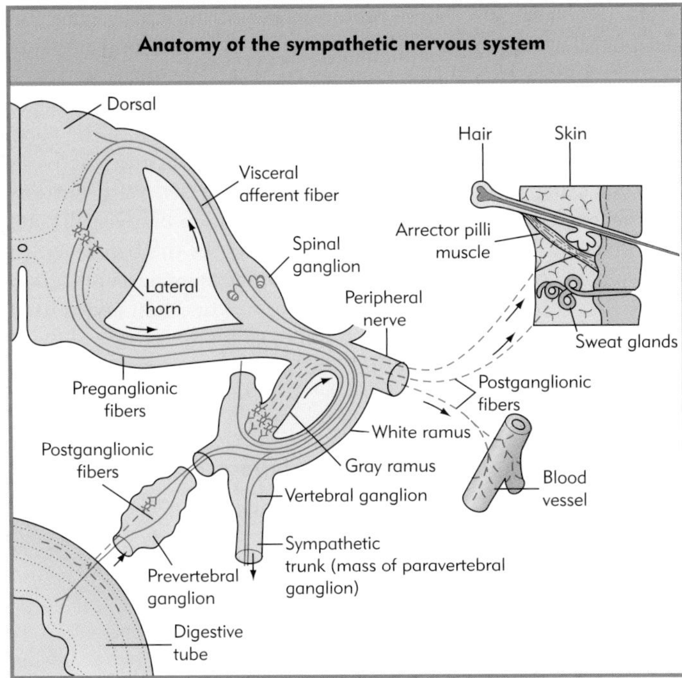

Figure 34.2 Anatomy of the human sympathetic nervous system at the spinal cord level. (Adapted with permission from Carpenter MB, Sutin J. The autonomic nervous system. In: Carpenter MB, Sutin J, eds. Human Neuroanatomy, 8th edn. Baltimore, MD: Williams & Wilkins; 1983:220.)

to a ganglion cell. Likewise, postganglionic fibers are the terminal fibers of a ganglion cell and synapse with appropriate end organs. However, some preganglionic fibers feed directly to peripheral ganglia before synapsing, and some make direct connections with the adrenal medulla. Because the adrenal medulla originates from neural tissue, it is analogous to the postganglionic nerve. There is considerable dispersion in the SNS: for every preganglionic fiber there are 20–30 postganglionic fibers. Moreover, the sympathetic terminal in a visceral organ or tissue is not a single terminal; rather, it is a multiple, branched series of endings called a *terminal plexus*. A single postganglionic nerve can innervate up to 25 000 effector cells via the terminal plexus. Finally, with elevated sympathetic activity the release of the postganglionic neurotransmitter norepinephrine (noradrenaline) may exceed the capacities of the reuptake and enzymatic breakdown systems that function to terminate its action. This excess norepinephrine (or spillover) can enter the circulatory system and can cause widespread humoral effects.

Historically, activation of the SNS has been considered a 'mass reflex' or response. Current understanding supports the selectivity of sympathetic responses, although the mechanism of this selectivity is not known. An example of the selectivity of the SNS can be observed in the activity recorded from skin and muscle sympathetic nerves in humans. Efferent sympathetic nerves to skin blood vessels, sweat glands, and piloerector muscles are generally silent during resting conditions and during blood pressure perturbations, but are activated by startle or an embarrassing question. In contrast, the efferent sympathetic nerves that supply skeletal muscle blood vessels show significant tonic activity that is inversely modified by changes in blood pressure via the baroreflex. This sympathetic activity is not altered by startle maneuvers.

In contrast to the parasympathetic nervous system, the sympathetic nervous system exhibits considerable dispersion: for each preganglionic fiber there are over 20 postganglionic fibers, each innervating up to 25 000 effector cells.

In the PNS, preganglionic fibers originate in two sites, the brainstem and the sacral spinal cord (Fig. 34.1). Preganglionic neurons from the dorsal motor nucleus of the vagus and the nucleus ambiguus send efferent signals to the head, heart, and abdominal viscera via cranial nerves III (oculomotor), VII (facial), IX (glossopharyngeal), and X (vagus). The vagus nerve controls most visceral function within the thorax and abdomen and accounts for as much as 75% of the parasympathetic nerve activity. The sacral parasympathetic nucleus originates in the intermediolateral cell column at sacral segments 2–4 and controls bladder, bowel, and penile erector function. Unlike the SNS, preganglionic fibers pass directly to ganglia that are close to or within specific organs. Very short cholinergic postganglionic fibers extend into the organ tissue. There are no interconnections between the components of the cranial and sacral outflows. In contrast to the SNS, there is very little dispersion of parasympathetic outflow; the ratio of pre- to postganglionic fibers is 1:1 to 1:3, which provides greater selectivity for the PNS. For example, salivation or micturition can occur without vagal-mediated bradycardia.

ANATOMY OF THE PERIPHERAL SYMPATHETIC NERVOUS SYSTEM

Although autonomic outflow is segmental and somewhat parallels the somatic outflow to skeletal muscle, it differs from the somatic system in that it is disynaptic. Preganglionic, autonomic, cholinergic neurons synapse to nicotinic receptors in peripheral ganglia and activate postganglionic neural fibers. In contrast, the somatic motor neurons have monosynaptic efferent pathways to nicotinic receptors on skeletal muscle. A useful principle is that the SNS 'disseminates' and 'amplifies' information related to maintenance of body homeostasis. Preganglionic sympathetic cell bodies in the intermediolateral cell columns of the spinal cord gray matter extend from spinal levels T1 to L3. Preganglionic, or B, fibers are myelinated, small (diameters less than 3 μm), and conduct at 2–14 m/s. Axons of these neurons leave the spinal cord in the ventral spinal roots along with somatic, α and γ neurons, then branch off in the white rami communicantes and enter the paravertebral ganglia comprising the 'sympathetic chain'. The fine myelination of these fibers is responsible for their white appearance. The paravertebral ganglia are arranged as a bilateral chain of ganglia running the length of the spinal column located anterolateral to the vertebral body.

The lumbar paravertebral ganglia are targeted for lumbar sympathetic block, which is used in the diagnosis and treatment of chronic pain states of the lower extremities.

The preganglionic fiber has several potential destinations once it enters a paravertebral ganglion (Fig. 34.2): it can synapse with one or more sympathetic neurons in the ganglion; ascend or descend in the paravertebral chain and synapse with neurons at other levels; synapse in the ganglion with a postganglionic fiber that leaves the paravertebral chain via gray rami communicantes to join a somatic nerve and travel to an effector site (e.g. blood vessels); or exit the sympathetic chain and synapse with an intermediate ganglion cell or with a prevertebral ganglion cell.

In addition to the 22 pairs of paravertebral ganglia referred to as the sympathetic chain, there are prevertebral, intermediate, and terminal ganglia. The intermediate ganglia are small structures, occasionally microscopic, that are located near the paravertebral chain. The prevertebral ganglia are composed of a network of pre- and postganglionic sympathetic fibers, parasympathetic fibers, and the ganglion cell bodies. The prevertebral ganglia most relevant to an anesthesiologist are the stellate ganglion (which is a fusion of the inferior cervical and first thoracic ganglia), the celiac ganglion, and the superior hypogastric (mesenteric) ganglion (Fig. 34.1). The stellate ganglion is the target of therapeutic and diagnostic blocks for chronic upper extremity pain syndromes. Interscalene and cervical plexus blocks often affect the stellate ganglion, resulting in Horner's syndrome (miosis, ptosis, anhidrosis, conjunctival injection). Other prevertebral ganglia include the superior and middle cervical ganglia, the aorticorenal ganglion, and the inferior mesenteric ganglion. The terminal ganglia lie in close proximity to their end organs (e.g. the urinary bladder and rectum). The postganglionic noradrenergic sympathetic fibers, or C-fibers, are largely unmyelinated and have diameters ranging from 0.3 to 1.3 μm and conduction velocities < 2 m/s. Like preganglionic fibers, one postganglionic fiber can synapse with a number of effector cells; however, a postganglionic fiber synapses with only one type of end organ. In other words, one postganglionic fiber can synapse with several vascular smooth muscle cells, but not simultaneously with a blood vessel, sweat gland, and piloerector muscle. The important end organs innervated by the SNS include eyes, secretory organs (including the sweat glands), heart, blood vessels, adrenal medulla, abdominal and pelvic viscera, and piloerector muscles.

Although the ANS has numerous functions, among the most important are temperature regulation and maintenance of blood pressure through baroreceptor-mediated reflex regulation of cardiac output and peripheral resistance. The autonomic reflexes play important roles in anesthesiology. Impairment of basal autonomic reflex function correlates with hemodynamic instability after induction of anesthesia. Reduced autonomic function may predict postoperative cardiac dysfunction, is associated with an increased risk of adverse cardiac events (especially malignant arrhythmias) after myocardial infarction, and has been implicated in prolonging myocardial ischemia in patients with angina. Because of these important relationships, the physiology of ANS reflexes will be reviewed.

THE BAROREFLEX AND OTHER NEURAL REFLEXES

Afferent signals from pressure sensors in central blood vessels are integrated in the CAN, predominantly the NTS, and directly influence ANS outflow to cardiovascular effectors (Fig. 34.3). Low-pressure cardiopulmonary baroreceptors are located primarily at the junction of the vena cavae and the right atrium, within the right atrium, and in pulmonary blood vessels. The function of these receptors is to monitor central blood volume. For example, when the cardiopulmonary baroreceptors detect slight decreases in central venous pressure, reflex increases of peripheral sympathetic activity are initiated and blood pressure is maintained. This reflex appears to be absent in heart transplant recipients. Arterial, or 'high-pressure', baroreceptor reflexes are mediated by pressure sensors located in the arch of the aorta and in the carotid sinus. Increased blood pressure increases afferent firing and, via CAN, stimulates increased vagal outflow and decreased sympathetic outflow, resulting in bradycardia and hypotension. Halothane profoundly attenuates the baroreceptor reflexes. In contrast, opioid–benzodiazepine anesthesia preserves these baroreceptor reflexes. For example, when fentanyl is used in combination with a benzodiazepine, reflex heart rate slowing in response to phenylephrine-induced hypertension is well maintained.

Halothane profoundly attenuates baroreceptor reflexes.

Vagally mediated bradycardia can result from a variety of stimuli and situations. Stretching the peritoneal cavity or other noxious visceral stimuli, pressure on the contents of the orbit, and volatile anesthetic mask induction in pediatric patients may cause increased vagal discharge and severe bradycardia. Reflex increases in vagal tone also may be associated with decreased sympathetic output, as in the carotid baroreceptor or Bezold–Jarisch reflex. The Bezold–Jarisch reflex involves afferent input from cardiac mechanoreceptors in the inferoposterior wall of the left ventricle; rapid pressure increases, mechanical distortion, and ischemia may serve as stimuli to produce bradycardia and hypotension. This mechanism has been used to explain bradycardia and hypotension induced by the tilt table test, neuraxial anesthesia, compression of the inferior vena cava by the gravid uterus, and anxiety-induced syncope. Asystole and cardiac arrest also may occur. Premedication to prevent these reflexes in normal subjects is controversial. Halting stimuli and increasing preload, followed by ephedrine, atropine, then low-dose epinephrine, appear to be appropriate responses to refractory, vagally mediated bradycardia that is progressing to asystole.

A number of other physiologic reflexes affect ANS tonic activity. One group involves hypoxic stimulation of chemoreceptors of the aortic and carotid bodies to excite the SNS and increase respiration. Another group involves direct stimulation of the CAN. For example, the Cushing reflex of bradycardia and hypertension in response to intracranial hypertension appears to be initiated by hypoxic or mechanical stimulation of the rostral VLM. Rapid changes in autonomic discharge should therefore be anticipated in states of shock, hypoxia, and from intracranial mechanical stimulation as occurs in tumor resection, brain trauma, or intracranial hemorrhage.

ANESTHETICS AND THE SYMPATHETIC NERVOUS SYSTEM

Because of the difficulty in quantifying efferent SNS activity in humans, there is a relative paucity of information relating to the direct effects of anesthetics on both basal sympathetic vasoconstrictor traffic and reflex regulation of the SNS. Sympathetic microneurography permits recording of vasoconstrictor impulses directed to blood vessels within skeletal muscle, and has been used to evaluate the effects of nitrous oxide in humans. An oxygen–nitrous oxide mixture (60/40%) induces a marked

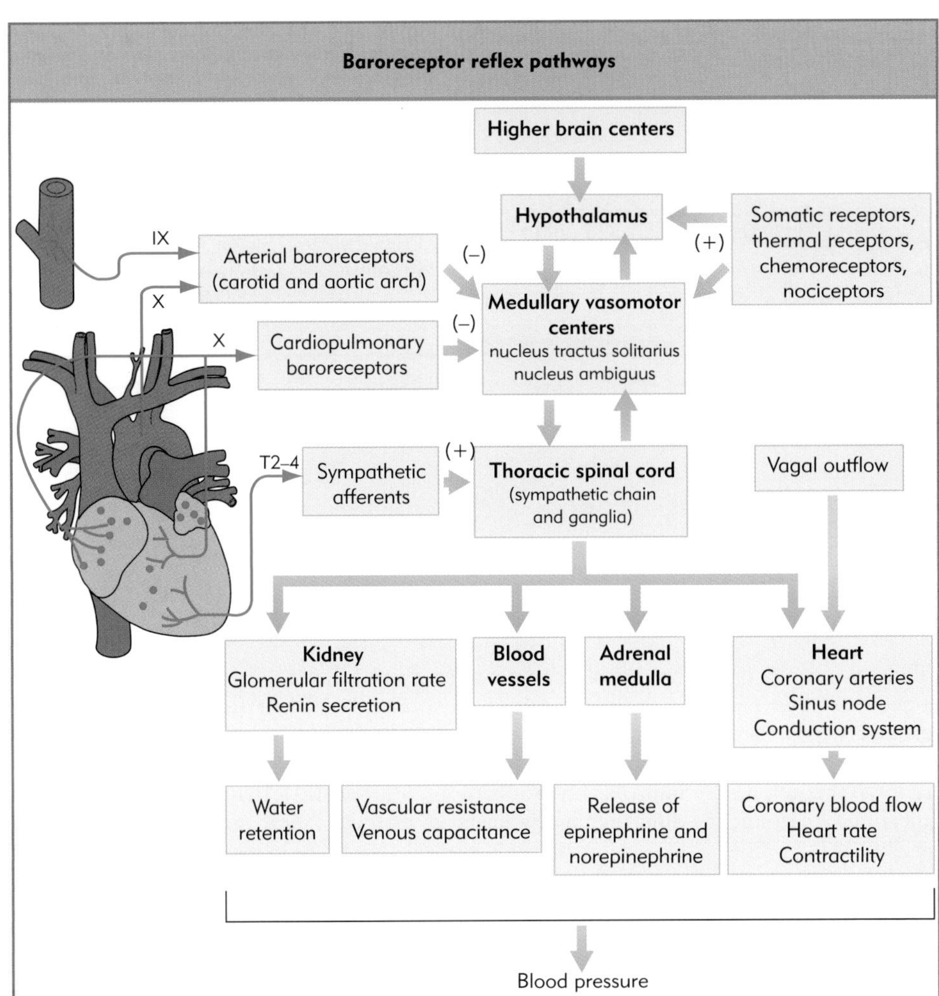

Figure 34.3 Baroreceptor reflex pathways. These pathways are modulated by higher brainstem centers and by other peripheral receptor systems. (Adapted with permission from Ebert TJ. Preoperative evaluation of the autonomic nervous system. Adv Anesth 1993;10:49–68.)

increase in sympathetic nerve traffic in healthy volunteers. Moreover, breathing nitrous oxide does not inhibit reflex sympathetic responses. Consequently, the enhanced sympathetic function permitted by adding nitrous oxide to an anesthetic regimen may at times provide an improved hemodynamic profile.

Both thiopental (thiopentone) and propofol result in near neural silence, as measured by microneurography, for several minutes following administration. Part of this sympathetic silence is related to the concomitant loss of consciousness, but both drugs also abolish the normal reflex sympathetic discharge response to hypotension. When etomidate is infused, basal sympathetic outflow and reflex sympathetic discharge are well maintained despite loss of consciousness, which results in a very stable blood pressure. In hypovolemic patients undergoing general anesthesia, thiopental and propofol can lead to precipitous declines in blood pressure that are mediated by reduced tonic levels of sympathetic outflow and inhibited reflex sympathetic discharge.

Intravenous anesthetics have marked differences in their effects on sympathetic tone and reflexes.

The volatile anesthetic desflurane has been associated with large increases in sympathetic activity and a generalized stress response when delivered at greater than 1 MAC (Fig. 34.4). The trigger for these responses is currently unclear, but two possibilities exist: desflurane may irritate airway receptors, thereby triggering a sympathetic response, or it may act centrally to disinhibit sympathetic outflow. This effect might occur with other volatile anesthetics also, but may only be apparent with desflurane because of its rapid uptake into central neural sites and the need to deliver it at high alveolar concentrations owing to its relative lack of potency.

AUTONOMIC PHARMACOLOGY

Parasympathetic nervous system

Acetylcholine (ACh) is a quaternary ammonium ester that is synthesized in the cytoplasm from choline and acetyl coenzyme A by choline acetyltransferase. It is stored in mass quantities within small synaptic vesicles at the nerve terminal, and released by exocytosis during nerve depolarization. Its actions in the neuroeffector junctions are rapidly terminated by acetylcholinesterase. ACh may coexist in synaptic vesicles with peptide cotransmitters (e.g. vasoactive intestinal peptide in the salivary gland). ACh has actions on two distinct receptor types: nicotinic and muscarinic (Chapter 20). ACh stimulates nicotinic receptors to result in rapid cell depolarization via increased channel permeability to Na^+. Nicotinic receptors are pentamers

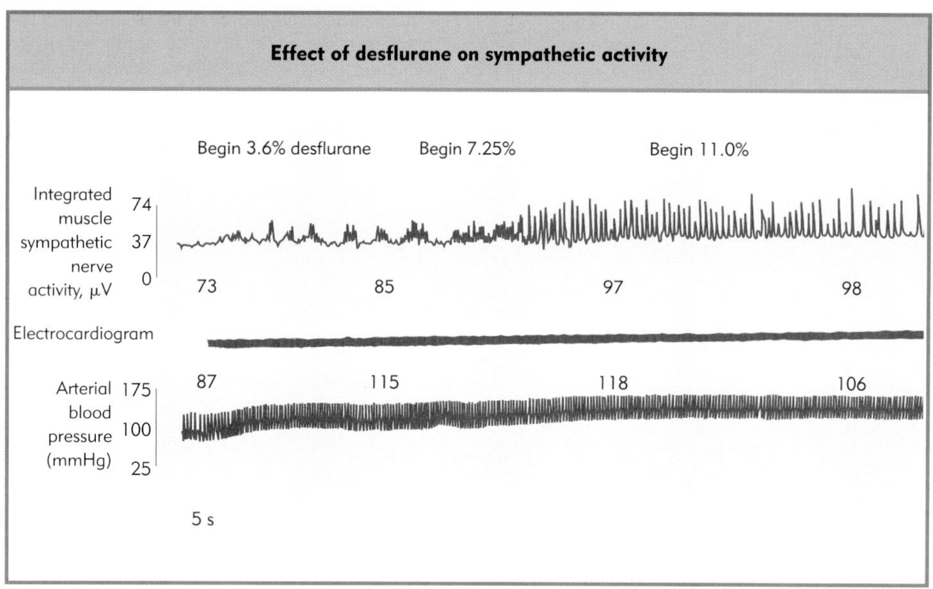

Figure 34.4 The effect of desflurane on sympathetic nerve activity, heart rate, and arterial pressure in a human volunteer following anesthetic induction with sodium thiopental (thiopentone). Sympathoexcitation occurred (top tracing) along with increases in heart rate and blood pressure. Heart rate and mean arterial blood pressure values are indicated over the electrocardiogram and blood pressure traces, respectively. (Adapted with permission from Ebert TJ, Muzi M. Sympathetic hyperactivity during desflurane anesthesia in healthy volunteers: a comparison with isoflurane. Anesthesiology 1993;79:444–53.)

of four subunit isoforms; they are located in skeletal muscle, on postganglionic neurons in autonomic ganglia, on adrenal chromaffin cells, and within the CNS. Muscarinic receptors are seven transmembrane domain proteins coupled to a family of G proteins that inhibit adenylyl cyclase activity (Chapter 3). Five muscarinic receptors with distinct chemical and anatomic properties have been defined pharmacologically: M1–5. The M1 receptors are located in autonomic ganglia, the CNS, and secretory glands. The M2 receptors exist in the sinoatrial and atrioventricular nodes of the heart, and modulate both the rate and the conduction of cardiac electrical activity. They also are found in atrial and ventricular myocardium, and can attenuate the contractility of cardiac muscle. The M3 receptors reside on select smooth muscle cells, where they mediate contraction and secretion at localized glands. In addition to PNS postganglionic junctions, muscarinic receptors exist on the presynaptic membrane of sympathetic nerve terminals in the myocardium, coronary vessels, and peripheral vasculature. When these receptors are stimulated the release of norepinephrine is inhibited, as occurs with presynaptic α_2-adrenoceptor stimulation. Muscarinic antagonism can enhance norepinephrine release and the augmentation of SNS activity. In this manner, atropine blockade of muscarinic receptors elicits not only vagal blockade but also sympathomimetic activity. Nicotinic antagonists that act at the neuromuscular junction may elicit tachycardia via a similar mechanism involving an antimuscarinic action.

Nicotinic receptors are ligand-gated ion channels, and muscarinic receptors are G protein-coupled receptors.

Parasympathetic agonists

Cholinergic agonists can act at nicotinic receptors, muscarinic receptors, or both. The nicotinic receptor agonists consist primarily of the depolarizing neuromuscular-blocking drugs (e.g. succinylcholine (suxamethonium) and hexamethonium), and some of these simultaneously stimulate autonomic ganglia (Chapter 37). Muscarinic receptor agonists are divided into a few general groups: the choline esters (ACh, methacholine (amechol), carbachol (carbamylcholine), bethanechol), the alkaloids (pilocarpine, muscarine, arecoline (arecholine)) that act directly, and the acetylcholinesterase inhibitors or anticholinesterases (physostigmine, neostigmine, pyridostigmine, edrophonium, echothiophate (ecothiophate)) that act indirectly. The direct-acting agonists have few clinical applications, with the exception of their topical use to produce miosis. In contrast, anticholinesterase drugs are frequently employed to reverse the action of nondepolarizing neuromuscular blocking drugs, to improve neuromuscular function in myasthenia gravis, for colonic pseudo-obstruction, and to improve mental functioning in Alzheimer's disease (involving newer drugs).

The diffuse action and rapid hydrolysis of ACh by acetylcholinesterase at the synapse, and plasma cholinesterase (or butyrylcholinesterase) in the plasma, make it virtually useless as a therapeutic agent. However, ACh may be used topically as a miotic agent during cataract extraction surgery when a rapid miosis is desired. Longer activity can be achieved with the synthetic drug methacholine, which contains a methyl group on the β position of choline. This modification prevents significant nicotinic receptor effects and slows acetylcholinesterase metabolism. Carbachol and bethanechol are long-acting synthetic parasympathetic agonists, the carbamic-linked ester moiety significantly reduces metabolism by acetylcholinesterase and plasma cholinesterase. Similar to methacholine, the methyl group on the β carbon of choline makes bethanechol specific for muscarinic receptors; it can be used orally or parenterally, as it has only minimal cardiac negative chronotropic and inotropic effects. Bethanechol can be a useful therapy for postoperative urinary retention and neurogenic bladder. Pilocarpine is derived from the South American shrub pilocarpa; it is a tertiary amine alkaloid with actions similar to those of methacholine. It is the only direct-acting cholinomimetic alkaloid used therapeutically. Clinical use includes treatment for xerostomia and glaucoma, where it is employed as a topical miotic to reduce intraocular pressure. Pilocarpine has minimal nicotinic effects unless given systemically, in which case hypertension and tachycardia may result.

The *anticholinesterase* drugs are ionized water-soluble agents that inhibit acetylcholinesterase at the synaptic cleft, thereby

Table 34.1 Commonly used anticholinesterases. (Adapted from Stoelting RK. Pharmacology in anesthetic practice. Philadelphia: JB Lippincott; 1987.)

Dose (mg/kg)	Elimination half-time (min)		Volume of distribution (L/kg)		Clearance (mL/kg/min)		% of renal contribution to total clearance	Speed of onset	Duration (min)	Recommended dose of atropine* (μg/kg)
	Normal	Anephric	Normal	Anephric	Normal	Anephric				
Edrophonium (0.5 mg/kg)	110	206	1.1	0.7	9.6	2.7	66	rapid	60	7
Neostigmine (0.043 mg/kg)	80	183	0.7	0.8	9.0	3.4	54	intermediate	60	15
Pyridostigmine (0.35 mg/kg)	112	379	1.1	1.0	8.6	2.1	76	slow	90	15

* Dose to be co-administered with anticholinesterase during reversal of neuromuscular blockade. (Adapted from Stoelting RK. Pharmacology in Anesthetic Practice. Philadelphia: Copyright © Lippincott Williams and Wilkins; 1987.)

increasing local concentrations of ACh. The anesthetist relies on anticholinesterases to reverse nondepolarizing neuromuscular blockade at the nicotinic ACh receptor (Chapter 37). Because anticholinesterase drugs also activate muscarinic receptors, the administration of a muscarinic receptor antagonist such as atropine or glycopyrrolate (glycopyrronium) can reduce the side effects of bradycardia, bronchospasm, or intestinal spasm (Table 34.1). The speed of onset of action for the commonly employed cholinesterase inhibitors is edrophonium > neostigmine > pyridostigmine.

The anticholinesterase physostigmine is a tertiary amine that has the ability to cross the blood–brain barrier and is sometimes employed to reverse the CNS effects of cholinergic receptor antagonists, e.g. atropine or scopolamine (hyoscine). Edrophonium, neostigmine, and pyridostigmine are quaternary amines that do not cross the blood–brain barrier. The common therapeutic application of neostigmine is for the reversal of neuromuscular blockade because it is the most potent anticholinesterase. It is also used to treat paralytic ileus, atonic distended urinary bladder, and myasthenia gravis. The slow onset of action of pyridostigmine limits its application for reversal of neuromuscular blockade, but its oral form is used to treat myasthenia gravis. Edrophonium has a rapid onset of action (peak effect in 1–2 minutes versus the 7–11-minute activation for neostigmine), a short duration (1–2 hours), and fewer cholinergic side effects than neostigmine. It also is used in the diagnosis of myasthenia gravis and to differentiate cholinergic crisis (excessive ACh) from inadequate therapy (insufficient ACh), which both result in weakness in myasthenic patients.

Irreversible anticholinesterases are usually organophosphate compounds such as parathion pesticide or sarin nerve gas. They form a phosphorylated enzyme that is resistant to attack by water. They readily pass into the CNS and are rapidly absorbed through the skin, hence their use as pesticides and in chemical warfare. The only therapeutic agent in this group is echothiophate, a long-acting, irreversible anticholinesterase that is instilled into the eye to lower intraocular pressure by decreasing the resistance to aqueous humor outflow. Echothiophate is absorbed into the circulation and can therefore prolong the duration of action of succinylcholine because of a reduction in plasma cholinesterase activity. The action of ester-based local anesthetics also may be lengthened in patients receiving echothiophate due to a slower metabolism of the local anesthetic. Enzyme activity may not return to normal for 4–6 weeks after discontinuation of chronic therapy.

Parasympathetic antagonists

Anticholinergic drugs (atropine, scopolamine, glycopyrrolate) competitively inhibit the action of ACh by reversibly binding to muscarinic cholinergic postganglionic receptors. They are selective for muscarinic ACh receptors at the doses usually employed clinically. Atropine and scopolamine are tertiary amines and can easily cross the placenta and the blood–brain barrier into the brain; glycopyrrolate is a quaternary amine and does not cross the blood–brain barrier. Atropinic drugs produce mydriasis and cycloplegia, and inhibit salivary, bronchial, pancreatic, and gastrointestinal secretions. They also relax bronchial smooth muscle to reduce airway resistance, increase heart rate, and act as gastrointestinal relaxants (Table 34.2). Atropine and scopolamine possess antiemetic properties and effectively control nausea induced by the vestibular apparatus; scopolamine skin patches are used to control motion sickness. Anticholinergic drugs have been used to reduce acid secretion in peptic ulcer disease; however, they also reduce lower esophageal sphincter tone and delay gastric emptying. These drugs should be used with caution in patients with cardiac tachyarrhythmias or severe coronary artery disease, and are contraindicated in narrow-angle glaucoma as they may increase intraocular pressure.

When bronchodilation without systemic side effects is desired, inhalation of anticholinergics is the most effective route of administration. Ipratropium, a derivative of methylatropine, is an inhaled anticholinergic drug with bronchodilator capabilities as effective as intravenous isoproterenol (isoprenaline), a potent β agonist. Low doses of ipratropium reduce airway size via preferential blockade of neuronal M2 muscarinic receptors, whereas large doses produce bronchodilation from blockade of M3 muscarinic receptors on airway smooth muscle. Anticholinergic drugs reduce airway secretions, but unlike atropine, ipratropium does not affect the mucociliary clearance of respiratory secretions. In chronic obstructive pulmonary disease (COPD) ipratropium is beneficial in improving pulmonary function without

Table 34.2 Comparison of antimuscarinic/anticholinergic drugs

Drug	Sedation	Heart rate	GI tone	Airway secretions	Mydriasis cycloplegia	Duration IV	Duration IM
Atropine	+	+++	−−	−	+	15–30 min	2–4 h
Scopolamine	+++	−/+	−	−−−	+++	30–60 min	4–6 h
Glycopyrrolate	0	++	−−−	−−−	0	2–4 h	6–8 h

−−−, markedly depressed; −−, moderately depressed; −, mildly depressed; 0, no effect; +, mildly increased; ++ moderately increased; +++, markedly increased; IM, intramuscular; IV, intravenous; GI, gastro-intestinal.

tachyphylaxis to long-term use. In acute asthma exacerbations, ipratropium may provide additional benefit when used with inhaled β agonists.

The naturally occurring anticholinergic drugs atropine and scopolamine are tertiary amines derived from the belladonna plant. Their anticholinergic function is due primarily to the L stereoisomer, although the drugs contain equal parts of both L and the D isomers. Low doses of atropine and scopolamine (up to 2 μg/kg) exert their effects within the CNS, augmenting vagal outflow, which may result in bradycardia. At the usual clinical doses (15–70 μg/kg) atropine acts at peripheral muscarinic receptors to block the action of ACh, thereby increasing heart rate and pupil size while reducing secretory gland activity, which results in both an antisialogogue effect and anhydrosis.

Scopolamine displays stronger antisialogogue and ocular activity but is less likely than glycopyrrolate or atropine to increase heart rate (Table 34.2). Scopolamine crosses the blood–brain barrier more effectively than atropine, to produce amnesia, drowsiness, fatigue, and nonREM sleep, and was often used in conjunction with sedatives and opioids for preanesthetic medication. A limitation of the central actions of scopolamine (and atropine) is an infrequent side effect termed the *central anticholinergic syndrome*. This consists of agitation, disorientation, delirium, hallucinations, and restlessness, but it may manifest as somnolence and needs to be considered in the differential diagnosis of delayed awakening from anesthesia. Physostigmine (15–60 μg/kg IV) can be administered for the treatment of central anticholinergic syndrome. As a quaternary amine, glycopyrrolate is unable to cross the blood–brain barrier and does not exert CNS side effects, but is more potent and longer acting at peripheral muscarinic receptors than atropine. It is used as an antisialogogue, to treat vagally mediated bradycardia, and to inhibit cardiac muscarinic receptor side effects when anticholinesterase agents are used to reverse the effects of muscle relaxants.

Sympathetic nervous system

The major neurotransmitters of the SNS are norepinephrine and epinephrine (adrenaline). Norepinephrine is released primarily from postganglionic neurons and epinephrine is produced in and released from the adrenal medulla. A number of cotransmitters may be released simultaneously with norepinephrine, including ATP and neuropeptide Y. In most vascular tissues ATP causes synergistic vasoconstriction with norepinephrine (α_1-adrenoceptors) via P_{2X} purine receptors, but in the coronary circulation ATP produces dilation via P_{2Y} receptors. In the adrenal medullary chromaffin cells epinephrine is released with ATP and norepinephrine, a precursor of epinephrine. Epinephrine is synthesized in four steps from the amino acid tyrosine: in the cytoplasm tyrosine is hydroxylated in the 3-position of the aromatic ring, then decarboxylated to form dopamine; in vesicles dopamine is hydroxylated on the β carbon into norepinephrine; and in the cytoplasm of the adrenal medulla the amine is methylated into epinephrine (Chapter 20). Corticosteroids increase expression of the enzyme responsible for norepinephrine methylation (phenylethanolamine-*N*-methyl transferase). The actions of catecholamines are terminated predominantly by local reuptake into nerve terminals, by diffusion, and by metabolism. Metabolism involves two major enzymes, monoamine oxidase (MAO-A and B isozymes) and catechol-O-methyltransferase (COMT). Although MAO is found in adrenergic neurons, COMT generally is not and its presence in the liver may be responsible for the initial metabolism of intravascular catecholamines. Intravascular metabolism is rapid (e.g. the plasma half-life of dopamine is 2 minutes). Owing to the complexities of catecholamine distribution and metabolism, even weight-based infusion may lead to significant variability in plasma concentration. For example, a 75-fold variation in plasma dopamine concentration can occur after weight-based infusion in healthy volunteers. A few rare disorders exist in the synthesis and metabolism of catecholamines, but they highlight the ability of the SNS to function in spite of some dysfunction in neurotransmitter synthesis and regulation.

Both α- and β-adrenoceptors are G protein-coupled receptors, each with multiple subtypes.

Most clinically employed catecholamines stimulate both α- and β-adrenoceptors; the exceptions are phenylephrine and methoxamine (pure α agonists) and isoproterenol (pure β agonist) (Fig. 34.5). Both α- and β-adrenoceptors are seven transmembrane domain G protein-coupled receptors. Adrenoceptors regulate intracellular signal transduction in a number of ways: in general, α_1- and β-adrenoceptors activate phospholipase C and adenylyl cyclase, respectively, and α_2-adrenoceptors inhibit adenylyl cyclase. Adrenoceptors are desensitized by continuous exposure to catecholamines: receptor phosphorylation and internalization may occur after minutes; downregulation may occur after hours. The α-adrenoceptors respond to catecholamines with an order of potency: norepinephrine ≥ epinephrine >> isoproterenol. Their order of potency on β-adrenoceptors is isoproterenol > epinephrine ≥ norepinephrine. Each catecholamine has distinct qualitative and quantitative effects on arterial and venous smooth muscle. Knowledge of their net

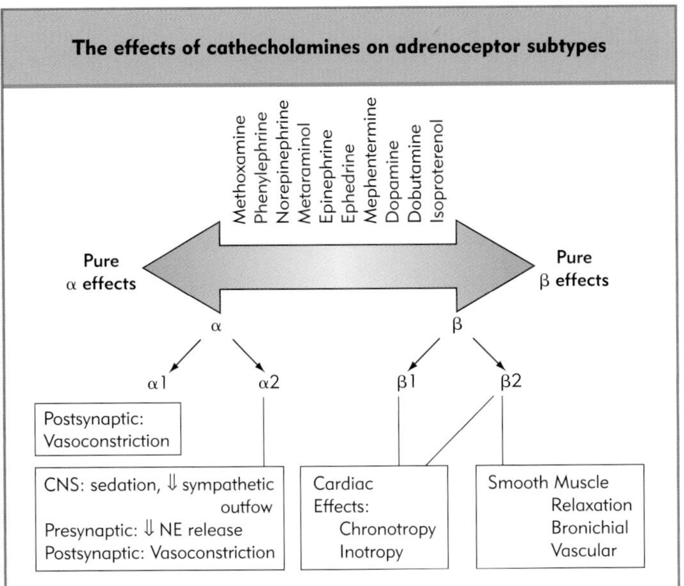

Figure 34.5 The effects of various catecholamines on adrenoceptor subtypes. Effects range from pure α agonist to pure β agonist. (Adapted with permission from Lawson NW, Wallfisch HK. Cardiovascular pharmacology: a new look at the 'pressors'. In: Stoelting RK, Barash PG, Gallagher TJ, eds. Advances in anesthesia. Chicago, IL: Year Book Medical Publishers; 1986:195. Copyright © Mosby Inc.)

effects in different vascular beds permits a better understanding of their effect on cardiac output. In addition to the direct effect of the catecholamine on inotropy, cardiac output is also influenced by effects on cardiac preload and afterload (Table 34.3).

The α-adrenoceptors

The α-adrenoceptors exist at both presynaptic and postsynaptic neuroeffector junction sites throughout the human body and are involved in cardiovascular regulation, metabolism, consciousness, and nociception. At least six subtypes of α-adrenoceptor have been identified, but this chapter will focus on the two 'primary' subtypes: α_1 and α_2. The α_1-adrenoceptors are characterized by stimulation by phenylephrine and methoxamine and inhibition by low concentrations of prazosin, whereas α_2-adrenoceptors are activated selectively by clonidine and dexmedetomidine and are blocked by yohimbine. Both α-adrenoceptor subtypes respond with an order of potency of norepinephrine ≥ epinephrine >> isoproterenol, but are distinguished by the greater potency of norepinephrine at α_1-versus the α_2-adrenoceptors. The α-adrenoceptors can also be differentiated by their regulation of intracellular Ca^{2+} and cAMP levels through specific G protein-coupled receptors. The α_1-adrenoceptors activate G_q, which stimulates phospholipase C hydrolysis of membrane phospholipids, increases cytoplasmic Ca^{2+} levels, and results in smooth muscle contraction. Stimulation of α_2-adrenoceptors activates G_i and results in decreased adenylyl cyclase synthesis of cAMP. Physiologic effects of α_2-adrenoceptor stimulation include contraction of vascular smooth muscle via postsynaptic receptors, and inhibition of norepinephrine release into the synaptic cleft via presynaptic receptors. Central effects include sedation, anxiolysis, analgesia, and modulation of sympathetic and parasympathetic outflow from the CNS.

Table 34.3 Relative potencies in humans of sympathomimetic amines as constrictors of resistance and capacitance vessels

Resistance Vessels		Capacitance Vessels	
Drug	***Relative potency***	***Drug***	***Relative potency***
Norepinephrine	1.000	Norepinephrine	1.000
Metaraminol	0.0874	Phenylephrine	0.0570
Phenylephrine	0.0684	Metaraminol	0.0419
Tyramine	0.0148	Methoxamine	0.0068
Mephentermine	0.0049	Ephedrine	0.0025
Ephedrine	0.0020	Tyramine	0.0023
Methoxamine	0.0018	Mephentermine	0.0023

(Data used with permission from Schmid PG, Eckstein JW, Abboud FM. Comparison of the effects of several sympathomimetic amines on resistance and capacitance vessels in the forearm of man. Circulation 1966;34:209.)

The β-adrenoceptors

Historically, β-adrenoceptors were pharmacologically differentiated based on their sensitivity to the agonists isoproterenol, epinephrine, and norepinephrine. The order of β_1-adrenoceptor sensitivity is isoproterenol > epinephrine ≥ norepinephrine, whereas that for β_2-adrenoceptors is isoproterenol > epinephrine >> norepinephrine (i.e. the potency of norepinephrine at the β_2-adrenoceptor is significantly less than that of epinephrine). Both β-adrenoceptor subtypes activate G_s and increase cAMP levels through activation of adenylyl cyclase. The β_1-adrenoceptors are located primarily in the sinoatrial and atrioventricular nodes, myocardium, ventricular conduction system, and adipose tissue. The β_2-adrenoceptors are more widespread, and are found in vascular smooth muscle (skin, muscle, mesentery, bronchi) and mediate vasodilatation and bronchial relaxation. Albuterol (salbutamol) is a selective agonist for β_2-adrenoceptors; there is no selective agonist for β_1-adrenoceptors. Atenolol, metoprolol, and esmolol are selective β_1-antagonists.

Endogenous catecholamines

The basic catecholamine structure is a phenylethylamine with two hydroxyl groups on the aromatic ring and a third on the β carbon (Table 34.4). Epinephrine and norepinephrine have a chiral center at the β carbon, where the L isomer is more active, and dopamine has no chiral center. Intravenous formulations of epinephrine and norepinephrine consist of the single L isomer; a racemic formulation of epinephrine is available for inhalation. The naturally occurring catecholamines act on both α- and β-adrenoceptors. More pronounced α activity is observed when minimal amino group substitutions occur, whereas increased β activity results as amino group substitutions increase. The dosage of catecholamines should be reduced if a patient is taking tricyclic antidepressants, which inhibit catecholamine reuptake, or monoamine oxidase inhibitors, which inhibit metabolism.

Table 34.4 Adrenoceptor activity of catecholamines

Drug, IV infusion dose (μg/min per kg)	Structure	Receptor site of activity				
		$\alpha_1$art	$\alpha_1$ven	β_1	β_2	DA
Epinephrine, 0.015	HO–C$_6$H$_3$(OH)–CHCH$_2$NHCH$_3$ (OH)	0	0	++++	++++	0
0.03–0.15		++	++	++++	++++	
0.15–0.30		++++	++++			
Norepinephrine, 0.1	HO–C$_6$H$_3$(OH)–CHCH$_2$NH$_2$ (OH)	+++++	+++++	++++	?+	0
Dopamine, 0.5–2	HO–C$_6$H$_3$(OH)–CH$_2$CH$_2$NH$_2$	0	++++			+++++
2–10		0	+++	+++	+++++	
10		++++	+++	+++++		

$\alpha_1$art = α_1 receptor, arerial; $\alpha_1$ven = $\alpha_1$receptor, venous; DA = dopamine receptors
0 = no effect; += slight effect; +++++ = potent effect

Dopamine

Dopamine is the immediate precursor to norepinephrine. Its receptors are located throughout the CNS, on SNS postganglionic nerve terminals, in the afferent and efferent arterioles of the nephron, and the adrenal glands. Dopamine receptors are G protein-coupled: D_1-like receptors stimulate adenylyl cyclase via G_s, and D_2-like receptors inhibit adenylyl cyclase via G_i. D_1-receptors are postsynaptic and agonism leads to coronary, renal, mesenteric, and peripheral arterial dilation. Fenoldopam is a selective D_1 agonist and is indicated for hypertensive emergencies. D_2 receptors occur at presynaptic and postsynaptic sites; presynaptic D_2 receptor activation leads to inhibition of norepinephrine release.

Dopamine has dose-dependent actions on both dopamine receptors and adrenoceptors (Table 34.4); dopamine can be converted into and stimulate net release of norepinephrine. At low doses (1–2 μg/min/kg body weight) vasodilatation of renal and mesenteric vasculature occurs and renal blood flow, glomerular filtration, and Na^+ excretion increase via D_1-receptor effects (Table 34.5). At doses of 2–10 μg/min/kg, β_1-adrenoceptor stimulation has positive inotropic and chronotropic effects. As dopamine doses reach 10 μg/min/kg, α_1-adrenoceptor activation causes peripheral vasoconstriction and can reduce renal blood flow. At the higher dosage range, titration of dopamine may be limited by tachycardia or dysrhythmias. Unlike dobutamine, dopamine may lead to increased myocardial work without a compensatory increase in oxygen delivery, resulting in ischemia.

Norepinephrine

Norepinephrine is the endogenous mediator of SNS activity. Exogenous administration results in dose-dependent hemodynamic effects on α- and β-adrenoceptors (Table 34.4). At low doses, β_1 actions predominate and cardiac output and blood pressure increase. Larger doses of norepinephrine cause further increases in blood pressure via arterial and venous smooth muscle contraction from α_1-adrenoceptor stimulation (Table 34.5). At these larger doses, heart rate and cardiac output may

Table 34.5 Cardiovascular and renal actions of catecholamines

Drug, IV infusion dose (μg/kg/min)	Cardiovascular effects					
	CO	***Inotropy***	***HR***	***Preload***	***TPR***	***RBF***
Epinephrine, 0.015	⇑–	⇑⇑	⇑⇑	⇑	⇑⇑	⇓–
0.03–0.15	⇑–⇓	⇑⇑	⇑⇑	⇑	⇑⇑⇑	⇓
0.15–0.30	⇑⇑	⇑⇑	⇑	⇑	⇑⇑	⇑
Norepinephrine, 0.1	–⇓	–	Reflex ⇓	⇑⇑⇑	⇑⇑	–⇓
Dopamine, 0.5–2	⇑	——	——	⇑	–⇓	⇑
2–10	⇑⇑	⇑	–⇑	⇑	–⇑	⇑
≥ 10	⇑–⇓	⇑⇑	⇑⇑	⇑	⇑⇑	–⇓

CO, cardiac output; HR, heart rate; TPR, total peripheral resistance; RBF, renal blood flow; –, no clear effect; ⇓, decreased effect; ⇑, increased effect.

decrease; myocardial ischemia can be exacerbated. Intravenous administration of norepinephrine causes marked arterial and venous vasoconstriction in most vascular beds; it is most often used therapeutically for the treatment of severe vasodilation (Table 34.5). Caution must be used in patients already exhibiting marked vasoconstriction, as norepinephrine administration may further increase vascular resistance such that limb and organ blood flow is compromised and ischemia occurs.

Epinephrine

Epinephrine is an endogenous catecholamine that is synthesized, stored, and released from the chromaffin cells of the adrenal medulla. Epinephrine actions at α- and β-adrenoceptors are dose dependent (Table 34.4). At low doses (0.015 mg/min/kg), β_1- and β_2-adrenoceptor actions predominate. Specifically, β_1-adrenoceptor stimulation produces predictable cardiac effects, including increased heart rate, cardiac output, contractility, and conduction. Stimulation of β_2-adrenoceptors causes relaxation of bronchial smooth muscle, an increase in liver glycogenolysis, and vasodilatation in most regional vascular tissue. This last effect results in a decrease in diastolic blood pressure and redistribution of blood flow to low-resistance circulations. At higher doses (0.15–0.30 mg/min/kg) α-adrenoceptors are activated, leading to vasoconstriction of the skin, mucosa, and renal vascular beds, and substantial blood flow redistribution away from these circulations (Table 34.5). Stimulation of α-adrenoceptors eventually decreases skeletal muscle blood flow, inhibits insulin secretion, and contracts mesenteric vascular smooth muscle.

In addition to improving cardiac function, exogenous administration of epinephrine is commonly used in conjunction with local anesthetics to prolong their duration of action. Epinephrine also is employed as treatment for anaphylactic shock, localized bleeding, bronchospasm, and stridor related to laryngotracheal edema. Subcutaneous doses of 0.2–0.5 mg can be used in early anaphylaxis in order to stabilize mast cells and reduce degranulation. As epinephrine stimulates cellular K^+ uptake via β_2-adrenoceptors, it can also be used to treat life-threatening hyperkalemia.

Synthetic β agonists

ISOPROTERENOL

Isoproterenol shows almost pure β-adrenoceptor activity as a consequence of the increased size of the alkyl substituent on the amino group (Table 34.6). Isoproterenol produces positive chronotropic and inotropic effects via β_1-adrenoceptor stimulation, and bronchodilatation and vasodilatation in vascular smooth muscle through β_2-activation (Table 34.7). The therapeutic role of isoproterenol is limited. It is rarely used as a bronchodilator owing to the availability of potent inhaled β_2 agonists, and is only used as a fourth-line chronotrope for severe bradyarrhythmias until an electrical pacemaker can be placed. Isoproterenol can promote tachyarrhythmias and causes mismatching of myocardial oxygen delivery and consumption. Isoproterenol reduces vascular resistance, so it is not used in vasodilatory shock.

DOBUTAMINE

Dobutamine consists of two enantiomers with direct-acting β_1-adrenoceptor agonism and competing α_1 agonism and antagonism. Dobutamine is employed clinically as a 'cardioselective' inotrope. Its predominant effect is β_1-adrenoceptor stimulation, resulting in positive inotropic effects but with smaller increases in heart rate than seen with isoproterenol (Table 34.7). It improves cardiac output without major adverse effects on the myocardial oxygen supply/demand ratio because heart rate is relatively stable and afterload is maintained.

EPHEDRINE

Ephedrine is a natural product of the *Ephedra* plant; it is a commonly used noncatecholamine sympathomimetic (Table 34.6). The action of ephedrine is considered indirect because it competes with norepinephrine for local reuptake, thus resulting in elevated concentrations of norepinephrine at receptor sites. Generally, the cardiovascular effects produced by ephedrine are similar to those of epinephrine but less potent and longer acting (Table 34.7). The primary mechanism for the increased myocardial performance associated with ephedrine is stimulation of β_1-adrenoceptors, although indirect α-adrenoceptor-mediated

Table 34.6 Adrenoceptor activity of synthetic α and β agonists

Drug, IV infusion dose	Structure	Receptor site of activity				
		$\alpha_1$art	$\alpha_1$ven	β_1	β_2	DA
Synthetic catecholamines						
Isoproterenol, 0.015 μg/min per kg	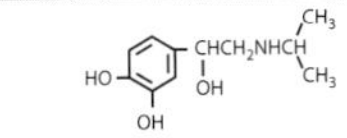 HO, OH, $CHCH_2NHCH(CH_3)_2$ (OH on side chain)	0	0	+++++	+++++	
Dobutamine, 5 μg/min per kg	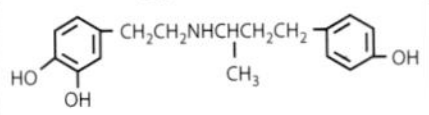 HO, OH, $CH_2CH_2NHCHCH_2CH_2$ (CH_3), OH	+	?	++++	++	0
Synthetic noncatecholamines						
Indirect acting						
Ephedrine, 5–10 μg IV push	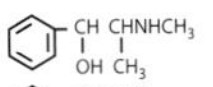 CH CHNHCH$_3$ (OH, CH$_3$)	++	+++	+++	++	0
Metaraminol, 0.5 μg/min per kg	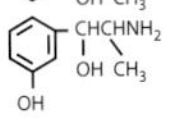 CHCHNH$_2$ (OH, CH$_3$), OH	+++++	++++	+++	0	0
Direct acting						
Phenylephrine, 0.15 μg/min per kg	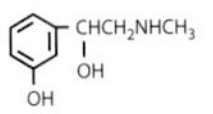 $CHCH_2NHCH_3$ (OH), OH	++++	+++++	0	0	0
Methoxamine, 5–10 mg IV push	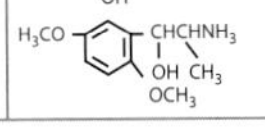 H_3CO, CHCHNH$_2$ (OH, CH$_3$), OCH_3	++++	0 -+?	0	0	0

$\alpha_1$art = $\alpha_1$receptor, arterial; $\alpha_1$ven = $\alpha_1$receptor, venous; DA = dopamine receptors
0 = no effect; += slight effect; +++++ = potent effect.

Table 34.7 Cardiovascular and renal actions of synthetic α and β agonists

Drug, IV infusion dose (μg/kg/min)	Cardiovascular effects					
	CO	***Inotropy***	***HR***	***Preload***	***TPR***	***RBF***
Synthetic catecholamines						
Isoproterenol, 0.015	⇑–⇓	⇑⇑⇑	⇑⇑⇑	⇓	⇓⇓	–⇑
Dobutamine, 5	⇑⇑	⇑⇑	–⇑	?	–	–⇑
Synthetic noncatecholamines						
Indirect acting						
Ephedrine, 5–10 mg IV push	⇑	⇑	⇑	⇑⇑	⇑	⇑–⇓
Metaraminol, 0.5	–⇓	⇑	Reflex ⇓	⇑	⇑⇑⇑	⇓⇓⇓
Direct acting						
Phenylephrine, 0.15	–⇓	–	Reflex ⇓	⇑⇑⇑	⇑⇑	–⇓
Methoxamine, 5–10 mg IV push	–⇓	–	Reflex ⇓	–	⇑⇑	⇓⇓

CO, cardiac output; HR, heart rate; TPR, total peripheral resistance; RBF, renal blood flow; –, no clear effect; ⇓, decreased effect; ⇑, increased effect.

venoconstriction has an important contribution through increasing preload and cardiac output. Intravenous ephedrine administration leads to increases in heart rate, systolic and diastolic blood pressure, cardiac output, and coronary artery blood flow. Ephedrine is therefore useful during general or regional anesthesia to treat hypotension.

Ephedrine can reduce bronchoconstriction by β_2 agonism. In addition, ephedrine decreases renal and splanchnic blood flow, stimulates the CNS (e.g. increases MAC), and is associated with tachyphylaxis after extended use. It is administered as a vasopressor during obstetrics because it has minimal effects on uterine blood flow. As with catecholamines, MAO inhibitors potentiate the pressor effects of ephedrine.

Amphetamines, methamphetamine, mephentermine, methylphenidate, and metaraminol are synthetic vasopressors with predominately indirect actions on α- and β-adrenoceptors. In particular, metaraminol produces a marked increase in both systolic and diastolic pressure through direct and indirect α-adrenoceptor-mediated vasoconstriction (Tables 34.6 and 34.7).

β_2 agonists

The β_2-adrenoceptor agonists selectively relax bronchial and uterine smooth muscle. Metaproterenol (orciprenaline), albuterol, salmeterol, and isoetharine (isoetarine) are inhaled, relatively selective β_2 agonists that decrease airway resistance and are indicated in the treatment of acute asthma and COPD. Side effects rarely occur at lower doses; the frequency of tachycardia is relatively low, as these drugs are inhaled and are 10 times less potent than isoproterenol at activating β_1-adrenoceptors. Prolonged use at higher doses typically causes tachyphylaxis. Terbutaline and ritodrine are tocolytic drugs that are frequently used to manage premature labor contractions because they stimulate β_2-adrenoceptors in the myometrium, resulting in relaxation (Chapter 68). These drugs stimulate both β_1- and β_2-adrenoceptors. They can be given orally or by subcutaneous, intramuscular, or intravenous injection. Side effects include hyperglycemia, hypokalemia, cardiac arrhythmias, tachycardia, and pulmonary edema.

β antagonists (blockers)

The typical β-blocker structure has an isopropyl alcohol group interposed between an amino group and an aromatic group that are attached via an ether linkage. The alcohol/amino structure confers β over α selectivity and the substituent aromatic group affects β_1 selectivity. β-blockers bind selectively to β-adrenoceptors and competitively inhibit the effects of endogenous and exogenous β agonists, which produces a rightward shift of the dose–response curve for β agonists. β-blockers produce negative chronotropic and inotropic effects and consequently are widely used for the treatment of cardiovascular disease. β-blockers also are helpful in the treatment of hypertension, but their mechanism of action is unclear and may involve several pathways, including reducing plasma renin concentrations.

Certain β-blockers (e.g. atenolol, esmolol, metoprolol) show a *relative selectivity* but not *specificity* for β_1-adrenoceptor subtypes, such that β_2-adrenoceptor antagonism may occur as blood levels increase (Table 34.8). The β antagonists can be further subdivided into either pure or partial blockers, based on the absence or presence of intrinsic sympathomimetic activity (ISA) (Table 34.8). Partial antagonists produce less myocardial depression and bradycardia than drugs without ISA, but are unable to preserve ventricular function. Despite the fact that the myocardial depression from volatile or intravenous anesthetics is additive to that of pure β-blockers, perioperative use of pure β-blockers reduces morbidity and mortality in patients with coronary artery disease. Clinically, both partial and pure antagonists are used in the treatment of hypertension and tachydysrhythmias, and both decrease mortality after myocardial infarction. However, drugs with ISA may be more useful in patients with bronchial asthma, compromised left ventricular function, and peripheral vascular disease. Labetalol, which is a combination of four enantiomers, has ISA from the R,R enantiomer on

Table 34.8 Antagonists of β-adrenoceptors

Drug	β_1 potency ratio[a]	Relative β_1 selectivity	Intrinsic sympathomimetic activity	Membrane stabilizing activity	Lipid solubility	Elimination half-life (h)	Total body clearance (mL/min)	Metabolism
Atenolol	1.0	++	0	0	low	6–9	130	renal
Carvedilol	10.0	0	0	++	moderate	7–10	0.6	hepatic
Esmolol	0.02	++	0	0	low	0.15	27 000	esterases[b]
Labetalol	0.3	0	+?	0	low	3–4	2700	hepatic
Metoprolol	1.0	++	0	0	moderate	3–4	1,100	hepatic
Nadolol	1.0	0	0	0	low	14–24	200	renal
Pindolol	6.0	0	++	+	moderate	3–4	400	renal/hepatic
Propranolol	1.0	0	0	++	high	3–4	1000	hepatic
Timolol	6.0	0	0	0	low	4–5	660	renal/hepatic

[a] β_1 Potency ratio is determined relative to propranolol (equal to 1).
[b] Red blood cell and nonspecific esterases.
0, no selectivity or activity; ++, significant selectivity or activity.

β_2-adrenoceptors; most other β-blockers used in the practice of anesthesia do not have ISA.

Perioperative use of β-blockers reduces morbidity and mortality in patients with coronary artery disease, despite their additive myocardial depression with volatile or intravenous anesthetics.

Although the clinical significance remains uncertain, certain β-blockers (e.g. propranolol, carvedilol) exhibit a membrane-stabilizing activity via the (+)-stereoisomer, which produces a local anesthetic-like effect on myocellular membranes. Withdrawal symptoms can occur as a result of discontinuing chronic β-blocker therapy. These hyperadrenergic symptoms include palpitations, tremors, and sweating. Relative contraindications to the use of β-blockers are reactive airway disease, atrioventricular heart block, or acute systolic cardiac failure. Although β-blockers may prevent appropriate hypoglycemic responses in diabetics, patients with both diabetes mellitus and coronary artery disease benefit from β-blocker therapy. β-blockers combined with non-dihydropyridine calcium channel blockers may significantly affect cardiac conduction, and when also combined with H_2-blockers severe negative inotropism may result.

PROPRANOLOL

Propranolol, a nonselective pure β-adrenoceptor antagonist, is the prototypical β-blocker (Table 34.8). It causes decreases in heart rate and cardiac output that are most pronounced during periods of SNS stimulation. Antagonism of β_2-adrenoceptors by propranolol can concomitantly increase peripheral and coronary vascular resistance (although this effect diminishes with chronic administration). In states of catecholamine excess this vasoconstriction may be dangerously magnified if α-blockade has not been achieved. Propranolol reduces myocardial oxygen consumption and reduces blood flow to major organs, except the brain.

Oral propranolol is useful therapeutically because it is lipid soluble and readily absorbed from the small intestine; however, because of extensive first-pass hepatic metabolism, larger oral doses are required to achieve clinical effects equivalent to those of intravenous doses. Prolonged use of propranolol may cause depression, nightmares, fatigue, and/or sexual dysfunction. Marked bradydysrhythmias may result when propranolol is used in conjunction with halothane or opioids.

ESMOLOL

Esmolol is a selective β_1-adrenoceptor antagonist with a low potency but a rapid onset and short duration of action. Its structure allows for rapid esterase degradation; the half-life of esmolol is only 9–10 minutes (Table 34.8). These properties make esmolol particularly useful to reduce the transient β-adrenergic stimulation that occurs in the perioperative period. Indeed, 50–100 mg intravenous esmolol administered only a few minutes prior to laryngoscopy and tracheal intubation can reduce or abolish the commonly observed tachycardia. As a consequence of its cardioselectivity and lack of β_2-adrenoceptor antagonism, minimal bronchial or vascular tone changes are observed. Esmolol is employed to manage short-duration tachycardia accompanied by hypertension, and supraventricular tachycardia, especially in patients with the potential for bronchial constriction or acute ventricular dysfunction. It can be used to produce controlled hypotension to reduce operative blood loss, and may be advantageous in reducing wall stress after repair of major arteries. An ultrashort-acting β_1-blocker, landiolol, may become available in the future; landiolol has an elimination half-life of 4 minutes and a β_1 potency ratio of 0.004.

LABETALOL

Labetalol has ISA on β_2-adrenoceptors and is considered a mixed antagonist because of its actions at both α- and β-adrenoceptors. Intravenous labetalol administration has an α:β antagonistic potency ratio of 1:7 compared with 1:3 after oral administration; these potency ratios are dependent, in part, on the four enantiomers present in labetalol. A lowered heart rate in the presence of lowered systemic blood pressure during labetalol therapy has certain advantages when employed in patients with coronary artery disease because the myocardial oxygen supply/demand ratio is improved. In addition, cardiac output is maintained because the decreased afterload compensates for reduced cardiac function. The peak hypotensive effect of labetalol occurs between 5 and 15 minutes and the duration of action is estimated to be 4–6 hours after a single intravenous dose.

α_1 agonists

Agonists of α_1-adrenoceptors exert vasopressor actions on arterial and venous vessels, thereby increasing mean arterial pressure, increasing preload, and redistributing flow in certain beds. In healthy individuals cardiac output is well maintained, and may improve because of increased preload. The concomitant increase in afterload can improve myocardial oxygen delivery via improved diastolic coronary blood flow. However, there is a potential for increased myocardial work and decreased organ blood flow through regional vasoconstriction. α_1 agonists may be used topically on nasal mucosa to produce decongestion and vasoconstriction.

PHENYLEPHRINE

Phenylephrine is a pure α agonist that is longer acting but considerably less potent than norepinephrine. Phenylephrine increases both venous and arterial resistance and often enhances preload (Tables 34.6 and 34.7). It is frequently employed in the perioperative period to treat hypotension accompanied by increased heart rate. It causes reflex slowing of the heart rate as blood pressure is increased. This vasopressor can be useful in reversing 'tet spells' (right-to-left shunt) in patients with tetralogy of Fallot; however, it does have some effect to increase pulmonary vascular resistance. Newer evidence suggests that phenylephrine is not detrimental to fetal oxygen delivery in pregnant patients who are hypotensive after neuraxial blockade.

METHOXAMINE

Methoxamine is a selective α_1 agonist similar to phenylephrine but without significant venoconstriction (Tables 34.3, 34.6, and 34.7). Its clinical uses are limited, except for the treatment of paroxysmal atrial tachycardia, where a single intravenous dose can counteract the tachycardia via baroreceptor reflex-mediated slowing of the heart.

α_2 agonists

Agonists of α_2-adrenoceptors include the imidazolines (clonidine), phenylethylamines, and oxaloazepines. They are utilized as antihypertensive agents because of their ability to decrease sympathetic outflow from the CNS and their ability to reduce local norepinephrine release at nerve terminals. Other actions of α_2 agonists include vasoconstriction via postsynaptic α_2-adrenoceptors, cardiac antiarrhythmic effects, decreased cerebral blood flow, and inhibition of insulin and growth hormone secretion. Side effects of α_2 agonists include bradycardia, sedation, and dry mouth. Bradycardia occurs through a centrally mediated enhancement of vagal outflow.

Preoperative administration of an α_2 agonist helps to diminish perioperative blood pressure variations, intraoperative plasma catecholamine levels, and the hemodynamic response to endotracheal intubation and surgical stimulation. The α_2 agonists lower the requirements for anesthetics and analgesics in the perioperative period via their sedative, analgesic, and anxiolytic properties. The ability of α_2 agonists to attenuate the sympathoadrenal stress response has been demonstrated during both general and regional anesthesia. Another attribute of α_2 agonists in the perioperative period is that their sedative effect is not accompanied by significant respiratory depression.

CLONIDINE

Clonidine is a selective α_2 agonist that has potent antihypertensive effects. Decreased blood pressure results from inhibition of preganglionic sympathetic fiber activity following α_2-adrenoceptor stimulation in the CNS. Small oral doses of clonidine (2 μg/kg) may reduce adverse myocardial events in patients with coronary artery disease having noncardiac surgery. Oral onset is 30–60 minutes, and clonidine is useful in treating hypertensive urgencies and emergencies; the sedative effect can be limiting. Abrupt discontinuation of clonidine can result in severe rebound hypertension; to avoid this, clonidine should be continued in the perioperative period. Another clinical application of clonidine has been neuraxial administration to treat acute and chronic pain; epidural clonidine (0.5 μg/kg/h) is indicated for the treatment of severe cancer pain. Clonidine is useful in treating the enhanced sympathetic activation of opioid withdrawal.

DEXMEDETOMIDINE

Dexmedetomidine, the (+)-stereoisomer of the imidazolidine compound medetomidine, is highly selective for α_2-adrenoceptors. It is seven times more potent for α_2- than α_1-adrenoceptors, and is considered a full agonist. When used with volatile anesthetics dexmedetomidine reduces the minimal alveolar concentration. It also reduces chest wall rigidity caused by opioids and lessens postanesthetic shivering. Dexmedetomidine has strong analgesic, sedative, and anxiolytic actions, and is indicated for sedation of mechanically ventilated patients in an intensive care setting. The recommended dosage is 1 μg/kg load and 0.2–0.7 μg/kg/h infusion; hypotension, bradycardia, and sinus arrest are potential side effects. Dosing may need to be reduced for hepatic dysfunction; it is not known whether renally excreted metabolites are active.

α antagonists

α-antagonists include the β-haloethylamines (phenoxybenzamine), imidazoline analogs (e.g. phentolamine), piperanzinyl quinazolines (e.g. prazosin), and indole derivatives (e.g. yohimbine) (Table 34.9). These agents exhibit either competitive or

Table 34.9 Antagonists of α-adrenoceptors

Drug	Type of antagonism	Receptor selectivity
Prazosin	Competitive	$\alpha_1 >> \alpha_2$
Phenoxybenzamine	Noncompetitive	$\alpha_1 > \alpha_2$
Phentolamine	Competitive	$\alpha_1 = \alpha_2$
Tolazoline	Competitive	$\alpha_1 = \alpha_2$
Yohimbine	Competitive	$\alpha_2 >> \alpha_1$

noncompetitive inhibition and have varying degrees of α_1 and α_2 selectivity. Important clinical actions of selective α_1 antagonists, such as prazosin, include reductions in blood pressure and preoperative treatment of catecholamine excess syndromes (e.g. pheochromocytoma); fatigue, reflex tachycardia, and first-dose orthostatic hypotension can be troublesome. Nonselective α antagonists are used less frequently: phenoxybenzamine is used preoperatively in treating pheochromocytoma and other catecholamine-secreting tumors; phentolamine is used intraoperatively in treating norepinephrine-secreting tumors and by subcutaneous injection to prevent skin necrosis secondary to catecholamine extravasation.

Key references

Berkowitz DE, Schwinn DA. Basic pharmacology of α- and β-adrenoceptors. In: Bowdle TA, Hovita A, Kharasch ED, eds. The pharmacological basis of anesthesiology. New York: Churchill Livingstone; 1994:581–606.

Carpenter MB, Sutin J. The autonomic nervous system. In: Carpenter MB, Sutin J, eds. Human Neuroanatomy, 8th edn. Baltimore, MD: Williams & Wilkins; 1983:220.

Ebert TJ. Preoperative evaluation of the autonomic nervous system. Adv Anesth. 1993;10:49–68.

Ebert TJ, Muzi M. Sympathetic hyperactivity during desflurane anesthesia in healthy volunteers: a comparison with isoflurane. Anesthesiology 1993;79:444–53.

Kinsella SM, Tuckey JP. Perioperative bradycardia and asystole: relationship to vasovagal syncope and the Bezold–Jarisch reflex. Br J Anaesth. 2001;86:859–68.

Robertson D, Low PA, Polinsky RJ eds. Primer on the autonomic nervous system. San Diego, CA: Academic Press; 1996.

Wood M. Cholinergic and parasympathomimetic drugs. Cholinesterases and anticholinesterases. In: Wood M, Wood AJJ, eds. Drugs and anesthesia. Pharmacology for anesthesiologists. Baltimore, MD: Williams & Wilkins; 1982:111.

Wood M. Drugs and the sympathetic nervous system. In: Wood M, Wood AJJ, eds. Drugs and anesthesia. Pharmacology for anesthesiologists. Baltimore, MD: Williams & Wilkins; 1982:407.

Further reading

Ahlquist RP. A study of the adrenotropic receptors. Am J Physiol. 1948;153:586–94.

Burnstock G. Integration of factors controlling vascular tone. Anesthesiology 1993;79:1368–80.

Ebert TJ, Harkin CP, Muzi M. Cardiovascular responses to sevoflurane: a review. Anesth Analg. 1995;81:S11–22.

Ebert TJ, Muzi M. Propofol and autonomic reflex function in humans. Anesth Analg. 1994;78:369–75.

Flacke WE, Flacke JW. Cholinergic and anticholinergic agents. In: Smith NT, Corbascia AN, eds. Drug interactions in anesthesia. Philadelphia, PA: Lea & Febiger; 1986:160.

Kamibayashi T, Maze M. Clinical uses of α_2-adrenergic agonists. Anesthesiology 2000;93:1345–9.

Lawson NW, Wallfisch HK. Cardiovascular pharmacology: a new look at the 'pressors'. In: Stoelting RK, Barash PG, Gallagher TJ, eds. Advances in anesthesia. Chicago, IL: Year Book Medical Publishers; 1986:195.

London MJ, Zaugg M, Schaub MC, Spahn DR. Perioperative β-adrenergic receptor blockade. Anesthesiology 2004;100:170–5.

Smiley RM, Kwatra MM, Schwinn DA. New developments in cardiovascular adrenergic receptor pharmacology: molecular mechanisms and clinical relevance. J Cardiothorac Vasc Anesth. 1998;12:80–95.

Ziegler MG. Antihypertensives. In: Chernow B, Lake CR, eds. The pharmacologic approach to the critically ill patient. Baltimore, MD: Williams & Wilkins; 1983:303.

SECTION 3

Muscle

Chapter 35

Voluntary motor systems – skeletal muscle, reflexes, and control of movement

Philip M Hopkins

TOPICS COVERED IN THIS CHAPTER

- **Types of muscle**
- **Structure of skeletal muscle**
- **Muscle contraction**
  - The motor unit and excitation–contraction coupling
  - Malignant hyperthermia
  - Regulation of the force of muscle contraction
- **Control of muscle contraction**
  - The muscle spindle and the stretch reflex
  - Efferent supply to the muscle spindles and control of muscle length
  - The motor response to nociceptive stimulation
  - Control of muscle tone
  - Motor programs for the generation of stereotyped patterns of movement
  - The basal ganglia
  - The cerebellum
  - Motor areas of the cerebral cortex
- **Drug treatment of movement disorders**
  - Parkinson's disease
  - Parkinsonian and other extrapyramidal reactions
  - Spasticity

TYPES OF MUSCLE

Muscles are the contractile tissues of the body. Morphologically, muscles can be described as striated or smooth, depending on the degree of organization of the contractile filaments. Both physiologically and pharmacologically, smooth muscles are a markedly heterogeneous group of tissues (Chapter 38). Striated muscles include cardiac and skeletal muscles. The skeletal muscles themselves are far from uniform. Examination of muscles from lower mammals reveals that some are pale in color whereas others are redder. Examples are the extensor digitorum longus (pale) and soleus (red) of the rat. The redness of the muscles reflects the amount of myoglobin in the muscle fiber. *Myoglobin* is the specialized heme-containing oxygen-storage protein of striated muscle. A high myoglobin content endows the fiber with a high capacity for aerobic metabolism. The fibers with the highest myoglobin content have a relatively slow rate of shortening; these 'slow-twitch' fibers are categorized as type I. Most 'fast-twitch' fibers have a low myoglobin content and are dependent on anaerobic metabolism (type IIb), whereas some have moderate myoglobin levels and aerobic capacity (type IIa).

All skeletal muscles in the human body contain a mixture of type I and type II fibers. However, whether through variations in the proportions of fiber type or through other factors, different human muscles show subtle differences in their physiologic characteristics. Different degrees of response to some drugs can be demonstrated in isolated muscle strips taken by biopsy from various regions of the body. The diaphragm is an especially interesting example, in that it shares some characteristics of cardiac muscle. This is presumably an adaptation to allow its continuous cycle of contraction and relaxation, as with the heart.

STRUCTURE OF SKELETAL MUSCLE

The skeletal muscles are the effector organs of voluntary movement. The muscle fibers are specialized, elongated excitable cells that range in diameter from 10 to 100 μm and in length from 0.5 to 12 cm. Most muscle fibers do not span the whole length of the intact muscle. At one end of the muscle the fibers extend from the tendon and end in long tapering points that interdigitate with other fibers. The fibers are tightly bound together by intrafascicular connective tissue, the endomysium (Fig. 35.1). Several lengths of bound muscle fibers are often required before the final fibers reach the tendon at the other end of the muscle. Functionally, however, muscles behave as if they are groups of fibers extending from tendon to tendon.

The integrity of individual skeletal muscles is maintained by a framework of connective tissue: that enclosing the whole muscle is termed the epimysium. Smaller and smaller bundles of muscle fibers are enclosed by sleeves of connective tissue – the perimysium – that are protrusions of the epimysium into the body of the muscle. The smallest bundles visible to the naked eye are termed muscle fascicles; these are made up of 12 or more fibers enclosed by their perimysium. In addition to holding the individual fibers together, the endomysium also provides the architecture to hold capillaries and nerves in place.

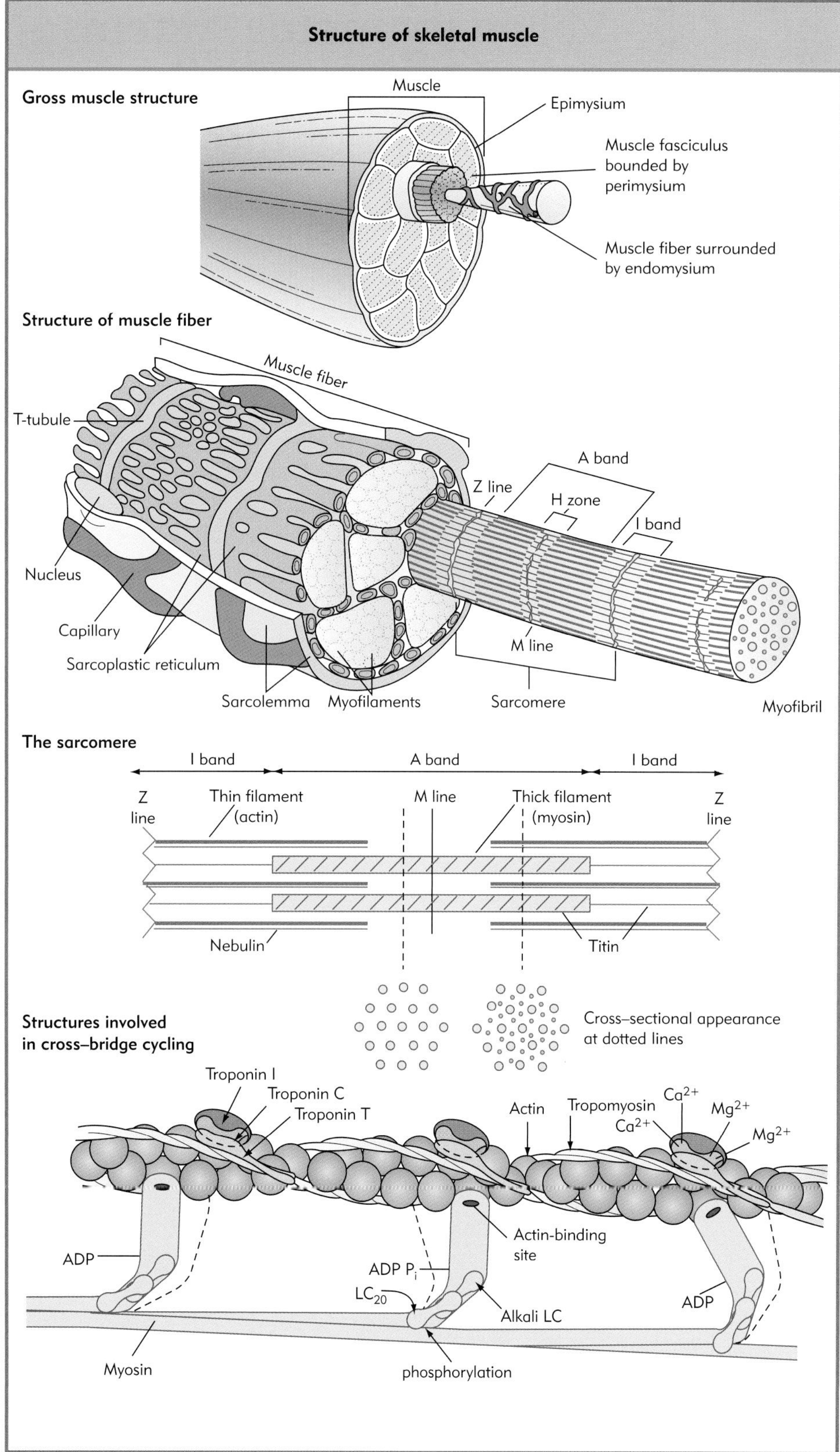

Figure 35.1 The structure of skeletal muscle. Note that within the muscle fiber the sarcoplasmic reticulum is arranged in parallel with the myofilaments, whereas the T-tubules are perpendicular. The organization of the major proteins constituting the thick and thin filaments within the sarcomere is maintained by several structural proteins, including nebulin and titin. The proteins forming the Z-line and M-line structures are closely related to actin. Each thick filament is surrounded by six thin filaments. The structural elements involved in cross-bridge cycling are shown. (With permission from Moffett et al., 1993.)

Movement of the skeleton is achieved by shortening, or contraction, of muscles. Each muscle fiber contains thousands of contractile units – myofibrils – made up of *sarcomeres* arranged in series in the long axis of the fiber. The myofibrils contain filaments of two types, thin and thick, which are arranged to form the lines and bands that are visible microscopically. The thin myofilaments consist of three major types of protein: *actin*, *tropomyosin*, and *troponin*. Actin, an α-helical protein, is an important structural protein in most cell types, but its organization in striated muscle enables a specialized role. Tropomyosin is a filamentous protein that lies in the groove of the actin helix. Troponin consists of three subunits, troponin I ('inhibitory'), troponin T (tropomyosin binding) and troponin C (Ca^{2+} binding). Troponin is found at every seventh actin subunit.

The thick myofilaments are formed from bundles of *myosin*, which consists of helical chains and a double globular head formed by the folding of the N-terminal regions of the chains. The tertiary structure of the head is maintained by myosin elastic light chain. Phosphorylation of another light chain protein, the LC_{20} or regulatory light chain, alters the angle between the helical rod and the globular head. There are several isoforms of myosin, which determine the twitch speed of the fiber.

MUSCLE CONTRACTION

Shortening of the sarcomere is achieved by the drawing together of opposing thin filaments by a ratchet-like effect of the thick filaments (Fig. 35.2). Pure actin and myosin will readily interact with each other. The actin filament has a series of myosin-binding sites that sequentially bind with increasing affinity to the head processes of the myosin molecule. In resting muscle, the

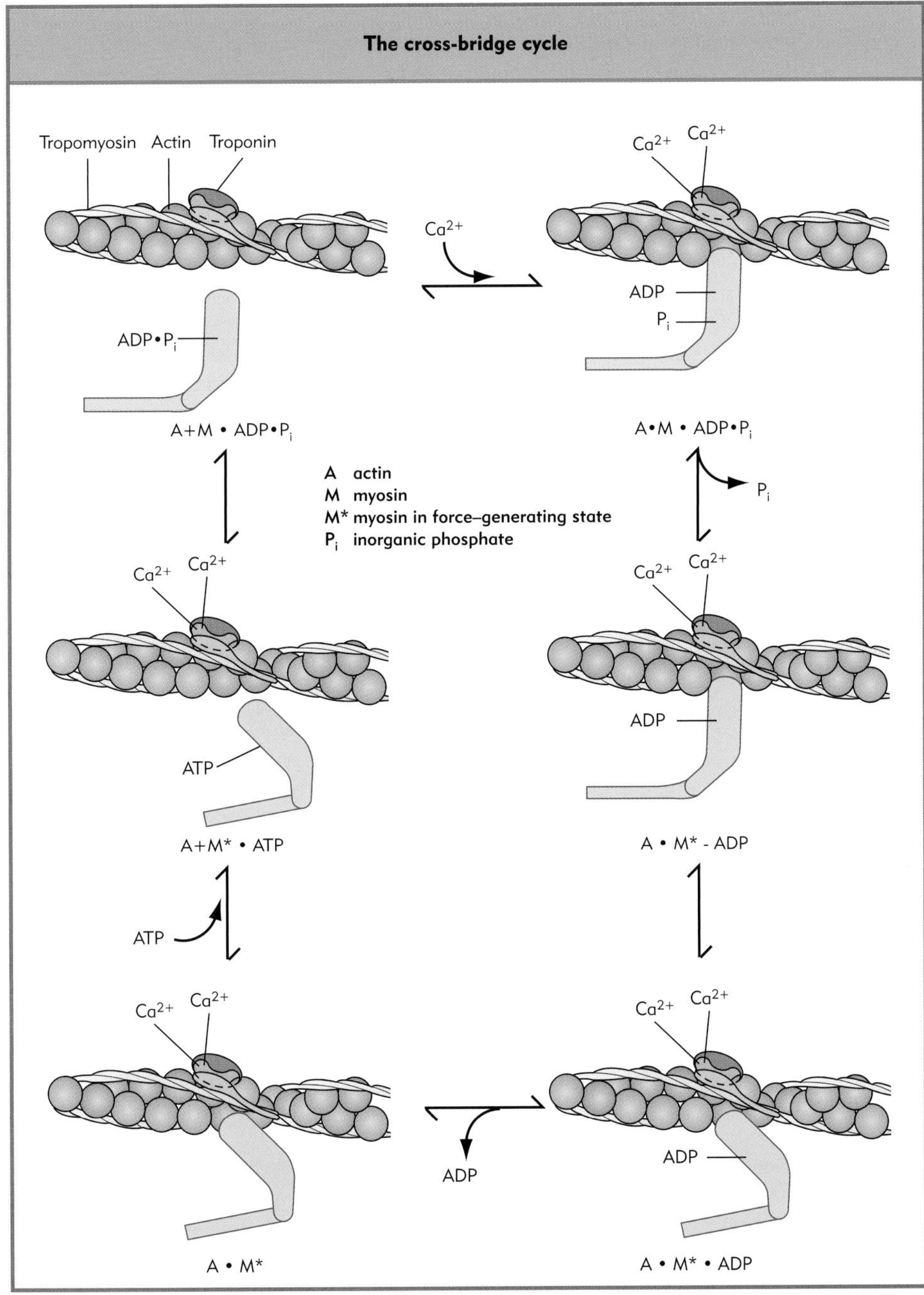

Figure 35.2 The biochemistry of the cross-bridge cycle. Activation starts with the addition of Ca^{2+} to the resting state (top left) and proceeds through various stages (in a clockwise direction here), returning to the resting state after hydrolysis of ATP.

myosin-binding sites of actin are covered by the tropomyosin filaments; as a result, the actin–myosin interaction is either weak or prevented completely. Tropomyosin is lifted clear from the myosin-binding sites on the actin molecule in response to a conformational change in troponin that is brought about by Ca^{2+} binding to troponin C. Increasing intensity of myosin binding – which at this stage is complexed with ADP and inorganic phosphate – to actin leads to dissociation of the inorganic phosphate from the myosin head. This stage is associated with a strongly bound cross-bridge between actin and myosin. This strong chemical bonding is a dynamic process, as it causes a conformational change in the myosin chain, leading to a swiveling of the myosin head in relation to the actin-binding sites, moving the myosin filaments against the actin. This is the basis of the contractile process. Once the conformational myosin change has occurred, ADP dissociates from the myosin head and the actin–myosin bond is subject to ATP-dependent hydrolysis, enabling a further interaction with a myosin-binding site further down the actin filament.

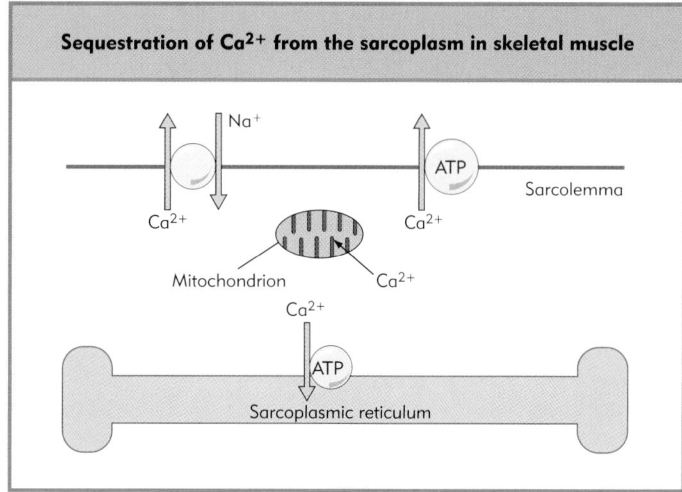

Figure 35.3 Mechanisms of sequestration of Ca^{2+} from the sarcoplasm of skeletal muscle.

In contrast to cardiac muscle, skeletal muscle contraction depends largely on intracellular Ca^{2+}.

The contractile process is dependent on the presence of Ca^{2+}. Indeed, regulation of muscle contraction is through control of the myoplasmic Ca^{2+} concentration. In contrast to heart muscle, skeletal muscle contraction is well maintained in the absence of extracellular Ca^{2+}, indicating that the source of Ca^{2+} for contraction in skeletal muscle is intracellular. The major internal store of Ca^{2+} in skeletal muscle is the sarcoplasmic reticulum (SR). In the SR, most Ca^{2+} is bound to a matrix formed by the low-affinity Ca^{2+}-binding protein calsequestrin, which is in equilibrium with the free, releasable Ca^{2+}. When muscle is stimulated, Ca^{2+} is released from the terminal cisternae of the SR through specialized Ca^{2+}-release channels (CRCs).

Following the release of Ca^{2+} from the SR, myoplasmic Ca^{2+} concentration remains high only while further Ca^{2+} release is taking place, as Ca^{2+} is continually sequestered from the myoplasm via the action of sarcolemmal and SR Ca^{2+} pumps, sarcolemmal Na^+/Ca^{2+} exchange, and mitochondrial uptake (Fig. 35.3). Therefore, when Ca^{2+} sequestration exceeds release, the muscle will relax. ATP is essential for both muscle contraction and relaxation as the immediate source of energy.

The motor unit and excitation–contraction coupling

The functional unit involved in skeletal muscle contraction is the motor unit. The motor unit comprises an α-motor neuron, the muscle fibers that it innervates, and the neuromuscular junctions that form the chemical synapse between the neuron and the muscle fiber. Each α-motor neuron branches at its terminus; as a result, it supplies from three to hundreds of muscle fibers. Stimulation of a muscle fiber follows the transduction of an action potential arriving at the terminal swelling of a motor neuron into an action potential at the postjunctional region of the neuromuscular junction (the motor endplate). This occurs through the action of acetylcholine (Chapter 36). An action potential generated at the motor endplate spreads across the sarcolemma and down the invaginations of this membrane, the *T-tubules*. The transduction of the electrical signal of the action potential in the T-tubule to produce physical interaction between the contractile proteins is known as excitation–contraction coupling (ECC). The contraction process is initiated by a rise in the myoplasmic Ca^{2+} concentration from a resting level of about 0.01 μmol/L to 5 μmol/L, and this rise is effected by the release of Ca^{2+} from the terminal cisternae of the SR. Here, the SR and the T-tubule are separated by a gap of only 12–14 nm, which is spanned at intervals by structures seen on electron microscopy as 'feet' (Fig. 35.4). These foot processes are large proteins that have affinity for the plant toxin ryanodine, and are therefore known as *ryanodine receptors*. Purified ryanodine receptors incorporated into planar lipid bilayers behave as Ca^{2+} channels, with identical properties to those of the CRC of isolated 'heavy' SR vesicles, indicating that the ryanodine receptor is the CRC of SR. High-power electron microscopy has revealed that this protein comprises four transmembrane subunits (M1–M4) (Fig. 35.4).

The T-tubular membrane also contains Ca^{2+} channels and has the greatest density of dihydropyridine-binding sites in the body. However, the passage of extracellular Ca^{2+} into the muscle cell is not essential for ECC. It now seems that these dihydropyridine 'receptors' (DHPRs) do not function as channels at all, but rather are the voltage sensors of the T-tubule, detecting the action potential and in so doing initiating intracellular events that lead to Ca^{2+} release from the SR. When the T-tubule is depolarized by the action potential, the intramembrane charge of the DHPR voltage sensor is shifted towards the external surface, causing a conformational change in a cytoplasmic loop of the DHPR (probably the loop between domains II and III; Fig. 35.4 and Chapter 6). At this point, the proximity of the DHPR cytoplasmic loop to the cytoplasmic N-terminal part of the SR CRC is so great that there is an induced conformational change in the CRC, probably mediated through charged amino acid residues. This in turn leads to a conformational change in the intramembranous channel-forming C-terminal region of the SR CRC, which results in opening of the channel and efflux of Ca^{2+} from the SR into the cytoplasm.

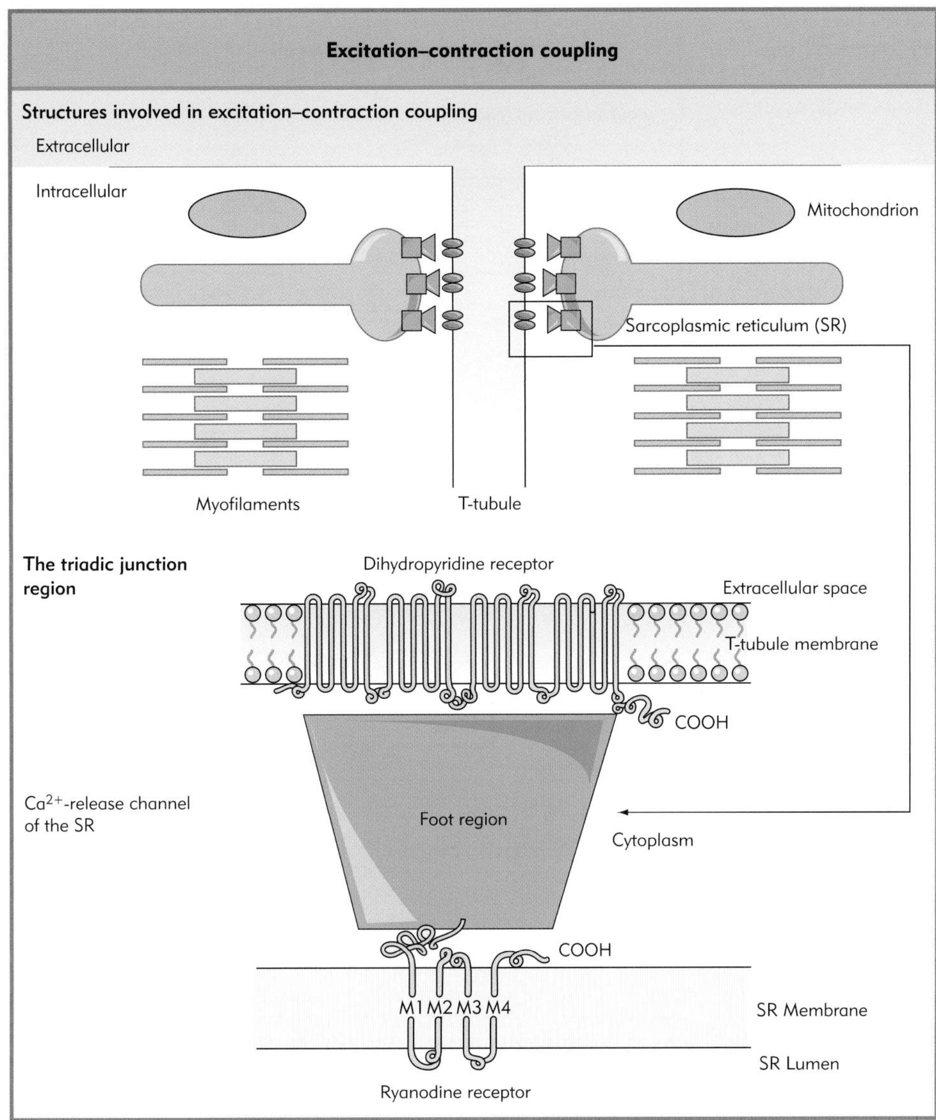

Figure 35.4 Excitation–contraction coupling. The structures involved in the coupling are shown (top), plus expansion of the triadic junction region to show the relationship of the dihydropyridine receptor voltage sensor and the SR Ca^{2+}-release channel (CRC). The foot process of the CRC is presumed to be the regulatory region.

Recent evidence suggests there are two populations of CRC, one where the cytoplasmic part is apposed to the T-tubule DHPR voltage sensors, and one where it is not. This has led to the suggestion that activation of the first population by conformational change in the DHPR voltage sensor leads to the local release of Ca^{2+}, which is the trigger for Ca^{2+}-induced Ca^{2+} release from the second population of CRC.

Malignant hyperthermia

Malignant hyperthermia (MH) results from a pathologic increase in skeletal muscle Ca^{2+} concentrations that is triggered by volatile anesthetics and depolarizing muscle relaxants. The susceptibility to MH is inherited in an autosomal dominant pattern. Molecular genetic studies have revealed that it is a genetically heterogeneous condition, that is, the same clinical disorder can be caused by abnormalities in one of several genes. Prime candidates for causative genes are those for the SR CRC and the DHPR voltage sensor. The gene coding the SR CRC is known as *RYR1* (after ryanodine receptor) and is the major gene implicated to date. More than 100 mutations and polymorphisms in *RYR1* have been reported, and more than 20 of these have been shown to have functional consequences consistent with our understanding of the pathophysiology of MH.

The clinical features of MH are secondary to increased myoplasmic Ca^{2+}, which causes muscle rigidity (increased myofilament interaction), hypermetabolism (secondary to increased demand for ATP and Ca^{2+}–calmodulin activation of glycolytic enzymes), and loss of integrity of the sarcolemma (lack of ATP and Ca^{2+} activation of membrane phospholipases).

Treatment of MH is dependent on early recognition of the developing reaction, withdrawal of trigger drugs, symptomatic treatment of the fever and metabolic disturbances, and the intravenous administration of dantrolene sodium, a drug that prevents the release of Ca^{2+} into the muscle cells. The site of action of dantrolene is disputed, but it either directly blocks the release of Ca^{2+} from the SR or reduces the stimulus to SR Ca^{2+} release following arrival of the action potential at the DHPR voltage sensors. Dantrolene is poorly soluble in water, and is therefore presented for intravenous use as a lyophilized powder containing a mixture of 20 mg dantrolene sodium, 3 g mannitol, and sodium hydroxide (to produce a pH of 9.5 when reconstituted with 60 mL sterile water). Dantrolene should be administered in intravenous doses of 1 mg/kg, repeated until a maintained response is seen. Up to 10 mg/kg has been required, but the usual total dose is 2–3 mg/kg. Side effects of dantrolene in the treatment of MH are usually unnoticed because of the severity of the MH reaction, although severe reactions, such as acute hepatic dysfunction, can occur.

MH can be avoided by using drugs that are known not to trigger the condition (intravenous anesthetics, opioids, nondepolarizing muscle relaxants, local anesthetics). Some authorities have proposed the use of dantrolene as 'prophylaxis' against MH in known susceptible individuals requiring surgery. Its short-term use provokes nausea, vomiting, and muscle weakness in a high proportion of recipients, as well as unpleasant CNS effects, including euphoria and disorientation. The use of prophylactic dantrolene is therefore not warranted as part of a 'belt and braces' approach. The relatively weak effects of dantrolene on cardiac and diaphragmatic muscle may also become significant in those patients with pre-existing cardiac or respiratory disease, respectively.

Regulation of the force of muscle contraction

When stimulated by a single action potential, the force developed by a muscle fiber depends on the sum of the myosin–actin interactions. The Ca^{2+} release is probably sufficient to fully saturate all the Ca^{2+}-binding sites of troponin C, but the Ca^{2+} concentration is not maintained sufficiently to achieve a steady-state (maximal) activation of all potential actin and myosin bonds. The number of myosin heads that are aligned with potential binding sites on the actin filaments, which is determined by the degree of stretch applied to the muscle fiber, is also important. This concept is best understood by considering the basic contractile units, the sarcomeres, and more specifically the consequences of changing sarcomere length (distance between adjacent Z-lines) (Fig. 35.5). Essentially, there is a relatively narrow range of length of muscle at which stimulation will lead to a maximal response. For maximum efficiency, therefore, muscle shortening should be limited. This is achievable, while still enabling a large range of joint movement, because most muscle insertions are relatively close to the joint. The negative feature of this arrangement is that there is a six- to eightfold reduction in the maximum tension generated that can be applied to a distal load.

The previous discussion concerned a single stimulus applied to a single muscle fiber. Consider now what happens if a second stimulus is applied a short interval after the first (Fig. 35.6). If the second stimulus is within 8 ms of the first, the plasmalemma will be electrically refractory and no second response will be seen. However, following the first stimulus, myoplasmic Ca^{2+} remains elevated for approximately 50 ms and tension does not return to the prestimulation level for a further 30 ms. Therefore, a second stimulus applied 8–80 ms after the first will have an additive effect, known as *summation*. Multiple stimuli at stimulation intervals of 40–80 ms will produce stepwise increases in tension, known as *steppe*. At stimulation intervals of less than 40 ms the steppes become fused to give a *tetanic* response. Physiologic rates of stimulation are invariably within this tetanic range, and these tetanic bursts give rise to a smooth, forceful contraction. Tension generated by the muscle fiber will increase as the intervals between these bursts are decreased, and will be maximal with continuous trains of stimuli.

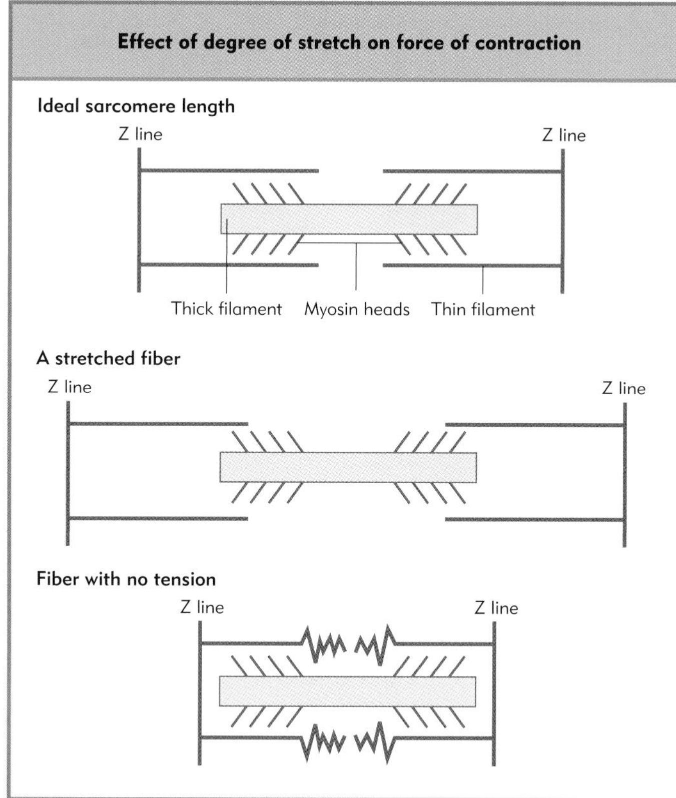

Figure 35.5 The effect of degree of stretch on the force of contraction. In the ideal situation, the sarcomere length is such that the thin and thick filaments overlap and align all the myosin heads adjacent to potential actin-binding sites; maximal force can then be generated if the fiber is stimulated. If the fiber is stretched so that the sarcomere length is increased, a point is reached where the ends of the thin filaments furthest from the Z-lines are pulled beyond the most centrally situated myosin heads. In this situation, if the fiber is stimulated there is redundancy of these myosin heads and the contractile response is submaximal. At the other extreme, if no tension is applied to the fiber its elastic nature minimizes sarcomere length, causing overlap of thin filaments attached to adjacent Z-lines. The response to stimulation would again be limited, as the most distal myosin heads would 'run out' of actin-binding sites as the thick filaments abutted onto the Z-line structures.

Several muscle fibers are innervated by a common motor nerve, and these fibers of the same motor unit will therefore contract simultaneously. However, not all motor units in the same muscle will contract at the same time. If a muscle at rest is required to increase its tension gradually, the smallest motor units will be activated first, with successively larger units being recruited as greater force is required. Thus *summation* of responses at the single fiber level and *recruitment* at the motor unit level combine to enable a continuum of tension development over a wide range.

The rate of cross-bridge formation, and consequently the force of contraction, varies according to the activation history of the fiber. The Ca^{2+} released as the result of one stimulus leads to a change in the position of the myosin heads by phosphorylation of LC_{20}, so that a succeeding stimulus may have a greater effect for the quantal release of Ca^{2+}. The mechanism involves the binding of four Ca^{2+} to calmodulin, which then activates myosin light-chain kinase (MLCK), which is similar to that contributing to the development of the latch state in smooth muscle (Chapter 38).

CONTROL OF MUSCLE CONTRACTION

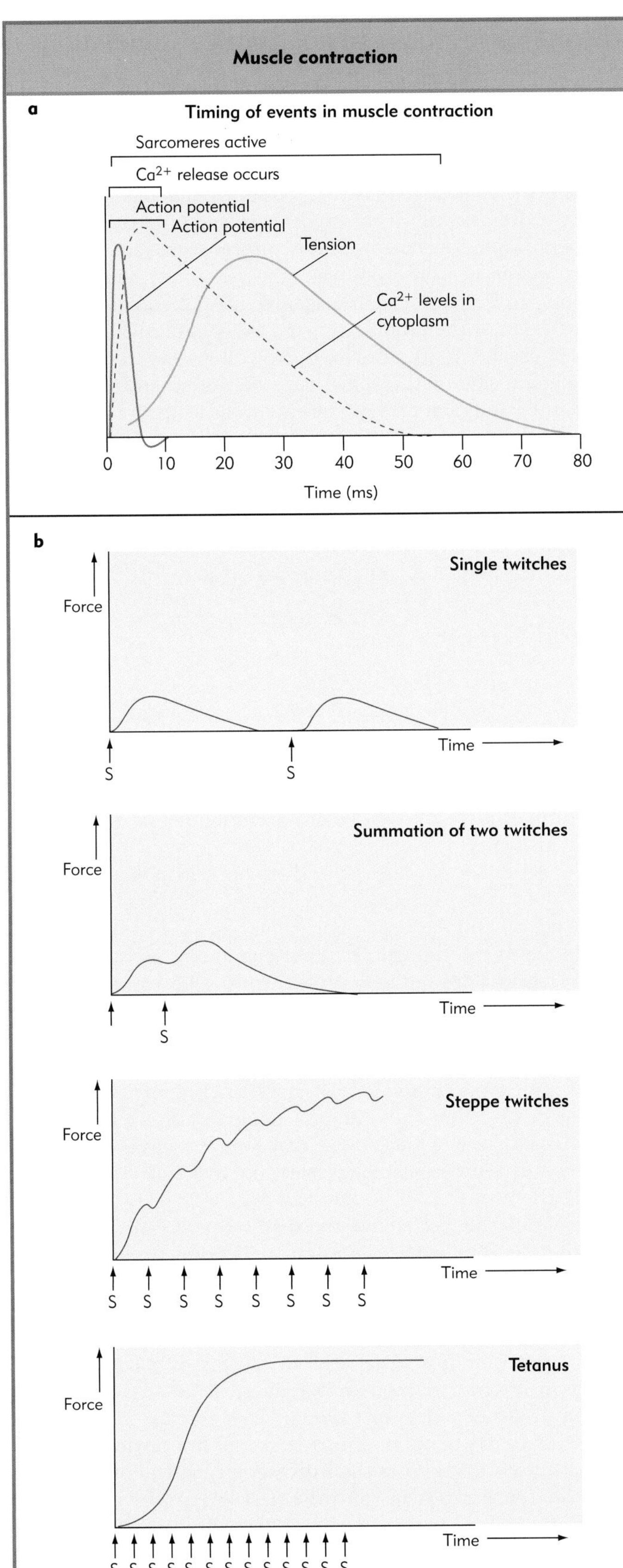

Figure 35.6 Muscle contraction. (a) The timing of events in muscle contraction. (b) The effect of stimulus interval on the force of contraction: single twitches; summation of two twitches; steppe twitches; and tetanus.

Control of skeletal muscle contraction is achieved at several levels, ranging from involuntary simple reflex responses to consciously initiated complex patterns involving many different muscle groups. In order to carry out a particular maneuver, the effectors (agonists) of the response need to be activated and, in addition, the muscles having the opposite effect (antagonists) need to be inhibited. In many movements, compensatory responses are required, for example to maintain posture and/or balance. As with any control system, feedback information is required if useful output is to be achieved. In the context of control of muscle contraction and movement of the skeleton, this feedback or sensory information is known as *kinesthesia*. Body position sense is a function of the proprioceptive receptors located in the joints, but there are also mechanisms for sensing the tension, length, and rate of shortening of the skeletal muscles. The receptors for detecting muscle tension are located in the tendons and are called the Golgi tendon organs. Afferent signals from the Golgi tendon organs are relayed up the spinal cord to higher centers, but also synapse at the spinal cord level to inhibit the efferent supply to the muscle via its α-motor neurons. The receptors for muscle length and change in length are found in the muscle spindle complexes.

The muscle spindle and the stretch reflex

Muscle spindles are encapsulated adapted muscle fibers orientated so that the enclosed intrafusal fibers are arranged parallel to the force-generating, or extrafusal, fibers. Muscle spindles are located throughout the body of muscles, being more numerous in muscles with higher proportions of small motor units. The structure of the muscle spindle and its innervation is illustrated in Figure 35.7. The spindle afferent fibers enter the spinal cord through the dorsal root and branch to make connections at their segmental level of innervation and to pass up the dorsal columns to higher centers. Among the segmental connections in the spinal cord are direct single synaptic connections with the α-motor neurons supplying the same muscle and its synergists. These are excitatory synapses, and it is this pathway that is responsible for the stretch reflex typified by the knee-jerk response to a tap on the patellar tendon (Fig. 35.8). The function of the stretch reflex is to maintain muscle length.

Efferent supply to the muscle spindles and control of muscle length

The muscle spindles are attached through the endomysium to the extrafusal fibers and are arranged so that intrafusal fibers are parallel to the extrafusal fibers. Contraction, relaxation, or passive stretching of the extrafusal fibers affects the tension of the intrafusal fibers, and the resulting afferent impulses from the sensory fibers of the muscle spindle are relayed in order to return the muscle to the required length. However, the required length is not fixed but can be constantly changed, depending on the desired movement or function. To enable appropriate sensory impulses from the muscle spindles, the degree of stretch of the central (sensory) regions of the intrafusal fibers can be controlled independently from the length of the extrafusal fibers by the action of γ-efferent neurons, which synapse on the peripheral regions of the intrafusal fibers. These regions contain contractile myofilaments; impulses from the γ-efferent neurons

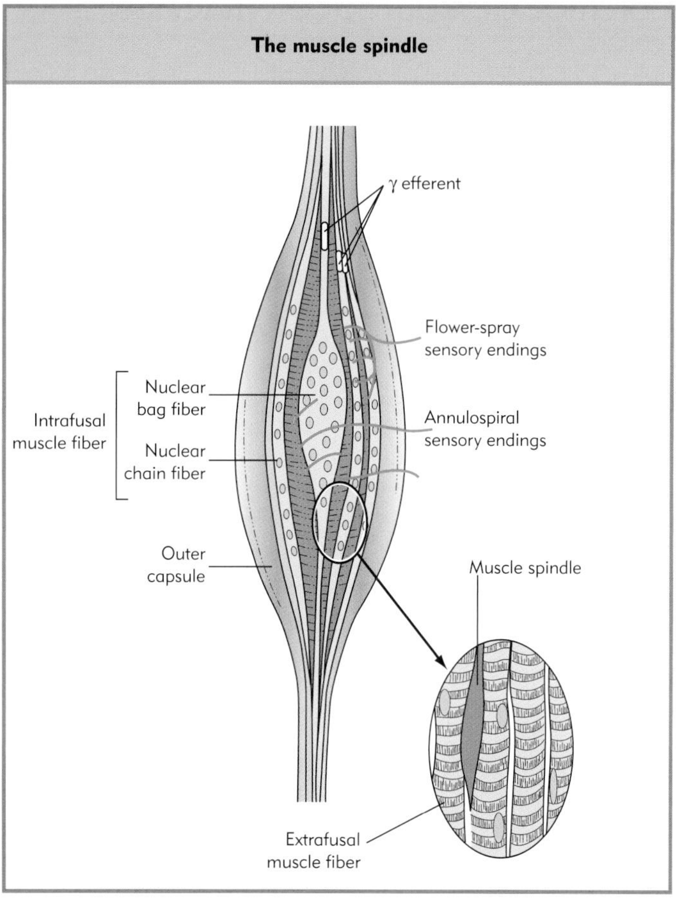

Figure 35.7 The muscle spindle. The intrafusal fibers have a central elastic portion with no myofibrils, making the nuclei prominent features. There are two types of intrafusal fiber: nuclear bag fibers, with a dilated central portion having annulospiral sensory endings; and nuclear chain fibers, with a more uniform diameter and flower-spray sensory endings at the central portion. Nuclear chain fibers detect muscle length, whereas nuclear bag fibers detect changing length or stretch. The neurons from both types of sensory ending are large myelinated fibers (Aα), which have high conduction velocities. (With permission from Moffett et al., 1993.)

cause their contraction, resulting in stretching of the central regions of the intrafusal fibers and increased sensory feedback.

During voluntary muscle contraction, the γ-efferent neurons are activated simultaneously with the α-motor neurons supplying the extrafusal fibers of the muscle. Therefore, if the desired response is a shortening of the muscle, and this occurs, the muscle spindle sensory feedback will not change because the reduction in stimulus, owing to shortening of the intrafusal fibers secondary to shortening of the extrafusal fibers, is balanced by the tendency to increase the stimulus by contraction of the end regions of the intrafusal fibers with subsequent stretching of the central regions. If, however, an excessive load prevents the desired shortening of the muscle, muscle spindle sensory feedback will increase because the stretching of the central regions of the intrafusal fibers caused by γ-efferent discharge will be unopposed. The increased sensory feedback results in greater excitatory stimulus to the α-motor neurons in the spinal cord, increasing the contractile effort to try to overcome the load in order to achieve the desired muscle length.

The motor response to nociceptive stimulation

A noxious stimulus applied to a limb results in withdrawal of the limb from the stimulus. This is another spinally mediated reflex response. In fact, two reflexes are implicated: the withdrawal reflex affecting the injured limb, and the crossed-extensor reflex affecting the contralateral limb. Nociceptive cutaneous afferents enter the dorsal horns of the spinal cord and send projections to interneurons in the cord. These interneurons are excitatory to the motor neurons supplying the flexors of the limb and inhibitory to the motor neurons supplying the extensors, resulting in flexion of the limb away from the stimulus. The nociceptive sensory afferents also have projections that cross to the contralateral side of the spinal cord before synapsing on interneurons. Stimulation of these interneurons leads to inhibition of the limb flexors and excitation of the extensors. The result of this crossed-extensor response is that the contralateral limb is made more rigid so that posture can be maintained during withdrawal of the stimulated limb. Other compensatory responses may also be activated, for example movements of the other two limbs to help to maintain posture and balance.

Control of muscle tone

Even at rest, most skeletal muscles are not completely flaccid. This resting tension, or muscle tone, can be markedly reduced by cutting the dorsal spinal roots, implicating the muscle spindle afferents as important determinants of muscle tone. Inputs to α-motor neurons from higher CNS centers can have facilitatory or inhibitory effects on the basal excitation from the muscle spindle afferents.

The reticular formation and brainstem nuclei provide facilitatory inputs to spinal motor neurons. The vestibular nuclei are specifically implicated in enhancing the tone of the postural muscles and are thought to coordinate actions to maintain posture against the influence of gravity. One example is the righting reflex, which is an ipsilateral extensor response to sudden tilting of the body to one side. A total spinal lesion, involving section of the spinal cord below the level of the vestibular nuclei, results in a flaccid paralysis. There is also a temporary loss of spinal reflexes below the level of section that recovers, possibly through the development of a denervation sensitivity of the spinal motor neurons, enabling a response to activation of muscle spindle afferents.

In contrast, section above the brainstem reticular formation (decerebration) in experimental animals dramatically increases muscle tone, especially in the postural and proximal limb muscles. Inhibition of the brainstem reticular formation is via the cerebellum and the basal ganglia, and it is through these centers that information from the cerebral cortex is relayed to the brainstem in order to make any reductions in postural muscle tone that are necessary for voluntary movements. Signals from the cortex to the peripheral muscle groups are carried in upper motor neurons that bypass the brainstem, running in the pyramidal tract (decussating in the medullary pyramids) and several extrapyramidal tracts.

Motor programs for the generation of stereotyped patterns of movement

Although the skeletal muscles are under voluntary control, most muscle activity is carried out at a subconscious level. In other

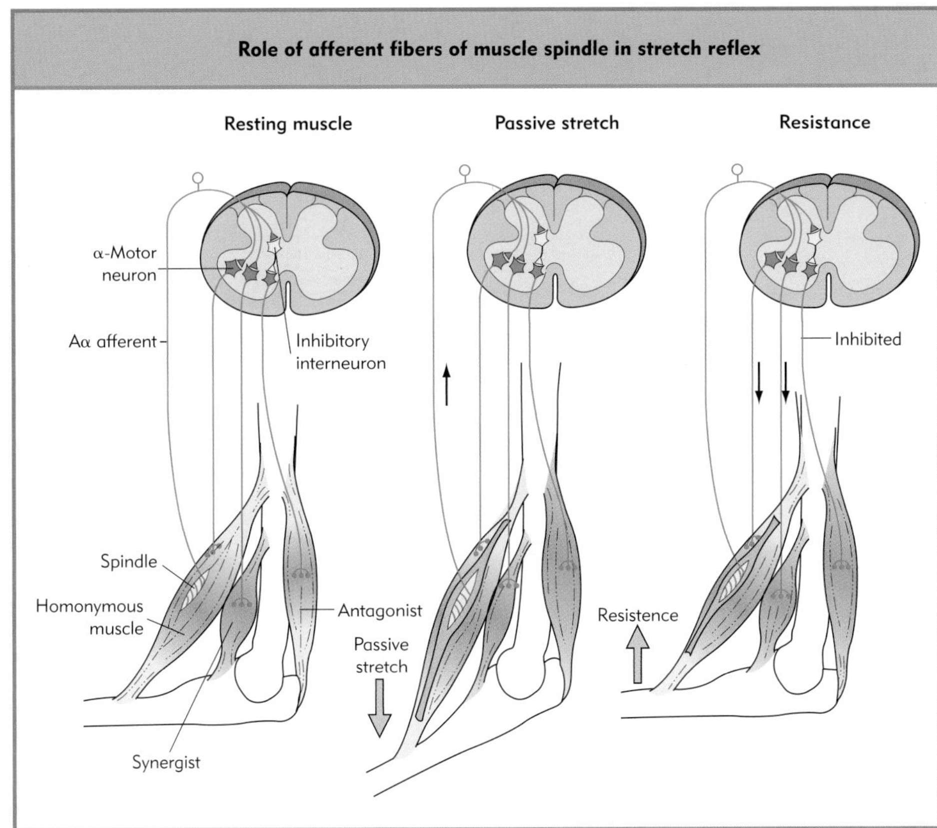

Figure 35.8 The role of the afferent fibers of the muscle spindle in the mechanism of the stretch reflex.

words, we do not have to think about each movement necessary to carry out a task, let alone the individual muscles that we need to contract and relax in order to generate each movement. Rather, the cortical function is to activate motor programs that have been learned and which from previous experience will result in the desired outcome. A motor program is defined as a set of commands that is generated in one area of the CNS before the onset of the relevant movement, and which causes activation or inhibition of motor units in an appropriately timed sequence.

There is evidence from lower mammals that motor programs can be generated at all levels of the CNS. For example, section of the spinal cord above and below the segmental innervation of the leg results in walking movements, an example of a spinal motor program. In humans, the basal ganglia are recognized to be important regions for motor program generation; this is evidenced by dyskinesias, which result from diseases affecting the basal ganglia or their connections. Dyskinesias are repeated inappropriate movements of whole muscle groups that appear to be caused by spontaneous activity of the diseased basal ganglia.

The basal ganglia

The basal ganglia consist of five subcortical nuclei (Fig. 35.9) that form one of the two major subcortical loops of the motor system; the other loop involves the cerebellum. The basal ganglia receive inputs from the entire cortex, which enter one of the two input nuclei, the caudate nucleus and putamen (collectively termed the striatum); these relay information back to the cortex via projections to the thalamus. These projections arise from one of the two output nuclei of the basal ganglia, the pars reticulata of the substantia nigra, or the internal segment of the globus pallidus.

Neurons of the output nuclei spontaneously discharge and cause a reduction of the excitatory output of thalamocortical neurons. Excitation of the input nuclei from the cortex leads, through the direct pathway of the basal ganglia, to inhibition of the tonic inhibitory fibers of the output nuclei, producing increased excitation of the cortex. There is also an indirect neural circuit of the basal ganglia via the input nuclei and the external segment of the globus pallidus, causing disinhibition of the subthalamic nucleus. Excitatory fibers from here project to the output nuclei, thereby causing increased inhibition of the thalamic output. The overall effect depends on the balance between the direct and indirect pathways. The pars compacta of the substantia nigra has an important modulatory role on the output of the basal ganglia. This is mediated by dopaminergic neurons synapsing in the input nuclei. The basal ganglia contain 80% of the dopamine present in the brain, and the more common movement disorders (e.g. Parkinson's disease) affect this system.

DOPAMINE RECEPTORS

Seven subtypes of dopamine receptor have so far been identified in the brain; D_1 and D_2 are by far the most abundant. These subtypes are principally found in the striatum (input nuclei) of the basal ganglia. The D_1 receptor is linked to a stimulatory G protein (see Chapter 3); activation leads to increased formation of cAMP by adenylyl cyclase. The resultant increased protein phosphorylation causes increased conductance of several types

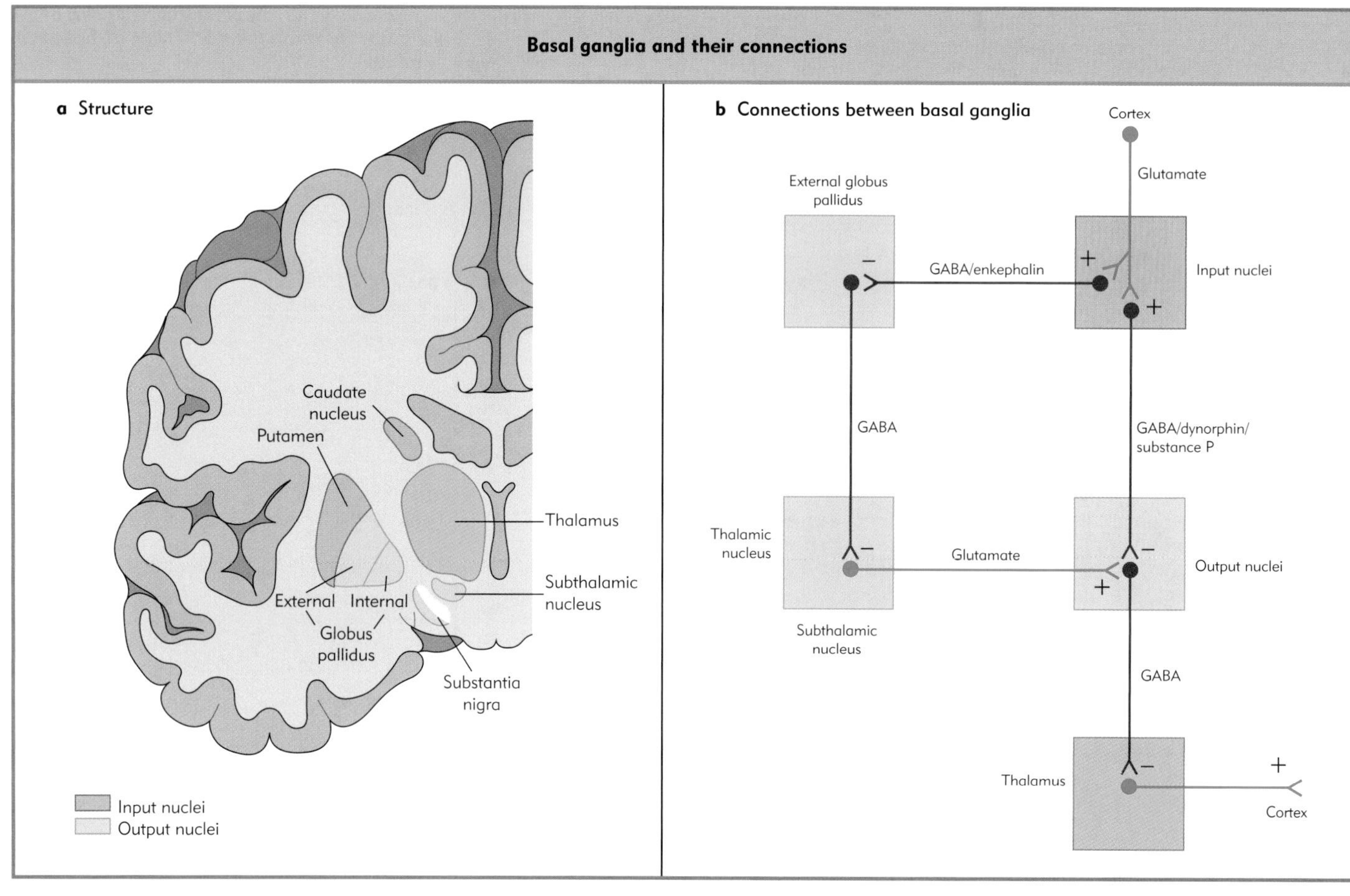

Figure 35.9 The basal ganglia and their connections.

of ion channel. Whether D_1 activation has an overall excitatory or inhibitory effect depends on the different ion channel populations and state of that particular cell. In the input nuclei of the basal ganglia, activation of D_1 receptors may lead to neuronal excitation or inhibition, depending on the subtype of the medium-sized spiny striatal neuron. Activation of D_2 receptors causes several cellular effects, including inhibition of cAMP formation via linkage to an inhibitory G protein, and increased production of the second messengers IP_3 and diacylglycerol. However, perhaps the most important mechanism whereby stimulation of D_2 receptors produces reduced neuronal excitability is through increasing the conductance of K^+ channels, which leads to hyperpolarization of the cell.

In the input nuclei of the basal ganglia dopamine activates the direct pathway via D_1 receptors and inhibits the indirect pathway via D_2 receptors. Both actions of dopamine lead to an increase in excitatory impulse transmission to the cortex. In Parkinson's disease there is a striatal dopamine deficiency resulting from the destruction of 70–90% of the dopaminergic neurons projecting from the pars compacta of the substantia nigra. This results in reduced cortical excitation, leading to rigidity through a reduction of the inhibitory cortical effect on the brainstem nuclei, and to bradykinesia through reduced corticospinal tract outflow.

The input nuclei of the basal ganglia also contain large cholinergic interneurons, stimulation of which opposes the effects of dopamine. The output of the basal ganglia tends to be phasic; damping of this variable output depends on the balance between dopaminergic and cholinergic activity. A resting tremor is another characteristic feature of Parkinson's disease.

The cerebellum

The cerebellum has two-way connections with the spinal cord, brainstem nuclei, the nuclei of the basal ganglia, and the cerebral cortex. The principal role of the cerebellum is in coordination of motor activity, especially rapid and fine movements. It also appears to be important in assimilating sensory information in order to predict future position of limbs in dextrous movements.

Motor areas of the cerebral cortex

The primary motor cortex lies anterior to the central sulcus. Stimulation experiments reveal that the primary motor cortex is highly organized with respect to the anatomic pattern of responses. As with the postcentral sensory gyrus, a motor homunculus indicates the areas of cortex controlling different muscle groups (Fig. 35.10). The size of the region in the homunculus represents the number of motor units in the innervated muscles.

The primary motor cortex is characterized by large neuronal cell bodies in cortical layer V, known as Betz cells, the axons of which run in the corticospinal (pyramidal) tracts. Smaller cells

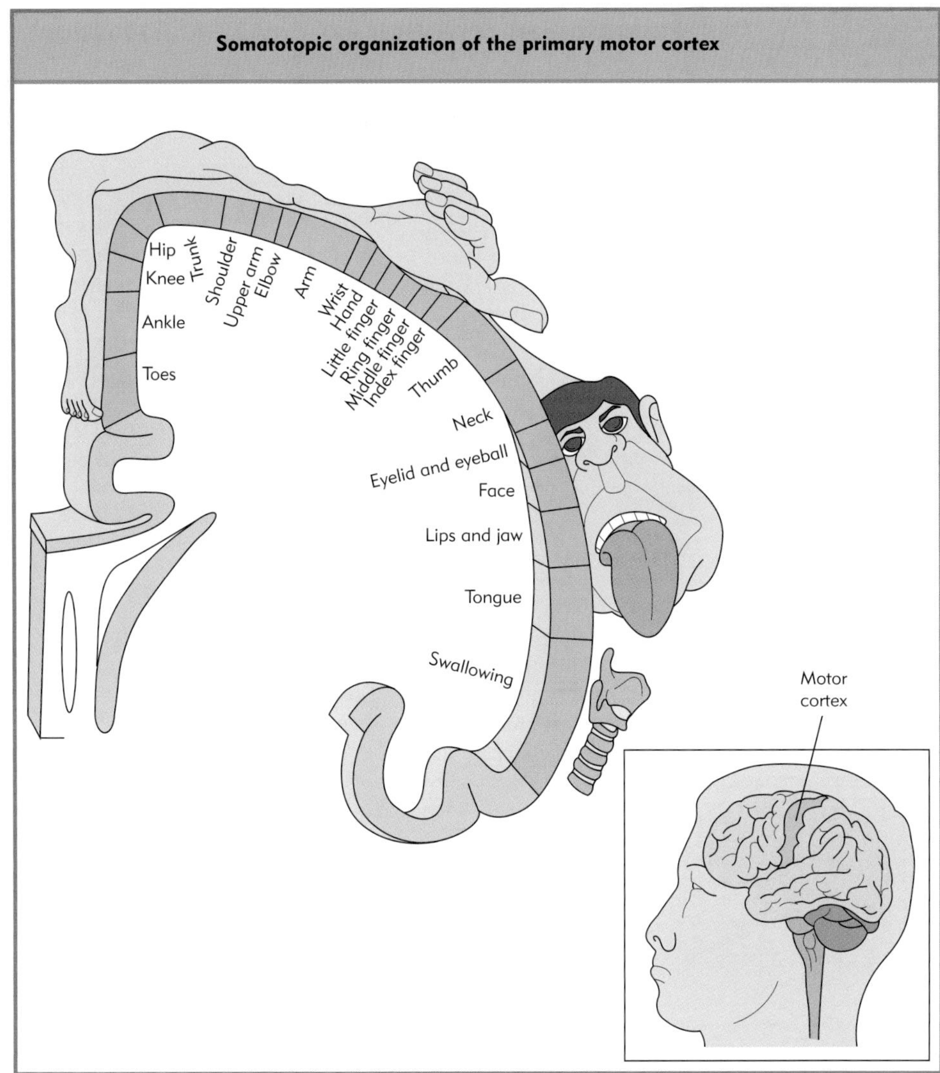

Figure 35.10 Somatotopic organization (motor homunculus) of the primary motor cortex. (With permission from Moffett et al., 1993.)

of layer V also contribute axons to the corticospinal tracts, as do neurons from the two premotor areas that lie anterior to the primary motor cortex. The primary motor cortex determines the force exerted in individual movements. The direction of movement is governed by a balance of the forces generated by a population of cells in this area with different vectors of force generation. The function of the premotor areas is to prepare the motor systems for movement. The medial and superior part of the premotor area, termed the supplementary motor area, programs motor sequences and coordinates bilateral movement. The lateral part of the premotor area, the premotor cortex, controls the proximal movements that project the arms to targets.

DRUG TREATMENT OF MOVEMENT DISORDERS

Parkinson's disease

Parkinson's disease, as described above, results from dopamine deficiency in the basal ganglia. Therapeutic approaches include the use of drugs to increase availability of dopamine, the use of dopaminergic receptor agonists, and the use of muscarinic cholinergic antagonists.

Levodopa (L-dihydroxyphenylalanine) is the amino acid precursor of dopamine but, unlike dopamine, it is absorbed in the intestine and crosses the blood–brain barrier. It is taken up into cells by an amino acid transporter coupled to Na^+ transport. In the basal ganglia it is converted into dopamine by DOPA decarboxylase. Decarboxylases are also found in many peripheral tissues; consequently, very little levadopa reaches the brain and the systemic dopamine production causes vomiting and hypotension. To increase availability of the drug to the brain, levodopa is administered in combination with *carbidopa,* a decarboxylase inhibitor that does not readily cross the blood–brain barrier. Side effects of levodopa/carbidopa combinations include nausea, vomiting, anorexia, postural hypotension, involuntary movements, and psychiatric disturbances.

Amantadine increases dopamine release from nerve terminals. Its principal use is in early disease before neuronal destruction is too advanced.

Selegiline is a selective inhibitor of monoamine oxidase B (MAO-B) and is effective in the treatment of Parkinson's disease. In humans, MAO-B is primarily responsible for the degradation of dopamine in the basal ganglia, whereas MAO-A predominates in other regions of the brain and the periphery. Inhibition of MAO-A in the gut leads to sympathomimetic effects from tyramine-containing foods, but the use of selegiline is associated with few side effects. There does not appear to be a dangerous interaction with opioids as there is with nonselective MAO inhibitors.

Bromocriptine and *pergolide* are dopamine agonists that act at D_1 and D_2 receptors, although they are more potent at the D_2 subtype. This profile of dopaminergic effects provides the optimal therapeutic response in Parkinson's disease. Peripheral dopaminergic effects can cause nausea and vomiting, which can be treated with domperidone. Other side effects include hypotension, especially postural, and psychiatric disturbance. Bromocriptine is one of the known causes of retroperitoneal fibrosis. Bromocriptine has also been advocated in the treatment of neuroleptic malignant syndrome, a rare reaction to major tranquillizers which is characterized by severe rigidity, hyperpyrexia, and rhabdomyolysis. *Apomorphine* is a potent dopamine agonist that has been used in refractory parkinsonism. Administration must be preceded by domperidone to limit the severe emetic response.

Cholinergic antagonists were the first group of drugs to be used with benefit in Parkinson's disease, although they have largely been superseded by levodopa/carbidopa. They are most effective in early disease where tremor is the predominant feature. Peripheral anticholinergic side effects include dry mouth, blurred vision owing to mydriasis, urinary retention, and constipation; confusion and agitation are central side effects. The two most commonly used drugs of this class are benzatropine and trihexyphenidyl, which have the additional beneficial action of blocking dopamine reuptake into nerve terminals.

Parkinsonian and other extrapyramidal reactions

Similar symptoms to the more common idiopathic Parkinson's disease can be caused by drugs with antidopaminergic effects, such as the major tranquillizers (phenothiazines, butyrophenones) and metoclopramide. Such drugs are commonly used in the prophylaxis and treatment of postoperative nausea and vomiting, where parenteral administration can lead to acute dystonic reactions in which there is simultaneous activation of opposing muscle groups. Dystonias can be localized, for example to produce an oculogyric crisis, or generalized, leading to painful, abnormal postures (opisthotonus). Anticholinergic drugs are the drugs of choice for drug-induced dystonic reactions and can be given parenterally (benzatropine, procyclidine, diphenhydramine) when the reaction is acute. Parkinsonism may also be secondary to encephalitis or arteriosclerosis. Treatment here is the same as for the idiopathic condition.

Spasticity

Spasticity is caused by chronic dissociation of lower motor neurons from upper motor neuron influences. Common causes include perinatal hypoxia, cerebrovascular insults, spinal cord lesions, and multiple sclerosis. Spasticity can result in chronic pain.

Benzodiazepines are effective centrally acting drugs in the treatment of increased muscle tone. *Baclofen* is also extensively used; this drug is an agonist at $GABA_B$ receptors. $GABA_B$ receptors are predominantly presynaptic receptors, activation of which inhibits the release of several neurotransmitters; they are particularly abundant in the brainstem and spinal cord. *Dantrolene*, a directly acting skeletal muscle relaxant (see above), may be beneficial in severe spasticity. Both baclofen and dantrolene can cause nausea, muscle fatigue, and, rarely, impaired liver function.

Key references

Carlsson A. The occurrence, distribution and physiological role of catecholamines in the nervous system. Pharmacol Rev. 1959;11:490–3.

Crowe A, Matthews PBC. The effects of stimulation of static and dynamic fusimotor fibers on the response to stretching of the primary endings of muscle spindles. J Physiol. 1964;174:109–31.

Huxley AF, Niedergerke R. Structural changes in muscle during contraction. Interference microscopy of living muscle fibers. Nature 1954;173:971–3.

Huxley HE. The mechanism of muscular contraction. Science 1969;164:1356–66.

Huxley H, Hanson J. Changes in the cross-striations of muscle during contraction and stretch and their structural interpretation. Nature 1954;173:973–6.

Lai FA, Erickson HP, Rousseau E, Lui QY, Meissner G. Purification and reconstitution of the calcium release channel from skeletal muscle. Nature 1988;331:315–19.

Moffett DF, Moffett SB, Schauf CL. Human physiology, 2nd edn. St. Louis: Mosby; 1993:290–323.

Renshaw B. Central effects of centripetal impulses in axons of spinal ventral roots. J Neurophysiol. 1941;9:191–204.

Rios E, Brum G. Involvement of dihydropyridine receptors in excitation–contraction coupling in skeletal muscle. Nature 1987;325:717–20.

Sherrington CS. Decerebrate rigidity, and reflex coordination of movement. J Physiol. 1898;22:319–32.

Further reading

Freund H-J. Motor unit and muscle activity in voluntary motor control. Physiol Rev. 1983;63:387–436.

Grillner S, Wallen P. Central pattern generators for locomotion, with special reference to vertebrates. Annu Rev Neurosci. 1985;8:233–61.

Halsall PJ, Hopkins PM. Inherited disease and anesthesia. In: Healy TEJ, Cohen PJ, eds. A practice of anesthesia, 7th edn. London: Arnold; 2003: 377–90.

Hopkins PM. Malignant hyperthermia: advances in clinical management and diagnosis. Br J Anaesth. 2000; 85: 118–28.

Huxley AF. Review lecture: muscular contraction. J Physiol. 1974;243:1–43.

Kandel ER, Schwartz JH, Jessel TM. Principles of neural science, 3rd edn. New York: Elsevier; 1991:Chs 35–42.

Marsden CD, Rothwell JC, Day BL. The use of peripheral feedback in the control of movement. Trend Neurosci. 1984;7:253–7.

Moss RL, Diffee GM, Greaser ML. Contractile properties of skeletal muscle fibers in relation to myofibrillar protein isoforms. Rev Physiol Biochem Pharmacol. 1995;126:1–63.

Robinson RL, Anetseder MJ, Brancadoro V et al. Recent advances in the diagnosis of malignant hyperthermia susceptibility: how confident can we be of genetic testing? Eur J Hum Genet. 2003;11:342–8.

Chapter 36

Neuromuscular junction physiology

Christopher B Prior and Ian G Marshall

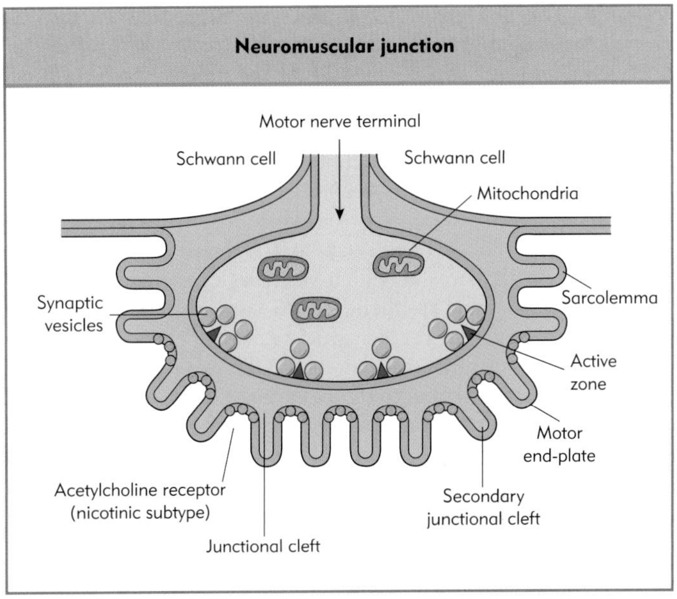

Figure 36.1 The neuromuscular junction, showing key structural features.

OVERVIEW

The neuromuscular junction is an intercellular relay structure designed for efficient communication between the motor axon and skeletal muscle fiber. It is perhaps the most studied and certainly the best understood mammalian neuroeffector junction. The neuromuscular junction is a chemical synapse and, as such, behaves as a pair of transducers, the motor nerve terminal and the muscle motor endplate, arranged in series (Fig. 36.1). As with any transducer, each has an input and an output signal. In the case of the motor nerve terminal, the input signal is a depolarizing wave produced by an action potential in the terminal part of the incoming axon. The output signal is the synchronous release of the chemical neurotransmitter acetylcholine into the junctional cleft of the neuromuscular junction. For the muscle motor endplate, the input signal is the presence of acetylcholine in the junctional cleft and the electrical output signal leads to an action potential in the skeletal muscle fiber membrane, resulting in muscle contraction. The entire functioning of the neuromuscular junction revolves around the efficient execution of these two transducer tasks. This complex signal transduction mechanism between the motor nerve and the muscle cell allows for signal amplification and modulation. There is insufficient energy in the nerve action potential in the relatively small mass of the nerve ending to excite the muscle fiber membrane directly, so some form of signal amplification is necessary. Alteration of the amount of acetylcholine released in response to motor nerve terminal depolarization, or of the sensitivity of the postjunctional muscle membrane to acetylcholine, can cause a reduction or enhancement of the process of neuromuscular transmission. This chapter describes the cellular structures and processes required for efficient neuromuscular transmission. The physiological processes involved in the functioning of the pre- and postjunctional elements of the system are described in detail, followed by a description of some of the evidence for the regulation of neuromuscular transmission.

PREJUNCTIONAL FEATURES OF NEUROMUSCULAR TRANSMISSION

Prejunctional morphology

As the motor nerve fiber (containing numerous axons) approaches a skeletal muscle, it branches extensively, sending terminal axons to many separate muscle fibers. A single motor nerve fiber and the group of muscle fibers it innervates are collectively termed a motor unit. The muscle fibers within any single motor unit are not grouped together but scattered throughout the muscle. All muscle fibers within a single motor unit contract simultaneously when its motor nerve fiber is activated. In mammalian skeletal muscle, as the terminal axon approaches the single muscle fiber it innervates, it loses its myelin sheath (Chapter 19) and branches into a number of bouton-like structures that lie in close apposition to the muscle fiber membrane. This structure is referred to as the *motor nerve terminal*. The boutons are compact structures that contain all the essential elements for the synthesis, storage, and release of acetylcholine (Fig. 36.1). The bulk of the motor nerve terminal cytoplasm is filled with numerous synaptic vesicles, spherical lipid bilayer membrane structures of approximately 60–100 nm in diameter that store acetylcholine. Synaptic vesicles are distributed throughout the motor nerve terminal but are particularly concentrated around electron-dense structures on the nerve terminal membrane, referred to as active zones. Active zones are thought to be the sites at which vesicular exocytosis of acetylcholine occurs; they are believed to comprise the molecular components required for synaptic vesicle docking and fusion with the nerve terminal cell membrane. Freeze-fracture electron microscopy reveals that active zones are not diffuse, disorganized structures but consist of an ordered arrangement of a number of electron-dense particles embedded within the nerve terminal membrane, called active zone particles. Each active zone is composed of four parallel lines of such particles. Within the active zone, the lines are arranged in two pairs. Given their dimension, the active zone particles are thought to be large, membrane-spanning proteins consisting of multiple subunits. One obvious candidate for this protein is the nerve terminal membrane voltage-gated Ca^{2+} channel, which is central to the evoked release of acetylcholine (Chapter 19 and below). Electron microscopy shows that synaptic vesicles close to the active zone are also arranged in a highly ordered fashion in a pair of parallel rows in line with the active zone particles (Fig. 36.2), which further implicates the latter in synaptic vesicle docking and fusion with the nerve terminal membrane.

Apart from synaptic vesicles, the only other major subcellular organelles present in the motor nerve terminal are mitochondria, which are necessary for the metabolic requirements of synthesis, storage, and release of acetylcholine (Fig. 36.3). The motor nerve terminal has no protein synthesis or Golgi processing apparatus; these processes take place within the cell body of the motor neuron in the spinal cord. The motor axon possesses a highly developed bidirectional axonal transport system that allows the facilitated movement of cellular components between the nerve cell body and the axon terminals. Synaptic vesicles do not move around freely within the terminal cytoplasm; throughout the nerve terminal there is an extensive network of intracellular filaments, composed mostly of actin. Microtubules, although present as a component of the axonal transport systems, do not extend to the nerve terminal membrane. The nerve terminal actin filaments are thought to be important in the anchoring of synaptic vesicles within the nerve terminal and in the ordered movement of synaptic vesicles towards and away from the active-zone release sites. Although initially created in the cell body, there is clear evidence that mature synaptic vesicles within the motor nerve terminal can undergo repeated cycles of filling and exocytosis.

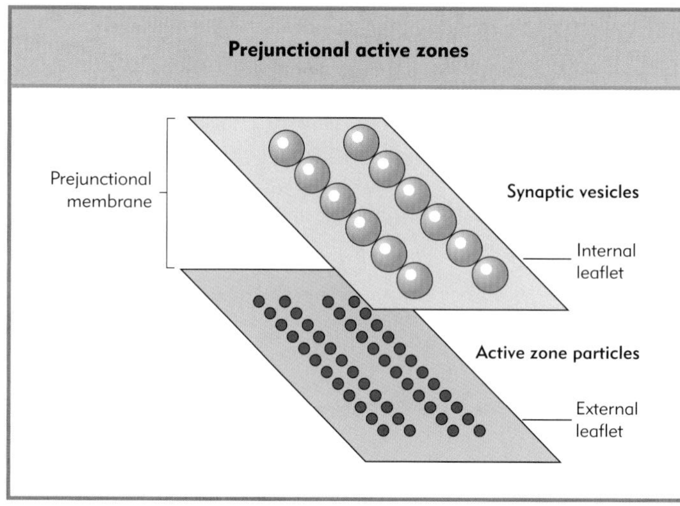

Figure 36.2 Structural organization of prejunctional active zones. Expanded view of the motor nerve terminal membrane showing the organization of synaptic vesicles and large intramembranous active zone particles, as revealed by electron microscopy.

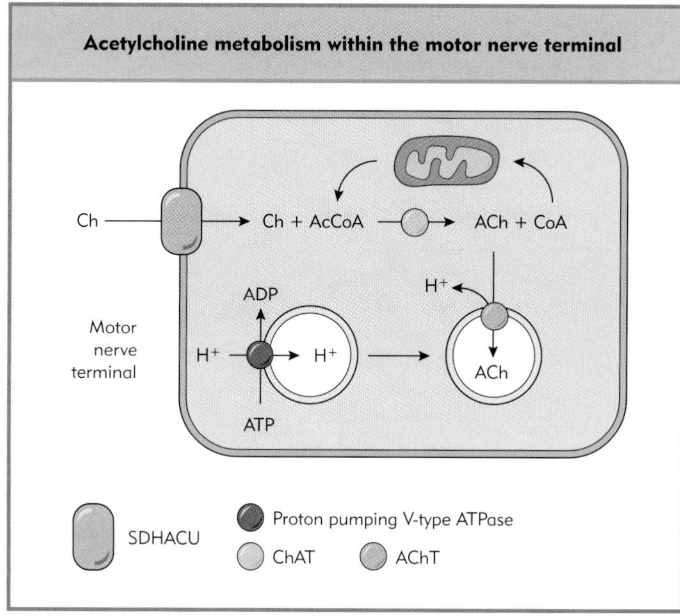

Figure 36.3 Acetylcholine metabolism within the motor nerve terminal. Choline is concentrated in the nerve terminal cytoplasm through the action of the plasma membrane sodium-dependent high-affinity choline uptake system (SDHACU). Cytoplasmic choline is acetylated by choline acetyl-*O*-methyltransferase, utilizing mitochondrially-derived acetyl-CoA as a substrate. Finally, a two-stage process loads acetylcholine into synaptic vesicles. The interior of the synaptic vesicle is made acidic as a result of H^+ entry through a proton-pumping ATPase. The acetylcholine transporter exchanges vesicular protons for cytoplasmic acetylcholine. Ch, choline; AcCoA, acetyl coenzyme A; AChT, acetylcholine transporter; ChAT, choline acetyl-*O*-methyltransferase.

Acetylcholine metabolism

In order for the motor nerve terminal to release acetylcholine in response to activation, metabolic processes must exist for the accumulation of choline by the terminals and for the synthesis and storage of acetylcholine (Fig. 36.3).

NERVE TERMINAL CHOLINE TRANSPORT

The main precursor of acetylcholine is the quaternary amine choline. Nerve cells of higher animals are unable to manufacture choline and so rely on external sources, such as the diet, or synthesis in the liver. Quaternary amines contain a nitrogen atom with a fixed positive charge. As such, these hydrophilic molecules are unable to move across lipid cell membranes by passive diffusion. They require a carrier mechanism to allow the charged molecule access to the interior of the nerve terminal. Two separate choline transport mechanisms have been described in nervous tissue. One system has a relatively low affinity for choline (K_m = 50 – 200 mmol/L), is widely distributed throughout all nervous tissue, and does not show marked energy dependence. The distribution of this low-affinity system does not correlate with the distribution of acetylcholine synthesis and is probably not related to neurotransmission. More likely it is concerned with the supply of intracellular choline for phosphatidylcholine and sphingomyelin metabolism. The second membrane choline transport system is far more selective in its distribution and far more specific in its functional role. The sodium-dependent high-affinity choline uptake (SDHACU) is found only in cholinergic nerve terminals, and consequently has a distribution in brain tissue that closely matches acetylcholine synthesis. Further, the normal functioning of the SDHACU system is a prerequisite for the efficient synthesis of acetylcholine by cholinergic nerve terminals. Under normal conditions, about half of the choline produced in the junctional cleft from the destruction of acetylcholine released from the nerve terminals is returned to the nerve terminal through the action of SDHACU.

SDHACU has a relatively high affinity for choline (K_m = 1 – 5 mmol/L) and a strict dependence on the presence of Na^+ in the extracellular environment. SDHACU can transport choline against its concentration gradient, going from approximately 10 mmol/L in the junctional cleft to around 30 mmol/L in the nerve terminal cytoplasm. As such, it can be classified as an active carrier-mediated transport system. In addition to having a relatively high affinity for choline, SDHACU will transport all the *N*-ethyl derivatives of choline but is unable to translocate the transmitter molecule acetylcholine itself. The exact mechanism underlying choline transport by SDHACU is unclear. Given the existence of a large transmembrane Na^+ concentration gradient, it is possible that choline uptake involves co-transport with Na^+ across the nerve terminal membrane.

Acetylcholine synthesis

Acetylcholine is synthesized in the nerve terminal cytoplasm by the addition of an acetyl group to choline in a reaction catalyzed by the enzyme choline acetyl-O-methyltransferase (ChAT). This enzyme is synthesized in the cell body of motor nerve cells and transported to the nerve terminal by axoplasmic transport involving neurofilaments. The localization of ChAT to cholinergic nerve endings is highly specific, and consequently this enzyme has been used as a specific marker for cholinergic neurotransmission in the CNS. The acetyl moiety required for the synthesis of acetylcholine from choline is derived from acetyl-CoA, which is synthesized by the decarboxylation of pyruvate within the matrix of the nerve terminal mitochondria. ChAT exists in the nerve terminal in unbound (soluble) and membrane-bound isoforms. The exact role of each isoform in the normal synthesis of acetylcholine by motor nerve terminals is unknown. Acetylcholine synthesis appears to be intimately linked to choline uptake by SDHACU. This could be as a result of a physical coupling between ChAT and SDHACU. Alternatively, it could reflect a rate-limiting kinetic interaction. The bulk of choline translocated by SDHACU is converted to acetylcholine; if SDHACU had a considerably lower rate than ChAT (i.e. if it was rate-limiting), then any change in the activity of SDHACU would result in altered acetylcholine synthesis.

Vesicular storage of acetylcholine

Once synthesized in the nerve terminal cytoplasm, acetylcholine is packaged into synaptic vesicles from which it can be released by exocytosis. Acetylcholine transport into synaptic vesicles is a process that is distinct from that of choline uptake mediated by SDHACU. The synaptic vesicle acetylcholine transporter is an exchange pump. The driving force for bringing acetylcholine into the interior of synaptic vesicles is a proton gradient across the vesicular membrane. The interior pH of cholinergic synaptic vesicles has been estimated to be 5.2–5.5. This is considerably lower than the cytoplasmic pH of around 7.0, and represents an ample energy gradient to drive acetylcholine accumulation via an acetylcholine/proton antiport. The acidic interior of the synaptic vesicle is produced by an Mg^{2+}-dependent vesicular membrane proton-pumping (V-type) ATPase. Thus, the uptake of acetylcholine by synaptic vesicles is a two-stage process utilizing ATP as its energy source. There is evidence suggesting that synaptic vesicle filling is a dynamic process. Thus, there is considerable passive leakage of acetylcholine from synaptic vesicles, and under certain conditions the acetylcholine content of cholinergic synaptic vesicles appears to be dependent on the level of free acetylcholine within the nerve terminal cytoplasm.

In addition to high concentrations of acetylcholine, cholinergic synaptic vesicles contain high concentrations of ATP and Ca^{2+}. The reason for the presence of the former is uncertain, although it has been suggested that ATP may act as a co-transmitter released along with acetylcholine. In this respect, ATP would have a very different role here from that at the sympathetic neuroeffector junction. At the neuromuscular junction ATP has no direct postjunctional excitatory or inhibitory effects. However, it is possible that either ATP or adenosine, enzymatically derived from ATP, could have modulatory effects on nerve terminal function, either to increase or to decrease transmitter release. The presence of a high concentration of Ca^{2+} in cholinergic synaptic vesicles suggests that synaptic vesicles may act as a Ca^{2+}-buffering system that removes Ca^{2+} from the nerve terminal cytoplasm via a vesicle membrane Ca^{2+}-pumping ATPase for subsequent extrusion to the extracellular space upon exocytosis.

Acetylcholine release

The release of acetylcholine from motor nerve terminals is quantal. At a typical mammalian neuromuscular junction, each time the motor nerve terminal is activated there is the Ca^{2+}-dependent synchronous release of 50–100 discrete packets (quanta) of acetylcholine, each comprising around 10 000 molecules. Each unit of released acetylcholine has been termed a quantum of transmitter, and this unit has been correlated with the exocytotic discharge of the entire content of a single synaptic vesicle. There are four identifiable phases involved in the synaptic vesicle exocytotic process. First, in order for the content of a synaptic vesicle to be released, the vesicle must be translocated to the release sites on the nerve terminal membrane (*mobilization*) and attached to these sites, so that the exocytotic release process can be initiated (*docking*). Once mobilized and docked, the contents of the synaptic vesicle can be released. The physical process of synchronous exocytosis of the contents of many synaptic vesicles is triggered by a nerve action potential. Subsequent to this, a number of specialized proteins on the synaptic vesicle (synaptobrevin) and nerve terminal membrane (syntaxin and SNAP-25) participate in the coupling of the synaptic vesicle to the nerve terminal plasma membrane and the formation of an exocytotic pore (*fusion pore formation*). Fusion pore formation leads to exocytosis and acetylcholine release. However, whether it leads inevitably to the total coalescence of the nerve terminal and synaptic vesicle membranes is uncertain. Following the depletion of the synaptic vesicle content, retrieval and refilling (*recycling*) of the spent synaptic vesicles occurs (Chapter 20).

The release of acetylcholine from motor nerve terminals following depolarization is highly dependent on the presence of extracellular Ca^{2+} – it is proportional to the fourth power of the extracellular Ca^{2+} concentration. The concentration of Ca^{2+} in the motor nerve terminal cytoplasm at rest is strictly regulated and very low (approximately 0.1 μmol/L, compared to around 1000 μmol/L in the extracellular space). A rise in the intracellular Ca^{2+} concentration is the trigger for exocytosis. The link between nerve terminal membrane depolarization and a rise in the intracellular concentration of Ca^{2+} is the nerve terminal membrane voltage-gated Ca^{2+} channel. In mammalian motor nerve terminals, these channels are P-type Ca^{2+} channels and are found in close apposition to the vesicular release sites, are opened in response to membrane depolarization, and allow Ca^{2+} access to the Ca^{2+}-dependent trigger mechanisms for exocytosis.

Molecular mechanisms of exocytosis

The molecular mechanisms involved in synaptic vesicular exocytosis are complex and highly regulated. The polar nature of the membrane surfaces of both synaptic vesicles and the nerve terminal plasma membrane means that there is a tendency for the two membranes to repel each other – i.e. there will be a considerable energy barrier, which has to be overcome before the two lipid membranes can fuse and an exocytotic opening can be formed between the inside of the synaptic vesicle and the junctional cleft. Thus, the process is energy dependent and can only take place at discrete membrane sites in a highly controlled fashion. The major steps in synaptic vesicle docking and fusion with the prejunctional membrane have been proposed to involve the formation and breakdown of 7S and 20S fusion core complexes. This model, known as the SNARE hypothesis, is outlined in Figure 36.4. The 7S complex is assembled from four proteins. Two of these, synaptotagmin and synaptobrevin (also known as VAMP, vesicle-associated membrane protein), are integral to the synaptic vesicle membrane, and two, syntaxin and SNAP-25 (synaptosomal-associated protein of 25 kDa), are integral to the nerve terminal plasma membrane. A further nerve terminal protein component, n-sec1, is believed to be involved in the regulation of the formation of the 7S complex. Syntaxin binds avidly to n-sec1 and the syntaxin–n-sec1 complex is unable to associate with SNAP-25 or synaptobrevin, and so the 7S complex cannot be formed. Once n-sec1 dissociates from syntaxin and the 7S complex is formed, synaptotagmin dissociates from the group, allowing the binding of a soluble component αSNAP (soluble NSF attachment protein) to syntaxin. In turn, the second soluble component, NSF (*N*-ethylmaleimide-sensitive factor), can bind to αSNAP and this results in the formation of the 20S complex. Because the synaptobrevin–SNAP-25–syntaxin complex binds αSNAP this complex is called the SNARE complex (SNAP receptor) and the three component proteins are referred to as SNAREs. Synaptobrevin is a v-SNARE (vesicle membrane SNARE) and syntaxin and SNAP-25 are t-SNAREs (terminal membrane SNAREs). The SNARE proteins are the cleavage sites for the *Clostridium* and tetanus neurotoxins, which are metalloproteases. Destruction of any of the three components of the exocytotic machinery by the neurotoxins leads to the inhibition of acetylcholine release. NSF is a homotrimeric ATPase, and it is the hydrolysis of ATP by NSF while bound in the 20S complex that leads to the disruption of the complex and the ultimate fusion of the vesicular and terminal membranes.

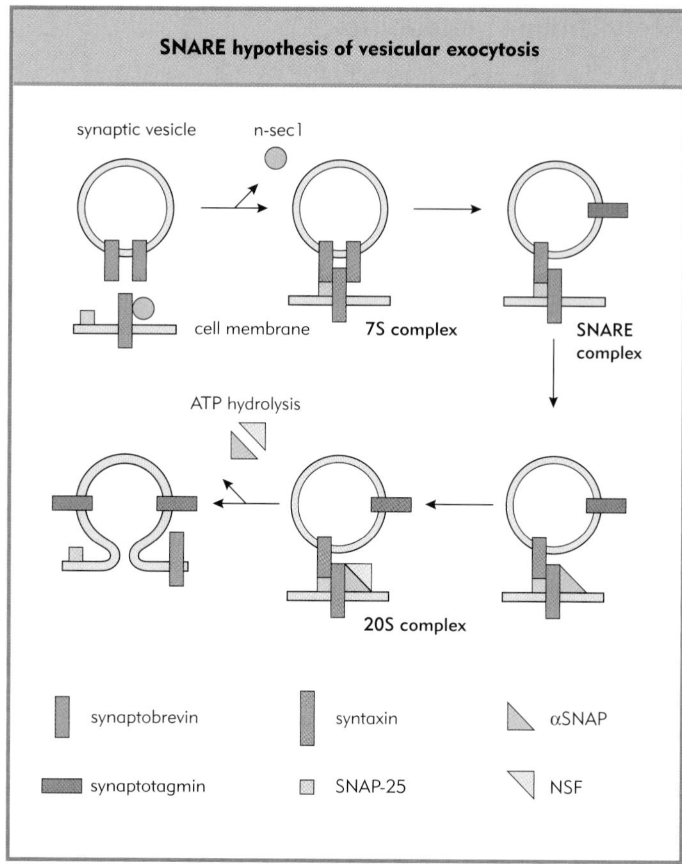

Figure 36.4 The SNARE hypothesis of vesicular exocytosis.

Although the SNARE hypothesis neatly accounts for many of the observed binding interactions between several of the nerve terminal protein components, it is very much incomplete. Many nerve terminal protein components, such as the synaptic vesicle proteins synaptophysin and the GTPase rab3A, and the terminal membrane proteins neurexin and GAP-43, are unaccounted for within this model. Further, it is not clear where the nerve terminal calcium channel fits into the SNARE hypothesis. Clearly, given the Ca^{2+} dependence of exocytosis, there must be a Ca^{2+} sensor within the exocytotic machinery. At low levels of quantal secretion there is a power relationship between the number of quanta of acetylcholine released and the extracellular Ca^{2+} concentration which indicates that, in mammalian species, a cooperative binding of three or four calcium ions is needed to trigger vesicular exocytosis. Thus there must be multiple binding sites for Ca^{2+} within the exocytotic machinery that allows the system to be activated. One possibility for the Ca^{2+} sensor/binding protein is synaptotagmin, which is known to possess multiple Ca^{2+}-binding sites. The binding of synaptotagmin and αSNAP to the SNARE complex is mutually exclusive, and if Ca^{2+} binding to synaptotagmin reduced its binding to the SNARE complex then this would promote 20S complex formation, and presumably exocytosis. One drawback with this notion is that genetic research has shown that exocytosis can take place even in the complete absence of synaptotagmin, although evoked exocytosis is highly impaired. Thus it is likely that other calcium triggers exist within the exocytotic machinery.

Synaptic vesicle recycling

Upon synaptic vesicle exocytosis there cannot be permanent and irretrievable merging of the synaptic vesicle and nerve terminal membranes. If this were to occur, the overall nerve terminal membrane area would be expected to increase following periods of sustained exocytosis. This only occurs when massive exocytotic release is triggered by neurotoxins such as α-latrotoxin (the active component of Black Widow spider venom). Two conjectures arise from this observation: first, that under normal conditions there is a relatively rapid recycling of synaptic vesicle membrane following exocytosis and, second that the mode of action of α-latrotoxin in triggering exocytosis somehow interferes with the normal membrane retrieval processes. Two forms of synaptic vesicle recycling have been proposed to exist within motor nerve terminals. In the classic model exocytosis is accompanied by complete membrane fusion and endocytosis takes place, at a site remote from the active zones, via the formation of clathrin-coated vesicles. In support of this, agents that inhibit the accumulation of acetylcholine by synaptic vesicles also inhibit the leakage of acetylcholine through the nerve terminal membrane. This suggests that the synaptic vesicle acetylcholine transporter is also present in the nerve terminal membrane – as would be expected if classic exo-/endocytosis were taking place. However, rapid synaptic vesicle recycling has also been observed in the absence of clathrin coating, and this has led to the concept of a local recycling of synaptic vesicles. In this model, acetylcholine release takes place via a 'kiss-and-run' mechanism and there is no coalescence of the two membranes. Whatever the mechanism, it is likely that following docking and activation a large pore is formed between the interior of the synaptic vesicle and the junctional gap. One candidate protein for this fusion pore is the vesicle-associated molecule synaptophysin. In the 'full-fusion' model formation of the fusion pore automatically leads to membrane convergence. In the 'kiss-and-run' model the acetylcholine escapes the synaptic vesicle through the fusion pore, the pore closes, and there is no membrane convergence.

Many questions remain as to the processes involved in synaptic vesicle recycling. Does a recycled synaptic vesicle have to be reprocessed through the early endosomal compartment before it can be refilled and released? Do endocytosed and locally recycled synaptic vesicle have different fates? In localized recycling, must a synaptic vesicle leave the active-zone site before being refilled and presented again for release?

POSTJUNCTIONAL FEATURES OF NEUROMUSCULAR TRANSMISSION

Postjunctional morphology

The motor endplate is the specialized region of the skeletal muscle fiber membrane that is chemically receptive to acetylcholine released from motor nerve terminals. In mammalian skeletal muscle there is a deep recess in the muscle fiber membrane – the junctional cleft – at the closest point of apposition of the terminal part of the motor nerve to the muscle fiber. The nerve terminal is essentially surrounded by the muscle fiber membrane and the terminal Schwann cell, which extends down to the muscle fiber membrane (see Fig. 36.1). The muscle fiber membrane in apposition to the nerve terminal is folded into deep clefts, called secondary junctional clefts. The junctional gap is narrowest (around 60 nm) at the peaks of the postjunctional folds, between the secondary clefts. These crests are opposite the release sites on the prejunctional membrane and are the main locations of postjunctional acetylcholine receptors (AChRs). These receptors are highly concentrated in the shoulder regions between the secondary clefts – in excess of 10 000/mm^2. This is a consequence of their being fixed both to each other and also to an underlying cytoskeletal matrix. During development, AChRs aggregate and anchor to appropriate sites; the mechanisms by which this occurs are poorly understood. The receptors are also found on muscle membranes outside the region of the motor endplate, but these receptors are sparsely distributed and have a much shorter half-life (20 hours) than the receptors at the motor endplate (several weeks). The AChR at the motor endplate is of the nicotinic subtype (nAChR), in that nicotine can mimic the effects of acetylcholine on this receptor.

The space between the muscle and nerve terminal membranes, the junctional cleft, is filled with a basement membrane material rich in collagen-like mucopolysaccharides. The basement membrane probably functions as a structural support, but it must also allow the free and rapid diffusion of acetylcholine through the junctional space. A second role of the basement membrane is to act as a trap for acetylcholinesterase, which has a strong affinity for the collagen-like components of the matrix (see below).

The acetylcholine receptor

The nAChR on the postjunctional membrane of the neuromuscular junction is the best-characterized member of a 'superfamily' of closely related ligand-gated ion channels (see Chapters 3 and 19). This receptor superfamily includes excitatory receptors such as all central and ganglionic nAChRs, the 5-hydroxytryptamine $5HT_3$ receptor, the AMPA-type (α-amino-3-hydroxy-5-methyl-4-isoxazole) glutamate receptor, and inhibitory receptors such as the $GABA_A$ (γ-aminobutyric acid type A) receptor and the glycine receptor. The general structure of the channels in the family is believed to be similar, although there are some important differences. The nAChRs are acetylcholine-activated nonselective cation channels. Each macromolecular complex contains two binding sites for acetylcholine which, when occupied, trigger a conformational change to open the channel pore through which Na^+, K^+, and, to a lesser extent, Ca^{2+}, but not chloride ions, can flow.

The nAChR at the neuromuscular junction is pentameric: it is composed of five individual protein subunits each with the same basic structure (Fig. 36.5a). The complex has a molecular weight of approximately 270 kDa. Each subunit is a single protein chain of 440–500 amino acid residues with both the N- and the C-terminal ends on the extracellular side of the cell membrane. The protein strand traverses the cell membrane four times; the hydrophobic transmembrane segments are designated M1, M2, M3, and M4. These membrane-spanning regions are believed to be α-helices, but there is now some evidence to suggest that they may be β-pleated sheets. There is a large (about 200 amino acid residues) extracellular segment at the N terminus; this region includes the acetylcholine-binding site. There is an intracellular loop of around 80–100 amino acid residues between M3 and M4 that contains several phosphorylation sites thought to be involved in receptor desensitization.

Four different subunits are found in each nAChR complex at the adult motor endplate. Two identical α subunits are combined with one each of the β, ε, and δ subunits (α2βεδ). The α subunits contain the bulk of the acetylcholine recognition sites. They are characterized by two disulfide-coupled cysteine residues at sites 192 and 193, which are thought to be involved in acetylcholine binding. In fetal muscle, denervated adult muscle, and in the electric organ of *Torpedo*, in which much of the original studies on acetylcholine receptor structure and function were performed, there is a γ subunit rather than an ε subunit (α2βγδ). In each nAChR complex the five subunits are arranged in a structure that resembles a goblet spanning the cell membrane, the cup being made from the N-terminal regions of each subunit (Fig. 36.5b,c). The stem of the goblet spans the cell membrane and forms the transmembrane cation channel. The ordering for the subunits around the pore is α-ε-α-β-δ (clockwise when viewed from the extracellular side), and the two acetylcholine-binding sites are thought to be located on the α subunits at the interfaces with the ε and δ subunits.

Site-directed mutagenesis has been used to show that the specificity of the nAChR for cations over anions is determined by the amino acid sequence of the M2; this region of each subunit lines the ion channel pore. In the inactive state of the channel, M2 regions of each of the five subunits are close together and the channel is closed. When two acetylcholine molecules bind to their binding sites, the receptor undergoes a conformational change that leads to the movement of the membrane-spanning regions relative to each other and the opening of the channel.

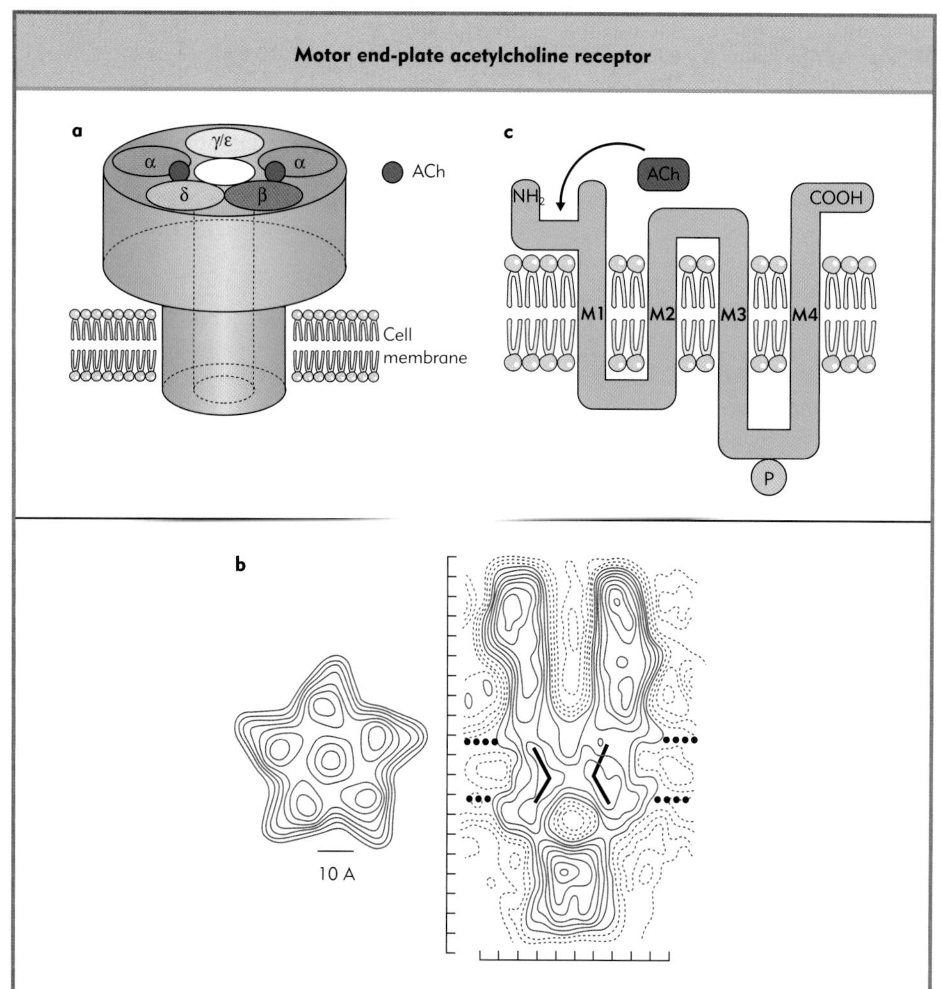

Figure 36.5 Motor endplate acetylcholine receptor. Structure of the nicotinic acetylcholine receptor (nAChR). The five protein subunits are arranged around the central ion channel pore. Two acetylcholine-binding sites (ACh) are shown at the interfaces of the α and ε subunits and the α and δ subunits. Note that the bulk of the receptor protein resides on the extracellular side of the cell membrane. (b) Electron-density maps of the *Torpedo* nAChR. High-resolution electron microscopy of the extracellular face (left) showing fivefold symmetry and a cross-sectional view (right) showing the extracellular portion and the likely gate (bent lines). Graduations are 1 nm. (With permission from Unwin, 1993, 1995.) (c) An individual subunit of the nAChR. The large N-terminal domain contributes to the ACh-binding site and there are several modulatory phosphorylation sites on the intracellular loop between M3 and M4.

Acetylcholinesterase

Acetylcholinesterase (AChE) catalyzes the hydrolysis of acetylcholine to choline and acetate. The enzymatic activity of AChE resides in a globular catalytic subunit. Hydrolysis of acetylcholine by the catalytic subunit involves the formation of an acetylated enzyme which, given the high catalytic efficiency of the enzyme, must be short-lived. Attack by water restores enzymatic activity, thereby liberating acetate. There is considerable diversity in the macromolecular assembly of AChE. At the neuromuscular junction, the principal form of AChE is the asymmetric or A12 species (Fig. 36.6). In this species of AChE, three groups of four catalytic subunits each are anchored by disulfide bonds to filamentous, collagen-containing structural subunits. The collagen-containing tail of the macromolecular complex is associated with the basal lamina of the postjunctional membrane, rather than with the postjunctional membrane itself. The macromolecular complex has the appearance of a bunch of flowers sprouting from the postjunctional motor endplate. The catalytic sites have good access to acetylcholine in the junctional cleft while being firmly anchored to the motor endplate region. A second class of cholinesterase enzyme (butyrylcholinesterase, pseudocholinesterase or plasma cholinesterase) exists that is encoded by separate genes and has different substrate specificity and tissue distribution. Butyrylcholinesterase is not present in the synaptic cleft of the neuromuscular junction but is present in plasma, being the enzyme responsible for the rapid hydrolysis of succinylcholine.

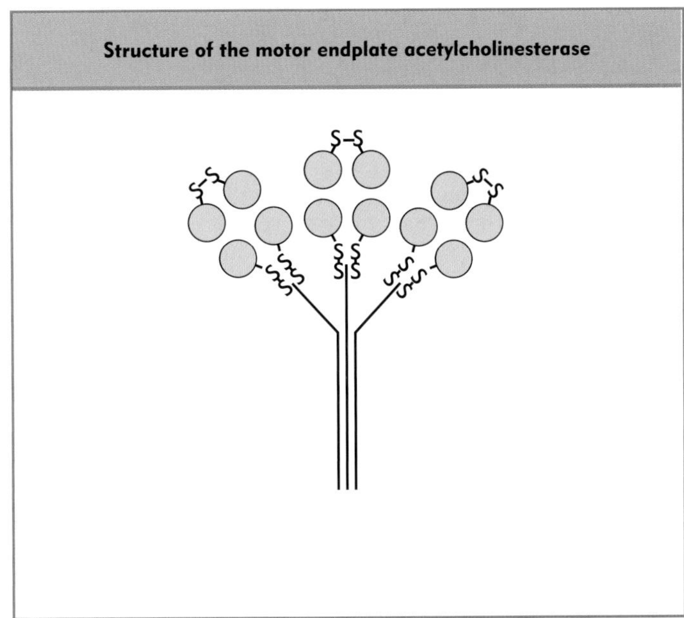

Figure 36.6 The structure of the motor endplate acetylcholinesterase. At this site, 12 globular catalytic acetylcholinesterase subunits are organized into an asymmetric (A12) macromolecular structure. The tail element of the macromolecular complex is largely composed of trihelical collagen and has a high affinity for the basal lamina within the junctional cleft of the neuromuscular junction.

Motor endplate excitation

When two molecules of acetylcholine interact with the binding sites on an nAChR there is a dramatic increase in the probability that the macromolecular complex will undergo a conformational change that opens a nonselective cation channel (Fig. 36.7). Current, in the form of cations, flowing through the channel leads to the generation of an endplate potential that eventually triggers an action potential in the muscle sarcolemma. In its resting state, the motor endplate is at the same potential as the rest of the muscle fiber membrane (approximately –80 mV in mammalian species). The opening of a nonselective cation channel allows Na^+ and K^+ to move across the sarcolemma down their respective electrochemical gradients. The electrochemical gradients are determined by the membrane potential and the distribution of the ions on either side of the membrane. Because the resting membrane potential is much closer to the K^+ equilibrium potential (about –90 mV) than to the Na^+ equilibrium potential (about +40 mV), the predominant movement of ions through the open channel is Na^+ into the muscle cell. However, as the membrane becomes progressively depolarized through Na^+ influx, K^+ will flow outwards.

The sequence of electrical events leading from single channel currents to the generation of muscle contraction is illustrated in Figure 36.7b. The ion flow at individual channels can be measured by patch-clamp techniques as single channel currents. Single channel currents are brief square-wave pulses, the duration of which represents channel open times and the amplitude

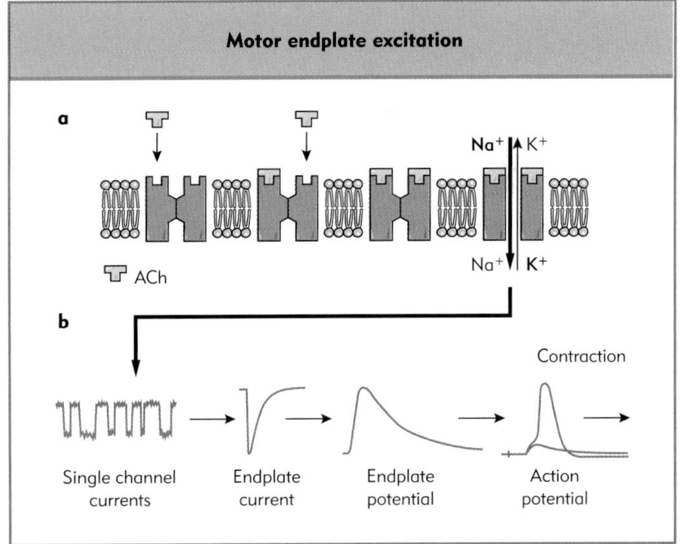

Figure 36.7 Motor endplate excitation. (a) Agonist binding results in current flow. In its resting state, the nicotinic acetylcholine receptor is closed and impermeable to ions. Following acetylcholine (ACh) binding to its recognition sites, the protein undergoes a conformation change that leads to the formation of a pore through the cell membrane through which cations can freely pass, driven by their transmembrane electrochemical gradients. (b) Single channel current leads to muscle contraction. Cations flowing through many thousands of individual receptor proteins lead to considerable electrical current flowing across the motor endplate. This inward current (depicted as a downward curve) depolarizes the endplate, which triggers a depolarizing action potential in the muscle fiber membrane (depicted as an upward curve). This propagating signal in turn leads to the activation of the muscle contractile machinery.

of which represents current flow (Chapter 6). The opening and closing of an ion channel are probabilistic events. Open times are exponentially distributed, such that there are many short openings and fewer longer openings. At the neuromuscular junction there are thousands of receptors available for interaction with released acetylcholine. The release of acetylcholine from an individual synaptic vesicle results in the near-simultaneous opening of hundreds to thousands of ion channels. The result is a miniature endplate current (MEPC), which represents the sum of all the single channel currents involved. Because of the exponential open-time distribution of single channel currents, the MEPC amplitude decays exponentially with time. The time course of this exponential decay is the same as the mean of the single channel open times. Each channel opening is an all-or-nothing event: the amplitude of the single channel current is independent of the acetylcholine concentration. However, the MEPC is a graded response, depending on the number of channel openings contributing to its occurrence. During normal evoked release tens of quanta of acetylcholine are released simultaneously. This results in the evoked endplate current (EPC) which, like the MEPC, can be measured under voltage-clamp conditions. As for the MEPC, the EPC amplitudes are directly related to the amount of acetylcholine interacting with receptors (i.e. how many channels are open). Although much valuable mechanistic information has been gained from patch-clamp and voltage-clamp recording techniques, in which the membrane potential is held constant to allow the current flow to be measured, normal neuromuscular transmission does not operate under such conditions. In the absence of a voltage-clamp, i.e. under normal conditions, the current changes described above result in changes in membrane potential, the miniature endplate potential (MEPP) and endplate potential (EPP), respectively. Like the EPC, the EPP amplitude is also graded according to the amount of acetylcholine released, although the relationship is not direct.

The single channel current, the EPC, and the EPP are all produced by the action of acetylcholine at the specialized chemically receptive area of the muscle membrane at the neuromuscular junction. The remainder of the muscle membrane does not normally express acetylcholine receptors, but it is electrically excitable. The trigger for the excitation of the muscle membrane adjacent to the motor endplate is the EPP. The EPP represents depolarization of the chemically excitable part of the muscle membrane (the muscle endplate) relative to the adjacent electrically excitable membrane. Whenever two adjacent areas of unequal potential exist, local circuit currents flow in an attempt to equalize the potentials, which depolarizes the electrically excitable area just surrounding the neuromuscular junction. If this is great enough (if it reaches the threshold potential for Na^+ channel activation), Na^+ channels open in the electrically excitable membrane, which initiate a self-propagating muscle action potential that activates the contractile mechanism by inducing Ca^{2+} release from the sarcoplasmic reticulum (Chapter 35). The margin of safety for neuromuscular transmission is determined by the size of the EPP compared with the action potential threshold. The muscle action potential is an all-or-nothing response, as is the contraction response in an individual muscle fiber. However, the gross muscle contraction is made up of the sum of the contractions of individual fibers; it can therefore be graded according to how many fibers are contracting in an all-or-nothing fashion. Therefore, the whole process, from single channel current to contraction, represents a series of either graded or all-or-nothing responses occurring in populations of structures. This is an important consideration when interpreting data from tension studies such as those used when monitoring neuromuscular transmission and neuromuscular block in humans.

REGULATION OF NEUROMUSCULAR TRANSMISSION

Prejunctional regulation

Neuromuscular transmission is a highly regulated phenomenon. One of the main ways in which the performance of the system can be either enhanced or depressed is through the modulation of the amount of acetylcholine released by the motor nerve terminal in response to activation. There is abundant evidence that the motor nerve terminal membrane contains receptors that can alter the evoked release of acetylcholine. Perhaps the best-characterized are those for acetylcholine itself (autoreceptors) and for adenosine. Others postulated to exist on motor nerve terminals include α_1- and β_1-adrenoceptors and receptors for ATP and calcitonin-gene-related peptide (CGRP).

Both muscarinic and nicotinic acetylcholine autoreceptors have been proposed to exist on motor nerve terminals. However, no clear picture has yet emerged as to the presence or role of these receptors. With respect to prejunctional nicotinic acetylcholine autoreceptors, some researchers claim a predominantly inhibitory role for these receptors, reducing acetylcholine release in response to activation, whereas others postulate the existence of excitatory feedback mechanisms whereby acetylcholine can boost its own release during times of nerve terminal stress. Indeed, it is even possible that multiple subclasses of prejunctional nicotinic autoreceptor may exist on the motor nerve terminal, and that both facilitatory and inhibitory control systems mediated by nicotinic acetylcholine receptors are present. Similarly, both facilitatory and inhibitory roles have been claimed for prejunctional muscarinic autoreceptors. Both excitatory and inhibitory prejunctional receptors have also been proposed for adenosine. The role of these receptors is generally less confusing than that of the acetylcholine receptors. Inhibitory adenosine A_1 receptors on the motor nerve terminals are activated by adenosine produced by the enzymatic destruction of vesicular ATP released from the nerve terminals. There is considerable – but less conclusive – evidence that there are also excitatory adenosine A_{2A} receptors on motor nerve terminals.

The process of vesicle mobilization increases the availability of synaptic vesicles for release. Mobilization is particularly important during times of high quantal output, because in the absence of an enhanced supply of synaptic vesicles to the release sites the per-impulse release of acetylcholine quanta cannot be sustained. Relatively little is known of the molecular mechanisms underlying mobilization at the neuromuscular junction; however, several candidate systems have been implicated. One of these involves the synapsins, a family of phosphorylated synaptic vesicle-associated proteins. Synapsin 1 interacts with synaptic vesicle-associated Ca^{2+}/calmodulin-dependent protein kinase II and the actin cytoskeletal matrix (Fig. 36.8). Binding of synaptic vesicles to the actin cytoskeleton via synapsin 1 would be expected to alter their availability for exocytotic release.

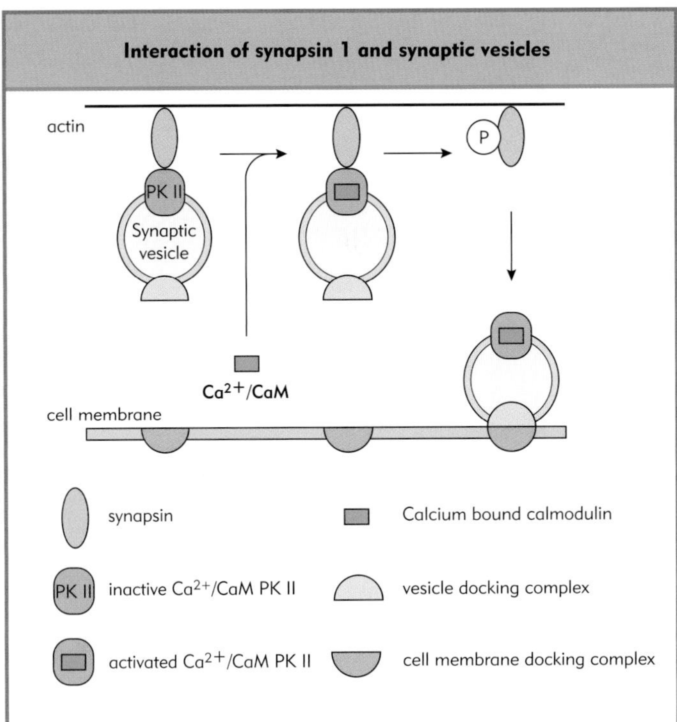

Figure 36.8 Interaction of synapsin 1 and synaptic vesicles. One possible calmodulin-dependent mechanism whereby synapsin 1 and PKII could act in concert to regulate the supply of synaptic vesicles for release. Alternative models propose that anchoring of synaptic vesicles to actin might facilitate, rather than depress, their availability for release.

Thus, it has been variously argued that this binding of synaptic vesicles to the actin cytoskeleton will decrease (through an anchoring effect) or increase (through a trafficking effect) the availability of synaptic vesicles for release. Whichever, it is clear that activation of Ca^{2+}/calmodulin-dependent protein kinase II by Ca^{2+}-bound calmodulin would lead to phosphorylation of synapsin 1, which causes it to dissociate from synaptic vesicles and hence would change the availability of synaptic vesicles for release (Chapter 19).

Postjunctional regulation

In addition to the prejunctional modulation of acetylcholine release, the efficiency of neuromuscular transmission is also influenced by the postjunctional modulation of nAChR function. The nAChR contains a number of potential phosphorylation sites, particularly on the M3–M4 intracellular loop of each of the five subunits. Various agents, including ATP and CGRP, can interact with their receptors on the muscle membrane at or near the motor endplate to influence the phosphorylation of the nAChR and modulate postjunctional sensitivity. Modulation by receptor desensitization often results from receptor phosphorylation activated by various intracellular signaling pathways. The fact that both pre- and postjunctional modulatory roles have been intimated for ATP is of considerable interest. It has been postulated that ATP has a genuine co-transmitter role at the neuromuscular junction but that, unlike sympathetic neuroeffector junctions, the ATP is modulatory rather than excitatory.

Key references

Bowman WC. Prejunctional mechanisms involved in neuromuscular transmission. In: Booji HDJ, ed. Fundamentals of anaesthesia and acute medicine: neuromuscular transmission. London: BMJ Publishing Group; 1996:1–27.

Donati F, Bevan DR. Postjunctional mechanisms involved in neuromuscular transmission. In: Booji HDJ, ed. Fundamentals of anaesthesia and acute medicine: neuromuscular transmission. London: BMJ Publishing Group; 1996:28–44.

van der Kloot W, Molgo J. Quantal acetylcholine release at the vertebrate neuromuscular junction. Physiol Rev. 1995;74:899–991.

Zimmermann H. Exocytosis and endocytosis. In: Synaptic transmission: cellular and molecular basis. Oxford: Thieme; 1993:54–67.

Further reading

Calakos N, Scheller RH. Synaptic vesicle biogenesis, docking, and fusion: a molecular description. Physiol Rev. 1996;76:1–29.

Holz RW, Fisher SK. Synaptic transmission and cellular signaling: an overview. In: Siegel GJ, ed. Basic neurochemistry: molecular, cellular, and medical aspects, 6th edn. New York: Raven Press; 1999:191–212.

Galzi JL, Revah F, Bessis A, Changeux JP. Functional architecture of the nicotinic acetylcholine receptor – from electric organ to brain. Annu Rev Pharmacol. 1991;31:37–72.

Kuhar MJ, Murrin LC. Sodium-dependent, high affinity choline uptake. J Neurochem. 1978;30:15–21.

Lindstrom J, Schoepfer R, Conroy WG, Whiting P. Structural and functional heterogeneity of nicotinic receptors. In: Marsh J, Bock G, eds. The biology of nicotine dependence. New York: John Wiley; 1990:23–52.

Parsons SM, Prior C, Marshall IG. Acetylcholine transport, storage and release. Int Rev Neurobiol. 1993;35:279–390.

Taylor P, Brown JH. Acetylcholine. In: Siegel GJ, ed. Basic neurochemistry: molecular, cellular, and medical aspects, 6th edn. New York: Raven Press; 1999:213–42.

Usdin TB, Eiden LE, Bonner TI, Erickson JD. Molecular biology of the vesicular ACh transporter. Trends Neurosci. 1995;18:218–24.

Chapter 37

Neuromuscular junction pharmacology

Cynthia A Lien and John J Savarese

Neuromuscular blocking agents have long been used as adjuncts to general anesthetics in order to facilitate endotracheal intubation, or to provide muscle relaxation to facilitate mechanical ventilation and surgery. Although the use of neuromuscular blocking agents has allowed for the development of modern surgical procedures, their use is not without risk. The sixfold increase in mortality associated with their early use, however, has been reduced with an increased understanding of their pharmacology and antagonism. The goals of ongoing research with neuromuscular blocking agents have been associated with improving the depth of monitoring of neuromuscular blockade, identifying agents that have a faster onset of effect and a shorter duration, and identifying alternative means of antagonizing neuromuscular block.

DEPOLARIZING NEUROMUSCULAR BLOCKERS

Succinylcholine (suxamethonium) (Fig. 37.1), introduced into clinical practice in 1952, is the most commonly used depolarizing neuromuscular blocking agent. In spite of a number of adverse side effects, it is commonly used because of its rapid onset of neuromuscular block or paralysis (60–90 seconds) and its short duration of action. Its rapid onset of effect is probably caused by its mechanism of action, a desynchronized depolarization of the muscle membrane (sarcolemma), resulting in disorganized muscle contractions called fasciculations. These are followed by a refractory period (relaxation). Its rapid onset of effect is also likely due to the typically used doses of the compound. Whereas its ED_{95} (or the dose that causes on average 95% suppression of neuromuscular response) is 0.3–0.6 mg/kg, doses of 1 mg/kg are recommended for rapid endotracheal intubation. Increasing the dose of the relaxant increases the plasma concentration of the compound and thus the driving force into the synaptic cleft of the neuromuscular junction, where the acetylcholine receptors are located. This increases the rate of onset, but also the duration of effect.

Succinylcholine binds to and activates the acetylcholine receptor (Chapter 36) but is not broken down by acetylcholinesterase. Therefore, it has a longer duration of action than acetylcholine. Succinylcholine is metabolized by butyrylcholinesterase (plasma cholinesterase, pseudocholinesterase), which is not found in the synaptic cleft. Therefore, it must diffuse out of the synaptic cleft into the plasma to be hydrolyzed. Until this occurs, it is available to bind repeatedly with the acetylcholine receptor. Its metabolite, succinylmonocholine, is a weak neuromuscular blocking compound and is metabolized slowly to succinic acid and choline. Patients with decreased levels of plasma cholinesterase activity, such as those with chronic disease, may have a slight prolongation in the duration of action of succinylcholine. In patients with an abnormal genetic variant for plasma cholinesterase, succinylcholine becomes a long-acting relaxant.

Succinylcholine remains in common use because of the rapid onset of its effect and its short duration of action.

Succinylcholine has a number of adverse effects, ranging from mild to catastrophic. Postoperative myalgia, which has been attributed to succinylcholine, is probably due to fasciculation of the muscles.

The cardiovascular effects of succinylcholine are quite varied because the compound stimulates autonomic cholinergic receptors (Table 37.1). Following the administration of small doses of succinylcholine, negative inotropic and chronotropic responses are seen. With larger doses, positive responses are

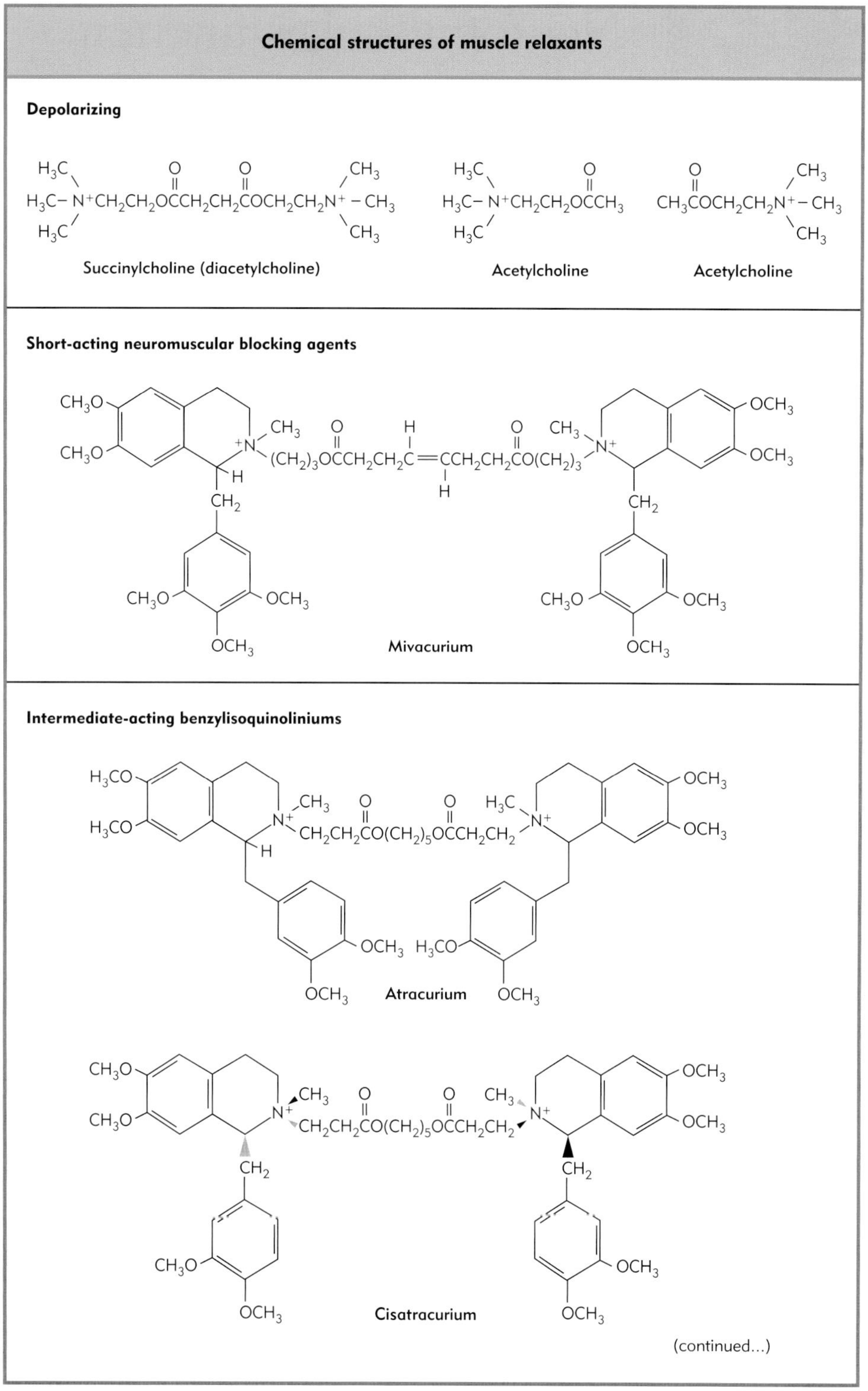

Chemical structures of muscle relaxants

Depolarizing

Succinylcholine (diacetylcholine)

Acetylcholine

Acetylcholine

Short-acting neuromuscular blocking agents

Mivacurium

Intermediate-acting benzylisoquinoliniums

Atracurium

Cisatracurium

(continued...)

Figure 37.1 Chemical structures of muscle relaxants. Two molecules of acetylcholine are shown for comparison with succinylcholine. Cisatracurium is one of 10 stereoisomers resulting from the four isomeric centers that occur in atracurium (the *1R-cis,1′R-cis* configuration).

seen. Stimulation of the muscarinic receptors in the sinus node, ganglionic stimulation, and direct myocardial effects are probably responsible for the bradycardia seen following the administration of succinylcholine. Bradycardia is most commonly observed in children who have not received atropine, owing to their predominantly vagal tone. It is also seen when a second dose of the drug is given to adults shortly after an initial dose.

Patients with muscular dystrophy and other neuromuscular diseases, extensive burns (sustained 1 day to 18 months prior to administration), trauma (sustained up to 60 days prior to administration), prolonged immobilization, or intra-abdominal infections are at risk of hyperkalemia following the administration of succinylcholine. The hyperkalemia can result in cardiac arrest. This exaggerated release of K^+ from muscle cells of

Figure 37.1, cont'd.

Chemical structures of muscle relaxants (cont.)

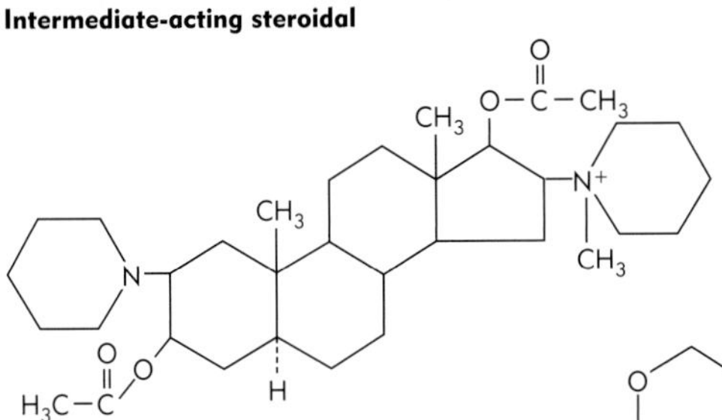

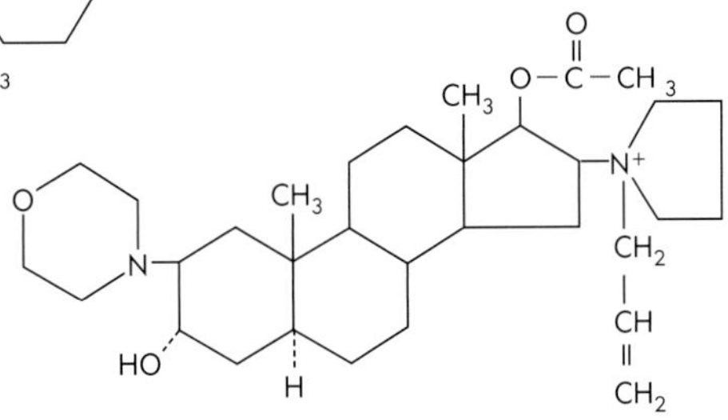

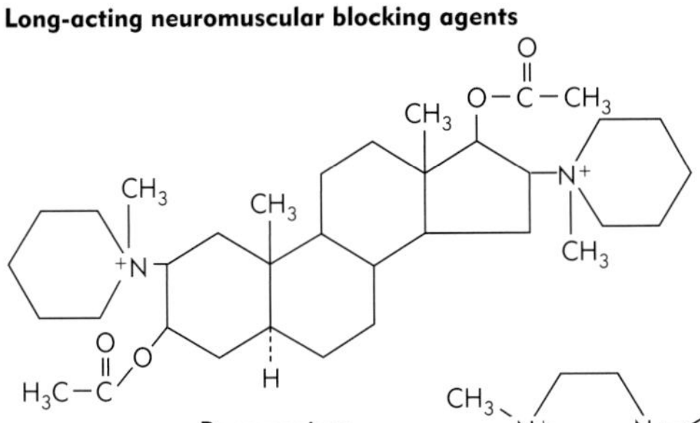

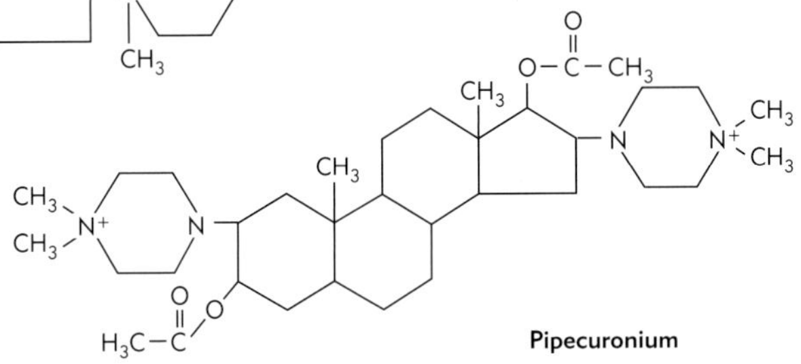

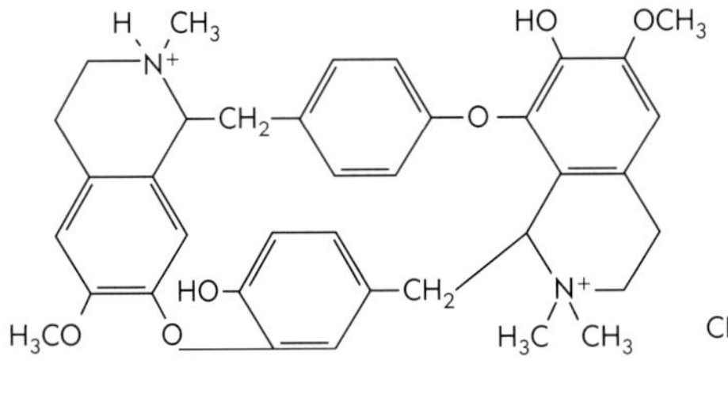

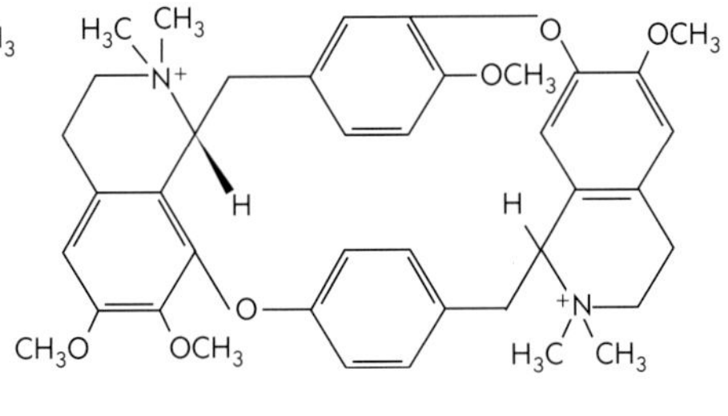

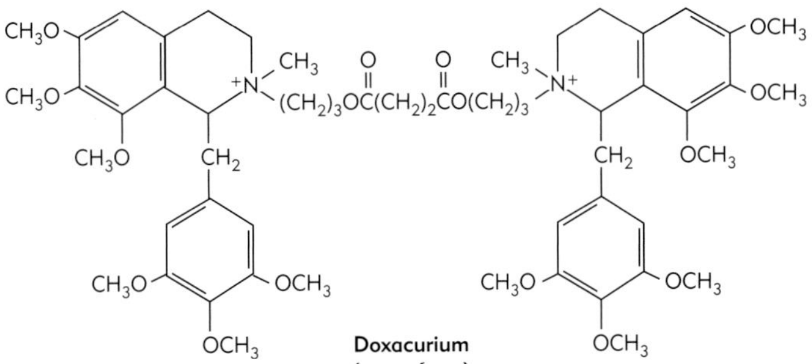

Table 37.1 Adverse effects of succinylcholine (suxamethonium)

Cardiovascular effects Arrhythmias Sinus bradycardia Junctional rhythms Ventricular arrhythmias: unifocal premature ventricular contractions, ventricular fibrillation Negative inotropic effect
Hyperkalemia secondary to burns, trauma, neuromuscular disease, closed head injury, intra-abdominal infections
Increased intraocular pressure
Increased intragastric pressure
Myalgias
Increased intracranial pressure
Masseter spasm
Malignant hyperthermia
Phase II neuromuscular block
Anaphylaxis: relatively high incidence of anaphylactoid reactions

immobilized patients is due to proliferation of extrajunctional nicotinic acetylcholine receptors (nAChRs). In contrast, healthy individuals and those with renal failure develop small increases (0.5 mEq/L) in serum K^+ concentration following the administration of succinylcholine. Succinylcholine is also a trigger for malignant hyperthermia (Chapters 10 and 35).

The increase in intraocular pressure seen following succinylcholine typically begins 1 minute after administration, peaks at 2–4 minutes, and subsides within 6 minutes. As a result, succinylcholine is relatively contraindicated in patients with an open anterior chamber. The increase in intraocular pressure may be attenuated by sublingual nifedipine, precurarization with a small dose of nondepolarizing muscle relaxant (note, however, that precurarization may compromise airway protection), or deepening anesthesia with a volatile agent.

Succinylcholine will cause increases in intracranial pressure. The mechanism of this phenomenon is not known, but may involve increased cerebral blood flow secondary to proprioceptive cortical neuron activation by muscle spindle afferents (Chapter 35). It can be attenuated by precurarization with a nondepolarizing relaxant, thiopental (thiopentone), or lidocaine (lignocaine).

With prolonged infusion or the administration of large doses of succinylcholine, a phase II block may develop. The characteristics of phase II blockade seen with monitoring are similar to those seen with nondepolarizing muscle relaxants. Fade occurs in response to tetanic stimulation and train-of-four stimulation (see below), and post-tetanic facilitation is present. Recovery, which otherwise proceeds quite rapidly (5–10 minutes), becomes more prolonged. Antagonism of succinylcholine-induced phase II block is controversial; administration of an anticholinesterase may hasten recovery.

Because of the adverse effect profile of succinylcholine, it is no longer recommended for the maintenance of neuromuscular block or for routine endotracheal intubation in pediatric patients. Research is ongoing to develop a nondepolarizing muscle relaxant with the favorable pharmacokinetic characteristics of succinylcholine in order to eliminate the need for depolarizing muscle relaxants and their attendant risks (massive K^+ efflux and malignant hyperthermia).

NONDEPOLARIZING NEUROMUSCULAR BLOCKERS

Nondepolarizing neuromuscular blocking agents act primarily by competitive inhibition of acetylcholine binding to the post-junctional nAChR. They block the ionic channel for periods of about 1 ms, which is longer than the normal lifetime of released acetylcholine. When either one or both of the two α subunits of the pentameric nAChR binds a nondepolarizing neuromuscular blocker at the acetylcholine-binding site, the ion channel of the receptor cannot open and the sarcolemma remains at its resting membrane potential. Acetylcholine competes in a concentration-dependent manner with nondepolarizing neuromuscular blocking agents for receptor sites. Relaxant concentration must decrease below a critical level (determined by its affinity for the receptor) before acetylcholine can bind and activate the receptor.

Nondepolarizing relaxants can also have presynaptic effects by interacting with presynaptic muscarinic and nicotinic cholinergic receptors. There they may reduce the release of acetylcholine from the nerve terminal, thereby enhancing their competitive postjunctional neuromuscular blocking potency. The specific presynaptic actions of nondepolarizing relaxants vary among agents.

Nondepolarizing neuromuscular blocking agents can be categorized based on a number of characteristics, including duration of action, means of elimination, side effects, and underlying chemical structure. They can also be classified on the basis of their cardiovascular effects. Their cardiovascular side effects result from their ability to cause histamine release, ganglionic blockade, or vagolysis, and are summarized in Tables 37.2 and 37.3.

Long-acting neuromuscular blockers

Long-acting muscle relaxants have a duration of action of 60–150 minutes. Included in this category are tubocurarine (D-tubocurarine), metocurine, doxacurium, gallamine, alcuronium, pancuronium, and pipecuronium (see Fig. 37.1). Following the administration of an intubating dose of muscle relaxant (typically twice the ED_{95}), at least 60 minutes are required for patients to recover to 25% of their baseline muscle strength. The long duration of action of these neuromuscular blocking agents results from their low clearance (1.5–3 mL/min/kg body weight). They are eliminated primarily through the kidney and undergo little or no metabolism (Table 37.2).

Of the long-acting neuromuscular blockers, only pancuronium undergoes significant metabolism. Whereas most of the compound is eliminated unchanged, primarily by renal mechanisms and secondarily by hepatic mechanisms, up to 20% is deacetylated in the liver at the 3-position. The metabolite is eliminated by the kidney and to a lesser extent by the liver. The 3-hydroxy metabolite is, like pancuronium, a neuromuscular blocking agent. Its potency is about 50% that of the parent compound and its elimination is similar to that of pancuronium.

Table 37.2 Long-acting neuromuscular blocking agents

Compound	ED_{95} (mg/kg)[a]	Dose for intubation[b]	Clinical duration of action (min)	Routes of elimination	Cardiovascular side effects	Chemical structure
D-Tubocurarine	0.5	1.0–1.2	60–100	Kidney, liver	Histamine release ganglionic blockade	Benzylisoquinolinium
Metacurine	0.3	1.0–1.3	60–120	Kidney	Mild histamine release	Benzylisoquinolinium
Doxacurium	0.025	2–3	90–150	Kidney, liver	None	Benzylisoquinolinium
Gallamine	3	1.3–2.0	90–120	Kidney	Strong vagolysis	Gallic acid derivative
Alcuronium	0.2	1.0–1.5	60–120	Kidney, liver	Ganglionic blockade, mild vagolysis	Toxiferine derivative
Pancuronium	0.06–0.07	1–2	60–120	Kidney, liver	Moderate vagolysis, sympathomimetic	Steroid
Pipecuronium	0.04–0.05	2–3	60–120	Kidney, liver	None	Steroid

[a]Effective dose for 95% of maximal blockade.
[b]Amount the ED_{95} should be multiplied by.

Table 37.3 Intermediate and short-acting neuromuscular blocking agents

Compound	ED_{95} (mg/kg)[a]	Dose for intubation[b]	Clinical duration of action (min)	Routes of elimination	Cardiovascular side effects	Chemical structure
Atracurium	0.25	2	30–45	Kidney: Hofmann elimination, ester hydrolysis	Histamine release ganglionic blockade	Benzylisoquinolinium
Cisatracurium	0.05	2–4	40–75	Liver, Hofmann elimination	None	Benzylisoquinolinium
Vecuronium	0.05	2	45–90	Liver, kidney	None	Steroid
Rocuronium	0.3–0.4	2–4	45–75	Liver, kidney	Mild vagolysis	Steroid
Mivacurium	0.07–0.08	3	15–20	Hydrolysis by plasma cholinesterase	Mild histamine release	Benzylisoquinolinium
Rapacuronium[c]	0.75–1.0	2	8	Kidney, liver	Mild hypotension, vagolysis	Steroid
430A	0.19	2–3	7	Chemical degradation	None	Chlorofumarate

[a]Effective dose for 95% of maximal blockade.
[b]Amount the ED_{95} (dose that, on avergage, causes 95% blockade) should be multiplied by.
[c]No longer available due to potentially severe bronchospasm.

Intermediate-acting neuromuscular blockers

The intermediate-acting muscle relaxants (Table 37.3) include atracurium, *cis*-atracurium, vecuronium (Fig. 37.2), and rocuronium. These compounds have a clinical duration of action (or recovery to 25% of baseline muscle strength) of 30–45 minutes, and spontaneous recovery of neuromuscular function occurs more quickly than it does with the long-acting relaxants. Their shorter durations of action are the consequence of their faster clearance rates (4–7 mL/min/kg). These compounds are eliminated by a variety of means: primarily by hepatic and secondarily by renal mechanisms (e.g. vecuronium and rocuronium), by Hofmann elimination and hydrolysis by esterases (e.g. atracurium, Fig. 37.3), or by Hofmann elimination alone (e.g. cisatracurium).

Vecuronium, a steroidal intermediate-acting relaxant, is the 2-desmethyl analog of pancuronium and is more extensively metabolized than pancuronium. As with pancuronium, 30–40% of a dose is deacetylated at the 3-position, to yield 3-desacetylvecuronium, which is 70% as potent as vecuronium

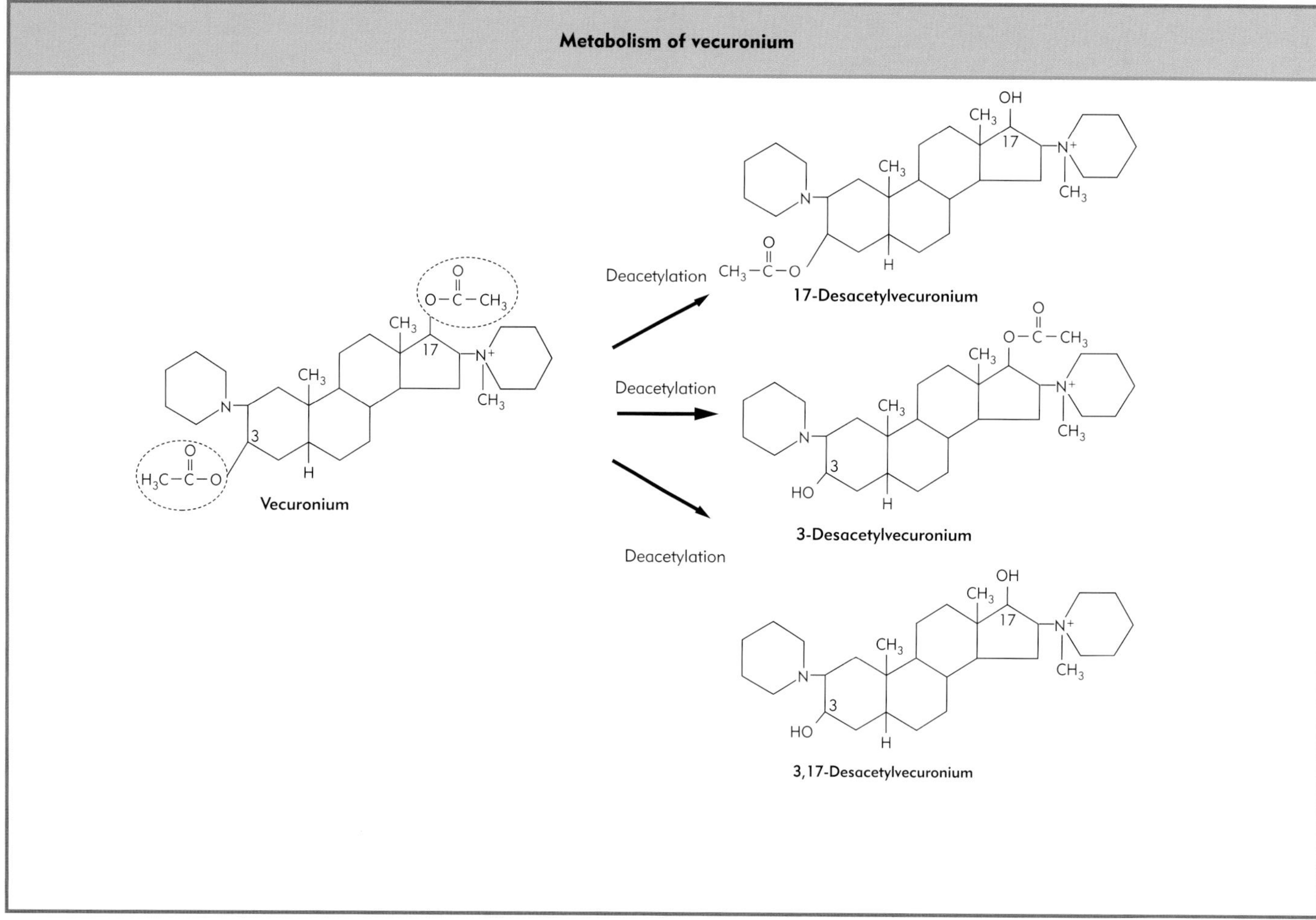

Figure 37.2 Metabolism of vecuronium. Vecuronium is deacetylated at the 3- and/or 17-positions to yield 17-desacetyl, 3-desacetyl-, or 3,17-desacetylvecuronium. Most deacetylation occurs at the 3-position.

(Fig. 37.2). It can also be deacetylated at the 17-position, to yield 17-desacetyl- or 3,17-desacetylvecuronium. In contrast to vecuronium, 3-desacetylvecuronium has a long duration of action. Its accumulation may account for the prolonged action of vecuronium in patients in the intensive care unit who have renal failure. Rocuronium, the other steroidal relaxant with an intermediate duration of action, does not undergo significant metabolism.

Both cisatracurium and atracurium depend on extensive degradation for their elimination from plasma. Cisatracurium is one of the 10 stereoisomers comprising atracurium. Both atracurium and cisatracurium undergo Hofmann elimination (Fig. 37.3), a chemical reaction in which a quaternary nitrogen atom is converted to a tertiary amine. This nonenzymatic reaction is base catalyzed and temperature dependent. Hofmann elimination of atracurium or cisatracurium yields laudanosine. This tertiary amine is excreted in the urine and bile and crosses the blood–brain barrier, where it is a potential CNS stimulant. Evidence of CNS excitement has been demonstrated in animals following the administration of extremely large doses of atracurium, but has not been reported in patients receiving the relaxant as an infusion in the intensive care unit. Even in patients with renal failure receiving an infusion of atracurium, plasma laudanosine concentrations reach a plateau that is substantially lower than those anticipated to cause CNS stimulation. In part because of its greater potency, the administration of cisatracurium results in less laudanosine formation than atracurium.

In addition to Hofmann elimination, atracurium undergoes ester hydrolysis to yield a quaternary alcohol and a quaternary acid (see Fig. 37.3). The esterase system that catalyzes this reaction is unrelated to plasma cholinesterase, which metabolizes succinylcholine and mivacurium. Less than 20% of atracurium or cisatracurium is eliminated unchanged through the kidney.

Short-acting neuromuscular blockers

The short-acting muscle relaxant mivacurium (see Table 37.3) exhibits rapid spontaneous recovery. Following administration of twice the ED_{95}, patients spontaneously recover to 95% of baseline muscle strength within 30 minutes. Rapid recovery results from its extensive metabolism by plasma cholinesterase, the same enzyme that metabolizes succinylcholine. Mivacurium is metabolized at about 80% the rate of succinylcholine, with a comparable K_m value; its plasma clearance is 60–100 mL/min/kg. Mivacurium metabolites are excreted in the urine and bile and do not appear to have pharmacologic activity (Fig. 37.4).

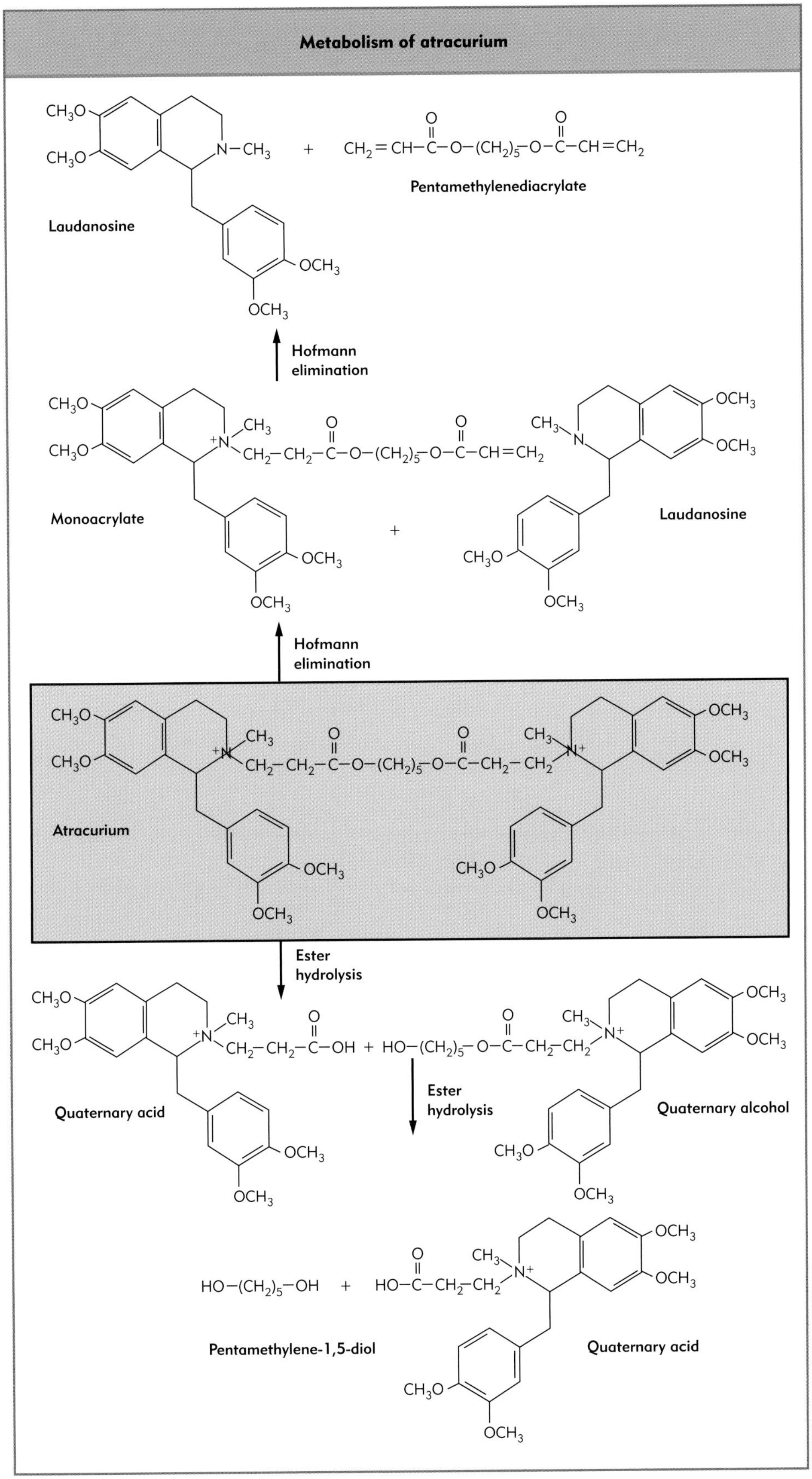

Metabolism of atracurium

Laudanosine + $CH_2=CH-C(=O)-O-(CH_2)_5-O-C(=O)-CH=CH_2$

Pentamethylenediacrylate

↑ Hofmann elimination

Monoacrylate + Laudanosine

↑ Hofmann elimination

Atracurium

↓ Ester hydrolysis

Quaternary acid + $HO-(CH_2)_5-O-C(=O)-CH_2-CH_2-N^+$ Quaternary alcohol

↓ Ester hydrolysis

$HO-(CH_2)_5-OH$ + $HO-C(=O)-CH_2-CH_2-N^+$

Pentamethylene-1,5-diol

Quaternary acid

Figure 37.3 Metabolism of atracurium. Atracurium undergoes Hofmann elimination to yield laudanosine and a monoacrylate, as well as ester hydrolysis to yield a quaternary acid and alcohol. A small amount is eliminated unchanged through the kidney.

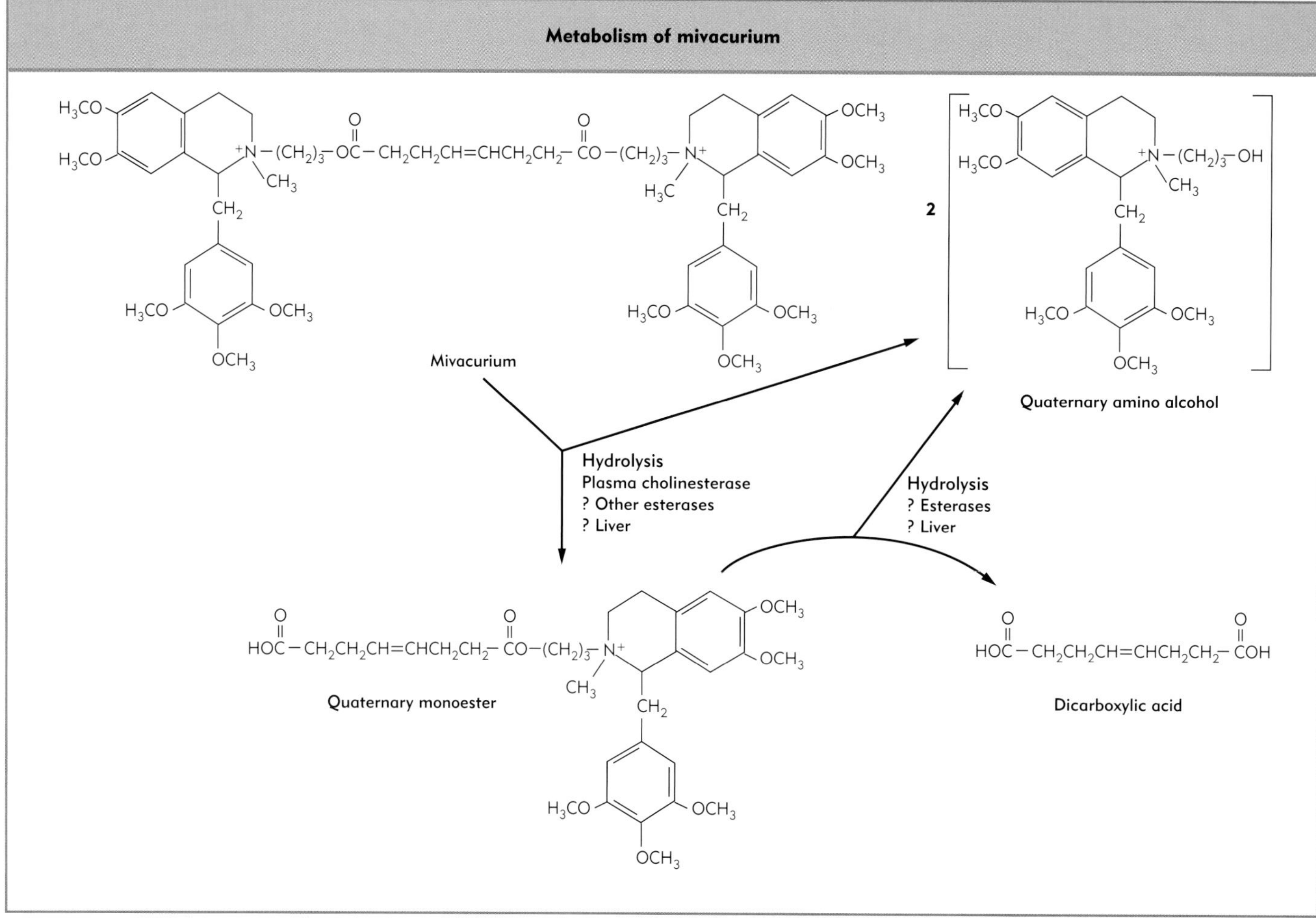

Figure 37.4 Metabolism of mivacurium. Mivacurium undergoes hydrolysis by plasma cholinesterase to yield a quaternary amino alcohol and a quaternary monoester.

The duration of action of neuromuscular agents is related to their clearance from the body. Long-, intermediate- and short-acting agents have clearances of approximately 2, 5, and 60 mL/min/kg, respectively.

Rapacuronium (ORG 9487), an analog of vecuronium, is a steroidal neuromuscular blocking drug recently removed from clinical practice. Its onset of effect is rapid, and intubating conditions following the administration of 1.5–2.0 mg/kg approximate or are equivalent to those of succinylcholine. In addition to having a fast onset of effect, rapacuronium is a short-acting nondepolarizing neuromuscular blocking agent. In the larynx spontaneous recovery to a twitch height of 75% of baseline occurs in approximately 6 minutes following 1.5 mg/kg and 17 minutes following 2.0 mg/kg.

Rapacuronium has a clearance of 7 mL/min/kg. It is metabolized in the liver to ORG 9488, its 3-desacetyl metabolite. This metabolite is a long-acting neuromuscular blocking agent that is primarily excreted unchanged in the urine. Its clearance is 1 mL/min/kg. Formation of this metabolite accounts for the increasingly prolonged duration of action of subsequent or larger doses of rapacuronium. Recovery of neuromuscular function following the administration of rapacuronium can be shortened, consistent with its nondepolarizing mechanism of neuromuscular block, by the administration of neostigmine.

Rapacuronium was removed from the market as it was felt to be responsible for severe bronchospasm that may have resulted in fatalities in pediatric and young adult patients. Studies of the compound reported that it caused bronchospasm in up to 10% of patients to whom it was administered. Rapacuronium-induced bronchospasm appears related to its antagonism at the muscarinic (M_2) receptor, increasing the airway resistance caused by stimulation of the vagus nerve.

430A (see Fig. 37.1), a nondepolarizing neuromuscular agent undergoing investigation in volunteers, is an asymmetrical mixed-onium chlorofumarate, a new class of relaxant. Its ED_{95} is 0.19 mg/kg and it has an ultrashort duration of action. Administration of 0.54 mg/kg results in 100% neuromuscular block in 60 seconds in the laryngeal adductors and 90 seconds at the adductor pollicis. These onset times are similar to those observed following administration of succinylcholine (1 mg/kg). Complete spontaneous recovery to a train-of-four ratio of 90% following administration of 0.54 mg/kg 430A requires 15 minutes at both the laryngeal adductors and the adductor pollicis. The times required for recovery from 5 to 95% of muscle strength and from 25% recovery of twitch height to a train-of-four ratio of 90% remain constant at 7 and 5 minutes, respectively, regardless of the dose of relaxant administered. This ultrashort duration of action and lack of accumulation are probably due to the compound's inactivation by cysteine adduction (Fig 37.5). Recovery from 430A-induced neuromuscular block can be further shortened by the administration of edrophonium.

ONSET OF NEUROMUSCULAR BLOCKADE

The onset of neuromuscular blockade is influenced by a number of factors, including muscle blood flow and the neuromuscular blocking potency as defined by intrinsic potency, the rate of equilibration between plasma and the biophase, and the plasma clearance.

Metabolism of 430A

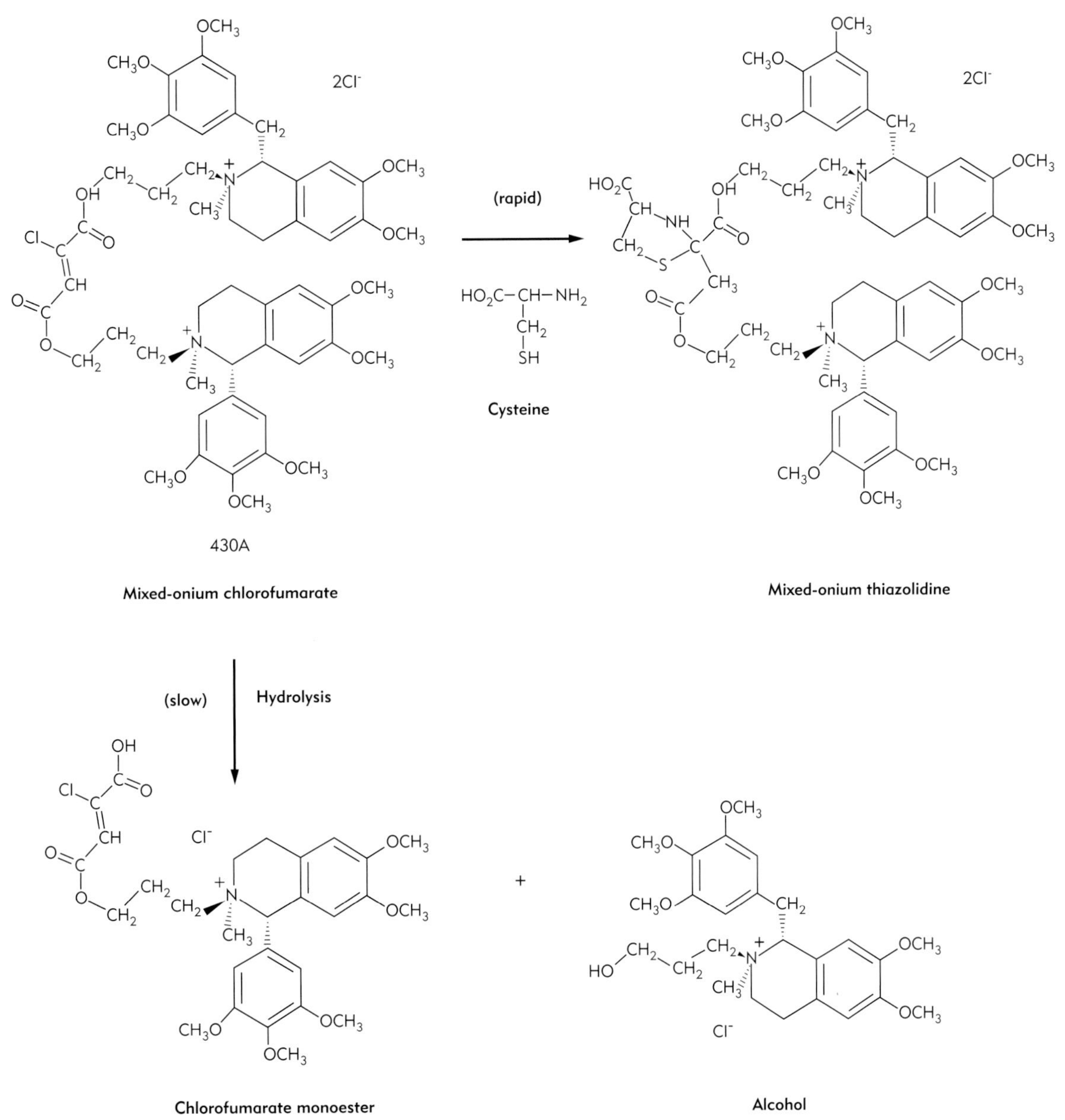

430A

Mixed-onium chlorofumarate

(rapid)

Cysteine

Mixed-onium thiazolidine

(slow) Hydrolysis

Chlorofumarate monoester

Alcohol

Figure 37.5 The metabolism of 430A. Cysteine is adducted to the molecule, rendering it inactive. 430A also undergoes a slower hydrolysis to an alcohol and a monoester.

The onset time of neuromuscular blockade is inversely related to molar potency. The least potent relaxants have the fastest onset both experimentally and clinically (Fig. 37.6). These observations led to the development of rocuronium, a structural modification of vecuronium made with the intention of lowering its neuromuscular blocking potency. The potency of rocuronium is reduced eightfold by modification of the acetoxy substitution at position 3 to a hydroxyl group, the position 2 substitution of piperidino by morpholino, and the position 16 substitution of piperidino with methyl quaternization by pyrrolidino with allyl quaternization. The reduced potency results in a significantly faster onset compared to vecuronium or other available nondepolarizing neuromuscular blocking agents.

The relationship between onset of block and potency can be explained by the practice of administering a greater number of molecules of the less potent compound to achieve the same degree of neuromuscular block as with the more potent compound. Because of this, more molecules are available to diffuse from the central compartment or plasma into the effect compartment, or neuromuscular junction, and the increased number of molecules increases the driving force for diffusion into the synaptic cleft. Once in the effect compartment, all molecules act promptly. So, when all other factors are equal, the increased rate of delivery resulting from the higher plasma concentration becomes the dominant element controlling onset time.

Onset of block is also affected by blood flow, and hence the delivery of relaxant, to the muscle group. Consequently, the musculature of the airway, with its greater blood flow than the adductor pollicis, has a faster onset of maximal effect than this peripheral muscle.

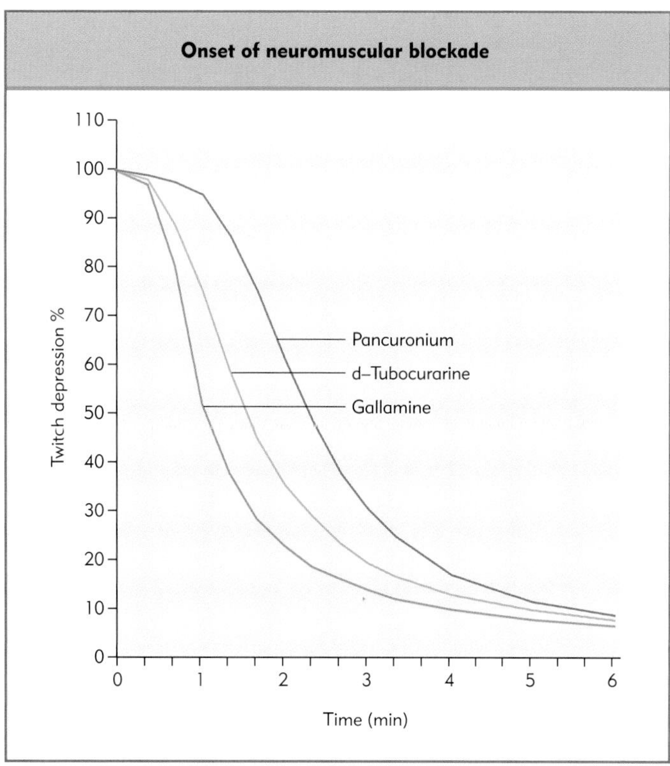

Figure 37.6 Onset of neuromuscular block with gallamine, pancuronium, or D-tubocurarine. Gallamine, which is the least potent of the relaxants tested, had the fastest onset. Pancuronium, the most potent of the three relaxants tested, had the slowest onset.

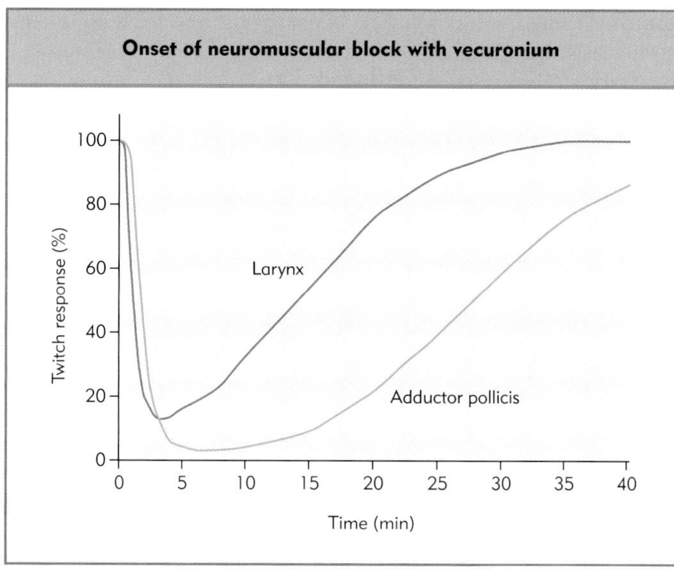

Figure 37.7 Onset of neuromuscular block with vercuronium in the larynx and in the adductor pollicis. Although onset of block (using 0.07 mg/kg vecuronium) occurs more quickly in the larynx, it is relatively resistant to neuromuscular block. Recovery also occurs more quickly in the larynx.

Complete neuromuscular block at the adductor pollicis is not required to ensure good conditions for endotracheal intubation, as onset of block at the larynx occurs more quickly.

The diaphragm and larynx are relatively resistant to neuromuscular blockers. In general, their dose–response curves are shifted to the right and larger doses of relaxants are required for the same degree of neuromuscular blockade as in a peripheral muscle such as the adductor pollicis. In spite of this relative resistance to neuromuscular blockade, block develops more quickly (Fig. 37.7). This may be important clinically for the timing of endotracheal intubation; it is not necessary to wait for complete loss of twitch of the adductor pollicis prior to laryngoscopy for good 'intubating conditions' (relaxed jaw, abducted vocal cords, and absence of diaphragmatic movement). In general, maximal blockade of airway musculature occurs 30–60 seconds earlier than in the periphery, a point where the adductor pollicis response to ulnar stimulation is decreased to 70% of baseline. The onset of neuromuscular blockade in the orbicularis oculi coincides closely with onset in the larynx. Therefore, monitoring of onset in this muscle group more closely reflects effects in the larynx.

RECOVERY OF NEUROMUSCULAR FUNCTION

Spontaneous recovery of neuromuscular function following administration of a nondepolarizing neuromuscular blocking agent involves diffusion of the relaxant away from the nAChR and the motor endplate, as well as its elimination from the body.

Recovery is facilitated in the presence of anticholinesterases, which increase acetylcholine concentration at the motor endplate. Recovery is also influenced by depth of neuromuscular block at the time of antagonism, the clearance and half-life of the relaxant used, and any factors that affect neuromuscular blockade (Table 37.4). Factors that affect the opening and closing times of the nAChR, alter resting membrane potential, or influence the release of acetylcholine from the presynaptic terminal may also affect neuromuscular block.

Anticholinesterases

Anticholinesterases (acetylcholinesterase inhibitors) effectively increase the concentration of available acetylcholine by inhibiting the action of acetylcholinesterase, the neuromuscular junction enzyme responsible for acetylcholine breakdown (Chapter 36). The increased concentration of acetylcholine at the neuromuscular junction increases the likelihood that an agonist rather than an antagonist will bind the nAChR.

Table 37.4 Factors potentiating neuromuscular blockade

Factors potentiating neuromuscular blockade
Drugs
Volatile anesthetics
Antibiotics: aminoglycosides, polymyxin B, lincomycin, clindomycin, neomycin, tetracycline
Dantrolene
Verapamil
Furosemide (frusemide)
Lidocaine (lignocaine)
Electrolyte and acid–base disorders
Hypermagnesemia
Hypocalcemia
Hypokalemia
Respiratory acidosis
Hypothermia

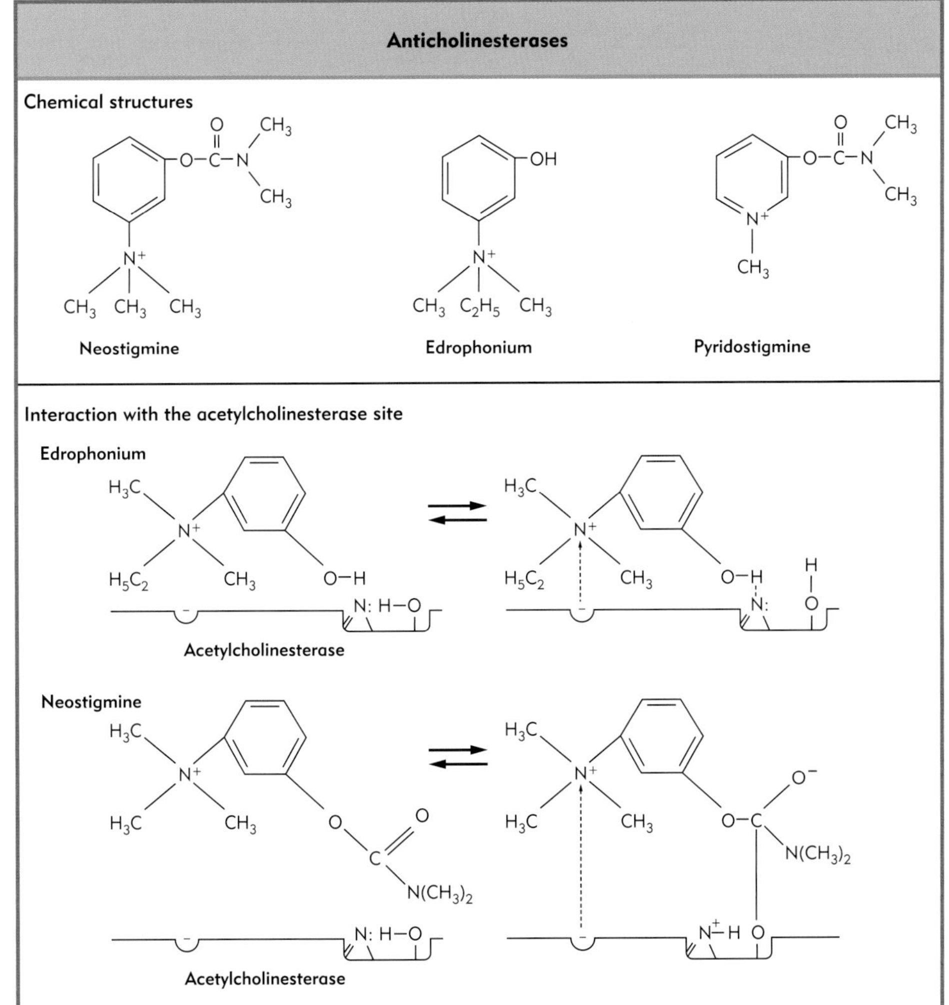

Figure 37.8 Anticholinesterases. The chemical structures of neostigmine, edrophonium, and pyridostigmine and the interaction of edrophonium and neostigmine with the acetylcholinesterase active site.

Recovery of neuromuscular function is determined by the elimination of the neuromuscular blocking agent from the body as well as the increased acetylcholine concentrations following administration of anticholinesterases.

Three anticholinesterases are used clinically to antagonize the effects of nondepolarizing neuromuscular blocking agents: edrophonium, neostigmine, and pyridostigmine (Fig. 37.8). The mechanisms by which neostigmine and pyridostigmine inhibit acetylcholine are identical (Fig. 37.8). The positively charged nitrogen atom in the anticholinesterase is attracted to the negatively charged anionic site at the acetylcholinesterase active site. Once bound to the enzyme, the anticholinesterase is slowly hydrolyzed and in the process its carbamate moiety binds covalently to (carbamylates) the catalytic site and inactivates the enzyme. The covalent bond can be cleaved by water (hydrolyzed) over the course of minutes, rendering the inhibition reversible. Edrophonium binds to acetylcholinesterase by electrostatic attraction; its presence in the active site denies acetylcholine access. Typical doses of neostigmine are up to 70 μg/kg and doses of edrophonium are up to 1 mg/kg, depending on the clearance of the relaxant and the depth of block to be antagonized.

When antagonizing moderate depths of neuromuscular block (three responses to train-of-four stimulation), the speed of action of the anticholinesterases is edrophonium > neostigmine > pyridostigmine. This ranking may be irrelevant at deep levels of neuromuscular block, where the faster action of edrophonium is lost. In fact, comparing large doses of edrophonium (1 mg/kg) with neostigmine (50 μg/kg), the latter more rapidly and more completely antagonizes profound levels of neuromuscular block than the former.

Acetylcholine and acetylcholinesterase both function at muscarinic as well as nicotinic sites. Administration of an anticholinesterase increases acetylcholine concentrations at these sites as well as at the neuromuscular junction, causing undesirable muscarinic side effects (e.g. bradycardia). In order to minimize muscarinic side effects, anticholinesterases are usually administered concomitantly with an antimuscarinic agent such as glycopyrrolate (10 μg/kg) or atropine (20 μg/kg).

Potential complications of administration of anticholinesterases include arrhythmias, bronchospasm, and nausea and vomiting.

Administration of doses of neostigmine greater than 2.5 mg is associated with an increased incidence of postoperative nausea and vomiting. Routinely not administering an anticholinesterase, however, results in a severalfold increased incidence of unacceptable neuromuscular block on admission to the postanesthesia care unit. Therefore, the decision not to administer anticholinesterases should not be made based only on the concern that patients will be nauseated postoperatively. A number of factors contribute to postoperative nausea and vomiting. In order to decrease the incidence following the administration of anticholinesterases, waiting for a greater degree of spontaneous recovery of neuromuscular function and then administering neostigmine – 2 mg or less - should be effective.

There is a limit to the depth of neuromuscular blockade that can be effectively antagonized by anticholinesterases. Anticholinesterases administered at any point after the administration of a nondepolarizing neuromuscular blocker will shorten the time required for recovery of neuromuscular function compared to spontaneous recovery. Recovery to clinically acceptable levels of neuromuscular function, however, occurs more quickly if the anticholinesterase is administered once a significant amount of spontaneous recovery has occurred and more acetylcholine receptors are available. In the case of neostigmine, the maximal effect of the anticholinesterase is observed approximately 7 minutes after its administration. Further recovery of neuromuscular function depends on ongoing elimination of the relaxant from the neuromuscular junction and the body.

The speed of antagonism of residual block is related to the depth of block at the time of administration of the anticholinesterase. Deeper levels of neuromuscular block require a longer time for the return of twitch strength to acceptable levels (train-of-four ratios ≥ 0.7, see later). The speed of antagonism of block by either tubocurarine or pancuronium depends on the dose of neostigmine administered: larger doses of anticholinesterase are required for more complete and faster recovery of neuromuscular function.

Following neostigmine antagonism of profound pancuronium-induced neuromuscular block there is an initial period of rapid but incomplete antagonism, which peaks within 10 minutes. Further recovery of neuromuscular function occurs relatively slowly; this second, slower stage of recovery appears to depend on the clearance of the relaxant. In the case of long-acting relaxants, with clearance values of 1.5–3.0 mL/min/kg and elimination half-lives of 1.5–2 hours, little drug is eliminated during the first 10 minutes after neostigmine administration, as this 10-minute period represents only about one-10th of one half-life. Consequently, during antagonism of long-acting relaxants the return of neuromuscular function to normal depends almost entirely on the antagonistic effect of the anticholinesterase. For relaxants with shorter half-lives (2–20 minutes), a larger fraction of the relaxant is eliminated during the 10-minute period following administration of the anticholinesterase. Therefore, antagonism of residual blockade in the latter represents a combination of the pharmacodynamic effect of the anticholinesterase and the pharmacokinetic effect of clearance of the relaxant. The net result is that antagonism of residual effect is more rapid and more complete with shorter-acting relaxants than with long-acting relaxants. This results in a higher incidence of residual weakness in the recovery room following the administration of long-acting nondepolarizing neuromuscular blockers compared with intermediate-acting drugs.

Factors rendering antagonism of residual neuromuscular block more difficult include an overdose of the nondepolarizing neuromuscular blocking agent, end-organ disease, volatile anesthetics, respiratory acidosis, and concomitant medications, such as aminoglycoside antibiotics.

Volatile anesthetics potentiate neuromuscular blockade and impede antagonism of residual neuromuscular blockade. For example, during neostigmine antagonism of residual vecuronium-induced block, the train-of-four ratio reached a mean of 0.85 within 15 minutes when isoflurane was discontinued at the time of neostigmine administration. If 1.25% end-tidal isoflurane was continued during the antagonism, the train-of-four ratio was only 0.7 within 15 minutes of neostigmine administration.

Volatile anesthetics can influence the depth of neuromuscular block and recovery of neuromuscular function by several possible mechanisms. These include alterations in local blood flow and interactions with Na^+ and Ca^{2+} channels.

Cholinesterases

Plasma cholinesterase is a blood glycoprotein produced in the liver; its physiologic role is not known. Blood transfusions and a purified form of the human enzyme may be given to patients homozygous for atypical plasma cholinesterase in order to shorten recovery times from succinylcholine or mivacurium. This speeds recovery of neuromuscular function by providing a means of metabolizing succinylcholine or mivacurium where none exists. The risk of transfusion-acquired infection usually makes this an undesirable alternative compared to conservative management. Human plasma cholinesterase has also been evaluated for the routine antagonism of mivacurium-induced block in patients with normal plasma cholinesterase activity. By increasing the enzymatic breakdown of the relaxant, recovery times can be shortened without exposing patients to the adverse effects of anticholinesterases, and antagonism of more profound levels of block may be possible.

Plasma cholinesterase deficiency

Approximately 5–10% of patients have decreased plasma cholinesterase activity. They may be heterozygous for an atypical plasma cholinesterase gene, a clear example of genetic control of drug metabolism (see Chapter 10), or they may have reduced plasma cholinesterase activity because of chronic disease, as in chronic renal or hepatic failure, where less enzyme is synthesized. Reduced activity can also be seen in the elderly, and in pregnancy. Rare individuals may also have up to a threefold higher than average cholinesterase activity.

Recovery from neuromuscular blockade induced with agents that are metabolized by plasma cholinesterase (succinylcholine, mivacurium) is slowed because of decreased clearance in patients with reduced plasma cholinesterase activity. When succinylcholine is administered to facilitate intubation, its effect may be prolonged by 7–10 minutes, which may pass unnoticed. However, if mivacurium is used to maintain muscle relaxation, the 5–95% recovery interval (defined by the recovery from 5 to 95% of baseline muscle strength), is increased from 10–13 minutes (normal) to 20–25 minutes. In about 5% of patients recovery from mivacurium is relatively slow; these patients can be identified by their response to an initial dose. In patients with normal plasma cholinesterase the interval between the return of the first and the third twitch in response to train-of-four stimulation is about 3 minutes. If prolonged recovery following the initial dose is observed, an anticholinesterase can be administered. Because neostigmine will inhibit plasma cholinesterase, edrophonium may a better choice for pharmacologic antagonism of mivacurium-induced block.

Rarely patients are homozygous for an atypical gene (incidence about 1 in 3000 in Caucasians). The duration of action of succinylcholine and mivacurium in these patients is markedly prolonged because the primary means of elimination is absent as a result of the absence or the reduced affinity (high K_m) of the enzyme for these substances. Elimination occurs through what would be secondary routes in genotypically normal individuals, such as the kidney and liver. In these rare individuals, mivacurium is the most potent, long-acting nondepolarizing muscle relaxant available. In patients homozygous for atypical plasma cholinesterase, a dose of 0.03 mg/kg, which is less than 50% of the ED_{95}, causes 100% neuromuscular block within 5 minutes, and the time for recovery to 25% of baseline muscle strength is 1–2 hours. Following a typical intubating dose of 0.2–0.25 mg/kg mivacurium, the duration of full paralysis is 2–4 hours, with complete spontaneous recovery in 4–8 hours. Once spontaneous recovery in these patients is demonstrable, the now long-acting neuromuscular blockade can be antagonized with neostigmine. In spite of pharmacologic antagonism, recovery from mivacurium block occurs more slowly than in patients with a normal genotype, and is similar to that following antagonism of a long-acting nondepolarizing blocker such as pancuronium. Although pharmacologic antagonism of mivacurium-induced block in such patients is recommended at the appropriate time, antagonism of succinylcholine block in these patients is not. Management of patients homozygous for the atypical gene who have received succinylcholine is conservative. These patients are sedated and mechanically ventilated until full spontaneous recovery to head lift has taken place.

Antagonism of residual neuromuscular block is possible with the administration of anticholinesterases (neostigmine, edrophonium, pryidostigmine), cyclodextrins and plasma cholinesterase.

ORG 25969

ORG 25969 (Fig. 37.9) is a novel type of antagonist for neuromuscular block induced with steroidal muscle relaxants. It is a γ-cyclodextrin that is water soluble and has a hydrophobic cavity.

Structure of synthetic γ-cyclodextrin

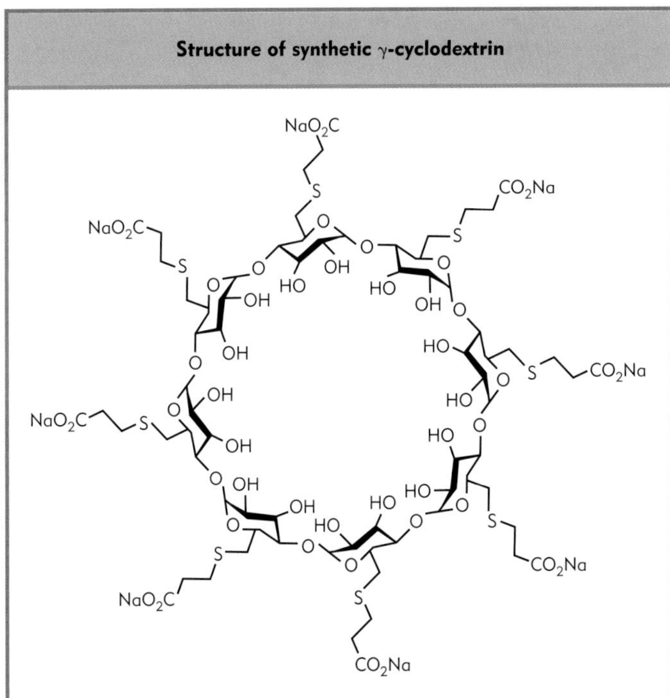

Figure 37.9 Structure of the synthetic γ-cyclodextrin (ORG 25969).

The hydrophobic cavity irreversibly encapsulates the steroidal neuromuscular blocking drugs, rendering them unable to bind with the nAChR. ORG 25969 has no effect on acetylcholinesterase. By effectively decreasing the amount of available nondepolarizing neuromuscular blocking agent, it can be administered within minutes of giving an intubating dose of a steroidal relaxant to rapidly restore neuromuscular function. The ORG 25969–relaxant complex is eliminated by the kidney. Its elimination, though, is not necessary for antagonism of neuromuscular block. In contrast to what is observed with anticholinesterases, the efficacy of ORG 25969 is not dependent on acid–base status.

MONITORING NEUROMUSCULAR FUNCTION

Activation or blockade of the nAChR depends upon the relative biophase concentrations of agonist and antagonist. Because the interaction of nondepolarizing relaxants with the acetylcholine-binding sites on the α subunit is competitive, blockade can be overcome by increasing the concentration of acetylcholine (or intensified by reducing it). This fundamental concept is important in clinical monitoring and reversal of neuromuscular blockade. A second fundamental concept is the economy of acetylcholine synthesis, storage, and release in the motor nerve terminal. The quantity of acetylcholine released per motor nerve action potential is inversely proportional to the number of action potentials reaching the nerve terminal per unit time – the stimulus frequency. For this reason, low concentrations of nondepolarizing relaxants block responses to high-frequency peripheral nerve stimulation. However, relatively high concentrations of relaxant are required to abolish responses elicited to low-frequency stimulation. The depth of blockade of evoked neuromuscular responses in the presence of nondepolarizing relaxants is directly proportional to the stimulus frequency. Consequently, stimuli of increasing frequency are able to detect increasingly subtle degrees of neuromuscular blockade. This provides a distinct advantage for evaluating the depth of nondepolarizing blockade, especially during recovery of neuromuscular function.

Peripheral nerve stimulation is employed at sites where motor nerve stimulation results in easily observed muscular contraction. The ulnar nerve/adductor pollicis response remains the most commonly observed and easily recorded response, and this is used in clinical studies of neuromuscular blockade or its antagonism. With single twitch stimulation at frequencies of 0.1 or 0.15 Hz, the evoked response is still present but markedly reduced during conditions of deep paralysis (95% blockade of the twitch). The problem with the use of this stimulus frequency in monitoring depth of block is that the responses are so infrequent that one cannot judge with any certainty the effect of the muscle relaxant. Train-of-four stimulation is a more useful method of peripheral nerve stimulation (Fig. 37.10). Four single stimuli are delivered at a frequency of 2 Hz for 2 seconds to elicit four twitch responses at 0.5-second intervals. This pattern may be repeated every 12-20 seconds. The train-of-four ratio is used to determine the degree of muscle relaxation; it is calculated by dividing the height or strength of the fourth response by that of the first response. The train-of-four ratio cannot be calculated clinically without instrumentation, but can be determined with precision by mechanomyography or electromyography. Clinically, evaluation of the number of responses present on train-of-four stimulation can be used to approximate the depth of neuromuscular blockade. The presence of only one visible twitch in response to train-of-four stimulation correlates with about 95% suppression of the single twitch response. The presence of two responses correlates with 80–85% suppression of twitch response. The presence of three twitches correlates with 75–80% neuromuscular blockade. The presence of four responses with an easily appreciable decrement in strength indicates recovery of the first twitch of the train-of-four response to at least 25% of control.

Until recently a train-of-four ratio of 0.7 was the standard for adequacy of return of neuromuscular function. The clinical utility of train-of-four monitoring is considerable. A control or baseline response is not needed and the stimulus pattern is not painful to the patient. It provides a good qualitative estimate of onset, depth, and recovery of block by simply counting the num-

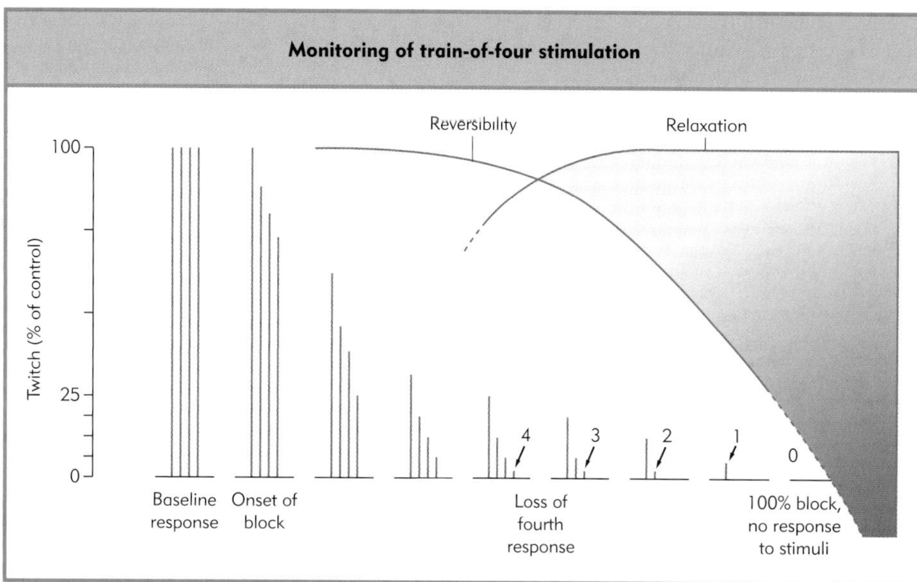

Figure 37.10 Monitoring of train-of-four stimulation. There is a 25% fade in the train-of-four with onset of neuromuscular block. With increasing depth of neuromuscular block, the fourth response is lost. At 100% block there is no response to stimulation. The greater the degree of spontaneous recovery, the quicker and more complete the pharmacologic antagonism. (See text for details of this method.)

ber of responses visible in the train and noting the presence or absence of fade in the response. In clinical use, though, when the train-of-four ratio has no apparent decrement in response, significant paralysis may still be present. Clinicians cannot reliably detect fade in the train-of-four ratio unless the ratio is < 0.4. It is not until the train-of-four ratio is greater than 0.7 that respiratory mechanical parameters such as inspiratory force and vital capacity have returned to 95% of baseline values.

Double burst stimulation (DBS) is another, perhaps better, method of stimulation to detect residual neuromuscular block during recovery of neuromuscular function. This pattern of stimulation applies two short tetanic bursts at an interval of 0.75 seconds. The most common pattern of DBS ($DBS_{3,3}$) applies stimulation at 50 Hz for three 60-ms impulses twice, separated by a 0.75-second interval, to produce two brief tetanic responses. If the second response is not as strong as the first, there is *fade*, which indicates a substantial degree of residual neuromuscular block. When the intensity of the second response is at least 60% of the first, fade is no longer detectable by either observation or palpation. This is important, as a DBS ratio of 0.6 or more is usually compatible with clinically acceptable neuromuscular function, such as the ability to lift the head for 5 seconds. In this way, DBS is more useful clinically than the train-of-four pattern of stimulation. Recently, even greater degrees of recovery have been described as being necessary to guarantee adequacy of recovery. Because the duration of action of anesthetics has become shorter, patients are more likely to be cognizant of the unpleasant effects of even subtle degrees of neuromuscular block (blurred vision, difficulty swallowing, malaise). Furthermore, patients are expected with increasing frequency to leave the hospital the same day as their surgery. Monitoring with a peripheral nerve stimulator is inadequate to guarantee recovery to a train-of-four ratio of 0.9. Studies are ongoing to determine the utility of the accelerograph at documenting the degree of residual neuromuscular block.

Depth of neuromuscular block can be monitored using electromyography, mechanomyography, and accelerography.

Maximum voluntary muscular tension development occurs at 30–50 motor nerve action potentials per second. Because motor nerve activation at rates higher than 50 Hz cannot be achieved voluntarily, external stimulation at 50 Hz is the highest rate of artificial stimulation consistent with normal physiology. Tetanic stimulation is usually applied at 50 Hz for 5 seconds during recovery from nondepolarizing block. The absence of easily visible or palpable loss of strength during tetanic contraction is an indicator of recovery of normal function. The most important aspect in monitoring of tetanic responses is the detection of fade. Considerable fade can occur within the first fraction of a second of a 5-second tetanic stimulus, following which the response is sustained at a substantially weaker level. This pattern may easily be misinterpreted as full recovery of function, when in fact considerable weakness may exist. For this reason, tetanic stimulation is seldom used.

Tetanic stimulation at 50 Hz for 5 seconds, followed 3 seconds later by a period of single twitch stimulation at a frequency of 1 Hz, is used to assess post-tetanic facilitation. This means of stimulation is useful to quantify profound depths of neuromuscular block. When twitch is elicited at 1.0 Hz following tetanus during very deep levels of neuromuscular blockade, the number of twitch responses following the tetanic stimulation can be counted. This is the post-tetanic count (PTC), and is a means of determining the depth of block when no response can be elicited with single twitch or train-of-four monitoring. Once the PTC is 2–3, the train-of-four response will begin to reappear within 20 or 30 minutes during pancuronium-induced block and within 7 to 8 minutes during vecuronium- or atracurium-induced block. When the PTC is 10–13, response to train-of-four stimulation should return promptly. The PTC is useful following the administration of the large doses of muscle relaxant given to facilitate endotracheal intubation. PTC can be used to predict when neuromuscular function has recovered to a point where either redosing is necessary or pharmacologic antagonism with anticholinesterase is possible.

Given the possibility of inadequate recovery of neuromuscular function, it is important to monitor depth of neuromuscular blockade carefully whenever muscle relaxants are administered. As monitors of neuromuscular blockade do not reliably detect subtle degrees of block, clinical tests of muscle strength should also be employed and the results of each test considered in conjunction with the others.

Key references

Ali HH, Savarese JJ. Monitoring of neuromuscular function. Anesthesiology 1976;45:216–49.

Bevan DR, Donati F, Kopman AF. Reversal of neuromuscular blockade. Anesthesiology 1992;77:785–805.

Donati F, Plaud B, Meistleman D. Vecuronium neuromuscular blockade at the adductor muscles of the larynx and at the adductor pollicis. Anesthesiology 1991;74:833–7.

Donati F. Onset of action of relaxants. Can J Anaesth. 1988;35:S52–8.

Kopman AF, Yee PS, Neuman GG. Relationship of train-of-four fade to clinical signs and symptoms of residual paralysis in awake volunteers. Anesthesiology 1997;86:765–71.

Naguib M, Flood P, McArdle JJ, Brenner HR. Advances in neurobiology of the neuromuscular junction: Implications for the anesthesiologist. Anesthesiology 2002;96:202–31.

Schiere S, Proost JH, Schuringa M, Wierda JMKH. Pharmacokinetics and pharmacokinetic-dynamic relationship between rapacuronium (ORG 9487) and its 3-desacetyl metabolite (ORG 9488). Anesth Analg. 1999;88:640–7.

Tramèr MR, Fuchs-Bader T. Omitting antagonism of neuromuscular block: Effect on postoperative nausea and vomiting and risk of residual paralysis. A systematic review. Br J Anaesth. 1999;82:379–86.

Further reading

Adam JM, Bennet DJ, Bom A et al. Cyclodextrin derived host molecules as reversal agents for the neuromuscular blocker rocuronium bromide: Synthesis and structure-activity relationships. J Med Chem. 2002;45:1806–16.

Ali HH, Utting JE, Gray TC. Quantitative assessment of residual antidepolarizing block (parts I and II). Br J Anaesth. 1971;43:473–85.

Belmont MR, Lien CA, Tjan J et al. The clinical pharmacology of GW280430A in human volunteers. Anesthesiology 2004;100: 768–73.

Bevan DR, Bevan JC, Donati F. Muscle relaxants in clinical anesthesia. Chicago, IL: Year Book Medical Publishers; 1988.

Boros EE, Bigham EC, Boswell GE et al. Bis-and mixed-tetrahydroisoquinolinium chlorofumarates: New ultra-short-acting nondepolarizing neuromuscular blockers. J Med Chem. 1999;42:206–9.

Donati F, Antzaka C, Bevan DR. Potency of pancuronium at the diaphragm and adductor pollicis muscles in humans. Anesthesiology 1986;65:1–5.

Engbaek J, Östergaard D, Viby-Mogensen J. Double burst stimulation (DBS). A new pattern of nerve stimulation to identify residual curarization. Br J Anaesth. 1989;62:274–8.

Kisor D, Schmith V, Wargin W et al. Importance of the organ-independent elimination of cisatracurium. Anesth Analg. 1996;83:1065–71.

Martyn JAJ, White DA, Gronert GA, Jaffe RS, Ward JM. Up-and-down regulation of skeletal muscle acetylcholine receptors: effects of neuromuscular blockers. Anesthesiology 1992;76:822–43.

Östergaard D, Jensen E, Jensen FS, Viby-Mogensen J. The duration of action of mivacurium-induced neuromuscular block in patients homozygous for the atypical plasma cholinesterase gene. Anesthesiology 1991;75:A774.

Viby-Mogensen J, Howardy-Hansen P, Chraemmer-Jorgensen B. Post-tetanic count (PTC): a new method of evaluating an intense nondepolarizing neuromuscular blockade. Anesthesiology 1981;55:458–61.

Yanez P, Martyn JAJ. Prolonged d-tubocurarine infusion and/or immobilization cause upregulation of acetycholine receptors and hyperkalemia to succinycholine in rats. Anesthesiology 1996;84:384–91.

White PF. Rapacuronium: Why did it fail as a replacement for succinylcholine? Br J Anaesth. 2002;88:163–5.

Chapter 38

Vascular smooth muscle

Xueqin Ding and Paul A Murray

TOPICS COVERED IN THIS CHAPTER

- **Vascular smooth muscle structure**
  - Regulation of $[Ca^{2+}]_i$
  - Mechanisms that increase $[Ca^{2+}]_i$
  - Mechanisms that decrease $[Ca^{2+}]_i$
  - Signaling pathways that regulate $[Ca^{2+}]_i$
- **Regulation of myofilament Ca^{2+} sensitivity**
  - Signaling pathways that regulate myofilament Ca^{2+} sensitivity
- **Regulation of contraction**
  - Neurohumoral regulatory mechanisms
  - Local regulatory mechanisms
- **Regulation of relaxation**
  - cAMP
  - Cyclic-GMP
  - K^+ channels

Vascular smooth muscle (VSM) tone is regulated by intracellular free Ca^{2+} concentration ($[Ca^{2+}]_i$) and myofilament Ca^{2+} sensitivity. Vasoactive stimuli can directly alter VSM tone by activating signal transduction pathways that either increase or decrease $[Ca^{2+}]_i$ and/or myofilament Ca^{2+} sensitivity. VSM tone can also be modulated by endothelium-derived relaxing and contracting factors (EDRFs and EDCFs). This chapter briefly summarizes the primary cellular mechanisms that mediate or modulate changes in VSM tone which are important in the control of blood pressure and organ perfusion.

VASCULAR SMOOTH MUSCLE STRUCTURE

VSM is comprised of a meshwork of individual smooth muscle cells. Each cell contains the major components needed to establish the membrane potential, and for contraction as well as relaxation. VSM cells are connected to each other by attachments to sheaths of connective tissue and specific junctions between muscle cells. VSM contracts more slowly, develops more force, and functions over a wider range of length than skeletal muscle. Another important property that differentiates VSM from skeletal muscle is the latch phenomenon. This refers to the fact that once VSM has developed full tension, the degree of activation can be reduced and the muscle will still maintain full tension. Furthermore, the energy consumed to maintain its full strength of contraction is less than that required for skeletal muscle. The importance of the latch mechanism is that it allows VSM to maintain prolonged tonic contractions (i.e. maintain a steady-state level of vasomotor tone) with very little use of energy.

The latch mechanism allows maintenance of a steady state of vasomotor tone with very little use of energy.

Myofilaments are cytoplasmic components of VSM. A large proportion of myofilaments are typical thin actin filaments, interspersed among which are a few myosin filaments. The arrangement of actin and myosin in VSM is not organized into distinct bands, as it is in skeletal and cardiac muscle. Instead, a network of intermediate filaments acts in place of the Z-bands (present in skeletal and cardiac muscle) to transmit the force of contraction from cell to cell. The functional equivalents of the Z-bands in VSM cells are dense bodies in the myoplasm, as well as dense areas that form bands along the sarcolemma. Intermediate filaments are interconnected via dense bodies to maintain cell shape and interconnectivity to other cells.

VSM sarcolemma contains an abundance of L-type Ca^{2+} channels, which when opened permit Ca^{2+} influx into the myoplasm. In addition to this pathway for increasing Ca^{2+} in the myoplasm, Ca^{2+} release from the sarcoplasmic reticulum (SR) is initiated via second-messenger pathways activated through sarcolemmal receptors (e.g. adrenergic receptors). As in striated muscle, contraction in VSM depends on an increase in $[Ca^{2+}]_i$. However, VSM lacks troponin, the regulatory protein that is activated by Ca^{2+} to cause skeletal muscle contraction. Instead, VSM cells contain a large amount of another regulatory protein called calmodulin (Fig. 38.1). Calmodulin is a small protein (16.7 kDa) which contains four Ca^{2+}-binding sites. When $[Ca^{2+}]_i$ increases, Ca^{2+} binds to calmodulin. The Ca^{2+}–calmodulin complex then activates myosin light-chain kinase (MLCK), an enzyme that is capable of phosphorylating myosin light chains (MLC) in the presence of ATP. MLC are 20 kDa regulatory subunits found on the myosin head. Phosphorylation of regulatory myosin light chains (rMLC) allows the binding of myosin to actin, which

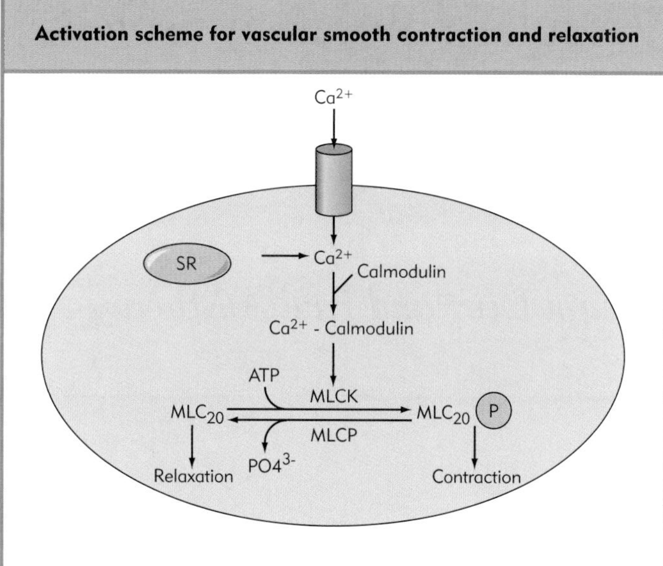

Figure 38.1 Activation scheme for vascular smooth contraction and relaxation. SR, sarcoplasmic reticulum; MLC, myosin light chain; MLCK, myosin light-chain kinase; MLCP, myosin light-chain phosphatase; ATP, adenosine triphosphate. (Adapted from Klabunde RE. http://www.cvphysiology.com/, 2004.)

increases actomyosin ATPase activity and causes VSM contraction. A fall in $[Ca^{2+}]_i$ inactivates MLCK and induces dephosphorylation of rMLC by myosin light-chain phosphatase (MLCP), thus deactivating actomyosin ATPase and causing VSM relaxation. Besides rMLC phosphorylation, the contraction of VSM is also regulated by thin filament-associated proteins such as caldesmon and calponin, which control actomyosin interactions.

Contraction of VSM is regulated by pharmacomechanical and electromechanical coupling mechanisms. Electromechanical coupling operates through changes in surface membrane potential, which results in changes in $[Ca^{2+}]_i$. A resting membrane potential of −40~−70 mV exists in VSM. More positive potentials (depolarization) open voltage-operated Ca^{2+} channels (VOCCs), causing Ca^{2+} influx to increase $[Ca^{2+}]_i$ and trigger contraction. A change to more negative membrane potentials (hyperpolarization) causes relaxation through inhibition of action potentials and a reduction of open-state probability of VOCCs.

Regulation of $[Ca^{2+}]_i$ is vital for VSM function.

Pharmacomechanical coupling operates through multiple cellular signaling mechanisms that change the degree of force without a change in membrane potential. The major mechanisms of pharmacomechanical coupling are Ca^{2+} release from the sarcoplasmic reticulum (SR) by inositol 1,4,5,-trisphosphate (IP_3), Ca^{2+} entry via receptor-operated Ca^{2+} channels (ROCCs), Ca^{2+} entry via store-operated Ca^{2+} channels (SOCCs), and changes in Ca^{2+} sensitivity of rMLC phosphorylation.

Regulation of $[Ca^{2+}]_i$

Regulation of $[Ca^{2+}]_i$ is vital for VSM function. Increases in $[Ca^{2+}]_i$ result from an influx of Ca^{2+} across the sarcolemma through plasma membrane channels, as well as Ca^{2+} release from the SR. The mechanisms for reducing $[Ca^{2+}]_i$ are the plasma membrane Ca^{2+}-ATPase (PMCA) and the Na^+/Ca^{2+} exchanger which contribute to Ca^{2+} extrusion, as well as the SR Ca^{2+}-ATPase, which provides a mechanism to sequester Ca^{2+} into the SR. In addition, several signaling pathways regulate $[Ca^{2+}]_i$.

Mechanisms that increase $[Ca^{2+}]_i$

TRANSARCOLEMMAL Ca^{2+} INFLUX

A number of transsarcolemmal Ca^{2+} influx pathways have been identified in VSM, including voltage-, receptor- and store-operated Ca^{2+} channels.

VOCCs play a central role in the regulation of vascular tone by altering membrane potential. Membrane depolarization opens VOCCs, whereas hyperpolarization closes these channels. Two types of VOCC, long-lasting (L-type) and transient (T-type) (Chapter 6), are found in VSM. L-type channels are the most numerous and the most important route of activating Ca^{2+} influx. VOCCs are modulated by several signaling pathways. Vasoconstrictors that activate the protein kinase C (PKC) pathway activate VOCCs, whereas vasodilators that stimulate the production of cAMP and activate protein kinase A (PKA) inhibit these channels. In addition, VOCCs are inhibited by increases in $[Ca^{2+}]_i$ and activation of cGMP-dependent protein kinase (PKG).

ROCCs denote a number of Ca^{2+}-permeable channels that are gated directly by binding of an agonist. ROCCs are triggered in response to activation of G protein-coupled receptors or tyrosine kinase-coupled receptors, which lead to Ca^{2+} entry into VSM (Chapter 3).

SOCC entry (also called capacitative Ca^{2+} entry, CCE) is another important route for Ca^{2+} entry. CCE is activated when intracellular Ca^{2+} stores are depleted. This depletion can be induced by different stimuli that release the stored Ca^{2+}, such as agonists, IP_3, ryanodine, the SR Ca^{2+}-ATPase inhibitors thapsigargin and cyclopiazonic acid, or incubating VSM cells in a Ca^{2+}-free medium. Multiple mechanisms for CCE are likely, but two general mechanisms have been postulated. Depletion of intracellular Ca^{2+} stores causes a conformational change in the IP_3 receptor, which could be conveyed directly to the plasma membrane by physically interacting with Ca^{2+} channels. Alternatively, signaling could occur through the action of a diffusible messenger released by the depleted intracellular Ca^{2+} store, which in turn acts on Ca^{2+} channels in the plasma membrane.

Ca^{2+} RELEASE FROM SR

The SR is the main intracellular Ca^{2+} storage site. There are two mechanisms that mediate Ca^{2+} release from the SR: Ca^{2+}-induced Ca^{2+}-release (CICR) via activation of the ryanodine receptor (RyR), and IP_3-mediated Ca^{2+} release via activation of the IP_3 receptor (IP_3R).

RyR is a large and complex molecule. It constitutes a Ca^{2+} channel in the SR with high-conductance for Ca^{2+}, and is responsible for the rapid Ca^{2+} release that activates contraction. This receptor has a central pore that permits the passage of Ca^{2+} and other divalent cations when activated. At least three isoforms of RyR have been cloned (RyR1–RyR3). RyR2 and RyR3 are the primary isoforms in smooth muscle cells. The RyR channels are modulated by numerous factors, including a number of physiological agents (e.g. Ca^{2+}, ATP, and Mg^{2+}), various cellular processes (e.g. phosphorylation, oxidation, etc.), and several pharmacological agents (e.g. ryanodine, caffeine, and ruthenium). Activation of the RyR Ca^{2+}-release channel is triggered by an increase in $[Ca^{2+}]_i$, producing the phenomenon known as Ca^{2+}-induced Ca^{2+} release (CICR). RyR may contribute to: 1) different types of intracellular Ca^{2+} wave generation, which allows activation of a cell without a requirement for bulk diffusion of Ca^{2+}; 2) agonist-induced amplification of the Ca^{2+} signal; and 3) the setting up of cytosolic Ca^{2+} oscillations, which may allow intracellular Ca^{2+} signals to be transmitted while reducing the risk of cell damage due to persistently high cytosolic Ca^{2+} levels.

Stimulation by a variety of agonists (norepinephrine, acetylcholine, serotonin) which results in binding to G protein-coupled receptors causes the activation of the enzyme phospholipase C (PLC), which induces the hydrolysis of phosphatidyl inositol bisphosphate (PIP_2) that leads to the formation of 1,2-diacylglycerol (DAG) and IP_3. IP_3 activates Ca^{2+} release via a second class of SR Ca^{2+} release channel, known as IP_3 receptors. IP_3R is a protein that consists of a tetrameric polypeptide with a molecular mass ~224 kDa. This receptor has binding domains for IP_3 and Ca^{2+}, and a central aqueous channel that permits the passage of Ca^{2+} from the lumen of the SR towards the cytosol. Following activation, IP_3R is capable of releasing large quantities of Ca^{2+} into the cytosol. This release is biphasic, with a fast release component followed by a slow release component. The interaction of IP_3 with its receptor is regulated by $[Ca^{2+}]_i$. A rise in $[Ca^{2+}]_i$ from basal levels to ~300 nM increases the efficacy of IP_3 to activate channel opening, but higher $[Ca^{2+}]_i$ reduces the effectiveness of IP_3. Thus, high levels of $[Ca^{2+}]_i$ provide negative feedback for the release of more Ca^{2+}. IP_3R is phosphorylated by various protein kinases, such as PKA and PKG, which inhibit IP_3-mediated Ca^{2+} release.

Mechanisms that decrease $[Ca^{2+}]_i$

PMCA

A major mechanism for Ca^{2+} extrusion is the PMCA, which produces Ca^{2+} efflux in exchange for $2H^+$ influx using the energy from ATP. PMCA is more abundant in VSM cells of large arteries than of large veins, and scarce or absent in smaller blood vessels. PMCA is activated by calmodulin, which increases its affinity for Ca^{2+} and the velocity of Ca^{2+} transport. PMCA is regulated by protein kinases. PKA, PKG, Ca^{2+}–calmodulin-dependent protein kinase II (CaMKII), and PKC can phosphorylate PMCA, which enhances the affinity of Ca^{2+} and the maximum Ca^{2+} uptake activity of PMCA. In addition, the activity of PMCA is modulated by some hormones and IP_3. Thyroid hormone and vitamin D can stimulate the PMCA pump, whereas IP_3 has the opposite effect.

Na^+/Ca^{2+} EXCHANGER

The Na^+/Ca^{2+} exchanger, an ion transport protein, extrudes Ca^{2+} in parallel with the PMCA pump. Ca^{2+} extrusion by this mechanism utilizes energy from the electrochemical gradient for Na^+, and transports three Na^+ into the cell while removing one Ca^{2+}. Na^+/Ca^{2+} exchanger activity is regulated by interconversions between active state and inactive state. High concentrations of cytosolic Na^+ or the absence of cytosolic Ca^{2+} promote the formation of the inactive state, whereas PIP_2 and cytosolic Ca^{2+} counteract the inactivation process.

SR Ca^{2+} ATPASE

Reuptake of Ca^{2+} into the SR is accomplished by a 105 kDa protein with high affinity for Ca^{2+}, the SR Ca^{2+}-ATPase, which is located in the SR membrane. It is also known as the SERCA pump. The SERCA pump utilizes the energy from ATP hydrolysis to translocate Ca^{2+} from the cytoplasm to the lumen of the SR. Within the SR lumen, Ca^{2+} is bound by several small hydrophilic proteins, including calreticulin and calsequestrin. These proteins can bind large amounts of Ca^{2+}. Ca^{2+} binding to these proteins causes a drop in free Ca^{2+} concentration in the SR lumen, which reduces the energy required to pump Ca^{2+} from the cytosol up its concentration gradient into the SR. SERCA pumps are regulated by phospholamban. Phospholamban is a small transmembrane protein of the SR. Regulation of SERCA occurs through an inhibitory association between phospholamban and the Ca^{2+}-ATPase, which can be relieved by phosphorylation via PKA or PKC. SR Ca^{2+}-ATPase operates in conjunction with the PMCA, and also with the Na^+/Ca^{2+} exchange system of the plasmalemma, to maintain low levels of $[Ca^{2+}]_i$.

Signaling pathways that regulate $[Ca^{2+}]_i$

There are several signal transduction mechanisms that regulate $[Ca^{2+}]_i$, and therefore the contractile state of VSM. Three different mechanisms will be briefly described: the phosphatidylinositol pathway, the G protein-coupled pathway (cAMP), and the nitric oxide–cGMP pathway (Fig. 38.2).

As noted above, agonists (such as norepinephrine, angiotensin II, and endothelin-I) bind to G protein-coupled receptors, which activate PLC. PLC induces the hydrolysis of PIP_2, which leads to the formation of IP_3 and DAG. IP_3 then stimulates the SR to release Ca^{2+}. DAG activates PKC, which increases Ca^{2+} influx by phosphorylating VOCCs.

The G protein-coupled pathway either stimulates (via G_s protein) or inhibits (via G_i protein) adenylyl cyclase (AC), which catalyzes the formation of cAMP. cAMP inhibits Ca^{2+} mobilization, including inhibition of IP_3 formation via inhibition of PLC or PLC-G-protein–receptor coupling, inhibition of Ca^{2+} release from the SR, stimulation of Ca^{2+} uptake and or/extrusion, and inhibition of Ca^{2+} entry.

A third mechanism that is very important in regulating VSM tone is the nitric oxide (NO)–cGMP system. Briefly, increases in NO activate guanylyl cyclase, causing increased formation of cGMP. cGMP activates PKG and decreases $[Ca^{2+}]_i$ via several mechanisms, including 1) activation of Ca^{2+} uptake by intracellular stores via phosphorylation of phospholamban and activation of the SR Ca^{2+}-ATPase; 2) increased Ca^{2+} efflux as a result of stimulation of the PMCA and Na^+/Ca^{2+} exchanger; 3) inhibition of Ca^{2+} release from intracellular stores via phosphorylation of the SR IP_3R by PKG; 4) membrane hyperpolarization induced by activation of K^+ channels; 5) inhibition of Ca^{2+} currents as a result of dephosphorylation of VOCCs.

REGULATION OF MYOFILAMENT Ca^{2+} SENSITIVITY

It is well established that the contractile state of VSM can be altered without a concomitant change in $[Ca^{2+}]_i$. This is achieved via a change in myofilament Ca^{2+} sensitivity. Several mechanisms have been proposed to mediate changes in myofilament Ca^{2+} sensitivity (Fig. 38.3), including 1) Ca^{2+}-dependent decreases in sensitivity (desensitization) induced by MLCK; 2) agonist-dependent increases in sensitivity (sensitization) via inhibition of MLCP; and 3) rMLC phosphorylation-independent

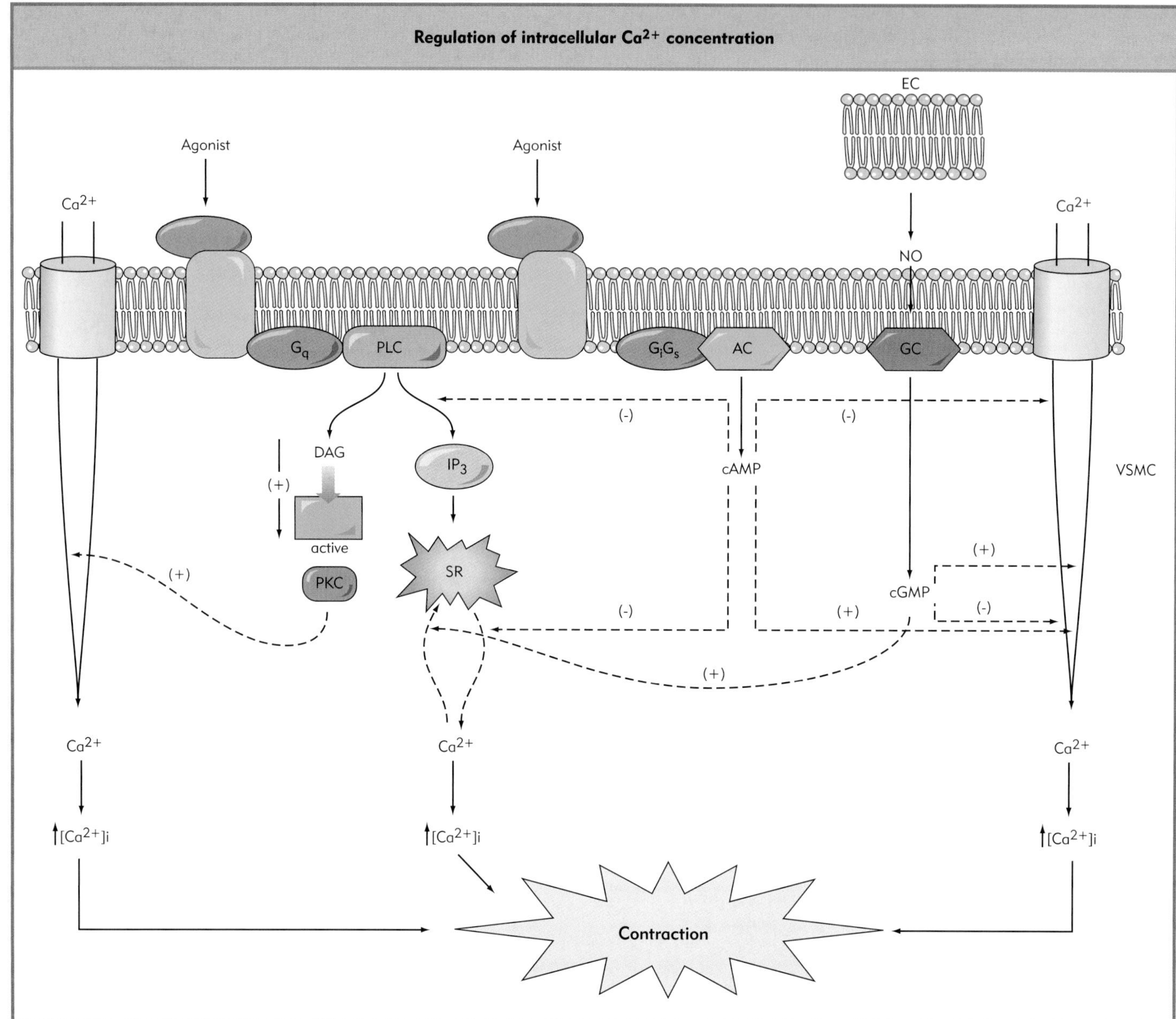

Figure 38.2 Regulation of intracellular Ca^{2+} concentration. EC, endothelial cells; VSMC, vascular smooth muscle cell; DAG, 1,2-diacylglycerol; PKC, protein kinase C; IP_3, inositol 1,4,5,-trisphosphate; PLC, phospholipase C; SR, sarcoplasmic reticulum; AC, adenylyl cyclase; NO, nitric oxide; GC, guanylyl cyclase; (+), stimulate; (–), inhibit; cGMP, 3′,5′-cyclic guanosine monophosphate; cAMP, 3′,5′-cyclic adenosine monophosphate; GPCR, G protein-coupled receptor.

regulatory mechanisms involving thin filament-associated proteins (caldesmon, calponin) and Na^+/H^+ exchanger. In addition, several signaling pathways may regulate myofilament Ca^{2+} sensitivity.

The contractile state of VSM can be altered without a concomitant change in $[Ca^{2+}]_i$ via a change in myofilament Ca^{2+} sensitivity.

MLCK

Desensitization of VSM occurs mainly as a consequence of phosphorylation of MLCK. Several kinases, including PKA, PKC, and CaMK II, are able to phosphorylate MLCK at a specific serine residue located in the region of the calmodulin-binding domain of MLCK. Phosphorylation of MLCK by CaMK II reduces its affinity for the Ca^{2+}–CaM complex, which results in a decrease in Ca^{2+} sensitivity of rMLC phosphorylation. This acts as a negative feedback mechanism to inhibit high levels of rMLC phosphorylation. PKA phosphorylates MLCK at two sites, A and B. Phosphorylation at site A, but not at site B, decreases the affinity of MLCK for the Ca^{2+}–calmodulin complex, and this is responsible for desensitization.

MLCP

Inhibition of MLCP is the main mechanism for Ca^{2+} sensitization. MLCP inhibition increases rMLC phosphorylation and hence the force developed by VSM at a constant $[Ca^{2+}]_i$. MLCP is a holoenzyme composed of three subunits: a 38 kDa catalytic

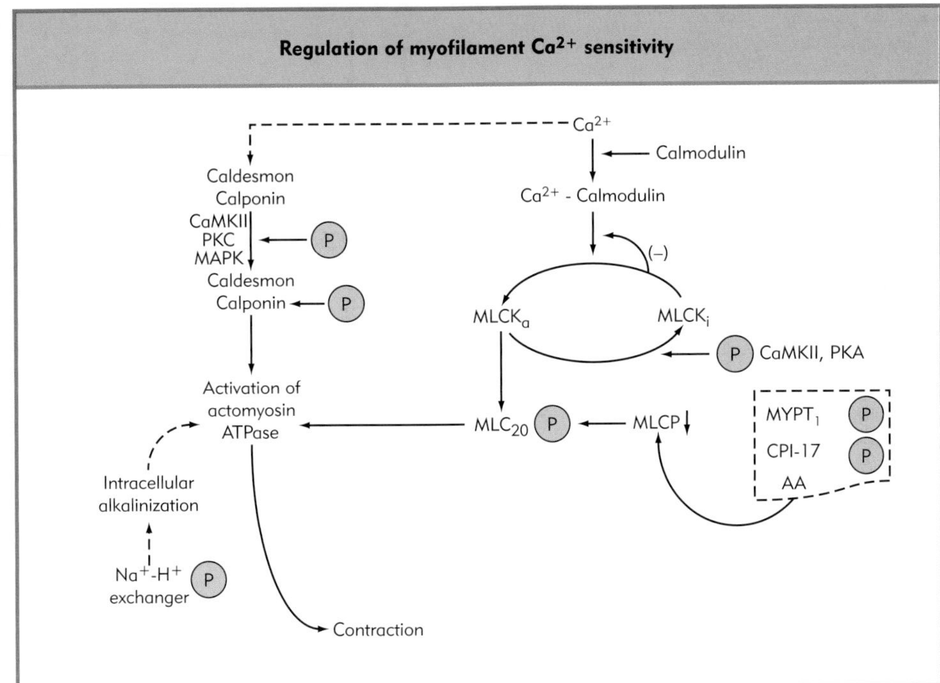

Figure 38.3 Regulation of myofilament Ca^{2+} sensitivity. MLCK, myosin light-chain kinase; MLCP, myosin light-chain phosphatase; a, active; i, inactive; AA, arachidonic acid; Ⓟ, phosphorylation; PKA, protein kinase A; CaMKII, Ca^{2+} calmodulin-dependent protein kinase II; MAPK, mitogen-activated protein kinase; PKC, protein kinase C.

subunit of type 1 protein phosphatase (PP1c), a large 110–130 kDa regulatory subunit (MYPT1), and a small 20 kDa subunit of unknown function. MYPT1 is the key subunit involved in binding to and activation of PP1c and in targeting myosin. Mechanisms that inhibit MLCP are: 1) phosphorylation of MYPT1; 2) inhibition by an endogenous, smooth muscle-specific phosphopeptide, CPI-17; and 3) dissociation of the holoenzyme by arachidonic acid.

THIN FILAMENT-ASSOCIATED PROTEINS

Smooth muscle thin filaments contain two specific regulatory proteins, caldesmon and calponin, both of which inhibit actomyosin ATPase activity. This effect is reversed by phosphorylation of these proteins.

Caldesmon is a typical actin-binding protein located on actin filaments. It contains sites of interaction with other contractile proteins distributed along the elongated caldesmon molecule. The functionally important actin- and calmodulin-binding sites are located in the C-terminal domain of caldesmon that is responsible for inhibition of myosin ATPase activation by actin. Caldesmon blocks the strong myosin-binding sites on actin, and thus prevents the actin filament from sliding over myosin, which is relieved by phosphorylation of caldesmon. Phosphorylation of caldesmon is mediated primarily by mitogen-activated protein kinase (MAPK) and PKC, which decreases the interaction of caldesmon with actin and by this means decreases the inhibitory action of caldesmon on the actomyosin ATPase activity.

Calponin is another actin- and calmodulin-binding protein that is relatively specific for VSM. Calponin is located on actin filaments and inhibits actomyosin ATPase and actin filament motility. It can be phosphorylated by PKC and CaMKII. This phosphorylation greatly decreases the affinity of calponin for actin, which reduces its ability to inhibit actomyosin ATPase. Therefore, phosphorylation of calponin has been considered as a mechanism of Ca^{2+} sensitization.

Na^+-H^+ EXCHANGER

Myofilament Ca^{2+} sensitivity can be altered by changes in intracellular pH. Intracellular alkalinization increases myofilament Ca^{2+} sensitivity by changing the pH dependence of the myofibrillar actomyosin ATPase activity. The Na^+/H^+ exchanger is an electroneutral transporter that mediates the 1:1 exchange of extracellular sodium for intracellular hydrogen ion. It is a ~110 kDa glycoprotein consisting of 10–12 putative transmembrane spanning regions followed by a hydrophilic cytoplasmic domain. In the basal state, the Na^+/H^+ exchanger is phosphorylated but not activated. Vasoconstrictors such as angiotensin II stimulate phosphorylation of the exchanger through PKC- and Ca^{2+}-dependent pathways, which results in intracellular alkalosis and an increase in myofilament Ca^{2+} sensitivity.

Signaling pathways that regulate myofilament Ca^{2+} sensitivity (Fig. 38.4)

(rho)-KINASE PATHWAY

The small GTPase (rho) is responsible for Ca^{2+} sensitization induced by agonist stimulation, and is thought to act by inhibiting MLCP. ρ-associated kinase ((rho)-kinase) plays a crucial role in Ca^{2+} sensitization. Agonists activate (rho) via G protein-coupled receptors. Activated (rho) interacts with (rho)-kinase, leading to its activation. The activated (rho)-kinase inhibits MLCP via phosphorylation of MYPT1 or CPI-17. Concomitantly, (rho)-kinase phosphorylates rMLC directly at the same site that is phosphorylated by MLCK. Thus, (rho)-kinase can increase myofilament Ca^{2+} sensitivity and contraction by two mechanisms (i.e. inhibition of MLCP and direct MLC phosphorylation).

PKC PATHWAY

Activation of PKC causes Ca^{2+} sensitization of rMLC phosphorylation. At least four PKC-mediated mechanisms have been

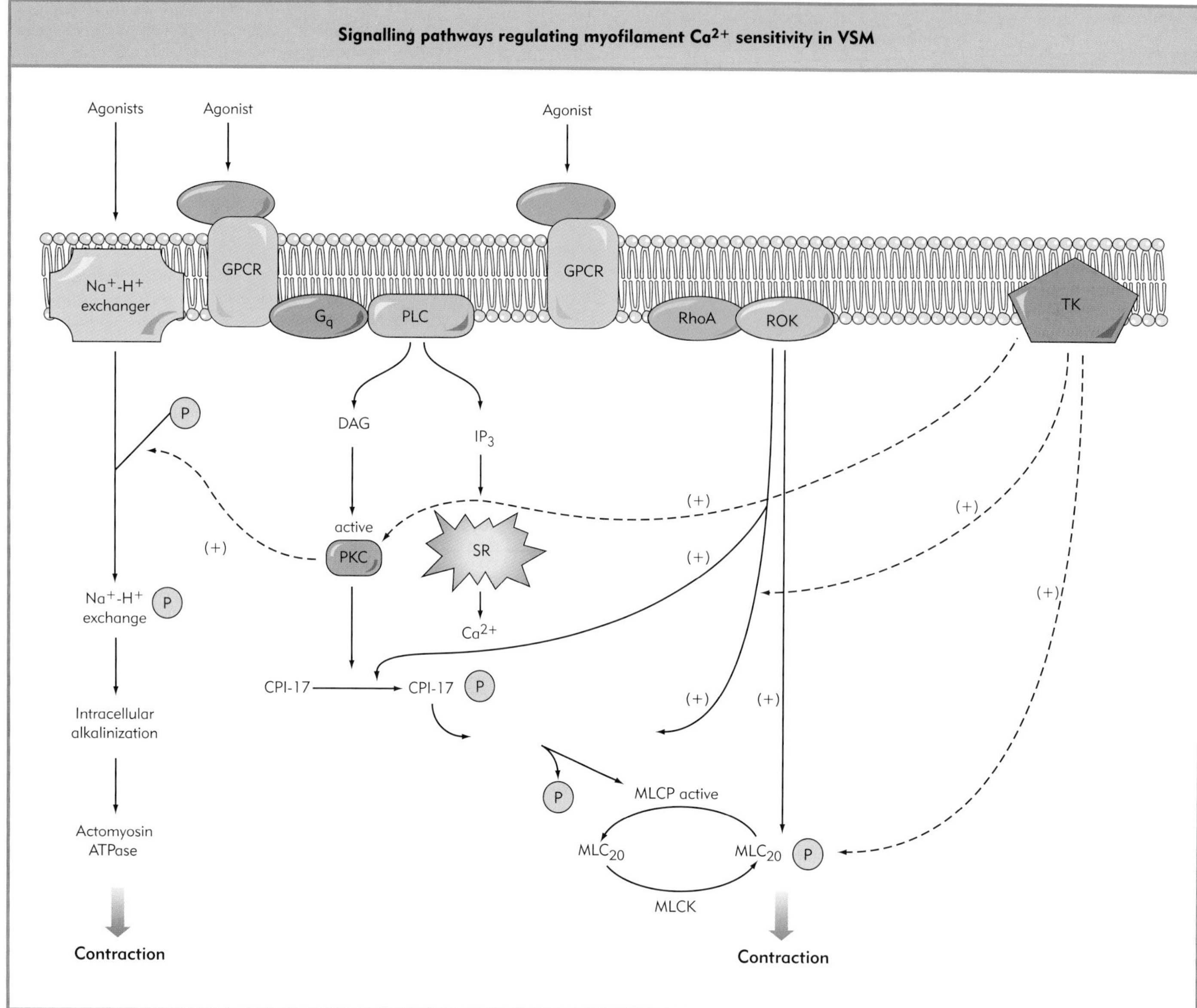

Figure 38.4 Signaling pathways regulating myofilament Ca^{2+} sensitivity in VSM. ROK, Rho-kinase; CPI-17, PKC-potentiated inhibitor protein of 17 kDa; MLCK, myosin light-chain kinase; DAG, diacylglycerol; PKC, protein kinase C; SR, sarcoplasmic reticulum; IP_3, inositol 1,4,5-trisphosphate; PLC, phospholipase C; Ⓟ phosphorylation; GPCR, G protein-coupled receptor; TK, tyrosine kinase; MLCP, myosin light-chain phosphate. Dash line is used to make figure clearer.

proposed: 1) PKC-dependent phosphorylation of the thin-filament accessory proteins, caldesmon and calponin; 2) PKC-dependent phosphorylation of CPI-17, which inhibits MLCP; 3) PKC-dependent phosphorylation of the contractile protein, MLC; 4) PKC-dependent activation of the Na^+/H^+ exchanger, resulting in intracellular alkalinization.

TYROSINE KINASE PATHWAY

Tyrosine kinases and phosphatases are present in large amounts in VSM and influence a number of processes crucial to contraction, including ion channel gating, Ca^{2+} homeostasis, and Ca^{2+} sensitization of the contractile process by phosphorylation of rMLC. Some vasoconstrictors (e.g. phenylephrine) are known to activate tyrosine kinases, which induces rMLC phosphorylation and contraction. In addition, tyrosine kinases are involved in the activation process of rho and PKC. Therefore, crosstalk among these different kinase pathways may be involved in the Ca^{2+} sensitization of VSM.

REGULATION OF CONTRACTION

The contractile state of the VSM is influenced by local (metabolic, autoregulatory, and endothelial), neural (autonomic nervous system), and humoral (angiotensin, epinephrine, and vasopressin) regulatory mechanisms.

Neurohumoral regulatory mechanisms

NOREPINEPHRINE AND EPINEPHRINE

In the periphery, catecholamines such as norepinephrine and epinephrine are stored and released from two primary sites. Postganglionic adrenergic neurons are the major source of norepinephrine, whereas epinephrine is released into the bloodstream mainly from the adrenal medulla. Norepinephrine and epinephrine produce their physiologic effects by activating α- and β-adrenoceptors on target tissues. α- and β-adrenoceptors are found on adrenergic nerve endings, VSM, and endothelial cells. Norepinephrine acts on postjunctional α_1-adrenergic receptors to cause VSM contraction. It can also activate α_2-adrenergic receptors on endothelial cells, which results in the release of NO and vasodilation. Epinephrine has similar effects on α-adrenergic receptors, although its most important effect is on β-adrenergic receptors that mediate relaxation. The net effect of these hormones depends on the relative distribution of α- and β-adrenergic receptors in the specific vascular bed.

ACETYLCHOLINE

Parasympathetic nerves are the major source of acetylcholine, which activates muscarinic cholinergic receptors. Muscarinic receptors are found on numerous end organs, including adrenergic nerve endings, VSM, and endothelial cells. Acetylcholine-induced activation of muscarinic receptors on VSM results in vasoconstriction. This response is more pronounced in veins than arteries. On the other hand, acetylcholine can also activate muscarinic receptors on endothelial cells, causing release of endothelium-derived relaxing factors (EDRF), which diffuse to VSM to cause vasorelaxation. This endothelium-dependent effect of acetylcholine is more prominent in arterial than in venous smooth muscle.

VASOPRESSIN

Vasopressin is formed in the hypothalamus and secreted by the posterior pituitary gland (neurohypophysis). Vasopressin exerts its effects by activating two subtypes of receptors: V_1-vasopressin receptors located in the blood vessel wall and V_2-vasopressin receptors located in the renal tubules and some vascular beds (e.g. pulmonary). Activation of V_1 receptors results in vasoconstriction, whereas V_2 receptor activation results in vasodilatation. Besides its direct VSM effects, vasopressin also interacts with pre- and postjunctional adrenergic receptors to facilitate the effects of adrenergic agonists.

OTHER VASOCONSTRICTORS

Angiotensin II has a powerful vasoconstrictor effect on VSM. Thromboxane and serotonin are constrictor paracrine agonists that are released by activated platelets. These vasoconstrictors bind to VSM receptors and activate PLC, which results in the production of second messengers that cause vasoconstriction by increasing $[Ca^{2+}]_i$ and/or myofilament Ca^{2+} sensitivity.

Local regulatory mechanisms

ENDOTHELIAL REGULATION (FIG. 38.5)

The vascular endothelium constitutes a single layer of thin cells that lines the intimal surface of blood vessels. Endothelial cells play an important role in the local regulation of VSM tone by producing vasodilator and vasoconstrictor substances termed

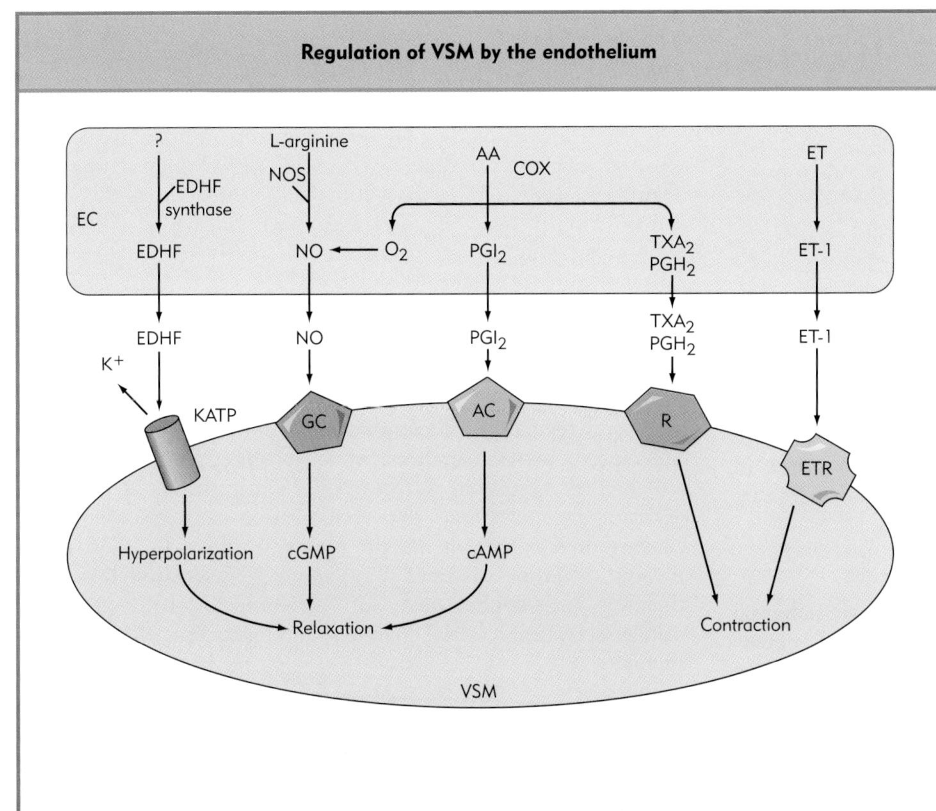

Figure 38.5 Regulation of VSM by the endothelium. AA, arachidonic acid; COX, cyclo-oxygenase; EDHF, endothelium-derived hyperpolarizing factor; ET, endothelin-1; O_2^-, superoxide anions; PGI_2, prostacyclin; NO, nitric oxide; NOS, NO synthase; TXA_2, thromboxane A_2; PGH_2, prostaglandin H_2; K^+, potassium ions; K_{ATP}, ATP-dependent potassium channel; GC, guanylyl cyclase; AC, adenylyl cyclase; R, YXA_2, PGH_2 receptors; cGMP, 3′,5′-cyclic guanosine monophosphate; cAMP, cyclic adenosine monophosphate; VSM, vascular smooth muscle cell; EC, endothelial cell; ETR, endothelin receptor.

endothelium-derived relaxing factor (EDRF) and endothelium-derived contracting factor (EDCF). Under normal circumstances the release of EDRFs appears to predominate. However, in certain blood vessels (peripheral veins and large cerebral arteries) the normal endothelium has a propensity to release EDCFs.

The major EDRFs are nitric oxide (NO), prostacyclin, and endothelium-derived hyperpolarizing factor (EDHF). NO is synthesized by oxidation of L-arginine by NO synthase, which is a Ca^{2+}–calmodulin-dependent enzyme. An increase in cytosolic Ca^{2+} is the stimulus for enhanced formation and release of NO. NO is released by endothelial cells in response to agonists such as acetylcholine, bradykinin, serotonin, substance P, thrombin, and vasoactive intestinal peptide (VIP). NO release by endothelial cells causes vasodilatation in adjacent VSM cells by stimulating soluble guanylyl cyclase, and thereby elevating the intracellular concentration of cGMP.

Prostacyclin (PGI_2) is a major product of arachidonic acid metabolism via the cyclo-oxygenase pathway. It inhibits platelet adhesion to the vascular endothelium and mediates relaxation through activation of adenylyl cyclase, which increases cAMP. As with NO, PGI_2 synthesis by endothelial cells is dependent on an increase in cytosolic Ca^{2+} triggered by endogenous mediators (bradykinin, thrombin, serotonin, and adenine nucleotides). Some drugs (Ca^{2+} channel antagonists, captopril, dipyridamole, nitrates, and streptokinase) can also stimulate its production.

EDHF is defined as the NO- and PGI_2-independent factor that exerts endothelium-dependent hyperpolarization of VSM cells. It is synthesized by a putative EDHF synthase and mediates its cellular effects by activating ATP-sensitive K^+ channels (K^+_{ATP}) in VSM to cause hyperpolarization and vasodilation.

Two well-described EDCFs are endothelin and vasoconstrictor prostaglandins. These contracting factors induce VSM contraction by increasing $[Ca^{2+}]_i$ and myofilament Ca^{2+} sensitivity via the activation of protein kinases such as PKC.

Endothelin exists as a family of three isoforms (ET-1, ET-2, and ET-3). ET-1 is the only isoform synthesized by endothelial cells. ET-1 acts through smooth muscle ET(A) and ET(B) receptors, which mainly mediate vasoconstriction. There are also endothelial ET(B) receptors, which oppose ET(A)- and ET(B)-mediated vasoconstriction by stimulating NO formation. Production of endothelin is stimulated by vasopressor hormones, platelet-derived factors, coagulation products, and cytokines, whereas endothelium-derived NO, prostacyclin, and a smooth muscle cell-derived inhibitory factor reduce endothelin production.

The endothelial cyclo-oxygenase pathway can produce thromboxane A_2, prostaglandin H_2, and superoxide anions. They are elicited by physical and chemical stimuli (i.e. hypoxia, pressure, and stretch), local factors, and circulating hormones. These mediators act directly on VSM to cause contraction. In addition, superoxide anions bind to NO, which inactivates its vasodilator effect.

METABOLIC REGULATION

Metabolites (e.g. adenosine, K^+) released from parenchymal cells act locally to relax VSM. The higher the rate of metabolism, the greater the rate of formation and release of these vasodilator substances. This provides a mechanism to match O_2 supply to the O_2 demand of the tissue. Changes in O_2 tension can also evoke changes in the contractile state of VSM. Increases in O_2 tension elicit contraction and decreases in O_2 tension elicit relaxation. In addition, increased metabolism increases CO_2 and body temperature, and decreases pH, which further enhances relaxation of VSM.

AUTOREGULATION

Increases in perfusion pressure directly stretch VSM, and the muscle contracts in response to the stretch. This is called myogenic autoregulation. Without autoregulation, the increased perfusion pressure would significantly increase blood flow. Thus, autoregulation ensures a constant blood flow in the face of changes in perfusion pressure. The opposite effect occurs when perfusion pressure decreases.

REGULATION OF RELAXATION

Direct relaxation of VSM may occur by one or more of the following mechanisms: 1) increased cytoplasmic concentration of cAMP; 2) increased formation of cGMP; and 3) hyperpolarization via activation of K^+ channels.

cAMP

Stimulation of plasma membrane receptors (e.g. β-adrenergic receptors) promotes the conversion of intracellular ATP to cAMP by the enzyme adenylyl cyclase. Adenylyl cyclase is coupled to plasma membrane receptors by a guanine nucleotide-binding protein. Two mechanisms have been suggested whereby cAMP can relax VSM: 1) decreasing $[Ca^{2+}]_i$ by enhancing Ca^{2+} pump activity and preventing the opening of VOCCs; and 2) decreasing the rate of myosin phosphorylation by phosphorylating MLCK via PKA. This latter effect results in a decrease in myofilament Ca^{2+} sensitivity.

Cyclic-GMP

cGMP is formed by the action of guanylyl cyclase and its effects are mediated by PKG. Relaxation is induced by the following mechanisms: 1) reduction of myofilament Ca^{2+} sensitivity, possibly via increased rMLC dephosphorylation; and 2) decrease in $[Ca^{2+}]_i$ by activating Ca^{2+} uptake, increasing Ca^{2+} efflux, inhibiting Ca^{2+} release, and inducing membrane hyperpolarization.

K^+ channels

K^+ channels are the dominant ion conductance pathways in VSM. Their activity importantly contributes to the establishment and regulation of membrane potential and vascular tone. The electrochemical gradient for K^+ ions is such that opening of K^+ channels results in diffusion of this cation out of the cells, resulting in membrane hyperpolarization and vasorelaxation. Closure of K^+ channels has the opposite effect. In VSM, there are four different classes of K^+ channel: ATP-sensitive K^+ (K_{ATP}) channels, large-conductance Ca^{2+}-activated K^+ (BK_{ca}) channels, voltage-activated K^+ (K_v) channels, and inward rectifier K^+ (K_{IR}) channels.

K_{ATP} CHANNELS

K^+_{ATP} channels play an important role in the response of VSM to a variety of pharmacological and endogenous vasodilators. K_{ATP}

channels consist of four inwardly rectifying potassium channel subunits (K_{IR}). Each K_{IR} subunit is associated with a larger regulatory sulfonylurea receptor (SUR). A hallmark and defining feature of K_{ATP} channels is that they are inhibited by micromolar concentrations of intracellular ATP. Nucleotide diphosphates, in the presence of Mg^{2+}, activate K_{ATP} channels. The inhibitory effect of ATP is due to binding of ATP to the K_{IR} subunit, whereas channel activation by Mg^{2+} dinucleotides occurs via interaction with the SUR. Another key distinguishing feature of K_{ATP} channels is the inhibition of channel activity by sulfonylurea agents (glibenclamide, tolbutamide). Activation of K_{ATP} channels causes membrane hyperpolarization, reducing Ca^{2+} influx through voltage-dependent Ca^{2+} channels and resulting in vasorelaxation. K_{ATP} channels mediate a portion of the vasodilator effects of many endogenous factors, such as calcitonin gene-related peptide, adenosine, prostacyclin, and NO. In addition, cAMP- and cGMP-mediated vasodilator pathways also involve activation of K_{ATP} channels.

OTHER K^+ CHANNELS

K_{IR} channels are activated by slight changes in extracellular K^+ and contribute to resting membrane potential. K_v channels are important regulators of smooth muscle membrane potential in response to depolarizing stimuli. BK_{ca} channels play a central role in the regulation of vascular tone owing to focal increases in subsarcolemmal Ca^{2+} due to Ca^{2+} release via ryanodine receptors in the SR.

SUMMARY

Contraction and relaxation of VSM is mediated by changes in $[Ca^{2+}]_i$ and/or myofilament Ca^{2+} sensitivity. Changes in $[Ca^{2+}]_i$ are achieved via transsarcolemmal Ca^{2+} influx (VOCCs, ROCCs, SOCCs) or efflux (PMCA, Na^+/Ca^{2+} exchange), or by SR Ca^{2+} release (RyR, IP_3R) and reuptake (SERCA pump). Ca^{2+}-dependent decreases in myofilament Ca^{2+} sensitivity are induced by phosphorylation of MLCK, whereas increases in sensitivity are mediated by inhibition of MLCP and phosphorylation of thin filament-associated proteins (caldesmon, calponin). Multiple signaling pathways (e.g. PKC, PKA, PKG, CaMKII, rho-kinase, tyrosine kinase) are involved in regulating the contractile state of VSM. In addition, neural, humoral, and local factors mediate or modulate changes in VSM tone.

Further reading

Damron DS, Kanaya N, Homma Y, Kim SO, Murray PA. Role of PKC, tyrosine kinases, and Rho kinase in alpha-adrenoreceptor-mediated PASM contraction. Am J Physiol Lung Cell Mol Physiol. 2002;283:L1051–64.

Doi S, Damron DS, Horibe M, Murray PA. Capacitative Ca^{2+} entry and tyrosine kinase activation in canine pulmonary arterial smooth muscle cells. Am J Physiol Lung Cell Mol Physiol. 2000;278:L118–30.

Doi S, Damron DS, Ogawa K, Tanaka S, Horibe M, Murray PA. K^+ channel inhibition, calcium signaling, and vasomotor tone in canine pulmonary artery smooth muscle. Am J Physiol Lung Cell Mol Physiol. 2000;279:L242–51.

O'Rourke ST, Vanhoutte PM. Vascular pharmacology. In: Loscalzo JL, Creager MA, Dzau VJ, eds. Vascular medicine: a textbook of vascular biology and diseases, 2nd edn. Boston: Little, Brown; 1996:117–41.

Pfitzer G. Regulation of myosin phosphorylation in smooth muscle. J Appl Physiol. 2001;91:497–503.

Sanders KM. Mechanisms of calcium handling in smooth muscles. J Appl Physiol. 2001;91:1438–49.

Somlyo AP, Somlyo AV. Signal transduction by G-proteins, Rho-kinase and protein phosphatase to smooth muscle and non-muscle myosin II. J Physiol. 2000;522:177–85.

SECTION 4

Cardiovascular system

Chapter 39

Cardiac physiology

Daniel Nyhan and Thomas JJ Blanck

CARDIAC STRUCTURE

Cardiac muscle is a unique type of striated muscle and resembles skeletal muscle in many of its basic features (Chapter 35). Myofibrils, which make up about half the volume of a cardiac myocyte, run parallel to the long axis of the cell. Myofibrils consist of ordered longitudinal arrays of interdigitating thick and thin filaments. The sarcomere is the repeating contractile unit found in each myocyte. The arrangement of the filaments gives rise to the lines and bands that can be seen on microscopy. Thick filaments are found in the center of the sarcomere and are made up of intertwined myosin molecules with myosin heads extending out from the longitudinal axis in opposite directions (Fig. 39.1). Thin filaments are made up of two chains of filamentous polymer actin intertwined to form a helical structure, and are attached to the Z line in the sarcomere. The I band consists of thin filaments surrounding the Z line; the A band is made up of the area of overlap of the thick filaments with the thin filaments. Titin, a huge cytoskeletal protein, ~3–4 MDa, is responsible for a significant portion of the passive tension generated by the cardiac myocyte. It is anchored at its N-terminal region to the Z line and actin (Fig. 39.2a). Titin molecules extend half the length of the sarcomere from the Z line through the I band and the A band to the M line, where its C terminus interacts with myosin-binding protein C.

Myocytes are joined together by specialized junctions known as intercalated disks. Actin filaments from adjacent cells insert into intercalated disks, as they do into Z lines (Fig. 39.1).

T-tubules, which are invaginations of the plasma membrane, are usually oriented transversely to the longitudinal axis of the myocyte; they allow closer access of the plasma membrane and extracellular fluid to the myocyte interior. The junctional sarcoplasmic reticulum (SR), which contains Ca^{2+}-release channels (CRC), is found in close apposition to the T-tubules. Voltage-gated Ca^{2+} channels (VGCC) are found within the T-tubular membrane. Upon depolarization, they open and allow extracellular Ca^{2+} to enter. The Ca^{2+} interacts with the CRC, resulting in Ca^{2+}-induced release of large amounts of Ca^{2+} from sarcoplasmic reticulum (SR) stores, which triggers contraction by a complex interaction with troponin and tropomyosin (Fig 39.2b–d). The tropomyosin molecule, a linear regulatory protein of 70 kDa, sits in the groove of the actin helix extended over seven actin monomers. The troponin complex is bound to the thin filament at the end of each tropomyosin and serves to transmit the intracellular Ca^{2+} signal to actin and myosin. The troponin complex consists of three proteins: troponin C, which binds two molecules of Ca^{2+} during each heartbeat, is complexed with troponin I, which inhibits the interaction of actin and myosin, and troponin T, which binds to tropomyosin. Binding of Ca^{2+} leads to a conformational change in troponin, resulting in repositioning of tropomyosin deeper into the groove between actin strands, and disinhibition of the actin–myosin interaction. The removal of tropomyosin from its inhibitory site allows the myosin head to bind to actin, resulting in the release of ADP, the binding and hydrolysis of ATP, and the utilization of ATP hydrolysis energy to allow the cycling of the myosin cross-bridge to another actin, and hence the shortening of the myocyte.

CARDIAC FUNCTION

The overall function of the cardiovascular system is to deliver oxygen and metabolic substrates to the tissues and to remove the products of metabolism. This requires the normal and integrated function of the systemic arterial and venous circulations, right heart, pulmonary circulation, and left heart. Most abnormalities of cardiac function arise in the left ventricle (LV). However,

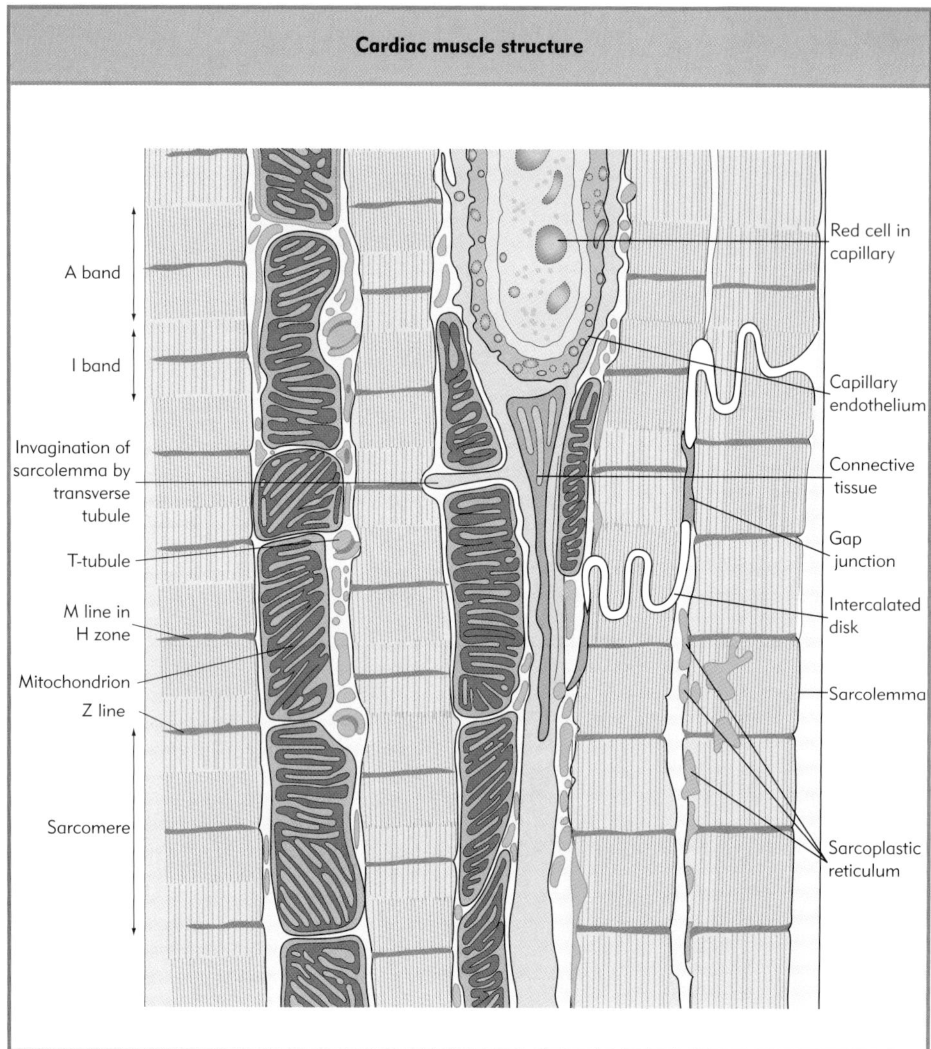

Figure 39.1 Cardiac muscle in longitudinal section. Cross-section showing cellular components. Mitochondria bordering the myofibrils are dark elliptical structures. The Z line demarcates the sarcomere, the repeating contractile unit. The dark structures in the cross-sectional view are myosin molecules, which form the thick filaments designated as the A band. The light I band on either side of the Z line consists of thin filaments composed of actin polymers. The T-tubule is a membranous invagination of the sarcolemma. (From Berne RM, Levy MN. Principles of physiology. Mosby; 1990:p215.)

normal and abnormal LV function is also critically influenced by interactions with both the systemic and the pulmonary circulations and with the other cardiac chambers. Cardiac pump function (specifically LV function) will be discussed in the context of its main determinants: systolic function, diastolic function, and heart rate. Loading conditions (preload and afterload, the latter encompassing arterial compliance, impedance, and the Anrep effect) and contractility will be discussed under systolic function. Heart rate (including the treppe or Bowditch effect) will be discussed briefly in the context of its effect on systolic function (Chapter 40 covers mechanisms of conduction and dysrhythmias). The concept of ascribing independent roles to preload, afterload, heart rate, and contractility in determining cardiac pump function is overly simplistic. These determinants of pump function are interrelated and have overlapping effects on the levels of cytoplasmic Ca^{2+} and/or on the Ca^{2+} sensitivity of the contractile elements (see below).

The cardiac cycle

Cardiac output is determined by heart rate and *stroke volume*. Normal stroke volume requires both normal systolic and normal diastolic LV function. Physiologists and cardiologists differ in their definitions of systole and diastole. Physiologic systole begins at the start of isovolumic contraction, when LV pressure exceeds atrial pressure (mitral valve closure occurs *after* this point), and extends to the peak of LV ejection. Physiologic diastole begins as LV pressure *starts* to fall. Aortic valve closure does not occur until LV pressure is less than or equal to aortic pressure. Cardiologists define systole as beginning with mitral valve closure and ending with aortic valve closure (both later in the cardiac cycle than the endpoints for physiologic systole). Depending on the circumstances, these are two operationally useful definitions of systole and diastole. However, the distinction is somewhat semantic when interpreted in the context of integrated pump function.

The effects of preload, afterload, heart rate and contractility on cardiac pump function are related to their overlapping effects on Ca^{2+} levels and Ca^{2+} sensitivity.

Both systole and diastole are active, energy-requiring processes. LV relaxation requires Ca^{2+} removal from troponin C, uptake by the SR and extrusion of Ca^{2+} across the sarcolemma. This results in reduced LV ejection, with LV pressure falling first below aortic pressure (with aortic valve closure) and then atrial pressure (with mitral valve opening and rapid ventricular filling).

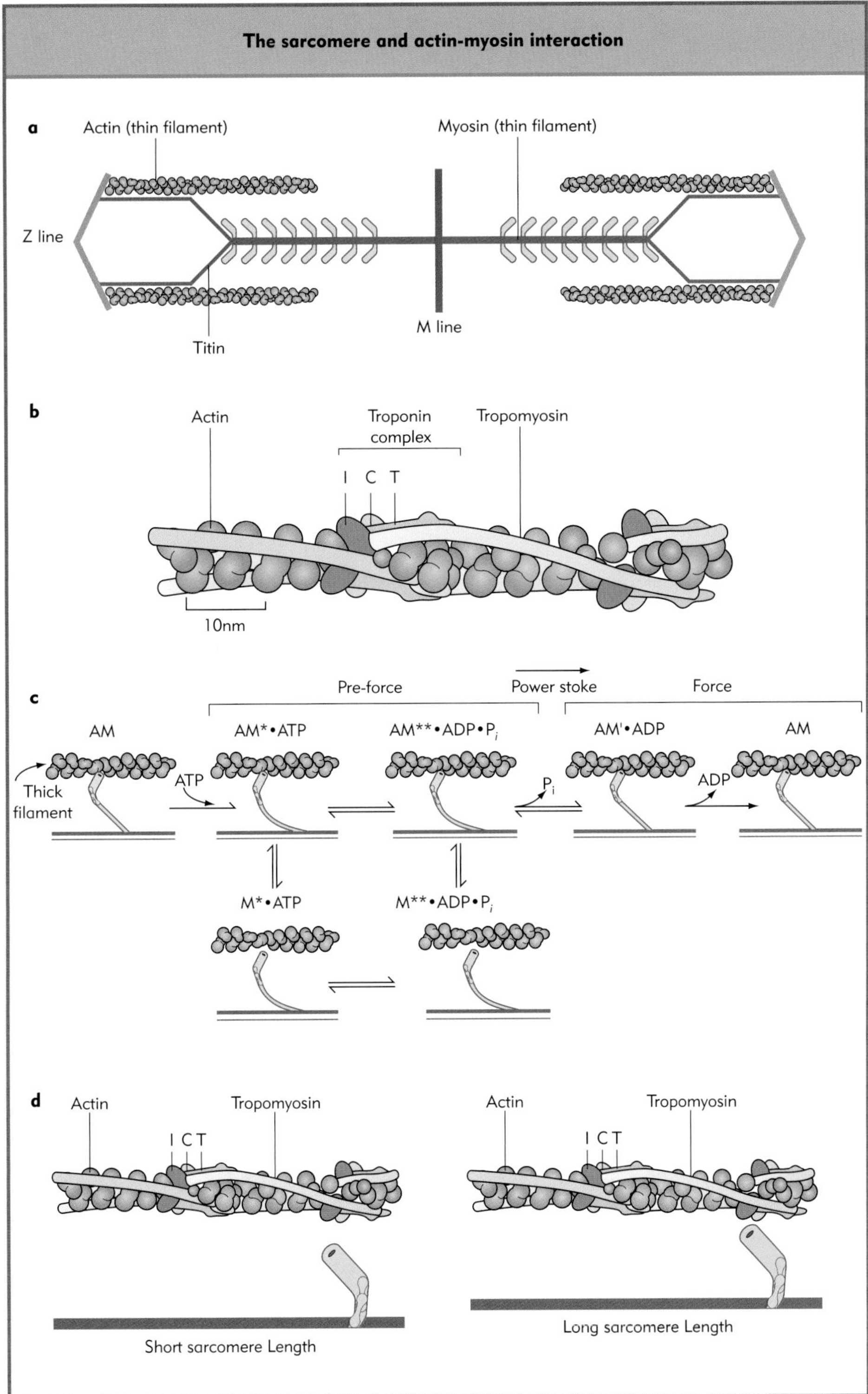

Figure 39.2 The actin filament and its interaction with the myosin head. (a) Diagram of the sarcomere showing approximate spatial relationships of thick and thin filaments and putative interactions of titin with the filaments, which would give rise to radial and axial restorative forces when the sarcomere is stretched. (b) Tropomyosin and troponin fit along the actin polymer in a muscle thin filament. Binding of Ca^{2+} to troponin C relieves the tropomyosin blockade of the actin–myosin interaction, initiating contraction. (c) Schema modified from the Rayment five-step model for interaction between the myosin head and the actin filament. The cycle starts with the rigor state, in which the myosin head is still attached to actin at the end of the power stroke. ATP binds to the ATP-binding pocket to cause the head to change conformation, reducing its affinity for actin and allowing it to move along the filament. Myosin ATPase activity splits the ATP into ADP and P_i (inorganic phosphate). As P_i is released, the power stroke occurs and the actin filament is moved by 5–10 nm, and the head returns to the rigor state. (d) Diagram of the thick and thin filaments illustrating the decrease in lateral separation at long lengths. The probability of cross-bridge interaction increases at increased length due to closer proximity to actin. M, M*, M**, represent different conformations of the myosin molecule; A represents actin.

At the level of the sarcomere, LV relaxation, an important but not a unique determinant of LV filling, begins even as blood is being ejected into the aorta. Normal pump function depends on normal filling, which is critically determined by an active process (LV relaxation) that begins during LV emptying.

Multiple parameters are used to evaluate cardiac function. These range from those that evaluate overall cardiac function (e.g. family of Frank–Starling curves) to those that evaluate one specific feature of cardiac function (e.g. maximal velocity of contraction, V_{max}) and maximal pressure change with time, dP/dt). The LV pressure–volume relationship (Fig. 39.3) is conceptually useful in discussing both systolic and diastolic function. The assessment of cardiac function by any of these determinants depends on their proper interpretation.

Systole and diastole are both active, energy-requiring processes.

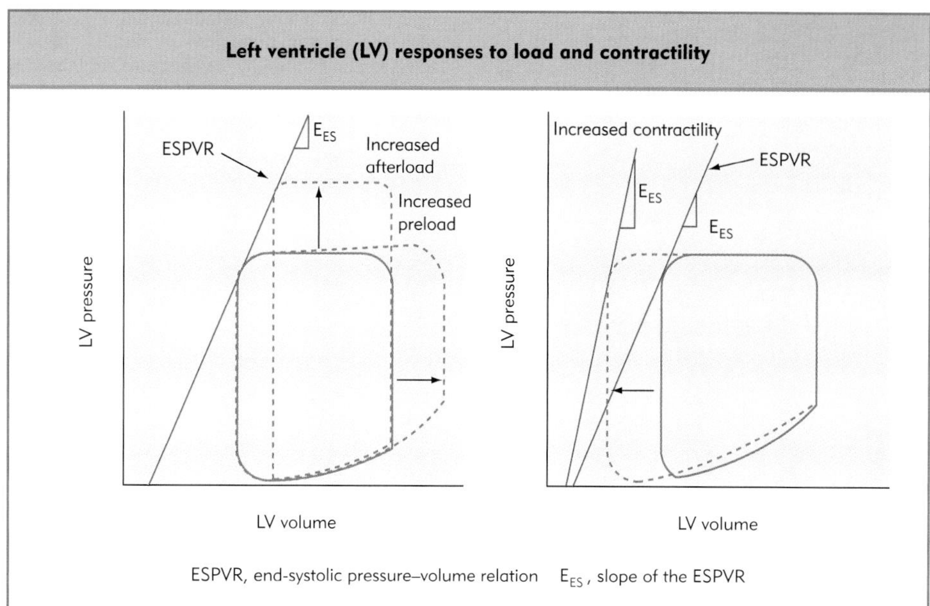

Figure 39.3 Left ventricle responses to load and contractility. The responses of the left ventricle to increased afterload, increased preload, and increased contractility are shown in the pressure–volume diagram.

Systolic function

Systolic function, defined as the ability of the LV to empty, is determined by the loading conditions of the heart (preload and afterload), contractility, and ventricular configuration. *Preload* (the load on the heart at the end of diastole, before contraction) is determined by ventricular volume. Starling's original descriptions detailed the influence of LV volume on cardiac output. The frequently used surrogates for LV volume (LV end-diastolic pressure, pulmonary capillary wedge pressure) are, even under normal circumstances, imprecise because of the curvilinear relationship between LV end-diastolic volume and pressure. Measurement of pressure–volume loops is one of the best methods available to assess cardiac function. However, it is limited by difficulties encountered with LV volume measurements throughout the cardiac cycle, and by criticism of the assumption that the LV end-systolic pressure–volume relationship (ESPVR) is linear outside the empirically measured range. The effects of increasing preload on LV end-diastolic volume, and hence on LV output, are readily discerned by inspection of the pressure–volume loop illustrated in Figure 39.3. At the level of the sarcomere, the phenomenon whereby increasing LV volume causes increased LV output (under conditions of constant contractility, afterload, and heart rate) has been ascribed to optimizing sarcomere length and overlap. However, extrapolation of this concept from skeletal to cardiac muscle is not justified. In cardiac muscle little (~10%) force is developed even when the muscle is at <80% of maximum length. Consequently, cardiac muscle has to develop almost all its force over a relatively small range of shortening near its maximal length. This feature (length-dependent activation) of cardiac muscle is incompletely understood. Increasing muscle length causes a decrease in lattice spacing between thick and thin filaments. Changes in cooperation in cross-bridge binding to actin and/or the elastic properties of titin with changes in length may contribute to length-dependent activation (see Fig. 39.2).

Afterload is the load on the contracting myocardium (at the start of contraction). The LV systolic wall stress is directly proportional to LV radius and afterload as defined by the law of Laplace:

$$\text{wall stress} = \frac{(\text{pressure} \times \text{radius})}{(2 \times \text{wall thickness})}$$

Systolic function is determined by preload, afterload, contractility, and ventricular configuration.

Normally, afterload is determined primarily by blood pressure. Abnormal vascular compliance (e.g. hypertension, atherosclerosis) exerts a proportionally greater influence on afterload. Aortic impedance is a related but more specific term; it is defined as the quotient of instantaneous aortic pressure and flow. A decrease in afterload (decreased blood pressure and/or increased arterial compliance) results in a decrease in the LV systolic wall tension required for ejection (or increased ejection if LV wall tension is constant and afterload is decreased). Conversely, increasing afterload reduces LV ejection if LV systolic wall tension remains unchanged. Importantly, increases in afterload can decrease ejection *without* changes in contractility (one simply moves to a different point on the same LV ESPV relationship; Fig. 39.3). However, sudden increases in afterload have a positive inotropic effect (Anrep effect), shifting to a different LV ESPV relationship. This is thought to result from activation of LV stretch receptors, which increase cytosolic Na^+; this in turn causes an increase in cytosolic Ca^{2+} via the Na^+/Ca^{2+} exchanger.

Heart rate, within a wide range, directly influences cardiac output, as long as filling during diastole is not compromised. Increased heart rate also has a positive inotropic effect in isolated papillary muscle strips (treppe or Bowditch effect). This results from enhanced Ca^{2+} cycling at rapid rates, resulting in an increase in the Ca^{2+} concentration to which the contractile elements are exposed.

Contractility is a major determinant of, but is not synonymous with, systolic function. Systolic function is also influenced by loading conditions and ventricular configuration. Ventricular emptying (systolic function) is effectively augmented by decreasing afterload or reduced by increasing afterload at the same level of contractility (Fig. 39.3). The pressure–volume loop in Figure 39.3 also illustrates how changing contractility (indicated in the pressure–volume loop as a change in the slope of the ESPVR) changes systolic function (ventricular emptying) under constant loading conditions. Increased contractility can be defined as a greater velocity of contraction that reaches a higher peak force when heart rate and loading conditions are kept constant. This definition is useful when analyzing in vivo or in vitro studies, but is limited at the subcellular level, where the mechanisms underlying the influences of preload, afterload, heart rate, and contractility overlap. The V_{max} of isolated papillary muscle is frequently used as an index of contractility, as the preparation is unloaded and can be stimulated at a constant rate. However, V_{max} is not measured directly but extrapolated from the force–velocity relationship, which may be nonlinear. Studies utilizing sarcomeres indicate that V_{max} is not independent of length at shorter sarcomere lengths but is independent (and thus can be used as an index of contractility) at longer sarcomere lengths. As indicated above, cardiac muscle functions at the upper end of its length– tension relationship.

At the molecular level it is not possible to separate the effects of heart rate, loading conditions, and contractility from each other. For example, inotropy is mediated by increased Ca^{2+} transients and/or increased sensitivity to Ca^{2+}; increasing heart rate results in increased cytosolic Ca^{2+} because of limited uptake of Ca^{2+} by the SR (treppe effect); increased preload causes length-activation mediated by increased sensitivity to Ca^{2+}, and increased afterload may increase cytosolic Ca^{2+} via stretch-sensitive channels.

Diastolic function

The importance of diastolic function to overall pump function is now well recognized. Normal ventricular diastolic function can be defined as ventricular filling sufficient to produce an adequate cardiac output without elevated filling pressures. Systolic dysfunction is the most common cause of diastolic dysfunction, in that systolic dysfunction results in elevated LV end-diastolic volume and filling pressures (Chapter 44). Diastolic dysfunction can also occur in the absence of systolic dysfunction. There are many causes of 'primary' diastolic dysfunction (Table 39.1), which can be classified into those that result from abnormalities proximal to the LV (dysfunction of the mitral valve, left atrium, and pulmonary veins), those extrinsic to the LV, and those intrinsic to the LV. Structural abnormalities and dysfunction at the mitral valve, left atrium, or pulmonary veins can cause elevated pulmonary pressures and pulmonary congestion without systolic dysfunction. Similarly, any other cause of diastolic dysfunction (either extrinsic or intrinsic to the LV) can cause pulmonary congestion and symptoms of cardiac failure without systolic dysfunction. The effects of some causes of primary diastolic dysfunction on the pressure–volume loop are illustrated in Figure 39.4.

Diastole is divided into four phases: isovolumic relaxation (when aortic and mitral valves are both closed), rapid ventricular filling, slow ventricular filling (diastasis), and atrial systole. During isovolumic relaxation, LV pressure decreases because of LV relaxation. However, LV pressure continues to decrease following mitral valve opening as a result of continued LV

Table 39.1 Determinants of left ventricular diastolic function and causes of dysfunction. (From Pagel PS, Grossman W, Haering JM, Warltier DC. Left ventricular diastolic function in the normal and diseased heart. Anesthesiology. 1993;79:836–54)

Myocardial relaxation and active elasticity
Residual cross-bridge activation during part or all of diastole
Slow relaxation (affects early diastolic filling)
Incomplete relaxation (affects compliance throughout diastole)
Recoil of elastic components compressed during systole
Intrinsic ventricular chamber characteristics
Passive ventricular elasticity (chamber stiffness)
Ventricular wall thickness (mass)
Ventricular wall compression (myocardial stiffness)
Viscoelasticity
Factors extrinsic to the ventricle
Pericardium
Right ventricular loading and function
Turgor of the coronary circulation
Compression by mediastinal or pulmonary masses
Pulmonary pathology or positive pressure ventilation
Left atrial structure and function
Preload
Wall thickness
Inotropic state
Pulmonary venous return
Mitral valve competency
Heart rate and rhythm

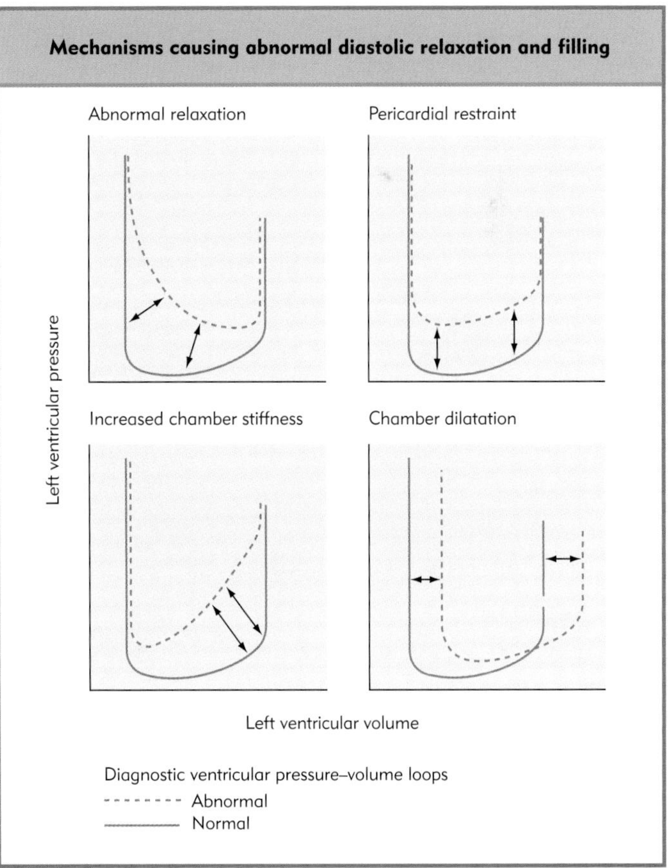

Figure 39.4 Mechanisms responsible for abnormal diastolic relaxation and filling.

relaxation, and also as a result of recoil of LV elastic and viscoelastic components. Relaxation requires the removal of Ca^{2+} from troponin C-binding sites. This allows actin and myosin to disassociate. Removal of cytosolic Ca^{2+} involves reuptake by the SR and the exchange of Ca^{2+} for Na^+ across the myocyte membrane (sarcolemma), both of which are active, ATP-dependent processes (the Na^+ gradient is maintained by the sarcolemmal Na^+, K^+-ATPase). Normally, Ca^{2+} is effectively removed by the SR and sarcolemma. Ineffective Ca^{2+} removal can result from insufficient time (excessive tachycardia), insufficient ATP (ischemia), or enhanced Ca^{2+} binding to troponin C, each of which can impair ventricular relaxation. Several invasive (isovolumic relaxation, early diastolic filling) and noninvasive (Doppler echocardiography) measurements are used to assess diastolic function, but their interpretation is difficult because diastolic function is influenced not only by variables confined to diastole, but also by variables that alter pump function during systole (loading conditions, heart rate, and contractility).

The heart is not a simple homogeneous pump, but a complex heterogenous organ.

Systolic and diastolic function can be interpreted in the context of wall stress. An increase in diastolic wall stress occurs if LV end-diastolic pressure increases for any reason, and an increase in systolic wall stress occurs with increases in heart rate, afterload, or contractility. An increase in wall stress from any cause leads to an increase in myocardial oxygen requirement (see below).

Cellular and subcellular aspects of cardiac function

Cardiac myocytes, which make up the vast majority of cells in the heart, work in coordination to propel blood through the body. Each cardiac myocyte has the ability to contract and relax, and to respond to positive and negative inotropic stimulation. An important feature of the heart that allows it to fulfill its pumping function is the integrated and coordinated action of billions of cardiac myocytes. The electrical impulse that initiates the heartbeat originates in specialized cells in the sinoatrial node of the right atrium. The impulse is transmitted through a specialized conduction system to individual atrial and ventricular myocytes.

Cardiac myocytes are cylindrical in shape, approximately 120 μm long, and 10–35 μm in diameter. The sarcolemma, or cell membrane of the myocyte, contains ion channels, ion pumps, substrate transporters, and receptors imbedded in its lipid bilayer, allowing communication with neighboring cells and the extracellular environment (Fig. 39.5). Low-resistance contact between myocytes is provided by gap junctions, which allow instantaneous transmission of electrical impulses from one myocyte to the next.

Voltage-gated Na^+ channels in the sarcolemma open in response to an electrical impulse and allow Na^+ entry, which depolarizes the cell and results in the opening of VGCC. These channels remain open for several milliseconds and result in the plateau phase of the action potential (Chapter 40). VGCC permit the entry of extracellular Ca^{2+} down a concentration gradient. The entry of Ca^{2+} to the myocytes (once thought to generate a

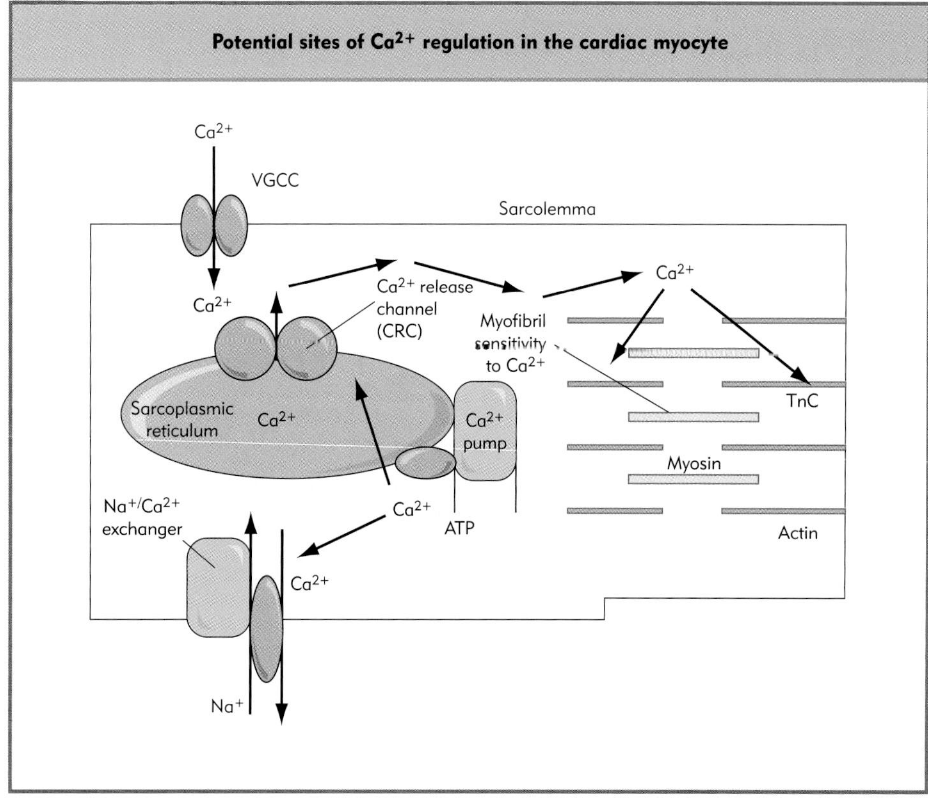

Figure 39.5 Schematic representation of a cardiac myocyte showing potential calcium regulatory sites in the cardiac myocyte. Myofibril sensitivity to Ca^{2+} can be either increased or decreased and the Ca^{2+} pump can sequester more or less Ca^{2+}, leading to changes in both systolic and diastolic function. The Na^+/Ca^{2+} exchanger is important for maintenance of Ca^{2+} homeostasis. VGCC, voltage-gated Ca^{2+} channels; TnC, troponin C.

common pool of Ca^{2+} that would activate the opening of multiple CRCs located in the junctional SR) is now believed to occur in small amounts in specific well-demarcated zones (adjacent to T-tubules), activating one or, at most, a few CRCs in the SR, resulting in a Ca^{2+} 'spark'. The opening of multiple L-type (long-lasting) VGCC results in the activation of many 'zones' and leads to the generation of many 'sparks' and a global increase in myoplasmic Ca^{2+} concentration, from 0.1 μmol/L (10^{-7} M) to 10 μmol/L (10^{-5} M).

Excitation–contraction coupling offers many potential sites for the regulation of contractile activity. Any site that Ca^{2+} passes through or binds to in the cardiac myocyte is a potential site at which contractility or relaxation (lusitropy) can be enhanced or depressed (Fig. 39.5). Negative or positive inotropy can result respectively from decreased or increased Ca^{2+} entry through the VGCC. The Ca^{2+} channel antagonists, such as nifedipine, diltiazem, or verapamil, decrease Ca^{2+} influx (Ca^{2+} current: I_{Ca}) and, consequently, contractility. Communication between the VGCC and the CRC via Ca^{2+} is another important site of regulation. Recent evidence demonstrates that SR free Ca^{2+} rarely goes below 50% of its maximal value after each beat and, although there still exists considerable thermodynamic driving force for Ca^{2+} release, Ca^{2+} release via the CRC is terminated. Furthermore, there is little limitation in Ca^{2+} availability in the junctional SR for the subsequent heartbeat, but rather a limitation in the availability of the CRC. Ca^{2+} in the junctional SR is rapidly replenished with a time constant (τ) of ~100 ms, whereas the recovery of the CRC has a τ of ~300 ms. The responsiveness of the CRC to a given amount of Ca^{2+} is decreased in myocytes isolated from hypertrophied hearts; in this situation, for a fixed I_{Ca} the CRC responds with less release of Ca^{2+}, and hence less Ca^{2+} is available to activate troponin C. Another important site at which contractility can be regulated is through the Ca^{2+} load in the SR. A decreased SR Ca^{2+} load, as occurs in heart failure, might lead to a decreased number of 'sparks', resulting in decreased 'contractility' because of the decrease in the number of troponin C molecules binding Ca^{2+}.

Excitation–contraction coupling involves the activation of sarcoplasmic reticulum Ca^{2+} release channels by the entry of extracellular Ca^{2+} through voltage-gated Ca^{2+} channels.

The regulation of Ca^{2+} (and, therefore, contraction) is linked to activation of β-adrenoceptors, which have multiple effects on Ca^{2+} handling at various sites in the myocyte (Fig. 39.6). Phosphorylation of VGCC via adenylyl cyclase stimulation and cAMP-dependent protein kinase activation increases the open time of the L-type VGCC and enhances I_{Ca}, resulting in greater stimulation of the CRC and an increase in the availability of Ca^{2+} for contraction. β-adrenoceptor activation results in the phosphorylation of at least two proteins that are involved in the positive lusitropic response: phospholamban and troponin I (TnI). Phospholamban is a pentameric protein found in the SR membrane that is linked to Ca^{2+}-ATPase function (Fig. 39.7). Phosphorylation of phospholamban leads to disinhibition of the SR Ca^{2+} pump, an enhancement in the rate of relaxation (lusitropic effect), and an increase in the amount of Ca^{2+} sequestered in the SR for subsequent contractions. Recent studies with a transgenic mouse model suggest that not all Ca^{2+}-ATPase molecules in the heart are linked to phospholamban, and therefore modulation of Ca^{2+} pump activity is only partial. Finally, removal of inhibition by phospholamban of Ca^{2+} pump activity results in a greater sensitivity of the Ca^{2+} pump to Ca^{2+}. Phosphorylation of TnI has a considerable positive lusitropic effect. TnI phosphorylation leads to a reduction in the affinity of TnC for Ca^{2+}; the unbinding of Ca^{2+} from TnC occurs more rapidly, allowing acceleration of the relaxation phase of the cardiac cycle.

Nitric oxide (NO) also modulates myocyte Ca^{2+} transients. Both the NOS3 (endothelial) and NOS1 (neuronal) isoforms of nitric oxide synthase (NOS) are expressed in cardiac myocytes, and are localized to specific organelles that regulate cellular function (NOS1 to the SR, NOS3 to the sarcolemma). NOS has also been localized in mitochondria, but the specific isoform(s) present is unclear. Precise regulation of cellular function requires not only localization within the cell but also specific protein–protein interactions. For example, NOS3 in membrane-bound caveolae produces NO that inhibits β-adrenoreceptor-induced inotropy and Ca^{2+} entry via L-type Ca^{2+} channels. In contrast, NO from SR NOS1 augments contractility.

ANESTHETIC EFFECTS ON CARDIAC FUNCTION

Contractile activity of the heart depends on extracellular Ca^{2+}. The negative inotropic activity of anesthetics appears to a large extent to be related to the interference with delivery to or response of myofibrils to Ca^{2+}. Figure 39.5 illustrates the major sites at which anesthetics could interfere with Ca^{2+} homeostasis and contractile activity. The two sites most affected by volatile anesthetics are the L-type VGCC and the SR CRC, also known as the ryanodine receptor. Many studies have supported the notion of a reversible, inhibitory alteration of the L-type VGCC in cardiac myocytes, leading to a decrease in the entry of Ca^{2+} and hence a smaller stimulus for Ca^{2+}-induced Ca^{2+} release.

The negative inotropic effect of volatile anesthetics results from reduced Ca^{2+} entry, reduced sarcoplasmic reticulum Ca^{2+} capacity, and reduced myofibril Ca^{2+} sensitivity.

The other major site of importance, the CRC, responds to the entry of activator Ca^{2+} with the release of larger amounts of Ca^{2+}, which can go on to activate the myofibrils. The SR capacity for Ca^{2+} appears to be reduced by volatile anesthetics, especially halothane. This effect is apparently related to an increased open time of the CRC, allowing Ca^{2+} to leak more or less continuously at a low level (i.e. a level not leading to a measurable increase in diastolic pressure, nor to increased inotropy). The final important site of potential negative inotropic activity is the myofibrils. The rate of cycling of actin–myosin cross-bridges is unaffected by halothane, enflurane, and isoflurane, and the force generated by each cross-bridge is the same in the presence or absence of anesthetic. However, the sensitivity of myofibrils and, in particular, troponin C, to Ca^{2+} appears to be decreased by volatile anesthetics, potentially contributing to their negative inotropic effect. Anesthetic agents are also important modulators of preconditioning in the heart. Anesthetic preconditioning is a phenomenon involving increased tolerance to ischemia

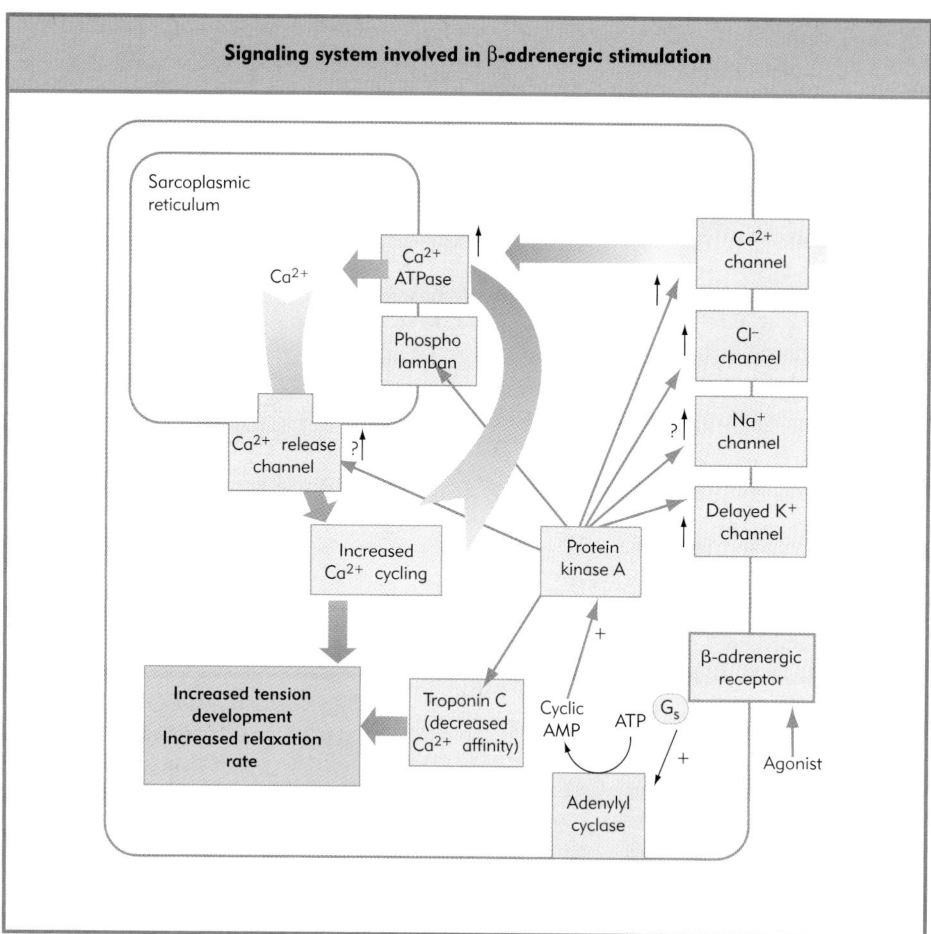

Figure 39.6 Signaling systems involved in positive inotropic and lusitropic (enhanced relaxation) effects of β-adrenergic stimulation. When β-adrenergic agonists interact with the β-adrenoceptor, the associated G protein (Gs) stimulates adenylyl cyclase, leading to a series of changes (increase in cAMP and activation of protein kinase A) that phosphorylate Ca^{2+} channels and stimulate metabolism. The result is an enhanced opening probability of the Ca^{2+} channel, thereby increasing Ca^{2+} entry through the sarcolemma of the T-tubule. In turn, increased intracellular Ca^{2+} stimulates the release of more Ca^{2+} from the sarcoplasmic reticulum and activates troponin C. Enhanced myosin ATPase activity explains the increased rate of contraction, with increased activation of troponin C causing increased peak force development. (With permission from Lynch, 1998.)

following pre-exposure to an anesthetic. The specific effect on preconditioning mechanisms is agent-specific, and this is a current area of intense investigation.

METABOLISM

The heart uses predominantly free fatty acids and glucose as its metabolic substrates. Following a meal with a carbohydrate load, glucose is the main substrate, whereas in the fasting patient elevated free fatty acids are the major substrate for aerobic metabolism. With exercise, lactate produced by skeletal muscle becomes the predominant energy substrate. The heart is an aerobic organ, as indicated by the large volume of the cell occupied by mitochondria (approximately 23% of total cell volume): 90% of cardiac metabolism is aerobic and 10% anaerobic. Contractile activity consumes 60% of the metabolic energy generated by the heart, whereas the SR Ca^{2+} ATPase consumes 15%. The Na^+ gradient is maintained by the Na^+/K^+-ATPase at the cell membrane; this process consumes 5% of available cellular energy. The 20% of energy remaining is used for basic cellular maintenance.

Xanthine oxidoreductase (XOR) is a key regulatory enzyme in myocyte metabolism. XOR exists in two interconvertible forms, xanthine oxidase (XO) and xanthine dehydrogenase (XDH). XOR is an essential enzyme in purine metabolism. Both XO and XDH convert hypoxanthine to xanthine, and xanthine to uric acid. XO and XDH differ in that XO reduces oxygen only, whereas XHD can reduce both oxygen and NAD^+. In the process, XO can produce reactive oxygen species (ROS). The levels of ROS produced and the efficacy of intrinsic antioxidant scavenging mechanisms determine the potential impact of the ROS. Purine metabolism occurs under physiological conditions, implying that the balance of ROS production/antioxidant defenses does not result in cellular injury. However, alterations in XOR and oxidant stress may underlie the development of heart failure.

CORONARY BLOOD FLOW

Coronary blood flow (CBF) is directly proportional to the pressure gradient and inversely proportional to the resistance of the vascular bed. Although extreme disturbances of coronary perfusion pressure can alter CBF, under normal conditions perfusion pressure is relatively stable and vascular resistance (including regional resistance) predominates as a determinant of CBF. The use of advanced techniques to study local or regional variations in CBF (small vessels including microvessels, subendocardium versus subepicardium, collateral versus noncollateral,

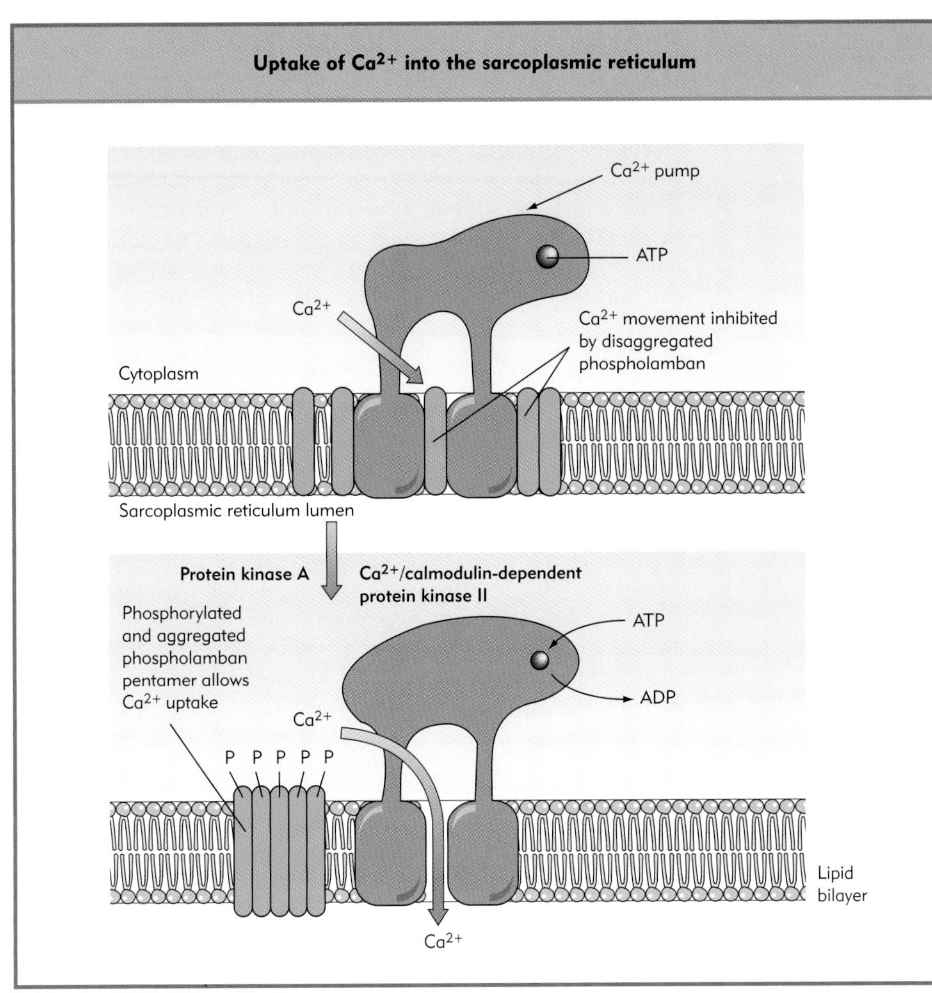

Figure 39.7 Uptake of calcium by the energy-requiring Ca^{2+} pump into the sarcoplasmic reticulum. Enhanced cytosolic Ca^{2+}or β-adrenergic stimulation results in phosphorylation of phospholamban at distinct sites. This removes the inhibition exerted by its unphosphorylated form. An increased rate of relaxation (lusitropy) follows because of the increased Ca^{2+} uptake. (With permission from Lynch C III, Vogel S, Sperelakis N. Halothane depression of myocardial slow action potentials. Anesthesiology. 1988;55:360–8.)

ischemic versus nonischemic) demonstrates the heterogeneity of the coronary vasculature. Different vessels relax or contract to a given stimulus with varying intensity, and may respond in opposite directions to the same stimulus. Whereas the coronary vasculature is subject to systemic influences, local control of coronary vascular resistance (and thus CBF) predominates in this as in other vital organs. The resistance of coronary vessels to flow is determined by compressive forces generated by contracting cardiac muscle and by a profuse, complex interacting array of local and systemic factors. Even under normal physiologic conditions, none of these factors exerts a uniform influence across the heart; this contributes to the regional heterogeneity observed in CBF. The presence of coronary disease adds additional variables to the control of CBF.

Under normal conditions with constant perfusion pressure, coronary vascular resistance is the major determinant of coronary blood flow.

The metabolic demands of the heart (i.e. a contractile pump with high energy and oxygen requirements) result in high basal oxygen extraction and low coronary sinus oxygen content. Therefore, increasing oxygen extraction is not an adequate mechanism for meeting increasing myocardial oxygen demand, which must be accommodated by increasing CBF. By extension, local mechanism(s) coupling oxygen supply to demand are pivotal in controlling local CBF. Clinically, the myocardial oxygen supply/demand ratio is optimized by manipulating global parameters (heart rate, afterload, contractility, preload), recognizing that the results of interventions may differ from one region of the myocardium to another. Results must also be interpreted in the context of both the direct and the indirect effects of an intervention. For example, α_1-adrenoceptor-mediated coronary vasoconstriction may be superseded by a concomitant increase in contractility, with metabolically induced coronary vasodilatation and increases in CBF. This is further complicated by the recent recognition that endothelial-cell α_2-adrenoceptor activation causes the release of endothelium-derived relaxant factor/nitric oxide (EDRF/NO), with resultant relaxation of underlying vascular smooth muscle.

Under normal conditions, the upstream pressure for perfusion of the coronary arteries is aortic diastolic pressure. As a result of myocardial compression, CBF to the LV ceases during parts of systole, especially in the subendocardium, where compressive forces are highest (Fig. 39.8). Flow in the right coronary artery may also be compromised under conditions of right

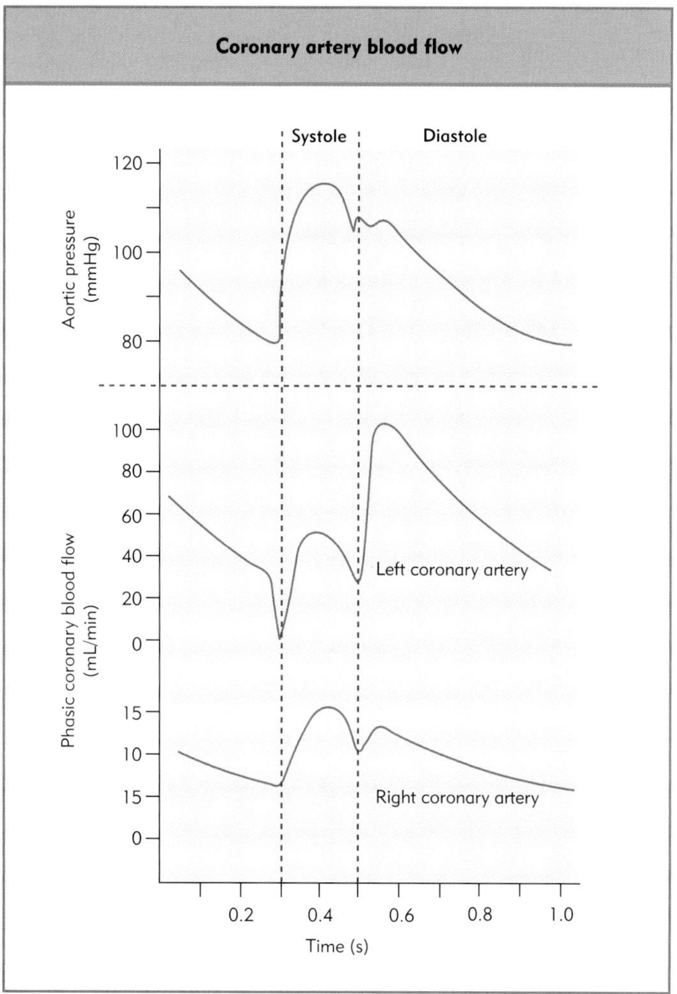

Figure 39.8 Blood flow in the left and right coronary arteries. The right ventricle is perfused throughout the cardiac cycle. Flow to the left ventricle is largely confined to diastole.

ventricular hypertrophy. The effective downstream or critical closing pressure in the coronary circulation is unclear. Because CBF to the LV occurs predominantly during diastole, it is unlikely that a 'vascular waterfall' occurs in the coronary circulation, and the effective downstream pressure will be close to the coronary sinus pressure. For the LV subendocardium, the LV end-diastolic pressure may be a more accurate reflection of the downstream pressure. The LV subendocardium is vulnerable to ischemia. Studies of transmural (endocardial versus epicardial) myocardial blood flow (and hence oxygen supply) and of indices of oxygen utilization (glycolytic pathway activity, high-energy phosphates, lactate) indicate that relative underperfusion of the subendocardium is the main reason for this vulnerability. The mechanism(s) responsible for this may be the greater systolic compressive force in the subendocardium causing increased compression and stretching (and hence resistance) in these vessels. In the ensuing diastole, a relatively greater perfusion pressure is required to open and maintain flow in these subendocardial vessels.

REGULATION OF CORONARY VASOMOTOR TONE

Coronary vasomotor tone is ultimately determined by contraction of vascular smooth muscle, which can be altered by systemic and local stimuli. It is difficult to determine which of these influences is important in controlling vasomotor tone in normal or diseased conditions. Assessing neural regulation of the coronary circulation is especially difficult because of both direct and indirect effects. When indirect effects (metabolism) are controlled, parasympathetic activation consistently causes coronary vasodilatation mediated by activation of muscarinic receptors on endothelial cells (Fig. 39.9), although the parasympathetic nervous system is not an important regulator of coronary vasomotor tone. However, defects in muscarinic receptor activation may be a manifestation of endothelial cell dysfunction. Similarly, the role of direct effects of α- and β-adrenoceptor activation (vasoconstriction and vasodilatation, respectively) in coronary vasoregulation is modest. α-adrenoceptor activation may divert CBF to areas of relatively greater oxygen need (e.g. the subendocardium in exercise, and to ischemic areas), as indicated by canine models. Studies in humans indicate that α-adrenoceptor activation can cause ischemia by constricting diseased vessels. Hormones (e.g. vasopressin, atrial natriuretic factor) or drugs that alter endogenously produced hormone levels (e.g. angiotensin-converting enzyme inhibitors) are not important regulators of coronary vasomotor tone. Potential mediators for metabolic regulation of coronary vasomotor effects (e.g. K^+, H^+, low oxygen carbon dioxide, and osmolarity) may act either directly on vascular smooth muscle or indirectly via endothelial cells. A complex interaction of local factors (which differ from region to region) regulates vasomotor tone and couples oxygen delivery to oxygen demand.

The factors controlling CBF are multifactorial, complex, and interactive, and determined by the net influence of local mechanical and vasoactive influences.

Temporary occlusion of coronary vessels causes an increase in CBF above baseline following the reinstitution of flow, indicating the presence of coronary reserve and *reactive hyperemia*. The absence of reactive hyperemia indicates that basal CBF is maximal and that vasodilator capacity has been exhausted. *Autoregulation* describes the phenomenon whereby CBF returns towards baseline following a change in coronary perfusion pressure and CBF. The mechanisms underlying reactive hyperemia and autoregulation are likely to be multifactorial, involving one or more of the mechanisms described above.

The influence of endothelial cells on vasomotor tone reflects the net effect of constrictors and dilators (Fig. 39.9). Endothelial cell dysfunction results in an imbalance favoring constrictors because of a relative deficit of vasodilator mediators. Moreover, atherodegenerative disease originates in the endothelium. Indeed, endothelial cell dysfunction (e.g. defects in acetylcholine-induced release of NO) is now interpreted as one of the earliest manifestations of the atherodegenerative process (Chapter 44).

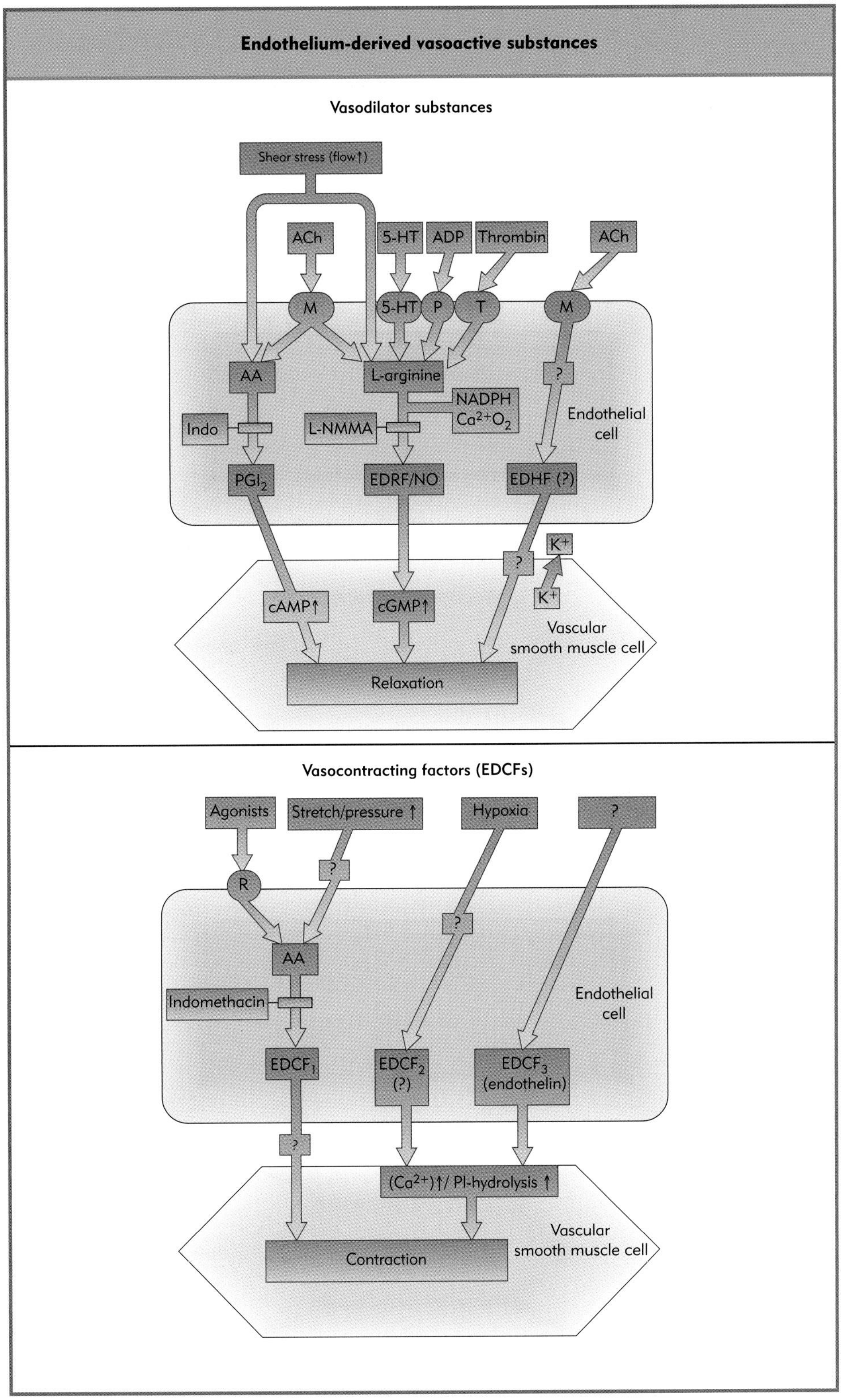

Figure 39.9 Endothelium-derived vasoactive substances. The endothelium produces both vasodilator and vasoconstrictive factors. Endothelium-derived vasodilator substances include prostacyclin. This is produced by the cyclooxygenase pathway, which can be blocked by indomethacin and aspirin. Endothelium-derived relaxing factor may be nitric oxide (NO) or a closely related compound. Its production can be blocked by arginine analogs, such as L-NMMA (Nγ-monomethyl-L-arginine). There are a number of endothelium-derived contracting factors (EDCFs). The release of $EDCF_1$ can be inhibited by cyclooxygenase inhibitors, such as indomethacin. $EDCF_2$ is released by hypoxia and is indomethacin insensitive. $EDCF_3$ is a potent vasoconstrictor peptide known as endothelin. 5-HT, serotonin; AA, arachidonic acid; PGI_2, prostacyclin; cGMP, cyclic GMP; cAMP, cyclic AMP; EDRF/NO, endothelium-derived relaxant factor/nitric oxide; M, muscarinic receptor; P, purinergic receptor; T, thrombin receptor; Indo: indomethacin; ACh, acetylcholine; PI, phosphatidylinositol; R, receptor; EDHF, endothelium-derived hyperpolarizing factor that hyperpolarizes the smooth muscle membrane.

Key references

Barouch LA, Harrison RW, Skaf MW et al. Nitric oxide regulates the heart by spatial confinement of nitric oxide synthase isoforms. Nature 2002;416:337–40.

Bassenge E, Busse R. Endothelial modulation of coronary tone. Prog Cardiovasc Dis. 1988;30:349–80.

Berry CE, Hare JM. Xanthine oxidoreductase and cardiovascular disease: molecular mechanisms and pathophysiological implications. J Physiol. 2004;555:589–606.

Fujimoto K, Bosnjak ZJ, Kwok W-M. Isoflurane-induced facilitation of the cardiac sarcolemmal K_{ATP} channel. Anesthesiology 2002;97:57–65.

Lynch C III. Myocardial excitation–contraction coupling. In: Yaksh et al., eds. Anesthesia: biologic foundations. Philadelphia, PA: Lippincott-Raven; 1997:1041–79.

Lynch C III, Vogel S, Sperelakis N. Halothane depression of myocardial slow action potentials. Anesthesiology 1988;55:360–8.

Marcus ML, Chilian WM, Kanatsuka H et al. Understanding the coronary circulation through studies at the microvascular level. Circulation 1990;81:1–7.

Massion PB, Feron O, Dessy C, Balligand J-L. Nitric oxide and cardiac function. Ten years after, and continuing. Circ Res. 2003;93:388–98.

Metzger JM, Westfall MV. Covalent and noncovalent modification of thin filament action. Circ Res. 2004;94:146–58.

Moss RL, Fitzsimons DP. Frank–Starling relationship. Long on importance, short on mechanism. Circ Res. 2002;90:11–13.

Nathan HJ. Coronary physiology. In: Kaplan JA, ed. Cardiac anesthesia. Philadelphia, PA: WB Saunders; 1993:235–60.

Olsson RA, Bunger R. Metabolic control of coronary blood flow. Prog Cardiovasc Dis. 1987;29:369–87.

Pagel PS, Grossman W, Haering JM, Warltier DC. Left ventricular diastolic function in the normal and diseased heart. Anesthesiology 1993;79:836–54.

Riess ML, Eells JT, Kevin LG, Camara AKS, Henry MM, Stowe DF. Attenuation of mitochondrial respiration by sevoflurane in isolated cardiac mitochondria is mediated in part by reactive oxygen species. Anesthesiology 2004;100:498–505.

Walker JS, de Tombe PP. Titin and the developing heart. Circ Res. 2004;94:860–2.

Further reading

Flavahan NA. Atherosclerosis or lipoprotein-induced endothelial dysfunction. Circulation 1992;85:1927–38.

Harrison DG, Bates JN. The nitrovasodilators: new ideas about old drugs. Circulation 1993;87:1461–7.

Hu G, Salem MR, Crystal GJ. Isoflurane and sevoflurane precondition against neutrophil-induced contractile dysfunction in isolated rat hearts. Anesthesiology 2004;100:489–97.

Luscher TF, Tanner FC, Tschudi MR, Noll G. Endothelial dysfunction in coronary artery disease. Annu Rev Med. 1993;44:395–418.

Moncada S, Higgs EA, Vane JR. Human arterial and venous tissues generate prostacyclin (prostaglandin X), a potent inhibitor of platelet aggregation. Lancet 1977; i:18–19.

Opie LH. Mechanisms of cardiac contraction and relaxation. In: Braunwald E, ed. Heart disease: a textbook of cardiovascular medicine. Philadelphia, PA: WB Saunders; 1997: 361–93.

Shibata T, Blanck TJJ, Sagawa K. Hunter W. The effect of volatile anesthetics on dynamic stiffness of rabbit papillary muscle. Anesthesiology 1988;70:496–502.

Tanaka K, Ludwig LM, Krolikowski JG et al. Isoflurane produces delayed preconditioning against myocardial ischemia and reperfusion injury. Anesthesiology 2004;100:525–31.

Chapter 40

Cardiac electrophysiology

Jeffrey R Balser and Annemarie Thompson

TOPICS COVERED IN THIS CHAPTER

- **Basics of cardiac electrophysiology**
  - Ion channels and the action potential
- **Structure and function of cardiac ion channels**
  - Function of voltage-gated ion channels
  - Na^+ channels inform long QT, Brugada, and conduction disease phenotypes
  - Cardiac Ca^{2+} channels serve as triggers for arrhythmias
  - I_{TO}, the transient outward current, is implicated in heart failure and arrhythmias
  - I_{Kr}, the rapid repolarizing current
  - I_{Ks}, the slow repolarizing current
  - Cardiac inward rectifiers
  - Pacemaker currents allow spontaneous depolarization
  - Other background currents
- **Tissue diversity and cellular arrhythmia mechanisms**
  - Tissue diversity, the conduction system, and adenosine
  - Cell-to-cell coupling
  - Re-entry and arrhythmogenesis
  - Automaticity and arrhythmia suppression
- **Common perioperative arrhythmias**
  - Perioperative atrial fibrillation
  - Ventricular arrhythmias
- **Pacing and cardiac electroversion**
  - Pacing and capture
  - Defibrillators
  - Electromagnetic interference

Cardiac arrhythmias, or irregular patterns of heart contraction, are a major cause of death (estimated at 400 000 annually in the USA). They also contribute to prolonged hospitalization in the perioperative period. Fortunately, the application of basic molecular science to the problems of cardiac excitability has yielded significant advances in our understanding of cardiac arrhythmias. The pioneering work of Hodgkin and Huxley in the 1950s unambiguously defined voltage-gated ion channels as the molecular entities that underlie membrane excitability. The development of 'patch-clamp' electrophysiological techniques by Sakmann and Neher in the 1980s allowed the measurement of ionic current through individual ion channels and exponentially increased our understanding of these proteins. Concurrent use of molecular biological methods to clone and sequence ion channels provided unparalleled insight into the basic structure of the cardiac ion channels and novel targets for antiarrhythmic drug therapy.

BASICS OF CARDIAC ELECTROPHYSIOLOGY

Ion channels and the action potential

The action potential represents the time-varying transmembrane potential of the cardiac cell during systole and diastole. Similarly, the surface electrocardiogram (ECG) represents the temporospatial average of the action potentials from all myocardial cells (Chapter 13). Figure 40.1 shows the approximate relationship between the action potential from a single ventricular myocyte and the ECG. The rate of upstroke of the action potential defines the time necessary for an individual cardiac cell to depolarize, whereas the duration of the QRS complex approximately represents the time necessary for the entire ventricle to depolarize. Similarly, the action potential duration defines the time required for a single cardiac cell to repolarize, and the QT interval represents the time required for complete ventricular repolarization.

The cardiac action potential can be divided into five phases that reflect time variation in the composition of ionic currents flowing during the cardiac cycle. These ionic currents arise mainly from passive movement of ions through ion channels, pore-forming transmembrane proteins in the cardiac cell membrane. In general, inward Na^+ and Ca^{2+} currents depolarize, whereas outward K^+ currents repolarize the membrane. In atrial and ventricular myocytes and Purkinje fibers, the initial depolarization period (phase 0) of the action potential results from inward Na^+ current (I_{Na}) through Na^+ channels. In the atrioventricular (AV) and sinoatrial (SA) nodal cells, inward Ca^{2+} currents (I_{Ca}) through T- and L-type Ca^{2+} channels produce a slower depolarizing upstroke. This heterogeneity in tissue excitability has profound implications (discussed below) for both cardiac arrhythmogenesis and antiarrhythmic drug therapy.

The QRS complex duration defines the time necessary for ventricular depolarization, whereas the QT interval reflects the time for ventricular repolarization.

The remaining phases of the action potential involve repolarization (Fig. 40.1). The earliest repolarization period (notch, phase 1) results from the transient outward K^+ current (I_{To}) and the inward Cl^- current (I_{Cl}). This is followed by a plateau (phase 2), during which repolarization is delayed, and depolarization is maintained primarily by inward I_{Ca}. The action potential is terminated (phase 3) by the rapid (I_{Kr}) and slow (I_{Ks}) components of delayed rectifier K^+ current (I_K). The duration of the action potential is determined by a delicate balance between these and many other smaller inward and outward currents from both ion channels and electrogenic pumps (e.g. Na^+/Ca^{2+} exchanger, Na^+,K^+-ATPase). $I_{Na/Ca}$ is the current carried by the Na^+/Ca^{2+} exchanger, and is the primary means of Ca^{2+} efflux. Phase 4 is the period when the action potential is maximally repolarized. In atrial and ventricular muscle, the resting potential is maintained near the K^+ equilibrium potential of –90 mV (E_K) by inward rectifier K^+ channels (I_{K1}) and the electrogenic Na^+,K^+-ATPase. In the absence of an applied stimulus (via conduction from a neighboring cell) or an injury that induces inward current (ischemia), these cells remain hyperpolarized and rarely fire action potentials spontaneously. Conversely, SA and AV nodal cells and Purkinje fibers possess inward pacemaker currents (I_f), background Na^+ current ($I_{Na/B}$), and electrogenic pumps (I_{pump}) that shift the resting membrane potential to more positive values (–50 to –70 mV), allowing spontaneous depolarization (pacemaking).

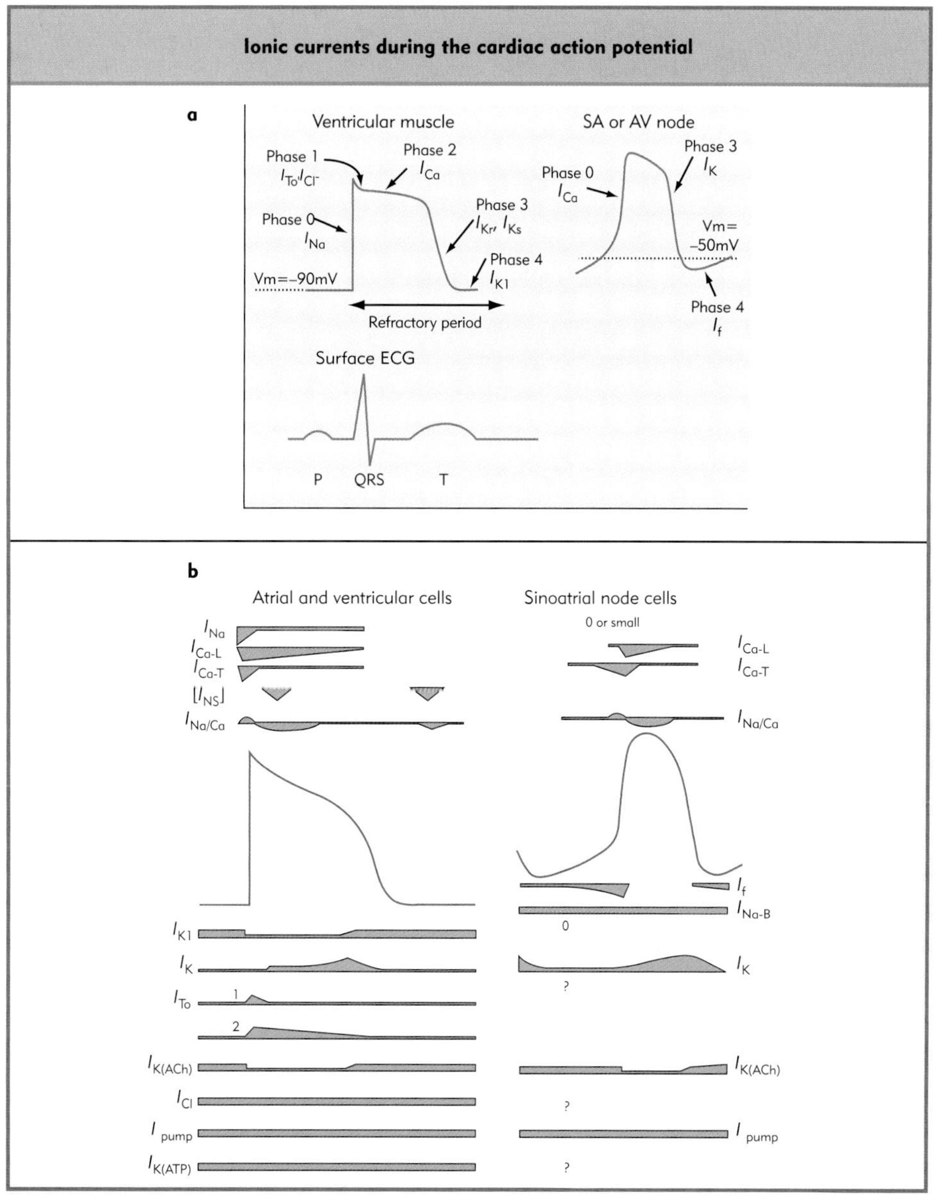

Figure 40.1 Ionic currents during the action potential. (a) The ventricular muscle action potential is shown in relation to the surface electrocardiogram (ECG). A sinoatrial (SA) or atrioventricular (AV) nodal action potential is also shown for comparison. The phases of the action potential (0–4) are shown along with the principal ionic currents (see text) flowing during each phase. Major tissue differences between phase 0 and phase 4 underlie the rationale for several antiarrhythmic therapeutic strategies. (b) The time course of a stylized action potential of atrial, ventricular, and sinoatrial node cells is shown with the various channels and pumps that contribute the currents underlying the electrical events. Where possible, the approximate time courses of the currents associated with the channels or pumps are shown symbolically without effort to represent their magnitudes relative to each other. The channels identified by brackets imply that they are active only under pathologic conditions. For the sinoatrial node cells I_{Na} and I_{K1} are small or absent. I_{NS}, nonselective. (From the Task Force of the Working Group on Arrhythmias of the European Society of Cardiology, 1991.)

STRUCTURE AND FUNCTION OF CARDIAC ION CHANNELS

Function of voltage-gated ion channels

Voltage-gated cation channels are the principal source of transmembrane ionic currents in the heart. The major pore-forming α subunits of these channels are members of a common gene family and possess striking sequence and structural homology (see Chapter 6). Figure 6.4 shows the α subunits of the three classes of voltage-gated cation channel as they are thought to reside in the cardiac cell membrane. The Na^+ and Ca^{2+} channels contain four homologous domains (I–IV), each composed of six transmembrane repeats (S1–S6). Similarly, many voltage-gated K^+ channels (Shaker/K_v families) resemble a single domain of an Na^+ or Ca^{2+} channel and assemble as tetramers to form functional ion-conducting channels.

Figure 40.2 shows a structural model of the outer pore of the voltage-gated Na^+ channel. Each of the four homologous domains contributes approximately 25% of the amino acids that form the outer pore. The structure of the pore is critical not only for conducting permeant ions (Na^+ in this case), but also for binding blocking ions, toxins, and drugs. Using *site-directed mutagenesis* (Fig. 40.2), single amino acid residues in the pore (or other sites) of the channel can be selectively replaced, and the permeation and binding characteristics after these manipulations re-evaluated using 'patch-clamp' single-channel recordings. Using these methods, the residues critical for 'normal' ion channel function may be determined. This hybrid approach, fusing single-channel electrophysiology with molecular biology, has greatly increased our knowledge of ion channel structure–function relationships.

Although voltage-gated ion channels conduct cations passively, they are nonetheless dynamic in nature, continuously opening and closing (gating) in response to changes in membrane potential. Channels open only transiently in response to membrane depolarization; hence the two gating processes critical to ion channel function are *activation* and *inactivation* (Fig. 40.3). Site-directed mutagenesis studies have defined specific regions of the channel critical to gating function; specific regions also appear to have consistent functional importance across the ion channel families. For example, in both Na^+ and K^+ channels the S4 domain contains highly conserved positively charged arginine residues that affect voltage-dependent channel activation during depolarization. By comparison, inactivation processes are more varied. For many K^+ channels the N-terminal domain 'swings' into the pore like a ball on a tether, occluding the pore from the

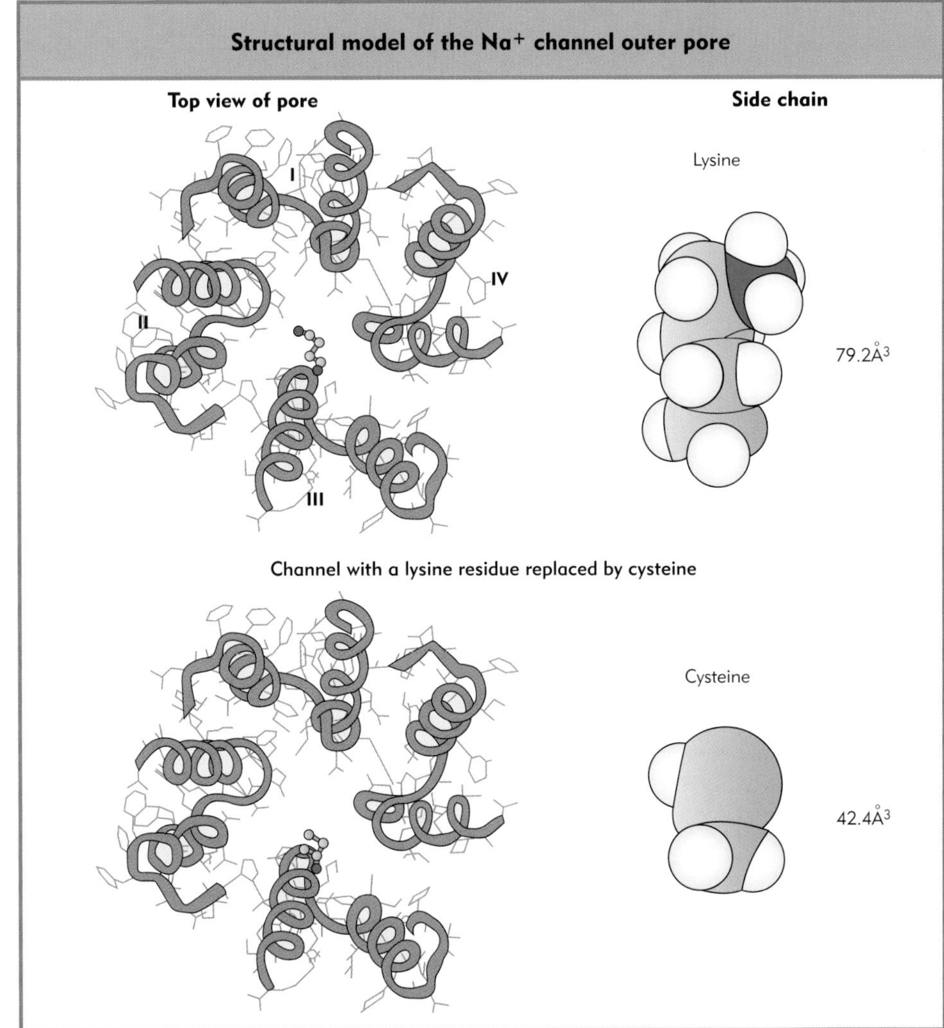

Figure 40.2 Structural model of the Na^+ channel outer pore. The channel is shown as viewed from outside the cell, looking longitudinally down the pore. Selective replacement of a lysine residue by a cysteine residue using site-directed mutagenesis induces changes in both cation block and ion permeation. (With permission from Pérez-Garcia et al. Mechanisms of sodium/calcium selectivity in sodium channels probed by cysteine mutagenesis and sulfhydryl modification. Biophys J. 1997;72:989-96.)

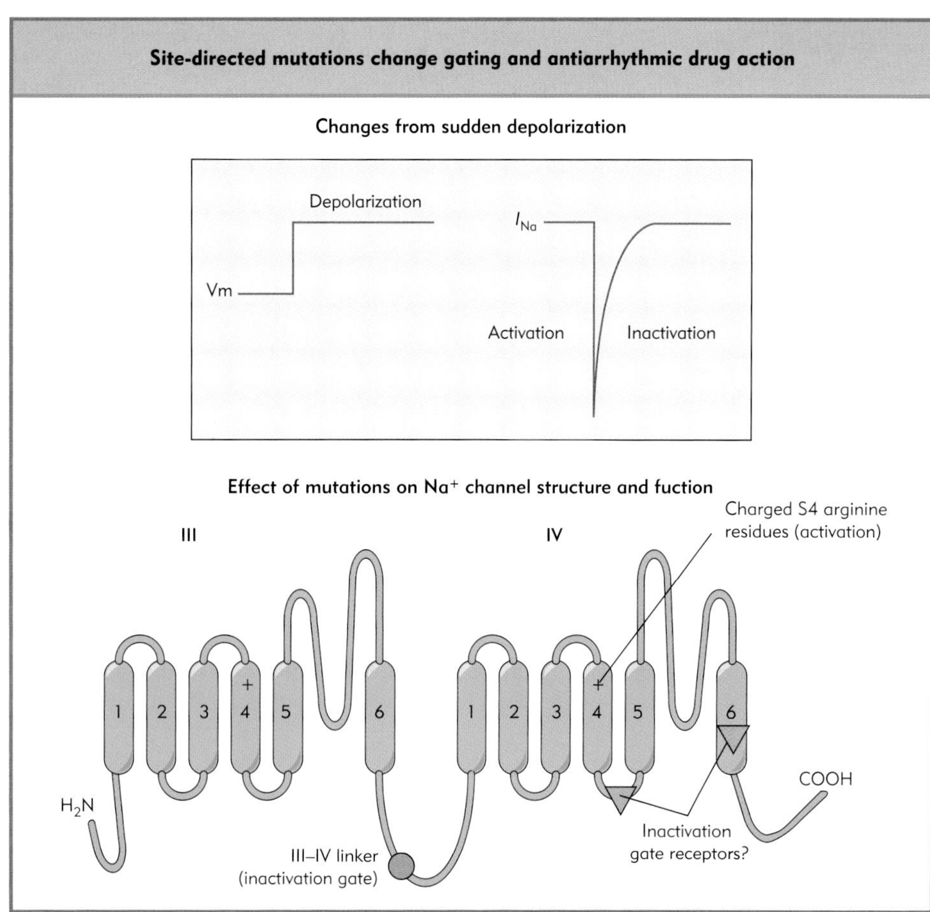

Figure 40.3 Site-directed mutations change gating and antiarrhythmic drug action. When suddenly depolarized, a transient inward Na^+ current (I_{Na}) flows into cardiac cells. This current rapidly activates (as single channels open) and then inactivates (as single channels close) during maintained depolarization (throughout the action potential plateau, phases 2 and 3 in Fig. 40.1). Mutations in specific locations alter gating functions (activation, inactivation) of Na^+ channels and may also attenuate antiarrhythmic drug action.

inside. In an analogous manner, the rapid inactivation process in Na^+ channels seems to involve movement of the domain III–IV linker over the cytoplasmic face of the channel (Fig. 40.3). Receptors for this 'hinged-lid' mechanism are disputed, but may reside on the cytoplasmic ends of the S5 and S6 segments. In addition, slower inactivation mechanisms that involve direct approximation of external pore-lining segments are described for K^+ channels and may also exist in Na^+ channels. Further, activation and inactivation gating may be mechanistically coupled. For example, covalent modification of the *external* S4 arginine residue in the Na^+ channel 'locks' the S4 segment in the outward configuration. This has the paradoxical effect of speeding inactivation, presumably by facilitating binding of the *internal* inactivation gate to its receptor. These coupled interactions emphasize the emerging view that ion channel gating processes involve the ensemble motion of multiple domains rather than individual amino acid residues.

With the cloning of individual ion channel genes it has been possible to unravel the details of cardiac ion channel structure and function. Structural biology has begun to provide high-resolution 3D structures of ion channels, such as the bacterial inward rectifier K^+ channel KcsA. These defined structures of noncardiac channels serve as powerful anchors for hypotheses regarding structure and function in the homologous cardiac ion channels. Table 40.1 indicates the genes encoding cardiac ion channels identified to date, organized to identify the gene products that underlie pharmacologically distinct ionic currents in the heart, many of which are illustrated in Figure 40.1. In some cases, α subunits (pore-forming) and a number of associated β subunits are listed. Some α subunits may be associated with multiple β subunits (i.e. mink/*I*sK). Studies are only now clarifying the key functional manifestations of these αβ subunit interrelationships, and the details of Table 40.1 should dramatically expand over the next decade.

New insights into the linkages between cardiac rhythm, ion channel structure, and the genetic code have emerged from the study of monogenetic cardiac arrhythmia syndromes. These include several varieties of the long QT syndrome (LQT), the idiopathic ventricular fibrillation syndromes (IVF), and genetic syndromes of conduction disease. Although these syndromes affect only small segments of the general population, it is clear that the mechanisms they reveal are fundamentally related to common acquired arrhythmia syndromes. For example, the inherited long QT syndrome is a model for drug-induced QT prolongation, whereas Brugada syndrome mutations may shed light on the mechanism of ischemia-induced re-entry and ventricular tachycardia.

Na^+ channels inform long QT, Brugada, and conduction disease phenotypes

Mutations in *SCN5A*, the gene encoding the cardiac Na^+ channel ($Na_v1.5$), cause a variant of the long QT syndrome (LQT-3), an autosomal dominant disorder in which patients exhibit prolonged ECG QT intervals and are at risk for the polymorphic ventricular tachycardia torsades de pointes. A

Table 40.1 Genes that encode cardiac ion channel α and β subunits. 'Common' names (usually first assigned) are given first, with the currently designated gene name in parentheses. Information obtained from NCBI website (http://www2.ncbi.nlm.nih.gov/), including LocusLink and OMIM, as well as the Human Genome Nomenclature database (http://www.gene.ucl.ac.uk/ nomenclature/). (From Roden et al. Cardiac ion channels. Annu Rev Physiol. 2002; 64:431–75.)

Current	α subunits		β subunits	
	Gene	***Human chromosomal location***	**Gene**	***Human chromosomal location***
Inward currents				
I_{Na}	*SCN5A* *$Na_v1.5$*	3p21	β_1*(SCN1B)* β_2*(SCN2B)*	19q13.1–q13.2 11q23
$I_{Ca\text{-}L}$	α_1*C (CACNL1A1)* *$Ca_v1.2$*	12pter–p13.2	β_1 *(CACNB1)* β_2 *(CACNB2)* $\alpha_2\delta$ *(CACNA2D1)*	17q21–q22 10p12 7q 21–22
$I_{Ca\text{-}T}$	α_1*H (CACNA1H)* *$Ca_v3.X$*	16p13.3		
Outward currents				
I_{Ks}	*KvLQT1 (KCNQ1)*	11p15.5	*minK/IsK (KCNE1)*	21q22.12
I_{Kr}	*HERG (KCNH2)*	7q36–q36	*minK/IsK (KCNE1)* *MiRP1 (KCNE2)*	21q22.12 21q22.12
I_{Kur}	*Kv1.5 (KCNA5)*		*Kv*β*1 (KCNAB1)* *Kv*β*2 (KCNAB2??)*	3q26.1 1p36.3
I_{K1}	*Kir2.1 (KCNJ2)* *Kir2.2 (KCNJ12)*	17q 17p11.1		
$I_{K\text{-}Ach}$	*GIRK1, Kir3.1 (KCNJ3)* *+GIRK4, Kir3.4 (KCNJ5)*	2q24.1 11q24		
$I_{K\text{-}ATP}$	*Kir6.2, BIR (KCNJ11)*	11p15.1	*SUR2 (ABCC9)*	12p12.1
I_{TO}	*Kv4.3 (KCND3)* *Kv1.4 (KCNA4)*	1p13.2 11p14		
I_f, I_h (pacemaker current)	*BCNG2, HCN2, HCN4*	19p13.3 15q24–q25		
I_{Kp}	*TWIK1 (KCNK1)* *CFTR (ABCC7)* *KvLQT1 (KCNQ1)*	1q42–q43 7q31.2 11p15.5	*MiRP1 (KCNE2)*	21q22.12

common mechanism is failure of fast inactivation gating, a so-called 'gain-of-function' mutation resulting in channels that exhibit recurrent openings throughout the action potential plateau. The small net depolarizing 'pedestal' of current through these channels is sufficient to upset the balance between inward and outward currents in the action potential plateau, and hence prolong action potential duration and consequently the QT interval. The first such defect identified was a 9-nucleotide deletion resulting in the deletion of three amino acids (ΔKPQ) in the III–IV linker of the channel (see Fig. 40.3). This finding is consistent with the prominent role of this region in normal fast inactivation. The next two mutations to be described, R1644H and N1325S, are both located in cytoplasmic S4–S5 linkers (Fig. 40.3), supporting a role for these regions as docking sites for the inactivation 'lid'. However, further studies in more kindreds have shown that mutations in other regions of the channel protein also result in defective inactivation. This reinforces the notion that primary sequence changes can exert prominent allosteric effects on distant regions of this large channel protein.

Inherited mutations in *SCN5A* that cause a marked loss of I_{Na} (in contrast to LQT3 'gain of function') cause a form of idiopathic ventricular fibrillation known as Brugada syndrome. Patients with Brugada syndrome experience sudden death in the absence of any detectable heart disease (and a normal QT interval), but do display an unusual electrocardiographic feature, J-point elevation in the right precordial leads. Some Brugada syndrome mutations result in a highly truncated, and therefore nonfunctional, protein, whereas others augment the inactivation gating processes (either fast or slow) to yield a loss of I_{Na}. A third phenotype associated with Na^+ channel mutations is conduction system disease. Computational modeling of these complex effects suggests a small degree of 'loss of function' is sufficient to provoke isolated cardiac conduction disease, whereas a more substantial loss of Na^+ channel function provokes more lethal tachyarrhythmias.

Mutations that impair cardiac Na^+ channel function cause idiopathic ventricular fibrillation. This may explain the enhanced proarrhythmic effect of potent Na^+ channel blockers in ischemia-induced Na^+ channel dysfunction.

The Brugada phenotype may provide insight into the proarrhythmic effects of potent Na^+ channel blockade in the Cardiac Arrhythmia Suppression Trial (CAST), where treatment with the potent Na^+ channel blocking drugs flecainide and encainide enhanced mortality (probably due to arrhythmias) in patients convalescing from acute myocardial infarction. Analysis of the CAST database indicated that the group at highest risk for an increase in drug-associated mortality were those at greatest risk for recurrent myocardial ischemia. Since CAST, studies have identified a reduction in Na^+ channel function in cardiac cells isolated from the ischemic border zone surrounding a cardiac infarct. The clinical observation that flecainide worsens the Brugada syndrome ECG phenotype may suggest a linkage between loss of Na^+ channel function (due to either ischemia or genetic predisposition) and proarrhythmic susceptibility to potent Na^+ channel blocking agents. Determining the extent to which DNA variants in *SCN5A* (or other ion channels) may produce little or no baseline clinical phenotype but nevertheless increase an individual's risk for ventricular arrhythmias on exposure to a range of stressors, including myocardial ischemia or drugs, is a critical future direction of arrhythmia research.

Cardiac Ca^{2+} channels serve as triggers for arrhythmias

Alternatively spliced forms of both the L- and the T-type Ca^{2+} channel have been described in cardiac tissue, and differences in both drug sensitivity and isoform expression in heart failure have been reported. Both L-type Ca^{2+} channel and Na^+ channel numbers are reduced in atrial myocytes from animals with atrial fibrillation, and it is believed that these changes perpetuate the arrhythmia. On the other hand, L-type Ca^{2+} channels have been implicated as a carrier of arrhythmogenic inward current. Prolongation of the action potential increases the amplitude of the intracellular Ca^{2+} transient, activating Ca^{2+}–calmodulin-dependent protein kinase (and thus enhancing L-type Ca^{2+} current and other arrhythmogenic inward currents), and thereby triggering arrhythmogenic early and delayed afterdepolarizations (EADs and DADs). Ca^{2+} channel blockers inhibit arrhythmogenic early EADs under these conditions, as does kinase inhibition. In animal models of hypertrophy, the amplitude of the T-type Ca^{2+} current is increased, reminiscent of the electrophysiologic phenotype observed in fetal cells (which exhibit large T-type currents), perhaps representing reversion to the fetal phenotype.

I_{TO}, the transient outward current, is implicated in heart failure and arrhythmias

A common finding in human heart failure is action potential prolongation, an effect that has been attributed in part to reduction of I_{To}. The extent of reduction of I_{To} and reduction in abundance of mRNA transcripts encoding Kv4.3 in human heart failure correlate, suggesting that heart failure reduces Kv4 channel expression. The mechanisms underlying this transcriptional regulation have not been elucidated, although action potential prolongation and consequent 'triggered' arrhythmias (EADs) as a hypothetical mechanism for sudden death during heart failure are under active investigation. Moreover, the gradient in I_{To} expression across the right ventricular free wall forms the basis of a leading theory for the ECG manifestations of the Brugada syndrome, and may form the basis for the proarrhythmic manifestations of Na^+ channel blockade.

Loss of function mutations in the rapid delayed rectifier K^+ channel and drugs that block it induce long QT syndromes.

I_{Kr}, the rapid repolarizing current

Mutations in *HERG*, the gene encoding I_{Kr}, cause a variety of the congenital long QT syndrome (LQT2), just as drugs that block I_{Kr} evoke the acquired form of the long QT syndrome. I_{Kr} suppression, due to either drugs or mutations, prolongs the cardiac action potential with 'reverse use dependence' (i.e. greatest action potential prolongation at slow rates), such that bradycardia increases the risk for torsades de pointes arrhythmias. A mechanism for this rate dependence may arise from the observation that the counterpart of I_{Kr}, termed I_{Ks} (see below), deactivates more slowly and incompletely at rapid heart rates. Hence, I_{Ks} accumulates at rapid heart rates and exceeds I_{Kr}, whereas at slow rates I_{Kr} is the dominant repolarizing current. Thus I_{Kr} block markedly prolongs the action potential and the QT interval at slow rates or after a long diastolic interval.

The development of excess QT prolongation and torsades de pointes during exposure to many I_{Kr}-blocking drugs is infrequent and largely unpredictable, but certain clinical risk factors can be identified. Similarly, patients with inherited forms of the long QT syndrome have relatively rare arrhythmia events. It is likely that genetic predisposition, drug exposure, hypokalemia, etc., interact to produce torsades de pointes. Thus, patients who develop excess QT prolongation upon drug exposure may have a 'subclinical' genetic defect that slightly impedes repolarization, causing a reduction in 'repolarization reserve'. Only when repolarization reserve is sufficiently impaired (by the addition of drug therapy) does torsades de pointes occur. This hypothesis is supported by reports of patients with inherited ion channel mutations who only present after drug challenge. These reports implicate two distinct mechanisms: 1) increased sensitivity of the *HERG* channel complex to drug block, with a normal baseline ECG but the development of torsade de pointes upon exposure to I_{Kr} blockers; and 2) reduction of I_{Ks} or another repolarizing current that is well tolerated until the superposition of I_{Kr} block. These findings suggest the possibility of genetic screening for patients susceptible to drug-induced arrhythmias. Pharmaceutical companies already screen promising compounds to rule out significant HERG channel blockade.

I_{Ks}, the slow repolarizing current

The Ik_s is mediated by two gene products, the pore-forming *KvLQT1* subunit, and the ancillary *minK* subunit. Autosomal dominant mutations in *KvLQT1* or *minK* evoke varieties of the long QT syndrome. Pharmacologic I_{Ks} block tends to produce homogeneous action potential prolongation in ventricular tissue;

however, β-adrenergic agonists such as isoproterenol evoke marked heterogeneity in action potential duration and arrhythmias. This experimental finding is consistent with the sensitivity of I_{Ks} to adrenergic stimulation, and with the observation that arrhythmias in patients with inherited *KvLQT1* or *minK* mutations usually arise during periods of adrenergic stress. Examination of currents generated by heterologous expression of KvLQT1 and minK channels with inherited mutations in divergent areas of the protein reveals a wide variety of defects that reduce I_{Ks} such as altered channel gating, or failure of the mutant channel to traffic to the cell surface.

The rare Jervell–Lange–Neilson (JLN) variant of the long QT syndrome, associated with congenital deafness, arises in children who inherit abnormal *KvLQT1* or *minK* alleles from both parents. The KvLQT1–minK complex is responsible for endolymph secretion in the inner ear, and its absence in JLN patients results in collapse of the endolymphatic space. This situation arises through consanguinity (i.e. the child inherits alleles each encoding the same abnormal protein), or occasionally by chance (in which case the child inherits alleles that encode different abnormal proteins). Although QT intervals are generally normal in these patients, sudden unexpected death, presumably due to long QT-related arrhythmias, can occur in the parents. This has obvious implications for family screening (and preoperative assessment) of a patient with JLN.

Cardiac inward rectifiers

The K^+ channels encoded by the K_{ir} superfamily (Table 40.1) are notable for the absence of a charged S4 segment (Fig. 40.3), and therefore exhibit less intrinsic voltage-dependent gating. Nonetheless, as their 'inward rectifier' name implies, these K^+ channels pass inward current in preference to outward current, and are primarily operative at hyperpolarized (rather than depolarized) potentials near the cell resting potential (the K^+ equilibrium potential, ~–85 mV). Hence, K_{ir} channels play a key role in 'setting' the myocyte resting potential. The inward rectification of these channels usually reflects block of outward current by intracellular constituents. For I_{K1}, Mg^{2+} alone appears sufficient, whereas for other members of this group polyamines (such as spermidine) have been implicated as further mediators of rectification.

The inward rectifier current I_{K1} probably represents expression of members of the Kir2.x family (Table 40.1). The acetylcholine-gated current ($I_{K\text{-}Ach}$) is recapitulated by coexpression of Kir3.1 and Kir3.4 (also termed GIRK1 and GIRK4), whereas the ATP-inhibited current ($I_{K\text{-}ATP}$) results from coexpression of a Kir6 channel with an ancillary protein, the sulfonylurea receptor (SUR). K_{ATP} channels are widespread and diverse in character, but the cardiac channel is recapitulated by coexpression of Kir6.2 with SUR2. SUR2 is a member of the ATP-binding-cassette (ABC) superfamily that includes the cystic fibrosis transport regulator (CFTR). Members of this family share a common structural motif, consisting of 12 putative membrane-spanning segments and two intracellular ATP-binding cassettes.

In addition to maintenance of the resting membrane potential, evidence supporting a role for Kir2.1/I_{K1} in the terminal phase of cardiac repolarization has come from the linkage of mutations in Kir2.1 with Andersen's syndrome, a neuromuscular disease whose manifestations include unusual forms of ventricular tachycardia. Acetylcholine activates $I_{K\text{-}Ach}$ via a G protein-delineated pathway, and activation of this channel is partly responsible for bradycardia and the slowing of AV conduction seen with vagal stimulation. ATP-sensitive K^+ channels also provide a link between the metabolic state of the cell and electrophysiologic activity. Several drugs activate these channels, but are not cardiac specific ('K^+ channel openers' such as nicorandil or pinacidil); cardiac-specific agents, on the horizon, may be useful to protect the myocardium against the deleterious effects of ischemia (including arrhythmias). ATP-sensitive channels are expressed not only on the cell surface, but also in mitochondria, where they may also be attractive targets for cardioprotection.

Pacemaker currents allow spontaneous depolarization

The cardiac rhythm is generated in sinus node cells by an inward current that continually depolarizes the cell toward its firing threshold during phase 4 of the action potential. Unlike other cardiac ionic currents activated by depolarization, this hyperpolarization-activated pacemaker current has been termed 'funny' (I_f) or 'hyperpolarization-activated' (I_h). The pacemaker channel superfamily includes cyclic nucleotide-binding domains in its C terminus, and pacemaker activity is regulated in vivo by cAMP-mediated adrenergic signaling pathways. Three members of this superfamily (HCN1, HCN2, and HCN4) have been found in mouse heart. Heterologous expression of these channels produces a hyperpolarization-activated current that, like I_h, displays only very weak selectivity for K^+ over Na^+, with a reversal potential of –35 mV. Although HCN channels display the typical six-membrane segment spanning architecture of voltage-gated K^+ channels, the mechanisms for their unusual hyperpolarization-activated gating and lack of selectivity may involve sequence differences in the S4 sensor and the selectivity filter regions of the pore.

The zebra fish mutant 'Smo' contains a mutation in a single HCN gene and displays marked heart rate slowing, but only partial loss of the I_h current (specifically, a fast kinetic component), suggesting that the total I_h current may represent an ensemble current from several different gene products. In addition to pacemaker cells, I_h current can be elicited by excessive hyperpolarization in ventricular muscle cells, suggesting that altered regulation of this current could underlie ventricular arrhythmias during pathologic conditions. The molecular basis of regulation of I_h by intracellular signaling systems has not been elucidated, nor have mechanisms to modify I_h function in bradyarrhythmias using pharmacologic agents, although this strategy may hold future promise as the molecular basis of I_h is elucidated.

Other background currents

In addition to currents that exhibit time- and voltage-dependent gating properties, voltage clamp studies of heart cells reveal additional currents that do not exhibit gating characteristics, known generally as 'background' currents. It has been suggested that expression of the twin-pore K^+ channel, known as TWIK-1, may underlie background current. Some data suggest that Cl^- channels (CFTR) may also underlie background current, as CFTR transcripts can be identified in heart. More generally, studies have identified Cl^- channels activated by changes in cell volume, as well as intracellular Ca^{2+}. Whether any background currents are appropriate targets for drug therapy is not yet known.

TISSUE DIVERSITY AND CELLULAR ARRHYTHMIA MECHANISMS

Tissue diversity, the conduction system, and adenosine

Diversity in the molecular basis for phase 0 among cardiac tissues figures critically in the physiology and pharmacology of cardiac arrhythmias (Fig. 40.1). The rate of the upstroke of the action potential is a determinant of conduction velocity through excitable tissue. Because I_{Ca} develops much more slowly than I_{Na}, impulses conduct through atrial and ventricular muscle far more rapidly than in the AV node. This tissue diversity protects the ventricle from fibrillation during very rapid atrial arrhythmias. Because β-blockers and Ca^{2+} channel blockers reduce Ca^{2+} current primarily (through G protein-mediated pathways and direct channel blockade, respectively), these agents slow conduction in the SA and AV node but not in ventricular myocardium. Hence, these agents slow the rate of ventricular stimulation during rapid atrial arrhythmias (a principal indication for their use), and may also terminate supraventricular rhythms that involve the SA or AV node primarily in a re-entrant pathway. Conversely, agents that selectively block Na^+ channels (local anesthetics) are not useful in these settings, but may be useful in terminating arrhythmias that arise in ventricular muscle, where I_{Na} predominates. Although β-blockers are effective in the *chronic* management of ventricular arrhythmias, the molecular mechanisms are ill defined and may ultimately involve voltage-gated ion channels indirectly through second-messenger systems. The acute effect of most agents that reduce I_{Ca} (β-blockers indirectly via G protein-coupled pathways, and Ca^{2+} channel blockers directly) in ventricular muscle is attenuation of the action potential plateau. This reduces intracellular Ca^{2+} and may induce negative inotropic effects (see Chapter 42).

Molecular diversity in the ion channels that mediate phase 0 and phase 4 depolarization between cardiomyocytes and AV and SA nodal tissue results in critical differences in physiology and pharmacology.

Phase 4, like phase 0, is another period where major differences exist between atrial and ventricular muscle and SA and AV nodal tissue (Fig. 40.1). Adenosine A_1 receptors exist in both atrial and nodal tissues and activate the K^+ current $I_{K(ACh.Ado)}$, which hyperpolarizes the cell membrane potential (transiently) to more negative potentials. This has less effect in atrial tissue (already at −90 mV), but drives pacemaker cells in the AV and SA nodes farther from the action potential firing threshold, slowing their rate. Adenosine also antagonizes adenylyl cyclase and thereby slows AV nodal conduction by a second mechanism: inhibition of I_{Ca}. Hence, adenosine has effects on supraventricular tachycardias that relate specifically to the tissue responsible for their generation.

It is mechanistically useful to group supraventricular arrhythmias by their responses to adenosine (Table 40.2). Supraventricular arrhythmias arising from re-entry in the atrium exhibit transient slowing of the ventricular rate in response to adenosine; however, the rate of atrial discharges (P waves) does not change significantly. Moreover, slowing the rate of QRS complexes in this manner may unmask P waves on the surface ECG and facilitate diagnosis. Atrial tachycardias resulting from abnormal phase 4 depolarization may transiently slow, or even stop, with adenosine if they are caused by cAMP-mediated triggered activity. Arrhythmias that involve AV nodal tissue in the re-entry pathway are terminated by adenosine. AV junctional rhythms (common during general anesthesia) have an inconsistent response to adenosine based on their variable etiology (re-entrant, automatic). Ventricular arrhythmias usually originate in tissues distal to the conduction system, and therefore exhibit no response to adenosine administration. Conversely, adenosine administration should induce some change (termination, ventricular rate reduction) in the R–R interval of wide

Table 40.2 Supraventricular tachyarrhythmias and their typical responses to bolus adenosine administration

Arrhythmia	Mechanism	Adenosine response
AV nodal re-entry	Re-entry within the AV node	Termination
AV reciprocating tachycardias	Re-entry involves AV node and accessory pathway (WPW)	Termination
Unifocal, multifocal atrial tachycardias	Re-entry in the atrium	Transiently slows QRS rate
Atrial flutter/fibrillation	Re-entry in the atrium	Transiently slows QRS rate
Other atrial tachycardias	Abnormal automaticity or cAMP-mediated triggered activity	Transient suppression or termination
Junctional rhythms	Variable	Variable

AV, atrioventricular; WPW, Wolff–Parkinson–White syndrome.

complex supraventricular rhythms. Diagnostic use of adenosine in this setting may prevent inappropriate therapy of ventricular tachycardia with Ca^{2+} channel blockers, which have longer elimination kinetics.

Cell-to-cell coupling

An intrinsic feature of cardiac excitability is cell-to-cell conduction of electrical impulses. As a result of this coupling, the electrical behavior of one cell heavily influences that of its neighbors. Coupling effects may even supersede the intrinsic electrical behavior of the cell. Quantitative models suggest that coupling is a critical factor in arrhythmogenesis. Spatial inhomogeneities in cardiac conduction are not essential for induction or the maintainance of arrhythmias; nonetheless, they make it easier to generate re-entrant arrhythmias. Such spatial inhomogeneities may result from either naturally occurring barriers to conduction (heart valves, tissue bundles) or from pathologic remodeling after myocardial infarction.

The structural correlate of cell-to-cell coupling is the gap junction, a macromolecular structure that interconnects cells with small channels and allows for the passage of ions. The distribution of gap junctions partly dictates the rate of conduction through tissue. For example, fast-conducting tissue (atrial and ventricular muscle, Purkinje fibers) has more extensive cell-to-cell coupling than slow-conducting tissue (SA and AV nodes). Each individual gap junction channel (known as connexons) comprises six connexin molecules, which co-assemble to form pores. It remains unclear whether primary abnormalities in the genes coding for these molecules form the basis of congenital disorders in conduction. The molecular substrates of cell-to-cell coupling may prove to be viable targets for pharmacologic or gene-therapeutic arrhythmia interventions.

Re-entry and arrhythmogenesis

Re-entry, which underlies most supraventricular and ventricular arrhythmias, involves the continuous movement of an impulse around a re-entrant loop (Fig. 40.4). The loop must be long enough to allow recovery of Na^+ and Ca^{2+} channels from inactivation (the refractory period) between passes. The 'excitable gap' refers to the time between recovery of tissue in the re-entrant loop and the arrival of the next impulse, and is related to the size and speed of conduction in the re-entrant loop. Anatomic sites for re-entry that can be affected by disease include the AV node (AV nodal re-entrant tachycardia), accessory pathways (Wolff–Parkinson–White syndrome, AV reciprocating tachycardia), and ventricular myocardium (ventricular scar after myocardial infarction: monomorphic ventricular tachycardias). These re-entrant pathways are thought to possess long excitable gaps. In contrast, a more *functional* form of re-entry occurs when an impulse propagates around a refractory core. During myocardial ischemia, re-entry may result from disparities in repolarization rates across tissues, both between normal and ischemic epicardium and between epicardial and endocardial layers. The electrical impulse finds the shortest circuit that allows tissue beyond the leading edge of excitability to recover, producing a short excitable gap. More sophisticated models of re-entry include the leading circle model, the figure-of-eight model, the anisotropic model, and the spiral wave model. Fibrillation in either the atrium or the ventricle may involve numerous coexistent functional re-entry circuits (micro re-entry).

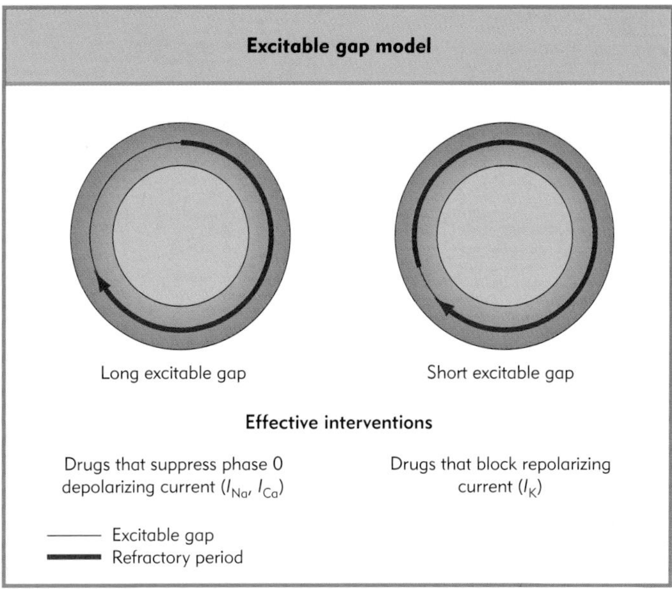

Figure 40.4 Excitable gap models for re-entry and pharmacologic intervention. Long-gap re-entry implies that the conduction loop is very long relative to the tissue refractory period, so there is a long period between complete recovery of tissue excitability and the next impulse. Short excitable gap re-entry implies the opposite: there is little time for the tissue to recover between impulses. Whereas fixed anatomic pathways for re-entry may have long excitable gaps (scar, accessory bundles), functional re-entry circuits are thought to possess short excitable gaps (fibrillating myocardium).

Our ability to relate mechanisms of re-entry to pharmacologic intervention is primitive; nonetheless, it is possible that re-entrant arrhythmias exhibit differential sensitivities to antiarrhythmic agents based on the length of their excitable gap. Drugs with Na^+ channel blocking activity should suppress currents responsible for the action potential upstroke in atrium and ventricle, and drugs with Ca^{2+} channel blocking effects should do the same in the SA or AV node. Hence, these drugs should provide antiarrhythmic action by slowing or blocking conduction. Re-entrant circuits with long excitable gaps may be most susceptible to this mechanism, as long excitable gaps may be insensitive to small changes in the refractory period. Alternatively, drugs that prolong repolarization (K^+ channel blockers) prolong the refractory period and might therefore extinguish the leading edge of impulse propagation in a re-entrant circuit with a short excitable gap. In support of this concept, agents that prolong the refractory period have been most successful in suppressing fibrillation of both the atrium and the ventricle.

Automaticity and arrhythmia suppression

Normally, atrial and ventricular tissues do not spontaneously undergo phase 4 depolarization. *Abnormal automaticity* or *depolarization-induced automaticity* refers to spontaneous depolarization caused by a pathophysiologic process, such as ischemia. Such automaticity may underlie unifocal and multifocal atrial tachycardias and ventricular tachycardias in the initial days following acute myocardial infarction. Maneuvers to hyperpolarize the atrial cell during phase 4 (adenosine) may be clinically effective. *Triggered automaticity* includes arrhythmias that arise from afterdepolarizations during or following complete repolarization. 'Early afterdepolarizations' (EADs) arise during phase

2 or 3, whereas 'delayed afterdepolarizations' (DADs) begin after completion of phase 3 and result from mechanisms distinct from EADs. The ion channels that underlie the depolarizing currents responsible for EADs and DADs are debated.

The major factor predisposing to EAD formation is action potential prolongation in the ventricle. Low serum K^+ concentrations, slow heart rates, and repolarization-prolonging antiarrhythmic drugs provoke EADs in vitro, and identical factors induce QT interval prolongation and torsades de pointes in patients. Ironically, these conditions are not pathologic in the atrium, and repolarization-prolonging drugs are the most common pharmacologic means of converting atrial fibrillation (Chapter 41). As discussed above, specific ion channel mutations induce congenital forms of the long QT syndrome which genetically predispose patients to torsades de pointes. One subtype (LQT-2), which results from a defect in the I_{Kr} component of repolarizing current, is enhanced by slow heart rates. Further, low K^+ concentrations reduce the magnitude of I_{Kr}. Notably, I_{Kr} is a target for most of the available antiarrhythmic agents that prolong repolarization. Therefore, the QT-prolonging effects of antiarrhythmic drug therapy appear to be analogous to the mechanisms involved in the congenital arrhythmias.

The major factor underlying DAD is an increase in intracellular Ca^{2+}. Although many conditions produce Ca^{2+} overload, digitalis toxicity and unopposed catecholamines are common causes. Catecholamines may underlie triggered activity during exercise, acute myocardial infarction, or perioperative stress. As such, DADs may underlie either supraventricular or ventricular tachycardias in perioperative patients who have no structural heart disease. Digitalis toxicity produces Ca^{2+} overload indirectly by inhibition of the Na^+ pump. Consequent high intracellular Na^+ limits the normal Ca^{2+} extrusion from the cell by the Na^+/Ca^{2+} exchanger. Catecholamines indirectly induce Ca^{2+} overload by increasing I_{Ca} through G protein-mediated pathways. DAD-induced arrhythmias may respond to maneuvers aimed at lowering intracellular Ca^{2+}, including Ca^{2+} channel blockade.

COMMON PERIOPERATIVE ARRHYTHMIAS

Perioperative atrial fibrillation

Atrial fibrillation is the most common perioperative tachyarrhythmia requiring pharmacologic intervention and it provides an opportunity to examine the relationship between arrhythmia mechanisms and drug selection. The agents most often used intraoperatively to control ventricular rate are the Ca^{2+} channel blockers, because of their effects on AV nodal conduction. These agents do not influence conduction in normal atrial tissue and therefore have little or no potential for converting atrial fibrillation. Nonetheless, in patients with accessory pathways these agents may paradoxically (either directly or indirectly) facilitate conduction through the accessory pathway and thereby induce malignant ventricular arrhythmias. Procainamide and amiodarone, agents that block both Na^+ and K^+ channels (Table 40.3), are most commonly used to attempt intravenous pharmacologic conversion of atrial fibrillation. Procainamide prolongs repolarization through both its own action and the action of its principal metabolite, *N*-acetylprocainamide. The efficacy of intravenous procainamide for conversion of atrial fibrillation is not well established. Largely owing to its repolarization-prolonging action, intravenous amiodarone is used to treat atrial fibrillation in patients where procainamide or other agents fail. The risk–benefit ratio for amiodarone in this setting has not been established, and valid concerns exist regarding potential pulmonary toxicity with perioperative use. As with procainamide, studies have not shown that intravenous amiodarone provides conversion to sinus rhythm at a rate exceeding that of placebo. Ibutilide is a potent, rapidly acting class III antiarrhythmic compound with 'pure' cardiac action potential-prolonging activity and few noncardiac side effects. Conversion rates for atrial fibrillation among nonsurgical patients have been remarkably high (~30% within 30 minutes), suggesting that selective K^+ channel blockade is an effective strategy for converting atrial fibrillation. Unfortunately, the pure repolarization-prolonging action of ibutilide manifests in the ventricle as well, and significant numbers of patients (>5%) receiving this agent experience torsades de pointes. It has been advised that this drug be used cautiously in patients in uncontrolled settings or those with underlying heart disease, and the risk–benefit ratio for its perioperative use is not yet clear. Because of this potential for inciting torsades de pointes, current strategies for therapeutic intervention in atrial fibrillation include the development of more selective K^+ channel blockers that may inhibit K^+ channel activity in the atrium but not the ventricle.

Table 40.3 Antiarrhythmic drug classification. These antiarrhythmic agents are available in intravenous form and used in anesthesiology and critical care. Agents are listed according to their preferred molecular target, but generally follow the original classification described by Vaughan Williams

Class[a]	Molecular target	Antiarrhythmic agents
IA	Na^+ and K^+ channels	Procainamide, quinidine, amiodarone[b]
IB	Na^+ channels	Lidocaine, phenytoin
II	β-adrenoceptors	Esmolol, propranolol, amiodarone
III	K^+ channels	Bretylium, ibutilide, amiodarone[b]
IV	Ca^{2+} channels	Verapamil, diltiazem, amiodarone

[a] Class IC agents (propafenone, flecainide) are potent Na^+ channel antagonists but are approved in the USA for oral administration only.
[b] While Amiodarone often prolongs the QT, it rarely causes forsades de pointes.

Atrial fibrillation is the most common perioperative tachyarrhythmia requiring pharmalogical intervention.

Some AV nodal blocking agents may also effect conversion to sinus rhythm. Intravenous Mg^{2+} effects conversion of atrial fibrillation at a rate exceeding that with either verapamil or amiodarone. In surgical and nonsurgical patients with recent onset atrial fibrillation, ventricular rate control with β-blockers produces a more rapid rate of conversion to sinus rhythm than rate control with Ca^{2+} channel blockers. Serum catecholamine levels are elevated following major surgery, and the arrhythmogenic potential of catecholamines in the human atrium is well established. Hence, unopposed β-adrenergic stimulation may be a factor contributing to atrial fibrillation in both perioperative and other settings. Because Mg^{2+}influences numerous voltage-gated ion channels and second-messenger systems in cardiac cells, the mechanism by which it accelerates conversion of atrial fibrillation is unclear. It may partly mimic β-blockade through reduction of catecholamine release from both peripheral and adrenal sources.

Ventricular arrhythmias

Coordinated ventricular contractions are essential for effective cardiac output from the ventricles. Ventricular arrhythmias are grouped according to their ECG morphology (Table 40.4). Because direct correlation between morphology and molecular mechanism is incomplete, the therapeutic principles are also somewhat empiric. Nonsustained ventricular tachycardias, including premature ventricular beats or runs of ventricular tachycardia lasting 30 seconds or less, often require no therapy. In fact, clinical studies in which patients were treated with class I antiarrhythmic drugs for nonsustained ventricular arrhythmias found death rates from proarrhythmic effects that exceeded those of placebo.

Sustained ventricular tachycardias may have either a monomorphic or a polymorphic morphology. In monomorphic ventricular tachycardia the amplitude of each QRS complex mimics its predecessor; the converse is true in polymorphic ventricular tachycardia, in which the QRS complex amplitude and axis change continuously in a sinusoidal or irregular pattern. Monomorphic ventricular tachycardia is thought to result from re-entry associated with scar tissue from a healed myocardial infarction. Although lidocaine is the traditional primary therapy for this arrhythmia, procainamide may be more effective. Our understanding of antiarrhythmic mechanisms and vulnerable parameters does not adequately explain why the addition of repolarization-prolonging activity with procainamide should markedly increase antiarrhythmic efficacy against monomorphic ventricular arrhythmias that presumably have a long excitable gap. If, in addition to the anatomic substrate, the re-entry loop involves tissue with inhomogeneous refractory periods (epicardial versus endocardial), and procainamide has differential effects on refractory period in these tissues, the agent may suspend re-entry by making repolarization more uniform.

When ventricular tachycardia is polymorphic, the mechanism of the arrhythmia profoundly influences the selection of antiarrhythmic therapy. Polymorphic ventricular tachycardia in the presence of corrected QT interval (QT_C) prolongation, whether acquired (e.g. from class IA or III antiarrhythmics or other drugs that prolong repolarization) or congenital, is torsades de pointes. Interventions for torsades de pointes are aimed at reducing the likelihood of EAD, and therefore include measures to increase heart rate and normalize QT_C (pacing, catecholamines, electrolytes). Conversely, polymorphic ventricular tachycardia without QT_C prolongation, common in settings of ischemia or structural heart disease, is managed with therapy similar to that for monomorphic ventricular tachycardia or ventricular fibrillation (Table 40.3). Randomized trials in ambulatory patients experiencing sudden death (VT/VF) suggest that amiodarone may be superior to lidocaine or placebo in supporting short-term survival. The most recent evidence-based recommendations by the American Heart Association have therefore changed the recommendation for lidocaine in VT/VF to 'indeterminate', below that for amiodarone and procainamide.

PACING AND CARDIAC ELECTROVERSION

Pacing and capture

Pacing has assumed a prominent place among the therapies for pathologic bradycardias and some tachycardias. Drug therapies are often limited in their ability to restore a hemodynamically effective cardiac rhythm in the face of sinus node dysfunction or severe conduction block. Temporary or permanent pacing can reduce the requirement for drug therapies, which often carry unwanted side effects. Pacemakers stimulate the heart by delivering a constant voltage (2.5–5.0 V) to the endocardial or epicardial surface of the atrium, the ventricle, or both. The amount of current that enters the myocardium depends on the impedance of the lead–tissue interface and the pulse characteristics (duration, strength). The minimum amount of current needed to stimulate and capture the myocardium (pacing threshold) is determined by both tissue and pacemaker variables.

Table 40.4 Classification of ventricular arrhythmias by electrocardiographic morphology

Arrhythmia	Usual substrate	Usual therapy
Nonsustained ventricular tachycardia (VT)	Normal ventricle	No drug therapy Search for reversible etiologies
Sustained VT Monomorphic VT[a]	Prior myocardial infarction (scar)	Lidocaine, then procainamide, bretylium or amiodarone
Polymorphic VT with normal QT interval	Acute ischemia, infarction, idiopathic cardiomyopathy	Defibrillation, same as for monomorphic VT
Ventricular fibrillation	Acute ischemia, infarction, idiopathic cardiomyopathy	Defibrillation, same as for monomorphic VT
Polymorphic VT with long QT interval (torsades de pointes)	Congenital, prior therapy with drugs prolonging repolarization	Mg^{2+}, pacing, lidocaine or phenytoin; consider amiodarone[b]

[a] Hemodynamically stable patients may respond better to procainamide than to lidocaine.
[b] Amiodarone induces polymorphic VT but is less proarrhythmic in this regard than other antiarrhythmics (class IA, IC, and II), and may be useful when other measures fail.

'Failure to capture' is a common difficulty with temporary pacing in the operating room, as well as with permanent pacemakers, and requires consideration of both pacemaker technology and the cellular events that underlie cardiac impulse propagation. Pacemakers stimulate the cardiac cell through cathodal stimulation; that is, the stimulating electrode injects current into the underlying cardiac tissue, causing direct depolarization of cells in its vicinity. This results in activation and opening of Na^+ channels, producing further intrinsic depolarization of these cells. Once an action potential is generated, the impulse spreads throughout the heart via cell-to-cell coupling through gap junctions. Inability to capture is caused by failure either to deliver stimulation or to depolarize sufficient myocardium for action potential propagation. Ongoing studies attempt to define novel mechanisms by which electrical stimulation may excite the heart (anodal and cathodal break stimulation, virtual cathode effects), and these may dramatically alter our approach to pacing.

Pacing failure usually results from mechanical factors (battery depletion, lead fracture or dislodgement, etc.), whereas depolarization and action potential propagation failure results from inflammation and fibrosis at the electrode–tissue interface. The latter process, termed 'lead maturation', is less problematic with the use of steroid-eluting electrodes. Loss of capture months to years after implantation, known as exit block, frequently results from failure of myocardial cells to propagate action potentials, and may be caused by a variety of conditions. Pathophysiologic states that cause cardiac tissue to depolarize, such as hyperkalemia, acidosis, and ischemia, induce Na^+ channel inactivation and prevent action potential generation (and propagation). Virtually all antiarrhythmic agents, especially those with class I activity, raise pacing thresholds. Similarly, drugs that impair conduction through other mechanisms (β-blockers) raise pacing thresholds. Inhalational anesthetics do not significantly affect pacing thresholds or impulse propagation. Drugs that enhance conduction, such as sympathomimetic agents, lower the pacing threshold, as do physiologic conditions that raise sympathetic tone, such as exercise and stress. Recognition of these important physiologic and pharmacologic variables is helpful in perioperative situations where pacing thresholds may change.

Defibrillators

Electroversion, through either external defibrillators or implanted (internal) cardioverter–defibrillators (ICD), involves the application of high-energy capacitor discharges to depolarize a large mass of myocardium simultaneously with the goal of abruptly terminating an abnormal rhythm. *Cardioversion* is utilized specifically for re-entrant tachycardias (either atrial or ventricular) and refers to the application of discharges that are synchronized with the QRS complex. Cardioversion terminates re-entrant arrhythmias by simultaneously depolarizing the entire re-entrant pathway, thus removing the arrhythmia substrate. Antiarrhythmic agents have limited efficacy for converting re-entrant arrhythmias and have undesirable side effects. Nonetheless, cardioversion may fail, either primarily or secondarily. Successfully cardioverted tachyarrhythmias may recur if the conditions inducing the re-entrant pathway are not corrected; hence, antiarrhythmic drug therapy may be a necessary supplement to cardioversion. Arrhythmias resulting from automatic or triggered automaticity may be resistant to cardioversion (ectopic atrial tachycardia, torsades de pointes).

Defibrillation refers to the asynchronous discharge of current to the myocardium and is indicated for pulseless ventricular arrhythmias, including ventricular fibrillation. The higher energy requirements for converting ventricular fibrillation reflect the involvement of the entire ventricle in multiple functional re-entry circuits (micro re-entry). With external defibrillation, the major factor determining success is transthoracic resistance, which is a function of not only tissue variables but also ventilatory phase and electrode size. Consequently, internal defibrillation, via either internal devices (internal cardioverter–defibrillators) or open thoracotomy, dramatically lowers the energy requirement. Most antiarrhythmic drugs raise the defibrillation threshold (bretylium and lidocaine are possible exceptions). Additionally, physiologic factors, including hypothermia, acidosis, or hypoxemia, may lower the success of defibrillatory shocks. As with cardioversion, antiarrhythmic drugs are useful as adjuncts to defibrillation in patients where ventricular fibrillation is recurrent and prompt elimination of the arrhythmia substrate is not feasible.

According to the updated ACC/AHA/NASPE Guidelines for implantation of ICDs, ICD insertion is a class IIa indication (weight of evidence/opinion in favor of usefulness/efficacy) for patients with an ejection fraction of ≤30% who are at least 1 month post myocardial infarction and 3 months post coronary artery revascularization surgery. This recommendation was based on a study where 1232 patients with a prior myocardial infarction and reduced left ventricular ejection fraction (≤30%) were randomized to receive an implantable defibrillator or conventional medical therapy. No electrophysiologic testing was required prior to randomization. There was a 31% reduction in the risk of death in patients receiving defibrillators compared to those receiving conventional medical therapy. This study is significant because in the United States alone 3–4 million patients have coronary artery disease and advanced left ventricular dysfunction, and there are 400 000 new cases annually. With the increase in patients who may benefit from defibrillator placement, the likelihood that these patients will present for noncardiac surgery also increases.

Electromagnetic interference

The major perioperative issue regarding pacemakers and ICDs is the risk of electromagnetic interference (EMI) from electrocautery or cardioversion. EMI can result in inhibition of pacemaker output, activation of a rate-responsive sensor resulting in increased pacing rate, ICD firing, and myocardial injury at the lead tip, resulting in failure to sense and/or capture. Improved pacemaker and ICD design, including the nearly universal use of bipolar leads and better shielding from EMI, has greatly reduced the probability of these adverse interactions. Except in urgent or emergency situations, management of pacemakers and ICDs in the perioperative setting begins with the preoperative visit, which should include documentation of cardiac history, including the type of device, indication, and date of device implantation. Because pacemakers and ICDs are programmable, obtaining the most recent interrogation report can be helpful in determining magnet response, and although definitive guidelines have yet to be established, it is recommended that ICDs be reprogrammed to suspend arrhythmia detection in cases where electrocautery is used, to prevent unintended therapy due to EMI. Magnet suspension of arrhythmia detection can also be used with most ICDs if the feature is programmed into the device, leaving the pacemaker function of some ICDs unaffected.

Key references

American Heart Asociation. Guidelines 2000 for Cardiopulmonary Resuscitation and Emergency Cardiovascular Care. Part 6: advanced cardiovascular life support: 7D: the tachycardia algorithms. The American Heart Association in collaboration with the International Liaison Committee on Resuscitation. Circulation 2000;102:I158–65.

Atlee JL. Perioperative cardiac dysrhythmias: diagnosis and management. Anesthesiology 1997;86:1397–424.

Engelstein ED, Lippman N, Stein KM, Lerman BB. Mechanism-specific effects of adenosine on atrial tachcycardia. Circulation 1994;89:2645–54.

Hondeghem LM, Katzung BG. Time- and voltage-dependent interactions of the antiarrhythmic drugs with cardiac sodium channels. Biochim Biophys Acta. 1977;472:373–98.

Roden DM, Balser JR, George AL Jr, Anderson ME. Cardiac ion channels. Annu Rev Physiol. 2002;64:431–75.

Tan HL, Bink-Boelkens MTE, Bezzina CR et al. A sodium channel mutation causes isolated cardiac conduction disease. Nature 2001;409:1043.

Yu FH, Catterall WA. Overview of the voltage-gated sodium channel family. Genome Biol. 2003;4:207.

Further reading

Bennett PB, Yazawa K, Naomasa M et al. Molecular mechanism for an inherited cardiac arrhythmia. Nature 1995;376:683.

Chen Q, Kirsch GE, Zhang D et al. Genetic basis and molecular mechanism for idiopathic ventricular fibrillation. Nature 1998;392:293.

Echt DS, Liebson PR, Mitchell LB et al. Mortality and morbidity in patients receiving encainide, flecainide, or placebo. New Engl J Med. 1991; 324: 781–8.

Gregoratos G, Abrams J, Epstein AE et al. ACC/AHA/NASPE 2002 guideline update for implantation of cardiac pacemakers and antiarrhythmia devices: summary article: a report of the American College of Cardiology/American Heart Association Task Force on Practice Guidelines (ACC/AHA/NASPE Committee to Update the 1998 Pacemaker Guidelines). Circulation 2002;106:2145–61.

Lukas A, Antzelevitch C. Differences in the electrophysiological response of canine ventricular epicardium and endocardium to ischemia: role of the transient outward current. Circulation 1993;88:2903–15.

Roden DM, Hoffman BF. Action potential prolongation and induction of abnormal automaticity by low quinidine concentrations in canine Purkinje fibers. Relationship to potassium and cycle length. Circ Res. 1985;56:857–67.

Sauguinetti MC, Jiang C, Curran ME, Keating MT. A mechanistic link between an inherited and an acquired cardiac arrhythmia: HERG encodes the I_{Kr} potassium channel. Cell 1995;81:299–307.

Spach MS, Heidlage JF. The stochastic nature of cardiac propagation at a microscopic level. Electrical description of myocardial architecture and its application to conduction. Circ Res. 1995;76:366–80.

Chapter 41

Cardiovascular pharmacology

David F Stowe

TOPICS COVERED IN THIS CHAPTER

- **Classification of cardiovascular drugs**
- **Positive inotropic and chronotropic drugs with secondary vascular effects**
  - Catecholamine agonists
- **Positive inotropic drugs with vasodilatory effects**
  - Phosphodiesterase III inhibitors
- **Positive chronotropic drugs**
  - Cholinergic receptor antagonists
- **Positive inotropic drugs**
  - Cardiac glycosides
- **Vasoconstrictor drugs**
  - Sympathomimetic α_1-adrenergic agonists
  - Non sympathomimetic vasocontrictor drugs
- **Vasodilator drugs**
  - Guanylyl cyclase activators
  - α_2-adrenergic receptor antagonists
  - Angiotensin-converting enzyme (ACE) inhibitors
  - Miscellaneous
- **Vasodilator drugs with negative inotropic and chronotropic effects**
  - β-adrenergic receptor antagonists
  - Calcium channel antagonists
- **Antidysrhythmic drugs with negative inotropic and chronotropic effects**
  - Class I–IV antidysrhythmics
  - Miscellaneous
- **Drugs with secondary cardiac and vascular effects**
  - Diuretics
  - Bronchodilators
  - Anticholinesterases
  - CNS and mild circulatory stimulants and depressants
- **Combining drugs to modulate cardiac and vascular effects**

CLASSIFICATION OF CARDIOVASCULAR DRUGS

There are many ways to classify drugs that alter cardiovascular system function: agonist or antagonist, natural or synthesized, endogenous or exogenous, principal receptor affected, enzyme activated or inactivated, autonomic or nonautonomic modulation, sympathetic or parasympathetic system (SNS, PSNS) mediated, preganglionic or postganglionic, organ targeted etc. Although most drugs that fall into a specific category have a generalized effect, e.g. autonomic nervous system (ANS) stimulation by catecholamines, there can be marked differences in the specific actions of these drugs. Unfortunately, many drugs that regulate the circulation have a multitude of effects on the heart and blood vessels. In addition, the selection of a drug to treat a circulatory condition often involves drugs with different mechanisms of action, e.g. diuretics or vasodilators to treat hypertension.

Expected and unexpected changes in blood pressure (BP) and heart rate (HR) can be due to a multitude of factors. The anesthesiologist is most often faced not with a class of drugs from which to choose, but rather with an immediate drug choice to rapidly correct BP or HR based on information about the cause of the change. For this review of cardiovascular drugs relevant to anesthesiology, the selection of drugs to treat given conditions, i.e. hypotension and bradycardia, is discussed, rather than a rigorous pharmacologic classification based on mechanism of action available in standard pharmacology texts.

Emphasis is placed on those cardiovascular drugs with a rapid onset of effect to treat urgent or emergent deleterious changes in cardiac contractility, HR, and vascular tone. These are drugs that will be given mostly by the intravenous (IV) route in the perioperative setting. Because the patient may also be taking other (oral) drugs that have longer-lasting effects on the heart and circulation, and which may interfere with the acute administration of shorter-acting drugs, a brief synopsis of other direct and indirect cardiovascular drugs is included. In general, primary indications for drug use are given first, followed by the secondary or less pronounced effects of the drug. It is often necessary to administer more than one of these agents to regulate cardiovascular function. Because many factors alter the circulation, dosages of most cardiovascular drugs are not fixed but are titrated to effect.

POSITIVE INOTROPIC AND CHRONOTROPIC DRUGS WITH SECONDARY VASCULAR EFFECTS

Catecholamine agonists

These drugs are natural or synthetic sympathomimetic catecholamines. Mechanisms of action are given in a simple fashion in Figure 41.1. All β_1 agonists increase HR and contractility (Table 41.1), but they also have variable agonist effects on other receptors (e.g. dopamine-1, β_2, and α_1) so that secondary effects on the vasculature are nearly as marked as the primary effect (Table 41.2). Selection is often based on the need to imitate or augment the natural ANS sympathetic response. It is useful, if not essential, to have information on cardiac output and systemic vascular resistance (SVR) as well as HR and BP in order to select the most useful of these drugs (Table 41.3).

Catecholamine agonists mimic the natural sympathetic response.

The adrenergic receptor agonist *dobutamine* is a synthetic catecholamine which, in addition to its strong β_1 effect has weaker β_2 and α_1 agonist effects, so that some vascular beds (e.g. coronary) are relatively more dilated and others (e.g. splanchnic) more constricted, depending on the concentration. Dobutamine is used primarily to treat acute moderate heart failure and to conduct a resting cardiac stress test. It is not as potent as epi-

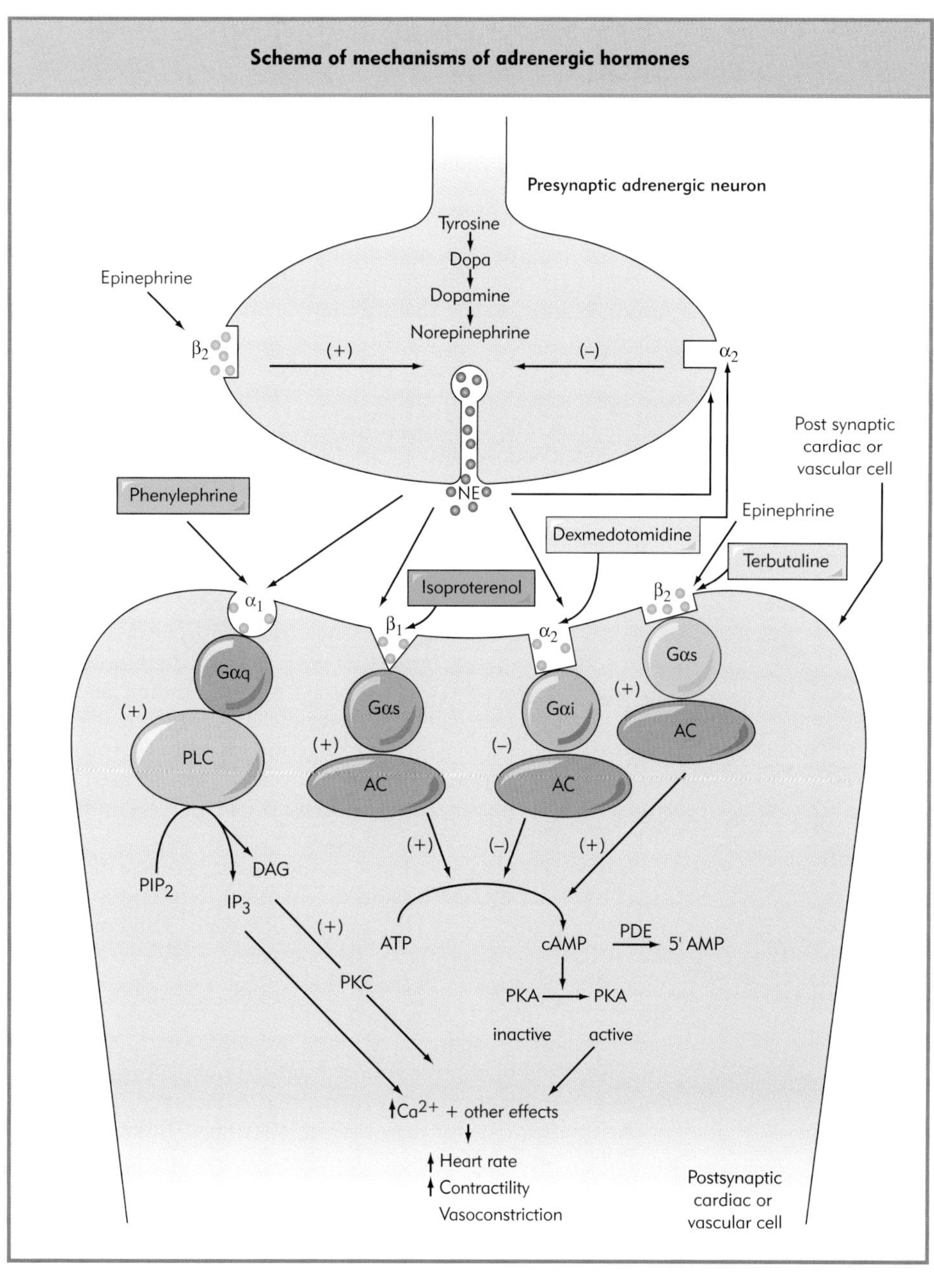

Figure 41.1. Simplified schema of mechanisms of adrenergic hormones to produce cardiovascular effects. The cardiac and vascular effects of noradrenaline (norepinephrine, NE) and adrenalin (epinephrine, E) depend on the pre- and post-synaptic receptors they occupy. Each post-synaptic neuron actually has only one receptor type; cardiac muscle tissue is innervated primarily by β_1 and β_2 receptors whereas vascular smooth muscle tissue is innervated primarily by α_1 and β_2 receptors. Most released NE is re-taken up by the presynaptic adrenergic neuron to terminate the post-synaptic effect of the neurotransmitter. Specific guanosine triphosphate-binding proteins (Gα subtypes) interact with specific receptor subtypes (α_1, β_1) to activate or inactivate the effectors phospholipase C (PLC), adenylyl cyclase (AC) and others. (+) and (–) refer to relative activation or inhibition. Downstream pathways diverge and converge, so effector pathways are not well understood. Receptor occupation may activate more than one class of G protein, which in turn activates many kinase pathways (such as protein kinase A (PKA), with different effects. Representative drugs (in blue) block at these receptor sites. PDE, phosphodiesterase; PIP_2, phosphatidyl inositol 4,5 bisphosphate; DAG, diacyglycerol; IP_3, inositol trisphosphate.

Table 41.1 General effects of β_1- vs β_2-adrenergic receptor stimulation

β_1	β_2
↑ Cardiac contractility	Arterial and venous dilation
↑ Heart rate	Bronchodilation
↑ Cardiac excitability	Uterine relaxation
↑ Plasma renin activity	Insulin secretion

Table 41.2 General effects of α_1- vs α_2-adrenergic receptor stimulation

α_1	α_2
Arterial vasoconstriction	Overall inhibited SNS activity
Venoconstriction	↓ Norepinephrine release
↓ Insulin release	Sedation (CNS postsynaptic)
Sphincter contraction	↓MAC/opioid requirement

nephrine (adrenaline) or isoproterenol in increasing contractility and HR, and does not stimulate dopamine receptors. Compared to norepinephrine it is not a good vasoconstrictor, and compared to dopamine it does not cause renal vasodilation at low concentrations. Onset of action is in minutes, and dosage is 0.5–30 μg/kg/min IV, which is a variable dose titrated to the desired cardiac and vascular effects.

Dopamine is a mixed effect natural sympathomimetic agent with a major direct effect on dopamine receptors and an indirect effect to stimulate the release of norepinephrine from presynaptic storage sites. Dopamine is used primarily to enhance contractility in heart failure and, at low concentrations (1–5 μg/kg/min IV) to decrease BP by promoting diuresis via renal vasodilation and tubular effects in acute renal failure. It is not as potent in increasing contractility and HR as are epinephrine and isoproterenol. At higher concentrations (5–50 μg/kg/min IV) it causes vasoconstriction by stimulation of α_1 receptors, and produces stronger cardiac effects. Onset of effect is 2–4 minutes. As with all sympathomimetic drugs there is an increased risk of supraventricular tachycardia (SVT) and ventricular tachycardia (VT).

The nonselective noncatecholamine sympathomimetic drug *ephedrine* directly stimulates α_1 and β_1 receptors to boost BP by its vasopressor and cardiac inotropic and chronotropic effects.

Table 41.3 Differential IV drug effects on pre- and postsynaptic adrenergic receptors

Receptor	β_1	β_2	α_1	α_2	**D_1**
Synaptic site	***Post***	***Pre/post***	***Post***	***Pre/post***	***Post***
Sympathomimetic agonists					
Dobutamine	+++	+	+	0	0
Dopamine[a]	++	++	++	+	+++
Ephedrine	+++	++	++	+	0
Mephentermine	+++	++	++	+	0
Epinephrine (adrenaline)	++	++	+++	+	0
Isoproterenol	+++	++	0	0	0
Norepinephrine (noradrenaline)	+	0	+++	++	0
α_1 Dominant adrenergic agonists					
Phenylephrine	0	0	+++	0	0
Methoxamine	0	0	+++	0	0
Metaraminol	++	0	+++	+	0
Other					
Fenoldopam[b]	0	0	+	0	+++
Terbutaline	+	+++	0	0	0
α_2 Dominant adrenergic agonists					
Clonidine[c]	0	0	++	+++	0
Methyldopa[c]	0	0	+	++	0
Dexmedetomidine[c]	+	0	0	+++	0

+ to +++ denotes receptor activation; 0 denotes a relative lack of effect on receptor activation. Actual efficacy on a specific receptor varies widely.

[a] Low dose causes vasodilation (D_1), high dose vasoconstriction (α_1).

[b] Vasodilation only (D_1).

[c] α_2 postsynaptic stimulation typically leads to vasodilation, and this effect may be enhanced by reduced central SNS activity.

Because it also has an indirect effect to release norepinephrine there are also enhanced β_1 and β_2 effects, the latter of which makes it a more effective bronchodilator than epinephrine. Onset is within minutes, and it is usually given in increments of 5–20 mg/min IV as needed when BP and HR are low. It can also be infused (50-200 μg/kg/min IV) as a less potent substitute for epinephrine. *Mephentermine* is a synthetic noncatecholamine sympathomimetic. It has both α_1- and β_1-adrenergic receptor agonist effects and so has vasoconstrictor and positive inotropic/chronotropic actions. Although it is more potent than ephedrine (dose is 4–100 mg/kg/min IV), it has little advantage over ephedrine and is seldom used.

Epinephrine (*adrenaline*) is a natural catecholamine sympathomimetic transmitter and hormone secreted primarily by the adrenal medulla with prominent rapid inotropic and chronotropic effects by β_1-adrenergic stimulation, and vasoconstrictive effects by its α_1 effects. It is given as a cardiac stimulant (1 mg every 3–5 min IV or intratracheal) for adult cardiac arrest with defibrillation from rapid (pulseless) VT or ventricular fibrillation. *Vasopressin* (40 units IV) is currently the drug of first choice for VF or VT, according to the revised ACLS protocol of the American Heart Association. For treatment of low cardiac output due to low HR and stroke volume with low to normal SVR, epinephrine is useful for inotropic support (infusion at 0.1–1 μg/kg/min IV). In much lower doses (0.1–0.5 mg sc, IM; 0.01 mg IV) its strong β_2 effect makes it useful as a bronchodilator and treatment for severe allergic reactions.

The synthetic sympathomimetic amine *isoproterenol* has dominant β_1 and secondary β_2 adrenergic receptor agonist effects and almost no α_1 effect. It is useful to increase HR with bradyrhythmias, and to treat complete heart block or carotid sinus hypersensitivity. It does not cause vasoconstriction. It is also a positive inotropic agent and bronchodilator, and is useful in treating shock and for resuscitation in cardiac arrest, particularly if SVR is high and α_1 adrenergic support is not needed. Its onset occurs within minutes and the dosage is 0.02–0.15 μg/kg/min IV, titrated to the desired effect.

Norepinephrine (*noradrenaline*) is a catecholamine sympathomimetic and the natural precursor molecule to epinephrine. Its dominant α_1 over β_1 effects make it a much more effective venous and arterial vasoconstrictor than epinephrine, with lesser – but effective – positive inotropic and chronotropic actions. Compared to other drugs in this class it is most useful when BP and SVR are low relative to cardiac contractility. Its onset is as rapid as that of epinephrine, and the dosage is 0.04–0.4 μg/kg/min IV as needed to maintain BP.

POSITIVE INOTROPIC DRUGS WITH VASODILATORY EFFECTS

Phosphodiesterase III inhibitors

Type III cAMP phosphodiesterase (PDE) inhibitors (bipyridine derivatives) are useful when the desired effect is to increase contractility and cardiac output without a marked increase in HR or vasoconstrictor effect. Unlike catecholamines, which stimulate cardiac β receptors, these drugs inhibit hydrolysis of cAMP, the ultimate product of β-receptor activation (Fig. 41.1). This prolongs the cardiac contractile (inotropic) and vasodilatory effects mediated by cAMP, hence the term inodilators. In cardiac cells this results in increased intracellular Ca^{2+}, and in smooth muscle cells results in decreased intracellular Ca^{2+}. An advantage of these drugs is that they are effective in the presence of α- and β-receptor blockade and catecholamine depletion.

Phosphodiesterase inhibitors act downstream of adrenergic receptors and thus are advantageous in the presence of receptor blockers.

The older of these drugs, *amrinone*, is given as a 0.75 mg IV load and then at 5–20 μg/kg/min. Thromobocytopenia can result from prolonged use. Amrinone has largely been supplanted by the newer drug *milrinone*, which is indicated for short-term treatment of acute uncompensated heart failure. Milrinone can initiate or exacerbate supraventricular tachycardia (SVT) and ventricular tachyarrhythmias, and its use should be limited to 48 hours. Loading dose is 50 μg/kg IV over 10 minutes, then 0.375–0.75 μg/kg/min IV. *Levosimendan* is a stereoselective drug in phase III trials; it has a PDE III inhibitory effect, in addition to a direct sensitizing effect on troponin to augment the contractile effect of a given intracellular Ca^{2+} concentration. Because of this action levosimendan may have a relatively better contractile effect than milrinone, particularly in patients with acute heart failure. Levosimendan also increases contractility, with a lesser increase in oxygen consumption than with milrinone.

POSITIVE CHRONOTROPIC DRUGS

Cholinergic receptor antagonists

Catecholamine-like agonists have mixed effects to increase HR, contractility, and vascular tone. In contrast, muscarinic cholinergic receptor antagonists primarily increase HR without other cardiovascular effects. *Atropine* is a belladonna alkaloid that blocks the postsynaptic effects of acetylcholine released from the vagus nerve as a nonselective competitive antagonist of all muscarinic (M) acetylcholine receptors. The main cardiac effect is to increase HR by blocking M_2 receptors on the SA nodal pacemaker. Often there is a transient and slight slowing of HR, probably due to a blockade of autoinhibitory presynaptic M_1 receptors. Atropine is used primarily to reverse asystole and to treat severe bradydysrhythmias due to sinoatrial (SA) and atrioventricular (AV) nodal block. It is also used as an adjunct to counteract the muscarinic effect of cholinesterase inhibitors, which cause bradycardia during reversal of neuromuscular blockade. Additional effects are reduced salivation and bronchodilation. Atropine is a tertiary amine, so at high doses it can cross the blood-brain-barrier to stimulate and then depress medullary and higher brain centers. Dosage is 0.4–1 mg IV or IM as a premedication, 0.25 mg/kg every 4–6 hours by inhalation for bronchoconstriction, and 0.5–1 mg IV, or 1–5 mg intratracheally, every 3–5 minutes for severe sinus bradycardia or cardiopulmonary resuscitation. Caution should be exercised in patients with tachydysrhythmias or acute myocardial infarction (MI).

Like atropine, *glycopyrrolate* is an anticholinergic drug; it is similarly used to stimulate HR, decrease secretions, counteract the muscarinic effects of acetylcholinesterase inhibitors, and treat bronchospasm. Unlike atropine, glycopyrrolate is a semisynthetic quaternary ammonium compound and so does not cross the blood–brain barrier to produce CNS effects. Dosage is 0.1–0.2 mg IV for vagolysis and secretions, and 0.4–0.8 mg every 8 hours by nebulizer for bronchospasm. Onset of action is slightly slower than for atropine, and the effects are longer lasting.

Glucagon, a peptide hormone secreted by pancreatic α cells, increases HR. Its major effect is to stimulate the conversion of glycogen to glucose, but it also increases cAMP levels in myocytes independent of adrenergic stimulation. It is used to treat hypoglycemia, and infrequently as an inotropic agent and to treat bradycardia (1–5 mg IV) due to β-blocker overdose. Its use may result in gastrointestinal side effects and hyperglycemia and/or hypoglycemia due to insulin release, and so must be used while carefully monitoring serum glucose.

POSITIVE INOTROPIC DRUGS

Cardiac glycosides

The cardiac glycosides (from *Digitalis* sp.) have been used for centuries as a tonic for congestive heart failure. These drugs block the Na^+, K^+-ATPase to cause less Na^+ to be pumped out of cells; the excess intracellular Na^+ reduces the Na^+ gradient for Ca^{2+} extrusion by the Na^+/Ca^{2+} exchanger so that intracellular Ca^{2+} increases, which enhances contractility independent of adrenergic stimulation or PDE III inhibition. Cardiac glycosides are still in use today to treat chronic heart failure, and to treat SVT (primarily atrial fibrillation) by decreasing SA nodal activity and by prolonging AV conduction. These drugs have a slow onset (in hours), and the duration of effect is days in fully digitalized patients. Digitalis-like drugs have a very narrow therapeutic index and patients must be followed for signs of toxicity. These include cardiac dysrhythmias (AV block, VT, VF), anorexia, nausea, vomiting, headache, drowsiness, and altered serum electrolytes. Toxicity can be enhanced by high serum Ca^{2+}, low K^+, or low Mg^{2+} levels, renal dysfunction, Ca^{2+} channel blockers, antibiotics and antidysrhythmic drugs, among others. It should not be given to patients in atrial fibrillation with Wolff–Parkinson–White (WPW) syndrome (accessory AV pathway) or wide QRS complexes as it may induce VF.

The toxicity of cardiac glycosides is enhanced by electrolyte abnormalities.

Digoxin is initially given as a 0.25–0.5 mg IV dose, followed in the next two 6-hour periods by doses of 0.125–0.25 mg IV, and thereafter 0.125–0.25 mg IV or orally every day for maintenance (therapeutic levels are 0.5–2 ng/mL). *Digitonin* is given only as an oral drug (0.8–1.2 mg orally, then 0.05–0.3 mg every day orally). For digoxin toxcity associated with low K^+, treatment is KCl 10–30 mEq/L IV slowly.

Another way to increase intracellular Ca^{2+} is to increase extracellular Ca^{2+}. Normal serum levels of Ca^{2+} (0.8–1.2 mM) are essential to maintain the contractility of cardiac and smooth muscle. *Calcium chloride* and *calcium gluconate* are used to enhance cardiac contractility if serum Ca^{2+} levels are low; they are also used to treat high serum levels of K^+ and Mg^{2+}, and to antagonize Ca^{2+} antagonist overdose. These drugs do not produce the profound contractile effects of catecholamines, are often given prophylactically (and controversially) at the end of cardiopulmonary bypass, and their effects are difficult to discern. Preparations of 10% calcium chloride provide three times more Ca^{2+} than 10% calcium gluconate, and are more irritating to veins when infused. It may be unwise to give these drugs to patients with stunned or infarcted myocardium because of the potential for enhanced ischemic damage. Dosage is 10 mg/kg IV over 10 minutes for calcium chloride, and 30 mg/kg IV over 10 minutes for calcium gluconate.

VASOCONSTRICTOR DRUGS

Sympathomimetic α_1-adrenergic agonists

These relatively pure vasoconstrictors are noncatecholamine sympathomimetic agents given temporarily to treat hypotension (see Table 41.3). Continued use can lead to organ failure, so these drugs are not a substitute for volume repletion or therapy for cardiac failure. *Phenylephrine* is a pure α_1-adrenergic receptor agonist used for rapid treatment of low BP secondary to volume depletion due to trauma or endotoxic shock and occasionally paroxysmal SVT. It is also added to local anesthetics to prolong their action. It should not be injected into terminal vascular beds such as the digits; it has no effect on cerebral vessels when the blood–brain barrier is intact. It is typically given as a bolus, 50–100 μg IV, or 10–200 μg/min IV infusion; onset of action is within 1 minute and effects last 15–20 minutes.

Methoxamine is similar to phenylephrine except that its effects are longer lasting (15–60 minutes). Because of the inability to titrate to BP, it is rarely used. Dosage is 1–5 mg every 15 minutes IV as needed. *Metaraminol* has β_1 effects in addition to its dominant α_1 action. It is used to treat low BP, as are the others in this group, but in addition can cause reflex bradycardia. Its withdrawal after long use can cause hypotension because of norepinephrine depletion. Dosage is 0.01 mg/kg IV, then 0.1–0.5 μg/kg/min; onset is within minutes and duration of effect is 30–90 minutes.

Non sympathomimetic vasoconstrictor drugs

Vasopressin, 8-arginine vasopressin, also known as *antidiuretic hormone*, is a peptide hormone released from the posterior pituitary. It is best known for its effect to increase renal resorption of water. It also acts on vasopressin receptors in the vasculature to mediate vasoconstriction, primarily in splanchnic, muscular, and cutaneous vessels; this can result in increased flow to coronary, pulmonary and brain circulations. Unlike epinephrine it is effective under conditions of hypoxia and acidosis and it has been shown to increase the hospital discharge rate for patients treated for asystole better than epinephrine. Vasopressin, 40 units i.v. once, is now the drug of choice for pulseless VT and VF in ACLS protocols. Vasopressin also exhibits hemostatic properties (pro-coagulant and platelet aggregation). *Desmopressin (DDAVP)* is a synthetic analogue of vasopressin that has less vasoconstrictor activity than vasopressin that is used primarily to treat diabetes insipidus and to maintain hemostasis in patients with hemophilia A and von Willebrand's disease.

VASODILATOR DRUGS

Guanylyl cyclase activators

The organic nitrates primarily dilate venous capacitance vessels to reduce BP. Their effects are caused by spontaneous or tissue-mediated release of nitric oxide (NO) from the drugs; NO, the first known gaseous local hormone, stimulates guanylyl cyclase in vascular smooth muscle to increase cGMP levels, which in turn decreases intracellular Ca^{2+} and causes arterial and venous vasodilation. Certain PDE inhibitors (especially type V), such as dipyridamole (Persantine) and sildenafil (Viagra), prolong the action of cGMP by inhibiting its hydrolysis and so may exacerbate the effects of the organic nitrates. *Glyceryl trinitrate* or *nitroglycerine* and *isosorbide dinitrite* are used acutely to treat hypertension and have a greater dilatory effect on capacitance than on resistance vessels. They are also anti-angina agents and are used to treat acute pulmonary edema and congestive heart failure; they can also induce uterine relaxation. Dosage is 5–200 μg/min IV or 0.1–4 μg/kg/min for reducing BP and relieving congestive heart failure. They are dissolved in dilute ethanol. Prolonged used leads to tolerance.

Nitroprusside has similar actions to the other nitrates but has equivalent arterial and venous vasodilatory effects. At low concentrations it produces a greater decrease in SVR than an increase in venous capacitance. It is useful in treating pulmonary hypertension, but its withdrawal can induce rebound systemic or pulmonary hypertension, especially in patients with congestive heart failure. Dosage is 0.1–8.0 μg/kg/min; onset is within 1 minute, and duration of effect is minutes.

Prolonged use of organic nitrates leads to tolerance of their vasodilatory effects.

Nitroprusside toxicity can occur owing to the release of cyanide ion (CN^-), a mitochondrial toxin that inhibits respiration despite adequate oxygen tension. Patients receiving more than 1 mg/kg over 12–24 hours are at increased risk for CN^- toxicity, manifested by tachyphylaxis to vasodilating effects, elevated mixed venous oxygen tension, and metabolic acidosis. Treatment is discontinuation of nitroprusside, correction of the acidosis, 100% inspired oxygen, and – importantly – sodium thiosulfate, 150 mg/kg IV bolus, to convert the CN^- to the much less toxic cyanomethemoglobin. Severe toxicity is treated additionally with either sodium nitrite, 5 mg/kg IV slow push, or amyl nitrite by inhalation.

Nitric oxide is an odorless, clear gas given by inhalation to treat adult respiratory distress syndrome (ARDS), acute or chronic pulmonary hypertension, and, in children, primary pulmonary hypertension of the newborn, congenital diaphragmatic hernia, and meconium aspiration. Like the organic nitrates that release NO, inhaled NO stimulates cGMP formation to effect vasodilation and bronchodilation. Dosage for ARDS is 1–20 ppm, and for primary pulmonary hypertension 20–40 ppm, titrated down to 5 ppm. Reactive pulmonary vasoconstriction may result from rapid discontinuation of NO.

α_1-adrenergic receptor antagonists

These drugs primarily inhibit α_1-adrenergic receptors to produce vasodilation when SNS stimulation is high. *Phenoxybenzamine* is an imidazoline that is more potent at α_1 than α_2 receptors, so the vasodilatory effect is greater than the effect of α_2 blockade to increase norepinephrine release by unopposed β_1 activity (Table 41.4). Its main indication is for long-acting chemical sympathectomy for pheochromocytoma. It is an oral medication (10 mg orally every 12 hours), and can cause direct and reflex tachycardia. *Phentolamine* has a similar effect to phenoxybenzamine, but in addition has mild β-blocking effects. *Prazosin* is a quinazoline derivative that has only postsynaptic α_1-blocking effects and thus does not increase HR directly via unopposed α_1 activity. It is an oral drug given at 1–5 mg b.i.d. or t.i.d. for the treatment of high BP.

Angiotensin-converting enzyme (ACE) inhibitors

These drugs block the conversion of angiotensin I to angiotensin II in the lung, so the Na^+-retaining effects of angiotensin II and aldosterone are blocked. This results in reduced BP due to Na^+ and water excretion. Block of angiotensin II also reduces the secretion of vasopressin from the posterior pituitary. As these drugs are also bradykininase inhibitors, increased bradykinin levels also produce vasodilation and can cause or exacerbate angioneurotic edema of the oral pharynx; they should not be used in pregnant patients. Only one, *enalaprilat*, is given intravenously: this is used to treat high BP, congestive heart failure, and to retard post-MI remodeling. Dosage is 0.625–1.25 mg IV every 6 hours slow push. Other ACE inhibitors are oral only: *captopril* 6.26–50 mg orally t.i.d.; *quinapril* 10–20 mg orally daily; and *lisinopril* 10–50 mg orally daily.

ACE inhibitors block formation of the vasoconstrict angiotensin II and degradation of the vasodilator bradykinin.

Table 41.4 Differential effects of adrenergic receptor antagonists

	β_1	β_2	α_1	α_2
Phenoxybenzamine	0	0		– –
Phentolamine	–	– –	– –	– –
Trimethaphan[a]	– –	– –	– –	– –
Esmolol	– – – –	–	0	0
Landiolol	– – –	0	0	0
Labetalol	– – –	– – –	–	0
Propranolol	– – –	– – –	0	0
Atenolol	– – –	–	0	0
Metoprolol	– – –	–	0	0

– to – – – – denotes relative activity to block receptor, leading to decreased effect (vasodilation and/or cardiac depression) of released norepinephrine from SNS postganglionic, presynaptic neurons, and epinephrine from the adrenal medulla. 0 denotes no effect on receptor.

[a] Acts at nicotinic preganglionic synapse to block postganglionic SNS activity.

Miscellaneous

Fenoldopam is a D_1 dopaminergic agonist (see Table 41.3); it is a rapid-acting vasodilator used for short-term control of severe malignant hypertension. The R(+) isomer is 200 times more efficacious than the S(−) isomer. It has much greater D_1 than α_1 effects, and no β-adrenergic, serotonergic, or D_2 dopaminergic activity. Dosage is 0.01–1.5 μg/kg/min IV; onset is 1–2 minutes, and half-life is 5 minutes. Metabisulfite in the formulation can trigger anaphylactoid reactions.

Terbutaline is a β_2 sympathomimetic adrenergic agonist with very few β_1 effects compared to epinephrine or isoproterenol (see Table 41.3). It is therefore a good drug to treat bronchoconstriction, to inhibit labor, and to treat anaphylactic shock. It is less potent than epinephrine or isoproterenol, but is useful if the β_2-agonist effect is desired without β_1 cardiac side effects.

Trimethaphan camsylate is unusual in that it is an ANS nicotinic ganglionic blocker (see Table 41.4); hence it blocks SNS postganglionic adrenergic activation. Its use is particularly as an indirect-acting vasodilator to control severe rapid-onset hypertension in malignant autonomic dysreflexia. Onset is rapid and the dosage is 3–30 μg/kg/min, titrated to effect.

Hydralazine is a direct-acting antihypertensive agent also used to reduce afterload in congestive heart failure. It acts primarily as a Ca^{2+} channel antagonist in arteriolar smooth muscle in fast-flow organs with little effect on capacitance vessels; it may also inhibit the peripheral conversion of dopamine to norepinephrine. It is rather slow acting (10–20 minutes for peak effect); dosage is 2.5–5 mg IV bolus every 15 minutes as needed, up to about 40 mg IV.

Diazoxide is a K^+ channel opener that causes earlier smooth muscle repolarization and lower Ca^{2+} influx to reduce arteriolar resistance with little venodilatory effect. It is a thiazide derivative but has no diuretic activity. At high doses it can cause hyperglycemia and act as an osmotic diuretic. Dosage is 1–3 mg/kg IV given slowly over 5–15 minutes, or 7.5–30 mg/min. It is rarely used because the effect is long lasting (3–15 hours) and is difficult to titrate.

Alprostadil is prostaglandin E_1. Like nitric oxide, it is used to maintain patency of the ductus arteriosus and to treat severe pulmonary hypertension and right heart failure; it is infused into the right atrium to minimize systemic vasodilatory effects. It also inhibits platelet aggregation and is given subcutaneously in the diagnosis and treatment of erectile dysfunction. The right atrial infusion dose rate for pulmonary hypertension is 0.05–0.4 μg/kg/min.

VASODILATOR DRUGS WITH NEGATIVE INOTROPIC AND CHRONOTROPIC EFFECTS

β-adrenergic receptor antagonists

β-blockers have variable effects to block β_2 (and for labetalol α_1 receptors), in addition to more potent β_1-adrenergic receptor antagonism (see Table 41.4). Hence they primarily block the stimulating effects of endogenous norepinephrine and epinephrine release that occurs with enhanced SNS activity.

Esmolol is highly selective for blocking β_1 rather than β_2 receptors. Esmolol has a rapid onset of action and is short acting. It is used to treat SVT, for prophylaxis of expected enhanced SNS activity with intubation, to decrease BP by producing myocardial depression, and occasionally to treat pheochromocytoma-induced tachydysrhythmias. Dosage is 500 μg/kg IV load, then 25–300 μg/kg/min titrated to HR and BP. *Landiolol* is a new β-blocker that is similar to esmolol but with greater β_1 over β_2 selectivity (250:1). It is ultrashort acting, with an elimination half-life of 4 minutes. It is used like esmolol but may be the choice to treat malignant hypertension (not due to autonomic dysreflexia) with tachycardia, as its effects are more easily titrated. It is generally safe for use in patients with pulmonary vascular obstructive disease. Dosage is 5–40 μg/kg/min IV.

Labetalol is used mostly as an acute antihypertensive treatment. It has nonselective β_1- and β_2-receptor antagonist effects and a mild α_1-blocking effect (β/α 7:1 when given IV). Caution should be exercised in patients with acute asthma and chronic obstructive pulmonary disease (COPD), congestive heart failure, heart block, severe bradyrhythmias, and cardiogenic shock. It is given at a dose of 2.5–20 mg IV slowly, or 0.5–2 mg/min.

Propranolol is an anti-anginal, antihypertensive, and class II antidysrhythmic agent. It is a nonselective β_1- and β_2-receptor antagonist. It is longer acting than esmolol or labetalol, and is not β_1 selective like esmolol. It decreases cardiac output and is used to treat high BP, SVT, VT, acute MI, thyrotoxicosis, pheochromocytoma, tremors, and for migraine prophylaxis. As with all β_2 antagonists it should be used cautiously in patients with COPD. It is not rapid acting and so is not useful for acute management of BP or refractory dysrhythmias. Dosage is 10–30 μg/kg IV every 5 minutes up to 50–150 μg/kg max; or 1–3 mg IV slow push.

Other β_1-selective antagonists are given either IV or orally on an acute or chronic basis. *Atenolol* is given chronically to treat high BP, angina, tachycardia, MI, and perioperatively to decrease myocardial ischemia and the morbidity and mortality related to cardiac disease. Dosage for acute MI is 5 mg IV repeat once after 5–10 minutes, then 50–200 mg orally every day. *Metoprolol* is used similarly. For acute MI the dose is 15 mg IV over 5 minutes, then orally 50 mg every 6 hours for 48 hours, then 100 mg orally every day. For control of BP the dosage is 50–200 mg orally every day.

Calcium channel antagonists

This class of drugs works by blocking L-type Ca^{2+} channels in a variety of cell types, with differential effects. Slowing Ca^{2+} influx generally leads to reduced cell activity. These drugs have common effects to promote arterial vasodilation in all vascular beds, including the coronary arteries; venodilatory effects are minimal. Reduced contractility may be offset by reduced afterload. Compared to nitrates, Ca^{2+} channel blockers can produce complete vessel dilation, there is no tachyphylaxis, and both large and small coronary vessels are dilated. However, reversal is much more difficult to achieve than with the nitrates. Calcium channel antagonists have differential effects on myocardial depression, and compensatory reflex SNS activation may occur. If myocardial depression by Ca^{2+} channel antagonism is excessive, treatment is with β_1 agonists, calcium chloride, or milrinone.

Nifedipine, a dihydropyridine Ca^{2+} channel blocker, is much more potent as a vasodilator than as a myocardial depressant; it is used to treat both classic and vasospastic angina, and for the treatment of hypertension and the suppression of preterm labor. Nifedipine has almost no effect to decrease HR or to slow cardiac conduction, but it can produce coronary steal. Its use with β_1-blockers does not typically lead to AV block. It is very light sensitive, so no IV form is available. Dosage is 10–40 mg t.i.d. sublingually. *Nimodipine* is a related drug that crosses the blood–brain barrier. It is used to treat cerebral vasospasm after subarachnoid hemorrhage. *Nicardipine* is typically given orally, but can also be used IV at 5–15 mg/h for short-term treatment of vasospasm after coronary artery bypass grafting, and for immediate but short-term hypertension and angina treatment.

Clevidipine is a new, short-acting Ca^{2+} channel blocker (phase III trials). It has a greater vascular selectivity in reducing arteriolar resistance than on increasing venous capacitance. It is ~50 times more potent in dilating vessels than inhibiting myocardial contractility or prolonging AV conduction time. It also has a natriuretic/diuretic effect, and is fast acting and rapidly metabolized with minimal reflex tachycardia. Dosage is 0.2–3 μg/min to lower BP 5–30%, and it is easy to titrate to effect.

Diltiazem, a benzothiazepine-type Ca^{2+} channel blocker, slows AV conduction and is used mostly to treat unstable angina and paroxysmal SVT or atrial fibrillation/flutter with a rapid ventricular response. It is also used to treat chronic hypertension, with minimal side effects. It preferentially vasodilates coronary vessels over other vascular beds. It is usually given orally (30–120 mg t.i.d. or q.i.d.), but is also available for IV dosing at 20–25 mg slow push. Its spectrum as a vasodilator, myocardial depressant, and antidysrhythmic agent lies between nifedipine and verapamil (see below).

ANTIDYSRHYTHMIC DRUGS WITH NEGATIVE INOTROPIC AND CHRONOTROPIC EFFECTS

Class I–IV antidysrhythmics

Antidysrhythmic agents (Tables 41.5 and 41.6) of the Vaughan Williams classification include class I Na^+ channel blockers/membrane stabilizers such as quinidine, disopyramide, and procainamide (class IA), lidocaine and phenytoin (class IB), and flecainide (class IC); class II β_1-blockers such as propranolol; class III drugs that prolong cardiac action potential duration (APD) such as bretylium and amiodarone; and class IV Ca^{2+} channel blocking drugs that shorten APD and slow AV conduction time, such as varapamil and diltiazem (see also Chapter 40). Each of these drugs has primary or secondary effects to reduce BP.

CLASS IA DRUGS

Procainamide, *quinidine* and *disopyramide* depress phase 0 depolarization and slow conduction in Purkinje fibers. They are useful in treating paroxysmal SVT, VT, and lidocaine-resistant VT and VF, as well as atrial fibrillation and WPW syndrome. They are no longer recommended for refractory VF, as amiodarone is more effective. Quinidine has effects like those of procainamide, but is seldom given IV because of its toxicity.

Table 41.5 Drug effects on cardiac electrophysiology

	Duration of refractory period			Atrial excitability	Ventricular excitability
	Atrial	*AV node*	*H-P*		
Procainamide[a]	–	–	+	–	–
Lidocaine[b]	0	0	–	0	–
Esmolol[c]	+	+	+	–	–
Bretylium	0	0	+	0	–
Amiodarone	+	+	+	–	–
Verapamil[d,g]	+	+	–	–	–
Digoxin[g]	–	+	–	–	–
Adenosine	+	+	0	–	0
Isoproterenol[e,f]	–	–	–	+	+
Atropine[f]	–	–	–	+	+

AV, atrioventricular; H-P, His-Purkinje
\+ denotes an increase; – denotes a decrease; 0 denotes no change.
[a] Also quinidine, disopyramide.
[b] Also phenytoin, flecainide.
[c] Also landiolol, propranolol.
[d] Also diltiazem.
[e] Also dopamine, ephedrine, epinephrine, norepinephrine.
[f] Effects depend on intrinsic SNS and PSNS activities.
[g] Used for ventricular rate control with AF. Drug effects at these sites are variable, dose related, or not well defined.

Table 41.6 Drugs used to treat acute dysrhythmias

	PSVT	AF	VE	VT	VF
Procainamide[a]	+	+	0	+	+
Lidocaine	0	0	+	+	+
Phenyltoin	0	0	0	+	0
Flecainide	+	0	0	+[d]	0
Propranolol	+	0	0	+[d]	0
Esmolol	+	0	0	+[d]	0
Bretylium	0	0	0	+	+
Amiodarone[e]	0	+[f]	0	+	+
Diltiazem[b]	+	+	0	+[d]	0
Verapamil[b]	+	+	+	+[d]	0
Digoxin[b]	+	+[f]	0	+[d]	0
Adenosine[c]	+	0	0	+[d]	0

PSVT, paroxysmal superventricular tachycardia; AF, atrial fibrillation/flutter; VE, ventricular ectopy; VT, ventricular tachydysrhythmia; VF, ventricular fibrillation. +, active, 0, not active, against type of dysrhythmia.
[a] Useful or [b] dangerous for WPW and related abnormal AV nodal re-entry pathways.
[c] Useful to differentiate SVT from VT.
[d] Secondary effect due to atrial slowing.
[e] Drug of choice for VT and pulseless VF.
[f] Slows ventricular response.

Procainamide, an amide local anesthetic, stabilizes membranes and, unlike the others, also blocks muscarinic cholinergic receptors; its loading dose is 10–50 mg/kg IV (100 mg every 2–5 minutes) and then up to 12 mg/kg. Disopyramide also antagonizes Ca^{2+} channels and is used orally.

CLASS IB DRUGS

Lidocaine, an amide local anesthetic, is a Na^+ channel antagonist for the treatment of VT and VF, for which it is now a second-line drug to amiodarone. It is also used to blunt reflex SNS activation with tracheal intubation, and for regional nerve conduction block. Dosage is 1 mg/kg IV for VT and VF, repeated if necessary, and then 20–50 μg/kg/min. *Phenytoin (diphenylhydantoin)* is used acutely to treat lidocaine-resistant VT, digitalis-induced toxic dysrhythmias, and chronically to treat congenital long QT syndrome, epilepsy, and for seizure prophylaxis. Rapid IV injection can cause hypotension and heart block. To treat ventricular dysrhythmias the dose is 1.5 mg/kg every 15 minutes up to 10–15 mg/kg maximum.

CLASS IC DRUGS

Flecainide, like procainamide, is used to treat paroxysmal SVT and VT. It acts primarily on the ventricles to slow AV conduction time, and may suppress preventricular excitations better than quinidine or disopyramide, but it can cause wide QRS complexes and induce new dysrhythmias. It is an oral drug only (100–200 mg orally every 12 hours).

CLASS II DRUGS

The β_1 antagonists, e.g. propranolol, are discussed above.

CLASS III DRUGS

Bretylium tosylate is used only for acute treatment of VT and VF. It works by markedly prolonging ventricular APD and refractory period. It also has a small positive inotropic effect owing to stimulated release of norepinephrine from adrenergic terminals. Loading dose is 5–10 mg/kg IV over 10 minutes, then 1–2 mg/min. *Amiodarone* also prolongs APD and is a potent vasodilator. It has properties consistent with all four Vaughan Williams classes, and is now preferred over lidocaine, bretylium, and procainamide as a first-line treatment for hemodynamically unstable VT or VF; for VF with defibrillation the dose is 300 mg IV followed by 150 mg IV. It should not be used to treat complete heart block or complete AV dissociation. Amiodarone has a rapid onset of action (minutes) but a very long (20–47 days) half-life after IV administration. Loading dose for tachy dysrthythmias is 150 mg over 10 minutes IV (15 mg/min), then 360 mg IV over 6 hours, or 1 mg/min IV, then 540 mg over 18 hours (0.5 mg/min IV).

CLASS IV DRUGS

These include diltiazem (above) and especially *verapamil*. This latter, a papaverine derivative, is a Ca^{2+} channel antagonist with a major effect to slow conduction and to stop dysrhythmias. It is used primarily to treat paroxysmal SVT, premature atrial depolarization, and, like digoxin, to control (slow) ventricular rate in atrial fibrillation and flutter. Verapamil should be used with caution or not at all in patients with WPW or wide QRS syndromes. It is also used to treat angina and high BP. It can cause severe AV dissociation, and must be used with caution in patients taking β_1 antagonists or cardiac glycosides. Dosage is 5–10 mg every 15 minutes IV for atrial dysrhythmias, and 2.5–10 mg IV for high BP.

Miscellaneous

Adenosine is an ultrashort-acting endogenous adenosine receptor agonist used to differentiate paroxysmal SVT from VT and to treat SVT. It slows conduction velocity through the AV node and may cease cardiac rhythm and lower BP briefly. It does not convert atrial fibrillation or flutter, and will not convert VT or VF. Dosage is 6–12 mg IV push, repeated if necessary 1–2 minutes later.

DRUGS WITH SECONDARY CARDIAC AND VASCULAR EFFECTS

Diuretics

There are many other drugs that have effects (mostly depressant) on the circulatory system. These include the diuretics, especially *furosemide* and *bumetanide,* which are fast-acting loop diuretics used to treat congestive heart failure and high BP, and to decrease intracranial BP by decreasing intravascular volume. Other diuretics that are antihypertensive agents are *ethacrynic acid* and *hydrochlorothiazide*. *Mannitol* is an effective osmotic diuretic.

Bronchodilators

Theophylline and *aminophylline* (85% theophylline) are methylated xanthines and PDE inhibitors that potentiate relaxation induced by β_2 adrenergic agonists, with effects mediated by cAMP. They are used as bronchodilators but can induce ventricular ectopy and tachycardia, and cause mild increases in cardiac output and BP.

Anticholinesterases

These drugs are used primarily to treat SVT and to reverse neuromuscular blockade; they are also used to diagnose and treat myasthenia gravis and postoperative ileus. They are combined with an anticholinergic drug to prevent bradycardia during reversal of skeletal motor blockade. Given alone they can cause severe bradycardia, but in smaller doses are used as adjuvants to treat SVT. *Neostigmine*, *edrophonium*, and *pyridostigmine* are quaternary amines and so have no CNS effects (Chapter 37). *Physostigmine* is a tertiary amine that enters the CNS. It is used to treat drug-induced anticholinergic CNS effects, and topically to treat glaucoma. It too can cause severe bradycardia.

CNS and mild circulatory stimulants and depressants

Several illegal drugs are used primarily for their CNS effects, but because they possess secondary stimulant effects on the heart and vasculature, the effects of primary cardiovascular drugs may be altered. Some of these are the Schedule I, II and III psychotropic drugs such as *amphetamines* and *phencyclidine*, which have no medicinal use, *marijuana*, which is used to treat anorexia and nausea, the topical local anesthetic and vasoconstrictor drug *cocaine*, and the phencyclidine derivative *ketamine* used as a general anesthetic. In general these drugs have acute CNS and ANS sympathomimetic effects. Chronically, they may cause downregulation of ANS receptors and cardiovascular depression.

Serotonin (5-hydroxytryptamine) is a CNS neurotransmitter that modulates the effects of other monamine transmitters, e.g. norepinephrine and dopamine. Partially selective serotonin receptor agonists such as *sumatriptan* and *metoclopromide* may augment sympathomimetic drug effects. Partially selective receptor antagonists such as *dolasetron* or *ondansetron* can augment the effects of vasodilators. Selective serotonin reuptake inhibitors (SSRIs) such as *fluoxetine* and *sertraline* may modulate the effects of monamine oxidase inhibitors (MAO) such as *phenelzine* (*Nardil*).

Clonidine is a central and peripheral α_1 and α_2 adrenergic agonist (see Table 41.3). It is used to treat opioid withdrawal syndrome and has mild antihypertensive effects. *Dexmedetomidine* is a relatively selective α_2 over α_1 (1620:1)-adrenergic receptor agonist used for continuous sedation in the intensive care setting. Presynaptic activation of α_2 receptors hinders the release of norepinephrine, and postsynaptic activation in the CNS causes sedation and inhibition of SNS activity, with a decrease in BP and HR. Dosage for sedation is 0.2–0.7 μg/kg/h.

Methyldopa produces a metabolite, α-methyl norepinephrine, that produces a clonidine-like α_2-agonist effect in cardiovascular control centers that results in reduced sympathetic outflow. It also reduces peripheral SNS effects by generating a false neurotransmitter and by reducing catecholamine synthesis. It is used primarily to depress overall SNS activity (HR, BP, SVR), but can also cause sedation, psychosis, and depression. It has very slow onset (4–6 hours) and a very long duration of action (10–16 hours), and so is seldom used to control BP. Dosage is 0.25–1 g IV, given over 60 minutes every 6 hours.

COMBINING DRUGS TO MODULATE CARDIAC AND VASCULAR EFFECTS

With the administration of an individual drug attention should be paid to its pharmacokinetics, receptor specificity, toxicity, receptor affinity, and efficacy, whether there is likely down- or up regulation of receptors involved, and the status of the ANS for the individual patient. Complicating outcome in the use of one drug is that cardiovascular drugs are seldom given alone. Often the approach is to treat several symptoms simultaneously with drugs from different groups. Although this may be necessary under certain circumstances, knowledge of the individual drugs and their interactions is essential. Drugs that are often given together are primary positive inotropic drugs with primary vasodilators or vasopressors. Examples are dopamine, dobutamine, or epinephrine with nitroprusside; nitroglycerine or milrinone to enhance cardiac preload and contractility and reduce afterload; and digitalis with a diuretic to treat congestive heart failure.

In summary, there are many drugs to treat a particular cardiovascular imbalance. Most of those discussed are short acting but have more than one effect, which may or may not be advantageous and can make drug selection more difficult. Along with the direct measure of arterial BP, HR, and urine output, prudent use of the pulmonary artery catheter can be helpful to assess cardiac output and pulmonary and systemic vascular resistances in patients with unstable or anticipated cardiovascular instability. With immediate hemodynamic information, the patient's history and medication list, and a thorough knowledge of cardiovascular pharmacology, the anesthesiologist or intensivist should be able to optimize drug selection to treat acute cardiovascular dysfunction.

Key references

Everly MJ, Heaton PC, Cluxton RJ Jr. Beta-blocker underuse in secondary prevention of myocardial infarction. Ann Pharmacother. 2004;38:286–93.

Hardman JG, Limbird LE, Gilman AG (eds) The pharmacologic basis of therapeutics, 10th edn. New York: McGraw-Hill; 2001: Chapters 6–11, 29–35.

Kloner RA, Rezkalla SH. Cardiac protection during acute myocardial infarction: where do we stand in 2004? J Am Coll Cardiol. 2004;44:276–86.

London MJ, Zaugg M, Schaub MC. Perioperative β-adrenergic blockade: Physiologic foundations and clinical controversies. Anesthesiology 2004;100:170–5.

Mangano DT, Layug EL, Wallace A, Tateo I. Effect of atenolol on mortality and cardiovascular morbidity after noncardiac surgery. Multicenter Study of Perioperative Ischemia Research Group. New Engl J Med. 1996;335:1713–20.

Further reading

Estafanous FG, Barash PG, Reves JG (eds) Cardiac anesthesia – principles and clinical practice. Philadelphia: JB Lippincott; 1994: Chapter 2.

Douglas SA, Ohlstein EH, Johns DG. Cardiovascular pharmacology and drug discovery in the 21st century. Trends Pharmacol Sci. 2004;25:225–33.

Eisenberg MJ, Brox A, Bestawros AN. Calcium channel blockers: an update. Am J Med. 2004;116:35–43.

Hensley FA Jr, Martin DE, Gravlee GP (eds) A practical approach to cardiac anesthesia, 3rd edn. Philadelphia: Lippincott Williams & Wilkins; 2003: Chapter 2.

Kaplan JA (ed) Cardiac anesthesia, 3rd edn. Philadelphia: WB Saunders; 1993: Chapters 3–6.

Sallach JA, Goldstein S. Use of beta-blockers in congestive heart failure. Ann Med. 2003;35:259–66.

Tamargo J, Caballero R, Delpon E. Pharmacological approaches in the treatment of atrial fibrillation. Curr Med Chem. 2004;11:13–28.

Toda N. Vasodilating beta-adrenoceptor blockers as cardiovascular therapeutics. Pharmacol Ther. 2003;100:215–34.

Chapter 42

Regulation and assessment of cardiac function

Paul M Heerdt and Marc L Dickstein

TOPICS COVERED IN THIS CHAPTER

- **Anatomy and cellular physiology**
  - Chamber geometry
- **Dynamic determinants of ventricular function**
  - Rate and rhythm
  - Preload
  - Afterload
  - Contractility
- **Clinical assessment of ventricular function**
  - Pulmonary artery catherization
  - Echocardiography
- **Ventricular–vascular integration**
  - Venous return model
  - Elastance matching
  - Pulsatility and wave reflection: caveats in models of mechanical coupling
  - Limitations of steady-state models
  - Models and reality: attempting to close the loop

During the course of an average lifespan the human heart beats over 2 billion times. Each heartbeat represents multiple electrical, biochemical, and mechanical events that occur over milliseconds, and translocate a volume of oxygenated blood into the peripheral circulation sufficient to meet the metabolic needs of the body. Regulation of contraction and relaxation of the heart and its performance as a pump involves acute and prolonged events that are both intrinsic and extrinsic to the heart proper.

ANATOMY AND CELLULAR PHYSIOLOGY

During organogenesis, multiple structures form individually and eventually fuse to form 'the heart'. Although regarded as a single organ, the heart actually represents two interdependent pumps (the right and left hearts) that are connected in series and contained in a common sac (the pericardium). Unlike the right ventricular (RV) inflow tract and the entire left ventricle (LV), which arise from the ventricular portion of the primitive cardiac tube, the RV outflow tract is derived from the bulbus cordis. In some phylogenetically lower animals this portion of the heart takes on specific functions; in sharks, for example, the bulbus is retained as a separate chamber involved with providing flow across the gills, and in turtles the RV outflow tract regulates the distribution of blood flow between the systemic and pulmonary circulations as it is ejected from an essentially common ventricle.

The atria are grossly similar in size and dimension, but the ventricles are quite different; the RV is crescent-shaped and largely wrapped around the interventricular septum, which represents the medial wall of the elliptical LV. Functionally the pattern of contraction varies between the LV and the RV. The LV contracts in a relatively homogeneous fashion, with both short and long axes shortening simultaneously. In contrast, the RV contracts sequentially from the inflow tract to the outflow tract. The mechanical significance of this sequential pattern of contraction is unclear, but the process is altered by sympathetic stimulation, positive inotropic drugs, total autonomic blockade, and volatile anesthetics. The myocardium of both ventricles is comprised of individual myofibrils, which are linked by specialized gap junctions to form a functional syncytium that allows for rapid conduction of electrical charge. Fundamentally, all myocytes display five basic characteristics: excitability (bathmotropy), conductivity (dromotropy), rhythmicity (chronotropy), contractility (inotropy), and relaxation (lusitropy).

At the center of cardiac mechanical function is the process of excitation/contraction coupling (Chapter 39). Myocyte depolarization leads to an influx of extracellular Ca^{2+} via voltage-gated Ca^{2+} channels and, to a lesser extent, electrogenic Na^+/Ca^{2+} exchange. This relatively small amount of Ca^{2+} functions primarily as 'activator Ca^{2+}', which stimulates the sarcoplasmic reticulum (SR) to release a larger amount of Ca^{2+} in a process known as Ca^{2+}-induced Ca^{2+} release (CICR). Storage and release of Ca^{2+} by the SR are relatively complex processes modulated by the high-capacity Ca^{2+}-binding protein calsequestrin and the ryanodine-sensitive Ca^{2+} release channel, respectively. Once myoplasmic Ca^{2+} concentration exceeds ~1 μM, Ca^{2+} binds to troponin C, producing a conformational change in tropomysin that allows interaction between actin and myosin myofilaments and mechanical shortening. As soon as the stimulus to release Ca^{2+} is terminated, reuptake of Ca^{2+} by the SR leads to a rapid decline in intracellular Ca^{2+} concentration that facilitates the dissociation of Ca^{2+} from troponin C and relaxation. Reuptake of Ca^{2+} into the SR is energy dependent, involving a Ca^{2+}-ATPase (the sarcoplasmic endoreticular ATPase subtype 2a, or SERCA2a) and its regulatory protein phospholamban. Most factors that influence the contractility of the heart – from pharmacologic manipulation to idiopathic failure – alter intracellular Ca^{2+} cycling.

Multiple factors intrinsic to the heart influence excitation–contraction coupling, the process of relaxation, and ultimately myocardial performance. In general, intrinsic processes influence initial sarcomere length, the number of active cross-bridges between actin and myosin, the rate of cross-bridge cycling, and the time course of activation and inactivation. However, in vivo the interaction between intrinsic and extrinsic regulators of myocyte function dictates the performance of the heart as a pump.

Chamber geometry

Although each myocyte is capable of contracting (changing length and developing tension), it is the association of millions of myocytes in a three-dimensional configuration that allows the heart to develop pressure and function as a pump. Consideration of the LV as a thin-walled sphere allows for relatively simple characterization of the relationship between intraventricular pressure (distending force at right-angles to the wall) and wall stress (tension per unit area, reflecting a shear force applied circumferentially) within the context of the law of Laplace (Equation 42.1) in which P = ventricular pressure; r = internal radius; σ = stress; and h = uniform wall thickness. Equation 42.1 can be simplified to Equation 42.2, as r>>h:

■ Equation 42.1

$$Pr = \sigma h\left(2 + \frac{h}{r}\right)$$

■ Equation 42.2

$$\sigma = \frac{Pr}{2h}$$

Application of the law of Laplace to a spherical model of the LV requires three assumptions: that wall thickness and internal radius remain constant; that the wall itself is thin relative to the internal radius, hence stress is constant throughout the wall; and that the chamber is at rest. In reality, the LV is more of an elongated ellipse than a sphere, and stress is not uniform across its wall. Nonetheless, the law of Laplace provides useful information in the qualitative assessment of pathophysiologic alterations in wall stress. For example, although both aortic stenosis and regurgitation increase LV wall stress, the concentric hypertrophy associated with stenosis can lead to a substantial increase in wall thickness that tends to reduce stress by offsetting increases in pressure and radius (Chapter 45). This is clinically important because of a direct relationship between wall stress and oxygen consumption.

In contrast to the LV, the complex geometry (essentially a crescent) and contraction pattern of the RV defies the simple application of spherical models. Although the general relationships between pressure and wall stress remain, it is difficult to incorporate global terms such as internal radius, and distribution of wall stress throughout the walls of the RV is probably even more heterogeneous than in the LV. Conceptually, if one considers that although RV systolic pressure is about 20% that of the LV, RV volume tends to be higher and the free wall thinner. Thus, RV wall stress during systole probably is not as different from that of the LV as would be anticipated from their differences in pressure. However, in the setting of a modest increase in afterload, RV wall stress increases to a greater degree than that of the LV because of a more prominent relative rise in both its pressure and its volume.

DYNAMIC DETERMINANTS OF VENTRICULAR FUNCTION

The fundamental determinants of ventricular pump function are generally regarded as *rate and rhythm*, *preload*, *afterload*, and *contractility*. Importantly, the concepts of preload, afterload, and contractility are largely derived from studies of isolated muscle, and as such are difficult to apply precisely to the intact heart. In isolated muscle experiments, for example, preload is defined as a weight attached to one end of the muscle that stretches it to a given length during diastole. With the preload weight just touching a support, a second weight termed the afterload is attached.

The fundamental determinants of ventricular pump function are: rate and rhythm, preload, afterload, and contractility.

Within this model afterload can be defined as the constant force an isolated muscle must develop during shortening sufficient to raise afterload weight. In the intact ventricle, a fair analogy for preload is the volume at end-diastole. In contrast, afterload has no direct analogy because the myocardial force generated by the ventricle changes constantly during ejection (i.e. muscle shortening). Nonetheless, with increased understanding of the complexities of cardiac physiology, improved techniques for determining intracavitary volume, and the widespread access to real-time images of the heart, these fundamental determinants of ventricular function – and their limitations – have assumed an expanded meaning to clinicians.

Rate and rhythm

Although the impact of heart rate and rhythm on cardiac pump performance is intuitive, there are subtle complexities. For example, when the contraction rate of a normal heart increases, so initially does the force of contraction (positive force–frequency relationship). In the setting of heart failure and abnormal myocardial Ca^{2+} cycling, however, an increase in heart rate can produce a decrease in contractile force (negative force–frequency relationship). Similarly, although the impact of arrhythmias on ventricular filling and ejection are easily visualized, subtle factors that alter the synchrony of regional ventricular contraction can influence cardiac pump performance. Indeed, selective pacing of specific areas within the ventricles, or resynchonization therapy, has recently emerged as a therapeutic intervention for some patients with severe chronic heart failure.

Preload

Representing the volume (and to a lesser extent the pressure) producing 'stretch' of myofibrils and determining sarcomere length prior to contraction, preload is directly related to end-diastolic wall stress. Limitations to measuring intracardiac volumes have traditionally led to reliance upon intracardiac pressures as an indirect indicator of preload. Recent advances in techniques for the measurement of intraventricular volume have greatly enhanced clinical appreciation of diastolic pressure–volume relationships and hence diastolic function. End-diastolic volume and pressure are determined by many processes that extrinsically affect venous return to the heart, and intrinsically influence relaxation and the ability of the heart to fill (Table 42.1). The ventricle normally has four phases of diastole: isovolumic relaxation, early rapid filling, diastasis, and atrial systole (Fig. 42.1). Of these phases, only isovolumic relaxation is an active process that requires the expenditure of energy by ventricular myocytes. Characterized as ventricular lusitropy, this active relaxation process can be quantified by the minimum value of the first derivative of ventricular pressure versus time (–dP/dt), or more precisely as a time constant of isovolumic pressure decline (τ). The calculation of τ is based on the monoexponential decline of pressure during the isovolumic phase of the cycle, i.e. from end-ejection (commonly defined as the point of peak –dP/dt) to opening of the mitral valve. Thus:

■ Equation 42.3

$$P = A^{-t/\tau}$$

where P = ventricular pressure, A = peak ventricular pressure –dP/dt, t = time after –dP/dt, and τ = relaxation time constant.

Owing to the relative lack of an isovolumic phase in the RV, calculation of τ is problematic. In the LV, two facets of τ calculation and interpretation are controversial: 1) precisely which portion of the LV pressure curve should be used and whether or not a 0 pressure asymptote should be assumed, and 2) the afterload dependence. Nonetheless, relaxation is delayed, and τ increased, in chronic processes such as hypertrophy or cardiomyopathy, or in acute processes such as ischemia or the use of negative inotropic drugs. In contrast, relaxation is enhanced, and τ reduced, by increases in heart rate and the administration of positive inotropic drugs.

Heart failure can result not only from impaired systolic function but also from diastolic dysfunction.

Rapid ventricular filling follows isovolumic relaxation and begins when ventricular pressure falls below atrial pressure. During this period, elastic recoil of the myocardium, together with continued relaxation, creates an atrial/ventricular pressure gradient (sometimes characterized as suction) that greatly facilitates ventricular filling. As the atrial/ventricular pressure gradient diminishes, the phase of diastasis (slow ventricular filling) begins, continuing until atrial systole. Early rapid filling normally accounts for 75–80% of ventricular end-diastolic volume; diastasis and atrial systole provide about 3–5% and 15–25%, respectively. Multiple processes can alter diastolic filling dynamics, most notably ectopy arising from the atrioventricular node and ventricular pacing (no atrial systole), and reductions in ventricular compliance (e.g. concentric hypertrophy). The characteristics of ventricular compliance in pathologic states can be quantified by measurements of chamber stiffness (the monoexponential relationship between chamber pressure and volume changes) and myocardial stiffness (a material property of the myocardium that reflects its resistance to stretching). The relationship between ventricular relaxation, chamber stiffness, diastolic filling, and sarcomere length reveals that heart failure, manifest as low cardiac output and pulmonary vascular congestion, can result not only from impaired systolic function but from impaired diastolic function as well (diastolic dysfunction).

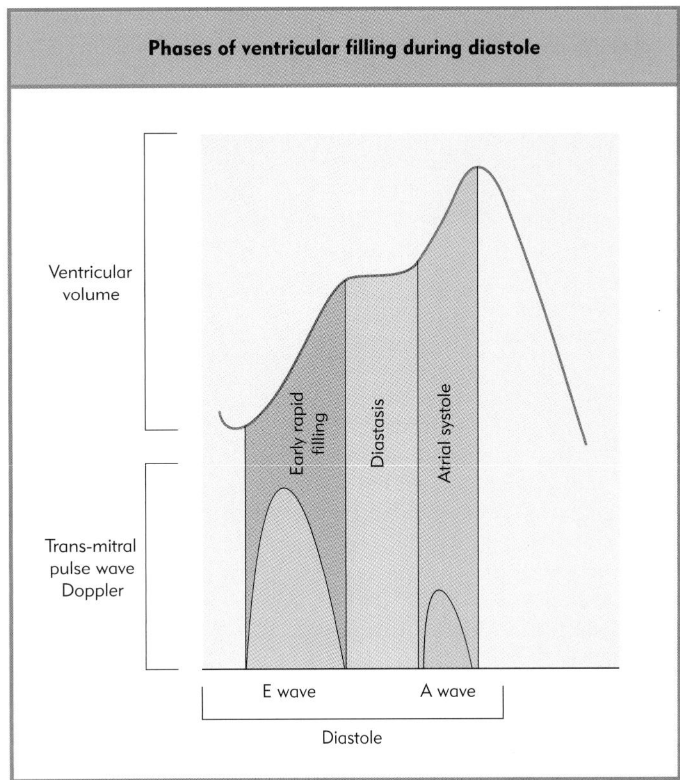

Figure 42.1 Phases of ventricular filling during diastole. Top depicts actual change in left ventricular volume. Bottom depicts pulsed-Doppler flow velocity patterns across the mitral valve corresponding with specific phases of ventricular volume change. E wave, early ventricular filling; A wave, atrial systole.

Table 42.1 Factors that influence ventricular compliance and filling

Extrinsic
Intrathoracic pressure
Pericardial inflammation or effusion
Intrapericardial mass
Intrinsic
Concentric hypertrophy (chronic hypertension or valvular stenosis)
Chronic cardiomyopathy
Acute ischemia
Infarction

Afterload

Despite the intuitive nature of the concept of afterload, it is actually difficult to apply precisely to the intact heart in that ejection is opposed by the variable hydraulic load imposed by the outflow circulation. Perhaps the closest parallel to afterload as defined in isolated muscle is instantaneous wall tension, but this parameter is difficult to quantify, particularly in the clinical setting. Accordingly, ventricular afterload is commonly summarized as the relationship between *mean* pressure and *mean* flow, expressed as systemic (SVR) or pulmonary (PVR) vascular resistance. Vascular resistance alone, however, is an incomplete expression of ventricular afterload, as the pressure and flow generated by the heart are not steady and continuous, but intermittent and pulsatile. Thus, in addition to steady-state resistive forces, ejection is opposed by elastic (large vessels are distended with each beat) and reflective (pressure waves reflected backwards) forces. In order to incorporate both pulsatile and nonpulsatile components into a single index of afterload, the concept of effective arterial elastance (the total change in aortic or pulmonary artery (PA) pressure divided by the volume change that occurs during a beat) has been proposed. Although this approach allows for quantification of total load, it does not dissociate pulsatile from nonpulsatile components. To achieve this, proximal aortic or PA pressure and flow characteristics can be resolved into individual frequency components (as each waveform actually represents the summation of forward and backward waves of multiple frequencies) and used to calculate input impedance (Z_{in}). This 'frequency domain' analysis of pressure and flow throughout the entire cardiac cycle allows for the creation of an impedance spectrum where the pressure/flow amplitude and phase ratios at each frequency are plotted over the range of 0 to about 25 Hz (Fig. 42.2). Specific components of the input impedance spectrum can then be used to represent different components of ventricular afterload, a) when analyzed to determine the location and magnitude of wave reflection; and b) when fit to a three-element model of the circulation that emulates an electrical circuit. This 'lumped parameter' model contains a *direct current (DC) component* (frequency independent) representing nonpulsatile load and characterized by Z at 0 frequency (Z_0), *an alternating current (AC) component* (frequency dependent) representing pulsatile load and described by the 'characterstic' Z (Z_C), defined as the average of values at 3 Hz and higher, and a *capacitor* (energy storage element), characterized by the compliance of the proximal aorta or PA, which through elastic recoil transmits energy downstream during diastole. This 'Windkessel' model is based upon similarities with early firehose systems that allowed water to be pumped by hand (pulsatile work, or AC component) into a distensible chamber (energy-storage element), which damped the pulsations and discharged the water as a continuous stream (steady-state, or DC component).

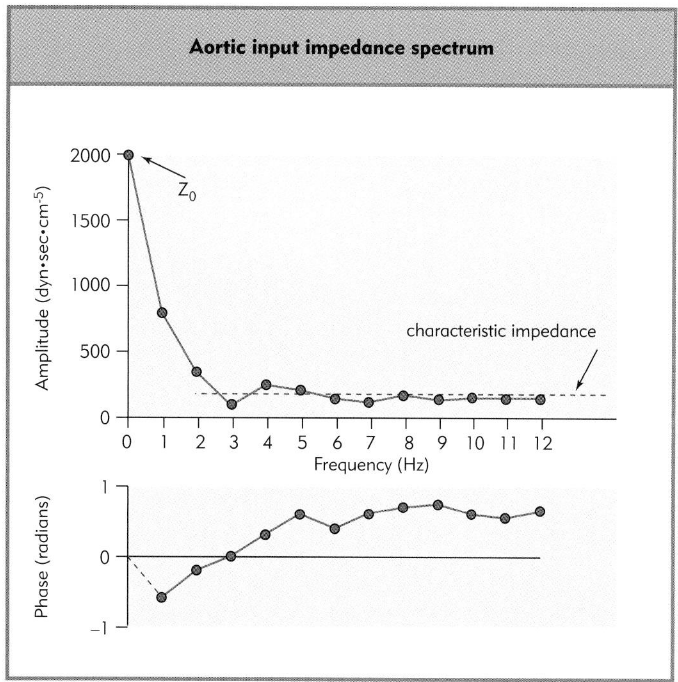

Figure 42.2 Aortic input impedance spectrum generated from pressure and flow recorded in the aortic root. Amplitude designates the ratio of pressure and flow at each frequency; Z_0 designates the ratio at 0 frequency, which is essentially equal to systemic vascular resistance and reflects the contribution of small resistance vessels to afterload. Characteristic impedance designates the average of values betweeen 3 and 12 Hz and reflects the contribution of afterload of large elastic vessels. Phase designates the phasic relationship between the pressure and flow wave at each frequency; when value is negative, flow precedes pressure. This information is useful in determining the characteristics of wave reflection.

Contractility

Contractility reflects the ability of the myocyte to generate tension in the face of a specific load; when the relationship is shifted such that tension is developed more rapidly and/or to a greater degree for the load, contractility is increased. Although this is relatively easy to quantify in isolated muscle systems or intact hearts beating isovolumically, where loading conditions can be strictly controlled, quantification of contractility in the ejecting heart is much more complex. Load-independent methods for assessing contractility in the intact heart have proved valuable in experimental preparations, but clinical application has not been uniformly successful. In general, indices of contractility can be derived from the phase of isovolumic contraction, the phase of ventricular ejection, the end-systolic pressure–volume relationship (ESPVR), or the relationship between stroke work and end-diastolic volume.

INDICES DERIVED FROM ISOVOLUMIC CONTRACTION

One of the most common and useful indices of contractility is the first derivative of developed pressure or dP/dt_{max}, which is sensitive for detecting acute alterations in contractility, easy to interpret, and relatively independent of afterload. Disadvantages include the need for high-fidelity measurements of pressure, distortion by wall properties and valve dysfunction, and a substantial influence by preload (Fig. 42.3).

Quantification of contractility in the ejecting heart is complex due to its dependence on load.

EJECTION PHASE INDICES

The most frequently used clinical index of global contractile function is ejection fraction (EF). Calculated as stroke volume divided by end-diastolic volume, the normal LVEF is 60–70%, and the normal RVEF is 45–50%. Both invasive and noninvasive techniques have been used to determine EF from image-based volume measurements (echocardiography, angiography, MRI, PET scanning) or indicator dilution techniques. Although EF provides useful information about systolic pump performance it is heavily influenced by afterload, which reduces its value as a specific index of contractility.

INDICES DERIVED FROM PRESSURE–VOLUME RELATIONSHIPS

Although often regarded as a relatively novel approach to assessment of cardiac function, ventricular pressure–volume loops were first constructed for frog hearts by Otto Frank in the late 1800s. Figure 42.4 depicts an LV pressure–volume diagram in

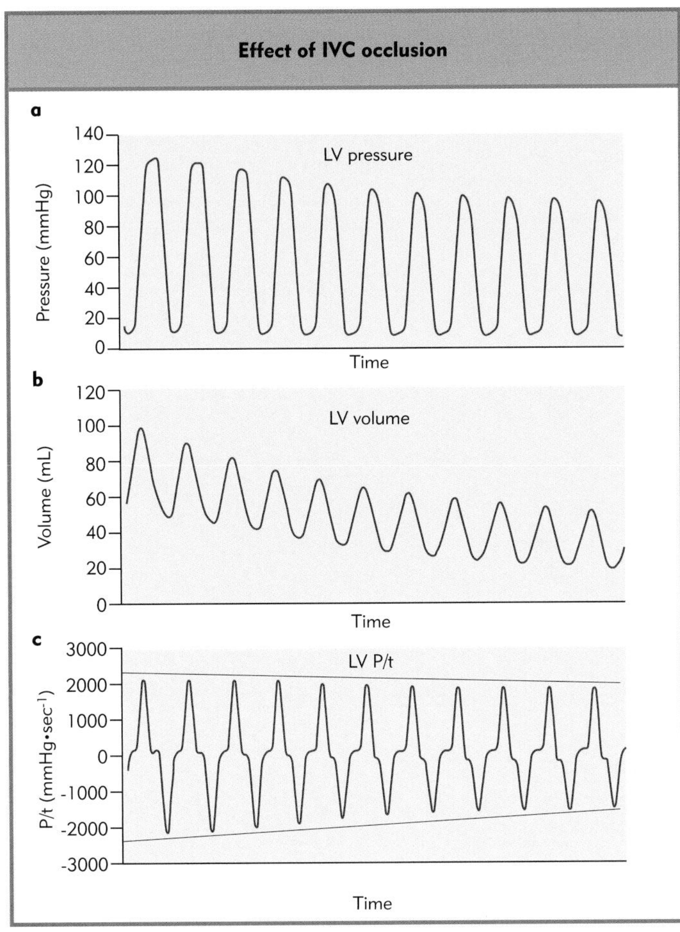

Figure 42.3 Left ventricular pressure, volume, and dP/dt during an acute reduction in preload (inferior rena cava (IVC) occlusion). (a) Left ventricular pressure, (b) volume, and (c) dP/dt. Despite no intrinsic change in contractility, dP/dt falls with the decline in volume, demonstrating the preload dependence of this index.

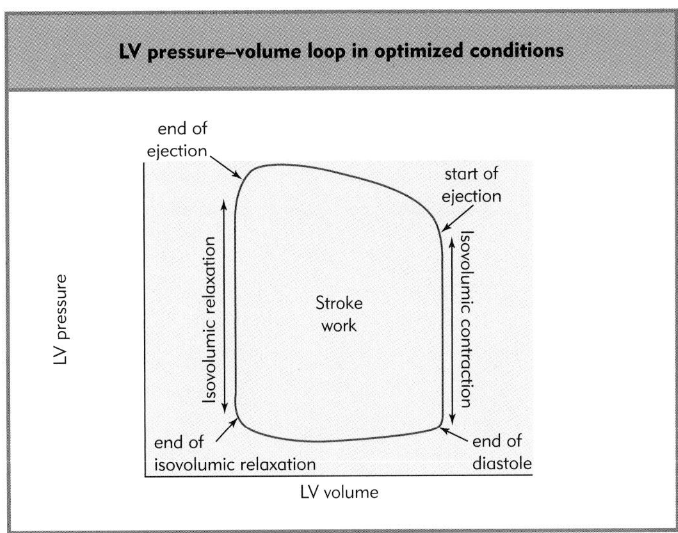

Figure 42.4 A left ventricular pressure–volume loop obtained under optimized conditions in an experimental animal. In general, the loop is rectangular with relatively well-defined phases corresponding to the beginning and end of ejection, and the beginning and end of filling.

which specific phases of the cardiac cycle are easily recognized. The upper left corner designates the relationship between pressure and volume at the end of systole (ejection), or the ESPVR, and the lower right corner denotes pressure and volume at the end of diastole (filling), or EDPVR. Although clear in the example, end-systole is not always so distinctly defined. This is evident in LV and RV pressure–volume loops obtained from the same experimental animal (Fig. 42.5). The RV loop is more triangular, with an ill-defined end-ejection point and a minimal period of isovolumic relaxation. In order to study regional myocardial function in conjunction with, or as an alternative to, global function, segmental dimension measurements can be obtained to create pressure–segment length loops. These loops are morphologically similar to pressure–volume loops (Fig. 42.5).

In the late 1970s Suga and Sagawa described the use of the ESPVR for characterizing ventricular contractility in a load-independent manner based on the concept of volume elastance (E), defined as $\Delta P/\Delta V$, or the inverse of compliance. If the empty heart is considered to behave like an elastic sac or balloon, as filling begins there is an initial increase in volume without significant pressure change. Eventually a volume is reached (V_0) at which contents go from being unstressed (no pressure) to stressed (under pressure), and pressure begins to rise as volume increases. If the subsequent pressure–volume relationship is

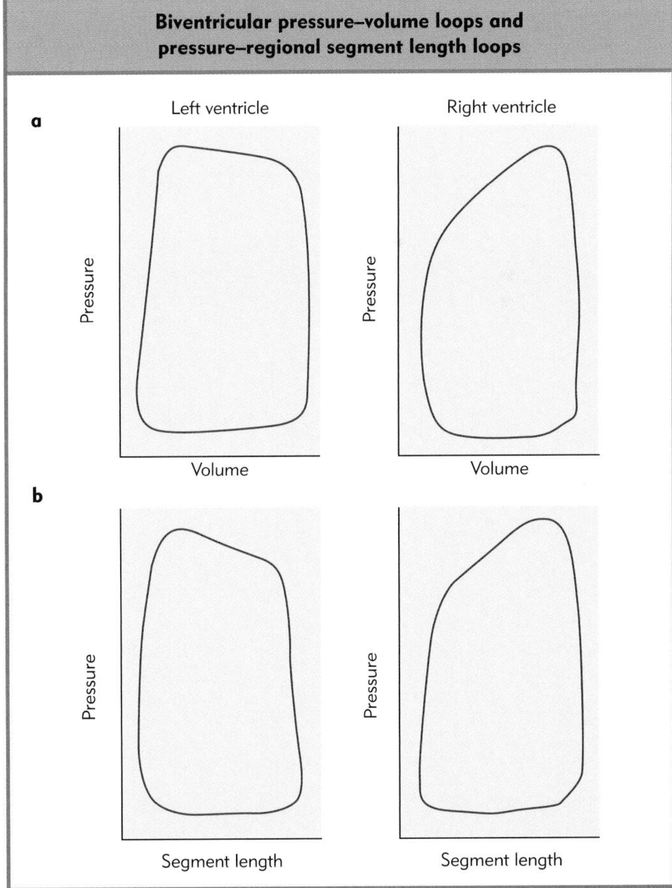

Figure 42.5 Comparison of left and right ventricular pressure–volume loops (a) and pressure/regional segment length loops (b) recorded simultaneously from the same heart. Under normal conditions, right ventricular loops tend to be more triangular with a poorly defined 'upper left corner'.

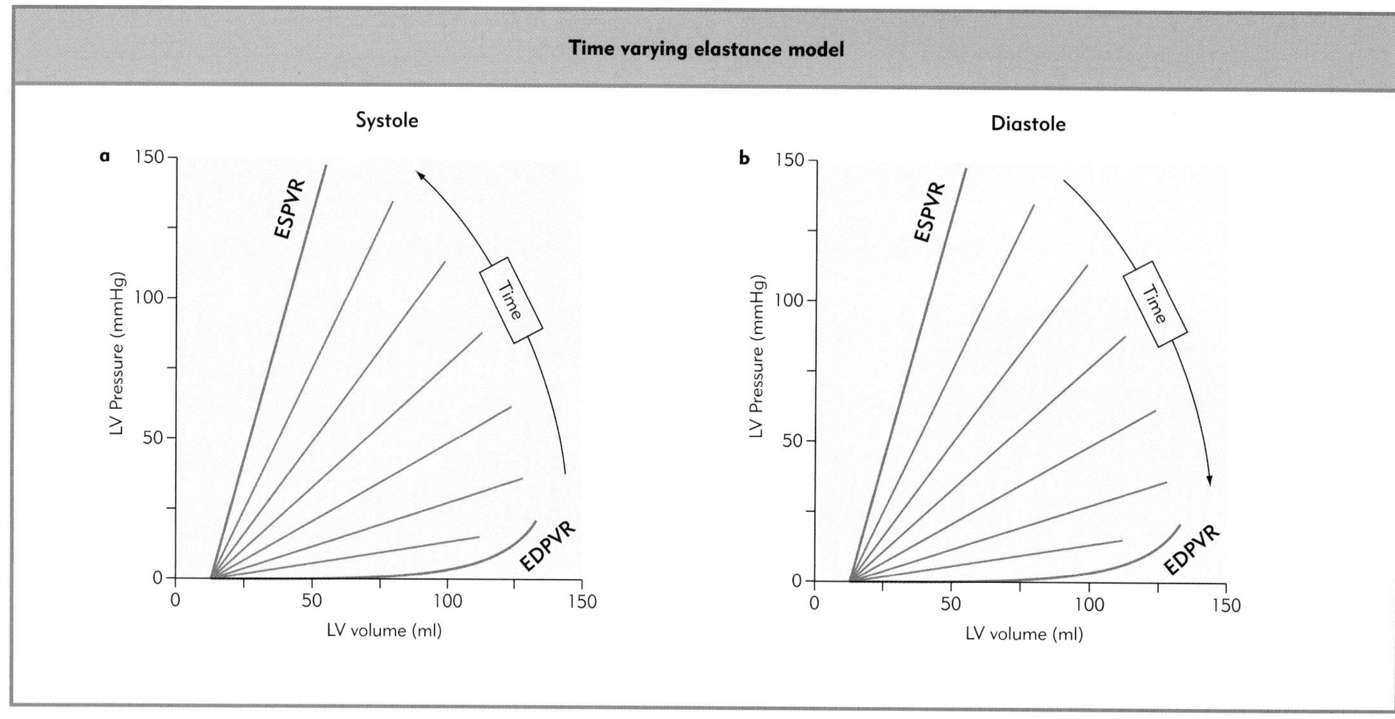

Figure 42.6 The time varying elastance model. (a) The change in the slope of the LV pressure–volume relationship (elastance) as the ventricle is contracting. The maximal elastance occurs at about the time of end-ejection; hence the steepest slope is termed the end-systolic pressure–volume relation. (b) As the ventricle relaxes during diastole, the slope of the pressure–volume relation decreases.

linear, then the slope of this line at any volume (V) is P/V–V_0, which represents E. However, unlike a balloon, the heart actively increases wall tension during contraction. As the wall stiffens the relationship between pressure and volume, and therefore E, changes. The pressure/volume ratio increases over the course of contraction to reach a maximum at the end of systole. This process has been conceptualized as the 'time-varying elastance model' (Fig. 42.6). Within this model, the ventricular pressure at any instant during ejection is linearly related to volume, with the slope of this time-varying elastance line progressively increasing until end-systole is reached. If contractility remains constant, the same time-varying elastance lines define the instantaneous relation between pressure and volume for both isovolumic beats and ejections over a range of loading conditions. In the intact left ventricle, maximal elastance (E_{max}) occurs essentially at end-systole and provides a load-independent index of contractility. Experimentally, E_{max} can be determined by varying loading conditions to provide a range of pressures and volumes, and regressing the point of end-systole for each beat; the slope of this regression is E_{max}, and the x (or volume) intercept is V_0 (Fig. 42.7). This method assumes that V_0 stays relatively constant and that the P/V–V_0 slope remains linear, which is valid under most physiologic conditions. However, acute alterations in contractility (e.g. the negative inotropic effect of volatile anesthetics) can alter both the slope and the volume intercept of the ESPVR (Fig. 42.7). In addition, E_{max} can be influenced by how end-systole is defined. The assumption is often made that end-ejection and the point of maximal P/V ratio occur at essentially the same time, but under some circumstances this is

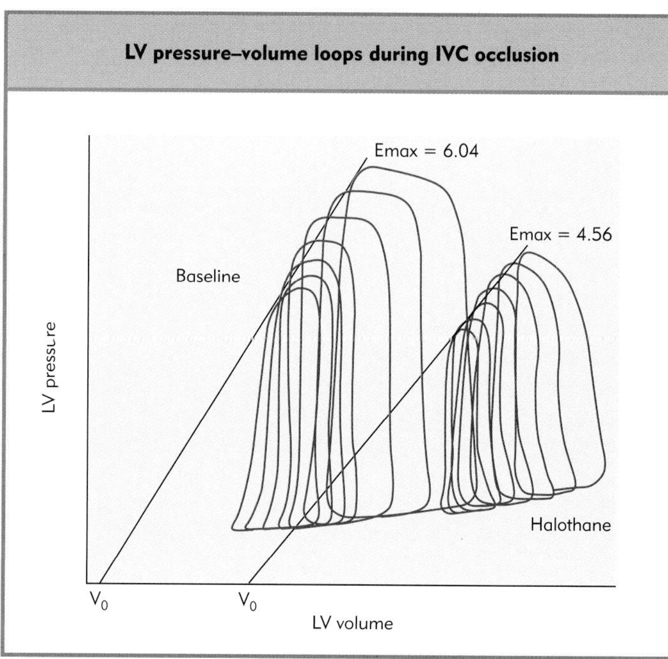

Figure 42.7 **Left ventricular pressure–volume loops obtained during an acute preload reduction (IVC occlusion).** Measurements were taken before and during administration of 1% halothane. Changes in both the slope of the end-systolic pressure volume relationship (E_{max}) and the volume intercept (V_0) were produced by halothane.

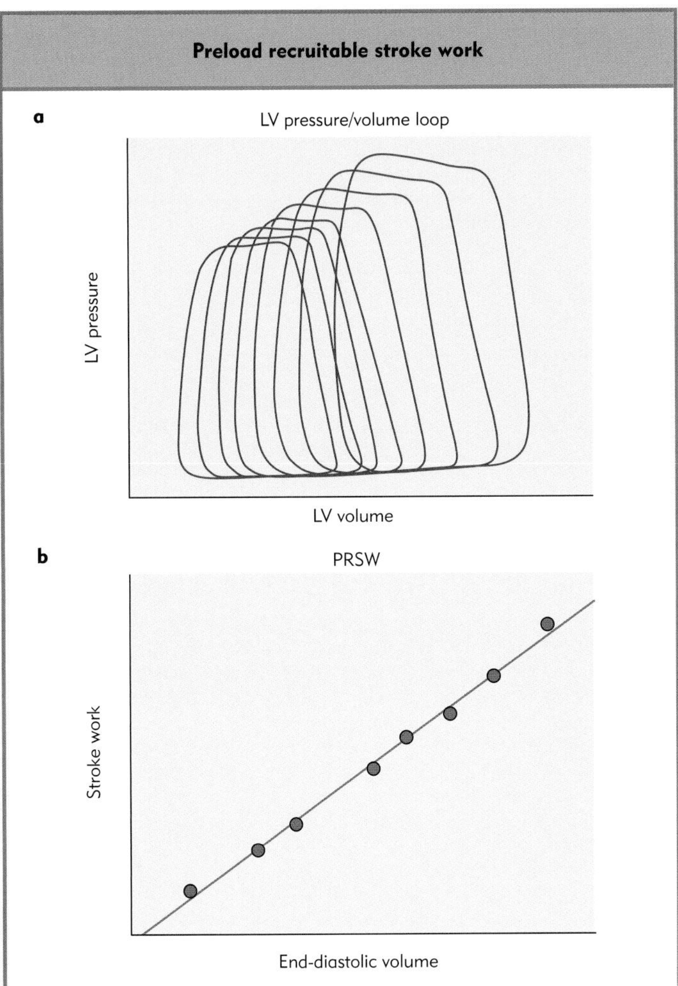

Figure 42.8 Preload recruitable stroke work (PRSW). (a) Left ventricular pressure–volume loops obtained during an acute preload reduction in an experimental animal. (b) The area of each loop (which represents stroke work) is plotted as a function of the end-diastolic volume to derive the preload recruitable stroke work (PRSW) as an index of contractility.

not so. Thus, many investigators use only the point of maximal P/V ratio when calculating E_{max}. An alternative to E_{max} is preload recruitable stroke work (PRSW), which essentially represents a linearization of the Frank–Starling relationship. To measure PRSW, venous return to the intact heart is acutely decreased and the area of each P/V loop, which represents the external work performed during the beat, is plotted as a function of the end-diastolic volume (Fig. 42.8). The slope of this relationship determines how much work the heart is capable of at any given preload. When contractility increases or decreases, the slope rises or falls as the heart performs more or less work for a given preload.

Several physiologic and pharmacological factors can directly alter contractility (Table 42.2), whereas others (e.g. nitroprusside, with its systemic vasodilation) produce indirect effects by stimulating regulatory autonomic responses. As the fundamental basis of contraction is Ca^{2+} binding to troponin C, the final common pathway of most processes is either intracellular Ca^{2+} availability or a change in sensitivity of troponin C to Ca^{2+} (Chapter 39). Alteration in contractility can be either acute or chronic, and a shift in the dose-response to most drugs occurs over time as a consequence of either changes in membrane receptor-binding affinity or number, or disruption of post-receptor events.

CLINICAL ASSESSMENT OF VENTRICULAR FUNCTION

Of the multiple techniques for evaluation of cardiac function, some are exclusively diagnostic whereas others are applicable for continuous monitoring at the bedside. A variety of methods for characterizing ventricular pump function based on estimates of volume have been described. Of these, chamber imaging techniques (angiography, echocardiography, magnetic resonance) are the most common. In general, the accuracy of the imaging techniques is far better for the LV than the RV, owing to the remarkably complex geometry of the RV. Alternative techniques that avoid the problems associated with complex geometry are radionuclide time–activity relationships (i.e. washout curves). These methods allow the determination not only of ejection fraction but also of indices of filling rates and ejection time, and thus have been widely used for perioperative evaluation of ventricular function.

Two main approaches to continuous perioperative evaluation of ventricular function are currently available: placement of a pulmonary arterial (PA) catheter, and transesophageal echocardiography (TEE). An additional technique that uses changes in thoracic bioimpedance to estimate stroke volume and cardiac output is available, but general experience with this method has not been favorable.

Pulmonary artery catherization

Since the introduction of the Swan–Ganz PA catheter to clinical use in the early 1970s, this device has become the mainstay for assessment of cardiac function in the critical care and perioperative settings. The PA catheter allows for direct measurement of right atrial, right ventricular, and PA pressure, indirect measurement of left atrial pressure, and indicator dilution-based calculation of cardiac output. Recent refinements have included the addition of fast-response thermistors, high-fidelity pressure transducers, fiberoptics for determination of mixed venous oxygen saturation, and miniaturized electronics located on the catheter for measurement of PA flow. Taken as a whole, a wide variety of variables can be derived from PA catheter data to characterize facets of biventricular function (Chapter 15).

PA BLOOD FLOW

A central feature of PA catheterization is measurement of cardiac output by the indicator (cold fluid) dilution technique. Because PA and aortic flows are matched at steady state, PA flow represents cardiac output. This thermodilution method of flow measurement utilizes a modification of the Stewart–Hamilton equation, which considers specific gravity, specific heat, and temperature of both cold injectate and blood, as well as injectate volume and a correction factor for warming of injectate along the catheter. In the denominator of the equation is the area under the curve for dilution of cold injectate back to baseline temperature. As other variables in the equation stay relatively constant, blood flow is inversely proportional to the area under the dilution curve. The accuracy and reproducibility of the thermodilution technique are dependent on the

Table 42.2 Factors affecting myocardial contractility

	Primary effect	Secondary effect	Contractility
Cardiac glycosides	Inhibition of Na^+, K^+-ATPase	Increase intracellular Ca^{2+}	Increase
β-adrenergic agonists, glucagon, histamine (H_2) agonists, phosphodiesterase III inhibitors	Increase cAMP, protein kinase A activation	Increase SR Ca^{2+} release, Increase troponin C Ca^{2+} affinity	Increase
α-adrenergic agonists, angiotensin II, endothelin	Phospholipase C activation → increase IP^3 and DAG, protein kinase C activation	Increase myofilament Ca^{2+} sensitivity, possibly increase SR Ca^{2+} release and reuptake	Increase
Myofilament sensitizers	Increase sensitivity to Ca^{2+}	+/– Inhibit phosphodiesterase III	Increase
Ca^{2+} channel agonists	Increase Ca^{2+} transient with depolarization	Enhance SR Ca^{2+} loading	Increase
Thyroid hormone	Mitochondrial stimulation Increase Na^+ transient Increase intracellular Ca^{2+} pool	Alteration in myosin isoenzymes Increase expression of β-adrenergic receptors	Increase
Hypoxia	Decrease ATP	Impair Ca^{2+} uptake into SR Increase resting level in myoplasm	Reduce Increase resting tension
Acidosis	Decrease intracellular Ca^{2+} transient Decrease myofilament Ca^{2+} sensitivity	Increase Na^+ entry secondary to enhanced H^+/Na^+ exchange	Reduce

characteristics of cold indicator injection (speed, proper volume, timing of respiratory cycle), complete and rapid mixing of the indicator in the RV, and proper calibration of the measuring system. When measurement conditions are strictly controlled, thermodilution measurements are remarkably accurate. However, variation in measurement technique, inappropriate injectate volume, and physiologic abnormalities such as tricuspid regurgitation can combine to produce significant error.

The ability to measure beat-to-beat changes in blood temperature with fast-response thermistors allows for estimation of RV ejection fraction from the difference between successive diastolic temperature plateaus. This measurement is used along with stroke volume (SV) to calculate end-systolic (ESV) and end-diastolic volumes (EDV) based on the relationships: EDV = SV/EF and ESV = EDV – SV. However, in that the technique is an indicator dilution method, clinical thermodilution measurements of RV ejection fraction are subject to error associated with catheter position, right heart dilation, and tricuspid regurgitation. Recently, thermodilution technology has been expanded to include automated measurement of cardiac output and RV ejection fraction via 'reverse thermodilution'. With this method, a coil on the PA catheter fractionally heats the blood passing over it, as opposed to cold injectate cooling the blood by the conventional technique. Finally, beat-to-beat measurements of flow have been obtained with a modified PA catheter. This device, which was once commercially available but failed in the marketplace, contains two Doppler transducers and two ultrasonic transit time transducers 12–13 cm from the tip. When positioned in the root of the PA, these transducers continuously measure blood velocity, catheter angulation, and the internal diameter of the vessel. The angulation-corrected diameter measurement is used to determine the cross-sectional area of the PA, which is then multiplied by the angulation-corrected velocity signal to yield instantaneous flow.

PRELOAD

Although preload is more a function of volume than pressure, RV preload can be indexed with measurements of mean right atrial and RV end-diastolic pressures. Right atrial pressures should be carefully interpreted in the context of pressure wave morphology. For example, a damped waveform may not accurately reflect RV end-diastolic pressure, and rhythm disturbances such as ectopy arising from the atrioventricular node may produce waveform distortion (cannon A-waves) and a mean right atrial pressure which is substantially higher than true RV end-diastolic pressure. Commonly, LV preload is assessed by measurement of pulmonary capillary wedge pressure (PCWP). Determined by measuring pressure distal to an occluding balloon in a branch of the PA, PCWP reflects left atrial pressure which has been transmitted back through the pulmonary venous, capillary, and distal arterial circulation. Thus, PCWP provides an index, but not a direct measure, of mean left atrial pressure, which itself is an index but not direct measure of LV end-diastolic pressure, which is an index but not a direct measure of LV end-diastolic volume. Given the indirect nature of PCWP as a monitor of preload, factors affecting the pulmonary circulation (i.e. lung injury, mechanical ventilation) can influence the utility of the absolute number. However, when measurement conditions are kept relatively consistent, changes in PCWP over time can provide useful trend information.

Preload is more a function of volume than pressure, so pressure indices of preload must be used cautiously.

AFTERLOAD

As noted above, LV and RV afterload are commonly expressed as SVR and PVR, respectively. Although these parameters express total afterload only incompletely, they remain useful clinical indices when considered in the context of their limitations. SVR is calculated as: (mean arterial pressure – right atrial pressure)/ cardiac output. PVR is calculated as (mean PA pressure – PCWP)/ cardiac output. In that right atrial pressure is usually quite small relative to mean arterial pressure, abnormalities in the waveform or absolute pressure frequently have little impact on SVR. In contrast, PCWP is usually much higher relative to mean PA pressure and can significantly influence the calculation of PVR. Additionally, PVR measurements are much more heavily influenced by flow than SVR, such that even in the absence of significant direct effects on the pulmonary circulation, a fall in cardiac output can produce a substantial increase in PVR. Refinements in PA catheter design now allow for characterization of RV afterload in terms of characteristic impedance and compliance calculated from internal measurements of PA diameter and flow. However, clinical use of these devices is not widespread.

CONTRACTILITY

Despite the utility of PA catheters, they provide little direct information regarding LV contractility. In contrast, owing to the direct access afforded to the right heart and pulmonary circulation, techniques have been described for the assessment of RV contractility. Two reported approaches to the assessment of RV contractility include the use of Doppler flow and PA pressure measurements to index RV power generation; and thermodilution-derived measurements of RV end-systolic and end-diastolic volumes to calculate preload recruitable stroke work.

Echocardiography

Both imaging and Doppler echocardiography have utility in perioperative monitoring of ventricular function. Transesophageal echocardiography (TEE) in particular is easily used in the operating room, and with standard transverse views provides reasonably clear images of biventricular morphology, structures, and both global and regional ventricular function (Chapter 17). When carefully and skillfully performed, TEE can provide much of the same information as a PA catheter.

BLOOD FLOW

Many techniques have been described for the calculation of cardiac output using Doppler measurements of blood velocity and ultrasonic transit time of vessel (or valve) cross-sectional area (flow = velocity × area). Because TEE is able to quantify blood velocity in the PA, across the mitral valve, through the LV outflow tract, and within the aortic root, cardiac output determinations from each of these areas have been described. However, because of anatomical variation and technical problems with optimal imaging, errors of up to 24% have been reported.

Transesophageal echocardiography clearly demonstrates that changes in end-diastolic dimensions are not always reflected in pulmonary capillary wedge pressure.

PRELOAD

The ability to continuously observe the cross-sectional area of the LV with TEE has enhanced appreciation of the fact that preload is a manifestation of end-diastolic volume, not just pressure. Indeed, TEE assessment of LV dimensions under variant intraoperative conditions clearly demonstrates that changes in end-diastolic dimension are not necessarily closely linked to alterations in PCWP. This highlights the importance of considering LV compliance in the assessment of diastolic function. In addition to direct imaging of the LV chamber, Doppler assessment of systolic pulmonary venous flow (both systolic and diastolic components) into the left atrium and visual inspection of interatrial septal motion can provide information about LV filling pressures which may be particularly valuable when interpretation of direct LV dimension data is complicated by significant regional wall motion abnormalities. In general, when the systolic component of pulmonary venous flow is less than 55%, or the interatrial septum does not exhibit paradoxical motion during the initial phase of exhalation following a positive-pressure breath, left atrial pressure is at least 15 mmHg. TEE also allows for evaluation of diastolic filling characteristics based primarily on transmitral flow patterns. Under normal circumstances, the majority of LV filling occurs during the early, rapid filling phase of diastole, with the remaining fraction being provided by atrial systole. Accordingly, transmitral flow patterns exhibit two velocity peaks, reflecting these filling intervals, designated as the 'E' (early) and 'A' (atrial systole) waves (Fig. 42.1). The ratio of these two waves provides a convenient means to evaluate LV filling dynamics; in the normal, compliant LV the E/A ratio is well over 1. In contrast, when compliance is reduced, atrial systole becomes much more important for filling and the ratio is less than 1.

AFTERLOAD

Vascular resistance is an incomplete index of afterload because it assumes the ventricle is a steady-state pressure–flow generator. TEE allows derivation of end-systolic wall stress from ventricular dimension, thickness, and pressure, thus potentially providing a more complete index of afterload.

CONTRACTILITY

Whereas continuous visual images of the contracting heart give the observer a general feel of contractility, reliable real-time quantification with TEE is lacking. Several techniques for offline assessment have been described, including the relationship between end-systolic wall stress and dimension or rate-corrected fiber shortening, but these indices are load sensitive. Similarly, ejection fraction reflects the forces of both contractility and afterload. The reported accuracy of EF predicted by TEE has not been as good as that determined by transthoracic echo, owing to limited imaging of the LV apex. An alternative TEE technique, LV fractional area change measured at the midpapillary level in the short-axis (cross-sectional) view is a reasonable approximation of EF and has become widely used.

The application of pressure–dimension or pressure–volume analysis techniques to echocardiographic images has been enhanced by the introduction of automated border detection software that allows the generation of a continuous LV dimension (and, by calculation, volume) waveform. With these data, pressure–volume loops similar to those generated by more invasive techniques have been generated and used to index contractility in a load-independent manner. To obviate the need for

LV pressure, some investigators have described the use of a peripheral arterial pressure and TEE-derived volume to construct loops that resemble the systolic portion of a true LV pressure–volume loop.

The introduction of tissue Doppler echocardiography has added a new tool for the quantification of regional ventricular function. Fundamentally, the Doppler beam is used to measure the velocity of systolic myocardial shortening with enhanced velocity mirroring an increase in ejection fraction. As with other ejection phase indices, systolic shortening is influenced by both preload and afterload. Recent extension of the methodology has focused on myocardial acceleration during isovolumic contraction and yielded promising data with regard to load-independent assessment of contractility.

VENTRICULAR-VASCULAR INTEGRATION

Whereas the concepts of preload, afterload, and contractility are fundamental to an understanding of ventricular function, consideration of the diverse interactions between the ventricles and their respective vasculatures is of paramount importance in understanding circulatory physiology as a whole. Perhaps the best example of this is the concept of afterload; as noted above, it is extremely difficult to precisely apply 'afterload' as derived from isolated muscle systems to the intact heart. Accordingly, although we tend to have a visceral appreciation of afterload as the forces that oppose ejection of blood from the heart, the reverse is actually true with regard to common clinical indices of afterload, such as vascular resistance, i.e. resistance is regulated by flow and pressure, not vice versa. A variety of models have been proposed to characterize interactions between the components of the cardiovascular system, each containing a volume of blood subjected to a pressure reflecting compliance (or the inverse, elastance) of that component. Importantly, even in the absence of cardiac contraction, pressure – and, for a period of time, flow – is maintained in both the arterial and venous systems because blood in each circuit is acted upon by the elastic character of the vasculature.

Venous return model

Guyton and colleagues proposed a model in which the circulation is summarized as a single vessel incorporating both the arterial and the venous system. For this model, the mean arterial (mAP) minus right atrial (RAP) pressure difference divided by the systemic vascular resistance (SVR) determines cardiac output, and the predominant variable regulating global cardiovascular performance is venous return (75% of blood volume is usually in the venous system). These investigators tested the hypothesis that the pressure difference driving blood through the arterial portion of the circulation is the difference between mAP and 'mean systemic pressure' (P_{ms}), a hypothetical distal pressure in the arterial bed dictated by the blood volume and compliance of the arterial bed. With this relationship, flow through the arterial bed (Q) is given by $Q = (mAP - Pms) / R_a$, where R_a is the arterial resistance. As steady-state flow through the arterial and venous beds is essentially the same (i.e. cardiac output = arterial flow = venous flow), cardiac output can also be expressed as total venous flow by $(P_{ms} - RAP)/R_v$, where R_v is the venous resistance. Thus, the P_{ms} – RAP difference is the pressure head for venous return.

In an elegant series of experiments using the right heart bypass model, Guyton demonstrated that increases in pump flow around the RV are matched by increases in left ventricular output (due to increased end-diastolic volume and pressure, and quantified by Starling curves). In addition, the experiments demonstrated that transient effects on venous return secondary to a range of changes in RAP can be used to construct linear venous return (Q_v) plots based on the relationship:

■ Equation 42.4

$$Q_v = -\frac{1}{R_v} \times RAP + \left[\frac{P_{ms}}{R_v}\right]$$

Within this relationship, P_{ms} is the pressure at which Q_v becomes zero, i.e. P_{ms} = RAP when $Q_v = 0$. By analogy, the zero-flow pressure within the pulmonary bed, termed mean pulmonic pressure (P_{mp}), is the upstream venous pressure driving blood flow to the left atrium. As with the systemic circulation, the pulmonary zero-flow pressure is dictated by both the volume of blood and the vascular compliance of the vasculature. Importantly, although the zero-flow pressure will be equal in each circulatory bed (assuming no effect of venous valves), the pressure at zero flow in the systemic and pulmonary beds is not necessarily equal because they are anatomically isolated. Ultimately, venous return concepts can be integrated with pressure–volume relationships for each ventricle to define the interaction between multiple hemodynamic components.

Elastance matching

Another approach to assessing ventricular–vascular interaction is based on the expression of both contractility and afterload in the common term of elastance. As noted above, the ventricular ESPVR can be used to summarize contractility as E_{max}, and the arterial ESPVR to describe total afterload as effective arterial elastance (E_a). When the E_a/E_{max} ratio is 0.5 (afterload low relative to contractility) the heart achieves maximal efficiency in terms of the amount of work performed for oxygen consumed. Alternatively, when the E_a/E_{max} ratio is 1.0, the heart is performing maximal stroke work; when the ratio exceeds 1 both efficiency and stroke work decline. As with each beat a pressure is generated by the ventricle sufficient to move a volume of blood into the circulation, which in turn accepts the blood at a certain pressure, it is possible to calculate ventricular EF from end-systolic elastance data as: $E_{max}/E_{max} + E_a$. When this relationship is considered in the context of optimal matching for stroke work occurring when the vascular/ventricular elastance ratio is 1.0, it is evident that optimal mechanical matching is associated with an EF of 50%.

Pulsatility and wave reflection: caveats in models of mechanical coupling

Because flow in the arterial tree is pulsatile, the load imposed by the vasculature on ventricular performance is affected by the nature of this flow. Put simply, the energy of pulsations represents energy lost in the form of work done by the blood on the vessel wall, and heat lost by friction. Therefore, changes in the vasculature (such as stiffening with aging) that result in greater pulsatility also decrease the efficiency of energy transfer from the ventricle to the vasculature. An extension of ventricular–vascular matching concepts based upon the product of pressure and flow, therefore, considers pump performance in both nonpulsatile and pulsatile (oscillatory) terms. This allows for characterization of how much work done (or power generated) by the system goes toward moving blood forward, and how much is lost to pulsatility (i.e. goes toward distending the system). Power output (W), which represents work performed per unit time, can be calculated by multiplying instantaneous pressure and flow, with the area under the waveform for each cardiac cycle representing the total power (W_T) for the duration of that beat. These values are averaged over a series of beats. If the mean pressure and flow over the same sequence of beats are multiplied, steady-state power (W_{SS}) is derived. In that W_T represents the sum of W_{SS} (that which goes toward providing forward flow) and oscillatory power (W_{OS}), the W_{OS} value (reflecting power lost to distending the system) can be calculated by subtraction.

As the oscillatory or pulsatile waves that are established by the heart in the vasculature have a finite velocity, the waveform of the arterial pulse is modified not only by vascular and blood properties, but also by the presence of reflected waves that collide with forward waves in the arterial tree. Through detailed analyses of pulsatile phenomena either in the time or the frequency domain (e.g. impedance spectra), the impact of alterations in wave reflections as a consequence of disease and aging may be appreciated. Although specific analysis of the site, magnitude, and consequence of wave reflection is relatively complex, a simpler manifestation of wave reflection can be found in visual inspection of the arterial waveform. When measured in a supine subject, systolic blood pressure in the dorsalis pedis artery is higher than that in the thoracic aorta. It is difficult to reconcile this observation with the notion that the large elastic arteries, like a simple Windkessel, serve to absorb and damp the energy of cardiac ejection and convert pulsatile input into steady flow at the level of the arterioles. What, then, accounts for an increase in peak pressure as the pressure wave travels distally in the arterial tree? The answer to this question is found in an analysis of the timing of reflected pressure waves colliding with forward waves and thus adding energy to the forward wave. In small distal arteries there is not much of a time delay and the reflected wave returns during the systolic peak. In the thoracic aorta, with much more distance to traverse to the main reflecting sites, the reflected wave returns later during diastole.

The increase in peak arterial pressure as the pressure wave travels distally in the arterial tree is due to reflected pressure waves, and results in systolic hypertension with age-related arterial stiffening.

With the stiffening of arteries that occurs with aging and arteriosclerosis, the speed of the traveling waves is greatly increased and reflected waves return during systole even in the thoracic aorta. This phenomenon contributes to systolic hypertension of aging and increases large vessel contributions to ventricular afterload. Stiffening of the arteries also contributes to a more rapid decline of blood pressure during diastole and a widening of the pulse pressure. Potential ramifications of this are a decreased pressure gradient for coronary perfusion, the majority of which usually occurs (for the LV) during diastole. Kass and colleagues studied the possible impact of aortic stiffening in an animal model and found that although diastolic coronary perfusion did decline, it was offset by increased perfusion in the latter stages of systole. This increased systolic perfusion is the result of reflected waves returning to the heart more quickly and accumulating in the proximal aorta to initiate a pressure gradient for coronary perfusion earlier in the cycle.

Limitations of steady-state models

Classically, it is taught that cardiac output is modulated by alterations in preload, contractility, afterload, and heart rate, whereas blood pressure is modulated by both cardiac output and vascular resistance. These variables are often presented as reasonably singular entities, but both cardiac output and blood pressure are determined by intrinsic and extrinsic processes that rapidly and continuously modify the interaction between the heart and the arterial and venous systems. A good clinical example is the simple intervention of an intravenous fluid bolus. Generally thought of as a singular means of increasing ventricular preload (end-diastolic volume) and hence stroke volume, this intervention will also increase afterload as a consequence of increased stroke volume, shift venous return characteristics, and modify autonomic nervous input to the heart and circulation, eliciting both direct (i.e. adrenergic stimulation) and indirect (i.e. cardiac force–frequency relationships and vascular production of endothelial substances) effects. This simple intervention may also lead to displacement of the intraventricular septum, with secondary alteration in left ventricular compliance and a shift in interventricular interaction.

Direct interventricular interactions occur throughout the cardiac cycle.

Although it has long been appreciated that the pressure in one ventricle directly affects the pressure in the other, understanding of the dynamic and mechanical interaction between the chambers has only recently become more complete. These direct *interventricular interactions* (IVIs) occur throughout the cardiac cycle, but are typically divided into systolic and diastolic. Given that the peak systolic pressure of the RV is normally one-fifth that of the left, the impact of a given change in pressure is much greater for the RV when viewed as a percentage of pressure generation. For example, up to 30% of RV pressure generation is dependent on LV pressure generation. In contrast, diastolic IVIs can impair filling at high contralateral ventricular preload, which confounds the issue of whether IVIs normally have a net positive or negative impact on overall cardiovascular performance. However, the loss of the LV contribution to RV systolic pressure is a significant factor in the pathophysiology of RV failure during left ventricular assist (when LV systolic pressures are suddenly reduced). Moreover, the reduction in LV diastolic compliance by leftward septal shift represents a clear example of the hemodynamic consequences of diastolic IVIs seen in acute RV failure.

Models and reality: attempting to close the loop

Computer modeling has begun to provide insight into a more broad and comprehensive view of cardiovascular performance. Expanded appreciation of the complexity of interactions (ventricular–vascular and interventricular) can be illustrated by

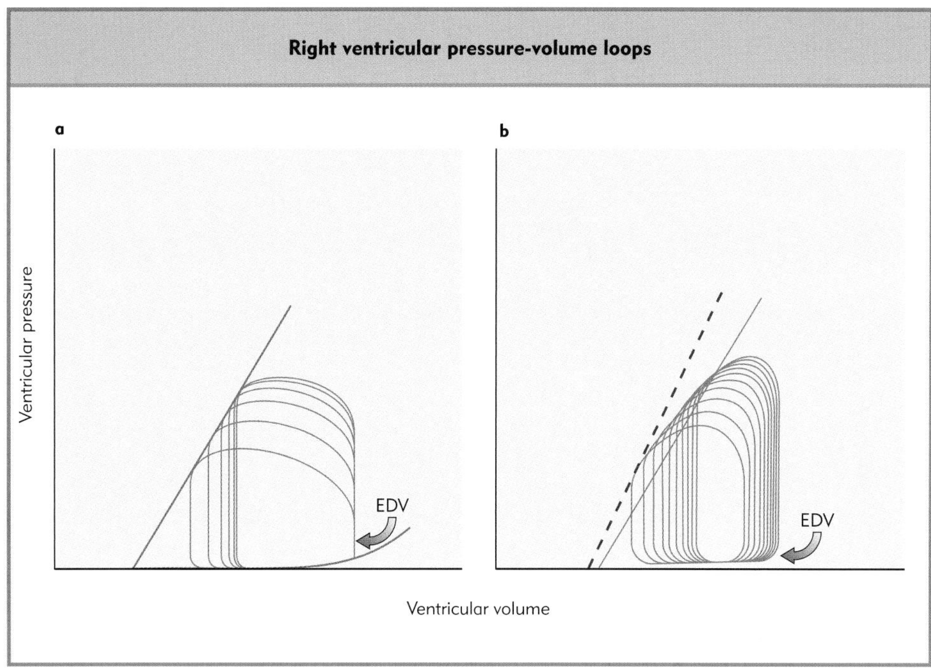

Figure 42.9 Right ventricular pressure–volume loops during the acute pulmonary vasoconstriction induced by protamine. (a) The commonly idealized response, in which RV pressure rises and stroke volume falls while end-diastolic volume (EDV) and contractility (ESPVR) remain constant. (b) The more realistic situation, in which the RV is allowed to interact (directly and in series) with the rest of the circulation. RV preload eventually decreases as a consequence of reduced LV filling, LV output, and therefore venous return (i.e. series interaction). As LV peak pressure decreases, the RV ESPVR is shifted downwards owing to the impact of LV pressure on septal function (i.e. direct ventricular interaction).

simulating clinical situations. For example, following cardiopulmonary bypass protamine administration elicits acute pulmonary hypertension and systemic hypotension. The clinical course suggests the deleterious response of marked pulmonary vasoconstriction, with the global impact on cardiovascular function manifest as an increase in RV afterload, a decrease in RV stroke volume, underfilling of the LV, and systemic hypoperfusion. The common idealized RV response to acute pulmonary vasoconstriction is shown in Figure 42.9a. Over a series of beats developed pressure rises while stroke volume falls. However, the consequences of this single change actually extend far beyond an increase in RV afterload (Fig. 42.9b). Although the reduction in RV output will cause a decrease in LV filling and thereby reduce LV stroke volume, this reduction causes a reduction in mAP and decreased flow across the systemic capillaries into the systemic venous system. After a period of equilibration venous return will decline, as predicted by Guyton, owing to a shift in the relationship between the hypothetical mean systemic pressure and RAP. Ultimately, RV end-diastolic volume (preload) will decline, further reducing RV stroke volume. In addition, the decrease in LV systolic pressure generation will decrease RV pump function via direct ventricular interactions as described above. Finally, the reduction in systemic arterial pressure may also reduce RV contractility via a reduction in coronary perfusion pressure. Accordingly, the interpretation of the hemodynamic response to a given event or intervention must be made within a framework that incorporates the multitude of interactions that occur in the cardiovascular system over a period of minutes, not seconds.

With each beat, the heart expends a certain amount of energy towards tension development to produce pressure, and myocyte shortening to produce flow. The balance between tension and shortening dictates the performance and efficiency of the heart as a pump. Although our ability to incorporate the profound complexity of intrinsic and extrinsic cardiovascular regulation into clinical practice is limited, a general understanding of the interaction between contractility and load – and a healthy respect for what we cannot measure – can be clinically important in the treatment of patients with compromised ventricular performance.

Key references

Burkhoff D, Sagawa K. Ventricular efficiency predicted by an analytical model. Am J Physiol. 1986;250:R1021–7.

Guyton AC, Lindsey AW, Abernathy JB, Richardson T. Venous return at various right atrial pressures and the normal venous return curve. Am J Physiol. 1957;189:609.

Kass DA, Kelly RP. Ventriculo-arterial coupling: concepts, assumptions, and applications. Ann Biomed Eng. 1992;20:41–62.

Sagawa K, Maughan L, Suga H, Sunagawa K. Cardiac contraction and the pressure volume relationship. New York: Oxford University Press; 1988:110–52.

Further reading

Damiano RJ, La Follette P, Cox JL et al. Significant left ventricular contribution to right ventricular systolic function. Am J Physiol. 1991;261:H1514–24.

Dickstein ML, Todaka K, Burkhoff D. Left-to-right systolic and diastolic ventricular interactions are dependent on right ventricular volume. Am J Physiol. 1997;272:H2869–74.

Heerdt PM Dickstein ML. Assessment of right ventricular function. Semin Cardiothorac Vasc Anesth. 1997;1:215–24.

Lang RM, Borow KM, Neumann A, Janzen D. Systemic vascular resistance: an unreliable index of left ventricular afterload. Circulation 1986;74:1114–23.

O'Rourke MF. Steady and pulsatile power energy losses in the systemic circulation under normal conditions and in simulated arterial disease. Cardiovasc Res. 1967;1:313–326.

Perrino AC, Harris SN, Luther MA. Intraoperative determination of cardiac output using multiplane transesophageal echocardiography. Anesthesiology 1998;89:350–7.

Saeki A, Recchia F, Kass DA. Systolic flow augmentation in hearts ejecting into a model of stiff aging vasculature. Influence on myocardial perfusion–demand balance. Circ Res. 1995;76:132–41.

Tuman KJ, Carroll GC, Ivankovich AD. Pitfalls in interpretation of pulmonary artery catheter data. J Cardiothorac Anesth. 1989;3:625–41.

Chapter 43 The peripheral circulation

Simon Howell and James Dodman

TOPICS COVERED IN THIS CHAPTER

- **Arterial system, venous system, and microcirculation**
  - Rheology: dynamics of blood flow
- **Cardiovascular regulatory mechanisms**
  - Baroreflex control
  - Intrinsic flow regulation
  - Regional blood flow
- **Intrinsic flow regulation**
  - Regional blood flow
- **Pharmacological control of blood pressure**
  - Vasodilators
  - Vasopressors
- **Hypertension and antihypertensive therapy**
  - β-adrenoceptor antagonists
  - ACE inhibitors
  - Angiotensin II antagonists
  - Diuretics
  - Calcium channel blockers
  - α_1-adrenoceptor antagonists
  - Hypertension and anesthesia

The primary role of the peripheral circulation is to deliver nutrients to and remove waste products from the tissues. However, blood vessels are not a passive conduit. They are structurally adapted to meet the differing needs of various tissues and are subject to complex regulatory mechanisms to control local and global blood flow.

ARTERIAL SYSTEM, VENOUS SYSTEM, AND MICROCIRCULATION

Apart from capillaries all blood vessels have the same basic three-layered structure (Fig. 43.1). The outermost layer, the adventitia, is a connective tissue sheath that holds the vessel loosely in place. The adventitia of the larger vessels, such as the aorta, pulmonary arteries, and iliac vessels, contains a plexus of small vessels, the vasa vasorum. These provide nourishment for the media of large vessels. In the largest arteries they penetrate into the outer two-thirds of the media.

The media is bounded by the inner and outer elastic laminae and consists of smooth muscle cells embedded in a matrix of collagen and elastic fibers. It provides the vessels with mechanical strength and contractile power.

The innermost layer is the intima; this is the main barrier to the passage of plasma proteins, but it is mechanically weak. It consists of a flat layer of endothelial cells lying on a thin layer of connective tissue. The intima synthesizes and secretes a number of vasoactive substances and has an important role in the local regulation of the circulation.

The intima synthesizes and secretes a number of vasoactive substances and has an important role in the local regulation of the circulation.

The pulmonary arteries, the aorta, and major branches such as the iliac vessels, have a tunica media rich in elastin and are classified as elastic arteries. During systole they expand to receive the blood ejected by the heart and then recoil during diastole, so smoothing the pulsatile ejection of blood by the heart into a more continuous flow. The medium and small arteries, such as the popliteal and radial arteries, act as low-resistance conduits. They have a tunica media that is thick relative to the vessel diameter and is rich in smooth muscle. These vessels have a rich sympathetic innervation and can contract. Their resistance is low, however, and consequently the pressure drop across them is small. Despite being unimportant in the regulation of blood flow, their thick walls help to prevent collapse at sharp bends such as the knee, and their ability to produce a profound contraction may prevent exsanguination from a severed vessel in the event of trauma.

The microcirculation consists of the fine plexus of vessels that ramify through the tissues and comprises arterioles, capillaries, and venules. The smallest arteries branch into first-order arterioles and then into second- and third-order arterioles, and finally into terminal arterioles. Arterioles are the main resistance vessels of the systemic circulation; they have the thickest walls of all arteries relative to the diameter of the vessel lumen, and the pressure drop across arterioles is greater than that in any other vessels in the systemic circulation (Fig. 43.3). The first-order arterioles are innervated by sympathetic nerves and are

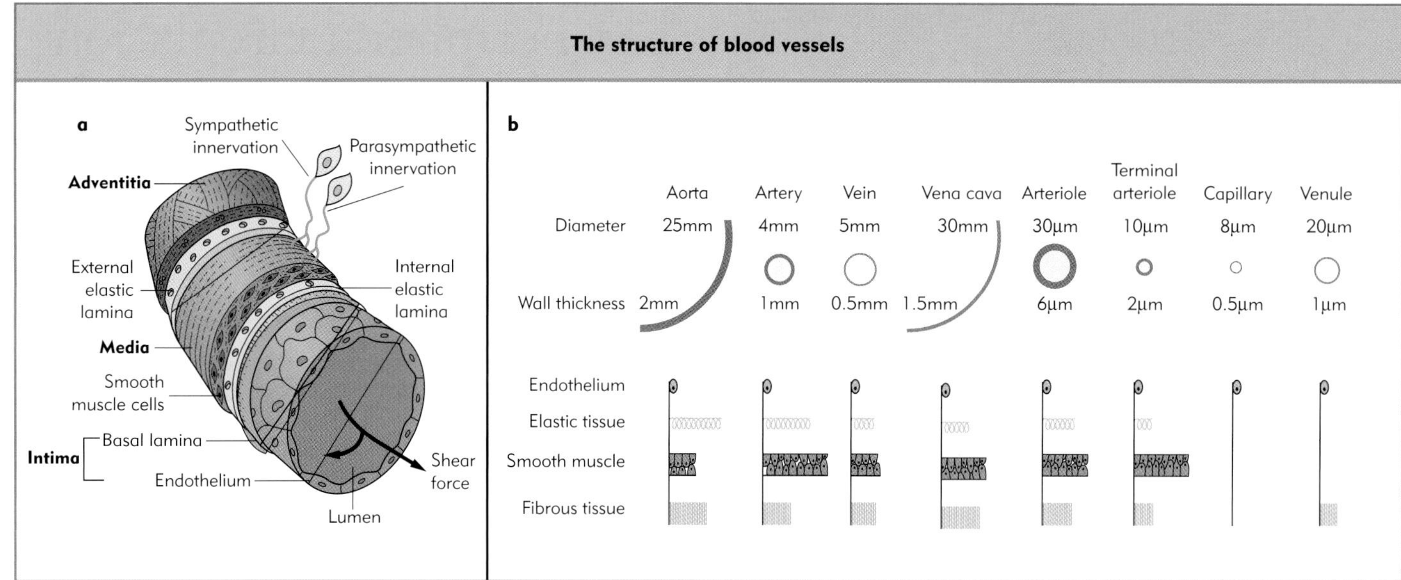

Figure 43.1 The structure of blood vessels. All blood vessels have the same general structure (a). Different vessels have varying internal diameters, wall thickness, and relative amounts of the principal components of the vessel walls (b). Cross-sections of the vessels are not drawn to scale because of the huge range from aorta and vena cava to capillary. (After Burton AC. Physiol Rev. 1954;34:619.)

subject to control by the sympathetic nervous system, whereas in the terminal arterioles control is dominated by local metabolites. Flow can be increased by increasing driving pressure or decreasing resistance. In general, blood pressure is tightly controlled, hence regulation of local blood flow occurs primarily by arteriolar vasoconstriction and vasodilatation. Each terminal arteriole gives rise to a cluster or module of capillaries. The smooth muscle tone of the terminal arteriole determines the extent to which the capillary module is perfused. In a few tissues, notably the mesentery, there is a ring of smooth muscle at the capillary entrance, the precapillary sphincter. The capillaries are devoid of smooth muscle and are effectively long thin tubes of endothelium 5–8 μm in diameter. Despite their small diameter the capillaries offer only a moderate resistance to flow. This is partly because of bolus flow (see below), and partly because the total cross-sectional area of the capillary bed is very large (Fig. 43.3). The distal ends of capillaries unite to form postcapillary (pericytic) venules whose walls contain pericytes but no smooth muscle. Smooth muscle reappears in the walls of venules 30–50 μm in diameter.

Regulation of local blood flow occurs primarily by arteriolar vasoconstriction and vasodilatation.

The wall of veins and venules (diameter 50–200 μm) follow the same three-layered structure seen in the arterial system. In the limbs the intima is formed into semilunar valves that prevent backflow. The venous media is thin and the vessels are easily collapsed and distended. Venules and veins outnumber arteries and arterioles, and the overall cross-sectional area of the venous system is greater than that of the arterial system, so that resistance to flow in the venous system is low. The venous system functions as a variable capacity reservoir which is capable of holding up to two-thirds of the circulating volume. Much of this capacity is located in small veins and venules, and sympathetically mediated vasoconstriction of these vessels can actively displace blood into the arterial circulation.

The venous system functions as a variable capacity reservoir which is capable of holding up to two-thirds of the circulating blood volume.

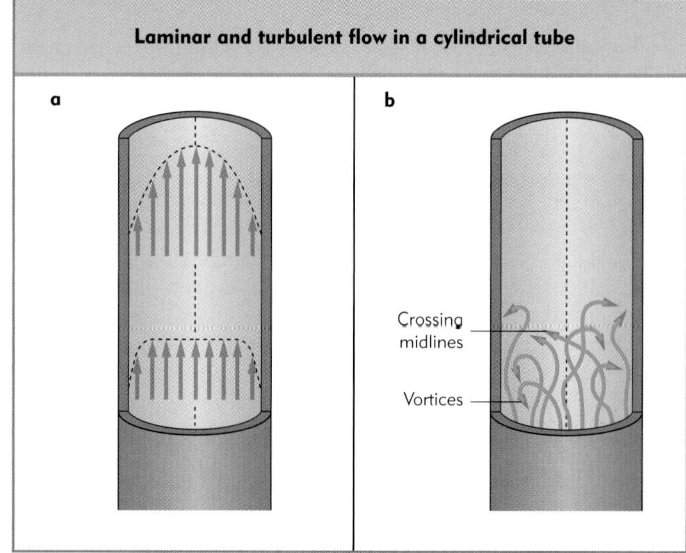

Figure 43.2 Laminar and turbulent flow in a cylindrical tube. The arrows indicate the velocity of flow, which increases from the edge to the center of the tube. Note that laminar flow takes some distance to become established and at the mouth of the tube a plug of fluid flows at uniform velocity. In laminar flow (a) all elements of the fluid move in streamlines (laminae) that are parallel to the axis of the tube; movement does not occur in a radial or circumferential direction. The layer of fluid in contact with the wall is motionless; the fluid that moves along the axis of the tube has the maximal velocity. In turbulent flow (b) the elements of the fluid move irreularly in axial, radial, and circumferential directions. Vortices frequently develop.

In many capillary modules blood flow waxes and wanes every 15 seconds or so. It may stop entirely for brief periods owing to spontaneous rhythmic contractions in the terminal arterioles (vasomotion). In well-perfused capillaries the transit time is typically 0.5–2 seconds. This may fall to 0.25 seconds during exercise.

In skeletal muscle capillary density provides an area available for the exchange of approximately 100 cm^2/g of muscle. In tissues where oxygen consumption is high and sustained, such as myocardium and brain, capillary density is greater and provides an area of about 500 cm^2/g tissue.

Rheology: dynamics of blood flow

The flow of fluid through tubes is governed by Darcy's Law of Flow. This is analogous to Ohm's law and states that flow in a steady state (Q) is linearly related to the pressure difference between two points ($P_1 - P_2$):

■ Equation 43.1

$$Q = K.(P_1 - P_2) = \frac{(P_1 - P_2)}{R}$$

where K = hydraulic conductance and R = hydraulic resistance. For the circulation this translates to cardiac output (CO) equals the difference between mean arterial and central venous pressure (P_a – CVP) divided by total peripheral resistance (TPR). Central venous pressure is close to zero compared to atmospheric pressure, and the expression may be simplified by omitting this term:

■ Equation 43.2

$$CO = \frac{(P_a - CVP)}{TPR} \approx \frac{P_a}{TPR}$$

Darcy's law is applicable only to laminar flow, in which the fluid flows in smooth streamlines and its velocity increases from the edge to the center of the tube. It takes several tube diameters from the tube entrance to establish laminar flow. In the entrance region a broad core of fluid flows at a uniform velocity (Fig. 43.2). This is the situation in the ascending aorta, and the near uniform velocity here allows the estimation of aortic flow by the Doppler method. With a particulate suspension such as blood the shearing of lamina against lamina tends to orientate red cells parallel to the direction of flow. Cells tend to be displaced a little towards the central axis (axial flow), leaving a thin, cell-deficient layer of plasma at the margins. This marginal layer is only 2–4 μm thick, but is important in the arterioles, where it leads to improved flow.

In the ascending aorta the near-uniform velocity allows the estimation of aortic flow by the Doppler method.

As the pressure difference across a tube is progressively raised a point is reached where laminar flow is lost and flow becomes turbulent. At this point Darcy's law breaks down and flow no longer increases linearly with pressure, but with the square root of pressure. Turbulent flow is encouraged by a high fluid velocity (v), large tube diameter (D), and high fluid density (ρ). Turbulence is discouraged by a high viscosity (η). These factors can be combined to give a dimensionless ratio called the Reynolds number (Re):

■ Equation 43.3

$$Re = \frac{v.D.\rho}{\eta}$$

For steady flow down a straight, rigid uniform tube turbulent flow begins at a Reynolds number of about 2000. Despite the fact that blood flow is pulsatile and the vessels are neither straight nor uniform, in most vessels flow is laminar. Turbulence occurs in the ventricles, where it helps to mix the blood and produce a uniform blood gas content. It also occurs in the human aorta during peak flow, where the Re reaches approximately 4600. Turbulence can also develop in arteries roughened by atheromatous plaques.

The resistance to laminar flow arises from the shearing between adjacent laminae. Because the lamina in contact with the tube is stationary it is not related to friction between the tube and the fluid. The resistance is affected by tube geometry because the radius of the tube affects the rate of shear of the laminae. The determinants of resistance for laminar flow of a newtonian fluid along a straight cylindrical tube are given by Poiseuille's equation. For a fluid of viscosity η traveling along a tube of length L and radius r, resistance R is given by the equation:

■ Equation 43.4

$$R = \frac{8.\eta.L}{\pi.r^4}$$

Resistance is inversely proportional to the fourth power of the radius. The increase in resistance from the human aorta, approximately 1 cm in radius, to an arteriole of radius 0.01 cm is 10^8. Further, vasoconstriction producing a 16% reduction in arteriolar radius doubles the resistance presented by that vessel. This is why the arterioles are the main site of resistance. The radius of a capillary is 3 μm, so it may seem at first sight that the capillaries should offer an even greater resistance to flow. However, there is a huge number of capillaries arranged in parallel. Also, blood in capillaries tends to move by bolus flow. The diameter of capillaries (5–6 μm) is less than the width of the human red cell (8 μm). Red cells therefore deform to enter the capillaries and travel through the capillary circulation in single file. Classic laminar flow is impossible, and the bolus of plasma trapped between each red cell is forced to travel along at uniform velocity. This is described as bolus or plug flow. Bolus flow eliminates some of the friction associated with laminar flow. The efficiency of bolus flow depends on the deformability of the red cell. In sickle cell anemia this is reduced. In hypoxic conditions the red cell adopts a rigid sickle shape that impairs capillary flow and causes tissue ischemia and damage (sickle cell crisis).

Blood is a nonnewtonian fluid, that is, its viscosity is affected by the diameter of the tube through which it is flowing. In tubes of diameter >1 mm its viscosity is independent of tube bore. However, in tubes of diameter <1 mm, viscosity starts to decrease. This is known as the Fahraeus–Lindquist effect. At a hematocrit of 47% human blood has a relative viscosity (to water) of ~ 4. In arterioles viscosity is reduced by the peripheral plasma stream produced by axial flow. Shear rates are highest peripherally and a reduction in friction at the margin has a marked effect. Consequently, relative viscosity falls to ~2.5. In capillaries bolus flow reduces viscosity to its lowest level of ~1.7. This decrease in viscosity reduces the driving (arterial) pressure required to perfuse the circulation and thus reduces cardiac work. The effect declines in wider tubes because the thickness of the marginal layer becomes insignificant relative to the tube diameter.

The viscosity of blood is affected by the diameter of the tube through which it is flowing.

Viscosity, and hence flow, is dramatically affected by hematocrit. Increases in hematocrit (polycythemia) lead to a decrease in flow. Decreased hematocrit (anemia, hemodilution) leads to increased flow. Plasma proteins have a smaller effect on viscosity, although increases in plasma proteins (e.g. in myeloma) will increase viscosity and thus decrease flow.

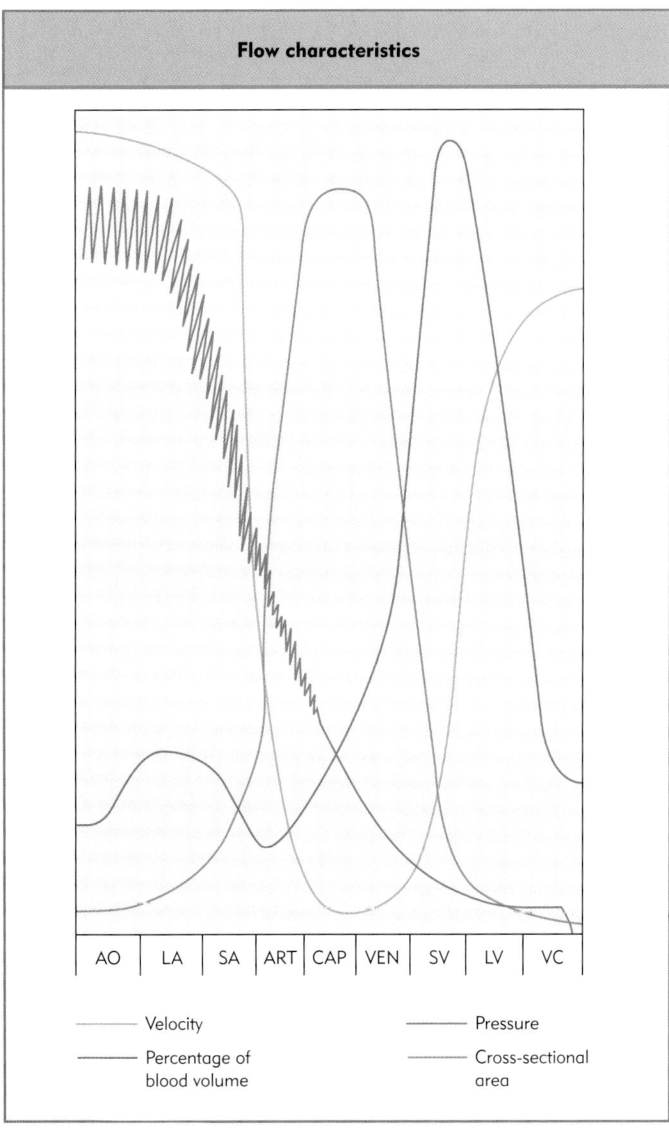

Figure 43.3 Flow characteristics in systemic vessels. The important features are the inverse relationship between velocity and cross-sectional area, the major pressure drop across the arterioles, the maximal cross-sectional area and minimal flow rate int he capillaries, and the large capacity of the venous system. The small but abrupt drop in pressure in the venae cava indicates the point of entrance of these vessels into the thoracic cavity and reflects the effect of the negative intrathoracic pressure. To permit schematic representation of velocity and cross-sectional area on a single linear scale, only approximations are possible at the lower values. AO, aorta; LA, large arteries; SA, small arteries; ART, arterioles; CAP, capillaries; VEN, venules; SV, small veins; LV, large veins; VC, vena cava.

CARDIOVASCULAR REGULATORY MECHANISMS

Long-term control of the circulation rests with a number of mechanisms that control the circulating volume. These mechanisms respond to a persistent elevation of arterial pressure by increasing salt and water output from the kidneys, and are described in detail elsewhere in this book (Chapters 57–59). They cause reductions in extracellular fluid volume, blood volume, and venous return. The reduction in venous return leads to falls in cardiac output and blood pressure. Over the following weeks the cardiac output returns to baseline, but a persistent reduction in systemic vascular resistance develops so that the lower arterial pressure is maintained.

Baroreflex control

In contrast to the renal mechanisms that control circulating volume the cardiovascular reflexes are mediated through the autonomic nervous system and are rapidly acting. They are concerned with the control of heart rate and vascular tone over a period of seconds to minutes, rather than days. Arterial baroreflexes enable rapid control of arterial pressure, buffering acute changes quickly. The sensors for this baroreflex, the arterial baroreceptors, are stretch receptors in the walls of the aortic arch and the carotid sinuses of the internal carotid arteries. Fibers from the carotid sinus baroreceptors travel in the carotid sinus nerves that join the glossopharyngeal nerves. Those from the aortic baroreceptors travel in the aortic nerves that join the vagus nerves. The fibers travel to a sensory area in the nucleus tractus solitarius in the medulla. From here, fibers project to the pressor and depressor areas in the medulla. The former lies in the anteriolateral portions of the upper medulla and the latter more medially in the lower medulla. There is a background tonic discharge from the baroreceptor afferents at normal arterial pressure. As the arterial pressure stretches the vessel wall the discharge rate of the baroreceptor afferents increases in proportion. The greater the arterial pressure, the greater the rate of discharge. Baroreceptors are also sensitive to rate of rise of pressure (dynamic sensitivity). They tend to adapt to sustained pressure changes, resetting to the previous background level of discharge.

On baroreceptor discharge, activity increases in the medullary depressor area and decreases in the pressor area. This results in an increase in vagal tone, which decreases the heart rate, and a reduction in the sympathetic outflow to the heart and peripheral vasculature, which produces a decrease in myocardial contractility and a reduction in vascular tone, causing a fall in systemic vascular resistance. The baroreflex has a particular effect on the splanchnic arterioles and venules. Vasodilatation of the latter reduces venous return. The opposite effects are seen in response to a fall in blood pressure, when a pressor response is elicited resulting in an increase in heart rate, an increase in myocardial contractility, and an increase in vascular tone. The primary effect of the arterial baroreflex is on heart rate and contractility. The effect on systemic vascular resistance is of secondary importance.

The arterial baroreflex does not have a role in the long-term regulation of blood pressure. Rather, the baroreflex resets to the new blood pressure in the face of long-term increases or decreases in blood pressure.

Decreased baroreflex responses are seen in hypertensive patients and with advancing age. Diseases such as diabetes and

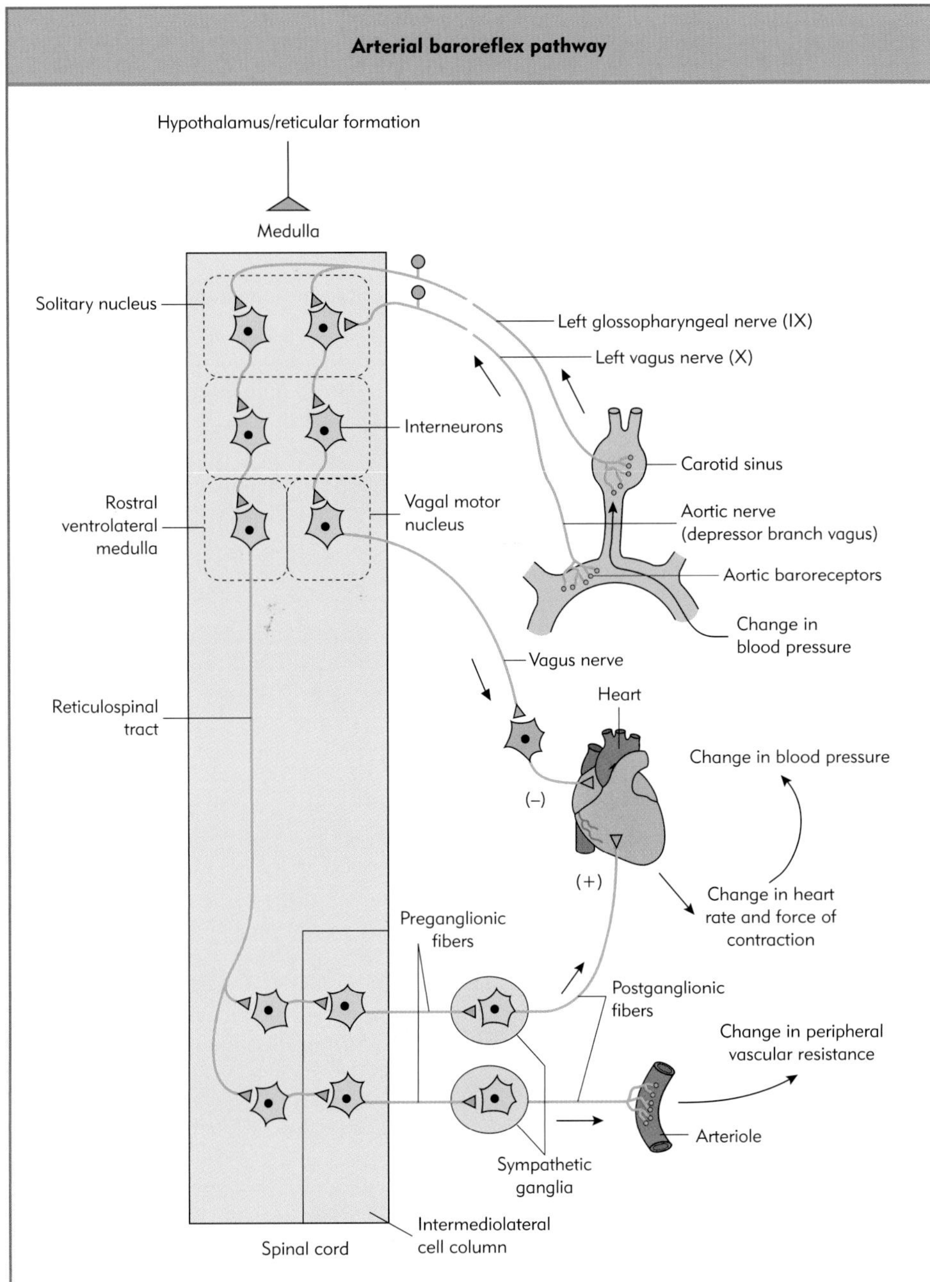

Figure 43.4 Schematic of the arterial baroreflex pathway. The afferent fibers travel in the glossopharyngeal (IX) and vagus (X) nerves, while the efferent fibers travel in the sympathetic nerves and vagus nerve.

Parkinson's disease that cause autonomic dysfunction may attenuate or abolish the arterial baroreflex, as may drugs that interfere with autonomic function. The baroreflex response is also depressed by most anesthetic agents.

Diabetes and Parkinson's disease and anesthetics may attenuate or abolish the arterial baroreflex.

The arterial baroreflex response is most effective in the pressure range 80–150 mmHg, and responds more vigorously to decreases in pressure than increases. It is important for the rapid regulation of blood pressure, for example in maintaining blood pressure when rising from the supine position.

Intrinsic flow regulation

Flow is locally controlled in certain vascular beds by a process known as autoregulation. This is defined as the ability of an organ to maintain relatively constant blood flow in the face of variations in perfusion pressure. At lower perfusion pressures there is vasodilatation, whereas higher perfusion pressures produce vasoconstriction. The result is a characteristic autoregulatory curve, as shown in Figure 43.5. Within the limits of autoregulation flow is constant despite variations in pressure. Outside the limits of autoregulation flow is directly dependent on driving pressure. Autoregulation is seen in the kidneys, brain, and heart. In the skin and lungs there is minimal autoregulation.

Autoregulation appears to be an intrinsic property that is seen even in denervated tissues. Two mechanisms mediate autoregulation, the myogenic response and vasodilator washout. The

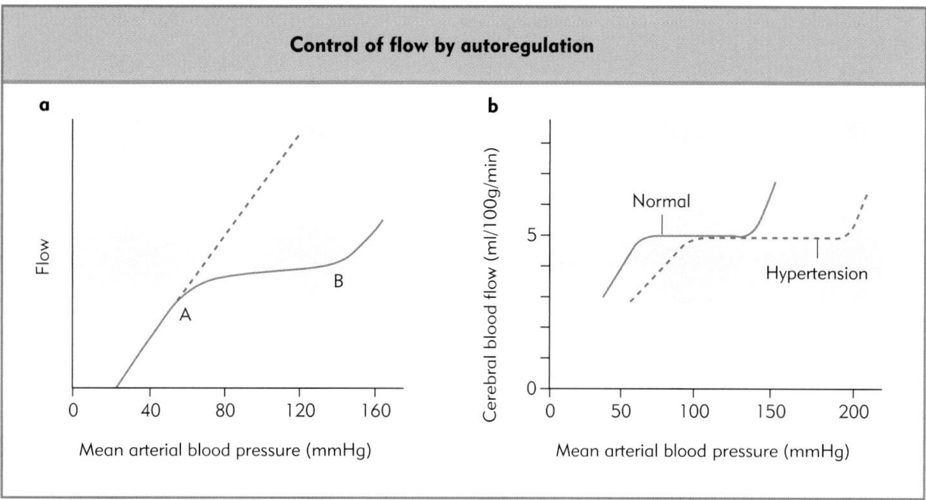

Figure 43.5 Pressure–flow curve showing autoregulation. Between A and B there is little change in flow with changes in perfusion pressure. Outside this range, flow increases approximately linearly with pressure.

myogenic response is a response of the vessel wall to stretch. Elevations in perfusion pressure stretch the smooth muscle cells in the vessel wall and cause contraction and vasoconstriction. A reduction in pressure and stretch of the smooth muscle leads to relaxation. The mechanism is not fully elucidated. However, it is understood that vessel distension activates the stretch-sensitive nonselective cation channels and chloride channels in smooth muscle. This produces depolarization, increasing the permeability of L-type calcium channels, increasing intracellular Ca^{2+}, and producing contraction. The vasodilator washout mechanism is summed up by its name! A reduction in perfusion pressure leads to a reduction in blood flow and causes a reduction in tissue PO_2 and an increase in tissue PCO_2 and other metabolites (lactic acid, adenosine, potassium, and hydrogen ions). The accumulating metabolites and the reduced PO_2 then directly cause vasodilatation. Conversely, high perfusion pressures increase flow, providing ample tissue oxygen and washing out metabolites. This causes vasoconstriction and a reduction in blood flow. Autoregulation appears to be controlled primarily by the myogenic mechanism in the brain, kidney, gut, liver, and spleen. The two mechanisms appear to be equipotent in skeletal muscle.

Nitric oxide has an important role in flow regulation. It is synthesized and released by endothelium, and acts as a vasodilator on neighboring myocytes. Nitric oxide release is stimulated by increased shear stress, the resultant vasodilatation and decrease in shear stress providing a negative feedback loop. Reduction in basal vascular tone during pregnancy is mediated by increased nitric oxide production, thus allowing a decrease in blood pressure despite an increase in cardiac output.

Blood flow is also regulated on a local level by the process of metabolic hyperemia. As oxygen demand to a region increases, vasodilator substances are released into the interstitial fluid and act upon arterioles to increase blood flow. The precise role of each mediator is unknown, but it is thought that acidosis, hypoxia, adenosine, potassium ions, and phosphate ions all contribute to the process.

Regional blood flow

HEART

Myocardial oxygen consumption is very high, of the order of 8 mL O_2/min/100 g of tissue. This is 20 times greater than in resting skeletal muscle. In exercise cardiac work can increase fivefold, and oxygen delivery must increase accordingly. Myocardial capillary density is correspondingly high, being 3000–5000 capillaries/mm^2. This provides a very large endothelial area for exchange and reduces the maximum diffusion distance to approximately 9 μm.

The myocardium extracts 65–75% of the oxygen from coronary blood, in contrast to the whole-body extraction of approximately 25% at rest. At high work rates extra oxygen is provided by increased blood flow. During light to moderate work coronary blood flow increases almost linearly with myocardial oxygen consumption. At high work rates blood flow lags behind somewhat and myocardial oxygen extraction increases. During exercise coronary oxygen extraction can rise to 90%. Myocardial arteries and arterioles are well innervated by sympathetic vasoconstrictor fibers whose tonic discharge contributes to arteriolar tone. This effect is overcome by metabolic vasodilatation with increasing myocardial work. The predominant vasodilator substance remains unclear, although adenosine is thought to be at least partly responsible. Autoregulation is well developed in the coronary circulation and is reset by metabolic vasodilatation to operate at a higher flow.

The branches of the coronary arteries within the myocardium are compressed during systole. This effect is most marked in the left ventricle during isovolumetric contraction, when pressure in the ventricular wall may reach 240 mmHg and coronary blood pressure is at its nadir, approximately 80 mmHg. Thus in the left ventricle coronary blood flow ceases briefly and may even reverse during systole. Flow is only fully restored during diastole, and 80% of left coronary blood flow occurs in diastole at basal heart rates.

Eighty per cent of left coronary blood flow occurs in diastole at basal heart rates.

LUNGS

The whole output of the right ventricle flows through the alveolar capillary bed. Thus, perfusion greatly exceeds needs and metabolic factors do not influence flow. There is an independent systemic bronchial circulation which meets the metabolic needs of the bronchi.

Pulmonary vascular resistance is about one-eighth of the systemic vascular resistance and pulmonary arterial pressure is

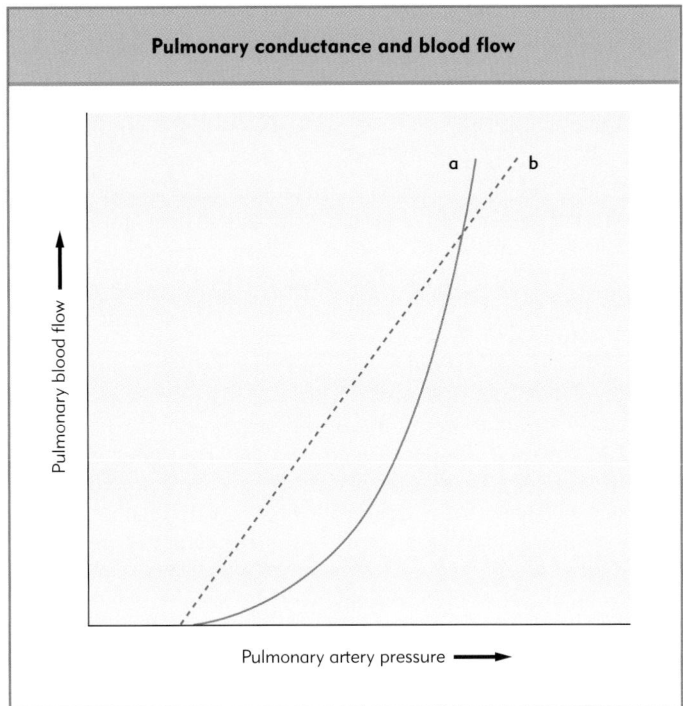

Figure 43.6 Graph showing increasing pulmonary conductance with increasing pulmonary blood flow. Curve A shows the observed nonlinear relationship between perfusion pressure and flow. Curve B shows the type of linear relationship that would be expected with constant pulmonary vascular resistance. (After Marshall BE, Marshall C. Active regulation of the pulmonary circulation. In: Will J, Dawson CA, Weir EK, Buckner CK, eds. The pulmonary circulation in health and disease. Orlando: Academic Press; 1987; 252.)

low, being 20–25 mmHg in systole and 6–12 mmHg in diastole. Pulmonary arteries and arterioles are shorter and thinner than systemic vessels. There is low basal tone in the pulmonary circulation and no autoregulation. Sympathetic motor nerves exist, but have an ill-defined role. Resistance is shared between the arteries, the microvasculature, and the veins. Consequently, pulmonary capillary pressure is approximately midway between mean pulmonary arterial pressure and left atrial pressure, i.e. 8–11 mmHg. Elevation of the left atrial pressure to 20–25 mmHg raises capillary pressure sufficiently to cause pulmonary edema. Vascular conductance increases with perfusion pressure (Fig. 43.6). This is probably due to vascular distension and to the recruitment of some vessels that were initially closed by airway pressure.

The pulmonary vessels also differ from systemic vessels in that they vasoconstrict in response to hypoxia (hypoxic pulmonary vasoconstriction). If the ventilation to a local region falls the alveolar oxygen content falls and carbon dioxide content increases. The small pulmonary arteries that pass close to the surface of small airways respond to this change by vasoconstriction, whereas the bronchial smooth muscle responds to airway hypercapnia by relaxation. These changes tend to maintain an optimal ventilation/perfusion ratio.

The pulmonary circulation can act as a blood reservoir. In a supine man pulmonary blood volume is about 600 mL. If intrathoracic airway pressure is raised by a Valsalva maneuver the external pressure on the blood vessels can expel up to half the blood content. On forced inspiration, which lowers intrathoracic pressure, pulmonary blood volume can increase to about

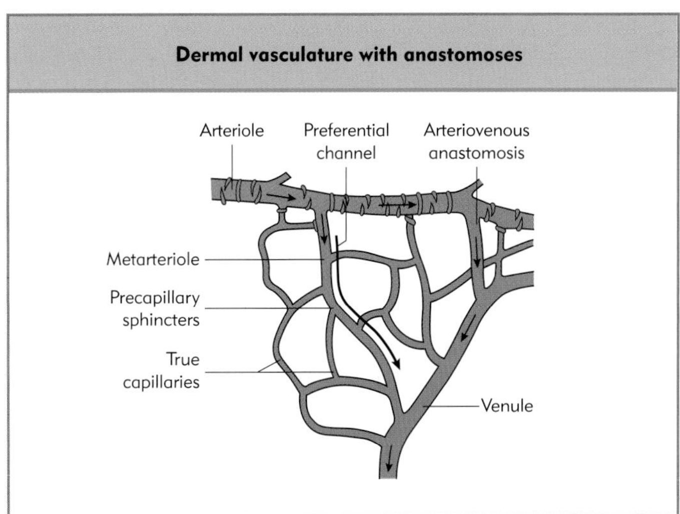

Figure 43.7 The dermal vasculature showing arteriovenous anastomoses. (After Levick JR. An introduction to cardiovascular physiology. Oxford: Butterworth–Heinemann; 1991: 211.)

1 L. The pulmonary capacitance vessels act as a transient source of blood for the left ventricle when output begins to increase at the start of exercise.

SPLANCHNIC CIRCULATION

The splanchnic circulation comprises the gastric, small intestinal, colonic, pancreatic, hepatic, and splenic circulations. They are arranged in parallel and fed by the celiac artery and the superior and inferior mesenteric arteries.

The resistance arterioles are the primary determinant of vascular resistance in the splanchnic circulation. Neuronal control of the mesenteric circulation is almost entirely sympathetic in origin. The parasympathetic fibers from the vagi have little effect on blood flow. Overall splanchnic blood flow requires about 25% of cardiac output. The splanchnic venous capacitance reservoir contains about one-third of the body's total blood volume. The sympathetic postganglionic fibers cause arteriolar vasoconstriction and decrease splanchnic perfusion. Sympathetic stimulation also contracts the smooth muscle of the capacitance veins in the splanchnic circulation, and may expel a large volume of pooled blood from the splanchnic into the systemic circulation. Autoregulation in the splanchnic circulation is less marked than in the cerebral, cardiac, or renal circulations. The response is present, however, and serves to restore blood follow to areas suffering hypoperfusion because of an acute reduction in perfusion pressure. The splanchnic circulation also responds to reduced perfusion pressure by the redistribution of blood flow within individual organs. For example, in hypovolemic shock perfusion usually favors the mucosa of the gut at the expense of the muscularis mucosa.

The liver is unique in that it has both an arterial and a venous afferent blood supply. In the resting adult the liver receives approximately 500 mL min of blood via the hepatic artery and a further 1300 mL min from the portal circulation. The hepatic microcirculation is described elsewhere.

KIDNEYS

The kidneys constitute less than 0.5% of body weight. They receive about 20% of the cardiac output, and this percentage can be increased further. Renal blood flow is regulated to maintain optimum delivery of filtrate to the nephrons and adequate reabsorption of fluid back into the vascular system. It is well beyond that required to supply the metabolic needs of the kidneys.

The renal vasculature has a sympathetic innervation. Both norepinephrine and epinephrine, released from the adrenal medulla, activate α_1-adrenoreceptors and cause renal vasoconstriction, which decreases renal blood flow and glomerular filtration. Dopamine is also released in the kidney. Activation of D_1 receptors in the kidneys causes significant increases in both cortical and medullary blood flow. Despite this, it has proved impossible to demonstrate concrete clinical benefit from so-called 'renal dose' dopamine infusions (Chapter 58).

The kidneys display autoregulation of blood flow over a range of perfusion pressure from 75 to 180 mmHg. Outside this range, flow is pressure dependent. Autoregulation is demonstrable in isolated kidneys, and is therefore assumed to be mediated by factors intrinsic to the kidney.

The kidneys display autoregulation of blood flow over a range of perfusion pressures from 75 to 180 mmHg.

The renin–angiotensin system has been described elsewhere. Angiotensin II is a potent vasoconstrictor. It vasoconstricts the afferent arterioles, but its primary effect appears to be on the efferent arterioles. Thus, it acts to maintain renal glomerular filtration even when renal plasma flow is reduced. Prostaglandins PGE_2 and PGI_2 are produced in the kidney during hemorrhagic hypovolemia. They cause vasodilatation of the efferent and afferent arterioles, and so help to prevent severe vasoconstriction and ischemia in the face of hypovolemia.

MUSCLE

The blood supply to skeletal muscle has to be able to supply metabolic needs that vary hugely between rest and vigorous exercise. Skeletal muscle constitutes 40% of adult body mass. The resistance of this large vascular bed has a substantial effect on blood pressure. The skeletal muscle vasculature also has a crucial role in the regulation of arterial blood pressure.

Skeletal muscle arterioles are innervated by sympathetic vasoconstrictor fibers whose tonic discharge maintains a high vascular tone in the skeletal muscle vasculature. This is essential if marked vasodilatation is to be possible during exercise. Further vasoconstriction is also possible.

During strenuous exercise muscle blood flow accounts for 80–90% of cardiac output. Muscle hyperemia is due almost entirely to a fall in vascular resistance as a result of metabolic vasodilatation. Blood flow increases almost linearly with local metabolic rate. The nature of the vasodilator agents is controversial. Initial vasodilatation appears to be due to local increases in interstitial potassium concentration and osmolality. These soon return to normal levels, leaving the cause of the vasodilatation during prolonged exercise unknown. Adenosine has been postulated as a mediator for this continued vasodilatation. Perfusion during exercise is also increased to some extent by the effect of the skeletal muscle pump, whereby the rhythmic massaging of the calf muscles on the deep veins assists limb perfusion.

Resting skeletal muscle extracts only 25–30% of oxygen from the blood. In strenuous exercise extraction can reach 80–90%. Despite this, in strenuous exercise intracellular oxygen tension may fall so low that anaerobic metabolism predominates, leading to the production of lactic acid and the incurring of an oxygen debt.

SKIN

Skin has a relatively constant metabolic rate. However, skin blood flow rate can vary between 1 mL/min/100 g and 200 mL/min/100 g, according to thermoregulatory requirements. This large variation in flow is controlled primarily by sympathetic vasomotor fibers whose activity is linked to temperature regulation. Certain skin areas possess abundant direct connections between dermal arterioles and venules called arteriovenous anastomoses (AVA) (Fig. 43.7). They occur at exposed sites with a high surface area/volume ratio; the fingers and toes, the palm and sole, and the lips, nose, and ears and are coiled muscular walled vessels of 35 μm average diameter. They are controlled almost exclusively by sympathetic vasoconstrictor fibers whose activity is controlled by a temperature-regulating center in the hypothalamus. When core temperature is high vasomotor drive is reduced and the AVAs vasodilate. They offer a low-resistance shunt pathway that increases cutaneous blood flow and heat delivery to the skin. Heat readily crosses the walls of the dermal venous plexus fed by the AVAs, and so skin temperature rises and heat loss increases. Conversely, under cold conditions AVAs constrict to conserve heat.

The cutaneous circulation participates in many cardiovascular reflexes. Hypotension reflexly elicits constriction of the cutaneous veins and arterioles, producing the pale cold skin characteristic of shock. The rise in cutaneous vascular resistance helps to support blood pressure, whereas the venoconstriction displaces blood centrally and helps to support central venous pressure.

Areas of skin may be subject to high pressures for long periods during sitting, standing, and lying, and this may compromise local blood flow. Ischemic damage is prevented by the high tolerance of the skin for hypoxia, reactive hyperemia on removal of the stress, and the onset of restlessness as metabolites accumulate and stimulate the skin nociceptors. The latter mechanism fails in patients such as paraplegics, the frail elderly, and of course patients under anesthesia and in the intensive care unit. If appropriate precautions are not taken such patients may suffer pressure necrosis (bed sores).

PHARMACOLOGICAL CONTROL OF BLOOD PRESSURE

Perioperative hypotension may compromise the perfusion of the heart, the brain, and other organs. Perioperative hypertension may put undue strain on the heart and lead to myocardial ischemia. Conversely, a degree of hypotension may be useful in some types of surgery. A number of vasoconstrictors and vasodilators that can be used in the manipulation of blood pressure are available (see also Chapter 41).

Vasodilators

Phentolamine binds reversibly to postsynaptic α_1-receptors and presynaptic α_2-receptors. Postsynaptic blockade causes marked arterial vasodilatation and a fall in blood pressure. This causes a compensatory tachycardia, to which the α_2-blockade contributes, and the fall in blood pressure is less than would otherwise be expected.

Phenoxybenzamine is a nitrogen mustard derivative that binds irreversibly to α_1- and α_2-receptors. Again it causes vasodilatation, but in this case the effect of a single dose may last for several days. The drug has a particular role in the preoperative preparation of patients undergoing surgery for pheochromocytoma (Chapter 52).

Prazosin is a selective competitive α_1-adenoreceptor blocker that reduces arterial and venous tone. α_2-Receptors are not blocked, the negative feedback of norepinephrine on its own release is not inhibited, and tachycardia does not occur. It has a greater affinity for α-receptors in veins than in arteries, and for this reason its effects resemble those of glyceryl trinitrate more than phentolamine or hydralazine.

Labetalol combines α_1-receptor blocking and nonselective β-receptor blocking activity. It produces a decrease in systemic arterial pressure because of simultaneous reductions in systemic vascular resistance and cardiac output.

Sodium nitroprusside (SNP) consists of a ferrous iron atom bound with five cyanide molecules and one nitric group. Contact with blood decomposes the molecule, releasing nitric oxide (NO). The NO binds to the Fe^{2+} moiety of guanylyl cyclase, with the subsequent production of cGMP. Increased levels of intracellular cGMP produce reduced levels of cytosolic Ca^{2+}, and cause dephosphorylation of myosin light chains and smooth muscle relaxation. SNP lowers blood pressure within 1–2 minutes and its effect dissipates within a few minutes of the infusion being stopped. The potential for cyanide and thiocyanate toxicity limits the dose and duration of use of SNP. The ferrous iron in SNP reacts with sulfhydryl groups in red blood cells and releases cyanide. This cyanide is reduced to thiocyanate in the liver and excreted in the urine. However, its half-life is 4 days, and this is considerably increased in renal failure.

The potential for cyanide and thiocyanate toxicity limits the dose and duration of use of SNP.

Organic nitrates such as glyceryl trinitrate, and isosorbide mononitrate and dinitrate also act via the release of NO. Unlike SNP, their dose and duration of use are not limited by cyamide accumulation.

Calcium channel blockers act by blocking membrane calcium channels. They inhibit transmembrane calcium influx and reduce smooth muscle tone, causing vasodilatation. The calcium channel blockers are discussed in detail elsewhere (Chapter 24).

Hydralazine is a potent vasodilator of arterioles. It has little or no effect on venous smooth muscle, and its precise mode of action is unclear. It is endothelium dependent, suggesting a role for nitric oxide. It also interferes with the mobilization of calcium in vascular smooth muscle. Its use is associated with a baroreflex-mediated increase in sympathetic activity causing increased heart rate and contractility and an increase in plasma renin activity. The drug has a slow onset, its effects taking 15–30 minutes to become apparent. The elimination half-life is about 4 hours, but the effective half-life is approximately 100 hours owing to the avid binding of the drug to smooth muscle. Because of this it is giving way to newer drugs for the short-term control of blood pressure.

Vasopressors

Vasopressors will raise blood pressure but their use is associated with a number of cardiac and regional hemodynamic effects. Peripheral vasoconstriction produces a reflex bradycardia and a reduction in cardiac output mediated via the baroreflexes. Increased preload (due to venoconstriction) and afterload (due to arteriolar constriction) increases myocardial oxygen demand. Vasoconstriction may be most marked in the renal, hepatic, and splanchnic beds, with the risk of severe hypoperfusion and organ failure. In anesthetic practice vasopressors are used to counteract the hypotension produced by sympathetic blockade during regional anesthesia, or that due to vasodilatation produced by general anesthesia. They are used to control perfusion pressure during cardiopulmonary bypass, and to support the circulation during cardiopulmonary resuscitation and the treatment of septic shock.

The sympathomimetic amines are the group of agents that are primarily regarded as vasopressors and are currently in clinical use. Vasoconstriction in response to sympathomimetic amines is mediated by stimulation of α_1-adrenoceptors. They may exert their effects directly on the receptors, or indirectly by displacing endogenous norepinephrine from adrenergic nerve terminals. These indirectly acting agents should be avoided or used with considerable caution in patients on monoamine oxidase inhibitors because of the potential for unpredictable hypertensive responses.

Phenylephrine is a potent α_1-adrenoceptor agonist with no activity at β receptors in clinical doses. Following a single dose mean arterial pressure rises, owing mainly to an increase in diastolic pressure. Systemic vascular resistance increases, and a baroreflex-mediated reduction in heart rate and cardiac output is observed. These effects are seen within about 1 minute of injection and last for about 10 minutes. Doses of 50–100 μg are usually given, and an infusion of up to 3 μg/kg/min may also be used.

Methoxamine is an α-adrenoceptor agonist with β-adrenoceptor blocking actions. It increases systolic and diastolic pressure by increasing systemic vascular resistance. A response is seen within about 1 minute of injection and lasts for about 20 minutes. Heart rate decreases because of the β-adrenoceptor blocking action and the baroceptor response to raised blood pressure.

Ephedrine has direct β_1- and β_2-adrenoceptor agonist effects and indirectly releases norepinephrine from adrenergic nerve endings. It increases myocardial contractility and heart rate, and thus increases cardiac output. Its vasoconstrictive effects tend to be counterbalanced by its tendency to cause β_2-mediated vasodilatation, and so there is usually little change in systemic vascular resistance. Diastolic and systolic pressure both increase. Doses of 3–6 mg titrated to effect are usually given, and its duration of action may be up to 20 minutes. It reduces uterine contractility and tends to restore and maintain uterine blood flow. It is therefore widely used in obstetric anesthetic practice.

Metaraminol acts both directly and indirectly and stimulates both α- and β-receptors. Like ephedrine, it tends to increase cardiac contractility and cardiac output. However, it also increases systemic vascular resistance and may produce a reflex bradycardia.

Vasopressin is an endogenous peptide produced by the hypothalamus and released from the posterior lobe of the pituitary gland. At normal plasma levels its main action is to promote water retention by the kidney. High concentrations are seen in hypovolemic hypotension, and at these levels vasopressin produces strong vasoconstriction in most tissues, helping to support arterial pressure. The cerebral and coronary vessels respond to vasopressin by vasodilation, producing a redistribution of the cardiac output to the brain and heart. Recent studies have suggested that there may be a clinical role for vasopressin in septic shock, where it may allow the dose of other vasopressors, such as norepinephrine, to be reduced.

HYPERTENSION AND ANTIHYPERTENSIVE THERAPY

Hypertension is common and is associated with considerable cardiovascular morbidity. People with persistently elevated blood pressure are at increased risk of cerebrovascular accident, coronary artery disease, and left ventricular hypertrophy and failure. Systolic and diastolic blood pressures are continuous variables. The relationship between blood pressure and cardiovascular events is continuous, consistent, and independent of other risk factors. Over recent decades the threshold at which treatment is initiated for hypertension has declined steadily as the population burden of disease engendered by so-called mild to moderate hypertension has become clear.

The Seventh Report of the Joint National Committee on the Prevention, Detection, Evaluation, and Treatment of High Blood Pressure (JNC VII) in the USA suggests that in patients over 50 years old a systolic blood pressure of greater than 140 mmHg is a much greater risk factor for cardiovascular disease than elevated diastolic blood pressure. Systolic blood pressure above 140 mmHg and diastolic blood pressure above 90 mmHg should be treated pharmacologically if it is unresponsive to lifestyle modifications. People with systolic blood pressure of between 120 and 139 mmHg should be classified as prehypertensive and advised about lifestyle modifications and risk prevention. The British Hypertension Society 2004 guidelines for the management of hypertension state that antihypertensive drug therapy should be initiated in patients with a sustained systolic blood pressure of 160 mmHg or greater or a sustained diastolic pressure of 100 mmHg or greater. Those patients with a sustained systolic pressure between 140 and 159 mmHg or a sustained diastolic pressure between 90 and 99 mmHg should receive treatment if they have evidence of target organ damage or cardiovascular complications of hypertension, are diabetic, or have a 10 year risk of cardiovascular disease of 20% or more calculated using the Joint British Societies cardiovascular disease risk assessment chart.

In 'white coat hypertension' subjects who have a normal blood pressure on ambulatory monitoring or self-administered home blood pressure examination have raised blood pressure when examined by a doctor or nurse. Pseudohypertension describes the condition whereby cuff readings of the blood pressure are consistently high and simultaneous intra-arterial readings are normal. It is not uncommon, and may lead to errors in treatment.

A specific cause for elevated blood pressure can be found in 6–8% of patients, this being secondary hypertension. The remainder of hypertension is described as primary or essential hypertension. The precise mechanism of hypertension is not fully understood. However, it is becoming clear that it is probably multifactorial and subject to both genetic and environmental influences. There is also increasing evidence for an effect of intrauterine growth on blood pressure in later life. It also appears that different mechanisms of hypertension may operate in different patients. A distinction is made between low-renin and high-renin hypertension. In the former, which is commoner in older patients, plasma renin activity is low, systemic vascular resistance is moderately elevated, and there is increased plasma volume and an elevated cardiac output. In high-renin hypertension, which is associated with younger patients, plasma renin activity is elevated and systemic vascular resistance is raised to a greater extent than in low-renin hypertension. Plasma volume and cardiac output are reduced and blood viscosity may be increased.

Hypertension produces structural changes in the cardiovascular system. In blood vessels there is endothelial dysfunction, smooth muscle replication or hypertrophy, intimal thickening, and migration of smooth muscles into the subintimal space. These changes are accompanied by alterations in collagen and elastin content. One result of these changes is an increased wall to inner radius ratio. This in turn results in exaggerated changes in luminal diameter for any given change in vascular smooth muscle tone.

Left ventricular hypertrophy (LVH) is found in up to 30% of unselected hypertensive patients and is produced by changes in myocyte size, shape, and number. It is an ominous sign, as mortality from ischemic heart disease is increased threefold in patients with LVH. It is not uncommon for LVH to progress to left ventricular failure. Stroke is a major cause of death in hypertensive patients. Indeed, the most marked benefit from the treatment of hypertension is a reduction in the incidence of cerebrovascular accidents. Hypertension may be a cause or a consequence of renal impairment, and adds considerably to the morbidity of renal disease.

Antihypertensive therapy has been shown to reduce the incidence of stroke, coronary events, congestive heart failure, and all-cause mortality. Systolic and diastolic blood pressures are continuous variables and there is no absolute agreement as to the level of blood pressure at which treatment should be initiated. Meta-analyses of blood pressure-lowering trials have shown that more, rather than less, intensive treatment of blood pressure lowers the rate of stroke and coronary events by up to 20%.

The British Hypertension Society 1999 guidelines recommend initial therapy with a thiazide diuretic or β-blocker unless there are specific indications for the other antihypertensive drugs. More recent BHS guidelines emphasize that many patients will need combination therapy. They point out that younger caucasians will usually have renin-dependent hypertension that responds well to ACE inhibitors, angiotensin (A) receptor blockade or β-blockers (B). Most other patients have low-renin hypertension that responds better to calcium channel blockers (C) or diuretics (D). These guidelines suggest 'A' + 'C' + 'D' as therapy for resistant hypertension. The JNC VII report suggests that patients with blood pressures of 140–159/90–99 mmHg unresponsive to lifestyle modifications will require therapy with a diuretic in most cases. Patients with pressures of ≥160 mmHg systolic or ≥100 diastolic will need combination therapy, for example with a diuretic and an ACE inhibitor.

β-adrenoceptor antagonists

β-blockers produce an initial reduction in blood pressure by reducing heart rate and cardiac output. Their long-term effect on blood pressure is due to reduced vascular tone produced in part by reduced renin release. The choice of a particular β-blocker will depend on characteristics such as the degree of β_1 selectivity, duration of action, side-effect profile, and so forth. Recent studies have suggested that perioperative β-adrenergic blockade may provide protection from perioperative cardiac events. The evidence for this is incomplete. At the time of writing there is only robust proof of benefit in the highest-risk patients. However, it would seem appropriate to select a β-blocker as first-line treatment for a newly diagnosed hypertensive patient who has other cardiovascular risk factors and in whom surgery is planned.

Recent studies have suggested that perioperative β-adrenergic blockade may provide protection from perioperative cardiac events.

ACE inhibitors

ACE inhibitors are useful for monotherapy or for combined therapy in the treatment of high-renin hypertension. Their acute hypotensive effect is due to a reduction in circulating angiotensin II. Their longer-term effect seems to depend on other mechanisms, including tissue angiotensin inhibition, degradation of bradykinin, or an increase in endothelium-dependent relaxation. The combination of β-adrenoceptor antagonists and ACE inhibitors may be of particular value in preventing vascular damage in high-renin patients.

Angiotensin II antagonists

Angiotensin II receptor antagonists are the newest major category of antihypertensive drug. Their prime target, like that of ACE inhibitors, is the renin–angiotensin system. However, they specifically block the angiotensin II subtype (1) receptor, which is responsible for the classic actions of angiotensin on the blood vessels, heart, adrenal glands, and sympathetic nervous system. Because angiotensin II receptor antagonists have no bradykinin potentiating effects they do not cause the troublesome side effect of cough that frequently occurs with ACE inhibitors. They do, however, have the same side-effect profile as ACE inhibitors in respect of sodium-depleted patients and those with critical renal blood flow.

Diuretics

Diuretics produce an initial reduction in blood volume, but with prolonged use circulating volume tends to return to normal. The persistent effects of these drugs are probably mediated by a reduction in the sodium content of smooth muscle increasing the efficiency of the Na^+/Ca^{2+} antiporter and consequently reducing the cytosolic Ca^{2+} concentration.

Calcium channel blockers

Calcium channel blockers bind to the L-type calcium channel in its inactive state and delay recovery of the channel to the excitable 'resting' state, thereby reducing calcium entry. They are effective for both chronic and acute hypertension. Sublingual nifedipine has been widely used for the acute control of blood pressure. However, there have been reports of fatal cerebral, renal, and myocardial events following the acute lowering of blood pressure with nifedipine and nicardipine, and this approach cannot be recommended.

There have been reports of fatal cerebral, renal, and myocardial events following the acute lowering of blood pressure with calcium channel blockers.

α_1-adrenoceptor antagonists

Prazosin is a potent α_1-receptor antagonist that lowers blood pressure by producing peripheral vasodilation. This does not produce a significant increase in heart rate because prazosin has no effect on α_2-receptors, but does act on the central nervous system to reduce sympathetic outflow. Cardiac output is not increased, despite the decreased afterload, because of the effect of prazosin on venous tone. Doxazosin and terazosin are highly specific α-receptor-blocking drugs with similar effects to prazosin, but have longer elimination half-lives and can be used for once-daily treatment.

Hypertension and anesthesia

It was established in the early 1970s that patients with treated hypertension exhibit smaller hemodynamic responses to anesthesia and awakening than untreated hypertensive patients (Fig. 43.8). The better stability of the treated patients suggests that all hypertensive patients should be properly controlled before

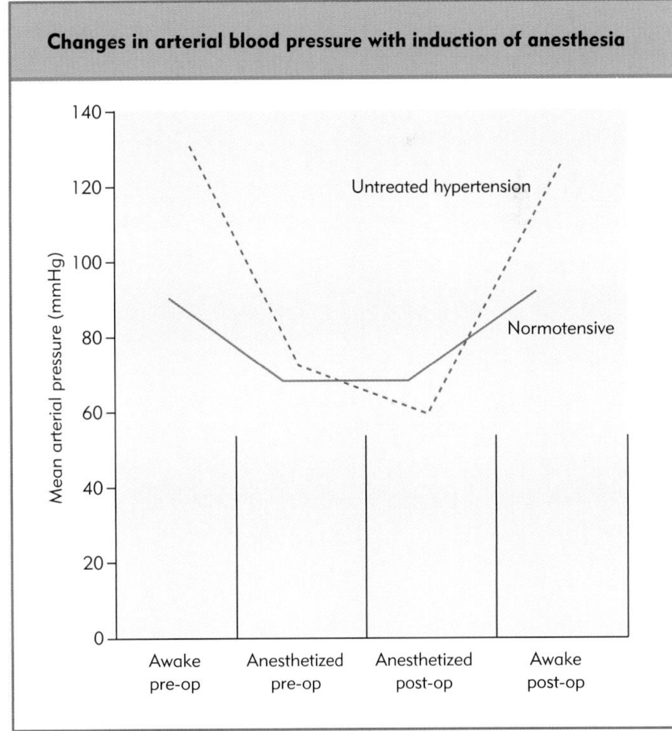

Figure 43.8 Changes in arterial blood pressure with induction of anesthesia in normotensive patients and patients with uncontrolled hypertension. Treated and untreated patients react differently to anesthesia. (Modified from Prys-Roberts C, Meloche R, Foëx P. Studies of anaesthesia in relation to hypertension I. Cardiovascular responses of treated and untreated patients. Br J Anaesth. 1971; 43:128.)

elective surgery. Such a policy results in a large number of operations being canceled, as even now a large proportion of such patients are untreated, and among those who are treated, many are not properly controlled, i.e. their blood pressure is still outside the normal range. The issue is further complicated by the fact that several epidemiological studies failed to identify hypertension as a significant predictor of adverse outcome. The majority of the available epidemiological evidence relates to patients with mild to moderate hypertension, and there are very few data on patients with markedly elevated admission blood pressure, above a level of 180/110 mmHg; an association between elevated admission blood pressures at levels up to this level and perioperative cardiac death is yet to be demonstrated. Further, as yet, no study has shown conclusively that treatment of hypertension prior to surgery brings about a significant improvement in perioperative outcome.

Key references

Boersma E, Poldermans D, Bax JJ et al. Predictors of cardiac events after major vascular surgery: Role of clinical characteristics, dobutamine echocardiography, and beta-blocker therapy. JAMA 2001;285:1865–73.

British Hypertension Society Website. http://www.bhsoc.org/

Chobanian AV, Bakris GL, Black HR et al. Seventh report of the Joint National Committee on Prevention, Detection, Evaluation, and Treatment of High Blood Pressure. Hypertension 2003;42.

Prys-Roberts C, Meloche R, Foëx P. Studies of anaesthesia in relation to hypertension I. Cardiovascular responses of treated and untreated patients. Br J Anaesth. 1971;43:122–37.

Williams B, Paulter NR, Brown MY et al. Guidelines for the management of hypertension: report of the fourth working party of the British Hypertension Society 2004 – BHS IV. Journal of Human Hypertension 2004:18;139–85.

Further reading

Brown MJ, Cruickshank JK, Dominiczak AF et al. Better blood pressure control: how to combine drugs. J Hum Hypertens. 2003;17:81–6.

Eagle KA, Berger PB, Calkins H et al. ACC/AHA guideline update for perioperative cardiovascular evaluation for noncardiac surgery. A report of the American College of Cardiology/American Heart Association Task Force on Practice Guidelines (Committee to Update the 1996 Guidelines on Perioperative Cardiovascular Evaluation for Noncardiac Surgery). 2002. American College of Cardiology Web site. Available at http./www.acc.org/clinical/guidelines/perio/driIndex.htm

Goldman L, Caldera DL. Risks of general anesthesia and elective operation in the hypertensive patient. Anesthesiology 1979;50:285–92.

Howell SJ, Sear YM, Yeates D, Goldacre M, Sear JW, Foex P. Risk factors for cardiovascular death after elective surgery under general anaesthesia. Br J Anaesth. 1998;80:14–19.

Howell SJ, Sear JW, Foëx P. Hypertension, hypertensive heart disease and perioperative cardiac risk. Br J Anaesth. 2004; 92:570–83.

London MJ, Zaugg M, Schaub MC, Spahn DR. Perioperative beta-adrenergic receptor blockade: physiologic foundations and clinical controversies. Anesthesiology 2004;100:170–5.

Varon J, Marik P. The diagnosis and management of hypertensive crises. Chest 2000;118:214–27.

Chapter 44

Ischemic heart disease and heart failure

Hugh C Hemmings Jr, Uday Jain and Stanton K Shernan

TOPICS COVERED IN THIS CHAPTER

- **Coronary artery disease**
- **Myocardial ischemia**
  - Coronary steal
  - Electrocardiography and echocardiography in diagnosis and monitoring
- **Myocardial ischemia–reperfusion injury**
  - Role of complement activation
  - Systemic inflammatory response syndrome
  - Treatment of myocardial ischemia–reperfusion injury
- **Myocardial preconditioning**
- **Myocardial infarction**
- **Heart failure**
- **Pericardial tamponade**
- **Pulmonary embolism**

Ischemic heart disease, including myocardial ischemia, infarction, and failure, is the most common cardiac disease in adults. More than 3 million patients with heart disease undergo anesthesia and surgery every year. Despite impressive innovations in pharmacological preventative therapy and surgical intervention, patients with cardiovascular disease have a significantly increased risk for perioperative morbidity and mortality (Table 44.1). This chapter reviews the pathophysiology of ischemic heart disease and heart failure and their relevance to anesthesiology.

CORONARY ARTERY DISEASE

The usual etiology of ischemic heart disease is coronary artery disease (CAD) due to coronary atherosclerosis. When myocardial oxygen demand exceeds delivery, limited myocardial blood flow and oxygen lead to ischemia and/or infarction. This can occur when demand is increased by increased contractility, afterload, and/or heart rate, or when supply is reduced by decreases in coronary perfusion pressure, tachycardia, plaque rupture and thrombus formation, embolism, or vasospasm.

Left coronary artery flow occurs primarily during diastole, whereas right coronary artery flow to the right ventricle (RV), which involves a lower downstream pressure, occurs in both systole and diastole (see Chapter 39). As the duration of diastole is reduced at higher heart rates, coronary perfusion is impaired. Left ventricular (LV) coronary perfusion pressure is the difference between aortic diastolic blood pressure and the back pressure (the higher of LV end-diastolic pressure LV (EDP) or coronary

Table 44.1 Clinical predictors of increased perioperative cardiovascular risk (myocardial infarction, congestive heart failure, or death)

Major
Unstable coronary syndromes
Recent myocardial infarction[a] with evidence of important ischemic risk based on clinical symptoms or noninvasive study
Unstable or severe[b] angina
Decompensated congestive heart failure
Significant arrhythmias
High-grade atrioventricular block
Symptomatic ventricular arrhythmias in the presence of underlying heart disease
Supraventricular arrhythmias with uncontrolled ventricular rate
Severe valvular disease
Intermediate
Mild angina pectoris
Prior myocardial infarction based on history or electrocardiographic changes
Compensated or prior congestive heart failure
Diabetes mellitus
Minor
Advanced age
Abnormal electrocardiographic findings (left ventricular hypertrophy, left bundle branch block, ST-T wave abnormalities)
Rhythm other than sinus (e.g. atrial fibrillation)
Low functional capacity (e.g. unable to climb one flight of stairs while carrying bag of groceries)
History of stroke
Uncontrolled systemic hypertension

[a] The American College of Cardiology National Database Library defines recent myocardial infarction as more than 7 days but less than or equal to 30 days.
[b] May include 'stable' angina in patients who are unusually sedentary.

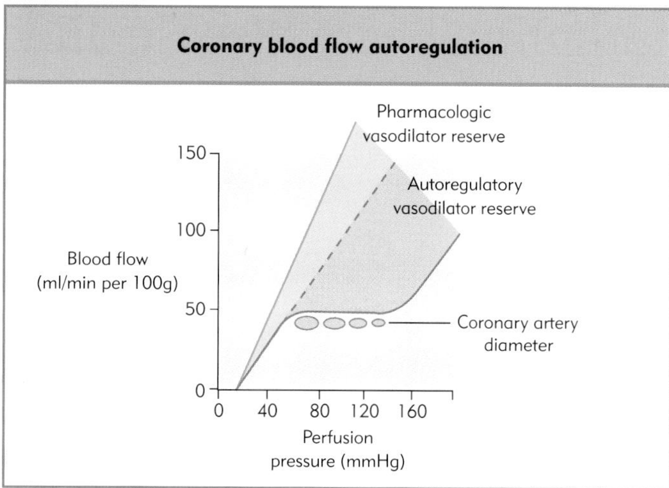

Figure 44.1 The variation of coronary blood flow with coronary perfusion pressure. Coronary blood flow is constant (autoregulated) over coronary perfusion pressures from 60 to 140 mmHg. At 60 mmHg there is maximal autoregulatory vasodilatation to maintain coronary blood flow. Further decreases in coronary perfusion pressure result in decreases in coronary blood flow. At pressures above 60 mmHg vasodilatation provides autoregulatory vasodilator reserve (coronary reserve). This provides the increased coronary blood flow necessary to meet increases in myocardial oxygen consumption, such as those induced by exercise. Infusion of vasodilators at perfusion pressures below the autoregulation range may further increase coronary blood flow. The flat (autoregulatory) portion of the curve is shifted up to higher flow levels by increases in the metabolic state of the heart and myocardial oxygen consumption.

sinus pressure). Coronary autoregulation maintains constant coronary blood flow for perfusion pressures of 60–120 mmHg by changes in coronary resistance, which is determined primarily by intramyocardial arterioles (Fig. 44.1). Plasma adenosine, Po_2, Pco_2, pH, and lactic acid and K^+ concentrations affect coronary vascular resistance and may mediate the close link between coronary blood flow and metabolism. An increase in perfusion pressure causes reflex coronary vasoconstriction (autoregulation). Acetylcholine, bradykinin, and prostaglandins release endothelium-derived relaxing factor (EDRF; nitric oxide), causing vasodilatation. Coronary vasodilatation is also caused by β_2-adrenoceptor stimulation, whereas vasoconstriction is caused by parasympathetic stimulation and α_1-adrenoceptor stimulation, which primarily affect large epicardial arteries. Interruption of coronary blood flow for as little as 1 second leads to a great transient increase in coronary flow, termed reactive hyperemia, through local myogenic responses.

Arrhythmias of many types are frequent complications of ischemia and infarction. Re-entry in the ischemic epicardium or ectopic foci in endocardial Purkinje fibers surviving in the infarct zone are frequent causes (Chapter 40). Ischemia and infarction of the inferior–posterior LV is associated with first-degree block, Mobitz type I second-degree block, and transient atrioventricular third-degree blocks. Ischemia and infarction of the anterior LV is associated with Mobitz type II second-degree block, occasional permanent infranodal block, and intraventricular conduction defects.

MYOCARDIAL ISCHEMIA

Normal myocardial oxygen consumption (MVO_2) is 6–8 mL/min/100 g tissue. Of this, about 20% is for basal metabolism, 1% for electrical activation, 15% for volume work, and about 65% for pressure work. If heart rate, pressure work, or contractility increases by 50%, myocardial oxygen consumption also increases by 50%. In addition, although an increase in volume work by 50% causes only about 5% increase in myocardial oxygen consumption, a similar increase in wall stress (chamber pressure × chamber radius/wall thickness) causes about a 25% increase in myocardial oxygen consumption.

Ischemia leads to contractile dysfunction. Even after adequate reperfusion is re-established, *myocardial stunning* associated with reversible contractile dysfunction may develop and persist for hours to days in the absence of necrosis. Alternatively, patients with ischemic heart disease may have chronic contractile dysfunction due to *myocardial hibernation*, which can be reversed by revascularization.

Prolonged ischemia results in a variety of cellular metabolic and ultrastructural changes that are initiated by the depletion of high-energy phosphates. In the absence of normal oxidative phosphorylation in mitochondria, concentrations of ATP and creatine phosphate diminish. Depletion of adenine nucleotides may persist for hours to days following severe ischemia, partially due to the limited capacity of myocardium for de novo purine synthesis. When ATP utilization exceeds the capacity of myocytes to resynthesize high-energy phosphates, degradation of adenine nucleotides results in the conversion of adenosine diphosphate (ADP) to adenosine monophosphate (AMP). Sustained reductions in ATP availability result in irreversible myocyte injury associated with sarcolemmal damage, acidosis, and cellular swelling as ATP-dependent ionic pump function becomes compromised, favoring extracellular leakage of K^+ and intracellular entry of Ca^{2+}, Na^+, and water. Myocardial ischemia is also associated with an accumulation of intracellular lactic acid, a decline in fatty acid oxidation, which normally provides 60–90% of myocardial energy requirements, and depletion of glutathione, an endogenous intracellular antioxidant. Characteristic changes in myocardial protein production and degradation can occur acutely following an ischemic insult or be delayed, suggesting a role for altered gene expression.

Perioperative myocardial ischemia is frequently silent (i.e. not associated with symptoms such as angina) and often occurs in response to known stimuli. During noncardiac surgery, ischemia is most common during emergence from general anesthesia and may result from a hyperdynamic circulation through pain, apprehension, or the administration of muscarinic anticholinergic agents in combination with cholinesterase inhibitors for reversing muscle relaxation. Stimuli during coronary artery bypass graft (CABG) surgery include manipulation of old grafts during reoperation, the administration of protamine, and an increase in myocardial oxygen consumption. Furthermore, perioperative coronary vasospasm and thrombosis may cause ischemia, which can progress to infarction. Episodes of ST segment deviation are most common in the first 8 hours after the release of aortic occlusion. Patients with perioperative ECG changes are more likely to have adverse cardiovascular outcomes after noncardiac or CABG surgery.

Coronary steal

Coronary steal is a reduction in perfusion to collateral-dependent myocardium following an increase in perfusion to myocardium from which the collaterals originate. Vasodilatation of coronary vessels, caused by anesthetics or other agents, in

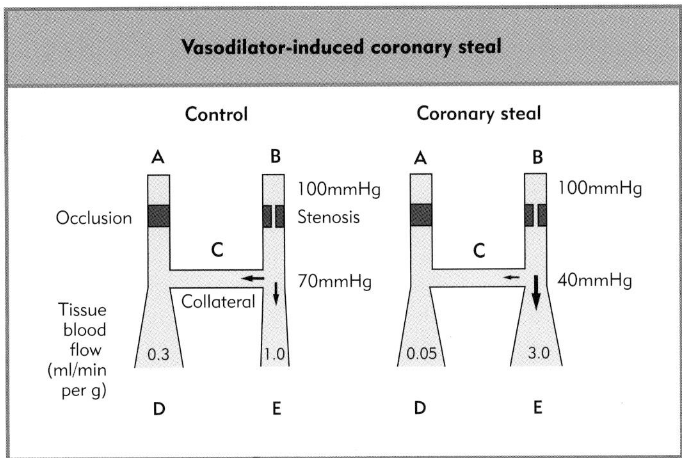

Figure 44.2 The mechanism of vasodilator-induced coronary steal in the coronary circulation. Collateral vessels (C) are maximally dilated in the control state and during coronary steal. During vasodilatation of E, perfusion pressure at the origin of the collateral vessels is reduced from 70 to 40 mmHg, resulting in decreased perfusion of ischemic tissue (D). In contrast, vasodilatation to areas distal to the stenosis causes an increase in blood flow to tissue (E) supplied by the stenotic artery, and coronary steal has occurred.

previously nonischemic myocardium increases total flow and leads to a greater reduction in pressure across an arterial stenosis. Lower pressure distal to the stenosis reduces flow to the ischemic myocardium as the distal vessels are already fully dilated (Fig. 44.2). Anesthetics rarely cause ischemia via this mechanism, partly because they also depress myocardial contractility, reducing oxygen demand. Transmural coronary steal involves increased subepicardial and decreased subendocardial perfusion, which can develop because subendocardial vessels are more dilated (have less vasodilator reserve) than subepicardial vessels in the resting state.

Electrocardiography and echocardiography in diagnosis and monitoring

A number of noninvasive tests are used for the detection of myocardial ischemia. Ischemia is provoked by increasing myocardial oxygen demand and possibly by reducing supply (e.g. via exercise, or the use of dobutamine). Alternatively, agents such as dipyridamole or adenosine are used to cause myocardial blood flow redistribution (steal) via collaterals from poorly perfused (flow restricted) to well-perfused areas, leading to ischemia. Ischemia or flow redistribution may be detected via EGG, TEE (transesophageal echocardiography), or scintigraphy.

Although ischemia may affect several features of the ECG, new ST segment deviation is used as a marker perioperatively because of its sensitivity and specificity (Chapter 13). The orthogonal leads III, V_2, and V_5 are suitable for recording ST segment depression and elevation in various regions of the heart during cardiac surgery. During noncardiac surgery, leads II and V_5 are adequate.

ST segment deviation may also have nonischemic causes. Fixed deviation may be caused by cardiac conduction changes and LV hypertrophy with strain. New deviations may be caused by changes in body position or acid–base and electrolyte status, hyperventilation, Valsalva maneuver, hyperglycemia, and pancreatitis. ST segment elevation observed on cooling at the beginning of cardiopulmonary bypass (CPB) and on electrical defibrillation after CPB is usually unrelated to ischemia. On termination of CPB, new ST segment deviation in association with a widened QRS complex may occur as a result of cardiac conduction abnormalities; it is usually of the opposite polarity to the terminal QRS complex. These cardiac conduction changes usually subside within a few hours after CPB but do indicate myocardial injury, even when transient. New postoperative ST segment elevation caused by pericarditis after cardiac surgery usually occurs in multiple leads and is associated with PR depression and J-point and concave-upward ST segment elevation with an upright T wave.

Perioperative myocardial ischemia is most common during emergence from anesthesia.

The modalities commonly used for perioperative ischemia detection include electrocardiography (ECG) and transesophageal echocardiography (TEE). The term ischemia usually refers to reversible ischemia; however, many changes observed perioperatively via ECG and TEE result from irreversible ischemia (i.e. infarction-in-evolution). Coronary vasospasm and thrombosis are frequent causes of ischemia that may progress to infarction. However, there are also nonischemic causes of changes in ECG, TEE, and pulmonary artery pressures that mimic those seen with ischemia.

A number of studies evaluating the utility of intraoperative TEE in cardiac surgical patients have focused specifically on the analysis of regional wall motion abnormalities (RWMA) and their relationship to postoperative morbidity and mortality. Although somewhat controversial, RWMA may be more sensitive indicators of myocardial ischemia than EGG changes, and may therefore be better predictors of adverse perioperative outcomes. However, ventricular pacing or acute changes in loading conditions can also be associated with RWMA in the absence of myocardial ischemia. In addition, ECG may be better for differentiating transmural ischemia and injury (often associated with ST segment elevation) from subendocardial ischemia (often associated with ST segment depression), because ischemia, infarction, or stunning may all lead to similar ventricular wall motion abnormalities and loss of systolic wall thickening detected by TEE.

MYOCARDIAL ISCHEMIA–REPERFUSION INJURY

Although prolonged myocardial ischemia alone jeopardizes cellular structural and biochemical integrity, oxygen deprivation limited to less than 20 minutes is usually associated with only transiently depressed myocardial contractility. Paradoxically, the restoration of blood flow following sustained myocardial ischemia beyond 45 minutes results in a phenomenon known as myocardial ischemia–reperfusion (I–R) injury, in which tissue injury is augmented in excess of that produced by ischemia alone. Perioperative myocardial I–R injury involves the generation of reactive oxygen species (ROS) upon the restoration of oxygen (O_2) delivery, and alterations in intracellular Ca^{2+} homeostasis. Activation of several proinflammatory pathways, including the complement, coagulation, and cytokine cascades, exacerbates tissue injury and functional impairment initiated by the original ischemic insult. Thus, myocardial I–R injury is a complex pathophysiological process that contributes significantly to perioperative cardiac dysfunction and the associated morbidity.

Reperfusion of ischemic tissues results in the formation of toxic ROS, including superoxide anions (O_2^-), hydroxyl radicals (OH^-), hypochlorous acid (HOCl), hydrogen peroxide (H_2O_2), and nitric oxide (NO)-derived peroxynitrite. Normally, hypoxanthine produced from AMP metabolism is further metabolized by xanthine dehydrogenase (XD) to xanthine. However, during ischemia XD is converted to xanthine oxidase (XO) by Ca^{2+}-dependent proteases. Unlike XD, which uses nicotinamide adenine dinucleotide (NAD) as an electron acceptor during oxidation of xanthine, XO uses O_2. During O_2 deprivation XO is unable to catalyze the conversion of hypoxanthine to xanthine, resulting in the accumulation of excess hypoxanthine. The reintroduction of O_2 during reperfusion permits the formation of ROS from XO-mediated conversion of this excess hypoxanthine. Although the human myocardium may not have significant quantities of XO, ischemia-induced ROS can be generated via other mechanisms, including the NADPH oxidase system located in polymorphonuclear leukocytes (PMN), dissociation of mitochondrial electron transport, catecholamine auto-oxidization, and free metal ions.

Reperfusion of ischemic tissues results in the formation of toxic reactive oxygen species that contribute to reperfusion injury.

ROS are potent oxidizing agents that directly damage cellular membranes, mitochondria, and the sarcoplasmic reticulum, resulting in depressed contractile function. Evidence of myocardial contraction-band necrosis on histological examination is the hallmark of ROS involvement in the 'oxygen paradox' associated with I–R injury. ROS also induce leukocyte activation and chemotaxis indirectly by Ca^{2+}-mediated activation of plasma membrane phopholipase A_2 to form arachidonic acid, an important precursor for eicosanoid synthesis. Furthermore, ROS can directly activate complement components and may be in part responsible for microvascular inflammation associated with an imbalance between endothelial cell production of NO and H_2O_2. Finally, ROS sustain I–R injury by stimulating endothelial cell adhesion molecule and cytokine gene expression via the activation of nuclear transcription factors such as nuclear factor (NF)-κB, which are in turn activated by oxidant stress. Thus, ROS play a significant direct role in early cellular damage during I–R injury, and indirectly stimulate proinflammatory mediators responsible for further sustained myocardial dysfunction.

A 'calcium paradox' may also be involved in myocardial I–R injury. Cytosolic Ca^{2+} and Na^+ concentrations increase during myocardial ischemia as ATP-dependent ionic pump function is impaired. Restoration of O_2 delivery and subsequent mitochondrial oxidative phosphorylation reactivates the Ca^{2+} pump (Ca^{2+}-ATPase) of the sarcoplasmic reticulum (SR) and the sarcolemmal Na^+ pump (Na^+,K^+-ATPase). The coordination of these major cation pumps with the sarcolemmal Na^+/Ca^{2+} exchanger normally helps to restore ionic gradients. However, in the presence of intracellular Ca^{2+} overload, excessive Ca^{2+} sequestration in the SR can cause spontaneous oscillations and cardiac muscle hypercontracture, especially when energy is concurrently restored to the myofibrils. Substantial cytoskeletal structural injury results in an irreversible state of hypercontracture-induced sarcomere shortening. Contractile elements become relatively insensitive to Ca^{2+} (i.e. 'calcium paradox'), resulting in overall depression of myocardial contractility. Sarcolemmal stability may also be compromised by excessive water influx and cellular swelling associated with a persistent cytosolic Na^+ overload in the presence of a rapidly normalizing extracellular osmotic load during reperfusion.

Although intracellular Ca^{2+} overload and ROS independently contribute to myocardial I–R injury, the pathophysiological mechanisms are not mutually exclusive. Intracellular Ca^{2+} overload is exacerbated during reperfusion by ROS, which interfere with Ca^{2+} flux at the level of the cell membrane or SR, directly compromise mitochondrial oxidative phosphorylation, and irreversibly inhibit anaerobic glycolysis. Ca^{2+}-dependent mechanisms also promote ROS production via protease-mediated XO activation and damage to the mitochondrial electron transport chain, which facilitates ROS leakage.

The endothelium plays an essential role in maintaining vascular homeostasis and is particularly vulnerable to the deleterious effects of both ischemia and reperfusion injury. Sustained hypoxia interferes with normal transcellular ion and water fluxes, thereby inducing ionic potential imbalances, cellular edema, and eventual damage to endothelial integrity. Following prolonged ischemia, endothelial production of certain bioactive agents (e.g. endothelin, thromboxane A_2 (TxA_2), and proinflammatory gene products (e.g. leukocyte adhesion molecules, cytokines) is enhanced. Endothelial production of other 'protective' gene products (e.g. constitutive NO, thrombomodulin) and bioactive agents (e.g. prostacyclin, NO) is concurrently suppressed. Thus endothelial ischemia induces a proinflammatory state.

Endothelial ischemia induces a proinflammatory state that further exacerbates reperfusion injury.

Normal endothelial cell function is further compromised following reperfusion via an exacerbation of the pathophysiological processes initiated during the initial ischemic insult (Fig. 44.3). ROS play a major role in the pathophysiology of endothelial I–R injury. Restoration of O_2 flow during reperfusion results in an accumulation of endothelial XO and the subsequent production of excessive O_2^- and H_2O_2 in addition to the ROS generated by locally activated leukocytes. In addition, Ca^{2+}-dependent endothelial NO synthase activity is reduced following I–R injury, leaving little NO to scavenge accumulating O_2^-. Diminished endothelial NO is responsible for impaired NO-mediated arteriolar smooth muscle relaxation, enhanced platelet aggregation, leukocyte endothelial cell adhesion, and promotion of the capillary filtration response to I–R injury. ROS are also involved in promoting leukocyte–endothelial cell interactions by mediating the expression of endothelial adhesion molecules, promoting the activation and deposition of complement on endothelial cell membranes, and enhancing phospholipase A_2-mediated production of leukotrienes (LTB_4) and platelet-activating factor (PAF).

Circulating leukocytes that have been activated systemically (e.g. multisystem organ dysfunction, circulatory shock, aortic occlusion–reperfusion, CPB) or remotely in combination with proinflammatory mediators (tumor necrosis factor-α, interleukin

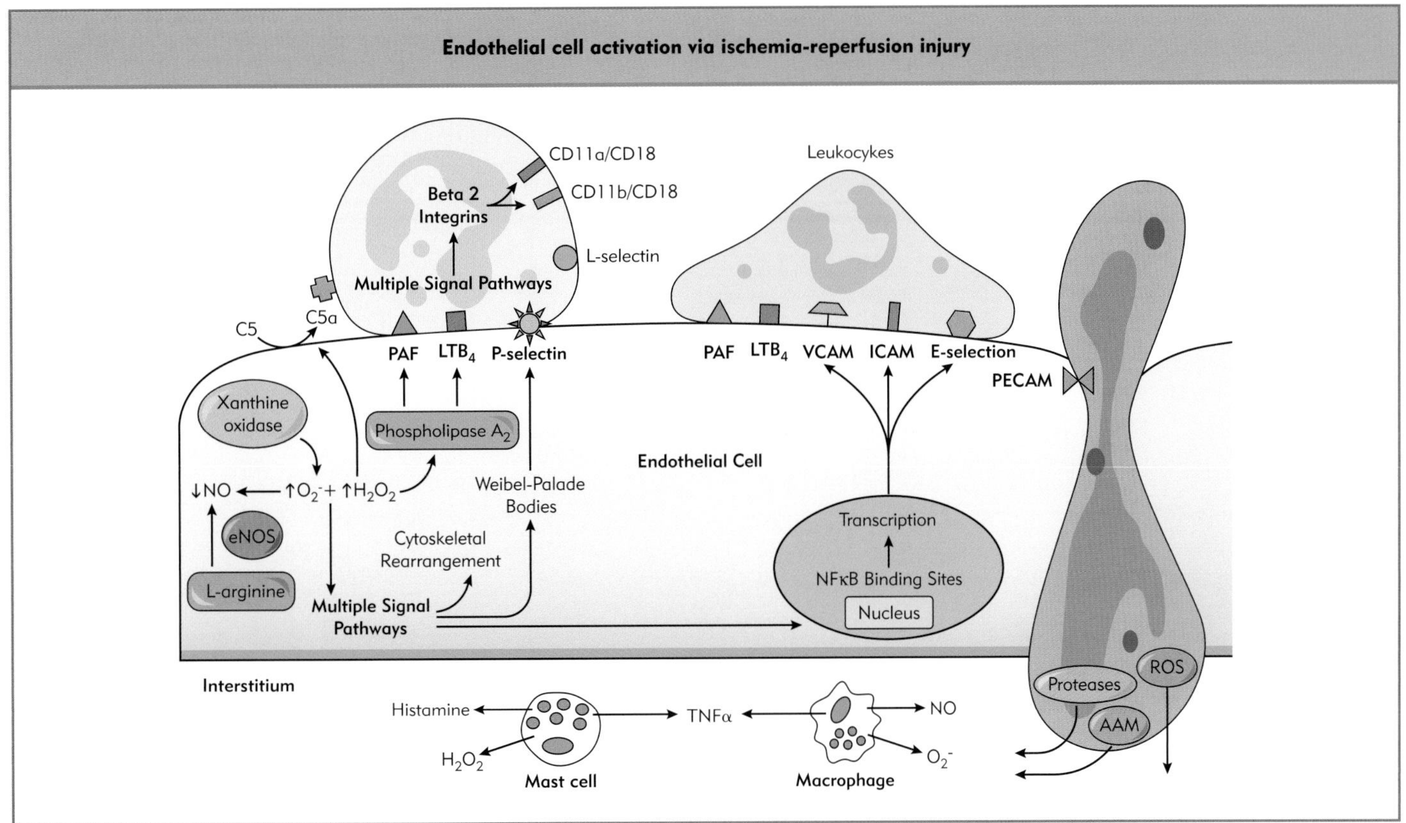

Figure 44.3 Endothelial cell–leukocyte interactions during ischemia–reperfusion (I–R) injury. Endothelial cell exposure to ischemia and the restoration of oxygen delivery (O_2) results in the intracellular production of reactive oxygen species (ROS: O_2^-; H_2O_2). Subsequent endothelial cell activation involves multiple signal pathways, resulting in decreased production of nitric oxide (NO), increased intracellular Ca^{2+}, and increased production of mediators, including platelet-activating factor (PAF), and leukotrienes (LTB_4). In addition, the surface expression of selectins (P-selectin, E-selectin) and intercellular adhesion molecules (ICAM, VCAM) is accelerated. Following activation by cytokines and activated complement components (C5a), leukocytes accumule at the endothelial cell surface and begin loosely adhering or 'rolling' via the interaction of the selectins (P-selectin, L-selectin). Firm adherence involves interactions between leukocyte β_2-integrins (CD11a/CD18; CD11b/CD18) and intercellular adhesion molecules. Leukocyte transmigration (diapedesis) within endothelial cell junctions is mediated by platelet–endothelial cell adhesion molecule (PECAM), and results in the release of destructive ROS, proteases, and arachidonic acid metabolites (AAM).

(IL)-1, thromboxane (TxB_2), activated complement fragments, PAF) may play a role in augmenting myocardial I–R injury. Local neutrophil *accumulation* at the site of myocardial I–R injury represents one of the most important components of the overall pathological process. Both neutrophils and vascular endothelium are involved in establishing a localized chemotactic factor concentration gradient involving complement fragment C5a, IL-8, transforming growth factor (TGF-α) and tumor necrosis factor (TNF).

Role of complement activation

The complement system is a major component of the humoral immune system that plays a major role in some of the inflammatory events occurring in myocardial I–R injury. This innate cytotoxic defense system is composed of a catalytic cascade involving approximately 20 intravascular proteins that utilize a variety of immunological processes to eliminate foreign cells, initiate inflammation, destroy pathogens, and disrupt cell membranes (Fig. 44.4). The complement system is subdivided into three pathways: the classical, the alternative, and the more recently described lectin complement pathway. Activation of these pathways occurs sequentially through the proteolytic cleavage and association of precursor molecules. The *alternative complement pathway* is an antibody-independent pathway activated by a variety of mechanisms, which leads to the formation of C3 convertase (C3bBb). *Classical complement pathway* activation occurs when antibody–antigen complexes interact with the first complement component (C1), and ultimately lead to the formation of the C3 convertase, C4b2a. The *lectin complement pathway* (LCP) is an antibody-independent pathway activated by binding mannose-binding lectin (MBL) to carbohydrate structures present on the surface of bacteria, yeast, parasitic protozoa, and viruses. In contrast to the classical complement pathway, activation of the LCP does not require antibody, C1, or C1q deposition, but instead relies on two serine proteases, MASP-1 and MASP-2, to cleave C2 and C4 to form the classical C3 convertase.

All three pathways merge at C3, which is cleaved by the respective C3 convertase into the anaphylatoxic peptide C3a and the opsonic fragment C3b. C3a is a mast cell and eosinophil chemoattractant and activator. Target cell attachment of C3b induces the formation of C5 convertase ($C3b_2Bb$ or C4b2a3b), which subsequently cleaves C5 into C5a and C5b. C5a promotes leukocyte chemotaxis, activation, and generation of inflammatory mediators. C5b initiates the formation of C5b-9, the membrane attack complex (MAC), which induces targeted endothelial cell production of chemokines (IL-8, monocyte chemoattractant protein-1) and the expression of proinflammatory selectins and

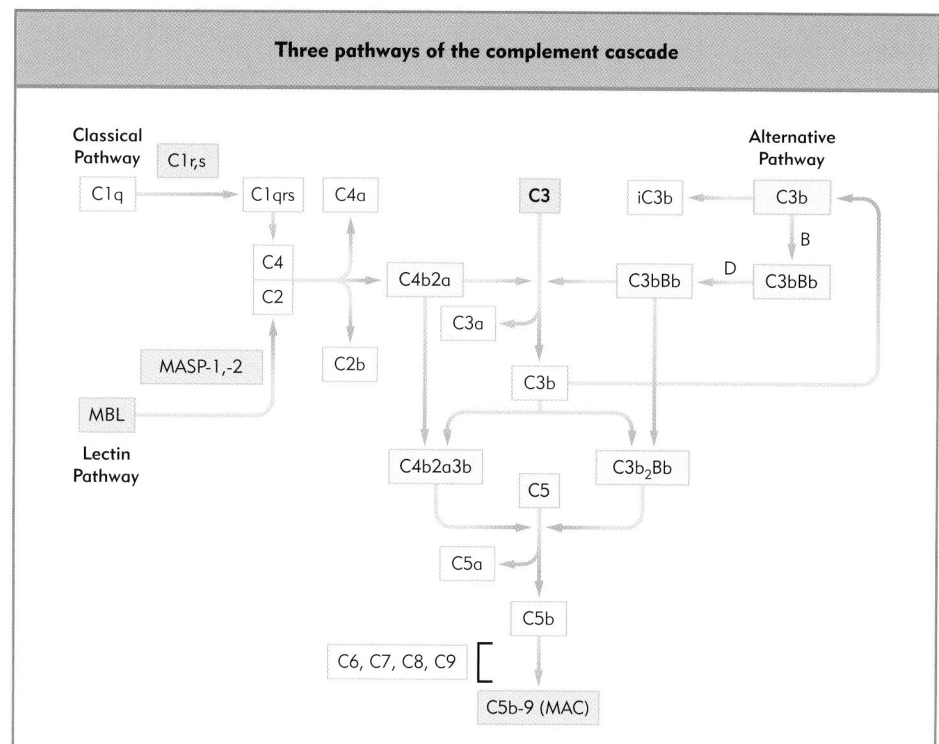

Figure 44.4 The three pathways of the complement cascade. The antibody-independent classical complement pathway, the antibody-dependent alternative pathway, and the lectin pathway all converge at C3 and lead to the production of terminal complement complex (C5b-9). MAC, membrane attack complex.

adhesion molecules. More importantly, multiple target cell 'hits' by the pore-forming C5b-9 promotes water, electrolyte, and small molecule transcellular fluxes, ultimately resulting in cell lysis and irreversible tissue injury.

Evidence for the role of activated complement components in myocardial I–R injury include both indirect effects of anaphylatoxins and direct effects of C5b-9 in modifying leukocyte responses, altering vascular homeostasis, and ultimately inducing tissue damage. Although reperfusion may further exacerbate the extent of complement-mediated myocardial injury, complement activation may actually be initiated during ischemia. During ischemia, disruption of myocyte membrane integrity may allow intracellular entry and activation of complement components. Exposed basement membranes, subcellular organelles, mitochondrial particles, cardiolipin, certain sensitizing antibodies, or the fibrinolytic system can directly activate the classical complement pathway. Activated complement components also play a role in modifying ROS production and Ca^{2+} flux that contribute to myocardial I–R injury. Ca^{2+} influx is also facilitated by complement activation via the formation and membrane insertion of C5b-9. Thus complement activation plays an important *early* role in modifying myocardial I–R injury.

Activation of complement pathways also plays an important role in the pathogenesis of myocardial ischemia–reperfusion injury.

Activated complement components are also particularly important facilitators of endothelial cell–leukocyte interactions and vascular injury. The anaphylatoxins C3a, C5a, and C4a act directly on smooth muscle to promote vasodilatation. In addition, anaphylatoxin-induced increases in vascular permeability are promoted via histamine release from mast cells and basophils, thereby facilitating neutrophil transmigration. C5a can independently promote neutrophil chemotaxis, aggregation, and the production of ROS, arachidonic acid metabolites, and proteolytic enzymes. C5a can also modify neutrophil adherence to endothelium by eliciting the release of PAF, which can subsequently activate neutrophils, upregulate β_2-integrins, and induce L-selectin shedding. Furthermore, C5a may amplify this inflammatory response by inducing cytokine production.

Complement activation associated with myocardial I–R injury may also result from antibody-independent activation of the classical complement pathway at the level of C2 and C4 via the LCP following binding of MBL to cell surface carbohydrates. Although MBL does not normally recognize the body's own tissues, oxidative stress may alter cell surface membrane glycosylation, leading to increased MBL deposition. Thus complement activation through any of the three delineated pathways may significantly contribute to the pathogenesis of myocardial I–R injury.

Systemic inflammatory response syndrome

During cardiac surgery requiring CPB, an imbalance in the *systemic* production of pro- and anti-inflammatory mediators can contribute to organ dysfunction initiated *locally* at the site of I–R injury. The pathophysiology of this systemic inflammatory response syndrome (SIRS) involves several interdependent pathways, including the contact system, coagulation–fibrinolytic cascades, complement cascades, and cytokine production (see also Chapter 73).

Several mechanisms are involved in the SIRS during cardiac surgery. Nonspecific activators of SIRS include surgical trauma, blood loss or transfusion, and hypothermia. Increased systemic concentrations of endotoxin associated with gut translocation following mucosal barrier injury due to splanchnic hypoperfusion can also indirectly activate the inflammatory response. Heparin–protamine complexes can systemically activate inflammatory mediators, including complement, histamine, thromboxane, NO and antibodies. Finally, inflammatory mediators generated locally at the site of I–R injury may contribute to those circulating systemically.

The SIRS is profoundly affected by the exposure of blood to bioincompatible surfaces in the CPB extracorporeal circuit, which results in the generation of factor XII and activation of the intrinsic pathway of the coagulation cascade via the contact system. The subsequent production of kallikrein activates the kinin–bradykinin system, stimulates C5a production, and leads to the generation of plasmin. Plasmin in turn activates the fibrinolytic system, generates additional contact activation proteins, and promotes C3 cleavage via the alternate complement pathway. The extrinsic pathway of the coagulation system is also activated in the perioperative period by the production of tissue factor from endothelium and muscle in response to surgical trauma, inflammatory stimuli, and oxidative or shear stress. Thrombin produced from both intrinsic and extrinsic coagulation pathways catalyzes the formation of insoluble fibrin from fibrinogen, which binds the platelet plug to initiate hemostasis.

The normal balance of hemostasis is often disturbed in cardiac surgical patients. The concomitant procoagulant activities of thrombin combined with the activation of fibrinolysis may become uncontrolled in the presence of significant vascular injury. In addition, several coagulation proteins, including thrombin and factor Xa, have proinflammatory properties. Subsequent disseminated intravascular coagulation and microvascular occlusion may contribute to multiorgan dysfunction syndrome. The combination of endothelial cell, platelet, and leukocyte activation with circulating cytokines and procoagulants associated with SIRS favors a systemic procoagulant/proinflammatory state which can exacerbate local I–R injury.

Treatment of myocardial ischemia–reperfusion injury

Myocardial I–R injury has been associated with transient reperfusion arrhythmias, myocardial stunning, and irreversible myocardial injury that can contribute to perioperative morbidity and mortality. Ideally, the morbidity can be diminished by limiting the duration and severity of the initial ischemic insult. However, aortic cross-clamping and CPB are still required for the majority of cardiac surgical procedures, thus subjecting patients to varying degrees of multiorgan I–R injury. Although extracorporeal circuit modification and CABG without CPB (OPCAB, or 'off-pump CABG') may reduce inflammatory mediator generation, neither procedure entirely prevents myocardial I–R and the associated perioperative morbidity. Modification of anesthetic techniques, including the use of thoracic epidural analgesia, can attenuate the perioperative stress response and myocardial injury following CABG. Several anesthetic agents, including sodium thiopental, propofol, opioids, midazolam, and volatile agents, have systemic anti-inflammatory effects. Myocardial gene delivery has been proposed as a potential myocardial protection technique. The remaining therapeutic strategies, many of them experimental, focus on preventing or treating reperfusion injury by administering pharmacological agents that target proinflammatory mediators associated with myocardial I–R injury.

Adenosine and adenosine-regulating agents can mitigate myocardial ischemia. The myocardial protective effect of adenosine is mediated through the K^+_{ATP} channel by a protein kinase C-mediated process. Acadesine is a purine nucleoside analog that selectively increases tissue adenosine concentrations during myocardial ischemia and has beneficial effects on post-reperfusion ventricular function and dysrhythmias, platelet adherence, and granulocyte accumulation. In addition, treatment with acadesine before and during CABG surgery has been shown to reduce the incidence of perioperative MI and cardiac death.

A variety of experimental therapies target proinflammatory mediators of myocardial ischemia–reperfusion.

Serine proteases play a central role in the amplification of the contact activation, coagulation, and complement cascades. Consequently, serine protease inhibition may limit the systemic generation of inflammatory mediators and similar processes related to local I–R injury in the perioperative period. *Aprotinin* is a nonspecific serine protease inhibitor that reduces blood loss and transfusion requirements in cardiac surgical patients. It also exhibits a variety of anti-inflammatory effects, including inhibition of platelet activation, leukocyte activation, and adhesion molecule expression, contact activation, proinflammatory cytokine production, and complement activation.

Anti-inflammatory effects of *corticosteroids* that may protect against myocardial I–R injury include reduced complement activation, diminished proinflammatory (TNF-α, IL-1β, IL-6, IL-8) and increased anti-inflammatory (IL-10) cytokine production, as well as attenuated leukocyte activation, adhesion molecule expression, and sequestration. Corticosteroids can improve cardiovascular performance and reduce perioperative morbidity. However, the theoretical risk for increased infection and poor wound healing, and controversy regarding efficacy and dosing regimens, limit their routine perioperative use.

Protective endogenous myocardial *antioxidants*, including glutathione reductase, superoxide dismutase, and catalase, can become depleted in the presence of overwhelming ROS generation, thereby reducing natural defenses and scavenging capacity. Thus, the use of exogenous free radical scavengers and antioxidants may ameliorate the deleterious consequences of I–R injury. Although a variety of antioxidants attenuate the sequelae of myocardial ischemia in experimental models, there are few data demonstrating clinical benefits.

Delineation of the complement cascade components and endogenous regulatory mechanisms provides the foundation for novel targeted pharmacological strategies to reduce myocardial I–R injury and morbidity. Most investigations of *complement inhibitors* have been limited to experimental models. Two complement inhibitors have been administered in large-scale clinical trials involving cardiac patients. *Soluble CR1* (sCR1), an inhibitor of C3/C5 convertases and cofactor of C3b and C4b inactivation, attenuates myocardial I–R injury in animals and reduces systemic inflammation following CPB. A recent trial involving the administration of a recombinant form of SCRI (TP10 Avant Immunotherapeutics, Inc., Needham, MA) demonstrated a potential benefit in reducing morbidity and mortality in male CABG patients. A humanized, single-chain *monoclonal anti-C5 antibody* (*Pexelizumab*; Alexion Pharmaceuticals, Cheshire, CT) has also been shown to attenuate complement activation, leukocyte activation, myocardial injury, blood loss, and cognitive dysfunction in a preliminary study. A therapeutic effect of this anti-C_5 antibody in ameliorating myocardial infarction or death in CABG patients has been suggested in more recent multicenter trials.

The Na^+/H^+ exchanger (NHE) is a sarcolemmal protein that facilitates the exchange of intracellular H^+ for extracellular Na^+. Myocardial ischemia results in an increase in intracellular H^+ that is exchanged for Na^+ by activation of the dominant myocardial NHE isoform (NHE-1). The subsequent increase in intracellular Na^+ promotes Na^+/Ca^{2+} exchange, resulting in the accumulation of intracellular Ca^{2+} as the ATP-dependent Na^+, K^+ pump becomes dysfunctional. NHE activity is usually self-limited during sustained ischemia once a transmembrane ionic equilibrium is achieved. However, reperfusion re-establishes an H^+ concentration gradient from the intracellular to the extracellular space, thereby promoting intracellular Ca^{2+} overload, myocyte hypercontracture, and cardiac dysfunction. Thus, NHE inhibitors, including *cariporide* and *eniporide*, may attenuate myocardial I–R injury by preventing excessive intracellular Na^+ and Ca^{2+} overload.

Gene–environmental interactions are being recognized for their role in the pathogenesis of cardiovascular disease. In the near future preoperative screening for polymorphisms in certain inflammatory and coagulation genes should contribute to a reduction of morbidity by permitting the identification of high-risk patients and introducing the opportunity for pharmacogenetic intervention and gene therapy.

MYOCARDIAL PRECONDITIONING

Ischemic preconditioning (IPC) refers to the phenomenon by which I–R injury can be diminished by prior exposure of the myocardium to brief periods of ischemia. Experimental investigation supports myocardial benefits of IPC, including reduced high-energy phosphate consumption, improved ventricular function, reduced myocyte apoptosis, and diminished neutrophil accumulation following I–R. Clinical trials employing IPC have demonstrated less myocardial ATP depletion, lower troponin T levels, and a protective effect on right ventricular contractility in patients undergoing CABG. However, the lack of consistency in the duration and number of IPC and reperfusion periods, the use of surrogate endpoints, ethical considerations involving the use of IPC in high-risk patients, and controversy over its benefit in 'cardioplegia-protected' myocardium have limited the widespread clinical use of IPC.

IPC mechanisms have been further delineated to reveal mechanisms of both 'early' and 'delayed' myocardial protection, as well as the development of pharmacological strategies that may provide a more practical means of myocardial preconditioning (Fig. 44.5). Activation of K^+_{ATP} channels by isoflurane, morphine-mediated δ_1 opioid receptor activation, adenosine, bradykinin, acetylcholine, catecholamines, and myriad other agents have been implicated as potential promoters of pharmacological myocardial preconditioning.

MYOCARDIAL INFARCTION

Myocardial ischemia can develop in the absence of coronary artery atherosclerosis (i.e. coronary artery spasm, congenital anomalies, direct or indirect trauma, emboli). However, the vast majority of myocardial infarctions occur after the rupture of a vulnerable intracoronary plaque and subsequent thrombosis (Fig. 44.6). Perioperative myocardial ischemia following noncardiac surgery usually begins shortly after surgery while the

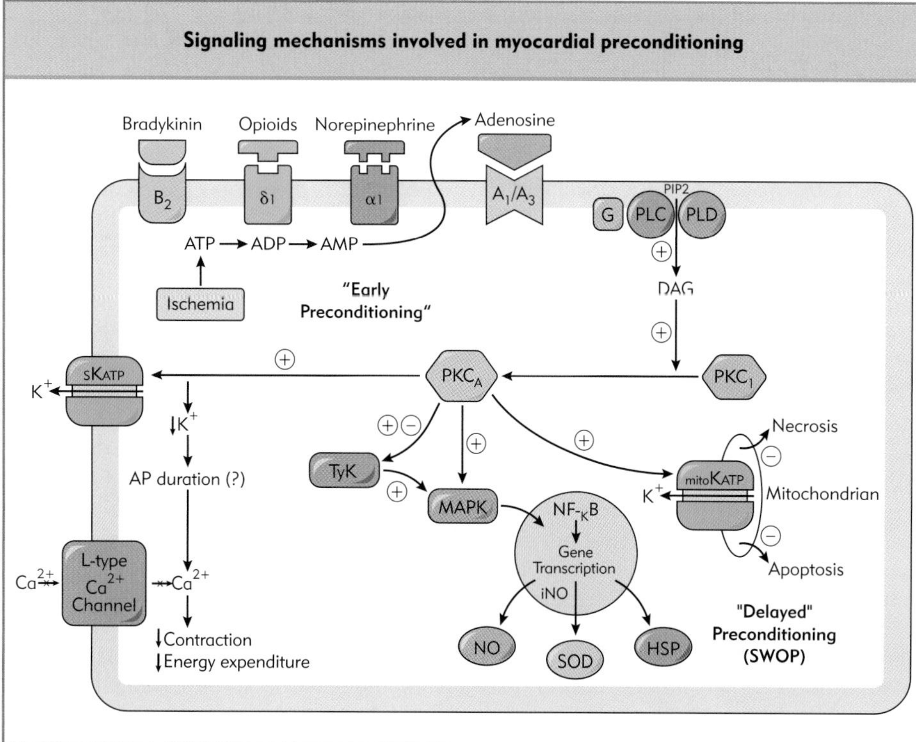

Figure 44.5 Signaling mechanisms involved in myocardial preconditioning. Ischemia-induced activation of adenosine A1-receptors, eventual K^+_{ATP} channel activation, and a decrease in intracellular calcium (Ca^{2+}), is responsible for the 'early preconditioning' (1–2-hour) phase of cardioprotection. Induction of new protein synthesis, including heat-shock proteins (HSP), nitric oxide (NO), and antioxidants (SOD: superoxide dismutase) via the promotion of gene transcription is responsible for a 'delayed, second window of myocardial protection' (SWOP), which reappears 12–24 hours after reperfusion. Receptor activation by several different agents (bradykinin, opioids, catecholamines, isoflurane) may permit pharmacological preconditioning through similar intracellular signaling mechanisms. ATP, adenosine triphosphate; ADP, adenosine diphosphate; AMP, adenosine monophosphate; B_2, bradykinin receptor type 2; δ, opioid δ receptor; α_1, α-adrenergic receptor type 1; A_1/A_3, adenosine receptor types 1 and 3; G, G regulatory protein; PLC/PLD, phospholipase C and D; PIP_2, phosphoinositolbisphosphate; DAG, diacylglycerol; PKC_I and PKC_A, protein kinase C inactive and active forms; sKATP, sarcolemmal ATP-dependent potassium channel; mKATP, mitochondrial ATP-dependent potassium channel; TyK, tyrosine kinase; MAPK, mitogen-activated protein kinase; NF-κB, nuclear factor-κB; iNO, inducible nitric oxide synthase. (From Chen V, Body S, Shernan S. Myocardial preconditioning: characteristics, mechanisms, and clinical applications. Sem Cardiothorac Vasc Anesth. 3:85–97, 1999.)

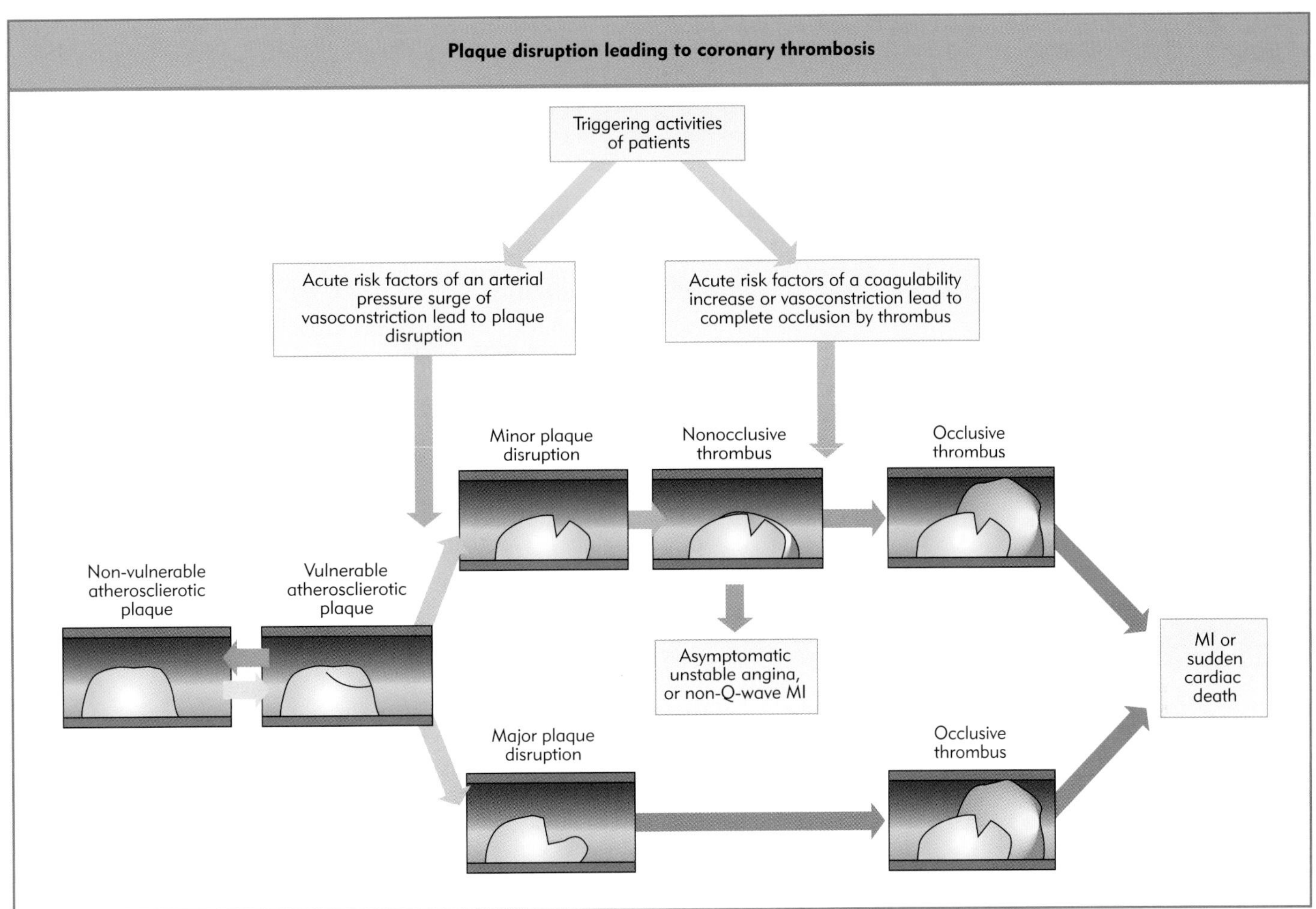

Figure 44.6 Hypothetical mechanisms by which hemodynamic changes leading to plaque rupture, increases in coagulability, and vasoconstriction trigger coronary thrombosis, unstable angina, myocardial infarction, and sudden cardiac death. (With permission from Muller JE, Abela GS, Nesto RW, Tofler GH. Triggers, acute risk factors and vulnerable plaques: the lexicon of a new frontier. J Am Coll Cardiol. 1994; 23:809–13.)

patient is emerging from anesthesia, during a period characterized by increased heart rate, blood pressure, sympathetic discharge, coronary tone, and procoagulant activity. Only half of patients experiencing a perioperative myocardial infarction have classic signs and symptoms of myocardial ischemia. The peak incidence of cardiac death following noncardiac surgical myocardial infarction is 1–3 days postoperatively. In a patient with CAD, perioperative myocardial infarction can occur after prolonged perioperative stress-induced ischemia even in the absence of plaque rupture and thrombosis.

The etiology of perioperative myocardial infarction following CABG surgery is variable. During CABG surgery the myocardium may be particularly susceptible to ischemia because of underlying CAD, perioperative hemodynamic instability, inadequate protection, coronary artery embolization, incomplete revascularization, graft spasm, or kinking. In addition, several proinflammatory pathways, including the complement, coagulation, and cytokine cascades, are activated by reperfusion of ischemic organs and exposure of blood to the bioincompatible surfaces of the extracorporeal circuit. The products of these pathways can promote recruitment and activation of leukocytes, resulting in the generation of additional inflammatory mediators and thereby exacerbating myocardial tissue injury and functional impairment.

The reported incidence of myocardial infarction after CABG surgery varies from 1 to 15%, reflecting the difficulty of establishing a uniform definition for irreversible perioperative myocardial injury. For example, 80–92% of post-CABG myocardial infarctions occur without clinical evidence of transmural infarction, suggesting that not all perioperative myocardial infarctions may be detected by new Q waves on ECG. Discrepancies in the incidence of postoperative Q waves and its value as an independent predictor of adverse outcome may reflect difficulties in ECG assessment in view of rhythm and conduction disturbances, pericardial inflammation, variable lead positioning, and unmasking of previous electrocardiographically silent infarcts.

The utility of cardiac isoenzymes in assessing postoperative myocardial injury has focused on troponin T and I levels. Although troponin I may ultimately be the myocardial injury marker of choice, controversy exists regarding its sensitivity, specificity, and correlation with perioperative outcome. Elevated postoperative creatine kinase (CK-MB) levels are also associated with increased postoperative ventricular wall motion abnormalities and decreased global left ventricular ejection fraction, which can persist for up to 9 months regardless of the presence of Q waves on ECG. Because postoperative CK-MB release can reflect skeletal muscle trauma and myocardial manipulation, even moderate CK-MB elevations do not necessarily indicate significant myocardial injury. However, greater CK-MB release (>10 times normal) correlates with increased morbidity, cost, and mortality. Consistent with the general consensus definition of acute infarction, a combination of new perioperative Q waves with a specific threshold of biochemical confirmation (cardiac enzyme release) may be required to improve the clinical predictive value of perioperative myocardial infarction in CABG patients.

HEART FAILURE

Despite many impressive innovations in pharmacological therapy and surgical intervention, congestive heart failure (CHF) remains an important therapeutic challenge. Among people over 65 years of age the incidence of CHF approaches 1 in 10 000, with a 5-year mortality of approximately 50%. CHF is a significant predictor of perioperative morbidity and mortality for both cardiac and noncardiac surgical patients.

CHF is often associated with systolic dysfunction or pump failure (Chapter 42). However, inherent in the definition of 'congestive' heart failure is the inability of the left ventricle (LV) to maintain an adequate stroke volume without an increase in end-diastolic pressure. Thus, CHF also represents an abnormality of diastolic function. Approximately half of patients who present with signs and symptoms or CHF have evidence of combined systolic and diastolic dysfunction. Interestingly, the remainder have normal ejection fractions and thus present primarily with isolated diastolic heart failure.

The classic signs and symptoms of CHF include fatigue, dyspnea, orthopnea, cough, weight gain, S3/S4 heart sounds, and evidence of pulmonary congestion on chest radiography. Clinical criteria alone often lead to a false positive CHF diagnosis. The incidence of classic signs and symptoms is similar for patients with either 'systolic dysfunction' or 'diastolic dysfunction'. Consequently, diastolic heart failure requires documentation of impaired relaxation or decreased compliance with a normal ejection fraction. Common diagnostic techniques for documenting the presence of diastolic heart failure include cardiac catheterization, radionucleotide ventriculography, cardiac MRI, echocardiography, and elevated brain natriuretic peptide (BNP).

Both myocardial contraction and relaxation are energy-dependent processes (Chapter 39). The increased cytosolic Ca^{2+} levels required for systolic contraction must be restored to presystolic levels to prevent slowing or incomplete LV relaxation. High-energy phosphates are required for actin–myosin disengagement, and restore cytosolic Ca^{2+} to presystolic levels by facilitating reuptake by the sarcoplasmic reticulum and trans-sarcolemmal efflux. Thus reductions in high-energy phosphates (e.g. with myocardial ischemia) lead to diastolic dysfunction. Decreased compliance and impaired relaxation also develop with both concentric and eccentric hypertrophic cardiomyopathy. Myocyte hypertrophy represents an initial normal adaptive response to increased load (i.e. systemic hypertension) in an attempt to preserve systolic function and reduce wall stress. However, chronic exposure eventually contributes to overall impaired cardiac performance by initiating diastolic dysfunction and exacerbating systolic failure. Interestingly, even after controlling for hemodynamic disturbances, adverse LV remodeling and progression of heart failure persist, suggesting systemic involvement (i.e. cardiorenal, neurohumoral, cytokines, genetic factors) that is also involved in the pathophysiology of CHF. The response to acute heart failure is to maintain circulation, though the chronic effects of heart failure are deleterious and increase myocardial oxygen consumption (Table 44.2).

An appreciation of the multifactorial model of CHF is important to guide therapeutic intervention. Therapy for chronic CHF begins with controlling risk factors (diet, exercise, alcohol intake, smoking). Pharmacological intervention includes the use of ACE inhibitors, angiotensin receptor antagonists, diuretics, β-blockers, aldosterone antagonists, digoxin, and BNP. Refractory CHF may require surgical intervention, including coronary revascularization, valve repair/replacement, ventricular resynchronization, intra-aortic balloon counterpulsation, ventricular assist device, surgical reverse remodeling, or heart transplantation.

Chronic heart failure remains an important predictor of perioperative morbidity for both cardiac and noncardiac surgical patients. Perioperative considerations include a comprehensive history and physical examination, maintenance of preoperative medications, a slow heart rate to optimize diastolic filling and reduce myocardial oxygen supply/demand, and avoiding excessive fluid resuscitation or dehydration. Anesthetic technique (i.e. regional versus general anesthesia) does not appear to influence adverse outcomes. Although several intravenous and volatile anesthetic agents cause varying degrees of diastolic dysfunction, their effects on diastolic function are probably not clinically significant.

Heart failure is an important predictor of perioperative morbidity.

Acute perioperative heart failure may develop in high-risk patients, including those with a history of cardiomyopathy, vascular surgery patients, thoracic surgery patients undergoing pneumonectomy, and orthopedic surgery patients following tourniquet release. The prevalence of preoperative diastolic dysfunction and the incidence of acute intraoperative diastolic dysfunction among cardiac surgical patients are especially significant. Cardiac surgical patients are particularly vulnerable to acute heart failure due to I–R injury, changes in loading conditions, metabolic disturbances, and β-receptor downregulation following CPB. Intraoperative echocardiography can be very valuable in diagnosing diastolic dysfunction, which has been associated with increased inotropic requirements and postoperative morbidity. Classic pharmacological therapy includes inotropic agents with lusitropic properties (i.e. β-adrenoceptor agonists, phosphodiesterase inhibitors). Although acute heart failure usually resolves with pharmacological intervention, occasionally intra-aortic balloon counterpulsation, or the insertion of a ventricular assist device, may be necessary.

PERICARDIAL TAMPONADE

Blood or other fluid in the pericardial space reduces the transmural pressure across the atria, limiting their filling and reducing stroke volume. When less than about 200 mL of fluid accu-

Table 44.2 Short- and long-term responses to heart failure

Response	Short-term effects (mainly adaptive), hemorrhage, acute heart failure	Long-term effects (mainly deleterious), chronic heart failure
Salt and water retention	Augments preload	Pulmonary congestion, anasarca
Vasoconstriction	Maintains blood pressure for perfusion of vital organs (brain, heart)	Exacerbates pump dysfunction (afterload mismatch), increases cardiac energy expenditure
Sympathetic stimulation	Increases heart rate and ejection	Increases energy expenditure
Desensitization	–	Energy sparing
Hypertrophy	Unloads individual muscle fibers	Deterioration and death of cardiac cells: cardiomyopathy of overload
Capillary deficit	–	Energy starvation
Mitochondrial density	Increase; helps meet energy demands	Decrease; energy starvation
Appearance of slow myosin	–	Increases force integral; decreases shortening velocity and contractility; energy sparing
Prolonged action potential	–	Increases contractility and energy expenditure
Reduced density of sarcoplasmic reticulum Ca^{2+} pump sites	–	Slows relaxation; possibly energy sparing
Increased collagen	May reduce dilatation	Impairs relaxation

mulates rapidly in a 70 kg person, central venous pressure (CVP) is usually 10–12 cmH_2O. Activation of the sympathoadrenal system leads to increased heart rate and constriction of capacitance vessels, causing augmentation of filling pressure, which maintains cardiac output. If pericardial fluid volume increases further, CVP increases and arterial blood pressure decreases, leading to shock followed by cardiac arrest. When pericardial fluid accumulates slowly, up to 400 mL may accumulate before symptoms occur. Trauma caused by catheters placed inside the heart and external trauma to the heart (e.g. rib fracture from blunt trauma or cardiopulmonary resuscitation) may cause tamponade. Localized tamponade may develop after cardiac surgery even though the pericardium is usually left open.

Signs and symptoms of tamponade include weakness, pulsus paradoxus (see below), and signs of right heart failure, including dyspnea, orthopnea, hepatomegaly, ascites, peripheral edema, jugular venous distension, and prerenal azotemia. Beck's triad consists of distant heart sounds, hypotension, and elevated CVP, usually up to 15 cmH_2O. Decreased urine output and Na^+ excretion occur as a result of reduced cardiac output, sympathetic activation, and a reduction in atrial natriuretic factor release subsequent to the lower atrial distending pressure. ECG shows low-voltage ST/T-wave changes, and P and QRS alternans. Widening of the cardiac silhouette is observed by chest radiography. Echocardiography is the most commonly used diagnostic technique. Transthoracic imaging is often adequate, though occasionally TEE is required. In the presence of a bloody effusion containing thrombi, identification of ventricular wall interface is difficult. Pericardial fluid may be observed as an echo-free crescent between the RV wall and the pericardium or the posterior LV wall and the pericardium. Two distinct echoes from the posterior wall may be caused by pericardial fluid.

With tamponade, the diastolic pressures in all cardiac chambers and the PCWP equalize with intrapericardial pressure. Reduced cardiac output and elevated CVP may result from tamponade or biventricular failure. If a large respiratory variation in blood pressure is also observed, tamponade is likely. The x descent during systole in the atrial pressure waveform is accentuated, whereas the y descent caused by opening of atrioventricular valves is depressed.

Pulsus paradoxus is a decrease of more than 10 mmHg in systolic blood pressure during quiet inspiration, accompanied by a greater than normal decrease in pulse pressure and heart rate. There is greater than normal blood flow into the right atrium during inspiration, which increases intrapericardial pressure. As the ventricular septum is displaced leftward, LV volume and blood pressure are reduced. The flow of blood from the right to the left heart is slowed and may occur during expiration.

The reduction of intrathoracic pressure during inspiration reduces blood pressure, and inspiration directly decreases LV contraction.

Volume loading and inotropic agents (e.g. isoproterenol or dobutamine) are used to maintain cardiac output. Pericardiocentesis is both diagnostic and therapeutic; it is falsely negative in about 20% of patients because of pericardial blood clots. If pericardiocentesis is not therapeutic, surgical drainage is performed. Cardiac performance often improves following pericardiotomy, though this is less likely in patients with constrictive pericarditis.

PULMONARY EMBOLISM

Pulmonary embolism (PE) is a common cause of perioperative heart failure and respiratory failure. Thrombi embolize most commonly from proximal deep veins of the lower extremities. Vascular damage, venous stasis, and hypercoagulability promote deep vein thrombosis (DVT). Risk factors for venous thromboembolism include previous venous thromboembolism, immobility, advanced age, malignancy, heart failure, use of oral contraceptives, obesity, and surgical procedures on the lower extremity, pelvis, and abdomen. Untreated proximal DVT is associated with a 50% risk of PE, resulting in death in approximately 1% of patients. Two-thirds of deaths occur during the first hour after PE, and the rest 4–6 hours later. Massive PE is defined as greater than 50% obstruction of pulmonary outflow, which may lead to RV failure and death. Hypoxic pulmonary vasoconstriction occurring with PE further accentuates pulmonary hypertension.

Signs and symptoms of PE are nonspecific. Mild PE may cause dyspnea, tachypnea, tachycardia, hemoptysis, and chest pain. Severe PE may cause dyspnea and circulatory collapse. Arterial blood gases may show hypoxia, high alveolar to arterial oxygen gradient, acidosis, and respiratory alkalosis caused by hyperventilation. Hypercapnia may occur in the presence of a large embolus. Pulmonary artery pressure is elevated, with normal PCWP and reduced cardiac output. Tachycardia, supraventricular arrhythmia (especially atrial fibrillation), incomplete right bundle branch block, and nonspecific ST/T-wave changes may be seen on EGG. Occasionally, a large S wave in lead I and large Q and T waves in lead III (S_1 Q_3 T_3) may be observed. Right precordial leads may reveal downward-sloping ST segment depression indicative of RV strain.

A ventilation/perfusion lung scan with xenon and technetium is the most common diagnostic test. The negative predictive accuracy of this scan is high, but its positive predictive accuracy is lower. After thoracic or cardiac surgery, which alter both ventilation and perfusion, a ventilation/perfusion scan is likely to show intermediate probability of PE. TEE can diagnose a saddle embolus that may be missed by a ventilation/perfusion scan, and can identify sources of emboli in the right heart. Pulmonary angiography is the gold standard for the detection of PE. Impedance plethysmography and duplex ultrasound evaluation of the deep veins may identify the source of emboli.

For prophylaxis, subcutaneous heparin or low-molecular-weight heparin and intermittent compression of the lower extremities may be used perioperatively. Patients should walk and perform lower extremity exercises as early after surgery as possible. Pulmonary vasodilators/inotropes, such as prostaglandin E_1 or isoproterenol, can be used to treat hemodynamic compromise. Ventilation may have to be supported. Fibrinolytic agents such as streptokinase, urokinase, or tissue plasminogen activator can be used to lyze emboli, as well as the underlying source. If anticoagulation is contraindicated, a filter (e.g. Greenfield filter) may be placed transvenously in the inferior vena cava to prevent further embolization. However, collaterals may develop over time and allow further embolization.

Key references

ACC/AHA Guidelines for the evaluation and management of chronic heart failure in the adult: executive summary a report of the American College of Cardiology/American Heart Association task force on practice guidelines (committee to revise the 1995 guidelines for the evaluation and management of heart failure). Circulation 2001;104:2996–3007.

Alpert J, Thygesen K. Myocardial infarction redefined – a consensus document of the joint European Society/American College of Cardiology Committee for the redefinition of myocardial infarction. J Am Coll Cardiol. 2000;36:959–69.

Chen V, Body S, Shernan S. Myocardial preconditioning: characteristics, mechanisms, and clinical applications. Semin Cardiothorac Vasc Anesth. 1999;3:85–97.

Griffin M, Hines R. Management of perioperative ventricular dysfunction. J Cardiothorac Vasc Anesth. 2001;15:90–106.

Hansson GK, Inflammation, Atherosclerosis and Coronary Artery Disease. New Engl J Med. 2005;352:1685–95.

Jessup M, Brozena S. Heart failure. N Engl J Med. 2003; 348:2007–18.

Laffey J, Boylan J, Cheng D. The systemic inflammatory response to cardiac surgery. Anesthesiology 2002; 97:215–52.

Landesberg G. The pathophysiology of perioperative myocardial infarction: facts and perspectives. J Thorac Vasc Anesth. 2003; 1:90–100.

Pagel P, Grossman W, Haering M, Warltier D. Left ventricular diastolic function in the normal and diseased heart. Parts 1 & 2. Anesthesiology 1993;79:836–54; 1104–20.

Shernan S. Perioperative myocardial ischemia–reperfusion injury. Anesthesiol Clin North Am. 2003;2:465–85.

Shernan SK, Collard CD. Role of the complement system in ischemic heart disease: potential for pharmacological intervention. BioDrugs 2001;15: 595–607.

Zaugg M, Schaub MC, Foex P. Myocardial injury and its prevention in the perioperative setting. Br J Anaesth. 2004;93:21–33.

Further reading

Bonnefoy E, Filley S, Kirkorian G, Guidolley J, Roriz R, Touboul P. Troponin I, troponin T, or creatine kinase-MB to detect perioperative myocardial damage after coronary artery bypass surgery. Chest 1998;114:482–6.

Hodakowski G, Craver J, Jones E, King S, Guyton R. Clinical significance of perioperative Q-wave myocardial infarction: the Emory Angioplasty versus Surgery trial. J Thorac Cardiovasc Surg. 1996;112:1447–54.

Lazar H, Bokesch P, van Lenta F et al. OBE and the TP10 Cardiac Surgery Study Group. Soluble human complement receptor 1 limits ischemic damage in cardiac surgery patients at high risk requiring cardiopulmonary bypass. Circulation 2004;110(Suppl II):II-274–9.

Mangano D. Effects of acadesine on myocardial infarction, stroke, and death following surgery: a meta analysis of the 5 international randomized trials. JAMA 1997;277:325–32.

Neumann F, Griesmacher A, Mohl W et al. Biochemical markers of perioperative myocardial ischemia in patients with coronary artery bypass grafting. Adv Clin Pathol. 1998;2:75–83.

Palda VA, Detsky AS. Perioperative assessment and management of risk from coronary artery disease. Ann Intern Med. 1997;127:313–28.

Theroux P, Chaitman B, Danchin N et al. Inhibition of the sodium–hydrogen exchanger with cariporide to prevent myocardial infarction in high-risk ischemic situations: main results of the GUARDIAN trial. Circulation 2000;102:3032–8.

Verrier E, Shernan S, Taylor K et al. for the PRIMO-CABG. Terminal complement blockade with pexelizumab during coronary artery graft surgery requiring cardiopulmonary bypass: PRIMO-CABG Randomized Trial. JAMA 2004; 291:2319–27.

Chapter 45

Valvular heart disease

Nikolaos Skubas and Stephen Thomas

TOPICS COVERED IN THIS CHAPTER

AORTIC INSUFFICIENCY

The normal aortic valve has three cusps (left, right, and noncoronary, named after their association with the respective coronary artery) and three sinuses of Valsalva (outpouching of the ascending aorta immediately above the corresponding cusp). Congenital anomalies (most commonly bicuspid aortic valve), infective endocarditis, collagen vascular disease, and rheumatic fever cause pathological changes in the aortic valve cusps. Marfan's syndrome, ankylosing spondylitis, and dilatation due to age change the proximal aortic root. Aortic insufficiency (AI) is caused by abnormalities of the aortic valve cusps or the aortic root. The association between hypertension and AI is debated. Acute AI may be caused by aortic valve cusp destruction from endocarditis, or by lack of support in aortic dissection.

Pathophysiology and clinical insights

The competent aortic valve shields the left ventricle from systemic blood pressure during diastole. In AI, the diastolic transvalvular pressure gradient (aortic pressure minus left ventricular diastolic pressure) drives blood into the left ventricle via the regurgitant orifice. The regurgitant volume is proportional to the pressure gradient, the size of the regurgitant orifice, and the duration of diastole. The regurgitant volume plus the normal, diastolic transmitral flow is ejected during systole. This enormous stroke volume creates wide pulse pressure and systolic hypertension. Chronic AI imposes a large volume overload on the left ventricle. Over time, cardiac myocytes respond by elongating and thickening in a way that effectively increases the size of the left ventricle with little or no increase in wall stress (eccentric hypertrophy: both size and thickness of the left ventricle are increased). The compliance of the left ventricle is increased in slowly progressive chronic AI, so that despite the large regurgitant volume the cardiac output and filling pressures remain normal. During this 'compensated' AI, the left ventricular contractility is preserved. A reduced ejection fraction reflects increased afterload rather than myocardial damage. When these adaptive mechanisms fail, myocardial dysfunction and left ventricular failure occur. This transition is often insidious, and frequently the patient remains asymptomatic until severe left ventricular dysfunction has developed (ejection fraction <0.5, LV end-systolic diameter >6 cm) because afterload remains low. In AI, myocardial oxygen demand is increased because of eccentric hypertrophy, whereas the oxygen supply is reduced secondary to the decreased diastolic perfusion gradient (diastolic aortic pressure minus left ventricular end-diastolic pressure). Sometimes patients may develop signs and symptoms of ischemia in the absence of coronary artery disease.

In acute AI there is no time for left ventricular enlargement to occur. Instead, the sudden regurgitant volume returns to a left ventricle of normal size and compliance. The sudden increase in diastolic volume raises the left ventricular end-diastolic and left atrial pressures rapidly and dramatically, whereas the forward stroke volume is decreased. Cardiac output may be maintained because of compensatory tachycardia, but stroke volume will continue to fall. Severe AI impairs cardiac output and reduces coronary blood flow and organ perfusion, leading to further myocardial deterioration. The effect of AI on the left ventricular pressure–volume relationship is shown in Figure 45.1.

Clinical diagnosis

The clinical presentation of chronic AI is characteristic of left heart failure: dyspnea on exertion, orthopnea, fatigue, and occasionally paroxysmal nocturnal dyspnea. Syncope and angina reflect decreased systemic perfusion. A prominent downward- and left-displaced apical pulse, a diastolic murmur at the left lower sternal border, and a pronounced carotid upstroke with rapid runoff (Corrigan's pulse) are created by the widened pulse pressure of AI. In acute AI many of the previous signs are modified or absent, and the patient frequently presents with pulmonary edema and/or cardiogenic shock.

Laboratory findings

In chronic AI the electrocardiogram (ECG) may manifest signs of left ventricular hypertrophy and conduction disorders, and the chest radiograph may reveal an increased heart size. Echocardiography will confirm the diagnosis and etiology, and grade the severity of AI, and diagnose the presence (and estimate the severity) of coexisting pulmonary hypertension (see Chapter 14 for basic information on echocardiography). Color-flow Doppler echocardiography images the AI regurgitant jet as it expands inside the left ventricular outflow tract (LVOT), with the ratio of the jet diameter over the LVOT width being used to grade the severity of AI (<30% mild, >60% severe) (Fig. 45.2). With increasing AI, the pulsed-wave Doppler duration and velocity of the normally observed diastolic flow reversal in the descending thoracic (or thoracoabdominal) aorta are increased (Fig. 45.3). The gradual equilibration between the aortic diastolic blood pressure and the LV diastolic pressures is reflected by the rate of the deceleration of the AI jet: the derived AI pressure half-time (PHT) is shorter when the AI is severe and the aorta 'empties' faster into the left ventricle (Fig. 45.4).

Anesthetic considerations

Anesthetic management in AI is aimed at preserving or augmenting the left ventricular forward flow by (a) maintaining adequate preload and contractility, (b) reducing afterload, and (c) minimizing the use of anesthetic agents with negative inotropic and/or chronotropic actions (however, they are indicated in the setting of acute AI secondary to aortic dissection) which counteract the compensatory mechanisms of AI. Patients with AI are at increased risk of myocardial ischemia because of decreased coronary artery perfusion pressure, so arterial blood pressure should be closely monitored. The hemodynamic management of AI is summarized in Table 45.1.

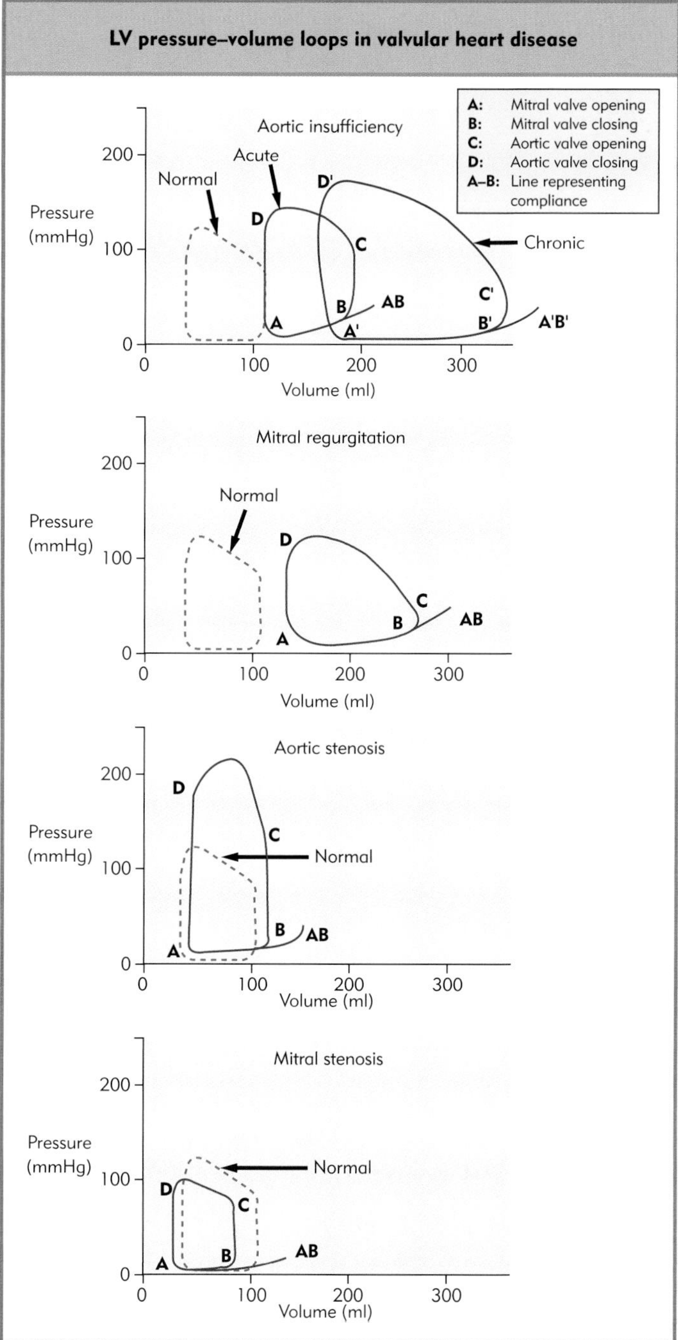

Figure 45.1 Left ventricular pressure–volume loops in valvular heart disease. Points A, B, C, and D correspond respectively to opening and closing of the mitral and aortic valves. Line AB represents the diastolic pressure–volume relationship corresponding to compliance. In aortic insufficiency there is a shift in the loop to the right that results in a low aortic diastolic pressure and early ejection of a large stroke volume. There is no period of isovolumic relaxation. In mitral regurgitation there is no period of isovolumic contraction as blood is ejected directly into the left atrium with the onset of systole; the ejection volume is normal. In aortic stenosis there is chronic pressure overload resulting from the reduced orifice, end-systole pressure is elevated, and there is reduced left ventricular compliance. Stroke volume is preserved. In mitral stenosis left ventricular filling and stroke volume are reduced.

AORTIC STENOSIS

Etiologies of aortic stenosis (AS) include 1) bicuspid aortic valve, a congenital lesion in which mechanical shear stress leads to injury and stenosis of the aortic valve orifice; 2) degeneration of

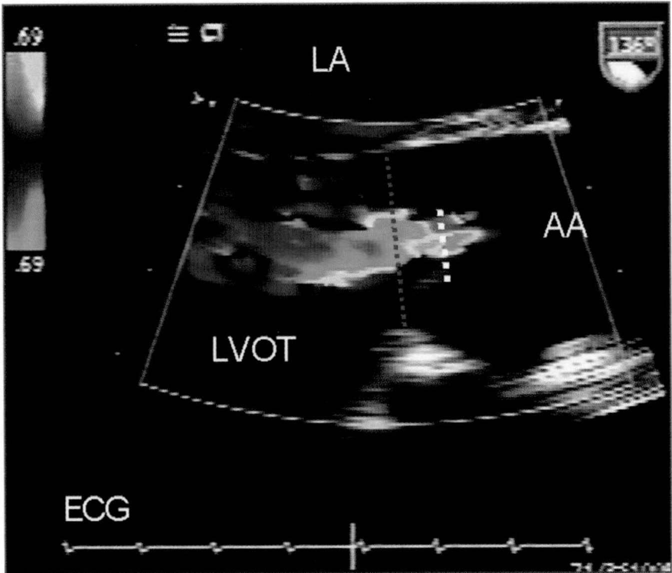

Figure 45.2 Aortic insufficiency: evaluation by transesophageal echocardiography. The ascending aorta (AA), the aortic valve, and the left ventricular outflow tract (LVOT) are visualized in the midesophageal long-axis view. Using color-flow Doppler, the AI regurgitant jet is visualized as it enters the LVOT during diastole (white marker on the ECG). The width of the AI jet (white dotted line) and the diameter of the LVOT (red dotted line) are measured. The AI jet/LVOT ratio correlates with the severity of AI: mild if <30%, severe if >60%. LA, left atrium.

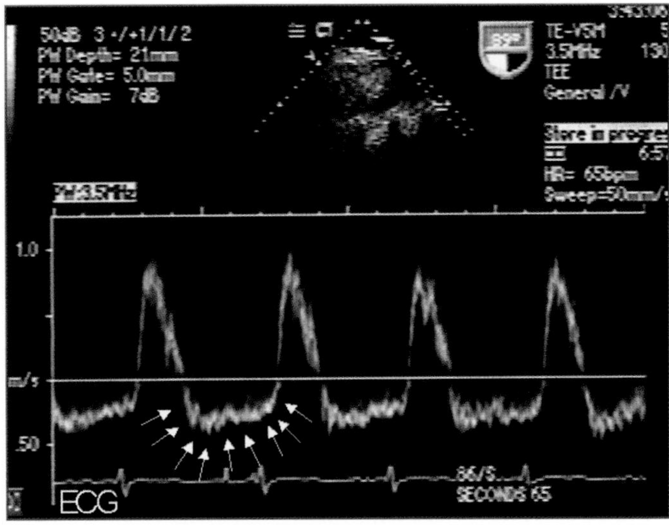

Figure 45.3 Aortic insufficiency: descending thoracic aorta flow. The distal descending thoracic aorta is visualized in the long-axis view, and the pulsed-wave Doppler cursor is placed either distally or proximally. In this pulsed-wave Doppler examination there is a positive (above the baseline) deflection occurring in systole, which represents the normal, forward aortic flow. The negative deflection (below the zero baseline, arrows) lasts for the entire diastole, is abnormal, and is caused by reversal of diastolic flow during severe AI.

the normal tricuspid aortic valve owing to autoimmune phenomena; 3) cardiovascular risk factors (hypercholesterolemia, male sex, smoking) that initiate a 'response to injury' similar to that of atherosclerosis; and 4) conditions associated with chronically elevated stroke volume and altered calcium metabolism (Paget's disease, hyperparathyroidism, renal failure associated with arteriovenous fistula). Rheumatic heart disease causes mixed AS and regurgitation, and coexists with mitral valve disease.

Pathophysiology and clinical insights

The normal aortic valve (AoV) area is 3–4 cm^2 at end-systole. Hemodynamic disturbances become apparent when the AoV area is less than 1.2 cm^2. Patients with critical AS (area <0.7 cm^2) are symptomatic because the left ventricle can no longer overcome the AoV obstruction. The presence of angina, syncope, or congestive heart failure is associated with death within 5, 3, and 2 years, respectively.

The stenosed AoV impedes left ventricular ejection and produces a systolic pressure gradient (usually >50 mmHg)

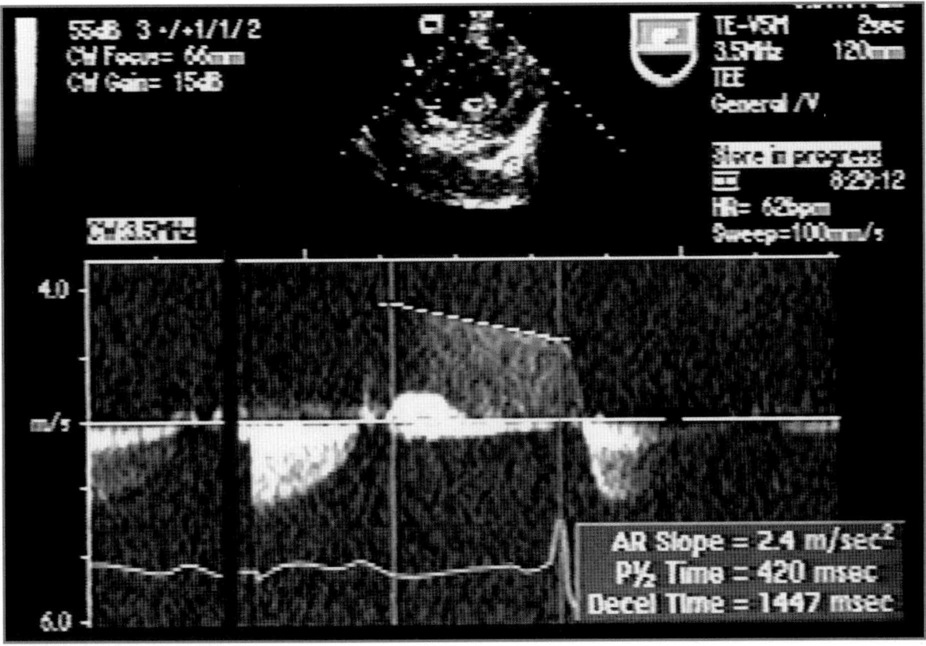

Figure 45.4 Aortic insufficiency: pressure half-time. The deep transgastric view of the left ventricular outflow tract (LVOT) is obtained with transesophageal echocardiography, and the continuous-wave Doppler sample volume is placed in the LVOT, just proximal to the aortic valve. The larger the aortic valve regurgitant orifice, the more rapidly the pressure gradient between aorta and left ventricle dissipates. Rapid dissipation leads to a sharp decline in the aortic insufficiency jet velocity across the aortic valve. By calculating the time that it takes for the peak pressure to decay by half (pressure half-time, $P_{(1/2)}$), an estimation of the severity is obtained. A Doppler half-time shorter than 400 ms indicates that moderate to severe aortic insufficiency is present.

Table 45.1 Management of valvular heart disease: hemodynamic goals

	AI	AS	MR	MS
Heart rate	↔ or ↑	↔ or ↓	↔ or ↑	↓ or ↔
Heart rhythm		Cardiovert if other than sinus		If AF: maintain slow ventricular rate
Preload	↔ or ↑	↔ or ↑	↔ or ↑	↔ or ↑
Afterload	↓	↔ to ensure perfusion pressure	↓	↔ (↑ will adversely affect pulmonary circulation)
Contractility	↓ may need augmentation in late stages	Usually adequate	↓ may need augmentation	Left ventricle may not handle increased preload
Myocardial O_2 balance	At risk because of low diastolic pressure	At risk if hypotension or tachycardia	± coronary artery disease	Usually not a problem

AI, aortic insufficiency; AS, aortic stenosis; MR, mitral regugitation; MS, mitral stenosis
↔ (normal), ↑ (elevated), ↓ (decreased), AF (atrial fibrillation).

across the AoV. Blood flow becomes turbulent, giving rise to the classic systolic ejection murmur of AS. However, the absence of murmur does not exclude the diagnosis of AS. According to the Gorlin equation (Equation 45.1), a patient with reduced left ventricular function and low cardiac output may have critical AS without a significant pressure gradient across the stenosed AoV. The chronically increased pressure work of the left ventricle leads to symmetric hypertrophy of the myocardial fibers, but the radius of the left ventricle remains unchanged (concentric hypertrophy or hypertrophic remodeling). This compensatory mechanism normalizes wall tension and maintains ejection fraction according to the law of LaPlace (Equation 45.2):

- Equation 45.1
  AoV area ~ cardiac output ÷ $\sqrt{\text{mean pressure gradient}}$
- Equation 45.2
  Tension [σ] = pressure × chamber radius ÷ [2 × wall thickness]

The left ventricle generates increased systolic pressure at a lower average wall stress than would occur in the absence of hypertrophy. However, because the cross-sectional area of the coronary vasculature does not increase to the same extent as muscle mass, the thickened myocardium has a reduced coronary blood flow reserve. This can lead to ischemia in the absence of anatomic obstruction of the coronary arteries. Angina develops because of inadequate coronary blood flow reserve and/or increased myocardial oxygen demand caused by high afterload. Left ventricular stiffness rises as collagen in the cardiac interstitium increases. Reduced compliance shifts the diastolic pressure–volume relation of the hypertrophied left ventricle upward, which leads to higher diastolic pressure and increases the potential for the development of pulmonary congestion. The clinical implication is that a 'normal' filling pressure may be associated with less than optimal left ventricular filling. The thickened myocardium of AS causes impaired relaxation of the 'stiff' left ventricle in early diastole, and the left atrial contribution to left ventricular preload increases. Patients with critical AS decompensate when they become tachycardic (the diastolic time is decreased) or with a rhythm other than sinus (i.e. junctional, rapid atrial fibrillation). The increased left ventricular systolic pressure may lead to functional mitral regurgitation. Conditions associated with decreased contractility or increased afterload can precipitate congestive heart failure and pulmonary edema. An exercise-induced decrease in total peripheral resistance can cause syncope, because stroke volume is fixed and cannot compensate for the reduced blood pressure. The effect of AS on the left ventricular pressure–volume relationship is shown in Figure 45.1.

Myocardial ischemia without coronary artery disease can occur with concentric myocardial hypertrophy in aortic stenosis and eccentric hypertrophy in aortic insufficiency.

Clinical diagnosis

The most common sign of AS is a systolic ejection murmur radiating to the neck, best heard over the aortic area. In mild AS the murmur appears early in systole, is associated with a thrill, and the carotid upstrokes are well preserved. As the disease progresses, the peak of the murmur occurs later in systole and is softer, whereas the carotid upstrokes are diminished and delayed in time (pulsus parvus et tardus). The second heart sound may become single as the aortic valve component is lost, or paradoxically split because of delay in left ventricular emptying.

Laboratory findings

The ECG often shows left ventricular hypertrophy with repolarization abnormalities. The echocardiographic examination is valuable for confirming the presence and severity of AS (thick, calcified, and echogenic cusps with reduced motility), determining left ventricular size and function, and ruling out other associated valve disease (Fig. 45.5). Cardiac catheterization is indicated before aortic valve replacement in patients at risk for coronary artery disease, and for AS assessment in symptomatic

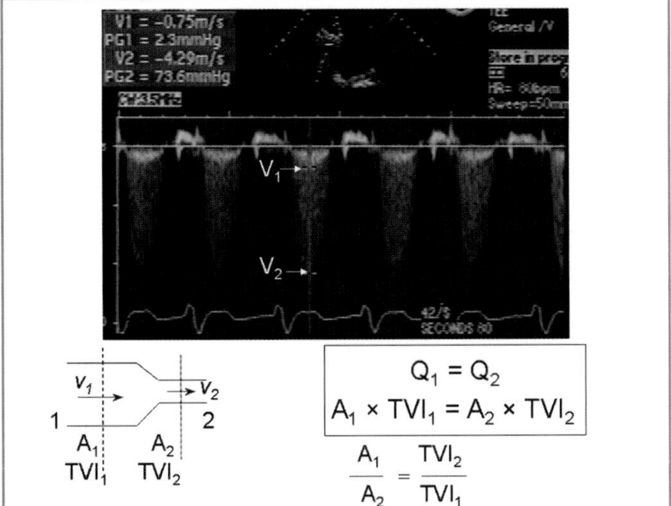

Figure 45.5 Aortic stenosis: calculation of the aortic valve area using the continuity equation. The continuity equation is used to calculate the orifice of a stenotic valve, using the concept of conservation of flow. The flow rate (or volume) across an orifice is the product of the orifice area and velocity (or time–velocity integral, TVI). The flow Q_1 across an orifice with surface A_1 has a velocity v_1 (or TVI_1) and is equal to flow Q_2 across an orifice with surface A_2, and velocity v_2 (or TVI_2). By rearranging the continuity equation, $A_2 = (A_1 \times TVI_1)/TVI_2$. If A_1 is the orifice of the left ventricular outflow tract (LVOT) and A_2 is the orifice of the aortic valve, $AVA = (LVOT \times TVI_{LVOT})/TVI_{AV}$. Because the flow duration across the LVOT and the aortic valve is the same, TVI can be replaced by velocity: $AVA = LVOT \times (V_{LVOT}/V_{AV})$. The AVA is inversely related to the TVI or peak velocity ratio of the LVOT and the aortic valve. In the transesophageal echocardiographic image, the left ventricle is imaged in the deep transgastric view, and the cursor line is placed through the calcified aortic valve. The continuous-wave Doppler mode demonstrates two velocities, with the faster (4.29 m/s) arising from the aortic valve, enveloping the slower (0.75 m/s) arising from the LVOT. The LVOT diameter was measured as 2.12 cm. The calculated AVA is 0.6 cm^2.

In patients with normal left ventricular systolic function and cardiac output, AS is usually severe when peak aortic velocity is ≥4.5 m/s, mean pressure gradient is ≥50 mmHg, AVA is ≤0.75 cm^2, and LVOT/AV TVI ratio is ≤0.25. (Reference: Maslow AD, Mashikian J, Haering M et al. Transesophageal echocardiographic evaluation of native aortic valve area: Utility of the double-envelope technique. J Cardioth Vasc Anesth. 2001;15:293–9.)

patients when the severity of AS cannot be determined by noninvasive techniques. Often, decreased cardiac output (secondary to increased wall stress/afterload) results in a modest pressure gradient (<30 mmHg) in spite of the presence of severe AS. Pharmacologic stress with dobutamine resolves the problem: if the stroke volume increases simultaneously with the transaortic pressure gradient, the AS is real, whereas if the stroke volume increase is greater than the transaortic pressure gradient increase (i.e. the AoV area becomes larger with higher cardiac output), the patient has 'relative' AS.

Anesthetic considerations

The anesthetic management of a patient with AS consists of maintaining sufficient myocardial O_2 supply by a) promptly treating any dysrhythmia and preserving normal sinus rhythm; b) ensuring that left ventricular preload is adequate, while bearing in mind that the pulmonary capillary wedge pressure underestimates the true left ventricular end-diastolic volume; c) preserving normotension, because coronary artery perfusion pressure depends on the gradient between diastolic arterial (aortic) pressure and LV end-diastolic pressure; and d) minimizing the use of anesthetic agents with myocardial depressant effects. The hemodynamic management of AS is summarized in Table 45.1.

MITRAL REGURGITATION

The normal mitral valve apparatus consists of an annulus that supports the two leaflets (anterior and posterior), and a subvalvular structure composed of the two papillary muscles (an anterolateral, supplied by the circumflex or the left coronary artery and a posteromedial, supplied by the right coronary artery), and their chordae tendinae attaching to the ventricular side of the leaflets. During systole, the mitral valve closes as the left ventricular-generated pressure exceeds the left atrial pressure, and the papillary muscles contract, preventing the leaflets from moving past their coaptation point. Contraction of the mitral annulus further promotes mitral valve competence and seals the left atrium from the left ventricle. During diastole, the mitral valve leaflets open and form a funnel extending from the mitral annulus to the papillary muscles.

Mitral regurgitation (MR) is primary when there is an abnormality of the mitral valve structure that leads to incompetence, and secondary when the leakage results from left ventricular disease that distorts the anatomy of the mitral valve. The causes of MR are mitral valve prolapse (the mitral valve leaflets are displaced into the left atrium during systole), ischemia (either global, which leads to left ventricular and mitral annulus dilation, or regional, when an ischemic papillary muscle does not contract), rheumatic heart disease (thickened and calcified leaflets and subvalvular apparatus with restricted motion, usually with coexisting mitral stenosis), and endocarditis (destruction of valvular tissue). In the elderly, MR may be due to annular calcification (preventing systolic contraction and closure).

Pathophysiology and clinical insights

In MR, flow during systole is both antegrade through the aortic valve (normal) and retrograde into the left atrium. The volume of regurgitant flow depends on the systolic transmitral valve pressure gradient (left ventricular systolic pressure minus left atrial pressure), the size of the regurgitant mitral valve orifice, and the duration of ejection.

In chronic MR, compensatory mechanisms maintain forward stroke volume and protect the pulmonary circulation. Chronic left ventricular volume overload induces compensatory dilatation of the left ventricle, maintaining forward cardiac output, so that left ventricular contractile function may be depressed without the development of clinical symptoms. The left atrium dilates and compliance increases (it can accommodate a larger volume without an increase in the left atrial and pulmonary capillary pressure). However, the gradual enlargement of the left ventricle causes the wall tension to increase. Progression to the decompensated symptomatic state varies from patient to patient, and may last from weeks and months to years. The forward failure is accompanied by pulmonary congestion. When left heart failure occurs, the risk of sudden death is increased. The reduced left ventricular contractility in MR is associated with loss of contractile elements and deficient production of cyclic adenosine monophosphate.

Acute MR, usually the result of rupture of a major chorda tendinae, is poorly tolerated because there is no time for compensation and the left ventricular size is unchanged. Therefore, forward stroke volume acutely decreases and the regurgitant volume enters a left atrium with normal compliance. The left atrial pressure increases rapidly, leading to pulmonary congestion and acute pulmonary hypertension. The effect of MR on the left ventricular pressure–volume relationship is shown in Figure 45.1.

Clinical diagnosis

In chronic MR, symptoms first appear when decompensation occurs. Symptoms may be precipitated by a superimposed hemodynamic stress, such as pregnancy, anemia, or infection. A holosystolic murmur is prominent and radiates to the axilla, and the cardiac impulse is displaced downward and to the left by ventricular dilation. The pulmonic component of the S_2 may be increased if pulmonary hypertension exists. The large left ventricular volume gives rise to an S_3. Palpitations because of atrial fibrillation and symptoms of congestive heart failure may accompany primary MR. Acute MR presents with dyspnea and orthopnea. The typical holosystolic murmur is rather soft, and an S_3 gallop is present.

Chronic left ventricular volume overload is compensated by ventricular dilation to maintain forward cardiac output until the increase in wall tension leads to failure.

Laboratory findings

Electrocardiographic and chest radiographic signs of enlargement of the left atrium or left ventricle are seen late in the course, and are not specific or sensitive for the diagnosis of MR. A careful two-dimensional echocardiographic examination should be able to define the mechanism of MR and yield clues to its severity (size of left atrium and left ventricle, leaflet(s) abnormality(ies), systolic function of left ventricle). Qualitative parameters used for grading the severity of MR include visual examination of the MR jet and evaluation of its size in relation to the size of the left atrium, and recognition of specific patterns of the transmitral and pulmonary vein flows. Quantitative parameters include the proximal isovelocity surface area, the vena contracta, and calculation of the regurgitation volume and fraction (Fig. 45.6).

Anesthetic considerations

When treating a patient with MR the acuity or chronicity of MR, the degree of left ventricular dysfunction, the presence or absence of atrial fibrillation, and associated coronary atherosclerotic disease must be considered. Augmenting forward stroke volume, diminishing the regurgitant volume (thus relieving congestive heart failure) by providing vasodilatation, and increasing heart rate (reducing the time for regurgitation by decreasing systolic ejection time) help maintain adequate mean arterial blood pressure. An arterial vasodilator with parasympatholytic effects, such as sodium nitroprusside, is appropriate provided the blood pressure is kept within acceptable limits. Otherwise,

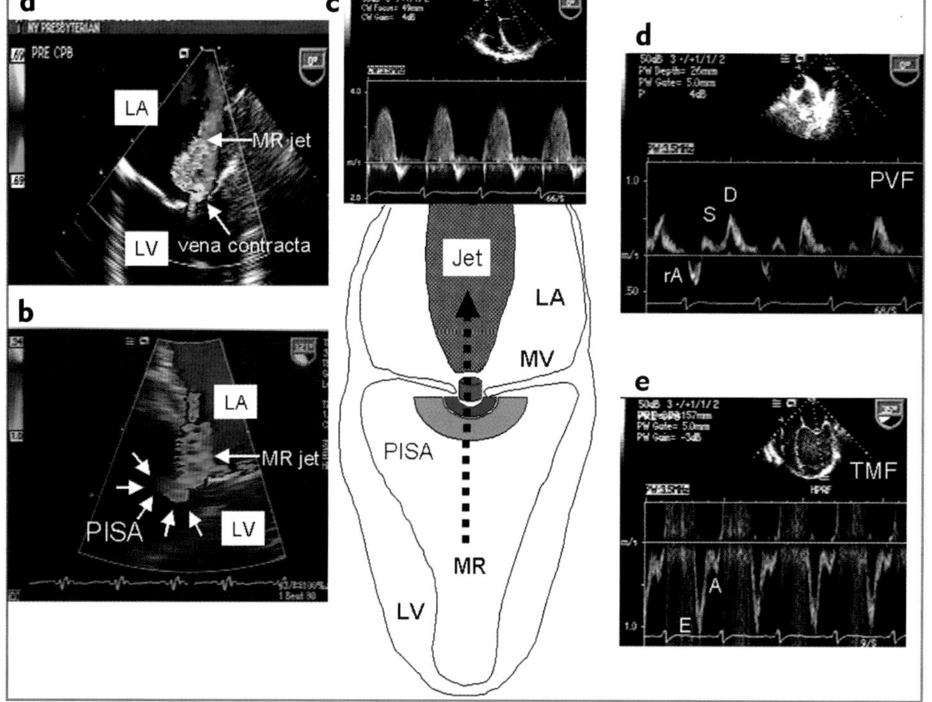

Figure 45.6 Echocardiographic evaluation of the severity of MR. (a) The visual examination of the MR jet is the most widely used method, but also the least accurate. The 'sizing' of the MR jet in relation to the area of the left atrium is rather cumbersome and time-consuming. The vena contracta is the width of the MR jet as it leaves the regurgitant orifice. A large central jet >10 cm^2 or >40% of LA area is consistent with severe (4+) MR. A vena contracta width >0.7 cm is found in severe MR. (b) The proximal isovelocity surface area (PISA) method is based on the principle of conservation of momentum: flow equals velocity × area. As flow approaches an orifice, it forms concentric isovelocity shells of decreasing surface area and increasing velocity. Doppler color flow mapping can depict such shells based on a selected velocity, or provide a range of isovelocity contours as a digital map. The flow through any such hemispheric shell (arrows) equals its surface area times the velocity that defines the shell ($2\pi r^2 \times$ [velocity]). The mitral valve regurgitant orifice is equal to PISA flow ÷ MR jet peak velocity. A regurgitant orifice >0.4 cm^2 is found in severe MR.(c) The maximal velocity and intensity of the MR jet are depicted with continuous-wave Doppler. An early-peaking triangular MR jet characterizes severe MR. (d, e) The hemodynamic effects of MR on LV filling are shown using pulsed-wave Doppler recording of the transmitral blood flow (TMF) and pulmonary venous flow (PVF). The increased filling gradient between the left atrium and the left ventricle at early diastole gives rise to accelerated blood flow (E), whereas the atrial contraction fails to generate adequate velocity (A), as it contracts against a full left ventricle, propagating retrograde into the pulmonary veins (rA). The left atrium fills from the left ventricle because of MR, and the systolic flow from the pulmonary veins towards the left ventricle is diminished during systole (S), whereas it remains intact during diastole, as the left atrium empties into the left ventricle (D). A blunted S (S<D) or a negative S wave correlates with severe MR. A high velocity (>1.2 m/s) E wave and an S/D ratio <1 correlate with moderate to severe MR (3+).

the addition of an inotropic agent such as dobutamine, or mechanical unloading of the LV with counterpulsation, may be employed. If arrhythmia is present, the ventricular rate should be controlled. The hemodynamic management of MR is summarized in Table 45.1.

MITRAL STENOSIS

Mitral stenosis (MS) is almost always a sequela of acute rheumatic fever, and rarely a consequence of inflammation or infiltrative processes. It affects women more frequently than men. There is usually an interval of 5–15 years before symptoms and signs of MS appear. The mitral valve leaflets are fibrosed, calcified, and fused, with limited motility.

Pathophysiology and clinical insights

MS produces pressure and volume overload proximal to and volume underload distal to the stenosed mitral valve. According to the Gorlin equation (Equation 45.1), the pressure gradient between left atrium and left ventricle during diastole is equivalent to (cardiac output ÷ diastolic time)^2 ÷ mitral valve area^2. Therefore, the fixed orifice of the stenosed mitral valve produces a pressure gradient, which is exponentially increased when the diastolic time is shortened, or when metabolic demands increase cardiac output (exercise, pregnancy, tachycardia). When the mitral valve area is less than 1.5 cm^2 or the pressure gradient across the mitral valve is >5 mmHg the thin-walled left atrium cannot overcome the increased flow resistance during diastole. It dilates, may undergo fibrotic changes, and loses its contractility. The pulmonary arterioles may react to the pressure overload with hypertrophy of their smooth muscle fibers, and pulmonary vascular resistance and pulmonary arterial pressure will increase. This leads to compensatory right ventricular hypertrophy and tricuspid regurgitation. The congested pulmonary vessels reduce lung compliance, increasing the work of breathing and leading to dyspnea. In addition, the normal distribution of blood from apex to base of the lungs is reversed, increasing the extent of ventilation/perfusion mismatch. Progressive dilatation of the left atrium often causes atrial fibrillation. This rhythm is particularly deleterious to patients with MS, as 1) the diastolic filling time is decreased when the ventricular rate is not controlled, leading to an increase in the transmitral gradient; 2) the left ventricle loses the volume attributed to the left atrial contraction (atrial kick); and 3) the sluggish blood flow inside the left atrium creates the environment for thrombus formation and systemic embolization. Atrial fibrillation develops in 30–40% of symptomatic patients and is associated with a 25% 10-year survival rate. Distal to the stenosed mitral valve the muscular left ventricle will be underfilled, which may lead to depressed contractile function. Left ventricular ejection fraction can be further decreased by a reflexive increase in systemic afterload. The effect of MS on the left ventricular pressure–volume relationship is shown in Figure 45.1.

Mitral stenosis produces pressure and volume overload proximal to the fixed valvular obstruction, which leads to pulmonary hypertension, reduced lung compliance, and ventilation/perfusion mismatch.

Clinical diagnosis

MS is diagnosed clinically by combining information from the history (exertional dyspnea, decreased exercise capacity, orthopnea, and paroxysmal nocturnal dyspnea) and physical examination (congested lungs, pronounced P_2 because of pulmonary hypertension, engorged jugular veins, hepatomegaly, peripheral edema). A loud S_1 and a diastolic rumble after a loud opening snap can be heard, provided the patient is not tachycardic. If cardiac output is low, the murmur is absent because the flow across the stenosed mitral valve during diastole is severely reduced.

Laboratory findings

Chest radiography may show enlarged atria and right ventricle, exaggerated pulmonary vasculature markings, and pulmonary edema, and electrocardiographic findings may consist of atial enlargement with biphasic P waves/or atrial fibrillation. Echocardiography provides information regarding the morphology of the stenosed mitral valve and the structural and hemodynamic consequences. Doppler flows may be used to assess the severity of MS (Fig. 45.7).

Anesthetic considerations

The anesthetic management of the MS patient entails the following goals: a) maintenance of adequate diastolic filling time (normal sinus rhythm, or controlled ventricular rate in atrial fibrillation with β-blockers and/or Ca^{2+} channel blockers); b) minimal anesthetic-related tachycardia; c) preservation of adequate preload; d) avoidance of factors that may precipitate pulmonary vasoconstriction and further increase right heart afterload, particularly if pulmonary hypertension exists; and e) maintenance of the contractile state and systemic and coronary artery perfusion pressure. After valvulotomy or mitral valve replacement, the chronically underloaded left ventricle may not handle the excessive increase in preload. Inotropes may be necessary, especially if right ventricular function is compromised. The hemodynamic management of MS is summarized in Table 45.1.

VALVULAR DISEASE IN PREGNANCY

The increased blood volume and cardiac output associated with normal pregnancy can accentuate the murmurs associated with stenotic heart valve lesions (MS, AS), whereas lowered systemic vascular resistance may attenuate murmurs of AI or MR. Labor and delivery are associated with an abrupt increase in cardiac output, and after delivery there is an increase in preload related to autotransfusion of uterine blood into the systemic circulation and to caval decompression. For example, during pregnancy many women will demonstrate MR by echocardiography, which is considered normal in the absence of valve pathology. Atrioventricular valve incompetence may be the result of annular dilation because of ventricular enlargement. Pregnant women with MS should continue antibiotic prophylaxis while being medically managed with diuretics and β-blockers in order to prevent tachycardia and optimize diastolic filling time. Patients with severe MS who are symptomatic before conception or those who develop symptoms of heart failure should undergo

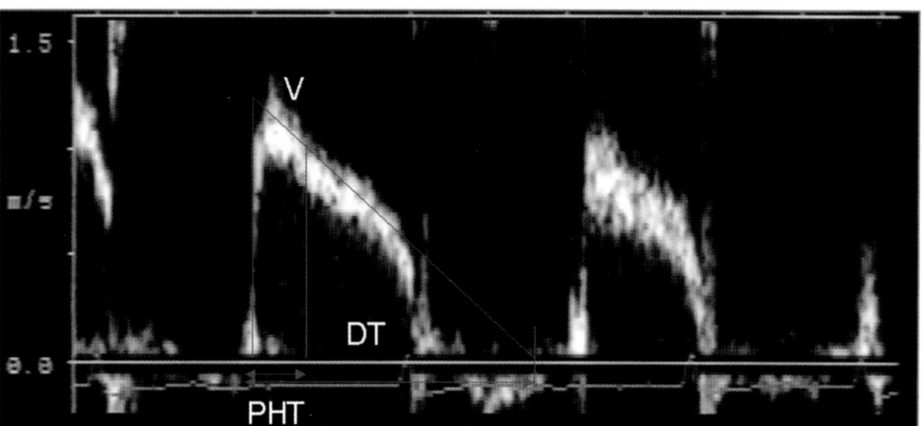

Figure 45.7 Evaluation of the severity of mitral stenosis using the pressure half-time method. Pressure half-time (PHT) is the time interval for the peak pressure gradient (at velocity V) to reach half maximal, and is the same as the interval for the peak velocity (V) to decline to a velocity equal to the peak velocity divided by $\sqrt{2}$ (1.4). PHT is proportionally related to deceleration time (DT), the time interval from peak velocity to baseline. PHT is 0.29 × DT. The mitral valve area (MVA) is calculated from PHT using the empiric formula MVA = 220/PHT. In the figure, V=1.12 m/s, PHT = 196 ms, DT = 676 ms, and MVA = 1.12 cm^2. With atrial fibrillation, as above, one should average the measurements of five to ten beats.

percutaneous balloon mitral valvulotomy or surgical closed mitral commissurotomy. Mitral regurgitation is mostly due to mitral valve prolapse. If the associated MR cannot be managed medically, surgery for mitral valve repair may be necessary. Aortic stenosis in pregnant women is associated with congenital bicuspid valve. It is better to delay pregnancy if the patient is symptomatic or if the transvalvular gradient is >50 mmHg. The association between bicuspid aortic valve and cystic medial necrosis may predispose to spontaneous aortic dissection, usually in the third trimester. Pregnant women with AI should be managed medically, with strict attention to volume status and blood pressure. Surgery is contemplated only if severe symptoms are present. Although patients with Marfan's syndrome and no identifiable cardiovascular abnormalities can safely become pregnant and have a normal vaginal delivery, those with an enlarged ascending aorta (>4 cm) are at high risk for spontaneous aortic dissection and/or rupture of the ascending aorta during the third trimester or at the time of delivery. Care should be taken to minimize pain and blood pressure fluctuation during labor and delivery. General anesthesia and cesarean section may allow more optimal hemodynamic control.

CONGENITAL HEART DISEASE

Bicuspid aortic valve

Bicuspid aortic valve is the most common congenital heart disease (2–3% of live births, predominately males). It is usually discovered in adolescence or adulthood at routine clinical examination, or when symptoms develop. The bicuspid valve has a single fused commissure and an eccentrically oriented orifice. Although not stenotic at birth, thickening, calcification, and immobility result from abnormal hemodynamic stress. Many patients have a coexisting abnormality of the media layer of the aorta above the valve, a predisposition for aortic root dilatation. Bicuspid aortic valves can be stenotic, regurgitant, or both. Left ventricular hypertrophy results from gradually worsening AS. The clinical features of AS are described above. Echocardiographic evaluation will demonstrate the valve anatomy, and the transaortic gradient can be calculated with Doppler interrogation. Those with Doppler gradients ≥70–80 mmHg, those who develop left ventricular repolarization abnormalities or ischemic changes in the ECG at rest or with exercise, and those with symptoms should undergo cardiac catheterization and possible balloon dilation.

Pulmonic stenosis

Pulmonic valve stenosis is an isolated congenital anomaly, or it may occur in association with ventricular septal defect. The commissures of the three pulmonic valve leaflets are fused and the valve is dome-shaped during systole. The patients are usually asymptomatic, and the condition can only be identified by auscultation of a loud systolic murmur. Pulmonic valve stenosis is considered severe when the valve area is less than 0.5 cm^2/m^2, the transvalvular gradient is more than 80 mmHg, or the right ventricular systolic pressure exceeds 100 mmHg. Right ventricular afterload is increased, which leads to right ventricular hypertrophy. Inability to increase cardiac output adequately with exercise manifests as dyspnea and fatigue, or retrosternal chest pain or syncope when the stenosis is severe. Eventually, right ventricular dilatation, tricuspid valve regurgitation, and right atrial dilatation develop. Peripheral edema and abdominal swelling occur when right ventricular failure develops, and the presence of cyanosis and clubbing signifies the presence of a patent foramen ovale, with right to left shunting of blood. The hypertrophic ventricular septum can change shape, from concave towards the left ventricle to flat or concave towards the right ventricle, affecting the filling and function of the left ventricle. A right ventricular impulse may be palpated at the left sternal border, and there may be a thrill at the second intercostal space. The S_2 is widely split, with a soft and delayed P_2. An ejection click precedes the murmur.

Right-sided axis and right ventricular hypertrophy are seen in electrocardiography in moderate or severe pulmonic stenosis. Chest radiography reveals diminished pulmonary vascular markings and an enlarged cardiac size if the patient has right heart failure or tricuspid regurgitation. Echocardiography will reveal the site of stenosis, right ventricular hypertrophy, and paradoxical ventricular septal motion, as well as calculation of the degree of stenosis by Doppler flow studies. Hemodynamic management should address both the right heart (adequate preload, control of heart rate and rhythm, maintenance of contractility) proximal to, and the pulmonary vascular bed (sufficient oxygenation and ventilation) distal to, the stenosis.

Ebstein's anomaly

In Ebstein's anomaly the septal and posterior leaflets of the tricuspid valve are displaced into the right ventricle. A portion of the anatomic right ventricle is atrialized, and the remaining functional right ventricle is small. The tricuspid valve is usually regurgitant, and 80% of patients have an interatrial communication (atrial septal defect or patent foramen ovale) with right-to-left blood shunting. The associated disruption of the right-sided bundle of His leads to right bundle branch block, and the presence of anomalous pathways increases the risk of paroxysmal atrial tachycardia. Right ventricular dysfunction may lead to right-sided congestive heart failure, frequently exacerbated by atrial tachyarrhythmias. Neonates present with severe cyanosis, which transiently improves as pulmonary vascular resistance falls, and worsens as the ductus arteriosus closes. Adolescents and young adults present with incidental findings of a systolic murmur or supraventricular arrhythmia. These arrhythmias may lead to cardiac failure, worsening of cyanosis, or syncope. A systolic murmur arising from tricuspid regurgitation is heard at the left lower sternal border. Hepatomegaly may also be present.

Right bundle branch block and tall and broad P waves are the electrocardiographic findings. A pre-excitation (δ) wave is found in 20% of patients. Chest radiography reveals a large heart, because of right atrial enlargement, and decreased pulmonary vascular markings when there is significant right-to-left shunt. Echocardiographic examination will reveal the anatomy of the lesion and the associated complications. The anesthetic management of Ebstein's anomaly is comparable to that of pulmonic stenosis, with the added consideration of the danger of paradoxic embolization.

Key references

Boon NA, Bloomfield P. The medical management of valvar heart disease. Heart 2002;87:395–400.

Carabello BA. Progress in mitral and aortic regurgitation. Prog Cardiovasc Dis. 2001;43:457–75.

Carabello BA. Aortic stenosis. N Engl J Med. 2002;346:677–82.

Irvine T, Li XK, Kenny A. Assessment of mitral regurgitation. Heart 2002;88(Suppl IV):11–19.

Rajamannan NM, Gersh B, Bonow RO. Calcific aortic stenosis: from the bench to the bedside – emerging clinical and cellular concepts. Heart 2003;89:801–5.

Further reading

Brickner ME, Hillis L, Lange RA. Congenital heart disease in adults. First of two parts. N Engl J Med. 2000;342:256–63.

Brickner ME, Hillis L, Lange RA. Congenital heart disease in adults. Second of two parts. N Engl J Med. 2000;342:334–42.

Reimold SC, Rutherford JD. Valvular heart disease in pregnancy. N Engl J Med. 2003;349:52–9.

Thibault GE. Studying the classics. N Engl J Med. 1995;333:648–52.

Zogbi WA, Enriquez-Sarano M, Foster E et al. Recommendations for evaluation of the severity of native valvular regurgitation with two-dimensional and Doppler echocardiography. J Am Soc Echocardiogr. 2003;16:777–802.

SECTION 5

Respiratory system

Chapter 46

Regulation of respiration

John R Feiner and John Severinghaus

TOPICS COVERED IN THIS CHAPTER

- **Brainstem structures**
- **Ventilatory responses**
  - Hypercapnic ventilatory response
  - Hypoxic ventilatory response
- **Altitude and acclimatization**
- **Sleep and sleep apnea**
- **Abnormalities of chemoreceptor function**

Ventilatory responses are important for maintaining normoxia and normocapnia. Mammalian pulmonary ventilation is driven by two types of chemoreceptor. Medullary receptors respond to changes in the blood partial pressure of carbon dioxide ($P\text{CO}_2$), and slowly to blood pH. Peripheral carotid body chemoreceptors respond primarily to changes in blood partial pressure of oxygen ($P\text{O}_2$), and also to pH and $P\text{CO}_2$. Wakefulness contributes a supratentorial drive to the medullary integrating centers where central and peripheral inputs are combined. During sleep, however, humans are largely dependent on chemoreceptor drive, and the absence of these systems can result in profound hypoventilation. During sedation or general anesthesia, ventilation may also be determined largely by chemoreceptor loops. Ventilatory responses also have significant effects on other aspects of human physiology. Hypoxic drive influences performance at high altitude, and in underwater and competitive swimming. The course of disease processes such as chronic obstructive pulmonary disease (COPD) and respiratory failure is also affected by ventilatory drive. Ventilatory responsiveness may be an important factor determining the way patients respond to anesthetic drugs.

Anesthesiologists are in a unique position to observe the functioning of the ventilatory control system. We alter ventilatory responses with anesthetics and analgesics, and then observe and measure these effects directly with pulse oximetry, end-tidal gas monitoring, or blood gas analysis. Anesthesiologists developed an early interest in these ventilatory control systems, and contributed much research to this area of physiology. This chapter focuses on human ventilatory control by O_2, CO_2 and H^+. The impact of anesthetic and other drugs used in surgery and intensive care on ventilatory control is covered in Chapter 51. Understanding these systems and their alteration by drugs is one of the most important and basic topics in anesthesia.

BRAINSTEM STRUCTURES

The structure and function of brainstem regions involved in the generation of the respiratory rhythm and its modulation have been identified in many animal studies. In vitro slice preparations can maintain a respiratory rhythm, which can be measured in efferent neurons. Pacemaker cells have been identified in the area of the ventrolateral medulla known as the preBötzinger complex (Fig. 46.1). This network of neurons appears responsible for the rhythmic output required for normal breathing. The pacemaker properties of the preBötzinger complex appear to be in the neurons themselves. Other areas of the brainstem may contribute different rhythm generation, including sighing and gasping, but the preBötzinger complex is most consistently associated with normal breathing. Various excitatory inputs and neuronal interconnections may modify and coordinate the behavior of pacemaker neurons. This area of the brainstem is intimately related to processing input from chemoreceptor and other afferent signals, and ultimately providing output to inspiratory, expiratory and airway muscles that results in coordinated breathing.

Many neuromodulators contribute to the function of brainstem neurons involved in respiration. These include substance P, norepinephrine (noradrenaline), acetylcholine, TRH, GABA, glycine, histamine and μ opioids. Pharmacologic agents commonly used in anesthetic practice can affect respiratory centers through a variety of these systems. μ opioid receptors are present on the neurons in the preBötzinger complex themselves, providing an inhibitory effect. Propofol exerts its influence primarily as a $GABA_A$ agonist, causing hyperpolarization in expiratory and preinspiratory neurons. Studies of volatile anesthetics on expiratory and inspiratory neurons have found that neural output is reduced primarily by decreased excitatory glutamatergic input. Volatile anesthetics also depress postsynaptic glutamatergic responses. Overall inhibitory input does not change substantially, although volatile anesthetics appear to enhance postsynaptic $GABA_A$ receptor responses whereas at the same time inhibitor input is blunted. The exact mechanism for decreased excitatory output is still unclear, as is the detailed mechanism of action of volatile anesthetics.

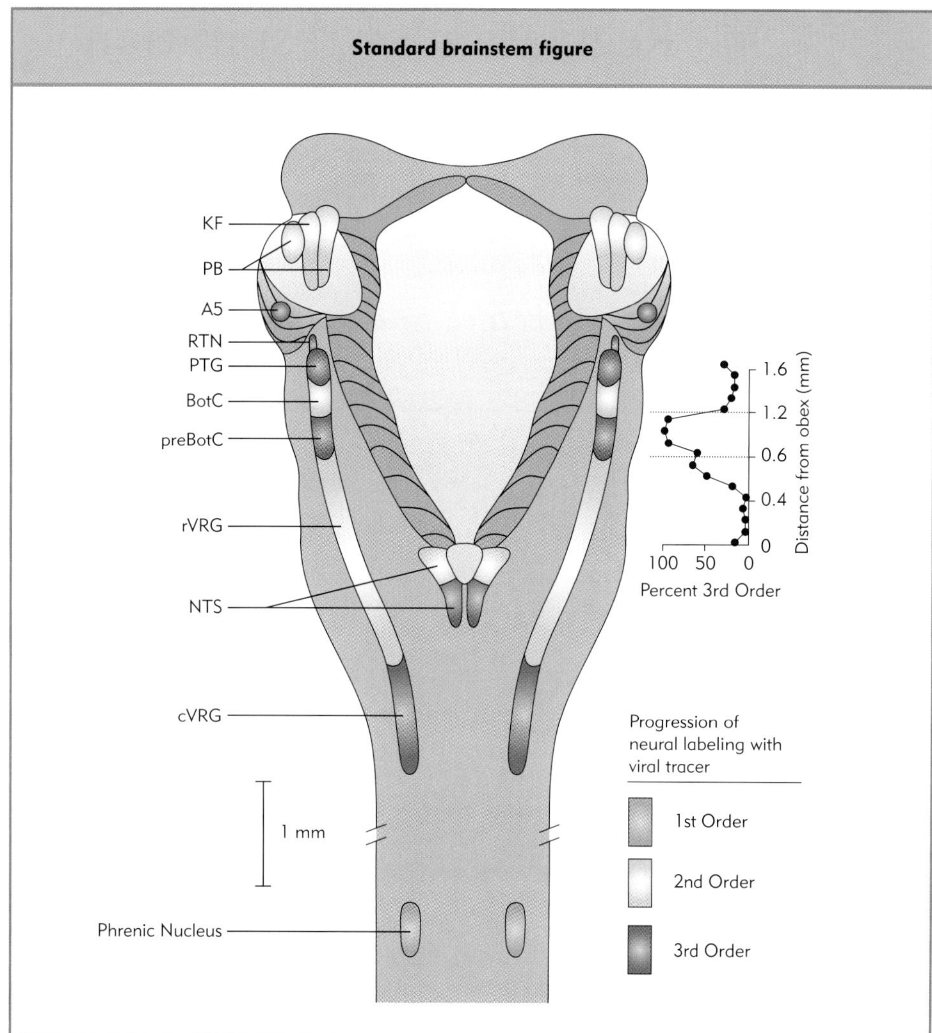

Figure 46.1 This is a dorsal view of the brainstem showing various structures involved in ventilatory control. VRG (r, rostral; c, caudal) is the ventral respiratory group. BötC is the Bötzinger Complex and preBötC is the preBötzinger Complex. Other brainstem nuclei include the nucleus tractus solitarius (NTS), parabrachial nuclei (PB), and the retrotrapezodial nucleus (RTN). The phrenic nerve nuclei are located in the upper cervical spinal cord. CO_2 chemoreceptor regions are on the ventral surface of the brainstem.

Additional investigations focus on multiple areas of the brainstem that may transduce signals from hypoxia and hypercapnia. Although the detailed receptor mechanisms involved in chemoreceptor signal transduction are unknown, the simplified view of central and peripheral chemoreceptors, with a central rhythm generator and signal integration, provides the clinical basis for understanding the basic ventilatory responses.

VENTILATORY RESPONSES

Ventilatory responses arise from many sources, but the most important are the central and peripheral chemoreceptors. Many other receptors provide input to ventilation, such as airways receptors and intrapulmonary receptors. Ventilatory response to CO_2 at high arterial partial oxygen pressure (P_aCO_2) (hypercapnic ventilatory response, HCVR), the hypoxic ventilatory response (HVR), and their synergistic interaction are commonly measured indices of ventilatory control.

Ventilatory responses arise from slower central and faster peripheral chemoreceptors responses.

Other studies emphasize the separation between the faster peripheral chemoreceptors and the slower central response. The reason for the latter distinction is that HCVR has both central and peripheral components, although studies are usually designed to measure the central chemoreceptor response. HVR is designed to measure the peripheral chemoreceptor response; however, it may include a component of central response from a depressant effect of hypoxia.

Hypercapnic ventilatory response

Awake P_aCO_2 is closely regulated to near 40 mmHg (5.3 kPa) by the medullary respiratory center. Exercise increases alveolar ventilation ($\dot{V}_A$, L/min) in proportion to whole-body CO_2 production ($\dot{V}CO_2$, L/min), keeping the fraction of CO_2 in expired alveolar air constant: $F_ECO_2 = \dot{V}CO_2/\dot{V}_A$, or approximately 0.05 [= (200 mL/min)/(4000 mL/ min)]. Under anesthesia, $\dot{V}_A$ is often altered without a change in CO_2 production, resulting in reciprocal changes in P_aCO_2. This relationship can be expressed (omitting factors such as barometric pressure) as:

$$\dot{V}CO_2 \approx \dot{V}_A \times P_aCO_2$$

CENTRAL CHEMORECEPTORS

While breathing air at sea level, about two-thirds of the ventilatory response to CO_2 arises from the stimulation of superficial chemosensitive neurons located near the ventral surface of the medulla, and the rest from the effect of P_aCO_2 (via pH) on the carotid bodies. Even when breathing oxygen, small amounts of peripheral chemoreceptor stimulation can still be detected. The central chemoreceptors respond primarily to the pH of the extracellular fluid (ECF), which varies (within 1–2 minutes) with P_aCO_2. Cerebrospinal fluid (CSF) and ECF bicarbonate concentration (HCO_3^-) are slowly altered (hours to days), either by primary metabolic acidosis/alkalosis or in compensation for abnormal P_aCO_2, as in COPD hypoventilation or hypoxic hyperventilation (e.g. altitude). These ECF HCO_3^- changes differ in both timing and magnitude from the blood changes, and affect ventilatory control in ways that can be understood only when the ECF HCO_3^- is determined.

While breathing air, two-thirds of the ventilatory response to CO_2 derives from central medullary chemoreceptors and one-third from the carotid bodies.

The relationship between P_aCO_2 and minute ventilation ($\dot{V}_A$) depends on the level of P_aCO_2 studied. In the awake state, reduction of P_aCO_2 may not reduce $\dot{V}_A$, and small rises result in little increase in $\dot{V}_A$ because of a 'wakeful drive' arising partly from visual input. This 'flat' portion is referred to as the 'dog leg' of the CO_2 response curve (Fig. 46.2). As P_aCO_2 increases (about 2–3 mmHg above normal), the relationship between P_aCO_2 and $\dot{V}_A$ becomes linear, defining HCVR as the slope ($\dot{V}_A/P_aCO_2$). At extremely high CO_2 levels ($P_aCO_2 \geq 80$ mmHg), the response flattens as maximum $\dot{V}_A$ is approached. In addition, in extreme hypercapnia CO_2 'narcosis' may alter ventilatory responsiveness. Normal HCVR varies widely, from 1 to 4 L/min/mmHg, even when normalized for body size.

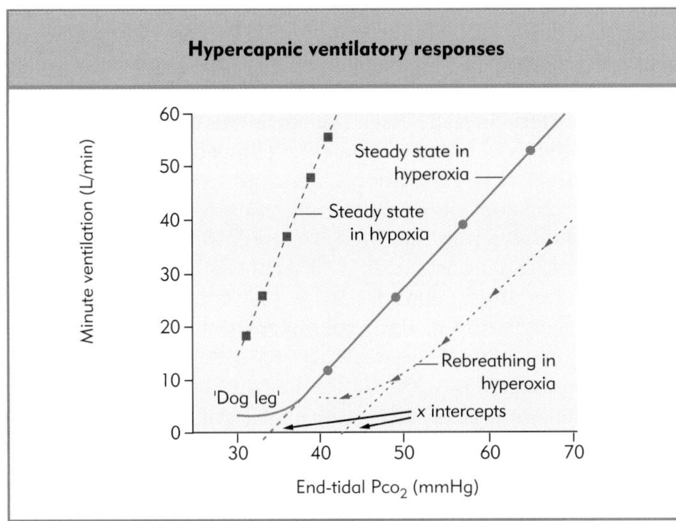

Figure 46.2 Hypercapnic ventilatory responses. Simulation of the relationship between end-tidal partial pressure of CO_2 ($P_{\acute{E}}CO_2$) and minute ventilation ($\dot{V}_A$) under different conditions. Ventilation does not continue to fall as $P_{\acute{E}}CO_2$ is lowered in awake subjects because of a 'wakeful' drive to breath; this gives rise to the 'dog leg'. In hypoxia (oxygen saturation (SaO_2) <75%), the steeper slope (approximately double) is caused by peripheral chemoreceptor stimulation. The CO_2 response obtained from rebreathing in hyperoxia has essentially the same slope as that obtained with the steady-state technique; however, the curve is shifted to the right because of the slow time constant of the central chemoreceptors, which yields a different *x*-intercept, the expected 'apneic' threshold. The slope ($\Delta\dot{V}_A/\Delta P_{\acute{E}}CO_2$) is determined from regression in the linear portion of the curve, as shown by the extrapolated line.

In sleeping or anesthetized normoxic or hyperoxic subjects, if $PaCO_2$ is reduced about 5 mmHg below the resting value, ventilation ceases. This $PaCO_2$ value is known as the 'apneic threshold'. Hypoxia can drive ventilation to lower $PaCO_2$. The HCVR slope is increased by hypoxia, typically being doubled at an arterial O_2 saturation (SaO_2) of 75% (Fig. 46.2). This increase in slope arises from the interaction of hypoxia and CO_2 in the peripheral chemoreceptors, and potentially from further processing in the medullary integrating centers.

Normal sleep slightly reduces the slope of the CO_2 response, but also shifts its position (defined as the intercept on the *x* axis) to a slightly higher $PaCO_2$ (1–4 mmHg). Most anesthetic agents reduce the slope in proportion to the depth of anesthesia, and also raise the *x* intercept.

MODIFICATION OF CENTRAL CHEMORECEPTOR SIGNALS

The zero-ventilation intercept of the CO_2 response curve (and, therefore, the apneic threshold) varies with changes in the metabolic acid–base status of blood; it also changes slowly as this alters CSF HCO_3^- levels. As acidosis stimulates breathing, the CO_2 response line shifts leftwards, reducing the intercept. At lower values of $PaCO_2$ each 1 mmHg rise in P_aCO_2 causes a larger pH fall (because of the log relationship of pH to P_aCO_2); as a result, HCVR increases slightly. Much of the interest in chemoreceptor physiology in anesthesia arises from the substantial changes in ventilatory responses caused by anesthetics, sedative hypnotics, and opioids (Chapter 51). The limited available evidence suggests that these agents depress the integrated respiratory center responses rather than the chemoreceptor sensitivities. For example, morphine does not block the activation by high P_aCO_2 of the ventral medullary chemoreceptor cells (as shown by a c-*fos* expression method).

DYNAMIC CHANGES

The central chemoreceptor responses are significantly slower than the carotid body responses. Although the circulatory delay from the lung to the brainstem is of the order of a few seconds, the 'wash-in' of a step rise of alveolar PCO_2 (P_ACO_2) into brain tissue is exponential, with a time constant of 1–2 minutes. The CO_2 response will therefore begin reasonably quickly, but it takes substantial time for $\dot{V}_A$ to reach its steady-state value. Figure 46.3 shows the change of $\dot{V}_A$ with time following a step increase in end-tidal PCO_2 ($P_{\acute{E}}CO_2$) from 40 to 55 mmHg. If this occurs in room air, 21% inspired oxygen, both central and peripheral chemoreceptor components are present. At a high fraction of inspired O_2 (F_IO_2) (not shown), the response is monoexponential, disclosing both the magnitude (gain) and the speed of the central chemoreceptor response.

MEASUREMENT

Two main techniques are used to measure HCVR. The most common is the Read rebreathing method. This involves rebreathing for about 6–8 minutes from a 5–7-L bag containing a mixture of 7% CO_2 in O_2; P_aCO_2 immediately jumps to approximately mixed venous level, and then rises at about 2–4 mmHg/min. $P_{\acute{E}}CO_2$ (substituting for P_aCO_2) is plotted against $\dot{V}_A$, and the slope is then determined by least-squares regression over the

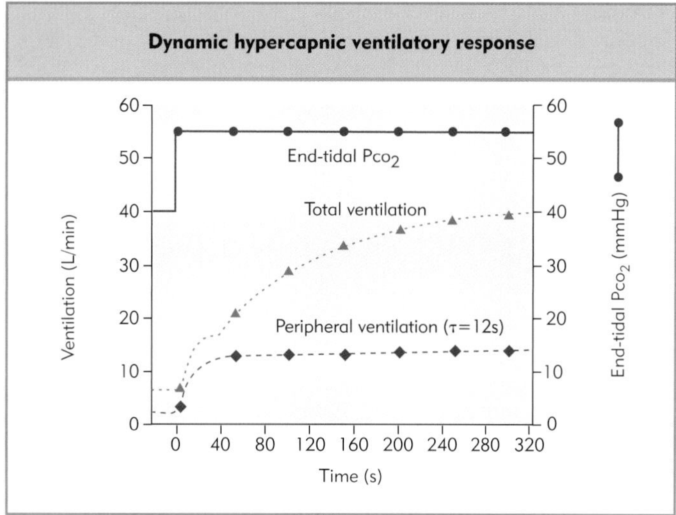

Figure 46.3 Dynamic hypercapnic ventilatory response. In the control period of this simulated response the end-tidal partial pressure of CO_2 ($P_{\acute{E}}CO_2$) was raised slightly above resting to ensure that ventilation was above the 'dog-leg' (see Fig. 46.1). $P_{\acute{E}}CO_2$ was then abruptly raised to 55 mmHg by the addition of inspired CO_2. When tested during normoxia, the rise in minute ventilation with a step increase in $P_{\acute{E}}CO_2$ has a small rapid component (~12-second time constant) arising in peripheral chemoreceptors (estimated by the dotted line), followed by a slightly delayed slow rise (~2-minute time constant, delay exaggerated here) as $P CO_2$ in the medullary chemoreceptors rises to a new equilibrium above arterial $P CO_2$. Peripheral chemoreceptor stimulation is responsible for approximately one-third of the total steady-state response, the slope of which is defined as the change in minute ventilation $\Delta \dot{V}_A/\Delta P_{\acute{E}}CO_2$ (2.0 L/min/mmHg in this example).

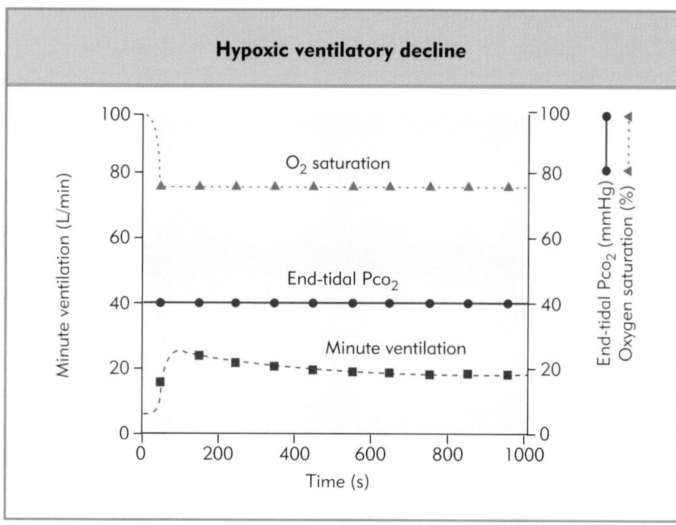

Figure 46.4 Hypoxic ventilatory decline (HVD). The development of HVD is shown for prolonged hypoxic exposure. After about 5 minutes of step hypoxia, HVD slowly eliminates about half of the hypoxic increase of ventilation. HVD is still poorly understood, but is of medullary, not peripheral, chemoreceptor origin. The HVD decrement is variable, eliminating all of the hypoxic response in some individuals.

linear portion of the plot (Fig. 46.2). This method cannot be used to determine the x-intercept. Alternatively, the steady-state technique employs a step increase in $P_{\acute{E}}CO_2$, which is then held constant at the chosen level until steady-state $\dot{V}_A$ is reached, as shown in Figure 46.3. This usually requires about 6 minutes, which is roughly three time constants. Inspired CO_2 must be increased abruptly to produce this step change, and must be continuously adjusted to maintain $P_{\acute{E}}CO_2$ constant while $\dot{V}_A$ increases. HCVR is the steady-state ratio of the change in $\dot{V}_A$ to the change in $P_{\acute{E}}CO_2$, and should be similar by the two methods. The rise in $P_{\acute{E}}CO_2$ or P_aCO_2 produced by anesthetics and adjuvant drugs is a qualitative way to demonstrate ventilatory depression. Most studies simply measure HCVR in the same individual before and after drug administration.

Hypoxic ventilatory response

Hypoxic ventilatory response is the slope of the increase of $\dot{V}_A$ plotted against the decrease of S_aO_2 ($\dot{V}_A/S_aO_2$). Moderate steady hypoxia (e.g. S_aO_2 70–90%) has a dual effect on breathing, stimulating ventilation via the carotid bodies within seconds (HVR); however, after about 5 minutes this initial response decays even at constant P_aCO_2, and after 20 minutes only about half the incremental ventilation persists (Fig. 46.4). This decay, believed to be a consequence of CNS hypoxia, is called hypoxic ventilatory decline (HVD). The absolute decrease in ventilation from the peak value is proportional to HVR, the initial response slope. The decline, expressed as a percentage of peak ventilation, is relatively consistent. Little or no decline or depression occurs in subjects with blunted HVR (see below), or in animals after peripheral chemoreceptor denervation. HVD appears to inhibit incoming peripheral drive.

Moderate hypoxia has a dual effect; stimulation of ventilation via the carotid bodies, followed by a decay in this response due to CNS hypoxia.

The mechanism of HVD is complex, and may be multifactorial. HVD occurs in mild hypoxia without any detectable effect on mental function in normal subjects, precluding a role of ATP production failure. However, in peripherally denervated animals ventilation is truly depressed by severe hypoxia, especially under anesthesia. At the onset of hypoxia, pH at the central chemoreceptor surface initially rises due to increased cerebral blood flow from hypoxia, but this is quickly followed by falling pH due to local lactic acid generation. Increased cerebral blood flow caused by hypoxia reduces the difference between tissue and arterial $P CO_2$, lowering the $P CO_2$ at the central chemoreceptors. This may explain a portion of HVD, but alone is not sufficient. HVD can be almost eliminated by minimizing hypoxic brain lactic acid generation in both volunteers and animals using the drug dichloroacetate. This acidification seems to be narrowly confined to a region near the location of the central chemoreceptors. Acidification is usually associated with stimulated ventilation, whereas in HVD it occurs in the context of ventilatory decrease. One possible mechanism is that ventilatory reduction occurs if intracellular acidosis exceeds extracellular acidosis; during ventilation stimulated with CO_2, extracellular acidosis is greater than intracellular because intracellular proteins buffer the rising $P CO_2$.

Several neurotransmitters and neuromodulators are known to depress ventilation. Endorphins seem a likely source of ventilatory decline; however, naloxone does not modify HVD in adults, and has only a small inconsistent effect in neonates. Adenosine probably plays some role in the process, as aminophylline partially blocks HVD in humans. Methylxanthines prevent neonatal apneic episodes, further suggesting an important link between adenosine, HVD, and clinical ventilatory response mechanisms.

HVD can also be reduced with γ-aminobutyric acid (GABA) receptor antagonists.

In neonates, both animal and human, HVD is prominent and hypoxia may cause apnea, especially before a substantial carotid body response has developed. Understanding the potential of hypoxia to cause ventilatory depression is important in pathophysiology. Anesthetic agents may block HVR, and even enhance HVD, contributing further to the depressant effects of hypoxia.

Hypoxia may cause apnea in neonates before the development of carotid body responses.

HVR AND THE PERIPHERAL CHEMORECEPTORS

The carotid bodies are located at the bifurcation of the carotid artery and are entirely responsible for hypoxic ventilatory stimulation in humans. The peripheral chemoreceptors have significant tone during air breathing. Inhalation of 100% O_2 reduces tidal volume for several breaths, until a rise in P_aCO_2 replaces the lost drive. Carotid body denervation leads to a permanent ~6 mmHg increase in P_aCO_2, which was originally thought to indicate that approximately 15% of normal $\dot{V}_A$ is a consequence of carotid body discharge. Further analysis, taking into account that chronic hypercapnia induces a compensatory rise in CSF and blood HCO_3^- sufficient only to restore CSF and arterial pH about halfway to normal, now suggests that the carotid bodies contribute about 30% of total ventilatory drive in resting normoxic humans.

The chemosensitivity of peripheral chemoreceptors is slowly modulated by chronic hypoxia. A few days to weeks at about 4000 m altitude causes a doubling of HVR through unexplained upregulation of responsiveness within the carotid bodies. Longer hypoxia eventually leads to enlargement of the carotid bodies (see below).

Carotid body neural output is proportional to arterial oxygen desaturation.

The carotid bodies are innervated by the carotid sinus nerve, a branch of the glossopharyngeal nerve (cranial nerve IX). Efferent sympathetic and parasympathetic nerves modify chemoreceptor responses by direct effects and by changes in vascular tone, which controls flow through the sinusoids. The carotid sinus nerve also transmits arterial baroreceptor information. The main functional cell in the carotid body is the type I or glomus cell, which contains many mitochondria, catecholamines, and inhibitory and excitatory neurotransmitters (including dopamine, norepinephrine, acetylcholine, serotonin, substance P, etc.). Carotid bodies are characterized by very high metabolic rate/O_2 consumption and very high blood flow, yielding an unusually small difference between arterial and venous PO_2. Anemia does not affect carotid body discharge, nor does carbon monoxide. These organs, therefore, 'sense' arterial not tissue PO_2 and do not sense arterial O_2 content or saturation. The relationship of nerve output to PO_2 is hyperbolic, approaching maximum output asymptotically at about 30 mmHg. This results in the approximately linear relationship of neural output to arterial O_2 desaturation rather than to PaO_2. The mechanism of detection of hypoxia is very complex, probably involving alteration of oxygen-sensitive K^+ channels, but the high O_2 consumption suggests that a diffusion limitation between blood and the detection mechanism in the type I cells is involved. Hypercapnia and increased H^+ are important stimuli of the peripheral chemoreceptors. Unlike the central chemoreceptors, the peripheral receptors are immediately accessible to and affected by metabolically derived H^+.

MODIFICATION OF PERIPHERAL CHEMORECEPTOR SIGNALS

Alteration of the ventilatory response to peripheral chemoreceptor signals may occur in both medullary and supramedullary integrating centers. For example, state of arousal, metabolic rate, and exercise all have a profound effect on HVR. Long-term hypoxia downregulates or 'blunts' the central response to incoming stimuli (see below). Most drugs that alter hypoxic responses do so mainly at the integrating centers. However, non-depolarizing muscle relaxants depress carotid chemoreceptor hypoxic sensitivity in proportion to their blockade of neuromuscular transmission. The conclusion that a drug produces a specific peripheral chemoreceptor effect is based on the experimental finding that drug-induced depression of HVR is substantially greater than the depression of HCVR. If similar depression of both HVR and HCVR occurs, as is the case with opioids, the integrating center is the presumed site of drug action.

Catecholamines are important modulators of the carotid body. Dopamine, which is secreted by the glomus cell, inhibits carotid body responses. Exogenously administered dopamine at clinical doses causes significant inhibition of peripheral chemoreceptor responses. Likewise, dopamine antagonists such as droperidol can augment HVR. Epinephrine and norepinephrine both stimulate responsiveness.

INTERACTION OF CENTRAL AND PERIPHERAL INPUTS

The ventilatory response to hypoxia is altered by CO_2. Understanding this effect is essential to understanding the function of the peripheral chemoreceptors. The interaction of CO_2 with hypoxia occurs in a synergistic, not an additive, manner. This means that the slope of the hypoxic response is steeper at higher levels of CO_2, not simply shifted upward and parallel, which would be an additive response. Conversely hypoxia increases the slope of the CO_2 response curve (see Fig. 46.2). Most of this interaction resides within the peripheral chemoreceptors. It is possible that central CO_2 responses also interact with peripheral chemoreceptor responses; however, most results indicate that the central hypercapnic response simply adds to the peripheral response. This interaction makes asphyxia (low P_aO_2, high P_aCO_2) the most potent stimulus of the peripheral chemoreceptors. At the other end of the spectrum, profound hypocapnia due to hyperventilation can reduce hypoxic responsiveness to nearly zero. Metabolic acid–base changes operate in a similar fashion.

The ventilatory response to hypoxia is altered synergistically by hypercarbia through interactions at peripheral chemoreceptors.

DYNAMIC CHANGES

One of the most distinguishing features of the peripheral chemoreceptors, compared with the central receptors, is their fast response time. The time constant is approximately 12 seconds, with a delay from lung to carotid body of only a few seconds. Figure 46.5 shows the rapid change of $\dot{V}_A$ in response

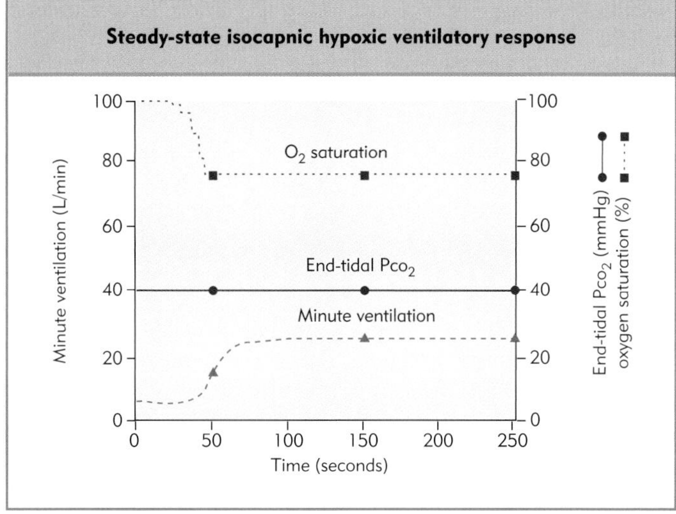

Figure 46.5 Steady-state isocapnic hypoxic ventilatory response. In this simulated example, oxygen saturation is lowered stepwise to 75% and ventilation rises rapidly as a result of stimulation of the carotid bodies. End-tidal partial pressure of CO_2 (P_{ETCO_2}) is kept constant by the addition of CO_2 to the inspired gas mixture (at an above-normal level, as in Fig. 46.2). Ventilation attains a plateau in about 2 minutes.

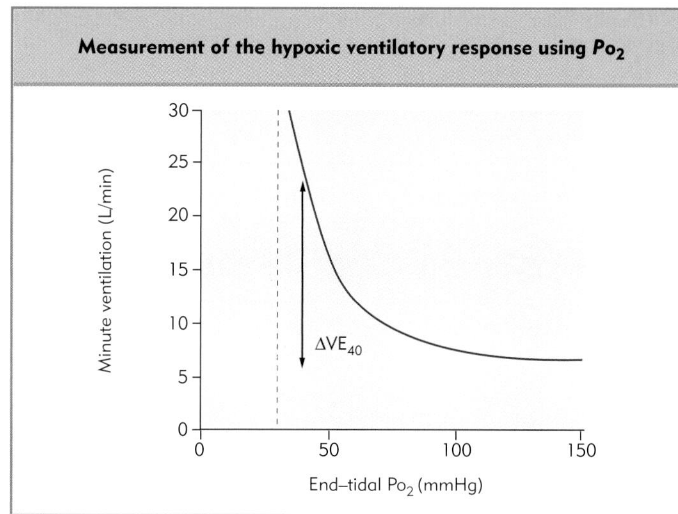

Figure 46.6 Measurement of the hypoxic ventilatory response (HVR) using O_2 partial pressure (P_{O_2}). The hypoxic response expressed relative to P_{O_2} is hyperbolic and is usually quantified using a sensitivity parameter A, where the minute ventilation is $A/P_{O_2} - 32$). Another measure of hypoxic response is $\Delta\dot{V}_{A40}$, the increase in ventilation when P_aO_2 is lowered from 200 to 40 mmHg ($A = 8\Delta\dot{V}_{A40}$). Using a rebreathing system with an adjustable CO_2 absorber to hold partial pressure of end-tidal CO_2 ($P_{\bar{E}}CO_2$) constant, a response curve similar to this can be obtained as P_{O_2} falls over about 5–10 minutes, although it may include some component of hypoxic ventilatory decline (HVD).

to decreased S_aO_2. Compare this rapid response with the slow increase in ventilation caused by stimulation of central chemoreceptors in Figure 46.3. The carotid body response is so fast that the output of the peripheral chemoreceptor changes phasically at a frequency equal to that of the respiratory rate, corresponding to the slight fluctuations in P_aO_2 and P_aCO_2 that occur with tidal breathing. The peripheral chemoreceptors are sufficiently fast and sensitive to detect these fluctuations. It is unclear whether this phasic activity contributes to the ventilatory response (e.g. in exercise).

MEASUREMENT

Peripheral chemoreceptor sensitivity can be measured by a variety of techniques. In animal preparations, the activity of nerve fibers from the carotid sinus nerve can be directly measured. In humans and in most animal experiments, $\dot{V}_A$ is the most useful measure. The hypoxic stimulus may be quantified by changes in either arterial P_aO_2 or S_aO_2 at constant P_aCO_2 ('isocapnic'). For clinical purposes, P_aO_2 is estimated from alveolar gas samples, as end-tidal P_{O_2} ($P_{\bar{E}}O_2$), which should be a close approximation under most circumstances. When expressed relative to P_{O_2}, the isocapnic hypoxic response appears hyperbolic with an asymptote at 32 mmHg (Fig. 46.6). A common way to quantify hypoxic response is to fit the data obtained at low P_{O_2} (40–60 mmHg) to a hyperbola: $\dot{V}_A = A/(P_{O_2} - 32)$, where A is extrapolated – but not measurable – ventilation at 33 mmHg P_{O_2} (incorrectly called a shape parameter). More usefully, A is eight times the increase in ventilation at PaO_2 40 mmHg, which can be measured directly. With the advent of pulse oximetry, most researchers have used SaO_2, with the near linear HVR slope of $\dot{V}_A$ vs S_aCO_2 (Fig. 46.7). With this method, the value of HVR may be determined at constant P_{CO_2} with a single measurement of the increase in ventilation caused by reduction to any low saturation (preferably between 70 and 85%).

The pattern of hypoxia has important effects on the values obtained in the measurement of HVR. Some investigators use a technique of rapid desaturation to a predetermined S_aO_2 and hold this level constant until the response reaches equilibrium over a period of 2–3 minutes. This steady-state technique is distinguished from a 'ramp' technique, where progressive hypoxia is produced, usually by rebreathing. During the ramp technique HVD occurs, yielding a lower value of HVR than the rapid

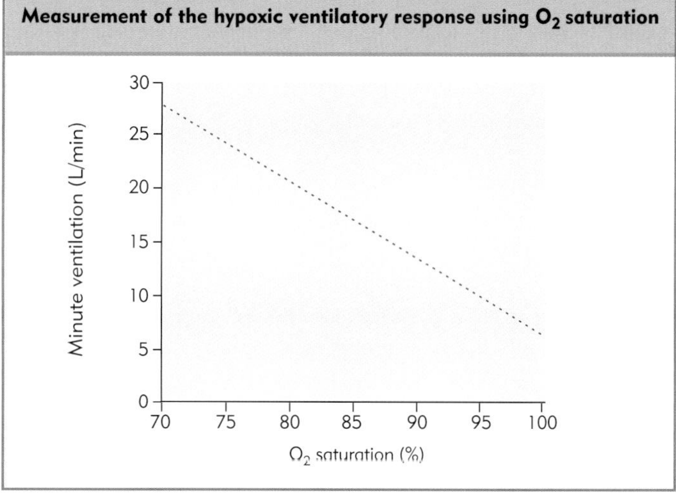

Figure 46.7 Measurement of the hypoxic ventilatory response (HVR) using arterial oxygen saturation (S_aO_2). The acute isocapnic steady-state ventilatory response to a step fall of S_aO_2 is a linear function of desaturation (between 65 and 90%), and may be quantified by a simple slope $\Delta\dot{V}_A/\Delta S_aO_2$ (HVR = 0.75 L/min/% O_2 saturation in this simulated example). The normal range of HVR is 0.2–1.0 L/min/% O_2 saturation.

steady-state technique in the same individual. The sudden change in F_IO_2 required by the steady-state technique is technically more difficult, and holding S_aO_2 constant during the increasing ventilation requires continued adjustment. During the rebreathing technique, the decline in S_aO_2 occurs naturally owing to oxygen consumption, and makes overshooting to extremely low S_aO_2 less likely.

Other measurements of peripheral chemoreceptor function may be used. The response to doxapram, a peripheral chemoreceptor stimulant, is simple, but it has not been shown to relate to HVR quantitatively either in different subjects or under different conditions. Carotid body sensitivity can be measured using single breaths of increased CO_2, or of 5% CO_2 in N_2, recording the transient response before the central chemoreceptors are stimulated. Another technique uses nonlinear regression to partition the ventilatory response to a step rise in P_aCO_2 into a fast time-constant component, representing peripheral chemoreceptors, and a slow time-constant component, representing the central chemoreceptors (see Fig. 46.3). With this technique, both the gain and the time constant of the central and peripheral chemoreceptors are determined in a single test, but the mathematical techniques are more complex.

Failure to perfectly control P_aCO_2 during the measurement of HVR is the single most important factor confounding the interpretation of research results on HVR. Because of the interaction between hypoxia and CO_2 within the peripheral chemoreceptors, most investigators consider maintaining isocapnia during measurement of HVR essential. If P_aCO_2 is allowed to fall, both central and peripheral chemoreceptor drives fall, more so in subjects with high HVR, introducing multiplicative error and scatter and minimizing the difference between individuals with high and low HVR. Even under perfect isocapnic conditions the HVR value depends on the exact value of P_aCO_2 used. Most studies are done at 'resting' P_aCO_2. However, subjects may become anxious and hyperventilate when exposed to unfamiliar apparatus used in the measurements, resulting in a low measured HVR. If P_aCO_2 is raised above the resting value by some constant but arbitrary amount in all subjects, the mean HVR is increased, but the error due to individual anxiety remains. When testing the effects of respiratory depressant drugs, it may be necessary to make control measurements at an elevated P_aCO_2 in anticipation of drug-induced elevation of P_aCO_2. Because individuals serve as their own controls in this type of study, the comparison is valid if the same P_aCO_2 is used in both control and after-drug measurements.

HVR varies considerably between subjects, with values of 0.2–1.5 L/min/% S_aO_2. About 10% of individuals have been reported to have very little response. Although some of these 'nonresponders' may have been misidentified by the use of a test P_aCO_2 that was too low, there is clearly a wide range in response. It is not known whether such abnormally low sensitivity is central or peripheral, but subjects with low values of both HCVR and HVR are more likely to have central integrative abnormalities.

ALTITUDE AND ACCLIMATIZATION

Events occurring at altitude help illustrate the mechanisms of ventilatory control and have therefore been widely studied. Hypoxia is the major underlying cause of acute mountain sickness (AMS). Low HVR should lead to lower P_aO_2 and worse performance at altitude. Such correlations have not been adequately confirmed, presumably because multiple factors, including gas exchange problems, contribute to hypoxemia and AMS. An association between low HVR and high-altitude pulmonary edema (HAPE) has been shown.

At altitude, P_aO_2, reduced by lower P_IO_2 due to lower ambient pressure, stimulates peripheral chemoreceptors, causing an increase in $\dot{V}_A$. Increased $\dot{V}_A$ lowers P_aCO_2, which reduces central chemoreceptor drive. In the initial new steady state this central chemoreceptor inhibition limits the rise of ventilation to about 10% at 4000 m altitude, and P_aCO_2 settles at about 35–36 mmHg. Over the first 8–24 hours P_aCO_2 gradually falls as the HCO_3^- levels in the CSF are reduced at the central chemoreceptors (via several mechanisms, which may include lactic acid production, active transport pH regulation, and diffusion from CSF to blood). After 24 hours, P_aCO_2 is typically about 30 mmHg at this altitude. If one then breathes enough O_2 to temporarily eliminate the hypoxic drive, ventilation remains elevated; P_aCO_2 rises only about 3–4 mmHg, a sign of the compensatory metabolic acidosis of the CSF. Arterial blood at this time is found to be alkaline, because renal compensation for the respiratory alkalosis is much slower. Over the subsequent days to weeks at this altitude, the carotid body drive slowly doubles (by 2 weeks), further increasing ventilation and reducing P_aCO_2.

Adaptations to high altitude include hyperventilation due to the hypoxic ventilatory response.

The higher $\dot{V}_A$ has substantial benefits in increasing P_aO_2. This is particularly true at levels corresponding to the steep portion of the oxyhemoglobin dissociation curve, where a P_aO_2 increase of several mmHg can lead to a significant improvement in oxyhemoglobin saturation. Additional adaptation at altitude includes increased HVR occurring over several days. However, HVD is also present at altitude.

Chronic altitude exposure (months to years) leads to different physiologic changes from those that occur in acute exposure. Whereas hypertrophied carotid bodies are believed to continue their intensified rate of stimulus, the integrating portions of the respiratory center appear to become less responsive. Hypoxic responses are depressed, P_aCO_2 is elevated and P_aO_2 is lower. In some individuals O_2 administration may actually increase ventilation through the release of HVD, where peripheral chemoreceptor responses are low. Carotid bodies themselves increase in size with prolonged exposure to altitude. Lower ventilatory responsiveness causing lower P_aO_2 is also a contributing factor to chronic mountain sickness. This reduced HVR is not reversible even after years at sea level.

SLEEP AND SLEEP APNEA

During sleep, humans are more dependent on chemical drive to breathe than during wakefulness, which provides supplementary stimulation. Subnormal chemoreceptor reflexes, which may not be evident while awake, can lead to devastating hypoventilation during sleep. The effects of sedatives and analgesics that cause respiratory depression may be far greater during sleep in subjects with abnormally low HVR and HCVR. This is probably a major factor in sleep apnea. Changes in ventilation and ventilatory control during sleep have important clinical consequences. Nocturnal disturbances of ventilation can lead to daytime somnolence and dysfunction. In the worst cases, cor pulmonale may develop as a result of pulmonary hypertension due to acute and chronic hypoxemia.

Differences may exist between ventilatory changes occurring in REM sleep and in other stages of sleep. One of the main differences is the irregular breathing patterns seen during REM sleep (Chapters 13 and 30). These patterns are probably mediated through central nonchemical drive, and include changes in respiratory rate, tidal volume, and even periods of apnea.

Chemical control of breathing may actually stabilize, not contribute to, this irregular pattern. Despite differences between REM and nonREM sleep, the following are generalizations that probably apply qualitatively to both.

Loss of wakefulness leads to a fall in $\dot{V}_A$ and a rise in arterial P_aCO_2. Without chemoreceptor responses, the decrease in $\dot{V}_A$ with sleep is even more pronounced. P_aO_2 may also drop during sleep. Alveolar hypoventilation, as described above, reduces alveolar and arterial P_aO_2. Increased ventilation/perfusion (V/Q) mismatching may also occur. In periodic breathing with apneic episodes, more profound arterial oxygen desaturation may occur. The extent of desaturation depends on the duration of apnea and the functional residual capacity. Apneic episodes are terminated by partial or complete arousal resulting from stimulation of chemoreceptors.

The effects of sedatives and analgesics that cause respiratory depression may be enhanced during sleep in individuals with subnormal chemoreceptor reflexes.

Periodic breathing may occur during the early stages of sleep owing to fluctuations in the state of CNS arousal. Breathing eventually develops a regular pattern during the deeper stages. Ventilatory responses to the increased P_aCO_2 and decreased P_aO_2 that occur during sleep may exaggerate the periodic breathing. The slope of ventilatory response to CO_2 is reduced during sleep. The curve is also shifted to a higher P_aCO_2, that is, the apneic threshold is higher. HVR also appears to be reduced. Although reduced, ventilatory control systems are still active, and the abolition of responses may result in an absence of breathing. Severe problems with periodic breathing can occur with apneic episodes during sleep and is probably the main form of central sleep apnea (CSA) (periodic breathing is covered below).

Obstructive sleep apnea (OSA) is caused by airway collapse, with partial or complete obstruction of breathing. Several poorly understood mechanisms affect the tone of airway muscles, and may be involved in the airway collapse that occurs during sleep. Poor airway anatomy and obesity are factors commonly contributing to OSA. Chemoreceptor function also modifies OSA. First, chemoreceptor tone affects airway muscle tone. Second, arousal from obstruction is mediated by chemoreceptor responses. The peripheral chemoreceptors are probably essential for this response. P_aCO_2 rises and P_aO_2 falls during apnea, which is the 'asphyxial' stimulus of the carotid body. Peripheral chemoreceptor sensitivity determines how low oxygen saturation falls during periods of airway obstruction and apnea.

ABNORMALITIES OF CHEMORECEPTOR FUNCTION

Several abnormalities of chemoreceptor function can occur in otherwise normal individuals, whereas others are unusual and represent disease states. Alterations in ventilatory control also provide an insight into the fundamental working of this regulatory system.

Periodic breathing occurs in a variety of circumstances, even in normal individuals. The best-defined type of periodic breathing is Cheyne–Stokes respiration, which is characterized by sinusoidally rising and falling tidal volumes with or without periods of apnea. Cheyne–Stokes breathing can occur in normal individuals during certain stages of sleep. During sleep at sea level the periodic breathing is most likely due to changes in the state of arousal, with changing ventilatory responses and apneic thresholds. Cheyne–Stokes breathing is well known to occur during sleep at high altitude. It also frequently occurs in such pathologic states as congestive heart failure.

Hypoxia predisposes to periodic breathing.

Certain conditions predispose to instability in the ventilatory response system to produce periodic breathing. Hypoxia is one of the most important factors promoting periodic breathing. The hypoxic stimulus of peripheral chemoreceptors results in increased ventilation. Increased ventilation decreases P_aCO_2, which decreases central chemoreceptor stimulation and the slope of the hypoxic response. Because of the shape of the oxyhemoglobin dissociation curve, increased ventilation can also markedly improve oxygenation, which will further change the output of peripheral chemoreceptors. During sleep, without the separate stimulus from wakefulness, this increase in ventilation can lead to such a sharp drop in peripheral chemoreceptor stimulation that apnea results. Apnea then leads to an increase in P_aCO_2 and a fall in S_aO_2. The resultant increased peripheral chemoreceptor stimulation and ventilation repeats this cycle.

Many factors influence whether these changes result in a continued unstable breathing pattern or stabilize with time. The circulatory delay to the chemoreceptors is one of the most significant factors leading to periodic breathing. An increased delay to both peripheral and central chemoreceptors is the primary reason that heart failure results in periodic breathing. Higher peripheral chemoreceptor responses also tend to increase periodic breathing. Almitrene, a drug that increases the gain of peripheral chemoreceptors, increases periodic breathing at high altitude.

Several diseases of chemoreceptor function are known. Ondine's curse (severe central sleep apnea) was initially described with loss of central chemoreception following surgery near the brainstem. During wakefulness individuals function well. However, during sleep profound hypoventilation or apnea can occur. Congenital forms have been described as 'primary alveolar hypoventilation syndrome'. Afflicted individuals appear to lack both peripheral and central chemoreceptor function. The defect most likely resides in areas of the brainstem above the entry of the peripheral and central chemoreceptor signals into the CNS. Affected individuals may require ventilatory support during sleep, and may experience significant hypoventilation or apnea during anesthesia and in the perioperative period.

Abnormal chemoreceptor function should be suspected in individuals with serious neurological abnormalities. Premature infants up to postconceptual ages of 50–60 weeks are at risk of apnea following anesthesia. The exact problem in chemoreceptor function has not been defined. Abnormal or immature chemoreceptor function has been implicated in sudden infant death syndrome (SIDS). Although prone sleeping and rebreathing of exhaled gases may be a factor in SIDS, lack of appropriate chemoreceptor arousal is probably contributory.

Key references

Berger A, Mitchell R, Severinghaus JW. Regulation of respiration. N Engl J Med. 1977;297:92–97, 138–43, 194–201.

Eyzaguiree C, Fidone SJ, Fitzgerald RS, Lahiri S, McDonald DM. Arterial chemoreception. New York: Springer-Verlag; 1990.

Forster HV, Dempsey JA. Ventilatory adaptations. In: Hornbein T, ed. Regulation of breathing, Part II. New York: Marcel Dekker; 1981:845–901.

Hickey RF, Severinghaus JW. Ventilatory adaptations: drug effects. In: Hornbein T, ed. Regulation of breathing, Part II. New York: Marcel Dekker; 1981:1251–312.

Loeschcke HH. Central chemosensitivity and the reaction theory. J Physiol. 1982;332:1–24.

McDonald DM. Peripheral chemoreceptors. In: Hornbein T, ed. Regulation of breathing, Part I. New York: Marcel Dekker; 1981:105–319.

Pietak S, Weenig CS, Hickey RF, Fairley HB. Anesthetic effects on ventilation in patients with chronic obstructive pulmonary disease. Anesthesiology 1975;45:160–6.

Severinghaus JW. Respiratory control related to altitude and anesthesia. In: Stanley TH, Sperry RJ, eds. Anesthesia and the lung. Vol 25. Dordrecht: Kluwer Academic; 1992:101–15.

Temp JA, Henson LC, Ward DS. Effect of a subanesthetic minimum alveolar concentration of Isoflurane on two tests of the hypoxic ventilatory response. Anesthesiology 1994;80:739–50.

Further reading

Cherniack NS, Widdicombe JG. The respiratory system. In: Fishman AP, ed. Handbook of physiology. Bethesda, MD: American Physiological Society; 1986.

Duffin J. The chemoreflex control of breathing and its measurement. Can J Anesth. 1990;37:933–42.

Feldman JL, Mitchell GS, Nattie EE. Breathing: rhythmicity, plasticity, chemosensitivity. Annu Rev Neurosci. 2003;26:239–66.

Neubauer JA, Melton JE, Edelman NH. Modulation of respiration during brain hypoxia. J Appl Physiol. 1990;68:441–51.

Nunn JF. Applied respiratory physiology, 4th edn. Oxford: Butterworth–Heinmann; 1993.

Chapter 47

Ventilation and perfusion

Marcus R Beadle and Andrew B Lumb

The main function of the lungs is to facilitate the exchange of oxygen and carbon dioxide between the air and blood. This chapter reviews the physiology of alveolar ventilation and the pulmonary circulation, before Chapter 48 considers how gas exchange occurs.

PULMONARY VENTILATION

Tracheobronchial anatomy

The adult trachea is typically 15 cm in length and 18 mm in diameter. It is made up of a series of 15–20 semicircular (C-shaped) cartilaginous rings, which are closed in their posterior border by a muscular layer (trachealis). The trachea bifurcates at the level of T4 and then branches irregularly to form 23 generations of airways, the numbers of which approximately double with each generation. Generations are termed major bronchi (generations 2–4), small bronchi (5–11), bronchioles (12–16), respiratory bronchioles (17–19) and alveolar sacs (20–23).

All the airway walls contain large amounts of elastin in their submucous layers to provide elastic recoil to the conducting system, and there is also a smooth muscle layer to facilitate the control of airway diameter. The cartilage rings become plates after the major bronchi, and become progressively less complete in more distal airways. In bronchioles and more distal airways there is no cartilage in the walls, these airways being entirely dependent on adjacent lung tissue recoil to hold them open.

As the airways divide, their diameter decreases and is typically less than 1 mm at the level of the bronchioles. However, because of the increasing number of airways with each division, the total cross-sectional area increases exponentially, with a resulting fall in velocity of gas flow and decrease in airway resistance in successive generations. As this occurs, airflow through the airways changes from turbulent to laminar at about the fifth generation of airway, and so a majority of airway resistance originates in the nose, pharynx, and major bronchi. At the level of the alveoli gas velocity is zero and movement of gases is predominantly by diffusion.

RESPIRATORY EPITHELIUM

The trachea is lined by columnar ciliated epithelium and numerous mucus-secreting goblet cells. The ciliated epithelia form a mucociliary escalator to clear particles that are deposited in the major airways (Fig. 47.1). In order to do this effectively, the cilia are bathed in a low-viscosity 'sol' layer, with just their tips embedded in a more viscous 'gel' layer above. Cilia beat at around 12–16 beats per second in a coordinated pattern to move the gel layer towards the larynx.

The majority of airway resistance originates in the nose, pharynx, and major bronchi.

The columnar epithelial cells seen in large airways become more cuboidal in small bronchi and bronchioles, and goblet cells become less frequent. On reaching the respiratory bronchioles the cuboidal epithelium becomes even thinner and merges with the alveolar type I pneumocytes described below.

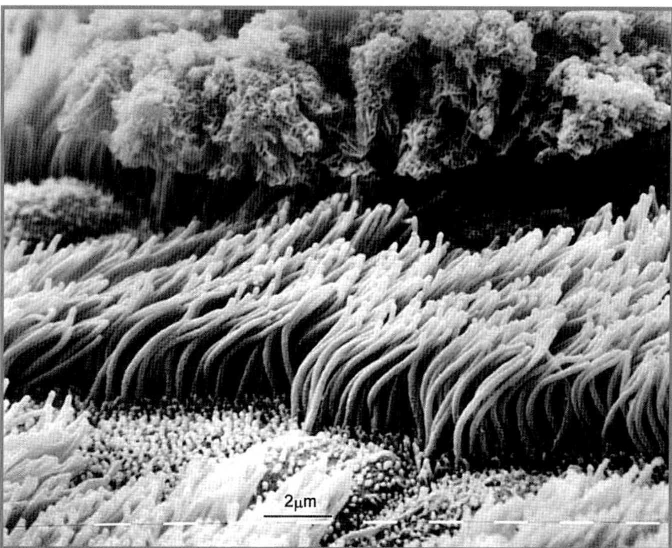

Figure 47.1 Respiratory epithelium. Scanning electron micrograph of ciliated epithelial cells in the respiratory tract. The cilia, with their tips embedded in the mucus above, beat in a coordinated fashion to transport mucus and debris away from the lower airways. (From Brewis et al. Respiratory Medicine. London: WB Saunders Company Ltd, 1995; 54-72, with permission.)

The alveoli have a mean diameter of 0.2 mm and are made up of three cell types:

- Type I pneumocytes make up 80% of the structure and are very thin to allow gaseous exchange to take place. Adjacent cells are joined by tight junctions to prevent fluid entering the alveoli.
- Type II pneumocytes are the stem cells from which type 1 cells arise, and are metabolically active cells manufacturing surfactant.
- Alveolar macrophages are an important defense against inhaled pathogens and responsible for the ingestion of any small inhaled dust particles that reach the alveoli.

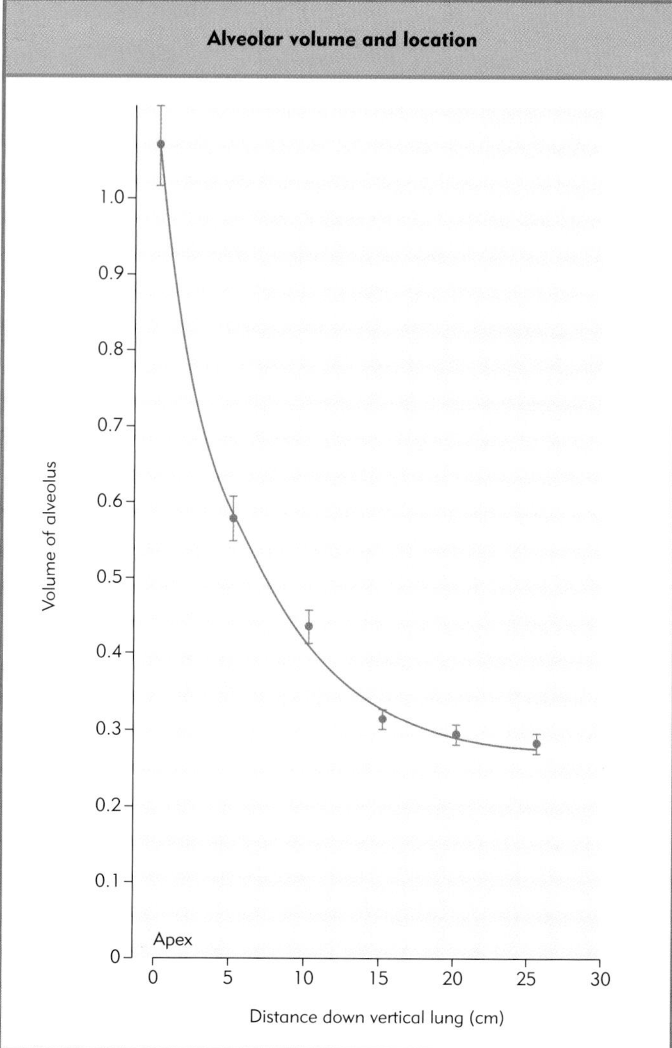

Figure 47.2 Alveolar volume according to location. Graph showing the fourfold change in alveolar volumes from the apex of the lung to the base. (With permission from Feldman S. Scientific foundations of anaesthesia, 3rd edn. London: Heinemann; 1982.)

Alveolar ventilation

Minute ventilation is the total volume of gas that enters and leaves the lung per minute, and is the product of tidal volume (V_T) and respiratory frequency. Minute ventilation is a function of both dead space and alveolar ventilation. The proportion of minute ventilation that reaches the alveoli (and is potentially able to undergo respiratory exchange) is known as the alveolar minute ventilation ($\dot{V}_A$) and is normally about 5 L/min. Dead space describes that part of each breath that does not take part in gas exchange, either because it remains within the conducting passages of the lung before being exhaled unchanged, or is distributed to alveoli with no – or only inadequate – perfusion. As described above, when inhaled gas reaches the alveolar sacs the tidal mass movement of gas has probably ceased, and oxygen and carbon dioxide movement is by diffusion.

REGIONAL DISTRIBUTION OF VENTILATION

During spontaneous respiration, dependent lung regions are better ventilated than the nondependent zones. This occurs irrespective of posture, such that when the subject is upright the lower zones receive more ventilation than the upper zones, but when supine the posterior zones are better ventilated. The inequality of ventilation occurs because the weight of lung tissue results in vertical gradients of intrapleural pressure adjacent to different lung regions. Alveolar size therefore must also vary, those at the apex being about four times the volume of basal alveoli in the upright posture (Fig. 47.2). Thus the alveoli in the basal area can expand their volume much more with each breath than those at the apex, which may already be almost fully inflated even during expiration. In a microgravity environment these variations in regional ventilation disappear almost completely.

Dead space

Dead space is made up of 'anatomic' and 'alveolar' dead spaces, the two combined being described as 'physiological' dead space.

Anatomic dead space includes the nasal passages, pharynx, larynx, and all the generations of conducting airways described above. Alveolar dead space is that part of each breath that passes through the conducting airways to the alveoli but which does not take part in gas exchange. Physiological dead space is the sum of anatomic and alveolar dead space, and represents all gas not taking part in gas exchange. The Bohr equation describes the physiological dead space.

■ Equation 47.1

$$\dot{V}_A = f\,(V_T - V_D)$$

where $\dot{V}_A$ is the alveolar minute ventilation, f is respiratory frequency, V_T is tidal volume and V_D is dead-space volume. A rearrangement of the above equation yields the dead space to tidal volume ratio V_D/V_T:

■ Equation 47.2

$$\frac{V_D}{V_T} = 1 - \frac{\dot{V}_A}{fV_T}$$

During expiration, assuming inspired CO_2 is zero, all eliminated CO_2 begins as alveolar CO_2 and subsequently becomes the CO_2 of mixed expired gas, so allowing $\dot{V}_A$ to be calculated. Finally, in the clinical situation, arterial CO_2 tension is almost identical to alveolar CO_2 tension, but is considerably easier to measure and is therefore substituted in the equation for alveolar CO_2. Equation 47.2 can then be refined to form the Bohr equation:

■ Equation 47.3

$$\frac{V_D}{V_T} = 1 - \frac{P_{\bar{E}}CO_2}{P_aCO_2}$$

where $P_{\bar{E}}CO_2$ is the CO_2 tension in mixed expired gas and P_aCO_2 is the CO_2 tension in arterial blood.

PULMONARY CIRCULATION

Vascular anatomy in the lung

The right and left pulmonary arteries follow the mainstem bronchi into the lung parenchyma, where they follow a branching pattern in parallel with the bronchi. The arteries give rise to arteriolar and capillary networks within the walls of alveolar ducts and alveoli, where the capillaries weave in and out of adjacent alveoli bulging into the alveolus air space (Fig. 47.3). The pulmonary venules, and then the veins, collect blood from the capillary network and return it to the left atrium, pursuing a course separate from those of the arteries and bronchi.

The pulmonary arteries and arterioles have three layers: adventitia, media, and intima. In pulmonary vessels the medial smooth muscle layer of arteries and arterioles is much less prominent than in systemic vessels of comparable size, and thins further as the vessels decrease in size to the microvessel level, where only an occasional pericyte represents the medial layer. In the intima, pulmonary endothelium is of the continuous type, with tight intercellular junctions. In the small arterioles, capillaries, and small veins that collectively make up the microcirculation, endothelial cells have very attenuated cytoplasm overlying the basement membrane to facilitate efficient gas exchange.

The pulmonary circulation receives the full cardiac output from the right ventricle at low pressures.

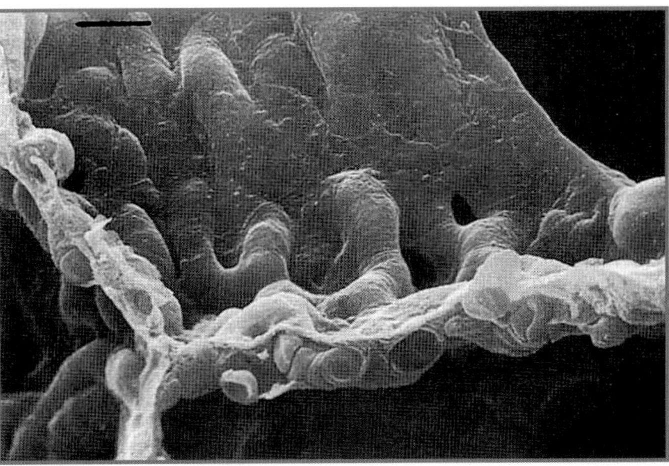

Figure 47.3 Alveolar capillaries. Scanning electron micrograph of the junction of three alveoli. Capillaries can be seen weaving between adjacent alveoli. Erythrocytes are seen in the front of the picture in the cut ends of the capillaries. (Reprinted by permission from the publisher from The Pathway for Oxygen: Structure and Function in the Mammalian Respitory System by Ewald R. Weibel, pp. 224, Cambridge, Mass: Harvard University Press, Copyright © 1984 by the President and Fellows of Harvard College.) The scale bar is 10 mm.

These anatomic features allow the pulmonary circulation to receive the full cardiac output from the right ventricle at low pressures and to provide adequate exchange of oxygen and carbon dioxide within the alveolar wall. During exercise, pulmonary blood flow can increase three- to fivefold without a significant increase in pressure as a result of distension of the arteries and veins and recruitment of additional capillary beds. Whereas the pulmonary arteries and arterioles comprise a surface area of about 2.5 m^2, the surface area of the capillary network is estimated at 50–150 m^2. About 150 mL of blood is contained in the arteries, only 80 mL in the capillaries, and 250–750 mL in the distensible veins. The normal capillary transit time across an alveolus of approximately 0.75 seconds allows for adequate exchange of oxygen and carbon dioxide. At very high pulmonary blood flow, for example during exercise, the capillary transit time may become so rapid that complete oxygenation is limited by the speed of diffusion of oxygen across the alveolar–capillary membrane. Because carbon dioxide is a more diffusible gas, its exchange is unaffected at high blood flow.

BRONCHIAL CIRCULATION

The lungs have a second circulation, the bronchial vasculature, which arises from the systemic circulation and receives about 1% of cardiac output. The bronchial arteries, usually two to four in number, have their origin at the aorta or, occasionally, from the intercostal arteries. At systemic pressures they perfuse the walls of the bronchi down to respiratory bronchioles, as well as the pulmonary arteries and veins, connective tissue, and pleura.

Pulmonary blood flow

Beyond the neonatal period the mean pressure within the pulmonary artery is low, about 15 mmHg. The pressure within the pulmonary veins is about 5 mmHg, and the microvascular pressure is intermediate. A Starling resistor model of lung blood flow is helpful in describing the pulmonary circulation. A Starling resistor is a collapsible tube (the microvessels) passing through a rigid box (the alveolar network) with variable upstream (pulmonary arterial) and downstream (pulmonary venous) pressures. West and colleagues used the Starling resistor model to describe three conditions of lung blood flow (Fig. 47.4). Alveolar pressure (P_A) acts as a Starling resistor to exert a resistance to flow through the collapsible pulmonary vessels. In zone 1, pressure at the pulmonary arterial end of the capillary is lower than alveolar pressure, so that blood flow cannot occur. In zone 2, arterial pressure (P_a) exceeds alveolar pressure, which is greater than venous pressure. Flow through zone 2 depends on the difference between arterial and alveolar pressures. Venous pressure (P_v) does not affect flow through zone 2; blood flow increases with vertical distance as the arterial–alveolar pressure difference increases. In zone 3, both arterial and venous pressures exceed alveolar pressure; as a result, flow is dependent on the difference between arterial and venous pressures and on distension of the microvessels within the alveolar wall. A fourth zone has been added to explain the reduction in flow in the most dependent parts of the lung as a result of increased interstitial pressure (P_i), where arterial pressure exceeds interstitial pressure, which exceeds alveolar and venous pressure ($P_a > P_i > P_A > P_v$).

REGIONAL LUNG PERFUSION

As for ventilation, the weight of blood leads to regional variations in pulmonary blood flow. West's model may be used to describe the effects of gravity on pulmonary blood flow. Zone 1 represents the uppermost portion of the lung, whereas zone 3 represents the most dependent portion. However, flow varies not only with gravity but also with resistance caused by branching, and with the variable diameter and length of the pulmonary vessels. The central and dorsal portions of human lungs are the best perfused, with a gradient of lower flow toward the periphery.

Factors affecting pulmonary vascular resistance

LUNG VOLUME

The additional zone in which interstitial pressures limit blood flow regardless of alveolar pressures highlights the importance of lung gas volume in determining blood flow and resistance. As lung volume increases, the larger, extra-alveolar vessels increase in diameter because they are tethered by the interstitium. At higher lung volumes, alveolar microvessels may be flattened. At low lung volumes extra-alveolar vessels diminish in diameter whereas alveolar vessels increase in size. The opposing effects of lung volume on extra-alveolar and alveolar vessel size and resistance are optimally balanced at functional residual capacity (FRC).

NEURAL CONTROL OF PULMONARY VESSELS

Pulmonary vessels have sympathetic, parasympathetic, and sensory innervation. At low resting vascular tone α_1- and α_2-adrenoceptor stimulation results in vasoconstriction, but there is little response to β_2-adrenoceptor stimulation. At increased basal vascular tone β_2-adrenoceptor stimulation causes vasodilatation and α-adrenoceptor stimulation causes constriction. Muscarinic cholinergic stimulation causes constriction when basal tone is low and vasodilatation when tone is high. Sympathetic and parasympathetic nerve fibers also contain vasoactive intestinal peptide (VIP) and substance P, which are vasodilators. The importance of these neurotransmitters in health and disease is unknown.

HUMORAL CONTROL OF PULMONARY VESSELS

There is now good evidence that in the resting state the pulmonary circulation is in a state of active vasodilatation, maintained by basal production of nitric oxide (NO). In response to shear stress or an agonist such as bradykinin, constitutive calcium-dependent nitric oxide synthase (cNOS) forms an NO radical from L-arginine in lung endothelial cells (Fig. 47.5). NO diffuses across the cell membrane into the adjacent smooth muscle, where it activates guanylyl cyclase to produce cyclic guanosine 3,5-monophosphate (cGMP) from guanosine 5-triphosphate (GTP). The cGMP interacts with cGMP-dependent protein kinase to cause a decrease in intracellular calcium ion concentration and smooth muscle relaxation. The effect is terminated by a phosphodiesterase that converts cGMP to GMP (Chapter 3).

A second, inducible calcium-independent nitric oxide synthase (iNOS) is produced in lung smooth muscle cells and macrophages. This isoform can produce large quantities of NO

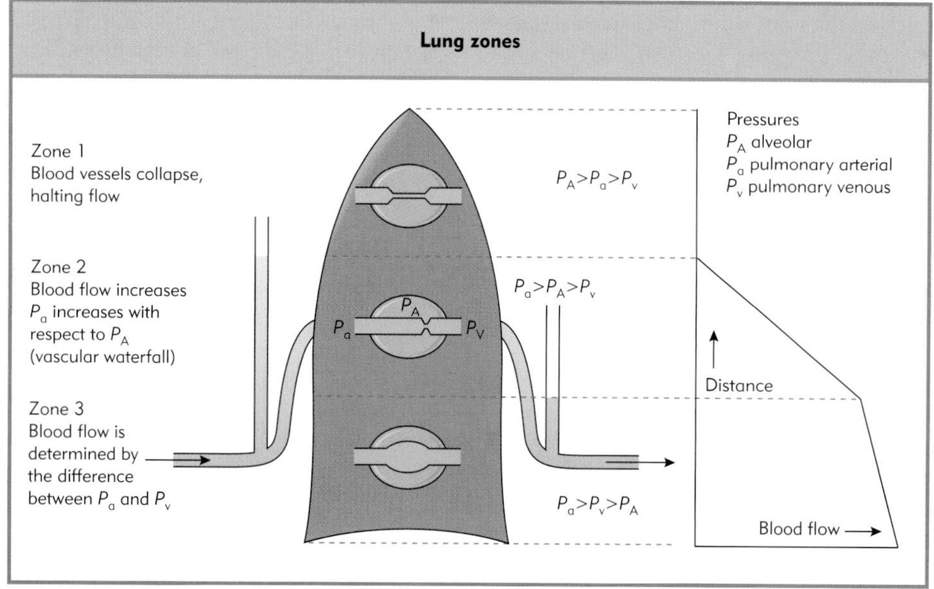

Figure 47.4 West's zones. A Starling resistor model showing the relationship between blood flow and vascular/alveolar pressures. See text for details (Adapted from West JB, Dollery CT, Maimark A. Distribution of blood flow in isolated lung: relation to vascular and alveolar pressures. J Appl Physiol. 1964; 19: 713–24.)

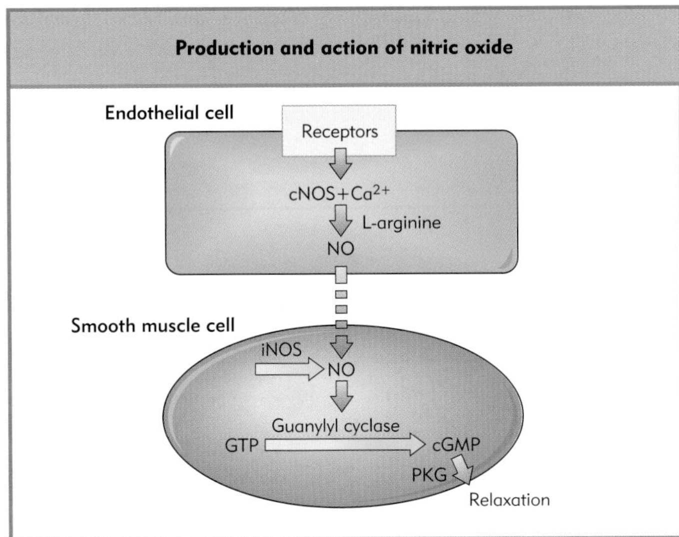

Figure 47.5 Cellular production of nitric oxide. Nitric oxide is pivotal in the control of pulmonary vascular resistance.

compared to endothelial cNOS. The cNOS isoform may be responsible for a steady, low rate of NO production and smooth muscle relaxation in the normal pulmonary circulation, whereas iNOS may produce increased NO in pathologic conditions. Acetylcholine is known to produce pulmonary vasodilation via an NO-dependent pathway. Nitroglycerin (glyceryl trinitate) and nitroprusside act as dilators in both the systemic and the pulmonary circulations by activation of guanylyl cyclase.

Inhaled NO is used therapeutically as a selective pulmonary vasodilator. With the exception of hyperoxia and alkalosis, conditions or drugs that dilate the pulmonary circulation also cause systemic hypotension. Because inhaled NO is delivered directly to its site of action in pulmonary smooth muscle cells and is then rapidly inactivated by binding to hemoglobin, it is effective as a pulmonary dilator without causing systemic dilation. It now has an accepted place in the treatment of persistent pulmonary hypertension of the newborn and severe acute lung injury in adults, and when used at appropriate doses has minimal adverse effects.

Nitric oxide is effective as a pulmonary vasodilator without causing systemic vasodilatation.

Endothelin-1 is a potent pulmonary vasoconstrictor and a vasodilator, depending on the dose and the age of the subject. It is a small peptide of 21 amino acid residues that is cleaved from the larger proendothelin-1 by endothelin-converting enzyme in endothelial cells. The hemodynamic effects of endothelin-1 are mediated by at least two distinct receptors, ET_A and ET_B. ET_A receptors are located on smooth muscle cells and mediate vasoconstriction, by phospholipase activation and the production of inositol trisphosphate and diacylglycerol, which increases intracellular Ca^{2+} concentration. ET_B receptors are found on endothelial cells and mediate vasodilatation via a mechanism that involves NO production. Interaction with platelet-activating factor (PAF), bradykinin, and prostanoids may all modulate the effects of endothelin-1.

Many lipid-derived mediators such as the prostaglandins, thromboxane, PAF, and leukotrienes are produced by endothelial cells and other cell types in the lung. Prostaglandins E_2 and $F_{2\alpha}$ are primarily vasoconstrictors but, depending on dose and underlying vascular tone, may have dilating effects. Prostaglandin E_1 is a vasodilator that is used clinically to maintain a patent ductus arteriosus as a bridge to surgery in some children with congenital heart disease. Prostacyclin is used as a vasodilator in the treatment of primary pulmonary hypertension. PAF is a proinflammatory agent with vasodilating properties at low concentrations and vasoconstricting properties at higher concentrations. The leukotrienes (LTC_4, LTD_4, and LTE_4) are mainly vasoconstrictors; LTB_4 is a neutrophil chemoattractant without vasoactive properties.

HYPOXIC PULMONARY VASOCONSTRICTION

Hypoxia increases pulmonary vascular resistance. When hypoxia involves a circumscribed area of lung, as in regional atelectasis, edema, or one-lung ventilation, blood flow is diverted away from this segment to other, better oxygenated, alveoli. This physiologic response of hypoxic pulmonary vasoconstriction (HPV) contrasts with that in vessels elsewhere in the body, which dilate in response to hypoxia. Low oxygen tension in both the alveoli and the microcirculation is the stimulus for constriction of the small arterioles and venules. The mechanism of HPV remains uncertain. Although HPV can be modulated by autonomic innervation and endothelium-derived factors, neither of these is essential for the reflex. For example, HPV is present in transplanted lungs. Inhibition of basal NO production may explain part of the response, and the production of endothelin-1 is stimulated by hypoxia. More recently, pulmonary vessels have been shown to have oxygen-sensitive potassium channels, activation of which by hypoxia could lead to changes in intracellular calcium levels in smooth muscle cells. Unfortunately, HPV is diminished in many forms of lung disease, such as acute lung injury, when inflammatory cytokines are thought to override the HPV, causing a further decline in oxygenation.

EFFECTS OF ANESTHETIC DRUGS

Both intravenous and inhalational anesthetics may have multiple effects on the autonomic nervous system, humoral mediators, prostanoid production, and the NO pathway. On balance, intravenous anesthetics, except for ketamine, do not alter pulmonary vascular tone. Ketamine increases pulmonary vascular tone and resistance in adults but leaves it unchanged in infants. Inhalational anesthetics minimally decrease pulmonary vascular tone, with the exception of nitrous oxide, which slightly increases tone. Drugs such as volatile anesthetics depress HPV in a dose-dependent fashion, though this effect is small at clinically used doses.

Transition from fetal to adult circulation

In the transition from fetal to neonatal life, the pulmonary circulation goes from accepting little blood flow to accepting all of the cardiac output. Prenatally, venous return of oxygenated blood from the placenta to the right atrium is shunted away from the lungs across the foramen ovale into the left atrium, and pulmonary arterial blood is shunted across the patent ductus arteriosus into the aorta (Fig. 47.6). Extensive muscularity of pulmonary arteries in the relatively hypoxic environment of the fetus produces high pulmonary vascular resistance, and the

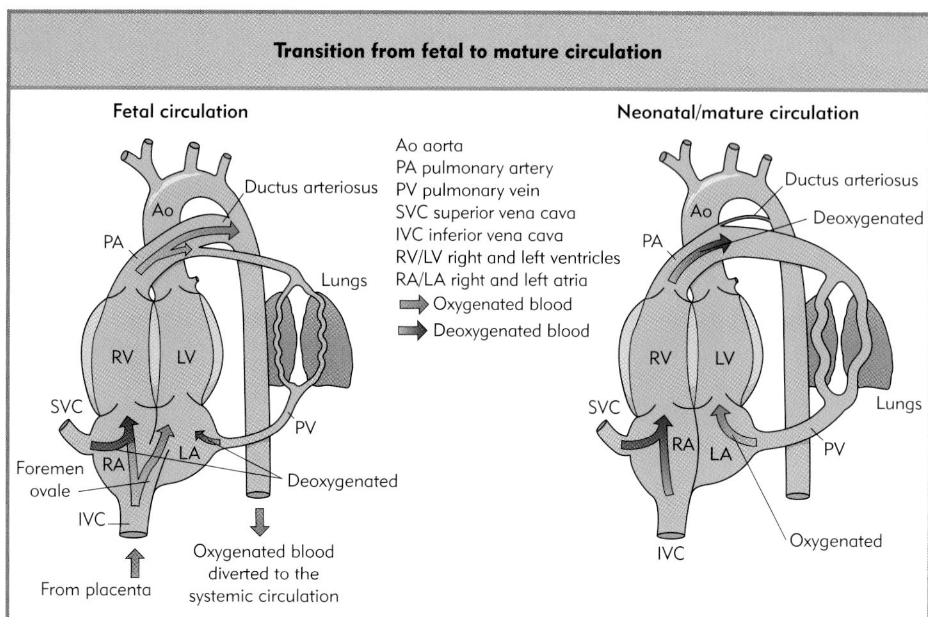

Figure 47.6 Transition from fetal to mature circulation. In the fetus (left), the presence of the foramen ovale allows some oxygenated blood to bypass the lungs. The ductus arteriosus and high pulmonary vascular resistance divert the majority of the rest of the blood to the systemic circulation. After birth, a dramatic reduction in pulmonary vascular resistance allows blood to enter the pulmonary circulation, and the ductus arteriosus and foramen ovale close.

patent foramen ovale and ductus arteriosus provide alternative routes for blood flow. In late gestation resistance begins to decrease, and at birth, with the onset of respiration, pulmonary vascular tone decreases dramatically. The foramen ovale and ductus close functionally. The process occurs rapidly, with pulmonary artery pressure decreasing from systemic levels in the fetus to 50% of systemic pressure at 3 days of life, and to low adult pressures by a week of life. The medial smooth muscle of the arteries involutes and the ductus and foramen ovale usually close permanently. An increase in NO production accompanies the decrease in pulmonary vascular resistance.

In addition to increasing pulmonary blood flow at birth, the neonate must clear significant amounts of alveolar and interstitial liquid that are residual from the fetal period. This is accomplished within the first 24 hours of extrauterine life, mainly by absorption into the pulmonary circulation, a process facilitated by sodium channels, possibly assisted by a membrane-bound protein, aquaporin, acting as a 'water channel'. Other important changes that occur early in life are the continued development of new alveoli and microvessels; this occurs mostly over the first 2 years, being complete by 8 years.

VENTILATION/PERFUSION RELATIONSHIPS

Almost all the cardiac output flows through the lungs, so pulmonary blood flow closely approximates to cardiac output (5 L/min). As $\dot{V}_A$ and cardiac output at rest are roughly the same, the overall (whole lung) ventilation ($\dot{V}$) to perfusion ($\dot{Q}$) ratio is close to 1. Previous sections of this chapter have described how both ventilation and perfusion of the lungs are greater in dependent regions, in such a way that regional ventilation and perfusion remain approximately matched irrespective of the posture of the subject. In the fairly extreme example of the upright posture, the gravitational effects on perfusion tend to be greater than on ventilation, and V/Q ratios are a little higher in the lung apices than in the bases.

When smaller units of lung tissue are considered, values for V/Q ratios in different regions become less uniform, ranging from 0.3 to 3 in a young healthy subject. This scatter of V/Q ratios becomes wider in older subjects, even in the absence of lung disease. Measurement of the scatter of V/Q ratios involves using the multiple inert gas technique, a research procedure that is not widely available. A slightly less precise approach is that adopted by Riley, whose model considers the lung as having only three V/Q ratio compartments: ventilated but unperfused alveoli (alveolar dead space, V/Q ratio of ∞); perfused but unventilated alveoli (pulmonary shunt, V/Q ratio 0); and appropriately perfused and ventilated 'ideal' alveoli (V/Q ratio 1) (Fig. 47.7). Though this is clearly not a true representation of the in vivo situation, Riley's model is helpful in the interpretation of clinical situations where V/Q ratios are abnormal.

The scatter of *V/Q* ratios becomes wider in older subjects, even in the absence of lung disease.

Alveolar dead space

In healthy subjects the alveolar dead space is too small to be measured reliably. However, any situation that reduces global or regional pulmonary blood flow will lead to areas of lung which are *relatively* underperfused for their ventilation, or not perfused at all, leading to an increase in alveolar dead space. An extreme example is pulmonary embolism. If the entire blood supply to one lung were to be completely occluded but that lung still underwent ventilation, then the entire ventilation to that lung would constitute alveolar dead space. Less extreme examples include a sudden fall in cardiac output in which perfusion to nondependent areas of lung decreases while their ventilation remains unchanged. During anesthesia with artificial ventilation, this will result in a dramatic reduction of the end-expiratory CO_2 as dead space suddenly increases. Positive-pressure ventila-

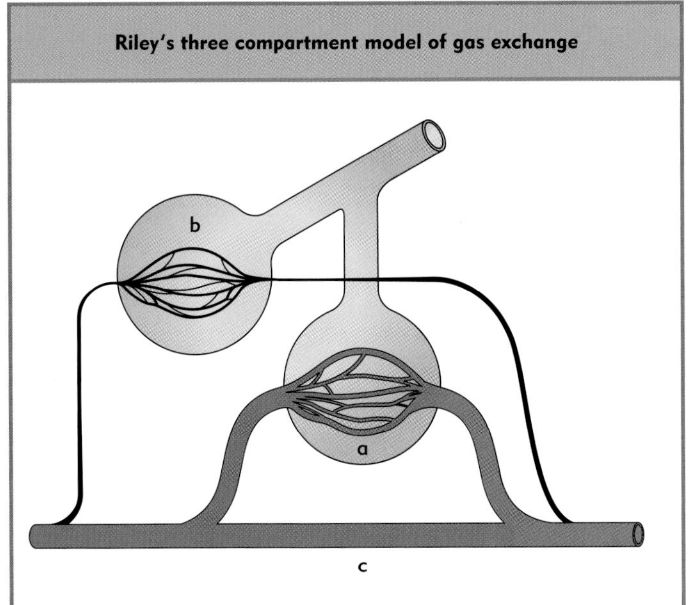

Figure 47.7 Riley's three compartment model of gas exchange. (a) The ideal alveolar unit (*V/Q* ratio 1); (b) the ventilated but unperfused unit (alveolar dead space, V/Q ratio ∞) and (c) the perfused, but unventilated unit (shunt, V/Q ratio 0).

tion also increases alveolar dead space, by causing preferential flow of gas to, and reducing pulmonary blood flow to, non-dependent portions of the lung, worsening *V*/Q mismatch.

Positive-pressure ventilation worsens *V/Q* mismatch.

Shunt

Not all blood returning to the left side of the heart from the pulmonary circulation has been fully oxygenated, and this blood is referred to as shunt. While the O_2 tension in an ideal alveolar capillary closely approximates that in the alveoli, venous blood returning from 'ideal' alveoli is diluted by poorly oxygenated or mixed venous blood from a number of sources as it reaches the left side of the circulation. Some shunt occurs from normal anatomic blood flow returning to the left side of the heart and is described as extrapulmonary shunt, for example venous return from bronchial and thebesian veins. Occasionally, venous admixture may result from abnormal anatomic variants, for example intracardiac shunting of blood from the right to the left side of the circulation, as occurs in some forms of congenital heart disease.

Intrapulmonary shunt involves blood flow through areas of lung with excessive perfusion for the amount of ventilation (low *V*/Q ratio) or through areas with no ventilation at all (*V*/Q = 0). General anesthesia, with or without paralysis, decreases FRC by relaxing the intercostal muscles and diaphragm, in many cases causing dependent areas of lung to collapse. These changes disturb the normal distribution of ventilation and perfusion sufficiently to cause an increased scatter of *V*/Q ratios, and the collapsed areas will constitute an intrapulmonary shunt with a *V*/Q ratio of 0. Surgery involving the abdominal or thoracic cavities will exacerbate the decrease in FRC by increasing diaphragmatic, chest wall, or retractor pressure on the lungs. In healthy humans, overall *V*/Q ratio increases from 0.8 before anesthesia to 1.3 during anesthesia with spontaneous ventilation, to 2.2 during positive-pressure ventilation, and to 3.0 with positive end-expiratory pressure (PEEP). Although PEEP decreases shunt by increasing FRC, it also decreases pulmonary blood flow, thereby decreasing the mixed venous oxygen partial pressure ($P_{\bar{v}}O_2$) and barely increasing that in the arteries (P_aO_2).

Shunt Equation

The shunt equation is used to calculate the proportion of blood passing through the lungs that is not participating in gas exchange. It follows Riley's model, and assumes that all blood has come either from alveoli with a normal *V*/Q ratio or from shunt carrying mixed venous blood. Blood that has come from regions of lung with low – but not zero – *V*/Q ratio will also contribute to the value obtained when using the shunt equation, but cannot be quantified. The shunt equation is based on the assumption that total O_2 flux through the pulmonary circulation is the sum of capillary and shunt O_2 flux.

■ Equation 47.4

$$(Cc'_{O_2} \times \dot{Q}c) + (C_{\bar{v}}O_2 \times \dot{Q}S) = Ca_{O_2} \times \dot{Q}T$$

where $Cc'O_2$ is pulmonary end-capillary blood oxygen content, $C_{\bar{v}}O_2$ is mixed venous blood oxygen content, CaO_2 is arterial blood oxygen content, $\dot{Q}c$ is pulmonary capillary blood flow, $\dot{Q}S$ is blood flow through the shunt, and $\dot{Q}T$ is total cardiac output.

This can be rearranged as:

■ Equation 47.5

$$\frac{\dot{Q}S}{\dot{Q}T} = \frac{C_{c'}O_2 - CaO_2}{C_{c'}O_2 - C_{\bar{v}}O_2}$$

where $\frac{\dot{Q}s}{\dot{Q}t}$ is the shunt fraction.

In order to use this clinically, it is necessary to derive $Cc'O_2$. Alveolar PO_2 may be calculated from the alveolar air equation (Chapter 48), and this value must then be converted to oxygen saturation by reference to the oxygen–hemoglobin dissociation curve. Finally, oxygen content is calculated using hemoglobin concentration, remembering to include a contribution from O_2 carried in blood in physical solution.

EFFECT OF SHUNT ON OXYGENATION

Shunt can result in severe arterial hypoxemia. Although the lung apex has a higher *V*/Q ratio than the base, it contributes less to total oxygenation because of its lower blood flow. This effect is further exacerbated by the sigmoid shape of the oxyhemoglobin dissociation curve: as hemoglobin cannot be more than 100% saturated, very high values of arterial PO_2 contribute relatively little to O_2 carriage in the blood compared to more moderate levels of arterial PO_2. For both these reasons, areas with high *V*/Q ratios cannot compensate for those areas with low *V*/Q ratio, and arterial PO_2 will fall.

For similar reasons, an increase in the inspired oxygen concentration will have limited success in correcting hypoxemia caused by *V*/Q mismatching. It will be highly beneficial in areas of the lung with low *V*/Q ratio, but will have no effect in areas with *V*/Q ratio of 0, as the extra oxygen cannot gain access to the blood flow through these regions.

An increase in the inspired oxygen concentration will have limited success in correcting hypoxemia caused by *V/Q* mismatching.

The effect of V/Q mismatching on arterial Po_2 may be exacerbated if cardiac output falls. With reduced cardiac output whole body O_2 delivery falls, and if O_2 extraction remains constant C_VO_2 will also fall. Where shunt is large, no matter how high the value of $Cc'O_2$, the mixing of venous blood with a low and falling O_2 content will result in reduced arterial Po_2. This effect is partly offset because a reduction in cardiac output results in a similar reduction in shunt fraction. Many investigators have observed that these two effects cancel each other out almost completely, except where shunt is very large, cardiac output is very low, or where shunt is a consequence of regional pulmonary atelectasis. There is reasonable evidence that the observed reduction in shunt is a consequence of HPV. This response is lost in severe acute lung injury; therefore, in this condition arterial oxygenation is often dependent upon cardiac output.

PULMONARY EDEMA

Under normal conditions the intact endothelial barrier allows the passage of small amounts of liquid into the interstitial space surrounding the vessel. Filtration occurs because the hydrostatic pressure is greater inside than outside the vessel. This filtrate contains small solutes such as sodium and chloride ions in isotonic concentrations, but the protein content is low compared to that of blood because the endothelium limits the passage of larger molecules. The liquid that leaves the normal microcirculation is reabsorbed from the interstitium by the protein osmotic (oncotic) pressure gradient into the microvessels downstream, where intravascular hydrostatic pressure is lower.

The passage of water and protein out of and into the microcirculation can be described by the Starling equation:

■ Equation 47.6

$$Jv = Lp.S(P_C - P_i) - s(p_C - p_i)$$

where Jv is the filtration rate across the microvascular endothelium, Lp is the hydraulic conductivity of the endothelium of surface area (S), $(P_c - P_i)$ represents the hydrostatic pressure gradient between the capillary (c) and the interstitium (i) driving the fluid out, and $(p_c - p_i)$ the osmotic pressure gradient favoring the passage of fluid back into the capillary. The constant s determines the physical properties of the membrane to allow the passage of proteins. Under normal conditions, a small amount of liquid is not reabsorbed into microvessels and moves from its initial perimicrovascular location in the alveolar wall to the extra-alveolar interstitium, where it is carried away from the lung by lymphatics. Lung lymph is returned to the blood via the thoracic duct, which empties into the right atrium.

Edema formation

The terms of the Starling equation differentiate 'hydrostatic' edema from 'permeability' edema. In hydrostatic edema, the driving forces $(P_C - P_i)$ and $(p_C - p_i)$ and the available surface area (S) for filtration are increased, favoring the outflow of liquid containing little protein into the interstitium. The terms Lp and s, which describe barrier characteristics, remain constant. In permeability edema, Lp increases and s decreases, signifying loss of barrier properties, and protein-rich liquid flows into the interstitium.

During hydrostatic pulmonary edema when endothelial and alveolar barriers are intact, microvascular reabsorption and lymphatic clearance can remove most of the liquid (Fig. 47.8). Excess liquid that is not removed by these mechanisms moves into the loose interstitial space surrounding bronchi and vessels. Clearance of protein-poor liquid from the interstitium occurs rapidly, over several hours. The capacity of the interstitial space has been estimated at 7 mL/kg: about 500 mL in a 70 kg human. This amount of pulmonary edema will be visible on a chest radiograph yet may not affect oxygenation because the alveoli are protected from the entry of edema liquid. Oxygenation decreases when liquid enters alveoli and blood passing by the walls of these alveoli cannot take on oxygen (i.e. shunt occurs). The alveoli are protected by the large capacity of the interstitial space and by tight junctions between alveolar epithelial cells.

The scenario of edema liquid movement just described occurs in the setting of intact endothelial (microvascular) and epithelial (alveolar) barriers. When either the endothelial or the epithelial barrier becomes more permeable, some protective mechanisms cease to operate. A damaged epithelium allows the easy passage of edema liquid, and the absorptive properties of the interstitium are less protective. Liquid can pass from interstitium to alveoli and back, depending on relative pressures in the two sites. Protein-rich edema liquid from the alveolar spaces may move into the larger airways, causing visible airway edema. Oxygenation deteriorates as alveoli become filled with fluid and alveolar hypoventilation occurs. Hypoventilation is caused by

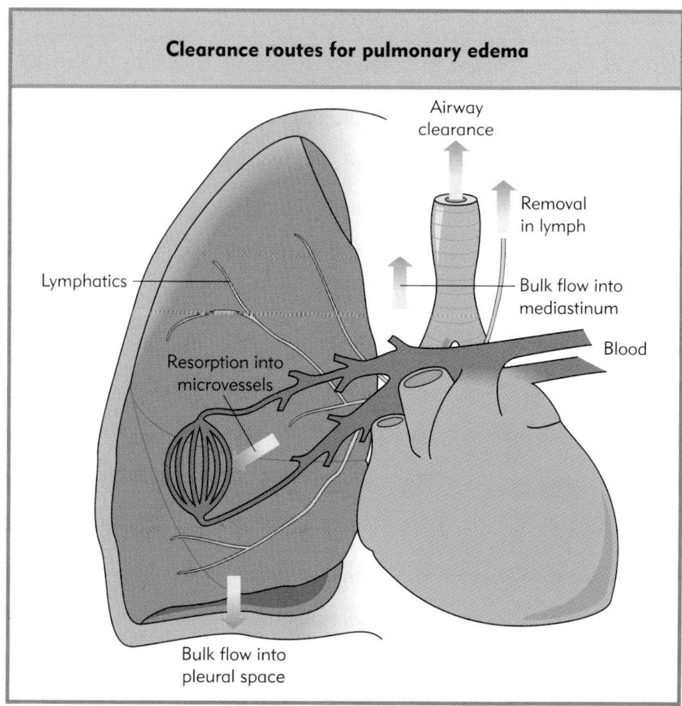

Figure 47.8 Clearance routes of pulmonary edema. Most edema fluid is cleared via microvascular reabsorption and lymphatic clearance, the rest by bulk flow into pleural space or mediastinum, and airway clearance.

the increasing work of breathing through edematous, noncompliant lungs.

Treatment

Because of this sequence of events in the formation of hydrostatic and increased permeability edema, current therapy is directed at lowering intravascular pressures and providing positive airway-distending pressures. First-line therapy is often aimed at lowering intravascular hydrostatic pressure with the use of loop diuretics and nitrates, which will favor the passage of water out of the interstitium back into the capillaries ($P_c - P_i$). Positive airway pressure, via either CPAP or artificial ventilation, will increase extravascular pressure, thereby preventing further fluid escaping into the airways as well as decreasing shunt and lessening the work of breathing. Therapy should also be aimed at treating the underlying problem leading to edema formation.

PULMONARY HYPERTENSION

Global hypoxia causes an increase in pulmonary vascular tone throughout the lung. The pulmonary hypertensive response to hypoxia is greatest in individuals with increased smooth muscle and collagen content in the medial layers of the arteries (e.g. in normal neonates and people living at high altitudes. In patients with long-term hypoxia secondary to chronic lung pathology pulmonary hypertension develops and leads to right heart failure and cor pulmonale. Known as secondary pulmonary hypertension, this can also occur with intermittent hypoxia from, for example, severe sleep apnea syndrome when hypoxia only occurs at night. Therapy with supplemental oxygen counteracts this effect, and delays the development of pulmonary hypertension. Primary pulmonary hypertension is a rare condition, often familial, in which there is proliferation of endothelial and smooth muscle cells in the pulmonary blood vessels. Most patients die in early adulthood, with many drug treatments being attempted but which are usually ineffective, leaving only lung transplantation as a realistic treatment option.

ASPIRATION PNEUMONIA

The passage of gastric contents into the larynx or oropharynx may lead to a form of acute lung injury. The syndrome seen is dependent on the quantity and nature of the substances inhaled and on the host's response. There are three components to the injury:

- Mechanical obstruction of the airways due to particulate material in the aspirate. This will lead to V/Q mismatching or collapse of the lung distal to the obstruction.
- Chemical injury may develop because of the acidic nature of gastric contents. The resulting aspiration pnuemonitis (Mendelson's syndrome) causes a chemical burn to the pulmonary parenchyma. As with any burn there is a biphasic response, the first a direct caustic effect on the cells of the lung, and the second, peaking 4–6 hours after the injury, is associated with cellular infiltrates and activation of inflammatory cells. The acute lung injury that results would then be indistinguishable from any other seen in intensive care, and is characterized by loss of surfactant, regional atelectasis, and V/Q mismatching.
- Infection develops if the material aspirated is colonized with bacteria, or when airway burns allow infection to develop from commensal pathogens. If the host's defenses are incapable of mounting a suitable response then a bacterial pneumonia will occur. It is this, along with the radiographic changes, that is classically referred to as 'aspiration pneumonia'.

Key references

Barker PM, Olver RE. Clearance of lung liquid during the perinatal period. J Appl Physiol. 2002;93:1542–8.

Barnes PJ, Liu SF. Regulation of pulmonary vascular tone. Pharmacol Rev. 1995;47:87–131.

Bhattacharya J. The microphysiology of lung liquid clearance. Adv Exp Med Biol. 1995;381:95–108.

Gurney AM. Multiple sites of oxygen sensing and their contributions to hypoxic pulmonary vasoconstriction. Respir Physiol Neurobiol. 2002;132:43–53.

Jeffery PK. Microscopic structure of normal lung. In: Brewis RAL, Corrin B, Geddes DM, Gibson GJ, eds. Respiratory medicine. London: WB Saunders, 1995;54–72.

Hedenstierna G. Atelectasis and its prevention during anaesthesia. Eur J Anaesthesiol. 1998;15:387–90.

Magnusson L, Spahn DR. New concepts of atelectasis during general anaesthesia. Br J Anaesth. 2003;91:61–72.

Marik PE. Aspiration pneumonitis and aspiration pneumonia. New Engl J Med. 2001;344:665–71.

Rubin LJ. Primary pulmonary hypertension. New Engl J Med 1997;336:111–q7.

Further reading

Cotes JE. Lung function. Assessment and application in medicine, 5th edn. Oxford: Blackwell Scientific, 1993.

Lumb AB. Nunn's applied respiratory physiology, 6th edn. Oxford: Elsevier; 2005.

West JB. Respiratory physiology – the essentials. Baltimore: Lippincott, Williams & Wilkins; 2004.

Chapter 48

Gas exchange

Mark C Bellamy and Simon Turner

TOPICS COVERED IN THIS CHAPTER

- **The composition of alveolar gas**
- **Gas transfer between alveolus and capillary**
- **Principles of oxygen transport**
- **Carbon dioxide transport**
- **Altitude and depth**
    - High altitude
    - Acute mountain sickness
    - High pressure and diving
- **Hyperbaric oxygen therapy**
- **Hypoxemia: mechanisms and systemic effects**
- **Oxygen therapy**
- **Extrapulmonary oxygenation**
    - IVOX, ECMO and the Novalung

Gas exchange and the transport of gases between the lung and tissues is a two-way process. Oxygen (O_2) passes from the atmosphere via the lungs, the bloodstream, extracellular fluid, and the interstitium into the cytoplasm of cells and ultimately into mitochondria. Metabolism of O_2 results in the production of high-energy phosphates in the cytoplasm and, predominantly, in the mitochondria. Consumption of O_2 results in the production of water and carbon dioxide (CO_2). Carbon dioxide is eliminated by a similar process 'in reverse'.

There is a gradient of O_2 partial pressures between atmospheric air, alveoli, and so on, down to the mitochondria (Fig. 48.1). The total O_2 available to tissues passing down this cascade is known as the 'O_2 flux' and it represents O_2 delivery (DO_2). Many factors have an impact on tissue DO_2, and these are discussed in physiologic sequence from the alveoli to the mitochondria.

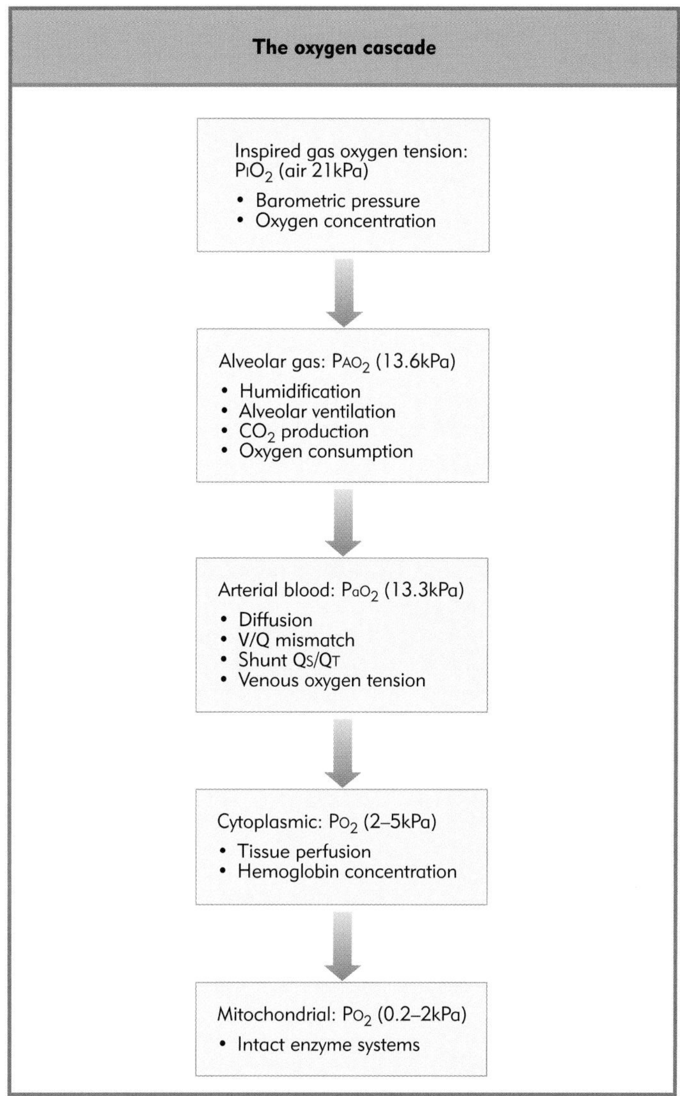

Figure 48.1 The oxygen cascade. Factors that contribute to the typical values are shown. Conversions: 21 kPa at sea level = 160 mmHg (1 atm = 100 kPa = 760 mmHg).

THE COMPOSITION OF ALVEOLAR GAS

The concentration of O_2 measured in the alveoli differs from that in inspired gas. First, inspired air is warmed and humidified through the upper airway. The nasal conchae and airway mucosa are important in this process. Warming and humidification of inspired gases continues down to the alveolar level. By the time gas reaches the alveoli, water vapor has been added at its saturated vapor pressure at body temperature. This is close to 6.3 kPa (1 atm = 100 kPa = 760 mmHg) and reduces the partial pressure of the components of inhaled gas. In the alveoli, O_2 is continuously diffusing down its concentration gradient into the blood, and is replaced by diffusion of CO_2 in the opposite direction. There is sinusoidal variation of the composition of alveolar gas through the respiratory cycle, but this is minimized because tidal alveolar ventilation is < 20% of functional residual capacity (FRC, the volume of gas in the alveoli at end-expiration). The alveolar partial pressure of O_2 (P_AO_2) is further reduced because the volume of CO_2 eliminated through the lungs is less than the net volume of O_2 taken up: this relationship is defined by the respiratory exchange ratio (RER). The major determinant of the RER is the respiratory quotient (RQ), which it equals at equilibrium, but the RER is also influenced by changes in ventilation, acid–base status and body temperature.

P_AO_2 may therefore be estimated by the following form of the alveolar gas equation:

■ Equation 48.1

$$P_AO_2 = P_IO_2 - \frac{P_ACO_2}{RER}$$

where P_IO_2 is the fractional inspired O_2 multiplied by (barometric pressure minus saturated water vapour pressure at body temperature).

The alveolar gas equation enables estimation of the alveolar partial pressure of O_2.

Derivation of this 'ideal' alveolar partial pressure of O_2 assumes that alveolar dead space (Chapter 47) is negligible. The value of RER also presents a possible inaccuracy, as measured values determine the RER of mixed expired gas, which is then assumed to closely approximate that of ideal alveolar gas. This version of the equation is sufficiently accurate for the approximation of P_AO_2 in many clinical situations, but it implies, when RER is not unity, that the FRC changes. Under most conditions the RER is less than 1, and the removal of more O_2 from, than the addition of CO_2 to, the FRC generates a pressure gradient for bulk flow of inspired gas from the anatomical dead space, thereby producing a concentrating effect of O_2 within the alveoli. This explains how PaO_2 is maintained during apneic oxygenation. The full form of the alveolar gas equation allows for this effect:

■ Equation 48.2

$$P_AO_2 = P_IO_2 - \frac{P_ACO_2}{RER}[1 - F_IO_2\,(1 - RER)]$$

where F_IO_2 is the inspired O_2 fraction.

An alternative form of the alveolar gas equation does not require calculation of the RER:

■ Equation 48.3

$$P_AO_2 = P_IO_2 - P_ACO_2\frac{(P_IO_2 - P_{\bar{E}}O_2)}{P_{\bar{E}}CO_2}$$

where $P_{\bar{E}}$ is the partial pressure of mixed expired gas.

Equation 48.2 fails to take account of changes in inert gas concentration, making no assumption about them and automatically compensating; consequently, if both versions of the equation are applied during periods of induction or recovery from nitrous oxide anesthesia they will produce different results. The difference between these results allows theoretic quantification of alveolar nitrous oxide concentration.

GAS TRANSFER BETWEEN ALVEOLUS AND CAPILLARY

Alveolar gases pass into pulmonary capillaries by passive diffusion according to their physicochemical properties. The extent to which this process occurs for O_2 is related to pulmonary capillary transit time. Under normal circumstances, O_2 transfer falls just short of equilibrium. Therefore, pulmonary blood flow, rather than the capacity for O_2 diffusion, normally limits pulmonary capillary oxygenation. This situation may differ in the face of pathologic processes or reduced inspired O_2 concentration (for example at low barometric pressure).

Oxygen in the alveolus is separated from capillary blood by a membrane. Outside the basement membrane are collagen and elastic fibers, though these are absent where alveolus and pulmonary capillary overlap. The capillary is separated from the alveolus only by a small tissue space. A single-cell layer of endothelium with basement membrane has a thickness of 0.2 μm, bringing the total thickness of the alveolar capillary membrane to 0.5 μm. The mean diameter of the pulmonary capillary is around 7 μm (i.e. similar to the diameter of a red blood cell). This arrangement forces red blood cells into close contact with the alveolar capillary membrane, which facilitates rapid uptake of O_2 into the cell.

The diffusing capacity for O_2 is the ratio between O_2 uptake and the alveolus-to-pulmonary capillary tension gradient driving uptake, which is difficult to quantify. In clinical practice, diffusing capacity is generally measured for carbon monoxide (CO). This is because the affinity of hemoglobin for CO is extremely high and the tension of CO in pulmonary capillary blood is, in effect, always zero. The formula for calculating diffusing capacity is thus simplified to:

■ Equation 48.4

$$\text{Diffusing capacity (CO)} = \frac{\text{CO uptake}}{P_ACO}$$

The elements in this equation are much more readily measured than those in the equivalent equation for O_2. A low value for CO diffusing capacity does not necessarily mean that there is thickening of the alveolar capillary membrane or impermeability (e.g. caused by fibrosis or edema formation) at this level. The lesion may be entirely functional. Furthermore, diffusing capacity may become abnormal where there is V/Q mismatching or a short capillary transit time. A reference value for CO transfer factor at steady state varies from laboratory to laboratory, but is around 113 mL/min/kPa, of which the most significant component is thought to relate to diffusing capacity across the membrane. The CO transfer factor varies considerably with body size, because although the alveolar-to-capillary tension gradients are similar irrespective of body size, gas volume and alveolar capillary membrane surface area vary greatly with size. Transfer factor (diffusing capacity) is therefore substantially greater when lung volume is large. Likewise, advancing age results in a reduction of diffusing capacity.

Interestingly, posture is also associated with changes in transfer factor. Diffusing capacity is considerably increased with supine posture. This may at first seem paradoxical, as supine posture is associated with reduced lung volume and increased *V*/Q mismatching. One explanation is that supine posture is also associated with more uniform pulmonary blood flow and an increase in total pulmonary blood volume. This may also be associated with reduced pulmonary capillary transit time, allowing greater time to equilibrium in those capillary beds where transit time is a limiting factor. Diffusing capacity is increased with exercise (up to a plateau), which again is likely to be related to elevated cardiac output and increases in both total pulmonary blood flow and $\dot{V}$A.

Diffusing capacity is increased with large lung volumes, with supine posture, but decreases in advanced age.

PRINCIPLES OF OXYGEN TRANSPORT

As can be seen from Figure 48.1, there is a cascade of O_2 tensions from alveolus to mitochondrion. At this level, O_2 functions as an electron acceptor in the energy-generating processes of oxidative phosphorylation and production of ATP (see Chapters 1 and 65). High-energy phosphate bonds in ATP are the fuel source for most biochemical and enzymatic processes of the cell. The delivery of O_2 to the tissues is the product of arterial O_2 content and cardiac output. The O_2 content of arterial blood is principally related to the O_2-carrying capacity of hemoglobin, although there is an additional component from dissolved O_2.

The delivery of O_2 to the tissues is the product of arterial O_2 content and cardiac output.

Hemoglobin is a tetramer of heme with four globin chains (two α and two β chains). Each hemoglobin molecule is capable of binding four molecules of O_2 to heme (Fig. 48.2). From this observation, and from the molecular weight of hemoglobin (around 63 500 Da) one can calculate that at 100% saturation 1.39 mL O_2 would combine with 1 g hemoglobin. The value measured in vivo is slightly less (1.34) as a result of forms of hemoglobin (carboxyhemoglobin, methemoglobin, sulphemoglobin) with reduced O_2 carrying capacity. Consequently, the bound O_2 in a given volume of blood is:

■ Equation 48.5

$$O_2 \text{ bound} = [Hb] \times SaO_2 \times 1.34$$

where [Hb] is hemoglobin concentration and SaO_2 is oxygen saturation. The dissolved O_2 in the same volume of blood can be calculated from P_aO_2 and the solubility constant (0.025 mL/kPa). Delivery of O_2 to the tissues is then given by:

■ Equation 48.6

$$DO_2 = \{([Hb] \times 1.34 \times SaO_2) + (P_aO_2 \times 0.025)\} \times \dot{Q}$$

where $\dot{Q}$ is cardiac output.

When O_2 is bound to hemoglobin, the conformation of the protein changes and the globin chains slide across each other (Fig. 48.2). When O_2 is unloaded the β chains pull apart. This allows the glycolytic metabolite 2,3-diphosphoglycerate (2,3-DPG) to slide between them and bind, resulting in lower affinity of hemoglobin for O_2. The well-known sigmoid shape of the oxyhemoglobin dissociation curve results from this cooperative or allosteric binding of O_2 (Fig. 48.3). The partial pressure of O_2 at which hemoglobin is 50% saturated is known as P_{50}, which is normally 3.55 kPa (26.6 mmHg). As O_2 affinity increases, the sigmoid curve is shifted to the left; in other words, P_{50} falls. Correspondingly, when O_2 affinity is reduced, the curve shifts

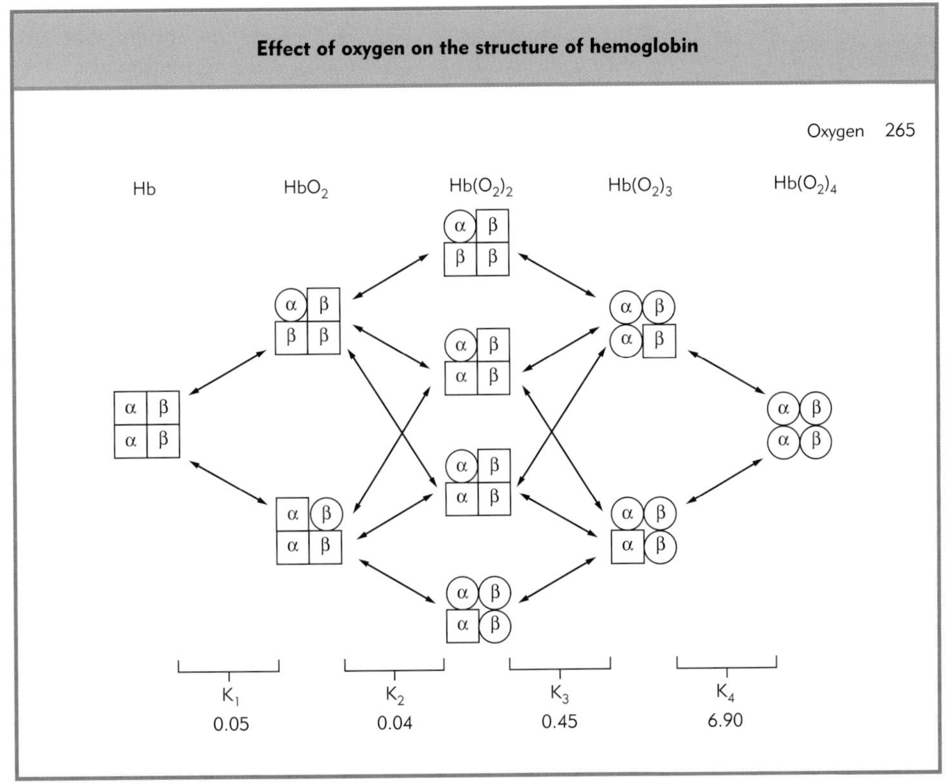

Figure 48.2 A schematic of the effect of oxygen on the structure of hemoglobin. The circles and squares symbolize two conformational states of the α- and β-globin chains of hemoglobin. The circles symbolize a low-affinity state and the squares a high-affinity state. The two states differ significantly in structure and in their subunit interactions, as well as in their O_2 affinities. The binding of one O_2 molecule to one subunit in the tetrameric protein alters the conformation of that subunit and alters subunit interactions. This strains the other subunit structures and induces them to undergo structural changes and assume the high-affinity state. This transition is responsible for the cooperative O_2-binding behavior of hemoglobin, leading to the sigmoid binding curve and cooperative O_2 binding. (With permission from Nunn JF. Nunn's applied respiratory physiology, 4th edn. Oxford: Butterworth Heinemann; 1993.)

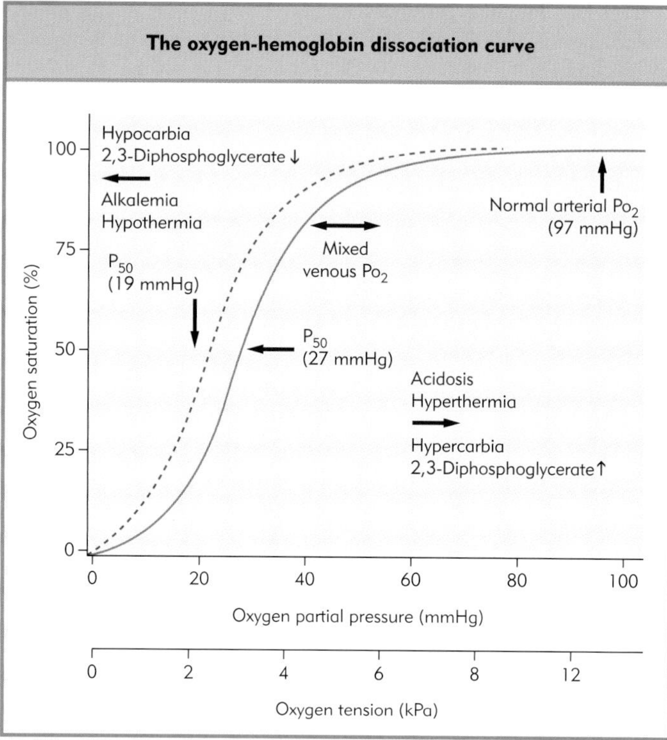

Figure 48.3 The oxyhemoglobin dissociation curve. The affinity of hemoglobin for oxygen is altered in either direction by the physiological variables indicated. Note that fetal blood is adapted to operate at a lower PO_2 than adult blood.

right and P_{50} rises. The normal P_aO_2 (97 mmHg or 13 kPa) is typically associated with an O_2 saturation of 98–100%. The O_2 saturation of mixed venous blood is around 75%: approximately 25% of O_2 delivered to tissues is used for metabolic processes, and the remaining 75% is returned to the heart and lungs still in combination with hemoglobin. This corresponds to a mixed venous value ($P_{\bar{v}}O_2$) between 40 and 50 mmHg (5.3 and 6.7 kPa). Typical whole body O_2 delivery is of the order of 650 mL/min/m^2, and typical O_2 extraction is around 160 mL/ min/m^2.

The shape of the oxyhemoglobin dissociation curve permits a high saturation at a range of arterial $Pa{O_2}$ values and unloading of O_2 at the tissues.

The oxyhemoglobin dissociation curve is shifted to the right by 2,3-DPG, increasing temperature, increasing acidosis, and increasing PCO_2 (the Bohr effect). The reverse of these processes causes a corresponding left shift. The usual stimulus for O_2 to be unloaded from hemoglobin is falling tissue PO_2. The more hypoxic and acidotic a tissue bed becomes, the more O_2 carried on hemoglobin becomes available. This results in a corresponding reduction in O_2 saturation (Fig. 48.3). Conditions associated with tissue hypoxia bring about right-shifting of the curve, with reduced oxygen affinity. In the lung and pulmonary capillary bed the opposite conditions pertain, which result in a left shift with increasing O_2 affinity and uptake. The capacity of P_{50} to change according to physiologic circumstances greatly enhances the ability of hemoglobin to load O_2 in the lung and unload it in (relatively) hypoxic tissues.

The sigmoid shape of the oxyhemoglobin dissociation curve has other important physiologic implications. Because the curve is roughly flat above a PO_2 of 80 mmHg (10.6 kPa), there is a relatively constant oxyhemoglobin saturation for arterial blood across the normal physiologic range, despite considerable variation in P_aO_2. The steep part of the oxyhemoglobin dissociation curve permits unloading of O_2 from hemoglobin even at relatively high PO_2 values. This favors the delivery of large amounts of O_2 into the tissues by diffusion.

Fetal hemoglobin differs structurally from adult hemoglobin. The β chains are replaced by γ chains. The fetal oxyhemoglobin dissociation curve is of a similar shape to that of the adult but is shifted to the left, resulting in a P_{50} of 20 mmHg. This means that fetal hemoglobin will load O_2 preferentially to adult hemoglobin, thus ensuring the effective transfer of O_2 across the placenta from maternal to fetal blood. Fetal hemoglobin is rapidly replaced by adult hemoglobin during the first year of life, except in conditions such as sickle cell disease, where a high concentration of fetal hemoglobin may persist throughout life.

Although the majority of hemoglobin present in the adult is HbA (two α and two β chains), a small proportion of abnormal hemoglobin may also be present. Around 2% is represented by HbA_2, which is composed of two α and two δ chains.

Hemoglobin can combine with molecules other than O_2; the most important of these is CO, which has an affinity for hemoglobin around 300 times greater than that of O_2. The formation of carboxyhemoglobin (HbCO) gives rise to a functional anemia and tissue hypoxia, as it is incapable of binding O_2. This is compounded by displacement of the oxyhemoglobin dissociation curve to the left, which further worsens tissue hypoxia by limiting the ability of hemoglobin to unload O_2. Displacement of CO from hemoglobin occurs slowly under normal clinical conditions, but can be accelerated by the administration of 100% O_2 or by treatment in a hyperbaric oxygen chamber. The criteria for treatment with hyperbaric O_2 include a carboxyhemoglobin concentration of >20%, neurologic dysfunction, or a history of loss of consciousness.

The iron molecules located within the heme ring are normally in the +2 oxidative state (ferrous). Oxidation of hemoglobin to the ferric (+3) oxidative state results in the formation of methemoglobin, causing functional anemia because of its poor O_2-binding characteristics. A number of oxidant drugs and stresses may give rise to methemoglobinemia, including acetominophen (paracetamol) toxicity and local anesthetic toxicity, most notably with prilocaine. These result in excess production of methemoglobin, which overwhelms the erythrocyte membrane-bound enzyme methemoglobin reductase. Treatment is with either ascorbic acid or methylene blue (1 mg/kg).

Oxygen delivery to the tissues is a function not only of the O_2 content of arterial blood and the physicochemical properties of hemoglobin, but also of tissue blood flow. Blood flow depends on the arteriovenous pressure gradient and vascular resistance (Chapter 43). As arterial and venous pressures are generally constant, the principal determinant of blood flow across a tissue bed is the vascular resistance of the bed. Recent evidence indicates that hemoglobin may also control blood flow by regulating vascular constriction and dilation. A major portion of nitric oxide in the blood binds to thiols of hemoglobin, forming *S*-nitrosohemoglobin (SNO-Hb), which on deoxygenation in the microcirculation releases NO and *S*-nitrosothiols, causing vasodilatation and increased blood flow. Moreover, viscosity and shear forces between blood and the vessel wall are now known to play an important role in regulating vascular tone to maintain perfusion in high-viscosity states.

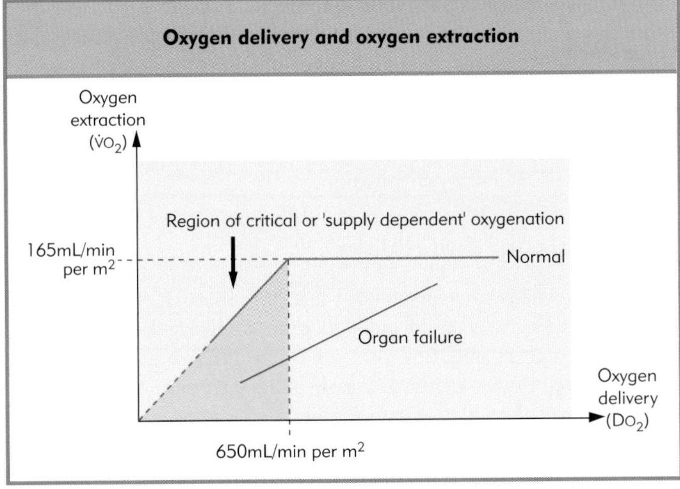

Figure 48.4 Relationship between oxygen delivery and oxygen extraction. See text for explanation.

The final stage of O_2 delivery to tissues is diffusion from capillary blood. This process is determined by the partial pressure gradient between the capillary and the cell. Oxygen utilization by tissues will increase the transcapillary O_2 tension gradient and (according to the shape of the oxyhemoglobin dissociation curve) the volume of O_2 unloaded to tissues. As long as the metabolic requirements of tissues are met, O_2 extraction is fairly constant, irrespective of DO_2. When DO_2 becomes flow limited, there is a linear relationship between O_2 delivery and O_2 extraction. This is known as flow-limited or critical O_2 delivery (Fig. 48.4). Pathologic disturbances of this relationship may occur in shock states and multisystem organ failure. Critical or inadequate DO_2 results in anaerobic metabolism, and the glycolytic pathway terminates in lactate production rather than further metabolism to the tricarboxylic acid cycle.

CARBON DIOXIDE TRANSPORT

As O_2 is consumed, CO_2 is produced. In general, the processes involved in CO_2 elimination are the reverse of those involved in O_2 absorption, as the same principles of partial pressure gradients and gas exchange apply. Carbon dioxide is much more soluble than O_2 in water and undergoes much more rapid tissue diffusion. Most CO_2 present in blood occurs as the bicarbonate ion. Generation of free CO_2 by metabolic processes rapidly results in the production of carbonic acid through the action of the catalytic enzyme carbonic anhydrase. This enzyme is present in large quantities in red blood cells. Carbon dioxide is transported in the circulation in three forms in dynamic equilibrium: the bicarbonate ion; free in physical solution; and as carbamino compounds (including those resulting from its binding to hemoglobin). As with O_2, physical solution is a relatively unimportant component, accounting for only about 6% of total CO_2 transfer. The solubility coefficient is around 0.23 mmol/L/kPa at body temperature.

Carriage as bicarbonate ion makes the greatest contribution to CO_2 transport (approximately 90%). Under the action of carbonic anhydrase, CO_2 combines with water according to the following equation (Chapter 60):

Carbon dioxide is transported in the circulation in three forms in dynamic equilibrium: the bicarbonate ion; free in physical solution; and as carbamino compounds.

■ Equation 48.7

$$CO_2 + H_2O \leftrightarrow H_2CO_3 \leftrightarrow H^+ + HCO_3^-$$

Carbamino compounds are formed by the reversible chemical reaction between CO_2 and terminal amino groups of protein chains or side-chain amino groups of lysine. The predominant site for formation of carbamino compounds in blood is hemoglobin. Reduced hemoglobin is at least three times more capable of binding CO_2 than is oxyhemoglobin. It is also less acidic than oxyhemoglobin. This facilitates its function as a proton acceptor, and in this way increases the solubility and production of bicarbonate ions. These two processes facilitate uptake of CO_2 in peripheral tissues. Hence the blood CO_2 tension/content values for arterial and venous blood differ, but only slightly. The reverse processes occur in the lung, promoting off-loading of CO_2 (Haldane effect). Additionally, CO_2 is transported by dissociation of carbonic acid to bicarbonate and hydrogen ions within red cells. The hydrogen ions are buffered by hemoglobin, and the bicarbonate diffuses out of the erythrocyte down a concentration gradient in exchange for chloride ions (the Hamburger shift). The reverse occurs in the lungs.

ALTITUDE AND DEPTH

High altitude

As altitude increases, barometric pressure falls. The concentration of atmospheric O_2 is a constant, at 21%. At sea level this represents 21 kPa, but this partial pressure is reduced with increasing altitude. A second phenomenon that comes into play at high altitude is reduced PO_2 secondary to dilution with water vapor. The saturated vapor pressure at body temperature is 6.3 kPa. Therefore, the PO_2 of inspired air reaching the lower airway is:

■ Equation 48.8

$$P_IO_2 = 0.21(\text{barometric pressure} - 6.3)\ \text{kPa}$$

Most commercial aircraft fly at an altitude of 9100 m (30 000 feet) and military aircraft at much greater altitudes. Such aircraft are pressurized to ~2400 m (8000 ft), and military aircraft use supplemental O_2. This is crucial, because at 19 000 m (63 000 feet), depending on weather conditions, barometric pressure is only 6.3 kPa, and therefore equals the saturated vapor pressure of water at body temperature. Hence P_AO_2 and P_ACO_2 become zero. In practice, asphyxiation would occur at lower altitudes.

Fortunately for mountaineers, there is also an effect of geographical location and latitude. Barometric pressure in the Himalayas is consistently slightly higher than that predicted from altitude alone. At the summit of Mount Everest, barometric pressure has been measured at 2.5 kPa greater than expected. This is crucial to the feasibility of ascents without supplemental O_2. At 9100 m (30 000 feet) the P_IO_2 is predicted to be 4.9 kPa. Up to approximately this height the use of 100% O_2 can restore P_IO_2 to the sea-level value. Lower P_IO_2 values will be obtained using supplemental O_2 at heights between

10 000 and 19 000 m (33 000 and 63 000 feet, respectively). At 19 000 m the saturated vapor pressure of water exceeds atmospheric pressure, and therefore body fluids (and water at body temperature) will begin to boil.

Rapid ascent to altitude from sea level, for example by an unpressurized aircraft, results in a number of physiologic and ventilatory changes: a rapid reduction in $P_{I}O_2$ reduces $P_{A}O_2$. The reduction in $P_{A}O_2$ is offset by hyperventilation (see Equations 48.1–48.3). This response is suboptimal, as the ventilatory response to hypoxia is attenuated by the resulting hypocapnia (Chapter 46). Where altitude is sustained for some days, acclimatization begins to occur. During this process, bicarbonate shifts in cerebrospinal fluid restore ventilatory drive. Early signs of hypoxia at altitude include impairment of night vision and impairment of mental performance. In the extreme form this can lead to loss of consciousness. This occurs on acute ascent to altitudes above 6000 m (20 000 feet). The time between attaining altitude and loss of consciousness varies according to the altitude reached. This is important to pilots in the event of acute cabin pressure loss. The shortest time to loss of consciousness is one lung–brain circulation time (this is similar to the well-known arm–brain circulation time in anesthesia) of 15 seconds. At heights below 16 000 m (50 000 feet) there is a longer interval before loss of consciousness.

Acute mountain sickness

Climbers who ascend to altitude slowly experience different effects from those that occur with rapid changes in altitude. This relates to a slower rate of ascent and much greater physical exertion. Acute mountain sickness has been divided into benign and malignant forms, but these conditions are probably only points on a pathologic spectrum, and benign forms may progress to malignant. Unacclimatized climbers develop breathlessness or exertional dyspnea at 2000 m (6600 feet). At greater altitudes, headache, nausea, and sleep disturbance develop. Above 5000 m (16 000 feet) climbers experience dysphoria, amnesia, and dizziness. Dyspnea is experienced at rest. Sleep apnea is also common at this altitude. Most commonly Cheyne–Stokes breathing occurs, punctuated by periods of apnea. This greatly exacerbates hypoxia. Cheyne–Stokes breathing and sleep apnea are related to hypoxic ventilatory drive and are relatively uncommon in those who live habitually at high altitude. There may also be a genetic component to adaptation to altitude.

Pulmonary edema can complicate acute altitude exposure. It is more commonly seen in unacclimatized climbers than in those ascending more slowly and allowing full acclimatization; nevertheless, it is idiosyncratic. The etiology has not been incontrovertibly established, but likely explanations include hypoxic pulmonary vasoconstriction and acute pulmonary hypertension. Cognitive dysfunction may be further complicated by cerebral edema. Papilledema has been observed.

As acute mountain sickness in its malignant form is often rapidly fatal, treatment should include descent from altitude, supplemental O_2, and treatment of fluid overload (for example with acetazolamide, a carbonic anhydrase inhibitor and diuretic).

Acute mountain sickness in its malignant form is often rapidly fatal: treatment should include descent from altitude, supplemental O_2, and treatment of fluid overload.

Acclimatization at altitude occurs over a period of days or months. Components of acclimatization include bicarbonate shift in the cerebrospinal fluid, which restores hypoxic drive; hemoglobin concentration rises secondary to increasing erythropoietin levels; and a left shift in the oxyhemoglobin dissociation curve at altitude (facilitating O_2 uptake) through changes in both pH and 2,3-DPG concentration.

High pressure and diving

Exposure to high pressure has a venerable history. Alexander the Great was lowered to the sea bed in a diving bell in 320BC. Saturation divers and one or two other groups of workers are exposed to environments where the atmospheric pressure approximates that of the sea outside their diving bell or pressure suit. Ventilatory requirements at high barometric pressures are similar to those at standard temperature and pressure, provided O_2 consumption is expressed at standard temperature and pressure and minute volume at body temperature and at the barometric pressure to which the diver is exposed. Confusion is best avoided by thinking in terms of the number of molecules – or moles – of O_2 consumed or CO_2 produced. These are essentially constant irrespective of depth. However, the volume that a mole of O_2 occupies at standard temperature and pressure is 22.4 L, whereas at 10 atm it is 2.4 L. The value for fractional concentration of alveolar CO_2 ($C_{A}O_2$) is given by its rate of production divided by $\dot{V}A$. Both gas volumes must be measured under the same conditions of temperature and pressure. Therefore, $C_{A}CO_2$ at 10 atm is about one-tenth of sea-level values (i.e. around 0.53%). Likewise, $P_{A}O_2$ can be calculated from the alveolar gas equation (see above). Hence at 10 atm, $C_{I}O_2$ of 21% reflects a $P_{I}O_2$ of 210 kPa and a $P_{A}O_2$ of 203 kPa.

The effects of increased pressure on breathing mechanics are also significant. The effects of weight loss that divers experience through buoyancy, together with pressure on the thoracic cage, significantly alter respiratory mechanics and distribution of pulmonary blood flow. Gas density increases proportionally with pressure. Therefore, at 10 atm inspired gas is 10 times as dense as it is at sea level. As can be seen from Poiseuille's formula (Chapter 50) and the Reynolds' number, this will have the effect of increasing resistance to flow while at the same time reducing the tendency to turbulent flow. The maximum breathing capacity at sea level is 200 L/min, but this is reduced to 50 L/min at 15 atm. In practice, at barometric pressures above 6 atm it is customary for divers to breathe a helium–oxygen mixture. This reduces the tendency to nitrogen narcosis and restores maximum breathing capacity because the helium has a much lower density than nitrogen (or air). Helium–oxygen mixtures can also allow lower $C_{I}O_2$ values because these are still compatible at depth with an adequate $P_{A}O_2$.

HYPERBARIC OXYGEN THERAPY

Hyperbaric therapy with air dates back to 1662, when a British clergyman pumped air into a chamber using bellows in the belief that raised pressure would cure a variety of ailments. After the second world war (when it was used medically with an increase in oxygen concentration to facilitate cardiac surgery) the advent of cardiopulmonary bypass saw a decline in its use.

Exposure to oxygen under increased pressure can occur not only in medical use but also in commercial and recreational

SCUBA (self-contained underwater breathing apparatus) divers and people working underground.

Ideal gases under pressure obey the gas laws (Chapter 11); Boyle's law states that at a constant temperature, the volume of a gas is inversely proportional to the pressure applied; Henry's law states that at a constant temperature the amount of a gas dissolved in a liquid is proportional to the partial pressure of the gas.

Owing to the shape of the oxyhemoglobin dissociation curve (Fig. 48.3), increasing the oxygen tension above atmospheric pressure does not result in a significant increase in the amount of oxygen carried by hemoglobin. However, it is possible to increase dissolved oxygen and thus improve tissue oxygen delivery. Furthermore, in pathologic states where there is a reduction in the caliber of capillaries (such as in tissue edema) below that of the diameter of erythrocytes, O_2-rich plasma may still perfuse the tissues. Technically this is achieved by delivering 100% oxygen at pressures above atmospheric in a pressurized chamber; for example, at pressures of 2 atm absolute the $Pa\text{O}_2$ approaches 200 kPa.

Hyperbaric oxygen increases the oxygen carried in solution in the plasma.

Established indications for the use of hyperbaric oxygen therapy (HBOT) include decompression sickness (the 'bends') and air/gas embolism. The mechanism of action is a reduction in size of the nitrogen bubbles owing to a direct pressure effect. Further indications according to the Undersea and Hyperbaric Medical Society 1999 Committee report are listed in Table 48.1.

HBOT is not without its associated problems. These include pressure-related problems – barotrauma to air-filled spaces (sinuses, ears and lungs); those relating to oxygen toxicity (seizures and visual disturbances); and practical considerations (scarcity of decompression chambers – "pots" – and hence the need to transfer critically ill patients). Limited access to patients once in the chambers may also preclude their use.

Table 48.1 Indications for the use of hyperbaric oxygen therapy
Carbon monoxide poisoning and carbon monoxide poisoning complicated by cyanide poisoning
Clostridial myositis and myonecrosis (gas gangrene)
Crush injury, compartment syndrome and other traumatic ischemias
Enhancement of healing in selected problem wounds
Exceptional blood loss (anemia)
Intracranial abscess
Necrotizing soft tissue infections
Refractory osteomyelitis
Delayed radiation tissue damage (soft tissue and bone necrosis)
Compromised skin grafts and flaps
Thermal burns

The effects of HBOT are seen in the central nervous (CNS), pulmonary, and cardiovascular systems, as well as air-filled cavities. In the CNS, as the $P\text{O}_2$ increases there is a reduction in cerebral blood flow and intracranial pressure. This has been used clinically. Although a $Pa\text{O}_2$ greater than 1500 mmHg causes an increase in blood pressure and a reflex bradycardia due to an increase in systemic vascular resistance, oxygen delivery is increased despite a reduction in blood flow. Patients are also informed at the stage of consent that their visual acuity may alter – typically they become more myopic after repeated treatments. Although this may benefit long-sighted patients, the underlying cause is not yet fully understood.

In the lung, hyperbaric oxygen rapidly results in oxidant stress as free radical scavenging is overwhelmed. Patients develop coughing and chest pain. Continual exposure may result in pulmonary fibrosis. The harmful effects of HBOT may be attenuated by limiting the exposure of the patient to either high pressure or 100% oxygen concentrations. Practically, therefore, in multiplace chambers (able to treat up to eight or more patients at once) only the patients are exposed to 100% O_2 via a hood. The health professional monitoring the patients during the dive breathes around 30% (due to a small amount of leakage from the hoods), both to reduce their exposure and to reduce the chance of a fire within the chamber. Chamber fires have been universally fatal to date. With this in mind, strict precautions are put in place to reduce the risk; for example, the patients wear cotton clothes (nylon risks static electricity and spark formation), facial make-up is prohibited (as it is frequently oil based), and electrical equipment (such as hearing aids and personal stereo equipment) is forbidden.

HYPOXEMIA: MECHANISMS AND SYSTEMIC EFFECTS

The definition of hypoxemia is a reduced oxygen tension in the blood. This is generally taken as occurring when the $P\text{O}_2$ is lower than 8 kPa, where the oxyhemoglobin dissociation curve begins to steepen. The term hypoxia refers to the lack of O_2 at the tissues. The reduction in oxygen delivery to the tissues, and specifically the mitochondria, may occur because of a reduction in the oxygen content of the blood (see above), or because of local and regional reductions in blood flow, as occur physiologically in the splanchnic bed with exercise and pathologically in the kidneys in septic shock, for example.

The oxygen-carrying capacity of the blood may be reduced by either low levels of hemoglobin (anemia) or by different species of hemoglobin, for example met- (MetHb) and carboxyhemoglobin (COHb), which have different affinities for oxygen. COHb, has a far greater affinity for oxygen (around 200 times), and this causes problems in that oxygen is not released to the tissues. Carbon monoxide is a colorless, odorless gas produced by incomplete combustion of carbon-based fuels, and accounts for around 3500 accidental deaths in the USA every year.

Finally, hypoxia may occur in situations where the tissues are presented with a plentiful supply of oxygen that the mitochondria cannot utilize, for example in the case of cyanide poisoning. Different tissues tolerate hypoxemia to different degrees, and the concepts of survival and revival times have been used (brain 1 minute versus 4 minutes, heart 5 versus 20, and liver/kidney 10 minutes versus 40 minutes).

Table 48.2 The nonpulmonary causes of hypoxia	
Stagnant hypoxia	Poor tissue perfusion owing to reduced blood flow or increased distance for diffusion, as in tissue edema
Histotoxic hypoxia	Cellular poisoning, e.g. cyanide, which uncouples oxidative phosphorylation within the mitochondria
Anemic hypoxia	Reduced red cell mass or hemoglobin concentration, or reduced O_2-carrying capacity of hemoglobin

Arterial hypoxemia may further result from pulmonary and nonpulmonary causes. Hypoxemia may result from a low inspired oxygen concentration (e.g. altitude – see above),hypoventilation, *V*/Q mismatch, and venous admixture (see Chapter 47). The nonpulmonary causes of hypoxia are described in Table 48.2.

OXYGEN THERAPY

The aim of oxygen therapy is to reverse hypoxia. Oxygen can be delivered by 'constant' or 'variable' performance systems. This division divides devices into those that deliver a constant fraction of inspired oxygen (F_IO_2) independent of the patient's ventilation (fixed performance) and those where the F_IO_2 is dependent on the patient's ventilation (variable performance).

Commonly used oxygen delivery devices include:

- nasal cannulae;
- the Hudson Mask;
- Venturi masks;
- anesthetic breathing systems of the Mapleson classification;
- noninvasive ventilation;
- invasive ventilation.

There are disadvantages to using dry gases at high flows: patient cooling, dehydration, and disturbance of the mucociliary functions of the upper airways such that normal host defenses are impaired.

Variable performing devices are generally open systems. They are simple, disposable, and provide low flows. Examples are the Mary Catterall (MC) masks (and moulded plastic descendents) and nasal cannulae. The former consists simply of a 'facial tent' whereby when the patient inhales at a greater inspiratory flow rate than that delivered by the wall-mounted flow meter: the patient will entrain air from the environment in an unmeasured manner. In this way the concentration of the piped oxygen is reduced. As the patient's inspiratory flow rate alters, so does the degree to which ambient air is entrained. The nasal cannula demands special consideration as it is often wrongly felt that a patient who mouth-breathes will gain no benefit from such a device. However, throughout ventilation the nasopharynx is filled with O_2 and acts as a reservoir, such that this O_2 will be entrained when air is breathed through the mouth.

This feature of entraining gases leads to the principles behind the fixed-performance Venturi mask. The Venturi consists of a narrowed aperture with side holes and relies on the Bernoulli effect. As gas passes through the constriction at a set rate its velocity increases. According to Newton's law of the conservation of energy, as the velocity of the gas (or its kinetic energy) increases, its pressure (or potential energy) must fall. Thus the area of low pressure causes gas to be entrained at a known rate (dependent on the size of the constriction, side holes, and driving gas flow) and at a far higher flow rate than the patient's maximal inspiratory flow rate. Therefore, the concentration of oxygen delivered is independent of patient effort.

The Venturi mask delivers a fixed concentration of oxygen, independent of patient effort.

The above devices are totally open to the atmosphere. The following are semi-open or closed:

- continuous positive airway pressure devices, i.e. CPAP nasal and facial masks;
- invasive devices, i.e. endotracheal and tracheostomy tubes (closed);
- mechanical ventilators: intermittent positive-pressure ventilation (IPPV); bilevel positive airway pressure (BiPAP), and many other modes may be employed.

EXTRAPULMONARY OXYGENATION

IVOX, ECMO and the Novalung

These three strategies share the common feature that the lungs may be 'rested' and allowed to recover while gas exchange occurs elsewhere. Thus the main indications have been surgical (i.e. cardiopulmonary bypass) or medical (i.e. providing a period of lung maturation and growth in congenital diaphragmatic herniae and acute respiratory distress syndrome).

EXTRACORPOREAL MEMBRANE OXYGENATION (ECMO)

ECMO was originated by Kolff and Berk, who noticed that blood became oxygenated as it passed through the cellophane chambers of their artificial kidney. In 1956 Clowes developed the first membrane oxygenator for use in cardiopulmonary bypass. Now, despite its infrequent use, ECMO is largely confined to children. Current indications for treatment are essentially that a patient has respiratory failure causing hypoxia, which responds to neither best-practice ventilatory support nor other measures that could be expected to improve ventilation/perfusion mismatch.

Practically, ECMO requires the insertion of an intravenous catheter (right internal jugular, femoral, or iliac veins) and systemic heparinization of the patient. Initially the catheters were inserted venoarterially, but this required permanent ligation of the vessels and the risk of reducing cerebral blood flow. For this reason, ECMO is now largely conducted in a venovenous manner via a double-lumen catheter placed in the internal jugular vein.

INTRAVENOUS OXYGENATION (IVOX)

IVOX relies on the placement of a hollow-fiber oxygenator mounted on a double-lumen catheter. The fibers are 200 μm in diameter and contain micropores that facilitate gas exchange. Containing many thousands of fibers and extending around 40–50 cm in length once inserted via the femoral or internal jugular routes, the system extends from superior to inferior vena cava across the right atrium. Oxygen is supplied via negative pressure to allow gas exchange to occur between the intraluminal gas phase and the extraluminal blood phase by diffusion.

Complications of use include those of central venous access, hemorrhage (in part due to the necessity for systemic anticoagulation), infection, deep venous thrombosis (due to a reduction in venous drainage from the lower limb following femoral venous placement), and reduction in the efficiency of the device due to thrombus formation within the fiber bundle.

IVOX was indicated for oxygenation of patients with severe acute respiratory distress syndrome (ARDS) to allow for less aggressive conventional ventilation in the hope of avoiding baro- and volutrauma to the lungs. However, partly because of an increase in the sophistication of current ventilators and a better understanding of the disease process, and partly because of the complexity and complication rate of IVOX, it has now fallen out of favor.

NOVALUNG

The Novalung (Novalung GmbH) is a new device whereby a membrane oxygenator is connected to the patient via cannulae inserted into the femoral artery and vein on opposite sides. Thus the pressure to drive blood through the oxygenator comes from the patient's own blood pressure. The device is impregnated with heparin and so systemic anticoagulation is not required. The manufacturers anticipate the Novalung being used in situations where ease of portability is of use, for example in inter-hospital transfers. The device can be instituted 'in the field'. However, potential disadvantages include those of instrumenting the femoral vessels, potentially restricting perfusion of the lower limbs, and disconnection leading to potentially fatal hemorrhage.

Key references

Bouachour G. Hyperbaric oxygen therapy in the management of crush injuries : a randomised double-blind placebo controlled clinical trial. J Trauma Injury Infect Crit Care 1996;41:2.

Cosgrove H, Bryson P. Hyperbaric medicine in soft tissue trauma. Trauma 2001;3:133–41.

Johnson AO, Page RL, Sapsford DJ, Jones JG. Flying and hypoxaemia at altitude. New method is more precise. Br Med J. 1994;308:474.

Lindberg P, Gunnarsson L, Tokics L et al. Atelectasis and lung function in the postoperative period. Acta Anaesthesiol Scand. 1992;36:546–53.

Milledge JS. Acute mountain sickness: pulmonary and cerebral oedema of high altitude. Intensive Care Med. 1985;11:110.

Nunn JF, Benatar SR, Hewlett AM. The use of iso-shunt lines for control of oxygen therapy. Br J Anaesth. 1973;45:711–8.

Riley RL, Lilienthal JL, Proemmel DD, Franke RE. On the determination of the physiologically effective pressures of oxygen and carbon dioxide in alveolar air. Am J Physiol. 1946;147:191–8.

Waldau T. Evaluation of five oxygen delivery devices in spontaneously breathing subjects by oxygraphy. Anaesthesia 1998;53:256.

Further reading

Lumb AB. Nunn's applied respiratory physiology, 5th edn. Oxford: Butterworth–Heinemann; 2000.

Stamler JS, Jia L, Eu JP et al. Blood flow regulation by S-nitrosohemoglobin in the physiological oxygen gradient. Science 1997;276:2034–7.

West JB. Ventilation: blood flow and gas exchange, 5th edn. Oxford: Blackwell Scientific; 1990.

Chapter 49

Respiratory mechanics

Andrew T Cohen and Alison J Pittard

TOPICS COVERED IN THIS CHAPTER

- **Anatomy**
- **Volumes and capacities**
- **Ventilatory muscles**
- **Forces**
  - Lung compliance: the lung elastic forces
  - Chest wall compliance: chest wall elastic forces
  - Nonelastic forces
- **Mechanical ventilation**
  - Intubation and establishing ventilation
  - Types of ventilator
  - Modes of ventilation
  - Invasive ventilation
  - Pressure support
  - BIPAP
  - Other modes of ventilation
  - Noninvasive ventilation
  - Newer modes of ventilation – protective lung strategies

ANATOMY

The respiratory system consists of two mechanical components, the lungs and the surrounding thoracic cavity.

The lung is comprised of conducting airways, parenchyma, and pleura. The airways are a system of branching tubes starting at the mouth and nose and ending at the terminal bronchioles. No gas exchange occurs above this point. The terminal bronchioles divide into the respiratory bronchioles, which have occasional alveoli branching off their walls. Respiratory bronchioles lead to alveolar ducts, which are lined with alveoli and make up the bulk of the parenchyma. The number of alveoli is variable and correlates with the height of the patient. The alveolar wall consists of two types of epithelial cell. Type I cells line the alveoli and form a thin sheet approximately 0.1 μm thick. Type II cells do not function as gas exchange membranes but are responsible for surfactant production. The pleura is in two parts: the parietal pleura, which coats the inner part of the thoracic cavity, and the visceral pleura, which surrounds the lung. In health the two layers of pleura are closely applied and move as one. The pressure in the potential space between them is called the intrapleural pressure and is usually subatmospheric, owing to the elastic properties of the lung. Commonly this subatmospheric pressure is referred to as a negative pressure (that is, relative to atmospheric pressure). The intrapleural pressure varies in upright humans from the apex of the lung to the base. It is less negative (higher) at the base owing to the weight of the lung.

The chest wall is a rigid expandable box that encases the lungs. The bony ribcage is reinforced by intercostal muscles. The diaphragm and abdominal contents function as a piston, forcibly aspirating gas into the lungs during inspiration and encouraging expiration by passive relaxation. Elastic forces tend to make the lung collapse to residual volume. This is prevented by the elasticity of the chest wall, which would otherwise expand (Fig. 49.1). The volume of chest and lung at the end of quiet expiration is a balance between these elastic forces.

Gas flows from high pressure to low pressure. Flow rate is determined by pressure difference and resistance. The relationship between pressure difference and flow depends on the nature of the flow, which may be laminar, turbulent, or transitional (see insets, Fig. 49.1). Gas movement in an unbranched cylinder below its critical flow rate is streamlined with a higher flow at the center than at the periphery. Laminar gas flow is inaudible. Under these circumstances the flow rate is directly proportional to driving pressure when the resistance is constant. The Poiseuille equation (Chapter 50) demonstrates the relationship between flow and the fourth power of the radius, and explains the importance of airway narrowing.

The Poiseuille equation demonstrates the relationship between flow and the fourth power of the radius, and explains the importance of airway narrowing.

The nature of the airway, as well as gas velocity, will determine whether flow remains streamlined or becomes turbulent. Turbulence is characterized by the irregular movement of gas in contrast to the smooth velocity profile seen in laminar flow. Flow in the trachea has a high velocity and will normally be turbulent, as the airways divide and the flow rate reduces, it is more likely to become laminar. In parts of the bronchial tree where branching and reduction in tube diameter occur eddies will be seen in the flow for some distance down the airway – this is

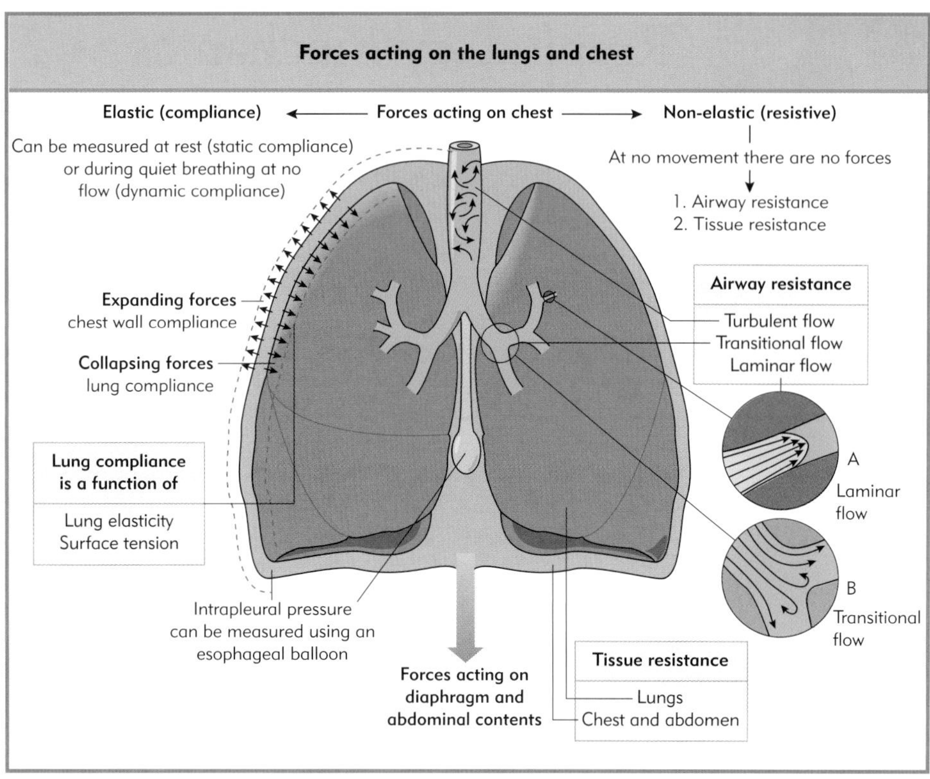

Figure 49.1 Forces acting on the lungs and chest wall during breathing – the left side details elastic forces, the right side nonelastic or resistive forces. Elastic forces are measured as compliance. The diagram shows the forces tending to cause chest wall expansion at rest balancing the forces tending to cause pulmonary collapse. In both cases the force is due to elastic recoil. This results in a negative intrapleural pressure, which can be monitored with an intraesophageal balloon. Compliance is measured as slope of the pressure–volume curve. The assessment of compliance should be made when there is no gas flow or tissue movement. Generally there are two ways of assessing compliance. *Static compliance*: a pressure–volume curve is plotted as a number of discrete points. Measurements are made after stabilization has occurred. *Dynamic compliance*: a pressure–volume curve is created from a pressure–volume loop obtained during breathing. It is the line joining the points of no flow at the start and end of inspiration.

Static compliance and dynamic compliance are merely two techniques to measure the same thing: compliance. It is important not to confuse the different information available from the pressure–volume loop obtained during breathing. It can be used to measure dynamic compliance as above; alternatively, the area of the loop gives information about resistive forces. Chest wall compliance is due to tissue elasticity. Lung compliance is due to lung elasticity and surface tension. In the lung, surface tension effects are the more important of the two, and would be significantly greater in the absence of surfactant. Nonelastic or resistive forces must be measured during movement and are due to airways resistance and tissue (or viscous) resistance. *Airways resistance* is determined by the nature of gas flow. In large airways where gas flow is high this is turbulent. It becomes laminar in smaller airways where gas flow has slowed, and is a mixture (or transitional) at junctions and branches. Transitional flow is seen in a large part of the airway. *Tissue (viscous) resistance* is due to the forces required to move the tissues of the lung, the chest wall, and the abdominal contents. Work is done against friction and heat is produced.

Inset A shows the parabolic velocity profile characteristically seen in laminar or streamlined flow. **Inset B** shows eddy currents commencing at a branch in the bronchial tree. Currents are carried some distance, resulting in transitional flow. This may revert to laminar or turbulent flow further down the airway, depending on other factors.

transitional flow. A substantial proportion of respiratory gas flow is transitional.

VOLUMES AND CAPACITIES

Lung volumes are measured indirectly or directly with a spirometer. Some are determined during quiet breathing, such as tidal volume, whereas others require the subject to perform maneuvers such as maximal inspiration and maximal expiration. A laboratory spirometer is an inverted U-shaped gas container suspended in a water bath by a wire which is attached to a counterbalance over low-friction pulleys. The spirometer is a gas volume-measuring system that is designed to be effectively frictionless and weightless. Figure 49.2 shows a trace obtained from a spirometer when a subject is asked to make a maximum expiration after a maximum inspiration. Lung capacity is the sum of two or more volumes. Residual volume and functional residual capacity (FRC) cannot be measured by spirometry; alternative techniques include an indicator dilution method using helium, or body plethysmography (Chapter 50).

Total lung capacity (TLC) is the volume of the lung at maximal inspiration. It contains the residual volume (RV) and vital capacity (VC). The residual volume is the volume remaining in the lungs at the end of maximum expiration.

The vital capacity contains the tidal volume (TV), the inspiratory reserve volume (IRV), and the expiratory reserve volume (ERV). The tidal volume is the volume of a normal quiet breath, and the inspiratory and expiratory reserve volumes are the amount of gas that can be inspired or expired after normal tidal flow.

The FRC contains the ERV and the RV. It is the volume of gas remaining in the lungs at the end of a normal expiration. If the lung emptied of air completely on expiration widespread alveolar collapse would occur, requiring additional forces for inspiration. The FRC protects against alveolar collapse occurring after each breath and provides a reservoir of alveolar gas to prevent major swings in arterial blood gases during the respiratory cycle. The inspiratory capacity (IC) and expiratory capacity (EC) are the tidal volume and the inspiratory or expiratory reserve volume, respectively.

The FRC protects against alveolar collapse occurring after each breath, and provides a reservoir of alveolar gas to prevent major swings in arterial blood gases during the respiratory cycle.

VENTILATORY MUSCLES

The muscles of ventilation are the diaphragm, intercostal, accessory, and abdominal muscles. The accessory muscles, including scalenus anterior and medius, sternocleidomastoid and trapez-

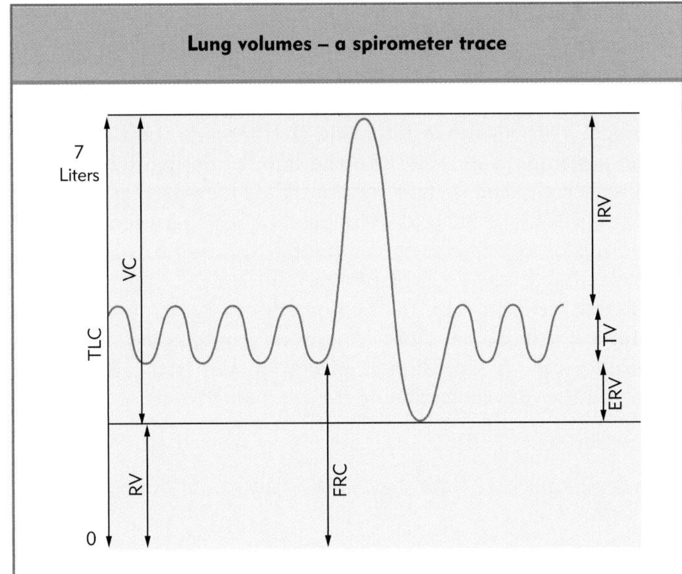

Figure 49.2 Lung volumes – a spirometer trace from a subject breathing quietly showing a maximum inspiration followed by a maximum expiration. Total lung capacity (TLC) contains the residual volume (RV) and vital capacity (VC). The residual volume cannot be measured by spirometry. Vital capacity contains the tidal volume (TV) the inspiratory reserve volume (IRV), and the expiratory reserve volume (ERV). The inspiratory capacity (IC) and expiratory capacity (EC) are the tidal volume and the inspiratory or expiratory reserve volumes, respectively. Functional residual capacity (FRC) contains the ERV and the RV. A capacity consists of two or more volumes.

ius, are recruited during periods of respiratory difficulty, aided by the abdominal musculature. Contraction of the external and internal intercostal muscles and the transversus thoracis muscle results in the ribs being raised and drawn closer to their neighbors, causing an increase in the diameter of the thoracic cavity. The diaphragm has a central muscular and a peripheral tendinous component. Contraction of the central muscle causes flattening and a further increase in thoracic volume.

The intercostal muscles receive their nerve supply from the intercostal nerves, whereas the diaphragm is supplied by the phrenic nerve. Respiratory drive is affected by many factors: for example, it is increased in acidosis or depressed by anesthetic drugs (Chapter 51). Muscle function itself can be compromised under certain circumstances, such as failure to reverse muscle relaxant drugs adequately. Muscle fatigue is a problem in the critically ill.

FORCES

A clear idea of the forces moving gas in and out of the chest helps an understanding of the effects of disease and artificial ventilation on pulmonary physiology. The physics of flows and factors involved in the transition from laminar to turbulent flow are covered in Chapter 43.

The SI unit of force is the Newton. This can be defined as the force required to accelerate 1 kg by 1 m/s^2, or:

$$\text{force} = \text{mass} \times \text{acceleration}$$

considering friction:

$$\text{force} = \text{velocity} \times \text{resistance}$$

where resistance is a measure of friction.

Considering elasticity:

$$\text{force} = \text{displacement} \times \text{stiffness}$$

where stiffness is a measure of distensibility.

Considering gas movement, force can be substituted by pressure and displacement substituted by volume. When a force acts, work is done. Energy is the ability to do work. Kinetic energy is due to the current state of motion of a body, whereas potential energy is the capacity to do work, such as the potential energy held in a tensioned clock spring. A gas possesses potential energy by virtue of its pressure and kinetic energy by virtue of its movement or flow.

The work done by moving gases can be expressed as follows:

$$\text{work} = \text{pressure} \times \text{volume}$$

At the end of expiration the lungs are at rest. The intrapleural space is mainly obliterated and the lung and chest wall move as one. During inspiration, work is done by the muscles of respiration to overcome:

- lung elastic forces;
- chest wall elastic forces;
- lung tissue resistive forces;
- chest wall resistive forces;
- airway resistive forces.

Resistive forces can only be measured during movement, as they have no value at rest. Elastic forces are present at all times, but are measured in the absence of resistive forces when there is no tissue movement or gas flow. Lung compliance is the relationship between volume displaced and pressure change, and can be measured by calculating the gradient of a graph of pressure versus volume. Anesthesiologists will be familiar with the difference in tidal volume delivered by the application of the same airway pressure in an adult and a child. This is because compliance is higher in the larger lung of the adult. It is possible to compensate for the volume effect by measuring specific compliance. This is compliance divided by lung volume. Static compliance is assessed by observing the relationship between lung volume and pressure at steady state. Generally this is performed in the laboratory by obtaining a number of readings at different static lung volumes. Dynamic compliance measurement is a way of assessing compliance during breathing. It is helpful to consider these forces individually.

Lung compliance: the lung elastic forces

The elastic property of lung is due to the nature of its connective tissue as well as its architecture. Lung expansion results in increasing tissue tension due to stretching and distortion of interwoven elastin and collagen fibers. Surface tension effects are also important, resulting in about 60% of the necessary force required to expand the lung.

Static lung compliance is measured in various ways. An isolated lung preparation can be inflated to known volumes and a static pressure–volume relationship plotted which is linear throughout most of its range. At high lung volumes, at the limit of distensibility, compliance is reduced and the curve flattened. The curve obtained during expiration does not overlap that of inspiration. Failure of stretched materials to return exactly to their relaxation length is seen in all elastic substances and is termed hysteresis.

Similar data can be obtained by placing an isolated lung in a jar and evacuating gas from around it. The curve now looks more physiological as the distending pressure is negative, simulating intrapleural pressure.

In humans it is not possible to measure intrapleural pressure directly, but it can be estimated from the pressure measured in a balloon placed at the lower end of the esophagus. It is not possible to validate absolute values measured, but the changes in pressure are considered accurate. Static lung compliance can be estimated by instructing a subject to breathe in a predetermined volume and measuring the esophageal pressure. If the glottis is open the force measured by an esophageal balloon is that required to stop the lung collapsing. This can be plotted against the change in lung volume to produce a compliance curve (Fig. 49.3, upper trace). These measurements are performed in an upright subject breathing from functional residual capacity.

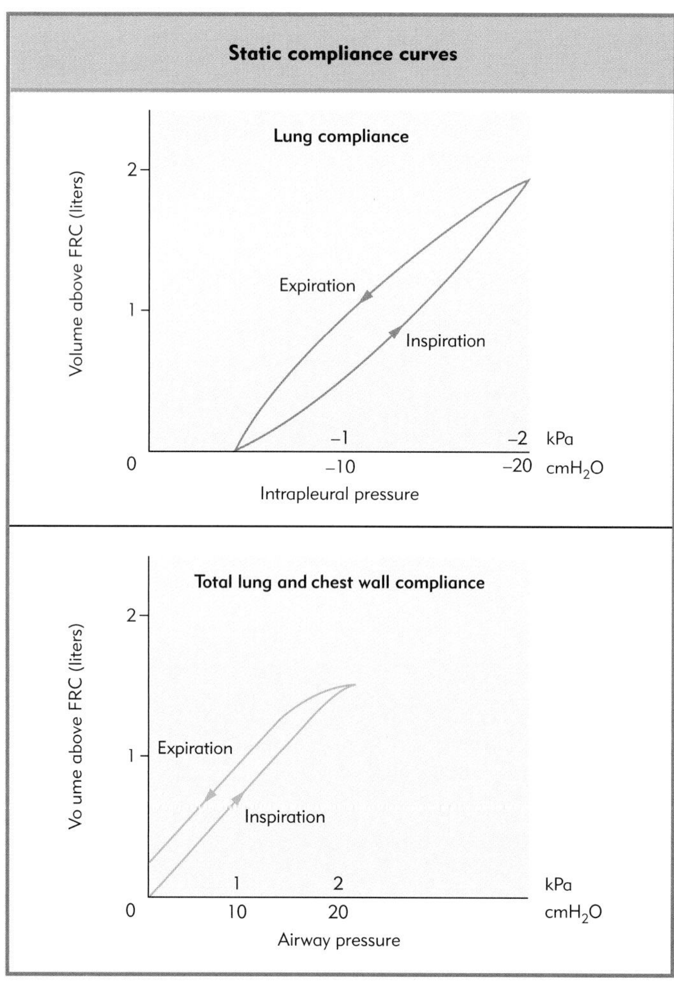

Figure 49.3 Static compliance curves: compliance can be assessed by measuring the slope of a pressure–volume curve. Upper curve is esophageal relaxation pressure and volume in a laboratory subject. Lower curve is plot of airway pressure and stepwise increase in volume in a ventilated patient. **Upper curve**: Lung compliance curve drawn by plotting static esophageal relaxation pressure against volume above FRC. Static lung compliance is the slope of the trace. The curve exhibits hysteresis, i.e. the expiratory curve does not overlap the inspiratory curve. At a given pressure the volume during expiration is higher than during inspiration. This phenomenon is caused by a number of factors, such as alveolar recruitment, surfactant, and the nature of elastic tissue. **Lower curve**: Total lung and chest wall static compliance can be obtained experimentally in a ventilated relaxed patient. Gas is administered from a large syringe in stages. A curve is plotted of volume injected and airway pressure.

SURFACE TENSION

Molecules of liquid are more closely approximated than they are in a gas, and so they are attracted to their neighbors with a greater force than they are to molecules of gas at a gas–liquid interface. This results in a tension that tends to pull molecules at the gas–liquid interface into the liquid, causing it to adopt a minimum area. The surface tension (T) is measured as force per unit length (L) of surface. The relationship between pressure and radius of a sphere such as a bubble or alveolus is important; for those interested an explanation follows.

Surface tension can be demonstrated quite easily in the laboratory. An oblong wire frame is constructed with one moveable side. A soap film is placed on the frame. The force acting on the moveable side of frame of length L is:

$$F = L \times T$$

However, the soap film has two surfaces, upper and lower, and so:

$$F = 2L \times T$$

The surface tension of water is 70 mN/m. In biological fluids such as plasma this is reduced to 50 mN/m. A bubble in a liquid, or a soap bubble in air, takes the shape having the minimum surface area, which is a sphere. The relationship between the pressure in a bubble and the tension in the wall is described by the Laplace relationship: $P \propto T/R$. This allows estimation of the pressure (P) above ambient required to prevent the collapse of a hollow curved object if the tension in the wall is T and the radius of curvature is R. This relationship can be explored further if it is imagined that the sphere is cut down the middle. The force acting on one half is the product of pressure and cross-sectional area, which is balanced by the force acting on the other side, which is the product of surface tension and length of circumference. In the case of a soap bubble there are two surfaces, and so the length is doubled:

$$\text{Pressure} \times \text{Area} = \text{Tension} \times 2 \times \text{Length}$$

or

$$P \times \pi \times R^2 = T \times 2 \times 2\pi R$$

or

$$P = 4T/R$$

Various factors affect the proportionality constant or numerator of this equation, such as the number of planes of curvature and the number of surfaces being considered. For an alveolus the equation reads:

$$P = 2T/R$$

This shows that as the radius of an alveolus becomes smaller the pressure required to balance the tension in the wall and so prevent collapse must rise. It also explains why, if two alveoli of different radii are connected together, theoretically the smaller one with the higher pressure should empty into the larger. The unique properties of pulmonary surfactant compensate for this phenomenon, and also prevent the surface tension increasing as the lung reduces in volume.

The importance of surface tension on static compliance can be demonstrated experimentally by plotting a compliance curve for an experimental lung inflated with saline. The absence of the air–fluid interface abolishes surface tension and results in a considerably more compliant lung.

SURFACTANT

Surfactant consists of phospholipids, which contain both hydrophobic and hydrophilic domains. The former project out into the alveolus, whereas the latter remain in the alveolar lining fluid. The most important constituent of surfactant is dipalmitoyl lecithin. Surfactants are detergents, which lower the surface tension in proportion to their concentration at the interface. Hence, as the alveolus expands during inspiration surfactant becomes less concentrated and surface tension increases. During expiration, however, the concentration of surfactant increases again and reduces surface tension, splinting open the alveolus and making it generally more stable. The surface tension in the alveoli is in the range of between 5 and 30 mN/m (Fig. 49.4).

During expiration surfactant reduces surface tension, splinting open the alveolus and making it generally more stable.

Lung compliance is affected in disease when there is a reduction in the production of surfactant or an alteration in elastic tissue or bronchial mucus. In pulmonary fibrosis elastic tissue is replaced by fibrous tissue, causing a reduction in compliance; alternatively, age or emphysema causes an increase in compliance from loss of elastic tissue. Pulmonary edema also causes a reduction in compliance. Surfactant is not normally produced until the late stages of gestation and in premature babies can be reduced, causing respiratory distress syndrome.

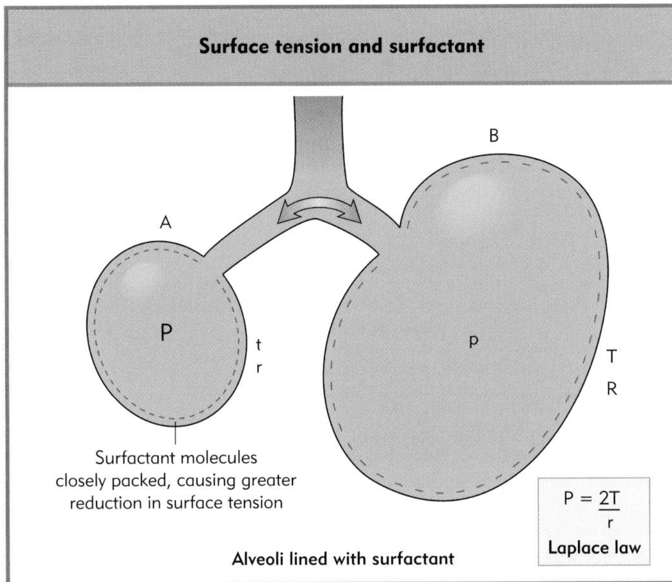

Figure 49.4 Surface tension and surfactant: effects on alveolar stability. Because of the Laplace relationship, if an alveolus acted like a bubble the pressure in a small bubble on the left, A (large PRESSURE, small radius), would exceed that in the large one on the right, B (small pressure, large RADIUS). If the two alveoli were connected A would empty into B. Surfactant not only reduces surface tension, its effect increases as the radius of the alveoli becomes smaller. This is due to the molecules being more closely packed as the radius falls. Thus bubble A has a lower surface tension, which reduces its tendency to empty into B. This effect helps stabilize the alveoli.

Absence of or a reduction in surfactant causes instability in alveoli, reduces compliance, and, by increasing surface tension, increases forces that can precipitate pulmonary edema.

Chest wall compliance: chest wall elastic forces

At end-expiration the elastic forces tending to cause the lung to collapse balance the forces tending to make the chest wall expand. This results in an intrapleural pressure which is less than atmospheric. Static chest wall compliance can be measured using appropriate relaxation pressures, but is often calculated (this is discussed below). Chest wall compliance can be reduced by obesity, by loss of skin elasticity for example due to scarring from burns, or by skeletal problems such as fusion of costochondral joints.

TOTAL COMPLIANCE (CHEST WALL AND LUNG)

The relaxation pressure for the whole respiratory system can be obtained by asking a subject to breathe in a quantity of air and then relax against an airway obstruction. This is a similar method to that described above, where the positive pressure required to expand an isolated lung is used to measure lung compliance. The pressure measured at the subject's mouth during relaxation is equal to the intra-alveolar pressure at that time. The gradient of volume of gas inhaled against the relaxation pressure represents total compliance. A problem with this method in an awake subject is the inability to completely relax the muscles of respiration.

Total compliance is related to lung and chest wall compliance as follows:

$$\frac{1}{\text{total compliance}} = \frac{1}{\text{lung compliance}} + \frac{1}{\text{chest wall compliance}}$$

Normal values in L/kPa:
Total compliance = 1
Lung = 2
Thorax = 2.

Clinically, for practical reasons compliance is usually assessed by measuring dynamic compliance, but a method has been described for measuring static total compliance in patients ventilated in intensive care. An automated gas delivery system is used based on a large syringe which injects gas into the airway in steps, allowing time for stabilization. By monitoring the accompanying changes in pressure, compliance can be calculated (see Fig. 49.3, lower trace).

DYNAMIC COMPLIANCE

The concept of dynamic compliance can be confusing, as all compliance measurements are made in the absence of gas flow. Dynamic compliance is measured in a similar way to static compliance, except that instead of the measurement being made when the lung is at rest after time for settling, it is measured by analyzing the slope of the line joining the zero-flow parts of a dynamic pressure–volume loop. Zero flow occurs as gas flow changes direction at the end of inspiration immediately prior to expiration, and again at the start of inspiration. It is important to realize that the shape of the dynamic loop does not affect compliance measurements, just the two points mentioned line OA in Figure 49.5 (inset represents reduced compliance). The width of the loop is due to the greater pressure differentials needed to

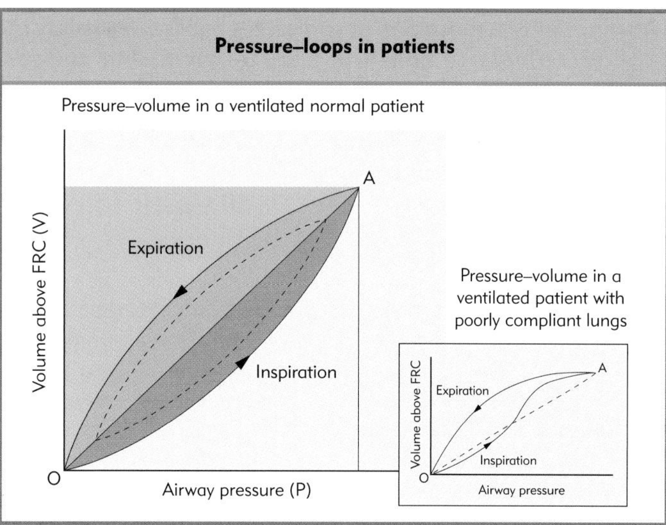

Figure 49.5 Diagrammatic representation of a dynamic pressure–volume loop obtained from a ventilated patient. The line is a pressure–volume loop obtained from a ventilated normal patient. It is a similar shape to that obtained from a subject breathing spontaneously. The green line OA connects the beginning of inspiration to the end of inspiration. It represents the dynamic compliance, as the flow is nominally zero at these points. Work done during inspiration against elastic forces is the sum of the areas shaded yellow + red. Work done during inspiration against resistive forces is the area shaded violet. Total work done during inspiration is the sum of the areas shaded yellow + red + blue. Work done during expiration against resistive forces is the area shaded red. Energy for expiration comes from potential energy stored in elastic tissue. An increase in resistive work as seen in bronchospasm would be shown by larger blue (inspiration) and red (expiration) areas. If a pressure–volume loop were plotted in a patient with poorly compliant lungs it would be more sloped towards the *x*-axis. The inset shows a loop taken from a patient with reduced compliance due to overdistension. At higher pressures there is no increase in lung volume. Dynamic compliance is represented by line OA. This loop represents a patient on the upper (violet) part of Figure 49.6.

work against frictional forces at any point than if measured at rest. The area of the loop reflects the tissue and airway resistance.

In the normal subject dynamic compliance measurements should yield similar figures to compliance measured statically, although they will never be identical. One reason for different values includes stress relaxation, which is seen in all elastic tissue owing to the tension of the stretched material reducing over time after stretching has occurred. Physiological reasons include varying tone of the pulmonary musculature, redistribution of blood, and the effects of alveolar time constants. These effects are more pronounced in lung disease.

LUNG STABILITY – INTERDEPENDENCE

The stability of lung units is a balance between collapsing forces such as surface tension and stabilizing forces that prevent collapse, such as airway pressure and surfactant. Stability is encouraged by the lung architecture, as each alveolus is supported by surrounding alveoli, alveolar ducts, and other airways. It is unlikely that alveoli of greatly varying diameters could exist side by side because they share septal walls. This mutual support, known as interdependence, is helped by other structures such as blood vessels and fibrous tissue that penetrate from the lung surface and add to lung stability.

TIME CONSTANTS

The alveolar time constant is the time that would be required for inflation if the initial gas flow were maintained throughout inspiration. It is the product of compliance and resistance. Compliance, resistance, and hence the time constant are dependent on lung volume. A poorly compliant alveolus has reduced capacity compared to its normal neighbor. Its maximum volume is not affected by respiratory pattern and it will achieve it quickly – it has a fast time constant. A second alveolus has a high airway resistance but a normal compliance. This alveolus takes some time to fill, but its capacity is not reduced as long as inspiration is long enough – it has a slow time constant. In disease, the lung is comprised of alveoli with a mixture of time constants. Those with fast time constants under certain circumstances may empty into those with shorter time constants. Differing time constants cause a reduction in dynamic compliance. This effect is exaggerated at high respiratory rates and associated short inspiratory times.

PEEP

PEEP (positive end-expiratory pressure) has many effects. In lung disease careful use of PEEP can cause an increase in compliance and an improvement in pulmonary function. The compliance curve in Figure 49.6 represents FRC to total lung capacity, a volume of approximately 4 L. This is significantly greater than

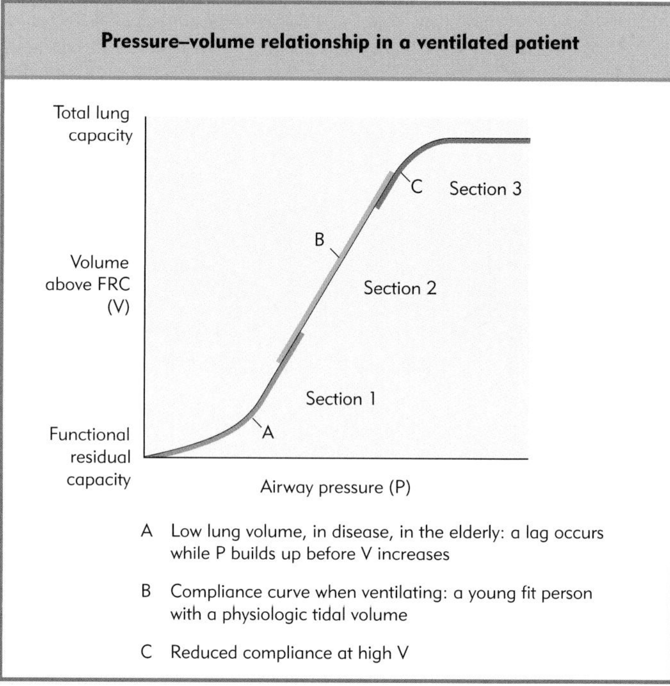

Figure 49.6 Diagrammatic representation of a pressure–volume curve in a ventilated patient. The slope at any point from FRC to TLC indicates total compliance (lung and chest wall). The curve has three distinct parts. **Orange** – at low lung volume, in disease and in the elderly, there is a lag while airway pressure builds up before lung volume starts to increase. This is due to the FRC being less than the closing capacity, allowing basal collapse to occur during expiration. **Green** – the center section represents the compliance curve seen when ventilating a young fit person with a physiological tidal volume. **Violet** – compliance is reduced at high lung volumes. This curve is flattened over the upper part, showing alveolar overdistension as a result of using a high tidal volume or excessive PEEP. Ideally, the tidal volume in a ventilated patient will sit on the yellow part of the trace, which represents optimal compliance. If a patient is on the blue curve it may be possible to increase compliance by reducing tidal volume or level of PEEP. If they are on the orange curve it should be possible to increase compliance by applying some PEEP. Point (A) represents the lower inflection point of the compliance curve, where the compliance suddenly increases. Ideally, PEEP should be set to match the pressure at point (A).

a normal tidal volume, which lies on part of the curve. If the tidal volume lies on the orange part of the curve the compliance will be reduced, but can be improved by increasing PEEP. Minor adjustments to PEEP can have a significant effect. Generally it is possible to optimize the respiratory effects of PEEP by setting the level to match the lower inflection point of the pressure volume loop (A). It is important to monitor the effect of PEEP on cardiovascular stability.

A tidal volume lying on the blue part of the curve represents overdistension (expressed as a dynamic loop in the inset of Fig. 49.5). Higher airway pressure is resulting in no increase in volume but increasing the risk of barotrauma. Reducing PEEP will increase compliance.

Nonelastic forces

An ideal lung would have elastic properties with no hysteresis and there would be no frictional or resistance effects. The relationship between intrapleural pressure and lung volume would be linear, inspiration overlapping expiration. In practice, such a graph plotted during breathing shows that intrapleural pressure is always more negative than this during inspiration and more positive during expiration. This is due to nonelastic (resistance or frictional) forces. The area of the loop generated is due to the work done against these forces. Generally resistance relates the forces producing movement to the movement produced. In the case of gases:

Resistance = pressure drop/flow
Total pulmonary resistance = airway resistance + tissue resistance.

TISSUE RESISTANCE

Energy is required to move the lung, chest wall, diaphragm, and abdominal contents during breathing to overcome tissue resistance even if there is no gas flow in the airway. Tissue resistance *cannot be measured directly* but has to be estimated by subtracting the measured airway resistance from the total pulmonary resistance. Quiet expiration is powered mainly by energy stored during stretching of elastic tissue during inspiration. If there is an increase in tissue resistance in disease, less energy will be available to overcome airway resistance and expiration will be prolonged.

Tissue resistance is normally about 20% of resistive forces. It is increased by conditions that cause pulmonary fibrosis, such as sarcoidosis and carcinomatosis. It can also be increased in musculoskeletal conditions that limit mechanical movement, such as kyphoscoliosis.

AIRWAYS RESISTANCE

Resistance to flow in the airways is affected by their radius and the flow characteristics of the gas. When flow is slow it is likely to be laminar. If flow increases or there is a change in airway characteristics, such as a constriction or branch, it loses the parabolic profile and is said to be turbulent. In many parts of the bronchial tree the flow pattern is transitional, which is a mixture of these two extremes.

In those parts of the respiratory tract where flow is laminar, flow is proportional to pressure drop:

$$\text{airway resistance} = \frac{8 \times \text{length} \times \text{viscosity}}{\pi \times \text{radius}^4}$$

Small reductions in radius have a marked effect on the resistance.

In the case of turbulence, flow is no longer directly proportional to pressure drop but rather to its square root. As this relationship is no longer linear, the resistance is not constant but varies with the flow. Turbulent flow is not affected by gas viscosity but is inversely proportional to the square root of the density, which is why breathing gas at high pressures increases airway resistance (density increases with increasing pressure). Similarly, helium, which has a low density, reduces the work of breathing and can be used to temporarily help patients with upper airway obstruction.

Measurement of airway resistance relies on the following relationship:

airway resistance = mouth–alveoli pressure drop/flow.

Alveolar pressure cannot be measured directly, but there are ways to estimate it. The *interrupter technique* relies on the assumption that if a shutter is intermittently closed at the mouth the pressure obtained as the airway is blocked and gas flow ceases equals alveolar pressure. This pressure is plotted against the gas flow immediately prior to the shutter closing.

The *body plethysmograph* (Chapter 50) relies on Boyle's Law to calculate the alveolar pressure. The patient is placed in an airtight box of known volume. During inspiration the chest expands and increases the box pressure in association with a fall in the intra-alveolar pressure. This allows the calculation of alveolar pressure, which can be related to measured gas flow, thereby allowing airway resistance to be estimated. Normal range is about 0.05–1.5 $cmH_2O/L/s$, or 0.005–0.15 kPa/L/s in adults. Using gas flow and the pressure in an esophageal balloon the total lung resistance can be obtained. This allows tissue resistance to be calculated by subtracting measured airway resistance.

Factors affecting airway resistance include the volume of the lungs. As the lung expands the airways become wider and longer, the overall effect being a reduction in airway resistance. Airway resistance is increased if the bronchi become narrowed due to bronchospasm, mucosal edema, mucous plugging, or epithelial desquamation. The parasympathetic system is of major importance in the control of bronchomotor tone. Afferents from the bronchial epithelium pass centrally to the vagus. Efferent preganglionic fibers also run in the vagus to ganglia located in the walls of small bronchi. Short postganglionic fibers lead to nerve endings that release acetylcholine to act on muscarinic receptors in the bronchial smooth muscle. Stimulation of any part of this reflex arc results in bronchoconstriction. Many drugs also affect the tone of the bronchial muscle.

All airways can be compressed by reversal of the normal transmural pressure gradient, which can occur during forced expiration. The cartilaginous airways have considerable structural resistance. The smaller airways have no structural rigidity and rely on elastic recoil of the lung tissue surrounding them. This results in expiratory flow limitation.

During anesthesia airway resistance can be increased by obstruction from a number of causes. The oropharyngeal airway can become obstructed, as normal pharyngeal reflexes are lost during anesthesia or in a comatose patient. It can also occur during REM sleep, particularly in the elderly. The lumen of the pharynx and larynx may become obstructed with foreign material, such as tumor, gastric contents, or blood. The larynx can also become obstructed by laryngeal spasm or subglottic edema.

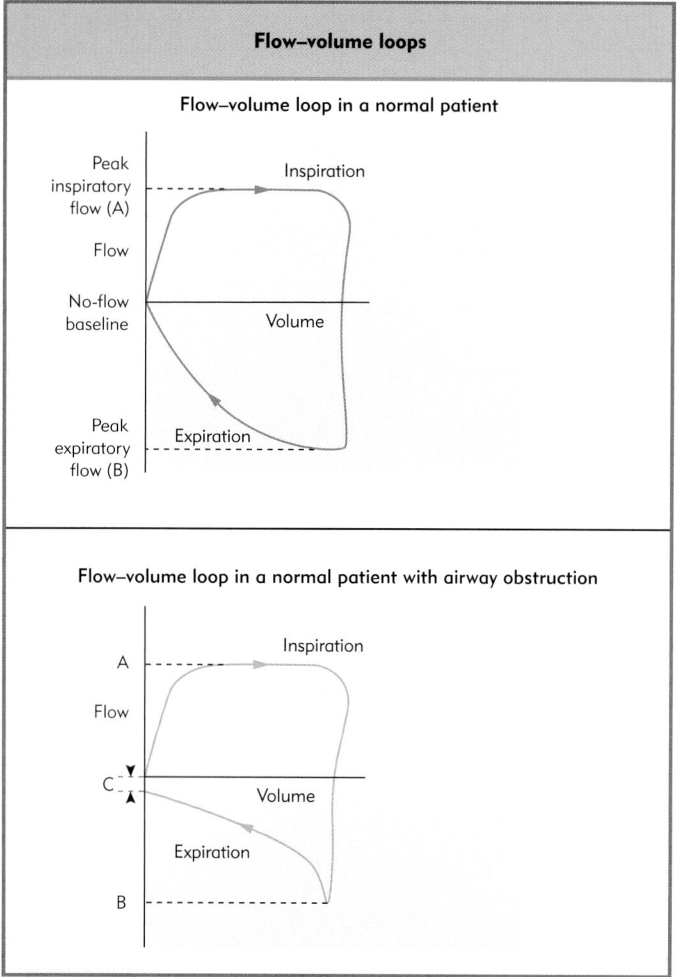

Figure 49.7 Flow–volume loops obtained during volume-controlled mechanical ventilation. The upper part of each loop is inspiration, point A is peak inspiratory flow, and point B peak expiratory flow. The upper trace is obtained from a normal patient. Flow pattern is affected by the mode of ventilation. In pressure-controlled ventilation the peak inspiratory flow is achieved early in inspiration and is followed by a decelerating pattern; expiration is unchanged. The lower trace has a lower peak expiratory flow (B), which drops off suddenly and ultimately has a flatter shape than the normal. This indicates expiratory flow limitation, as seen in bronchospasm. This loop is also incomplete: the expiratory curve does not reach the no-flow baseline indicated by line C. This can be due to air-trapping and incomplete expiration, or to gas leakage from the circuit.

Airway obstruction can be detected by analyzing a flow–volume loop (Fig. 49.7).

WORK OF BREATHING

During inspiration work is done against elastic and resistive forces. That done combating the resistive forces is dissipated as heat. Energy used in displacing elastic tissue can be compared to that used in stretching a spring. It is stored as potential energy, which is available to power expiration. In mechanically ventilated patients and in the healthy at rest, expiration is passive. Expiratory work is not normally important.

The energy used by muscles of respiration can be calculated by measuring oxygen cost. In a resting healthy individual this is small, being less than 2% of the total oxygen uptake. Respiratory efficiency is expressed as a percentage, and is the actual work done divided by the calculated energy used multiplied by 100. It is normally less than 10%, the majority of the energy being lost as heat generated within muscles.

Work is performed when a force moves its point of application. In terms of the lungs it is measured using pressure and volume changes. Pressure–volume loops monitored during mechanical and spontaneous ventilation supply information about many aspects of lung mechanics, as well as the work of breathing. The work of breathing can be assessed by analyzing different areas of the loops. Figure 49.6 is a diagrammatic representation of a pressure–volume loop obtained during breathing. By analyzing the colored areas elastic and resistive work can be calculated. The slope of the line OA that joins the origin to the end of inspiration allows the calculation of dynamic compliance.

Further information can be obtained by observing the pattern of the flow–volume loop, which can be displayed on many modern intensive care ventilators. Figure 49.7 represents two flow–volume loops obtained during conventional volume-controlled mechanical ventilation. The upper part of each loop is inspiration, point A is peak inspiratory flow, and point B peak expiratory flow. Reductions in peak flow rates imply increased airway resistance. In pressure-controlled ventilation the peak inspiratory flow is achieved early in inspiration, and is followed by a decelerating pattern to baseline at end-inspiration; expiration is unchanged. The upper trace is obtained from a normal patient. The lower trace has a lower peak expiratory flow (B) that drops off suddenly and which ultimately has a flatter shape than the normal. This indicates expiratory flow limitation, as seen in bronchospasm. The flow–volume loop should finish where it starts, with the flow being zero at the end of expiration. The loop in the lower trace is incomplete. This can be due to air-trapping and incomplete expiration, or to gas leakage from the circuit.

Patients tend to optimize their respiratory pattern to match compliance and airway resistance. The work of breathing is increased if either compliance is reduced or airway resistance is increased. When compliance is reduced, increased work is done against elastic forces. It is possible to compensate by reducing the tidal volume and increasing respiratory rate. Conversely, patients with high airway resistance reduce the resistive component of the work of breathing by reducing respiratory rate and increasing tidal volume. If the work of breathing becomes too great, some assistance may be required.

MECHANICAL VENTILATION

There are many indications for artificial ventilation, ranging from patients undergoing intra-abdominal surgery necessitating muscle relaxation to those admitted to the critical care unit with hypoxia or ventilatory failure. The basic principles used are the same in each case, e.g. maintenance of adequate oxygenation, efficient carbon dioxide removal, and the avoidance of iatrogenic damage; however, the mode of ventilation and hence the choice of ventilator used in different indications will vary.

Causes of acute respiratory failure include:

- Lung pathology
  - Infection
  - Obstruction (bronchospasm/foreign body)
  - Smoke inhalation
  - Chest trauma (pneumothorax)

- Breathing problems
  - Muscle weakness (nerve/muscle/neuromuscular junction disorders)
  - Decreased consciousness level/respiratory drive (drugs, head trauma, hypercapnia)
- Cardiovascular pathology
  - Myocardial infarction resulting in decreased cardiac output
  - Congestive cardiac failure
  - Pulmonary emboli.

Intubation and establishing ventilation

Once the decision to ventilate a patient has been made, access to the airway should be obtained by a trained operator with skilled assistance. It should be performed in a safe environment with all the necessary equipment available, including adjuncts for use in a patient who is difficult to intubate. Full monitoring, as recommended in guidelines published by the Association of Anaesthetists (GB and Ireland) and ASA (USA), should be established, including end-tidal carbon dioxide monitoring. Initial ventilator settings may be based on normal physiological parameters and then adjusted in response to information from pulse oximetry, airway pressure, measured volumes, and arterial blood gases.

Types of ventilator

Machines can be classified in many ways, for example how each breath is generated (flow or pressure) and cycled (volume, time, or flow). Beyond this there is little standardization regarding terminology.

Flow generators are designed to maintain a constant flow throughout inspiration. Airway volume and pressure rise linearly until a preset volume (volume cycled) is reached when inspiration ends and expiration begins. Alternatively, time cycling may be used. These machines have the advantage of producing a constant tidal volume in the presence of varying compliance, such as a patient breath-holding during emergence from anesthesia. This is at the expense of varying airway pressure, which may rise alarmingly if compliance falls (and risk causing barotrauma) (Fig. 49.8).

Pressure generators (Fig. 49.9) produce a constant pressure during inspiration using an inspiratory flow pattern that falls exponentially as volume rises. Inspiration ends after a preset time has passed. Some systems cycle inspiration to expiration when a preset flow rate has been reached. Pressure generators are less likely to cause barotrauma, as peak airway pressure is controlled. Tidal volume will be maintained despite small leaks in the breathing circuit (hence their preferred use in pediatrics, where uncuffed endotracheal tubes are used). Earlier filling of the lung in this mode may result in superior gas exchange.

Modes of ventilation

In mechanical ventilation a breath initiated by a ventilator is called mandatory. Any breath initiated by the patient, whether mechanically assisted or not, is called spontaneous. Mandatory breaths are generally delivered intermittently to allow some spontaneous breathing by the patient (intermittent mandatory ventilation, IMV). Most ventilators will attempt to *synchronize* the mandatory breaths with the patient's respiratory effort, allowing the patient to initiate breaths wherever possible (synchronized intermittent mandatory ventilation, SIMV).

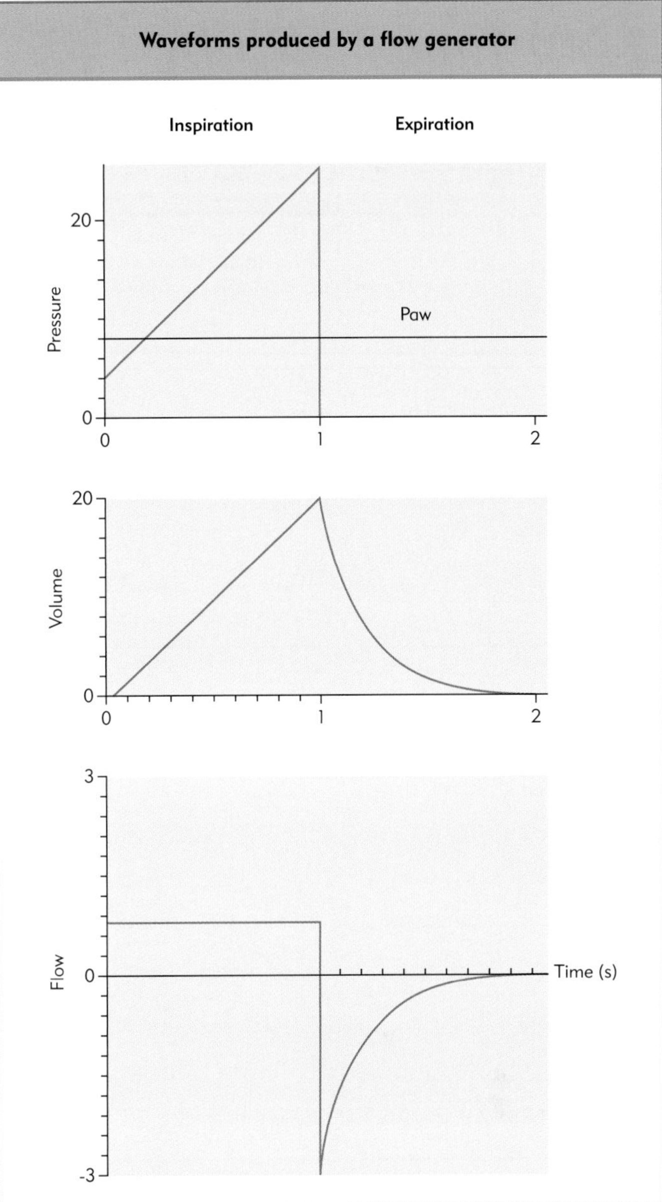

Figure 49.8 Waveforms produced by a flow generator (volume-controlled ventilation).

The respiratory cycle can be divided into four parts:

- the change from expiration to inspiration;
- inspiratory phase;
- the change from inspiration to expiration;
- expiratory phase.

Each phase uses a variable (pressure, volume, flow, time) to initiate, sustain, and end it (cycle). In the case of inspiration, initiation is known as triggering.

Basic descriptions can be used for the various modes of ventilation that are available. First, consider the variable being controlled during each mandatory breath (pressure or volume) and then the pattern of breathing (spontaneous, mandatory,

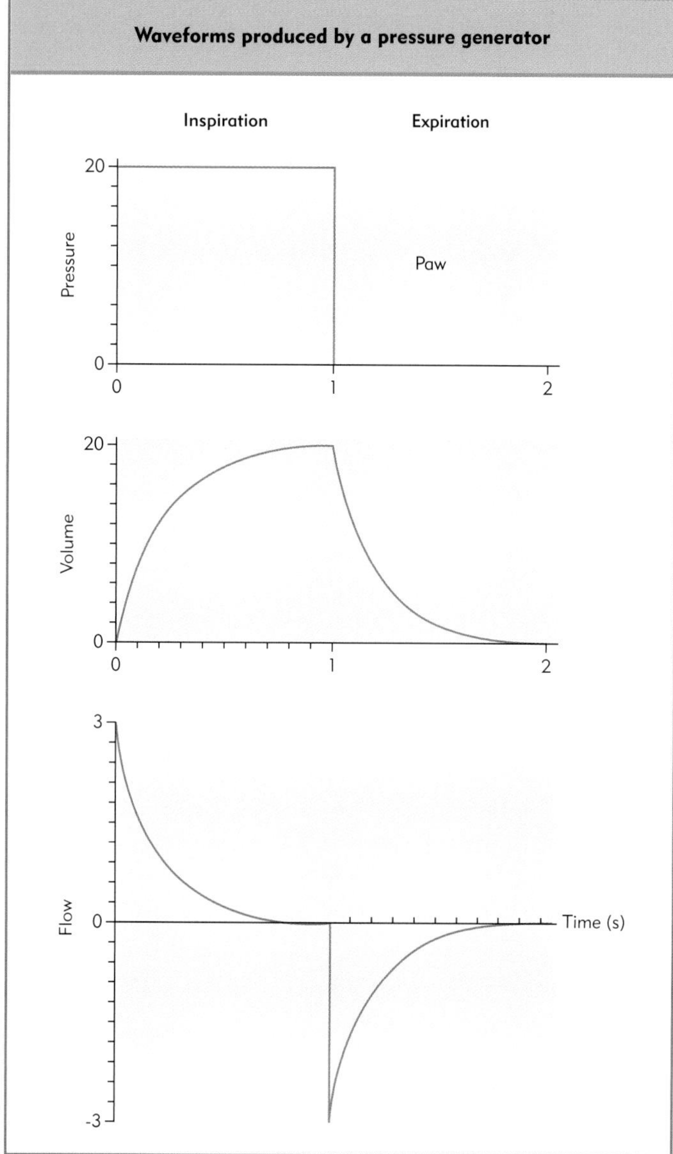

Figure 49.9 Waveforms produced by a pressure generator (pressure-controlled ventilation).

intermittent mandatory, or synchronized mandatory). In modern equipment the pressure or volume delivered by the ventilator is controlled by an internal feedback mechanism. If a preset level is not reached the ventilator will adjust the output in an attempt to correct this. Simple ventilators, such as transport ventilators, do not make use of feedback; this has the advantage of keeping the ventilators small and relatively inexpensive, but can result in patients being under- or overventilated.

If detailed descriptions of types of ventilator are needed, the variables used to trigger, limit, and cycle each breath are used, along with any automatic features used to switch between different breathing patterns.

Invasive ventilation

Where oxygenation is critical or airway protection is required, such as in unconscious patients, endotracheal intubation is necessary. The declining use of muscle relaxants in critical care and the trend to keep patients lightly sedated means they are more likely to take spontaneous breaths. To ensure that lung damage is kept to a minimum, SIMV is now used. Should a spontaneous breath occur the ventilator delays its mandatory breath and assists the patient-triggered breath. This also ensures a minimum mandatory minute ventilation. The inspiratory trigger may be a change in flow or pressure. This will result in a set pressure being generated (PCV) or a set flow rate developing (volume control ventilation, VCV). To avoid the risks of both barotrauma (pressure damage) and volutrauma (overdistension) the delivered volume can be limited in PCV and pressure limited in VCV. The sensitivity of the trigger can be altered depending on the patient's respiratory effort. The change in flow/pressure required to trigger the ventilator should be as small as possible (high sensitivity) to limit self-triggering while ensuring that the patient receives a breath as soon as there is any inspiratory effort. More ventilators now employ a continuous base flow in association with flow triggering. In these systems there is a constant flow of air during expiration. When the patient starts to inspire the flow return in the expiratory limb will be lower than that in the inspiratory limb, and the ventilator is immediately triggered.

Pressure support

In this mode the ventilator is patient triggered; a positive pressure is applied during inspiration. The level of pressure support can be set to reduce the work of breathing for the patient. This improves gas exchange and maintains active respiratory muscle activity. A degree of continuous positive airway pressure (CPAP) will usually also be employed to increase functional residual capacity and prevent atelectasis. CPAP is used in a spontaneously breathing patient and pressure is applied throughout the respiratory cycle. Positive end-expiratory pressure (PEEP) is pressure exerted only at the end of expiration (in a ventilated patient).

Breathing circuits and endotracheal tubes provide resistance to breathing. This can be compensated for by the application of pressure support. Newer ventilators can calculate the compensatory pressure support required and automatically adjust the pressure; this is known as tube compensation.

BIPAP

There are various forms of BIPAP (biphasic positive airway pressure). The generic form is based on the principle of ventilation using time to cycle between two levels of pressure (P_{insp} and PEEP) and allowing the patient to breathe at both levels; it is well tolerated. If the patient is not taking any spontaneous breaths this mode functions as PCV. The tidal volume is not fixed and depends on lung compliance. This mode of ventilation was once restricted to noninvasive ventilators, but is now being incorporated into mechanical ventilators used for invasive ventilation in critical care.

Other modes of ventilation

The aim of high-frequency jet ventilation and oscillation is to reduce peak airway pressure by reducing tidal volume. The normal relationship between physiological parameters and ventilator settings does not exist, and therefore skilled operators are required if it is to be used safely. It is difficult to show convincing proof of advantage over more conventional modes of ventilation.

Noninvasive ventilation

In some situations, particularly chronic obstructive pulmonary disease, it can be shown that avoiding intubation can reduce the mortality associated with acute exacerbation. Avoidance of tracheal intubation has led the impetus for the development of noninvasive methods of mechanical ventilation. The technique involves the use of a tight-fitting facial or nasal mask and a pressure generator (pressure-controlled ventilation, PCV), which will compensate for small leaks. The choice of cycling variable differs depending on the manufacturer.

CPAP and BIPAP are the commonest modes used, but noninvasive positive-pressure ventilation (NIPPV) is used in patients who have little respiratory drive. Synchronization is not used and each breath is mandatory. Noninvasive ventilators have the advantage of being small, relatively cheap, and portable, and are designed for use at home. They use an electric motor to drive a blower, which delivers a continuous flow along a single tube to the patient. A small orifice is sited close to the mask where gas continuously leaves the circuit.

Newer modes of ventilation – protective lung strategies

It has become apparent in recent years that conventional modes of ventilation can cause lung damage. This leads to an increase in morbidity and mortality. High pressures were often used to distend collapsed alveoli and maintain normocapnia, resulting in barotrauma, including pneumothorax. Initially strategies to keep the lung on the steepest part of the compliance curve were used, as described earlier. These involved prolonging inspiratory time to keep the alveoli open and reducing expiratory time to prevent end-expiratory collapse (inverse ratio ventilation). High intrathoracic pressures and long inspiratory times can result in reduced venous return and hypotension; therefore, patients must be closely monitored, be adequately volume replete, and be monitored for the adverse effects.

The reduced expiratory time may lead to hypercapnia, although provided the pH remains above 7.2 it is doubtful that this results in any significant morbidity. Accepting a higher $Pa\text{CO}_2$ (permissive hypercapnia) will allow lower inspiratory pressure to be used. If the expiratory time is inadequate air-trapping may occur, leading to an increase in end-expiratory pressure (known as auto-PEEP). This may also result in barotrauma.

ARDS is the most severe form of acute lung injury (ALI). Although the pathophysiology is understood the underlying cause can be variable, as can the clinical course. There is disruption to respiratory epithelium, which results in decreased surfactant production and to the alveoli filling with a protein-rich fluid. Clinically this is seen as poorly compliant lungs and hypoxia. The damage to the lung is nonhomogeneous, and there will be areas of relatively normal lung next to abnormal lung. Traditionally high pressures were used to ventilate the lung effectively, but this can result in barotrauma. Overdistension of normal lung and repetitive opening and collapsing of abnormal alveoli will cause damage due to stretching, and ultimately breaking, of interalveolar supportive tissue (volutrauma). The 'open lung' strategy employs a short period (5–30 minutes) of high inflation pressure (35–60 cmH_2O) to open (or recruit) collapsed alveoli, and then high levels of PEEP (10–15 cmH_2O) are applied to prevent end-tidal collapse once the pressures are reduced to more normal levels. This model has been shown to reduce both barotrauma and volutrauma.

Key references

Artigas A, Lemaire F, Suter P, Zapol W (eds). Adult respiratory distress syndrome. Edinburgh: Churchill Livingstone; 1992.

Lumb AB. Nunn's applied respiratory physiology, 5th edn. Oxford: Butterworth-Heinemann; 2000.

Scurr C, Feldman S, Soni N. Scientific foundations of anaesthesia: the basis of intensive care, 4th edn. Oxford: Heinemann Medical; 1990.

West JB. Respiratory physiology – the essentials, 5th edn. Baltimore: Williams & Wilkins; 1995.

Chapter 50

Lung function testing

Roger Hainsworth

Although the principal role of the lungs is the exchange of respiratory gases between the blood and the atmosphere, lungs do have other functions, some which may impinge on their respiratory role. One of the most important secondary functions is that of a blood filter, trapping emboli returning from the systemic circulation and preventing them from blocking vital parts of the circulation. Clearly, pulmonary vessels blocked by microemboli can no longer function for gas exchange, and excessive embolization results in pulmonary hypertension and impairment of respiratory function. The lungs are also a reservoir of blood that can change in volume, for example to allow the cardiovascular system to adjust to the sequestration of blood in dependent veins during standing. In the supine position, the increased volume of blood in the pulmonary vessels and in the chambers of the heart reduces the volume of air that can be accommodated in the alveoli. The lung also has metabolic functions, perhaps the best known of which is the conversion of angiotensin I to angiotensin II. However, it is the respiratory function of the lung that is of main interest in this chapter.

Respiratory function refers to the uptake of oxygen and the elimination of carbon dioxide by the body; this should be adequate to maintain normal levels of blood gases both at rest and at all levels of exercise. The ideal lung is able to achieve this with a minimum expenditure of work, both against elastic forces and against the resistance to gas flow in the airways. A minimum amount of ventilated air should be wasted in the conducting airways and in poorly perfused regions of the lung. Each breath should effectively exchange the pulmonary alveolar gases; this requires that the volume remaining in the lungs after each expiration (the functional residual capacity, FRC) be not excessively large. Finally, the distribution of the pulmonary blood flow and the ventilation of the alveoli should be as even as possible, and there should be a minimal barrier to the diffusion of gases.

The overall function of the lungs can really only be assessed by determining the effects of exercise on arterial blood gases and ventilation. This, however, is time consuming and requires medical supervision; therefore, it is applicable only to selected patients. Most lung function tests are carried out by technicians and examine various specific aspects of lung function. The simplest level of study is spirometry, which not only allows the measurement of vital capacity and its subdivisions, but may also permit expiratory and possibly inspiratory flow rates to be assessed. Laboratories specializing in lung function assessment also have facilities for the measurement of lung volumes by inert gas dilution or, possibly, the nitrogen washout method, and probably also possess a body plethysmograph. Pulmonary gas transfer can be assessed by the single-breath carbon monoxide method. Larger respiratory units are equipped for more specialized investigations, including exercise tests, compliance studies, and studies of ventilatory control.

SPIROMETRY

Spirometer types

A spirometer is a device for measuring the volumes of air that can be breathed. If the volume signal is differentiated, either electronically or by manual measurements from the volume–time traces, spirometers can also be used to derive the gas flow rates. The most accurate type of spirometer is the *water-sealed bell spirometer*. This is an inverted bell, sealed under water and

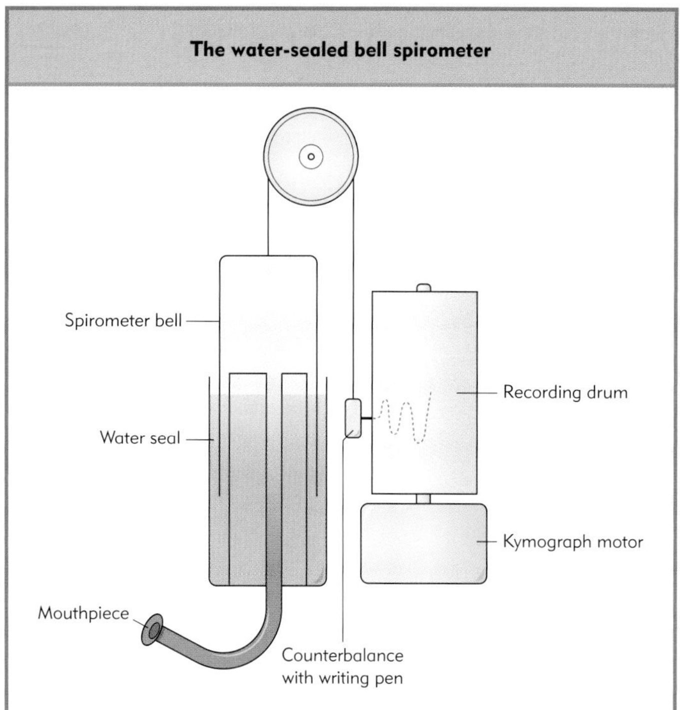

Figure 50.1 The water-sealed bell spirometer. The kymograph indicates rate of change of volume in the spirometer bell and hence the expiratory and inspiratory flow rates.

counterbalanced (Fig. 50.1). Assuming the bell is a perfect cylinder, the displacement of the counterweight and the attached pen is directly related to the change in volume. If the recording kymograph is set to move rapidly, it is possible to determine the rate of change of volume and hence the expiratory and inspiratory flow rates.

Although this type of spirometer is inherently very simple, there are a number of precautions relating to its use. Generally, the bell will have a diameter to match the calibration on the recording device or the supplied paper. Nevertheless, a check should be made by injecting known volumes of gas. The readout gives volumes at ambient pressure and temperature, although the volumes actually within the lung are at body temperature and atmospheric pressure saturated with water vapor (BTPS). This is usually about 10% greater than the measured volume, and should be corrected accordingly by applying the gas laws or by the use of appropriate tables.

For accurate measurements of high flow rates the spirometer bell and counterweight should have minimum inertia, and bells constructed of lightweight plastic materials are preferred. Another problem may be leaks in the system; these can easily be checked by occluding the connecting tubing and applying a weight on the top of the bell. The bell should not continue to move.

Water-filled spirometers have the disadvantages that they are heavy, subject to spillage, and that electronic outputs are not directly obtained. In attempts to solve these problems, various other devices have been introduced. One widely used device that is convenient and readily transported is the *bellows* or *wedge spirometer*. As gas moves into the bellows, the bellows move about the hinge and a pointer tracks over moving paper to define the expiratory volume–time trace. It does not, however, record tidal volume or inspiratory volumes. Bellows spirometers need to be carefully calibrated, with particular attention paid to the linearity of the readings.

Because spirometry is used to assess the volumes of the gas breathed and flow is derived from the rate of change of volume, an alternative approach is actually to determine flow and then derive volume by integration. Some caution, however, is required with this approach, as integration over relatively long time periods, such as may occur in patients with severe obstructive lung disease, tends to be unstable. Accurate flow-measuring devices and high-quality electronic circuits are therefore required. One widely used and accurate flow-measuring device is the *Fleisch pneumotachograph*, in which flow is determined from the pressure difference across a small resistance. It is based on Poiseuille's equation, which states that the flow through a tube is directly proportional to the pressure difference across it. This relationship applies only to laminar flow, which depends on the critical value of Reynold's number not being exceeded (see Chapter 11). Because Reynold's number is directly related to the diameters of the tubes through which the gas flows, the Fleisch pneumotachograph uses a bundle of tubes of small diameter instead of one large tube to provide the resistance. Condensation in the device is prevented by a heating element.

A very simple lightweight device that determines the peak flow rate is the *Wright peak flowmeter*. The expired gas passes through an orifice and moves a lever against a spring by an amount calibrated to read the peak flow. This device is not as accurate as most other spirometers, but it is simple, cheap, and convenient, and may be used by patients at home.

Lung volumes

The divisions of the lung volumes (and common abbreviations used for these entities) are illustrated in Figure 50.2. Note that the various subdivisions, by convention, are termed as volumes, and combinations of subdivisions are capacities. Spirometry can only determine the volumes and capacities that are actually ventilated: that is, the vital capacity and its subdivisions.

Vital capacity may be determined in three ways: from a single expiratory effort; from a single inspiratory effort; or from the sum of expiratory reserve volume and inspiratory capacity. In healthy subjects there should be little difference between these methods, but in patients with obstructive disease the measurement from the single expiratory maneuver may be lower, owing to air-trapping, and inspiratory measurements provide higher values.

Expiratory reserve volume and inspiratory capacity may be used to derive residual volume and total lung capacity from measurements of FRC.

Maximal flow rates

Flow of any fluid through a tube or system of tubes may be given by Poiseuille's equation:

■ Equation 50.1

$$F = \frac{\pi}{8} \times \frac{(P_1 - P_2)}{\eta l} \times r^4$$

where $P_1 - P_2$ is the pressure gradient across the resistance, η is the viscosity of the fluid, and r and l are terms relating to the radius and length of the tube, respectively. Resistance to flow is expressed by analogy with Ohm's Law as $(P_1 - P_2)/F$ and is

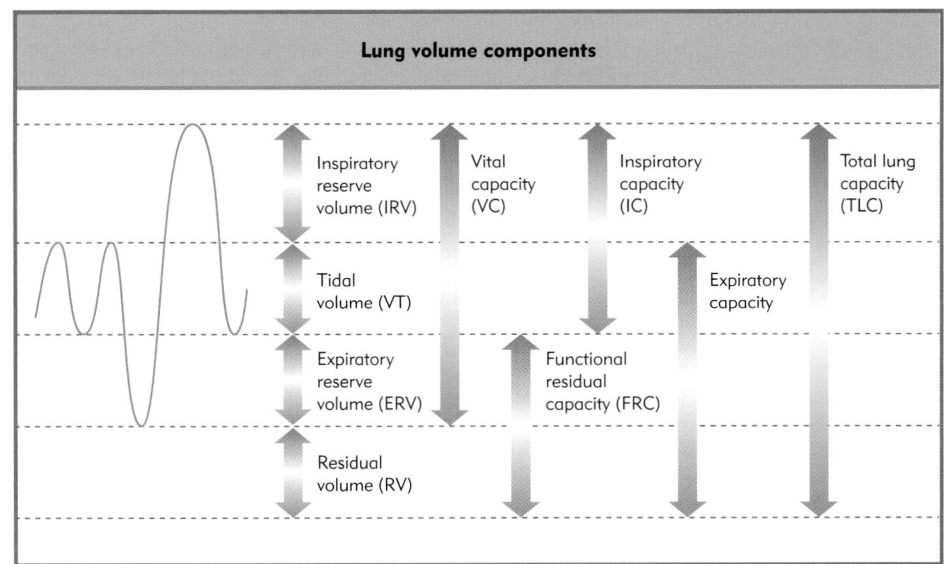

Figure 50.2 Lung volume components. The total lung capacity can be divided into various subdivisions (called volumes) and combinations of subdivisions (called capacities).

proportional to $1/r^4$. Therefore, changes in r, which in the lung relate to the radius of the airways, have a major impact on the flow. Assessments of airway resistance by spirometry are based only on the flow part of the expression and ignore pressure. Patients with fibrotic lung disease, in which the elastic recoil of the lung is exceptionally large, have particularly large expiratory flow rates. It might also be expected that the maximum flow achieved would be critically dependent on the effort made by the subject. However, the flow remains relatively unaffected by effort because high levels of intrathoracic pressure have the effect of compressing the unsplinted intrathoracic airways. As air flows along the system of airways, the pressure falls from maximal at the alveolar end to atmospheric at the mouth. The positive pressure within the thorax compresses the alveoli to drive the air out, but it also compresses the airways, and at some stage there will be a point – called the equal pressure point – at which the external and internal airways pressures balance; just beyond this point, airways close and flow is limited. Flow is therefore dependent largely on the elastic properties of the lung and the diameters of the airways, and only to a smaller extent on the effort made by the subject.

Flow may be assessed from the forced expiratory spirogram. Several measurements may be made from this. The most commonly used is the *forced expiratory volume in the first second*, (FEV_1); other measurements include $FEV_{0.75}$, the volume expired in three-quarters of a second; and the *maximum mid-expiratory flow rate*, the volume expired between 25% and 75% of vital capacity divided by time. *Peak expiratory flow*, the instantaneous maximum, is sometimes used because it can readily be estimated using Wright's peak flowmeter, and may be abnormal when FEV_1 is relatively normal in people with large airway obstructions (see below).

Flow–volume loops provide an alternative method for evaluating airways resistance. Instead of plotting volume against time, as in the expiratory spirogram, flow is plotted against either absolute lung volume or change in volume. This may be obtained for both expiration and inspiration. The normal expiratory curve (Fig. 50.3) is roughly triangular in shape. The highest flow is at the onset of expiration, when the elastic recoil is maximal and the diameter of the airways is maximal because of

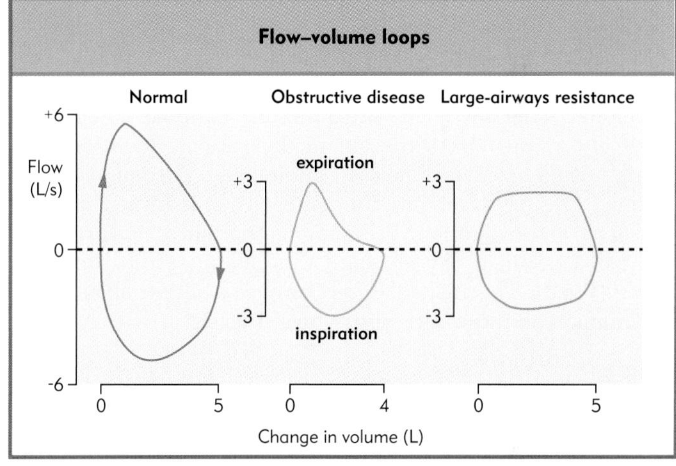

Figure 50.3 Flow–volume loops. Flow (expiration upwards) is plotted against change in volume for normal individuals (left), in obstructive disease (center), and in patients with diseases such as goiter compression or tracheal stenosis, who have large-airways resistance (right).

the negative intrathoracic pressure distending them. The inspiratory part of the loop is dependent on the inspiratory muscles and is normally more even. Patients with obstructive disease have a lower peak expiratory flow, and this declines more rapidly with reducing volume, resulting in a concave shape (Fig. 50.3). This is particularly apparent in patients with emphysema, who also have reduced elastic recoil.

In most patients flow–volume loops do not provide much more information than the expiratory spirogram. However, they are of use in assessing the effects of large-airways resistance, such as that occurring in tracheal stenosis or goiter compression. In these conditions, the high peak flow velocities cause the Reynold's number to exceed the critical value and flow becomes turbulent. When flow is turbulent, it becomes a function of the square root of pressure instead of pressure, and this effectively limits flow. This causes reduction and flattening of both expiratory and inspiratory flow rates (Fig. 50.3). Inspiratory flow is dependent on inspiratory muscle effort and is reduced when the muscles are weakened, for example following diaphragmatic paralysis.

FUNCTIONAL RESIDUAL CAPACITY

The FRC is the volume of gas in the lung at the end-expiratory point. It is the sum of residual volume and expiratory reserve volume, and cannot be determined by spirometry. Three main methods are available for the estimation of FRC: inert gas dilution, nitrogen washout, and body plethysmography.

Inert gas dilution

An inert, insoluble, readily detectable gas is required. The principle of the method is that the subject breathes from a closed-circuit system containing the gas until there is complete equilibrium between the lungs and the circuit. Assuming that the subject is switched into the circuit (Fig. 50.4) at the end-expiratory point, FRC is calculated from the dilution of the tracer gas. The main constituents are a mouthpiece attached to a tap, a soda lime canister to absorb carbon dioxide, a pump for circulating the gas to prevent a large dead-space effect, a spirometer, a gas analyzer, and an inlet for oxygen to replace that which is taken up from the lungs. Usually helium is used, and the circuit is initially filled with a mixture of about 20% helium in air and oxygen, with the tap to the patient closed and the pump turned on to mix the gases thoroughly. The initial helium reading, FHe1, is taken and the patient then is turned into the circuit at end-expiration. Rebreathing continues, with replacement of consumed oxygen, until the helium reading becomes stable (FHe2). This may take 3 minutes in healthy subjects, but much longer in those with obstructive disease.

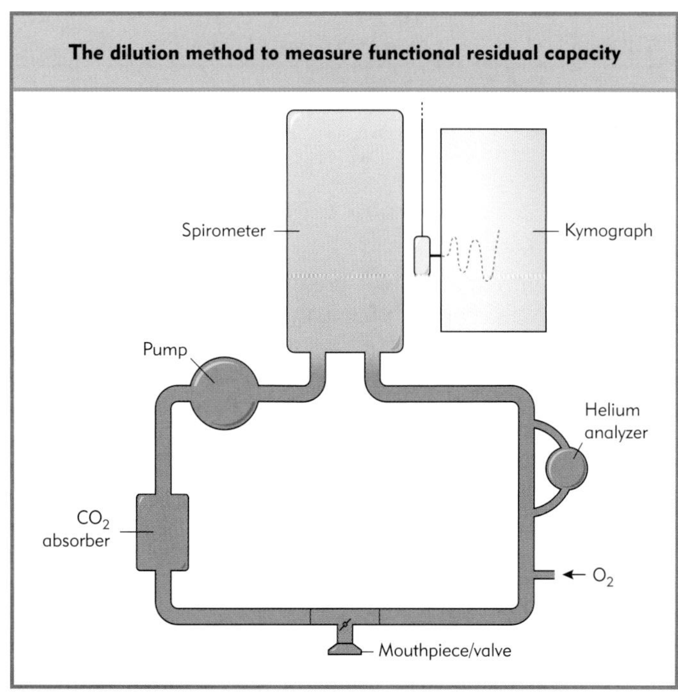

Figure 50.4 Measurement of functional residual capacity (FRC) by the inert gas dilution method.

After mixing, the volume of helium in the circuit V_{He} is equal to V_C FHe1, where V_C is the volume of the circuit. Therefore, $V_C = V_{He}/\text{FHe1}$. After rebreathing, the same volume of helium becomes equilibrated through both circuit and lung, so that:

$$V_{He} = (V_C + \text{FRC})\text{FHe2}$$

Solving these equations gives:

■ Equation 50.2

$$\text{FRC} = V_{He}\left[\frac{\text{FHe1} - \text{FHe2}}{\text{FHe1} \times \text{FHe2}}\right]$$

The main limitation of this method is that in patients with obstructive disease, and especially those with emphysema, in which ventilation of regions of the lung is very poor, FRC is likely to be underestimated. The patient may need to rebreathe for up to 10 minutes before a steady value of the helium concentration is obtained, and even then distribution of the gas throughout the lung is likely to be incomplete.

Nitrogen washout

The principle of the nitrogen washout method is that the patient breathes 100% oxygen and breathes out into a spirometer, with monitoring of the nitrogen in the expired gas until all is washed out. Allowance needs to be made for washout of dissolved nitrogen from other body compartments. The estimate of FRC is made from the volume of collected gas and its nitrogen concentration by calculating the volume that would have initially contained the nitrogen washed out. The disadvantages of this method are that washout takes a long time and, like the helium-rebreathing method, it does not estimate the volume of poorly ventilated regions of the lung. It is also very sensitive to the accuracy of the nitrogen analysis and to any small leak that may occur, for example at the mouth, during the prolonged washout period.

Body plethysmography

Body plethysmography applies Boyle's Law to the gas in the thorax and derives an estimate of its volume. This is usually called thoracic gas volume (VTG) to distinguish it from the value derived by helium dilution or nitrogen washout. It determines the total gas volume, whether ventilated or not, and may also be used to determine airways resistance (or its reciprocal, conductance).

The subject sits in an airtight box, the plethysmograph (Fig. 50.5), inserts a mouthpiece, and applies a nose clip. The mouthpiece is connected to a flowmeter, for example a Fleisch pneumotachograph, and a shutter. Mouth pressure is recorded. At the end-expiratory point, detected by the flowmeter, the shutter is closed and the subject is asked to pant gently against the shutter. As no gas enters or leaves at the mouth, the mouth pressure is equal to that in all gas-containing regions of the lung, whether adequately ventilated or not. Because the total mass of gas and its temperature are constant throughout the respiratory effort, Boyle's Law can be applied:

$$\begin{aligned} P_1V_1 &= P_2V_2 \\ P_B\text{VTG} &= (P_B - \Delta P)(\text{VTG} + \Delta V) \\ &= P_B\text{VTG} + P_B\Delta V - \Delta P_B\text{VTG} - \Delta P\Delta V \end{aligned}$$

where P_B is barometric pressure; ΔP and ΔV are the changes in lung pressure and volume, respectively, occurring with the

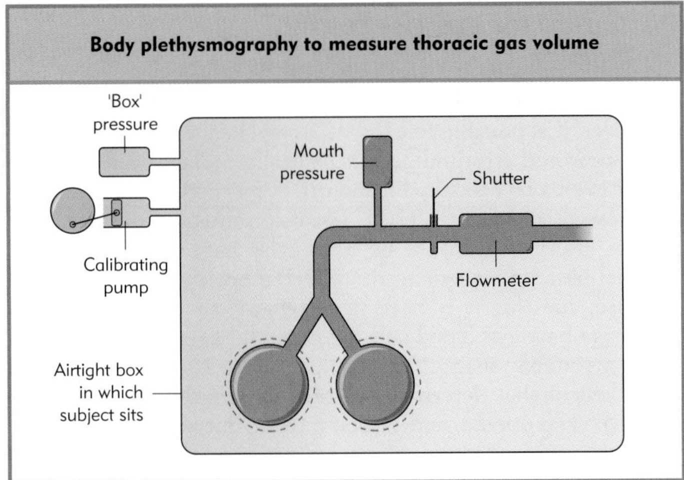

Figure 50.5 Body plethysmography to measure thoracic gas volume. This method measures the thoracic gas volume (VTG) as the total volume, whether ventilated or not. It can also be used to determine airways resistance or conductance. Alveolar volume is shown as spheres, with change in inspiration shown by dashed outlines.

inspiratory effort. Because both ΔP and ΔV are relatively small, their product can be ignored. Thus:

■ Equation 50.3

$$\mathrm{VTG} = \frac{P_B \Delta V}{\Delta P}$$

The value of ΔP is determined from the change in mouth pressure and ΔV is determined from the plethysmograph, either by use of a very sensitive volume recorder or, usually, by determining changes in plethysmograph pressure and converting that to volume by use of a calibrating pump that induces a measured pressure change for a known volume change.

The body plethysmograph can also assess *airways resistance*. The output from plethysmograph pressure, P_{BOX}, can be plotted against either the mouth pressure or the flowmeter output, F. These alternatives can be switched automatically when the shutter is opened or closed. When the shutter is open and the subject pants, recordings are obtained of F/P_{BOX}. With the shutter closed (as when determining thoracic gas volume), we obtain PA/P_{BOX}, where PA is alveolar (equal to mouth) pressure. By dividing these two tangents, $(\mathrm{PA}/P_{BOX})/(F/P_{BOX})$, we obtain PA/F, which is airways resistance. This is often expressed as its reciprocal, airways conductance (F/PA), or as specific conductance, which is obtained by dividing by thoracic gas volume.

TRANSFER FACTOR

The primary function of the lungs is the transfer of the respiratory gases. The transfer factor test was designed to provide a noninvasive method of assessing the efficiency of this process. Carbon dioxide is much more soluble and diffusible than oxygen, and the only factor likely to prevent its elimination is inadequate alveolar ventilation. Oxygen, however, may not cross the lung at a rate sufficient for full oxygenation of hemoglobin. Information about oxygen transfer requires arterial blood sampling and is discussed in the next section. Information on the likely efficiency of oxygen transfer can be obtained from the rate of transfer of carbon monoxide. Carbon monoxide has similar solubility and diffusibility to oxygen, but the affinity of hemoglobin for carbon monoxide is over 200 times greater than that for oxygen, so even at very low concentrations carbon monoxide is readily taken up by the pulmonary capillary blood.

Measurement

Transfer factor may be determined by a steady-state method that assesses the rate of uptake of carbon monoxide by analyzing its inspiratory and end-tidal concentrations. However, more commonly used now is the single-breath method. The subject takes a vital capacity breath of a gas containing a small concentration of carbon monoxide, holds it for a known period, and then rapidly exhales it. The rate of carbon monoxide transfer can be determined from the difference between the volumes of carbon monoxide inspired and expired and the breath-holding time.

In practice, there are a number of complications to this simple concept. To work out the amount of carbon monoxide transferred, we need to know the concentrations and volumes of the gas in the lung at the start and end of breath-holding. The concentration at the start is not the same as that in the inspired gas because it is diluted by residual volume. For this reason, an inert indicator such as helium is added to the inspired gas, which would typically consist of 0.3% carbon monoxide, 15% helium, 25% oxygen, and the balance as nitrogen. This gas fills a bag inside an airtight box, which has a connection to a spirometer, so the spirometer can indirectly record changes in volume in the bag. The subject takes a maximal inspiration from the bag and the volume is recorded by the spirometer. After the breath-hold (usually 10 seconds), expiration is initially to the spirometer to washout dead-space gas before a mixed alveolar sample is collected and analyzed to determine FAHe and FACO.

Helium is not taken up by the lungs, and its dilution would initially be the same as that of the carbon monoxide, so that carbon monoxide at the start of the breath hold is FICO (FAHe/FIHe). The alveolar volume, which in healthy subjects is equal to total lung capacity, is VI (FIHe/FAHe). The rate of transfer of carbon monoxide declines during the breath-holding period because its alveolar partial pressure decreases as it is taken up. This introduces a logarithmic function:

■ Equation 50.4

$$\text{Transfer factor} = \frac{f \times V\mathrm{I} \times \mathrm{FIHe}}{t \times \mathrm{FeHe}} \times \log_{10}\left[\frac{\mathrm{FICO} \times \mathrm{FAHe}}{\mathrm{FACO} \times \mathrm{FIHe}}\right]$$

For units of mL/min/mmHg f is 160, and for units of mmol/min/kPa f is 53.6.

Transfer coefficient is sometimes determined. This is simply transfer factor divided by total lung capacity.

Membrane diffusing capacity and *alveolar capillary volume* are believed to be the two factors that determine the total diffusing capacity or transfer factor. The following equation links them:

■ Equation 50.5

$$\frac{1}{\mathrm{TL}} = \frac{1}{D_m} + \frac{1}{(\theta V_c)}$$

where T_L is the transfer factor of the lung, D_m is membrane diffusing capacity, V_c is pulmonary capillary volume, and θ is the reaction rate of carbon monoxide with hemoglobin, which depends on the oxygen tension. Transfer factor is determined at normal oxygen tension, then after breathing 100% oxygen and breathing in the test gases mixed with oxygen rather than oxygen and nitrogen. This procedure yields two values for transfer factor. The reaction rates θ are determined knowing the oxygen tensions during both estimates, and T_L and D_m can then be solved using simultaneous equations.

Interpretation

The significance of the transfer factor can best be appreciated by considering the stages in the passage of carbon monoxide from alveoli to pulmonary capillary blood. The first and most important consideration is that the alveoli containing the gas should be adequately supplied with capillaries containing blood. Although the gas must diffuse across the alveolar–capillary membrane, this rarely is a limiting factor unless there is very severe thickening or advanced pulmonary congestion and edema. Transfer factor is, therefore, mainly dependent on the quantity of hemoglobin present in the pulmonary capillaries, and on the close and even distribution of ventilated alveoli and perfused capillaries. Transfer factor would be expected to be high when pulmonary blood volume is increased, as in the supine compared with the upright posture, and during physical exercise. During pulmonary congestion the increased blood volume in the lung may result in a very high transfer factor, although in advanced disease with lung damage the transfer factor may become low.

Low values of transfer factor are found in anemia, and correction factors may be applied. Low values are also associated with lung diseases involving pulmonary capillaries and alveoli. These include fibrosing alveolitis, in which there is uneven obstruction of both alveoli and capillaries. Multiple pulmonary microemboli usually cause only a modest reduction in transfer factor unless the degree of embolism is sufficient to cause pulmonary hypertension. Obstructive lung disease, asthma, and bronchitis are not usually associated with marked reductions in transfer factor. However, in emphysema, transfer factor is greatly reduced because of the marked destruction of pulmonary vessels and alveoli and the gross unevenness of ventilation and perfusion.

ASSESSMENT OF PULMONARY FUNCTION DURING EXERCISE

The main symptom in respiratory disease is breathlessness, and except in very severe conditions this only becomes a problem during exercise. It is therefore necessary to study lung function during exercise to make an effective evaluation. Exercise tests may be carried out for several reasons. In some people, exercise may provoke bronchospasm. In the investigation of these patients a moderately severe bout of exercise is undertaken followed by serial estimates of expiratory flow rates for up to 30 minutes afterwards. Exercise tests may also be used to evaluate a patient's exercise tolerance. For this purpose, an incremental exercise program may be used, for example the Bruce protocol. Exercise is continued until either exhaustion or the age-related maximal heart rate is reached. The other purpose of exercise testing is to stress the cardiorespiratory system by causing increases in pulmonary blood flow and decreases in pulmonary arterial oxygen levels. The lungs then have the problem of transferring more oxygen in a shorter time. This stress should unmask defects that may not be apparent at rest.

Procedure for exercise testing

Ideally, a motorized treadmill with controllable speed and gradient, or an electrically braked cycle ergometer is used. However, it is possible to exercise using cheaper devices, such as a self-powered treadmill, a mechanically braked cycle ergometer, or even a box to step on and off. A method of collecting the gas is essential. Ideally a 120 L Tissot spirometer would be used, but an alternative would be a Douglas bag and a gas meter. Arterial blood gas needs to be collected both at rest and during exercise; for this it is necessary to have an arterial catheter. Analysis of arterial blood and the expired gas can be carried out using a suitable analyzer. Some laboratories may be equipped with devices that determine ventilation, expired gas concentrations, oxygen uptake, and carbon dioxide output automatically.

The exercise protocol selected depends on the purpose of the study and the ability of the patient. Initially, after insertion of the arterial catheter and allowing sufficient time for stabilization, the mouthpiece is inserted and, after flushing the spirometer (or bag) with expired gas, a timed collection is made. Values obtained at rest tend to be of limited value as the presence of a mouthpiece frequently causes the patient to overbreathe or, occasionally, to underbreathe. For this reason, it is useful to take a resting blood sample before inserting the mouthpiece. To assess the various aspects of respiratory function it is not always necessary for the patient to attempt maximal exercise, and much useful information can be obtained from measurements at rest and in light and moderate exercise, these levels being selected for the particular patient. The calculations assume that the blood and the gas samples are taken at the same time. To achieve this, blood samples should be withdrawn halfway through a gas collection period. Gas collections may be taken for 2 minutes during rest and in the third or fourth minute of each level of exercise. This period is chosen to allow the subject to reach a steady state, which is necessary for the blood and the expired gas measurements to be related.

Calculations

The measurements made at rest and each level of exercise are volume of gas expired per minute ($\dot{V}_E$), average respiratory rate over the collection period, arterial blood gases and pH, and mixed expired concentrations of oxygen and carbon dioxide, $F_{\bar{E}}O_2$ and $F_{\bar{E}}CO_2$.

Oxygen uptake $\dot{V}O_2$ may be determined from the difference between the volume of oxygen inspired and that expired per minute:

$$\dot{V}_{\bar{E}}O_2 = \dot{V}_E \times F_{\bar{E}}O_2$$

and

$$\dot{V}_IO_2 = \dot{V}_I \times F_IO_2$$

Inspired volume is not precisely known, but may be calculated on the assumption that the volume of nitrogen (and other inert gases) remains unchanged.

$$\dot{V}_{\bar{E}}N_2 = \dot{V}_E\,(1 - F_{\bar{E}}O_2 - F_{\bar{E}}CO_2)$$
$$\dot{V}_IN_2 = \dot{V}_{\bar{E}}N_2$$
$$V_I = V_{\bar{E}}N_2/0.79$$

so that

$$\dot{V}IO_2 = \dot{V}EN_2 \times 0.265 = \dot{V}E\,(1 - F_{\bar{E}}O_2 - F_{\bar{E}}CO_2)\,0.265$$

■ Equation 50.6

Subtracting:

$$\dot{V}O_2 = \dot{V}_E\,[(1 - F_{\bar{E}}O_2 - F_{\bar{E}}CO_2)0.265 - F_{\bar{E}}O_2]$$

Note that $\dot{V}E$ is usually expressed at standard temperature and pressure, dry (STPD).

Carbon dioxide output is a more simple calculation:

$$\dot{V}_{\bar{E}}CO_2 = \dot{V}_E\,F_{\bar{E}}CO_2$$

The *respiratory exchange ratio* (RER) is $\dot{V}_{\bar{E}}CO_2/(\dot{V}O_2)$.

Alveolar–arterial oxygen tension difference ($P_AO_2 - PaO_2$) is calculated using the alveolar gas equation. The air inspired into the alveoli is saturated with water vapor at body temperature, leaving the tension of oxygen that would exist in the absence of gas exchange as $(P_B - w)FIO_2$ where $P_B - w$ is barometric pressure minus water vapor pressure. As the gas equilibrates in the alveoli, some of the oxygen is replaced by carbon dioxide. This would leave the alveolar oxygen tension as the saturated inspired level minus the alveolar carbon dioxide tension if each oxygen molecule were precisely replaced by one carbon dioxide. This occurs only when RER = 1. When RER does not equal 1, it is necessary to correct for this. The full form of the alveolar gas equation is:

■ Equation 50.7

$$P_AO_2 = FIO_2\,(P_B - w) - \frac{PACO_2}{RER} + \frac{PACO_2}{RER} \times FIO_2\,(1 - RER)$$

The term on the right is relatively small and is often ignored. P_ACO_2 may be substituted by $PaCO_2$ (partial pressure of carbon dioxide in arterial blood). The alveolar to arterial oxygen tension difference is obtained by subtracting the value of PaO_2 taken at the same time as the gas collection from the value of PaO_2 derived above. The alveolar tensions determined using this method assume an 'ideal' lung. Errors are likely to occur in patients with lung disease, particularly those associated with significant amounts of ventilation–perfusion mismatch.

Wasted ventilation or *'physiologic' dead space*, the sum of the anatomic dead space and the alveolar dead space (inadequately perfused alveoli), can also be determined from the data obtained in these studies. Dead space can be defined as the portion of tidal volume that does not take part in gas exchange (i.e. no carbon dioxide is evolved). The volume of carbon dioxide evolved to each breath is assumed to come only from functioning alveoli. Thus:

$$V_T \times F_{\bar{E}}CO_2 = (V_T - V_D)F_ACO_2$$

where V_T and V_D are tidal volume and dead space volume, respectively. By rearranging this equation and using $PECO_2$ to substitute for $FECO_2$, and P_ACO_2 (or better, $PaCO_2$) to substitute for $FACO_2$, the equation becomes:

■ Equation 50.8

$$VD/VT = (P_aCO_2 - PECO_2)/P_aCO_2.$$

The value of VT is determined from the minute ventilation and the respiratory frequency, and dead space is calculated by subtracting the dead space volume of the breathing valve and mouthpiece.

Interpretation

Severe exercise associated with lactic acidosis increases ventilation disproportionately and results in lower values P_aCO_2 and higher pH. Otherwise, blood gases and pH should be little changed, particularly during mild and moderate exercise. Hyperventilation lowers P_aCO_2 and raises pH. If the patient was hyperventilating chronically before the study, the pH would probably have reverted to near normal via renal compensation. Until the onset of acidosis, minute ventilation normally increases linearly with the increase in $\dot{V}O_2$. Oxygen uptake is approximately 4% of minute ventilation. This may vary to some extent, depending on the type of exercise, and tends to be less in older subjects. Nevertheless, a significant departure from this value, to less than about 3%, suggests an abnormally high minute ventilation as a consequence of either hyperventilation or an abnormally large dead space; in the latter, alveolar ventilation would not be abnormally large and $PaCO_2$ would not be low.

Exercise testing with arterial blood gas analysis can provide information on the matching of ventilation and perfusion throughout the lungs (Fig. 50.6). Even in healthy subjects in the upright position, there is considerable unevenness of both ventilation and perfusion (Chapter 47). Because of gravity, pulmonary blood flow increases from the apex to the base of the lung. Gravity also causes the lung to be stretched more at the apical part, and consequently the compliance also increases from apex to base, with a resulting increase in basal ventilation. Nevertheless, even though both ventilation and perfusion increase from apex to base, the ventilation/perfusion ratio is highest at the apex and

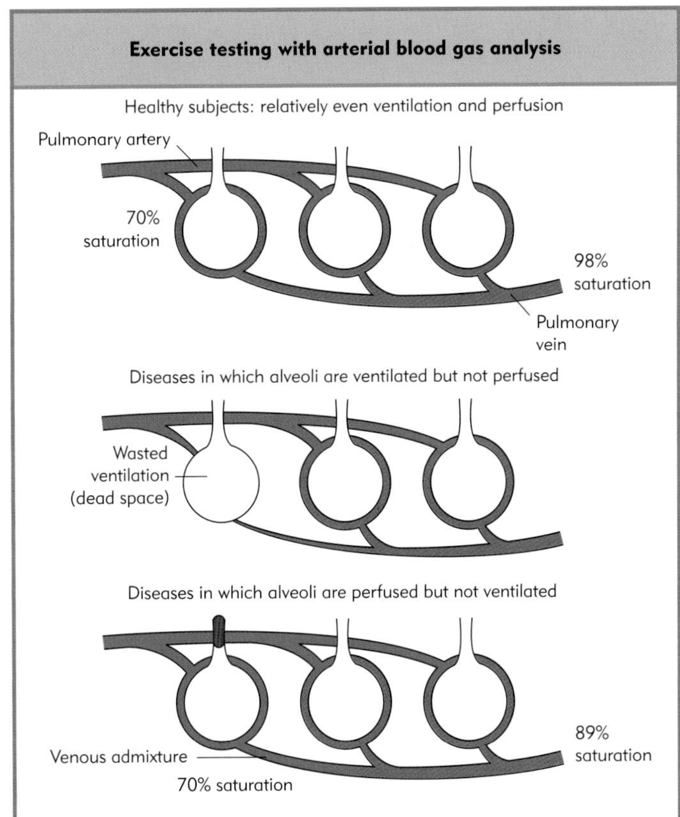

Figure 50.6 Exercise testing with arterial blood gas analysis. Even in normal individuals there is some unevenness in ventilation and perfusion. In patients with diseases invading the alveoli or the pulmonary capillaries there is more unevenness, with some alveoli inadequately ventilated and others inadequately perfused. The former results in wasted ventilation (dead space), the latter in venous admixture.

decreases progressively towards the base. In patients with diseases involving the alveoli and pulmonary capillaries there is much more unevenness, with some alveoli inadequately ventilated and others inadequately perfused (Fig. 50.6). Alveoli that are ventilated and not perfused contribute to the wasted ventilation (alveolar dead space). A pure increase in dead space would have little effect on the blood gases because normal exchange would take place in functioning alveoli. Alveoli that are perfused but not ventilated have a completely different effect and result in venous admixture. This is effectively an intrapulmonary shunt. Shunting caused by ventilation/perfusion imbalance can be distinguished from permanent shunts, for example caused by cardiac defects, because if the patient with lung disease is given 100% oxygen to breathe the blood becomes fully saturated.

Normally wasted ventilation is no more than one-third of tidal volume at rest, and this proportion decreases with exercise as tidal volume increases. The alveolar–arterial oxygen difference is normally less than 2 kPa (15 mm/Hg). The difference results from differences in ventilation/perfusion ratios and blood entering the left atrium from the thebesian and bronchial veins.

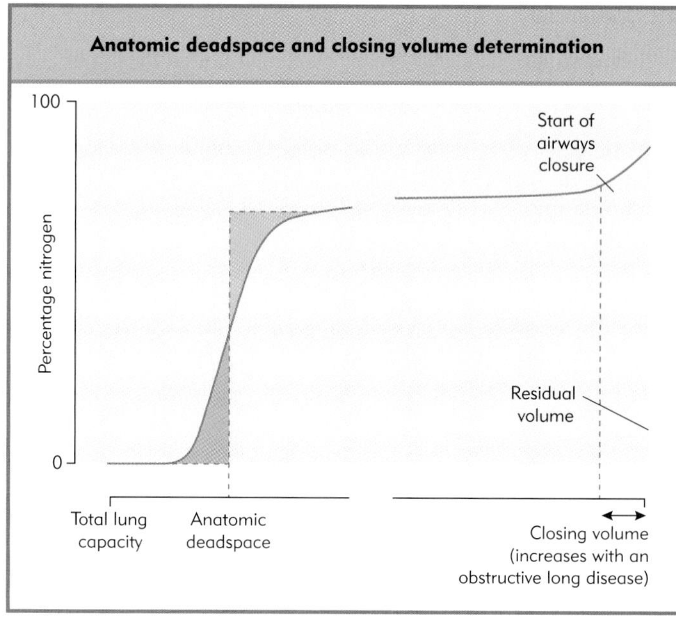

Figure 50.7 Assessment of the anatomic dead space and closing volume. In Fowler's method, a single vital capacity inspiration of oxygen is followed by exhalation into a spirometer with continuous measurements of nitrogen concentration (*y*-axis) and volume (*x*-axis). The anatomic dead space is estimated at the middle of the rising phase of the nitrogen curve, i.e. by equating shaded areas. Closing volume starts when the nitrogen level rises again and the total volume in the lung at that time is closing capacity (closing volume + residual volume).

ANATOMIC DEAD SPACE AND CLOSING VOLUME

Anatomic dead space is defined as the volume of the conducting airways, where no gas exchange takes place (Fig. 50.7). *Closing volume* is the volume towards the end of a forced expiration, after which some airways have effectively closed and more of the expired gas comes more from the relatively poorly ventilated regions of the lung. *Closing capacity* is the volume of gas within the lungs at the point at which airways closure begins. It is the sum of closing volume and residual volume.

These values can be determined using the technique described by Fowler, which involves a single breath of pure oxygen. The method requires a rapidly responding nitrogen meter, a recording spirometer, and an *X–Y* plotter to relate the expired nitrogen concentration to the expired volume. The procedure is for the subject to make a maximal exhalation to atmosphere, then take a vital capacity inspiration of 100% oxygen. The subject then exhales to residual volume into the spirometer, during which continuous recordings of nitrogen concentration and volume are made. Initially, the expired gas comes from the dead space and is nitrogen free. There is then a mixing phase; anatomic dead space is determined by bisecting the line of mixing. As the breath continues, alveolar gas is expired; if ventilation is even, the plateau rises only slowly. A steeper rise during the plateau phase can be used as a measure of uneven ventilation. Towards the end of the exhalation the nitrogen concentration may show a secondary rise. This is because the airways in the more compliant regions of the lung (bases) have closed and the exhalate comes from the apical part, which, because of its lower compliance, received less oxygen during the initial inspiration. The volume expired after the start of this secondary increase in nitrogen is the closing volume. It is small in young healthy subjects but increases with age, and is particularly large in the presence of obstructive lung disease.

COMPLIANCE

Compliance is the relationship between the change in volume of the lungs, chest wall, or both, and the changes in the relevant distending pressure. *Static compliance* is the value obtained when all measurements are made at times when there is no gas flow. *Dynamic compliance* is measured by relating volume and pressure during very slow breathing (Chapter 49). Dynamic compliance is likely to be less than the static value, particularly in patients with obstructive disease, because of the increased pressure gradients required to cause gas flow. Generally, subjects with larger lungs have similar pressure changes; consequently, their compliance is likely to be greater. For this reason we usually normalize compliance by dividing it by total lung capacity. This is the *specific compliance*.

Lung compliance is a measure of the elastic forces acting on the lung and other factors impeding its expansion. It is therefore increased when the lung becomes stiff, as in fibrotic disease, and reduced when the fibrous and elastic tissues are destroyed, as in emphysema. It is also influenced by surface tension at the alveoli, so it is low when surfactant is depleted. Compliance is also reduced by bronchial smooth muscle contraction, as well as when the pleurae are thickened. Compliance and its measurement are discussed in detail in Chapter 49.

Key references

Bates DV. Respiratory function in disease, 3rd edn. Philadelphia: WB Saunders; 1989.

Cotes JE. Lung function, assessment and application in medicine, 5th edn. Oxford: Blackwell Science; 1993.

Darkin J, Kourtelli E, Winter R. Making sense of lung function tests. London: Arnold; 2003.

Hughes JMB, Pride NB. Lung function tests: physiological principles and clinical applications. London: WB Saunders; 2000.

Lumb AB. Nunn's Applied respiratory physiology, 5th edn. Oxford: Butterworth–Heinemann; 2000.

Further reading

Forster RE, DuBois AB, Briscoe WA, Fischer AB. The lung. Chicago: Year Book Publishers; 1986.

Nunn JF. Applied respiratory physiology, 4th edn. Oxford: Butterworth-Heinemann; 1993.

West JB. Respiratory physiology: the essentials, 5th edn. Baltimore: Lippincott, Williams & Wilkins; 1999.

Chapter 51

Drugs affecting the respiratory system

Keith H Berge and David O Warner

TOPICS COVERED IN THIS CHAPTER

- **Effects on ventilatory function**
  - Normal physiology
  - Drug effects
- **Effects on airway function**
  - Normal physiology
  - Pathophysiology
  - Drug effects
  - Perioperative management of the patient with asthma
- **Effects on pulmonary vasculature**
  - Normal physiology
  - Pathophysiology
  - Drug effects

Many drugs used in clinical anesthesia have profound effects on respiratory function, both beneficial (e.g. the relief of bronchospasm in asthmatic patients) and harmful (i.e. impairment of pulmonary gas exchange). This chapter reviews the actions of anesthetic drugs and adjuvants on the striated skeletal muscles responsible for the bellows function of ventilation, the smooth muscle that determines airway caliber, and the vascular smooth muscle that regulates blood flow within the pulmonary vasculature. Although many of these agents affect more than one of these components, the discussion focuses on that area where the drug in question exerts its greatest effect, and only mentions it again briefly if it appears in the other areas.

EFFECTS ON VENTILATORY FUNCTION

It is fortunate that respiratory muscle function is relatively well maintained during ether anesthesia; indeed, this property was crucial in permitting the safe use of inhaled anesthetics before the advent of assisted ventilation. Modern inhaled anesthetic drugs have many advantages, but unfortunately they profoundly depress the function of both the bellows muscles of the chest wall (e.g. the diaphragm) and the muscles responsible for maintaining upper airway patency. Although anesthetic techniques have evolved to address this depression, alterations in respiratory function caused by anesthesia constitute a major source of morbidity and mortality in modern anesthetic practice.

Normal physiology

Although its complexity is often not appreciated, even quiet breathing requires the integration of medullary respiratory centers to coordinate the activity of multiple muscle groups. This activity may be voluntarily controlled, but is most often automatically regulated to maintain the partial pressure of arterial carbon dioxide (P_aCO_2) within a very narrow range in response to variable metabolic demands. Respiratory muscles must simultaneously serve both ventilatory and nonventilatory functions, such as speech and the maintenance of posture. The control systems regulating such a complex system are complicated and highly susceptible to disruption by anesthetic drugs. The level of consciousness itself is an important variable affecting ventilatory control, especially of the upper airway muscles.

The neural control of coordinated breathing is highly susceptible to disruption by anesthetic drugs.

In awake human subjects, consistent phasic (i.e. intermittent) electromyographic (EMG) activity is observed in the diaphragm, the parasternal intercostal muscles, and the scalenes during inspiration. As a result of this phasic activity, the diaphragm descends and the ribcage expands, thereby generating airflow. Expiration during quiet breathing is primarily passive, caused by relaxation of the diaphragm and the passive recoil of the elastic tissues of the respiratory system. Active expiration, utilized during exercise-induced hyperpnea, is produced by contraction of the abdominal muscles, as well as the transversus thoracis and internal intercostal muscles in the lateral ribcage. In upright postures, abdominal muscles are tonically active to support the abdominal contents against gravity and to prevent shortening of the diaphragm, which would impair its efficiency. Tonic activity has also been reported in the diaphragm and intercostal muscles, but the presence of this activity is controversial.

Several upper airway muscles demonstrate phasic EMG activity during inspiration, which helps maintain upper airway patency during the negative upper airway pressures generated by inspiratory flow. This activity is of critical importance; in its absence, even modest negative upper airway pressures can markedly narrow the upper airway. To overcome this collapse, active muscle contraction causes the glottis to widen during inspiration and narrow during expiration. Phasic and tonic activity is also present in several other upper airway muscles to maintain airway patency.

Drug effects

GENERAL ANESTHETICS

At doses producing surgical anesthesia, most general anesthetics (with the possible exception of ketamine) decrease resting minute ventilation, thereby increasing the P_aCO_2 maintained during spontaneous breathing (Fig. 51.1). Most agents also impair the response of minute ventilation to hypercarbia. These effects are partially offset by surgical stimulation. At equipotent combinations, these effects can also be ameliorated by the substitution of nitrous oxide for a portion of volatile anesthetic. The difference between that level of P_aCO_2 that will support spontaneous ventilation and that which will result in apnea is only 4–5 mmHg, regardless of the depth of anesthesia. Thus, efforts to assist ventilation result in only a minimal reduction of hypercarbia before apnea results. For this reason, controlled ventilation is commonly used to maintain normocarbia in anesthetized patients. General anesthetics also have important depressing effects on the activity and coordination of the muscles surrounding the upper airway that may compromise airway patency.

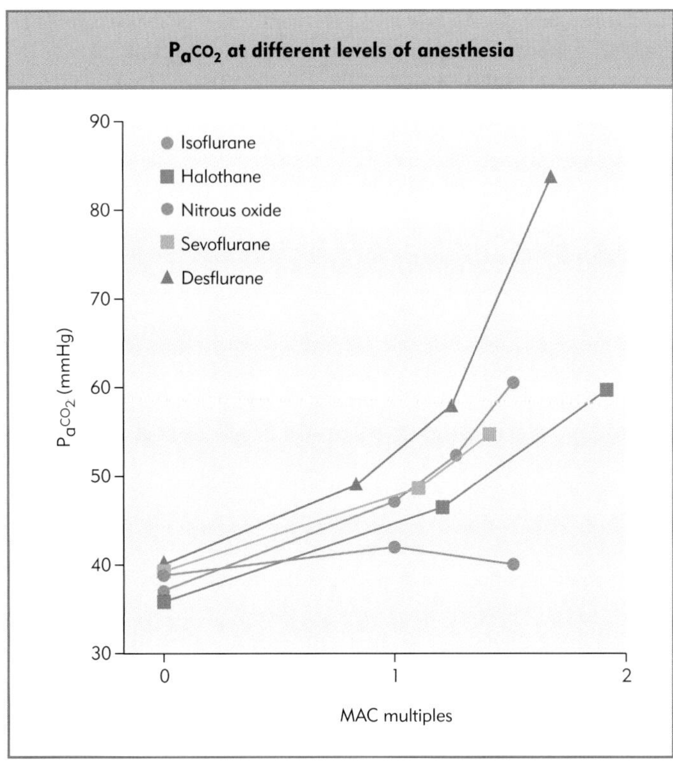

Figure 51.1 Partial pressure of arterial carbon dioxide maintained during spontaneous breathing at different levels of anesthesia, expressed as multiples of minimal alveolar concentration (MAC). Note that at equivalent anesthetic depth desflurane is the most potent respiratory depressant.

Anesthetic effects occur at multiple levels: medullary control, airway and chest wall muscles, and lung function.

The mechanisms by which anesthetics affect breathing are poorly understood. At high concentrations all anesthetics produce a global depression of respiratory motor neuron function and apnea, presumably by direct depression of medullary function. At surgical levels of anesthesia these effects are considerably more complex. For example, halothane anesthesia has differential effects on various respiratory muscle groups, depressing activity in the parasternal intercostal muscles but actually increasing activity in muscles with expiratory actions, such as the transversus abdominis. Halothane anesthesia also enhances the response of neural drive to the diaphragm during carbon dioxide rebreathing. Thus, it appears that at modest depths of surgical anesthesia halothane and other anesthetics produce respiratory depression by altering the distribution and timing of neural drive to the respiratory muscles, rather than by producing a global depression of activity (Fig. 51.2). Hypoxic ventilatory drive arising from carotid chemoreceptors is also depressed by the volatile anesthetics. The anesthetic concentration necessary for this effect is controversial. Some studies find clinically significant effects at very low concentrations, whereas in others depression is significant only at surgical depths of anesthesia. The upper airway muscles appear to be more susceptible to anesthetic-induced depression than the diaphragm.

Anesthetics have other important effects on the respiratory muscles in addition to hypoventilation. Disruption of normal upper airway muscle activity can produce airway obstruction, and changes in the position and motion of chest wall structures alter underlying lung function. Lung changes produced by deformation of the chest wall include a decrease in the functional residual capacity and atelectasis in dependent lung regions (Fig. 51.3), changes that significantly impair pulmonary gas exchange. This impairment can usually be overcome by increasing the inspired fraction of oxygen intraoperatively, but changes in chest wall function may persist into the postoperative period and produce significant postoperative morbidity.

OPIOIDS

These commonly used anesthetic adjuvants cause hypoventilation by dose-dependent depression of the brainstem respiratory centers, producing a decrease in both respiratory rate and tidal volume. Both the slope and the intercept of the ventilatory response to hypercarbia are altered. Similar effects are observed after intravenous, intramuscular, epidural, and intrathecal administration, albeit at different doses. As with the anesthetics, opioid effects are modulated by the level of consciousness. For example, patients may maintain adequate ventilation when aroused, but not when allowed to fall asleep. The partial agonist or mixed agonist/antagonist agents are less commonly associated with profound hypoventilation, but also have limitations in analgesic properties due to a ceiling effect (see Chapter 31). Some opioids, such as morphine, can release histamine and thereby exacerbate bronchospasm in susceptible patients. The potent synthetic opioids, such as fentanyl and its derivatives, can produce chest wall muscle rigidity sufficient to render ventilation impossible in the absence of neuromuscular blockade. This rigidity is typically associated with advanced age and the rapid administration of a large dose (e.g. up to 80% of patients receiv-

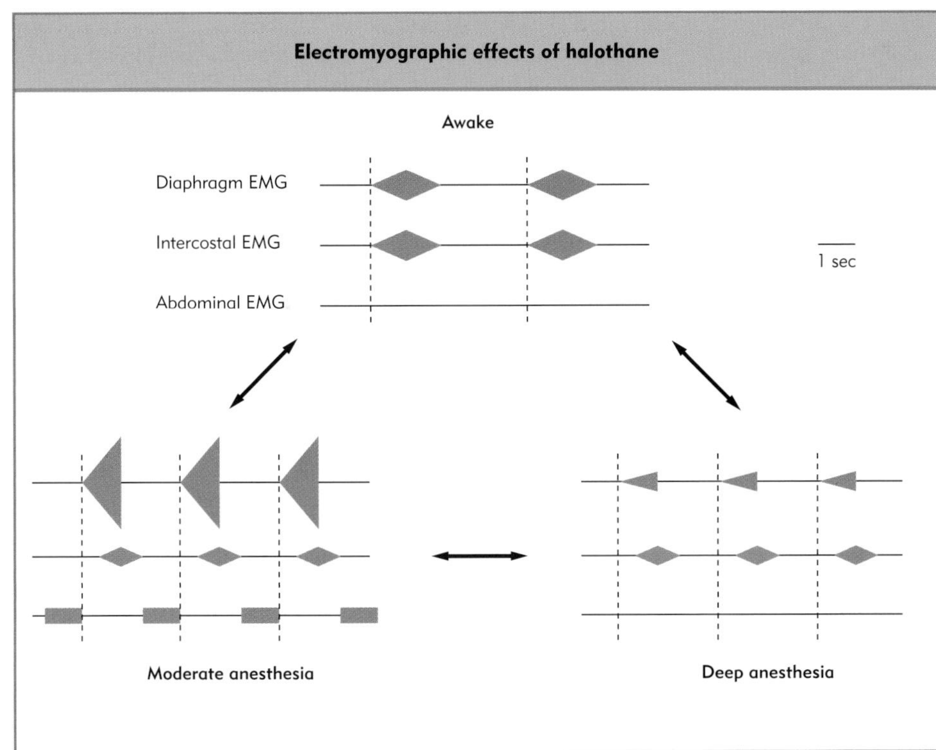

Figure 51.2 Effects of an anesthetic on EMG activity. Diagrammatic representation of the typical effects of halothane on the pattern of electromyographic activity in a human subject lying supine in three muscles with respiratory actions: the diaphragm and intercostal muscles, which have inspiratory actions, and the abdominal muscles, which have expiratory actions. While awake, the diaphragm and intercostal muscles are active during inspiration and synchronous, and the abdominal muscles are not active. With moderate anesthesia the pattern of activity is changed, with changes in timing (increased breathing frequency and asynchrony between the diaphragm and intercostals), intensity of activity (decreases in intercostal activity and increases in diaphragm activity), and the appearance of new activity (expiratory activity in the abdominal muscles). These changes in respiratory muscle coordination promote inefficiency of the bellows function of the chest wall and result in hypoventilation and increases in $P_{a}CO_2$. At deep levels of anesthesia there is global depression of all respiratory muscle function.

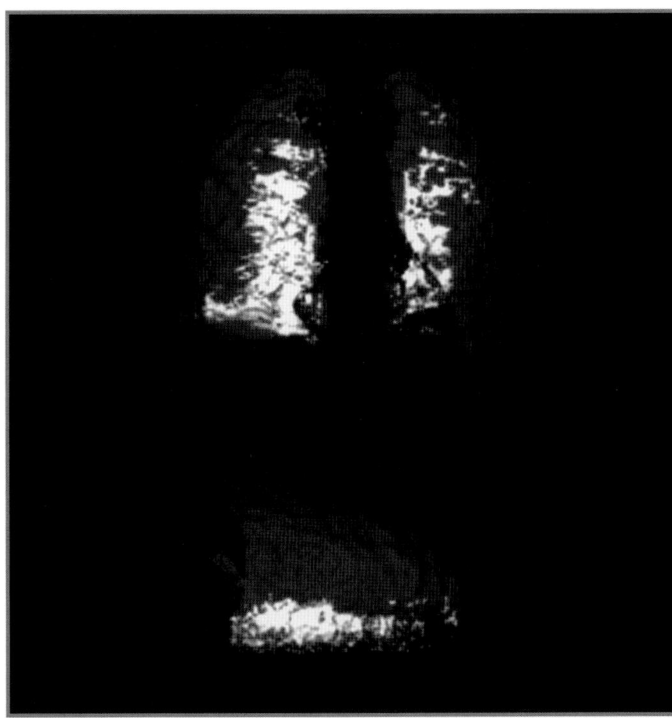

Figure 51.3 Two-dimensional representation of a lung volume image in a supine halothane-anesthetized subject obtained by fast three-dimensional computed tomography. The surface of the lung is shown in shades of gray with areas of lung atelectasis shown in white. Conceptually, this represents the view of a gray transparent three-dimensional model of lung shape, with a superimposed opaque white model of atelectasis. In the top pane, this anteroposterior view clearly shows the right and left lungs, with a visible cardiac shadow. The lateral view in the bottom panel demonstrates that the atelectatic areas are located in the most dependent lung regions. In this view, down is posterior and left is caudad. (From Warner DO, Warner MA, Ritman EL. Atelectasis and chest wall shape during halothane anesthesia. Anesthesiology 1996; 84:309–21.)

ing fentanyl 30 μg/kg), although it is occasionally seen with much lower doses.

BENZODIAZEPINES

These drugs do not generally cause significant respiratory depression when used alone in modest doses. Reported effects on hypercapnic responses are variable: some studies show moderate effects, and others no effect. When combined with fentanyl, benzodiazepines may produce profound depression of resting breathing, although the combination has no greater effect on hypercapnic sensitivity than fentanyl alone.

α_2 AGONISTS

First developed for the treatment of hypertension, drugs such as clonidine and dexmedotomidine possess hypnotic and analgesic properties that are useful in clinical anesthesia. When administered either intravenously or into the central neuraxis, they have only modest effects on resting breathing, similar to those occurring during natural sleep, and little effect on hypercapnic responses. They may thus prove quite useful in providing sedation with minimal respiratory depression in a variety of settings.

VENTILATORY STIMULANTS

Doxapram is an antiepileptic agent that causes an increase in the depth and rate of respiration, presumably via stimulation of either brainstem nuclei or carotid body chemoreceptors. Although this is effective in the short term to promote a return to adequate ventilation during recovery from anesthesia, its use has become uncommon, as mechanical ventilation, either invasive or noninvasive, is safer and more reliable. Methylxanthine drugs, a class that includes theophylline and caffeine, can increase skeletal muscle performance. These drugs improve diaphragmatic contractility, although it is unclear whether this effect is responsible for their reduction of subjective dyspnea in patients with chronic obstructive pulmonary disease (COPD). Although considered to be a ventilatory stimulant, theophylline actually has little effect on hypercapnic responses, but may augment hypoxic responses and resting breathing.

EFFECTS ON AIRWAY FUNCTION

Normal physiology

The airways, from the nasal passages to the terminal alveoli, are highly responsive to neural and humoral input. As such, their functioning can be profoundly altered by drugs, exogenous allergens, and circulating factors such as cytokines. Normal airway reflexes include protective cough reflexes, vasomotor regulation of nasal airflow resistance, and regulation of lower airway resistance via alteration of the smooth muscle tone of the conducting airways. A variety of receptors are distributed throughout the airways to mediate the afferent limb of these responses. Effectors include the skeletal muscles of the chest wall and upper airways, and the smooth muscle lining the trachea and bronchi. In humans, the predominant innervation of airway smooth muscle is via cholinergic fibers in the vagus nerve that synapse with ganglia in the airway wall (Fig. 51.4). Stimulation of these parasympathetic pathways produces bronchoconstriction, mucous secretion, and vasodilatation of bronchial vessels. The abundant β_2-adrenoreceptors in the human airway are not innervated by sympathetic nerves, but rather are activated by circulating epinephrine. Other neural systems that inhibit airway smooth muscle, termed nonadrenergic noncholinergic systems, are less well defined; candidate neurotransmitters include nitric oxide and vasoactive intestinal peptide. Cholinergic neurotransmission in the vagus nerve can also be modified by a variety of mechanisms, including prejunctional inhibition by muscarinic and opioid receptors.

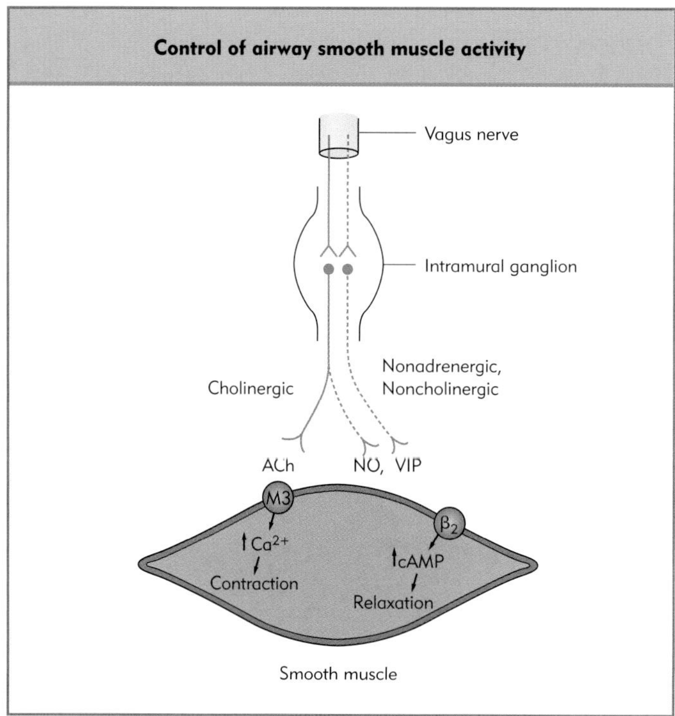

Figure 51.4 Systems controlling airway smooth muscle activity in humans. Note that β_2-adrenergic receptors on airway smooth muscle are not innervated. It is not known whether the nonadrenergic noncholinergic system utilizes distinct neural pathways (depicted by dashed lines) or whether its putative mediators nitric oxide (NO) or vasoactive intestinal peptide (VIP) are co-transmitters released with acetylcholine (ACh) from postganglionic nerves. (Adapted with permission from Warner DO. Airway pharmacology. In: Benumof J, ed. Airway management: principles and practice. St Louis: Mosby Yearbook; 1995.)

Pathophysiology

Many drugs targeting the airways are used principally in the therapy of reactive airways diseases such as asthma. Asthma is one of the few chronic diseases in the developing world with an increasing prevalence, despite improved knowledge of its pathogenesis and treatment. Theories of its pathogenesis have shifted from an underlying defect in smooth muscle reactivity to a view of asthma as a chronic inflammatory disease. The histologic alterations seen in the airway of asthma sufferers, i.e. patchy epithelial desquamation, thickening of the collagen layer of the basement membrane, and smooth muscle hypertrophy, appear to be the result of ongoing inflammatory changes. These changes result in chronic airway mucosal infiltration by activated eosinophils, lymphocytes, and mast cells. The characteristic changes in smooth muscle reactivity are thus a consequence of chronic exposure to inflammatory mediators. Therefore, the primary pharmacotherapy of asthma is aimed at quelling this chronic inflammatory response.

Asthma is a chronic inflammatory disease.

Drug effects

GLUCOCORTICOIDS

Based on the understanding of asthma as an inflammatory disease, corticosteroids have assumed a primary role in its treatment. These drugs bind to specific receptors in the cytoplasm and then are translocated to the nucleus, where they regulate the function of several genes, generally decreasing the production of inflammatory mediators such as cytokines. The advent of inhaled corticosteroids, which are poorly absorbed into the systemic circulation, has represented a significant advance in asthma therapy, minimizing the undesirable side effects associated with chronic corticosteroid use, such as significant adrenal cortical suppression or osteoporosis. There are few significant adverse side effects resulting from systemic absorption at doses adequate to control symptoms in the majority of patients. Adverse local side effects include thrush and dysphonia, presumably from deposition of the drug on the oropharynx and vocal cords. Adrenal suppression can be detected by sensitive measures in patients receiving high-dose inhaled therapy, but is rarely of clinical significance. Patient compliance may be an issue, as there is little perception of immediate benefit from treatment and concern about the side effects of steroid therapy. In patients with severe asthma systemically administered corticosteroids, with their attendant risks of adverse effects, may be required.

SYMPATHOMIMETIC AGENTS

These agents bind to β-receptors on the smooth muscle cell membrane, stimulating adenylyl cyclase and increasing the intracellular concentration of cAMP. This action can prevent or reverse the bronchoconstriction that results from provocative substances such as leukotrienes, acetylcholine, bradykinin, prostaglandin, and histamine. They may also modulate cholinergic neurotransmission, affect inflammatory cells, and stimulate mucociliary transport. Although β_2 agonists are effective when administered systemically via the intravenous or subcutaneous route, inhaled administration is convenient and minimizes undesirable systemic side effects. Inhaled short-acting β_2 agonists such as albuterol and terbutaline provide rapid symptomatic relief, whereas long-acting agents such as salmeterol and formeterol are of slower onset but provide a more sustained effect useful in those who suffer nocturnal exacerbations of asthma. Recently, concern has arisen that excessive use of long-acting inhaled β_2 agonists might increase the risk of morbidity and mortality from asthma, although the increased usage noted prior to an adverse event might simply be a marker for increasingly unstable asthma. It has been suggested that chronic use of only β_2 agonists may relieve symptoms without treating the underlying inflammatory process. For this reason, many recommend that these drugs be used episodically for acute exacerbations of symptoms, rather than as chronic therapy.

CROMOLYN AND NEDOCROMIL

These drugs inhibit the release of inflammatory mediators from several types of cells. They are generally more effective in prophylaxis than in the treatment of bronchospasm. Efficacy varies widely among patients, but because of their relative safety a therapeutic trial is often indicated.

METHYLXANTHINES

These agents have several mechanisms of action to relieve bronchospasm. Theophylline was thought to act by inhibiting phosphodiesterases that metabolize cAMP, thereby increasing intracellular cAMP concentration and causing bronchodilation. However, the drug concentrations necessary to demonstrate this effect in vitro exceed therapeutic levels in vivo. Other possible mechanisms of action include antagonism of adenosine, stimulation of endogenous catecholamine release, anti-inflammatory actions, and cardiovascular effects. Once the mainstay of chronic asthma therapy, the methylxanthines have been eclipsed by inhaled corticosteroids. However, when properly used, these drugs remain safe and efficacious for the management of patients with asthma and chronic obstructive pulmonary disease (COPD).

MUSCARINIC ANTAGONISTS

Drugs such as ipratropium bromide act as competitive antagonists of acetylcholine at the M3 subtype muscarinic receptor, which mediates parasympathetic bronchoconstriction. They also inhibit mucous secretion in the airway. These drugs generally have limited usefulness in the chronic therapy of asthma, perhaps reflecting a minor role for cholinergic motor tone in the pathogenesis of asthma. They appear to be more effective in the management of patients with COPD.

LEUKOTRIENE RECEPTOR ANTAGONISTS

This novel class of antiasthma drug targets an inflammatory mediator that may contribute to airway reactivity in asthma. Pranlukast, approved for marketing in Japan in 1995, represents the first specific competitive antagonist of leukotriene receptors to reach the marketplace. The results of several large clinical trials worldwide show pranlukast to be both safe and effective in decreasing concomitant bronchodilator and corticosteroid use while improving peak expiratory flow rate and decreasing symptom severity scores (Fig. 51.5). These agents have proved very useful in the chronic therapy of asthma.

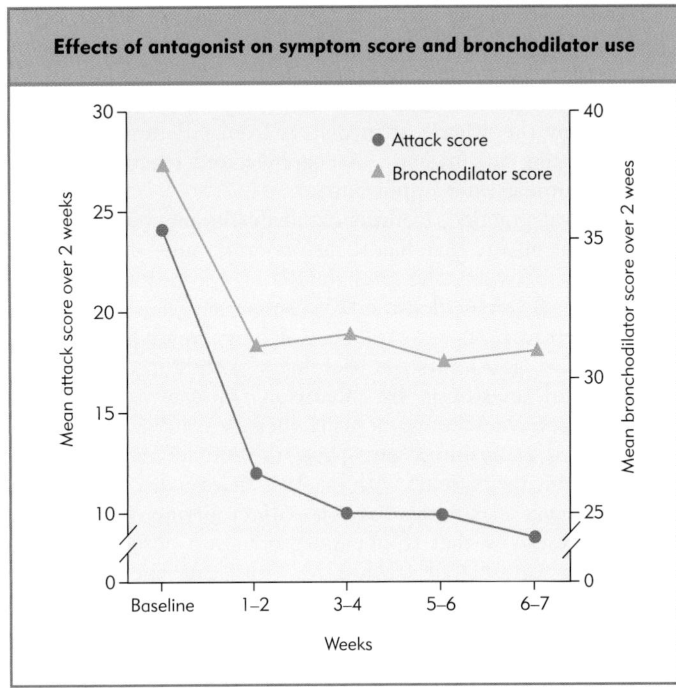

Figure 51.5 Effects of the leukotriene antagonist prankulast on symptom score and bronchodilator use score. Use of prankulast significantly improved these measures of asthma severity during an 8-week clinical trial. (Data taken with permission from Barnes NC, de Jong B, Mizamoto T. Worldwide clinical experience with the first marketed leukotriene receptor antagonist. Chest 1997; 111:52S–60S.)

Leukotriene receptor antagonists represent a novel therapy for asthma.

ANESTHETIC DRUGS AND ADJUVANTS

Volatile anesthetics are potent bronchodilators and reduce responses to bronchoconstricting stimuli, including endotracheal intubation, in both humans and animals. Because of these bronchodilating effects, volatile anesthetics have been used to treat status asthmaticus, although their efficacy in this condition is anecdotal.

Volatile anesthetics attenuate reflex bronchoconstriction in part by depressing the neural pathways that mediate these reflexes at multiple sites. This action has been localized in the vagal motor pathway to a depression of parasympathetic ganglionic transmission and, at higher concentrations of volatile anesthetics, attenuation of acetylcholine release from postganglionic nerves. Volatile anesthetics also directly relax airway smooth muscle by at least two mechanisms. They decrease intracellular calcium concentration during both the initiation and maintenance of airway smooth muscle contraction, and may decrease the force developed by the smooth muscle for a given level of intracellular calcium (i.e. the 'calcium sensitivity'). The relative importance of neurally mediated versus direct smooth muscle relaxant effects of volatile anesthetics depends on the mechanism producing bronchoconstriction. During reflex bronchoconstriction, such as that produced in response to noxious stimuli such as airway instrumentation, depression of neural pathways is of greatest importance. During bronchoconstriction produced by the release of mediators from inflammatory cells, such as during anaphylactic or anaphylactoid reactions, direct effects assume greater importance.

In clinical practice, isoflurane and desflurane are more irritating to the airway than halothane or seroflurane, although few differences between the bronchodilating properties of most volatile agents can be identified experimentally. This stimulation of airway nociceptors can produce coughing, breath holding, and laryngospasm, and limits the usefulness of these agents for the induction of anesthesia by inhalation. In contrast to other volatile agents, desflurane actually increases airway resistance when added to inspired gas. Thus, desflurane may not be a suitable agent for patients with reactive airways disease.

Intravenous anesthetics may also affect airway reactivity. In vitro studies show that thiopental produces a dose-dependent constriction of isolated trachea by promoting the release of thromboxane A_2. This finding is not observed with oxybarbiturates such as methohexital. Thiopental has also been reported to cause bronchospasm by releasing histamine, although other studies have not demonstrated an association between bronchospasm and barbiturate administration. Although thiopental releases histamine from skin mast cells, this effect has not been experimentally demonstrated in lung. Ketamine depresses neural airway reflex pathways and directly relaxes airway smooth muscle by decreasing intracellular calcium concentration. Ketamine-induced release of endogenous catecholamines may also contribute to its bronchodilating effects. Propofol apparently blunts airway reflexes, as propofol induction of anesthesia permits insertion of the laryngeal mask airway without apparent reflex responses such as laryngospasm. The incidence of wheezing during induction is reduced during propofol induction compared with barbiturates, suggesting its usefulness in patients with reactive airways.

Perioperative management of the patient with asthma

Preoperative preparation is directed towards minimizing airway inflammation and reactivity, with continuation of anti-inflammatory agents and bronchodilators until immediately before surgery. Firm data to support the traditional preference for regional anesthesia in these patients are lacking, although it seems reasonable to avoid the stimulation of airway manipulation when feasible. The volatile anesthetics remain the foundation of general anesthetic techniques, with little difference in clinical outcome observed among the available agents when utilized after intravenous induction. Propofol would appear to be the intravenous drug of choice for induction. If airway instrumentation is necessary, prior adequate anesthesia of the airway is essential. This can be provided by a period of ventilation with a volatile anesthetic following intravenous induction. In addition, both β_2 agonists and muscarinic antagonists blunt increases in respiratory system resistance associated with endotracheal intubation. Lidocaine may also be useful, with intravenous administration preferred, as airway irritation by nebulized lidocaine may actually increase airway resistance in asthmatic subjects.

Volatile anesthetics are the rational choice for asthma and bronchospasm.

If bronchospasm develops, it is of primary importance to first firmly establish the diagnosis of bronchospasm, as many other processes, such as mechanical obstruction of the endotracheal tube, may produce signs mimicking bronchospasm. Once the diagnosis is confirmed, anesthesia should be deepened utilizing a volatile anesthetic. Other drugs to deepen anesthesia, such as propofol and fentanyl, may also be useful. The role of intravenous aminophylline is controversial, as in experimental animal models of asthma it has no benefit beyond that provided by volatile anesthetics. In contrast, β_2 agonists provide further bronchodilation under such circumstances, and are definitely indicated. If given via inhalation repeated doses may be necessary, as the efficiency of nebulized drug delivery is decreased through endotracheal tubes, especially in the setting of severe bronchospasm. In severe cases, intravenous administration of β-adrenergic agonists may be necessary.

EFFECTS ON PULMONARY VASCULATURE

Normal physiology

The caliber of the pulmonary vasculature is regulated by several factors, including the mechanical stresses associated with gravity and changes in lung volume, neural control via autonomic nerves, vasoactive substances released from the vascular endothelium, and factors intrinsic to vascular smooth muscle, such as hypoxic pulmonary vasoconstriction. These factors are normally integrated to optimize the balance between regional ventilation and perfusion, and hence gas exchange (Chapter 47). The fact that pulmonary vessels comprise a low-pressure system makes gravitational effects relatively important in determining blood flow, according to well-described lung zones. However, recent evidence suggests that intrinsic regional differences in vascular conductance not related to gravity are also important. There is abundant sympathetic and parasympathetic innervation of pulmonary vessels. Sympathetic stimulation increases pulmonary vascular resistance, primarily via stimulation of α_1-receptors. The effect of parasympathetic stimulation varies with species and with the level of pre-existing vascular tone. The physiologic role of this neural innervation remains unclear. A variety of endogenous peptides, amines, and lipid mediators affect vascular tone, including angiotensin II, bradykinin, vasopressin, atrial natriuretic peptide, endothelin, acetylcholine, histamine, serotonin, and eicosanoids. Many of these mediators, such as nitric oxide, are produced in the vascular endothelium. As with neural innervation, the exact physiologic role and interactions of these compounds are unknown. Finally, small pulmonary arteries respond to local hypoxia by increasing their tone (hypoxic pulmonary vasoconstriction, HPV). HPV serves to direct blood flow away from relatively hypoxic areas of the lung, thereby better matching local ventilation to local perfusion and limiting the amount of hypoxemia resulting from atelectasis. Although the mechanism responsible for HPV remains unknown, it is not neurally mediated as it remains intact in denervated transplanted lungs, and appears to be intrinsic to vascular smooth muscle.

Hypoxic pulmonary vasocontriction is intrinsic to lung vascular smooth muscle.

As a consequence of the large surface area of the pulmonary capillaries (approximately 70 m^2 in the adult human lung), a significant amount of fluid and accompanying solutes leaves the microcirculation and enters the interstitium by processes dependent on the relative balance of hydrostatic and oncotic forces. Fluid is normally returned to the circulation by lymphatics. A safety factor exists in the system such that pressure in pulmonary capillaries can increase three- to fourfold before lung interstitial volume increases.

Pathophysiology

Several chronic disease states result in hypertension in the pulmonary arterial circulation. These include increases in pulmonary flow resulting from congenital cardiac disease, increases in outflow pressure from cardiac failure or valvular disease, increased tone from chronic hypoxia, loss of the vascular lumen from thromboembolism, parenchymal disease, or idiopathic disease (e.g. primary pulmonary hypertension). Many of these chronic conditions produce vascular remodeling, characterized by increased concentric smooth muscle mass, endothelial cell injury, and intimal proliferation. The overall physiologic result of these responses to lung injury is not only impairment of the gas-exchanging ability of the lung, but right ventricular strain, which may ultimately result in heart failure and death.

Acute pulmonary hypertension may result from acute lung injury (ALI), a pathologic lung response sustained by activated inflammatory cells, predominately polymorphonuclear leukocytes. The generalized inflammation of the lung seen in this disorder creates increased pulmonary vascular tone and pulmonary hypertension by altering the reactivity of the pulmonary vasculature to both endogenous and exogenously administered vasoactive substances. As an example of the disruption of normal function, ALI generally inhibits HPV. Lung fluid balance is also affected by ALI, producing a flooding of the alveoli, which is worsened by the increased hydrostatic pressure gradient due to pulmonary hypertension. Surfactant function, important for maintaining the architectural integrity of the lung, is also impaired in ALI. A bewildering variety of inflammatory mediators may contribute to the changes seen in ALI, which may be acute with rapid resolution or result in chronic impairment from fibrotic changes.

Drug effects

INHALED ANESTHETICS

Volatile anesthetics affect pulmonary vascular pressures to only a small degree in the absence of underlying pulmonary disease. As in the systemic circulation, they appear to interfere with the normal response of the pulmonary vasculature to dilating factors released from the endothelium. Nitrous oxide can increase pulmonary vascular resistance when administered to patients with coexisting pulmonary hypertension. Inhaled anesthetics directly inhibit HPV in isolated lung models; however, halothane and isoflurane have only minimal further effects on oxygenation in anesthetized patients undergoing one-lung ventilation, presumably as a consequence of other compensatory mechanisms. For example, decreases in cardiac output produced by anesthetics may actually tend to enhance the effectiveness of HPV and offset concurrent direct inhibition.

RESPIRATORY GASES

Responses to increases in arterial carbon dioxide and oxygen partial pressures can be difficult to predict, as both local and systemic factors interact. However, in general, both act as vasodilators within physiologic ranges in most vascular beds. Chronic inhaled oxygen therapy has been shown to reverse or at least impede progressive worsening of pulmonary hypertension in patients suffering from hypoxia-inducing lung diseases such as COPD. Oxygen is a drug with a definite therapeutic window. Too little oxygen in the inspired mixture, or too low an inspired partial pressure, as may occur at high altitude, results in pulmonary hypertension via HPV, and ultimately in the possibility of tissue hypoxia. High inspired partial pressures of oxygen are directly toxic to the lung parenchyma. Such conditions might occur when breathing concentrated oxygen for prolonged periods, or when breathing room air under hyperbaric conditions. Oxygen in such concentrations overwhelms the body's normal antioxidant defense mechanisms, such as superoxide dismutase, glutathione peroxidase, and catalase, rendering the tissues susceptible to damage by free radicals such as superoxide, hydroxyl, and singlet oxygen. Although hyperoxia is toxic to all tissue beds, the respiratory system is most at risk because of its exposure to the highest concentrations, and will manifest symptoms and histologic changes after as little as 6 hours of exposure to 100% oxygen. Ultimately, with continued exposure these changes result in systemic hypoxemia by disrupting efficient gas exchange.

VASODILATORS

Systemically administered vasodilators, such as the nitrovasodilators, β_1 agonists, Ca^{2+} channel antagonists, or prostacyclin produce a response in all vascular beds, including the pulmonary vasculature. Unfortunately, many currently available intravenously administered agents tested in dose ranges sufficient to reduce pulmonary pressure result in systemic vasodilation and hypotension to a degree that renders them useless for selective pulmonary vasodilation. In addition, intravenous vasodilators such as nitroprusside, prostacyclin (PGI_2), prostaglandin E_1, or isoproterenol interfere with HPV, increasing venous admixture and further worsening arterial hypoxemia. As a consequence, systemic therapy has little role in the therapy of pulmonary hypertension, except perhaps for the Ca^{2+} channel blockers, which, despite interfering with HPV, improve survival in a responsive subgroup of patients with primary pulmonary hypertension. Nebulized administration of prostaglandins is a promising approach that may confer a degree of pulmonary selectivity.

NITRIC OXIDE (NO)

NO is a vasodilating substance with an extremely short half-life which is produced principally by endothelial cells. In addition to regulating local vascular tone, NO regulates other physiologic functions, such as platelet aggregation, neurotransmission, and antitumor and antimicrobial activity. NO diffuses out of the endothelial cell and into adjoining vascular smooth muscle cells, causing relaxation and vasodilation via a cyclic GMP messenger system. The short half-life of NO, and therefore the limitation of its effect to the immediate locale of its formation, is due to

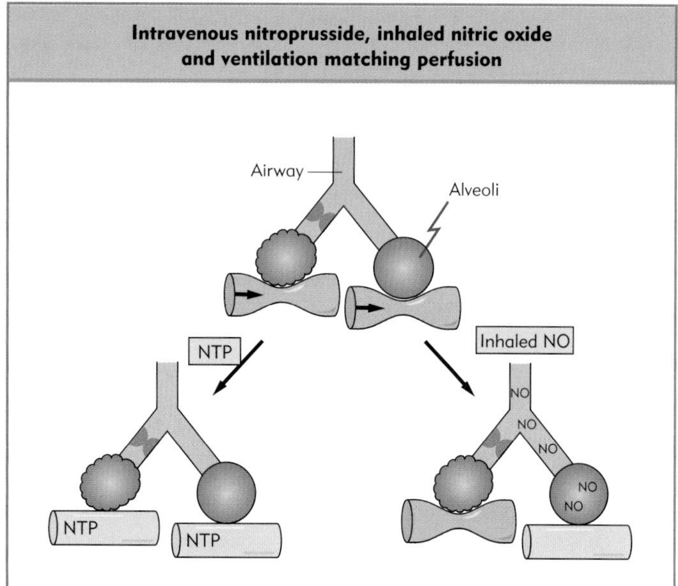

Figure 51.6 Schematic of the effects of intravenous nitroprusside (NTP) and inhaled nitric oxide (NO) on ventilation/perfusion matching. Two alveoli with accompanying pulmonary capillaries are shown, one with normal ventilation (right) and one with no ventilation due to airway obstruction or atelectasis (left); NTP dilates all pulmonary arteries, which may worsen mismatching of ventilation to perfusion. Inhaled NO dialates only arteries associated with ventilated alveoli, which may improve matching of ventilation to perfusion. (Adapted with permission from Lunn RJ. Inhaled nitric oxide therapy. Mayo Clin Proc. 1995;70:247–55.)

its rapid binding to hemoglobin. The nitrovasodilators sodium nitroprusside (SNP) and nitroglycerine (NTG) act in part by the release of NO through spontaneous or enzymatic breakdown, although other mechanisms of action may also be important. That SNP is a more potent arteriolar vasodilator and NTG a more potent venodilator most likely reflects regional differences in the uptake or breakdown of these drugs, and the subsequent release of NO.

Inhaled NO therapy produces selective pulmonary vasodilation.

Inhaled NO therapy has been advocated as a method of producing selective pulmonary vasodilation to treat pulmonary hypertension. Although toxic in higher concentrations, inhaled NO in a concentration range of 60 ppb to 60 ppm (cigarette smoke contains up to 1000 ppm) results in selective pulmonary vasodilatation with minimal systemic vasodilation. A possible additional benefit of the inhalation route is that NO is delivered directly to those vascular beds providing flow to the lung regions that are best ventilated, thus not worsening venous admixture and arterial hypoxemia as do the intravenously administered agents (Fig. 51.6). NO has proved useful in improving gas exchange or pulmonary artery pressures in neonates following the correction of cardiac anomalies, in persistent pulmonary hypertension of the newborn, and in adult respiratory distress syndrome. However, several randomized controlled clinical trials have been unable to demonstrate that NO improves outcomes in most patient populations.

SUMMARY

Many anesthetics and adjuvants have significant effects on the respiratory system that require active intervention by the anesthesiologist, especially the profound depression of respiratory muscle function. Some of these effects, such as bronchodilation, are fortuitously quite beneficial in selected patients.

Key references

Drummond GB. Upper airway reflexes. Br J Anaesth. 1993; 70:121–3.

Froese AB, Bryan AC. Effects of anesthesia and paralysis on diaphragmatic mechanics in man. Anesthesiology 1974; 41:242–55.

Greenberger PA. Corticosteroids in asthma. Rationale, use, and problems. Chest 1993; 101:418S–21S.

Pizov R, Brown RH, Weiss YS et al. Wheezing during induction of general anesthesia in patients with and without asthma. Anesthesiology 1995; 82:1111–16.

Nandi PR, Charlesworth CH, Taylor SJ, Nunn JF, Dore CJ. Effect of general anaesthesia on the pharynx. Br J Anaesth. 1991; 66:157–62.

Warner DO, Warner MA, Ritman EL. Atelectasis and chest wall shape during halothane anesthesia. Anesthesiology 1996; 84: 309–21.

Westbrook PR, Stubbs SE, Sessler AD, Rehder K, Hyatt RE. Effects of anesthesia and muscle paralysis on respiratory mechanics in normal man. J Appl Physiol. 1973; 34:81–6.

Further reading

Barnes PJ. Modulation of neurotransmission in airways. Physiol Rev. 1992; 72:699–729.

Iscoe SD. Central control of the upper airway. In: Mathew OP, Sant'Ambrogio G, eds. Respiratory function of the upper airway. New York: Marcel Dekker; 1988:125–92.

Warner DO. Airway pharmacology. In: Benumof J, ed. Airway management: principles and practice. St Louis: Mosby Yearbook; 1995.

Warner DO. Respiratory muscle function. In: Biebuyck JF, Lynch C III, Maze M, Saidman LJ, Yaksh TL, Zapol WM. Anesthesia: biologic foundations. Vol. II, Part 3. Respiratory system. New York: Raven Press; 1997:1395–415.

Zapol WM, Bloch KD. Nitric oxide and the lung. New York: Marcel Dekker; 1997.

SECTION 6

Pathological sciences

Chapter 52

Blood constituents and transfusion

Mark C Bellamy and Dafydd Thomas

BONE MARROW, BLOOD CELLS, AND PLASMA CONSTITUENTS

In fetal life, the yolk sac is the main site for hemopoiesis until 6 weeks of gestation. From 6 weeks until 7 months, the liver and spleen play the major role. Both liver and spleen continue to produce red blood cells until 2 weeks after birth, although the principal site of hemopoiesis from 7 months of fetal life onwards throughout normal childhood and adult life is bone marrow. In infants, practically all bones are involved. In adults, hemopoiesis is confined to vertebrae, ribs, sternum, skull, sacrum, pelvis, and proximal femur. Under extreme conditions there can also be expansion of hemopoiesis into other long bones. The phenomenon of extramedullary hemopoiesis (liver and spleen) is also occasionally seen.

A common, pluripotential stem cell gives rise to all cells of the hemopoietic line. After a number of divisions and early differentiation, the pluripotential stem cell differentiates into progenitor cells for the three main marrow cell lines: erythroid, granulocytic (including monocytes), and megakaryocytic. Progenitor cells are capable of responding to a number of stimuli, with increased production of one or other cell lines according to need. Transplanted hemopoietic cells seed successfully to the marrow, but fail to survive at other sites. This is the basis for bone marrow transplantation.

Red blood cells

The pronormoblast is the earliest red blood cell recognizable in the marrow. Progressively smaller normoblasts result from cell division. As this process of maturation proceeds, cells develop a progressively greater hemoglobin content. There is progressive loss of RNA and protein-synthesizing apparatus from the cytoplasm, and the cell nucleus is extruded from late normoblasts. This results in a cell known as a reticulocyte, which initially resides in bone marrow and has low levels of cytoplasmic RNA (but is still capable of synthesizing hemoglobin). Hemoglobin-synthesizing capability is lost when the cell enters the circulation as a mature erythrocyte. The mature cell is a biconcave disc with no nucleus. At times of hemopoietic stress, reticulocytes may also appear in the peripheral circulation.

Erythropoiesis is predominantly governed by the hormone erythropoietin. Relative renal hypoxemia gives rise to expression of a nuclear transcription factor that causes increased expression of the erythropoietin gene. Erythropoietin increases the number of stem cells committed to erythropoiesis.

The mature red blood cell has a diameter of 8 μm and a lifespan of 120 days. It is extremely flexible, and can pass through vessels in the microcirculation with a minimum diameter of only 3.5 μm. It is capable of synthesizing adenosine triphosphate (ATP) and the reduced form of nicotinamide adenine dinucleotide (NADH) by the anaerobic glycolytic pathway. The red cell membrane-associated enzyme methemoglobin reductase is associated with the glycolytic pathway and NAD^+/NADH metabolism. Function of this enzyme is important for maintaining the ferrous (Fe^{2+}) oxidative state of iron in hemoglobin. Oxidation to the ferric state (Fe^{3+}) results in methemoglobin, which is ineffective as an oxygen carrier. Many drugs can induce significant oxidative stress and thus result in methemoglobin production. These include acetaminophen (paracetamol) and most local anesthetic agents, notably prilocaine.

Many drugs, including acetaminophen and prilocaine, can induce methemoglobin production.

Red cell production in the marrow is a process requiring many precursors to synthesize the new cells and their proteins, including hemoglobin. Essential substances known as hematinics include vitamins (vitamin B_{12}, folate, vitamin C (ascorbic acid), D-α-tocopherol (vitamin E), vitamin B_6, vitamin B_1 (thiamine), vitamin B_2 (riboflavin), pantothenic acid, metals (iron, manganese, cobalt) and essential amino acids.

Deficiencies can result in failure of erythropoiesis, with characteristic anemias. Megaloblastic (i.e. large, immature cells) anemia results from deficiencies of vitamin B_{12} or folate. Iron-deficiency anemia results in small, hypochromic cells. Anemia may also occur with amino acid or androgen deficiency, although this may be simply an adaptive response to reduced tissue oxygen consumption rather than a direct effect of the 'hematinic' deficiency. The anemias of chronic disease fall into this category.

HEMOGLOBIN

Hemoglobin is a red cell protein that facilitates oxygen and carbon dioxide transport (Chapter 48). There are approximately 640 million molecules of hemoglobin in each red blood cell. Hemoglobin consists of four polypeptide chains (two α and two β chains). Each of these chains is associated with a heme prosthetic group. Each hemoglobin chain has a molecular weight of 68 kDa. Adult blood contains traces both of hemoglobin F (fetal hemoglobin) and hemoglobin A_2. These contain α chains, but the β chains are replaced with γ and δ chains, respectively. Most hemoglobin (65%) is synthesized at the erythroblastic stage and the remainder at the reticulocyte stage. Heme synthesis (predominantly in the mitochondrion) begins with the condensation of glycine and succinyl coenzyme A. Vitamin B_6 is a coenzyme for this process. A ring structure is formed (protoporphyrin) that then combines with iron to form heme. Each heme molecule associates with a globin chain manufactured on the polyribosomes. A tetramer forms comprising two α and two β chains, each with its associated heme molecule.

White blood cells

Leukocytes may be divided into two broad groups: phagocytes and lymphocytes. Phagocytes include neutrophils (polymorphonuclear cells or polymorphs), eosinophils, basophils and monocytes. Neutrophils have a diameter of 12–15 μm and a characteristic dense multilobular (two to five lobes) nucleus. The cytoplasm is characterized by numerous fine azurophilic granules. Mature polymorphs contain two types of granule, both derived from lysozymes. Primary granules contain myeloperoxidase and acid phosphatase. Secondary granules contain alkaline phosphatase and lysozyme. The earliest recognizable neutrophil precursor is the myeloblast, which is seen in bone marrow but not in peripheral blood; this divides to form myelocytes, with a distinct myelocyte for the eosinophil and the basophil cell lines. The myelocytes divide to form metamyelocytes, which further mature to take on the multilobular form of the mature polymorph. Intermediate nuclear morphologies are known as 'band' or 'juvenile' forms. At times of high neutrophil production (infection), immature band forms may be seen in the peripheral circulation.

Lymphocytes are small cells (7–15 μm in diameter) produced in both marrow and thymus. Larger lymphocytes may be seen following antigenic stimulation. The immune response is a function of both T and B lymphocytes (Chapter 54).

Platelets

Platelets are produced in bone marrow from megakaryocytes, which are derived from the pluripotential stem cell. Each megakaryocyte undergoes rapid nuclear replication without cell division. With the addition of further nuclei, there is an increase in cytoplasm and cell size. When the cell reaches the eight-nucleus stage, replication ceases. The cytoplasm becomes progressively more granular and produces microvesicles, which coalesce to form platelet demarcation membranes. Fragmentation of megakaryocyte cytoplasm then follows, with the release of platelets. Each megakaryocyte releases about 4000 platelets. Young, immature platelets spend 24 hours in the spleen before entering the circulation. Platelets have a lifetime of 10–15 days.

Plasma

Blood cells are suspended in plasma, a solution of electrolytes, proteins such as albumin, globulins and clotting factors, lipids, and lipoproteins. Plasma acts as a vehicle for nutrient transport and the immune system and plays a key role in coagulation and hemostasis.

BLOOD GROUPS

Red blood cells possess over 300 antigen systems expressed on the cell surface. These antigen systems are genetically determined. They are important in the recognition of 'self' as opposed to 'nonself'. The surface antigens are of clinical relevance in blood transfusion compatibility, and to some extent in compatibility of transplanted organs. The transfusion of cells of a different antigenicity to the patient's can result in lysis by endogenous antibodies, or the production of new antibodies with this potential.

The main group of cells involved is the red blood cell. Some antigenic systems are known as blood group systems. A blood group results from expression of alleles at a single locus or at closely linked loci. There are 18 important blood group systems. Together with their number of potential antigens, these include ABO (4), Rhesus (45), MNS (38), P (1), Lutheran (18), Kell (21), Lewis (3), Duffy (6), Kidd (3), and others. By convention, the genotype is distinguished from the phenotype by the use of italic script. For example, *A1* is a genotype, but A1 is a phenotype.

Most red blood cell antigens are expressed and readily detectable by the age of 2 years. Thereafter they remain stable throughout life. Many components of the genotype are inherited together because of linkage on the same chromosome. However, some degree of recombination (Chapter 4) is possible because of the phenomenon of crossover. This occurs after the first meiotic division. Crossover is more likely where alleles are located remotely on the chromosome. Most blood group systems follow simple mendelian inheritance.

ABO and transfusion

Important among blood group systems is the ABO system. Inheritance of this system is characterized by codominance and silent genes (amorphs). Silent genes have no observable phenotypic expression. Many blood group genes result directly in expression of a protein antigen: the Rhesus system is an example of this. Other blood group systems, such as the ABO system, are characterized by a carbohydrate antigen. Expression of the gene encoding for carbohydrate antigens is dependent on the presence of appropriate substrate or enzyme systems. These may in turn rely on the presence of another gene. The ABO system relies on the presence of the H gene to produce necessary substrate: in those rare individuals (Bombay) who lack this gene, carbohydrate antigens of the ABO system are not expressed. Red blood cells of these individuals appear to be group O by phenotype, whereas they may be other blood groups by genotype.

The ABO blood group system is the most important. It is fully expressed by 6 months of age, and by this time most individuals have antibodies directed against any antigens to the ABO system that are not present in the host. These antibodies, endogenously present, will destroy incompatible cells in vivo. Prior to blood transfusion, grouping using sera against A_1, A_2, B, or A+B as appropriate, is used. Incompatibility results in agglutination.

Because of the presence of antibodies in incompatible transfusion recipients, donor red cells have the potential to be rapidly broken down. Therefore, only red cells against which an endogenous antibody is not present may be transfused. Thus blood for transfusion must generally be ABO compatible (Table 52.1). Possible exceptions to this include the transfusion of group O blood to other blood groups (universal donor), and the ability of patients with group AB blood to receive donations from all other blood groups (universal recipient). During blood cross-matching, ABO compatibility is established first.

Group O blood can be considered as 'universal donor', whereas patients with group AB blood can be considered as 'universal recipients'.

This is accompanied by antibody screening. Once potential suitable donor units have been identified, cross-matching is then possible. Patients who have received a blood transfusion should have a new cross-match performed after 48 hours if further transfusions are required. This is because of the potential of the first transfusion to stimulate new antibody production during this timespan. Where massive blood transfusions are administered, for example an exchange transfusion (10 units or more)

Table 52.1 ABO compatibility: antigens and antibodies in the ABO system

Group	Subgroup	Antigens on red cells	Antibodies in serum
O		None	anti-A anti-A_1 anti-B anti-AB
A	A_1 A_2	A+A_1 A	anti-B anti-B
B	–	B	anti-A anti-A_1
AB	A_1B A_2B	A+A_1+B A+B	none

within a period of a few hours, further compatibility testing is academic until a 48-hour period has elapsed. This is because of the diversity of antigens present and washout of host-derived antibodies.

Patients who have received a blood transfusion should have a new cross-match performed after 48 hours if further transfusions are required.

Rhesus system

The Rhesus system is the second most important blood group system. The antibody against the most important antigen, Rhesus D, is not endogenously present. However, it is rapidly formed after exposure to the Rhesus D antigen (for example following transfusion or during pregnancy). The antibody against Rhesus D is clinically important because of the facility with which it can cross the placenta and cause hemolytic disease of the newborn. Other important antigens in the Rhesus system are the C and E antigens. It is thought that these are encoded at a single locus.

Rhesus D antibody can cross the placenta and cause hemolytic disease of the newborn.

TRANSFUSION THERAPY

In the 1940s, blood transfusion was considered a surgical procedure. We now live in an era of separate stored products and the future will include bioengineered substitutes. Raw materials for blood transfusion come from a variety of sources: volunteer, paid, or conscripted donors. There has been interest in related blood donors and autologous transfusion (self-donation).

Whole blood is collected from the donor into an anticoagulant solution. Anticoagulant solutions are generally citrate based, chelating calcium ions and thus interfering with clotting. Donations from different donors can be pooled, or apheresis can be used to produce quantities of blood components from a single/few donor(s). Apheresis ('taken away') extracts a portion of the blood, for example plasma or platelets, and retransfuses the remainder back into the donor (Fig. 52.1). This technique limits the number of donors to which the recipient of a multiple-unit donation is exposed. Donor blood is tested for hepatitis viruses (A, B, and C), human immunodeficiency virus (HIV) 1 and 2, *Treponema pallidum* (syphilis), ABO and Rhesus compatibility, and cytomegalovirus. Some transfusion services also test for HTLV I and II. Collected samples are processed into red cells, platelets, and plasma. Plasma can be stored as fresh frozen plasma or prepared into albumin solutions, usually in a concentration of 5 or 20% albumin. Various clotting factors can be prepared individually or as a cryoprecipitate of slowly thawing frozen plasma.

Red cells are stored at 4°C and tested for compatibility prior to release for transfusion. Platelets are pooled into units of four or more, stored at 22°C, and gently agitated through their shelf life to prevent adherence to plastics. Plasma is stored at –20°C and transfused within 4 hours of thawing to room temperature, or fractionated, to make a number of pooled blood products. Guidelines for the use of fresh frozen plasma (FFP) now

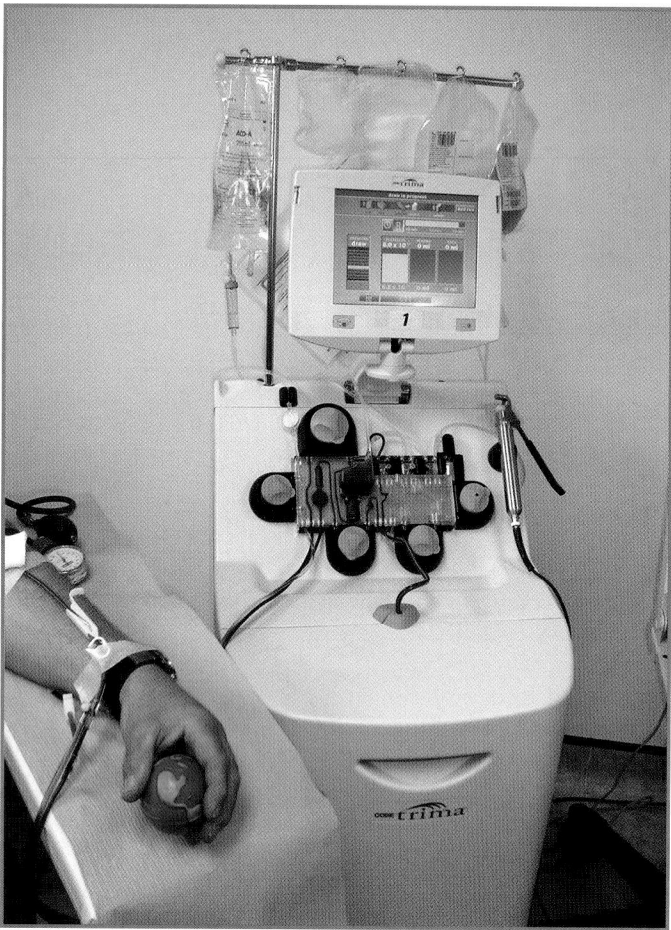

Figure 52.1 Apheresis machine collecting platelets from a previously tested regular donor. The equivalent volume of three adult doses can be collected in a little over an hour.

recommend that, provided the thawed FFP is maintained at 4°C, it can be kept for 24 hours (UK) or 5 days (USA) prior to infusion.

Blood-giving sets should normally include a 170 μm filter. Microaggregate filters should be avoided and never used for platelet transfusion. Blood products should only be mixed with isotonic saline (avoid solutions such as Hartmann's, Ringer's lactate, and other calcium-containing solutions, as these may cause coagulation of the product). Before administration, the product should be checked for hemolysis within the bag (pink supernatant). Blood products may be presented cold from the fridge; if these are to be transfused rapidly, it is necessary to use appropriate warming devices. It is important to avoid overheating blood, as this results in hemolysis, cytokine release, and serious adverse reactions. There is a risk of bacterial infection in units that have been open for more than 4 hours.

The 'group and save' or 'type and screen' procedure reduces the need for unnecessary expensive cross-matching. It can be performed hours or days in advance, and documents the ABO and Rhesus type of the patient's blood. Screening may also be performed for 'unexpected' red cell antibodies. This means that a suitable unit of donor blood can be selected and rapidly cross-matched within 10–15 minutes. In emergency situations group-specific blood may be issued without the need for cross-matching if the previous antibody screen did not identify problems.

Blood components

WHOLE BLOOD

Whole blood is prepared from a single donation and consists of 450 mL of blood with 63 mL anticoagulant (typically citrate). The hematocrit varies between 0.35 and 0.45. It contains no functional platelets, and levels of factors V and VIII are 20% of normal. Albumin and other clotting factors are normal. Whole-blood transfusion is indicated for replacement of blood loss where clotting factors are also required. In general, this means hemorrhage exceeding 50% of the patient's blood volume.

RED CELL CONCENTRATE

Red cell concentrates (packed red cells) are prepared from a single donor and consist of 220 mL of packed cells and 80 mL of plasma. The hematocrit lies between 0.65 and 0.75. This product is used for red cell replacement in anemia. It is also available in a leukocyte-depleted form, in which 70–90% of platelets and white blood cells are removed in the preparation of red cell concentrates. This may also be referred to as buffy coat-poor blood. In the UK, New Zealand, and a number of European countries all blood components are leukoreduced by filtration of the collected blood prior to storage. A four-log reduction of the white cell numbers results, i.e. 99.99% of the white cells are removed. The removal prior to storage is intended to remove most of the white cells, which degranulate during storage with the release of various bioactive substances, e.g. cytokines. Leukoreduction reduces the risk of transmission of cytomegalovirus, and more recently the process has been employed to reduce the potential risk of vCJD transmission. Red cell concentrates, particularly if leukodepleted, cause fewer white blood cell febrile transfusion reactions than does whole blood.

An added solution of 50–80 mL saline adenine glucose (SAG) or SAG-M (with mannitol) can be substituted for the residual plasma as a red cell nutrient, producing a hematocrit between 0.5 and 0.7.

PLATELETS

Platelets are produced either as single or pooled donor (4–6) units. Each donation consists of 40–70 mL of plasma with platelet suspension equivalent to 5.5×10^{10} platelets (UK); the exact number of platelets per donation is described by national standards and varies considerably between countries. The ideal platelet transfusion should be ABO and Rhesus compatible, especially in young women. A transfusion of 5–6 units of platelets produces an increment in platelet count of between 20×10^9 and 40×10^9 cells/L. Platelets may also be produced by single-donor apheresis. Between 150 and 500 mL of plasma are produced with around 3×10^{11} suspended platelets.

FRESH FROZEN PLASMA

FFP is produced as a single-donor product. Units of FFP consist of 250–500 mL of separated plasma frozen at –20°C. It includes both labile and stable factors, albumin, γ-globulin, fibrinogen, and factor VIII. Fresh frozen plasma can transmit hepatitis viruses and HIV; virologic safety relies on donor screening. Transfused units of FFP should be ABO compatible. The dose is usually between 2 and 5 units according to the results of clotting tests (prothrombin time or thromboelastogram). Very occasionally FFP may cause anaphylaxis.

CRYOPRECIPITATE

Cryoprecipitate is collected in packs containing between one and six single-donor units. It is collected by harvesting the precipitate that forms during slow thawing of frozen plasma. The resulting precipitate is resuspended in 10–20 mL of plasma. Each unit contains 150 mg fibrinogen, 150 IU factor VIII, and fibronectin. Between 6 and 18 units are required in hemophilia, DIC, and fibrinolytic states to raise plasma fibrinogen level by 1 g/L.

ALBUMIN

Albumin is produced by fractionation of a large plasma pool followed by pasteurization at 60°C for over 10 hours, which is thought to produce complete viral inactivation, although it may not inactivate prion proteins. Albumin solutions are presented as 5% solution and 20% sodium-depleted (salt-poor) solution. Albumin is indicated in the treatment of shock states, hypoproteinemia, and liver disease.

FACTOR CONCENTRATES

A number of factor concentrates are available, including separated freeze-dried factors VIII and IX (250 IU/vial) and both pure and impure forms of factors VII, IX, and XI. These factors have been associated with viral transmission. In recent years there has been a shift towards the production of factor concentrates using human recombinant techniques. Human recombinant factor VIII is now standard in the treatment of hemophilia in most countries, following experience in the late 1970s and 1980s with hepatitis and HIV transmission.

Risks of blood transfusion

The most common risk of blood transfusion is the unavailability of appropriate blood when it is needed. Transfusion of the wrong blood accounts for over 50% of all transfusion-related clinical incidents and 70% of transfusion-related deaths. This is generally as a result of inaccurate labeling of the patient's blood sample or the blood for transfusion, or failure to check patient and product identities. The confidential reporting of transfusion incidents can highlight areas of clinical transfusion practice where improvement in safety can be achieved by greater vigilance and ongoing education of personnel involved (Fig. 52.2).

Transfusion of the wrong blood is most usually a result of inaccurate labeling of the patient's blood sample or the blood for transfusion, or failure to check patient and product identities.

Viral transmission is a real but rare problem. Recent figures suggest that the risk of HIV transmission in the UK is approximately 1 per 8 million donor exposures. The risk of transmission of hepatitis viruses, particularly B and C, is higher than this. As yet, the risk of transfusion of prion proteins (causing variant Creutzfeldt–Jakob disease) is unknown, but may be lymphocyte dependent. All blood components in the UK have been universally leukoreduced since October 1999. In many

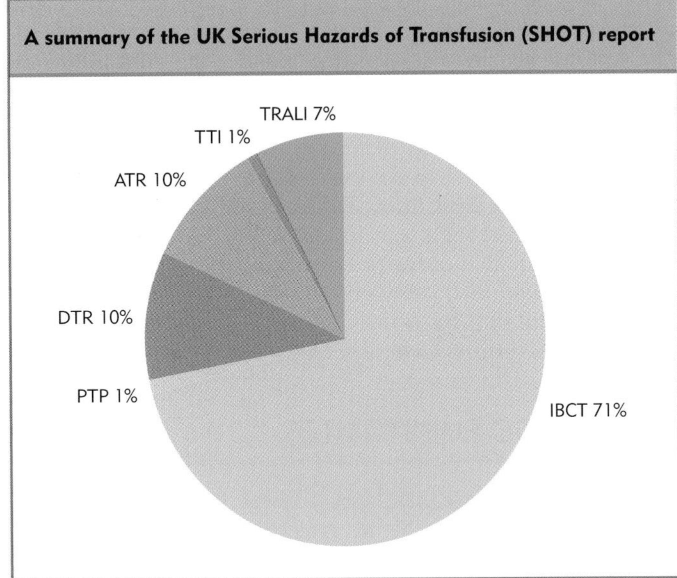

Figure 52.2 A summary of the UK Serious Hazards of Transfusion (SHOT) report. TRALI, transfusion-related acute lung injury; TTI, transfusion-transmitted infection; ATR, acute transfusion reaction; DTR, delayed transfusion reaction; PTP, post-transfusion purpura; ICBT, incorrect blood component transfused.

countries of the Western world where vCJD is not considered a risk, the debate continues concerning the benefit of such leukoreduction. Opinion is divided about the expense of producing 4 log-reduced leukodepleted blood components. The additional clinical benefits, compared to those of 90% leukoreduced components achieved by buffy coat removal only, are considered in some countries to be too minimal to warrant the additional expense of universal provision. Remaining risks relate to febrile white cell reactions, hyperkalemia, hemolyzed blood, and bacterial contamination.

Complications of blood transfusion include acid–base and electrolyte changes. Although stored blood is acidic, transfusion rapidly corrects metabolic acidosis in the shocked anemic patient. Hyperkalemia rarely occurs in blood that has been stored for less than 2 weeks. Blood transfusion using citrate-anticoagulated products may cause a rapid reduction in plasma-ionized calcium, resulting in systemic anticoagulation and myocardial depression. There is a risk of hypothermia when cold blood is transfused rapidly.

Acute transfusion reactions are relatively uncommon. These include hemolytic reactions, 75% of which are caused by ABO incompatibility. Anaphylactic reactions occur occasionally. These are a consequence of antibodies to IgA in IgA-deficient patients. Febrile white blood cell reactions are common and are caused by antibodies to leukocyte antigens. These antibodies can also give rise to noncardiogenic pulmonary edema. Approximately 1–2% of transfusions result in histamine release and urticaria. Post-transfusion purpura is an uncommon complication of blood transfusion.

When emergency transfusion is given there is controversy as to whether group O or group-compatible blood should be used. Group O blood has the advantage that there is no risk of ABO incompatibility, and errors in patient identification do not pose a problem. It is rapidly available, and can be held in a flying squad refrigerator for immediate use. ABO-compatible blood has the advantage that it does not deplete stocks of group O blood. There is no problem of changing blood group for follow-on transfusions and little risk of hemolysis in the patient from antibodies in transfused plasma. The decision on which to use should be based on locally defined protocols.

Transfused blood has the capacity to carry oxygen almost immediately after transfusion. Evidence for this is presented by the fact that exchange transfusions with bank blood do not generally result in massive acidosis, multiple organ failure, or even a reduction in mixed venous oxygen content. Transfused blood has reduced intracellular 2,3-diphosphoglycerate, but this is offset by the effects of local acidosis and hypoxia.

NEW BLOOD SUBSTITUTES

For many years there has been a quest for appropriate and effective substitutes for blood transfusion. Traditionally much reliance has been placed on the use of artificial colloid solutions (modified fluid gelatin, starches, etc.). These are effective as plasma expanders and hence improve tissue oxygen delivery. They do not carry oxygen (apart from in solution, which contributes a very small proportion compared to carriage by hemoglobin). More recently, there has been much interest in the development of oxygen-carrying substances. Initial work on perfluorocarbons appeared promising, but at present there are no commercially available compounds.

Stroma-free hemoglobin solutions seem much more promising and are currently in phase III clinical trials. The most likely to enter clinical practice are those based on recombinant 'human' blood, although a bovine version has also been produced. Production of human stroma-free hemoglobin is from hemoglobin harvested from expired pooled donor units, heat-treated for viral inactivation, and as a genetically engineered product. As free hemoglobin would pass rapidly across the glomerulus and give rise to renal failure, a larger version of the molecule is required. A number of approaches have been used. The most favored is polymerization (or dimerization) of the molecule using an inorganic crosslink, for example the difumarate bond. The resulting dimer has an oxygen 50% saturation pressure (P_{50}) similar to that of blood, and therefore has similar oxygen carriage and offloading characteristics. It differs from blood in that it is less viscous and is stroma free (i.e. it has no cellular material). This means that shelf life may be prolonged. There are no surface antigens present, hence there is no need for cross-matching. Stroma-free hemoglobin solutions are effective as oxygen carriers and very effective at delivering oxygen to the tissues. There may be an uncoupling of supply-dependent oxygen extraction, leading to further spectacular improvements in tissue oxygenation. Moreover, these compounds appear to bind nitric oxide and may have a vasopressor effect, as well as an effect on limiting tissue ischemia reperfusion injury. As with the perfluorocarbons, no such products are commercially available for human use.

BLOOD CONSERVATION

Increasing clinical demand for allogeneic blood, combined with various threats to the continued supply of blood components, has meant that it is necessary to develop conservation strategies to ensure that blood components are used appropriately.

It may seem strange that such a policy is necessary, as it may be assumed that blood has been used in the past in a rational and appropriate manner. Unfortunately, repeated audits and studies examining the ways in which blood components are used has shown wide variance in clinical transfusion practice. This variance appears to have been as a result of personal bias rather than as a result of scientific evidence on transfusion need. The published audits have shown a degree of overtransfusion, with no clinical detriment if transfusion is withheld in stable patients. This has been particularly obvious in patients in the perioperative period, where it seems that allowing a lower hemoglobin does not affect outcome in terms of mortality or morbidity. In fact, the contrary seems to be true, with patients experiencing better outcome if they avoid transfusion but keep their hematocrit at around 0.30.

It has been shown that the transfusion of whole blood results in a change in the immune status of the recipient. The effects include an increase in perioperative infection, and it has been postulated that cancer recurrence may also be increased following blood transfusion. Although the latter has not been confirmed by prospective randomized controlled trials, the incidence of perioperative infection is certainly reduced in those patients not receiving a transfusion.

In an attempt to conserve blood stores a more vigilant culture has developed where ongoing audit of blood usage has allowed the collection of data that can help assess the appropriateness of blood component transfusion. In this climate there has been a gradual and conscious change in transfusion practice, leading to the withholding of transfusion unless there is a clinical need, and the increased use of alternatives to allogeneic blood (Table 52.2). The slow development of artificial oxygen carriers has meant that the only alternative available has been autologous blood. Increased interest has developed for these methods, which utilize the patient's own blood to minimize allogeneic blood transfusion.

Autologous transfusion

The three main methods include red cell salvage (which can be undertaken during the operation – intraoperative cell salvage (ICS) – or postoperatively, postoperative cell salvage (PCS)); acute normovolemic hemodilution (ANH); and predeposit autologous donation (PAD).

The promotion of autologous transfusion, particularly in the USA in response to the HIV epidemic, resulted in a widespread use of such techniques. The evaluation of such techniques followed rather than preceded this development. The implementation of measures to reduce viral transmission via blood transfusion has been very successful, and the current risks of HIV transfusion from allogeneic transfusion are minimal. Many researchers have tried to evaluate the cost-effectiveness of such methods, and as a result it has become apparent that PAD is an expensive method of autologous transfusion. The cost of testing and storing autologous blood is more expensive than the routine collection of allogeneic blood, and it has been shown that 50% of the collected units are not reinfused to the patient as there is no clinical need at the time of operation. As has been stated above, transfusion of an incorrect blood component is one of the most frequently made errors and is as likely to be made with autologous blood as with allogeneic blood. In addition, the patient may present for surgery with a lower hemoglobin and red cell mass than they would have had without predeposit. Patients are in fact at a higher risk of requiring a blood transfusion than if

Table 52.2 Blood conservation strategies to minimize transfusion of allogeneic products

Strategy	Clinical considerations	Equipment required
Better operative hemostasis	Education of surgical team that hemostasis is a priority	Diathermy, harmonic scalpels, ultrasonic and laser resection, maintenance of normothermia, epidural anesthesia, hypotensive anesthesia
Preoperative autologous donation	Raise awareness among patients, surgeons, and referring clinicians; adherence to clinical guidelines	Suitable clinic or ward for donation; staff for collection and monitoring; laboratory staff for processing and storage
Isovolemic hemodilution	Adequate starting Hb; surgical and anesthetic awareness; anticipated blood loss large enough to justify the process	Adequate vascular access to enable blood collection; collection bag with anticoagulant; clamp to isolate collected blood and prevent entrainment of air
Intraoperative cell salvage	Anticipated blood loss sufficient to warrant transfusion; awareness among operating team; staff trained to operate apheresis machine	Apheresis machine; disposable collection and processing circuit; heparinized saline
Postoperative cell salvage	Sufficient postoperative drainage to warrant collection	Trained ward staff to enable reinfusion of collected blood – whether washed or unwashed process used
Pharmacological agents	Preoperative consideration and anticipated blood loss; prior preparation/availability of the agents	Aprotonin; tranexamic acid; DDAVP; recombinant factor VIIa
Pre- or postoperative hematinics	Preoperative check of Hb and iron studies; awareness by staff preparing patients for surgery	Iron, oral or IV; recombinant erythropoietin
Withholding transfusion unless clinically necessary	Tolerated well in young fit patients; caution in patients with cardiopulmonary disease	None – a clinical decision

they had been left alone. Additional drawbacks include the need for repeated venesections in the weeks preceding surgery, which mean that a fixed operating date needs to be agreed. The mild hypovolemia and anemia induced may be problematic for certain groups of patients.

Acute normvolemic hemodilution can be undertaken immediately prior to surgery or anesthesia. The collection of the blood can be via one of the intravascular cannulae required for the anesthesia and surgery. Blood is collected into standard venesection bags containing citrate, and weighed to prevent overfilling. Once collected and labeled with the patient's identification labels, the collected blood can be kept at room temperature in close proximity to the patient, offering added safety to the technique. After completion of the surgery – or at least when the risk of significant bleeding has passed – the collected blood can be reinfused to restore the hemoglobin level to a concentration that is above an agreed trigger for transfusion. The principle is to decrease the red cell loss even if the volume of operative blood loss remains the same, as blood of a more dilute nature is lost. Mathematical models have been described to calculate the amount of blood that is needed to be venesected to save one unit of red cells. The fact that these models have required four units to be removed before one unit of red cells is saved has tended to reduce enthusiasm for the technique.

Red cell salvage has advantages over other techniques as it can never be used unless the patient is bleeding at the time of operation. This principle ensures that there is a high collection to transfusion ratio and that the blood is close to the patient. Additional benefits include the fact that the blood is fresh, with a good 2,3-DPG content, and does not require expensive testing, as it is not stored. Disadvantages have been listed as the need for trained operators and the fact that the capital equipment is relatively expensive. These are not serious considerations when blood shortages are a reality. The lack of stores of allogeneic blood would seriously inhibit surgical programs. In these circumstances all of the above techniques may become necessary if we are to continue to try and develop surgical programs to tackle orthopedic, cardiac, and cancer illnesses.

Strategies to minimize blood transfusion

In the climate of blood conservation a number of strategies can be employed to delay or indeed avoid allogeneic transfusion altogether. Apart from the use of autologous techniques it is essential that an integrated approach is developed in all clinical areas where transfusion is currently deemed a possibility. Many strategies are already employed by some religious groups who object to or refuse to receive a blood transfusion. Jehovah's Witnesses, for example, will not accept any form of allogeneic transfusion, and have a very well organized network to help their members obtain information on alternatives. Most of the methods are well described in the medical literature, and it is rare that clinicians have not heard of or indeed used these techniques. What is exceptional is the way in which transfusion can be avoided if all blood-saving techniques are employed in a coordinated manner. Audit of blood transfusion continues to show wide variances in practice. Hospitals that approach blood conservation in a focused way can reduce allogeneic blood use without altering clinical outcome. At a time when blood demand is threatening to outstrip supply, all those working in transfusion medicine are obliged to ensure that they are using the donated allogeneic blood in the most appropriate way. To be able to demonstrate that this is occurring there is a need to ensure that clinical audit is in place to look at blood usage by specialty at all hospitals. Audit can also ensure comparisons are made between hospitals and between practitioners at those hospitals in terms of blood usage. It is only by continued vigilance the we can seriously address a narrowing of the variance in transfusion practice and make the use of blood components more focused and more appropriate.

Further reading

Consensus Statement – Autologous transfusion 3 years on: What is new? What has happened? Transfusion Med. 1999;9:285–6.

Crosby ET. Perioperative hemotherapy: I. Indicators for blood component transfusion. Can J Anaesth. 1992:39:695–707.

Crosby ET. Perioperative hemotherapy: II Risks and complications of blood transfusion. Can J Anaesth. 1992;39:822–37.

Department of Health. (2002) Better blood transfusion: appropriate use of blood. HSC 2002/009.

Goodnough LT, Brecher ME, Kanter MH, Aubuchon JP. Transfusion medicine. Part 1. New Engl J Med. 1999;340:438–47.

Goodnough LT, Brecher ME, Kanter MH, Aubuchon JP. Transfusion medicine. Part 2. New Engl J Med. 1999;340:525–33.

Goodnough LT, Shander A, Brecher ME. Transfusion medicine: looking to the future. Lancet 2003;361:161–9.

Hebert PC, Wells G, Blajchman MA et al. A multicenter randomized controlled clinical trial of transfusion requirements in critical care. New Engl J Med. 1999;340:409–17.

Hoffbrand AV, Petite JE. Essential haematology, 3rd edn. Oxford: Blackwell Scientific; 1993.

Irving GA. Perioperative blood and blood component therapy. Can J Anaesth. 1992;39:1105–15.

Salem MR. Blood conservation in the surgical patient. Baltimore: William & Wilkins; 1996.

Scottish Intercollegiate Guidelines Network (2001) Perioperative blood transfusion for elective surgery: a national guideline. (available from: http://www.sign.ac.uk/guidelines/fulltext/54/index.html).

SHOT Committee. Serious hazards of transfusion annual report, 2001–2002. Manchester: SHOT Steering Group; 2003.

Chapter 53

Hemostasis and coagulation

Andrew Quinn and Mark C Bellamy

TOPICS COVERED IN THIS CHAPTER

- **Coagulation**
  - Platelet function
  - The coagulation cascade
  - Vessel wall
  - The fibrinolytic system
- **Drugs affecting coagulation and platelet function**
  - Heparin
  - Other agents used to inhibit thrombin
  - Oral anticoagulants
  - Platelet drugs
  - Hemostatic drug therapy
  - Impaired coagulation in sepsis
- **Hemostatic defects and bleeding disorders**
- **Evaluation of coagulation**
  - Bleeding time
  - Prothrombin time
  - Activated partial thromboplastin time
  - Thrombin time
  - Thromboelastography®
  - Specific tests

Patients undergoing surgery can develop derangement of the hemostatic pathway and fibrinolysis. These changes require active support from the anesthesiologist, and demand a clear understanding of the pathophysiology and basic clinical principles. This chapter covers the physiology, pharmacology, and pathophysiology of hemostasis and coagulation.

COAGULATION

Coagulation is one of a group of homeostatic mechanisms that prevent ongoing bleeding following tissue injury. It results from the interaction between damaged tissue, plasma clotting factors, and platelets. The coagulation cascade is balanced by the fibrinolytic cascade, which regulates the breakdown of fibrin and fibrinogen and prevents excessive formation of thrombi. Normal clotting and hemostasis represents a dynamic interaction between the coagulation cascade, the fibrinolytic cascade, and platelet function.

Platelet function

The principal role of platelets is the formation of mechanical plugs during hemostasis. Key functions in this process include adhesion, release (platelet degranulation), aggregation, fusion, and platelet procoagulant activity. After blood vessel injury, platelets are exposed to subendothelial connective tissues. This promotes platelet adhesion, which is dependent on the presence of the plasma protein von Willebrand factor (vWF), part of the main fraction of factor VIII (factor VIII-related antigen, VIIIR:AG). The rate of adhesion depends on surface membrane glycoproteins (absent in the Bernard–Soulier syndrome).

Exposure to collagen at sites of vascular injury, or the presence of activated thrombin, results in platelet degranulation. Platelet granules contain adenosine diphosphate (ADP), serotonin, fibrinogen, lysozyme, and heparin-neutralizing factor (also known as platelet factor 4, PF4). The release process is dependent on prostaglandin synthesis (Fig. 53.1). Platelet membrane peroxidation results in the synthesis of thromboxane A_2. Thromboxane A_2 reduces the level of cyclic adenosine

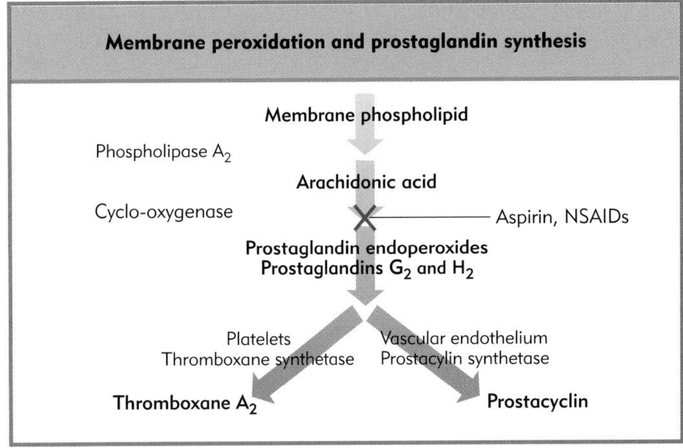

Figure 53.1 Processes involved in membrane peroxidation and prostaglandin synthesis. (NSAIDs, nonsteroidal anti-inflammatory drugs.)

monophosphate (cAMP) and initiates the release reaction. Thromboxane A_4 potentiates platelet aggregation and is a potent vasoconstrictor. Hence, compounds affecting levels of platelet cAMP affect the release reaction. The vasodilator prostaglandins, such as prostacyclin, synthesized by vascular endothelium, stimulate adenylyl cyclase. Prostacyclin has an important role in limiting clot formation and in preventing adhesion of platelets to normal vascular endothelium.

Platelet aggregation requires thromboxane A_2 and follows ADP release. Adenosine diphosphate causes platelet swelling and facilitates a reaction whereby membranes of adjacent platelets stick to each other. This initiates a positive feedback loop in which further ADP and thromboxane A_2 are released, resulting in secondary platelet aggregation. This self-fueling process results in the aggregation of a sufficiently large platelet mass to plug the breach in the vascular endothelium.

Platelets have a procoagulant activity. Following aggregation and release, platelet membrane phospholipid, platelet factor 3 (PF3), is exposed. This exposed surface provides a suitable template for the concentration and orientation of proteins involved in the coagulation cascade.

The glycoprotein (GP) IIb/IIIa receptor is the most prevalent receptor on the platelet surface and represents the final common pathway for platelet aggregation. In the presence of platelet activation, previously inactive GP IIb/IIIa receptors on the platelet membrane surface undergo structural modification and activation. This enables the binding of fibrinogen and vWF, which act to crosslink platelets and promote the generation of a platelet mass.

Membranes of adjacent platelets fuse in the presence of high concentrations of ADP and enzymes liberated in the release reaction. This process is further potentiated by thrombin. Fibrin formation reinforces the stability of the evolving platelet plug and eventually results in clot retraction and stabilization. Platelet degranulation (release reaction) may also promote vascular endothelial healing via the release of specific growth factors.

The coagulation cascade

Historically, the coagulation system was divided into two initiating pathways, the tissue factor (extrinsic) and the contact factor (intrinsic) pathway, which met in a final common pathway (see also Chapter 44). This traditional concept of separate and common coagulation pathways has validity in describing the processes of coagulation in vitro and relates well to laboratory tests of clotting. In vivo, a newer, unified concept describes the processes more usefully. In this there are three major steps: *initiation*, *amplification*, and *propagation*. This differs from the traditional 'waterfall' hypothesis. It can be interpreted as extrinsic and intrinsic pathways occurring simultaneously on different cell surfaces, with mutual interaction.

Factor XII is not included because patients with isolated factor XII lesions do not have bleeding disorders.

INITIATION

Clotting is initiated through a sequence of events broadly analogous to the 'extrinsic pathway'. Cells outside blood vessel walls differ from vascular endothelium in that they express a cell membrane protein known as 'tissue factor', a glycoprotein consisting of extracellular, transmembrane, and cytoplasmic domains. Tissue factor is located at the cell surface in vessel subendothelium, organ capsules, epithelial surfaces, and within the nervous system. It is not found free in the circulation.

Initiation occurs when injury results in the exposure of tissue factor to circulating coagulation proteins. Tissue factor binds activated factor VII (VIIa) (Fig. 53.2), small quantities of which are normally found free in the circulation. Binding of VIIa activates small quantities of factors IX and X. Factors IXa and Xa (in the presence of Va bound to tissue factor) generate a priming quantum of thrombin (IIa). This thrombin primer is responsible for the 'initiation' of the coagulation process proper. Thrombin activates platelets and promotes the assembly of coagulation factors on the platelet surface (Fig. 53.3).

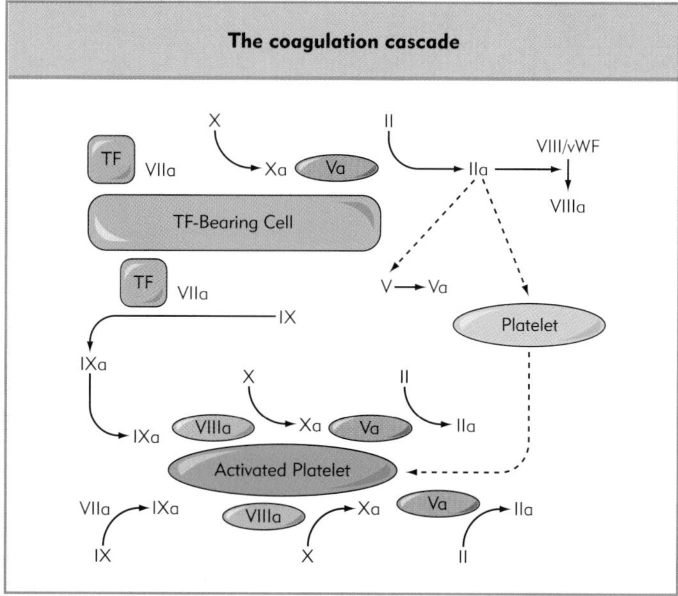

Figure 53.2 The coagulation cascade. See text for details. TF, tissue factor; vWF, von Willibrand factor.

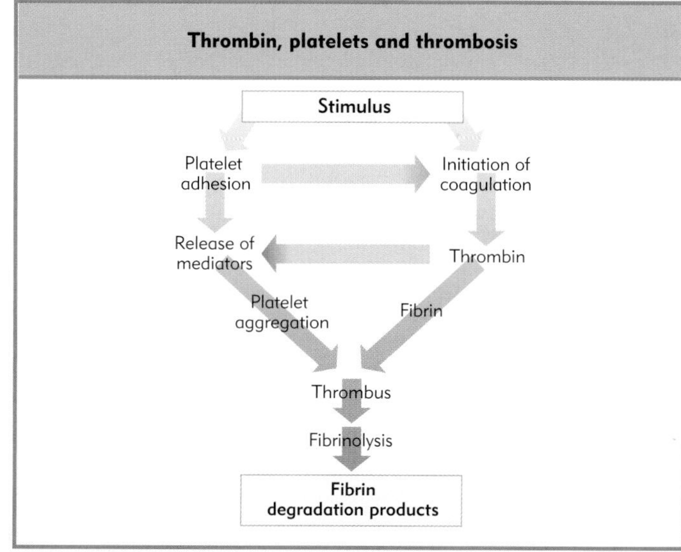

Figure 53.3 Thrombin and platelets and their interaction in thrombosis.

AMPLIFICATION

Until now the quantities of thrombin generated are inadequate to trigger significant cleavage of fibrinogen to fibrin. The process of amplification involves several feedback mechanisms. First, the generation of activated VIIa is increased by positive feedback on its own production. This means that factor VII bound to tissue factor is 'activated' (in the presence of factors VIIa, IXa, and Xa) to activated VIIa. Second, thrombin activates the nonenzymatic cofactors, factor V and factor VIII. These accelerate the process by which Xa cleaves prothrombin to thrombin (IIa). They also enhance mutual amplification between IXa and Xa. In a final feedback loop, thrombin activates factor XIa, which further enhances production of factor IXa.

PROPAGATION

During propagation, large amounts of factor X associate with factor VIIIa on the surface of the activated platelet, resulting in activation of the factor X to Xa. This reaction requires platelet factor 3 (platelet phospholipids) and calcium ions. In the presence of these cofactors there is a 20-fold increase in production of Xa. This in turn, together with Va on the activated platelet surface, forms prothrombinase complex, which rapidly cleaves prothrombin (factor II) to thrombin (factor IIa). Finally, thrombin cleaves fibrinogen to fibrin.

Stabilization of the fibrin clot is required to complete the process. After the formation of fibrin monomer there is maximum thrombin generation. Consequently, there is sufficient thrombin to activate factor XIII to crosslink soluble fibrin monomers to a stable fibrin matrix. Furthermore, thrombin activates the thrombin-activatable fibrinolysis inhibitor (TAFI), which maintains clot stability.

Factors XII, XI, IX, X, and VII and prothrombin circulate in the plasma as inactive precursors (zymogen) and are all activated by proteolytic cleavage. The activated clotting factors are themselves serine proteases, that is, they have a serine residue at their active centers that is involved in the hydrolysis of peptide bonds.

Factor VIII is a large protein (1.5–2.0 MDa) consisting of two components. The larger component (VIIIR:AG) is involved in platelet-related activities, including platelet adhesion to exposed subendothelial connective tissue and platelet aggregation. Von Willebrand factor (VIII:WF) is part of factor VIIIR:AG. The remaining component, factor VIII coagulant (VIII:C), is noncovalently bound to VIIIR:AG.

Fibrinogen has a molecular weight of 340 kDa. It consists of three pairs of polypeptide chains, α, β, and δ, crosslinked by disulfide bonds. Thrombin releases fibrinopeptide A and B from α and β chains of fibrinogen by proteolysis. This forms fibrin monomer, consisting of the crosslinked α, β, and δ chains. Hydrogen bonds then form spontaneously between molecules of fibrin monomer, giving rise to fibrin polymer. Factor XIII is activated by thrombin. Activated XIII stabilizes fibrin polymer by introducing Glu–Lys isopeptide bonds between adjacent fibrin monomers.

Vessel wall

The hemostatic response results from interaction between the clotting cascade, platelet activity, and the blood vessel wall. Following vascular injury there is immediate constriction of the damaged vessel, with reflex constriction of adjacent small arteries and arterioles. In massive injury this immediate reflex prevents exsanguination. Reduction in blood flow velocity permits contact activation of platelets and the coagulation cascade. These processes are accompanied by the release of vasoactive amines, thromboxane from platelets, and fibrinopeptides liberated by fibrin formation. These all potentiate local vasoconstriction at the site of injury. This process is potentiated by VIII:WF. Activation of platelets and the coagulation cascade, as described above, results in definitive hemostasis when fibrin formed by coagulation combines with the platelet mass to produce a retractile clot.

However, if coagulation were to continue unchecked there would be widespread vascular occlusion, leading to tissue ischemia. Localization of coagulation to the area where the original platelet plug is formed is achieved by two methods. First, the cascade of reactions that leads to clot formation is programmed to occur – and is most efficient – when restricted to a surface such as platelet phospholipid. Second, there is a series of inhibitors that restrict the reaction to the site of injury. These inhibition processes include circulating factors, such as antithrombin and heparin cofactor II, those derived from endothelium, such as the protein tissue factor pathway inhibitor (TFPI), and the thrombomodulin system, which converts prothrombotic thrombin to an anticoagulant through the activation of circulating protein C.

When small quantities of thrombin have been generated thrombin may bind and activate TFPI. The thrombin–TFPI complex then inactivates previously formed factor VII–tissue factor complexes, thus inhibiting further synthesis of factors IXa and Xa. In effect this is a negative feedback system. Heparin potentiates the action of TFPI two- to fourfold by binding TFPI and TF–VIIa complex, bringing them closer and increasing their interaction. Heparin also triggers the release of endothelial stores of TFPI.

Antithrombin is a protein synthesized in the liver and endothelial cells that binds and directly inactivates thrombin and the other serine proteases (factors Xa, VIIa, IXa, and XIa) by the formation of peptide bonds with the active serine sites. The uncatalyzed reaction between the serum proteases and antithrombin is relatively slow, but in the presence of heparin the reaction is virtually instantaneous, resulting in the immediate blockage of fibrin formation. Endothelial cells express heparin sulfate, which binds antithrombin, resulting in inactivation of any nearby serine proteases and preventing the formation of fibrin in undamaged areas. Activated coagulation factors and other procoagulants are filtered by the reticuloendothelial system, in particular hepatic Kupffer cells.

The hemostatic response results from interactions between the clotting cascade, platelets and the blood vessel wall.

Proteins C and S are both vitamin-dependent inhibitors of the procoagulant system and are produced in the liver. Protein C circulates in the blood as a zymogen and is activated to a serine protease by the binding of thrombin to thrombomodulin. Protein S markedly enhances the activity of protein C. By inactivating factors Va and VIIa, proteins C and S reduce the speed of thrombin generation.

Thrombomodulin is an endothelial cell receptor that binds thrombin. When thrombomodulin and thrombin form a complex, the conformation of the thrombin molecule is changed so that it readily activates protein C while losing platelet-activating and protease activity. On binding to thrombomodulin, thrombin switches role from a potent procoagulant into an anticoagulant. In the normal physiological state this is important because endothelial cells produce thrombomodulin that binds any circulating thrombin, preventing clot formation in undamaged vessels.

Patients who have homozygous protein C deficiency develop widespread intravascular coagulation, resulting in blindness due to retinal artery occlusion, stroke, and coagulopathy through disseminated intravascular coagulation (DIC). Such patients rarely survive infancy. In the heterozygous form of the disease, patients survive into adult life but may develop multiple systemic thromboses, including pulmonary embolus or the Budd–Chiari syndrome. These complications are exacerbated by pregnancy or the oral contraceptive pill, which reduce circulating levels of protein C. Paradoxically, anticoagulants such as warfarin may increase the tendency of these procoagulant phenomena by inhibition of the formation of vitamin K-containing clotting factors, and hence further inhibition of protein C activity.

Surgical procedures often disturb the natural balance of the coagulation system, leading to either a thrombotic or a bleeding tendency. Many perioperative factors interfere with coagulation, such as hypothermia, metabolic acidosis, volume expanders, and extracorporeal circulation. Other clinical factors that interfere with coagulation include immobility, infections, cancer, or drugs, as well as the operative procedure itself. During the first several hours after surgery there is a marked increase in tissue factor, tissue plasminogen activator (t-PA), plasminogen activator inhibitor-1 (PAI-1), and von Willebrand factor (vWF), leading to a hypercoagulable and hypofibrinolytic state.

Surgery leads to a hypercoagulable and hypofibrinolytic state.

The fibrinolytic system

In addition to the regulatory mechanisms described above that limit activation of the clotting cascade, there is also a biologic cascade (amplification) system for limitation of clot size and dissolution of stable fibrin – the fibrinolytic cascade (Figs. 53.4 and 53.5). Excessive fibrinolysis becomes a clinical problem for anesthesiologists in the areas of cardiac, vascular, and transplantation surgery; it may also occur during sepsis. Fibrinolysis occurs as a result of digestion of fibrin by proteolytic enzymes.

Plasmin is the key serine protease involved in fibrinolysis. Plasminogen is activated to plasmin by two plasminogen activators: tissue type (t-PA) and urokinase (u-PA); t-PA is active when bound to fibrin. Endothelium also produces a rapid t-PA

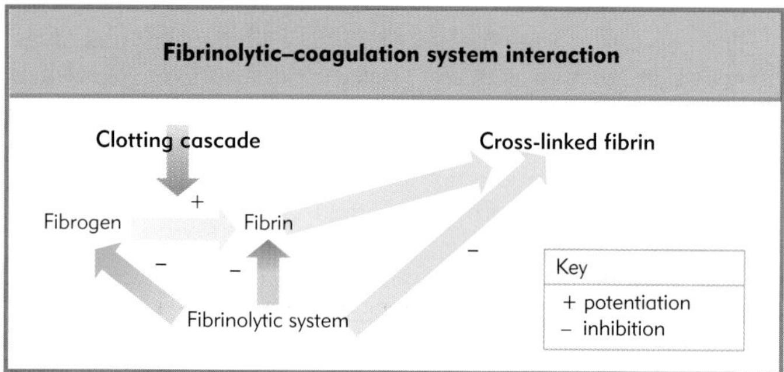

Figure 53.4 Interaction between the fibrinolytic and coagulation systems.

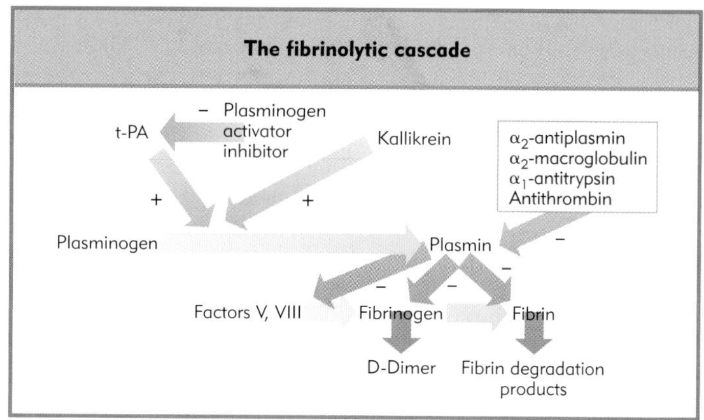

Figure 53.5 The fibrinolytic cascade. t-PA, tissue plaminogen activator.

inactivator, plasminogen activator inhibitor (PAI). There are three subclasses of this inhibitor, although most effects appear to be attributable to PAI-1. Platelets stimulated by thrombin also produce PAI. Consequently, platelet aggregation limits fibrinolysis. There are a number of complex interactions. Activated protein C (an anticoagulant in the clotting cascade) also reduces endothelial production of PAI. Hence, protein C is also a promoter of the fibrinolytic process by increasing circulating levels of t-PA. Factor XII activation (secondary to endothelial damage) promotes kallikrein release and hence activation of fibrinolysis. Once plasminogen has been activated to plasmin, it triggers the complement cascade.

Plasminogen is adsorbed on to fibrin at specific lysine-binding sites. Fibrins (but not fibrinogen) also have t-PA-binding sites. The fibrin molecule constitutes an environment that facilitates the presentation of t-PA to plasminogen and cleavage of this zymogen to plasmin. Plasmin digests fibrin to fibrin degradation products (FDP) (fibrin split products, FSP); plasmin is then released from lyzed fibrin and returns to the circulation. Normally, free plasmin is rapidly inactivated by α_2-macroglobulin and antithrombin. When present in excess, free plasmin cleaves fibrinogen, producing D-dimer, and can inactivate factors V and VIII; this occurs in DIC.

Processes that regulate fibrinolysis display anatomic variation. Fibrinolysis is more active in the arterial than in the venous system, in deep than in superficial veins, and in the upper than in the lower limbs. In pregnancy both fibrinogen and plasminogen levels are increased, but t-PA levels are reduced. At the same time α_2-antiplasmin levels are increased; overall fibrinolysis is reduced. Hormones involved in the neurohumoral stress response (corticosteroids, catecholamines, vasopressin) cause a transient increase in fibrinolytic activity. Hence, there is increased fibrinolysis during surgery, and possibly during venous occlusion. This latter effect may also be as a consequence of reduced PAI. Increased fibrinolysis in venous occlusion may explain the mechanism of action of calf compression devices in preventing deep venous thrombosis during surgery.

DRUGS AFFECTING COAGULATION AND PLATELET FUNCTION

A number of drugs affect coagulation and platelet function. They may exert their effect by potentiating the naturally occurring inhibition of coagulation, particularly at the level of factor Xa and thrombin (e.g. the heparins). The venom of the Malayan pit viper (*Ancrod*) promotes intravascular conversion of fibrinogen to fibrin and subsequent breakdown to FDPs, which are in themselves antifibrinolytic. Several anticoagulants (the oral anticoagulants) exert their effect by antagonizing vitamin K and hence suppressing the synthesis of vitamin K-dependent clotting factors: factors II, VII, and X (half-lives 60, 80, and 36 hours, respectively), protein C, and other proteins. Fibrinolysis may be either enhanced (t-PA, streptokinase, urokinase), or inhibited (aprotinin, tranexamic acid, ε-aminocaproic acid). Also, there are drugs that can alter the normal physiology of platelets, thereby interfering with coagulation.

Heparin

Unfractionated heparin is a naturally occurring negatively charged sulfated water-soluble mucopolysaccharide organic acid (Fig. 53.6). Unfractionated heparin has a molecular weight ranging from 3000 to 30 000 Da. It is present in high concentrations in liver, lungs, and intestines in the granules of mast cells and basophils. It exerts its anticoagulant effect by binding with antithrombin. This brings about a change in conformation that substantially enhances antithrombin binding and inhibits factors XIIa, XIa, IXa, and Xa and thrombin by 100 times (see Fig. 53.3). Following the reaction between the active site of the protease and the reactive site of antithrombin, a further conformational change in antithrombin occurs that causes it to envelop the protease. This change reduces the affinity of antithrombin for heparin, which is released to participate in further antithrombin–protease reactions. Heparin can also activate the other major circulating antithrombin, heparin cofactor (HCII). Activation of HCII is thought to be a nonspecific effect relating to the total charge on the molecule, rather than acting via a specific receptor. Lastly, heparin can stimulate the release of TFPI, which reduces prothrombinase production. Plasma TFPI concentrations increase two- to sixfold following heparin injection. This increase occurs with both unfractionated and low molecular weight heparin.

Standard preparations of heparin are unfractionated and derived from either porcine intestine or bovine lung as either calcium or sodium salts. As heparin is derived from several biologic sources, its activity may vary per unit weight; consequently, heparin dose is expressed in standard international units (IU). The plasma concentrations of heparin are not uniformly related to the anticoagulant effect produced, and there is a wide variability in dose–response effects in patients. More than 50% of heparin circulates bound to certain proteins. Raised levels of these proteins may account for the heparin resistance seen in malignancy and inflammatory disorders. Heparins do not significantly cross the placenta.

Indications for heparin include anticoagulation during cardiopulmonary bypass, treatment and prophylaxis of deep vein thrombosis, treatment of pulmonary embolism, and protection of the patency of intravascular catheters and extracorporeal systems (e.g. in renal dialysis). Heparin given intravenously exerts its effect immediately. The peak effect after subcutaneous injection occurs after 30 minutes. Heparin is not active orally and is metabolized in the liver and excreted by the kidney; it has an elimination half-life between 2 and 3 hours. The effect of heparin is monitored by activated partial thromboplastin time (aPTT), a measure of the intrinsic coagulation cascade. The therapeutic range of aPTT is 60–100 seconds (1.5–2.5 times normal).

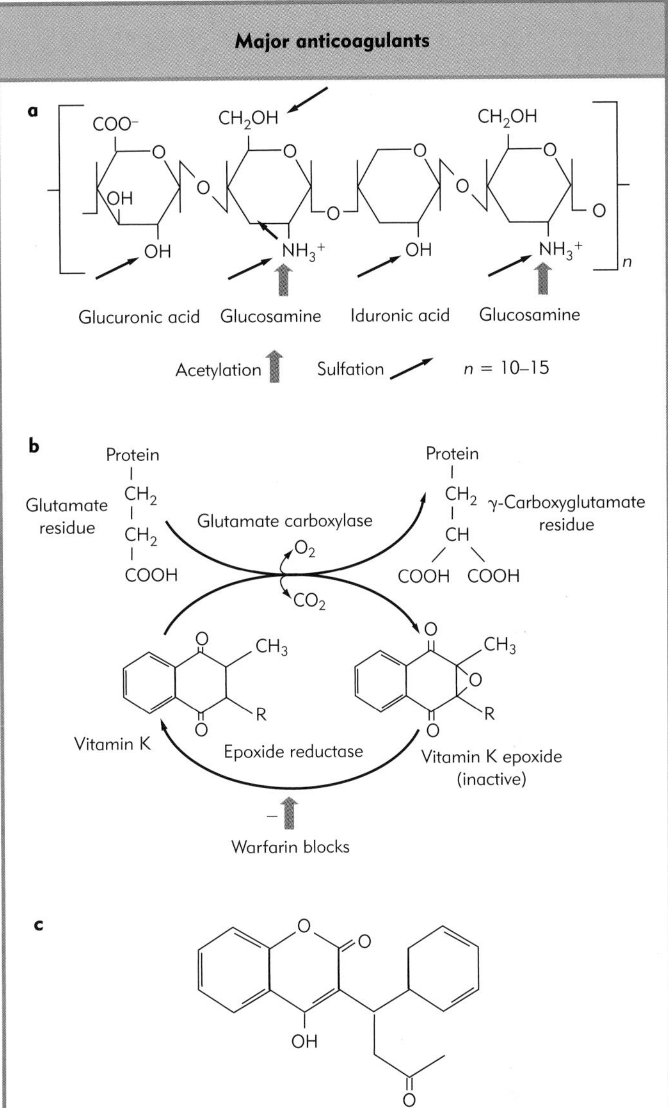

Figure 53.6 Major anticoagulants. (a) The repeating structure of heparin has a high affinity for antithrombin. (b) Vitamin K is involved in the conversion in the liver of glutamate residues in certain plasma proteins to γ-carboxyglutamate (GLA) residues. (c) Warfarin and other coumarin derivatives block the reduction of vitamin K epoxide formed in this reaction back to its active form.

ADVERSE EFFECTS

Heparin has a number of adverse effects, the most common of which is hemorrhage. This is unusual where aPTT is maintained within the therapeutic range. Some patients are at particular risk for heparin-induced bleeding (e.g. patients who have vitamin K deficiency (antibiotic therapy, liver disease) or who have had recent surgery). There is evidence for increased – and more prolonged – bleeding after emergency cardiac surgery in patients who have received platelet-active drugs such as abciximab, clopidogrel, or ticlopidine. Although therapeutic doses of heparin may represent a relative contraindication to regional anesthetic blockade, low-dose heparin prophylaxis (5000 IU twice daily subcutaneously) is not a contraindication to central neural blockade. Patients on long-term heparin therapy may develop a reduction in antithrombin activity to 10–20% of normal levels, and may exhibit 'heparin resistance', requiring an increased dose. Heparin resistance can result in paradoxic thrombosis. Antithrombin levels are restored by the administration of fresh frozen plasma or antithrombin concentrate.

Heparin-induced thrombocytopenia can result from prolonged therapy due to immune-mediated platelet aggregation.

A complication of prolonged heparin therapy (typically 5 days or more) is heparin-induced thrombocytopenia. This occurs more frequently when bovine lung heparin is used than with porcine heparin. In type 1 heparin-induced platelet deficiency there is a transient self-limiting fall in platelet count to 50×10^9 cells/L, probably as a result of direct heparin-induced platelet agglutination. Type 2 deficiency is more severe and overlaps with heparin-associated thrombosis. It occurs in around 6% of patients. Platelet count falls to 10×10^9 cells/L and is associated with thromboembolic phenomena. Thrombocytopenia results from immune-mediated platelet aggregation triggered by immunoglobulins G and M antibodies against platelets. The condition generally resolves rapidly on discontinuation of heparin, although occasionally it may persist for 1–2 months; in this case, intravenous immunoglobulin therapy is used. Reintroduction of heparin can be catastrophic.

LOW MOLECULAR WEIGHT HEPARINS

Low molecular weight heparins (LMWH, e.g. enoxaparin, tinzaparin) have a relatively specific effect against factor Xa compared with other clotting factors. Both unfractionated and low molecular weight heparins possess a pentasaccharide sequence which binds to antithrombin III (ATIII), but only the unfractionated heparins have the adjacent ternary sequence which is necessary for potentiation of the interaction between ATIII and factor IIa. This sequence is not necessary for potentiation of the interaction between ATIII and factor Xa, hence the relative specificity shown by LMWH for Xa. A 20 mg dose of enoxaparin has an effect on factor Xa that is the equivalent of 2000 IU of heparin. The affinity of plasma proteins for LMWHs is much less than for unfractionated heparin (UFH), so that only 10% is protein bound. LMWHs are not subject to the rapid degradation that UFH suffers, as they are not inactivated by platelet factor 4 and do not bind to endothelial cells or macrophages. This produces almost complete bioavailability, compared to 40% for low-dose subcutaneous UFH, and this gives a more predictable anticoagulant action. Low molecular weight heparins in prophylactic doses do not affect prothrombin time (PT), aPTT, platelet aggregation, or binding to fibrinogen. They are rapidly absorbed after subcutaneous injection, as maximum activity is seen within 1–4 hours. The half-life of enoxaparin is between 4 and 5 hours. It is excreted renally (largely intact), although there is some hepatic conjugation. The available LMWHs differ in the distribution of molecular weights, in vitro potency, bioavailability, anti-Xa activity, and consequently their pharmacodynamic behavior, recommended dose regimen, and efficacy/safety ratio.

HEPARIN REVERSAL

The effects of unfractionated heparin wear off rapidly so that an antagonist is rarely required, except after high doses, e.g. in cardiopulmonary bypass. Protamine is a basic protein extracted from fish sperm that combines with heparin to form a stable, inactive complex. Protamine has a high arginine content, which makes it strongly basic (cationic) and enables it to form a stable complex with the highly negatively charged heparin molecule. In general, 1–2 mg protamine is necessary to neutralize 1 mg (100 IU) heparin. Protamine has several adverse effects; these include hypotension and flushing, which are probably related to histamine release and which can be minimized by giving protamine very slowly. There is a high incidence of anaphylactic and anaphylactoid reactions to protamine; these are most common in patients who have fish allergy and in diabetics receiving protamine-based insulin. Protamine activates complement and releases platelet thromboxane A_2, which may lead to severe pulmonary vasoconstriction and bronchoconstriction. Pretreatment with a cyclo-oxygenase inhibitor (aspirin) may offset this effect. With LMWHs, protamine is able to neutralize the anti-IIa but not the anti-Xa action of heparin, because of its inability to bind the smaller heparin molecules.

Therapeutic anticoagulation is a contraindication to central nerve blockade. The risks associated with epidural or spinal anesthesia in patients receiving heparin prophylaxis is a controversial subject. Published guidelines have stated that the minimum delay between last dose and the placement or removal of an epidural catheter is 4 hours for unfractionated heparin and 12 hours for LMWHs.

Other agents used to inhibit thrombin

Hirudin is a polypeptide originally obtained from the medicinal leech. The molecule is now manufactured by recombinant technology. The recombinant hirudin preparations are available for postoperative DVT prophylaxis and alternative anticoagulant use in patients with heparin-induced thrombocytopenia. Hirudin acts by irreversible binding to the active site of thrombin. The major clinical disadvantage of hirudin preparations is their mode of excretion by renal clearance, leading to a plasma half-life of 14 hours. The promise of direct thrombin inhibitors as a replacement for heparin has not yet been borne out in large-scale randomized trials.

Arginine analogs have been used in laboratory-based medicine as direct inhibitors of thrombin, but they are too toxic for use in humans.

Oral anticoagulants

The commoner oral anticoagulants are coumarin derivatives that resemble vitamin K in structure. They include warfarin and the dicoumarides (e.g. phenindione) (Fig. 53.6). The anticoagulant effect of these drugs is related to their ability to interfere with the production of biologically active vitamin K-dependent clotting factors (II, VII, IX, X). The anticoagulant effect of warfarin is seen 8–12 hours after either oral or intravenous administration, with the peak effect at 3–5 days (this corresponds with the nadir levels of vitamin K-dependent factors). Warfarin has a half-life of 24–36 hours. It is metabolized in the liver to a number of inactive derivatives that are conjugated and excreted in both bile and urine. In clinical practice warfarin is used principally to reduce the incidence of thromboembolism associated with prosthetic heart valves and atrial fibrillation. Dosage is monitored and adjusted according to PT, which is very sensitive to a reduction in factors VII and X. As factor VII has a very short half-life (7 hours), its concentration falls the earliest. A therapeutic PT is 1.5–4 times the normal value. An excessively prolonged PT cannot be easily corrected merely by omitting a dose of warfarin, because the drug has a long elimination half-life and the synthesis of vitamin K-dependent factors may be delayed. Similarly, a subtherapeutic PT needs correction by several doses of warfarin over a period of 3–4 days.

Warfarin should be discontinued 3–4 days prior to elective surgery to allow the PT to normalize. Clot formation on prosthetic heart valves is life threatening and requires urgent cardiopulmonary bypass. Anticoagulation should therefore be maintained perioperatively in patients who have prosthetic valves and in others at high risk of thromboembolism. In these patients, intravenous heparin is substituted as the warfarin is tailed off. Heparin is preferable in these circumstances as its effects are more readily controllable because of its shorter half-life, and because its effects can be reliably reversed with protamine. Reversal of the effects of warfarin can be attempted prior to emergency surgery using vitamin K (10–20 mg IV) and fresh frozen plasma. Because warfarin is highly protein bound, many drugs that displace it from its binding sites may substantially potentiate its anticoagulant effect (e.g. co-trimoxazole, metronidazole, amiodarone, quinidine, and tolbutamide). Cimetidine inhibits the cytochrome P450 system and hence reduces hepatic warfarin clearance. Some drugs (e.g. the barbiturates and rifampin (rifampicin)) increase the activity of hepatic microsomal enzymes, which reduces the anticoagulant effect of warfarin. In theory, volatile anesthetic agents may displace warfarin from protein-binding sites and hence prolong its anticoagulant effect; this has been demonstrated for halothane.

Platelet drugs

Many drugs interact with platelets, either to potentiate or to inhibit function. Desmopressin (1-deamino-8-D-arginine vasopressin, DDAVP), an analog of arginine–vasopressin, is frequently used in patients who have platelet dysfunction (e.g. in renal failure) to promote platelet activity. The nature of this effect is not fully understood, although it is probably related to its ability to release vWF from vascular endothelium, which then interacts with platelets to promote adhesion.

Antifibrinolytic drugs also potentiate platelet function, in part by promoting crosslinking of fibrin and platelet adhesion to fibrin, and in part by preserving the functional activity of platelet surface glycoproteins, including Ib and IIa. Drugs in this category include tranexamic acid and ε-aminocaproic acid. The primary effect of these drugs is inhibition of fibrinolysis, mediated through binding of these molecules to lysine residues on free plasmin. Hence, these drugs function as pharmacologic mimics of α_2-antiplasmin and α_2-macroglobulin.

Another antifibrinolytic drug that potentiates platelet function is aprotinin. This drug is now well established in both cardiac surgery and liver transplantation. Aprotinin is a nonspecific serine protease inhibitor. It is active against kallikrein, plasmin, trypsin, and thrombin. It also has a direct effect on platelet function, enhancing the integrity and function of surface glycoproteins and enhancing the platelet release reaction. In cardiac surgery aprotinin has been shown to reduce blood loss in high-risk patients, particularly where aspirin has been given preoperatively. Its use in liver transplantation is more controversial. Antifibrinolytic drugs have been associated with an increased risk of arterial thrombosis.

Nefamostat mesylate is a new synthetic protease inhibitor. It has a short half-life and has been used as an anticoagulant for plasma. Its use in cardiopulmonary bypass significantly reduces blood loss and is associated with platelet preservation and reduced fibrinolysis. Etamsylate (ethamsylate) also promotes enhanced platelet activity, acting by stimulating platelet aggregation.

Drugs that inhibit platelet function include the arachidonic acid derivative prostacyclin (epoprostenol). Prostacyclin is produced by endothelial cells. It inhibits platelet aggregation through activation of adenylyl cyclase and is a potent vasodilator. Nonsteroidal anti-inflammatory drugs (NSAIDs), including aspirin, inhibit cyclo-oxygenase activity and prostacyclin production. Prostacyclin is rapidly degraded to 6-ketoprostaglandin $F_{1\alpha}$, which is devoid of biologic activity.

Aspirin differs from other NSAIDs in that it is an irreversible rather than a reversible enzyme inhibitor (Chapter 32). Nonsteroidal anti-inflammatory drugs block prostaglandin synthesis, and the production of both thromboxane A_2 and prostacyclin is inhibited. Aspirin has an irreversible effect; consequently, thromboxane synthetase is inhibited for the lifetime of the platelet and there is a prolonged effect on production of the prothrombotic prostaglandin thromboxane A_2. However, its effect on the vascular endothelium is more transient because the nucleated endothelial cells can rapidly regenerate functional enzyme. Overall, the effect of a dose of aspirin is prolonged inhibition of thromboxane A_2 production and an antiplatelet (anticoagulant) effect that may last days or weeks, with only transient inhibition of prostacyclin. By contrast, other NSAIDs show a reversible effect on prostaglandin synthetase enzymes, and their antiplatelet effect is generally limited to the duration of action of the drug.

Dipyridamole, originally introduced as a vasodilator, acts as a phosphodiesterase inhibitor in vascular smooth muscle, increasing platelet cAMP and inhibiting aggregation. Dipyridamole does not affect cyclo-oxgenase activity directly, and thromboxane A_2 and prostacyclin formation are unchanged. In thromboembolic conditions where platelet lifespan is reduced, dipyridamole tends to restore it.

Newer anti-platelet drugs target the ADP receptor and GPIIb/IIIa receptor.

ADP is a key cofactor of platelet aggregation. Three separate families of membrane-bound ADP receptors have been proposed. Clopidogrel and ticlopidine are thienopyridine derivatives and are licensed for the secondary prevention of vascular events in patients with established atherosclerotic disease. Neither drug has antiplatelet activity in vitro but requires metabolism by the hepatic cytochrome P450 system. Their antiplatelet effect appears to result from the noncompetitive antagonism of a platelet ADP receptor. About 70% of ADP receptors on a platelet are sensitive to the effects of thienopyridines. These are the low-affinity receptors responsible for platelet aggregation and adenylyl cyclase inhibition. Thromboxane production is normal, indicating that prostaglandin synthase is unaffected. Recovery occurs only with the generation of a new population of platelets. Spontaneous bleeding is less frequent in patients treated with thienopyridines than in those treated with aspirin. The plasma half-life of ticlopidine is 30–55 hours, and that of clopidogrel is 20–50 hours. These times are two to three times longer in the elderly. It is therefore recommended that clopidogrel is stopped 7 days prior to surgery and ticlopidine 10–14 days beforehand. Animal studies have shown that high-dose corticosteroids and aprotinin will partially reverse the effects of thienopyridines on the bleeding time, but there has been nothing to confirm this in humans.

The platelet GPIIb/IIIa receptor plays an important role in platelet aggregation. A mouse-derived monoclonal antibody directed against the GPIIb/IIIa receptor caused inhibition of the fibrinogen–platelet interaction and subsequent platelet aggregation. Abciximab (Reopro) is the chimeric form of this antibody. Two other receptor blockers are available: eptifibatide and tirofiban. All of these are given intravenously with a continuous intravenous infusion after a loading dose. Results with all agents suggest that monotherapy is not as effective as combination treatment. Moreover, there is further potentiation in the presence of heparin. The recommended dose regimen of abciximab produces 80–90% receptor blockade. Unless the patient is also receiving heparin or there is thrombocytopenia, spontaneous bleeding is uncommon. There has been concern regarding surgical bleeding with the new antiplatelet agents. When abciximab is discontinued, there is a gradual reduction in receptor blockade. Twelve hours after discontinuation about 70% of the receptors are still blocked, but a nearly normal bleeding time has been reported. Eptifibatide and tirofiban have a slightly more rapid offset of action. There is limited specific therapy to reduce bleeding with these agents. The therapy with the best supporting evidence is to administer platelets. Although free abciximab may not be circulating, that bound to the native platelets redistributes among the total pool, resulting in an overall smaller percentage of blocked receptors.

Hemostatic drug therapy

Specific therapies – DDAVP and antifibrinolytic drugs – have already been discussed. Although not yet approved for indications other than bleeding in hemophiliacs, the most recent promising hemostatic drug is recombinant activated factor VII (FVIIa; NovoSeven). Factor VIIa is the only hemostatic drug that does not only substitute a missing factor, but actively initiates and promotes coagulation. The hemostatic effect of factor VIIa is based on its property to bind to tissue factor and activated platelets, which rapidly activates factor II to thrombin and factor X to Xa. The result is the generation of a localized thrombin burst, enabling feedback activation of intrinsic coagulation, further platelet activation, and finally the generation of fibrin. A major advantage of FVIIa is that this procoagulant effect does not occur in the systemic circulation but is limited to the site of vessel injury (i.e. tissue factor exposure).

Impaired coagulation in sepsis

In sepsis, the normal compensatory mechanisms that prevent excessive activation of the coagulation cascade are suppressed and cannot adequately counteract fibrin deposition. Inflammatory cytokines and thrombin can impair the generation of plasmin, and therefore the lysis of fibrin, by stimulating platelets and the endothelium to release plasminogen activator inhibitor-1, and also limiting the availability of tissue plasminogen activator. Thrombin can also stimulate inflammatory pathways and further reduce the body's fibrinolytic capabilities by activating thrombin-activatable fibrinolysis inhibitor to suppress the activity of plasmin. As mentioned earlier, the regulation of thrombin formation involves three anticoagulant systems: protein C, antithrombin, and tissue factor pathway inhibitor. Activated protein C inactivates factors Va and VIIIa, thereby inhibiting thrombosis and promoting fibrinolysis. The derangement of coagulation and fibrinolysis in sepsis is mediated by several proinflammatory cytokines, such as TNF-α, IL-1, and IL-6. The principal mediator of coagulation activation in sepsis is IL-6. Activated protein C has anti-inflammatory effects on monocytes and granulocytes, reducing leukocyte activation and cytokine production. It also limits the rolling of monocytes and neutrophils on injured endothelium by binding to cell adhesion molecules. This effect is distinct from its regulatory role in coagulation.

Activation of protein C in severe sepsis may be inadequate because of reduced thrombomodulin levels on endothelial cell surfaces due to endothelial injury. In the PROWESS trial, 1690 patients with severe sepsis were given human activated protein C (Drotrecogin α (activated)) 24 μg/kg/h for 96 hours. This reduced 28-day mortality from 30.8% to 24.7%. Serious bleeding was commoner in the treatment than the control group, but despite this, activated protein C seems a promising strategy in severe sepsis.

HEMOSTATIC DEFECTS AND BLEEDING DISORDERS

Bleeding disorders may result from abnormalities of the vasculature, of platelet function, or from disorders of the coagulation cascade. 'Vascular' bleeding disorders are a mixed group of conditions characterized by easy bruising and spontaneous bleeding from small vessels. The underlying abnormality is either in the vessel wall or in perivascular connective tissue. In general, these conditions are not severe. Standard clotting tests and screening tests are often normal, although the Ivy bleeding time may be prolonged.

Acquired vascular defects may result in abnormal bleeding. These include senile purpura, purpura of infections, Henoch–Schönlein syndrome, steroid purpura, and scurvy.

Abnormal bleeding caused by thrombocytopenia or abnormal platelet function is characterized by mucosal hemorrhage, spontaneous purpura, and prolonged bleeding from surgery or trauma. Causes of thrombocytopenia include failure of platelet production and increased destruction of platelets. Failure of platelet production may result from selective depression of megakaryocytes, for example by drugs (azathioprine, ranitidine), chemical toxicity, or viral infection (e.g. cytomegalovirus). Platelet production may be depressed as part of generalized bone marrow failure (e.g. aplastic anemia, leukemia, myelosclerosis, marrow infiltration by tumor, cytotoxic drugs).

Causes of increased platelet destruction include autoimmune thrombocytopenic purpura (acute or chronic). Idiopathic thrombocytopenic purpura (ITP), seen predominantly in young women, may occur in conjunction with systemic diseases, such as lupus erythematosus. Platelet sensitization with autoantibodies (IgG) results in early clearance of platelets from the circulation by the reticuloendothelial system. In severe disease, mean platelet survival may be reduced to less than 1 hour. Platelet transfusion may be relatively ineffective. Treatment is based on immunosuppression, as fewer than 10% of patients recover spontaneously. Acute thrombocytopenia occurs most frequently in children. Most cases follow viral infection or vaccination. Spontaneous remission is the rule.

Drug-induced immune thrombocytopenia is a cause of increased platelet destruction. Several drugs, including quinine, quinidine, sulfonamides, and rifampicin may produce immune thrombocytopenia. The drug induces the formation of antibody directed against a drug–plasma protein hapten. Circulating immune complexes are adsorbed on to the platelet. Consequently, platelet damage is coincidental to the underlying process. The damaged platelet is removed by the reticuloendothelial system. Treatment is discontinuation of suspected drugs. Recovery is generally rapid (see heparin adverse effects, above).

Disorders of platelet function may be present in patients who have skin or mucous membrane hemorrhage in whom bleeding time is prolonged despite a normal platelet count. Thromboelastography (see below) is likely to reveal a reduced maximum amplitude. Hereditary disorders of platelet function are rare. There is defective platelet adhesion (as well as coagulopathy) in von Willebrand's disease.

Acquired platelet dysfunction may be secondary to drugs (NSAIDs, aspirin, dipyridamole) or systemic disease. Such conditions include Waldenström's hypogammaglobulinemia associated with multiple myeloma and renal failure (see below).

Disseminated intravascular coagulation (DIC) is a disorder of platelets and clotting factors. It complicates many disease processes, including sepsis, trauma, and malignancy (Fig. 53.7). It generally presents as an acute disorder, although there is also a chronic form. Disseminated intravascular coagulation is characterized by activation of the clotting cascade with the formation of small thrombi throughout the microcirculation, which leads to vascular occlusion and ischemic damage, particularly in the kidney and splanchnic bed. Fibrinogen, coagulation factors, and platelets are rapidly consumed (consumptive coagulopathy). This leads to rapid worsening of clotting. Platelet plugs and fibrin in the microcirculation trigger the fibrinolytic cascade. These have an anticoagulant effect, prolonging thrombin time. All clotting tests (PT, aPTT, and thrombin time) are abnormal. Characteristically, fibrinogen levels are reduced and both FDP and D-dimer levels are raised. Perhaps the best laboratory correlate of clinical disease course is the fibrinogen level.

The management of DIC is focused on controlling any predisposing condition. Treatment of the coagulopathy is likely to be ineffective until the underlying disorder has been treated. Fresh frozen plasma, cryoprecipitate, and platelets are used as directed by both laboratory tests and clinical endpoints (hemorrhage). Historically, heparin was used to prevent consumption of clotting factors. This practice has now largely been abandoned because of the risk of exacerbating bleeding, but may sometimes be required where arterial thrombosis is a major feature. Antifibrinolytic drugs are not used, as fibrinolysis in DIC is generally a secondary phenomenon.

Coagulation disorders (disorders of the clotting cascade) may be either hereditary or acquired. Hereditary disorders affecting each of the 10 coagulation factors are described. The most common are hemophilia (factor VIII) and Christmas disease (factor IX). Von Willebrand's disease is a disorder of factor VIIIR:AG.

Although all of these conditions are rare, hemophilia A is the least rare. It is an X-linked disorder, although up to one-third of patients have no family history and may represent new mutations. The incidence is 1 in 10 000. The lesion is low or absent factor VIII:C activity as a consequence of abnormal structure or absence of the factor. In general, factor VIIIR:AG and vWF are quantitatively and qualitatively normal. Perioperative and traumatic hemorrhage is potentially life threatening. Whole-blood clotting time is prolonged. Activated partial thromboplastin time is likewise prolonged, and factor VIII is reduced. Bleeding time and PT are normal. Bleeding episodes can be treated with factor VIII concentrates or cryoprecipitate. Fresh frozen plasma contains factor VIII, but is rarely used as the increment in factor VIII levels is small for each unit. Spontaneous hemorrhage is uncommon unless factor VIII is below 20% of normal. During major surgery, factor VIII should be maintained between 60 and 100% of normal values.

Christmas disease (hemophilia B) is caused by factor IX deficiency. Its clinical presentation and inheritance closely resemble those of hemophilia A. The incidence is 1 in 50 000. Hemorrhage and surgery are treated with factor IX concentrates. As factor IX is relatively stable, fresh frozen plasma is also effective in the treatment of this condition.

Von Willebrand's disease results from a defect in the synthesis of the major fraction of factor VIII: VIIIR:AG. The platelet effect of vWF (promotion of platelet adhesion to subendothelial tissue) results from a specific abnormal configuration of the VIIIR:AG molecule. The condition is characterized by perioperative hemorrhage and bleeding from mucous membranes. Laboratory investigation shows a prolonged bleeding time and low levels of VIII:C and VIIIR:AG. Platelet aggregation in response to ADP is normal, but is defective in response to ristocetin (ristomycin). Bleeding episodes are treated with cryoprecipitate or concentrates of factor VIII.

Several disease states lead to acquired bleeding disorders. The coagulopathy of liver disease is multifactorial. Because of biliary obstruction there may be reduced absorption of fat-soluble vitamins (A, D, E, K) and a selective reduction in synthesis of vitamin K-dependent clotting factors (II, VII, IX, X). Progressive deterioration of hepatocellular function leads to reduced synthesis of the remaining clotting factors, with the exception of factor VIII, which is produced by endothelial cells. Patients who have cirrhotic liver disease show enhanced fibrinolysis. This is because of reduced clearance of t-PA and reduced synthesis of the antifibrinolytic globulins α_2-antiplasmin and α_2-macroglobulin. Platelet function and numbers decline as hepatic synthetic function fails. The liver constitutively produces thrombopoietin, the cytokine responsible for signaling platelet synthesis, and patients who have liver failure and cirrhotic liver disease often suffer portal hypertension and hypersplenism, which lead to abnormal platelet production, sequestration, and pooling.

Patients who have renal disease likewise suffer abnormal hemostasis through an acquired disorder of platelet function secondary to uremia. Accumulation of middle molecules and metabolic acids interferes with vWF and subsequent platelet aggregation. Platelet dysfunction is proportional to uremia and is restored following dialysis or transplantation. The platelet dysfunction of renal disease may be corrected (at least in part) by desmopressin.

EVALUATION OF COAGULATION

Abnormal bleeding may result from thrombocytopenia, platelet function disorders, or abnormalities of the clotting cascade. The most common cause of abnormal bleeding is thrombocytopenia. Therefore, initial investigation should include a full blood count and blood film examination.

Bleeding time

Bleeding time is one of several measures of platelet plug formation in vivo and may detect abnormalities of platelet function where blood count and platelet numbers are normal. The commonly used method uses the Ivy template. Bleeding should stop spontaneously after 3–8 minutes. Bleeding time is prolonged with thrombocytopenia or platelet dysfunction.

Prothrombin time

The PT tests the extrinsic and common pathways (see Fig. 53.3). Both factor VII and factors common to both systems are evaluated. Tissue thromboplastin (extracted from brain) and calcium ions are added to plasma, and a clot should form within 10–14 seconds.

Activated partial thromboplastin time

The aPTT is a measure of the intrinsic system. Hence, factors XII, XI, IX, and VIII are tested, in addition to factors common to both systems. A surface activator (e.g. kaolin), phospholipid, and calcium ions are added to plasma, which should produce a clot within 30–40 seconds. Both PT and aPTT are normally correctable by adding normal plasma to the plasma being tested. Failure of this maneuver to correct PT or aPTT suggests that an inhibitor of coagulation is present (e.g. FDPs, heparinoids).

Thrombin time

Fibrinolysis may be suspected on the basis of a reduced fibrinogen, prolonged thrombin time, or the presence of D-dimer or FDPs. Thrombin time is assayed by adding thrombin to plasma and observing the time to fibrin formation, normally 10–12 seconds.

Thromboelastography®

In perioperative thromboelastography (TEG)® a sample of fresh blood (0.3 mL) is placed in a small well at 37°C and gently rotated. A piston connected to a recorder is suspended in the sample well. As fibrin strands begin to form, the piston begins to oscillate with the movement of the well. The evolving TEG trace produces a dynamic clot fingerprint that progressively describes activation of the clotting cascade, fibrin formation, the fibrin–platelet interaction (clot stability), clot retraction, and fibrinolysis (Fig. 53.7).

The thromboelastogram

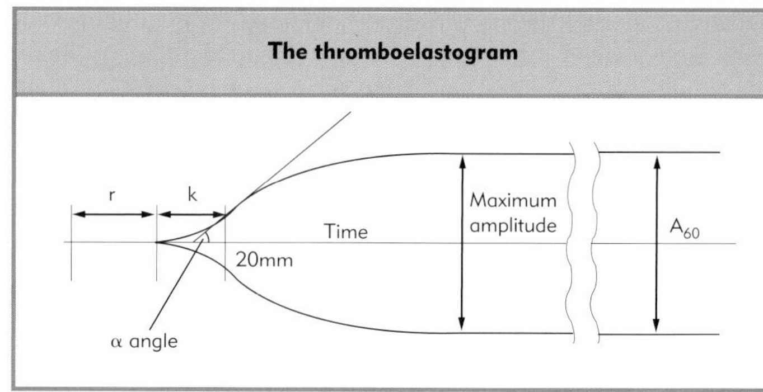

Figure 53.7 Schematic representation of the thromboelastogram. The diagram is discontinuous, as A60 – the amplitude at 60 minutes – would otherwise be far to the right of the figure.

Thromboelastography correlates only loosely with the results of standard coagulation tests. This reflects the interdependency of TEG variables rather than reliance on independent endpoints. Thromboelastography is more sensitive than standard tests of clotting at detecting subtle changes in balance between coagulation, fibrinolysis, and related hemostatic pathways. A prolonged reaction time gives evidence of a defect in the early part of the clotting cascade, perhaps implying a need for fresh frozen plasma. A reduced α angle is related to a reduced rate of clot propagation, suggesting a need for fibrinogen (cryoprecipitate). Maximum amplitude relates to clot tensile strength. This reflects platelet numbers and function as well as the effectiveness of fibrin crosslinking.

Specific tests

Most clotting factors may also be assayed by specific tests, including radioimmunoassay, enzyme-linked immunosorbent assay (ELISA), or specific factor assays based on aPTT or PT in which all factors except the one to be measured are present in reagent plasma. This requires a supply of plasma from patients who have known hereditary deficiencies of the factor in question. Factor levels in test plasma are assessed by the degree to which test plasma corrects the prolonged clotting time of substrate-deficient plasma.

Key references

Dahlback B. Blood coagulation. Lancet 2000:355:1627–32.

Hoffbrand AV, Pettitt JE, Moss PAH. Essential haematology, 4th edn. Oxford: Blackwell; 2001.

Hoffman M. Remodeling the blood coagulation cascade. J Thromb Thrombolysis 2003;16:17–20.

Further reading

Booth NA. The laboratory investigation of the fibrinolytic system. In: Thomson JM, ed. Blood coagulation and hemostasis, 4th edn. Edinburgh: Churchill Livingstone; 1991:115–49.

Dettinmeier P, Swindell B et al. Role of activated protein C in the pathophysiology of severe sepsis. Am J Crit Care 2003;12:518–24.

Dzik WH, Arkin CF, Jenkins RL, Stump DC. Fibrinolysis during liver transplantation in humans: role of tissue-type plasminogen activator. Blood 1988;71:1090–5.

Ferguson J, Waly H, Wilson J. Fundamentals of coagulation and glycoprotein IIb/IIIa receptor inhibition. Am Heart J. 1998;135:S35 –S42.

Irving GA. Perioperative blood and blood component therapy. Can J Anaesth. 1992;39:1105–15.

Kovesi T, Royston D. Is there a bleeding problem with platelet-active drugs? Br J Anaesth. 2002;88:159–63.

Levi M, Cate H, van der Poll T. Endothelium: interface between coagulation and inflammation. Crit Care Med. 2002;30:S220–4.

Veldman A, Hoffman M, Ehrenforth S. New insights into the coagulation system and implications for new therapeutic options with recombinant factor VIIa. Curr Med Chem. 2003;10:797–811.

Walker CPR, Roysten D. Thrombin generation and its inhibition: a review of the scientific basis and mechanisms of action of anticoagulant therapies. Br J Anaesth. 2002;88:848–63.

Webster N. Inflammation and the coagulation system. Br J Anaesth. 2002;89:216–20.

Yassen KA, Bellamy MC, Sadek SA, Webster NR. Tranexamic acid reduces blood loss during orthotopic liver transplantation. Clin Transplant. 1993;7:453–8.

Chapter 54

The immune system

Helen F Galley and Nigel R Webster

The extremely adaptable and complex immune system is able to recognize and eliminate a variety of foreign cells and molecules. The immune system has both the function of recognition and that of response. The recognition component is remarkably specific: it can discriminate between self and nonself, and also can identify the subtle chemical differences that distinguish one pathogen from another. The *recognition response* is then converted to an appropriate *effector response* to enable the neutralization or elimination of the particular organism, cancer cell, or foreign tissue. Subsequent exposure to the same antigen induces a *memory response*, characterized by a rapid enhancement of immune reactivity.

INNATE IMMUNITY

Immunity is the only state of protection from infectious disease and consists of both specific and nonspecific components. Nonspecific, or *innate immunity*, is the pre-existing resistance to disease and comprises four types of defensive barrier: anatomic, physiologic, phagocytic/endocytic, and inflammatory. Anatomic barriers prevent microorganisms from entering the body and include the skin and mucus secretions. Intact skin prevents the penetration of most pathogens; a low skin pH also inhibits bacterial growth. The conjunctivae and the alimentary, respiratory, and urogenital tracts are covered by mucus membranes, which are protected by saliva, tears, and mucus. In the gastrointestinal tract, for example, organisms trapped in mucus are propelled out of the body by ciliary action. Physiologic barriers include temperature, pH, and a variety of soluble factors, including lysozyme, *interferons* (IFNs), and complement. *Lysozyme*, found in mucus, cleaves the peptidoglycan layer of bacterial cell walls. The IFNs are produced by virus-infected cells and bind to nearby cells, inducing a generalized antiviral state. The *complement* system is a multicomponent-triggered enzyme cascade that results in membrane-damaging reactions that destroy pathogenic organisms and facilitate their clearance.

Complement

The complement system is a group of serum proteins activated in a sequential enzymatic cascade; they have an important role in antigen clearance. There are two pathways of complement activation: the *classic pathway*, which is activated by specific immunoglobulin molecules, and the *alternative pathway*, which is activated by a variety of microorganisms and immune complexes. Each pathway involves the activation of different complement proteins but results in a common endpoint, the generation of a *membrane attack complex* (MAC), which is responsible for cell lysis. This complex inserts itself into cell membrane phospholipid and makes large transmembrane channels in the target cell, disrupting the membrane and causing cell lysis. Complement components also amplify antigen–antibody reactions, attract phagocytic cells to sites of infection, augment phagocytosis, and activate B lymphocytes. The complement system is nonspecific and will, in theory, attack host cells as well as foreign cells. To prevent host cell damage, regulatory mechanisms, including spontaneous hydrolysis of complement components and inactivating proteins, restrict complement reactions to designated targets (see Chapter 44 also).

Phagocytosis

Ingestion of extracellular macromolecules and particles is achieved via *endocytosis* and *phagocytosis*, respectively. In endocytosis, macromolecules in extracellular fluid are internalized by invagination of the plasma membrane to form endocytic vesicles (Chapter 2). *Pinocytosis* is nonspecific, whereas in *receptor-mediated endocytosis* macromolecules bind selectively to membrane receptors. The ingested material is degraded by enzymes of the endocytic processing pathway. Phagocytosis involves the ingestion of particles, including whole microorganisms, via expansion of the plasma membrane to form a *phagosome*. Virtually all cells are capable of endocytosis, but phagocytosis occurs in only a few specialized cells (Fig. 54.1). Dedicated phagocytes include polymorphonuclear neutrophils, mast cells, and macrophages; "nonprofessional" phagocytes such as endothelial cells and hepatocytes also have phagocytic potential. Cells infected with viruses and parasites are killed by large granular lymphocytes termed natural killer (NK) cells, and by eosinophils.

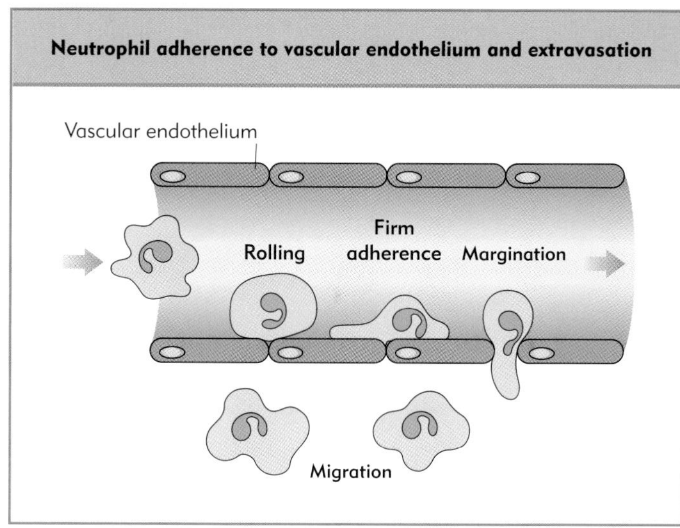

Figure 54.2 Process of neutrophil adherence to, and extravasation across, the vascular endothelium.

The inflammatory response

The *inflammatory response* to tissue damage or invasion by pathogenic organisms results in vasodilatation, increased capillary permeability, and influx of phagocytic cells. Movement of phagocytic cells involves a complex series of events, including *margination*, or adherence of cells in the bloodstream to the endothelial cell wall; *extravasation*, or movement of phagocytes between capillary endothelial cells into the tissue; and *chemotaxis*, the migration of phagocytes through the tissue to the site of inflammation. The process of leukocyte margination is a carefully regulated process involving specific adhesion molecules. These comprise three structurally dissimilar groups of molecules and are located on the extracellular portion of the cell membrane of both endothelial cells and leukocytes. Examples include E-selectin, intercellular cell adhesion molecule (ICAM), and vascular cell adhesion molecule (VCAM). These molecules cause circulating leukocytes to slow down and then roll along the endothelium. Firm adherence and transmigration then occur (Fig. 54.2). The inflammatory response is initiated by a series of interactions that involve several chemical mediators produced by the invading organisms or damaged cells and the cells of the immune system and plasma enzyme systems. These include complement, C-reactive protein and other *acute-phase proteins*, *histamine*, *kinins*, and bacterial cell wall products such as *endotoxin* and *exotoxin*.

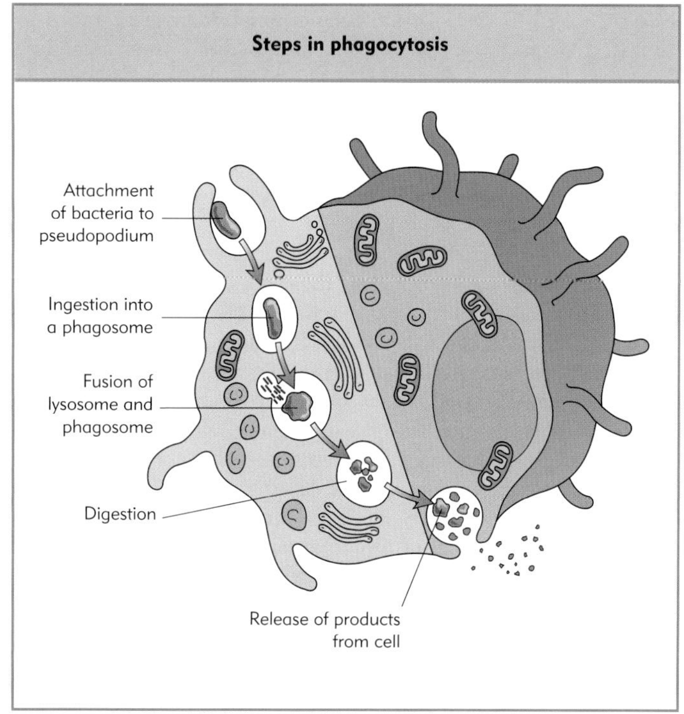

Figure 54.1 Phagocytosis of bacteria. The steps in phagocytosis.

Severe infection with Gram-negative organisms leads to the appearance of endotoxin or lipopolysaccharide (LPS) in the bloodstream which interacts with LPS-binding protein (LBP) and binds to CD14 receptors, transducing signals via Toll-like receptors, which culminate in the activation of nuclear factor κ B (NF-κB). NF-κB is a redox-sensitive transcription factor that regulates, in part, gene expression of many cytokines, growth factors, adhesion molecules, and enzymes involved in immune and inflammatory responses. It is maintained in a nonactivated state in the cytoplasm by association with an inhibitor subunit, IκB (Fig. 54.3). Proteolysis of IκB in response to activation stimuli, including LPS and cytokines, reveals a nuclear recognition site. This then prompts the NF-κB to move into the nucleus, where it binds to target DNA and results in mRNA expression. NF-κB activation leads to increased gene expression of several important mediators involved in the inflammatory response, including chemokines, cytokines, and adhesion molecules. Although some cells (e.g. endothelial cells) do not themselves express CD14, LPS can activate these cells via interaction with soluble CD14 and LBP present in the circulation.

Toll-like receptors (TLRs) are pathogen-associated molecular pattern receptors for a variety of diverse molecules derived from bacteria, viruses, and fungi. To date, 10 TLR family members have been identified. TLR2 is crucial for the propagation of the inflammatory response to components of Gram-positive and Gram-negative bacteria and mycobacteria, such as peptidoglycan, lipoteichoic acid, bacterial lipoproteins, lipopeptides, and

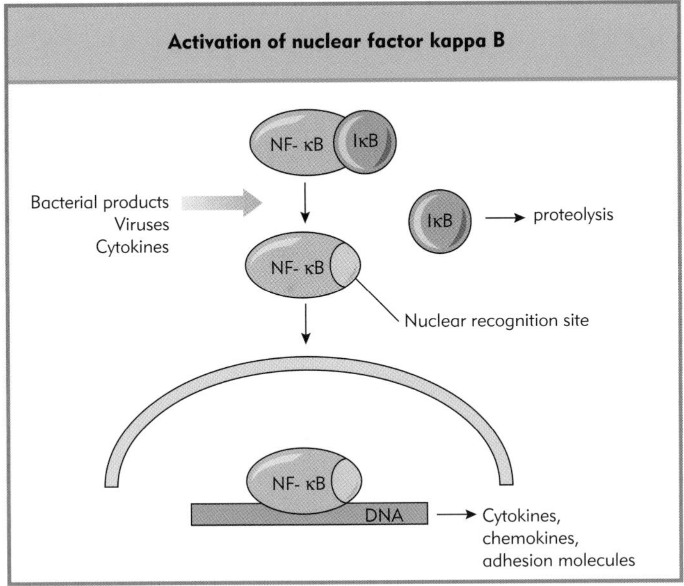

Figure 54.3 Activation of nuclear factor-κ B (NF-κB). See text for explanation.

lipoarabinomannan. TLR2 is predominantly expressed in the cells involved in first-line host defense, including monocytes, macrophages, dendritic cells, and neutrophils, but some expression is also seen in endothelial cells. TLR4 has been identified as the receptor for LPS and lipoteichoic acid.

Another receptor important for host responses to infection has been described recently, called triggering receptor expressed on myeloid cells (TREM-1). It is expressed on blood neutrophils and a subset of monocytes. In vitro studies have shown that TREM-1 is upregulated in response to Gram-positive and Gram-negative bacteria, mycobacteria, and bacterial cell wall components, including both LPS and lipoteichoic acid. Triggering of the TREM-1 receptor induces neutrophils to secrete inflammatory cytokines (see below).

ACQUIRED IMMUNITY

Specific or *acquired immunity* targets microorganisms that are not destroyed by the innate immune system. Specificity, diversity, memory, and the ability to discriminate self from nonself are key features of acquired immunity. Acquired immunity is intricately involved with the innate immune response. Cells of the phagocytic system activate specific immune responses and modulate the production of soluble mediators that orchestrate the inflammatory response and the interplay involved in the elimination of a foreign organism.

The immune response can also be classified into humoral (from body fluid) and cell-mediated processes. The humoral component involves the interaction of B cells with antigen, and the proliferation and differentiation of the B cells into antibody-secreting plasma cells. Antibody is the effector of the humoral response; it binds to antigen, which neutralizes the antigen and facilitates its removal. The complex of antibody and antigen is known as the immune complex. B-cell activation also activates the complement system, resulting in lysis of the foreign organism. Effector T cells generated in response to antigen are responsible for cell-mediated immunity. Cytokines secreted by T cells activate various phagocytic cells, enabling the killing of intracellular bacteria. Cytotoxic T cells (Tc cells) are important in the recognition of altered self cells (i.e. virus-infected cells or tumor cells).

MAJOR HISTOCOMPATIBILITY COMPLEX

The major histocompatibility complex (MHC) is a tightly linked cluster of genes located on chromosome 6 and associated with intercellular recognition and self/nonself discrimination. MHC molecules play a major role in the acceptance of self (histocompatible) or rejection of nonself (histoincompatible). The MHC complex encodes immune mediators and antigens (human lymphocyte antigens or HLA), which play an important role in antigen recognition by T cells, and determines the response of an individual to infectious antigens and hence their susceptibility to disease. The MHC genes are organized into those encoding three classes of HLA molecule (Table 54.1): class I (regions A, B, and C), class II (region D), and class III (regions C4, C2, Bf). Class I genes encode glycoproteins expressed on the surface of most nucleated cells and present antigens for the activation of specific T cells. Class II genes encode glycoproteins expressed mainly on antigen-presenting cells, including macrophages and B cells, where they present antigen to other defined T-cell populations. Class III genes encode several different immune products, including complement system components, enzymes, and tumor necrosis factors (TNF); they have no role in antigen presentation.

CELLS OF THE IMMUNE SYSTEM

Leukocytes (white blood cells) develop from a common pluripotent stem cell during hematopoiesis and proliferate and differentiate into different cells in response to hematopoietic

Table 54.1 Simplification of the organization of the major histocompatibility complex (MHC)

	HLA							
***MHC* Complex class**	***II***			***III***		***I***		
Region	DP	DQ	DR	C4, C2, Bf		B	C	A
Gene products	DPαβ	DQαβ	DRαβ	Complement proteins	Tumor necrosis factors, TNF-α, TNF-β	HLA-B	HLA-C	HLA-A

Table 54.2 Cells of the immune system

Cell type	Function	Mediator production
Monocytes and macrophages	Phagocytosis, antigen presentation, cytokine release, activation of Th cells, secretion of complement proteins, secretion of hydrolytic enzymes, secretion of reactive oxygen species	Interleukin (IL)-1β, 1L-6, IL-8, IL-12, interferon (IFN)-α, transforming growth factor (TGF)-β, tumor necrosis factor (TNF)-α
Neutrophils	Phagocytosis, cytokine release, secretion of hydrolytic enzymes, secretion of reactive oxygen species	IL-1β, IL-6, IL-8
Natural killer cells	Nonspecific tumor cell cytoxicity, antibody-dependent cytotoxicity	IFN-γ, IL-3
T lymphocytes Helper subset 1 (Th1) Helper subset 2 (Th2) Cytotoxic (Tc)	Antigen recognition on presenting cells, cytokine release	IL-2, IL-3, IL-4, IL-5, IL-9, IL-13, IFN-γ, TNF-β, IL-6, IL-10 IFN-γ, TNF-β
B lymphocytes	Antigen recognition, antibody production, cytokine release	IL-1β, IL-12
Eosinophils	Phagocytosis, parasitic killing	IL-1β, IL-3, IL-5, granulocyte–macrophage colony-stimulating factor (GM-CSF)
Basophils	Role in allergic reactions	–
Mast cells	Role in allergic reactions, histamine release, cytokine release	IL-1β, IL-3, IL-6, GM-CSF, TGF-β, TNF-α

growth factors, a process that is balanced by programmed cell death or *apoptosis*. The *lymphocyte*, the only cell to possess specificity, diversity, memory, and recognition of self/nonself, is the central line of the immune system. *Monocytes, macrophages*, and *neutrophils* are accessory immune cells specialized for phagocytosis. This process is facilitated by *opsonins* (e.g. complement and antibody), which increase the attachment of antigen to the membrane of the phagocyte (Table 54.2). Macrophages are also important in antigen processing and presentation in association with a class II MHC molecule, and for the secretion of interleukin-1 (IL-1). Lymphocytes constantly recirculate between blood, lymph, and tissues, mediated by interactions between cell adhesion molecules on the vascular endothelium and receptors for the adhesion molecules on the lymphocyte surface.

Different maturational stages of lymphocytes can be distinguished by their expression of surface antigens that can be identified by particular monoclonal antibodies. A particular surface molecule that is identifiable by one or more monoclonal antibodies (several different antibodies may bind to one surface antigen, reacting at different parts of the molecule) is called *cluster of differentiation*, or CD, antigen.

Antigen processing and presentation

Antigens are substances such as proteins, carbohydrates, and glycoproteins that are capable of interacting with the products of a specific immune response. An antigen that is capable of eliciting a specific immune response by itself is called an immunogen. Foreign protein antigens must be degraded into small peptides and complexed with class I or II MHC molecules in order to be recognized by a T cell. This is called antigen processing. Whether complexing occurs with class I or II MHC molecules seems to be determined by the route by which the antigen enters the cell. Mature immunocompetent animals possess large numbers of antigen-reactive T and B lymphocytes. Their specificities are determined prior to contact with antigen by random gene rearrangements in the bone marrow during cell maturation. When antigen interacts with and activates mature antigenically committed T and B cells, it brings about the expansion of the particular population of cells with the given antigenic specificity for that antigen. This is called *clonal selection* and *expansion*. This process explains both specificity and memory attributes. Specificity is implicit, as only those lymphocytes possessing appropriate receptors will be clonally expanded. Memory occurs because there is a larger number of antigen-reactive lymphocytes present after clonal selection, and many of these lymphocytes have a longer lifespan (and are therefore termed *memory cells*). The initial encounter of antigen-specific lymphocytes with an antigen induces a *primary response*; subsequent encounters are more rapid and intense (*secondary response*). Self/nonself recognition is achieved by clonal elimination during the development of lymphocytes bearing self-reactive receptors, or functional suppression of these cells in adults.

Antibody structure

Antibodies or immunoglobulins are lymphocyte-produced protein molecules that combine specifically with antigens. Antibody molecules consist of two identical light chains and two identical heavy chains joined by disulfide bonds. Each heavy and each light chain has a variable amino acid sequence region and a constant region. The unique heavy-chain constant region sequences determine the five classes or *isotypes* of immunoglobulin: IgM, IgG, IgD, IgA, and IgE. These isotypes vary in their effector function, serum concentration, and half-life. IgG is the most common isotype and the only immunoglobulin to cross the placenta. IgM exists as a pentamer and is most effective in viral neutralization, bacterial agglutination, and complement activation. IgA is the predominant isotype in external secretions, including breast milk and mucus. IgD and IgE are the least abundant isotypes; IgD and IgM are the major isotypes on mature B cells, and IgE mediates mast cell degranulation.

Monoclonal antibodies are laboratory-manufactured homogeneous antibodies with identical antigenic specificities. These antibodies are produced by cloned *hybridoma* cells, which are manufactured by fusing normal lymphocytes with myeloma cells. The clone retains the normal antibody functions and receptors of lymphocytes together with the immortal growth characteristics of myeloma cells. Monoclonal antibodies provide an indefinite supply of antibody with a highly defined antigenic specificity that recognizes a single antigenic determinant or *epitope*. Monoclonal antibodies are under investigation as therapeutic agents in sepsis (Chapter 73) and immunosuppression (see below).

Cytokines

The orchestration of immune and inflammatory responses depends upon communication between cells by soluble molecules. These molecules are given the generic name cytokines and include chemokines, ILs, growth factors, and IFNs. Cytokines are low-molecular-weight secreted proteins that regulate both the amplitude and the duration of the immune inflammatory responses (Table 54.3). They have a transient action that is tightly regulated. Cytokines are extremely potent, combining with small numbers of high-affinity cell-surface receptors and producing changes in the patterns of RNA and protein synthesis. They have effects on growth and differentiation in a variety of cell types, with considerable overlap and redundancy between them, partially accounted for by the induction of synthesis of common proteins. Interaction may occur in a cascade system in which one cytokine induces another, through modulation of the receptor of another cytokine, and through either synergism or antagonism of two cytokines acting on the same cell. Cytokines should not be categorized as growth stimulators or inhibitors, or pro- or anti-inflammatory. Rather, their specific actions depend on the stimulus, the cell type, and the presence of other mediators and receptors (Fig. 54.4).

Chemokines are a family of small proinflammatory molecules characterized by four conserved cysteine residues. The α-chemokines have two pairs of cysteine residues separated by a variable amino acid sequence and are chemotactic for neutrophils (e.g. IL-8, platelet basic protein, epithelial neutrophil-activating peptide), whereas β-chemokines have two adjacent pairs of cysteine residues and are chemotactic for monocytes/macrophages (e.g. platelet factor 4, monocyte chemotactic protein 1, macrophage inflammatory protein 1) and T cells (e.g. RANTES). Chemokines have been described as having more restricted actions than cytokines, but this is more likely to be a consequence of differential expression of receptors. The IFN family, IFN-α, -β, and -γ, are broad-spectrum antiviral agents that also modulate the activity of other cells, particularly IL-8 and platelet-activating factor (PAF) production, antibody production by B cells, and activation of cytotoxic macrophages. Growth factors regulate the differentiation, proliferation, activity, and function of specific cell types. The best-known are colony-stimulating factors, which cause colony formation by hematogenic progenitor cells (e.g. granulocyte–macrophage colony-stimulating factor, or GM-CSF). Other examples include factors that regulate the growth of nerve cells (NGF), fibroblasts (FGF), epidermis (EGF), and hepatocytes.

In addition to the low-molecular-weight protein mediators, there are also lipid mediators of inflammation, for example PAF and arachidonic acid metabolites. PAF is a labile alkyl phospholipid released from a variety of cells in the presence of antigen and leukocytes in response to stimulation by immune complexes. In addition to its platelet effects, the actions of PAF include the priming of macrophages to respond to other inflammatory mediators, and altering microvascular permeability. Arachidonic acid metabolites include the prostaglandins, leukotrienes, and eicosanoids (hydroxyeicosatetraenoic acids (HETEs) and hydroxyperoxyeicosatetraenoic acids (HPETEs)), all of which have profound inflammatory and vascular actions and may regulate, and be regulated by, other cytokines.

TNF-α and TNF-β have a vast range of similar effects and are usually referred to as inflammatory cytokines. They have a central role in initiating the cascade of other cytokines and factors that make up the immune response to infection, and play a key role in sepsis (Chapter 73). Their wide variety of effects is attributable to the ubiquity of their receptors, their ability to activate multiple signal transduction pathways, and their ability to induce or suppress an array of genes, including those for growth factors, cytokines, transcription factors, receptors, and acute-phase proteins. Although both TNFs have similar biological activities, regulation of their expression and processing is quite different.

Receptors and antagonists

The biological activities of cytokines are mediated by specific cellular receptors. Often these receptors comprise multiple subunits that provide phased stages of activation and biological action. For example the IL-2 receptor complex consists of three subunits, IL-2Rα, IL-2Rβ, and IL-2Rγ. Although the IL-2Rα/β combination can bind IL-2, IL-2Rγ is also required for high-affinity binding, ligand internalization, and signaling, all of which are required for maximal effect. Other cellular receptors exist in more than one type that act alone but have different binding affinities for different forms of a cytokine protein (e.g. IL-1 receptor type I binds IL-1α better than IL-1β, and IL-1 receptor type II has more affinity for IL-1β). Binding of a cytokine to one type of receptor may result in interactions with another receptor; the two receptors for TNF, for example, use ligand passing, in which TNF binds transiently to receptor type I, with full signal transduction, but may then move on to the type II receptor with activation of another signal for apoptosis.

Soluble cytokine receptors have been identified that compete with membrane-bound receptors for cytokines, thus regulating cytokine signals. Exceptions to this are soluble receptors for IL-6 and ciliary neurotropic factor, which act as agonists rather than antagonists. Such soluble receptors may be membrane-bound receptors that are shed into the circulation either intact or as truncated forms (e.g. soluble TNF receptors, sTNF-R), or may begin as related precursor molecules that are enzymatically cleaved (e.g. IL-1R). Soluble receptors may appear in response to stimuli as part of a naturally occurring independent regulatory process to limit the deleterious effects of a mediator (e.g. sTNF-R), but some have little binding activity and may represent superficial and unimportant losses of cellular receptors (e.g. the

Table 54.3 Sources and biological effects of immune mediators

Mediator	Source	Biological activity	Effects on other cells
Interferon (IFN)-α, β	T cells, B cells, macrophages, fibroblasts	Pyrogenic, cytotoxic	Macrophages: increases class I MHC antigens, IL-1, PAF production; B cells: proliferation, differentiation; T cells: proliferation, chemotactic
IFN-γ	Th1, Tc, NK cells	Pyrogenic, antiviral, cytotoxic antitumor effect, mimics septic shock, causes release of NO and ODFRs, upregulates IL-1 and PAF production	Macrophages: increases class 1 MHC antigens, IL-1, and PAF production, downregulates IL-2-mediated IL-8 mRNA production; B cells: proliferation and differentiation; chemotactic for monocytes; stimulates formation of adhesion molecules
Tumor necrosis factor (TNF)-α, β	Neutrophils, lymphocytes, endothelial cells, smooth muscle cells, macrophages, mast cells	Pyrogenic, cytotoxic, antitumor effect, mimics septic shock, promotes angiogenesis, causes release of NO and ODFRs, induces or suppresses gene expression for cytokines, receptors, and acute-phase proteins	Wide variety of effects through ability to regulate gene expression, important role in host resistance to infection as immunostimulant and mediator of the inflammatory response, promotes hematopoiesis
Interleukins IL-1α, β	Macrophages, endothelial cells, fibroblasts, hepatocytes B cells, mast cells, eosinophils	Pyrogenic, cytotoxic, antitumor effect, promotes angiogenesis, causes release of NO and ODFRs, induces prostaglandin synthesis, initiates the acute-phase response	Macrophages: TNF and IL-6 production; B cells: proliferation, differentiation; T cells: proliferation; chemotaxis; formation of adhesion molecules; hematopoiesis
IL-2	Th1 cells	Pyrogenic, antitumor effect, mimics septic shock, causes release of ODFRs	B and T cells: proliferation, differentiation, release of IgG from activated B cells; chemotaxis, augments neutrophil and macrophage function; formation of adhesion molecules
IL-4	Th2 cells	Cytotoxic, antitumor effect, inhibits induction of NOS, inhibits release of superoxide by macrophages, numerous anti-inflammatory effects	Macrophages: suppresses activation, upregulates class II MHC antigens, inhibits IgG receptor expression, inhibits expression of IL-1, IL-6, IL-8, TNF; stimulates IL-1ra expression; B and T cells: proliferation, differentiation, enhances antigen-presenting capacity; chemotaxis; formation of endothelial cell adhesion molecules; hematopoiesis
IL-6	Th2 cells, macrophages, endothelial cells, fibroblasts, hepatocytes, mast cells	Cytotoxic, antitumor effect, mimics septic shock, causes release of ODFRs, induces hepatic acute-phase proteins	B cells: differentiation, antibody production; T cells: activation, proliferation, differentiation, induces IL-2 production; formation of adhesion molecules; hematopoiesis
IL-8	Macrophages, endothelial cells, hepatocytes, neutrophils, fibroblasts	Angiogenic, leukocyte infiltration in septic shock and adult respiratory distress syndrome (ARDS)	Neutrophils: activation; upregulates cell adhesion molecules; chemotactic for polymorphonuclear neutrophils
IL-10	Th2 cells	Inhibits induction of NO, suppresses synthesis of ODFRs, may be immunostimulatory or immunosuppressive	Macrophages: inhibits antigen-presenting capacity, downregulates class II MHC antigen expression, suppresses prostaglandin E_2, TNF, IL-1, IL-6, IL-8 production; B cells: induces IgA synthesis, enhances survival, upregulates IL-2 receptors; T cells: inhibits IFN; neutrophils: inhibits proinflammatory cytokine synthesis, upregulates IL-1 receptor antagonist expression

IgA, immunoglobulin A; IgG, immunoglobulin G; MHC, major histocompatibility complex, NK, natural killer cells; NO, nitric oxide; NOS, nitric oxide synthase; ODFRs, oxygen-derived free radicals; PAF, platelet activating factor.

Table 54.3 cont'd Sources and biological effects of immune mediators

Mediator	Source	Biological activity	Effects on other cells
Granulocyte colony-stimulating factor (G-CSF)	Macrophages, endothelial cells	Proliferation, differentiation and activation of neutrophils; mimics septic shock; causes release of ODFRs	Neutrophils: proliferation, prolongs survival, enhances antibody-dependent cytotoxicity and superoxide anion production; chemotactic for granulocytes and monocytes
Granulocyte–macrophage colony-stimulating factor (GM-CSF)	T cells, B cells, macrophages, endothelial cells, fibroblasts, mast cells, eosinophils	Proliferation, maturation and function of hematopoietic cells; causes release of ODFRs	Neutrophils: proliferation, differentiation, prolongs survival, increases superoxide, leukotriene, PAF, and arachidonic acid release, enhances phagocytic activity, inhibits IL-8 production and neutrophil migration; monocytes: proliferation, differentiation, induces IL-1, IL-8 and TNF release; chemotaxis; formation of adhesion molecules; angiogenesis; hematopoiesis
Transforming growth factor (TGF)-β	Platelets, fibroblasts, monocytes, mast cells	Stimulatory or inhibitory effects on proliferation and differentiation of many cells types, modulates cellular and humoral immune responses, suppresses chemokine-mediated NO release	Lymphocytes: suppresses B- and T-cell proliferation, inhibits NK activity, inhibits IgG and IgM secretion, upregulates B-cell IgA secretion; macrophages: induces secretion of growth factors; chemotactic for macrophages
IL-1 receptor antagonist (IL-1ra)	Macrophages, endothelial cells, neutrophils, fibroblasts	Blocks the biological activity of IL-1 by competing for the IL-1 receptor	–
Platelet activating factor (PAF)	Macrophages, endothelial cells, neutrophils	Activates and aggregates platelets, mimics endothelial alterations of septic shock, induces release of ODFRs	Macrophages (enhances IL-1, IL-2 and TNF production); intracellular messenger in neutrophils; causes release of lysosomal enzymes; chemotactic for neutrophils; formation of adhesion molecules

IgA, immunoglobulin A; IgG, immunoglobulin G; MHC, major histocompatibility complex, NK, natural killer cells; NO, nitric oxide; NOS, nitric oxide synthase; ODFRs, oxygen-derived free radicals.

soluble form of the IL-2Rα). Soluble cytokine receptors not only mediate biological activity but also control desensitization to ligands. This can be achieved by reducing the availability of ligands, decreased signaling, and stimulating cellular mechanisms that can prevent activity.

The biological actions of some cytokines are also regulated by receptor antagonists. The receptor antagonist for IL-1 (IL-1ra) competes with receptors for IL-1, but when bound does not induce signaling. IL-1ra binds to cell receptors much more avidly than to soluble receptors; consequently, soluble receptors have little effect on the inhibitory action of IL-Ira. The appearance of IL-1ra is independently regulated by other cytokines as part of the inflammatory process.

Lymphocytes

Acquired immune defenses against specific microorganisms (antigen) form the second component of the immune response. Antibodies activate the complement system, stimulate phagocytic cells, and specifically inactivate microorganisms. Lymphocytes, which form the basis of the acquired immune defense system, consist of antibody-producing plasma cells derived from B lymphocytes and T lymphocytes, which control intracellular infections. Binding of microorganisms to antibodies on the cell surface of B cells leads to preferential selection of these antibody-producing cells. This is termed *priming*, and subsequent responses are faster and amplified; this is the basis of vaccination. T cells exploit two main strategies to combat intracellular infections: the secretion of soluble mediators that activate other cells to enhance microbial defense mechanisms, and the production of cytolytic T cells that kill the target organism. The NK cells have an important role in tumor cell destruction. They are large granular lymphocytes that do not exhibit immunologic memory and are nonspecific in their recognition of tumor cells.

Regulation of MHC gene expression (e.g. by cytokines; see Table 54.3) plays a fundamental role in the immune system, as alterations of cell surface expression of class I or II molecules can affect the efficiency of antigen presentation. T lymphocytes consist of two subsets: T helper (Th) cells, which are $CD4^+$, recognize class II MHC molecules, and produce IFN-γ and other macrophage-activating factors; Tc cells are $CD8^+$ and recognize both specific antigens and class I MHC molecules on the surface of infected cells.

Circulating Th cells are capable of unrestricted cytokine expression and are prompted into a more restricted and focused

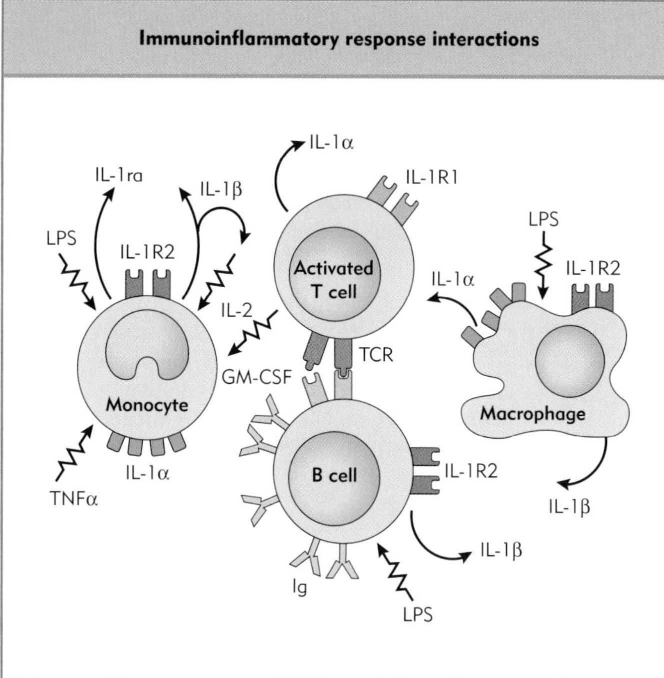

Figure 54.4 The interaction between monocytes, macrophages, and activated T and B cells during the immunoinflammatory response. See text for abbreviations. (From Galley HF, Webster NR. The immuno-inflammatory cascade. Br J Anaesth. 1996;77:11–16. © The Board of Management and Trustees of the British Journal of Anaesthesia.)

pattern of cytokine production, depending on signals received at the onset of infection. The cells can be classified according to the pattern of cytokines they produce. Th1 cells secrete a characteristic set of cytokines associated with cellular immunity (cellular cytotoxicity). Th2 cells are associated with humoral or antibody-mediated immunity. Typically, Th1 cells secrete IL-2, IFN-γ, TNF-β, and transforming growth factor β (TGF-β), whereas Th2 cells secrete IL-4, IL-5, IL-6, IL-9, IL-10, and IL-13, and also help B cells to produce antibodies. Both cell types produce IL-3, TNF-α, and GM-CSF. IL-12 and IL-4 are early inducers of Th1and Th2 responses, respectively; therefore, the local balance of these cytokines is an important determinant of subsequent immune responses.

HYPERSENSITIVITY REACTIONS

A localized inflammatory reaction called *delayed-type hypersensitivity* (DTH) can occur when some subpopulations of activated Th cells encounter certain antigens. Tissue damage is usually limited, and DTH plays an important role in defense against intracellular pathogens and contact antigens. Development of a DTH response requires a prior sensitization period when Th cells are activated and clonally expanded by antigen presented along with the required class II MHC molecule on an appropriate antigen-presenting cell. A further antigen contact induces an *effector* response, where the expanded clonal T-cell population can respond immediately by producing a variety of cytokines (Fig. 54.5), leading to the recruitment and activation of macrophages and other nonspecific inflammatory cells. The activated T cells are generally Th1. A DTH response becomes apparent about 24 hours after secondary antigen contact, peaking at 48–72 hours. The delay occurs because of the time required for cytokines to activate and recruit macrophages. A complex and amplified interaction of many nonspecific cells occurs, with only about 5% of the participating cells being antigen specific. The macrophage is the primary effector cell of DTH responses and the influx and activation of these cells provides an effective host response against intracellular pathogens. Generally, the pathogen is cleared with little tissue damage, but prolonged DTH responses can themselves be damaging, ultimately leading to tissue necrosis in extreme cases.

Immediate hypersensitivity reactions occur within 8 hours of secondary *allergen* exposure and are not cell mediated but humoral in nature, and depend on the generation of antibody by secreting plasma cells and memory cells. The hypersensitivity reactions can be classified into type I (IgE dependent), type II (antibody-mediated cytotoxicity), type III (immune complex-mediated hypersensitivity), and type IV (DTH) (Table 54.4). Type I reactions are mediated by IgE antibodies, which bind to receptors on mast cells or basophils, leading to degranulation and the release of mediators. The principal effects are smooth muscle contraction and vasodilatation; these can result in asthma, hayfever, eczema, and serious life-threatening systemic anaphylaxis. Type II hypersensitivity reactions occur when antibody reacts with antigenic markers on cell surfaces, leading to cell death through complement-mediated lysis or antibody-dependent cytotoxicity. Type II reactions include hemolytic (Rh) disease of the newborn and autoimmune diseases such as Goodpasture's syndrome and myasthenia gravis. Type III reactions are mediated by antigen–antibody reactions or *immune-complex deposition* and subsequent complement activation. Deposition of immune complexes near the site of antigen entry can cause the release of lytic enzymes from accumulated neutrophils and localized tissue damage. The formation of circulating immune complexes contributes to the pathogenesis of a number of conditions, including allergies to penicillin, infectious diseases (e.g. hepatitis), and autoimmune diseases (e.g. rheumatoid arthritis).

TRANSPLANTATION IMMUNOLOGY

Transplantation is the transfer of cells, tissues, or organs from one site to another. Tissues that are antigenically similar or histocompatible do not elicit rejection; the reverse is termed histoincompatible. There are many antigens that determine histocompatibility, but those loci responsible for the most vigorous rejection reactions are located within the MHC. Graft rejection is an immunologic process involving cell-mediated responses, specifically T cells. The immune response is mounted against tissue antigens on the transplanted tissue that differ from those of the host. The most vigorous of these reactions are associated with the MHC (the HLA in humans). However, even with identical HLA antigens, differences in minor histocompatibility loci outside the MHC can contribute to graft rejection. Graft rejection can be divided into the sensitization and the effector stages. During sensitization, leukocytes derived from the donor migrate from the donor tissue into lymph nodes, where they are recognized as foreign by Th cells; this stimulates Th cell proliferation. This is followed by migration of the effector Th cells into the graft and rejection. Graft rejection can be suppressed by both specific and nonspecific immuno-

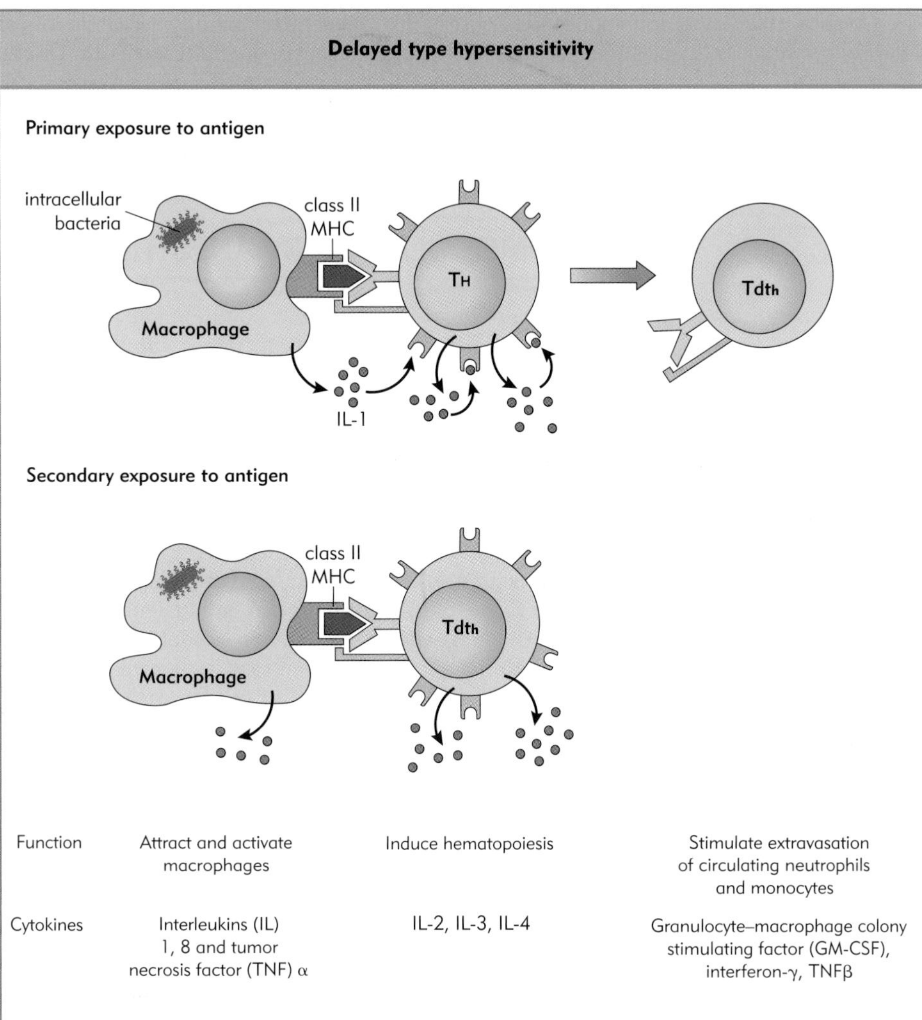

Figure 54.5 Overview of the delayed-type hypersensitivity response. In the sensitization phase following primary contact with antigen, Th cells proliferate and differentiate into Tdth cells. Following secondary contact with antigen, Tdth cells secrete a variety of cytokines that have three primary functions.

suppressive agents. Nonspecific agents include purine analogs, corticosteroids, cyclosporin A, total lymphoid irradiation, and antilymphocyte serum. Specific approaches, such as blocking the proliferation of activated T cells using monoclonal antibodies to the IL-2 receptor, or the depletion of T-cell populations with anti-CD3 or anti-CD4 antibodies, have also been used.

CANCER IMMUNOLOGY

Tumor cells display surface structures that are recognized as antigenic and elicit immune responses. Macrophages mediate tumor destruction by lytic enzymes and the production of TNF-α. NK cells recognize tumor cells via an unknown mech-

Table 54.4 Classification of hypersensitivity reactions

Type	Name	Time	Mechanism	Manifestations
I	IgE mediated	20–30 min	Antigen binding to IgE induces release of vasoactive mediators	Systemic and local anaphylaxis
II	Antibody-mediated cytotoxic	5–8 h	Antibody to cell surface antigens activates complement and antibody-dependent cytotoxicity	Blood transfusion reactions, autoimmune hemolytic anemia
III	Immune-complex mediated	2–8 h	Immune-complex deposition induces complement activation	Systemic lupus erythematosus, rheumatoid arthritis, glomerulonephritis
IV (delayed reaction)	Cell mediated	24–72 h	Sensitized Tdth cells release cytokines	Contact dermatitis; graft rejection

anism. They can either bind to antibody-coated tumor cells, a process known as *antibody-dependent cell-mediated cytotoxicity* (ADCC), or they can secrete a factor that is apparently cytotoxic only for tumor cells. Tumor cell antigens also often elicit the generation of specific serum antibodies, which can activate the complement system, producing the MAC. However, some tumors are able to endocytose the MAC pore and repair the tumor cell membrane before lysis occurs. Complement products can also induce chemotaxis of macrophages and neutrophils and the release of toxic mediators. Ironically, antibodies to tumor cells may also enhance tumor growth, possibly by masking tumor antigens and preventing recognition by NK cells.

Cancer immunotherapy

A number of experimental immunotherapy regimens have been used in the treatment of cancer. Injections of cytokines, including IFN-γ and TNF-α, are beneficial in some cancers. However, cytokine therapy may also result in unwanted side effects, including fever, hypotension, and decreased leukocyte counts. In vitro activation of lymphocytes with irradiated tumor cells in the presence of IL-2 has also been used. This approach results in the induction of *lymphokine-activated cells* (LAK cells), including cytotoxic lymphocytes and NK cells, which can then be reinfused into the patient, providing enhanced tumor-killing capacity. Monoclonal antibodies to CD3 that activate T lymphocytes in vitro and reduce nonspecific T-cell activation in vivo reduce tumor growth in mice, but human studies have not been performed. Gene therapy, in which cells from patients with cancer are genetically altered to increase immune responses, is a recent development in cancer immunotherapy. Specifically, trials in patients with melanoma, in which melanoma cells are transfected to produce IFN-γ and TNF-α, are under way. In addition, patients with lung cancer are being given gene therapy to introduce two genes, one that suppresses tumor cell growth, and another antisense gene that blocks activation of a gene that allows the proliferation of tumor cells. Genetic therapy is likely to be the way forward in cancer immunotherapy.

HUMAN IMMUNODEFICIENCY VIRUS

Human immunodeficiency virus (HIV) is the causative agent for acquired immunodeficiency syndrome (AIDS). The virus infects host cells by binding to CD4 molecules on cell membranes. Upon entry into the cell, the virus copies its RNA into DNA with a viral reverse transcriptase (Chapter 4). The viral DNA then integrates into the host chromosomal DNA, forming a provirus, which can remain in a dormant state for varying lengths of time. Activation of an HIV-infected $CD4^+$ T cell triggers activation of the provirus, leading to destruction of the host cell plasma membrane and cell death; this leads to severe immunosuppression. Because only about 0.01% of the $CD4^+$ T cells are infected by HIV in an HIV-infected individual, the extensive depletion of the Th cell population implies that uninfected $CD4^+$ cells are also destroyed. Several mechanisms have been proposed for this, including complement-mediated lysis, apoptosis, or antibody-mediated cytotoxicity. Early immunologic abnormalities include loss of in vitro proliferative responses of Th cells, reduced IgM synthesis, increased cytokine synthesis, and reduced DTH responses. Later abnormalities include loss of germinal centers in lymph nodes, marked decreases in Th cell numbers and functions, lack of proliferation of HIV-specific B cells and lack of anti-HIV antibodies, a shift in cytokine production from Th1 to Th2 subsets, and a complete absence of DTH responses.

IMMUNE MODULATION BY ANESTHETICS

Increased susceptibility to infection is common in postoperative patients. Although trauma, surgical stress, and endocrine responses modify the immune response, anesthetic agents also modulate immune function, as shown by in vitro studies of the responses of immunologically important cells to clinically relevant concentrations of anesthetic agents. Volatile and intravenous anesthetic agents and opioids such as morphine and fentanyl suppress a variety of functions essential to the recruitment and activity of neutrophils, including respiratory burst activity, polarization, chemotaxis, and hydrogen peroxide production. Halothane and sevoflurane also induce leukocyte adhesion to endothelium, shown recently in a sophisticated study using intravital microscopy in vivo in rats. In contrast, a similar study found that lidocaine (lignocaine) decreased leukocyte adhesion in vivo. Lymphocyte function, as indicated by mitogen stimulation of T-cell proliferation, is attenuated by some intravenous anesthetics. Interferon-stimulated NK cell activity is inhibited by halothane and isoflurane anesthesia in mice. In patients anesthetized with large doses of fentanyl, a prolonged anesthesia-associated suppression of NK cell activity was found.

There have been a few studies on the effect of anesthetic agents on cytokine production. Anesthesia with ketamine decreased TNF-α production by peritoneal macrophages in mice, both in vitro and ex vivo. Propofol and midazolam reduce IL-8 release from stimulated human neutrophils at the post-translational level in vitro, probably by altering the way in which the cytokine is transported from the cell. However, a previous in vitro study found that propofol and ketamine increased mononuclear cell IL-Iβ, TNF-α, IL-4, and IFN-γ production. The anti-inflammatory mediator IL-Ira was increased by clinically relevant concentrations of fentanyl in isolated human monocytes. Propofol is formulated in a 10% soybean emulsion (Intralipid), which itself may affect in vitro neutrophil respiratory burst activity and chemotaxis and IL-2-dependent lymphocyte responses. However, neutrophil polarization and T-cell proliferation are unaffected. In vivo infusion of Intralipid, however, caused increased ex vivo T-cell proliferation but decreased chemotactic migration of leukocytes. Consequently, the modulatory effects of anesthetics on cytokine responses remain unclear.

Although many studies have shown marked effects of a variety of anesthetic and analgesic agents on neutrophil, monocyte, and lymphocyte function, and also on cytokine responses to mediator stimulation, the clinical relevance of the observed degrees of immunosuppression in a previously healthy population is likely to be negligible. However, anesthesia-induced effects on specific components of the immune system may be relevant in vulnerable patient populations, including the elderly, pediatric patients, the critically ill, and those who are immunocompromised. Further investigations are necessary to determine the contribution of choice of anesthetics on morbidity and mortality.

Key references

Cohen J. TREM-1 in sepsis. Lancet 2001;358:776–8.

Farrar MA, Schreiber RD. The molecular biology of interferon-gamma. Annu Rev Immunol. 1993;11:571–611.

Milstein C. Monoclonal antibodies. Sci Am. 1980;243:66–7.

Rose-John S, Heinrich PC. Soluble receptors for cytokines and growth factors: generation and biological function. Biochem J. 1994;300:281–90.

Sheeran P, Hall GM. Cytokines in anaesthesia. Br J Anaesth. 1997;78:201–19.

Stevenson GW, Hall SC, Rudnick S, Seleny FL, Stevenson HC. The effect of anesthetic agents on the human immune response. Anesthesiology. 1990;72:542–52.

Tami JA, Parr MD, Thompson JS. The immune system. Am J Hosp Pharm. 1986;43:2483–93.

Further reading

Galley HF, Webster NR. The immuno-inflammatory cascade. Br J Anaesth. 1996;77:11–16.

Morisaki H, Suematsu M, Wakabayashi Y et al. Leukocyte–endothelium interaction in the rat mesenteric microcirculation during halothane or sevoflurane anesthesia. Anesthesiology 1997;87:591–8.

Chapter 55

Microbiology

Andrew T Hindle

Anesthesiologists are involved in the care of patients who are either at risk or have been infected with a microbial agent. This chapter focuses on those areas where anesthesiologists must have knowledge of microbes, antimicrobials, and other means by which infection can be prevented or treated.

MICROORGANISMS

Bacteria are single-celled prokaryotic organisms consisting of an outer cell wall and a cell membrane. Bacteria can be classified by their staining characteristics as well as their shape (Table 55.1). Analytical techniques designed to identify and classify bacteria use the biochemical and genetic characteristics of the bacteria. The staining pattern of bacteria is determined by staining the bacterial cell wall with a Gram stain, the majority of bacteria being defined as either Gram-positive or Gram-negative.

Table 55.1 Classification of bacteria by their staining characteristics

Bacterium type	Staining characteristics	Shape	Names of bacteria
Bacilli	Positive	Rod	B. antharacis C. diptheriae Clostridia
Bacilli	Negative Acid fast	Rod	Shigella *E. coli* *Salmonella* *Mycobacterium*
Cocci	Positive	Sphere	*Staphylococcus* *Streptococcus* *Neisseria*
Vibrio	Negative	Comma	*Vibrio cholera*
Spirochete	Negative	Corkscrew	*Treponemus pallidum*
Mycoplasma	Negative		*M. pneumonia*

The cell wall of Gram-positive bacteria contains 90% peptidoglycan arranged in polymeric layers connected by amino acid bridges. The cell wall of Gram-negative bacteria is much thinner, containing only 20% peptidoglycan. Gram-negative bacteria also differ in that they contain a periplasmic space that surrounds the plasma membrane, and a lipopolysaccharide located next to the peptidoglycan layer. The lipopolysaccharide is similar to the cell wall in construction, in that it contains phospholipids and is connected to the peptidoglycan layer by lipoproteins. The lipid portion contains lipid A, which is responsible for many of the toxic effects of Gram-negative bacteria.

Fungi

Fungi are simple eukaryotic organisms that can occur as yeasts, single-celled colonies, molds, or a tangle of filaments (attached cells). Fungi are normal inhabitants of the human body, but may cause disease when the bacteria that normally keep them in check are compromised by either antibiotic use or a failure in the host immune system. These conditions allow the proliferation of fungi and the development of an opportunistic infection.

Protozoa

Protozoa are single-celled eukaryotic organisms. They include *Entamoeba histolytica*, *Giardia lamblia*, *Toxoplasma gondii*, and malarial parasites *(Plasmodium spp.)*.

Viruses

Viruses contain genetic information in the form of DNA or RNA but must enter a living cell/host to replicate. The virus uses the host protein-synthesizing apparatus and some of the cell's enzymes to generate virus proteins; these assemble to form infectious virus, which can leave the cell to infect other cells. A virus consists of a capsid core, DNA or RNA, and, sometimes, an envelope (Fig. 55.1). The capsid is the outer shell of the virus that protects the genetic material within.

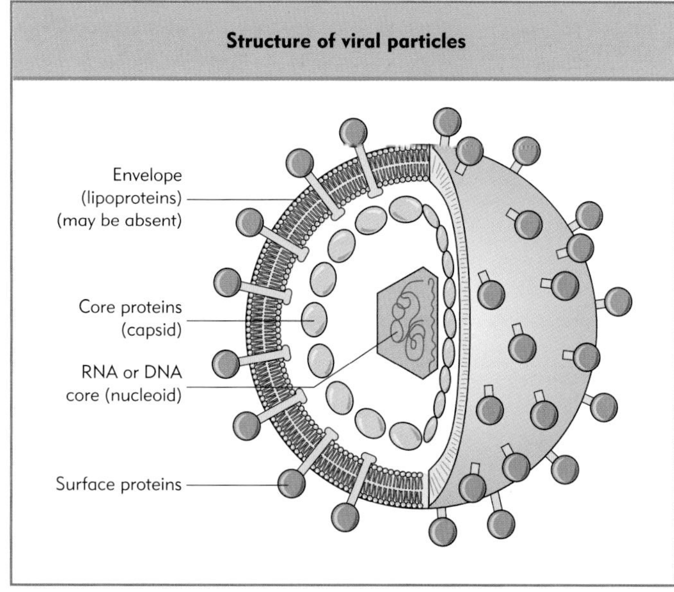

Figure 55.1 Basic components of virus particles.

All viruses attach to a specific structure on the host cell surface (adsorption) and subsequently enter the cell. The virus coating is digested and the nucleic acids are released. The virus material acts within the cell to synthesize viral parts, which assemble into complete viruses. These leave the cell by one of two processes: budding, or lysis. The arrangement and type of viral genetic material are used for subclassification of viruses. An example of a human double-stranded DNA virus is the Epstein–Barr virus (EBV). Influenza virus type A is a human single-stranded RNA virus; the *human immunodeficiency virus* (HIV) is a retrovirus (RNA-based genetic material).

Human cells secrete interferons in response to viral infection; these interact with adjacent cells to make them more resistant to attack by virus. The immune system takes over and begins to fight the infection by removing the virus on the outside of the cells, as well as the virus-infected cells. HIV is an exception to this situation because HIV infects cells of the immune system itself, leading to an immunocompromised state (Chapter 54).

Antiviral drugs are limited in their ability to treat or prevent viral illnesses. No agents actually 'kill' viruses. However, there are drugs that inhibit viral replication. Acyclovir inhibits the replication of herpes virus by inhibiting DNA polymerase. Azidothymidine (zidovudine, AZT) inhibits HIV replication by inhibiting viral DNA polymerase and by competitive inhibition of viral reverse transcriptase (the latter is probably more important). Dideoxyatidine (zalcitabine, ddC), which acts synergistically with AZT against HIV, inhibits reverse transcriptase and is a DNA chain terminator.

Prions

Prions are thought to be small infectious proteins that are conformational variants of a protein normally found in the brain. Brain prion protein is degraded at a sufficient rate that its concentration does not build up to an unacceptable level. The infectious protein is less amenable to degradation, resulting in accumulation and disease. The diseases most commonly associated with prions are neurologic illnesses resulting from 'slow virus' infection. These include Creutzfeldt–Jakob, kuru, scrapie, and bovine spongiform encephalopathy.

ANTIBIOTICS

Antibiotics are the most commonly prescribed nonanesthetic drugs administered by anesthesiologists, usually as prophylaxis against perioperative infection or in the management of critically ill patients in the intensive care unit (ICU). Antibiotics have a number of important sites of action to inhibit growth (bacteriostatic) or kill (bacteriocidal) bacteria (Fig. 55.2). Synergistic combinations often target multiple sites of action.

The five general mechanisms of antimicrobial action are inhibition of cell wall synthesis; outer membrane damage; modification of nucleic acid/DNA synthesis; modification of protein synthesis (at ribosomes); and modification of energy metabolism within the cytoplasm (at the folate cycle).

Antibiotics affecting cell wall synthesis

Bacteria rely on their cell walls to protect them from the hypotonic environment. The bacterial cell wall is unique to bacteria and distinguishes them from mammalian cells. It is therefore a

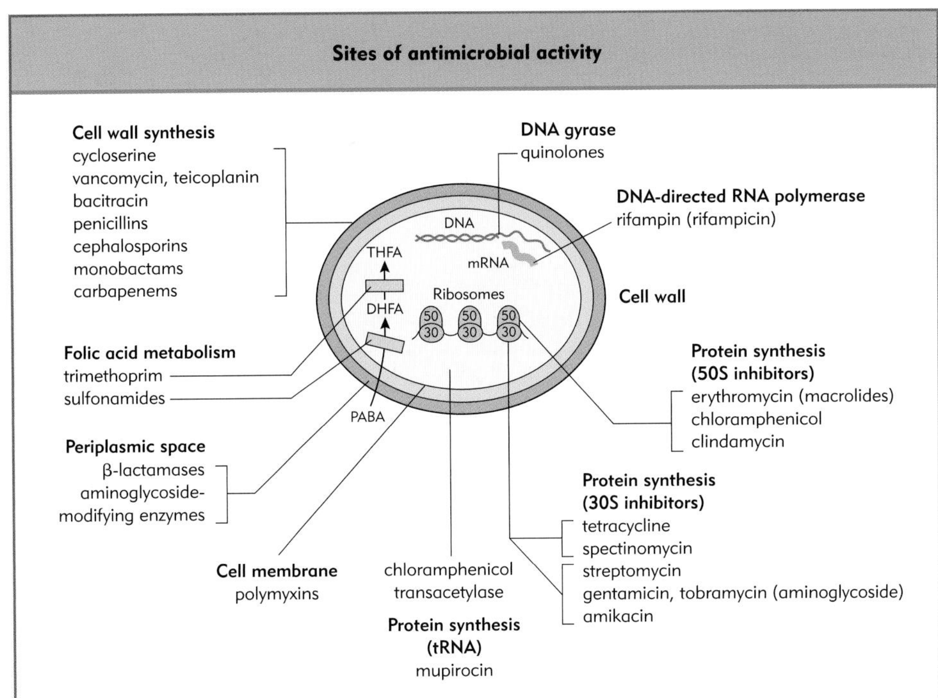

Figure 55.2 Sites of bacteriocidal or bacteriostatic action on microorganisms. The five general mechanisms of antimicrobial actions are (1) inhibit synthesis of cell wall, (2) damage outer membrane, (3) modify nucleic acid/DNA synthesis, (4) modify protein synthesis (at ribosomes), and (5) modify energy metabolism within the cytoplasm (at folate cycle). DHFA, dihydrofolate; PABA, *p*-aminobenzoic acid; THFA, tetrahydrofolate.

potential target for drugs that will only affect the growth of the bacteria. Antibiotics that interfere with cell wall synthesis include the glycopeptides (vancomycin), cephalosporins, and teicoplanin. The relevant points of attack are outlined in Figure 55.3.

Antibiotics modifying nucleic acid synthesis

Metronidazole, which belongs to the nitroimidazole group, is an inactive prodrug; its reduced metabolites act to prevent the replication of bacterial DNA, causing strand breakage (Fig. 55.4).

Antibiotics affecting nutrient supply

Bacteria cannot absorb folate and so must use p-aminobenzoate to synthesize tetrahydrofolate. The latter is necessary for the ultimate synthesis of DNA, RNA, and bacterial cell proteins. The *sulfonamides* and *trimethoprim* interfere with this pathway (Fig. 55.5).

Antibiotics affecting cytoplasmic membranes

Polymixins *(polymyxin B, colistin)* act by displacing Mg^{2+} and Ca^{2+} from membrane phosphate groups. This disrupts the membrane and essential ions, which can subsequently leak from the cell. Polymyxins have a preferential effect on the cytoplasmic membranes of Gram-negative bacteria and have been used in the selective decontamination of the gut (discussed below).

Fungi

The membranes of fungal cells, unlike those of bacteria and mammals, contain sterols, which are targeted by antifungal drugs. Polyene antibiotics (amphotericin B (amphotericin), nystatin) bind to membrane sterols to form a complex that creates a pore in the membrane. Essential constituents of the fungus (sugars, K^+, phosphate esters) leak outwards and cell death rapidly follows. Part of the damage to the cell membrane caused by amphotericin B may occur through inhibition of the Na^+/K^+ ATPase pump and enhancement of nitrite synthesis. Imidazole compounds *(miconazole, ketoconazole, fluconazazole)* inhibit the formation of sterols by blocking the synthesis of ergosterol, probably by interfering with the demethylation of lanosterol, a precursor of ergosterol.

INDICATIONS FOR ANTIBIOTICS

Currently, there are no universally accepted policies regarding the prescription of antibiotics for either prophylaxis or treatment of infection. Common indications for prophylaxis and treatment are outlined below.

Prophylaxis

Prophylaxis is defined as the administration of an antibiotic in order to prevent infective complications in a patient who has no underlying infection. The anesthesiologist is frequently asked to administer prophylactic antibiotics and should therefore demonstrate the requisite knowledge in this area. The Canadian Infectious Disease Society has outlined the following requirements for the use of prophylactic antibiotics in surgery:

- High serum levels immediately prior to surgery;
- Serum levels sustained throughout the procedure;
- Activity against most organisms that can contaminate the operative site.

WHEN TO ADMINISTER

Antibiotic infusions should be completed 30 minutes before surgical incision. The incidence of infection rises proportionally if administration is delayed following the start of surgery.

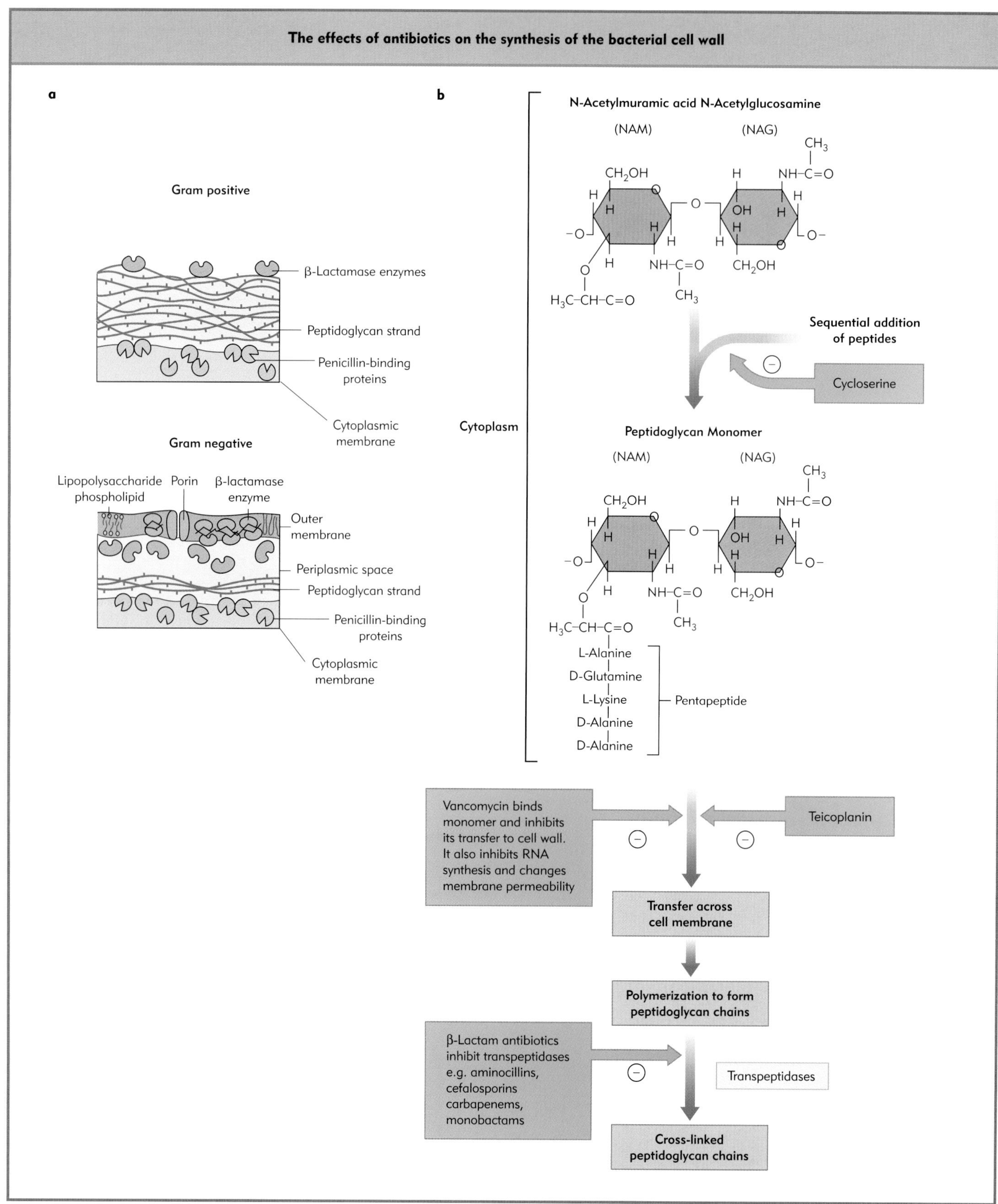

Figure 55.3 Antibiotic action on cell wall synthesis. (a) Gram-positive bacteria have a thick outer coating and Gram-negative bacteria have a thinner (three to five strands) rigid peptidoglycan structure with an added outer membrane. (b) The β-lactam drugs act by inhibiting the synthesis of the rigid peptidoglycan part of the cell wall. Other antibiotics have effects on various stages in the synthesis of the bacterial cell wall. The multiplicity of actions of vancomycin is the reason why bacterial resistance to vancomycin is low. Penicillin-binding proteins may signal the induction of β-lactamases, which destroy penicillin and have caused significant problems by increasing the development of resistant bacteria.

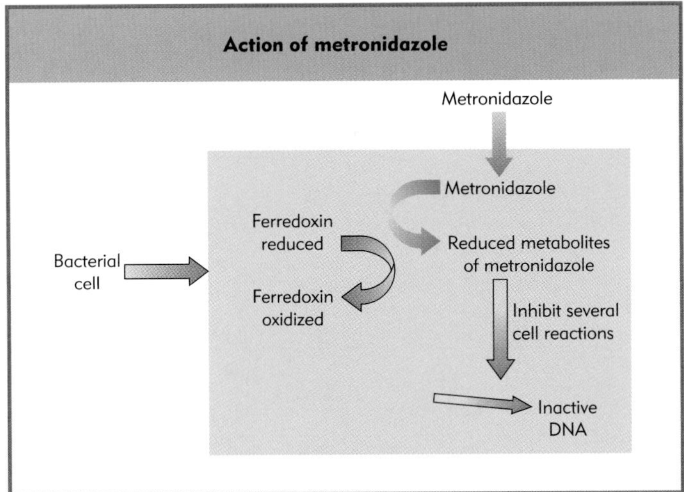

Figure 55.4 Mechanisms of action of metronidazole. The extent of the bacterial reactions inhibited by metronidazole is still uncertain.

Conversely, if antibiotics are administered too early (>2 hours before surgery) there is a significant increase in postoperative surgical wound infection.

The decision to administer antibiotics will depend upon the risk of infection, the consequences of infection, and the consequences of administering antibiotics

METHOD OF ADMINISTRATION

Antibiotics should be administered intravenously because the reduction in number of bacteria required to cause infection is higher with this route than others. A single dosing regimen is usually adequate, but repeated doses may be required if a procedure lasts more than 4 hours, there is blood loss sufficient to require transfusion (>1 L), or the duration of surgery is more than twice the elimination half-life of the chosen antibiotic.

The highest risk for infections is generally thought to occur at wound closure, and so effective concentrations of antibiotic should be maintained in the wound for up to 4 hours after the surgical procedure. Some clinicians would argue that it is justifiable to continue with the antibiotics throughout the postoperative period if the patient is being monitored invasively or has undergone major complex surgery. However, the above suggestions have been countered by some authors, who suggest that prolonging the duration of prophylaxis into the postoperative period provides no benefit and indeed serves only to increase the emergence of resistant strains of bacteria.

PENICILLIN ALLERGY

Patient reports of allergy to penicillin are extremely unreliable: patients tested for penicillin allergy are only positive in 15% of cases. The correct diagnosis is important, because the alternative use of vancomycin is expensive and may increase the prevalence of vancomycin-resistant bacteria.

SURGICAL PROCEDURES REQUIRING ANTIBIOTIC PROPHYLAXIS

Traditionally, the administration of prophylaxis has been limited to prosthetic implants in 'clean surgical' procedures. However, the incidence of infection in clean nonprosthetic surgery may have been underreported. The reasons underlying this may include the fact that 50% of all complications occur in the community after the patient has been discharged home. There is now evidence that patients receiving single-dose prophylaxis in clean nonprosthetic surgery have a lower rate of infection than those who do not.

ELECTIVE MAJOR ORTHOPEDIC SURGERY

The incidence of infection following major joint replacement is approximately 1%. Infections may be prevented during orthopedic surgery by systemic antibiotic therapy. Cefuroxime administered as a single dose at induction, followed by three further doses, has been shown to be effective. However, it has been recently demonstrated that a single dose of cefazolin is equally effective as multidosing regimens.

The spread of bacteria may also be reduced by the use of exhaust suites and clean air filtration systems. However, some researchers working in conventionally ventilated theaters claim infection rates comparable to that achieved by Charnley, who was responsible for pioneering such systems. Antibiotic-impregnated cemented implants have now gained widespread acceptance and further enhance systemic antimicrobial prophylaxis.

Staphylococcus aureus is the commonest infecting organism of prosthetic implants, with an incidence up to 30%, whereas

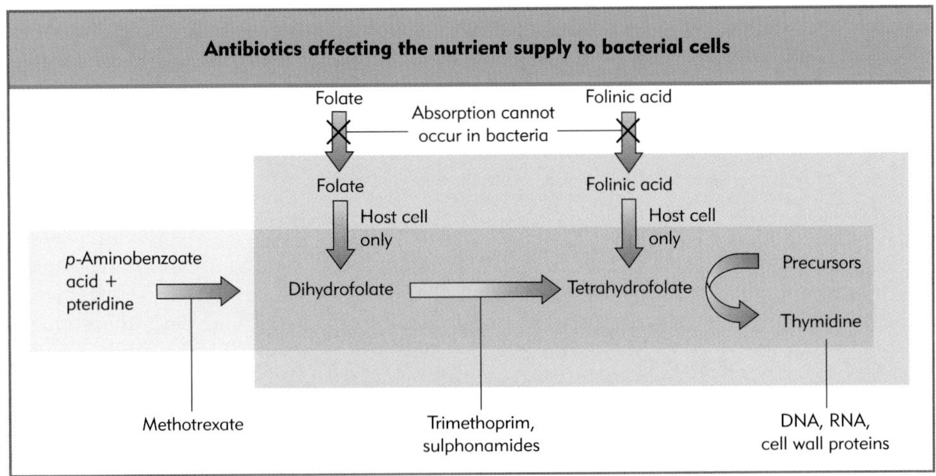

Figure 55.5 Antibiotics affecting the supply of nutrients to bacterial cells. Host cells can produce thymidine from folate. Bacteria cannot absorb folate and must synthesize it from *p*-aminobenzoic acid.

Table 55.2 Antimicrobial prophylaxis before surgery (Data from Harrison G, Weed HG. Med Clin North Am. 2003;87:9–755)

Procedure	Likely pathogen	Antimicrobial
Cardiac surgery including pacemaker insertion	Staphylococcus, *Corynebacterium*, Gram– bacilli	Cefazolin/cefuroxime Vancomycin
Gastrointestinal		
Appendix	Anaerobes, enterococcii	Cefoxitin
Biliary tract	Enteric Gram– bacilli	Cefoxitin, cefazolin
Colorectal		Neomycin + erythromycin base/cefoxitin or cefazolin
Gastroduodenal/esophageal	Enterococcii Gram+ bacillii	Cefazolin
Genitourinary	Enterococci Enteric Gram– bacilli Staphylococcus Coagulase-negative staphylococcus	Ciprofloxacillin Trimethoprim-sulfamethoxazole
Gynecological Abortion – first and second trimesters Cesarian – high-risk only Hysterectomy (vaginal/abdominal)	Anaerobes, enterococci Enteric Gram– bacilli Group B streptococcii	Cefazolin or cefoxitin
Head and neck	Anaerobes, Staphylococcii enteric Gram– bacilli	Ampicillin or clindamycin + gentamicin
Neurosurgery	Staphylococci	Cefazolin or vancomycin
Ophthalmic	Staphylococcii, streptococci, *Pseudomonas aeruginosa*, enteric Gram– bacilli	Topical eye drops over 24 h Gentamicin, tobramycin or ciprofloxacillin
Thoracic	Staphylococcii, streptococci Enteric Gram– bacillii	Cefazolin, vancomycin
Vascular prosthetic repair	Staphylococci, streptococci	Cefazolin or vancomycin
Vascular groin incision	Enteric Gram– bacilli Staphylococci, streptococci, clostridia	

Gram-negative bacteria cause 10–30% of infections. Approximately 10–15% of infected prostheses have no identifiable infecting organism. The commonest infecting organisms for deep joint infections are coagulase-negative staphylococci.

PROPHYLAXIS IN TRAUMA

Prevention of infection has been achieved in the treatment of penetrating abdominal wounds, open fractures, and early wounds that can be adequately debrided and closed. Prophylactic antibiotics do not prevent infection in wounds where treatment has been delayed. Continuing contamination is the primary reason for ineffectiveness in these situations, and the prolonged use of prophylactic antibiotics only serves to increase the likelihood of antibiotic-resistant strains emerging. It is recommended that antibiotics are not administered to patients undergoing closed fracture reduction.

VASCULAR AND CARDIAC SURGERY

The choice and duration of antibiotic cover for the prevention of graft infection in vascular bypass surgery has been controversial. Cephalosporins such as cefuroxime or ceftriaxone are the most popular choices, with reduction in wound infections from 6–25% without prophylaxis to 0–3% with prophylaxis. Furthermore, the success of antibiotic-impregnated artificial grafts is also debatable. The peak time for graft exposure to bacteria occurs at approximately 7–10 days, and this may influence the prescribed duration of systemic antibiotic cover. However, prolonging the duration of cover may result in the development of multiresistant organisms. Currently there are no agreed guidelines for antibiotic prophylaxis in adult cardiac surgery. In a recent audit carried out across the United Kingdom it has been shown that approximately 96% of units use either one or two agents for prophylaxis (Table 55.2).

Nonpharmacological causes of postoperative infection

- **Temperature** Supplemental warming can reduce the incidence of postoperative infection from 19% to 6%.
- **Diabetes control** It is claimed that aggressive insulin treatment can reduce the incidence of hospital infection and overall hospital stay by 34%.
- **Oxygen therapy** Patients randomized to receive 80% inspired oxygen therapy demonstrated an overall reduction in infection at 2 weeks follow-up from 11.2% to 5.2%. However, this effect has not been reproduced in a more recent trial which showed that high perioperative F_IO_2 was detrimental.

Prophylaxis against endocarditis

Anesthesiologists regularly manage patients with heart valve lesions who are to undergo cardiac and noncardiac surgery, and they must know when to administer prophylactic antibiotics. These procedures can cause bacteremia, which may infect heart valve lesions, with catastrophic consequences. It is extremely difficult to estimate the relative risk of endocarditis developing after a particular procedure, just as it is difficult to establish the relative success of prophylaxis within the confines of the current guidelines. The rationale for using antibiotics to prevent endocarditis is not based on data from well-conducted clinical trials but on a consensus view of what is likely to be effective. The reader is directed to an excellent review on the subject by Dajani et al. for the American Heart Association.

CLEANING, DISINFECTION, AND STERILIZATION

The anesthesiologist is responsible for ensuring that equipment is safe and clean. Although some equipment, such as endotracheal tubes, are single use and are discarded after use, there are certain items that are reusable. Cross-contamination between patients as a result of reusing equipment must be prevented.

Decontamination

Anesthetic equipment, such as laryngeal masks, facemasks, and Guedel airways, collects debris as a result of being in contact with patient secretions; this debris should be removed by washing before the item is disinfected and/or sterilized. There has been a trend in recent years to use single-use masks and airways, with obvious cost implications for healthcare providers

Disinfection

This involves the removal of nearly all microbes apart from spores and may be achieved by the use of chemical disinfectants or pasteurization.

CHEMICAL DISINFECTANTS

- **Chlorhexidine alcohol** This solution may be used for cleaning facemasks that might perish during the pasteurization process (see below). Items exposed to a 0.05% solution of chlorhexidine may be left for 30 minutes, but if a 0.5% solution is combined with 70% ethanol, the disinfection time is reduced to only 2 minutes. Facemasks and oropharyngeal airways should be decontaminated and disinfected prior to use. Chlorhexidine and alcohol solution may be used for cleaning the external surfaces of the anesthetic machine and ventilator.
- **Glutaraldehyde (Cidex)** This is not recommended for routine use. However, it is very popular for cleaning endoscopic equipment such as fiberoptic laryngoscopes and bronchoscopes. Glutaraldehyde requires bicarbonate (0.3%) to be added for activation. It kills bacteria during a 30-minute immersion, but spores require exposure for 3 hours.

Pasteurization

Pasteurization involves heating to a temperature of 80°C for 10 minutes. This has been shown to cause very little damage to perishable items such as laryngeal masks and red rubber tubes, the latter still being used in some centers.

Sterilization

Sterilization ensures the killing of all bacteria, *including spores*. Anesthetic equipment is exposed to steam under high pressure and at a temperature in excess of the boiling point of water. The process is called autoclaving, and cannot be used to sterilize perishable items such as facemasks and plastic items.

DRY HEATING

Equipment is exposed to temperatures of 150–170°C for 30 minutes. The method is not suitable for plastics or rubber, as they can perish at these temperatures. The use of ethylene oxide or propylene oxide requires a special sterilizer. The process is expensive and prolonged.

INFECTION RISK TO THE ANESTHESIOLOGIST

Patients with hepatitis B or C and HIV represent a serious infectious risk to the anesthesiologist. The risk of contracting hepatitis B can be reduced by prophylactic immunization, and all healthcare workers should receive routine prophylactic hepatitis B vaccination. The take-up of vaccination for hepatitis B is in excess of 80%, but there are anxieties that some healthcare workers do not return for necessary booster doses. Unfortunately, there is no vaccine for hepatitis C or HIV.

When patients are admitted for routine elective or emergency surgery there is no information on their hepatitis or HIV status. It is therefore safer to take precautions and assume that all patients are potential carriers of HIV or hepatitis B/C. Less than 20% of anesthesiologists take a history in order to screen out patients who may constitute a risk for the passage of hepatitis or HIV. Governments have been reluctant to adopt hepatitis or HIV screening procedures for all patients.

The risk of contracting HIV is small (0.4%) following an inoculation injury. However, the risk of seroconversion following exposure to a hepatitis B antigen-positive patient is much higher (30%). The risk of inoculation both from patients known to be infected and from those whose hepatitis and HIV status is unknown can be reduced if simple precautions are taken.

Transmission of infection can be reduced by wearing protective gloves and goggles, not resheathing needles, and the placement of sharps in bins designated specifically for that purpose.

TREATMENT OF ESTABLISHED INFECTIONS

This section will focus on those areas in which the anesthesiologist is involved in managing established infections. These include infections secondary to the insertion of monitoring equipment or devices for the management of pain relief, as well as infections on the intensive care unit.

Central venous catheter infections

It has been estimated that there is a 10–20% mortality rate from intravascular catheter-related infections. A number of factors are important in determining the likelihood of patients developing central venous catheter (CVC)-related infections:

- Poor aseptic technique
- Migration of organisms from insertion site
- Catheter hub infection
- Contaminated infusate
- Distant infection source
- Catheter type – infections are more common with polyvinyl chloride or polyethylene.

Short-term catheters are most likely to become infected as a result of skin commensals, which cause up to 65% of catheter-related infections, *Staphylococcus* being the commonest infecting organism.

There is general agreement that the longer catheters stay in the more likely the patient is to develop a catheter-related infection. There is less clarity as to the length of time that catheters should be left in situ before the incidence of infection rises, causes clinical concern, and the catheter should be replaced. There has been argument concerning the 'replacement' of catheters over guidewires using the track of the original catheter. There is now evidence that the replacement of catheters over guidewires does not produce any greater risk of infection than resiting the catheter at a different site.

Catheter-related infections are diagnosed by catheter tip culture. Only 15–25% of catheters are microorganism positive in suspected cases. Diagnosis can be difficult because it is unusual to find any signs of infection at the insertion site. Bacterial and fungal infections are usually attributed to a catheter when other sources have been eliminated. If infection is suspected the catheter should be removed, the tip sent for culture, and the patient commenced on blind antibiotic therapy. Subsequent therapy should be based upon known sensitivities. For the non-immunocompromised patient antibiotic therapy should be continued for 10–14 days if catheter infection is suspected.

Epidural catheter infections

The number of epidurals used to manage postoperative pain is increasing, and there is also a rising trend in chronically implanted epidural catheters for cancer pain in the community. The incidence of epidural abscesses is extremely low, the incidence being estimated at 0.2–1.2 per 10 000 hospital admissions, 1 in 1930 and 1 in 5000 patients catheterized with epidurals. Reports of infection have been limited to retrospective surveys and case reports. Although the risk of abscess is low, there can be disastrous consequences if it remains undetected and not treated.

MECHANISM OF INFECTION

This is usually via bloodborne spread, skin contamination of the catheter placement site, or intraluminal infection via the epidural infusate.

Prospective audits have demonstrated that almost 29% of catheter tips can become colonized, the commonest infecting organism being coagulase-negative staphylococci. The incidence of colonization is higher in obstetric and trauma patients, where it may be as high as 66%. Given that the incidence of epidural abscess is rare, it is apparent that the incidence of colonization does not predict the development of an epidural abscess.

The most effective way of preventing catheter colonization and subsequent abscess formation is by strict asepsis, disinfection with chlorhexidine-containing solutions, inspection of epidural catheter sites at least once daily, and further disinfection if inflammation or infection is suspected.

Skin preparation

It is unknown whether antibiotics protect against infection, as most elective surgical patients receive antibiotic prophylaxis as a routine measure prior to surgery.

Disinfecting the skin before catheter insertion has been shown to influence the incidence of septicemia. Interestingly, 18% of needles can become colonized despite the strictest aseptic precautions. There have been a number of suggestions as to the best chemical for preparing the skin prior to catheter insertion.

POVIDONE-IODINE

This may not eliminate bacteria, and there is suggestion that previously opened bottles for repeated use may support bacterial growth and result in reduced activity against skin flora. For this reason some manufacturers are now supplying single-use povidone-iodine packages in epidural trays.

CHLORHEXIDINE

The general view appears to be that chlorhexidine with alcohol is preferred to povidone-iodine as a means of reducing the colonization of catheters and microbial regrowth following insertion. The addition of alcohol has been shown to increase the quality and duration of the antibacterial effect. The presence of alcohol has to be balanced against the risk of flammability, which has been suggested if alcohol-containing solutions are used as skin preparation when surgical diathermy is going to be used.

The effectiveness of these solutions in reducing epidural abscess formation is more difficult to assess, because abscess formation is so rare that it would be difficult to design a study of sufficient statistical power to establish meaningful conclusions as to the best skin preparation solution.

Patients with epidurals must be monitored with at least once-daily inspection of the catheter exit site. Early diagnosis and treatment improve outcome in cases of established epidural abscess. If infection is suspected, the skin should be disinfected, the catheter removed, and the tip sent for culture. The presence of neurological signs, including radicular pain and progressive motor block, is indicative that the patient must be referred for nuclear magnetic resonance imaging, with possible surgical intervention and appropriate antibiotic therapy.

There has been some debate as to whether there is a relationship between the duration of catheterization and infection rates. The literature appears to support the view that if the catheter is kept in for more than 3 days the infection risk increases. There is no justification in sending off epidural catheter tips for routine analysis.

INFECTIONS IN THE INTENSIVE CARE UNIT

This section is devoted to issues surrounding the treatment and prophylaxis of infections in the intensive care unit (ICU). Patients who are admitted to the ICU acquire their infections from either the community (community-acquired infections, CAI) or the ICU itself (nosocomial infections, NI).

Nosocomial infections

Nosocomial infections occur in almost 10% of ICU admissions. They are increasing in number, owing to the greater number of trauma patients who would not previously have survived their pathology, the growing number of immunocompromised patients in the hospital population, the number of patients with multiple organ failure, and the increased use of antimicrobials with the concomitant problems of multiply antibiotic-resistant organisms. A survey of European ICUs showed that 45% of patients were infected, 21% acquiring their infections on the ICU. The sources of ICU infection are outlined in Table 55.3.

Table 55.3 Incidence and source of infection in the ICU

Source of infection	Percentage of patients infected
Enteric Gram-negative	30–70
Gram-positive	15–40
Polymicrobial	30–40
**Ps. Aeruginosa, Acinetobacter* spp.	50–65

* Microbes causing VAP in patients in receipt of antibiotics in the last 14 days.

VENTILATOR-ASSOCIATED PNEUMONIA

Ventilator-associated pneumonia (VAP), the most common nosocomial infection in the ICU, occurs in 15–20% of patients, resulting in an estimated 30–70% mortality and, at best, an extended stay in the ICU. This mortality has been ascribed to, in part, delays (>24 hours) in appropriate therapy, and in a recent multivariate analysis such delays proved to be the strongest predictor of mortality. However, the use of prophylactic antibiotics against ventilator-associated pneumonia can result in the development of more virulent bacteria with a higher mortality rate. A number of different strategies have been proposed in an attempt to minimize the use of inappropriate antibiotics:

- Bronchoscopic protected brush specimen;
- Bronchoscopic broncheolar lavage;
- Endotracheal aspirates;
- Clinical pulmonary infection score.

The microbiological organisms that most commonly infect the respiratory tract are outlined in Table 55.3.

FUNGAL INFECTIONS

The incidence of nosocomial fungal infections has risen substantially and they are now the fourth most common nosocomial infection in ICUs. Their proportion of all bloodstream infections has risen from 2.5 to 7.1%, with a concomitant rise in pneumonia from 3.9 to 4.4%. Disseminated candidiasis has risen tenfold in patients with HIV and malignancy. Deep candidal infections are difficult to diagnose and carry a mortality of 40%, and postmortem studies have suggested that fungal infections were the most common findings previously not suspected prior to the death of the patient.

Precise species identification by antifungal sensitivity testing is crucial prior to commencing appropriate antibiotic therapy. Patient groups at risk include both neutropenic and nonneutropenic groups. Patients undergoing general surgery, for example those with recurrent gastrointestinal leaks and perforation, are at risk from invasive candidiasis, but the risk can be reduced by using prophylactic fluconazole. Some intensivists are beginning to advocate routine fungal prophylaxis as part of the empirical antibiotic regimen. However, the long-term effects of such a strategy in terms of the development of antibiotic resistance has yet to be elucidated.

Antimicrobial resistance in the ICU

Intensive care clinicians are faced with a dilemma in the use of antibiotics. Antibiotics are known to treat infection and reduce mortality, yet their overuse can lead to increasing numbers of antibiotic-resistant organisms, with important consequences for patient care, hospital costs, and length of stay. A number of factors can promote the development of resistance to antimicrobials in the ICU, and they are outlined below.

CROSS-INFECTION

A number of factors contribute to the incidence of cross-infection in the ICU:

- **Patient factors** Intensive care patients have suppressed immunity, malnourishment, and severe underlying disease. They are also likely to have multiple invasive devices during their stay on the ICU. Furthermore, ICUs are becoming increasingly crowded with patients, leading to reduced spacing between patients and the potential for microbial transfer from one to another.
- **Antibiotics** The source of infection is often unknown on admission to the ICU, and 'blind therapy' is commonly instituted in an attempt to cover the most likely infecting organisms. Almost 90% of these patients are prescribed empirical antibiotics as 'best-guess' cover for the infecting organism. The decision to use an antibiotic at a specified dose is based on careful consideration of the known local strains of resistant bacteria, the history, clinical findings, radiology, specimen culture, the pharmacokinetics of the antibiotic, as well as the renal and hepatic function of the patient.

PREVENTING CROSS-TRANSMISSION

Preventing cross infection is important if one is to reduce not only the promotion of resistant organisms, but also the transmission of nonresistant organisms.

Handwashing is the most important preventative measure against cross-infection. Many studies have demonstrated poor compliance with handwashing. Some use plain soaps, whereas others prefer to use alcohol-based hand rubs. The effect of the latter on multiresistant organisms needs to be evaluated.

The use of gloves appears to be synergistic with handwashing in reducing the incidence of cross-infection. In cases of multiresistant organisms the use of gloves between patients may reduce contamination and cross-infection when carers are handling infected biological fluids and coming into contact with skin surfaces.

The use of gowns has been recommended to prevent the spread of MRSA (methycillin-resistant *Staphylococcus aureus*). Their effect on the prevention of cross-contamination by other microbes is less well defined. The use of gowns should be based on documented evidence that they reduce cross-infection.

Facemasks have been used to prevent infection of hospital workers by patients with pulmonary tuberculosis. They have not been shown to be of any benefit to preventing cross-contamination by antimicrobial-resistant bacteria.

There is good evidence that the isolation of patients prevents cross-infection. Patients should be isolated when diagnosed with a multiresistant organism and remain isolated until they are no longer colonized.

Antibiotics and renal support therapy

Some patients in the ICU will require modification of the antibiotic dose in order to achieve effective plasma concentrations. Dosing depends upon the half-life, clearance, and volume of distribution of the drug (see Chapter 8). Prescription of drugs in patients with renal failure is aimed at achieving effective plasma concentrations while avoiding toxicity.

Apart from gentamicin and vancomycin, most antibiotics do not require any alteration of dose at creatinine clearance in excess of 50 mL/min. These two antibiotics must have their dose reduced when creatinine clearance is less than this. In addition, the antitubercular drugs ethambutol, rifampicin, and pyrazinamide need reduced dosing in renal failure. Some patients in the ICU depend on artificial support in order to maintain fluid and electrolyte balance: methods used include dialysis, or one of the various forms of hemofiltration and dialysis.

HEMODIALYSIS/HEMOFILTRATION

The dosing of antibiotics can be extremely difficult in patients receiving renal support, with only a few antibiotics being measured on and off dialysis or during hemofiltration. The removal of drugs by dialysis depends on dialysate, drug, and patient factors. Many antibiotics are removed during dialysis; consequently, administration should take place after dialysis. However, for patients with particularly severe infections it may be advantageous for antibiotics to be administered before dialysis. Antibiotic kinetics during the various forms of continuous hemofiltration and dialysis are highly variable. The reader is directed to a review by Cotterill for further information on antibiotic dosing schedules during dialysis and hemofiltration techniques.

SIDE EFFECTS OF ANTIBIOTICS

Antibiotics cause a number of side effects, including gastrointestinal, renal, and anaphylactic reactions. It is easier to diagnose side effects in patients not residing in the ICU, but the complexity of the clinical picture in the ICU can make the diagnosis of an antibiotic-related side effect extremely difficult.

Anaphylactic and anaphylactoid reactions

Anaphylactic and anaphylactoid reactions are potentially the most serious that anesthiologists can expect to see following the administration of antibiotics. Anaphylaxis is mediated by antigen (IgE) following prior exposure to that antigen (see Chapter 54). A cephalosporin should not be administered to patients who have a documented hypersensitivity reaction to penicillin; vancomycin is a suitable alternative. Cross-reactivity with cephalosporins in people who are allergic to penicillin ranges from 5.4 to 16.5%. There is also significant cross-reactivity between the cephalosporins and the newer carbepenems such as imipenem. Vancomycin is recommended in patients who are allergic to penicillin if dermal testing confirms they are also allergic to cephalosporins. Skin testing is potentially hazardous because it can result in anaphylaxis and may not always diagnose true allergy. Allergic reactions to vancomycin are extremely rare, but a rapid infusion of vancomycin over less than 30–45 minutes may cause reddening of the skin over the face, neck, and hands. This so-called 'red man' syndrome may be distinguished from anaphylaxis by the lack of associated features of anaphylaxis, and reversibility on terminating the infusion.

Gastrointestinal side effects

Approximately one-third of patients develop gastrointestinal symptoms following antibiotic administration. This may be because of alterations in bowel flora following prolonged antibiotic therapy. Patients receiving single-dose regimens are subject to a lower incidence of symptoms than those receiving multiple doses.

Interactions with other drugs

An increased sensitivity of patients to warfarin has been described during the use of cefamandole as prophylaxis in cardiac surgery. The mechanism for this is unknown, as is the case with erythromycin. Penicillins have been reported to decrease the anticoagulant effect of warfarin; again, the mechanism is not known.

Hepatic side effects

Penicillins can cause cholestasis, and macrolides (erythromycin) and quinolones cause cholestatic hepatitis. Cephalosporins cause little in the way of hepatotoxicity.

Neuromuscular blockade

Antibiotics interacting with the neuromuscular junction or neuromuscular blocking agents include the aminoglycosides, especially neomycin. The neuromuscular blocking effects of these antibiotics appear to be presynaptic as well as postsynaptic. The effects seem to be related, at least in part, to the blockade of Ca^{2+} channels. Both N- and P/Q-type Ca^{2+} channels are blocked by vecuronium, the effects not being reversed by anticholinesterases. Antibiotics interact with neuromuscular blocking drugs, and it has been demonstrated that gentamicin and tobramycin prolong recovery from vecuronium.

Renal side effects

Renal toxicity following antibiotics is manifest physiologically by increased renal vascular resistance, reduced renal blood flow, and reduced glomerular filtration rate. Altered tubular function may occur, with increased membrane permeability to K^+, H^+, Ca^{2+}, and Mg^{2+}. Aminoglycosides are selectively concentrated by the kidneys, where they bind to and damage intracellular phospholipid target sites. The β-lactams are concentrated by the kidney and cause toxicity via lipid peroxidation and depression of mitochondrial function.

Key references

Borgers M. Antifungal azole dcrivativcs. In: Greenwood D, O'Grady F, eds. The scientific basis of antimicrobial therapy. Cambridge: Cambridge University Press; 1985:133–53.

Bouza E, Burillo A, Munoz P. Catheter related infection: diagnosis and intravascular treatment. 2001;13:224–33.

Cotterill S. Antimicrobial prescribing in patients on haemofiltration. Antimicrob Chemother. 1995;36:773–80.

Dajani AS, Taubert KA, Wilson W et al. Prevention of bacterial endocarditis. Recommendations by the American Heart Association. American Medical Association 1997;277:1794–801.

Harrison G, Weed HG. Antimicrobial prophylaxis in the surgical patient. Med Clin North Am. 2003;87:59–75.

Lalla F. Surgical prophylaxis in practice. J Hosp Infect. 2002; 50:S9–S12.

Marcus R. Surveillance of health care workers exposed to blood in patients infected with the human immunodeficiency virus. New Engl J Med. 1988;319:1118–23.

Scott D, Imahara BS, Avery B, Nathens. Antimicrobial strategies in critical care. Curr Opin Crit Care 2003;9:286–91.

Scott K, Fridkin, Robert P. Anitmicrobial resistance in intensive care units. 1999;20:303–15.

Vincent JL, Bihari DJ, Suter PM et al. The prevalence of nosocomial infection in intensive care units in Europe. Results of the European Prevalence of Infection in Intensive Care (EPIC) Study. EPIC International Advisory Committee. JAMA 1995;274:639–44.

Further reading

Greif R, Akça O, Horn E-P, Kurz A, Sessler DI, et al, for the Outcomes Research Group. Supplemental perioperative oxygen to reduce the incidence of surgical-wound infection. *N Engl J Med.* 2000;342:161-167

Pryor KO, Fahey TJ 3rd, Lien CA, Goldstein PA. Surgical site infection and the routine use of perioperative hyperoxia in a general surgical population: a randomized controlled trial. *JAMA.* 2004;291:79-87

Chapter 56

Ischemic brain injury

Nina J Solenski, Robert E Rosenthal and Gary Fiskum

TOPICS COVERED IN THIS CHAPTER

- **Focal ischemia and infarction**
- **Cerebral blood flow**
  - Metabolic coupling
  - Ischemic penumbra and core
  - Cerebral autoregulation
  - Etiology of focal ischemic stroke
  - Etiology of hemorrhagic stroke
  - Surgical risk and ischemic stroke
  - Preoperative evaluation – risk stratification
- **Global cerebral ischemia**
- **Cardiopulmonary resuscitation**
  - Blood flow
  - Total circulatory arrest
  - Ventilation following ischemia
  - Therapeutic hypothermia
- **Pathophysiology of ischemic brain injury**
  - Focal versus global ischemia
  - Neurotic and apoptotic cell death
  - Excitotoxicity
  - Ischemic acidosis
  - Reperfusion injury and oxidative stress
  - Inflammation

FOCAL ISCHEMIA AND INFARCTION

Focal cerebral ischemia is the most common cause of stroke in humans. Stroke is caused by either a blockage or rupture of an extra- or intracranial artery, leading respectively to either infarction or hemorrhage. The term 'ischemic stroke' implies blockage, whereas 'primary hemorrhagic stroke' implies rupture of an artery (Fig. 56.1). The treatments for these two types of stroke are radically different, and selecting the wrong treatment could worsen rather than improve brain damage. Rapidly distinguishing between these two causes of cerebral ischemia is therefore essential. Focal ischemia differs from global ischemia in that focal cerebral infarction results in pan-necrosis within one or more specific arterial territories.

Ischemic strokes occur when an artery is blocked, depriving the brain of oxygen and glucose, and slowing the removal of metabolic wastes. The brain is at special risk for ischemia because there is insufficient redundancy in the arterial supply to maintain adequate blood flow, and the storage of energy substrate is limited. Neuronal cell death can occur within minutes, depending on the severity and duration of ischemia.

An ischemic stroke can evolve into a hemorrhagic stroke as a consequence of damage to the integrity of the vascular tree distal to the occlusion. In this setting a 'bland' infarction is converted into a hemorrhagic one; usually this results in small 'petechial' and *asymptomatic* hemorrhages. Approximately 40–70% of ischemic embolic strokes result in some type of hemorrhagic conversion. Occasionally larger symptomatic hemorrhages occur as a result of hemorrhagic conversion, particularly in the setting of anticoagulation use.

The internal carotid arteries supply ~70% of cerebral blood flow (CBF) and vertebrobasilar arteries supply ~30% of CBF. For this reason, anterior circulation strokes are more common. Region-specific anterior circulation symptoms depend on the particular vessel occluded.

Primary hemorrhagic strokes are typically produced by intracranial arterial rupture. Bleeding can occur within the brain ('parenchymal' hemorrhage) and, if severe enough, can rupture into the ventricles; or around the brain within the subarachnoid space (subarachnoid hemorrhage). The blood produces injury by multiple mechanisms, including by compressing and tearing the surrounding brain tissue (including its blood vessels), by increasing intracranial pressure, or by toxic effects, mainly from blood products. Following a subarachnoid hemorrhage extravasation of blood can lead to secondary cerebral arterial vasospasm and new ischemic strokes.

Ischemic strokes may be preceded by *transient ischemic attacks* (TIA); as many as 20% of stroke patients report one or more prior TIAs. A TIA is defined as a brief episode of neurological deficit due to brain or retinal ischemia lasting less than 24 hours. This more classic definition, based on an arbitrary 24-hour time limit, is now in question based on newer concepts of brain ischemia and treatment options. Because transient ischemic symptoms can result in *permanent* brain damage or 'stroke' in some cases, stroke experts are now proposing that a TIA is a neurological deficit lasting less than 1 hour and without

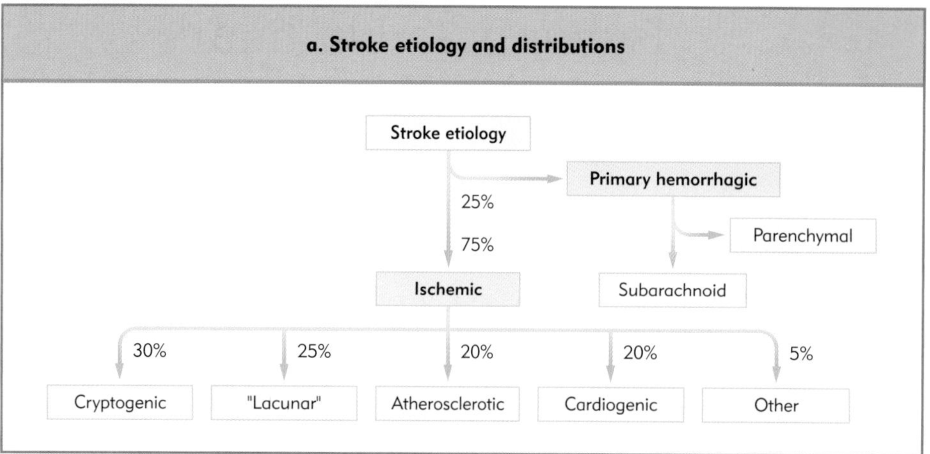

Figure 56.1 a. Stroke etiology and distributions. Distribution of the two major types of stroke types, ischemic and primary hemorrhagic, by etiology. Ischemic strokes represent the majority. Note that in nearly one-third of ischemic strokes no easily identifiable etiology is found ('cryptogenic').

b. Region-specific ischemic patterns

Occluded cerebral artery	MRI territory	Neurologic deficits	Clinical comments
MCA proximal		Contralateral: weakness/sensory loss visual field deficit Head/eye deviation Global aphasia (dominant side)	Observe closely for signs of increased cerebral edema with neurological deterioration Risk of hemorrhagic conversion
MCA superior		Contralateral: weakness > sensory loss visual field deficit	Oral motor dysfunction leads to increase aspiration risk
MCA inferior		Contralateral: sensory loss visual field deficit apraxia (neglect)	If nondominant side neglect can significantly impede rehabilitation
ACA		Contralateral: leg weakness +/- apraxia mild leg sensory loss Apathy, abulia, incontinence	Behavioral changes can result in significant morbidity requiring education of the family of its organic nature
PCA		Contralateral: visual field deficit	

b. Region-specific ischemic patterns. The middle cerebral artery (MCA) can be occluded either proximally (occluding both the superior and inferior branches) or more distally at the individual branches (superior, inferior). Less common occlusion pattern involve the anterior cerebral artery (ACA) and the posterior cerebral artery (PCA). Shown are correlative transaxial cranial MRI images of the ischemic brain. Neurologic deficits occur contralateral to the side of infarction.
MCA, middle cerebral artery; ACA, anterior cerebral artery; PCA, posterior cerebral artery.

evidence of acute infarction. Transient large artery occlusions may cause permanent cell injury without clinical symptoms, even with brief occlusions lasting only a few minutes. The major acute complications of ischemic stroke are summarized in Table 56.1.

The risk of stroke is highest during the first month: approximately 15–30% of subsequent strokes occur during the first month following a TIA, and 40–50% occur during the first year. The 90-day risk of stroke after TIA has been estimated to be almost 10%, with half of these occurring in the first 2 days after the TIA. In patients experiencing a TIA resulting from an internal carotid stenosis, the 90-day stroke risk is 20–25%.

CEREBRAL BLOOD FLOW

Metabolic coupling

Although the brain represents only 2% of total body weight it accounts for 20% of the resting oxygen consumption. Therefore, in order to meet this high demand for oxygen and glucose the brain requires a high level of perfusion. The brain receives approximately 800 mL of blood per minute, resulting in a regional blood flow of 40–60 mL/100 g/min. Rising metabolic demand is rapidly met by local increases in CBF, which provides increased substrate delivery. This relationship between metabolic demand and CBF is referred to as a regional flow–metabolism coupling.

One clinical implication of flow–metabolism coupling is that most volatile anesthetics are cerebral vasodilators and reduce cerebral metabolic demand while preserving metabolic coupling. In patients where uncoupling has occurred (i.e. stroke, ICH), anesthesia can induce relative cerebral hyperemia, possibly complicating neurosurgical procedures particularly if maintaining hemostasis is critical.

The relationship between CBF and metabolic demand is reflected in the measurement of the cerebral metabolic rate for oxygen ($CMRO_2$). $CMRO_2$ can be expressed as the oxygen extraction factor (OEF) by taking the difference between the cerebral arterial and venous oxygen contents. Under normal physiological conditions CBF and $CMRO_2$ are matched and OEF is normal. These relationships can, however, become deranged under clinical conditions such as ischemic stroke and severe traumatic brain injury. For example, under conditions of cerebral ischemia OEF is increased; the term 'misery perfusion' has been used to describe the condition of mild ischemia, and can pertain to the 'penumbra' regions in the brain (see below).

In severe ischemia OEF is maximal but cannot overcome the poor delivery of substrates due to low CBF, and thus brain tissue damage will be irreversible. Conditions of extreme hyperemia result in 'luxury perfusion', which can be deleterious as OEF is decreased. During hypothermic conditions brain OEF remains normal, but there is significant reduction in CBF and $CMRO_2$. These concepts are summarized in Figure 56.2.

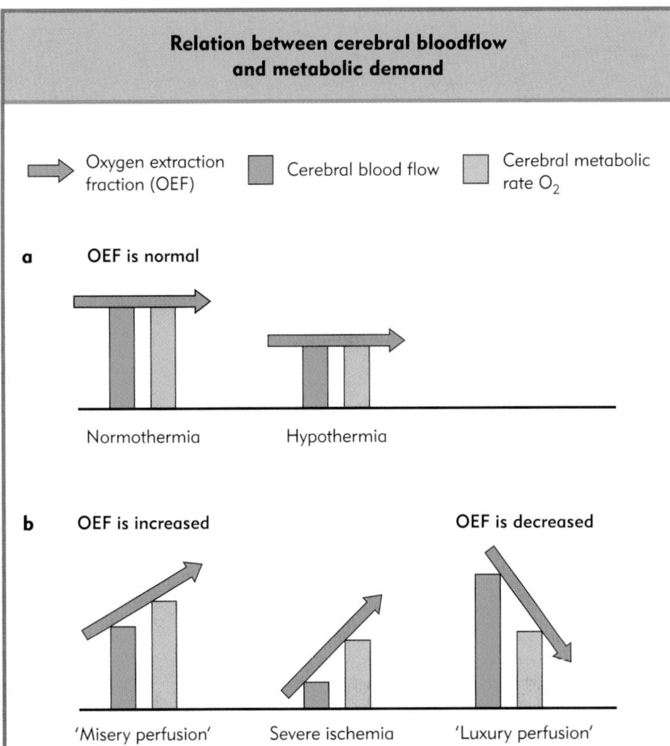

Figure 56.2 Relationship between cerebral blood flow and metabolic demand

Table 56.1 Major acute complications of ischemic stroke

Neurologic
Extension of stroke – stenosis becomes an occlusion
Recurrent stroke – new territory from a cardioembolic source
Cerebral edema – maximal 24–72 hours; larger strokes more prone to be symptomatic
Hemorrhage – transformation of a bland stroke with or without hematoma formation; associated with the use of anticoagulation therapy, and with early edematous large infarctions
Cardiovascular
Hypotension – due to aortic dissection, primary cardiac arrhythmia, ischemia or acute failure
Hypertension – due to 'hypertensive crisis', increased intracranial pressure, dysautonomia due to full bladder
Myocardial ischemia or infarction
Respiratory
Aspiration – airway obstruction

Ischemic penumbra and core

CBF below 20 mL/100 g/min is often used to define 'ischemia' which, if persistent, leads to neuronal death. This concept is based on traditional studies with carotid artery clamping in humans, estimating the 'penumbra' threshold to be around 20 mL/100 g/min for the whole brain. Current imaging studies confirm the existence of the penumbra in acute ischemic stroke, but also allow for a better physiological definition. Data from PET studies indicate that the penumbra is characterized by reduced CBF, increased OEF, and relatively preserved $CMRO_2$. In addition, brain MRI studies provide evidence of an ischemic penumbra based on a theory of 'diffusion/perfusion mismatch'.

The zones of cerebral ischemia are conceptually divided into 'viable', 'reversible' (or 'salvageable') and 'infarcted' regions. The relative severity and duration of the ischemia are important determinants of tissue death (Fig. 56.3). Other factors, such as the development of collateral flow and the extent of reperfusion, also determine the evolution and extent of infarction.

There are important differences in cellular biochemistry and morphology in the ischemic core versus the better-perfused 'penumbra' region. In the ischemic core there is electrical silence, with permanent depolarization and membrane failure. With loss of the membrane ionic pump mechanism there is a massive cellular influx of Na^+, Cl^-, and Ca^{2+}, and efflux of K^+. In the ischemic penumbra there is recurrent anoxic depolarization with ionic cycling. Overall membrane function is preserved but impaired. If no reperfusion occurs the penumbra becomes part of the expanding ischemic core (Fig. 56.4).

Cerebral autoregulation

Regional cerebral blood flow is maintained fairly constant over a wide range of systemic blood pressures owing to an intrinsic autoregulation of perfusion pressure (Chapter 30). The exact mechanisms of autoregulation are the subject of vigorous

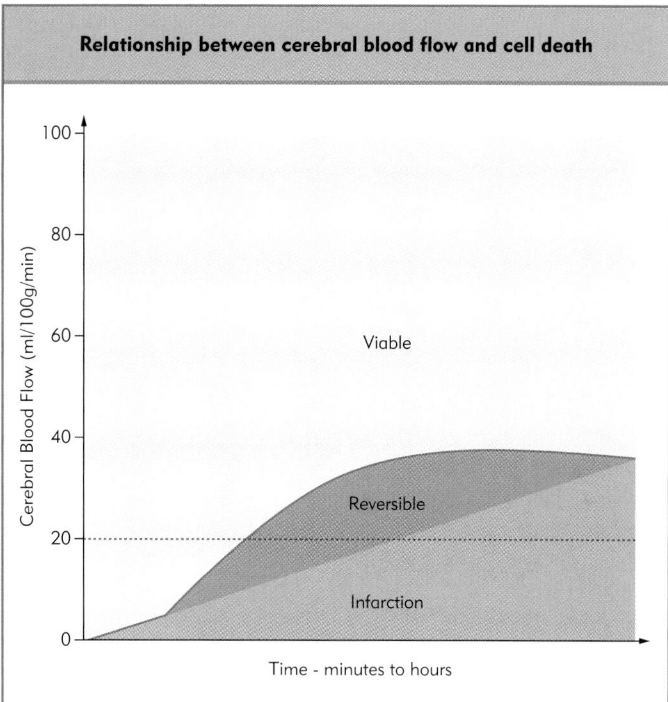

Figure 56.3 Relationship between cerebral blood flow and cell death following ischemic stroke. Neuronal cell damage and its potential reversibility is dependent on the severity and duration of reduced CBF. The ischemic penumbra region can evolve into an infarction if reperfusion does not occur rapidly and the region remains ischemic over time. (Adapted with permission from Fisher M. Clinical atlas of cerebrovascular disorders. London: Wolfe;1994.)

investigation, and include myogenic and endothelial responses, metabolic factors, neural regulation, and activation of K^+ channels. There is increasing recognition of neuronal-induced changes in astrocytic Ca^{2+} response, which probably represents a novel mechanism of CBF regulation. Under normal conditions, as systemic arterial blood pressure increases, perfusion pressure remains constant. Under ischemic and other abnormal conditions, autoregulation is deranged (Fig. 56.5), and a more passive linear relationship between CBF and cerebral perfusion pressure (CPP) exists. The exact cause of autoregulation failure is unknown. Because autoregulation failure occurs at brain sites distant to the local injury, simple explanations of increased local acidosis are probably too simplistic. The derangement of normal cerebrovascular autoregulation response can have critical implications for blood pressure control during the induction and maintenance of anesthesia. Furthermore in the patient with chronic uncontrolled hypertension, the normal relationship between CBF and CPP is shifted to the right (Fig. 56.5). The clinical implication is that lowering the blood pressure could produce cerebral ischemia compared to the normotensive patient.

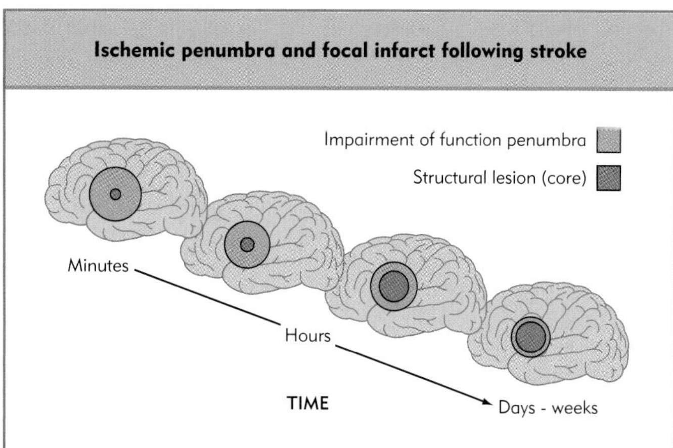

Figure 56.4 Ischemic penumbra and focal infarct following stroke. Clinical symptoms typically correspond to the combined ischemic penumbra and core regions. Over time, the core can expand to include more of the penumbra region, depending on the presence or efficacy of reperfusion. (Adapted from Dirnagl U, Iadecola C, Moskowitz MA. Pathobiology of ischaemic stroke: an integrated view. Trends Neurosci. 1999;22:391–7, with permission.)

Precipitous drops in systemic arterial blood pressure during ischemic conditions, which would normally be tolerated, may result in worsened cerebral ischemia.

Etiology of focal ischemic stroke

LARGE-VESSEL THROMBOSIS

Atherosclerotic lesions form at regions of turbulent blood flow, including bifurcations and curves of large vessels. As an atherosclerotic plaque grows the vessel becomes increasingly stenotic, and total occlusion usually results from in situ thrombus formation. Cerebral ischemia or frank infarction is more often the result of the thrombus formation rather than being due to a direct hemodynamic compromise.

Significant hemodynamic occlusion occurs at a vascular luminal cross-sectional reduction of 75–80%. The North American Symptomatic Carotid Endarterectomy Trial (NASCET) analyzed the role of carotid endarterectomy (CEA) on stroke

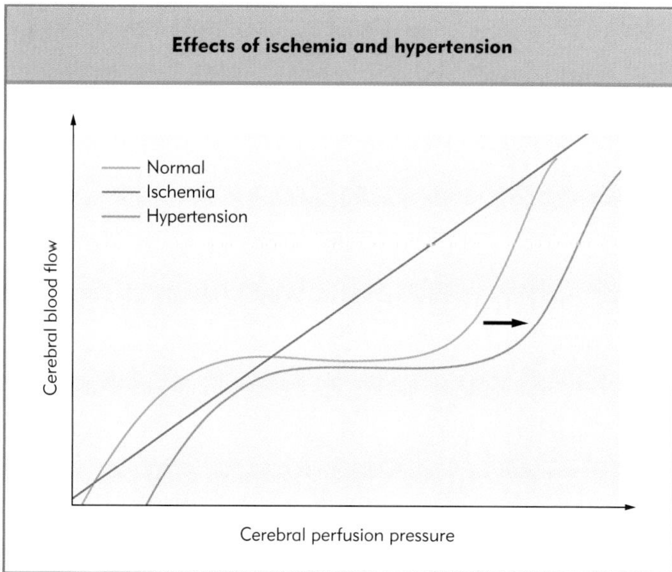

Figure 56.5 Effects of ischemia and hypertension on the relationship between cerebral blood flow and cerebral perfusion pressure. Under normal conditions CBF is maintained (plateau region in figure) over a relatively wide range of arterial blood pressures owing to intrinsic autoregulation of the cerebral blood vessels. However, during severe cerebral ischemia a passive linear relationship between CBF and cerebral perfusion pressure (CPP) exists.

outcome in patients with carotid artery stenosis disease. A significant improvement in stroke outcome was observed in patients undergoing CEA with greater than 70% stenosis; this number is commonly used to define a 'hemodynamically critical stenosis'.

EMBOLIZATION

Thromboembolic

Ischemia and infarction also result when thrombotic material from an atherosclerotic lesion embolizes to a distal cerebral vessel; this is referred to as 'artery to artery' embolization. This can occur from any of the major intracranial cerebral arteries, and also from a totally occluded carotid artery 'stump'. There is a strong association between aortic plaques (atheroembolic source) and ischemic stroke, as demonstrated in large autopsy case–control studies.

Cardioembolic

Fifteen to 70% of ischemic strokes occur from a cardioembolic source. The heart can be a nidus for clot formation due to atrial fibrillation, severe cardiomyopathy, valvular disease (mitral and aortic valves in particular), or infrequently primary congenital lesions (i.e. atrial septal defect and aneurysm). The middle cerebral artery (MCA) is the most commonly involved vessel, presumably owing to its flow mechanics, including its relatively large lumen, rapid blood flow, and curving course off the internal carotid artery. In approximately half of the cases of MCA embolic stroke, recanalization of the clot is seen. Predicting the extent of endogenous clot lysis is difficult, and there is currently no reliable means to determine whether and to what extent this will occur in any individual patient.

'Small vessel' or lacunar infarctions

About 25% of cerebral ischemic events are related to small vessel disease. Small vessel disease refers to vascular pathology in the small (approximately 40–800 μm diameter) perforating arteries of the brain. Perforating arteries that emerge from the proximal portion of the MCA are called the lenticulostriate vessels and are an important blood supply to the deeper structures of the brain, including the basal ganglia and the internal capsule (major motor-sensory tracts). Perforating vessels emanating from the basilar artery (the paramedian vessels) and from the posterior cerebral artery (the thalamoperforating branches) are essential for blood flow to critical brainstem nuclei and the thalamus. The actual vascular pathology involved in obstruction of 'small vessels' in the creation of 'lacunar infarction' is not well understood. Microatheromata stenosing or occluding a penetrating artery are commonly associated with chronic hypertension. In extreme hypertension leading to disordered cerebrovascular autoregulation fibrinoid necrosis prevails, involving destruction of the connective tissue portion of the small vessels. The most common risk factors associated with this disease are hypertension, diabetes, and in some series cigarette smoking. In general, the clinical course following a small vessel ischemic stroke is favorable, with improvement usually occurring sometimes within weeks.

LOW-PERFUSION STATE OR 'WATERSHED' ISCHEMIA

The term 'watershed' refers to cerebral ischemia that occurs in the border zone between different arterial territories. This occurs most commonly as a consequence of large vessel disease and poor collateral flow. An example is severe cardiomyopathy with low cardiac output and poor perfusion across a stenotic carotid artery. A second example is severe hypotension, usually in the setting of significant carotid stenosis, which can result in a border-zone cerebral infarction. This etiology can be diagnosed by neuroimaging, which demonstrates a classic pattern with infarction in the high cortices (ACA–MCA border zone) or in the interface between ACA–MCA or MCA–PCA arterial territories.

Etiology of hemorrhagic stroke

SUBARACHNOID HEMORRHAGE

Primary subarachnoid hemorrhage (SAH) most commonly occurs as a consequence of head trauma or rupture of a congenital aneurysm. Neurologic morbidity is related both to the initial damage to brain tissue from the hemorrhage and to secondary ischemic deficits due to delayed vasospasm. A variety of grading systems for SAH exist which can assist in the preoperative evaluation; the most commonly used is the modified Hunt and Hess grading scale. In general, patients with grades I and II do well, whereas those with grades III or IV have high morbidity and mortality and are more likely to have elevated intracranial pressure (ICP) and vasospasm.

Vasospasm occurs in up to 25% of patients following SAH. The resulting cerebral ischemia is the major cause of morbidity and mortality in this disease, making aggressive identification and treatment imperative. Vasospasm can be identified at the bedside with the use of transcranial Doppler ultrasonography, which demonstrates increased velocities in blood flow. The gold standard for identification of vasospasm, however, is cerebral angiography, which can identify vasospasm in multiple territories.

Up to 15–20% of SAH patients experience symptomatic obstructive hydrocephalus with increased ICP. Significant improvement can occur with timely placement of an intraventricular catheter for cerebrospinal fluid drainage. Rebleeding is also a serious complication, with an associated mortality as high as 50%.

Significant medical complications can occur following SAH, including hyponatremia, cardiac arrhythmias and pulmonary dysfunction. Cardiac arrhythmias are usually benign but infrequently can include torsades. In high grade SAH, serious pulmonary complications can occur including acute neurogenic pulmonary edema and Acute Respiratory Distress Syndrome.

Cerebral ischemia resulting from vasospasm is the most common morbidity in subarachnoid hemorrhage.

INTRAPARENCHYMAL OR INTRACEREBRAL HEMORRHAGE

Except for trauma, the most common cause of intracerebral hemorrhage (ICH) is uncontrolled hypertension, with bleeding and hematoma most commonly occurring within the deeper structures of the brain. Large lobar hemorrhage is rarely caused by primary hypertension, and is more commonly associated with vascular anomalies such as arteriovenous malformations (AVM) or with amyloid angiopathy.

Surgical risk and ischemic stroke

CAROTID ENDARTERECTOMY (CEA)

Based on the NASCET results, 2% of patients undergoing CEA for symptomatic carotid stenosis had a disabling stroke. Pooled estimates of risk, however, demonstrate an operative risk of stroke and death for asymptomatic stenosis of 2.8%, and of 5.1% for symptomatic carotid stenosis. Factors that increase the risk of stroke include female gender, age >75 years, contralateral carotid occlusion, carotid ulceration, intraluminal thrombus, severe hypertension, and symptomatic rather than asymptomatic carotid stenosis. Factors associated with an unacceptably high risk of stroke include recent large cerebral infarction, hemorrhagic infarction, progressing stroke, alteration in consciousness, and unstable medical conditions. Most strokes associated with the CEA procedure are believed to occur from embolization during manipulation of the carotid artery prior to cross-clamping, and less commonly are due to hypoperfusion, failure to shunt, or to a prolonged period of hypotension.

Preoperative evaluation – risk stratification

The main patient population undergoing a CEA is elderly and therefore typically possess multiple co-morbidities which significantly increases the risk of neurologic and cardiopulmonary complications following CEA. In one large retrospective study involving 22,000 patients undergoing CEA between 1988 and 1992, independent risk factors for perioperative stroke and death included congestive and ischemia heart disease, and diabetes mellitus. These medical factors should be carefully evaluated in the overall risk stratification schema for each patient. Risk stratification schemes such as presented in Table 56.2 can assist in the preanesthestic assessment of the patient. According to this schema, a patient's risk is determined based on a combination of medical, neurologic, and angiographic findings.

Table 56.2 Risk stratification for carotid endarterectomy

Risk group	Risk profile	% M & M
1	-Neuro, -Med, -Angio	1
2	-Neuro, -Med, +Angio	2
3	-Neuro, +Med, +/-Angio	7
4	+Neuro, +/-Med or +/-Angio	10
Type risk	**Characteristics**	
+Medical	angina, myocardial infarction, congestive heart failure, severe hypertension (>180/110), COPD, advanced age, severe obesity	
+Neurologic	new deficit (< 24hrs), progressive deficit, frequent daily ischemic attacks, multiple cerebral infartions	
+Angiographic	contralateral carotid artery occlusion, ICA siphon stenosis, proximal or distal plaque extension, high carotid bifurcation, presence of soft thrombus	

%M & M – mortality and morbidity; Neuro. – neurologically, Med. – medically, Angio – angiographically; COPD – chronic obstructive pulmonary disease; ICA – internal carotid artery

Adapted from Sundt TM Jr., Sandok BA, Whisnant JP: Carotid endoarterestocmy:complication and preoperative assessment of risk Mayo Clin Pro. 50:301-306, 1975.

CORONARY ARTERY BYPASS SURGERY (CABG)

CABG is associated with overt strokes in an estimated 1–3% of patients. In patients with a history of stroke or TIA, the perioperative stroke risk is increased as high as 8.7%. Other associated stroke risk factors include advanced age, prolonged cardiopulmonary bypass, recent myocardial infarction, left main coronary artery disease, smoking, and impaired renal function. Carotid stenosis may be correlated with a higher risk of stroke following CABG, but it may simply be a marker of systemic atherosclerotic disease. There is strong positive correlation between aortic arch disease and stroke after CABG. This increased risk may be in part related to the cannulation of the aorta while extracorporeal circulation is initiated.

In addition to frank strokes following CABG, up to one-third of patients experience a decrease in level of alertness or encephalopathy, which may be partly due to a cerebral hypoxic–ischemic injury. In large prospective study, perioperative encephalopathy was twice as common as stroke (respectively about 7% vs 3%). Encephalopathy was defined as confusion, agitation, delirium, or cognitive changes within 24 hours of the procedure. Suggested causes include microemboli or hypoperfusion in addition to more recognized medication- or renal-related causes. These data indicate that ischemia can be a critical part of the observed post-CABG encephalopathy.

Atheromatous embolization due to carotid artery and aortic manipulation is associated with stroke in CEA and CABG.

Off-pump CABG is becoming a popular alternative technique to conventional CABG. Meta-analysis of the combined end-points of death, myocardial infarction, and stroke (occurring during the first 30 days postoperatively) in off-pump versus on-pump CABG suggests only a trend toward reduced risk with off-pump CABG.

GLOBAL CEREBRAL ISCHEMIA

Global cerebral ischemia (GCI) occurs when blood flow to the entire brain is greatly reduced or stopped completely. The most common clinical scenario is cardiac arrest, in which blood flow to the brain ceases as a result of cardiac arrhythmia. Unlike focal cerebral ischemia, GCI produces an insult to the *entire* brain, which begins during the ischemic period but continues long after normal blood flow is restored.

Each year in the United States, over 700 000 people die as a result of cardiac disease; 460 000 of these deaths occur as a result of unexpected sudden cardiac death (SCD) either in an emergency department (120 000) or before reaching hospital (340 000).

The modern era of cardiopulmonary resuscitation (CPR) began in 1960, when Kouwenhoven described the technique of closed chest cardiac massage as an alternative to open chest CPR, which until that time had been the standard resuscitative technique. Widespread clinical experience with standard CPR, however, has failed to reproduce the 70% long-term survival rate initially reported. Various studies of hospital inpatients who underwent resuscitative efforts following cardiac arrest report hospital discharge rates of only 18–24%. Worse outcomes have been reported for victims of out-of-hospital cardiac arrest.

Survival to hospital discharge, however, is not the only measure of long-term CPR success. In order to prevent neurologic injury, any resuscitative technique must provide the brain with at least 20–30% of baseline cerebral cortical blood flow. However, standard external CPR is incapable of providing adequate cerebral perfusion to prevent postischemic neurological injury, and neurologic sequelae are frequent complications of initially successful resuscitation. In a study of 262 initially comatose survivors of cardiac arrest, 79% died within 1 year; cerebral failure was the cause of death in 37% of cases. Only 14% of patients were either neurologically normal or only slightly disabled at 12 months. Another review of an additional 459 survivors of out-of-hospital cardiac arrest indicated that 61% regained consciousness, but 39% never regained consciousness. Sixty-seven per cent of those regaining consciousness demonstrated complete neurologic recovery, 27% showed mild deficits, and 11% had severe motor and sensory deficits. Permanent significant brain damage due to ischemia/reperfusion contributes substantially to the mortality and neurological morbidity of cardiac arrest survivors.

Global cerebral ischemia occurs with severe reduction in blood flow to the entire brain, as in cardiac arrest and circulatory arrest.

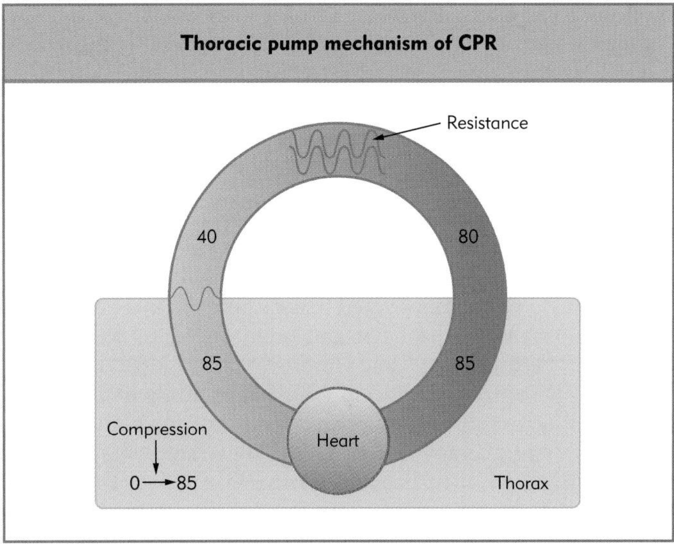

Figure 56.6 Thoracic 'pump' mechanism of blood flow during CPR. Representative pressures recorded during conventional CPR compression with forward carotid flow indexed from esophageal pressures. There is no significant pressure gradient across the heart. The extrathoracic arterial pressure is similar to the intrathoracic aortic pressure. The extrathoracic venous pressure is markedly lower than the intrathoracic venous (right atrial) pressure. The extrathoracic arteriovenous pressure gradient results in forward flow. (Adapted from Weisfeldt ML, Chandra N. Physiology of cardiopulmonary resuscitation. Annu Rev Med. 1981;32:435–42, with permission.)

CARDIOPULMONARY RESUSCITATION

Blood flow

For CPR to be effective, chest compressions must provide adequate circulation to perfuse vital organs (brain and heart) until the resumption of a spontaneous circulation. In order to maintain cerebral viability during cardiac arrest, CPR must provide 20–30% of baseline cerebral blood flow. CPR is more effective if started early during cardiac arrest, as superior flows are generated in the earliest phases of CPR. A recent human study indicates better quality of life outcomes after early access, immediate resuscitation, early defibrillation, and early advanced care. Standard external CPR cannot be considered a means of providing effective prolonged (more than several minutes) circulatory support during cardiac arrest.

Disappointing early clinical results with CPR led to a re-evaluation of the basic mechanism of generating blood flow during closed-chest compressions. It had originally been postulated that forward blood flow during CPR is generated through direct compression of the heart between sternum and spine, in the presence of a closed mitral and a patent aortic valve during left ventricular compression. Echocardiographic examination of patients during CPR failed to support this 'heart pump' mechanism, as no change in ventricular size is noted during compression: both mitral and aortic valves remain patent during compression and relaxation. Rather, CPR appears to generate forward blood flow through a 'thoracic pump' mechanism, i.e. chest compressions appear to produce a generalized increase in intrathoracic pressure which is differentially transmitted to extrathoracic arteries and veins, the net result being forward flow (Fig. 56.6).

IMPROVING FLOW/RESUSCITABILITY

Assuming that forward flow is generated during CPR by elevations in intrathoracic pressure, not by direct cardiac compression, any modification that increases intrathoracic pressure during compression should increase forward flow as well as augment end-organ perfusion. Modifications of standard CPR include CPR with simultaneous compressions and ventilations (SCVCPR), CPR using a specially designed compressive vest (vest CPR), CPR with ventilation at high airway pressures, and others. One technique that has received attention in the lay press in recent years is active compression/decompression (ACD) CPR. The ACD device is a handheld device with a suction cup to attach to the chest that creates a vacuum in the thorax with each chest wall decompression. By combining ACD with an inspiratory impedance threshold device (ITD, which impedes influx of inspiratory gas during chest wall decompression) the amplitude and duration of the vacuum within the thorax is augmented. Experimentally, ACD + ITD CPR results in a greater than threefold increase in blood flow to the heart and brain compared to standard CPR. Compared to standard CPR, ACD + ITD CPR significantly improved short-term (1- and 24-hour) survival rates for patients with out-of-hospital cardiac arrest.

Pharmacologic enhancement

Epinephrine has been routinely used as the vasoactive drug of choice in cardiac arrest because of its potency as a vasopressor, and because of the need to perfuse the coronary arteries in order to achieve successful resuscitation. Because epinephrine, as well as other vasporessors, loses much of its efficacy in acidotic, hypoxic environments, the use of higher-dose epinephrine was proposed as an alternative to standard-dose resuscitative therapy. Animal models demonstrated superior myocardial and cerebral blood flow with high doses; resuscitation rates following ventricular fibrillation cardiac arrest were also improved. However, human studies have not demonstrated improved survival or neurologic outcome with higher-dose epinephrine administered during resuscitation.

In the 1990s endogenous vasopressin levels were found to be higher in cardiac arrest survivors, suggesting that vasopressin might be used as an alternative agent during CPR. Subsequent preclinical studies demonstrated that vasopressin increases blood flow and oxygen to the heart and brain, increases the rate of successful resuscitation, and improves neurologic outcome. Based on these studies, a recent randomized study of 1219 out-of-hospital arrest victims compared vasopressin to epinephrine for vasopressor therapy during CPR. The results showed that the effects (survival to hospital admission, survival to hospital discharge) of vasopressin were similar to those of epinephrine in the management of ventricular fibrillation and pulseless electrical activity, but vasopressin was superior to epinephrine in patients with asystole. Additionally, vasopressin followed by epinephrine may be more effective than epinephrine alone in the treatment of refractory cardiac arrest. Although the effect of vasopressin on neurologic outcome has not been reported in humans, the positive results of this study support the addition of vasopressin to standard pharmacotherapy during resuscitation from cardiac arrest.

Total circulatory arrest

Total circulatory arrest (TCA) with deep hypothermia is a method of support for vital organs that is often used during the repair of complex congenital heart abnormalities in infants, and during repair of the aorta in adults. Hypothermia is induced prior to circulatory arrest in an effort to slow the metabolic rates of vulnerable organs and prevent end-organ injury, especially to the heart and brain. Despite the addition of hypothermia, patients undergoing TCA may still suffer significant neurologic injury. Serum markers of brain injury, especially S-100B (elevated primarily following astroglial stress or injury) are profoundly elevated in pediatric patients undergoing TCA. Similarly, in adults, S-100B levels were higher in complex aortic operations, and were significantly greater in patients requiring a period of TCA. In children, heart surgery performed with TCA as the predominant support strategy is associated with a higher risk of delayed motor development and neurologic abnormalities at 1 year than is surgery with low-flow bypass as the predominant support strategy. In adults, reduction of higher cognitive function occurs in some patients who undergo cardiac surgery using deep hypothermic TCA. Although hypothermia provides significant neuroprotection during TCA, the potential role for additional pharmacologic neuroprotection is under investigation.

Ventilation following ischemia

Hyper- or hypoventilation can greatly affect neurologic outcome following cerebral ischemia. Despite the absence of human studies to support the practice, prophylactic controlled hyperventilation is often recommended for patients resuscitated from cardiac arrest. This practice, following cardiac arrest and other neurologic injuries, is based on two premises: 1) elevations of intracranial pressure result in worsening of neurologic outcome. Hyperventilation, through its vasoconstrictive effects, may lower cerebral blood volume and ICP; and 2) cerebral lactic acidosis is commonly seen following cardiac arrest, and is correlated with poor neurologic outcome. Because CO_2 passes freely through the blood–brain barrier hyperventilation should diminish cerebral CO_2, thereby increasing pH and reversing acidosis.

Human studies of cerebral blood flow in patients with brain lesions or head injury suggest that controlled hyperventilation-induced vasoconstriction may acually aggravate ischemic brain injury. In the only randomized clinical trial of hyperventilation published to date 113 patients with severe head injury (GCS <8) were studied. Patients were then randomly assigned to one of three treatment regimens: 1) controlled physiologic ventilation 2) hyperventilation, or 3) hyperventilation plus THAM (a buffer used to replace bicarbonate buffer lost in the CSF during hyperventilation.) At three and six months after injury the number of patients with a favorable outcome was significantly lower in the hyperventilated patients than in either the control or hyperventilation plus THAM groups. It was concluded from this study that prophylactic hyperventilation may be deleterious in selected groups of patients with severe head injuries. (Muizelaar JP, et al. J Neurosurg 1991;75:731–39.

The conflicting results presented above make it difficult to recommend a rational approach to the ventilation of the patient suffering from ischemic/anoxic brain injury. In light of very compelling human data suggesting that marginally ischemic areas of the brain may be rendered more ischemic by hyperventilation, and in the absence of positive human trials, it seems that routine hyperventilation should be avoided. Careful attention should be paid to the development of increased intracranial pressure, so that therapeutic (not prophylactic) hyperventilation, as well as other measures to lower ICP, can be employed if this complication of neurologic injury develops.

Hyperventilation and hyperoxia may aggravate neuronal damage in cerebral ischemia.

The proper method of oxygen administration after cerebral ischemia is similarly unclear. Several preclinical models of global cerebral ischemia suggest that even transient hyperoxia following resuscitation can aggravate oxidative neuronal injury and worsen clinical neurologic outcome. Results are less clear-cut for focal ischemia and traumatic brain injury, however, as some animal models suggest that increased inspired oxygen can actually promote neurologic recovery during critical periods of ongoing ischemic injury seen following stroke and trauma.

Therapeutic hypothermia

Whereas many drugs are reported to provide neuroprotection in animal models of global cerebral ischemia, preclinical expectations of preventing brain injury through pharmacologic intervention have not been translated into human neuroprotection. No increased survival or neuroprotection among survivors was demonstrated in humans through the use of glucocorticoids, thiopental, or two different calcium channel antagonists, lidoflazine or nimodipine. Similarly, several large clinical trials failed to demonstrate a role for high-dose epinephrine. Many more drug trials for neuroprotection following focal cerebral ischemia (stroke) have also failed in humans.

In contrast to the disappointing neuroprotective drug trials, the recent results of two prospective randomized trials of moderate hypothermia following cardiac arrest in humans provide optimism that neuroprotective intervention is possible. Therapy with moderate hypothermia was attempted because several previous animal studies had demonstrated that mild or moderate hypothermia markedly mitigates brain damage after cardiac arrest in dogs, although the exact mechanism remains unclear. In two studies comparing cardiac arrest survivors randomized to standard post-resuscitative therapy or moderate induced hypothermia, patients receiving hypothermia demonstrated an improved neurologic outcome and reduced mortality. These results led the International Liaison Committee on Resuscitation to recommend that: 1) unconscious adult patients with spontaneous circulation after out-of-hospital cardiac arrest should be cooled to 32–34°C for 12–24 hours when the initial rhythm was ventricular fibrillation; and 2) cooling may also be beneficial for other rhythms or in-hospital cardiac arrest.

Although several studies have shown that various pharmacological agents improve outcome after experimental stroke (focal ischemia), no study has demonstrated significant neuroprotection in humans. Similar to global ischemia, however, induced hypothermia appears to show great promise as part of a neuroprotective strategy following focal cerebral ischemia. Laboratory studies have shown that intraischemic hypothermia is more protective than postischemic hypothermia, and more benefit is conferred with temporary than with permanent occlusion models. The efficacy of postischemic hypothermia is critically dependent on the duration and depth of hypothermia and its timing relative to ischemia.

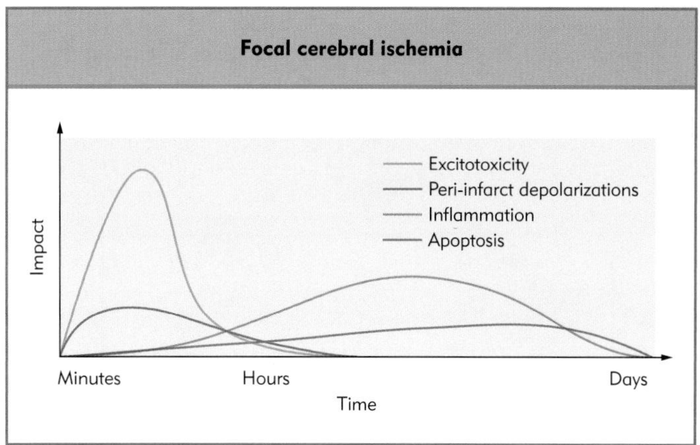

Figure 56.7 Temporal course of disrupted cellular mechanisms in focal cerebral ischemia. Excitotoxic mechanisms predominate in the early stages of cerebral ischemia, damaging neurons and glia. Delayed mechanisms are equally lethal, and include inflammation and programmed cell death (apoptosis). (Adapted from Dirnagl U, Iadecola C, Moskowitz MA. Pathobiology of ischaemic stroke: an integrated view. Trends Neurosci. 1999;22:391–7, with permission.)

PATHOPHYSIOLOGY OF ISCHEMIC BRAIN INJURY

The brain is the most vulnerable of all major organs to deprivation of blood flow. This unique sensitivity is due to the extremely high energy demand of neurons, caused by the rapid cycling and active transport of Na^+ and Ca^{2+} across their membranes. During brain ischemia there is a massive release of glutamate and other excitatory neurotransmitters. This leads to neuronal de-energization and a rise in intraneuronal Ca^{2+} that is more rapid than that of other cells, including the myocyte. Beyond these general characteristics, the pathophysiology of ischemic neural cell death is multifactorial and varies considerably based on the clinical condition that precipitates the ischemia.

Focal versus global cerebral ischemia

The neuropathology resulting from focal and global cerebral ischemia is significantly different. Focal ischemia caused by occlusion of small or large blood vessels results in primarily necrotic death of neurons and other cells within the core of the eventual infarct, evident morphologically within an hour. Neuronal cell death within the area termed the penumbra that surrounds this necrotic core occurs over several days to weeks, and eventually contributes to 50% or more of the final infarct volume (Fig. 56.7). Blood flow within the penumbra varies from critically low to near normal. This fluctuating gradient of fuel and oxygen is accompanied by an equally variable concentration of ATP. Neurons within the penumbra are the primary cells salvageable by thrombolytic improvement of blood flow or through neuroprotective interventions. The extensive and localized cell death accompanying a stroke elicits a powerful localized inflammation reaction that contributes to delayed cell death and disruption of the blood–brain barrier.

In contrast to stroke, neural cell death following global cerebral ischemia is highly selective and occurs throughout many regions of the brain, from the cortex to the brainstem. Although neurons are the primary neural cells that die following global ischemia, oligodendrocytes and astrocytes also succumb. The pattern of neuronal cell death varies considerably with the duration of ischemia and with other factors. For instance, poor outcome is associated with preischemic hyperglycemia or elevated body temperature. Neurons in the deep layers of the frontal cortex and within the CA1 region of the hippocampus are the most vulnerable, and demonstrate morphological signs of severe damage and death within 1 to several days after as little as 5 minutes of normothermic global ischemia. As the period of ischemia increases to 10 minutes or more, neuronal death is more widespread and is very evident within 24 hours. As global ischemia culminates in few if any discernable infarcts, the contribution of inflammation to delayed neural cell death is less than that of focal ischemia. Successful cardiopulmonary resuscitation is, however, associated with a 'sepsis-like' syndrome, characterized by elevated levels of plasma cytokines and endotoxin, which could exacerbate neuronal injury.

Necrotic and apoptotic cell death

Ischemic cell death is viewed as a continuum between necrosis and apoptosis, two distinctly different forms of cell death. In contrast to the generalized destruction of cell membranes, organelles, and macromolecules that occurs during necrosis, apoptosis is a programmed form of cell death, normally active during brain development and dependent on the expression of a large number of specific gene products. Whereas necrosis tends to be more rapid than apoptosis, necrotic neuronal death can occur for many days after cerebral ischemia. Molecular markers of apoptosis are evident in the brain following ischemia alone, although they change much more within minutes to days of

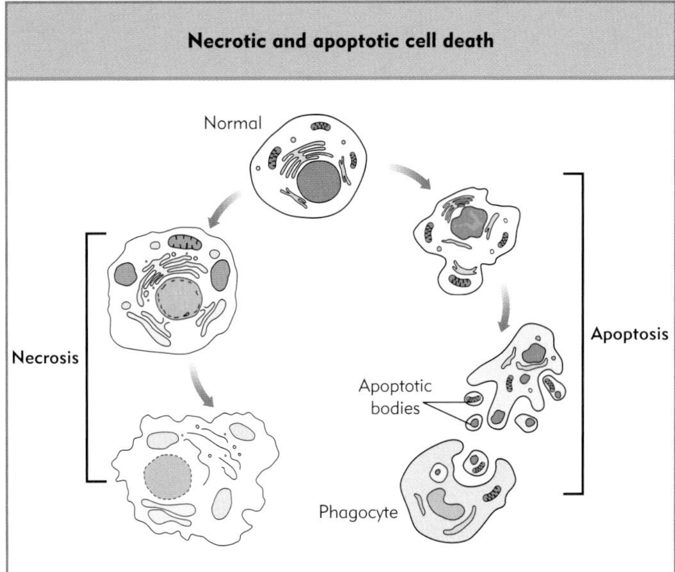

Figure 56.8 Morphological changes associated with necrotic and apoptotic cell death. (Adapted from Saikumar P, Dong Z, Mikhailov V, Denton M, Weinberg JM, Venkatachalam MA. Apoptosis: definition, mechanisms, and relevance to disease. Am J Med 1999;107:489–506, with permission.)

reperfusion. Apoptotic cell morphology is distinct from necrotic autolysis, and eventually the apoptotic cell disperses as numerous small vesicular bodies, ultimately engulfed by phagocytes (Fig. 56.8). The appearance of apoptotic cells is therefore transient, and not nearly as obvious as that of ghost cells generated by necrotic disruption of cell membranes and the release of intracellular contents into the extracellular milieu. Release of intracellular proteins is largely responsible for the inflammatory reaction readily apparent during the maturation of focal ischemic infarcts. Whereas apoptosis contributes little to inflammation, cytokines released by inflammatory and other cells are potent initiators of apoptotic cell death.

Neurons within the penumbra of a focal infarct are potentially salvageable by thrombolysis or neuroprotective interventions.

Necrotic and apoptotic cells also differ in regard to the molecular mechanisms that execute the respective pathways. Necrosis always involves at least an early transient if not a sustained loss of ATP that results in loss of cellular ionic homeostasis. In particular, the rise in intracellular Ca^{2+} activates numerous degradative enzyme activities. These, as well as other processes described below, ultimately cripple cellular energy metabolism and destroy membrane integrity. These alterations are accompanied by swelling of intracellular organelles and loss of identifiable nuclear morphology. In contrast, apoptosis is a relatively ordered series of events that are typically triggered by the activation of particular apoptosis-specific proteases termed 'caspases' that act on targets throughout the cell, resulting in shrunken nuclei, chromatin condensation, and cytoskeletal alterations that allow for plasma membrane blebbing and the formation of vesicular apoptotic bodies without the nonspecific release of cellular proteins.

Apoptosis is activated by either 'intrinsic' or 'extrinsic' pathways; evidence indicates that both contribute to ischemic cell death (Fig. 56.9). The intrinsic pathway involves the release of multiple proteins from the mitochondria into the cytosol. The first of these proteins identified was cytochrome c, a peripheral inner membrane protein that is also located free in solution between the mitochondrial inner and outer membranes. Supranormal accumulation of Ca^{2+} in mitochondria, as occurs during and following cerebral ischemia, is only one of many triggers that release cytochrome c. Pathologic insults ranging from oxidative stress to deprivation of cellular trophic factors elevate levels and promote mitochondrial translocation of proapoptotic proteins, e.g. Bax. This protein increases the permeability of the mitochondrial outer membrane directly, allowing for the dispersion of cytochrome c and other intermembrane

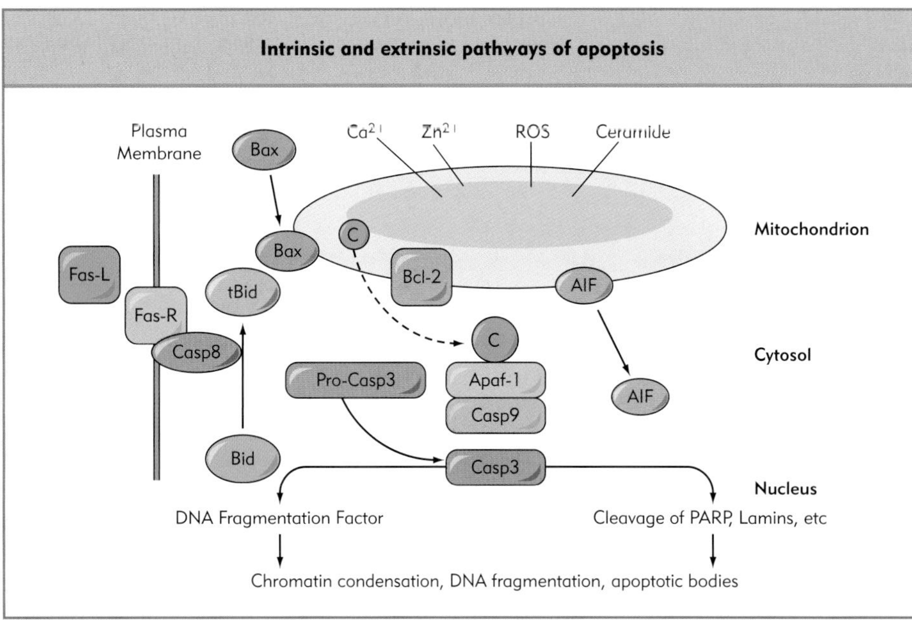

Figure 56.9 Intrinsic and extrinsic pathways of apoptosis. The intrinsic pathway of apoptosis is initiated by the release of cytochrome c (C) and other proteins from the mitochondrion into the cytosol. Activation of caspase 9 (Casp9) in the 'apoptosome' results in cleavage and activation of caspase 3 (Casp3), which mediates many of the molecular events that are characteristic of apoptosis. Caspase 8 (Casp8) is activated upon binding to the Fas receptor complex (Fas-R) following receptor binding by Fas ligand (Fas-L). The extrinsic pathway of apoptosis occurs when caspase 3 is directly activated by caspase 8. Caspase-independent apoptosis can occur when apoptosis-inducing factor (AIF) translocates from the mitochondria to the nucleus, where it mediates chromatin condensation and DNA fragmentation. ROS, reactive oxygen species.

proteins. Once released through the outer membrane, cytochrome c binds to Apaf1 in the cytosol. In the presence of ATP, an additional protein, caspase 9, is recruited into the macromolecular complex termed the apoptosome. Formation of the apoptosome activates caspase 9, which in turn proteolytically activates caspase 3. This key apoptotic protease, together with additional caspases it activates, targets a multitude of cellular proteins, ultimately leading to many cellular alterations, including degradation of nuclear DNA and disruption of the cytoskeleton.

The extrinsic apoptotic pathway can activate caspase 3 independently of the mitochondrion and the apoptosome. Certain 'cell death ligands', e.g. TNF-α and Fas ligand, bind to their respective cell surface receptors, specifically activating caspase 8, which in turn cleaves and activates caspase 3. Binding of ligands to these receptors, which often occurs in response to inflammation, can also activate the intrinsic pathway through caspase 8-mediated cleavage of the protein Bid, which then binds to Bax, causing it to permeabilize the mitochondrial outer membrane. Interfering with any of these steps in both the intrinsic and the extrinsic apoptotic pathways affords protection against cell death, including that observed following cerebral ischemia. Although specific antiapoptotic drugs are not in current use for neuroprotection, some are in development for clinical trials.

Excitotoxicity

Excitotoxic glutamate receptor activation is a primary mediator of neuronal injury and death following hypoxic–ischemic insults. Failure to maintain the normal transcellular Na^+ gradient results in reversal of the Na^+-dependent glutamate uptake transporter and massive release of glutamate into the extracellular space. Maximal binding of glutamate to several ionotropic receptors results in sustained neuronal influx of Na^+ and Ca^{2+}, exacerbated by influx through voltage-gated ion channels and uncompensated by energy-dependent efflux. The intracellular Ca^{2+} concentration rises from a normal basal level of approximately 0.1 μM to more than 30 μM within several minutes of complete ischemia, accompanied by a qualitatively similar rise in cytosolic Na^+ and a reduction in K^+.

The abnormal rise in intracellular Ca^{2+} elicited by ischemic activation of glutamate receptors activates numerous Ca^{2+}-sensitive enzymes, including phosphatases, proteases, phospholipases, and endonucleases. Together, the abnormally high activity of these enzymes results in degradation of metabolic and structural proteins, e.g. the cytoskeletal protein spectrin, membrane phospholipids, and DNA. These events are largely responsible for the *acute* necrotic cell death that occurs within the core of the infarct generated by ischemic stroke (Fig. 56.10). During cerebral ischemia, glutamate present within synaptic vesicles is also released, accompanied by Zn^{2+} that is also concentrated in these vesicles. Evidence suggests that the uptake of Zn^{2+} in postsynaptic neurons contributes to their damage. In clinically relevant scenarios involving global cerebral ischemia, the duration of initial excitotoxicity may only last 5–15 minutes, yet this period is sufficient to trigger *delayed* necrotic death within 1 to many days. Although glutamate receptor antagonists, e.g. ketamine, are powerful neuroprotectants when administered prior to the onset of ischemia, their effectiveness is reduced or lost when added following cardiac arrest or stroke, at times when their use is clinically feasible.

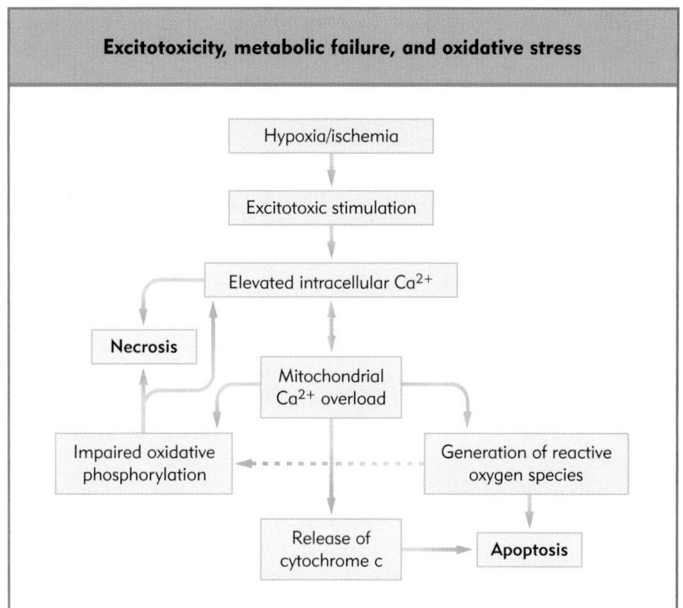

Figure 56.10 Relationships between excitotoxicity, metabolic failure, and oxidative stress. Severe anoxia or ischemia releases excitatory neurotransmitters from neurons and astrocytes. Binding of glutamate to ionotropic receptors causes massive neuronal Ca^{2+} influx that can lead directly to necrotic cell death through prolonged activation of degradative enzymes. Reperfusion, if initiated early enough, allows for cellular re-energization and lowering of intracellular Ca^{2+}. Respiration-dependent uptake of Ca^{2+} by mitochondria can, however, impair their ability to generate ATP and promote mitochondrial production of reactive oxygen species. High intracellular Ca^{2+} during early reperfusion also promotes the formation of reactive oxygen species by activation of specific enzymes, e.g. cyclooxygenase and nitric oxide synthase. The release of cytochrome c caused by mitochondrial Ca^{2+} overload, together with oxidative stress, is a potent activator of apoptosis.

Glutamate receptor antagonists such as ketamine are powerful neuroprotectants against excitotoxicity when given prior to the onset of ischemia.

Ischemic acidosis

During severe anoxia and ischemia a profound reduction in intracellular and tissue pH occurs, caused by the generation of protons during the hydrolysis of ATP and creatine phosphate, and due to accelerated lactate production by anaerobic glycolysis. Within 10 minutes of cardiac arrest intracellular pH can fall to 6.5 in normoglycemic individuals, and to 6.0 in those who are hyperglycemic. This highly abnormal environment contributes to tissue injury following both global and focal cerebral ischemia, as evidenced by worse outcomes in hyperglycemic patients. Acidosis adversely affects many aspects of cell function and activates certain degradative enzymes, e.g. lysosomal cathepsin protesases, that contribute to necrotic cell autolysis. Careful management of blood glucose is therefore imperative in both stroke and cardiac arrest patients.

Reperfusion injury and oxidative stress

Reperfusion of ischemic tissue is necessary for any chance of recovery and survival. Replenishment of oxidizable fuel and oxygen often results in normalization of intracellular ATP within minutes, followed by normalization of ionic homeostasis soon thereafter. Cellular re-energization does not, however, necessarily indicate that cell function is normal, as indicated by the finding that brain electrical activity is often absent – or at least severely depressed – for hours after resuscitation from cardiac arrest. Measurements of cerebral energy metabolism, including rates of glucose utilization, the formation of metabolic intermediates, and oxygen utilization, indicate that energy metabolism, and aerobic energy production in particular, are impaired for hours to days after global or focal cerebral ischemia. This phenomenon led to the concept of '*reperfusion injury*', referring to events occurring during reperfusion that either exacerbate the damage caused by ischemia alone or that induce new forms of injury. We now know that activation of apoptotic signal cascades constitutes one form of reperfusion injury. The histopathology of neuronal death that occurs in selectively vulnerable brain regions after global ischemia or in the penumbra following ischemic stroke is, however, primarily necrotic in appearance, or exhibits characteristics of both necrosis and apoptosis. Considerable evidence supports the concept that reperfusion-dependent delayed neural cell death is largely the consequence of oxidative stress, possibly a consequence of abnormal Ca^{2+} sequestration by mitochondria upon activation of respiration during reperfusion (Fig. 56.10).

The primary reactive oxygen and nitrogen species thought to mediate oxidative damage to lipids, proteins, and nucleic acids are the hydroxyl radical and peroxynitrite. Both of these are products of superoxide anion radicals (Fig. 56.11). Superoxide is a product of many normal reactions, including several involved in prostanoid metabolism, e.g. those catalyzed by cyclooxgenases. Another important source of superoxide is the mitochondrion, possessing sites within the electron transport chain and the tricarboxylic acid cycle strongly implicated in oxidative stress associated with reperfusion injury and neurodegenerative diseases, e.g. Parkinson's disease. Normally, the vast majority of superoxide so produced is detoxified by reactions catalyzed by superoxide dismutases, present in mitochondrial, cytosolic, and extracellular compartments, generating hydrogen peroxide (H_2O_2). Hydrogen peroxide is further metabolized to water and oxygen via the enzymes catalase and glutathione peroxidase. If, however, the rate of superoxide production exceeds the rate of dismutation, it may react spontaneously with nitric oxide to form the highly reactive and toxic peroxynitrite anion. Although nitric oxide is produced normally and is an important regulator of blood flow, increased production of it, along with superoxide, during reperfusion appears responsible for much of the oxidative alterations to lipids, proteins, and nucleic acids that is well documented following cerebral ischemia. Another purported culprit in reperfusion injury is the hydroxyl radical formed when the production of hydrogen peroxide exceeds the activities of catalase and glutathione peroxidase to metabolize hydrogen peroxide to water and oxygen. The generation of hydroxyl radical from hydrogen peroxide is catalyzed by nonbound reduced iron (Fe^{2+}), known to increase during reperfusion and under acidic conditions. Evidence that iron-catalyzed hydroxyl radical production plays an important role in reperfusion injury includes the neuroprotection observed in animal models with the administration of iron chelators.

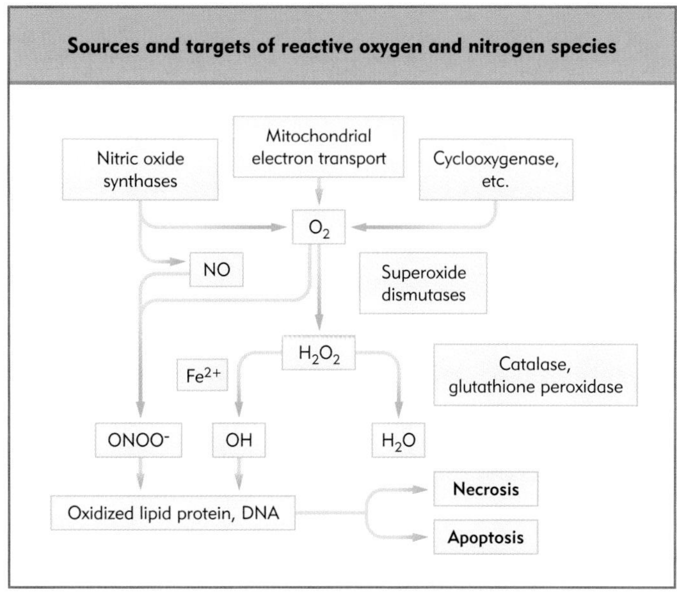

Figure 56.11 Sources and targets of reactive oxygen and nitrogen species. Numerous reactions produce reactive oxygen and nitrogen species during reperfusion. These reactions include those catalyzed by nitric oxide synthases, mitochondrial dehydrogenases, and electron transport chain components, and various oxidases and oxygenases, e.g. cyclo-oxygenase. Abnormally high rates of H_2O_2 production and metabolism can deplete cells of glutathione, causing a state of oxidative stress. Small levels of free iron (Fe^{2+}) are capable of catalyzing the reduction of H_2O_2, forming the highly toxic hydroxyl radical (OH·) that, together with peroxynitrite, mediates much of oxidative damage during reperfusion.

As peroxynitrite and hydroxyl radical oxidatively modify all classes of molecule, it follows that they affect almost all aspects of cell function. For instance, mitochondrial energy metabolism is very sensitive to oxidative stress, owing to the dependence of oxidative phosphorylation on the activity of many proteins and on structurally normal mitochondrial membranes. In addition, by depleting cells of glutathione, which maintains protein sulfhydryl groups in a reduced state, reactive oxygen species can indirectly increase or decrease the activity of certain enzymes, channels, and transporters. This shift in cellular redox state may in fact be at least partially responsible for the secondary rise in intraneuronal Ca^{2+} that occurs after anoxia and excitotoxicity. Oxidative damage to DNA is one of the most potent initiators of apoptosis, stimulating the expression of numerous proapoptotic proteins.

Although the results of the few stroke clinical trials that tested antioxidants were disappointing, this therapeutic approach is still considered viable. Protection against oxidative stress appears to be at least partially responsible for the neuroprotective effects of estrogen, and may explain why female stroke patients have a lower level of oxidized lipids in their CSF than do male stroke victims. Excessive brain oxygenation beyond what is necessary to support oxidative energy metabolism may contribute to reperfusion injury, suggesting the need for clinical studies comparing the effects of different postischemic ventilatory oxygen levels on outcome following cardiac arrest and stroke.

Inflammation

Inflammation not only plays an important role in ischemic neuronal injury following stroke, but also appears critical in the chain of events leading up to focal cerebral ischemia. Current data indicate that inflammation serves to fuel atherosclerosis and can act as the link between atherosclerosis and atherothrombosis. The accumulation of inflammatory cells, mainly monocytes/

macrophages, within the vascular wall starts early during atherogenesis. During later disease stages their activation can lead to plaque rupture and thrombus formation, increasing the likelihood of stroke. Stroke risk has been linked to serologic markers of inflammation, such as C-reactive protein (CRP) and soluble intercellular adhesion molecule (SICAM). The exact triggering mechanism of stroke is unclear, but may include such factors as endothelial activation, infectious disease, proinflammatory interactions between vessel walls and circulating blood elements, as well as others (see Chapter 44).

Inflammation plays an important role in cerebral ischemia and during reperfusion.

Soon after the onset of blood vessel occlusion, ischemic injury triggers inflammatory cascades in the parenchyma that further amplify tissue damage. Animal models demonstrate that reactive microglia, macrophages, and particularly leukocytes are soon recruited into the ischemic brain; additional inflammatory mediators are then generated by these cells, or by neurons or astrocytes. In contrast to data relating to experimental ischemia, direct histological evidence of leukocyte recruitment in human stroke is limited to a few small necropsy studies. Newer imaging tools also have provided indirect evidence of leukocyte recruitment in human stroke. Little information is available, however, about the temporal profile of human leukocyte migration, especially during the earliest phases following focal cerebral ischemia, where therapeutic intervention appears most promising. In animal models, interruption of neuroinflammatory mechanisms has proved very effective in limiting infarct size after experimental focal cerebral ischemia. However, two large recent human trials of treatment aimed at neutrophil adhesion have been unsuccessful.

The pathogenic role of inflammation following global cerebral ischemia and reperfusion is much less defined. Inflammation appears to increase the risk of sudden cardiac death or cardiac arrest. Patients who had sudden cardiac death had higher levels of CRP in their blood and in cardiac plaque than those who died from noncardiac disease. These results suggest that measuring CRP as part of the routine physical examination may identify individuals at risk for cardiac arrest, myocardial infarction, or stroke.

Unlike focal ischemia, there is little evidence at present to suggest a pathologic role for white blood cell infiltration into the brains of cardiac arrest survivors. This does not suggest, however, that inflammation does not play a significant role after resuscitation from cardiac arrest. In fact, there appears to be a systemic inflammatory response syndrome in patients who are successfully resuscitated from cardiac arrest. On admission, high levels of plasma IL-6, IL-8, IL-10, and soluble TNF receptor type II can discriminate between survivors and nonsurvivors. The precise importance of inflammation on global cerebral ischemic injury, however, remains to be determined.

Key references

Astrup J, Siesjo BK, Symon L. Thresholds in cerebral ischemia – the ischemic penumbra. Stroke 1981;12:723–5.

Ferguson GC, Eliasziw M, Bar HWK et al. The North American Symptomatic Carotid Endarterectomy Trial: Surgical results in 1415 patients. Stroke 1999;30:1751–8.

Johnston CS. Transient ischemic attack. New Engl J Med. 2002;347:1687–92.

Lo EH, Dalkara T, Moskowitz MA. Mechanisms, challenges and opportunities in stroke. Nature Rev Neurosci. 2003;4:399–415.

Roach GW, Kanchuger M, Mangano CM et al. Adverse cerebral outcomes after coronary artery bypass surgery. Multicenter study of the Perioperative Ischemia Research Group and the Ischemia Research and Education Foundation Investigators. New Engl J Med. 1996;335:1857–63.

Sundt TM Jr, Sandok BA, Whisnant JP. Carotid endarterectomy: complications and preoperative assessment of risk. Mayo Clin Proc. 1975;50:301–6.

Further reading

Bernard SA, Gray TW, Buist MD et al. Treatment of comatose survivors of out-of-hospital cardiac arrest with induced hypothermia. New Engl J Med. 2002;346:557–63.

Hypothermia After Cardiac Arrest Study Group. Mild therapeutic hypothermia to improve the neurologic outcome after cardiac arrest. New Engl J Med. 2002;346:549–56.

Krieger DW, Yenari MA. Therapeutic hypothermia for acute ischemic stroke: what do laboratory studies teach us? Stroke 2004;35:1482–9.

Maier CM, Steinberg GK. Hypothermia and cerebral ischemia: mechanisms and clinical applications. Totowa, NJ: Humana Press; 2003.

Mohr JP, Choi DW, Grotta JC, Weir B, Wolf PA. Stroke: pathophysiology, diagnosis and management, 4th edn. Philadelphia: Churchill Livingstone; 2004.

Ropper AH. Neurological and neurosurgical intensive care, 4th edn. Philadelphia: Lippincott Williams & Wilkins; 2004.

Wenzel V, Krismer AC, Arntz R, Sitter H, Stadlbauer KH, Linder KH. A comparison of vasopressin and epinephrine for out-of-hospital cardiopulmonary resuscitation. New Engl J Med. 2004;350:105–13.

Wolcke BB, Mauer DK, Schoefmann MF et al. Comparison of standard cardiopulmonary resuscitation versus the combination of active compression–decompression cardiopulmonary resuscitation and an inspiratory impedance threshold device for out-of-hospital cardiac arrest. Circulation 2003;108:2201–5.

SECTION 7

Renal system

Chapter 57

Renal physiology

H Thomas Lee, Mladen Vidovich and Salim Mujais

TOPICS COVERED IN THIS CHAPTER

- **Anatomy**
- **Production of filtrate**
  - Renal blood flow
  - Autoregulation
  - Glomerular filtration
- **Tubular processing of filtrate**
  - Overall function of the proximal tubule
  - Specific proximal tubule functions
  - Regulation of proximal tubule transport
  - Thin limb of the loop of Henle
  - Thick ascending limb of the loop of Henle
  - Distal convoluted tubule
  - Collecting duct
  - Mechanisms of tansport
  - Hormonal effects
- **Regulation of urine tonicity**
  - Formation of dilute urine
  - Formation of concentrated urine
- **Measurement of renal function**
- **Neuroendocrine regulation**
- **Kidney transplantation**

The kidneys play a major role in regulating both the composition and the volume of body fluids. Renal function can be divided conceptually into two complementary processes: 1) production of a plasma ultrafiltrate by the glomeruli, and 2) processing of this filtrate by the tubules. The first process is minimally selective in that it separates plasma proteins and cellular elements from plasma water but has no effect on solutes. The second process is more complex and involves the controlled retrieval or excretion of a variety of solutes. This task is accomplished along the length of the tubule, with the varied requirements met by specialized morphology and function (Fig. 57.1).

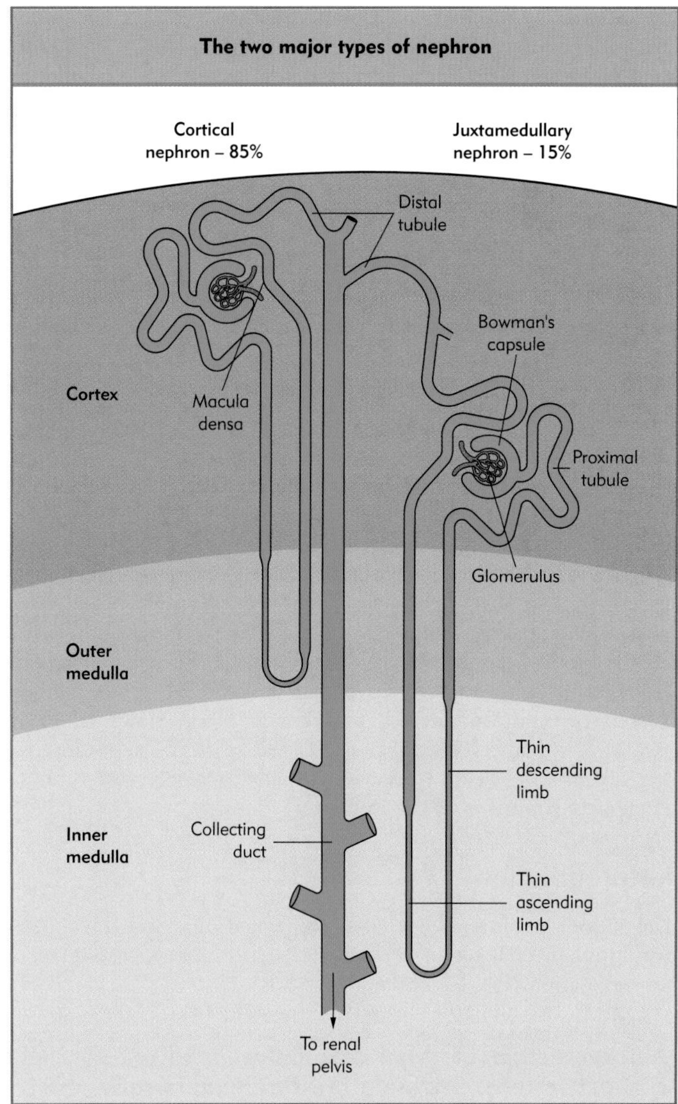

Figure 57.1 The structure and location of the two major types of nephron.

ANATOMY

Each human kidney weighs about 150–200 g and is located retroperitoneally just below the diaphragm. The renal artery originates from the aorta to supply each kidney; however, approximately one-third of the population has multiple renal arteries supplying one kidney. The kidney is anatomically divided into cortex, medulla, pyramids, calyces and pelvis, and ureter. The medulla is further divided into inner and outer zones.

Nephrons are the functional units of the kidney, each kidney containing more than 1 million nephrons. The renal tubules commence in the cortex of the kidney, where a hollow, funnel-like structure, Bowman's capsule, surrounds the capillary bed of the glomerulus. The glomerular filtrate captured in Bowman's capsule flows into the proximal convoluted tubule (PCT), from where it goes into the hairpin-shaped loop of Henle. Most nephrons (~85%) have a short loop of Henle that passes from the cortex to the outer medulla and returns to the cortex, where it continues as the distal convoluted tubule (DCT). These are cortical or short-loop nephrons. The remaining 15% of nephrons are juxtamedullary or long-loop nephrons, so called because their Bowman's capsule is closer to the outer medulla than those of the cortical nephrons, and the loop of Henle passes through the outer medulla and deep into the medulla before returning again to form the DCT in the cortex. The collecting tubules penetrate the outer and inner medullae as collecting ducts, where they start to coalesce, eventually to form the renal pelvis (Fig. 57.1).

PRODUCTION OF FILTRATE

Renal blood flow

Under resting conditions in the adult approximately 20% of cardiac output passes through the kidneys, which constitute only approximately 0.5% of body mass. This rate of blood flow (400 mL/100 g of tissue per minute) is much greater than that in other vascular beds ordinarily considered to be well perfused, including brain, heart, and liver. From this enormous blood flow only a small quantity of urine is formed. The kidney is unique in that blood flow dictates oxygen consumption. This characteristic differs from other major organs such as heart and brain, where oxygen consumption drives how much blood flows to each organ. The clinical significance is that a global nonselective increase in renal blood flow may actually increase renal tubular oxygen consumption in the ischemic kidney.

Autoregulation

The kidney maintains a relative constancy of blood flow rates during major changes in perfusion pressure, a property termed autoregulation (Fig. 57.2).

Autoregulation of renal blood flow involves parallel changes in renal perfusion pressure and vascular resistance involving intrinsic mechanisms.

Autoregulation implies that vascular resistance changes in a direction that matches the perfusion pressure. The changes in renal vascular resistance that accompany graded reductions in renal perfusion pressure are demonstrable in innervated, denervated, and isolated kidneys. This implies that autoregulation of renal blood flow is an intrinsic property of the kidneys. Several hypotheses have been proposed to explain this autoregulation:

- **Myogenic hypothesis** According to this hypothesis, arterial smooth muscle contracts and relaxes in response to increases and decreases in vascular wall tension. Thus an increase in perfusion pressure, which initially distends the vascular wall, is followed by contraction of resistance vessels, thereby resulting in recovery of blood flow from an initial elevation to a value comparable to the control level.
- **Tubuloglomerular feedback (TGF) hypothesis** Increased perfusion pressure leads to increased blood flow and glomerular capillary hydraulic pressure, thereby increasing glomerular filtration rate and distal tubule flow rate. Increased distal delivery (variations of NaCl concentration in the macular densa region between ~20 and 60 mM/L) is sensed by the macula densa, which activates effector mechanisms that increase preglomerular resistance, thereby reducing renal blood flow, glomerular pressure, and filtration rate. Several substances have been proposed to play a role in TGF, including ATP, adenosine, prostaglandins, and the renin–angiotensin system. Recent evidence with genetically engineered mice demonstrated that adenosine is the key autoregulatory molecule (see below).
- **The metabolic hypothesis** predicts that a decrease in organ blood flow results in the accumulation of vasodilator metabolites that restore blood flow to its previous level. In the kidney, however, metabolism is determined by Na^+ reabsorption, which in turn is roughly proportional to GFR (glomerular filtration rate). As GFR frequently varies directly with renal blood flow, it follows that metabolism should also vary with RBF.

The range of perfusion pressures over which renal blood flow is held constant (the autoregulatory range) is reset in hyper-

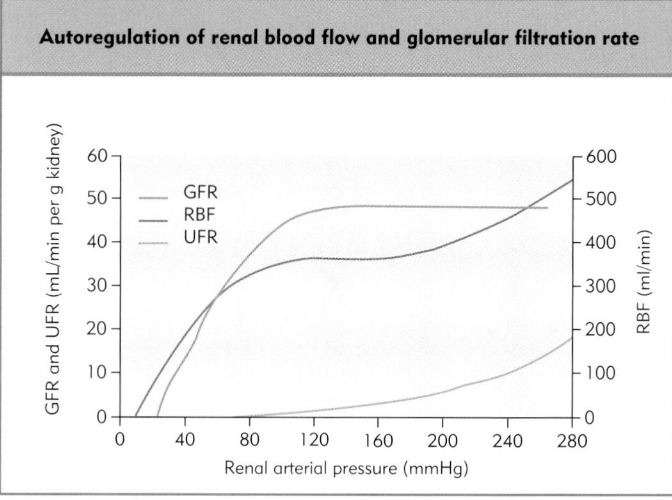

Figure 57.2 Autoregulation of renal blood flow (RBF) and glomerular filtration rate (GFR). Renal arterial pressure in dogs varies from 20 to 280 mmHg; autoregulation of RBF and GFR is observed between about 80 and 180 mmHg. UFR, urine flow rate.

tension, and blood flow will decline at apparently adequate perfusion pressures. In diseased kidneys this autoregulatory advantage is lost and flow becomes dependent on perfusion pressure, hence the greater vulnerability of the diseased kidney to reductions in perfusion pressure. This highlights the need for more careful monitoring and maintenance of blood pressure in patients with underlying renal disease. It is not uncommon to see intraoperative and postoperative oliguria and azotemia in such patients resolve when blood pressure is increased.

Glomerular filtration

Glomerular filtration is the initial step in renal function. The glomerulus is a specialized capillary bed with two important characteristics: 1) it is located between two arterioles, hence it is capable of operating at higher hydrostatic pressures, and capable of varying this pressure by varying the respective resistances of the afferent and efferent arterioles; and 2) it has a very high hydraulic permeability, allowing large volumes to be filtered. The glomerular ultrafiltrate is identical in composition to plasma, except that it is relatively free of large protein and protein-bound ions.

Glomerular filtration rate (GFR) is determined by three main factors: 1) the balance of pressures acting across the capillary wall, 2) the rate at which plasma flows through the glomeruli, and 3) the permeability and the total surface area of the filtering capillaries. These determinants of GFR are, in turn, subject to the influence of a number of factors, including local and circulating hormones. Na^+ delivery to the distal tubule itself modulates GFR by a process of tubuloglomerular feedback.

DETERMINANTS OF GLOMERULAR ULTRAFILTRATION

The driving forces that control ultrafiltration across the glomerular capillary wall are the same as those that determine fluid movement across other capillaries. At any point along the glomerular capillary network, the net forces favoring ultrafiltration (ultrafiltration pressure, PUF) is given by the difference between the transcapillary hydraulic pressure (ΔP), which favors filtration, and the corresponding difference in colloid osmotic pressure ($\Delta\pi$), which opposes it:

■ Equation 57.1

$$\text{PUF} = \Delta P - \Delta\pi$$

The transcapillary filtration pressure is the difference between the mean hydraulic pressure in the glomerular capillary (P_{Glom}) and the mean hydraulic pressure in Bowman's space, which is equal to the pressure in the lumen of the proximal tubule (P_{Tubule}):

■ Equation 57.2

$$\Delta \text{P} = \text{P}_{\text{Glom}} - \text{P}_{\text{Tubule}}$$

The mean transcapillary oncotic pressure is the difference between the oncotic pressure of plasma in the glomerular capillary (π_{Glom}) and that of the filtrate in Bowman's space (π_{Tubule}). Because the filtrate is practically protein free, π_{Tubule} is negligible and $\Delta\pi$ is essentially equal to π_{Glom}.

The local rate of ultrafiltration is equal to the product of PUF (the net driving pressure) and the local effective hydraulic permeability of the capillary wall (k). For the entire capillary network, a surface factor (S) accounts for the surface area of the glomerulus. The product of the surface area (S) and the hydraulic permeability (k) is termed K_f, the ultrafiltration coefficient. Hence, the single nephron glomerular filtration rate (SNGFR) can be written:

■ Equation 57.3

$$\begin{aligned}\text{SNGFR} &= \text{PUF} \times K_f \\ &= (\Delta \text{P} - \Delta\pi) \times K_f \\ &= [(P_{\text{Glom}} - P_{\text{Tubule}}) - (\pi_{\text{Glom}} - \pi_{\text{Tubule}})] \times K_f\end{aligned}$$

Changes in SNGFR can be evoked by alterations in the ultrafiltration coefficient (K_f) or in the net driving force for ultrafiltration (PUF), which in turn is determined by the mean transcapillary hydraulic pressure difference (ΔP), the oncotic pressure of the glomerular network (π_{Glom}), and the initial glomerular plasma flow rate (QA).

SNGFR varies linearly with plasma flow rate up to a plateau beyond which further increases in flow are without effect. Clinically, this translates into a dependence of GFR on renal plasma flow and renal perfusion pressure within the limits of autoregulation. Ultrafiltration of fluid across the walls of the glomerular capillary occurs only when the local transcapillary hydraulic pressure difference, ΔP, exceeds the opposing difference in oncotic pressure, $\Delta\pi$. Therefore, at mean values of ΔP less than approximately 20 mmHg (the normal average value for $\Delta\pi$), the net driving force for filtration is nonexistent and SNGFR is zero. As ΔP increases above this threshold value, SNGFR also increases, but in a nonlinear manner. This nonlinearity is due in part to the fact that as ΔP increases the formation of ultrafiltrate causes a concurrent, although smaller, rise in glomerular plasma oncotic pressure that partially offsets the increment in ΔP. A decline in the value of ΔP leads to a parallel reduction in SNGFR, whereas a rise in ΔP results in a relatively minor increase in SNGFR.

AUTOREGULATION OF SNGFR

The kidney has the ability to maintain relatively constant blood flow despite marked declines in mean arterial pressure (MAP). In addition to renal blood flow, GFR is also autoregulated. Graded reductions in mean arterial pressure from 120 to 80 mmHg result in only modest falls in mean values for glomerular plasma flow (QA) and SNGFR. Further reduction in MAP to 60 mmHg causes steeper average declines in QA and SNGFR, indicating that the autoregulatory ability of the kidney has been exceeded. Autoregulation of GFR is largely the consequence of autoregulation of renal plasma flow.

TUBULOGLOMERULAR FEEDBACK (TGF)

TGF maintains the composition of the tubule fluid in the macula densa region within narrow limits by controlling GFR. Variations of NaCl concentration between ~20 and 60 mM/L cause inverse changes in GFR that, for the most part, are the result of a progressive increase in the afferent arteriolar resistance and a subsequent fall in the glomerular capillary pressure. The reductions in capillary pressure and GFR are rapidly inducible and reversible. This mechanism has been studied in micropuncture experiments, in which measurements of glomerular function are made while microperfusion techniques are used to alter the rate of flow through the loop of Henle. In these experiments, when the loop of Henle flow rate is increased, SNGFR generally declines.

Since the 1970s, adenosine has been proposed as the mediator of TGF based on the pharmacological data. Recently, this has been confirmed by the use of mouse strains with knockout mutations in the adenosine A_1-receptor gene. Mice lacking A_1 adenosine receptors have a complete lack of TGF.

TUBULAR PROCESSING OF FILTRATE

The human kidney produces approximately 150–180 L of protein-free filtrate per day. The renal tubules process this large volume to conserve essential nutrients (glucose, amino acids etc.), to eliminate potentially toxic substances (organic bases and acids, excess K^+, acid), and to reduce the quantity of salt and water excreted in the final urine to less than 1% of that filtered. The tubule portion of each nephron is divided into segments arranged in series; each segment has unique morphologic characteristics and transport functions (Table 57.1).

Overall function of the proximal tubule

The main function of the proximal tubule is bulk conservation of water and necessary solutes in a selective fashion. It is a very high-capacity segment that responds to changes in delivery. Because of the magnitude of its transport functions, its oxygen consumption is high.

The single active process is the Na^+/K^+-ATPase pump located at the basolateral membrane of all renal segments (Fig. 57.3). This pump lowers intracellular Na^+ concentration to levels between 10 and 20 mEq/L, thus creating a gradient between luminal and intracellular Na^+ concentration. By positioning passive transporters that are driven by the Na^+ gradient at the luminal side of the cell, this segment can carry out several transport processes. The passive transporters driven by the Na^+ gradient include a glucose–Na^+ cotransporter, an amino acid–Na^+ cotransporter, and Na^+–hydrogen ion exchangers (NHE).

The Na^+ pump located in all tubular cells is the single active process that drives the reabsorption of Na^+ and other solutes via the resulting Na^+ electrochemical gradient.

The above processes create an osmotic gradient between the lumen and the hyperosmotic intercellular space, thereby driving water reabsorption via water channels (aquaporins).

The proximal tubule can be functionally and morphologically divided into three distinct segments, termed S_1, S_2, and S_3. These are characterized by descending mitochodrial density, luminal surface area, and endoplasmic reticulum development. This morphologic simplification parallels decreasing contribution to fluid absorption and glucose and amino acid reclamation. The

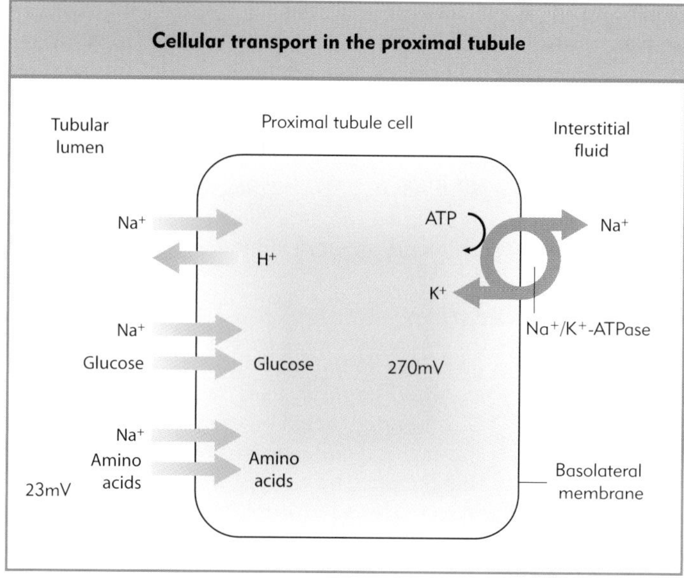

Figure 57.3 Cellular transport model for the proximal tubule. The Na^+/K^+-ATPase transports Na^+ from the interior of the cell across the basolateral membrane, creating a low intracellular Na^+ concentration and a negative intracellular electrical potential, which cause Na^+ to diffuse from the tubular lumen into the cell through the brush border. Glucose and amino acids are cotransported with Na^+ through the brush border of the tubular epithelial cells, followed by facilitated diffusion through the basolateral membranes. Hydrogen ions are antitransported with Na^+ from the interior of the cell across the brush border membrane and into the tubular lumen. Movement of Na^+ into the cell, down an electrochemical gradient established by the Na^+/K^+-ATPase on the basolateral membrane, provides the energy for transport.

S_3 segment in particular (located near the level of loop of Henle) is the most vulnerable part of the kidney in the face of ischemia and reperfusion injury owing to its precarious (im)balance between O_2 supply and demand.

Specific proximal tubule functions

Transport of Na^+ in the proximal convoluted tubule involves two phases: entry into the cell via the luminal membrane, and exit via the basolateral membrane. The latter process is effected primarily by the Na^+/K^+ pump. The transport of glucose, phosphate, sulfate, carboxylic acid, and amino acids is intimately linked to luminal Na^+ entry. In addition to these cotransport

Table 57.1 Segmental distribution of solute reabsorption along the nephron (95% of filtered)

Segment	**Na^+**			**HCO_{3-}**	**Ca^{2+}**	**PO_4^{2-}**
	Normal	*High ECV*	*Low ECV*			
Proximal tubule	67	50	80	85	70	80
Thick ascending limbs	20	30	14	10	20	–
Distal convoluted tubule	7	12	4	–	5–10	10
Collecting duct	5	2	2	5	5	–
Urine	1	6	0	0	1	10

ECV, extracellular volume.

mechanisms, Na^+ also enters the proximal tubular cell in a 1:1 exchange for hydrogen ion by the NHE (Fig. 57.3).

GLUCOSE REABSORPTION

Luminal entry of glucose is mediated by a Na^+–glucose transporter with 1:1 coupling. It is driven by the Na^+ gradient, and is delivery responsive but saturable, with a tubular maximum which, when exceeded, results in glucosuria.

AMINO ACID REABSORPTION

Luminal entry of amino acids is mediated by Na^+–amino acid transporters with 1:1 coupling. It is driven by the Na^+ gradient, and is delivery responsive but saturable, with a tubular maximum that is much higher than the corresponding glucose tubular maximum, hence amino aciduria is not readily observed even with very high plasma levels of amino acids. Detection of aminoaciduria is an indication of proximal tubular damage.

BICARBONATE RECLAMATION

The glomerular ultrafiltrate has a pH of 7.25, a $P\text{CO}_2$ of 60 mmHg and an HCO_3^- concentration of 24 mEq/L. In the proximal convoluted tubule (PCT), the tubule fluid is acidified to approximately pH 6.7. This acidification is accompanied by a decrease in the HCO_3^- concentration to 8 mEq/L. Together with the removal of ~50% of the filtered water in the PCT, this decrease in HCO_3^- concentration reflects reabsorption of ~75% of filtered HCO_3^-, such that the PCT reclaims the majority of filtered HCO_3^-. Further HCO_3^- reabsorption occurs in the proximal straight tubule (S_3). The proton secretory capacity, however, is far less in this segment than in the PCT. As a consequence of the decline in luminal pH in the proximal tubule, titratable buffers are titrated to their acid form, and ammonia is trapped in the tubule fluid. Hydrogen ions enter the lumen in exchange for Na^+. This process is carrier mediated by the NHE, is Na^+ dependent (high affinity) and is driven solely by *combined gradients* of the two cations. The process has an apparent tubular maximum (Tm) dependent on volume status.

WATER TRANSPORT

Water transport in the proximal tubule occurs mainly via transcellular pathways. Fluid reabsorption is iso-osmotic and driven by solute gradients. Because of the 'leakiness' of the epithelium in this nephron segment, most volume reabsorption can be driven by osmotic pressure differences of 2–3 mmol/kg. Water flow occurs mainly through vasopressin independent water channels traversing the membrane.

CALCIUM TRANSPORT

Approximately 10 g of Ca^{2+} are filtered across the glomerulus every day. This amount is many times greater than the total ECF Ca^{2+} content. Of the 10 g that are filtered, more than 98% is reabsorbed at various sites in the renal tubules, 70% in the proximal tubule. At this site, Ca^{2+} reabsorption does not appear to be under hormonal regulation. The reabsorption is linked to Na^+ reabsorption and is determined at least in part by volume status. When volume is depleted, Na^+ and Ca^{2+} reabsorption at this site are enhanced. Approximately 20% of the filtered Ca^{2+} is reabsorbed in the ascending limb of the loop of Henle.

PHOSPHATE TRANSPORT

Serum phosphate is approximately 85% filterable. Tubular transport mechanisms maintain phosphate homeostasis through the regulation of its reabsorption along the entire nephron, but concentrated in the proximal tubule. Under conditions of a normal phosphorus diet, approximately 85% of the filtered load of phosphate is reabsorbed by the proximal tubule. Na^+–phosphorus cotransport in the brush border membrane is energized by the electrochemical gradient for Na^+ and appears to be the rate-limiting step in reabsorption. A large number of factors, such as ECF volume, systemic acid–base balance, plasma phosphate, various hormones (parathyroid hormone, growth hormone, calcitonin, vitamin D), and pharmacologic agents, influence the renal excretion of phosphate.

MAGNESIUM TRANSPORT

The renal handling of Mg^{2+} involves filtration and partial tubular reabsorption. In humans, 3.5 g of Mg^{2+} are filtered over a 24-hour period, and only 3% of this amount is excreted in urine (100–150 mg/day), an amount equal to the daily net intestinal absorption. Twenty to 30% of filtered Mg^{2+} is reabsorbed in the proximal tubule. Although the fractional reabsorption of Mg^{2+} is only half that of Na^+, it changes in parallel with that of Na^+ in response to changes ECF volume.

URATE TRANSPORT

The renal excretion of urate is a complex process in humans, as there is a pronounced heterogeneity of urate transport within the proximal tubule. Bidirectional transport (reabsorption and secretion) occurs simultaneously within the proximal tubule. Urate is absorbed by a process that extends along the entire length of the proximal tubule. However, the influence of this absorptive movement is modified by the coexistent operation of a secretory mechanism throughout the proximal tubule. There is no evidence for active tubule transport of urate beyond the proximal tubule. The amount excreted in the final urine is only approximately 6–8% of that filtered.

Regulation of proximal tubule transport

The proximal tubule accounts for the reabsorption of two-thirds of the filtered Na^+ and is thus a prominent regulator of body Na^+. Systemic pH or its determinants ($P\text{CO}_2$, HCO_3^-) significantly affect proximal reabsorption of HCO_3^-. Reabsorption of HCO_3^- is directly related to proton concentration in the circulating blood; an increase in proton (a decrease in pH) enhances HCO_3^- reabsorption. *Angiotensin II* is the main hormonal regulator of Na^+ reabsorption in the proximal tubule by its control of the NHE. Angiotensin II in the physiologic range enhances Na^+ and fluid reabsorption in this segment. *Parathyroid hormone* inhibits fluid and HCO_3^- reabsorption; the decrease in fluid reabsorption is a consequence of the decrease in HCO_3^- transport. The primary effect of the hormone is probably inhibition of the NHE by a cAMP-dependent mechanism. *Catecholamines* increase reabsorption directly. The rich innervation of the proximal tubule and this direct effect highlight the importance of the renal nerves in regulating volume absorption. *Dopamine* inhibits proximal NaCl reabsorption. Renal denervation induces a natriuresis and renal nerve stimulation leads to Na^+ conservation through α-adrenoceptors.

The proximal tubules mediate the reabsorption of most filtered Na^+, which is regulated by angiotensin II.

Thin limb of the loop of Henle

The thin limb of the loop of Henle is composed of the thin descending limb (DLH) and the thin ascending limb (ALH). The DLH and ALH contribute importantly to the process of urinary concentration and dilution, primarily by passive transport of water and NaCl, respectively. The remarkable separation of passive water reabsorption in the DLH and passive NaCl reabsorption in the ALH is attributed to the abrupt change of the passive permeability properties of these segments at the tip of the loop of Henle.

The thin descending limb (DLH) begins at the end of the proximal tubule at the junction of the outer and inner stripes of the outer medulla. The thin descending limb is permeable to water but impermeable to Na^+ and Cl^-. This leads to water exit into a hypertonic interstitium and gradual concentration of the luminal solutes as water is progressively reabsorbed. The ascending thin limb (ALH) begins at the bend of the loop in long-looped nephrons. Short-looped nephrons have no ALH. The ALH is similar to the DLH in that it has a flat endothelial-like epithelium with minimal Na^+/K^+-ATPase activity. Therefore, it does not transport solutes actively. In contrast to the DLH, the ALH is water impermeable, moderately urea permeable, and highly NaCl permeable. As a result of these differences in permeability, the osmolarity of the tubular fluid can be passively decreased as the fluid moves from the bend of the loop of Henle towards the medullary thick ascending limb.

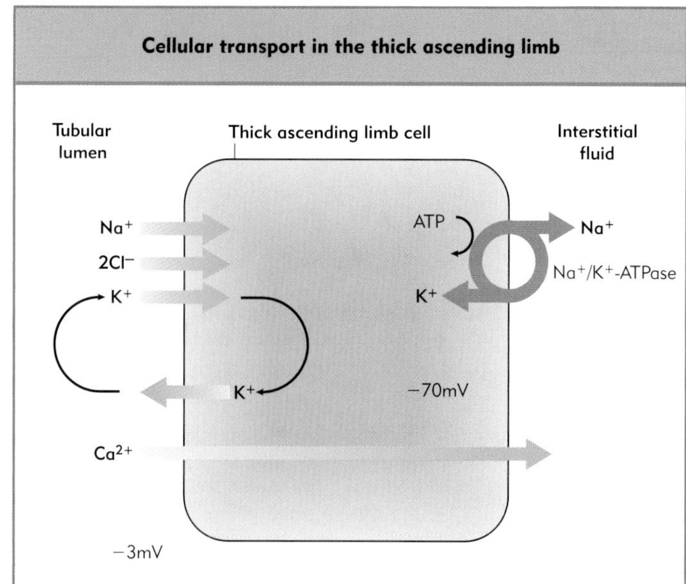

Figure 57.4 Cellular transport model for the thick ascending limb of the loop of Henle. The $Na^+/K^+/2Cl^-$ cotransporter in the luminal membrane transports these ions into the tubular cell using the potential energy provided by the Na^+/K^+-ATPase. Ca^{2+} is reabsorbed by all nephron segments through transcellular and paracellular routes.

Thick ascending limb of the loop of Henle

The thick ascending limb of the loop of Henle reabsorbs approximately 30% of the NaCl filtered at the glomerulus. This segment is responsible for the ability of mammals to dissociate the excretion of salt and water. It permits the dilution of urine by its ability to reabsorb solutes while being water impermeable, and assists the concentration of urine by its contribution to the creation of a hypertonic interstitium.

The basic mechanisms of Na^+ transport are similar in the medullary and cortical thick ascending limbs of the loop of Henle despite morphologic and permeability differences. Thick ascending limbs reabsorb NaCl at a rapid rate. The mechanism can again be best understood by separating this reabsorptive process into luminal plasma membrane entry and basolateral exit phases (Fig. 57.4). At the latter membrane the mechanism of Na^+ exit is mediated by Na^+/K^+-ATPase, as in other nephron segments.

At the luminal side, Na^+ entry is effected by means of a transporter that couples the entry of one Na^+ ion and one K^+ ion to two Cl^- ions for a stoichiometry of 1Na:1K:2Cl. This cotransporter is electroneutral and is driven by the concentration gradient for Na^+ created by the active transport of Na^+ at the basolateral membrane by the Na^+/K^+-ATPase. The transported Cl^- exits from the cell via basolateral pathways, either a Cl^- channel or a KCl cotransporter. Potassium re-enters the lumen via conductive pathways along the luminal membrane. The recycling of K^+ (positive charge) back to the lumen and the basolateral negative Cl^- current create a positive voltage inside the lumen. This positive transepithelial voltage, along with high permeability for cations, drives the passive transport of Ca^{2+}, Mg^{2+}, and ammonia. The large reabsorptive fluxes for Ca^{2+} and Mg^{2+} in this region of the nephron account for a major part of their total renal tubular reabsorption. Sodium reabsorption along these segments has another role: it dilutes the tubular fluid by removing solute, whereas water remains within the lumen because of its low water permeability. The ascending limb also provides the driving force for the generation of the osmotic gradient that is maintained by the countercurrent mechanism, and thus is responsible for the ability to concentrate the urine. Thus, interference with Na^+ transport in the thick limbs can alter water handling by the kidneys. The Na:K:2Cl transporter is the target for loop diuretics.

Increased delivery of fluid from the proximal tubule is associated with increased absolute Na^+ reabsorption in the loop of Henle. Thus, the loop of Henle is capable of reabsorbing most of the increase in load delivered from the proximal tubule. The effect of such increases in reabsorptive capacity would then be to minimize increases in delivery to the distal tubule and collecting duct.

Distal convoluted tubule

The distal convoluted tubule (DCT) is a morphologically and functionally heterogeneous segment that extends from the macula densa to the early branching of the cortical collecting tubule. The DCT possesses the highest activity of the basolateral Na^+/K^+-ATPase of any of the nephron segments. At the luminal membrane, a thiazide-sensitive NaCl cotransporter is responsible for Na^+ transport. Sodium reabsorption in the distal convoluted tubule is mineralocorticoid independent and results in a luminal negative potential difference. Active Ca^{2+} reabsorption occurs in this segment and is modulated by parathyroid hormone (Fig. 57.5). By inhibiting Na^+ reabsorption in the DCT, thiazides lower cellular Na^+ concentration and inhibit the lumen negative potential. This enhances Na^+ entry into the cell by Na^+/Ca^{2+} exchanger across the basolateral membrane, favoring basolateral Ca^{2+} exit. The resultant decrease in cell Ca^{2+} favors luminal

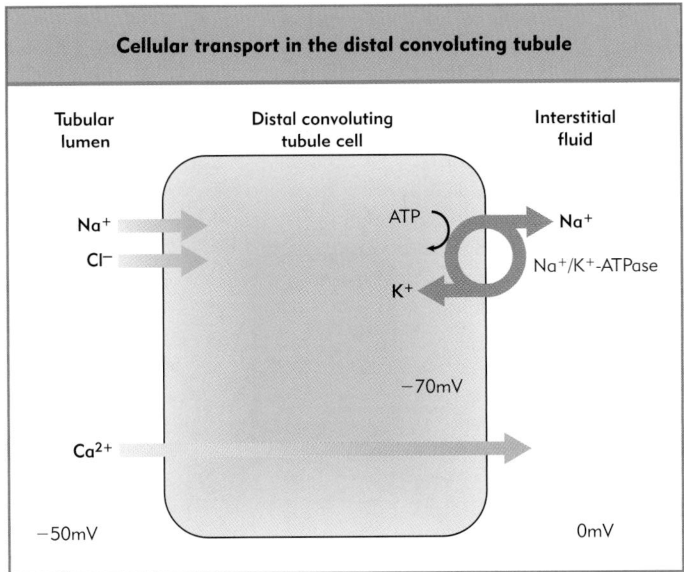

Figure 57.5 Cellular transport model for the distal convoluted tubule (DCT). The basolateral membrane Na^+/K^+-ATPase maintains a low intracellular Na^+ concentration; Na^+ is absorbed from the lumen through a luminal membrane Na^+/Cl^- cotransporter. Active Ca^{2+} reabsorption occurs in this segment.

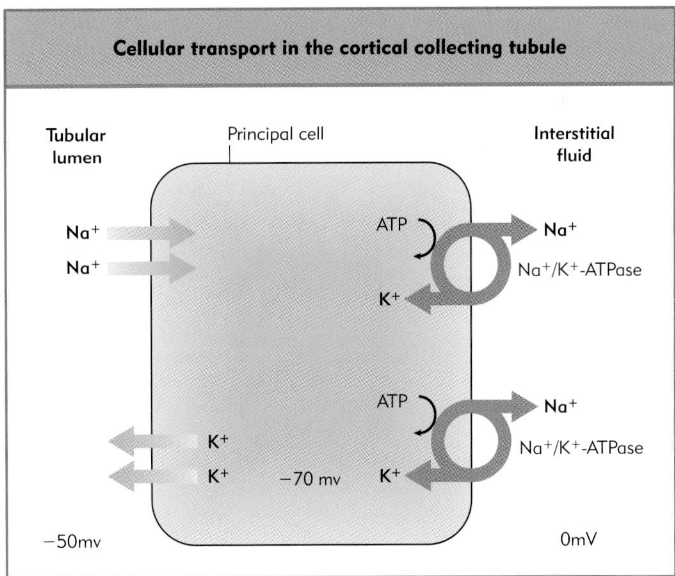

Figure 57.6 Cellular transport model for the cortical collecting tubule. The Na^+/K^+-ATPase maintains a high intracellular K^+ and low intracellular Na^+, favoring their passive diffusion across the luminal membrane through specific channels.

Ca^{2+} entry. The net effect is enhanced Ca^{2+} reabsorption by the DCT.

Collecting duct

The collecting duct consists of the cortical collecting tubule (CCT), the outer medullary collecting tubule (MCT), and the inner medullary collecting duct (IMCD). The collecting duct is the final regulator of excretion of many solutes. It fine-tunes the functions of the upstream segments. This is facilitated by the small volume that is delivered to it, and by the operation of multiple cell types with specialized functions. In general, this segment determines the excretion of K^+ and acid, and regulates the concentration of urine.

Mechanisms of transport

Transport in the CCT is driven primarily by basolateral Na^+/K^+-ATPase. Sodium entry occurs at the luminal membrane. The reabsorption of Na^+ is mineralocorticoid sensitive and generates a lumen with negative voltage that enhances K^+ exit via K^+ conductive pathways in the luminal membrane, and hydrogen ion secretion via a proton-translocating ATPase located at the luminal membrane. Potassium and hydrogen ion secretion in this segment can be enhanced by increased Na^+ delivery and inhibited by blockade of Na^+ transport (Fig. 57.6). The MCT has no appreciable Na^+ transport; its transport function is mostly related to hydrogen ion secretion and water transport. The IMCD reabsorbs NaCl through amiloride-sensitive conductive channels at the luminal membrane. The reabsorption of Na^+ is mineralocorticoid sensitive, and is inhibited by atrial natriuretic peptide (ANP).

The cortical collecting tubule is the major site of K^+ excretion and determinant of K^+ balance.

The CCT is the major site of K^+ excretion in the nephron. Because most of the filtered K^+ is reabsorbed in proximal portions of the tubule, K^+ secretion in the CCT becomes the major determinant of K^+ balance. The secretion of K^+ in this segment is achieved by a series of interlocked processes that can best be visualized by following their workings from the basolateral to the luminal membranes. Potassium entry at the basolateral membrane is achieved by the Na^+/K^+-ATPase, which maintains a high intracellular K^+. Potassium exit at the luminal membrane occurs through K^+ channels and is dependent on luminal voltage charge and flow. Luminal voltage is dependent on Na^+ reabsorption that creates a negative charge. Enhanced K^+ excretion occurs with enhanced Na^+/K^+-ATPase activity, enhanced K^+ channel permeability, and increased luminal negativity. The increase in Na^+/K^+-ATPase activity in the CCT described above is the crucial mechanism of K^+ adaptation; this increase in activity is aldosterone dependent.

Hormonal effects

Aldosterone receptors have been identified in the cortical and medullary collecting tubules, and the direct effects of the hormone are generally restricted to these segments. At the level of the CCT aldosterone has three major effects: enhanced Na^+ permeability of the luminal membrane by increasing synthesis of Na^+ conductive pathways; stimulation of basolateral Na^+/K^+-ATPase activity; and increased production of ATP. All of these effects are geared to increase Na^+ transport (reabsorption) in this segment. This leads to an increased negative lumen potential difference that potentiates the secretion of K^+ and hydrogen ions. At the level of the medullary collecting tubule, aldosterone enhances acidification; this is Na^+ independent and may be facilitated chronically by stimulation of the proton-ATPase.

Approximately 85% of ingested K^+ is eliminated in the urine and the remainder (<15%) is excreted in the feces. The predominant site of K^+ regulation is the collecting duct system.

A number of factors modify K^+ transport by the distal nephron to alter the rate of K^+ excretion. High plasma K^+ stimulates K^+ secretion by the distal nephron, and low concentrations impair it. K^+ secretion by the CCT varies directly with the rate of fluid delivery. Vasopressin stimulates Na^+ reabsorption and K^+ secretion by both the DCT and the CCT. Aldosterone stimulates K^+ secretion by the CCT by altering the conductance of the apical membrane to both Na^+ and K^+, and by increasing the number of Na^+/K^+-ATPase pumps in the basolateral membrane. Increased excretion of poorly permeant anions such as sulfate is accompanied by kaliuresis. Acute acidosis inhibits K^+ secretion by the distal nephron and alkalosis stimulates it.

ACIDIFICATION

Fluid delivered to the distal nephron is normally low in HCO_3^- (5–7 mEq/L) and pH (6.5–6.7). The distal nephron reabsorbs the remaining HCO_3^- and further lowers the luminal pH in order to titrate filtered buffers and trap ammonia. Acidification of the urine finally excreted depends largely on distal secretory mechanisms, which titrate nonreabsorbed inorganic phosphate to a pH as low as 4.5. This process is limited by the availability of phosphate in the urine. A larger portion of total acid excretion results from the titration of available ammonia to ammonium ion, a process that can be modulated more flexibly and which increases in the presence of acidosis. Acidification is enhanced in the presence of systemic acidosis, hypokalemia, and increased mineralocorticoid levels, and is decreased by alkalosis, low mineralocorticoid levels, and reduced luminal buffer availability.

REGULATION OF URINE TONICITY

Formation of dilute urine

The tubular fluid presented to the loop of Henle is iso-osmotic with plasma, as water is reabsorbed passively down the osmotic gradient caused by the active reabsorption of solute. In the thick ascending limb of the loop of Henle and the distal collecting duct, however, solute is actively reabsorbed, but water does not follow because these segments are almost impermeable to water. The tubular fluid here is hypotonic (see Fig. 57.5). In the absence of vasopressin, the final part of the DCT, the connecting tubule, and the collecting tubules are impermeable to water and the tubular fluid remains hypotonic, producing dilute urine.

Formation of concentrated urine

The production of concentrated urine depends on the long loops of Henle of the juxtaglomerular nephrons passing through the increasing hypertonic renal medulla (Fig. 57.7). The generation of the increasing solute concentration gradient through the medulla depends on the differential permeability to urea and NaCl of the thin ascending limb of the loop of Henle and the collecting tubule. Because of the low permeability to urea of the thin ascending limb, the tubular fluid presented to the collecting tubule has a high concentration of urea relative to the interstitial fluid. The collecting tubule is permeable to urea, which passes out of the collecting tubule in its course through the medulla. This raises the osmolarity of the interstitium of the medulla, and hence water passes passively out of the descending limb of the loop of Henle. As fluid passes down the descending limb, less water passes from the tubule to the interstitium because the tubular fluid becomes progressively concentrated as the water leaves. This generates a concentration gradient down the medulla, as the interstitial solutes become less diluted by water leaving the descending limb as it progresses from the outer to the inner medulla. When the tubular fluid reaches the thin ascending limb of the loop of Henle, which is permeable to NaCl, NaCl passes out of the tubule down its concentration gradient, which becomes progressively smaller from inner to outer medulla as the fluid ascends the loop of Henle. This differential reabsorption of NaCl up the ascending limb serves to increase the concentration gradient down the medulla, and hence the loop of Henle has been termed a countercurrent multiplier. In the presence of vasopressin the collecting tubules are permeable to water, which flows out of the tubules down the concentration gradient as they pass through the medulla, thus producing concentrated urine.

Another countercurrent mechanism is involved in supplying blood to the medulla without destroying the concentration gradient necessary for the production of concentrated urine. The vasae rectae are the peritubular capillaries that accompany the loops of Henle as they penetrate and then return through the medulla. The capillary loops of the vasae rectae allow passive countercurrent exchange of solute and water between descending and ascending blood as it follows the hairpin course of the loops of Henle.

MEASUREMENT OF RENAL FUNCTION

Renal clearance is the volume of plasma completely cleared of a substance by the kidney per unit time (units are mL/min). The clearance of a substance can be calculated from the equation $C = UV/P$, where U and P are the concentrations of the substance in urine and plasma, respectively, and V is the rate at which urine is produced. For a substance that it is relatively filtered at the glomeruli and which is neither secreted nor absorbed by the renal tubules, the clearance will equal the GFR. Such a substance is inulin, which is a plant polysaccharide. An endogenous alternative to inulin is creatinine, a metabolite of muscle creatine. Creatinine is not reabsorbed or metabolized by the kidney and its rate of secretion by the tubules is clinically negligible. Clearance of these substances gives a measure of GFR. The renal plasma flow can be estimated from the renal clearance of a substance that is completely eliminated in its first pass through the kidney. This requires that the substance be filtered at the glomeruli and secreted extremely efficiently by the tubules. Para-aminohippuric acid (PAH) meets these criteria. Like creatinine, it is an endogenous substance, being the end-product of metabolism of aromatic amino acids. Having calculated the renal plasma flow, the RBF can be calculated from the hematocrit. Another measure that is sometimes of interest is the filtration fraction, which is the ratio of the GFR to the renal plasma flow. The filtration fraction can be calculated from the creatinine and PAH clearances.

Clearance of creatinine, a metabolite of muscle creatine that is filtered but not reabsorbed, metabolized or secreted by the kidney, reflects glomerular filtration rate.

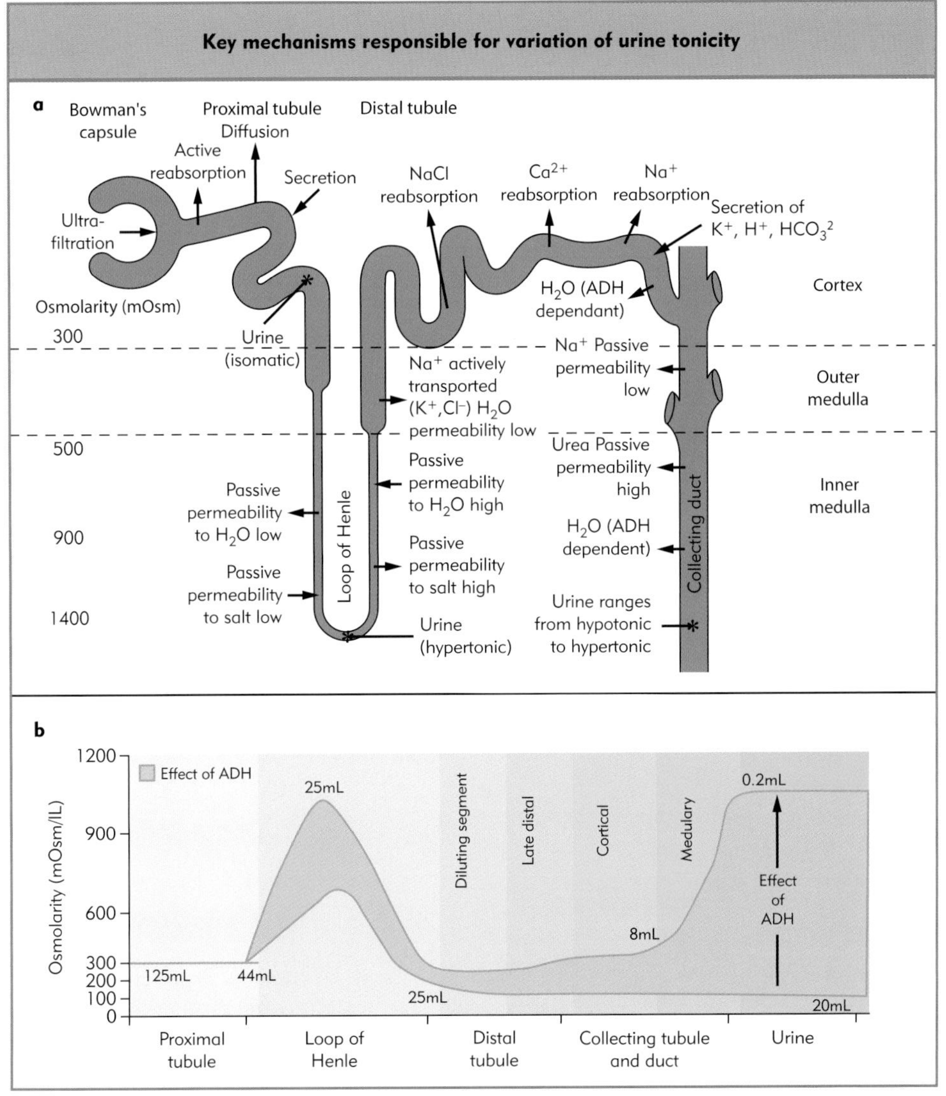

Figure 57.7 Key mechanisms responsible for variations of urine tonicity. Differences in permeability to Na^+, Cl^-, urea, and water in the loop of Henle and collecting duct (a) generate an increasing osmotic gradient from cortex to medulla and produce hypotonic urine in the distal convoluted tubule (b). In the presence of vasopressin, water is reabsorbed from the terminal distal convoluted tubule and collecting ducts, concentrating the urine. In the absence of vasopressin (or ADH), the permeability of the distal convoluted tubule and collecting ducts to water is low and the urine remains hypotonic. Volumes indicate approximate flow through each tubular segment in mL/min. ADH, antidiuretic hormone.

NEUROENDOCRINE REGULATION

The physiology of urine formation and the reabsorption of filtered Na^+ and water is determined by both intra- and extrarenal factors. Major extrarenal factors are aldosterone, catecholamines released via the sympathetic nervous system, antidiuretic hormone (ADH/vasopressin), and atrial natriuretic peptide (ANP). Osmoreceptors located primarily in the hypothalamus sense increases in blood osmolarity above a threshold of 280 mmol/L. Increases in effective osmolarity enhance the electrical activity of osmoreceptor cells, which in turn increase the release of vasopressin from the posterior pituitary gland (neurohypophysis). Vasopressin release is inhibited by increased stretch of atrial baroreceptors with an increase in preload. Therefore, changes in both osmolarity and intravascular volume regulate its release. A 1% increase in blood osmolarity can reduce urine flow to one-third and increase urine concentration threefold. Vasopressin acts primarily on V_2 receptors in the cortical collecting tubules and medullary collecting ducts to increase water permeability, leading to increased water reabsorption and the production of small-volume highly concentrated urine. An inability to produce vasopressin or defects in V_2 receptor results in *diabetes insipidus*, a disease characterized by the production of large-volume low-concentration urine and persistent thirst. Increased release of vasopressin in the syndrome of inappropriate ADH release (SIADH) results in impaired water excretion accompanied by hyponatremia and hypo-osmolality. Whereas low levels of vasopressin leads to increased RBF and renal medullary washout, vasopressin at high concentrations binds to V_1 receptors in vascular smooth muscle and mesangial cells and leads to powerful vasoconstriction, increased arterial blood pressure, and reduced renal blood flow and GFR.

Vasopressin increases water permeability in the collecting tubules to increase water reabsorption from urine; disorders result from increased (SIADH) and reduced (diabetes insipidus) release.

The renin–angiotensin–aldosterone system is a critical part of the neuroendocrine response to regulate Na^+ and K^+ homeostasis and blood pressure (Fig. 57.8). Renin is released from the granular cells of the juxtaglomerular apparatus in response to activation of the sympathetic nervous system, stimulation of

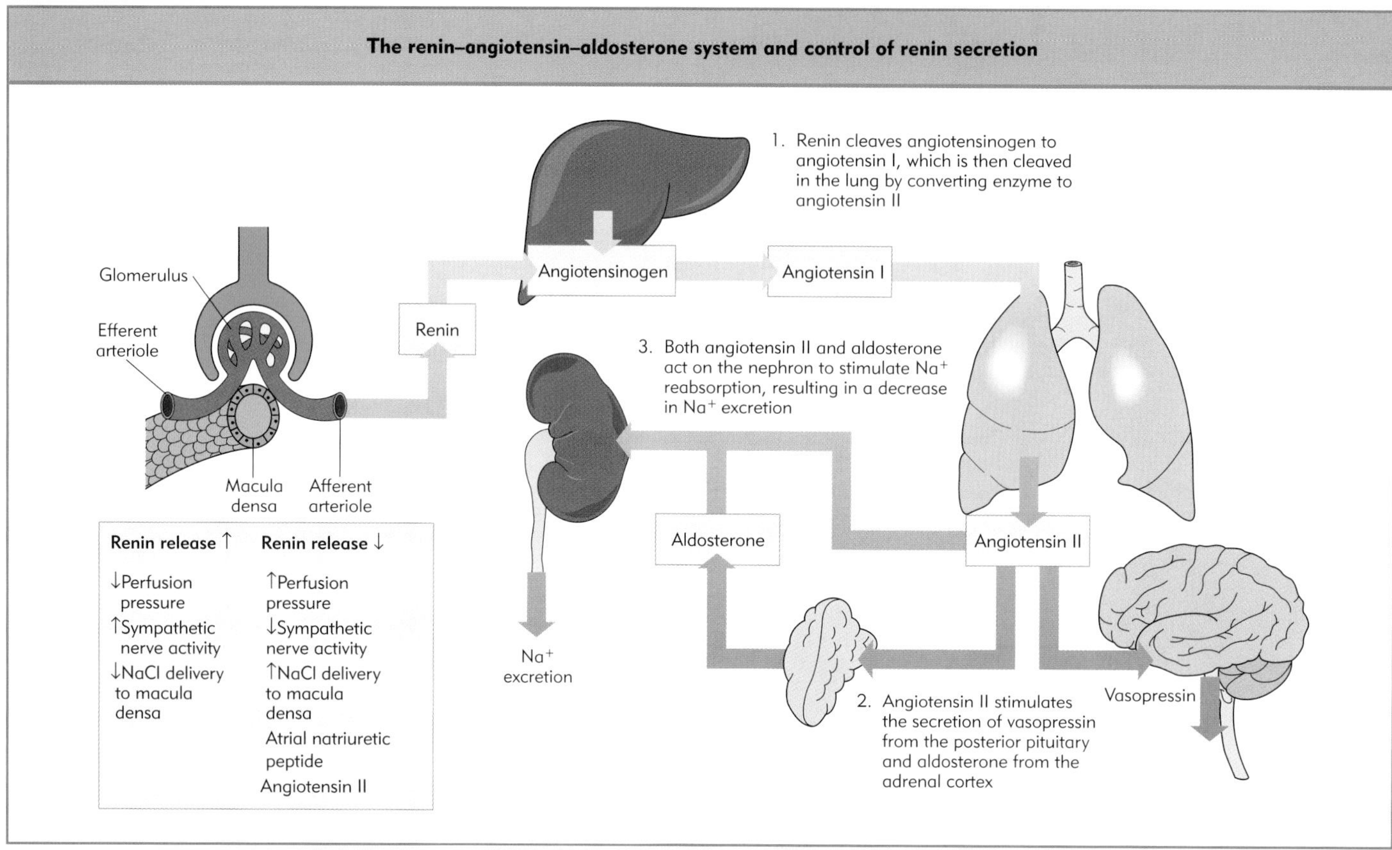

Figure 57.8 The renin–angiotensin–aldosterone system, and factors that control the secretion of renin. (Reproduced with permission from Berne RM, Levy MN. Principles of physiology. St Louis, MO: Mosby; 2003.)

intrarenal baroreceptors, or reduced delivery of NaCl to the macular densa. Renin catalyzes the proteolysis of angiotensinogen to angiotensin I in the systemic circulation. Angiotensin I is converted to angiotensin II by angiotensin-converting enzyme (ACE) in the lungs. Angiotensin II stimulates the release of aldosterone from adrenal cortex. Aldosterone acts in the distal tubules and collecting ducts to regulate the excretion of Na^+ and K^+.

ANP, originally found in cardiac atria and subsequently in other tissues such as brain, is released in response to increases in intravascular volume. It acts on the arterial and venous systems, adrenal gland, and kidneys to decrease intravascular volume and reduce blood pressure. Actions include vascular smooth muscle relaxation, sympathetic tone reduction, and inhibition of renin and aldosterone secretion, resulting in reduced Na^+ retention.

KIDNEY TRANSPLANTATION

Kidney transplantation is increasing, partly because of an increased number of living donor transplants. Uremic end-stage renal disease has many causes (diabetes mellitus, immune-mediated kidney destruction, hypertension, chronic infection, etc.) and results in fluid overload, electrolyte imbalance, and acidosis. Even patients on dialysis therapy develop secondary systemic dysfunction, such as peripheral neuropathy, coagulopathy, pleural effusions, osteodystrophy, and immune dysfunction.

The ischemic tolerance of the kidney is longer than that of other visceral organs; this allows sufficient time for ABO matching, cross-matching of recipient serum with donor lymphocytes, and HLA tissue typing. If indicated, patients should be dialyzed before the operation to correct acidosis, hyperkalemia, and volume overload.

Mannitol and sometimes furosemide are routinely given immediately before the removal of the donor kidney. Subsequently, there is brisk diuresis in the living donor, requiring aggressive hydration before kidney removal and during the early postoperative period. The rationale for diuretic therapy is to maintain tubular perfusion and filtration of the donor kidneys. Mannitol may also protect against reperfusion injury by scavenging free radicals.

Rejection of a transplanted kidney is a devastating complication. Recently, anti-T-lymphocyte antibody has been utilized in transplant recipients to reduce the incidence of delayed graft function. The rationale for this is to prevent T-lymphocyte-mediated tissue injury in promoting rejection and reperfusion injury.

The rationale for dopamine use in renal protection is based on its diuretic properties and its effects on renal perfusion and blood flow. However, a global increase in renal blood flow per se may not be beneficial and may actually worsen renal ischemia, as dopamine increases both cortical and medullary blood flow. Agents that selectively increase medullary blood flow without systemic hemodynamic perturbation are not yet clinically available. Dopamine may be beneficial in maintaining systemic perfusion pressure for the newly implanted kidney. Patients with end-stage renal disease are routinely hypertensive preoperatively, and maintenance of blood pressure is critical for preservation of kidney perfusion and organ function.

Key references

Berne RM, Levy MN. Principles of physiology. St Louis, MO: Mosby; 2003.

Brown R, Ollerstam A, Johansson B et al. Abolished tubuloglomerular feedback and increased plasma renin in adenosine A_1 receptor-deficient mice. Am J Physiol Regul Integr Comp Physiol. 2001;281:R1362–7.

Koeppen BM, Stanton BA. Renal physiology. St Louis, MO: Mosby; 2001.

Schnermann J. Adenosine mediates tubuloglomerular feedback. Am J Physiol Regul Integr Comp Physiol. 2002;283:R276–7.

Vander AJ. Renal physiology. New York: McGraw-Hill; 1994.

Further reading

Lieberthal W, Nigam SK. Acute renal failure. II. Experimental models of acute renal failure: imperfect but indispensable Am J Physiol Renal Physiol. 2000;278:F1–F12.

Salahudeen AK. Cold ischemic injury of transplanted kidneys: new insights from experimental studies. Am J Physiol Renal Physiol. 2004;287:F181–7.

Schwiebert EM, Kishore BK. Extracellular nucleotide signaling along the renal epithelium. Am J Physiol Renal Physiol. 2001;280:F945–63.

Chapter 58

Renal pathophysiology

Manuel L Fontes, Susan Garwood and Solomon Aronson

TOPICS COVERED IN THIS CHAPTER

- **Acute renal failure**
    - Pathogenesis of acute renal failure
- **Hypertensive renal disease**
- **Management of perioperative renal failure**
    - Dopamine
    - Mannitol
    - Furosemide
    - Atrial natriuretic peptide
    - Calcium channel blockers and other agents
    - Perioperative oliguria

In patients with renal disease, optimal perioperative management is demanding because the recognition of subtle change is difficult. As our understanding of renal disease evolves, traditional answers have turned into new questions. Recent insights include the intrarenal actions of intrinsically produced vasogenic substances, and the involvement of inflammatory mediators, both humoral and cellular, in the pathogenesis of renal dysfunction.

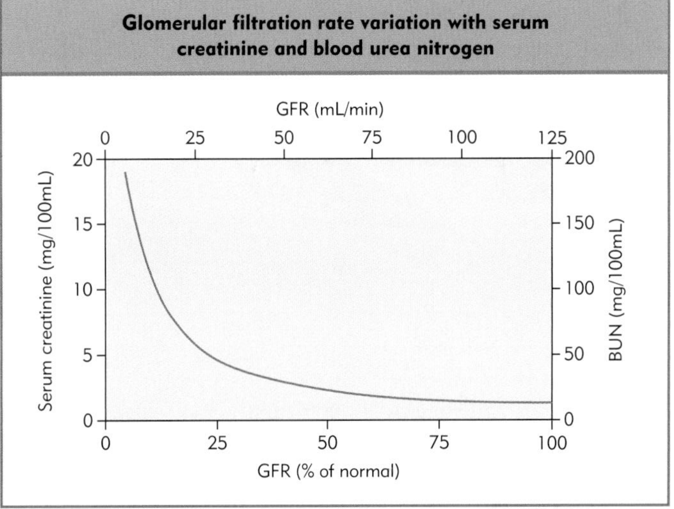

Figure 58.1 Relationship between the rate of glomerular filtration (GFR) and the serum creatinine concentration or the blood urea nitrogen (BUN) concentration. Absolute values for the GFR, as determined by inulin clearance, refer to measurements in healthy adults and from patients who are in nitrogen balance on a normal protein intake. Although there is considerable scatter of these values among individuals, a single average curve has been drawn; however, for a particular person whose GFR has been reduced by, for example, 50%, the serum creatinine concentration could lie anywhere between about 1.4 and 3.0 mg/dL.

ACUTE RENAL FAILURE

Symptoms of renal failure typically are not detected until less than 40% of normal functioning nephrons remain, and uremic symptoms do not occur until less than 5% of normal functioning nephrons remain (Fig. 58.1). Acute renal failure (ARF) is attributed to several mechanisms involving tubular, vascular, and/or glomerular effects. Typically, an early compensatory phase of normal renal adaptation (e.g. pre-prerenal failure) progresses to ARF (Fig. 58.2). Depending on renal function reserve, this may occur over a period of hours to days. At this point, the decline in renal function results in retention of nitrogenous end products of metabolism and an inability to maintain fluid and electrolyte homeostasis.

With wide variations in the definition of 'acute renal failure' in the literature and with no consensus on biochemical markers of renal dysfunction, the design of therapeutic trials and interpretation of results is difficult. For example, ARF in the perioperative period has been defined as the need for postoperative dialysis, or as a postoperative serum creatinine level exceeding a predetermined preoperative value (e.g. an increase of 0.5 mg/dL (440 μmol/L) or an increase of >50%). Oliguria (urine output of < 400 mL/day, or <20 mL/h) is a common marker of ARF, but it too lacks both sensitivity and specificity.

Perioperative ARF heralds a poor prognosis because of the loss of renal function and because of the life-threatening associated complications, including sepsis, gastrointestinal hemorrhage, and CNS dysfunction. The incidence of renal dysfunction following certain high-risk surgical procedures is as high as 50% (depending on the population analyzed and the methods used to define ARF). It is estimated that perioperative renal failure leads to 50% of acute renal replacement therapy. The associated

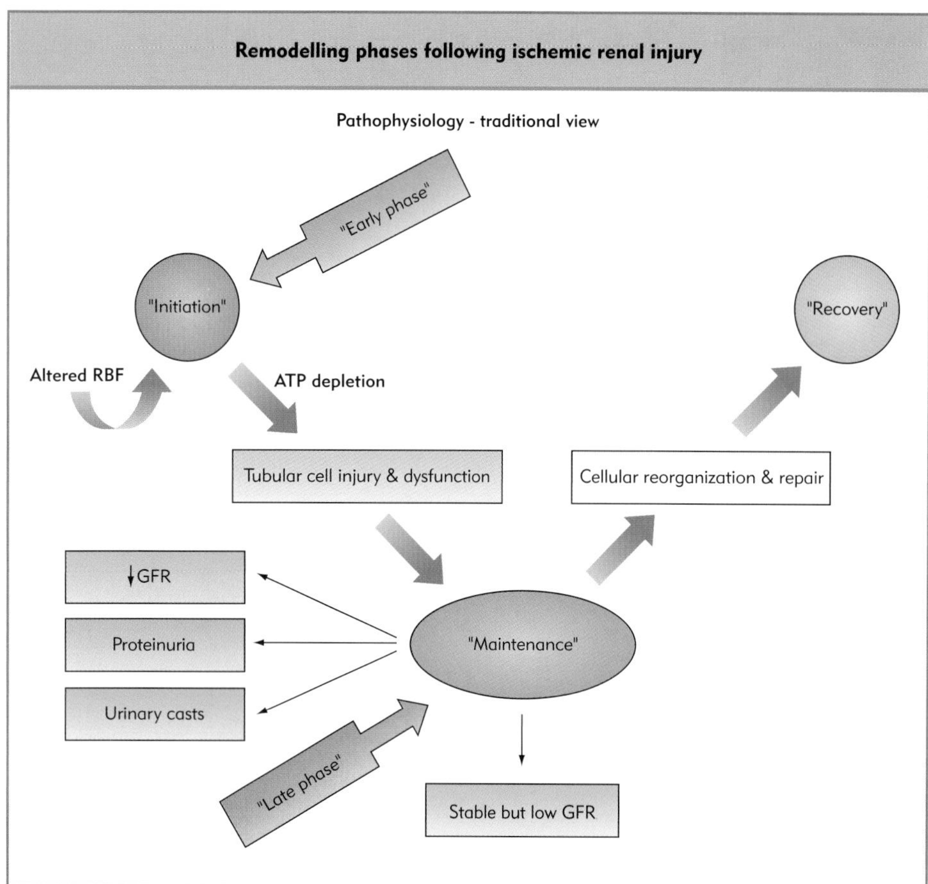

Figure 58.2 Remodeling phases following ischemic renal injury. Following an ischemic insult, multiple functional and structural changes take place at both the microcellular and the macrocellular levels. The first of these changes is referred to as the 'initiation phase' or the 'early phase', marked by loss of high-energy phosphates, lactic acidosis, and cellular swelling. Next, tubular dysfunction occurs, with inability to concentrate solute, increasing proteinuria, the presence of backleak, and varying degree of glomerular impairment. A late phase then follows, whereby the peak injury is reached, with stabilization of GFR reduction and commencement of structural remodeling. In an adaptive remodeling state cellular repair occurs, with eventual normalization of GFR and renal clearance, i.e. the 'recovery phase'.

mortality is excessive, with 20–90% of affected individuals dying postoperatively. Despite major improvements in surgical techniques, perioperative monitoring, and adjuvant therapies aimed at mitigating renal dysfunction, neither morbidity nor mortality related to renal events has diminished over the past few decades. The related costs for treatment of renal failure are prohibitive and have a tremendous impact on resource utilization, doubling intensive care unit stay and quadrupling overall hospital stay.

Pre-existing renal insufficiency, detected or undetected, is an important risk factor for perioperative acute renal failure.

With inadequate renal blood flow, injury is commonly caused by drugs that alter intrarenal distribution of blood flow, abnormal hemodynamics, or pre-existing disease (Table 58.1). Patients who have pre-existing renal insufficiency are especially prone to ARF during cardiovascular surgery. Patients who have diabetes mellitus and renal insufficiency are especially vulnerable to radiocontrast agents. Clinical conditions such as heart failure alone do not cause renal failure on the basis of decreased renal blood flow. Renal dysfunction follows heart failure only in the presence of other nephrotoxic factors, such as radiocontrast agents, nonsteroidal anti-inflammatory drugs, antibiotic agents, or hypoxemia. Acute tubular necrosis is believed to occur in this environment as a result of the combined effects of heart failure-induced vasoconstriction, enhanced reabsorptive activity and oxygen demand, and mismatch between local and circulating vasodilating agents (prostaglandins and nitric oxide) and potent vasoconstrictors (endothelin-1, vasopressin, and norepinephrine). Evidence for this comes from animal models of heart failure that demonstrate preservation of renal function and morphology prior to exposure to known nephrotoxins. It is believed that heart failure alone induces upregulation of renal endothelial nitric oxide synthase (eNOS) as well as induction of prostaglandin synthesis inclusive of the inducible cyclo-oxygenase-2 (COX-2) isoenzyme. These compensatory vasodilators play an important role, particularly in the medulla. With heart failure such compensatory responses to acute renal insult are markedly reduced, resulting in significant rise in both creatinine and plasma urea. Upon histologic inspection, the outer medulla shows extensive necrosis. Similarly, in humans the pathologic findings in ARF are extremely variable. Patients with limited reserve are most sensitive to further renal injury, but certain individuals are more susceptible as a result of genetic tendencies.

Risk factors augment the risk of ARF (Table 58.2). In coronary bypass surgery, the following perioperative risks have been identified: pre-existing renal dysfunction, prior cardiac surgery, diabetes, hyperglycemia (glucose >300 mg/dL just prior to surgery), acute congestive heart failure, and low cardiac output requiring multiple inotropic support or the use of intra-aortic balloon counterpulsation. The interaction of various acute risk factors appears to be central in the pathogenesis of ARF. In noncardiac surgery, recognizable predictors of postoperative ARF include pre-existing renal dysfunction that is most often undetected preoperatively because both physiologic and biochemical markers in clinical practice are generally insensitive.

Table 58.1 Causes of renal hypoperfusion associated with acute renal failure

Intravascular volume depletion (hypovolemia)
Major trauma, burns, crush syndrome Fever Hemorrhage Diuretic use Pancreatitis, vomiting, diarrhea, peritonitis, dehydration, bowel preparation
Decreased cardiac output
Congestive heart failure or low-output syndrome Pulmonary hypertension, massive pulmonary embolism Positive-pressure mechanical ventilation
Increased renal/systemic vascular resistance ratio
Renal vasoconstriction: α-adrenoceptor agonists, hypercalcemia, amphotericin B (amphotericin), cyclosporin A (ciclosporin) System vasodilation: afterload reduction (vasodilators), antihypertensive medications, anaphylactic shock, anesthesia, sepsis
Renovascular obstruction
Renal artery: atherosclerosis, embolism, thrombosis, dissecting aneurysm, vasculitis Renal vein: thrombosis, compression
Glomerular and small vessel obstruction
Glomerulonephritis Vasculitis Toxemia of pregnancy Hemolytic uremic syndrome Disseminated intravascular coagulation Malignant hypertension Radiation injury
Increased blood viscosity
Multiple myeloma Macroglobulinemia Polycythemia
Interference with renal autoregulation
Prostaglandin inhibitors with congestive heart failure, nephrotic syndrome, cirrhosis, hypovolemia Angiotensin-converting enzyme (ACE) inhibitors in presence of renal artery stenosis or congestive heart failure

Table 58.2 Risk factors for the development of acute renal failure

Acute
Volume depletion Aminoglycosides Radiocontrast dye exposure Nonsteroidal anti-inflammatory drugs Septic shock Hemoglobinuria or myoglobinuria
Chronic
Pre-existing renal disease Hypertension Congestive heart failure Diabetes mellitus Advanced age Cirrhosis of the liver
Intraoperative
Aortovascular surgery Biliary tract surgery Cardiopulmonary bypass and cardiac surgery Unstable hemodynamics Aortorenal vascular resistance maldistribution

Under normal physiologic conditions, homeostasis may be maintained despite substantially reduced renal function. Thus, impaired functional reserve capacity becomes evident only when perioperative stress severely comprises renal function.

Intrinsic renal causes of ARF are described according to the primary lesion (i.e. tubular, interstitial, vascular, or glomerular). Tubular injury is the most common dysfunction seen during the perioperative period, and is usually ischemic in origin. This is evident in aortic surgery, in which the ischemic burden is much more severe following suprarenal cross-clamping rather than infrarenal cross-clamping (Fig. 58.3). Glomerular function rapidly deteriorates during the first few hours postoperatively, and, depending on the duration of ischemia and other associated risks, may or may not normalize. Prerenal azotemia and acute tubular necrosis represent extreme examples of the same problem. Most cases of ischemic renal failure are reversible, although irreversible critical necrosis can occur if ischemia is prolonged and severe. Direct toxicity is the second most common cause of perioperative ARF. Ischemia and toxicity often combine to cause ARF in high-risk patients. Common toxins encountered during the perioperative period include aminoglycoside antibiotics, radiocontrast agents, and chemotherapeutic agents (e.g. cisplatin). Acute interstitial nephritis, secondary to an acute allergic reaction, is another less frequent cause of perioperative renal failure.

Pathogenesis of acute renal failure

Normally, renal blood flow (1–1.25 L/min) far exceeds renal intrinsic oxygen requirement. Essentially, all blood passes through the glomeruli, and about 10% of renal blood flow is filtered (a glomerular filtration rate (GFR) of 125 mL/min in the normal adult). The basal normal renal blood flow is 300–500 mL/min/100 g tissue, which is greater than that in most other organs. This primarily reflects blood flow to the cortical glomeruli, as perfusion to the inner medulla and papilla is only about 10% of total flow. Because the renal cortex contains most of the glomeruli and depends on oxidative metabolism for energy, ischemic hypoxia initially injures cortical structures, particularly the pars recta of the proximal tubules. As ischemia persists, glucose, glycogen, and other energy substrates are consumed, and the medulla, which depends to a greater extent on glycolysis for its energy sources, is also affected.

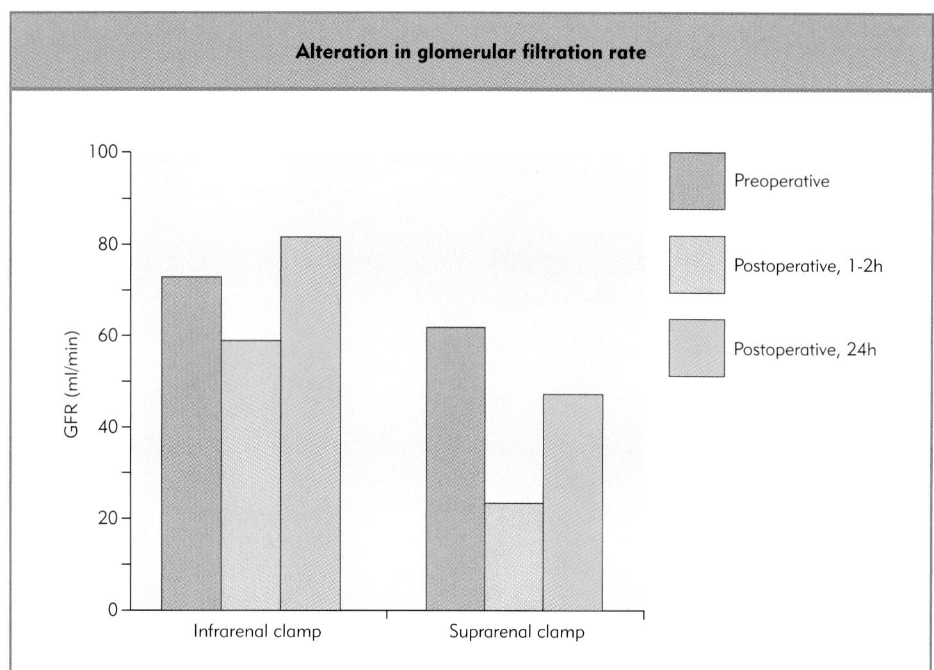

Figure 58.3 Alteration in glomerular filtration rate (GFR) in response to surgery. The extent of ischemic injury varies according to risk factors, the duration of ischemia, and the type of surgery. In abdominal aortic surgery the GFR is markedly reduced by 2 hours following a suprarenal aortic cross-clamp, with residual reduction at 24 hours postoperatively. In contrast, infrarenal lesions undergo only a small decrement in GFR that is very transient, returning to baseline by the following day after surgery.

Renal clearance is determined by the delivery of waste products to the kidney (i.e. renal blood flow) and the ability of the kidneys to extract them (GFR). A series of systemic and renal compensatory responses is activated initially to preserve ultrafiltration and renal clearance. The hallmark of experimental models of hemodynamically mediated ARF is a reduction of renal blood flow (generally >50%) for at least 40–60 minutes. Once a decrease in renal perfusion is established, GFR is disproportionately depressed compared to the decline in blood flow. When renal blood flow is decreased sufficiently to depress GFR to less than 5% of normal, blood flow may only be depressed by 25–50% of normal. Hence, although decreased renal blood flow is the initiating event, most of the time there are clearly other factors (tubular pathology) that account for abnormal filtration.

The response to renal hypoperfusion involves three major regulatory mechanisms that support renal function: afferent arteriolar dilatation increases renal perfusion; efferent arteriolar resistance increases the filtration fraction; and hormonal and neural responses improve renal perfusion pressure by increasing intravascular volume, thereby indirectly increasing cardiac output (Fig. 58.4). The afferent arterioles react to reductions in perfusion pressure by smooth muscle relaxation to decrease renal vascular resistance. This property represents a relaxation response or myogenic reflex to reduced transmural pressure across the arteriolar wall.

The kidney also possesses a tubuloglomerular feedback mechanism to maintain salt and water excretion. Decreased solute delivery to the macula densa in the cortical portion of the thick ascending limb of the loop of Henle results in relaxation of the juxtaposed afferent arteriolar smooth muscle cells, thereby improving glomerular perfusion and filtration.

Reduced delivery of Na^+ to the macula densa also causes the release of renin from the granular cells of the juxtaglomerular apparatus. Renin catalyzes the cleavage of angiotensin I from

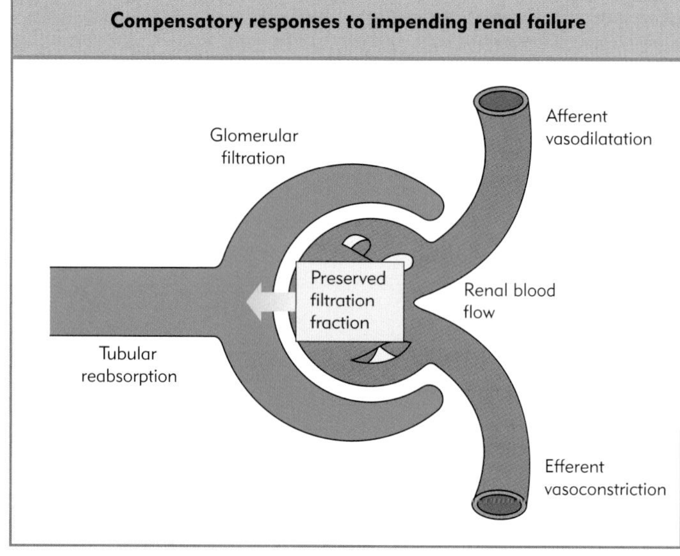

Figure 58.4 Compensatory responses to impending acute renal failure.

angiotensinogen. Angiotensin I is then transformed into angiotensin II in the lungs by angiotensin-converting enzyme (ACE). Angiotensin II stimulates the production of aldosterone, which stimulates the reabsorption of Na^+ and water, primarily in the distal tubule and collecting ducts (Chapter 57). Initially, angiotensin II exerts a selective vasoconstrictive effect on the efferent arteriole. This occurs in part because the kidney synthesizes prostaglandins during hemodynamic instability and increased adrenergic stimulation. Prostaglandin E_2 (PGE_2) reduces the vasoconstrictive effect of angiotensin II (a very potent vasoconstrictor) on the afferent arteriole and thereby preserves renal blood flow. Prostaglandin synthesis is inhibited when hydration, renal perfusion, and Na^+ balance are normal; in these circumstances it does not affect renal function.

A selective increase in efferent arteriole resistance decreases glomerular plasma flow, thereby preserving GFR. Glomerular filtration is augmented because capillary pressure upstream from the site of vasoconstriction rises. This mechanism enables the kidney to offer high vascular resistance to contribute to the maintenance of systemic blood pressure without compromising its filtration function. Efferent arteriolar resistance is changed largely through the action of angiotensin II.

The mechanisms that influence efferent arteriolar vasoconstriction ultimately overwhelm the system and cause afferent arteriolar vasoconstriction as well. The resulting decrease in filtration fraction is a hallmark of ischemic ARF. Histopathologic data indicate that the proximal tubules bear the brunt of the initial injury. As renal blood flow decreases and compensatory mechanisms fail, necrotic tubular cell debris is incorporated into occluding casts that lodge within the tubule lumen and cause obstruction. This obstruction causes an increase in tubular pressure, which further decreases filtration fraction and promotes backleak upstream. Early cell changes are reversible, such as the swelling of cell organelles, especially in the mitochondria. As ischemia progresses, lack of ATP inhibits the Na^+,K^+-ATPase; water, Na^+, and Cl^- accumulate in tubular cells; intracellular K^+ falls; and tubular cells begin to swell. In experimental models of ARF, the following pathologic changes occur. Swelling of tubular epithelial cells leads to the formation of bullae, which protrude into the tubular lumen. Necrosis of tubular cells results in abnormal membrane permeability. Structural changes in the glomerular epithelium decrease glomerular filtration. Finally, constriction of intrarenal arteries and arterioles further reduces glomerular blood flow.

The onset of tubular damage in experimental models of ARF is usually within 25 minutes of ischemia; at this point the microvilli of the proximal tubular cell brush borders begin to change. Within an hour they slough off into the tubular lumen, and membrane bullae protrude into the straight portion of the proximal tubule. After a few hours, intratubular pressure rises and tubular fluid backflows passively. Within 24 hours, obstructing casts appear in the distal tubular lumen. Even if renal blood flow is completely restored after 60–120 minutes of ischemia, the GFR may not immediately improve. Ischemic tubular damage may be exacerbated further by an imbalance between oxygen supply and demand. Most vulnerable to the imbalance are cells of the thick ascending tubule of the loop of Henle in the medulla. In ischemia-induced ARF lesions are unevenly distributed among the nephrons, probably reflecting variability in blood flow. Experiments of this nature have served to change our view of the progression from a renal insult to renal failure. Traditionally, the paradigm for the pathophysiology of postoperative renal failure emphasized an ischemic event or noxious injury which culminated in tubular epithelial injury and dysfunction; an initiation and a maintenance phase or an early and late phase are thus described, ultimately followed by a recovery phase (see Fig. 58.2). However, it has become clear that additional mechanisms, including renal vascular endothelial injury and vasomotor dysfunction, extend the tubular injury phase and orchestrate ongoing injury. Thus, an 'extension' phase has been added to the paradigm, during which cortical blood flow normalizes, but continued hypoxia in the corticomedullary junction and activation of vascular endothelial cells and an inflammatory response ensues. As the extension phase progresses glomerular filtration rate falls, even though renal blood flow in the cortex returns to baseline and proximal tubular cells in the outer cortex undergo repair and regeneration. Inflammatory cells migrate into the outer medullary region, increasing the inflammatory response via the release of cytokines and chemokines. Preliminary work in animal models has demonstrated that the inflammatory cascade in the outer medulla can be interrupted at a number of points, improving outcome in ischemic renal injury.

Activation of an inflammatory cascade in the renal medulla due to ischemic renal failure contributes to sustained renal dysfunction despite normalized renal blood flow, and may be an effective target for therapy.

In cardiac surgery, the blood–polymer contact during cardiopulmonary bypass (CPB) produces a systemic inflammatory response that varies appreciably from patient to patient. CPB activates polymorphonuclear neutrophils (PMN), rapidly increasing their surface expression of CD11b, the β_2-integrin whose activation-induced changes permit leukocyte adhesion to endothelial cells and vascular egress. Activated PMN have been linked to renal injury in other clinical settings. Syndromes characterized by a systemic inflammatory response such as sepsis and the adult respiratory distress syndrome (ARDS) are frequently complicated by renal injury even in the absence of overt hypotension, suggesting that subtle intrarenal ischemia may be aggravated by the presence of coexisting inflammatory pathologies. Animal models of ischemia/reperfusion indicate that circulating inflammatory mediators can exacerbate primary ischemic insults. When an isolated kidney is subjected to mild-to-moderate ischemia, subsequent reperfusion with activated PMN converts an otherwise recoverable renal insult into irreversible renal injury. Thus, episodes of renal hypoperfusion and/or ischemia that are insufficient independently to cause renal injury can lead to significant damage if the kidneys are subsequently subjected to activated PMN. Blockade of PMN infiltration by preventing leukocyte CD11b–endothelial cell intercellular adhesion molecule (ICAM) adhesion can rescue renal function. Additional support for this hypothesis comes from human studies demonstrating that patients with ARF are more likely to recover renal function if dialysis is performed with biocompatible membranes, thereby inducing less systemic inflammatory response.

The kidney has a distinct susceptibility to ischemic injury. The reason for this is not readily apparent, as renal blood flow is normally high and oxygen supply far exceeds requirements. Although the kidneys receive nearly 25% of the cardiac output and extract relatively little oxygen, the discrepancy between cortical and medullary blood flow and oxygen consumption is marked. The apparent abundance of blood flow to the cortex maximizes flow-dependent functions, such as glomerular filtration and tubular reabsorption. In the medulla, blood flow and oxygen supply are restricted by a tubular vascular anatomy specifically designed for urinary concentration (Fig. 58.5). Normally, 90–95% of blood flow is delivered to the cortex, compared with 5–10% to the medulla. The selective vulnerability of cells in the thick ascending limb of the loop of Henle is thought to result from their high oxygen consumption. Average blood flow is 500 mL/min and 3 mL/min per 100 g of tissue for the cortex and medulla, respectively, whereas the oxygen

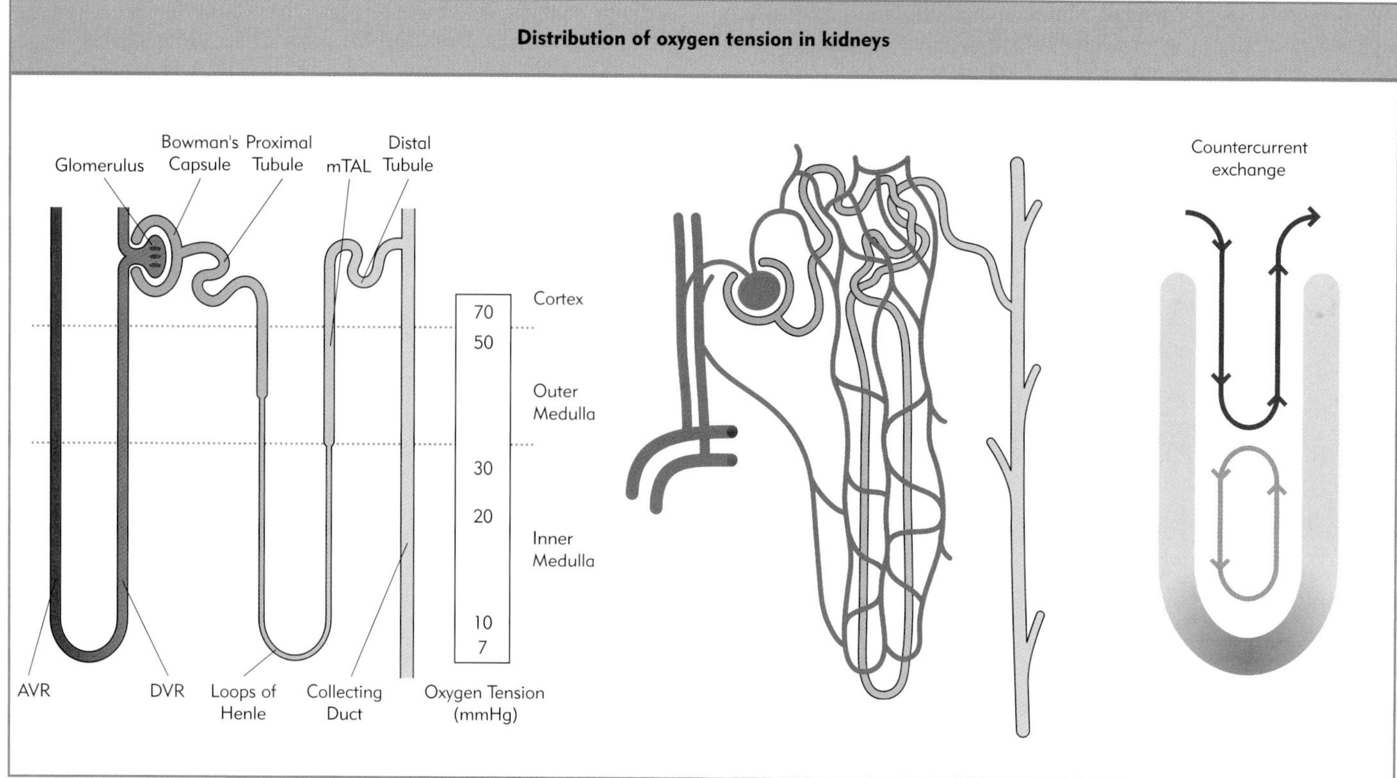

Figure 58.5 Distribution of oxygen tension in the kidneys. Oxygen tension is highest in the cortex and progressively declines through the inner structures of the medulla. AVR, ascending vasa recta; DVR, descending vasa recta.

extraction ratio (i.e. oxygen consumption over oxygen delivery) is 0.18 and 0.79 for the cortex and medulla, respectively. Normally the partial pressure of oxygen is about 55 mmHg in the cortex and 8–15 mmHg in the medulla, making the medullary thick ascending limb of the loop of Henle most vulnerable to tissue hypoxia. Therefore, severe hypoxia may easily develop in the medulla with what otherwise would seem to be adequate total renal blood flow.

Oliguria may protect against acute renal failure by reducing ultrafiltration and energy-requiring tubular functions.

The initial response to decreased renal blood flow is increased Na^+ absorption in the ascending limb of the loop of Henle, which increases oxygen demand in the region most vulnerable to decreased oxygen delivery. To compensate for this, sympathoadrenal mechanisms cause cortical vasoconstriction and oliguria, which tend to redistribute blood flow away from the outer cortex to the inner cortex and medulla. This cortical-to-medullary redistribution of renal blood flow protects the vulnerable medullary oxygen balance. At the same time, decreased Na^+ delivery to the macula densa causes afferent arterial constriction. With afferent arterial vasoconstriction, glomerular filtration decreases, after which solute reabsorption in the loop of Henle and oxygen consumption are reduced. The severity of cellular injury appears to be related to the degree of imbalance between cellular oxygen supply and demand. In the hypoperfused kidney preparation, oxygen-enriched perfusion reduces cellular damage and hypoxic perfusion increases it; complete cessation of perfusion (GFR zero, preventing ultrafiltration) is associated with less cellular injury than is hypoxic perfusion. Modulation by various drugs or compensatory mechanisms can reduce tubular workload and prevent medullary hypoxic cellular injury. Among the compensatory mechanisms that reduce cellular injury are reduced tubular transport or reduced glomerular filtration. Afferent arterial vasoconstriction and consequent oliguria may be a protective response to acute tubular injury. By reducing ultrafiltration, energy-dependent ischemic injury to medullary tubular cells is prevented, even at the cost of retaining nitrogenous waste. Thus, in some cases the oliguria may protect against ARF.

HYPERTENSIVE RENAL DISEASE

Hypertension is a leading cause of renal failure. Diastolic hypertension is linked to microvascular injury that becomes progressive over decades, ultimately leading to renal replacement therapy. More recently, increase in pulse pressure (difference between systolic and diastolic blood pressure) has emerged as a stronger predictor of renal failure, as well as mortality from renal causes. Whereas these findings relate to ambulatory settings, individuals with increased pulse pressure presenting for coronary bypass surgery are at significant risk of developing postoperative renal dysfunction, including dialysis-dependent renal failure. The pathogenesis of renal injury in relation to pulse pressure is unclear, but may involve reduced perfusion pressure from a low diastolic pressure and other cofactors, including advanced age, diabetes, and peripheral vascular disease.

Elevated serum creatinine (1.5–2.9 mg/dL (133–257 μmol/L)) is a risk factor for decreased survival when associated with essential hypertension. Control of hypertension is critical in modifying the rate of progression of renal insufficiency. Hypertension associated with CRF may be accompanied by reversible sympathetic activation, which appears to be mediated by an afferent signal arising in the failing kidneys. The increased sympathetic nerve discharge is unrelated to age, antihypertensive medication, total body volume, erythropoietin levels, or norepinephrine levels.

Although antihypertensive therapy has reduced mortality and morbidity from congestive heart failure and stroke, a reduction in end-stage renal disease (ESRD) has not been clearly established. The best antihypertensive medication to slow the progression of renal insufficiency is not clear; however, it is accelerated if hypertension is treated only with a diuretic. Reasons for the failure of antihypertensive treatment regimens to prevent ESRD caused by hypertension are inadequate control of blood pressure (i.e. target pressure too high), or that antihypertensive drugs reduce systemic blood pressure but not intraglomerular blood pressure, as preglomerular resistance vessels are dilated. Therapy with ACE inhibitors can decrease proteinuria and preserve GFR in patients who have diabetes mellitus independently of changes in systemic blood pressure. Calcium channel antagonists may have a similar effect, but their long-term influence on the progression of renal failure is not known.

MANAGEMENT OF PERIOPERATIVE RENAL FAILURE

Important considerations for the anesthesiologist treating patients with chronic renal failure (CRF) include extracellular volume status, anemia, acid–base and electrolyte abnormalities, platelet dysfunction, susceptibility to infection, hypertension, left ventricular dysfunction, pericarditis, and neurologic dysfunction. Most of the fluid, electrolyte, acid–base, neurologic, and platelet abnormalities improve with dialysis. Anemia is well tolerated because tissue blood flow increases with decreased blood viscosity and increased cardiac output. Rightward shift of the oxyhemoglobin dissociation curve as a result of metabolic acidosis and an increased concentration of diphosphoglycerate also aid tissue oxygenation. Adverse drug reactions occur in renal failure through decreased renal excretion, decreased renal metabolism, decreased hepatic metabolism, and altered volume of distribution owing to decreased protein binding and lipid solubility. Reduced protein binding and uremia-induced alterations in the blood–brain barrier in renal disease may result in the need for lower induction doses of intravenous drugs. Accumulation of morphine glucuronides may account for the prolonged depression of ventilation observed in some patients who have renal failure. Drug interactions and altered end-organ responses also contribute to abnormal drug reactions.

Dopamine

In single-nephron isolated kidney and animal experiments, stimulation of renal dopamine receptors increases renal blood flow, GFR, and excretion of salt and water. Furthermore, in animal models dopamine can prevent acute renal failure if given before a renal insult. In normal volunteers, dopamine increases effective renal plasma flow, an effect that plateaus at 3 μg/kg/min. Consequently, the introduction of dopamine into clinical practice in general, and cardiac surgery in particular, was heralded with great enthusiasm. Low-dose or renal-dose dopamine is widely used, often routinely or selectively in higher-risk patients, in the hope of preventing renal dysfunction. However, the experimental success did not appear to translate to clinical renal protection. Based on meta-analysis of clinical studies comparing dopamine versus placebo, the rates for mortality, ARF, and need for replacement therapy were 4.7% vs 5.6%, 15.3% vs 19.5%, and 13.9% vs. 16.5%, respectively. This review concluded that the 'use of low-dose dopamine for the treatment or prevention of acute renal failure cannot be justified on the basis of available evidence and should be eliminated from routine clinical use'.

Although theoretically attractive as a renal protective agent, dopamine has not demonstrated a consistent protective effect in clinical trials.

In cardiac surgery, earlier reports indicate that dopamine increased urinary flow rates as well as the excretion of Na^+ and K^+ above that accounted for by cardiovascular changes (increase in cardiac output), confirming that it had a specific renal action. However, randomized trials demonstrated that dopamine did not perform better than placebo for a number of renal parameters. None of these studies was large enough to detect a difference in serum creatinine. By analyzing both functional and structural markers of renal tubular function, such as low molecular weight urinary proteins (retinol-binding protein, RBP; α- and β_2-microglobulin) and urinary enzymes (*N*-acetyl glucosamine, NAG), it was shown that dopamine actually increased excretion of these markers, suggesting that it may cause subclinical tubular injury. Thus dopamine does not prevent ARF after cardiac surgery when used in a routine or prophylactic manner.

Mannitol

Mannitol is an osmotic diuretic that promotes free water diuresis by acting as a nonreabsorbable solute (primarily in the proximal tubule). Mannitol effectively expands extracellular volume by shifting fluid from the intracellular to the extracellular compartment, with consequent increases in renal blood flow, GFR, and renal tubular flow. Mannitol also affects renal pressure–flow relationships, such that higher blood flow occurs at similar (or lower) levels of renal perfusion pressure by unclear mechanisms. The effect of mannitol on renal blood flow is thought to be secondary to the release of intrarenal prostaglandins or atrial natriuretic peptide (ANP), decreased intravascular cell swelling or decreased renin production, and/or an increase in intravascular volume. Although it is reasonable to assume that increasing renal blood flow is beneficial, especially when oxygen and nutrient delivery is compromised, it may not necessarily be so. Another critical question is what effect mannitol has on intrarenal blood flow distribution. The inner cortex and medulla would stand to benefit the most from increases in oxygen and nutrient delivery when the kidney is susceptible to hypoxic injury, whereas decreases in renal blood flow to the outer cortex may tax the kidney at a time when it can least afford it.

The theoretic benefits of mannitol can be predicted from its other actions, coupled with an understanding of the pathophysiology associated with acute perioperative renal failure. Mannitol reduces reabsorption of NaCl, K^+, phosphate, and water in the proximal tubule, NaCl in the thick ascending limb of the loop of Henle, and water in the collecting duct. These are all energy-consuming processes. In addition to preserving oxygen balance by decreasing demand, mannitol may relieve the vascular congestion and endothelial cell edema that may result from hypoperfusion of the medulla. Given the paucity of clinical data demonstrating the benefit of mannitol in preserving renal function, one must carefully weigh its risks (i.e. intravascular volume depletion following acute volume overload, hyperosmolarity, hypokalemia, and hyponatremia) with its theoretic benefit.

Furosemide

Although furosemide protects the kidney against ischemic injury in animals, most clinical studies have failed to demonstrate efficacy in the prevention or treatment of ischemic or toxic ARF. Both mannitol and loop diuretics, if administered early in the course of ischemic ARF, can convert oliguric to nonoliguric renal failure, although there is little evidence that this reduces mortality. Patients who respond to diuretics may have less severe baseline renal damage than those with no response.

Increased renal blood flow and solute load associated with dopamine and diuretics in the setting of depleted energy stores may explain the lack of renal protection by these agents.

In at-risk surgical patients the maximal increase in serum creatinine above baseline was twice as high with furosemide as with either dopamine or placebo, whereas the incidence of acute renal injury (defined as a maximal increase in serum creatinine of > 0.5 mg/dL) occurred most frequently with furosemide. These negative effects have not been fully accounted for. Activation of the renin–angiotensin system and a regional redistribution of intrarenal blood flow have been suggested. As with dopamine, it is likely that cellular ATP stores are depleted by the increased energy demands caused by the solute load distally. The fact that the increased renal blood flow associated with dopaminergic drugs is accompanied by an increased workload that may outstrip the available cellular energy is an important experimental finding that may shed light on our consistent failure to promote renal protection by trying to increase renal blood flow. Finally, diuretics can be detrimental in ARF induced by radiocontrast agents. Currently, the use of loop diuretics can only be justified to increase urine output for fluid management, with no clear evidence for improved outcome.

Atrial natriuretic peptide

Natriuretic peptides are released from many tissue types: atria (atrial natriuretic peptide, ANP) and in some cases ventricles, brain (brain natriuretic peptide, BNP), vascular endothelial cells, and kidneys. ANP is most often released in response to atrial stretch seen in congestive heart failure, or from other conditions that result in both acute and chronic volume expansion. ANP has an interesting pharmacodynamic profile, acting as both a direct vasodilator and a diuretic, increasing Na^+ elimination by renal and from extrarenal effects. Renal effects include increases in GFR and in Na^+ excretion (mainly by diminishing Na^+ reabsorption in the medullary collecting tubules), possibly mediated by an increase in peritubular capillary hydraulic pressure and/or local release of dopamine.

The increase in GFR caused by ANP is associated with little or no change in renal blood flow, suggesting that ANP produces both afferent arteriolar dilation and efferent arteriolar constriction. The direct tubular effect, in comparison, appears to be mediated by a cGMP-dependent protein kinase, which closes Na^+ channels through which luminal Na^+ normally enters the cell. In addition to these tubular and glomerular effects, ANP has a variety of other actions that also promote increased secretion of Na^+ and water. For example, it can reduce basal renin release, inhibit angiotensin II- and K^+-induced aldosterone secretion (the latter primarily via a direct action on the adrenal gland), inhibit proximal Na^+ reabsorption and aldosterone release induced by angiotensin II, and diminish the collecting tubular response to ADH. Thus, the fall in activity of the renin–angiotensin–aldosterone system seen with volume expansion may be mediated in part by ANP.

Doses of ANP in animals insufficient to cause profound vasodilatation generally do not improve renal outcomes after injury. However, larger doses in combination with dopamine to support systemic blood pressure improve GFR. Urodilatin is a renal natriuretic peptide with greater natriuretic potency than ANP. In the setting of ischemic ATN urodilatin in nonhypotensive doses in combination with dopamine and mannitol resulted in almost complete restoration of GFR. In clinical trials in patients with established ATN, ANP treatment improved creatinine clearance by 8 hours up to 24 hours; as in animal models, both mannitol and dopamine were used concomitantly. Despite a trend towards reduced renal replacement therapy in the ANP group, mortality was comparable to that in the placebo group. In a much larger study in patients with ATN, ANP offered no advantage over placebo. The use of ANP in the setting of radiocontrast agent-induced nephropathy has been similarly investigated in patients with stable chronic renal failure, but no efficacy was found. The administration of urodilatin for postoperative ARF showed a trend towards lower peak creatinine, but the incidence of dialysis and hyperkalemia was comparable to that of placebo. In all, the use of ANP both to treat and to prevent ARF is unwarranted.

Calcium channel blockers and other agents

Calcium channel blockers have been advocated as renovascular vasodilators. Vasoconstriction occurs, in part, as a consequence of increased free Ca^{2+} levels within vascular smooth muscle. In renal transplantation, Ca^{2+} channel blockers reduce the incidence of tubular necrosis and delayed graft dysfunction. Calcium channel blockers reduce the vasoconstrictive effect of cyclosporin A and may prevent the vasoconstrictive effects of radiocontrast agents. However, indiscriminate use of calcium channel blockers may be associated with systemic hypotension and low renal perfusion. Calcium channel blockers are not therefore recommended or justified in most forms of ARF.

Perioperative oliguria

Premedication and anesthetic drugs may increase or reduce catecholamines, alter renal vascular resistance, depress the myocardium and hence renal blood flow, or have a direct nephrotoxic effect on renal tubular function. Surgery in general, aortic cross-clamping and declamping in particular, trauma, and stress also may influence urine formation by changing myocardial function, sympathetic activity, neuronal or hormonal activity, intravascular volume, or systemic vascular resistance. During general anesthesia, ureteral peristalsis may affect the rate of urine output. General anesthetics decrease the frequency and force of ureteral contraction and hence urine delivery. All anesthetic agents alter renal function by changing blood pressure and cardiac output so that renal blood flow in the inner cortex is redistributed, causing Na^+ and water conservation (i.e. decreased urine formation). Regional anesthesia above level T4 reduces sympathetic tone to the kidney, making renal blood flow and filtration depend directly on perfusion pressure.

Monitoring urine output as a sign of the adequacy of renal perfusion is based on the assumption that patients who have diminished renal perfusion excrete a low volume of concentrated urine. Urinary flow rate and volume are indirect markers of renal function because of the many nonrenal factors that also influence renal function. Urine flow (regardless of the amount) indicates blood flow to the kidney because glomerular filtration and the generation of urine can only occur if perfusion occurs. Many studies show no correlation between urine volume and histologic evidence of acute tubular necrosis, reduction in GFR or creatinine clearance, or changes in blood urea (BUN) or creatinine in patients who have burn injuries, trauma, cardiovascular surgery, or shock states.

Reduced renal perfusion initiates a series of systemic and renal compensatory responses that preserve ultrafiltration. At this stage, glomerular filtration and renal blood flow are maintained by increased distribution of blood flow to the kidney, selective afferent vasodilatation, efferent vasoconstriction, and increased Na^+ and water conservation. If these protective mechanisms fail and renal blood flow decreases further, afferent arterial vasoconstriction ensues and reduces capillary hydrostatic pressure and ultrafiltration. As this happens, blood flow and glomerular filtration in the outer cortical nephrons decline because redistribution of renal blood flow protects the vulnerable medullary oxygen balance. Decreased glomerular filtration during compromised flow therefore appears to be protective because decreased urine delivery to the tubules requires less reabsorptive work and prevents further oxygen supply-and-demand imbalance.

Modulation by various drugs or compensatory mechanisms can reduce tubular workload and prevent medullary hypoxic cellular injury. Among the compensatory mechanisms that reduce cellular injury are reduced tubular transport and glomerular filtration. Consequently, in some patients selective vasoconstriction may protect against ARF. The beneficial effect of renal vasodilators depends on the regional effects these agents have within the kidney. If vasodilatation causes an increase in renal blood flow and consequent glomerular filtration at a time when the kidney can least afford it because of reduced oxygen delivery, then damage can be potentiated rather than diminished. This paradox highlights the difficulties of renal failure management and may indicate why our management record is so dismal.

Key references

Alpen SL, Lodish HF. Molecular biology of renal function. In: Brenner BM, Rector FC Jr, eds. The kidney, 4th edn. Philadelphia: WB Saunders; 1991:132–63.

Badr KF, Ichikawa I. Prerenal failure: a deleterious shift from renal compensation to decompensation. New Engl J Med. 1988;319:623–9.

Charlson ME, MacKenzie CR, Gold JP, Shires GT. Postoperative changes in serum creatinine. When do they occur and how much is important? Ann Surg. 1989;209:328–33.

Kellum J, Levin N, Bouman C, Lameire N. Developing a consensus classification system for acute renal failure. Curr Opin Crit Care 2002;8:509–14.

Lameire N, Vanholder R. Pathophysiology of ischemic acute renal failure. Best Practice Res Clin Anesthesiol. 2004;18:21–36.

Myers BD, Moran SM. Hemodynamically mediated acute renal failure. New Engl J Med. 1986;314:97–105.

Novis BK, Roizen MF, Aronson S, Thisted RA. Association of preoperative risk factors with postoperative acute renal failure. Anesth Analg. 1994;78:143–9.

Rinder C, Fontes M, Mathew J, Rinder HM, Smith BR. Neutrophil CD11b upregulation during cardiopulmonary bypass is associated with postoperative renal injury. Ann Thorac Surg. 2003;75:899–905.

Shusterman N, Strom BL, Murray TG, Morrison G, West SL, Maislin G. Risk factors and outcome of hospital-acquired acute renal failure. Clinical epidemiologic study. Am J Med. 1987;83:65–71.

Valtin H. Renal dysfunction: mechanisms involved in fluid and solute imbalance. Boston, MA: Little, Brown;1979.

Further reading

Kellen M, Aronson S, Roizen MF, Barnard J, Thisted RA. Predictive and diagnostic tests of renal failure: a review. Anesth Analg. 1994;78:134–42.

Kharasch ED. Metabolism and toxicity of the new anesthetic agents. Acta Anaesthesiol Belg. 1996;47:7–14.

Sladen RN. Effect of anesthesia and surgery on renal function. Crit Care Clin. 1987;3:373–93.

Thadhani R, Pascual M, Bonventre JV. Acute renal failure. New Engl J Med. 1996;334:1448–60.

Chapter 59

Regulation of blood volume and electrolytes

Abhiram Mallick and Andrew R Bodenham

TOPICS COVERED IN THIS CHAPTER

The volume and composition of circulating blood volume and body fluid compartments in health are tightly regulated within normal limits. Disturbances or adaptation of normal mechanisms are commonly seen in disease or under conditions of physiologic stress. A basic understanding of the dynamics of the fluid compartments is essential for fluid management in patients undergoing anesthesia and major surgery or requiring intensive care.

BODY FLUID COMPARTMENTS

There are two principal body fluid compartments (Fig. 59.1): *intracellular fluid* (ICF) and *extracellular fluid* (ECF). The ECF consists of *interstitial fluid* (ISF) in a compartment between the capillaries and cells, and *plasma volume* (PV). The ICF constitutes approximately two-thirds of total body water (28 L in a 70 kg young adult). The ECF is about a third of total body water (14 L), including 11 L of interstitial fluid and 3 L of plasma. Blood volume is approximately 5 L, of which 3 L is plasma and another 2 L is red cell volume. Although it is intravascular, the red cell volume is technically a part of the ICF.

Total body water (TBW) is approximately 60% of total body weight (i.e. 42 L in a 70 kg young adult). Fat tissue has a lower water content. Therefore, the fraction of TBW to body weight is slightly lower in women (55%) and substantially lower in obese people and the elderly. In infants and young children, TBW is about 80% of the body weight, of which ECF volume is up to 40%, almost half of the TBW. Body sodium balance primarily regulates ECF volume, whereas body water balance regulates the ICF volume.

Composition of fluid compartments

The volume and composition of each fluid compartment are determined by the quantities, concentrations, and movements between the compartments of water, plasma proteins, and electrolytes, especially sodium. Electrolyte and protein concentrations differ markedly in the fluid compartments (Fig. 59.2). The composition of ICF varies somewhat depending on the nature and the function of the cell. Sodium concentration primarily determines both the tonicity and the osmolality of ECF, with nearly equal concentrations in both ISF and PV, but the ICF contains little Na^+. The plasma proteins, albumin and globulins,

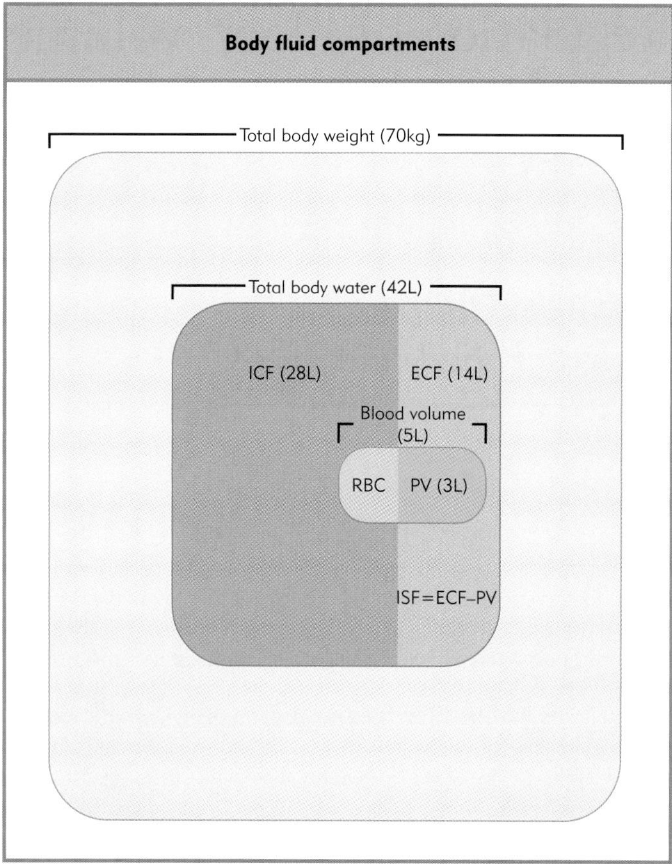

Figure 59.1 Schematic diagram of body fluid compartments. The interstitial fluid (ISF) volume is calculated as the difference between the extracellular fluid volume (ECF) and the plasma volume (PV). ICF, intracellular fluid; RBC, red blood cell volume.

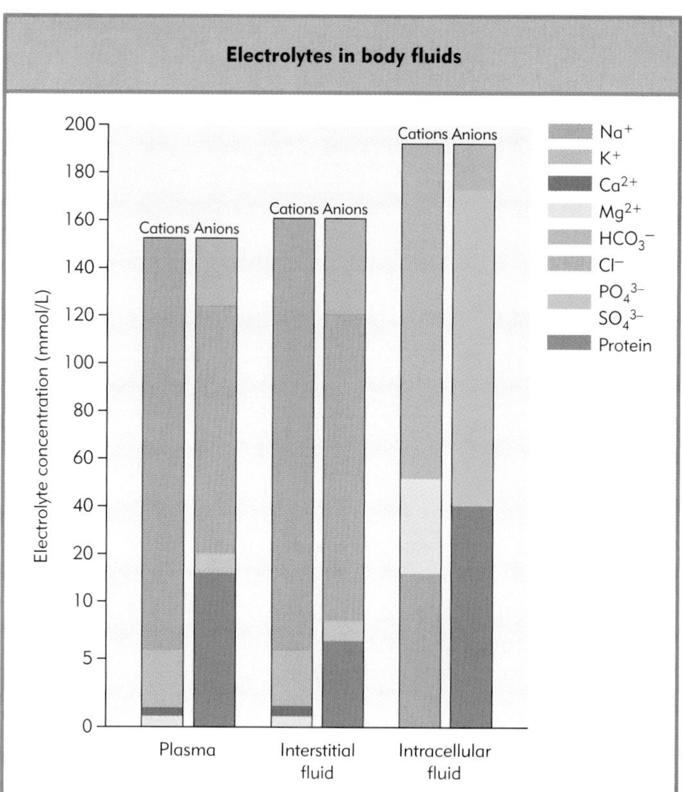

Figure 59.2 Electrolytes in intracellular fluid, interstitial fluid, and plasma. Note nonlinear scale.

determine the plasma colloid oncotic pressure, which in turn maintains adequate PV. There are other osmotically active constituents such as urea, but they are equally distributed throughout the TBW. Albumin does not pass easily across the capillaries into the ISF despite a significant concentration gradient because of its large size compared to electrolytes. Albumin, which in health escapes in small quantities into the ISF, is returned via lymphatics into the plasma. It is therefore highly concentrated in the circulating blood volume. The protein concentration gradient between plasma and ISF is principally responsible for maintaining the proportions of circulating PV and ISF volume.

Movement of water between ICF and ECF

OSMOSIS

Osmosis is defined as the movement of water between compartments through a semipermeable membrane, which occurs when the concentrations of solutes on either side of the membrane are not equal. The cell membrane is freely permeable to water, and the movement of water between compartments is governed by their relative osmotic pressure gradients. Water diffuses towards the side of the membrane where the concentration of osmotically active solutes is greater. The pressure needed to oppose exactly the movement of water down a solute concentration gradient across a membrane is called the *osmotic pressure*. Each molecule or ion dissolved in water causes osmosis of water directly proportional to the concentration of that molecule or ion. The osmotic pressure is proportional to the number of molecules or ions, not their molecular weight.

OSMOLALITY

The osmolarity of a solution quantifies the forces determining the distribution of water, and refers to the number of osmotically active particles per liter of solution. In contrast, osmolality is a measurement of the number of osmotically active particles per kilogram of solvent. Therefore, the osmolarity is affected by the volume of the solution and temperature, whereas osmolality is not. Osmotically active solutes depress the freezing point of fluids. The freezing point of normal human plasma is about −0.54°C, which corresponds to an osmolality of 290 mmol/L. All the body fluid compartments have the same osmolality as plasma, and hence they are in equilibrium.

CALCULATION OF OSMOLALITY

The osmolality of plasma can be calculated approximately according to the following formula:

■ Equation 59.1

$$\text{Osmolality} = (\text{serum Na}^+ \times 2) + \text{blood glucose} + \text{blood urea (mmol/kg)}$$

where Na^+, glucose, and urea are expressed in mmol/L. Sugars, alcohols, and X-ray contrast solutions may increase the osmolality but falsely lower the calculated value, generating an increased osmolality gap between the calculated and measured values. A hyperosmolar state occurs when the concentration of osmotically active particles is high. For example, raised blood urea, hyperglycemia, and hypernatremia can increase serum osmolality.

TONICITY

Tonicity is a term used to describe the osmolality of a solution relative to plasma. Solutions that have the same osmolality as plasma are said to be isotonic; those with higher osmolality are hypertonic; and those with lower osmolality are hypotonic. All solutions for intravenous administration that are initially iso-osmotic with plasma would remain isotonic if it were not for the fact that some solutes diffuse into cells, some are excreted by the kidneys, and others are metabolized. Thus, a 0.9% saline solution remains isotonic because there is no net movement of osmotically active particles into the cells. By comparison, a 5% dextrose solution is isotonic when initially infused, but as dextrose is metabolized the net longer-term effect is that of infusing a hypotonic solution.

Movement of water between plasma and ISF

COLLOID ONCOTIC PRESSURE

The capillary endothelium has a pore size of 6.5 nm and is freely permeable to small molecules and electrolytes, but not to large protein molecules. Plasma proteins, especially albumin, are largely confined to the intravascular compartment and exert a colloid osmotic pressure (COP) of about 25 mmHg or 1.2 mosmol/kg. The plasma COP opposes fluid filtration across the capillary membrane as a result of the hydrostatic pressure in the vascular system.

STARLING FORCES

It is at the capillary level that fluid interchange between the plasma and the ISF takes place. The major determinants of fluid movement are the so-called Starling forces (Fig. 59.3). The net fluid movement is proportional to the difference between the hydrostatic and osmotic pressure gradient across the capillary wall.

The reflection coefficient (σ) indicates the capillary permeability to albumin, with a value of 0 representing free permeability and a value of 1 complete impermeability. The reflection coefficient for albumin ranges in health from 0.6 to 0.9 in various capillary beds. As a result, fluid moves into the tissues whenever the hydrostatic gradient increases or when the osmotic gradient decreases. If COP is reduced, fluid accumulates in the ISF, and if the lymphatic clearance is exceeded, edema develops. The effects of Starling forces can be seen during surgery: the face and eyes of patients placed in the head-down position for long periods become edematous (i.e. through an increase in capillary hydrostatic pressure (P_c)), whereas more generalized edema is common in patients given large volumes of crystalloid (low plasma COP (π_c)). The value of π_c is equal at arterial and venous ends of the capillary bed, whereas the P_c results in fluid being forced out of the arterial end of the capillary and reabsorbed in the venous end. Overall, there is a net efflux of fluid out of capillaries into the ISF, which is removed by the lymphatic circulation.

The balance between capillary filtration and lymphatic drainage determines the ISF volume; homeostatic mechanisms can accommodate only a limited amount of excess fluid. P_c, the most powerful factor favoring fluid filtration, is determined by capillary flow, arteriolar resistance, venous resistance, and pressure. Increased capillary filtration can alter the balance of Starling forces at equilibrium. When coupled with increased lymphatic drainage, preservation of the oncotic pressure gradient limits the accumulation of ISF. As increasing ISF volume results in decreasing concentration of proteoglycans and glycosaminoglycans, fluid drains more freely into the lymphatics. If P_c is increased when lymphatic drainage is maximal, edema is formed.

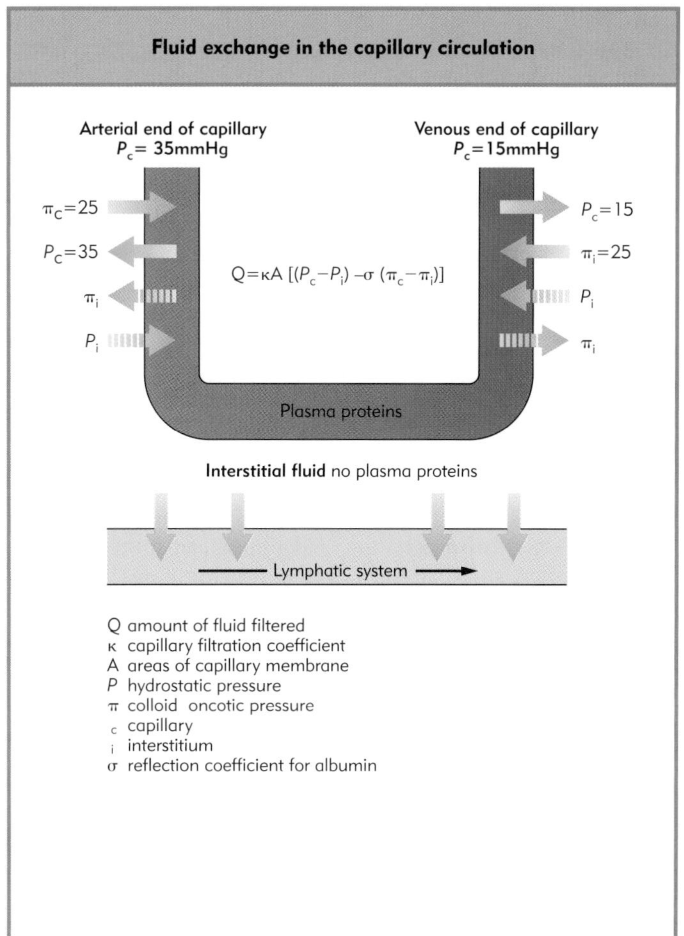

Figure 59.3 Fluid exchange in the capillary circulation. A schematic representation of the Starling forces.

Lymphatic system

Up to 3 L/day of intravascular fluid is lost from plasma to the ISF, and if this fluid were not returned to the bloodstream via the lymphatic system this would lead to hypovolemia. The lymphatic system regulates the ISF volume by draining excess interstitial fluid back to the systemic circulation. The fluid carried by the lymphatics, which contain proteins, lymphocytes, and macrophages, is called lymph. The lymphatic circulation starts from blind-ended lymphatic capillaries in the ISF compartment. These converge to form larger lymphatics, which drain into the thoracic duct and right lymphatic duct to end at the junction of internal jugular and subclavian veins. They branch and interconnect freely, and extend into almost all tissues in parallel with the systemic capillaries, with the exception of the central nervous system, eyes, and certain cartilage structures. These anatomical areas have other forms of fluid circulation, in the form of the cerebrospinal fluid, the aqueous and vitreous humors in the eye, and the synovial fluid of joints, respectively.

The lymphatic system plays an important role in absorption of lipids from the intestine. Absorbed lipids, i.e. chylomicrons, fatty acids, and trigycerides, from the gut, together with lymph, form *chyle* in the mesenteric lymphatics, the cisterna chyli, and the thoracic duct. Other functions of the lymphatic system include its role in immune function and the absorption of drugs following subcutaneous administration. Edema results when interstitial fluid accumulates faster than the lymphatics can remove it. The generalized tissue edema seen in critically ill patients results from expansion of the ISF compartment. Ascites, pericardial, and pleural effusions are formed in a similar fashion as localized collection of protein-rich edema fluid. Multiple factors are involved, including increased capillary permeability, altered Starling forces, and decreased lymphatic transport.

REGULATION OF BLOOD VOLUME

Blood volume represents the sum of red cell volume and plasma volume. Red cell volume and plasma volume can change independently of each other to alter blood volume. Physical exercise, environmental stresses, trauma, and illness can influence each of these volumes. Expansion of red cell volume usually occurs slowly over many weeks to months, whereas plasma volume expansion can occur rapidly over several hours or days. A principal factor regulating red cell production is the hormone erythropoietin. Reduced tissue oxygen tension (renal) is the primary factor stimulating erythropoietin synthesis. Other factors, such as iron, folic acid, vitamin $B_{12,}$ bone marrow function, and general health status are also important determinants of red cell synthesis.

Plasma volume is regulated through complex mechanisms that include reflexes mediated by the sympathetic nervous system (Chapter 34), renal mechanisms (Chapter 57), and humoral factors such as vasopressin (antidiuretic hormone, ADH), natriuretic peptides, and the renin–angiotensin–aldosterone axis (Fig. 59.4). Renal mechanisms modulate renal blood flow, glomerular filtration, and tubular reabsorption of sodium and water. The integrated responses to increased and decreased blood volume are summarized in Figure 59.5. The exact interplay between these systems in health and disease are still inadequately understood.

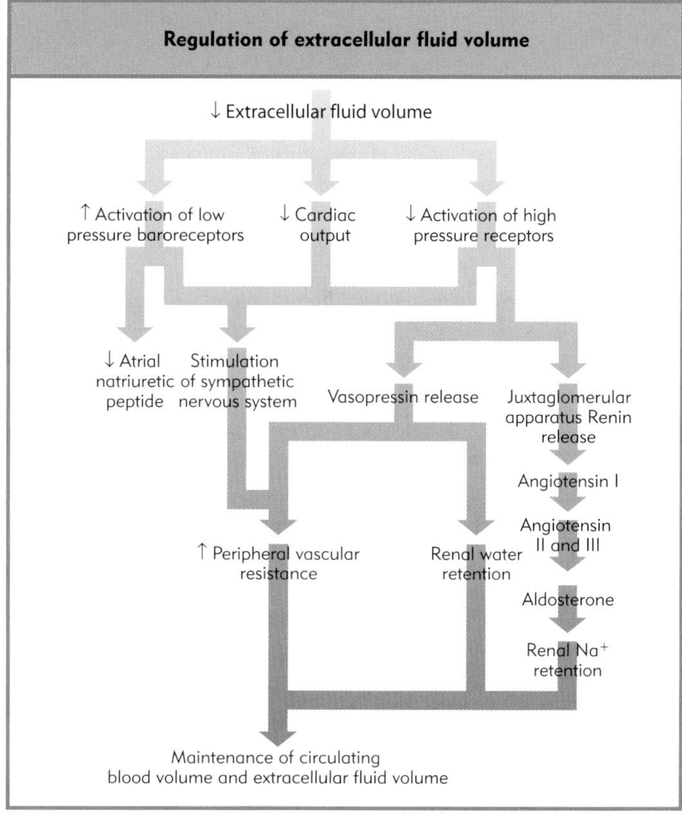

Figure 59.4 Regulation of extracellular fluid volume.

Renin–angiotensin–aldosterone axis

The renin–angiotensin–aldosterone (RAA) axis plays a vital role in the regulation of ECF and blood volume through coordinated effects on the heart, blood vessels, and kidneys. In volume-depleted states glomerular filtration rate (GFR) and sodium delivery to the distal nephron decrease, causing the release of renin by the afferent arteriolar cells of the juxtaglomerular apparatus of the kidney (Chapter 57). Renin catalyzes the cleavage of plasma angiotensinogen to angiotensin I. Angiotensin I has little effect on blood pressure. The angiotensin-converting enzyme in the lungs converts angiotensin I to the active hormone angiotensin II. Angiotensin II is destroyed rapidly (half-life 1–2 minutes). The known effects of angiotensin II include vasoconstriction, aldosterone release from the adrenal cortex, vasopressin release, adrenergic tone modulation, and the generation of thirst. Angiotensin II is a potent vasoconstrictor that produces a rise in both systolic and diastolic blood pressure. Angiotensin III, a metabolite of angiotensin II, also acts directly on the adrenal cortex to increase the secretion of aldosterone.

From the early concept of a circulating renin–angiotensin system, knowledge has evolved with the identification of the chemical machinery for the formation of angiotensin peptides in the interstitial compartment of diverse tissues, and the suggestion that angiotensin II synthesis may occur within the cell itself. Clinically, angiotensin antagonist drugs have proved beneficial in retarding or even reversing the cardiovascular sequelae of hypertensive disease, and may even interfere with the mechanisms by which atherosclerosis develops or progresses. They are the only drugs that have been proved to reduce mortality in heart failure.

Aldosterone regulates Na^+ reabsorption in the distal nephron: high concentrations of aldosterone may reduce urinary Na^+ excretion to almost zero. Aldosterone is the most important regulator of total extracellular Na^+ and therefore of ECF volume and blood volume. Aldosterone acts primarily on the renal collecting ducts to stimulate reabsorption of Na^+ and the secretion of K^+ and H^+ (Chapter 57). It binds with intracellular receptors in the nucleus that stimulate the expression of several genes modulating the activity of ionic transport systems located in the apical and basolateral membranes of target epithelial cells. Drugs that block the formation of angiotensin II (angiotensin-converting enzyme inhibitors) or block aldosterone receptors (spironolactone) will enhance Na^+ and water loss and may reduce plasma volume.

Vasopressin

Vasopressin is secreted from the posterior pituitary in response to osmoreceptor stimulation. The osmoreceptors are located in the wall of the third ventricle in the hypothalamus and sense a rise in osmolality as small as 1–2%. Acute arterial hypotension

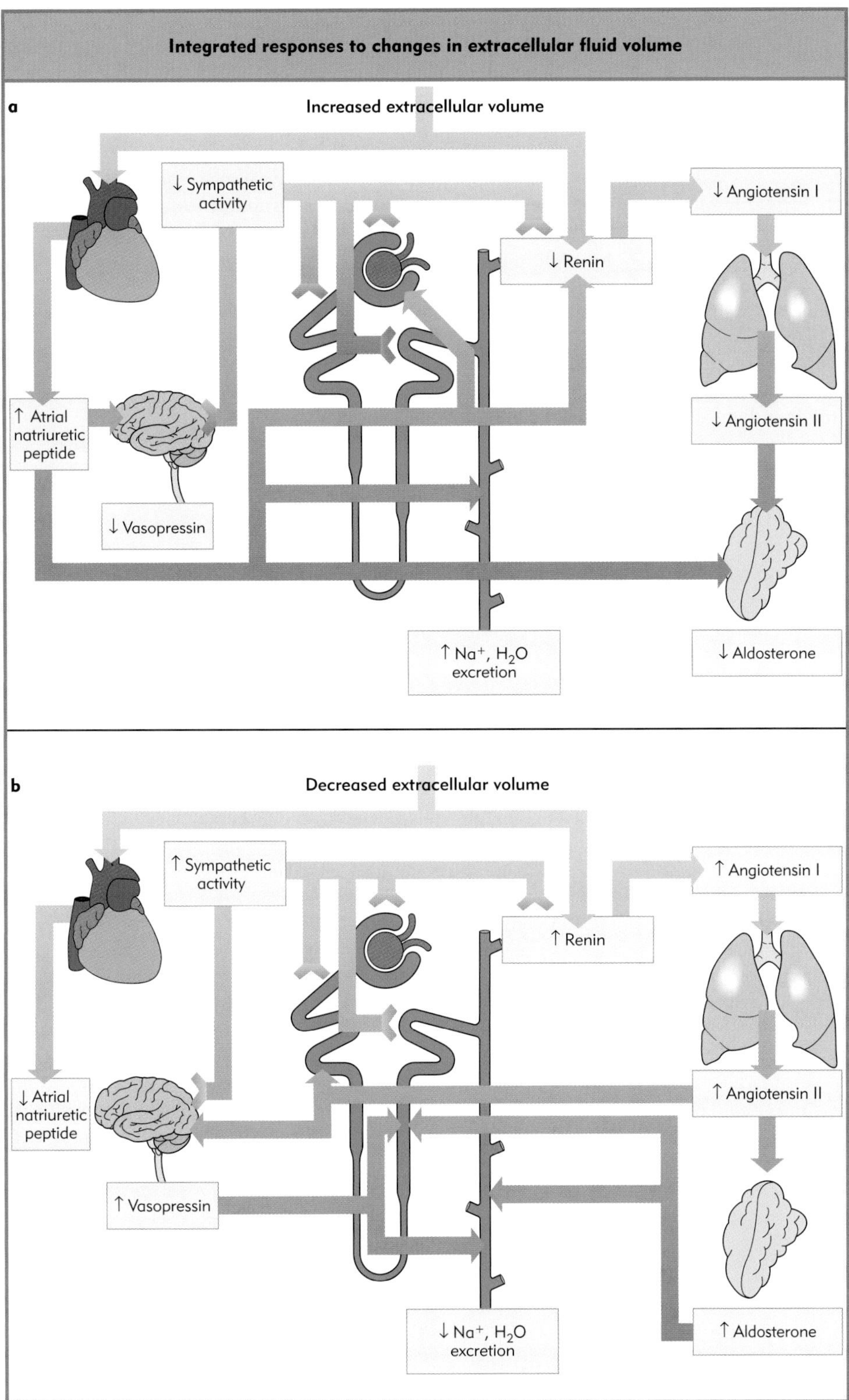

Figure 59.5 Integrated responses to changes in extracellular fluid (ECF) volume. The renal responses to increased ECF volume (a) include an increase in glomerular filtration rate and reduced Na^+ reabsorption in the proximal tubule, loop of Henle, and collecting duct. The mechanisms for reduced Na^+ and water excretion in response to decreased ECF volume are essentially the opposite (b). (With permission from Berne RM and Levy MN. Principles of Physiology. St Louis, IL. Copyright © Mosby 1990.)

and hypovolemia (a 10% decrease in blood volume) also increase vasopressin secretion. Vasopressin directly stimulates vascular V_1 receptors to produce constriction of both veins and arteries, thereby increasing total peripheral resistance and blood pressure.

High endogenous levels of vasopressin (syndrome of inappropriate antidiuretic hormone secretion) in nonshock states do not produce a rise in blood pressure. However, vasopressin infused at very low doses increases blood pressure in shock states by stimulation of vascular V_1 receptors. Vasopressin is increasingly used as an option to raise blood pressure in patients with septic shock and to wean the traditional vasopressors already in use. An inappropriately low level of serum vasopressin is found in septic shock secondary to exhaustion of neurohypophyseal stores due to intense and prolonged stimulation and blunted baroreflex mediated vasopressin release. Low doses of vasopressin targeted to achieve serum vasopressin levels similar to that present in cardiogenic shock, have been shown to produce a significant rise in blood pressure in septic shock. The effect of vasopressin on clinical outcome is unknown. It is thought a high dose of vasopressin may subject patients to a greater risk of splanchnic and coronary artery ischemia.

To preserve plasma volume, vasopressin acts primarily on the renal collecting ducts to increase water permeability, apparently by increasing the expression of water channels (aquaporins); this results in greater water reabsorption. The importance of vasopressin is seen when the pituitary or hypothalamus is damaged, leading to failure to secrete vasopressin. Diabetes insipidus follows, with excretion of up to 20 L of dilute urine daily. Both aldosterone and vasopressin levels can increase as a part of the stress response to surgery and critical illness, independent of the changes in blood volume. This may reduce the usefulness of urine flow as an indicator of volume status and renal perfusion.

Natriuretic peptides

Since their discovery 20 years ago, natriuretic peptides have been shown to play an important role in the regulation of ECF and blood volume. It is now appreciated that the heart is an important endocrine organ. This peptide family consists of four peptides: atrial natriuretic peptide (ANP), brain natriuretic peptide (BNP), C-type natriuretic peptide (CNP), and Dendroaspis natriuretic peptide (DNP). These peptides are structurally similar but genetically distinct peptides that have diverse actions in cardiovascular, renal, and body fluid homeostasis.

ATRIAL NATRIURETIC PEPTIDE

Atrial natriuretic peptide (ANP), a polypeptide hormone of 28 amino acids, is produced in the cardiac atria and to a lesser extent in the ventricles, and is released in response to increased wall tension. Although other tissues produce ANP, including the lungs, aortic arch, brain, kidneys, adrenals, gastrointestinal tracts, thymus, and eye, the concentrations are thought to be too low to be clinically significant.

BRAIN NATRIURETIC PEPTIDE

Brain natriuretic peptide (BNP) was discovered in porcine brain and subsequently found to be produced in greater quantity in human heart, primarily by the left ventricle. It is released in response to increased ventricular wall stress. Serum concentration of BNP has recently been clinically used as a biomarker to assist in the diagnosis and prognostic assessment of patients with suspected heart failure.

BNP is used for treatment of and as a biomarker for evaluation of heart failure.

The physiologic actions of natriuretic peptides involve the kidneys, vasculature, heart, sympathetic nervous system, and RAA axis. ANP and BNP exert similar actions in humans. Natriuretic peptides regulate fluid volume homeostasis through their natriuretic and diuretic effects. They dilate the afferent arterioles and constrict the efferent arterioles, leading to increased glomerular filtration while maintaining a constant renal blood flow. They also exert an effect on the collecting ducts to inhibit tubular water transport by antagonizing the action of vasopressin. In the heart, natriuretic peptides reduce intracellular calcium concentration by a protein kinase-mediated pathway and promote relaxation. The hemodynamic effects of therapeutic BNP include a reduction of both preload and afterload and a consequent improvement in cardiac performance. The FDA has recently approved recombinant BNP for the treatment of refractory heart failure.

Natriuretic peptides reduce sympathetic tone in the peripheral vasculature. This is accomplished through dampening of baroreceptors, suppressing the release of catecholamines from autonomic nerve endings and inhibiting sympathetic outflow from the central nervous system. These peptides also reduce the activation threshold of vagal efferents and thereby blunt the extent of tachycardia and vasoconstriction that typically results from a drop in blood pressure.

MEASUREMENT OF FLUID COMPARTMENTS

The volume of the body fluid compartments can be measured by estimating the 'volume of distribution' of a substance that will be distributed in only one compartment after injection. The volume of distribution (see Chapter 8) is equal to the amount of substance injected (minus any that has been metabolized or excreted during the time allowed for mixing) divided by the concentration of the substance. Although the principle appears simple, there are a number of factors that must be considered: the substance to be used must be nontoxic; it must mix evenly throughout the compartment being measured; it should remain unchanged in the body during the mixing period; and its concentration should be relatively easy to measure. Such techniques have been used as research tools but are too cumbersome for clinical use.

Blood volume

Plasma volume can be measured by using Evans blue dye, which binds to plasma proteins, or by injecting serum albumin labeled with radioactive iodine. The average PV in a normal 70 kg adult is approximately 3.5 L (50–55 mL/kg). If the PV and hematocrit are known, the blood volume can be calculated as PV/(1 – hematocrit) and is approximately 70–80 mL/kg in healthy adults. Infants by the age of 1 year have a blood volume of 85–90 mL/kg, and that of a neonate is relatively greater, at 95–105 mL/kg. The red cell volume can be measured by injecting chromium-labeled red cells and, after mixing, measuring the fraction of the red cells that are labeled. These methods can be used in healthy individuals for research purpose. In critically ill and postoperative patients these methods have limited value, as in these patients plasma volume and red cell volume can vary depending on vascular tone and capillary permeability.

Extracellular volume

It is difficult to measure ECF volume, as the limits of this space are ill defined and few substances mix rapidly in all parts of the space while remaining exclusively extracellular. The lymphatic system cannot be separated from the ECF and is measured with it. Many substances enter the cerebrospinal fluid slowly through the blood–brain barrier. Substances that distribute in the ECF appear in glandular secretions and in the contents of the gastrointestinal tract. However, ECF volume can be approximately measured by using radiolabeled [^{14}C] inulin. This measurement has a limited value in clinical practice.

Intracellular volume

The ICF cannot be measured directly but can be calculated by subtracting the ECF volume from the TBW. Total body water is measured by the dilution technique used to measure the other fluid compartments. Deuterium oxide (D_2O, heavy water) is most frequently used.

DISTURBANCES OF BLOOD VOLUME

Hypovolemia

Hypovolemia is common in surgical, trauma, and critically ill patients. Hypovolemia is defined as a depletion of the effective circulating blood volume. It is due to losses either from the body or into body cavities – so-called 'absolute hypovolemia' – or to sequestration of fluid within the body as a result of generalized diffuse capillary leak, so-called 'relative hypovolemia' (Table 59.1). Large fluid deficits become obvious in systemic inflammatory states (e.g. sepsis syndrome), characterized by panendothelial injury and increased capillary permeability with loss of proteins and fluids from the intravascular to the ISF. Therefore, the effective circulating volume is low with an expanded ECF volume in many conditions, such as sepsis or sepsis syndrome, liver disease, and anaphylaxis. Absolute or relative hypovolemia can be accentuated during anesthesia because sympathetic reflexes are blunted. Anesthetic drugs themselves, including volatile and intravenous agents, may contribute to relative hypovolemia by causing further vasodilatation. Spinal and epidural anesthesia produces relative hypovolemia by blocking efferent sympathetic vasomotor signals resulting in venous pooling.

During hypovolemia the body tries to perfuse the vital organs, including the heart and the brain, by sustained vasoconstriction at the expense of other organs such as the gut, liver, and kidneys. In severe protracted hypovolemia systemic perfusion and the function of the microcirculation are impaired. This then triggers a vicious cycle of progressive tissue damage that may finally lead to the development of multiple organ failure. The primary objective of fluid therapy is to restore and maintain adequate intravascular blood volume in order to restore oxygen delivery, organ perfusion, and microcirculatory flow, and to avoid the activation of a complex series of damaging mediators.

Table 59.1 Causes of hypovolemia

Absolute hypovolemia: fluids leave body	
Gastrointestinal	Bleeding Vomiting Diarrhea Fistula Tube drainage
Renal	Diuresis Osmotic diuresis Diabetes insipidus
Skin	Burns Large exudative lesions
Trauma	Fractured long bones Ruptured spleen Hemothorax
Surgical	Blood loss
Relative hypovolemia: fluids redistribute within body	
Internal fluid shift	Third-space loss Nephrotic syndrome Cirrhosis
Capillary leak	Anaphylaxis Sepsis or sepsis syndrome
Sequestration	Intestinal obstruction Peritonitis

Edema

Edema, a clinical sign of an excess accumulation of fluid within the ISF, manifests as tissue swelling, pericardial and pleural effusions, ascites, or pulmonary edema. It can occur with fluid overload, decreased fluid excretion (as in renal failure), and expansion of the ISF due to increased capillary permeability and/or reduced plasma COP. Retention of salt and water by the kidneys in response to body regulatory mechanisms contributes to the edema seen in chronic conditions such as congestive heart failure and liver disease. The exact pathophysiology of edema in these conditions is poorly understood. Consideration of the variables of the Starling equation (see Fig. 59.3) allows the mechanisms of edema formation to be characterized as related to hydrostatic pressure, increased capillary permeability, or lowered COP (Table 59.2). In clinical practice, more than one of these mechanisms may operate at the same time.

Lymphedema

Lymphedema is defined as the accumulation of lymph in the extracellular space owing to lymphatic blockade or dysfunction. Most cases are seen as a chronic disorder of the limbs or scrotum. The early edema seen in surgically transposed free flaps or transplanted visceral organs, e.g. bowel, lung, heart, is partly due to the accumulation of lymph as a result of transected lymphatics.

In the western world chronic lymphedema is usually seen as a complication of radical cancer surgery or radiotherapy. In

Table 59.2 Causes of edema

Hydrostatic pressure effect	Fluid overload, cardiac failure, neurogenic pulmonary edema, loss of autoregulation, renal failure
Reduced oncotic pressure (low albumin)	Malnutrition, critical illness, pre-eclampsia, nephrotic syndrome, cirrhosis
Increased capillary permeability	Acute lung injury, brain injury, sepsis or sepsis syndrome, burns, reperfusion injury

tropical and subtropical countries filariasis, a parasitic infection, is responsible for the majority of cases of lymphedema. Lymph slowly accumulates in the tissues distal to the site of damage over weeks, months, or years. In the initial stage the edema is soft, pitting, and temporarily reduced by elevating and compression bandages. Pain may occur due to stretching of soft tissues, and be related to conditions such as infection, thrombosis, and nerve entrapment syndromes. If left untreated an inflammatory state develops, with collagen deposition and soft tissue overgrowth. At this stage the tissue becomes less pitting, more firm or brawny, and elevation of the limb no longer results in reduction of edema.

Hypoalbuminemia

Albumin is a naturally occurring plasma protein with a molecular weight of 69 kDa and a degradation half-life of about 18 days. Hepatocytes synthesize albumin at a rate of 9–12 g/day to maintain a normal plasma concentration of 30–40 g/L. Albumin accounts for 60–80% of plasma COP. The albumin concentration of the ISF is variable, depending on the capillary permeability. Albumin from the ISF returns to the circulation via lymphatic vessels.

Marked alterations in the concentrations of albumin can occur after major surgery, trauma, burns, sepsis, and critical illness as sustained losses secondary to increased capillary permeability. Long-term hypoalbuminemia is a marker of malnutrition or liver disease. Dilutional hypoalbuminemia is frequently secondary to the administration of excess intravenous fluids. Renal loss of albumin is significant in pregnancy-induced hypertension and nephrotic syndrome. In most acutely ill patients, low albumin levels should be considered as a marker of disease severity rather than as a pathology in their own right.

Low serum albumin is a common finding in critically ill patients. The threshold and overall value of replacing albumin by intravenous infusion is contentious. Most clinicians administer albumin when the serum concentration is less than 15 g/L, or when there are continuing losses.

ASSESSMENT OF BLOOD VOLUME AND HYPOVOLEMIA

The clinical measurement of blood volume is not easy. Techniques such as the dilution technique using either Evans blue dye or labeled red cells are clinically impractical. Surrogate markers for blood volume have been used to guide fluid therapy, including clinical assessment, biochemical markers, invasive cardiac filling pressures, cardiac output, and end-diastolic volume measurements. A marked swing in direct arterial pressure waveforms with respiration or mechanical ventilation gives an indication of inadequate intravascular volume. Over the years there has been considerable interest in targeting filling pressures for fluid therapy, including central venous and pulmonary artery occlusion pressures. Targeting filling pressures is sometimes difficult, as left ventricular filling depends on factors other than such pressure. These include left ventricular compliance, intrathoracic pressure, and pulmonary vascular resistance (see Chapter 15). Fluid therapy guided by filling pressures may have a deleterious effect on lung function and gas exchange by increasing pulmonary capillary leak in the presence of acute lung injury.

Clinical assessment

Conventional clinical assessment includes capillary refill, skin turgor, thirst, urine output, heart rate, and blood pressure. The physical signs of hypovolemia, such as oliguria, hypotension, and tachycardia, are nonspecific and insensitive. Normovolemic patients may be oliguric because of renal failure or stress-induced endocrine responses. Supine and orthostatic hypotension reflects a blood volume deficit greater than 30% and 20%, respectively. Hypovolemia is often unmasked under anesthesia and sedation because of a decrease in sympathetic tone. Intermittent positive-pressure ventilation and positive end-expiratory pressure can impede venous return, suggesting hypovolemia even in normovolemic patients.

Hypovolemic individuals normally show an increase in heart rate of more than 20 beats/min and a postural drop in systolic blood pressure greater than 20 mmHg on assuming an upright position. However, there is a high incidence of false-positive and false-negative findings. Young healthy subjects can withstand acute blood loss of 20% of blood volume while exhibiting only postural tachycardia and variable postural hypotension, whereas 20–30% of elderly patients may demonstrate orthostatic changes in blood pressure despite a normal blood volume.

Biochemical markers

Physical signs of low intravascular volume may be further confirmed by laboratory tests demonstrating high levels of urea, a high plasma osmolality, low urine Na^+, high urine osmolality, and metabolic acidosis including raised serum lactate (Table 59.3). These markers are nonspecific and take time to develop. Blood urea is raised in hypovolemia but may be elevated by high protein intake, gastrointestinal bleeding, accelerated catabolism, and renal failure. Severe hypovolemia may result in lactic acidosis owing to compromised tissue perfusion.

Central venous pressure

Central venous pressure (CVP) is commonly measured in the critically ill as an indicator of circulating blood volume. However, there are a number of pitfalls. CVP is dependent on

Table 59.3 Laboratory findings of hypovolemia

Test	Normal range	Suggests hypovolemia
Blood urea nitrogen (mmol/L)	2–14	>15
Serum creatinine (μmol/L, mg/L)	>50 (>6)	>150 (>17)
Urinary sodium (mmol/L, mg/L)	>30 (>690)	<15 (<345)
Urinary osmolality (mmol/kg)	400–800	>800
Serum lactate (mmol/L, mg/L)	<1.5 (<135)	>2.0 (>180)

venous return to the heart, right ventricular compliance, peripheral venous tone, and posture. A normal CVP does not always exclude hypovolemia. It is not reliable in the presence of pulmonary vascular disease, valvular heart disease, right ventricular dysfunction, and chronic airflow limitation. The absolute value of CVP is sometimes difficult to interpret, as CVP may be maintained through peripheral venoconstriction. It is unreliable in the presence of right ventricular dysfunction or chronic airflow limitation. A single reading of CVP is difficult to interpret in critically ill patients. Therefore, it is usual to look for a trend of changes in CVP in response to fluid challenge in critically ill patients.

Pulmonary artery occlusion pressure

The pulmonary artery (PA) catheter has been used for the last 25 years to measure pulmonary artery occlusion pressure (PAOP) as a surrogate indicator of blood volume and left ventricular preload. Like CVP, the absolute level of PAOP does not confirm or exclude hypovolemia. Impairment of left ventricular function may increase PAOP even in the presence of adequate circulating volume. The interpretation of PAOP also requires caution in mechanically ventilated patients. It is now well established that use of the PA catheter is frequently associated with inaccurate measurements. Even when measurements are accurate, benefits can only be obtained when appropriate treatment decisions are made based on these measurements. Many randomized prospective trials have recently shown that treatment protocols based on PA catheter measurements do not translate into better clinical outcomes. Right ventricular end-diastolic volume index measured using a PA catheter fitted with a fast-response thermistor has been used as a preload measure to guide intravenous fluid therapy, but this technique has not shown any extra benefit compared to traditional PA catheters. The continued routine use of PA catheters may not be justified, particularly as there are now less invasive techniques to provide the same measurements.

Esophageal Doppler monitoring

This is a relatively noninvasive method of measuring stroke volume and cardiac output. An esophageal probe of 6 mm diameter is inserted into the esophagus to measure the descending aortic blood flow velocity using high-frequency ultrasound waves of 2–4 MHz. The Doppler frequency shifts are displayed as velocity–time waveforms. The integral area under each waveform equates to the stroke volume flowing down the descending aorta. By applying a correction factor from a nomogram incorporating the patient's age, height, and weight, an estimation of left ventricular stroke volume can be made. The flow time can be corrected for heart rate by dividing it by the square root of cycle time (FTc). A short FTc may be due to hypovolemia or excessive arterial vasoconstriction. FTc is predominantly affected by the changes in preload. Therefore, both stroke volume and FTc are monitored in response to fluid challenge.

Intrathoracic blood volume

Pulse contour cardiac output (PiCCO) has been developed as a new technique to measure cardiac output, intrathoracic blood volume, and extravascular lung water. PiCCO can be used in any patient who has central venous and arterial catheters. This method uses the principle of transpulmonary thermodilution, in which room-temperature injectate is injected via the central line and the changes in blood temperature are measured by a thermistor within the arterial catheter. The measured intrathoracic blood volume provides a guide to preload and acts as guide to fluid administration. There is a growing body of evidence that volume-based assessment of intravascular filling with a continuous cardiac output may provide a better prediction of cardiac output changes in response to fluid therapy. Practitioners familiar with both PAC and PiCCO find themselves abandoning PAC in favor of the PiCCO system, because the data on intrathoracic blood volume and extravascular lung water may be more physiologically and clinically relevant, and there is no added risk to the patient, who already has a central venous catheter and an arterial catheter in place.

Cardiac output

Cardiac output is conventionally measured by a thermodilution technique with the help of a PA catheter. There are also less invasive techniques for determining cardiac output using Doppler and bioimpedance principles. Continuous estimation of cardiac output is now possible using the PiCCO and the LidCO techniques. LidCO uses a lithium dilution principle, in which a small dose of lithium is injected via a central line and detected by the lithium-sensitive electrode in the arterial catheter. This method appears similar to the PiCCO technique.

Fluid challenge

The absolute value of cardiac output does not confirm hypovolemia, but the response of cardiac output to a fluid challenge may provide an indication to the intravascular volume. Small boluses of fluid (e.g. 250 mL of a colloid) are administered to produce a small and rapid increase in blood volume, with assessment of changes in cardiac output, CVP, and PAOP at each addition. In the absence of cardiac output measurements a sustained increase in CVP or PAOP of more than 3 mmHg in response to a fluid challenge represents a significant increase and is probably indicative of an adequate circulatory volume.

Concept of fluid responsiveness

Cardiac filling pressures or cardiac end-diastolic volumes have been used as markers of left ventricular preload during fluid therapy. These measurements have been demonstrated to be of poor value in detecting volume responsiveness in critically ill patients. In only half of patients does cardiac output appear to increase after a fluid challenge, and these patients may be considered as responders to fluid therapy. Therefore, there is a need to distinguish the responders who can benefit from fluid administration from nonresponders, for whom further fluid administration can be detrimental. Recently some dynamic variables, including systolic pressure variation (SPV), pulse pressure variation (PPV), and stroke volume variation (SVV), have been shown to be good predictors of volume responsiveness in critically ill patients. The presence of a large respiratory variation in these hemodynamic indices would encourage the physician to decide to give fluid as a first choice, rather than inotropes or vasopressors. These indices need further evaluation in spontaneously breathing hypovolemic patients.

Tissue perfusion

The ultimate goal of fluid therapy is to maintain or restore tissue perfusion and organ function. Restoration of depleted intravascular volume should improve tissue perfusion, but simple robust monitors of tissue perfusion in individual organs are not available. Global tissue perfusion is therefore indirectly assessed by systemic hemodynamic measurements, skin color, capillary refill, core–peripheral temperature difference, urine output, and surrogate markers of anaerobic metabolism, including arterial pH, base excess, mixed venous oxygen saturation, and blood lactate. These global perfusion indices are to be nonspecific markers of the volume status. Assessment of regional perfusion is more difficult. However, many methods have been developed, including monitoring of gastric mucosal CO_2 as an indicator of splanchnic perfusion, the jugular vein oxygen saturation (SjO_2) and cerebral oximetry for cerebral perfusion, tissue oxygen electrodes, sublingual tonometry, hepatic vein oxygen saturation, and microdialysis catheters. These methods need further clinical evaluation.

FLUID THERAPY

Hypovolemia and dehydration should be corrected by the administration of fluids. Healthy individuals will correct the deficits with oral intake of water and food. Oral rehydration solutions containing sodium and glucose in water are used worldwide in conditions of massive fluid loss, e.g. diarrhea. Administration of intravenous fluids is very common in the hospital setting. The rationale of intravenous fluid therapy is to replace fluid losses and to prevent or rapidly correct relative or absolute deficiencies in circulating blood volume. Two broad categories of fluids are available: crystalloids and colloids. The crystalloids include 5% dextrose, 4% dextrose in 0.18% saline, Hartmann's (Ringer's lactate) solution, and 0.9% saline. Albumin is a natural colloid, whereas artificial colloids are synthesized from gelatin, starches, and dextrans. The carrier solution for colloids is usually saline. Both crystalloids and colloids are administered for volume replacement, whereas the former are generally used for maintenance fluid requirements.

Daily requirements of fluids and electrolytes

WATER

A healthy adult requires approximately 2.5 L of water daily to replace losses, e.g. gastrointestinal loss of 100–200 mL/day, insensible losses of 500–1000 mL/day (half of which is respiratory and half cutaneous), and urinary loss of 1500 mL/day. Changes in body or environmental temperature can vary the amount of insensible loss. In patients with raised body temperature there is about a 7% increase in insensible losses per degree centigrade rise in temperature. There can also be a massive increase in insensible losses with physical exertion and sweating, particularly in humid environments.

ELECTROLYTES

An adult requires on average 1.73 g (75 mmol) of sodium daily to maintain sodium balance. Sodium reabsorption by the renal tubules is a very efficient process. Normal kidneys can reduce daily sodium excretion to less than 230 mg (10 mmol) in hypovolemic states, and can also excrete excess sodium efficiently with increased intake. Consequently, patients who have a normal cardiac and renal reserve can tolerate intravenous administration of Na^+ far in excess of normal daily requirements. In contrast renal reabsorption and excretion of K^+ is less efficient. The daily K^+ requirement slightly exceeds 1.6 g (40 mmol). A diuresis typically induces an obligate K^+ loss of at least 400 mg (10 mmol) for every liter of urine passed. Other electrolytes, such as Cl^-, Ca^{2+}, and Mg^{2+}, require no short-term replacement, but must be supplemented during long-term intravenous fluid therapy if enteral feeding is either contraindicated or not possible.

GLUCOSE

Glucose-containing intravenous fluids have been traditionally used to limit sodium load, to prevent hypoglycemia, and to limit catabolism. Hyperglycemia is common during major surgery and in the perioperative period because of the surgical stress response. Most patients do not require glucose-containing fluids, apart from infants and patients receiving insulin or drugs that interfere with glucose synthesis, who are at risk of hypoglycemia. Iatrogenic hyperglycemia can limit the effectiveness of fluid resuscitation by inducing an osmotic diuresis. Hyperglycemia may aggravate global and focal organ (e.g. heart, brain) ischemic injury. Tight glycemic control in postoperative patients using an insulin sliding scale has recently been shown to improve the outcome of patients undergoing major surgery. Glucose administration is indicated in patients with hepatic failure where hypoglycemia is likely to occur, and in hypernatremic conditions to replace water deficits. Dextrose–saline (4% dextrose in 0.18% saline) with potassium 20–40 mmol/L is commonly used as a maintenance fluid.

Crystalloids

Crystalloids are solutions of sodium chloride or glucose or both in water. They are usually isotonic, but can be hypotonic or hypertonic. In addition, other electrolytes, including potassium, calcium, and lactate, are added to make the composition of the intravenous fluid closer to that of plasma. The constituents of commonly used crystalloids are shown in Table 59.4. Following administration, such fluids disappear rapidly from the intravascular compartment to distribute throughout the ECF. A 1 L infusion of isotonic crystalloid results in less than 250 mL expansion of blood, but the remaining 750 mL will expand the ECF compartment. Excess use of these fluids during volume resuscitation is likely to cause pulmonary and/or tissue edema. These fluids are generally used to meet the maintenance fluid requirements and as first-line fluids during resuscitation.

Colloids

Colloid solutions contain high molecular weight molecules suspended in saline. The composition of commonly used colloids, including albumin, modified gelatin, hydroxyethyl starches, and dextrans, is shown in Table 59.4. Colloids are also termed plasma expanders because they exert oncotic pressure and hence retain fluid in the intravascular compartment, provided the capillary membrane function is intact. The carrier solution is typically 0.9% saline. The duration of intravascular retention of such solutions depends on the size of the molecules, their overall oncotic effect, and their plasma half-lives.

Colloids are increasingly used for replacement of depleted plasma volume. However, doubts remain as to which colloid is best. Differences in molecular weights and other characteristics

Table 59.4 Composition of some intravenous fluids

Fluid	Constituents				
	Glucose (g/L; mmol/L)	*Na^+ (g/L; mmol/L)*	*Cl^- (g/L; mmol/L)*	*Lactate (g/L; mmol/L)*	**Osmolality (mmol/kg)**
Crystalloids					
Dextrose 5% (D5W)	50 (278)	0	0	0	252
Dextrose 10% (D10W)	100 (555)	0	0	0	505
Hartmann's/Ringer's	0	3.0 (130)	3.87 (109)	2.52 (28)	273
Saline 0.9%	0	3.54 (154)	5.47 (154)	0	308
Hypertonic saline 7.5%	0	29.4 (1280)	45.4 (1280)	0	2560
$NaHCO_3$ 8.4%	0	23.0 (1000)	0	0	2000
D5W/0.33% saline	50 (278)	1.3 (56)	1.99 (56)	0	365
Colloids					
Hydroxyethyl starch 6%	0	3.54 (154)	5.47 (154)	0	310
Gelofusine 3.5%	0	3.45 (150)	4.44 (125)	0	310
Albumin 5%	0	3.54 (154)	5.33 (150)	0	310
Dextran 10%	0	3.45 (150)	5.33 (150)	0	310
Albumin 25% (salt poor)	0	1.38 (60)	2.13 (60)	0	1200

determine their safety and efficacy. Adverse effects of clinical importance include the effect on the platelet and coagulation system, anaphylactic or anaphylactoid reactions, and the effect on the reticuloendothelial system.

ALBUMIN

Albumin is relatively expensive compared to synthetic colloids. Albumin 4.5% in saline is iso-oncotic, whereas 20% albumin – so-called 'salt-poor' albumin (Na^+ 138 mg/dL; 60 mmol/L) – provides a very high COP and can expand the plasma volume by up to five times the volume administered by drawing fluid in from the ISF. The intravascular half-life of albumin is variable because of leakage into the interstitial space, and varies greatly with changes in the patient's condition. In normal individuals, approximately 4–5% of infused albumin escapes from the IVF per hour, equivalent to a plasma half-life of about 16 hours.

GELATINS

Gelatins are polypeptides with a molecular weight of approximately 35 kDa prepared by hydrolysis from chemically modified bovine collagen. Three preparations of modified gelatin are currently in use, including succinylated (Gelofusine), urea crosslinked (Haemaccel), and oxypolygelatin (Gelifundol). The only major difference between these preparations is in ionic composition, especially chloride and calcium. Gelatins provide isovolemic volume replacement. They have poor intravascular retention, with plasma half-lives of 1–2 hours. Therefore, reinfusions are necessary for prolonged volume support. Gelatins do not appear to influence hemostatic mechanisms, apart from a dose-dependent dilution of clotting factors. The incidence of severe anaphylactoid reactions no longer appears to be a problem with succinylated gelatin. The risks of anaphylactoid reaction are slightly greater with urea-crosslinked gelatins. Although widely used elsewhere, gelatins are not approved for clinical use in the USA.

DEXTRANS

Dextrans are highly branched polysaccharide molecules. Dextrans are commonly described by their number-averaged molecular weight (MWn, arithmetic mean of molecular weights): dextran 40 and dextran 70 have MWns of 40 and 70 kDa, respectively. The kidneys eliminate dextran 40, but dextran 70 passes into tissues and undergoes hydrolysis. Dextrans have numerous effects, including plasma volume expansion, improved microcirculatory flow, and antiplatelet and antifibrin activities. Dextran 40 improves microcirculatory flow secondary to reduced blood viscosity and red cell aggregation, and may be useful for patients undergoing vascular surgery and graft reconstruction procedures. Dextrans also induce an acquired von Willebrand's state (Chapter 53) by reducing the levels of both the components of factor VIII: VIIIR:Ag (factor VIII-related antigen) and VIII:C (factor VIII coagulant). With reduced VIII:C, there is reduced binding to platelet membrane receptor proteins GPIb and GPIIb/IIIa, which results in decreased platelet adhesion. In the past, the clinical use of dextrans has been associated with severe hypersensitivity reactions. Currently dextrans are not routinely used during fluid resuscitation.

HYDROXYETHYL STARCH

Hydroxyethyl starches (HES) are produced by hydroxyethyl substitution of amylopectin, a D-glucose polymer obtained from sorghum or maize. The pattern of hydroxyethyl substitution on glucose units reduces the susceptibility to hydrolysis by nonspecific amylases in the blood. The different HES products are commonly described by their weight-averaged molecular weight (MWw; the number of molecules at each weight multiplied by the particle weight divided by the total weight of all the molecules). HES products have molecules of different sizes with mean MWw ranging from 70 to 450 kDa. They are also described by their degree of hydroxyethyl substitution: hetastarches (C2/C6 ratio 0.6–0.7), pentastarches (C2/C6 ratio 0.5) and tetrastarches (C2/C6 ratio 0.4). Very small molecules tend to leak out of the intravascular space, and very large molecules can affect blood coagulation.

The duration of plasma volume expansion depends on the chemical characteristics of particular HES solutions and varies from 6 to 24 hours. Hydroxyethyl starches are comparable to 4.5% albumin in plasma volume expansion. HES usage varies between countries. First-generation hetastarches with high molecular weights (>450 kDa) presented in saline (Hespan) or in a lactate-buffered glucose containing balanced electrolyte solution (Hextend) are used clinically in the USA. In the UK medium molecular weight (220 kDa) pentastarches (second generation) are commonly used, and in Europe lower molecular weight (130 kDa) tetrastarches (Voluven) are favored. Long-term use of HES products leads to storage of HES molecules in the reticuloendothelial system. HES molecules remain detectable in lymph nodes even 10 months after administration. Intense prolonged debilitating pruritus has been reported following HES administration (especially the high molecular weight compounds), an effect that is unique to HES colloids. HES molecules are known to affect platelet function and the normal coagulation cascade in the blood, resulting in an acquired coagulation disorder – i.e. a von Willebrand's-like syndrome. HES molecules also can cause structural alteration in the renal tubules. Because of its side effects the dose of administered HES product is usually limited to 15–20 mL/kg. The side effects appear to be less in incidence with third-generation low molecular weight HES products (Voluven).

Hyperchloremic metabolic acidosis

Several recently published studies have suggested that saline, both when used alone and as a component of colloids in large quantities, can cause a hyperchloremic metabolic acidosis. This is probably not seen with the use of Hartmann's solution. It was initially thought to be a dilutional effect on plasma concentration of bicarbonate, but this was later ruled out as there was no change in plasma volume as measured both pre- and post-operatively by the Evans blue dye dilution technique. Instead, it has been shown that there is a strong relationship between total chloride given and base excess changes. Several hypotheses have been postulated.

The administration of saline, which has equal amounts of sodium and chloride, raises plasma chloride by a larger amount as its initial level is lower in plasma. The rise in plasma chloride increases the dissociation of water, resulting in more free hydrogen ions, as measured by a fall in pH. This has also been attributed to a reduced 'plasma strong ion difference' (SID). The ions in plasma can be broadly grouped into three classes: a) the respiratory group, bicarbonate and carbon dioxide; b) the weak acids such as albumin and phosphate, which are not completely dissociated; and c) the strong ion group, which are completely dissociated: sodium, chloride, potassium, calcium, magnesium, and lactate. The difference between the cations (Na^+ K^++ Ca^{2+}+ Mg^{2+}) and the anions (lactate + Cl^-) of the strong ion group is known as the strong ion difference. The SID is normally around 40 in health and it makes the blood alkaline. When excess saline is infused into blood, the chloride concentration goes up more than the sodium concentration, which increases the amount of H^+. To preserve the electrical neutrality water dissociates, thereby raising the free hydrogen ion concentration.

The effect of this hyperchloremic metabolic acidosis on morbidity and outcome is not clear. Hyperchloremic acidosis is not encountered with infusions of Hartmann's solution. Randomized double-blind studies comparing saline with Hartmann's following major surgery have not shown any difference in duration of mechanical ventilation, intensive care stay, hospital stay, or incidence of complications, including raised urea, raised creatinine, and subsequent renal failure.

Hypertonic fluids

The need to deliver fluid resuscitation in prehospital settings led to the development of hypertonic solutions. Hypertonic saline is thought to restore blood pressure by causing an osmotic fluid shift from the intracellular to the extracellular compartment, and from extracellular to intravascular compartment. For 1 L of blood loss, 250 mL of hypertonic saline (7.5%) appears to provide the same volume effect as 3 L of isotonic saline (0.9%). Therefore, it is called small volume resuscitation, e.g. 4–5 mL/kg. Small volume resuscitation has been shown to reduce intracranial pressure and to improve the cerebral perfusion pressure in patients with traumatic brain injury. In general there are insufficient data in the literature to conclude that hypertonic is better than isotonic crystalloid resuscitation. A colloid component including dextran or starch has been added to hypertonic saline to make it hypertonic–hyperoncotic in order to preserve the gained volume and hence hemodynamic stability for a longer time.

REGULATION OF ELECTROLYTES

Sodium

Sodium is the principal extracellular cation. Serum Na^+ concentration is an index of TBW rather than total body Na^+ under normal conditions. This ion principally maintains serum osmolality and ECF volume. Sodium plays a crucial role in the generation of cell membrane action potential. Disorders of Na^+ concentration – hypernatremia or hyponatremia – usually result from a relative deficit or excess of water, respectively.

SODIUM REGULATION

Serum Na^+ concentration (135–145 mmol/L) and total body Na^+ are closely regulated by renal function. Sodium is easily filtered by the glomeruli of the kidneys, and most of it is reabsorbed by the renal tubules. Several hormones, including aldosterone, ANP, and vasopressin, control the reabsorption of sodium and water in the renal tubules to maintain the amount of total body Na^+. Aldosterone is responsible for renal Na^+ reabsorption in exchange for K^+ and H^+ in the distal convoluted tubules and the collecting ducts of the kidneys. Atrial natriuretic peptide has an opposing effect by increasing renal excretion of Na^+; it tends to decrease PV. Normally, changes in serum Na^+ and osmolality lead to an appropriate change in vasopressin release by the posterior pituitary, which in turn can vary renal free water excretion (urine osmolality 50–1400 mmol/kg) in order to maintain serum Na^+ within the normal range. Increased vasopressin secretion in response to either raised plasma osmolality or hemodynamic stimuli results in reabsorption of water by the kidney and subsequent dilution of serum Na^+. Inadequate vasopressin release results in renal free water excretion, which can produce hypernatremia in the absence of adequate water intake. The end result of these physiologic processes is that in situations with Na^+ loss, for example diarrhea or excessive sweating, renal Na^+ conservation is high and urinary Na^+ concentration falls to extremely low levels. However, when Na^+ intake is excessive, decreased renal tubular reabsorption results in loss of more sodium in the urine.

Clinically, hyponatremia is more common than hypernatremia. Treatment of hyponatremia depends on whether it has developed acutely (<48 hours) or is chronic (>48–72 hours). For symptomatic hyponatremia some authorities advocate the administration of hypertonic saline (3%) during the first few hours to reduce brain edema, followed by a slow correction limited to 10 mmol/L over the next 24 hours to avoid the development of osmotic demyelinating syndrome. In patients with asymptomatic hyponatremia slow correction is the appropriate approach. Hypernatremia usually reflects dehydration. This requires correction of the underlying problem and replacement of the water deficit, either by increasing oral intake or by intravenous infusion of 5% dextrose.

Potassium

Potassium, the major intracellular cation, normally has an intracellular concentration of 150 mmol/L, about 28 times of that of ECF (3.5–5 mmol/L). Total body K^+ in a 70 kg adult is approximately 4256 mmol (166 g), of which 4200 mmol (164 g) is intracellular (98%) and 56 mmol (2 g) is extracellular (2%). Potassium plays an important role in the functioning of excitable cells such as muscles and neurons (Chapter 6). It is also involved in the maintenance of resting cell membrane potential. Therefore, changes in extracellular K^+ strongly influence excitation of the myocardium.

POTASSIUM REGULATION

Total body K^+ and serum K^+ concentrations are closely regulated by the renal tubules, so that potassium excretion is usually equal to daily potassium intake. There are several hormones, including aldosterone, epinephrine (adrenaline), and insulin, that have effects on plasma K^+ concentration. Aldosterone facilitates sodium reabsorption in exchange for potassium, resulting in an increased renal excretion of K^+. Epinephrine and insulin can alter plasma K^+ concentration by shifting K^+ into cells. Plasma K^+ is also influenced by acid–base balance. Assuming a plasma K^+ of 4 mmol/L and a normal glomerular filtration rate of 180 L/day, a total of 720 mmol (28 g) K^+ is filtered daily. Most is reabsorbed in the proximal tubules, but only the amount ingested (normally 40–120 mmol (1.5–4.7 g) daily) is lost in urine. Excretion of K^+ depends primarily on secretion by the distal nephron, and is increased by aldosterone, hyperkalemia, diuretics, and the presence in tubular fluid of nonreabsorbable anions such as phosphates and sulfates.

Hyperkalemia results from renal insufficiency in critically ill patients. Glucose and insulin reduce plasma potassium; insulin promotes potassium entry into cells by a mechanism separate from glucose entry, and glucose is required to prevent hypoglycemia. In patients with established acute or acute-on-chronic renal failure, hyperkalemia reflects a generalized metabolic disturbance and is an indication to start renal replacement therapy. Hypokalemia is common in critically ill patients. Potassium should be replaced in conjunction with correction of underlying causes and abnormalities.

Calcium

Calcium is found primarily in bone (99%) and the ECF (1%). Serum calcium is approximately 40% protein bound, especially to albumin, 10% chelated to serum anions, and 50% is in free ionized form. Normal concentration of ionized Ca^{2+} in the ECF is 1.0–1.5 mmol/L, whereas that in ICF is about 50 nmol/L. The free ionized fraction is the physiologically active component responsible for many cellular processes, including neuromuscular transmission, excitation–contraction coupling in muscles, release of hormones and neurotransmitters, enzyme activation, blood coagulation, and bone structure. Calcium is an intracellular messenger and is required for the activity of phosphoinositides and cAMP. Calcium is also important in the generation of the plateau phase of the cardiac action potential.

Alterations in serum albumin, common in critically ill patients, can change total serum calcium concentration by as much as 30%. Additionally, free fatty acids and intravenously administered lipids in the critically ill may increase calcium binding by forming additional calcium-binding sites. Although there are formulae to correct total serum calcium for albumin concentration and pH, they are poor predictors of ionized Ca^{2+}. Measurement of ionized Ca^{2+} is therefore essential for the accurate diagnosis of hypocalcemia in critically ill patients.

CALCIUM REGULATION

Calcium is regulated via two primary hormones: parathyroid hormone (PTH) and 1,25-dihydroxy-vitamin D (Chapter 66). Both of these are secreted in response to a decrease in serum ionised Ca^{2+}. Metabolites of vitamin D exert a major role in long-term control of circulating Ca^{2+}. Vitamin D, following ingestion or manufacture in the skin under the stimulus of ultraviolet light, is hydroxylated at the 25-position in the liver and the 1-position in the kidney, giving the active metabolite 1,25-dihydroxy vitamin D. Both PTH and 1,25-dihydroxy vitamin D stimulate Ca^{2+} release from bone and Ca^{2+} absorption from renal tubules and the intestine; hence, they can maintain a normal circulating Ca^{2+} within narrow limits even in the absence of dietary intake.

Hypocalcemia is a common disorder in ICU patients and diagnosed by measurement of ionized calcium rather than total calcium concentration. Acute hypocalcemia should be treated urgently to bring serum ionized calcium back to normal, and definitive treatment is required for the underlying disorder.

Phosphate

Phosphorus, in the form of phosphate, is found mostly inside the cell. Bone accounts for 85% of body phosphate. The normal serum phosphate level ranges from 0.8 to 1.3 mmol/L (7.6–12.3 mg/dL) in adults. Serum phosphate level is regulated by renal excretion. Therefore the most common cause of hyperphosphatemia is renal failure. Phosphate plays a vital role in oxidative phosphorylation of carbohydrate, fat, and protein metabolism. Phosphate is a structural component of nucleic acids, phospholipids, and the cell membrane. It is also essential for intracellular second-messenger systems, including cAMP and phosphatidoinositol. As a part of 2,3-diphosphoglycerate (2,3-DPG), it helps in the offloading of oxygen from hemoglobin in the tissues.

Low serum phosphate is more common in up to one-third of long-stay ICU patients. Mild to moderate hypophosphatemia has not been conclusively linked with significant clinical symptoms, including muscle weakness. Low phosphate levels are seen as a part of refeeding syndrome in ICU patients. Low phosphate levels have been implicated as a cause of failure to wean from ventilatory support, although it appears unlikely to be a significant factor on its own. Intravenous phosphate is administered in form of potassium phosphate infusion 20 mmol over 4–6 hours, with monitoring of its levels.

Magnesium

Magnesium is found mostly in the ICF and in bone. Of total body Mg^{2+}, 99% is intracellular and only 1% is extracellular. Of the normal serum Mg^{2+} (0.8–1.2 mmol/L; 1.9–2.9 mg/dL), free 'ionized' Mg^{2+} (50%) is physiologically active. Serum Mg^{2+} is regulated primarily by renal excretion. Free Mg^{2+} is an essential cofactor for ATP-requiring enzymes such as the cell membrane Na^+/K^+-ATPase and more than 300 enzymes involved in energy metabolism. Normal adult requirements are 0.4 mmol/kg/day (5 mg/kg/day) orally or 0.1 mmol/kg/day parenterally. These requirements are increased up to three times in critical illness. Hypomagnesemia is very common in critically ill patients and many therapeutic interventions, including catecholamine infusions, diuretics, and aminoglycoside antibiotics, can reduce it further. Hypomagnesemia is commonly associated with hypokalemia, because the function of the Na^+/K^+-ATPase pump is impaired, resulting in renal potassium wasting and intracellular potassium depletion.

Symptoms of hypomagnesemia are nonspecific and variable. The incidence of serious arrhythmias is higher in patients with hypomagnesemia. Magnesium replacement has been shown to prevent arrhythmias after myocardial infarction. Moreover, magnesium administration has been shown to be useful in treating supraventricular and ventricular arrhythmias even in patients with normal levels of Mg^{2+}. Alcoholic patients in the intensive care unit are particularly prone to hypomagnesemia. Magnesium has a proven role in the management of eclampsia. Magnesium is administered as an infusion of magnesium sulfate (40 mmol over 4 hours), with monitoring of its level following the infusion.

Key references

Finfer S, Bellomo R, Myburgh J, Norton R. Efficacy of albumin in critically ill patients. Br Med J. 2003;326:559–60.

Kreimeier U, Messmer K. Small volume resuscitation: from experimental evidence to clinical routine. Advantages and disadvantages of hypertonic solutions. Acta Anaesthesiol Scand. 2002;46:625–38.

Mallick A, Bodenham AR. Disorders of the lymph circulation: their relevance to anaesthesia and intensive care. Br J Anaesth. 2003;91:265–72.

Stephens R, Mythen M. Optimising intraoperative fluid therapy. Curr Opin Anaesthesiol. 2003;16:385–92.

Further reading

Bellomo R, Shigehiko U. Cardiovascular monitoring tools. Curr Opin Crit Care 2003;9:225–9.

Bunn F, Alderson P, Hawkins V. Colloids solutions for fluid resuscitation. Cochrane Database Syst Rev. 2003; 1: CD001319.

Decaux G, Soupart A. Treatment of symptomatic hyponatremia. Am J Med Sci. 2003;326:25–30.

Mosa MM, Cheng DCH. Oxygen therapeutics (blood substitutes) in cardiac surgery. Curr Opin Anaesth. 2003;16:21–6.

Rivers E, Nguyen B, Havstad S et al. Early goal directed therapy in the treatment of severe sepsis and septic shock. New Engl J Med. 2001;345:1368–77.

Squara P, Bennett D, Perret C. Pulmonary artery catheter: does the problem lie in the users. Chest 2002;121:2009–15.

Waters JH, Gottileb A, Schoenwald P et al. Normal saline versus lactated Ringer's solution for intraoperative fluid management for intraoperative fluid management in patients undergoing abdominal aortic aneurysm repair: an outcome study. Anesth Analg. 2001;93:817–22.

Wilkes MM, Navickis RJ. Patient survival after human albumin administration – a meta-analysis of randomized control trials. Ann Intern Med. 2001;135:149–64.

Chapter 60

Acid–base homeostasis

Andrew P Gratrix and Simon M Enright

TOPICS COVERED IN THIS CHAPTER

- **Definitions**
  - Acid and base
  - pH and pKa′
  - Buffer
  - Anion gap
  - Acidosis and acidemia
  - Alkalosis and alkalemia
- **Normal physiology**
  - Henderson–Hasselbalch equation
  - Production of acids
  - Buffering systems
- **The role of the lungs**
- **The role of the kidney**
  - Bicarbonate reabsorption
  - Bicarbonate generation
  - Urinary buffers
- **The role of the liver**
  - Lactate
  - Ammonia, glutamine, and urea
- **Disturbances of hydrogen ion homeostasis**
  - Metabolic acidosis
  - Metabolic alkalosis
  - Respiratory acidosis
  - Respiratory alkalosis
- **Interpretation of laboratory values**
  - Oxygen measurement
  - Carbon dioxide measurement
  - pH measurement
  - Acid–base diagrams
- **The effect of temperature on arterial blood gas interpretation**
  - α-stat
  - pH-stat

Intracellular and extracellular hydrogen ion (H^+) concentrations are normally kept within narrow limits. However, disturbances in the homeostatic mechanisms that maintain a normal H^+ environment are commonly encountered in anesthesia and intensive care. In this chapter both the basic science of acid–base physiology in normal and abnormal situations and a reasoned approach to the interpretation of arterial blood gas analysis are described.

DEFINITIONS

Acid and base

According to the Brönsted–Lowry concept an acid is a compound that dissociates in water to release H^+ (protons) (Equation 60.1). A base is a compound that can accept H^+ (Equation 60.2).

■ Equation 60.1

$$HA \leftrightarrow H^+ + A^-$$

■ Equation 60.2

$$B + H^+ \leftrightarrow BH^+$$

pH and pKa′

pH is a useful means of expressing H^+ concentration ($[H^+]$, where the square brackets designate 'concentration of ') – pH is the negative logarithm to the base 10 of $[H^+]$ in moles/liter (mol/L). As acidity increases, the pH decreases. Neutral pH is the pH at which the concentrations of H^+ and OH^- are equal ($[H^+] = [OH^-]$). Water is more ionized at body temperature than at room temperature, so neutral pH at body temperature is 6.8; this is the average intracellular pH. Normal extracellular pH (7.4) is slightly alkaline. p*K*a is the pH at which a compound is 50% ionized.

Buffer

A buffer is a substance with the capacity to bind or release H^+ and thus minimize changes in $[H^+]$ or pH. Buffers consist of a mixture of a weak acid and its conjugate base. A buffer is most effective at its p*K*a, at which it is 50% ionized. Most of the buffering capacity (80%) occurs in the range of −1 to +1 pH units around the p*K*a. The effectiveness of a buffer also depends on the ability of the body to remove H^+, for example as CO_2 in the bicarbonate system.

Anion gap

On the basis of electroneutrality, the total serum cation concentration is equal to the total serum anion concentration (Equation 60.3).

■ Equation 60.3

$$[Na^+] + [K^+] + [Ca^{2+}] + [Mg^{2+}] = [HCO_3^-] + [Cl^-] + [PO_4^{3-}] + [SO_4^{2-}] + [\text{protein}] + \text{organic acid anions}$$

To simplify Equation 60.3, the minor serum cations (K^+, Ca^{2+}, and Mg^{2+}) are considered unmeasured cations (UC) and the minor serum anions (PO_4^{3-}, SO_4^{2-}, protein, and organic acids) are considered unmeasured anions (UA); this gives Equation 60.4:

■ Equation 60.4

$$Na^+ + UC = HCO_3^- + Cl^- + UA$$

The anion gap (AG) is the difference between the unmeasured anions and cations (Equation 60.5). The normal range for the anion gap is 12 ± 4 mmol/L, which is of use in classifying different types of metabolic acidosis.

■ Equation 60.5

$$AG = UA - UC = Na^+ - HCO_3^- - Cl^-$$

Acidosis and acidemia

Acidosis is an abnormal condition that tends to decrease blood pH. Acidemia is a blood pH less than 7.35.

Alkalosis and alkalemia

Alkalosis is an abnormal condition that tends to increase blood pH. Alkalemia is a blood pH greater than 7.45.

NORMAL PHYSIOLOGY

Henderson–Hasselbalch equation

The relationship between pH and buffer p*K*a may be calculated by the Henderson–Hasselbalch equation:

■ Equation 60.6

$$pH = pKa + \log_{10}\frac{[\text{base}]}{[\text{acid}]}$$

The most important buffering system in extracellular fluids is the carbonic acid–bicarbonate system, and so extracellular pH can be described by Equation 60.7:

■ Equation 60.7

$$pH = pKa + \log_{10}\frac{[HCO_3^-]}{[H_2CO_3]}$$

As H_2CO_3 is in equilibrium with the amount of dissolved CO_2 ($P\text{CO}_2$), this equation can be rewritten as the modified Henderson–Hasselbalch equation (Equation 60.8), in which the p*K*a of the system is 6.1 and *S* is the solubility coefficient of CO_2 in plasma:

■ Equation 60.8

$$pH = 6.1 + \log_{10}\frac{[HCO_3^-]}{(S \times P\text{CO}_2)}$$

When $P\text{CO}_2$ is expressed as mmHg, $S = 0.03$; when $P\text{CO}_2$ is expressed in kPa, $S = 0.23$. The Henderson–Hasselbalch equation can be transformed into the Henderson equation (Kassirer–Bleich modification), which has no logarithms (Equation 60.9):

■ Equation 60.9

$$[H^+] = 23.9 \times \frac{P\text{CO}_2}{[HCO_3^-]}$$

It is the ratio of $P\text{CO}_2$ to HCO_3^-, and not the absolute values of either, that determines the extracellular $[H^+]$ and pH. Intracellular pH is maintained at 6.8 ($[H^+]$ =160 nmol/L). The normal range of pH in extracellular fluids is 7.35–7.45 (35–45 nmol/L of H^+). Thus, a fourfold concentration gradient occurs for H^+ from inside to outside the cell. This is counterbalanced by the intracellular potential of –70 mV, which tends to attract H^+ into the cell. In clinical practice we are unable to measure or manipulate intracellular pH.

Production of acids

Normal metabolism produces H^+ and CO_2. Around 50–100 mmol/day of H^+ are released from cells into the extracellular fluid. Aerobic metabolism of organic compounds produces water and CO_2. The latter is an essential component of the extracellular buffering system, and control of CO_2 depends upon normal lung function. The main sources of H^+ are:

- metabolism of amino acids – conversion of amino nitrogen into urea in the liver, or of sulfhydryl groups of some amino acids into sulfate (e.g. methionine and cysteine), releases equimolar concentrations of H^+;
- incomplete metabolism of carbon skeletons of organic compounds – anaerobic carbohydrate metabolism produces lactate and anaerobic metabolism of fatty acids and ketogenic amino acids produces acetoacetate; both processes release equimolar concentrations of H^+, either directly or indirectly.

Buffering systems

Buffering systems are present in both extra- and intracellular fluids (extracellular groups are discussed here, as these can be measured and manipulated). The main extracellular buffers in blood are H_2CO_3/HCO_3^-, the hemoglobin (Hb) system (HHb/Hb^- and $HHbO_2/HbO_2^-$), proteins (histidine residues), and phosphate ($H_2PO_4^-/HPO_4^{2-}$). The main intracellular buffers are proteins, phosphate, organic phosphate, and HCO_3^-.

The efficacy of a buffer system depends on:

- the concentration of the buffer;
- the p*K*a of the system (80% of buffering activity occurs within p*K*a ± 1 unit; Fig. 60.1);
- whether the system is 'open' or 'closed'.

OPEN (PHYSIOLOGICAL) AND CLOSED (CHEMICAL) BUFFERING SYSTEMS

The bicarbonate system has the advantage of being an open system, which means that it is not constrained by the p*K*a and a

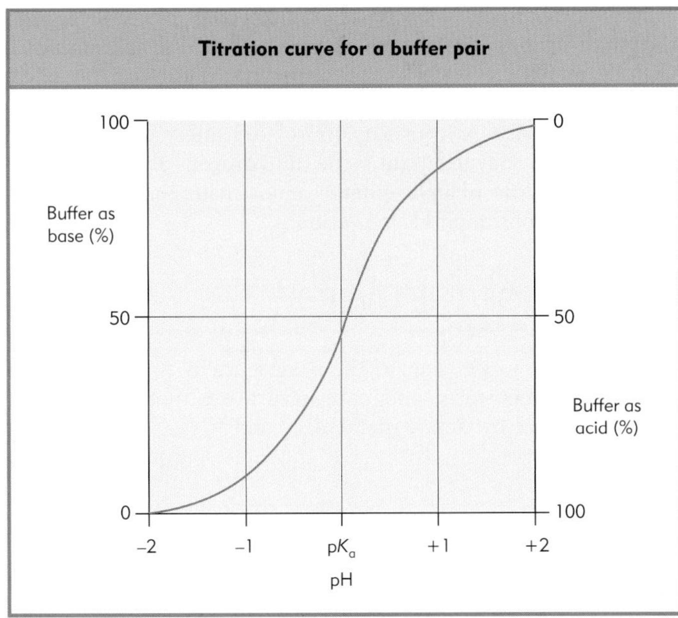

Figure 60.1 Titration curve for a buffer pair. Around 80% of the buffering capacity occurs within −1 to +1 pH units of the p*Ka*. The p*Ka* of the bicarbonate system is 6.1, so its buffering capacity within the physiological range is limited.

limited amount of buffer; the result is relatively independent control of CO_2. Thus, altering minute ventilation gives the flexibility to adjust CO_2 concentrations back to normal levels. This gives the system up to 20 times the buffering capacity of a closed system, in which the total amount of buffer remains constant.

The major extracellular systems can be divided into the bicarbonate buffer system and the nonbicarbonate buffer system.

Bicarbonate buffer system

Most CO_2, a potentially toxic product of aerobic metabolism, is lost via the lungs, but some is converted into bicarbonate that contributes to the total extracellular buffering capacity. An ideal physiological buffer has a p*Ka* around 7.4, but that of the H_2CO_3/HCO_3^- system is only 6.1. This may seem a disadvantage, but HCO_3^- is still the most important extracellular buffer for the following reasons:

- it accounts for around 60% of the total blood buffering capacity;
- its presence is necessary for efficient buffering by Hb, which accounts for most of the rest of the total capacity;
- it is necessary for H^+ secretion by the kidney.

Normally, arterial P_{CO_2} is kept within narrow limits at about 40 mmHg (5.3 kPa). This value depends on the balance between the rate of CO_2 production and its removal, and is controlled by chemoreceptors in the respiratory center in the medulla of the brainstem and in the carotid and aortic bodies.

The components of the bicarbonate buffer system are in equilibrium (Equation 60.10). The initial step is catalyzed by the enzyme carbonic anhydrase, which is present in high concentrations in erythrocytes and renal tubular cells. As these cells have the ability to remove H^+, this reaction favors the production of HCO_3^-. The generation of HCO_3^- is accelerated if $[CO_2]$ rises, $[HCO_3^-]$ falls, or $[H^+]$ falls because it is buffered by erythrocytes or excreted by renal tubular cells. Therefore, an increase in intracellular P_{CO_2} or a decrease in intracellular $[HCO_3^-]$ in erythrocytes and renal tubular cells maintains extracellular $[HCO_3^-]$ by accelerating the production of HCO_3. This minimizes changes in the HCO_3^-/P_{CO_2} ratio and therefore changes in pH.

■ Equation 60.10

$$CO_2 + H_2O \leftrightarrow H_2CO_3 \leftrightarrow H^+ + HCO_3^-$$

Hemoglobin

Hemoglobin is an important blood buffer, but only works effectively with the bicarbonate buffer system. Buffering by hemoglobin depends on the imidazole group of histidine, which dissociates less (p*Ka* increases) when hemoglobin is deoxygenated. Thus, oxygenated hemoglobin is a stronger acid than deoxygenated hemoglobin. Deoxygenated hemoglobin is a better buffer than oxygenated hemoglobin, and each molecule can accept 0.7 mmol of H^+ for 1 mmol of oxygen (O_2) released without a change in pH. Intracellular metabolism in erythrocytes does not produce CO_2, which enters from the plasma along a concentration gradient. Inside the cell, carbonic anhydrase catalyzes the production of carbonic acid, which dissociates into H^+ and HCO_3^-.

Most of the H^+ produced is buffered by hemoglobin, and the HCO_3^- diffuses out of the cell along a concentration gradient – electrochemical neutrality is maintained by inward diffusion of chloride ions (chloride shift). The increase in P_{CO_2} in venous blood is accompanied by an increase in HCO_3^- production in erythrocytes, which thus minimizes change in the HCO_3^-/P_{CO_2} ratio and changes in pH.

Nonbicarbonate buffer systems

The phosphate system (HPO_4^{2-} and $H_2PO_4^-$) has a p*Ka* of 6.8 and so has theoretic advantages over the bicarbonate system. However, the concentration of phosphate is only around 1 mmol/L (3.1 mg/dL), and it can only operate as a closed system. It is of greatest importance in the intracellular compartment and in urine.

Plasma proteins contain titratable groups (primarily histidine) and have the ability to buffer H^+. Plasma proteins only have around 15% of the buffering power of hemoglobin, and therefore buffer around 5% of all extracellular H^+.

THE ROLE OF THE LUNGS

The lungs are responsible for the excretion of respiratory acid (CO_2). Around 16 mol of CO_2 is produced per day (360 L). Unless respiratory depression or disease is present, the lungs are able to rapidly compensate for changes in acid–base status (especially acidosis) by changes in minute volume. Stimulation and limitation of minute volume is controlled by neurons in the medulla oblongata and pons, which form the respiratory center. Chemosensitive areas of the center are able to detect blood concentrations of CO_2 and H^+. Acidosis and increases in CO_2 both cause stimulation, and the effect is to increase minute volume, thus CO_2 is eliminated, bringing pH back towards normal.

THE ROLE OF THE KIDNEY

The H^+ produced by the body is mostly removed by ventilation, because it reacts with HCO_3^- to form CO_2, which is exhaled. Therefore, HCO_3^- is lost from the body as CO_2, and the main function of the kidney in acid–base homeostasis is to conserve and produce additional HCO_3^-. The normal plasma concentration of HCO_3^- is 22–30 mmol/L, which is freely filtered at the glomerulus. The transport maximum for HCO_3^- reabsorption is close to the amount filtered at normal plasma concentration. Therefore, the response to a high HCO_3^- is continued excretion until the plasma concentration falls to normal levels.

From the renal tubular cells H^+ is secreted into the lumina, where it is buffered by constituents of the glomerular filtrate. Urinary buffers are constantly replenished by continuous glomerular filtration and reabsorption. Other buffering systems are only useful in the short term, and the kidneys provide the only route for elimination of most of the excess acid produced. The two renal mechanisms that control HCO_3^- are reabsorption and generation (see also Chapter 57).

Bicarbonate reabsorption

Normal urine is almost free of HCO_3^-. Bicarbonate is filtered at a concentration of about 25 mmol/L, and an amount equivalent to that filtered is returned to the body by tubular cells. The filtered HCO_3^- combines with H^+, which is secreted by tubular cells, to form H_2CO_3. The H_2CO_3 dissociates to form water and CO_2 (catalyzed by carbonic anhydrase in the brush border); CO_2 diffuses into tubular cells along its concentration gradient and, once intracellular, combines with water to form H^+ and HCO_3^- (again under the influence of carbonic anhydrase). The H^+ is secreted into the tubular lumen in exchange for Na^+. As the intracellular concentration of HCO_3^- rises, it diffuses into the extracellular fluid accompanied by Na^+.

Most of the reabsorption occurs in the proximal tubule (around 90%). No direct transport of HCO_3^- occurs, but there is luminal conversion of HCO_3^- into CO_2. This cycle reclaims buffering power that would be lost by glomerular filtration. The secreted H^+ is derived from cellular water and is incorporated into water in the lumen, with no net loss of H^+. As such, this mechanism only preserves the status quo.

Bicarbonate generation

This process helps to correct acidosis and involves increased activity of carbonic anhydrase with loss of H^+ and generation of HCO_3^-. Carbonic anhydrase is stimulated by:

- a rise in $P\text{CO}_2$, which is caused indirectly by a rise in extracellular $P\text{CO}_2$ and a reduction in the CO_2 concentration gradient between inside and outside the tubular cell; and
- a fall of extracellular HCO_3^-, which causes an increase in concentration gradient between inside and outside the cells, and leads to a fall in intracellular HCO_3^-.

The ability of the kidneys to excrete excess H^+ depends on the presence of filtered buffer bases other than bicarbonate (which is totally reclaimed). Loss of H^+ and buffer base (as Hb) occurs. Bicarbonate formed in the tubular cells diffuses into the extracellular fluid, and therefore a net gain of bicarbonate results.

Urinary buffers

The two important urinary buffers are phosphate and ammonia/ammonium (NH_3/NH_4^+ are considered in the role of the liver).

The p*K*a of the phosphate buffer system is 6.8, so at pH 7.4 most is in the form HPO_4^{2-}. Phosphate is the most important urinary buffer because the p*K*a is similar to the pH of urine, and the concentration of phosphate increases from 1.2 to 25 mmol/L (3.7–77 mg/dL) as water is reabsorbed in the tubular lumen. In mild acidosis, phosphate is released from bone to allow this buffering activity. At a urinary pH of 5.5, most of the filtered phosphate is converted into the dihydrogen phosphate and, therefore, at low pH phosphate cannot maintain the essential buffering of continued H^+ secretion.

THE ROLE OF THE LIVER

The liver is no longer seen as the passive 'slave' to the kidney in acid–base homeostasis, and may have a coordinating role. Its main effects are by lactate metabolism and NH_3–glutamine–urea metabolism.

Lactate

Normal production of lactate is around 1400 mmol/day from the skin, gut, muscle, brain, and erythrocytes. The protons produced titrate local HCO_3^- and most of the lactate (70%) is removed by the liver (30% via the kidneys and heart), in which it is converted into CO_2 and water by oxidation and gluconeogenesis. Bicarbonate is reformed by gluconeogenesis, which replaces that lost to titration in the periphery. Production and removal of lactate are therefore normally in balance. Lactate enters hepatocytes via two main routes:

- Semispecific monocarboxylate transporter, which is pH sensitive and activated by a pH gradient of acid (outside) to alkaline (inside). Increased activity occurs in starvation and diabetes. Normal lactate concentration in the blood is 0.5–1 mmol/L. The transporter becomes saturated at serum lactate >2.5 mmol/L.
- Simple diffusion of un-ionized lactic acid, which takes over from the above route at higher serum lactate concentrations. Simple diffusion is not limited by saturation.

Once inside the hepatocyte, the main pathway of lactate disposal is via gluconeogenesis with concomitant bicarbonate regeneration (Equation 60.11). The H^+ is provided by ionization of water ($2H_2O \leftrightarrow 2H^+ + 2OH^-$), and the hydroxyl ion produces bicarbonate ($2OH^- + 2CO_2 \leftrightarrow 2HCO_3^-$). Glucose is produced by the intermediates pyruvate and oxaloacetate (intracellular acidosis inhibits the formation of oxaloacetate from pyruvate).

■ Equation 60.11

$$\underset{\text{(Lactate)}}{2CH_3CHOCOO^-} + 2H^+ \leftrightarrow \underset{\text{(Glucose)}}{C_6H_{12}O_6}$$

In mild acidosis (e.g. exercise, mild blood loss) there is increased activity of the lactate transporter and increased diffusion of lactate to hepatocytes, with removal of excess lactate and HCO_3^- regeneration. In more severe acidosis (such as shock), an increased peripheral production of lactate and H^+ is accompanied by decreased liver blood flow. When liver blood flow reaches a critical point (around 25% of normal), saturation of the transporter (at lactate concentration of 2 mmol/L) and inhibition of gluconeogenesis at the pyruvate–oxaloacetate stage cannot be overcome by increased lactate entry into the cell. Failure of gluconeogenesis causes the intracellular pH to fall, which further inhibits lactate uptake and removal. This sets up a vicious circle of increasing lactic acidosis.

Ammonia, glutamine, and urea

As blood pH falls, urine pH falls and the urine contains more NH_4^+. Increased NH_4^+ excretion appears to allow continued H^+ excretion after urinary buffers such as phosphate have been depleted in acidosis. Normally, around 40 mmol/day of NH_4^+ is excreted, but this may increase to 400 mmol/day in severe acidosis.

The traditional model is that glutamine is taken up by renal tubular cells and deaminated by glutaminase to produce NH_3. This diffuses into the tubular fluid, where it buffers H^+, secreted by the tubular cells, to form NH_4^+, which is excreted in the urine. The drawback of this model is that cellular deamination of glutamine leads not to NH_3 but to NH_4^+ production, which is unable to buffer further H^+. Consequently, a new theory has emerged in which the liver has a central regulatory role, NH_4^+ is not a buffer, and the kidneys do not simply act as proton excretors.

The liver performs three interrelated functions that affect acid–base homeostasis:

- Deamination-oxidation of amino acids;
- Urea production; and
- Glutamine production.

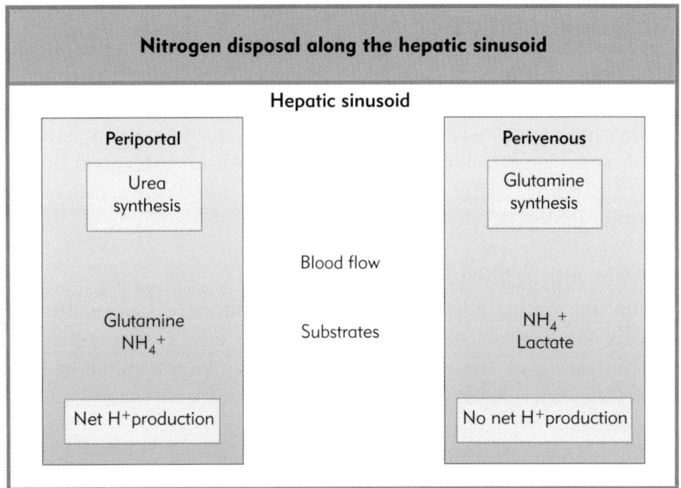

Figure 60.2 Organization of nitrogen disposal mechanisms along the hepatic sinusoid.

Amino acids are dipolar molecules at physiological pH and contain an amino group (NH_3^+) and a carboxyl group (COO^-). Deamination and oxidation in the liver leads to the production of NH_4^+ and bicarbonate (100 g of neutral amino acid yields 1000 mmol of HCO_3^- and 1000 mmol of NH_4^+). This bicarbonate load cannot be excreted by the kidney and would rapidly lead to alkalosis. However, oxidation–deamination is closely linked to the energy-dependent formation of urea in the urea cycle, which occurs exclusively in the liver (Equation 60.12).

■ Equation 60.12

$$CO_2 + 2NH_4^+ \leftrightarrow \underset{\text{(Urea)}}{CO(NH_2)_2} + H_2O + 2H^+$$

Most of the NH_4^+ formed by deamination of amino acids is converted into urea, which is excreted in the urine. For each mole of urea produced, 2 moles of H^+ are formed. This H^+ titrates the bicarbonate formed from deamination of amino acids. Conversion of the NH_4^+ from neutral amino acids (containing one carboxyl and one amino group) into urea leads to H^+ production, which exactly neutralizes HCO_3^- production from deamination. In addition, another pathway is available for the disposal of NH_4^+, in which NH_4^+ is incorporated into glutamine by the enzyme glutamine synthetase. The glutamine route for NH_4^+ disposal does not carry the physiological penalty of proton production, and therefore leads to a net production of HCO_3^-.

Urea synthesis occurs mainly in the periportal cells of the liver sinusoid (Fig. 60.2). Glutamine synthesis is located in one or two cells at the end of the sinusoid, which are close to the centrilobular vein. These cells have no urea cycle activity and are the only ones that contain glutamine synthetase. Any NH_4^+ not converted into urea by the periportal cells passes to perivenous cells and is vigorously scavenged to produce glutamine. At normal pH a net uptake of glutamine by the liver occurs, but in acidotic conditions there is net production and release of glutamine. Glutamine therefore serves as a nontoxic transport form of NH_3^+ to the kidneys. It is now obvious that the extent to which bicarbonate (produced by amino acid metabolism) is titrated by H^+ produced during urea synthesis depends on the proportion of amino nitrogen that is converted into either urea or glutamine. By switching the urea cycle on and off, the liver can exert control over acid–base homeostasis. For example, in acidosis the urea cycle is inhibited, net bicarbonate is generated from amino acid metabolism, and NH_4^+ excretion by the kidneys is increased.

DISTURBANCES OF HYDROGEN ION HOMEOSTASIS

Normal $[H^+]$ is low (35–45 nmol/L) compared to other ions (e.g. $[Na^+]$ is 140 mmol/L). However, the small size of H^+ permits high reactivity with protein-binding sites, and small changes in $[H^+]$ can have significant effects on protein function (e.g. enzyme activity). When there is an imbalance between H^+ production and H^+ removal, $[H^+]$ and pH deviate from normal, but the range of extracellular pH compatible with life is narrow (6.8–7.7, which corresponds to $[H^+]$ 20–160 nmol/L).

The clinical effects of acidemia and alkalemia may be direct or indirect (alterations in blood flow or humoral effects). The principal effects of acidemia include:

- generalized depression of function;
- decreased myocardial contractility, cardiac output, blood pressure;
- dilatation of blood vessels (not responsive to constrictors);
- tendency to fibrillation and other arrhythmias (especially in the presence of hypercapnia); and
- depression of central nervous system that leads to coma.

The principal effects of alkalemia include:

- lower plasma $[K^+]$ and arrhythmias;
- reduction in cardiac output and cerebral blood flow; and
- lowered unbound $[Ca^{2+}]$, neuronal irritability, and tetany.

The four major types of acid–base disturbance are now considered – metabolic acidosis, metabolic alkalosis, respiratory acidosis, and respiratory alkalosis.

Metabolic acidosis

Metabolic acidosis occurs when a primary decrease in extracellular bicarbonate causes a fall in pH below 7.35. The causes of metabolic acidosis can be divided into those with a normal anion gap (hyperchloremic) and those with an increased anion gap (Fig. 60.3). Some important causes of metabolic acidosis are given in Table 60.1.

NORMAL ANION GAP (<12 MMOL/L)
If the anion gap is normal, loss of bicarbonate has occurred, usually via the gastrointestinal tract or kidneys. The result is concentration of the other major measured extracellular anion, chloride, which leads to hyperchloremia.

INCREASED ANION GAP (>12 MMOL/L)
If the anion gap is increased, strong acids have been added to the system that buffers bicarbonate. This may result from retention of endogenous acids produced in excess, such as lactic acid (from tissue hypoxia), or by the addition of exogenous acids.

LACTIC ACIDOSIS
Lactic acidosis is of importance to anesthetic and intensive care practice and is a result of tissue hypoxia caused by hypotension, hypovolemia, or sepsis. Lactic acidosis should be suspected when an increased anion gap acidosis cannot be accounted for by renal failure or ketone production. The normal lactate level is around 1 mmol/L. Severe lactic acidosis is associated with levels >5 mmol/L.

Compensation in metabolic acidosis

The compensatory response to metabolic acidosis is an increase in ventilation (usually via an increased tidal volume – 'Kussmaul' breathing), but this is only partial and does not return the pH to normal.

Table 60.1 Causes of metabolic acidosis

Cause	Examples
Normal anion gap	
Gastrointestinal loss of bicarbonate	Diarrhea, fistulae, ureterosigmoidostomy
Renal loss of bicarbonate	Renal tubular acidosis (types I–IV), carbonic anhydrase inhibitors
Other	Administration of NH_4Cl and other Cl—containing compounds, hyperalimentation, dilution
Increased anion gap	
Increased acid production	Diabetic ketoacidosis, starvation
Exogenous acid	Methanol, salicylate, ethylene glycol
Lactic acidosis	Shock, sepsis, exercise, inborn errors of metabolism
Reduced acid secretion	Acute and chronic renal failure

Treatment of metabolic acidosis

Treatment of metabolic acidosis includes correction of the underlying disorder and specific alkali therapy. Initial therapy is directed against the cause of the disorder (e.g. improved oxygen delivery and tissue perfusion in lactic acidosis, insulin therapy in diabetic ketoacidosis, and fluid therapy in hypovolemia). Alkali therapy is reserved for severe acidosis (pH <7.25) that is not responsive to general measures, especially when cardiovascular instability is present. Sodium bicarbonate is most commonly

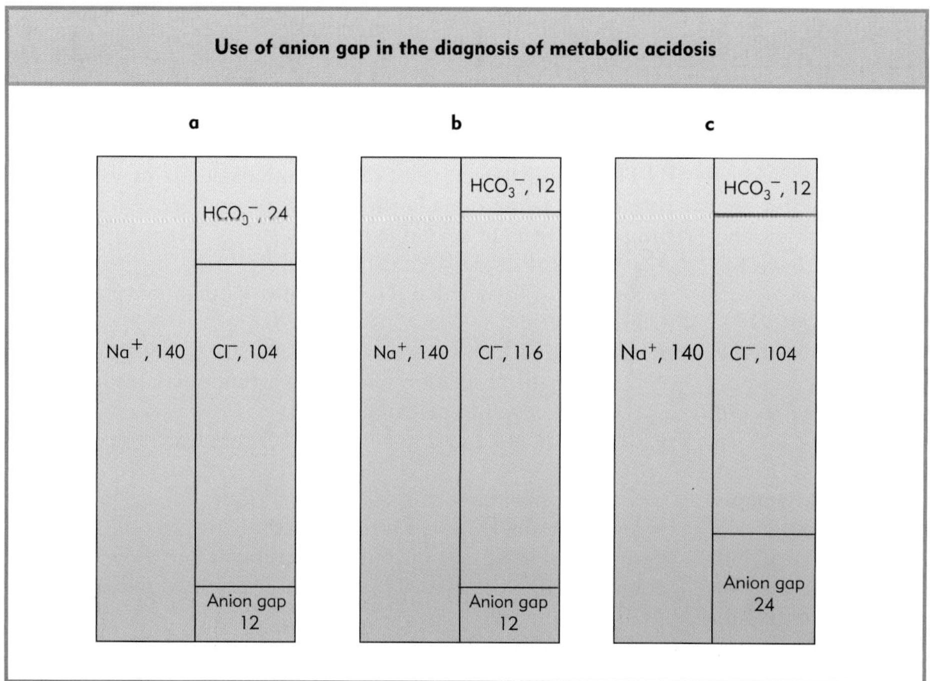

Figure 60.3 Diagram showing the use of anion gap in the diagnosis of metabolic acidosis. (a) Normal pH. (b) Metabolic acidosis – normal anion gap. (c) Metabolic acidosis – increased anion gap. (All concentrations in mmol/L).

used, but has potential drawbacks that include CO_2 production, which leads to hypercapnia and worsening of intracellular acidosis, hypernatremia, and hyperosmolality. Bicarbonate is thus used with caution, and only with reference to arterial blood gas status. A simple method to correct the acidosis is based on a half-correction of the base excess. The amount of bicarbonate to be given is calculated by Equation 60.13, in which 0.3 × body weight represents the extracellular fluid volume.

■ Equation 60.13

$$\underset{(mmol)}{HCO_3^- \text{ dose}} = 0.3 \times \underset{(kg)}{\text{body weight}} \times \underset{(mmol/L)}{\text{base excess}} \times 0.5$$

Bicarbonate is given slowly, especially when ventilation is impaired, and via a central intravenous catheter. Newer agents such as tromethamine (THAM) and carbicarb (Na_2CO_3 and $NaHCO_3$) have not been shown to reduce mortality in metabolic acidosis.

Metabolic alkalosis

A primary increase in bicarbonate that leads to a pH above 7.45 results in metabolic alkalosis. This can develop in conditions that cause loss of H^+ or gain of HCO_3^-. The special case of pyloric stenosis is considered in detail below. Some important causes of metabolic alkalosis are given in Table 60.2.

Compensation occurs by hypoventilation, but this is limited by the presence of hypoxic drive at lower $Pa\text{O}_2$.

PYLORIC STENOSIS

Pyloric stenosis is a relatively common cause of metabolic alkalosis, and is of prime importance to the pediatric anesthesiologist. The condition occurs mainly in males, typically within 2–4 weeks of birth. Unexplained pyloric hypertrophy leads to gastric outlet obstruction that results in repetitive vomiting. There is loss of H^+ (accompanied by Cl^-), which is secreted into the gastric lumen by parietal cells, whereas bicarbonate formed by these cells returns via venous blood, leading to systemic alkalosis. The response of the kidneys is a bicarbonate diuresis with accompanying urinary loss of Na^+ and K^+, which leads to hypovolemia and hypokalemia. As extracellular fluid volume continues to fall, elevated aldosterone promotes further loss of K^+ and H^+, and worsens the hypokalemia and alkalosis. Treatment consists of slow rehydration with intravenous fluids (saline solution with K^+) and gradual correction of the metabolic alkalosis and electrolyte disturbances, prior to definitive surgery.

TREATMENT OF METABOLIC ALKALOSIS

For diagnostic and therapeutic purposes it is useful to classify the causes of metabolic alkalosis into two groups, chloride responsive and chloride resistant (Table 60.3).

Treatment of the majority of metabolic alkaloses (chloride sensitive) is by administration of saline solution. Alkalosis is usually accompanied by hypokalemia, which may be severe, therefore K^+ supplementation (10–40 mmol/h) is given with the saline, and frequent electrolyte determination is carried out. For more severe forms of alkalosis (chloride resistant), therapeutic options include carbonic anhydrase inhibition (causing a brisk bicarbonate diuresis), intravenous NH_4Cl (not recommended in hepatic failure because of the release of NH_3), or HCl (0.1 or 0.2 mol/L in saline given via a central catheter slowly with reference to the base excess). The most effective treatment of metabolic alkalosis caused by renal impairment is dialysis.

Respiratory acidosis

Respiratory acidosis occurs when an acute or chronic rise in arterial CO_2 reduces pH to <7.35.

ACUTE RESPIRATORY ACIDOSIS

The major causes of acute respiratory acidosis are given in Table 60.4. In acute respiratory acidosis a compensatory increase in serum bicarbonate may or may not occur, depending on the duration of the precipitating event. Therapy consists of treatment of the underlying cause and improvement in alveolar ventilation (by either respiratory stimulation or, more commonly, artificial ventilation). An inverse relationship exists between arterial $P\text{CO}_2$ ($P_a\text{CO}_2$) and alveolar ventilation (Equation 60.14).

■ Equation 60.14

$$P_a\text{CO}_2 = \frac{\text{metabolic rate}}{\text{effective alveolar ventilation}}$$

The decision to instigate mechanical ventilation is based on clinical grounds (duration of illness, exhaustion, prognosis) and laboratory investigations (arterial blood gases, ABG). Unless significant cardiovascular failure and tissue hypoxia are present, sodium bicarbonate is not required. Some evidence indicates that bicarbonate therapy may improve the efficacy of bronchodilating drugs, such as β_2-receptor agonists, in bronchospastic disorders.

Table 60.2 Causes of metabolic alkalosis

Cause	Example
Loss of H^+	Gastrointestinal: persistent vomiting, nasogastric suction Renal: diuretics (thiazides, loop), excess mineralocorticoid (exogenous – steroid therapy; endogenous – Cushing's disease)
Gain of HCO_3^-	Exogenous alkali (HCO_3^-, citrate, lactate)
Maintenance	Renal failure, hypokalemia, chloride depletion

Table 60.3 Chloride-sensitive and chloride-resistant metabolic alkalosis

Cause	Examples
Chloride-sensitive (urinary Cl^- <10 mmol/L)	Gastric losses, diuretic therapy, low Cl^- intake, intestinal losses
Chloride- resistant (urinary Cl^- >10 mmol/L)	Renal artery stenosis, Cushing's syndrome, primary aldosteronism, exogenous mineralocorticoids, severe K^+ deficiency

CHRONIC RESPIRATORY ACIDOSIS

With chronic respiratory acidosis, for example in a patient who has chronic obstructive airways disease, renal compensation results in an increased reabsorption of bicarbonate, which leads to increased plasma levels, increased base excess, and a return of plasma pH towards normal. These patients may present with acute-on-chronic respiratory acidosis from infective exacerbations, and artificial ventilation may be required because of ventilatory failure from exhaustion or CO_2 narcosis (loss of hypoxic drive with excess O_2 administration). These patients may also develop a metabolic alkalosis as a result of diuretic therapy, which leads to depression of ventilation and further increases in P_aCO_2.

Respiratory alkalosis

Respiratory alkalosis is caused by a primary decrease in P_aCO_2 that leads to a pH >7.45. The major causes are given in Table 60.4.

Respiratory alkalosis caused by overzealous intermittent positive-pressure ventilation under anesthesia can result in a decrease in cardiac output and hypotension, left shift of the oxyhemoglobin dissociation curve, hypokalemia and myocardial irritability, decreased cerebral blood flow, bronchoconstriction, post hyperventilation hypoxia, and loss of central respiratory drive. Treatment of respiratory alkalosis is directed at the underlying cause. Long-standing respiratory alkalosis leads to renal compensation via increased excretion of bicarbonate, which results in lower plasma levels and a decrease in pH.

INTERPRETATION OF LABORATORY VALUES

The mainstay of assessment of acid–base status of a patient is analysis of arterial blood gases (ABGs) (Table 60.5). The blood gas analyzer directly measures PO_2, PCO_2, and pH. Other variables are derived from the Henderson equation and from graphic representations such as the Siggard-Andersen nomogram.

Table 60.4 Causes of respiratory acid–base disturbances

Cause	Examples
Respiratory acidosis	
Pulmonary disease	COAD, asthma, chest trauma
Central nervous depression	Drugs – opioids, trauma, tumor, infection
Peripheral nervous depression	Myasthenia, polio, neuromuscular blockers
Respiratory alkalosis	
Psychological	Hysteria, pain, anxiety
Respiratory	Pulmonary embolus, asthma, pneumonia
Shock	Sepsis, cardiac, hypovolemic
Central nervous system	Cardiovascular event, tumor
Drugs	Aspirin, aminophylline
Miscellaneous	Positive-pressure ventilation, pregnancy, altitude

COAD, chronic obstructive airways disease.

Table 60.5 Significant values of ABG and other variables in acid–base status

Variable	Normal range
pH	7.4 (7.35–7.45)
Pa_{O_2}	75–100 mmHg (10–13.3 kPa)
Pa_{CO_2}	35–45 mmHg (4.7–6 kPa)
$[HCO_3^-]$	22–26 mmol/L
Base excess	−2 to +2 mmol/L
[Lactate]	0.7–2.1 mmol/L

Standard HCO_3^- and base excess assume a Pa_{CO_2} of 40 mmHg (5.3 kPa.).

Oxygen measurement

This is based on the electrochemical reduction of oxygen at a cathode using electrons generated at the anode. For each O_2 molecule reduced four electrons move between the electrodes. This electrical current is proportional to the concentration of oxygen present.

OXYGEN ELECTRODE (POLAROGRAPHIC ELECTRODE, CLARKE ELECTRODE)

This consists of a gold or platinum cathode and a silver/silver chloride anode in a potassium chloride solution. A DC voltage of 0.6 V is applied across the electrodes. Electrons are produced by

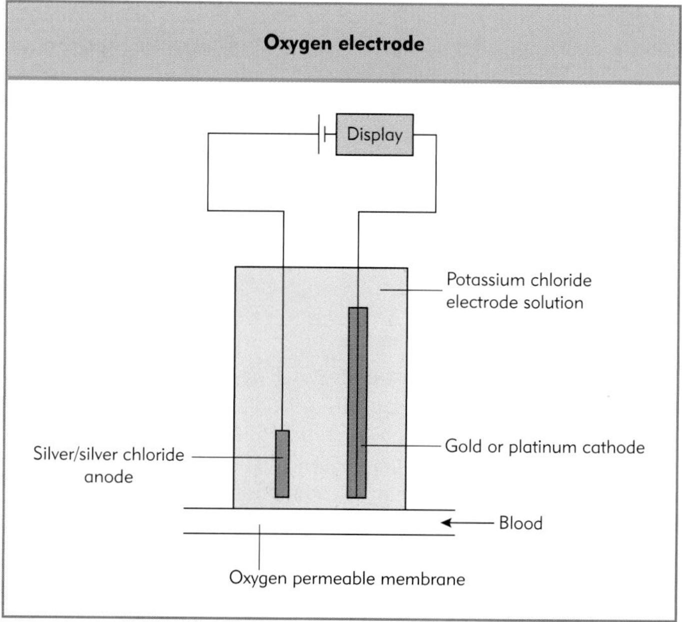

Figure 60.4 Oxygen electrode.

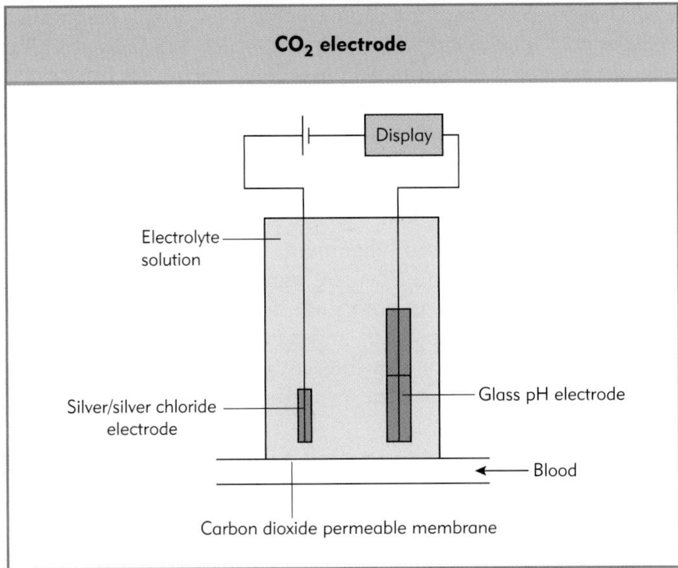

Figure 60.5 CO_2 electrode.

the silver/silver chloride anode and reduce oxygen molecules, as in Equation 60.15.

■ Equation 60.15

$$O_2 + 2H_2O + 4e^- \rightarrow 4(OH)^-$$

The current flow between the electrodes is measured by a galvanometer and displayed as a measure of oxygen concentration (Fig. 60.4).

Carbon dioxide measurement

CO_2 ELECTRODE

This consists of a glass pH electrode and a silver/silver chloride reference electrode. Both electrodes are enclosed within a membrane which is permeable to CO_2, and impermeable to blood cells, plasma and hydrogen ions. Buffer solutions of known pH are used to establish the relationship between pH and CO_2. This is dependent on the carbonic acid equation (Equation 60.16):

■ Equation 60.16

$$H_2O + CO_2 \leftrightarrow H_2CO_3 \leftrightarrow H^+ + HCO_3^-$$

The diffusion of CO_2 across the membrane causes Equation 60.16 to move to the right. This produces H^+ and a fall in pH proportional to the concentration of CO_2 (Fig. 60.5).

pH measurement

pH ELECTRODE

This consists of a silver/silver chloride electrode and a mercury/mercury chloride electrode. The pH electrode responds to the activity of H^+ rather than the concentration, and the electrodes must be calibrated with solutions of known pH (Fig 60.6).

When faced with a set of ABG measurements it is important to have a scheme for interpretation:

- pH (normal, acidosis, or alkalosis);
- Primary disorder (either metabolic, respiratory, or both, determined by assessing $P\text{CO}_2$ and HCO_3^-); and
- Compensation, which occurs via respiratory mechanisms (changes in ventilation) in a primary metabolic disorder, or via a metabolic mechanism (renal excretion and/or retention of HCO_3^-) in a primary respiratory disorder. In general, compensation is never complete and overcompensation does not occur.

Acid–base diagrams

In mixed disorders an acid–base diagram can be used to aid diagnosis. These represent the behavior of the whole body during acid–base disturbances and show responses to therapeutic intervention or compensation. They generally involve a graphic representation in which two variables (from pH, $P\text{CO}_2$, and HCO_3^-) are plotted on the x and y axes, and the third is represented by isobars.

An example is the Davenport diagram (Fig. 60.7), in which plasma $[HCO_3^-]$ is plotted against pH. The normal buffer curve shows changes in normal blood when $P\text{CO}_2$ is altered. In uncompensated respiratory disorders, patients move up (acidosis) or down (alkalosis) the normal buffer curve. Patients who have an uncompensated metabolic disorder move down (acidosis) or up (alkalosis) the 40 mmHg isobar. The diagrams can be used to show compensations for primary acid–base disturbances.

Siggard-Andersen nomograms use measured values of pH and $P\text{CO}_2$ to calculate the bicarbonate concentration, base excess or deficit, and total buffer base. The Siggard-Andersen curve nomogram (Fig. 60.8) has pH on the x axis and log $P\text{CO}_2$ on the y axis. Points to the right of a vertical line through pH 7.4 represent alkalosis, and points left of that line represent acidosis. Points above and below the horizontal line through $P\text{CO}_2$ = 40 mmHg represent hypo- and hyperventilation. The CO_2 titration line passes from the point at which $P\text{CO}_2$ = 40 mmHg and pH = 7.4 to the 15 g/dL point on the hemoglobin scale. As hemoglobin decreases, the slope of this titration line decreases, which illustrates a reduction in total buffering power of the blood. The CO_2 titration line is plotted for a given blood sample after measuring the pH and then equilibration of the sample with gas mixtures of known $P\text{CO}_2$. Standard bicarbonate

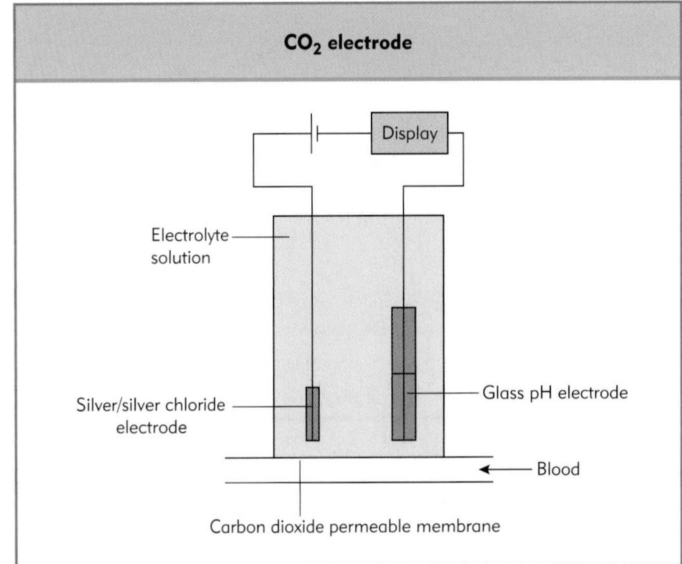

Figure 60.6 pH electrode.

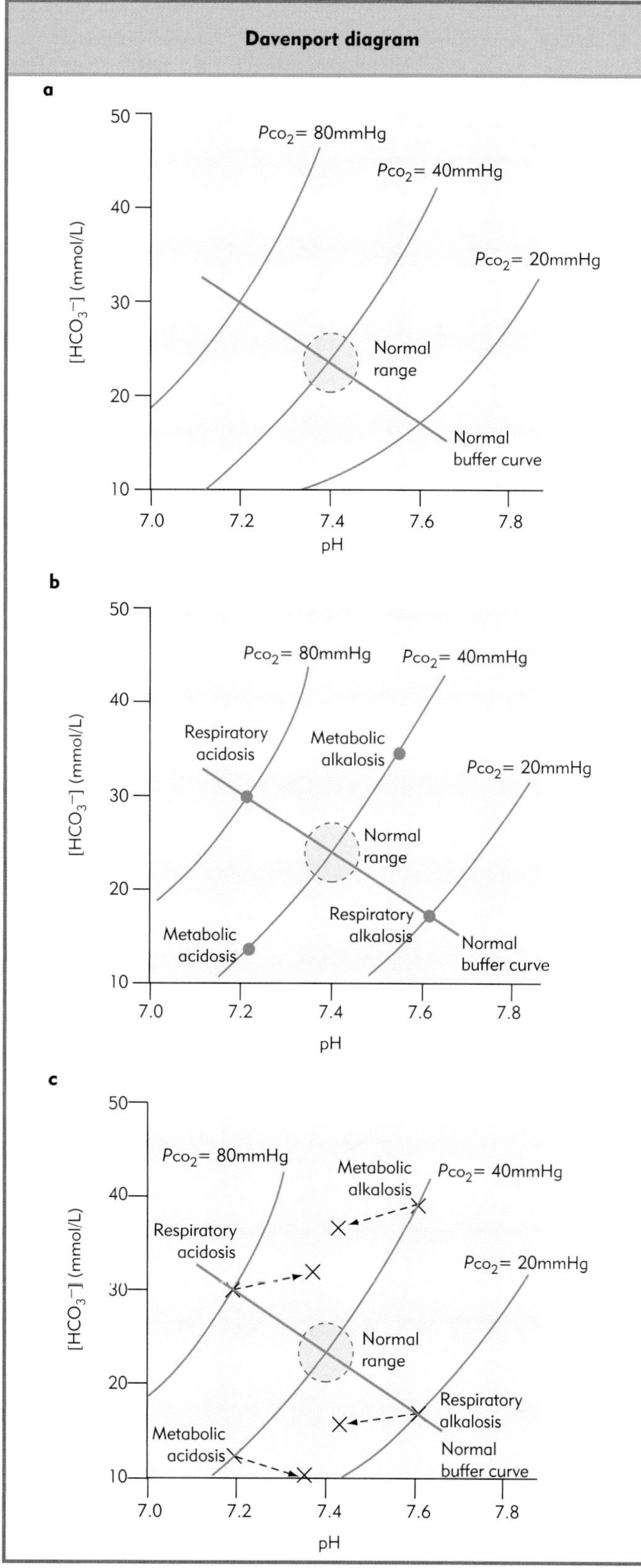

Figure 60.7 Davenport diagrams. (a) For normal changes with altered arterial Pco_2. (b) For primary respiratory disorders (shown along the normal buffer curve) and primary metabolic disorders (shown along the Pco_2 40 mmHg (5.3 kPa) isobar). (c) For compensation of primary disorders. (*x*) represents lines of compensation. (Reproduced with permission from Shoemaker et al. Textbook of critical care. Philadelphia: WB Saunders; 1989.)

(bicarbonate concentration after the removal of any respiratory component) is read from the point at which the CO_2 titration line crosses the standard bicarbonate line (horizontal from PCO_2 = 40 mmHg). The point at which the CO_2 titration line crosses the lower curved scale is the base excess, and the point where the line crosses the upper curved scale shows total buffer base concentration (which includes bicarbonate, hemoglobin, and protein buffers).

The Siggard-Andersen alignment nomogram is shown in Figure 60.9. The pH and PCO_2 are measured directly and a line is drawn between these points on the nomogram. The base excess, standard bicarbonate, and total plasma CO_2 are read from the intersection of this line with the relevant scales. The base excess scale is dependent on the hemoglobin concentration.

THE EFFECT OF TEMPERATURE ON ARTERIAL BLOOD GAS INTERPRETATION

Temperature affects both PCO_2 and the pH of blood. As blood is cooled, CO_2 becomes more soluble, which results in a reduction of PCO_2 by around 4.5% per degree centigrade. The pH of blood varies inversely with temperature, the coefficient being –0.015 units per degree centigrade (the pH of in vitro human blood at 77°F (25°C) would be around 7.6). The reasons for this include the increased dissociation of water at higher temperature (H^+ increases and pH decreases) and the increased buffering of H^+ by the α-imidazole of hemoglobin as temperature falls. These pH changes are seen in human blood in vitro, and also when the temperature in poikilothermic ('cold blooded') animals changes in vivo. Within the range of normal practice (body temperature 95–104°F, 35–40°C), these small changes are unlikely to affect acid–base management significantly, and temperature correction is of limited value. However, in clinical situations in which body temperature is far from normal (although blood gas analysis is carried out at 98.6°F, 37°C), for example extreme hypothermia associated with drowning, or active cooling during cardiopulmonary bypass (with the reduction of temperature to around 82.4°F, 28°C), corrections are necessary.

There are two types of management of acid–base status in these situations, 'α-stat' and 'pH-stat'.

α-stat

α-stat management seeks a blood pH of 7.4 when measured at 37°C, independent of patient temperature. This means that the actual pH would be much higher (e.g. if temperature was 25°C the actual pH must be 7.58 to have a pH of 7.4 at 37°C). This type of management is simple because no temperature correction is necessary when interpreting a set of blood gases, as these are always measured at 37°C. The α-stat hypothesis of pH control is based on the finding that in vivo blood pH of exothermic animals varies inversely with temperature. However, exotherms and endotherms have basically similar enzymes, receptors, and transport proteins.

pH-stat

pH-stat regulation aims for a pH of 7.4 when expressed at patient temperature. Thus, a pH of 7.4 at 25°C, when measured at 37°C, would appear extremely acidotic.

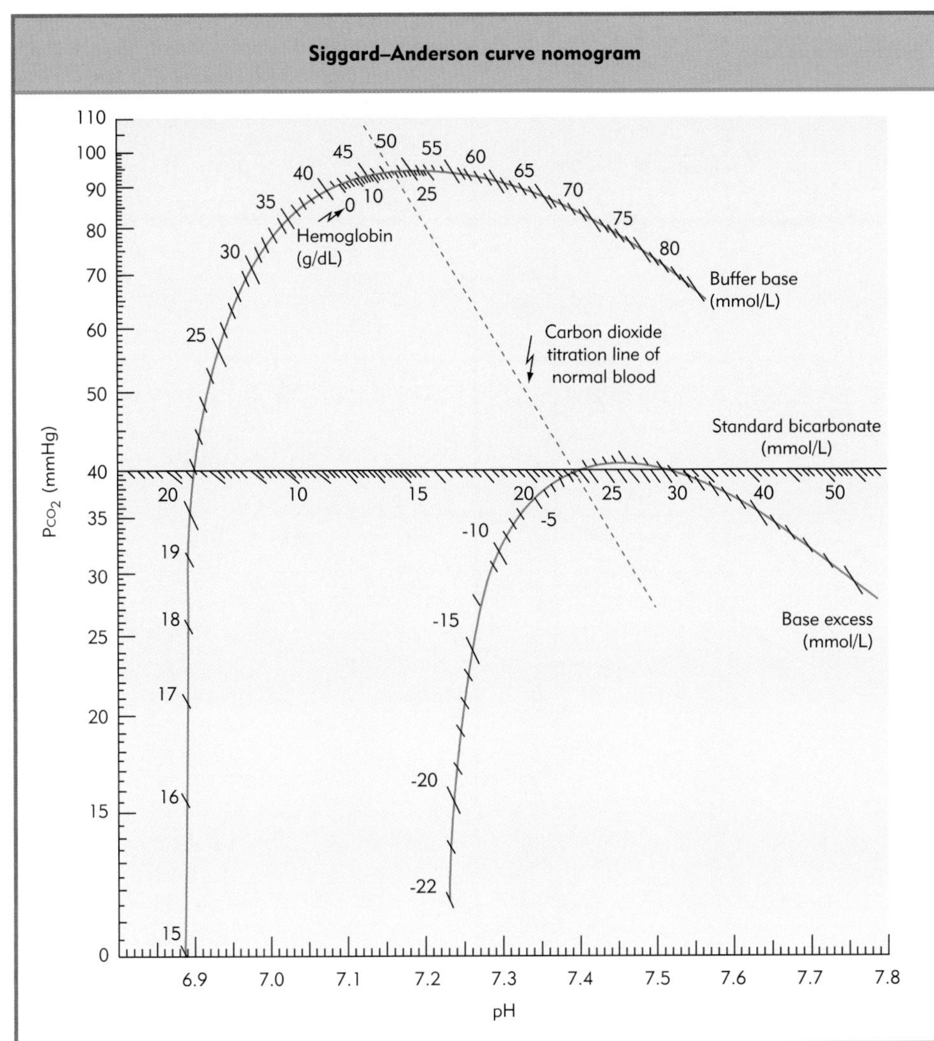

Figure 60.8 The Siggard-Andersen curve nomogram. This shows the carbon dioxide titration line, which is constructed from equilibration of arterial blood with two gas mixtures of known P_{CO_2} and hemoglobin concentration. Standard bicarbonate, base excess, and total buffer base are read from the nomogram. (Copyright © Radiometer, Copenhagen, Denmark. Reproduced with permission.)

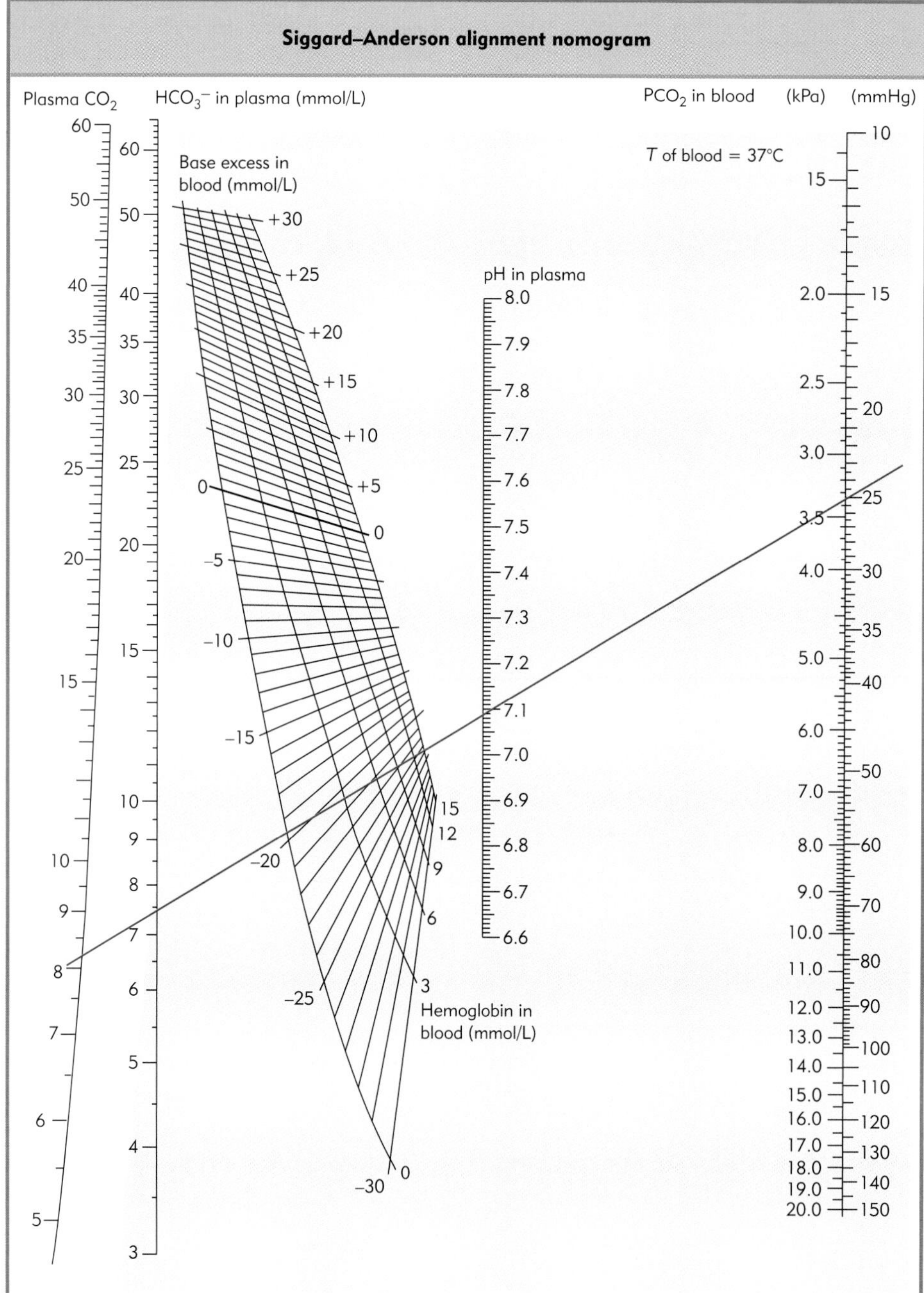

Figure 60.9 Siggard-Andersen alignment nomogram (for blood temperature of 37°C). A line is shown to depict a patient with P_{CO_2} of 25 mmHg (3.3 kPa) and pH of 7.1. (Copyright © Radiometer, Copenhagen, Denmark. Reproduced with permission.)

Key references

Astrup PB, Severinghaus JW. The history of blood gases, acids and bases. Copenhagen: Munksgaard; 1986.

Cohen RD. Roles of the liver and kidney in acid base regulation and its disorders. Br J Anaesth. 1991;67:154–64.

Davenport HW. The ABC of acid base chemistry, 6th edn. Chicago: University of Chicago Press; 1974.

Grogono AW. Acid–base balance. Int Anaesthesiol Clin. 1986; 24.

Rose BD. Clinical physiology of acid–base and electrolyte disorders, 4th edn. New York: McGraw-Hill; 1984.

Siggard-Andersen O. An acid–base chart for arterial blood with normal and pathophysiological reference areas. Scand J Clin Lab Invest. 1971;27:239–45.

Siggard-Andersen O, Engel K. A new acid–base nomogram. An improved method for the calculation of the relevant blood acid base data. Scand J Clin Lab Invest. 1960;12:177.

Further reading

Cohen RD, Simpson R. Lactate metabolism. Anaesthesiology 1975;43:661–73.

Maloney DG et al. Anions and the anaesthetist. Anaesthesia 2002;57:140–54.

Nattie EE. The alpha stat hypothesis in respiratory control and acid base balance. J Appl Physiol. 1990;69:1201–7.

Shapiro BA, Peruzzi WT, Kozlowski-Templin R. Clinical Application of Blood Gases. Mosby 5th ed. 1994.

Sirker AA et al. Acid–base physiology: the traditional and the modern approaches. Anaesthesia 2002;57:140–54.

Williams JJ, Marshall BE. Editorial: A fresh look at an old question. Anaesthesiology 1982;56:1.

SECTION 8

Gastrointestinal system and metabolism

Chapter 61

Gut motility and secretions

David J Rowbotham, Peter M Kimpson and Howard M Thompson

The primary function of the gut is to extract water and nutrients from food. This involves the processes of *digestion*, whereby food is broken down, and *absorption* of its constituents by the intestinal mucosa into the portal circulation.

Both chemical and physical factors are important in digestion. Prior to swallowing, food is chewed and mixed with salivary amylase in the mouth. In the stomach, it is softened and disintegrated into smaller particles, first by the action of gastric acid and enzymes, and second by mechanical churning via the muscular contractions of the stomach wall. Salivary amylase and gastric pepsin start the enzymatic breakdown of nutrients, which continues in the small intestine with the addition of pancreatic enzymes. The result is the formation of a liquefied residue called chyme.

Gastric chyme is ejected incrementally through the pylorus into the duodenum. Biliary and pancreatic secretions are added and thoroughly mixed with the intraluminal contents by gut wall contractions. Eventually, the products of digestion are brought into contact with the absorptive surfaces of the small intestine. Undigested matter is passed into the large intestine prior to voiding by defecation.

A high degree of control is required to allow the secretory processes and various motility patterns to occur in an orderly and efficient manner. Such control and coordination are achieved by a complex interplay of neural and humoral influences that occur as food passes through the gut.

BASIC ANATOMY

Essentially, the gut is a long muscular tube lined with epithelial mucosa, that extends from the oropharynx to the anal sphincter. Although the structure of the gut wall varies in different regions of the tract, generally it comprises an outer longitudinal and an inner circular layer of smooth muscle (Fig. 61.1). Anatomically and physiologically it is divided into four distinct regions: esophagus, stomach, small intestine (duodenum, jejunum, and ileum), and large intestine (cecum, colon, and rectum).

REGULATION AND INTEGRATION OF GUT FUNCTION

The function of the gut is coordinated by a complex interplay between the autonomic nervous system (neurocrine secretion), paracrine secretion, and endocrine (hormonal) activity.

Nervous system

The gut is innervated by the autonomic nervous system, which comprises extrinsic (to the gut), sympathetic, and parasympathetic elements together with an intrinsic network called the enteric nervous system (ENS). The ENS is organized into a number of anatomically distinct networks, of which the best described are the *myenteric (Auerbach's) plexus* and *submucosal (Meissner's) plexus* (see Fig. 61.1). The myenteric plexus is located between the circular and the longitudinal layers of smooth muscle, and extends the length of the gut, including the upper esophagus, where the muscle is striated. The myenteric plexus has an essential role in the generation of peristaltic

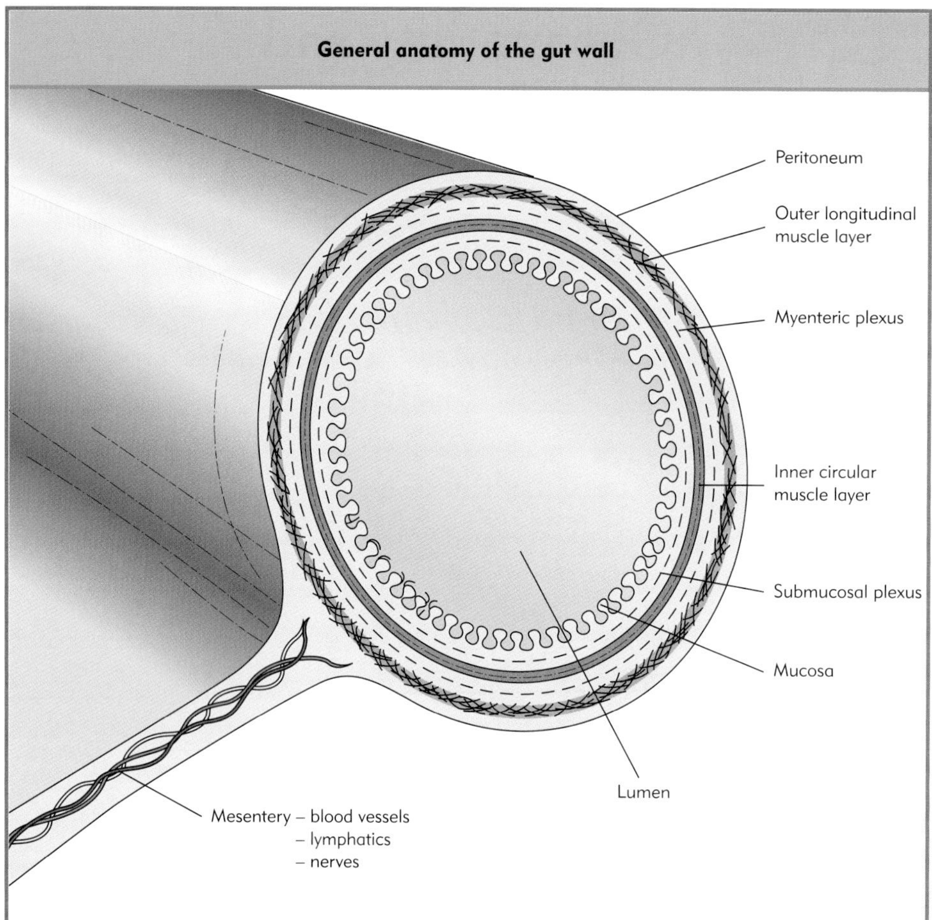

Figure 61.1 General anatomy of the gut wall. The gut is a muscular tube that extends from the oropharynx to the anus and consists of two muscle layers, an inner layer of circular muscle, and an outer layer of longitudinally arranged fibers. The luminal surface is lined with mucosa and the outer surface is invested with visceral peritoneum. The enteric nervous system consists of two main networks: the myenteric plexus lies between the longitudinal and circular layers of smooth muscle, and the submucosal plexus lies between the circular smooth muscle layer and the mucosa. Blood vessels, lymphatics, and nerves reach the gut by means of the mesentery.

activity. The submucosal plexus is located between the circular smooth muscle layer and the mucosa. It is most developed in the small intestine, where it is involved in secretory control.

Extensive afferent and efferent communication occurs between the sympathetic and parasympathetic systems and the ENS. Activity in the ENS results in the release of neurotransmitters (neurocrines), which have effects on other nerve cells, smooth muscle cells, paracrine cells, and endocrine cells. The number of identified neurotransmitters of the ENS continues to rise (Table 61.1) – more than 20 have now been identified in enteric neurons, with most neurons containing several of them. *Acetylcholine* (ACh) and *tachykinins*, such as *substance P*, cause smooth muscle contraction. *Vasoactive intestinal peptide* (VIP), *nitric oxide* (NO), and *adenosine triphosphate* (ATP) are inhibitory to smooth muscle. *5-Hydroxytryptamine* (5-HT) is released by stimulation of the mucosa and involved in the initiation of the peristaltic reflex.

Paracrines

Paracrines are chemicals that diffuse through interstitial fluid to exert an effect close to their site of release. Although paracrines exert only a direct local action, they may bring about more widespread effects, either because the cells from which they are secreted are scattered over a wide area of mucosa, or because they influence the release of gut hormones from endocrine cells. Histamine and somatostatin are important gut paracrines. Enterochromaffin-like (ECL) cells secrete histamine by decarboxylation of histidine; histamine is involved in the control of gastric acid secretion. Somatostatin is found throughout the gastric and duodenal mucosa and in the pancreas. It reduces gut secretions by exerting an inhibitory effect on all of the gut hormones and a direct inhibitory effect on parietal cells. Octreotide, a synthetic analog of somatostatin, inhibits the secretion of many gastrointestinal and pituitary hormones, including growth hormone, serotonin, gastrin, insulin, motilin, and VIP. It is currently licensed for the treatment of acromegaly, pancreatic fistulae, metastatic carcinoid tumors, and VIPomas.

Hormones

Gut hormones are released from endocrine cells into the bloodstream to exert remote actions by means of specific receptor interaction in a target tissue. As with the neurocrines, many substances have been identified as having potential gut hormone activity. Five peptide hormones are recognized as being most important (see Table 61.1): gastrin, cholecystokinin (CCK), secretin, gastric inhibitory peptide (GIP), and motilin.

Gastrin and CCK share the same sequence of five C-terminal amino acids (-Gly-Trp-Met-Asp-Phe), which results in a degree of cross-receptor activity. Some gut hormones demonstrate heterogeneity – gastrin, CCK, and secretin exist in more than

Table 61.1 Chemical mediators in the gut and their physiologic actions. Several chemical mediators (neurotransmitters (neurocrines), paracrines, and gut hormones (endocrines)) identified in gastrointestinal nerve, paracrine, and endocrine cells have established physiologic actions. Many other potential mediators have been identified, but as yet their physiologic effects are not fully elucidated

Neurotransmitter	Main physiologic functions
Gastrin-releasing peptide (GRP)	Vagal stimulation of gastrin secretion
Acetylcholine (Ach)	Smooth muscle contraction, peristalsis
Substance P	Smooth muscle contraction, peristalsis, possible visceral nociception
Vasoactive intestinal peptide (VIP)	Smooth muscle contraction, peristalsis, relaxation of sphincters, vasodilation
Nitric oxide (NO)	Smooth muscle relaxation, peristalsis
Adenosine triphosphate (ATP)	Smooth muscle contraction, peristalsis
5-Hydroxytryptamine (5-HT)	Activation of peristalsis, generation of nausea
Calcitonin gene-related peptide	Possible role in visceral nociception
Somatostatin	Inhibition of release of gut hormones, inhibition of gut secretions
Paracrine	
Histamine	Stimulation of gastric acid secretion
Somatostatin	Inhibition of release of gut hormones, inhibition of gut secretions
Gut hormone	
Gastrin	Stimulation of gastric acid secretion Stimulation of peptide secretion Maintenance of gastrointestinal mucosal integrity
Cholecystokinin (CCK)	Stimulation of gallbladder contraction Stimulation of pancreatic exocrine secretion Inhibition of gastric emptying Trophic action on exocrine pancreas
Secretin	Inhibition of gastric acid secretion Stimulation of pepsin Stimulation of pancreatic alkaline secretion Stimulation of biliary alkaline secretion Trophic action on exocrine pancreas
Gastric inhibitory peptide (GIP)	Stimulation of insulin release Inhibition of gastric acid secretion
Motilin	Generation of the migrating motor complex

one molecular form. Many factors influence the release of these hormones, of which vagal stimulation, gut distension, and the presence of intraluminal acid and nutrients are physiologically the most important (Table 61.2).

Gut endocrine cells are widely distributed throughout the gastrointestinal mucosa, and belong to the group of secretory cells known as *amine precursor uptake* and *decarboxylation (APUD) cells*. Gastrin is released from G cells located in the gastric antral mucosa and to a lesser extent in the duodenum. Cells that secrete CCK, secretin, GIP, and motilin are located in the small intestine, particularly in the duodenum and jejunum.

GASTRIN

The main role of gastrin is the stimulation of gastric acid and pepsin secretion. Acid itself has an inhibitory influence on gastrin release, thereby providing a negative feedback system. Gastric distension, the presence of products of protein digestion in the stomach, and vagal stimulation cause gastrin release. Vagal

Table 61.2 Physiologic stimulants for the release of gut hormones

Vagal stimulation	Peptides, amino acids	Fatty acids	Carbohydrate	Hydrogen ions	Gastric distension
Gastrin	Stimulation			Inhibition	Stimulation
CCK		Stimulation	Stimulation		
Secretin				Stimulation	
GIP		Stimulation	Stimulation		
Motilin	Stimulation				

innervation of the G cell is unusual in that it is not cholinergic, but involves *gastrin-releasing peptide (GRP)*.

CHOLECYSTOKININ

Not only does CCK cause contraction of the gallbladder and stimulate secretion of enzymes and alkaline fluid by the exocrine pancreas, it also inhibits the rate of gastric emptying. The main stimulus for CCK secretion is the presence of peptides, amino acids, and fatty acids (chain length >10 carbon groups) in the duodenal lumen.

SECRETIN

Secretin is released when duodenal pH falls below 4–5. It inhibits gastric acid secretion and at the same time promotes the secretion of biliary and pancreatic alkaline fluid. In this way, secretin neutralizes the acidity of gastric fluid as it enters the duodenum.

GASTRIC INHIBITORY PEPTIDE

When GIP was first identified it appeared to cause inhibition of gastric secretions and was therefore named 'gastric inhibitory peptide'. This inhibitory effect is now thought to be less important at normal physiologic concentrations of GIP. Carbohydrate and fat in the duodenum cause its release, after which it acts as a stimulus for insulin release in preparation for the imminent arrival of absorbed substrate from the gut.

MOTILIN

Motilin is involved in the regulation of interdigestive gut motility. It is released in a cyclic manner during fasting, with a periodicity of 1–2 hours. It stimulates a burst of peristalsis, the migrating motor complex, which starts in the stomach and then sweeps through the small intestine, clearing it of undigested matter and other debris in preparation for the next meal.

Trophic effects

In addition to their influence on gut motility and secretions, some gut hormones also exert important *trophic* effects. Gastrin is an essential factor in maintaining gastrointestinal mucosal integrity, and CCK and secretin are involved in growth of the exocrine pancreas.

PERISTALSIS

Peristalsis is the reflex propagation of a wave of muscular contraction along the gut wall. It is an important component of gut motility, as it creates a tendency for the intraluminal contents to be propelled along in the normal anterograde manner. Peristalsis is an inherent property of the gut that continues even when the gut is denervated from its extrinsic autonomic connections. The ENS, particularly the myenteric plexus, has a pivotal role in the generation of peristaltic waves. Extrinsic autonomic influence modulates activity – parasympathetic activity tends to increase peristalsis and sympathetic activity to inhibit it.

Distension of the gut wall and the release of 5-HT (because of mucosal stimulation) initiate the peristaltic reflex (Fig. 61.2). Activity in sensory afferents stimulates cholinergic interneurons that pass both proximally and distally in the myenteric plexus. Proximally, the release of ACh and substance P from excitatory motor neurons mediates the contraction of circular smooth muscle. At the same time, distal smooth muscle relaxation is brought about by the release of VIP, NO, and ATP from inhibitory motor neurons. A 'ring' of contraction develops behind the food bolus to propel it along the gut. The same pattern of reflex activity is then activated in a more distal segment of gut, and thus the wave of peristalsis is propagated forward.

SWALLOWING

Swallowing, or deglutition, takes place after food has been chewed, or masticated, in the mouth. Saliva, secreted from the parotid, submandibular, and sublingual glands during chewing, is mixed with food to act as a lubricant. Saliva also has an antibacterial action, helps buffer any gastric acid that may regurgitate into the esophagus, and initiates carbohydrate digestion by way of its amylase content.

The esophagus is a continuation of the pharynx. In its proximal third it comprises striated muscle, and in this region innervation of the motor endplate by efferents from the myenteric plexus is uniquely mediated by NO. Striated muscle is gradually replaced by smooth muscle, such that by the distal third of the esophagus all the muscle is smooth. There is the typical arrangement of outer longitudinal and inner circular muscle layers. At the pharyngoesophageal junction the muscle is thickened to form the upper esophageal sphincter (UES). At the gastroesophageal junction the lower esophageal sphincter (LES) is found. In the resting state both the UES and LES are closed, and resting tone is considerably higher than in the adjacent esophagus.

Swallowing can be initiated by voluntary action, but once under way proceeds as an involuntary reflex. It is triggered by afferent impulses in the trigeminal (V), glossopharyngeal (IX), and vagus (X) cranial nerves. Integration of the reflex takes place in the nucleus ambiguus and the nucleus of the tractus solitarius, with efferent innervation via the trigeminal (V), facial (VII), vagus

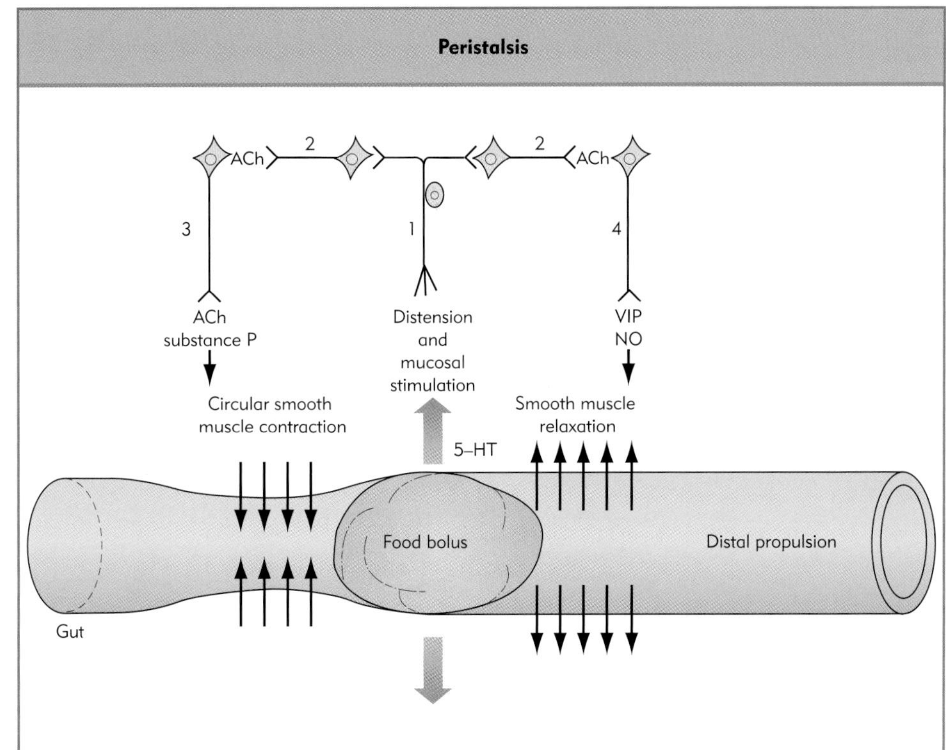

Figure 61.2 Peristalsis. The peristaltic reflex is initiated by distension of the gut wall and the release of 5-HT by mucosal stimulation. Elements of the ENS are involved in the coordination of this reflex. Stimulation of sensory afferents (1) causes a biphasic response in fibers of the myenteric plexus. Proximal to the site of stimulus, cholinergic interneurons (2) relay the signal to excitatory motor neurons (3), which cause ACh- and substance P-mediated contraction of the circular muscle layer. Simultaneously, other cholinergic interneurons (2) relay the signal to distal inhibitory motor neurons (4). Here, the release of VIP, NO, and ATP mediates the relaxation of smooth muscle. In this way, the food bolus is propelled forward to initiate the same pattern of neuronal activity distally, thus propagating the peristaltic wave.

(X), and hypoglossal (XII) nerves. Chewed food is formed into a bolus and propelled backward into the oropharynx by the tongue. Upward displacement of the soft palate and contraction of the superior constrictor muscle prevent retrograde passage of food into the nasopharynx. Sequential contraction of the superior, middle, and inferior constrictor muscles propels the food bolus into the esophagus. As the food passes through the oropharynx reflex closure of the larynx and inhibition of respiration occurs. Upward movement of the larynx and folding back of the epiglottis protect the laryngeal inlet.

A peristaltic ring of contraction transports the food bolus distally down the esophagus at a velocity of 2–4 cm/s. Thus, it takes approximately 10–15 s to pass through the 30 cm esophagus and enter the stomach. Coordinated relaxation of the UES and LES occurs as the food bolus passes. This sphincteric relaxation may be mediated by NO.

Any food that fails to be swept into the stomach with the *primary peristaltic wave* causes *secondary peristalsis* by way of mechanical stimulation of the esophagus. Secondary peristalsis also occurs whenever esophageal reflux of gastric juice occurs.

GASTRIC MOTILITY AND SECRETIONS

In the stomach, food is temporarily stored while the process of digestion begins. Digestion is achieved by the action of acid and enzymes together with gastric motility patterns that churn up the food and break it down into smaller particles, which eventually become liquefied into gastric chyme.

Gastric juice

The normal stomach secretes approximately 2 L of gastric juice per day. This consists of four main components: hydrochloric acid, pepsin, mucus, and intrinsic factor.

Hydrochloric acid is necessary to activate *pepsin*, from its proenzyme *pepsinogen*; pepsin initiates protein digestion. Low gastric pH is also important to prevent microbial growth. *Mucus* is an essential component in mucosal cytoprotection against the effects of acid, pepsin, and mechanical damage. *Intrinsic factor* is required for the efficient absorption of vitamin B_{12} in the terminal ileum.

Oxyntic glands (Fig. 61.3) play a central role in the production of gastric juice and are located in the main body and fundus of the stomach. These complex structures contain several cell types, including *parietal cells, peptic (or chief) cells*, and *mucus-secreting cells*. The parietal cells secrete hydrochloric acid and intrinsic factor, and the peptic cells secrete pepsinogen.

Control of gastric acid secretion

The human stomach contains one billion parietal cells, each one capable of secreting three billion hydrogen ions (H^+) per second to produce gastric acid with a pH <1. At the cellular level three chemical mediators are important in the control of gastric acid secretion (Fig. 61.4): bloodborne *gastrin* from G cells, *ACh* from vagal efferents, and *histamine* from ECL cells.

G cell-derived gastrin is secreted into the bloodstream, in which it equilibrates with interstitial fluid. In the gastric mucosa, gastrin binds to specific surface receptors on both parietal and histamine-secreting ECL cells. Thus, gastrin has two actions: it directly stimulates the parietal cell to secrete acid, and it simulates the release of histamine from ECL cells. The histamine has a paracrine effect and diffuses through interstitial fluid to nearby parietal cells, at which interaction with H_2 receptors activates acid secretion.

Increased *vagal tone* causes acid secretion by stimulation of G cell, ECL cell, and parietal cell types. The neurotransmitter at the ECL cell and parietal cell is ACh, via an M3 receptor, whereas GRP serves this role at the G cell. Thus vagally mediated acid

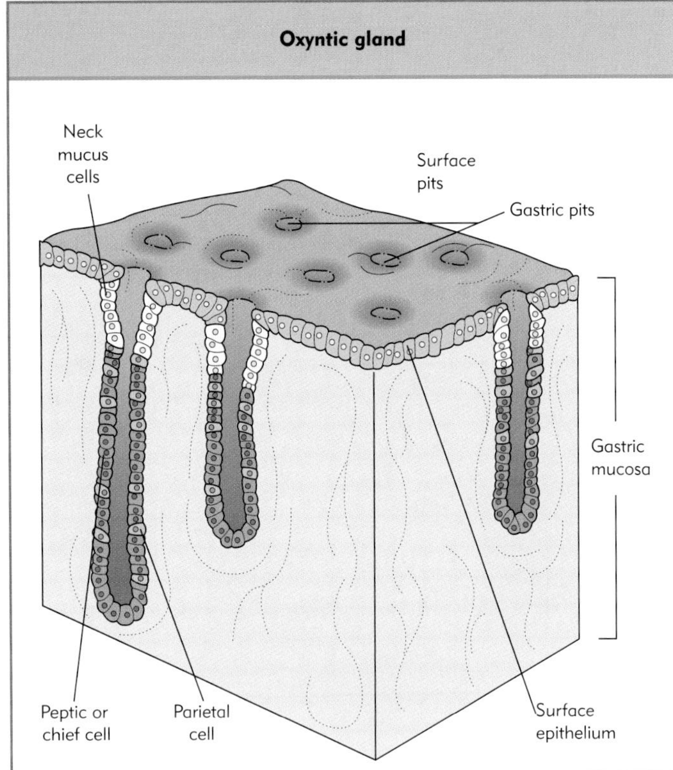

Figure 61.3 Oxyntic gland. Oxyntic glands are found in the main body and fundus of the stomach. They are complex structures that contain several specialized epithelial cell types. Parietal cells secrete hydrochloric acid and intrinsic factor. Peptic (or chief) cells secrete pepsinogen, which is converted into pepsin in the gastric lumen. Mucus cells at the neck of the gland secrete soluble mucus, which mixes with the gastric chyme to act as a lubricant. Oxyntic glands open on to the luminal surface of the stomach to form gastric pits.

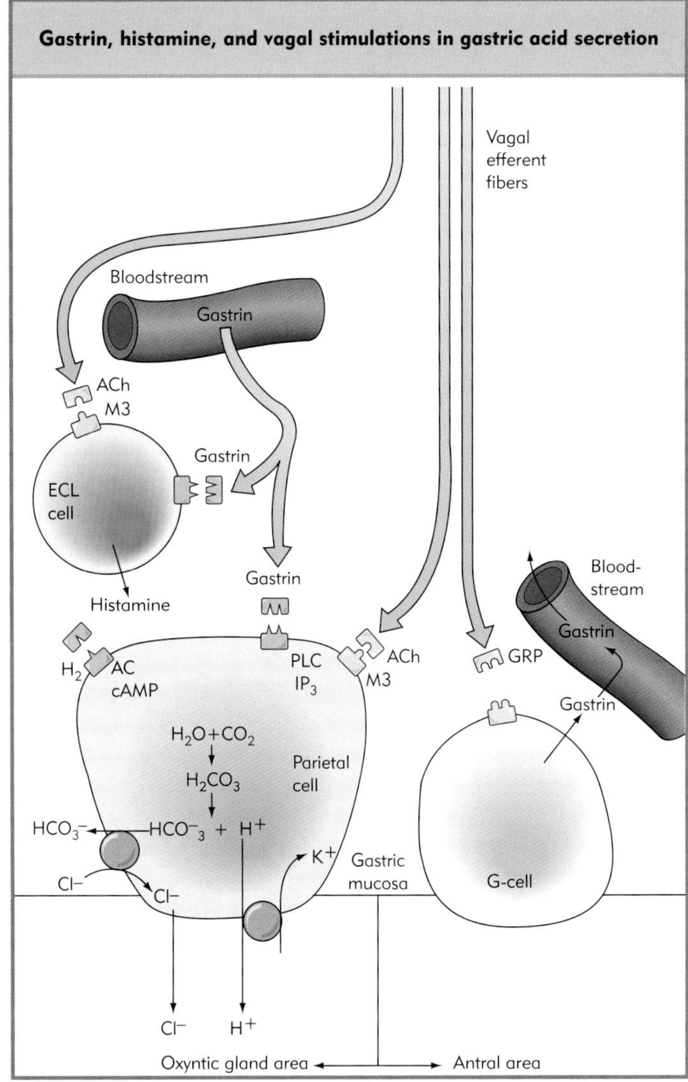

Figure 61.4 Gastrin, histamine, and vagal stimulation in gastric acid secretion. Several factors, including vagal stimulation, activate G cells to secrete gastrin into the bloodstream to act as a gut hormone. Gastrin interacts with receptors on the parietal cell and histamine-secreting ECL cell surface membranes. In this way, gastrin stimulates acid secretion both directly from the parietal cell, and indirectly via histamine release. Histamine acts as a paracrine effector by binding to nearby parietal cells at histamine type 2 (H_2) receptors to cause acid secretion. Both the parietal cell and the ECL cell are stimulated by ACh from vagal efferents. Vagal stimulation is mediated by GRP at the G cell. Thus, increased vagal tone brings about acid secretion by stimulating all the elements of this system. Carbonic anhydrase (CA) catalyzes the formation of carbonic acid (H_2CO_3) from carbon dioxide and water in the parietal cell. This dissociates to liberate H^+, which is 'pumped' into the gastric lumen by membrane H^+,K^+-ATPase. Bicarbonate is extruded from the cell in exchange for chloride, which diffuses into the gastric lumen down its concentration gradient. (AC, adenylyl cyclase; cAMP, cyclic adenosine monophosphate; PLC, phospholipase C; IP_3, inositol trisphosphate.)

secretion is brought about directly by stimulation of the parietal cell, and indirectly by gastrin and histamine release.

In the parietal cell, two second-messenger systems are activated to bring about the synthesis and release of H^+. Gastrin and ACh activate the phospholipase C–inositol trisphosphate (PLC–IP_3) system, whereas histamine activates the adenylyl cyclase–cyclic adenosine monophosphate (AC–cAMP) system.

The final common pathway is activation of the luminal membrane H^+, K^+-ATPase, the so-called 'proton pump', which actively transports H^+ into the gastric lumen in exchange for extracellular K^+. The energy required to pump H^+ against the four million-fold concentration gradient (parietal cytoplasm pH is 7.3, versus the luminal pH of <1) is provided by mitochondria that occupy a high proportion of the cytoplasmic volume in the parietal cell. In the resting state, H^+, K^+-ATPase is not in the apical membrane, but in the membranes of tubulovesicles contained within the cytoplasm. When the parietal cell is stimulated to secrete acid, these tubulovesicles fuse with the apical membrane, which increases its surface area greatly and exposes H^+, K^+-ATPase to the gastric lumen.

The generation of H^+ within the parietal cell (see Fig. 61.4) starts with the formation of carbonic acid (H_2CO_2) from carbon dioxide (CO_2) and water (H_2O) catalyzed by carbonic anhydrase (CA). Carbonic acid disassociates into bicarbonate (HCO_3^-) and H^+.

The physiologic influences that control gastric acid production (Fig. 61.5) may be considered in terms of cephalic factors (those that involve the brain), gastric factors (those produced by the presence of food in the stomach), and intestinal factors (those that arise from the transit of food into the duodenum).

Gastric acid secretion starts before food enters the stomach as a consequence of *cephalic factors*. Anticipation, sight, smell, taste, and the acts of chewing and swallowing all initiate, and then perpetuate, acid secretion by stimulation of vagal efferents via the vagal nuclei in the brainstem.

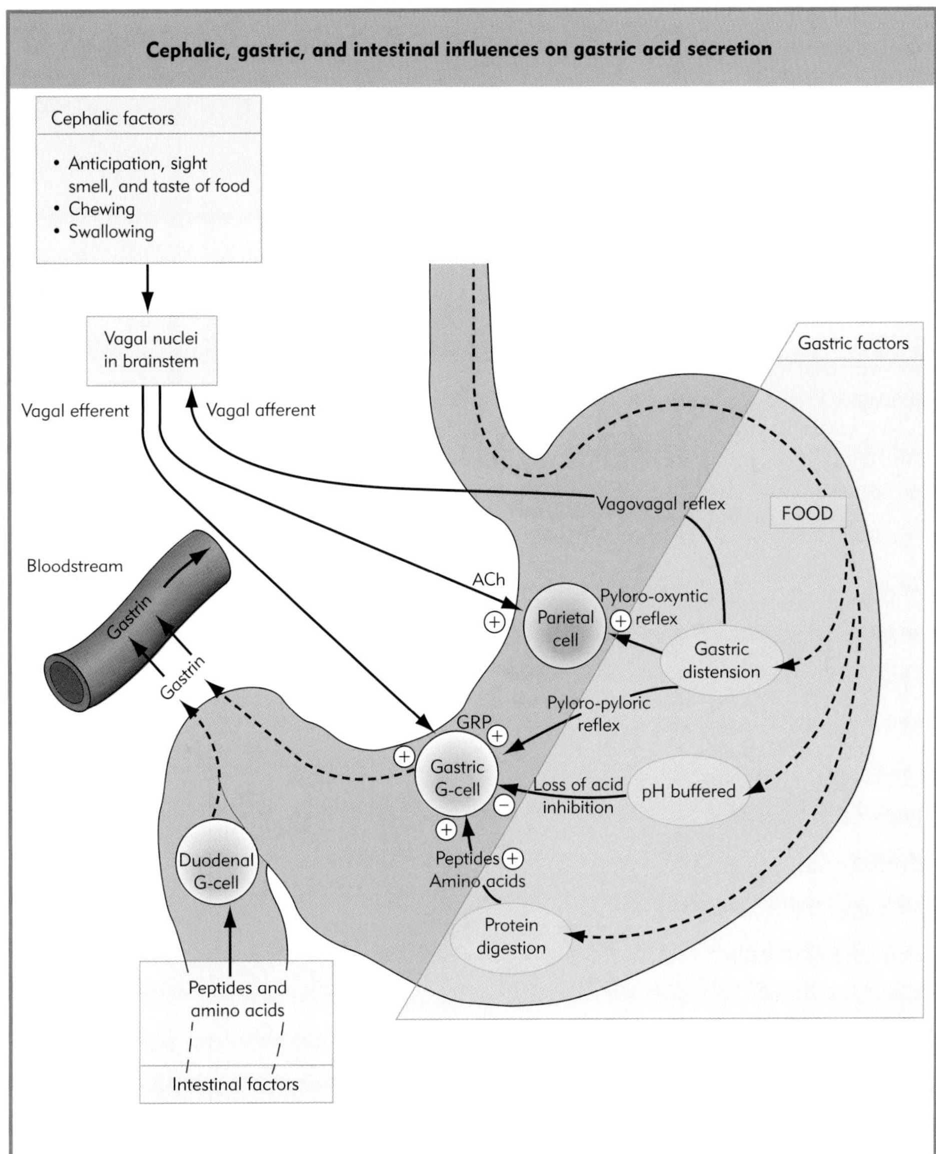

Figure 61.5 Cephalic, gastric, and intestinal influences on gastric acid secretion. *Cephalic factors* – anticipation, sight, smell, and taste of food together with the acts of chewing and swallowing – result in vagally mediated acid secretion. *Gastric factors* – buffering of acidic gastric pH – stops the inhibition of gastrin release from G cells at pH <3; distension of the stomach wall initiates vagovagal, pyloropyloric, and pyloro-oxyntic reflexes, which results in activation of G cells and parietal cells; peptides and amino acids directly stimulate G cells in the stomach. *Intestinal factors* – protein digestion products – directly stimulate G cells in the duodenum.

In the *gastric phase*, entry of food into the stomach results in acid secretion in a number of ways. In the empty stomach, low gastric pH (<3) reduces gastrin release from G cells by a direct inhibitory action. Food buffers the low pH and arrests this inhibition. Distension of the stomach by ingested food results in a number of neuronally mediated reflexes to increase acid secretion. Mechanoreceptor activation in the stomach wall sends sensory information via vagal afferents to the brainstem. Stimulation of the vagal nuclei results in efferent vagal activity that leads to acid secretion. As both afferent and efferent limbs of this reflex are vagal, it has been called the *vagovagal reflex*. In addition, two local distension reflexes occur. Localized stretching of the stomach causes gastrin release from G cells (*pyloropyloric reflex*) and acid secretion from parietal cells (*pyloro-oxyntic reflex*). Finally, peptides and amino acids from protein digestion have a direct effect on G cells in both the gastric antrum and duodenum to stimulate gastrin secretion. This intestinal factor is of relatively minor importance compared to cephalic and gastric factors.

Physiologic inhibition of acid secretion

As gastric emptying proceeds and during the interdigestive phase, several factors reduce gastric acid secretion to basal levels. The loss of cephalic factors at the end of a meal reduces vagally mediated acid secretion. As the stomach empties, 'gastric factors' diminish. The pH is buffered less, which allows it to fall, with consequent G-cell inhibition. Mechanoreceptor activation is also less, and so G-cell and parietal cell activation by neural reflexes is reduced.

Specific paracrine and endocrine factors slow gastric acid secretion. The primary paracrine inhibitor of acid secretion is somatostatin, which is released when gastric pH falls below 3. Somatostatin-secreting D cells are located in close proximity to gastrin cells and thus exert a continuous inhibitory restraint on the secretion of gastrin. Release of the gut hormones secretin and, to a lesser extent, GIP reduces acid secretion by inhibition of parietal and G cells. Secretin release occurs in response to the acidification of duodenal chyme as gastric emptying progresses.

The presence of carbohydrate and fatty acids in the duodenal lumen releases GIP. Secretin also stimulates pancreatic and biliary alkaline secretion to neutralize duodenal luminal pH. Some prostaglandins inhibit acid secretion as part of the mucosal cytoprotection mechanism.

Drugs reducing acid secretion

The most widely used drugs of this type are the *H_2 receptor antagonists* (H_2RA, e.g. cimetidine, ranitidine) and the *proton pump inhibitors* (PPI, e.g. omeprazole, lansoprazole). Another group, the *prostaglandin analogs* (e.g. misoprostol), also inhibit gastric acid secretion, and in addition increase mucosal blood flow and enhance mucus and bicarbonate production. These are not usually used as sole agents, but rather in association with nonsteroidal anti-inflammatory drugs in an attempt to prevent the antiprostaglandin gastric side effects (e.g. peptic ulceration) associated with their use (Chapter 32).

H_2 RECEPTOR ANTAGONISTS

Since their introduction, H_2RAs have become among the most widely prescribed of all drugs and have revolutionized the management of peptic ulceration. They inhibit acid secretion by competitive and reversible inhibition of H_2 receptors on the parietal cell surface membrane (Fig. 61.6). In this way they directly block the action of histamine in acid secretion and indirectly inhibit the synergistic influences of gastrin and cholinergic vagal stimulation on acid secretion normally mediated via histamine release.

Prompt symptomatic relief is provided by H_2RAs, and they heal 80–95% of peptic ulcers within 6–8 weeks of initiating treatment. Unfortunately, the relapse rate is high, with 80% of patients suffering a recurrence of the ulcer in the first year after treatment. The overall 5-year relapse rate falls to around 20% with half-dose maintenance therapy. The circadian rhythm of acid secretion has a peak secretion in the early hours after midnight, which is a critical time for peptic ulcer formation, as the buffering effects of saliva and food are absent; hence maintenance therapy is administered in the evening.

PROTON PUMP INHIBITORS

The final common pathway of acid secretion is blocked by PPIs through inhibition of H^+, K^+-ATPase in the apical membrane of the parietal cell. Therefore, PPIs have the potential to achieve a greater degree of acid inhibition than H_2RAs, which is reflected in their clinical efficacy. Two subunits form H^+, K^+-ATPase: the α subunit, with 8–10 membrane-spanning domains, which is the site of energy-producing phosphorylation, and a smaller β subunit of unknown function. The PPIs, such as omeprazole and lansoprazole, are benzimidazole sulfoxides, which inactivate H^+, K^+-ATPase by irreversible covalent binding to cysteine groups on the extracellular face of the α subunit (see Fig 61.6). Thus, it is necessary for the drug to diffuse out of the parietal cell to exert its pharmacologic effect. On the luminal side of the parietal cell apical membrane the drug is converted in the acid medium from sulfoxide into sulfenamide, which is the active form. Deactivation of the enzyme is total and permanent; synthesis of new H^+, K^+-ATPase is required for further acid secretion.

Omeprazole provides significantly faster ulcer healing in the first 2 weeks of therapy than do H_2RAs, as well as better symptomatic relief. Of the antacid drugs, PPIs are the most effective for refractory peptic ulcers, reflux esophagitis, and the Zollinger–Ellison syndrome.

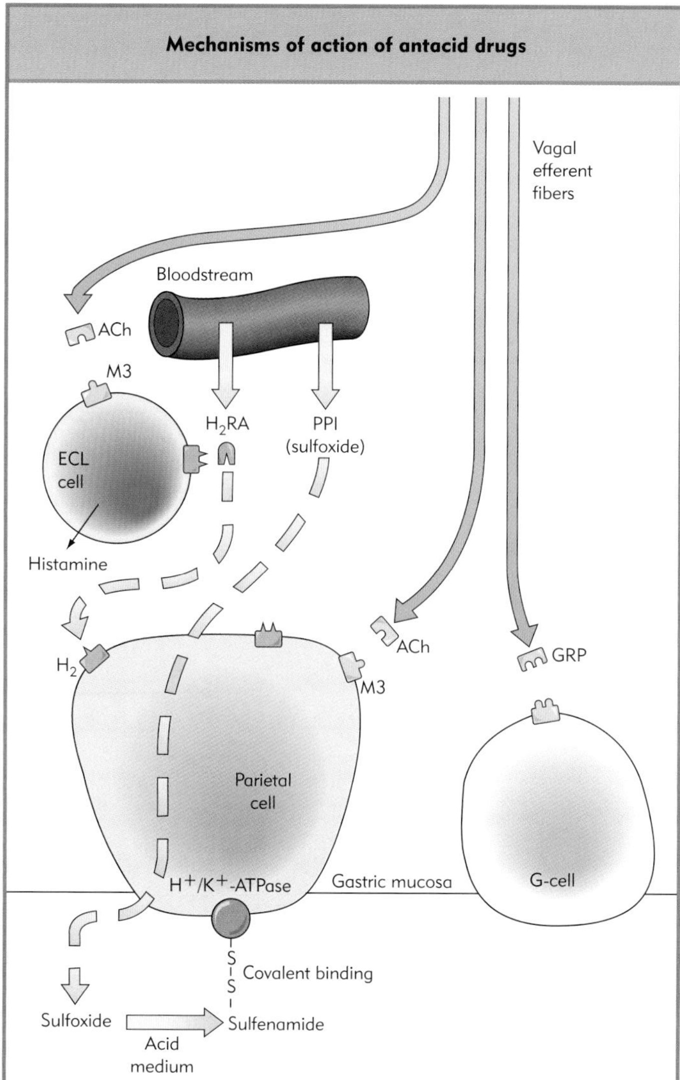

Figure 61.6 Mechanisms of action of antacid drugs. Acid secretion is inhibited by H_2RAs through competitive and reversible inhibition of H_2 receptors on the parietal cell surface membrane (see Fig. 61.4). In this way they directly block the action of histamine in acid secretion, and indirectly inhibit the synergistic influences of gastrin and cholinergic vagal stimulation, normally mediated via histamine release. An acid environment is required for the conversion of PPIs into active sulfenamide before they can irreversibly inactivate H^+, K^+-ATPase. This is achieved by diffusion across the parietal cell into the gastric lumen. Covalent bonds develop between the sulfenamide and cysteine groups on the extracellular face of the α subunit of the enzyme.

It is now recognized that many peptic ulcers are caused by the growth of the organism *Helicobacter pylori* in the gastroduodenal mucosa. Both H_2RAs and PPIs suppress the growth of this organism, which may be a factor in their ability to heal peptic ulcers. Curative treatment for peptic ulcer disease is now possible by antibiotic eradication of *H. pylori*, and has very low recurrence rates.

PEPSIN

Pepsinogen is secreted from peptic (or chief) cells in the oxyntic gland. Some pepsinogen is also secreted from mucosal cells in the gastric antrum and the duodenum. In the presence of gastric acid this proenzyme is converted into active pepsin, which itself catalyzes further conversion from pepsinogen. The main stimulus for pepsinogen release is the increased vagal activity seen in the cephalic and gastric phases of acid secretion. Gastric acid itself initiates a local cholinergic reflex that triggers pepsinogen secretion from peptic cells. Entry of acidic gastric chyme into the duodenum stimulates the release of secretin. This, together with gastrin, causes further pepsinogen secretion.

MUCUS

Two forms of mucus are secreted by the gastric mucosa, soluble and insoluble. Surface mucus cells secrete *insoluble mucus* and bicarbonate, which together with sloughed mucosal cells form a protective barrier over the mucosal surface. Insoluble mucus has an important role in the protection of the mucosal surface against acid, pepsin, and mechanical damage. Prostaglandins stimulate this secretion as part of the mucosal cytoprotection. *Soluble mucus* is a mucoprotein secretion from oxyntic neck mucus cells and occurs in response to vagal stimulation. It mixes with gastric contents and functions primarily as a lubricant.

Motility of the stomach

The arrangement of muscle in the stomach wall is more complex than in other parts of the gut, with circular, longitudinal, and oblique elements. The LES occurs at the gastroesophageal junction and the pyloric sphincter at the gastroduodenal junction. The stomach exhibits several types of motility pattern – receptive relaxation and contraction, peristaltic propulsion and mixing, and the migrating motor complex.

During feeding, the smooth muscle in the wall of the proximal stomach undergoes relaxation to make room for the incoming meal. This *receptive relaxation* allows the stomach to accommodate food with little increase in intragastric pressure. This is followed by low-amplitude long-lasting rhythmic contractions that reduce the size of the stomach as gastric emptying occurs. In the proximal part of the stomach, food can remain relatively undisturbed for up to an hour. During this time, digestion of carbohydrate takes place by salivary amylase.

In the mid and distal parts of the stomach more vigorous muscular activity takes place following the ingestion of a meal. *Peristaltic contractions* are generated in the region of the mid-stomach and pass distally toward the pylorus at a rate of about three per minute (Fig. 61.7). In this way, food is propelled toward the gastric outlet. The speed of propagation increases as the pylorus is approached, to a point at which the peristaltic wave 'overtakes' the intraluminal contents, which results in a combination of forward propulsion of some of the gastric contents through the pylorus, and retropulsion of the remainder back into the body of the stomach. Thus, mixing of food with gastric juice and mechanical reduction of particle size occurs. The role of the pyloric sphincter in controlling the passage of gastric chyme into the duodenum is unclear. The origin of these peristaltic waves lies in the intrinsic electrical activity of the smooth muscle cells, which undergo spontaneous rhythmic depolarization to generate so-called slow waves. These are generated in the mid-stomach and pass distally toward the pylorus, but do not necessarily generate peristaltic waves of contraction. Only when the amplitude of these waves reaches a certain threshold does muscular contraction begin. The greater the slow wave potential above the threshold, the greater the force of

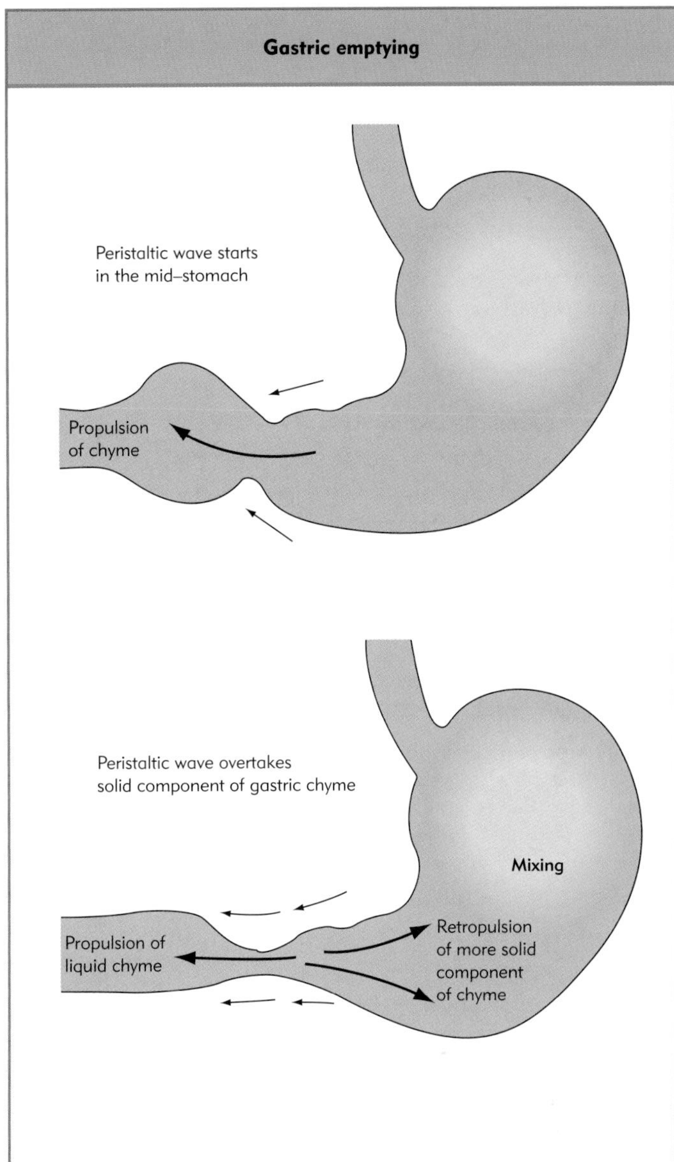

Figure 61.7 Gastric emptying. Food is disintegrated into smaller particles and eventually liquefied into gastric chyme by the actions of acid, enzymes, and muscular activity. The contractions involved are peristaltic in nature and pass from the mid-stomach distally. As the wave of contraction approaches the pylorus, its rate of propagation increases. In this way it overtakes the more solid component of chyme, which undergoes 'retropulsion' back into the body of the stomach. Liquid chyme stays ahead of the contractile wave and is transported into the duodenum.

muscular contraction. Vagal stimulation and gastrin increase gastric peristalsis, whereas sympathetic stimulation, secretin, GIP, and somatostatin depress activity.

It normally takes several hours for the stomach to empty following a meal. The speed at which substances empty from the stomach depends on their physical state and chemical composition. Liquids empty rapidly, whereas solids take longer (during which time they are broken down and liquefied in gastric juice). The delivery of nutrients to the duodenum from the stomach results in a negative feedback inhibition on gastric emptying. This 'duodenal brake' allows time for further digestion and absorption in the small intestine. Chemoreceptors in the duodenum are sensitive to the chemical composition of the chyme

Table 61.3 Perioperative causes of delayed gastric emptying

Physiologic
Pain
Anxiety
Elderly (liquids only)
Pregnancy (some patients only)
Pathologic
Gastrointestinal tract obstruction
Acute gastritis
Migraine
Electrolyte imbalance
Diabetes
Raised intracranial pressure
Certain muscle disorders
Polymyositis
Dermatomyositis
Systemic sclerosis
Pharmacologic
Opioids
μ agonists
Partial agonists
Mixed agonist/antagonists
Anticholinergics
Sympathomimetics
Dopamine
Ganglion blockers
Aluminum and magnesium hydroxides

being ejected from the stomach. Hypertonicity, fatty acids, and H^+ activate the secretion of CCK, secretin, and GIP, which inhibit gastric emptying. During the interdigestive period the *migrating motor complex* is initiated in the proximal stomach.

Several factors can delay gastric emptying in the perioperative period, as summarized in Table 61.3.

Drugs enhancing gastric emptying

Metoclopramide and *domperidone* are antidopaminergics and effective gastric prokinetics. However, at the doses commonly in use they do not effectively reverse opioid-induced delay. *Erythromycin* promotes gastric motility. Erythromycin analogs that have agonistic activity at the motilin receptor but no antibacterial action are now available and undergoing clinical trials.

Gastroesophageal reflux disease

Reflux of gastric fluid into the esophagus is common, occurring in normal individuals about once an hour without signs or symptoms of tissue damage. Such reflux is rapidly cleared by stimulation of esophageal peristalsis. In some circumstances reflux becomes pathologic, causing symptoms and leading to complications from chronic esophageal injury. Classically, the sensations of 'heartburn' and 'dyspepsia' occur, which may be associated with 'acid' regurgitation into the pharynx. In severe cases, persistent pulmonary aspiration of gastric fluid results in the development of respiratory symptoms and disease. Not infrequently, esophageal chest pain mimics myocardial ischemia; this causes anxiety in the patient and diagnostic difficulties for the clinician. In the early stages of the disease endoscopic and histologic findings may be normal despite significant symptomatology. In such patients, however, 24-hour esophageal pH monitoring demonstrates increased exposure of the mucosa to gastric juice.

The LES normally provides a barrier between the esophagus and the stomach. The sphincter-like function is related to the architecture of the muscle fibers as the esophagus enters the gastric pouch. Under normal circumstances the LES remains closed and relaxation occurs only as part of the swallowing reflex as the wave of esophageal peristalsis approaches. Several neural and humoral factors modulate the inherent myogenic tone of the LES. α-adrenergic stimulation, gastrin, motilin, enkephalin, and substance P increase tone, whereas β-adrenergic stimulation, CCK, secretin, GIP, and VIP decrease it. Metoclopramide, domperidone, neostigmine, succinylcholine, and metoprolol increase tone; anticholinergics (e.g. atropine, glycopyrrolate), volatile anesthetic agents, opioids, dopamine, sympathomimetics, Ca^{2+} channel blockers, diazepam, theophylline, caffeine, glyceryltrinitrate (GTN), and alcohol tend to decrease tone.

The causes of gastroesophageal reflux disease (GERD) may be categorized as mechanical incompetence of the LES, inappropriate relaxation of the LES, inefficient clearing of refluxed gastric juice, and abnormalities of the gastric reservoir.

Mechanical incompetence is the most common cause of GERD (accounts for about two-thirds of cases). Such incompetence occurs when the anatomy of the LES becomes distorted, as with hiatus hernias and gastric dilation, or when a primary abnormality of myogenic function causes low sphincter pressure.

In some patients increased episodes of reflux occur because of *inappropriate relaxation of the LES*. Abnormal coordination of the components of the swallowing reflex, upon which the vagus nerve has an important controlling influence, may be a significant factor. Hence, if a pharyngeal swallow is not followed by a wave of esophageal peristalsis, reflex relaxation of the LES may occur and allow reflux of gastric juice into the esophagus.

Esophageal clearance is an important component of the human antireflux mechanism. Under normal circumstances swallowing clears any refluxed gastric fluid by means of the primary peristaltic wave. Any residual refluxate stimulates secondary peristaltic waves by distending the esophagus. Acid in the esophagus also stimulates smooth muscle contraction, but this is less organized than the peristalsis initiated by distension. Thus, acid in the esophagus may disrupt normal peristalsis and so impede the clearance of refluxate.

Abnormalities of the gastric reservoir may contribute to pathologic reflux, including elevated intragastric pressure, delayed gastric emptying, and increased acid production. Elevated intragastric pressure may result from gastric outlet obstruction, or backing up from a more distal intestinal obstruction. In diabetic autonomic neuropathy, failure of active relaxation of the stomach causes raised intragastric pressure. Subsequent dilation of the stomach distorts the anatomy of the LES, shortening its effective length and reducing its resistance to reflux. Delayed gastric emptying that results in a persistent gastric reservoir may occur in conditions such as gastric atony caused by myotonic abnormalities (e.g. advanced diabetes). Gastric hypersecretion exacerbates the disruption of esophageal motility because of acid reflux, as discussed above.

Several components of the refluxate may cause damage to the esophageal mucosa – gastric acid and pepsin are the main injurious agents in gastric juice. If an element of duodenogastric reflux is also present, the situation becomes more complex. In a patient who has high gastric acid production, reflux of alkaline duodenal fluid may have a beneficial effect by neutralizing gastric acidity. In addition, bile salts inhibit pepsin and gastric acid inhibits pancreatic trypsin. However, in a patient who has low gastric acid secretion or who has a high degree of duodenogastric reflux, alkaline duodenal fluid and pancreatic enzymes become injurious agents in their own right. In such patients antacid therapy may worsen the situation.

Persistent pathologic reflux causes recurrent damage and repair cycling, with the eventual development of the complications of GERD. This usually takes the form of a benign stricture formation that causes dysphagia or metaplastic transformation of native squamous epithelium into columnar epithelium, characteristic of the so-called Barrett's esophagus. This columnar epithelium is more resistant to acid and associated with a reduction in symptoms of heartburn. Peptic ulcer or malignant disease may further complicate Barrett's esophagus. Pulmonary complications may also follow chronic regurgitation and pulmonary aspiration. Nocturnal cough, wheezing, recurrent infections, and progressive pulmonary fibrosis can all occur.

The aim of treatment is to prevent the tendency to reflux by the suppression of acid production (e.g. H_2 antagonists, PPIs) and surgical correction of a mechanically defective LES (e.g. Nissen fundoplication). Symptomatic relief may be achieved using antacids, alginate, and prokinetic drugs. The most effective drugs, in terms of both symptom relief and healing of esophagitis, are PPIs. Treatment of complications includes dilation of strictures and surveillance for neoplastic change.

MOTILITY PATTERNS IN THE SMALL INTESTINE

In the small intestine, digestion continues with the addition of exocrine pancreatic secretions and bile, which enter the duodenum via the sphincter of Oddi. Secretin stimulates the secretion of alkaline fluid from these sources to neutralize chyme from the stomach. The exocrine pancreas also secretes a range of enzymes that are essential for digestion. These include proteases, which, like pepsin, are secreted as proenzymes, together with lipase and amylase, which are secreted in their active forms. Bile contains bile salts, which together with phospholipids and cholesterol, form micelles that take part in the digestion and absorption of lipids. Bile salts are themselves absorbed in the small intestine to be recycled by the liver for bile synthesis.

Motility patterns in the small intestine serve to mix intraluminal contents with digestive secretions, expose digested nutrient subunits to the absorptive surfaces, propel intraluminal contents in a distal direction, and prepare the small intestine for the next meal.

During the digestive period, *stationary segmenting contractions* occur to divide the small intestine into segments (Fig. 61.8). After a short period relaxation occurs, followed by further contractions in adjacent parts of the gut wall to form new segments. Unlike peristaltic waves, the contraction is not propagated along the gut wall. In this way, the intraluminal contents are pummeled, mixed, and exposed to mucosal surfaces. Distal propulsion may occur with this motility pattern if the stationary segmenting contractions occur in a proximal to distal sequence. Normal *peristalsis* (see Fig. 61.2) also transports intraluminal contents through the gut. Slow waves occur in both the small and large intestine and are similar to those seen in the stomach. They appear to be important in setting the frequency of contractions, with neurohumoral influences interacting to determine the degree of smooth muscle activity. Increased vagal activity stimulates intestinal motility, as do gastrin, CCK, and insulin. Sympathetic stimulation, secretin, and glucagon inhibit smooth muscle activity. The exact role of each of these mediators in the control of motility is unclear. During the interdigestive phase, migrating motor complexes sweep through the small intestine to clear it of undigested matter in preparation for the next meal (see above).

MOTILITY PATTERNS IN THE LARGE INTESTINE

In the large intestine, water and electrolytes are extracted from the intraluminal contents so that semisolid feces are formed as the distal colon and rectum are approached. Storage takes place in the distal colon until voluntary emptying occurs by defecation.

The large intestine consists of the cecum, the ascending, transverse, descending, and sigmoid colon, and the rectum. It is anatomically distinct from the small intestine in that the outer longitudinal muscle is concentrated into three flat bands, called teniae coli. The parasympathetic supply to the descending colon, sigmoid colon, and rectum is from cholinergic parasympathetic elements in the pelvic nerves that originate from sacral roots 2, 3, and 4. As the anal canal is approached, the circular smooth muscle layer thickens to form the internal anal sphincter. Overlapping and slightly distal to the internal anal sphincter are layers of striated muscle that comprise the external anal sphincter.

The passage of intraluminal contents from the small to the large intestine occurs intermittently and is regulated in part by a sphincteric mechanism at the ileocecal junction. The restriction to flow imposed by this periodically relaxes to allow ileal peristalsis and migrating motor complexes to propel intraluminal contents through. Several motility patterns occur in the large intestine: stationary segmental contractions, mass movement, and defecation.

Stationary segmental contractions similar to those in the small intestine occur throughout the colon and rectum. They last about a minute, which is considerably longer than those in the small intestine, and are probably responsible for the haustrations in the large intestine. Functionally, these contractions expose intraluminal contents to the mucosal surface for efficient extraction of water and electrolytes. In the descending colon, sigmoid colon, and rectum the frequency of segmenting contractions increases. This acts as a brake on distal flow as feces approach the rectum. Passage through the colon is slow (normally several days). This passage occurs intermittently in a motility sequence that drives feces distally, called *mass movement*, which occurs about three times per day.

The rectum is normally empty or nearly empty and the anal canal is closed due to internal sphincter contraction. Entry of feces into the rectum during a mass movement causes distension. Rectal distension has two effects: it causes the sensation of the urge to defecate, and it activates the rectosphincteric reflex, which causes relaxation of the internal sphincter. The urge to defecate can be overcome by voluntary contraction of the external sphincter. Relaxation of the internal sphincter is transient, as

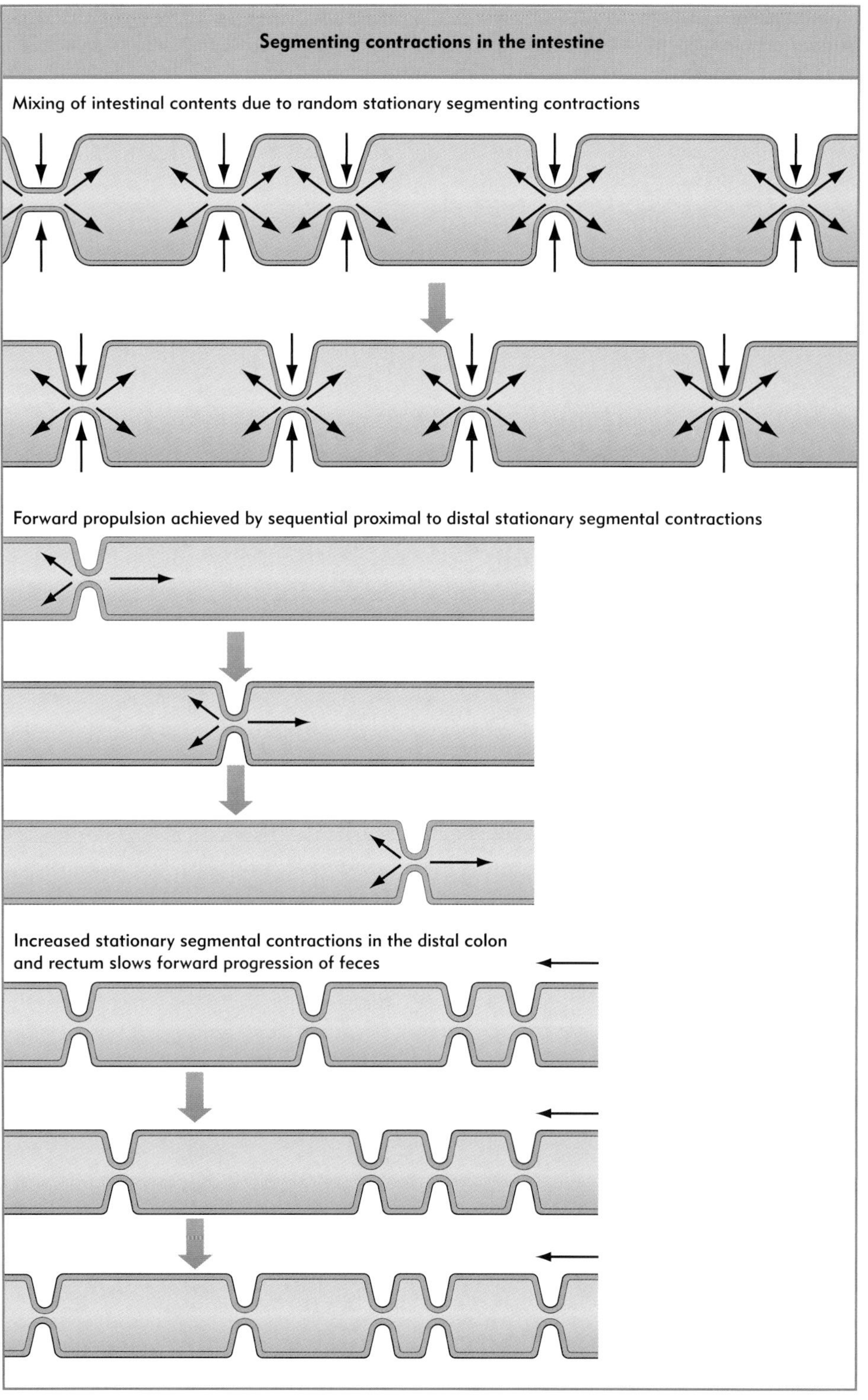

Figure 61.8 Segmenting contractions in the intestine. Stationary segmenting contractions divide the small intestine into short lengths. Subsequent relaxation is followed by a new set of ring contractions that create new segments. Thus, intraluminal contents are mixed with digestive fluids and exposed to the absorptive mucosal surfaces. In the small intestine, sequential patterns of segmenting contractions serve to propel intraluminal contents distally. In the distal large intestine an increase in the frequency of segmenting contractions acts as a brake on the transport of feces as the rectum is approached.

stretch receptors within the rectal wall accommodate to the stimulus of distension and the internal sphincter regains its tone. If defecation is convenient it is initiated by voluntary action and involves contraction of the distal colon and rectum together with relaxation of the internal and external anal sphincters. Often voluntary acts such as 'Valsalva-type' maneuvers and contraction of the abdominal wall can raise intra-abdominal pressure. The gastrocolic reflex promotes defecation following food ingestion and is most prominent in children.

ABNORMAL GASTROINTESTINAL MOTILITY: POSTOPERATIVE ILEUS

Postoperative ileus may be defined as the temporary impairment of bowel motility after surgery or injury. It is especially common after open intraperitoneal surgery. It is characterized by a lack of passage of flatus and stool, and results in unpleasant symptoms such as nausea, vomiting, and abdominal distension, as well as delaying the resumption of normal diet and nutrition. Distal bowel motility is slowest to return to normal after a surgical insult, so the clinical duration of ileus will depend mostly on the duration of colonic paralysis. The pathophysiology is complicated and only partially characterized. Neural, endocrine, and inflammatory factors probably all play a role. Inhibitory reflex activity involving the spinal cord is the most important neural pathway, although ultrashort reflexes within the gut wall and short reflexes confined to the prevertebral ganglia also contribute to the inhibition of bowel activity in response to noxious stimuli. The afferent arm of the spinal reflex originates in the visceral and parietal peritoneum in response to injury or bowel manipulation. This is important because it is possible to block this afferent activity by thoracic epidural analgesia using local anesthetics. The effect of the neuroendocrine stress response to surgery is compounded by the release from the gut of numerous hormones, such as motilin, VIP, and substance P, that are capable of acting locally and systemically to inhibit motility. An increase in systemic catecholamine release will tend to decrease gastrointestinal perfusion, which may impair motility. The inflammatory response in the injured tissue may contribute to the persistence of ileus mediated by leukocyte-derived nitric oxide, with its relaxant effect on smooth muscle.

Opioid analgesia has a profound inhibitory effect on gastric emptying and gut motility. This is mediated via agonist action at the μ-receptor causing nonpropulsive smooth muscle contraction. This results in increased oral–cecal transit time, constipation, and increased common bile duct pressure due to increased tone of the sphincter of Oddi. Methylnaltrexone, a quaternary opioid antagonist with limited ability to cross the blood–brain barrier, has shown promise in reversing the inhibitory gastrointestinal effects of morphine without affecting analgesia.

Epidural analgesia using local anesthetics has been shown to reduce the duration of ileus in numerous studies where appropriate segmental blockade was demonstrated. In abdominal surgery this means thoracic epidural anesthesia must be used to block the visceral afferents and sympathetic efferents. Although the addition of opioids to epidural local anesthetic may improve analgesia, this is at some detriment to the reduction of ileus compared to local anesthetic-only regimens.

Clinical experience with pharmacological prokinetic agents has been disappointing in postoperative ileus. More promising is the use of early enteral feeding after laparotomy. Traditional surgical practice has been to withhold oral feeding until ileus has resolved, but there is now good trial evidence to show that early oral feeding has benefits in reducing the duration of ileus, and earlier discharge from hospital. The presence of food in the gut stimulates the release of prokinetic gut hormones and reflex gut motility as well as maintaining gut mucosal barrier integrity.

In conclusion, there is now good evidence that the global disorder of motility and secretion that results in ileus can be minimized by a multimodal approach involving epidural anesthesia and postoperative analgesia using local anesthetics, together with opioid-sparing techniques and early enteral feeding.

Key references

Ching CK, Lam SK. Drug therapy of peptic ulcer disease. Br J Hosp Med. 1995;54:101–6.

Goyal RK, Hirano I. The enteric nervous system. N Engl J Med. 1996;334:1106–15.

Johnson LR. Gastric secretion. In: Johnson LR, ed. Gastrointestinal physiology, 5th edn. Chicago: Mosby; 1997: 69–87.

Helander HF, Keeling DJ. Cell biology of gastric acid secretion. Clin Gastroenterol. 1993;7:1–22.

Hellström PM. Motility of the small intestine: a case of pattern recognition. J Intern Med. 1995;237:391–4

Holte K, Kehlet H. Postoperative ileus: a preventable event. Br J Surg. 2000;87:1480–93.

Peters JH, DeMeester TR. Gastroesophageal reflux. Surg Clin North Am. 1993;73:1119–44.

Shamburek RD, Schubert ML. Pharmacology of gastric acid inhibition. Clin Gastroenterol. 1993;7:23–54.

Weisbrodt NW. Motility of the small and large intestine. In: Johnson LR, ed. Gastrointestinal physiology, 5th edn. Chicago: Mosby; 1997: 43–58.

Further reading

Mythen MG. Postoperative gastrointestinal tract dysfunction. Anesth Analg 2005;100:196–204.

Ogilvy AJ, Smith G. The gastrointestinal tract after anaesthesia. Eur J Anaesthesiol. 1995;12(Suppl.10):35–42.

Chapter 62

Nutrition, digestion, and absorption

Iain T Campbell

DIGESTION AND ABSORPTION

Nutrients are absorbed from the gastrointestinal tract, which consists of the mouth, pharynx, esophagus, stomach, and large and small intestines. Accessory structures outside the digestive system, but associated with digestion and absorption, are the salivary glands, pancreas, liver, and gallbladder (Fig. 62.1). Their secretions pass into the digestive tract via their ducts. Blood that drains the gastrointestinal tract passes via the portal vein and carries the absorbed products of digestion to the liver, where they are metabolized before these products of hepatic metabolism circulate to the cells of the rest of the body. The splanchnic circulation receives about 25% of the cardiac output, and is at its maximum after a meal.

Various substances and enzymes are excreted by the wall of the gut and the exocrine glands that empty into its lumen. These include a variety of inorganic molecules, such as hydrochloric acid in the stomach and bicarbonate from the pancreas. Amylase is synthesized and excreted by the salivary glands, pepsinogen by the stomach, amylase, proteases and a variety of other digestive enzymes by the pancreas, and bile by the liver. The various enzymes are secreted in response to stimuli; water and inorganic ions follow passively. The nature of the secretions may be modified by the ducts as they pass into the intestine.

Digestion

The large complex molecules of carbohydrates, proteins, and triglycerides are degraded for absorption into simple sugars, small peptides, amino acids, free fatty acids (FFA), and monoglycerides. Digestion starts with saliva and continues in the stomach and small intestine, where it is completed and most of the absorption takes place. Some excretory components, such as water and inorganic ions, pass from the bloodstream through the enterocyte by a variety of transport mechanisms, whereas others are synthesized in the cells and are stored there until an appropriate nervous or hormonal signal stimulates secretion. Significant amounts of water and inorganic salts are absorbed by the large intestine. A variety of specialized transport systems function in the wall of the gut and transfer specific products of digestion from the lumen into the bloodstream. Others move passively along concentration gradients, and are affected by molecular size and lipid solubility.

Motility and excretion are highly regulated functions with regulation by a variety of stimuli that stimulate excretion, from the sight and smell of food to the vestibular apparatus that may induce vomiting via the vomiting center. In contrast, few mechanisms normally affect digestion and absorption, other than the food itself.

The *innervation of the gastrointestinal tract* is via 'short' and 'long' nerves. The short nerves make up the plexi contained within the walls of the digestive tract and give it a degree of autonomous function. The long nerves control function via the central nervous system; the parasympathetic vagus nerve is the major motor nerve and its impulses are excitatory and cholinergic. The parasympathetic sacral outflow (S2–4) supplies the motor nerves for the rectum and lower colon. The sympathetic nerves provide the principal sensory input via the splanchnic nerves. Sympathetic stimulation is mainly inhibitory.

The *salivary glands* contain three types of excretory cell. Serous cells excrete a watery solution which mixes with mucin from mucous cells to form the mucus that lubricates the bolus of food. Amylase is excreted in response to parasympathetic stimuli. It digests starch to produce maltose and oligosaccharides. Digestion by salivary amylase continues for some time after the swallowed bolus enters the stomach.

The *stomach* produces hydrochloric acid secreted by exocrine glands in its body and fundus. The three types of secretory cell

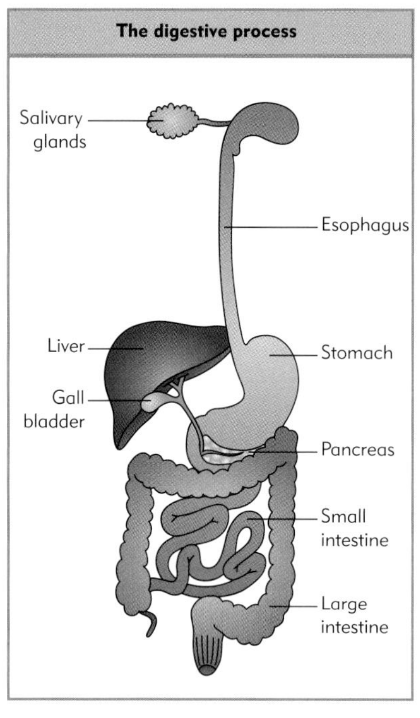

Digestive organ functions

Organ/gland	Secretion	Substrate/ function	Products
Salivary glands	Salivary amylase Mucus	Starch	Oligo- and disaccharides Lubrication
Stomach	Hydrochloric acid Pepsinogen → Pepsin	Antibacterial Protein	Denatured protein Polypeptides
Gallbladder	Bile salts	Lipids	Emulsion
Pancreas	Trypsinogen→ trypsin Chymotrypsinogen → chymotrypsin Amylase Lipase and Phospholipase	Proteins Polypeptides Starch and oligosaccharides Lipids and phospholipids	Peptides and amino acids Dextrins and disaccharides Free fatty acids and monoglycerides
Small intestine Brush border	Aminopeptidase Dipeptidase Disaccharidase	Peptides Dipeptides Disaccharides	Amino acids Amino acids Monosaccharides
Large intestine	Digestion/absorption of endogenous proteins, cellular debris, plasma		

Figure 62.1 The digestive processes. (Adapted with permission from MacBurnie M, Wilmore DW. Rational decision making in nutritional care. Surg Clin North Am. 1981;61: 571–82.)

are chief cells, parietal cells, and mucous cells. Chief cells secrete pepsinogen, the inactive precursor of pepsin, and parietal cells hydrochloric acid, which converts pepsinogen into pepsin and provides the optimium pH for pepsin activity. It also kills ingested bacteria and contributes to the breakdown of ingested connective tissue by denaturing protein. The mucus provides a protective covering for the gastric mucosa.

Hydrochloric acid is secreted by H^+, K^+-ATPase in the luminal membrane and Na^+/Cl^- cotransport in the basolateral membrane of parietal cells. Its secretion is stimulated by vagal mechanisms. These vagal stimuli act also via the nerve plexi within the stomach wall to stimulate gastrin-secreting cells in the wall of the antrum. The gastrin in turn stimulates the body and the fundus of the stomach via the bloodstream to secrete more hydrochloric acid. Histamine is also involved in hydrochloric acid release. The secretion of hydrochloric acid is inhibited when it contacts the antral mucosa, and when food passes into the duodenum.

Pepsinogen secretion by the chief cells is stimulated by acetylcholine released from the vagus nerve. It is converted into the active enzyme pepsin by hydrochloric acid and by pepsin itself. Pepsin is a protease that hydrolyzes protein into short chain peptides (chains of amino acids).

The *exocrine pancreas* consists of clusters of cells or acini that secrete enzymes into intercalated ducts which converge before opening into the duodenum. The epithelial cells lining the ducts secrete a relatively large volume of fluid rich in bicarbonate, which neutralizes the acid that enters the duodenum from the stomach and thus provides the optimum pH for the pancreatic digestive enzymes to work.

The pancreas secretes a rich mixture of digestive enzymes that can digest the whole diet. These include the proteolytic enzymes trypsinogen and chymotrypsinogen. Enterokinase is excreted from the epithelial lining of the small intestine and activates trypsinogen to give trypsin, which itself activates both chymotrypsinogen and trypsinogen. Procarboxypeptidase, secreted by the pancreas, is converted into caboxykinase by trypsin and hydrolyzes terminal amino acids from proteins and peptides.

The lipid digestive enzymes are lipase (which hydrolyzes triglycerides into FFA and monoglycerides), phospholipase, and cholesterol esterase. Amylase, similar to salivary amylase, degrades starch to give oligosaccharides (principally maltose), and ribonuclease and deoxyribonuclease hydrolyze nucleic acids.

Four hormones – gastrin, cholecystokinin, secretin, and gastroinhibitory peptide – are released in the gastrointestinal tract in response to intraluminal stimuli that act directly on endocrine cells in the luminal lining. In addition to its action on the stomach, stimulating acid and pepsin release, gastrin has a generalized trophic action on the gastrointestinal tract. It also stimulates insulin secretion after a protein meal. Secretin and cholecystokinin are hormones released from the duodenal mucosa.

Secretin stimulates the excretion of bicarbonate from the duct cells of the pancreas. Cholecystokinin stimulates both the secretion of pancreatic digestive enzymes and contraction of the gallbladder. Gastroinhibitory peptide is produced in the mucosa of the duodenum and jejunum, and it too stimulates insulin secretion. There are numerous other gastrointestinal hormones – neurotensin, grehlin, substance P, motilin, etc. – for the interested reader, but their detailed discussion is beyond the scope of this chapter.

Bile salts are intimately involved in the digestion and absorption of fat. The stimulus to the excretion of bile is the absorption of bile salts from the terminal ileum via the portal vein and the enterohepatic circulation. Secretin also stimulates the secretion of water and inorganic ions, principally bicarbonate, into the duodenum. Bile salts help in the digestion of lipid. They are amphipathic molecules with both lipid-soluble (steroid nucleus) and polar (–OH and –COOH) domains that surround lipid molecules presenting their polar parts to the aqueous environment of the gut. They thus form an emulsion of micelles, each of which contains about 20 lipid molecules. These diffuse in aqueous solution and render the fat molecules more susceptible to the action of lipase, which breaks them down to give FFA and monoglycerides. These are absorbed along the length of the intestine. Cholesterol and fat-soluble vitamins are also absorbed by the same mechanisms.

SMALL INTESTINE

When the gastric contents move into the small intestine and are broken down further they become hyperosmotic. Water moves into the gut from the bloodstream and from the various mucosal endocrine glands, and the contents of the small intestine become iso-osmotic with blood. Absorption occurs along the whole of the small intestine and is normally complete by halfway, so there is a significant reserve of absorptive area. Some water and sodium chloride enter the large intestine, where their absorption is completed.

The absorptive surface of the small intestine is highly folded and convoluted, with fingerlike projections or villi that greatly increase the absorptive area (Fig. 62.2). Each villus has its own lymph drainage and arterial and venous supply. In addition, the luminal surface of the cells of the intestinal epithelium consists of a series of projections, the so-called brush border, which contains a number of enzymes and transport systems involved in the movement of the products of digestion from the lumen into the circulation. Some molecules also pass down concentration gradients that depend on their lipid solubility.

Water and electrolytes

About 2 L of water enters the small bowel each day from the stomach and another 7 L from the various secretions in the bowel, of which about 500 mL enter the large intestine and

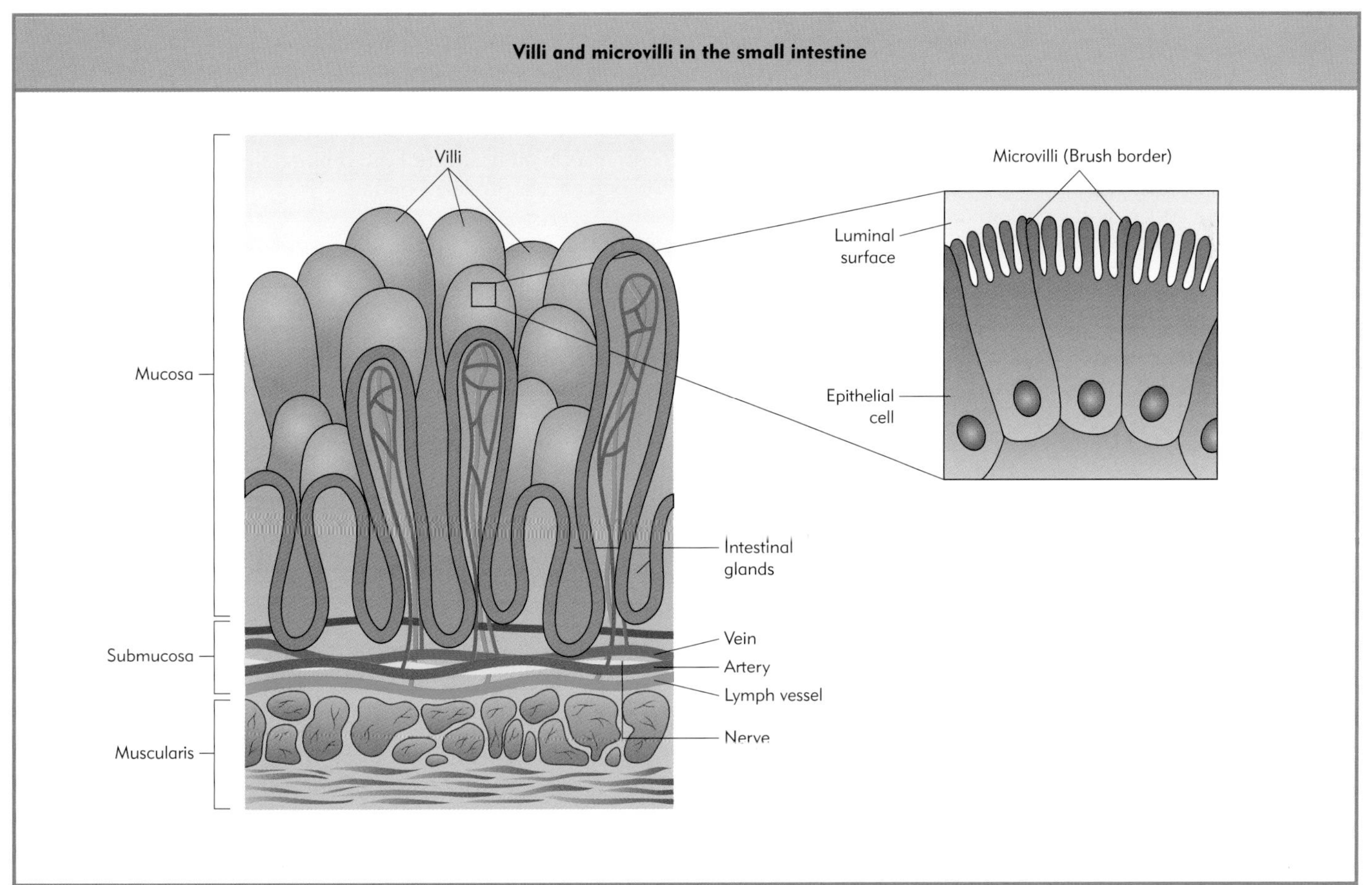

Figure 62.2 Villi and microvilli in the small intestine.

100 mL are excreted in the feces. Water absorption occurs mostly by osmosis following the various products of digestion. Sodium plays a major role in this process: it diffuses through the brush border into the enterocyte, and is actively pumped into the circulation by a Na^+, K^+-ATPase in the basal membrane of the cell. Other ions are absorbed by a mixture of active and passive processes, but there are specific transport mechanisms for iron and Ca^{2+}.

Absorption of nutrients

CARBOHYDRATE

Starch is hydrolyzed into oligosaccharides by salivary and pancreatic amylase and broken down by oligosaccharidases in the brush border of the enterocyte to give monosaccharides. Cellulose, or fiber, is excreted in the feces. The various monosaccharides are absorbed by a variety of mechanisms: fructose passes by facilitated diffusion, and glucose and galactose by a carrier-mediated mechanism coupled with Na^+ that requires energy.

PROTEIN

Protein in the digestive tract consists not only of dietary protein, but also of endogenous peptides derived from digestive enzymes, epithelial cells, and plasma proteins that leak into the lumen. The peptides are hydrolyzed by brush border peptidases and the amino acids are absorbed by carrier-mediated transport systems coupled with Na^+ that consume energy. There are specific carriers for different groups of amino acids. Some absorption of di- and tripeptides occurs.

LIPID

The degradation of triglyceride into monoglyceride and FFA and the formation of micelles are discussed above, along with the role of bile salts in the absorption of these substances into the enterocyte. Once in the enterocyte, monoglycerides and FFA are resynthesized into triglycerides. These are aggregated, phospholipid and protein added, and a chylomicron formed which enters the lymphatic system and the general circulation.

THE COLON

The principal absorptive function of the large intestine is to absorb Na^+, accompanied normally by about 400 mL of the 500 mL of water that enters it from the ileum. Some vitamins are also synthesized in the large bowel, and the bacterial fermentation of indigestible carbohydrates produces flatus, which consists of nitrogen, carbon dioxide, hydrogen sulfide, and methane. The colonic mucosa also produces mucus and excretes K^+ and bicarbonate. The mucus protects the epithelium from trauma and the bicarbonate neutralizes acids, but when large volumes of fluid are lost in the feces significant K^+ depletion can occur.

NUTRITIONAL (MACRONUTRIENT) REQUIREMENTS

Protein and energy requirements are met by oxidation of carbohydrate, fat, and protein. The principal hormones that control the metabolism of these substances are insulin and glucagon. Insulin is an anabolic hormone; its secretion is stimulated by glucose, but also by some amino acids. When insulin falls secondary to a decrease in blood glucose, glucagon rises. Glucagon stimulates glycogenolysis, lipolysis, and gluconeogenesis. This releases glucose from liver glycogen, free fatty acids from adipose tissue, and stimulates the formation of glucose in the liver and kidney from the gluconeogenic precursors, i.e. glycerol, amino acids, and lactate. Insulin is the principal anabolic hormone. It stimulates the storage of glucose as glycogen, inhibits lipolysis, and stimulates protein synthesis. A lack of insulin, as is seen in diabetes mellitus or in the acute response to trauma, and in exercise, results in a breakdown of body protein.

Assessment of protein and energy requirements

Basal energy expenditure can be calculated from age height and weight using one of the standard formulae (see Chapter 65), and the value increased by a percentage to take into account activity and, in hospital patients, severity of illness and temperature. Alternatively, basal or resting energy expenditure can be measured by indirect calorimetry. Unless the calorimeter is built into a ventilator, in which case energy expenditure can be measured throughout the 24 hours, basal expenditure is normally measured over a limited period of up to 30 minutes and the results extrapolated to 24 hours, with an appropriate percentage added to allow for activity as described above. In acute illness energy expenditure is also elevated in a relatively predictable fashion, the precise percentage being dependent on the type of illness (Table 62.1).

Provision of macronutrient requirements

In a healthy individual about 10–15% of energy requirements are provided by protein oxidation and the remainder split roughly 50:50 between oxidation of carbohydrate and fat. The precise proportions in health are unclear, the concerns being the long-term effects on health (elevated blood lipids, atheroma, etc.) of the percentage provided by fat.

PROTEIN

In health, lean body mass is relatively constant and the protein ingested equals that oxidized and excreted as various waste products in the urine, principally as urea, plus that lost in the feces and in shed skin. This stability of lean body mass is a dynamic one in which protein synthesis and protein breakdown occur simultaneously. For a stable body mass these are in equilibrium, with a proportion equal to the protein intake being

Table 62.1 Predicted elevation in energy expenditure above basal (stress factors) produced by a variety of conditions (Adapted from MacBurney M, Wilmore DW, 1981)

Condition	Stress factor
Postoperative	1.00–1.05
Cancer	1.10–1.45
Peritonitis	1.05–1.25
Long bone fracture	1.15–1.30
Severe infection/multiple trauma	1.30–1.55
Burns	1.50–2.00

oxidized. The minimum protein requirement is about 0.5 g/kg/day, so a recommendation of 1 g/kg/day covers the requirements of a healthy individual. Any protein intake above this is oxidized to CO_2 and water, the nitrogen being excreted in the urine as urea. The only factors that promote protein retention and an increase in lean tissue are exercise, or drugs such as anabolic steroids. In trauma and sepsis there is an increase in gluconeogenesis, which results in increased oxidation and a rise in urinary nitrogen excretion.

The standard method used to assess protein metabolism is the measurement of urinary nitrogen excretion and nitrogen balance. However, outside a metabolic ward a 24-hour urine collection is extremely difficult to make accurately. Another method used to assess protein metabolism is with isotopic tracers: isotopes of various amino acids labeled with ^{13}C or ^{15}N are infused and their appearance is tracked in blood, urine, tissue, and exhaled air. From the dosage administered and the rates of appearance and disappearance of the isotopes in blood, urine, or exhaled air, rates of whole-body protein synthesis breakdown and oxidation can be quantified.

In sepsis and trauma the relationship between protein synthesis and breakdown is disturbed. After a relatively minor stimulus such as elective surgery protein synthesis is depressed and protein breakdown unaltered, but the net result is an increased breakdown of protein and a loss of lean tissue. In severe trauma, sepsis, and multiple organ failure both synthesis and breakdown are elevated, but breakdown is elevated more than synthesis, so that net protein catabolism is even worse. Using tracer techniques the maximum protein intake that a septic or injured patient can tolerate has been estimated at about 1.5–2 g/kg/day. Provided energy requirements are covered by carbohydrate and fat, this rate of protein provision stimulates protein synthetic rate to its maximum. Any protein intake over and above this is oxidized.

Net catabolism due to gluconeogenesis persists in trauma and sepsis despite adequate nutritional intake.

The cause of this net catabolism in trauma and sepsis is gluconeogenesis, which persists despite an apparently adequate nutrient intake. Why this occurs is unclear, but it is certainly caused in part by elevation of the classic counterregulatory hormones glucagon, cortisol, and the catecholamines, but the inability to produce negative nitrogen balance of this severity by infusing these hormones into normal volunteers indicates that other factors must also be involved. The most obvious ones are the cytokines. Their precise mechanism of action is not really known, but is probably a combination of action on both hepatic and peripheral tissues. In severe catabolic illness nutritional support alone will not preserve lean tissue. To do so in these patients, pharmacological methods of modifying metabolism are needed.

Nature of the protein intake

Proteins differ in their composition depending on the amino acids that are present. The 'standard' protein has usually been taken as whole egg protein, but evidence is now accumulating that in critical illness amino acid requirements differ from this standard. Amino acid solutions enriched or supplemented with glutamine, arginine, and branched-chain amino acids are beneficial in trauma and sepsis. This is because of their actions in stimulating immune function and regulating protein metabolism. Glutamine is the energy substrate for the lymphocyte and the enterocyte. Glutamine and the branched-chain amino acids also have a pivotal role in interorgan substrate transfer. Supplementation of parenteral nutrition in critically ill intensive care patients has been shown to have a favorable influence on outcome 6 months after discharge. Glutamine has been described as a 'conditionally essential' amino acid in trauma and sepsis. In contrast to trauma and sepsis, malnourished patients are avid retainers of nitrogen: nutritional supplementation is at its most effective in these individuals.

GLUCOSE

Glucose intake or infusion stimulates insulin secretion. Insulin stimulates glucose oxidation, glucose storage, and protein synthesis, and inhibits lipolysis. At lower rates of glucose provision (and insulin response) most of the glucose is oxidized to provide energy. At higher rates (and a higher insulin response) a greater percentage of the glucose provided is stored as glycogen. The amount oxidized does not increase at intakes beyond 4–5 mg/kg/min. When the glycogen stores have been filled, infused or ingested glucose is converted to fat. For a 70 kg (154 lb) adult this maximum rate of glucose intake or infusion corresponds to a daily glucose intake of about 500 g, which amounts to 2000 kcal (8.4 MJ).

In trauma and sepsis, in the stage immediately after injury insulin secretion is inhibited by catecholamines, but glycogenolysis is stimulated. There is a surfeit of available circulating glucose, but an impairment in the ability to use it. In the recovery phase insulin concentrations are high relative to blood glucose levels, which indicates a degree of insulin resistance. This represents the inability to store glucose, rather than an impairment of the ability to oxidize it.

LIPID

On absorption, fat is presented to peripheral tissues as chylomicrons, triglycerides, and following assimilation as lipoproteins, and is metabolized as fatty acids. Some fats – linoleic and linolenic – are 'essential' for growth and development. However, the predominant role of fat in metabolism is to provide the energy requirements not covered by glucose. The rate of fatty acid oxidation is normally proportional to its concentration in the blood, which in turn is controlled by the lipolytic hormone glucagon (with a reciprocal action to insulin) and, under stress, catecholamines. Following injury insulin secretion is inhibited and the intense adrenergic discharge stimulates lipolysis, which raises the circulating concentrations of FFAs. In these circumstances the healthy tissues of the body then derive their energy requirements from fat oxidation. High circulating concentrations of FFA also inhibit glucose utilization.

The provision of fat in artificial nutritional support has traditionally been as long-chain fatty acids (16–18C), but over the past decade or so it has been recognized that medium-chain fatty acids (8–12C) have significant advantages. They are absorbed by the portal blood as opposed to the lymphatics when taken orally, and are metabolized more rapidly than long-chain fatty acids as they do not need carnitine to enter the mitochondria (see Chapter 65). Long-chain n-3 fatty acids in fish oil also have certain biological advantages over the more commonly used n-6 fatty acids, having a damping effect on inflammatory responses, less thromboxane, and more prostacyclin (prostaglandin I_3) production, reduced blood viscosity and enhanced immune function, and are now starting to be included in artificial feeding preparations.

ARTIFICIAL NUTRITIONAL SUPPORT – PARENTERAL AND ENTERAL FEEDING

Nutritional support may be enteral via a nasogatric or nasoenteral tube, or via a feeding enterostomy, which can be inserted at operation or via an endoscope. If the gastrointestinal tract is not functioning the nutritional support may be given intravenously (parenterally). The biochemical and physiologic implications of the two routes are quite different, and the use of the gastrointestinal tract is now considered to have certain advantages in terms of its effect on the metabolic response to trauma.

Enteral feeding

Enteral feeding is the preferred route of nutritional support as it is cheaper and more physiological than parenteral. Food is absorbed via the portal vein and passes through the liver, which has a close association with the pancreas, whose two hormones have fundamental effects on anabolism and catabolism. These are released directly into portal vein blood, so the liver is exposed to higher concentrations of insulin and glucagon than are other tissues.

One advantage of enteral feeding is that more 'natural' nutrients can be given, with polypeptides or even whole protein with all the vitamins and minerals – substances that have to be added to parenteral feeds under strict sterile conditions. Another advantage is the potential to maintain the integrity of the gastrointestinal tract. The intestinal mucosa normally obtains its nutrient requirements from the lumen. Its nutritional and immunological health depends on its continued exposure to various nutrients and substances presented by the luminal contents, such as food antigens. In starvation – but also to an extent with elemental diets, and also in response to hypoperfusion states such as shock, hemorrhage, and sepsis – the intestinal mucosa becomes permeable and bacteria and endotoxin translocate to the regional lymph nodes and to the portal and systemic circulations. In shock the mucosa is actually disrupted. A lot of evidence from animal studies indicates that this mechanism may be the cause of the 'inflammatory response syndrome'. Inflammatory mediators are released, particularly from macrophages in the liver (Kupffer cells), and multiple organ dysfunction and organ failure may ensue. Little direct evidence supports this contention in humans, but early postoperative enteral feeding after severe abdominal injury, and even after elective abdominal surgery, is associated with fewer postoperative complications, particularly septic complications, than in patients treated conventionally by initial abstention, then gradual resumption of oral intake. This beneficial effect is more marked with 'immunologically enhanced' enteral feed containing glutamine, arginine, and n-3 fatty acids after abdominal trauma and major surgery.

Early postoperative enteral feeding is associated with fewer complications.

The main disadvantages of enteral feeding are mechanical, with the unpredictable ability of the gastrointestinal tract to tolerate and absorb enough nutrients to fulfil nutritional requirements. It is common practice to infuse nutrients continuously, as this facilitates the tolerance of large volumes, but if the infusion is into the stomach the normal mechanisms of maintaining gastric acidity are overwhelmed and the upper gastrointestinal tract, including the pharynx and esophagus, can become colonized with commensals. This may be associated with a higher incidence of nosocomial pneumonia. Aspiration pneumonia is also a potential problem. Diarrhea is a common complication, along with nausea, vomiting, and abdominal distension. In severe illness gastric emptying may also be delayed, which predisposes to the dangers of vomiting and aspiration. Direct infusion of nutrients into the jejunum via a needle jejunostomy or one inserted at operation may solve this problem, but this procedure has its own complications. All of this makes it more difficult to fulfil a patient's full energy and protein requirements using the enteral route compared with the parenteral route, particularly with patients who need nutritional support for prolonged periods, such as those in multiple organ failure on intensive care. Evidence is emerging, however, that in terms of clinical outcome a degree of underfeeding in these patients may not be a bad thing.

Parenteral feeding

The principal difference metabolically between parenteral and enteral feeding is that the gastrointestinal tract and the liver are bypassed, so the regulatory, buffering, and protective effects of these organs on the absorption of nutrients are missing. Nutrients are placed directly into the bloodstream, so the patient is exposed to a variety of complications and problems such as thrombosis, hyperglycemia, and infection that do not exist when nutritional support is given via the gastrointestinal tract.

Parenteral feeding bypasses the regulatory, buffering and protective effects of the gastrointestinal tract and liver.

Traditionally, intravenous feeding has been given via a central vein because of the hyperosmolar nature of the solutions and the danger of thrombosis. Peripheral intravenous feeding has, however, been carried out successfully in many centers, sometimes with the help of nitroglycerin patches to promote vasodilatation and maintain the patency of the vein. Dilute solutions (e.g. 20% dextrose instead of 50%) tend to avoid the problem of thrombosis, but larger volumes have to be given and problems of fluid overload may arise, particularly in critically ill patients. The morbidity and mortality associated with intravenous feeding maintained for less than a week, or given to well nourished individuals (i.e. people who essentially do not need it), are greater than the benefit gained.

More metabolic problems occur with intravenous than with enteral feeding. Substances administered intravenously have to be well defined chemically and pharmaceutically, so the patient's requirements must also be extremely well defined. Since the advent of parenteral feeding the importance of many substances has come to be appreciated after patients developed signs of deficiency. These are now given routinely, and include essential fatty acids, phosphates, zinc, copper, selenium, chromium, etc.

Other complications of intravenous feeding result mostly from the consequences of glucose being placed directly into the vascular system. Intravenous glucose infusion bypasses the regulatory and buffering functions of gastrointestinal absorption and the liver, and control of blood glucose is more fragile. The insulinemic response may be less than adequate for the prescribed amount of glucose, particularly in septic and seriously injured patients, such that exogenous insulin is needed. This is given into the venous system, whereas normally it would appear in the portal vein. Similarly, if a glucose infusion prompts a vigorous insulin response (or exogenous insulin is given) and the infusion is stopped abruptly, the excess insulin in the circulation can produce hypoglycemia.

Hypergylcemia itself can induce a hyperosmolar nonketotic diuresis and, in severe cases, coma. Malnourished patients who are being nutritionally repleted with glucose, and particularly with added insulin, shift their extracellular phosphate into cells as lean tissue is laid down, which may produce hypophosphatemia unless adequate supplementation is given. Symptoms include paresthesia, confusion, and coma. The same applies to K^+ and Mg^{2+}; hypokalemia and hypomagnesemia both predispose to arrhythmias.

Hyperglycemia also predisposes to infection, with a suppressant effect on lymphocyte function. Recent work with critically ill patients has shown that by keeping tighter control of blood glucose concentrations by infusing insulin (i.e. maintaining blood glucose concentrations around 5–6 mmol/L, rather than letting it rise to 10–12 mmol/L), mortality could be improved. Whatever the cause, the ready availability of bedside glucose monitors now facilitates the easy and tighter control of blood glucose levels, although such a technique does still predispose to the potential dangers of hypoglycemia.

Excessive quantities of glucose raise carbon dioxide production and the respiratory quotient and so increase ventilation, which can be a problem in the presence of respiratory impairment. High levels of glucose and insulin also stimulate the sympathetic nervous system via an action on the hypothalamus that affects blood pressure and heart rate and rhythm. The potential for this to happen is obviously greater when these substances are infused directly into the circulation than when given enterally.

Complications from the intravenous infusion of fat include the deposition of lipid in the lungs and reticuloendothelial system and impaired leukocyte function, but with modern lipid emulsions these problems are less likely than in the past. Hypertriglyceridemia is sometimes a problem, but usually clears when feeding is slowed or stopped for a while. Administration of heparin and insulin has been suggested if lipemia persists. Heparin stimulates lipoprotein lipase activity and the release of FFA, and insulin encourages their deposition in adipose tissue.

Hepatic dysfunction and the elevation of liver transaminases is a common feature of parenteral feeding. The administration of excessive quantities of intravenous feed, usually glucose based, is associated with deposition of fat in the liver (insulin promotes fat synthesis from glucose). The precise cause of these abnormalities is not known, although they may be related to lack of enteral stimulation. Inhibition of gallbladder emptying, commonly seen with intravenous feeding, certainly is, and in many patients biliary sludge may form.

When amino acids are given at rates greater than they can be utilized in protein synthesis the excess is deaminated and the patient may become uremic. This should be monitored for and the rate of amino acid provision adjusted accordingly. The respective advantages and disadvantages of the enteral and parenteral routes are summarized in Table 62.2.

Table 62.2 Advantages and disadvantages of enteral and parenteral routes of nutritional support

Parenteral or intravenous feeding	
Advantage	Better control of intake, ensuring that nutrient requirements are met
Disadvantages	Potential for fluid overload Venous thrombosis Systemic infections Unnatural route of delivery, bypassing the gut and the liver Intake has to be chemically and pharmaceutically well defined Fragile blood sugar control Osmotic diuresis Hypophosphatemia Sympathetic stimulation Excess CO_2 production Hepatic dysfunction
Enteral feeding	
Advantages	More 'natural' food and easier to provide a 'balanced' diet Intake is processed by gut and liver Maintains integrity of gastrointestinal tract Cheaper and more physiologic
Disadvantages	Gastrointestinal intolerance Distension, vomiting, diarrhea, etc, may limit quantities fed Nosocomial pneumonia Aspiration pneumonia

STARVATION

Starvation is defined as an inadequacy or absence of exogenous energy substrate, depending on whether the starvation is partial or complete. The work of Keys and colleagues in the latter part of the Second World War – the so-called Minnesota study – on normal volunteers provided most of what is known about the whole-body physiological aspects of starvation. The endocrine–substrate relationships seen in starvation were defined in the 1960s, and in the last 20 years we have come to appreciate that many hospital patients are malnourished, that admission to hospital often results in a decline in nutritional status, and that this may have an adverse effect on outcome. Malnutrition increases the risk of virtually all the complications to which patients undergoing major surgery are routinely exposed – wound and anastomotic breakdown, infection, thrombosis (due to diminished activity), etc. Malnourished patients have a reduced respiratory drive and tolerate higher degrees of hypoxia and hypercarbia than normal individuals.

Adaptation to starvation

Apart from its mineral and water content the body is composed of carbohydrate, fat, and protein. The oxidation of these endogenous nutrients provides the starving individual with energy, but the stores of these energy substrates are finite. There are no 'stores' of protein, so protein loss is associated with a decline in function, be it muscle strength, immune function, or the ability to digest normal food if and when intake is resumed.

The adaptive responses to starvation have two overriding themes, conservation of energy and conservation of protein (nitrogen) (Table 62.3).

Table 62.3 Metabolic adaptations to starvation

Energy conservation	Protein conservation
Decrease in spontaneous activity	Glucose required for brain, red cells, renal medulla, wound tissue
Decrease in metabolic rate	Glycogen stores exhausted after 24–48 hours
Loss of metabolically active tissue	Glucose normally obtained from glucogenic amino acids with loss of lean tissue
Decrease in sympathetic activity	Ketones synthesized by liver from free fatty acids Peripheral tissues adapt to using ketones instead of glucose

ENERGY CONSERVATION

The body conserves energy in two ways, one behavioral, the other biochemical. Behaviorally, voluntary and spontaneous activity decreases. The individual does not move unless he or she has to. Responses to external stimuli are diminished, and in extreme cases responses may be elicited only if survival itself is threatened. Biochemically, basal or resting metabolic rate declines. In absolute terms a decline in metabolic rate of 30% was described in the Minnesota study, but when normalized to body size (to take account of the loss of body mass) the real decrease was only 15%. This decrease in energy expenditure arises partly from a decrease in mass of the metabolically most active tissues – the liver decreases in size by 40%, the gastrointestinal tract by 30%, and the kidneys and heart by about 20% each. The mucosa of the gastrointestinal tract decreases in mass and in function, such that if refeeding is started with a normal diet after a prolonged period of adaptation to starvation the diet is not tolerated and the subject is unable to digest it. In addition, a decrease in sympathetic nervous activity and a decline in thyroid activity occur, both of which lead to a decrease in metabolic rate.

PROTEIN AND NITROGEN CONSERVATION

The basic problem is the ongoing needs of some tissues for glucose and their inability, at least initially, to metabolize anything else. Glucose stores are limited, and when they are exhausted within the first 48 hours the principal alternative source of glucose is synthesis from the gluconeogenic amino acids that make up the body protein. The main consumer of glucose is the brain, but red blood cells and the adrenal medulla also need it as they derive their energy requirements from glycolysis. In the injured or septic individual the wounded and septic tissue obtain their energy from glucose, also by glycolysis. Wound tissue does not have the ability to oxidize glucose.

The biochemical changes that occur in starvation keep the brain supplied with glucose, but at the same time minimize the rate at which lean tissue is lost. Adaptation of substrate utilization and oxidation in starvation follow three well recognized and sequential phases, the glycogenolytic phase, the gluconeogenic phase, and the ketogenic phase (Fig. 62.3).

Glycogenolysis

Glucose is stored as glycogen in liver and muscle. Glycogen acts as a store or buffer of glucose to cover the relatively brief periods (8–12 hours in humans) when the organism does not eat. Glucose is released from glycogen into the bloodstream, and enough glycogen is present to maintain blood glucose for about 24 hours. Glycogen is also stored in muscle in quantities greater than that in liver because of the greater muscle mass. Muscle glycogen does not contribute to blood glucose, as muscle lacks glucose-6-phosphatase, but normally provides energy for muscle contraction. However, when oxygen (and energy) demand outstrips supply, such as in severe exercise, or in shock, when glycogenolysis is stimulated by epinephrine (adrenaline), glucose is metabolized to pyruvate and converted into lactate. Lactate can pass into the circulation and, as a gluconeogenic precursor, is synthesized into glucose by the liver.

Gluconeogenesis

When glucose stores run out the glucose requirements of the brain, erythrocytes, and renal medulla are obtained from gluconeogenesis, the precursors being lactate, glycerol, and the gluconeogenic amino acids obtained from body protein. Nitrogen passes to the liver and kidney; the kidney is also a site of gluconeogenesis. Nitrogen is transferred largely as alanine and glutamine. Branched-chain amino acids have a specific role in this: they are deaminated to their corresponding oxo (keto) acids, which are oxidized in muscle. The amino group is transferred to either pyruvate, the end-product of glycolysis, to form alanine or 2-oxoglutarate (α-ketoglutarate) – a constituent of the Krebs cycle – to form glutamate. Glutamate may combine with a further amino group to form glutamine. About 50% of the amino groups leave muscle as alanine and glutamine, which pass to the liver and kidney, respectively, for gluconeogenesis.

Ketogenesis

The largest energy store in the body is adipose tissue, in which fat is stored as triglycerides. Ultimately, in prolonged starvation the body obtains most of its energy from fat oxidation. Ketones are synthesized in the liver from fatty acids and substitute for glucose in the peripheral tissues. The brain continues to metabolize glucose, but some metabolic adaptation occurs and eventually the brain derives about half its energy requirements from ketones. As it does so the rate of consumption of amino acids diminishes; nitrogen excretion, the ultimate index of protein oxidation, declines from 10–12 g/day to about 2–6 g/day.

Fat is oxidized and ketones are synthesized in the mitochondria. To enter the mitochondria the long-chain fatty acids require carnitine and its associated enzymes. The synthesis of carnitine requires a methyl group obtained from the amino acid methionine, so that even for fat to be used as fuel there is an ongoing requirement for the breakdown of lean tissue.

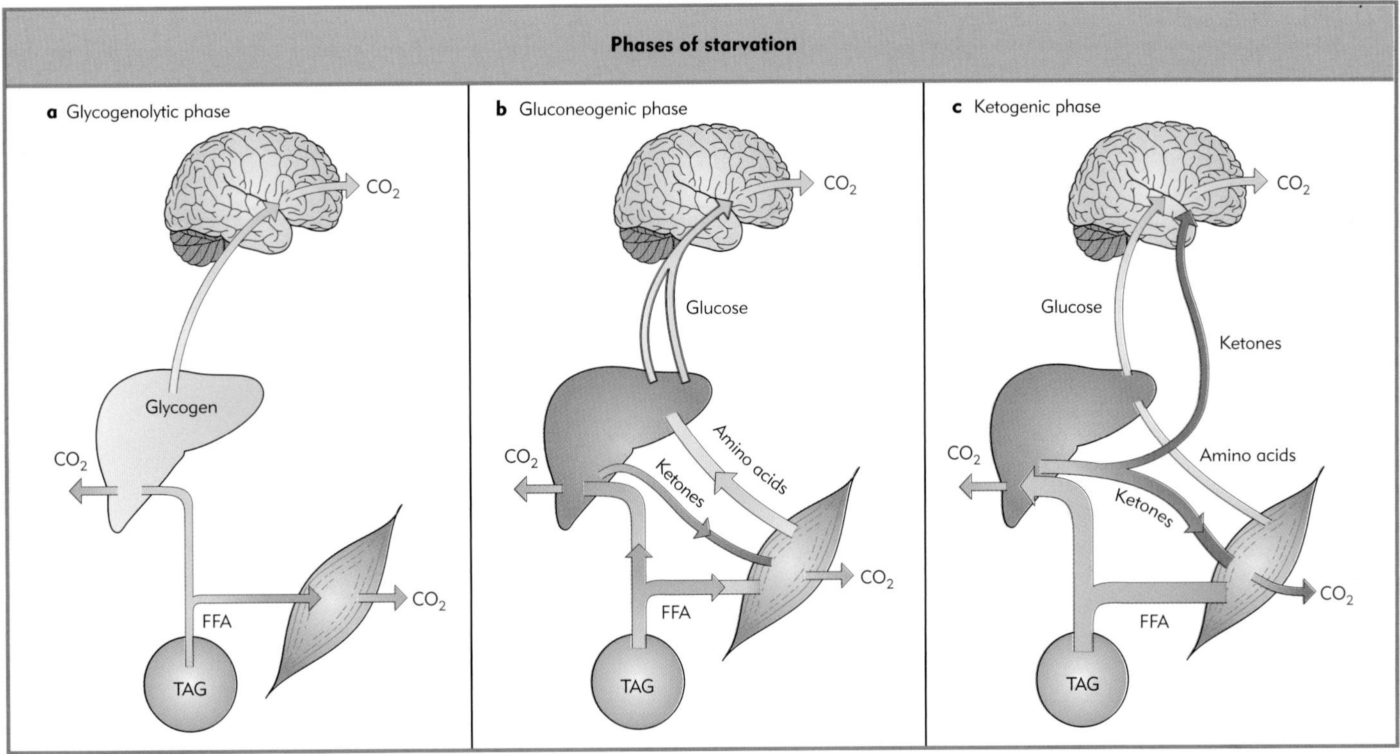

Figure 62.3 The glycogenolytic, gluconeogenic, and ketogenic phases of starvation. (a) Glycogen stores in the liver provide glucose for the brain. Peripheral tissues oxidize both FFA from adipose tissue (triglyceride, TAG) and glucose from glycogen stores. Glycogen is still present in the muscle, but does not contribute to blood glucose other than indirectly as lactate. (b) In the gluconeogenic phase glucose is obtained predominantly from amino acids in lean tissue, and the use of FFA by peripheral tissue is increased. (c) In the ketogenic phase (fully adapted) the brain derives about 50% of its energy requirements from ketones. Gluconeogenesis continues but is much diminished.

When the fat stores eventually run out a 'premortal' rise in nitrogen excretion occurs as protein oxidation increases just before death. The time an individual can survive without food depends on his or her energy (fat) stores. Some pathologically obese individuals have fasted under medical supervision, receiving mineral and vitamin supplements, for over a year, but in people of normal body size and composition death usually occurs at 60–70 days.

Key references

Calder PC. Immunonutrition may have beneficial effects in surgical patients. Br Med J. 2003;327:117–18.

Green CJ. Existence, causes and consequences of disease-related malnutrition in the hospital and the community, and clinical and financial benefits of nutritional intervention. Clin Nutr. 1999;18(Suppl 2):3–28.

Jensen MB, Hessov I. Nutrition and rehabilitation after discharge from hospital: accelerating the rehabilitation with nutrition and physical training. Nutrition 2000;16:619–21.

Lewis R, Egger PJ, Sylvester PA, Thomas PD. Early enteral feeding versus 'nil by mouth' after gastrointestinal surgey: systematic review and meta-analysis of controlled trials. Br Med J. 2001;323:773–6.

MacBurnie M, Wilmore DW. Rational decision making in nutritional care. Surg Clin North Am. 1981;61:571–82.

MacFie J. Enteral versus parenteral nutrition: the significance of bacterial translocation and gut barrier function. Nutrition 2000;16:606–11.

Martinez-Riquelme AE. Allison SP. Insulin revisited. Clin Nutr. 2003;22:7–15.

Shaw JHF, Wilbore M, Wolfe RR. Whole body protein kinetics in severely septic patients. Ann Surg. 1987;205:288–94.

Streat SJ, Beddoe, AH, Hill GL. Aggressive nutritional support does not prevent protein loss despite fat gain in septic intensive care patients. J Trauma 1987;27:262–6.

Van den Berghe G, Wouters P, Weeks F et al. Intensive insulin therapy in critically ill patients. New Engl J Med. 2001;345:1359–67.

Further reading

Frayn KN. Metabolic regulation. A human perspective, 2nd edn. Oxford: Blackwell Science; 2003.

Ganong WF. Review of medical physiology, 21st edn. New York: Lange Medical Books/McGraw Hill; 2003.

Hill GL. Disorders of nutrition and metabolism in clinical surgery. Edinburgh: Churchill Livingstone; 1992.

Payne-James J, Grimble G, Silk D, eds. Artificial nutritional support in clinical practice. London: Greenwich Medical Media; 2001.

Chapter 63

Physiology and pharmacology of nausea and vomiting

Kirsty Forrest and Karen H Simpson

TOPICS COVERED IN THIS CHAPTER

The elimination of ingested toxins by emesis has clear survival advantages, but its role in perioperative situations is less obvious. The effective control of emesis is facilitated by research concerning neuronal pathways and transmitters. Animal studies have limitations, e.g. nausea in animals is impossible to confirm, and not all animals can vomit. Animals incapable of vomiting may have developed an adequate system of preingestion toxin detection that may involve nausea. The feeding habits of many animals that can vomit suggest that they need a postingestion toxin detection system that is linked to a means of eliminating the contents of the upper gastrointestinal tract (GIT). However, animals that can vomit display species differences in neuroanatomy and in susceptibility to emetogens (e.g. apomorphine). Humans have both pre- and postingestion systems for detecting toxins. Higher cognitive activity can also recruit nausea and vomiting as a response to many circumstances, e.g. sights, smells, and psychological changes such as anxiety.

DEFINITIONS

Nausea is a subjectively unpleasant sensation associated with awareness of the urge to vomit. Retching refers to the labored rhythmic activity of the ventilatory muscles that usually precedes vomiting. Vomiting or emesis is the forceful expulsion of upper gastrointestinal contents via the mouth, caused by the powerful sustained contraction of the abdominal muscles. Nausea, retching, and vomiting are often, but not invariably, related. An emetogen is a stimulus to emesis, and an emetic is a chemical capable of inducing emesis.

INITIATION AND CONTROL OF VOMITING

Initiation of vomiting

Physical, pharmacological, physiological, psychological, and pathophysiological stimuli can trigger vomiting:

- dilatation of the stomach (e.g. obstruction or overeating);
- gastric mucosal irritation (e.g. alcohol or drugs);
- higher cognitive activity (e.g. unpleasant sights, smells, or ideas);
- pharyngeal mucosal stimulation;
- vestibulocochlear stimulation (e.g. motion sickness);
- pregnancy;
- pain (e.g. renal colic, migraine);
- poisons, toxins, and medications (e.g. chemotherapy, analgesic, and anesthetic drugs);
- therapeutic radiation;
- raised intracranial pressure, intracerebral hemorrhage, and tumors.

Neurophysiology of vomiting

A toxin recognized by color, smell, or taste causes rejection of the food and the development of a learned aversion that may include nausea. Postingestion detection may occur before or after absorption of the toxin into the blood. The vagus nerve mediates preabsorption detection, particularly in the upper GIT (Figs 63.1 and 63.2). Splanchnic afferent stimulation may play a role, particularly after vagotomy. There are bare vagal nerve endings in the gut wall, most of which terminate in the nucleus of the tractus solitarius (NTS). A few fibers end in the area postrema (AP) and dorsal motor vagal nucleus (DMVN). The NTS has connections with the AP, and most information from the gut probably takes this route. Potential neurotransmitters

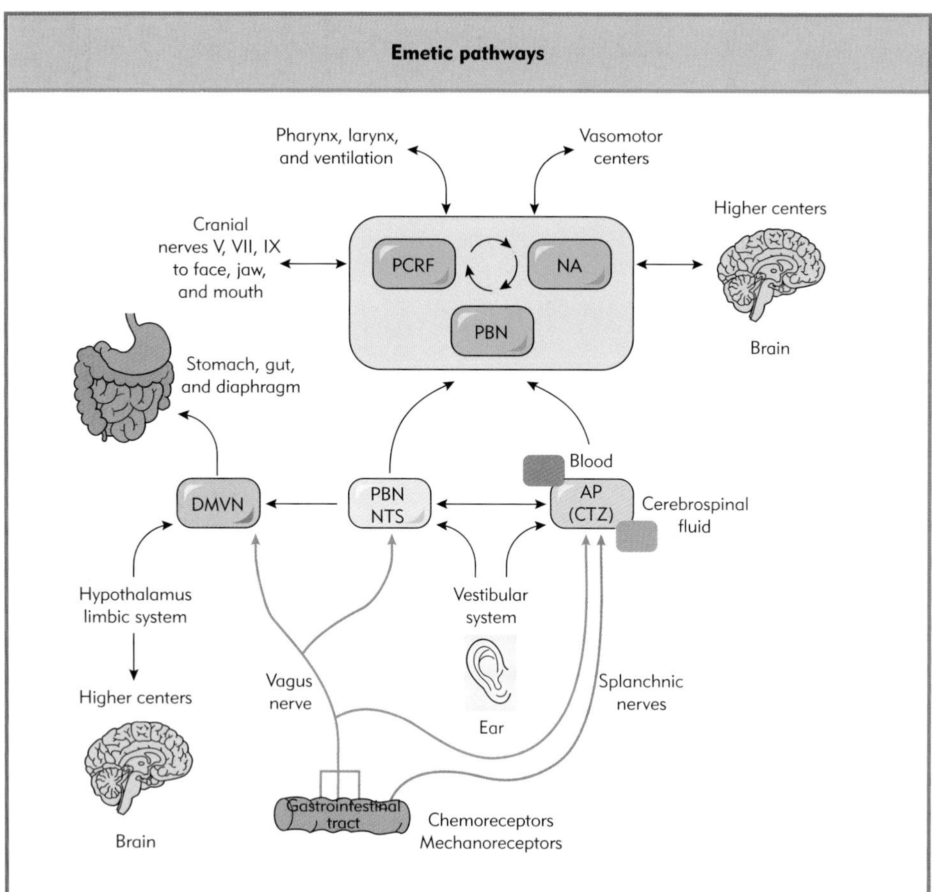

Figure 63.1 Emetic pathways. The control of emesis within the brain and gastrointestinal tract. AP, area postrema; CTZ, (chemoreceptor trigger zone) DMVN, dorsal motor vagal nucleus; NA, nucleus ambiguus; NTS, nucleus of tractus solitarius; PBN, parabrachial nucleus; PCRF, parvicellular reticular formation.

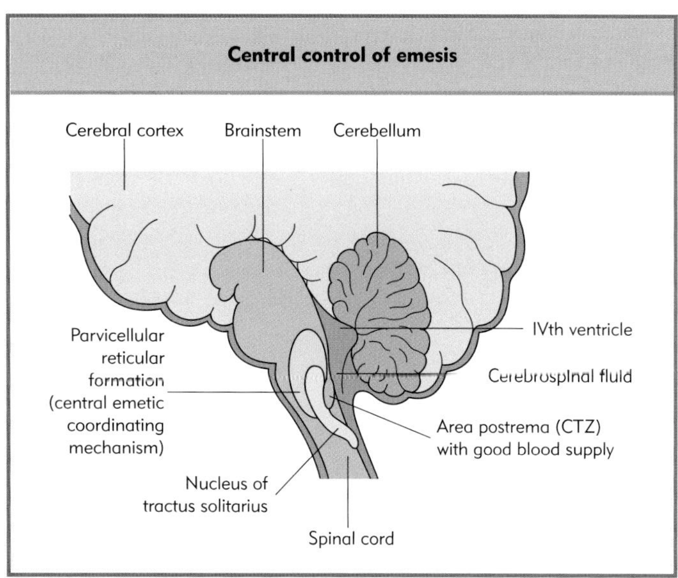

Figure 63.2 Central control of emesis. The structures within the brain involved in the control of emesis.

here include thyrotropin-releasing hormone, catecholamines, enkephalin, substance P, vasopressin, and somatostatin.

Mucosal afferents are responsible for the emetic response to luminal toxins. Stimuli to mucosal afferents include hypertonic solutions such as saline or copper sulfate, 5-hydroxytryptamine (5-HT), cholecystokinin (CCK), plant alkaloids, and invertebrate toxins. Secondary sensory cells in the gut mucosa may respond to changes in the luminal environment, and they release a transmitter that causes the discharge of afferent fibers. Irradiation, cytotoxic drugs, and gut ischemia may produce emesis by releasing 5-HT from the gut mucosa, and by stimulating vagal afferent fibres. Antagonism of 5-HT_3 and CCK_A receptors does not prevent mucosal afferents from responding to stimuli such as hypertonic saline or luminal acid. Therefore, mucosal afferents are sensitive to both 5-HT and CCK, but these pathways are not essential mediators in the emetic pathway. Muscular afferents are tension receptors in the gut wall that respond to distension and contraction. They facilitate smooth digestion by monitoring gut content and propagation. Abnormal gut distension or contractility can stimulate vomiting.

Postabsorption detection occurs in the AP (chemoreceptor trigger zone, CTZ), which is a vascular area on the surface of the caudal end of the floor of the fourth ventricle. The blood–brain barrier is incomplete in this area, so agents in both blood and cerebrospinal fluid can gain access to the AP. This area receives afferents from the NTS, vagus nerve, splanchnic nerves, and vestibular labyrinth. If the AP is destroyed vomiting can still occur, so it is clearly not essential for the process.

Emesis is mediated by what was previously called the 'vomiting center' (VC), although no such single brain area has ever been identified. The VC should be regarded as a central pattern generator or a medullary control system; a number of brainstem nuclei are involved. The VC coordinates the action of various autonomic and somatic nuclei that collectively mediate vomiting.

The NTS receives afferents from the vagus and AP. It sends efferents to all the nuclei involved in vomiting, and to the hypothalamus and limbic system. The parvicellular reticular formation (PCRF) may regulate ventilation during vomiting via connections with the parabrachial nucleus (PBN) and nucleus ambiguus (NA). The PCRF connects with trigeminal (V), facial (VII), and hypoglossal (IX) cranial nerve nuclei, controlling the tongue, mouth, and jaws during emesis. The NA controls laryngeal and pharyngeal musculature, and some aspects of ventilation. It connects with the PBN. The interaction between the two, possibly regulated by the PCRF, may be the mechanism responsible for retching and vomiting. Inputs from the vagus, hypothalamic, and limbic systems reach the DMVN, and it sends afferents back to these areas. Cortical activity may influence the processing of gastrointestinal afferent information, or initiate vomiting, via these connections. The DMVN is responsible for motor outputs to the GIT. The efferent limb of the vagal reflex in the vomiting pathway originates from the DMVN. Excitatory cholinergic and inhibitory nonadrenergic noncholinergic (NANC) pathways back to the GIT mediate the efferent part of the pathway. Nuclei in the ventrolateral medulla regulate sympathetic outflow from the spinal cord.

MECHANICS OF VOMITING

Prodromal emetic phenomena include nausea, salivation, tachycardia, altered breathing, pallor, sweating, and pupillary dilatation. Brainstem nuclei act to integrate the motor components of vomiting.

Visceral events

The contents of the small intestine are returned to the stomach and the gastric contents are confined by a number of visceral events. A reduction in electrical control activity inhibits gastrointestinal motility in the proximal bowel. The proximal stomach relaxes, and a retrograde giant contraction (RGC) is initiated or antiperistalsis occurs in the jejunum. This returns small intestinal contents to the relaxed stomach. Phasic contractions occur in the stomach antrum and small intestine, with inhibition of small intestinal activity that lasts for several minutes. Striated esophageal muscles contract, shortening the intra-abdominal esophagus toward the diaphragm. The cardia and gastroesophageal sphincter dilate to enable the gastric contents to pass easily into the esophagus once retching commences. Residual esophageal contents are cleared by secondary peristalsis and closure of the lower esophageal sphincter once active vomiting has ceased.

Somatic events

Rhythmic inspiratory movements against a closed glottis characterize retching. The mechanisms that are designed to limit gastroesophageal reflux are overcome. There is synchronized contraction of the diaphragm, abdominal muscles, and internal intercostal muscles. This causes simultaneous large pressure changes (100 mmHg) that are negative in the thorax and positive in the abdomen. The upper esophageal sphincter relaxes during a retch. It is pulled open by raising of the hyoid bone and larynx, allowing gastric contents to reflux upwards. The esophageal sphincter contracts again between retches to prevent expulsion. During vomiting, the diaphragm does not contract but is fixed in the inspiratory position. The glottis is closed, and the soft palate lifts to close the posterior nares. Contraction of the abdominal muscles produces a pulse of positive pressure, transmitted from the abdomen to the thorax. Relaxation of the cardia and esophagopharyngeal sphincter and elevation of the soft palate then occurs, allowing gastric contents to pass from the stomach to the mouth.

MEDIATORS OF EMESIS

Investigating the emetic pathway

Many neurotransmitters have been implicated in the mediation of emesis. Identification of agonist and antagonist ligands can influence the development of therapies. The emetic pathways have been investigated using animal models and human studies, including vagotomy and ablation of the AP. The actions of unknown substances or receptors have been studied using ligands whose mode of action is understood. For example, any agent that inhibits apomorphine-induced vomiting may be acting as a D_2 antagonist in the AP, as this is how apomorphine exerts its effect. Intracerebroventricular (ICV) injections of agonist and antagonist ligands have also been used to investigate the site of action of different compounds. Radioligand-binding studies have also been used to identify central and peripheral receptors. The c-*fos* gene is rapidly expressed in response to many kinds of neuronal activation. Administering multiple potent emetic agents and then looking for expression of the c-Fos protein product throughout the brain has been used to map some of the central neuronal circuits responsible for vomiting. Anatomical areas responsible for vomiting can also be mapped using electrical stimulation, usually in decerebrate cats.

Antiemetics and receptors

Antiemetics can be classified by their actions at various receptors (Table 63.1).

DOPAMINE

The classic AP receptor involved in emesis is the D_2 dopamine receptor. Other receptors in the AP may also exert their effects by releasing dopamine (e.g. 5-HT_3 receptors). Dopamine receptors are present in the NTS and DMVN. Dopamine agonists, such as bromocriptine and apomorphine, produce emesis. Dopamine antagonists, such as metoclopramide, droperidol, and prochlorperazine, are useful antiemetics but have extrapyramidal side effects that can limit their use, particularly in children. Domperidone is a D_2 antagonist with reduced brain penetrance.

5-HYDROXYTRYPTAMINE

The use of 5-HT_3 receptor antagonists has improved the prevention and treatment of nausea and vomiting associated with chemotherapy and radiotherapy. These agents are also useful in the management of postoperative nausea and vomiting (PONV). The 5-HT_3 receptors are distributed centrally (in the AP, NTS, cerebral cortex, and hippocampus) and peripherally (in the gut mucosa, nerve endings, and primary afferent nerve fibers). They act at ligand-gated cation-selective ion channels (see Chapters 3 and 20). Activation allows ion channel opening, which increases

Table 63.1 Receptor site affinities of antiemetic drugs

	Receptor site affinity				
Drug group	***Dopamine (D_2)***	***Muscarinic (cholinergic)***	***Histamine (H_2)***	***Serotonin (5-HT_3)***	***NK_1***
Phenothiazine					
Fluphenazine	++++	+	++	–	
Chlorpromazine	++++	++	++++	+	
Prochlorperazine	++++				
Butyrophenone					
Droperidol	++++	–	+	+	
Haloperidol	++++	–	+	–	
Domperidone	++++				
Antihistamine					
Diphenhydramine	+	++	++++	–	
Promethazine	++	++	++++	–	
Anticholinergic					
Scopolamine	+	++++	+	–	
Benzamide					
Metoclopramide	+++	–	+	++	
Antiserotonin					
Ondansetron	–	–	–	++++	
Granisetron	–	–	–	++++	
Zacopride	–	–	–	++++	

++++, high affinity; –, low affinity.

the conductance to sodium and potassium ions; this results in membrane depolarization and neuronal excitation. Nonselective agonists include 2-methyl-5-HT and phenyl biguanide. Selective antagonists include ondansetron, granisetron, zacopride, MDL 7222, and ICS 205930. These agents have no effect on apomorphine-induced vomiting. Animal studies show that 5-HT causes emesis by acting on 5-HT_3 receptors located centrally and within the small intestine. 5-HT receptors also affect gastric emptying and gut transit time. MKC-733, a selective 5-HT_3 receptor agonist, delays liquid gastric emptying in association with relaxation of the proximal stomach, stimulates fasting antroduodenal migrating motor complex activity, and accelerates small intestinal transit time.

Some cytotoxic drugs may release 5-HT from neurons near the hindbrain structures that are involved in the emetic reflex. In contrast, the emetic effect of cisplatin is mainly at the gut receptor, rather than at the AP. Cisplatin causes emesis by damaging the intestinal mucosa and releasing 5-HT from the enterochromaffin cells. This increased release of 5-HT is reflected by increased concentrations of its principal metabolite 5-hydroxyindoleacetic acid (5-HIAA) in plasma and urine. Antagonism of 5-HT_3 receptors can prevent the emesis that follows increased local 5-HT concentrations. The 5-HT released from the gut undergoes extensive first-pass metabolism, so it does not produce more generalized effects. Reducing 5-HT production might have an antiemetic effect. Inhibiting 5-HT synthesis and depleting endogenous stores can achieve this. Tryptophan hydroxylase is the rate-limiting enzyme in the synthesis of 5-HT. It can be inhibited by *p*-chlorophenylalanine (*p*-CPA). Animal and human studies have shown that treatment with *p*-CPA reduces basal and cisplatin-evoked increases in urinary excretion of 5-HIAA and attenuates emesis.

The 5-HT_{1A} receptors are located primarily on presynaptic nerve terminals in the cerebral cortex, raphe nucleus, NTS, and hippocampus, and in arterioles. Activation leads to a reduction in cyclic AMP (cAMP) and hyperpolarization of the cell membrane that inhibits neuronal firing. Agonists such as 8-OH DPAT (8-hydroxy-2-(di-*N*-propylamino)tetralin), flesinoxan, and buspirone produce anxiolysis and hypotension. Antagonists include pindolol, cyanpindol, and spiperone. Animal studies show that 5-HT_{1A} agonists block the effects of different classes of emetogen, including cisplatin, morphine, and oral copper sulfate, and they are active in motion and conditioned-vomiting models. The mechanism of antiemetic action is speculative. Its broad spectrum suggests an action on a convergent structure in the CNS. Preclinical data suggest that behavioral side effects may limit its use. Buspirone is an anxiolytic, but is only a weak partial agonist at 5-HT_{1A} receptors and has little antiemetic efficacy.

Characterization of the 5-HT_4 receptor is derived from cumulative evidence from several sources, rather than from identification of any particular ligand. This receptor has been difficult to study because there is no suitable radioligand. A pharmacological profile is available. The 5-HT_4 receptor is widely distributed within the cerebral cortex, superior colliculi, GIT, and myocardium. Activation increases intracellular cAMP and results in membrane depolarization. Receptor activation in the gut causes the release of acetylcholine in the myenteric plexus. This relaxes the esophagus and sphincter and increases gastric motility and emptying. Receptor activation also causes cerebral activation and tachycardia. Agonists include the benzamides (metoclopramide and cisapride), the benzimidazolones (BIMU-1 and BIMU-8), and some indole derivatives (5-methoxytryptamine). Antagonists include the benzamide SDZ 205,557, the benzimidazolone DAU 6215, and the indole GR113808. The 5-HT_4 receptor does seem to influence emesis, but animal studies have produced conflicting results. Oral agonists (zacopride and 5-methoxytryptamine) provoke vomiting, but administration of the highly potent, selective antagonist GR125487 does not prevent emesis.

ACETYLCHOLINE

Acetylcholine is the agonist at muscarinic and nicotinic cholinergic receptors in the parasympathetic nervous system (see Chapter 34). Muscarinic cholinergic receptors are found in the NA, NTS, and DMVN. Central acetylcholine receptors mediate the vestibular initiation of motion sickness. Therefore, drugs that penetrate the blood–brain barrier are needed to alleviate this. Acetylcholine receptors are also found peripherally, where they mediate the gastrointestinal motor correlates of vomiting. Atropine, scopolamine (hyoscine hydrobromide), and glycopyrrolate are the anticholinergic drugs commonly used in anesthesia. Glycopyrrolate is a quaternary ammonium compound that does not cross the blood–brain barrier and so has no useful antiemetic activity. Anticholinergic drugs are antiemetic owing to a combination of central blocking of motion sickness, peripheral reduction of salivary and gastric secretions, motor (antispasmodic) activity, and prevention of relaxation of sphincters. The central potency of scopolamine is around 10 times that of atropine. This probably accounts for its success in the prophylaxis and management of motion sickness. Scopolamine is poorly absorbed enterally, but can be absorbed transdermally and sublingually. Side effects include drowsiness and confusion; this is a particular problem in the elderly.

OPIOIDS

Opioids have both emetic and antiemetic actions. The emetic effect may be via stimulation of opioid (probably μ) receptors in the AP; ablation of the AP abolishes the emetic response to opioids. The μ or δ type receptors may be responsible for the antiemetic effect of opioids, particularly in high doses.

ADRENERGIC AGENTS

α-adrenoceptor agonists initiate vomiting in many animal studies. Agonists such as xylazine, epinephrine (adrenaline), and norepinephrine (noradrenaline) evoke vomiting in cats and dogs by their action at α_2-adrenoceptors in the AP. Antagonists such as yohimbine, tolazoline, and phentolamine act to block this effect. In humans clonidine (an α_2 agonist) may be antiemetic. Methoxamine-induced vomiting is probably mediated by central α_1-adrenoceptors, most likely acting on postsynaptic cells in the AP. In conditions where adrenoceptors are a factor in causing vomiting, e.g. in pheochromocytoma and endotoxic shock, α_2-adrenoceptor antagonists may have a role as antiemetics.

ENKEPHALIN

The AP is rich in enkephalin receptors. Local tissue concentrations of enkephalin seem to alter the susceptibility of the AP to excitatory stimuli. Enkephalin also increases dopamine release.

CHOLECYSTOKININ

The gastrointestinal mucosa contains CCK, which causes activation of vagal afferents in a similar manner to 5-HT. A specific CCK_A receptor antagonist, devazepide, blocks this effect.

NEUROKININS

The mammalian tachykinin (TK) peptides and their three neurokinin receptors represent an effector system with wide-ranging actions on neuronal, airway smooth muscle, mucosal, endothelial, immune, inflammatory, and remodeling cell function. Recent data suggest pathophysiological relevance for TKs in various diseases, including asthma, emesis, and depression. Animal studies have shown that CP99,994 [(+)-(2*S*,3*S*)-3-(2-methoxybenzylamino)-2-phenylpiperidine], which is an antagonist of substance P at a neurokinin (NK_1) receptor, is effective against a broad range of emetogens. It affects a number of emetic mechanisms: release of 5-HT, vagal stimulation (radiation and cisplatin), dopamine D_2 receptors (apomorphine), and opioid receptors (morphine). It is also active against nicotine (a centrally acting emetogen), gastric irritants (copper sulfate), and a clinically used emetogen (ipecacuanha). Clinical activity has been observed using single and/or dual NK receptor antagonists in emesis trials. Randomized control clinical trials have shown an antiemetic effect of the NK_1 receptor antagonist GR205171 (compared with placebo) for established PONV.

Aprepitant is the first available drug from of the neurokinin NK_1 receptor antagonist group. Oral aprepitant, in combination with other agents, is indicated for the prevention of acute and delayed chemotherapy-induced nausea and vomiting associated with highly emetogenic chemotherapy in adults. In three randomized double-blind placebo-controlled trials comparing aprepitant plus standard therapy (intravenous ondansetron and oral dexamethasone) with standard therapy plus placebo, overall complete responses were seen in significantly more patients in the aprepitant group. The TK–NK receptor interactions and incompletely overlapping functions mediated by each NK receptor may indicate added therapeutic benefit of using multiple NK receptor blockade.

σ-RECEPTOR MODULATORS

The σ receptors are distributed throughout the brain, including in the cranial nerve nuclei, hypothalamus, hippocampus, red nucleus, septum, and cerebellum. The role of σ receptors is poorly defined because of lack of a selective ligand. A large and chemically diverse range of compounds binds to σ receptors, e.g. opioids, steroids, and antipsychotic drugs. The ligand usually used to study σ activity (*N*-allylnormetazocine) is not specific and it produces many of its effects via interactions with other receptors. More selective σ agonists have been described, including 1,3-ditolylguanidine (DTG), amitriptyline, and *cis*-*N*-[2-(3,4-dichlorophenyl)ethyl]-*N*-methyl-2-(1-pyrrolidinyl) cyclohexylamine (BD737). Antagonists include haloperidol and the putative antipsychotic agent a-(4-fluorophenyl)-4-(5-fluoro-2-pyrimidinyl)-1-piperazinobutanol (BMY 14802). Agonists such as DTG produce emesis that is blocked by antagonists such as haloperidol and BMY 14802. Studies in pigeons have shown that antagonists with higher affinity for the σ site have a higher potency in blocking agonist-induced emesis. Studies in rats have produced conflicting results.

γ-AMINOBUTYRIC ACID

Benzodiazepines potentiate the inhibitory γ-aminobutyric acid (GABA) interneurons that are most densely located in the hippocampus, cerebellum, and cortex. Some studies suggest that benzodiazepines decrease the incidence of PONV and chemotherapy-induced emesis. The mechanism of action may be by anxiolysis, hypnosis, retrograde amnesia, or a specific effect on the GABA pathways involved in emesis.

CALCITONIN

Calcitonin is a polypeptide hormone derived from thyroid C cells that regulates plasma calcium concentration (see Chapter 66). Treatment with synthetic calcitonin is associated with nausea and vomiting; the mechanism of this is unclear. Some evidence in dogs suggests that calcitonin leads to central vagal blockade that may be relevant.

HISTAMINE

Histamine (H_1) receptors are concentrated in the NTS and DMVN. Centrally acting antihistamines that often possess anticholinergic activity, e.g. cyclizine and diphenhydramine, are used in the management of motion sickness and PONV. They have a relatively high therapeutic index and few side effects (drowsiness and anticholinergic effects). Their antiemetic effects are mediated via either H_1 or acetylcholine receptors.

CANNABINOIDS

Cannabis is derived from resin of the plant *Cannabis sativa*. The major active constituent is a Δ^9-tetrahydrocannabinol. The body has endogenous cannabinoids with central and peripheral receptors. An endogenous ligand anandamide is a derivative of arachidonic acid. The antiemetic activity of cannabis may be related to its psychotropic effects in the forebrain that inhibit the emetic pattern generator via descending pathways. The synthetic derivative nabilone has antiemetic effects and has been used in cancer chemotherapy. The psychoactive nature of the drug and social issues have limited research into its therapeutic potential. Adverse effects include euphoria, dysphoria, sedation, incoordination, and fetal toxicity.

CAPSAICIN

Capsaicin is a sensory neurotoxin causing desensitization of vagal afferent C fibers (see Chapter 22). Resinferatoxin (RTX) is a naturally occurring analog that is 1000 times more potent than capsaicin and which does not have its profound cardiorespiratory side effects. In animals, RTX blocks emesis induced by copper sulfate (gastric irritation), irradiation (5-HT release and vagal stimulation), and loperamide (a centrally acting emetogen). RTX may induce depletion of a neurotransmitter, possibly substance P or calcitonin gene-related peptide, at a central point in the emetic pathway, possibly in the NTS.

GLUTAMATE

Animal studies have shown that glutamate antagonists, particularly nonNMDA (*N*-methyl-D-aspartate) receptor antagonists NBQX and CNQX, can block cisplatin-induced emesis. Their site of action may be in the AP.

GINGER

The powdered rhizome of *Zingiber officinale* (the common ginger root) is a traditional treatment for gastrointestinal complaints. It is regarded as a carminative and spasmolytic agent. The active ingredient in ginger root and its mechanism of action is unknown. A local effect on the GIT has been proposed. Its efficacy in the treatment of nausea and vomiting is unproven. Some studies have demonstrated that oral premedication with ginger is as successful as metoclopramide for PONV, but metoclopramide is not always efficacious and so the significance of this is questionable. It has been suggested that ginger is equivalent to vitamin B_6 in reducing nausea, retching, and vomiting for women in early pregnancy. A systematic review of randomized controlled trials of ginger showed that the absolute risk reduction for PONV was not significant.

ACUPUNCTURE

The traditional Chinese method of acupuncture or acupressure at the P6 (Nei Guan) point is an effective treatment for nausea and vomiting. It is useful in managing emesis due to pregnancy, chemotherapy, radiotherapy, and PONV in adults and children. It is probably most effective in the conscious patient. It is often ineffective if administered during general anesthesia. It was an effective treatment for emesis in a double-blind randomized control trial of acupuncture versus placebo during spinal anaesthesia for cesarean section. The mechanism of acupuncture antiemesis is unclear. It has been suggested that it may increase gastric motility.

STEROIDS

The addition of dexamethasone is efficacious in patients with chemotherapy-induced emesis where 5-HT_3 antagonists are not completely successful. The same has been shown for PONV. Morphine administration by patient-controlled analgesia (PCA) is often associated with nausea and vomiting. A study has shown that the minimum effective dose of dexamethasone for reducing this complication is 8 mg. This is as effective as adding droperidol 0.1 mg/mL to the morphine PCA, without causing drowsiness, restlessness, or arrhythmias. Dexamethasone as a single dose has few serious side effects. The mechanism of antiemetic action of corticosteroids is unknown. They may decrease central and peripheral prostaglandin production. They may lead to an anti-inflammatory action that reduces stimuli from the operative site and/or blocks 5-HT release from the gut.

POSTOPERATIVE NAUSEA AND VOMITING

PONV has been called 'the big little problem'. In the 'ether era', 75–80% of patients experienced PONV. It still occurs in 20–30% of patients even with modern anesthesia and novel antiemetics, and it is intractable in 0.1% of cases. PONV varies between the patients of individual (experienced) anesthetists, between different institutions, and between countries. The United Kingdom has the highest incidence of PONV in western Europe and Germany has the lowest. Patients are often more worried about PONV than about pain. Emesis was responsible for dissatisfaction in 71% of patients in a survey of patients undergoing day-case (ambulatory) surgery. Complications can occur from PONV, e.g. inhalation of gastric contents, wound dehiscence, bleeding, wound hematomas, dehydration, and electrolyte disturbances.

Predisposing factors

Risk factors that predispose to PONV can be related to the patient, the anesthetic regimen, surgical procedures, and postoperative factors (Table 63.2).

PATIENT FACTORS

- **Anesthetic history**. The risk of emesis increases threefold if there has been previous PONV.

Table 63.2 Risk factors for developing postoperative nausea and vomiting (PONV)

Predisposing patient factors
Female gender (perimenstrual > preovulatory)
Motion sickness
Vestibular problems
Morbid obesity
Early pregnancy
Nonsmoking status
Increased gastric volume
Excessive anxiety
Ingestion of solid food
Delayed gastric emptying
Anesthetic agents
Inhalational – volatiles, nitrous oxide
Intravenous – ketamine, etomidate, thiopental
Opioid analgesics – agonists, agonist–antagonists
Surgical procedures
Laparoscopy
Lithotripsy
Strabismus correction
Tonsillectomy (and/or adenoidectomy)
Middle-ear operations
Orchidopexy
Postoperative factors
Severe pain
Hypotension/dehydration
Premature ambulation
Forcing oral fluid intake

- **Gender**. There is no difference between the sexes in childhood (<11 years) or late adulthood (>70 years); otherwise, the incidence of PONV is two to three times greater in females than in males. Females have more severe vomiting. There may be hormonal influences, as the incidence of PONV peaks during the third and fourth weeks (luteal phase) of the menstrual cycle.
- **Age**. PONV is least common in infants (<1 year), with an incidence of approximately 5%. It increases to 20% in children (<5 years). It reaches a maximum of 35–50% in late childhood (6–16 years). It decreases throughout adulthood, and is lowest by the eighth decade.
- **Delayed gastric emptying**. PONV increases when gastric motility and emptying are retarded.
- **Motion sickness**. A history of motion sickness may predispose to PONV.
- **ASA status**. Patients who are ASA 1 and 2 are at greater risk than those who are 3 and 4.
- **Smoking**. Smoking seems to confer some protection from PONV. This may be due to the inducement of the cytochrome P450 enzymes, leading to a faster elimination of emetic anesthetic agents. Developing specific inducers for these enzymes may prove to be a novel way of reducing PONV.
- **Anxiety**. The influence of mood on PONV is not confirmed.
- **Body habitus**. Obese patients may be more susceptible to PONV.

ANESTHETIC FACTORS

A number of studies have examined the particular effects of different anesthetic agents. The use of benzodiazepines for premedication may reduce PONV. Thiopental, etomidate, and ketamine are all emetogens. There is some evidence that propofol may be antiemetic. In a meta-analysis of 84 randomized controlled trials involving 6069 patients, the use of propofol for maintenance of anesthesia reduced the incidence of PONV by 20%. However, this effect was only seen for the first few hours after surgery. Propofol was antiemetic only in those patients with a high incidence of PONV, such as those having pediatric strabismus or undergoing major gynecologic surgery. When used as an induction agent alone, propofol had a statistically significant but less clinically relevant effect on PONV. Propofol has been used as a low-dose infusion (1 mg/h/kg body weight) to treat chemotherapy-induced emesis that was previously resistant to 5-HT_3 antagonists. Its mechanism of action is not clear. Propofol has little effect on endogenous 5-HT_3 receptors; it has no antidopaminergic activity, and it does not alter apomorphine-induced vomiting. It may act by suppression of the AP, vagal nuclei, and/or other central sites. Some studies have shown that benzodiazepines such as midazolam have antiemetic actions. The effect of subhypnotic doses of both propofol and midazolam on PONV outlasts the sedative effects of these drugs.

The use of nitrous oxide for the maintenance of anesthesia has been suspected of contributing to PONV because nitrous oxide increases gut distension and middle-ear pressure, but this remains unproven. Omission of nitrous oxide as part of a standard anesthetic technique may increase the risk of awareness and outweigh the antiemetic effect. Most volatile anesthetics have been implicated in emesis. Total intravenous anesthesia reduces the incidence of PONV compared with inhalation anesthesia when nitrous oxide is excluded. Sevoflurane with propofol infusion may produce less immediate PONV than occurs with halothane.

A number of other factors related to anesthesia can also influence PONV.

- **Opioid analgesics**. Intraoperative opioids are a major cause of PONV.
- **Reversal of neuromuscular blockade**. The use of neostigmine may be associated with more PONV than if neuromuscular block is allowed to reverse spontaneously.
- **Postoperative analgesia**. Opioids after surgery are associated with higher rates of PONV. The use of local and regional anesthetic techniques and adequate doses of nonopioid analgesia reduce opioid requirements and hence PONV. Acetominophen (paracetamol) or nonsteroidal anti-inflammatory or COX-2 inhibitors have all been shown to be opioid sparing.
- **Perioperative fluid regimens**. Adequate hydration reduces PONV. A randomized controlled trial has shown that supplemental preoperative fluid administration reduces PONV. A larger reduction in emesis was seen than with intraoperative fluid administration. Fluid may need to be given preoperatively to increase gut perfusion and prevent the gut ischemia and serotonin release associated with anesthesia.
- **Experience of the anesthetist**. Inexperienced anesthetists have more cases of PONV.
- **Supplementary perioperative oxygen** decreases PONV in abdominal procedures, perhaps by ameliorating intestinal

ischaemia. Supplementary oxygen does not affect the incidence of PONV in nonabdominal operations.

PREOPERATIVE SURGICAL FACTORS

Patients presenting for emergency procedures with a full stomach or with GIT obstruction or stasis have an increased risk of PONV. Other emergency patients seem to have a lower risk of emesis than do elective patients. Vomiting often accompanies some surgical conditions, notably peritonitis, bowel obstruction, and raised intracranial pressure. Gastric decompression using a nasogastric tube may relieve the nausea associated with gastric distension, but it can replace it with nausea resulting from stimulation by the tube. The use of a perioperative nasogastric tube to empty the stomach does not alter the incidence of PONV, even if the tube is inserted and removed while the patient is anesthetized.

OPERATIVE PROCEDURE

Some procedures are emetogenic. About 36–76% of patients experience emesis after adenotonsillectomy. This may be a consequence of blood in the esophagus and stomach stimulating vagal afferents, trigeminal nerve stimulation, and the use of opioids. Other surgery associated with a high risk of PONV includes otoplasty, middle-ear surgery, strabismus surgery, and gynecologic procedures (especially when the cervix is dilated). Intra-abdominal operations often involve direct stimulation of gut vagal afferents, causing emesis. GIT ischemia leads to 5-HT release and PONV. Surgery of increasing duration may lead to increased emesis. In a study of more than 6000 patients, anesthesia lasting less than 60 minutes had an odds ratio of 1.0 for patients developing PONV, surgery of 60–120 minutes had an odds ratio of 1.5, and surgery longer than 120 minutes had an odds ratio of 2.04.

POSTOPERATIVE FACTORS

There are a number of postoperative factors associated with PONV.

- **Relief of postoperative pain reduces PONV**. Antagonism of opioid analgesia by naloxone increases PONV.
- **Hypotension**. Patients with low blood pressure often feel nauseated, perhaps as a result of reduced medullary blood flow to the AP. Treatment of hypotension with volume replacement, vasoconstrictors, or inotropes usually cures the nausea.
- **Ambulation**. Motion and changes in position, such as the turning of a supine patient into the recovery position, can precipitate PONV via cholinergic and, perhaps, histaminergic input to the AP from the vestibular apparatus. Opioids may sensitize the vestibular system to motion-induced nausea and vomiting.
- **Oral intake**. Early oral fluid intake can increase PONV. Patients having day-case procedures, who are required to ingest fluids before discharge, have significantly more emesis than patients who are fluid restricted.
- **Opioids**. Opioids are the major culprit in PONV. There is little difference in emetogenicity between the intramuscular, intravenous patient-controlled analgesia (PCA), intrathecal, and epidural routes.

Studies of postoperative nausea and vomiting

There are many studies on PONV, but poor design often compromises their interpretation. Various patient, anesthetic, surgical, and postoperative factors must be considered in the design of the research. Appropriate exclusion criteria should be used. Studies should be double-blind, randomized, and controlled design. The sample size must be large enough to detect a significant difference in groups, if one exists; this often requires big groups. The required number of subjects for a clinical trial is related to power, significance, and the size of the difference between the success criteria of the two treatment groups, which should be determined before the trial (see Chapter 18). Logistic regression analysis has been used to identify the relative contribution of individual factors and combinations of factors to PONV. This is expressed by the relative odds of developing PONV for a particular factor or combination. Gender, history of PONV, opioids, and interaction between gender and history of PONV are significant, independent, fixed patient factors that have been identified as risk factors. A history of motion sickness was only weakly associated with PONV.

The measured events and endpoints must be defined. Vomiting is relatively straightforward to assess. Most studies use the number of episodes of vomiting to grade severity. Assessment of nausea is more difficult. Duration of symptoms, subjective assessments, or a visual analog score can be used. The data obtained are nonparametric and appropriate statistical analysis is required. The timing of assessment must be standardized. It is often performed in the postanesthesia care unit, and then on the ward for inpatients. In day surgery, the time intervals are necessarily different and should include telephone follow-up or a postal questionnaire. Important endpoints in day surgery include time to first fluid intake, time to discharge from hospital, and unanticipated readmissions to hospital with reasons.

Treatment

The 'antiemetic for all seasons' remains elusive, despite many studies of PONV; this relates to the multifactorial nature of the problem. The results of trials comparing antiemetics are difficult to interpret. Seemingly similar studies often reach different conclusions. A large European multicenter trial comparing the use of the three antiemetics droperidol, dexamethasone, and ondansetron has confirmed previous findings. The conclusion was that the efficacy of prophylactic antiemetic drug therapy is dependent on the patient's overall risk of developing PONV.

No currently available drug blocks all the receptor types involved in the initiation and mediation of PONV. The drugs studied were found to have the same efficacy. Sequential therapy is additive and not synergistic, as originally thought. The conclusion was that the cheapest drug therapy should be used first, because with each successive therapeutic intervention the incremental antiemetic benefit diminishes. This trial results should lead to questions about the common use of giving two antiemetics simultaneously to high-risk patients at the time of surgery. Adverse effects associated with low-dose droperidol (0.125–0.5 mg) are apparent. Its use, especially in day-case anesthesia, could be questioned. It is effective in reducing PONV associated with morphine for PCA, although adverse effects such as dysphoria and akathisia occur. Its use has markedly reduced because of concerns about cardiovascular side effects. Metoclopramide does not perform well in a large proportion of clinical trials. Antihistamines remain first-line drugs in many centers for safety reasons and their low cost. Cyclizine is as effective as droperidol when mixed with morphine for PCA. In some institutions, premixing of drugs in syringes is limited by pharmacy because of concerns about stability and sterility. Prochlorperazine, a dopamine D_2 antagonist, is a common second-line choice. The 5-HT_3 antagonists are often used as third-line agents. Nonpharmacological techniques such as acupuncture are not in widespread use at present. Pediatric patients deserve special consideration, as PONV is common and often disregarded in this group. Prophylactic antiemetics are effective in children.

It is appropriate to give high-risk patients a prophylactic drug to antagonize the proposed mechanism of emesis, rather than to have departmental protocols determining standard first- and second-line antiemetics. The same is true of treatment of established PONV. The cost of prophylactic treatment of all patients has to be weighed against the benefits. All currently available drugs have side effects that limit their indiscriminate use. Many patients would rather accept pain than have the emesis associated with opioids, or the dysphoria that can occur with the treatment of opioid-induced nausea. The time of administration of prophylactic antiemetics may be important. Many drugs give better results when given near the end of surgery rather than before anesthesia. It is recognized that perioperative factors, such as fluid hydration and increased oxygen therapy, prevent the development of PONV. These are simple strategies that could be cheaply and widely applied and they have few adverse effects. The development of future drugs, such as NK_1 receptor antagonists and cytochrome P450 enzyme inducers, is awaited, but these will not be a panacea. The concept of 'balanced antiemesis' makes clinical and scientific sense.

Key references

Ali SZ, et al. Effect of supplemental pre-operative fluid on postoperative nausea and vomiting. Anaesthesia 2003;58:780–4.

Apfel C et al. A factorial trial of six interventions for the prevention of postoperative nausea and vomiting. New Engl J Med. 2004;350:2441–51.

Grundy D, Reid K. The physiology of nausea and vomiting. In: Johnson LR, ed. Physiology of the gastrointestinal tract, 3rd edn. New York: Raven Press; 1994:879–901.

Heffernan A, Rowbotham D. Editorial. Postoperative nausea and vomiting – time for balanced antiemesis? Br J Anaesth. 2000;85:675–7.

Joris JL et al. Supplemental oxygen does not reduce postoperative nausea and vomiting after thyroidectomy. Br J Anaesth. 2003;91:857–61.

Sweeney B. Editorial II. Why does smoking protect against PONV? Br J Anaesth. 2002;89:810–13.

Further reading

Koivuranta M, Laara E, Snare L, Alahuhta S. A survey of postoperative nausea and vomiting. Anaesthesia 1997;52:443–9.

Rose JB, Watcha MF. Postoperative nausea and vomiting in paediatric patients. Br J Anaesth. 1999;83:104–17.

Strunin L, Rowbotham D, Miles A (eds) The effective prevention and management of post-operative nausea and vomiting. UK Key Advances in Clinical Practice Series. London: Aesculapius Medical Press; 2003.

Chapter 64

Physiology and pharmacology of the liver

Raymond M Planinsic and Ramona Nicolau-Raducu

TOPICS COVERED IN THIS CHAPTER

- **Anatomy, physiology, and blood flow**
- **Metabolic and synthetic functions**
- **Excretory functions**
- **Drug metabolism and excretion**
- **Liver function tests**
  - Test for hepatocellular injury
  - Cholestasis tests
  - Synthetic function tests
  - Quantitative tests of liver function
- **Pathophysiology of liver disease**
  - Serology of viral hepatitis
  - Cardiovascular system
  - Pulmonary system
  - Central nervous system
  - Renal system
  - Hemostatic system
  - Portal hypertension
- **Effects of anesthesia and surgery**
- **Liver transplantation**
- **Hepatic toxicity**

ANATOMY, PHYSIOLOGY, AND BLOOD FLOW

Although the liver is the largest organ in the fetus, it does not mature fully until after birth. On the 18th day of gestation the hepatic diverticulum forms from the ventral floor of the distal foregut thickening. Over the next few days, the hepatic diverticulum protrudes into the mesenchyme of the septum transversum, forming sheets and cords of hepatoblasts along the sinusoidal vascular network from tributaries of the vitelline veins. The portal vein develops from fusion of the vitelline veins, which then ramifies within the liver along the mesenchymal channels into the portal tract. The hepatic artery is derived from the celiac axis, and arterial sprouts grow into the hepatic primordium along the portal tract. After 8 weeks, hepatoblasts adjacent to the mesenchyme of the portal tracts differentiate into a single circumferential layer of biliary epithelial cells known as the ductal plate. The ductal plate begins to reduplicate, forming a double layer of cells around the portal tract. The peripheral biliary tubular structure forms between the two cell layers of the ductal plate. Beginning with the 11th week of maturation, the intrahepatic biliary tree develops into the mature architecture of the biliary tract from the hilum of the liver outward, and continues after birth for several months. Bile acid synthesis begins at 5–9 weeks of gestation and bile secretion at 12 weeks. Thus, from the earliest stages of hepatocellular bile formation there is a patent passage for bile to the alimentary canal. By week 16, the architectural organization of the liver is well established (Fig. 64.1).

The development of living donor liver transplantation has made a major contribution to our understanding of segmental liver anatomy. The division of the liver into right and left lobes is based on the location of the main scissura (fissure), which contains the middle hepatic vein (Fig. 64.2). The right portal scissura contains the right hepatic veins and divides the right liver into two sectors: anterior and posterior. The falciform ligament defines the medial margin of the lateral segment. According to Hjortsjo, the anterior segment fissure, in which a hepatic vein traverses, divides the anterior segment into two subsegments. Embryologically, the liver develops from four buds. The right bud develops into two lateral lobes, segments VII anterior and VI posterior, and the left bud develops into segment II. A central bud develops along the biliary axis and gives rise to the median lobe, which forms segments IV, V, and VIII. The deep central portion of the liver is comprised of the caudate lobe with segment I to the left of the inferior vena cava (IVC), and segment IX to the right of the IVC. On the anterior surface, the dorsal sector is comprised of segments IV, VIII, and VII (Fig. 64.3).

The portal vein divides at the hepatic hilum into the right and left pedicles (the left portal vein is longer than the right) on which the right and the left lobes of the liver are based. The caudate lobe is most commonly vascularized by the left branch of the portal vein. The common hepatic artery supplies the liver with arterial blood through its right and left hepatic branches, whose origins most commonly arise from the superior mesenteric artery and the left gastric artery, respectively. The venous drainage of the liver is through three main hepatic veins that drain into the suprahepatic portion of the IVC and many accessory

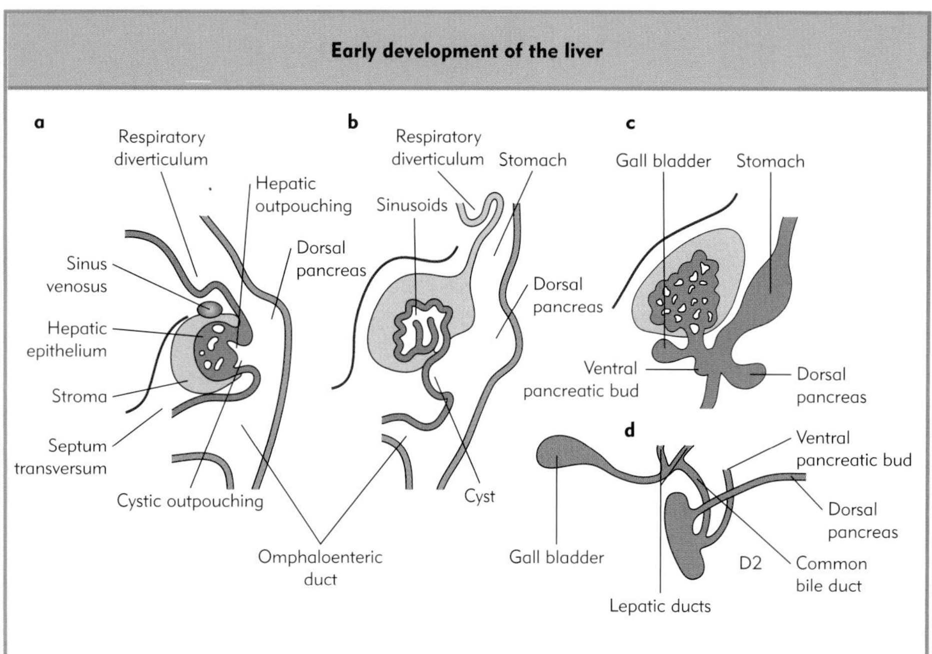

Figure 64.1 Early development of the liver. (a) Hepatic and cystic separations as hepatic epithelium and stroma grow into the septum transversum before 4.5 weeks' gestation. (b) Continued growth and presence of liver sinusoids and stomach at 4.5 weeks of gestation. (c) Gallbladder and ventral pancreatic bud are clearly defined at 5 weeks. (d) Further development of the biliary tract, with hepatic ducts, common bile duct, and second part of the duodenum (D2) present at 6 weeks of gestation. (With permission from O'Rahilly R, Müller F. Human embryology and teratology, 2nd edn. New York: John Wiley; 1996.)

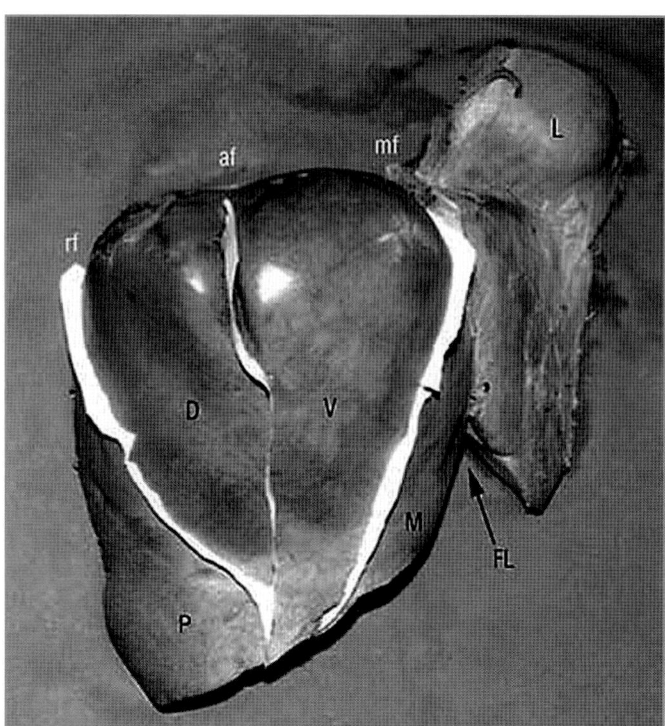

Figure 64.2 Three portal fissures (splits) relating to the anterior segment. rf, right portal fissure; af, anterior segment fissure; mf, main portal fissure; L, lateral segment; D, dorsal area of the anterior segment; V, ventral area of the anterior segment; P, posterior segment; M, medial segment; and FL, falciform ligament. (With permission from Kogure K, Kuwano H, Fujimaki N, Ishikawa H, Takada K. Reproposal for Hjortsjo's segmental anatomy on the anterior segment in human liver. Arch Surg. 2002;137:1118–24.)

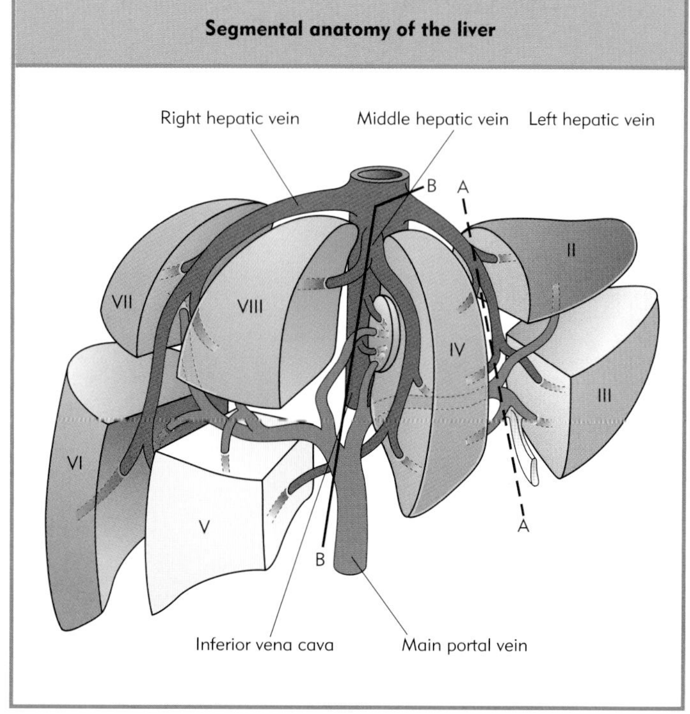

Figure 64.3 Segmental anatomy of the liver with the planes of liver splitting. (A–A) Plane of a conventional split into left lateral segment and (extended) right lobe. (B–B) Plane of a split into left and right lobes along the border of the middle hepatic vein. (With permission from Deshpande RR, Heaton ND, Rela M. Surgical anatomy of segmental liver transplantation. Br J Surg. 2002; 89:1078–88.)

hepatic veins that drain into the retrohepatic vena cava. The right hepatic vein is single in more than 90% of cases, and is formed by the convergence of the anterior trunk, which drains mainly segments V and VI, and a posterior trunk, which drains segment VII. The middle hepatic vein usually forms a common trunk with the left hepatic vein and drains segments IV on the left and segments V and VIII on the right. The left hepatic vein drains segments II and III, and receives a contribution from segment IV. Short accessory right hepatic veins drain the dorsal sector of the liver (segments VI and VII) and empty directly into the retrohepatic IVC. The caudate lobe drains predominantly on the left. In addition there are up to 20 small short venules attaching the caudate lobe to the retrohepatic vena cava.

At the cellular level the liver is organized into hepatic lobules, which consist of hepatocytes organized in plates approximately two hepatocytes thick. Lobules are separated by a fibrous septum and venous sinusoids. The sinusoids receive arterial blood from the hepatic arterioles and venous blood from the terminal portal venules. The sinusoids drain into the central vein. The organizational unit of the human liver is also known as an acinus, as first described by Rappaport. Three concentric zones surround the portal triads. Portal triads consist of a portal venule, hepatic arteriole, and bile ductule. Zone 1 cells are closest to the afferent blood vessels and are thus the first cells in the sinusoids to receive blood. Zone 2 and 3 cells are located further from the afferent blood vessels and therefore receive blood which is partially deoxygenated. Thus zone 2 and 3 cells are more susceptible to ischemic damage. Bile flows in a direction opposite to that of blood, draining into intralobular bile ductules and forming a countercurrent system similar to that in the kidney.

The liver contains 12% of total blood volume, has a large compliance, and plays an important role in regulating cardiac filling. It is relatively protected in low gut blood flow states because of a dual blood supply from the hepatic artery (~25% of total hepatic blood flow) and the portal vein (~75% of total hepatic blood flow). Despite dual vascularization and a high flow (25% of cardiac output, or 20–30 mL/min/kg body weight), hepatic perfusion pressure is low (<5 mmHg from the terminal portal venules to the hepatic vein). Hepatic arterial blood flow compensates for decreased portal venous blood flow by increasing flow up to 20–30% (hepatic arterial buffer response). However, the compensation for oxygen delivery is much greater because of the higher oxygen content in the hepatic artery (~45% of total hepatic oxygen supply) compared to the portal vein (~55% of total hepatic oxygen supply). The hepatic arterial buffer response is a dynamic interaction between hepatic arterial and portal venous blood flow, which tends to maintain total hepatic blood flow and oxygen delivery when portal blood flow decreases. Adenosine is involved in the underlying physiological mechanism of the hepatic arterial buffer response.

The hepatic arterial buffer response tends to maintain total hepatic blood flow and oxygen delivery when portal blood flow decreases.

Liver blood flow is also regulated through endothelial cell control of local vascular tone. Endothelial mediators that may control hepatic blood flow under physiologic and/or pathologic conditions include nitric oxide and carbon monoxide, which exert a local vasodilator effect, and endothelin, a peptide responsible for vasoconstriction.

METABOLIC AND SYNTHETIC FUNCTIONS

The parenchyma of the liver is composed of hepatocytes, which are responsible for the complex functions of absorbing digestive material from portal venous blood and secreting metabolites into bile. They synthesize plasma proteins, glucose, cholesterol, fatty acids, and phospholipids. In addition, they metabolize, detoxify, and inactivate exogenous and endogenous compounds and play a role in the immune system. Nonparenchymal cells consist of endothelial, Kupffer, hepatic stellate, and pit cells. Endothelial cells line the hepatic sinusoids, providing a permeable barrier for the exchange of molecules between the blood and hepatocytes. Kupffer cells are hepatic macrophages. Hepatic stellate cells play an important role in fibrogenesis in various liver diseases. Pit cells are also known as natural killer cells and are perhaps involved in antitumor defense of the liver.

Carbohydrate metabolism is divided into three phases: absorptive, postabsorptive, and fasting. The degree of hypoglycemia or hyperglycemia determines whether the liver produces or stores glucose. During the absorptive phase, glucose is distributed directly from intestine to tissues. In perivenous hepatocytes glucose is used to synthesize and saturate glycogen stores. In the postabsorptive phase glycogen is degraded to glucose in periportal hepatocytes. Depletion of stored glycogen occurs after 24 hours. Then, endogenous gluconeogenesis produces glucose from amino acids, lactate, and glycerol. Oxidation of fatty acids, stored as triglycerides in adipocytes, produces ketones. These two utilizable substrates, glucose and ketones, provide energy for the brain.

The liver synthesizes plasma proteins, primarily albumin. Most other plasma proteins secreted by the liver are glycoproteins, involved in many biologic functions, such as hemostasis. Periportal cells convert NH_3 to urea via the ureagenesis cyle. Additional ammonia is converted to glutamine by perivenous hepatocytes.

The liver plays an important role in lipoprotein and cholesterol metabolism. Lipids are insoluble in plasma and require carrier proteins (apoproteins). Lipoproteins are formed from absorbed lipids and are divided into four classes: chylomicrons, very low-density (VLDL), low-density (LDL), and high-density (HDL) lipoproteins. Cholesterol synthesis begins with acetyl-CoA and is stored as the esterified form in the periportal cells. Hepatocytes are the only cells in the body that convert cholesterol to bile acids, which facilitate fat absorption from the intestine.

EXCRETORY FUNCTIONS

Red blood cells are destroyed by the reticuloendothelial system (spleen, bone marrow, liver) and the released hemoglobin is split into globin and heme. Heme is reduced by microsomal enzymes to bilirubin, which is released into the plasma, combines with albumin, and is transported to the liver. In hepatocytes, bilirubin is esterified with monosaccharides – mainly glucuronic acid – which is then excreted into the bile. However, bacterial enzymes convert bilirubin into urobilinogens, which are eliminated in the feces. Small amounts of urobilinogen are reabsorbed and undergo enterohepatic circulation, and are then excreted in the urine. Liver excretory function is assessed by measuring the amounts of free and conjugated (esterified) bilirubin. Patients become jaundiced when serum bilirubin exceeds 2–3 mg/dL.

DRUG METABOLISM AND EXCRETION

The duration and intensity of drug effects are determined by their blood concentration as a function of time (pharmacokinetics; Chapter 8) and by the end-organ response to a given drug concentration (pharmacodynamics; Chapter 7). When a drug is administered orally, the liver metabolizes a fraction absorbed before it reaches the systemic circulation. This is known as the first-pass effect. The drug fraction that reaches the systemic circulation is known as its bioavailability. Propanolol and lidocaine are drugs with a high hepatic extraction ratio, and as a consequence have a low oral bioavailability.

Drugs are eliminated from the body by excretion of the unchanged form or through biotransformation. The liver has a major role in this biotransformation, via either oxidation (phase I reactions) or conjugation (phase II reactions) of compounds, making them more water soluble (hydrophilic) and hence more easily secreted in bile or filtered by the kidneys. The main determinants of drug elimination by the normal liver are intrinsic clearance, blood flow, and plasma protein binding. These characteristics lead to a classification of drug elimination based on the hepatic extraction ratio. Intrinsic clearance is the main excretion route for drugs with low hepatic extraction ratios (< 0.3). For drugs with high extraction ratio (> 0.7) clearance is determined mainly by liver blood flow. For drugs with intermediate extraction ratios clearance depends on both intrinsic clearance and blood flow.

Portosystemic shunts increase the bioavailability of hepatically cleared oral medications.

In patients with cirrhosis, drug elimination is delayed by reduced intrinsic clearance and/or by portosystemic shunts. For substances with a low extraction ratio, the reduction in drug-metabolizing enzyme activity is responsible for impaired intrinsic clearance. In contrast, for substances with a high extraction ratio, such as propranolol, an impaired cellular influx due to altered hepatic microcirculation explains the decreased clearance. The systemic elimination of highly extracted drugs, such lidocaine, is not normally related to hepatic blood flow, but appears to be related to intrinsic clearance. The presence of portosystemic shunts increases the systemic bioavailability of the drug by bypassing the liver. The combined effect of these factors can produce important alterations in drug metabolism and bioavailability that should be taken into account whenever drugs are given to patients orally.

Glucuronidating enzymes are located within hepatic microsomes and are less susceptible to liver injury. In addition, extrahepatic glucuronidation explains why the metabolism of drugs such as oxazepam, lorazepam, chloramphenicol, and morphine are not significantly affected by intrinsic liver disease. Oxidative metabolism of drugs by hepatic cytochrome P450 enzymes are variably affected by liver disease, depending on whether the cytochrome P450 system is induced (phenobarbital) or impaired.

Pharmacodynamic changes in liver disease are more difficult to assess than pharmacokinetic changes. There is evidence that the sensitivity of the brain to sedatives and the response of the kidney to diuretics are altered in cirrhosis. In chronic liver disease without cirrhosis, cellular injury can range from minimal to severe. Under these circumstances, drug elimination is well maintained when cellular injury is mild and becomes impaired only late in the evolution of chronic liver disease.

LIVER FUNCTION TESTS

Tests for hepatocellular injury

Measurements of aminotransferase enzymes are used to indicate hepatocellular necrosis. Aspartate aminotransferase (AST) and alanine aminotransferase (ALT) catalyze the transfer of the α amino groups of aspartate and alanine to the α keto group of ketoglutaric acid to form glutamine. AST and ALT are located primarily in the liver, but AST is also present in heart, skeletal muscle, kidney, and brain. An AST:ALT ratio >2 strongly suggests a diagnosis of alcoholic liver disease.

Cholestasis tests

Markers used to identify cholestasis are alkaline phosphatase (ALP) and γ-glutamyltranspeptidase (GGT). These enzymes are distributed in bone, liver, intestine, and placenta. GGT is useful in differentiating whether an elevated ALP is secondary to hepatobiliary disease or whether its origin is extrahepatic.

Serum bilirubin is predominantly found in an unconjugated form reflecting a balance between production and hepatobiliary excretion. Unconjugated bilirubin increases in hemolysis, resorption of hematoma, and muscle injury. Conjugated hyperbilirubinemia occurs in parenchymal liver disease and biliary obstruction as excretory function is impaired.

Synthetic function tests

Approximately 10 g of albumin is synthesized and secreted daily by the liver. Plasma albumin concentration is decreased in severe acute or chronic liver disease, and is one of the criteria used in the Child–Pugh classification of cirrhosis (Table 64.1). Albumin levels depend on several factors, such as nutritional status, catabolism, hormonal status, and urinary and gastrointestinal losses.

Synthesis of the coagulation factors is an important function of the liver, except for factor VIII, which is produced by endothelial cells and megakaryocytes. The prothrombin time (PT) measures the extrinsic pathway of the coagulation cascade (factors II, V, VII, and X, which are vitamin K dependent). A prolonged PT can be due to hepatocellular disease or fat malabsorption. This can be differentiated by the administration of vitamin K, which will correct coagulopathy due to fat malabsorption. The International Normalized Ratio (INR) is a standardized method of reporting of PT that eliminates variability in measurements for different laboratories.

Quantitative tests of liver function

Owing to limitations in the sensitivity and specificity of 'traditional' liver function tests (AST, ALT, bilirubin, ALP, GGT), more sensitive quantitative tests of liver function are required. Investigators have suggested following the metabolism of several drugs as indicators of liver function. These are currently limited mainly to research, and include indocyanine green clearance, C-aminopyrine breath test, antipyrine clearance, galactose elimination capacity, C-caffeine breath test, phenacetin breath test, methacetin breath test, diazepam breath test, erythromycin

Table 64.1 Modified Child–Pugh classification of hepatic cirrhosis

Class	A	B	C
Serum bilirubin (mg/dL)	< 2.0	2.0–3.0	> 3.0
Serum albumin (mg/dL)	> 3.5	3.0–3.5	< 3.0
Ascites	None	Well controlled	Poorly controlled
Encephalopathy	None	Minimal	Advanced/com
Nutrition status	Excellent	Good	Poor/wasting
Prothrombin time (seconds prolonged)	1–4	4–6	>6

breath test, phenylalanine breath test, and hepatic lidocaine metabolism.

PATHOPHYSIOLOGY OF LIVER DISEASE

Hepatitis is a generalized inflammation of the liver and may be caused by drugs, viral agents, and toxins such as alcohol. Viral hepatitis is the major cause of chronic liver disease and cirrhosis worldwide. The most common viral agents responsible for chronic liver disease are HBV and HCV. Other etiologies include sclerosing cholangitis, autoimmune hepatitis, nonalcoholic steatohepatitis (NASH), and cryptogenic hepatitis. Liver biopsy is used to confirm the diagnosis of chronic hepatitis and to exclude other diagnoses, such as Wilson's disease, hemochromatosis, or α_1-antitrypsin deficiency. It is also an important tool in establishing the severity of liver injury and the stage of fibrosis. Fibrosis can vary from minimal fibrosis to portal expansion, bridging fibrosis, and cirrhosis. Although the Child–Pugh classification for patients with liver disease (Table 64.1) was first described to predict operative outcome, it does not assess all of the pathophysiologic effects on the various organ systems. Understanding these effects is necessary for optimal intraoperative management.

Serology of viral hepatitis

Six major viruses (A, B, C, D, E and G) are the agents responsible for viral hepatitis (Table 64.2). Enzyme linked immunoassay (ELISA) and molecular biologic (polymerase chain reaction, PCR) diagnostic tests are important tools to test for viral antigen, antibody, DNA, or RNA in serum and body secretions. Serological markers depicting the typical clinical course for acute hepatitis A and B viral infections are shown in Figure 64.4.

Cardiovascular system

Patients with end-stage liver disease (ESLD) have a hyperdynamic cardiovascular system manifested by an elevated cardiac index (often >3.5 L/min/m^2), hyperkinetic left ventricular function, and low systemic vascular resistance. This is a result of peripheral vasodilatation, the etiology of which may be related to mediators not cleared by the diseased liver, and arteriovenous shunting.

Table 64.2 Viral hepatitis serology

Hepatitis type	A	B	C	D	E	G
Size	*27 nm*	*42 nm*	*30–60 nm*	*35 nm*	*37 nm*	*30–60 nm*
Genome	ssRNA	dsDNA	ssRNA	ssRNA	ssRNA	ssRNA
Antigens	HAAg	HBsAg HBeAg HBcAg	HCAg	HDAg	HEAg	None available
Antibodies	Ig G/Ig M anti-HAV	IgM Anti-HBc Anti-HBc Anti-HBs Anti-HBe	Anti-HCV	IgM anti-HDV	Anti-HEV	None available
Viral markers	HAV RNA	HBV DNA DNA polymerase	HCV RNA	HDV RNA	None	HGV RNA

HAV, hepatitis A virus; HBV, hepatitis B virus; HBsAg, HBV surface antigen; HBcAg HBV core antigen; HBeAg, HBV envelope; HCV, hepatitis C virus; HDV, hepatitis D virus or delta; HEV, hepatitis E virus. (With permission from Bacon BR, DiBisceglie AM. Liver disease: diagnosis and management. In: Rose H, Keeffen E, eds. Evaluation of abnormal liver enzymes, use of liver tests, and the serology of viral hepatitis. Edinburgh: Churchill Livingstone; 2000: Chapter 3.)

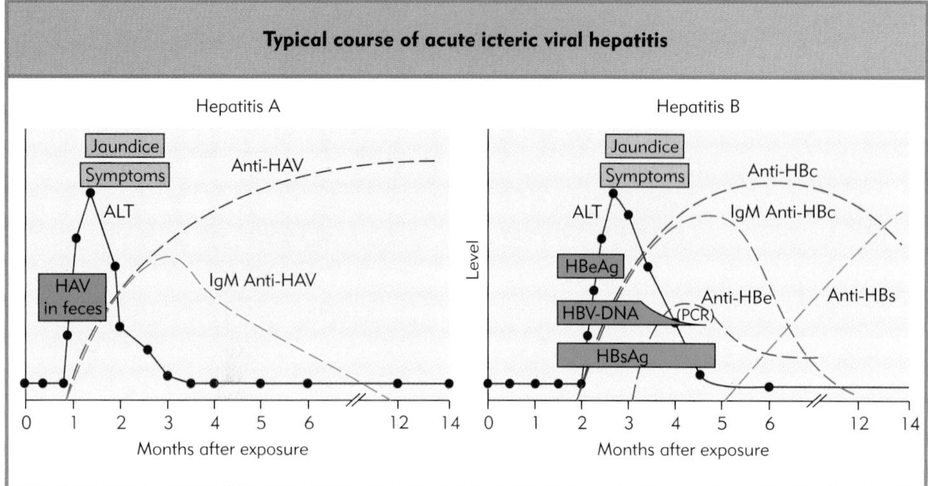

Figure 64.4 Typical course of acute icteric viral hepatitis, type A and B. See Table 64.2 for abbreviations. (With permission from Hoofnagle JH, Di Bisceglie AM. Serologic diagnosis of viral hepatitis. Semin Liver Dis. 1991;11:73–83.)

End-stage liver disease is characterized by elevated cardiac output and low systemic vascular resistance.

Conduction abnormalities leading to arrhythmias and/or cardiomyopathy may develop as a result of copper deposition in patients with Wilson's disease. Iron deposition results in similar problems in patients with hemochromatosis. Arrhythmias and myocardial dysfunction associated with acute alcoholic intoxication may also occur. Transthyretin Met 30-associated familial amyloid polyneuropathy is a rare form of amyloidosis and has been characterized by progressive autonomic neuropathy, with amyloid deposits found in the myocardium, the conduction system, and the sympathetic and parasympathetic nervous systems.

Pulmonary system

Arterial hypoxemia may occur in patients with ESLD due to intrinsic pulmonary disease such as asthma or COPD, or restrictive lung disease, often the result of pleural effusions or ascites. Other considerations include interstitial fibrosis, cystic fibrosis, or α_1-antitrypsin deficiency, which may be associated with ESLD. The hepatopulmonary syndrome (HPS) consists of arterial hypoxemia (P_aO_2 <55 mmHg on room air) in the setting of liver disease due to shunting through intrapulmonary vascular dilatations. Patients with HPS experience an improvement of hypoxemia when changing position from upright to supine (orthodeoxia), and an improvement in symptoms of shortness of breath when rising from the recumbent position (platypnea). Chest radiography and pulmonary function tests are usually normal, apart from a reduced diffusion capacity of carbon monoxide.

Portopulmonary hypertension (PPH), associated with ESLD, carries with it a significant risk for intraoperative mortality. Diagnostic testing should include right and left heart catheterization to evaluate pulmonary artery pressure (PAP) and cardiac output, and echocardiography to evaluate right ventricular function. A vasodilator, such as intravenous epoprostenol, adenosine, or inhaled nitric oxide, to determine the reversibility of PPH can be given at the time of catheterization. A decrease in mean PAP (mPAP) by more than 10 mmHg with either no change or an increase in cardiac output suggests a significant degree of reversibility. For patients with a positive response during the vasodilator trial, chronic oral vasodilator therapy with calcium channel blockers (diltiazem or nifedipine) or phosphodiesterase inhibitors (sildenafil) can be initiated. In liver transplantation, prognostic guidelines are based on mPAP, and include mild (mPAP ≤ 25–35 mmHg), moderate (mPAP 35–50 mmHg), and severe (mPAP ≥ 50 mmHg) PPH. Patients with severe PPH should not undergo transplantation, given the very high mortality rate. Patients eligible for transplantation must have normal right ventricular function, cardiac index ≥3.5 L/min/m^2, no evidence of thromboembolic disease, and must respond to a pulmonary vasodilators (e.g. epoprostenol).

Central nervous system

Hepatic encephalopathy (HE) is a potentially reversible neuropsychiatric syndrome that occurs in patients with significant liver dysfunction. It is characterized by an altered sleep–wake cycle, varying degrees of confusion and disorientation, asterixis, hyperreflexia, and slowing of the dominant rhythm on electroencephalography. The clinical stages of HE are: stage 1, mild confusion, euphoria or depression, decreased attention, mental slowing, untidiness, slurred speech, irritability, reversal of sleep pattern, possible asterixis; stage 2, drowsiness, lethargy, gross mental slowing, personality changes, inappropriate behavior, intermittent disorientation, lack of sphincter control, asterixis; stage 3, somnolent but arousable, unable to perform mental tasks, persistent disorientation, amnesia, occasional attacks of rage, incoherent speech, pronounced confusion, asterixis probably absent; and stage 4, coma.

The etiology of this encephalopathy is unknown; possible factors include endogenous ammonia, altered cerebral metabolism, changes in blood–brain barrier permeability, abnormal neurotransmitter balance, impaired neuronal Na^+, K^+-ATPase activity, and an increase in endogenous activators of GABA receptors. Factors that worsen the syndrome include gastrointestinal bleeding, infection, diuretic drugs, acid–base and electrolyte imbalance, and anesthesia. Administration of flumazemil (benzodiazepine antagonist) and reduction of ammonia levels with diet (low proteins) and lactulose are treatment options.

Renal system

Renal dysfunction is not an uncommon complication of ESLD. Patients often exhibit prerenal azotemia due to diuretic use, paracentesis, or hypovolemia. Nephrotoxic drugs such as intravenous contrast dyes used in radiographic studies, immunosuppressants such as cyclosporin, or antibiotics such as aminoglycosides may lead to acute tubular necrosis.

Renal insufficiency in patients with ESLD may be associated with the hepatorenal syndrome (HRS). In HRS, renal failure is a result of renal vasoconstriction in response to marked splanchnic and systemic vasodilatation.

Administration of terlipressin, a splanchnic and systemic vasoconstrictor, may improve renal function. Reduced urine output, very low urinary Na^+ levels (<5–10 mEq/dL), and a high urine:plasma creatinine ratio are characteristic of HRS. HRS patients usually do not respond to volume challenges with an increase in urine output. Renal insufficiency associated with HRS has been shown to be reversible with orthotopic liver transplantation.

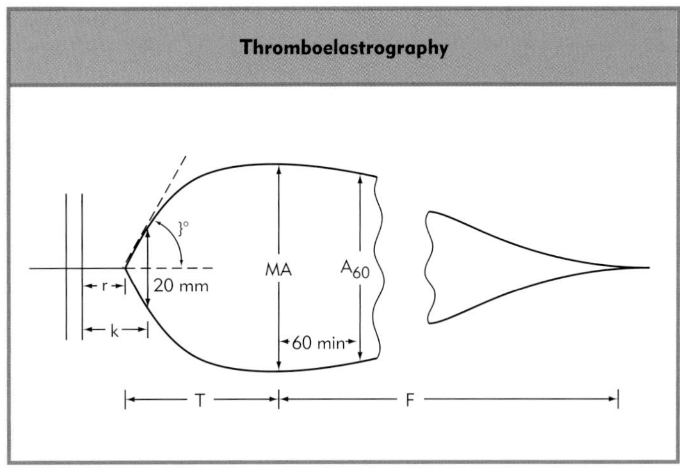

Figure 64.5 Thromboelastography (TEG). Measured parameters and normal values. r = reaction time 10–14 min; r+k = coagulation time 13–20 min; α = clot formation rate 53–67°; MA = maximum amplitude 59–66; A_{60} = amplitude 60 min after MA; A_{60}/MA × 100 = whole blood clot lysis index > 85%; F = whole blood clot lysis time > 300 min.

Hemostatic system

Patients with ESLD manifest derangements in hemostasis. Decreased synthesis of vitamin K-dependent clotting factors (II, VII, IX, and X) due to impaired protein synthetic function and malabsorption of vitamin K in cholestatic disease will lead to coagulopathy. The presence of coagulation defects such as antithrombin III deficiency and proteins C and S, factor V Leiden, or factor II mutations and antiphospholipid syndrome must all be considered, especially in the patient with known portal vein thrombosis.

Traditional clotting studies, such as prothrombin time (PT), partial thromboplastin time (PTT), platelet count, fibrinogen level, or fibrin degradation products, may also aid in the treatment of coagulopathy. Some centers monitor the coagulation system by thromboelastography (TEG). This provides rapid information on the interactions between platelets, clotting factors, and the thrombolytic system, allowing treatment to be started immediately (Fig. 64.5).

Portal hypertension

Cirrhosis of the liver is the most common cause of portal hypertension, in which the intraluminal portal venous pressure is >12 mmHg. As a result of increased pressure in the portal system, portosystemic bypasses may develop in the vicinity of the rectum (hemorrhoids), gastroesophageal junction (esophageal varices), retroperitoneum, and falciform ligament (periumbilical and abdominal collaterals). The most common complication of portal hypertension is upper gastrointestinal bleeding caused by ruptured esophageal varices. Portal hypertension may also induce splenomegaly. Hypersplenism, immunologically mediated platelet destruction, and decreased platelet production can all lead to thrombocytopenia. Medical management may include β-blockers, which reduce portal pressure. Refractory patients may undergo transjugular intravascular portosystemic shunts (TIPS) or surgical shunts (splenorenal shunts) to relieve portal hypertension.

Pathophysiological mechanisms proposed to explain the formation of ascites in decompensated cirrhosis include decreased oncotic pressure secondary to reduced albumin production, lymph overproduction, secondary hyperaldosteronism with Na^+ retention, and increased concentration of antidiuretic hormone. Treatment consists of diuretic therapy (spironolactone with or without furosemide). For massive, tense ascites, paracentesis under a sterile technique is usually required. Proper fluid volume replacement with albumin or colloid is required to prevent the development of hepatorenal syndrome caused by diminished 'effective blood volume'.

EFFECTS OF ANESTHESIA AND SURGERY

Surgical procedures cause significant stress for patients with advanced liver disease. Even simple interventions are accompanied by extremely high perioperative morbidity and mortality. The surgical stress response is usually followed by the release of catecholamines, renin, angiotensin, and vasopressin, which act on the splanchnic circulation to reduce hepatic blood flow. Function in a cirrhotic liver may be further compromised when hepatic blood flow is reduced. The degree of hepatic injury and the increase in hepatic enzyme concentrations depend on the type of surgery rather than the type of anesthesia. Hepatic blood flow may be further decreased depending on the type of procedure (upper abdominal versus extremity). Different types of anesthesia administered for similar surgical procedures may produce different effects on hepatic circulation. The degree to which a subarachnoid block affects liver blood flow is greater with higher levels of block. In contrast to halothane, isoflurane increases hepatic blood flow in the range of 1–2 MAC.

All intravenous anesthetics can be used in patients with advanced liver disease when titrated to effect. For albumin-bound drugs such as thiopental, the volume of distribution is decreased and therefore the dose should be decreased. Succinylcholine can be safely used in patients with liver disease despite a decrease in plasma cholinesterase levels. Nondepolarizing muscle relaxants can be chosen to facilitate tracheal intubation, but the volume of distribution is high for the majority of these drugs (D-tubocurarine, pancuronium, atracurium, etc.). The effective dose is increased, but clearance of drugs depending on hepatic metabolism or renal excretion is decreased.

All anesthetics, especially volatile agents, reduce hepatic blood flow to a variable degree. Halothane should be avoided, as it is accompanied by a significant reduction in hepatic blood flow and oxygen supply during surgery, which can cause severe postoperative hepatic dysfunction. Enflurane or isoflurane are the volatile anesthetics of choice for inhalation anesthesia. Experience is lacking with the newer volatile anesthetic agents sevoflurane and desflurane. The potential for the production of Compound A from sevoflurane with possible renal toxicity may be problematic. Nitrous oxide has been used for many years in patients with advanced liver disease, and has not been implicated in postoperative hepatic complications. Opioids can be used in patients with hepatic disease, despite its decreased clearance and prolonged half-life. Fentanyl is considered the opioid of choice because it does not decrease the hepatic oxygen and blood supply to the liver. Opioids can induce spasm of the sphincter of Oddi, which can be treated with atropine, naloxone, or glucagon. Anesthesia with isoflurane alone or in combination with fentanyl may provide conditions that will allow adequate hemodynamic stability and minimal derangements in hepatic blood flow.

All anesthetics reduce hepatic blood flow, particularly halothane.

If patients are not coagulopathic, regional anesthesia can be considered. However, epidural blockade reduces hepatic blood flow by increasing splanchnic vascular resistance. The metabolism of local anesthetics is altered in patients with ESLD. Plasma clearance is reduced, and the half-life of all local anesthetics is prolonged in cirrhotic patients. If amide local anesthetics are used, ropivacaine, which is less cardiotoxic than bupivacaine, should be considered. Spinal epidural abscess is an uncommon complication; however, chronic liver disease has been reported as a predisposing condition.

LIVER TRANSPLANTATION

Candidates for adult orthotopic liver transplantation (OLT) are listed and ranked for transplantation based on their bilirubin, INR, and creatinine levels. For liver transplant candidates under the age of 18, ranking is based on bilirubin, INR, albumin, growth failure, and age factors that better predict mortality in children. The transplant procedure is divided into three stages: stage I, preanhepatic; stage II, anhepatic; and stage III, neohepatic. In stage I, patients are vasodilated and occasionally hypovolemic. After incision, with the release of potential ascites, this may become more evident. The goal during stage I is to correct volume deficits, and to maintain euvolemia and stable hemodynamics. Surgical dissection with associated blood loss and vascular compression can lead to hemodynamic instability. The use of inotropes may be necessary, and options include low-dose dopamine or epinephrine infusion. Maintenance of normal acid– base balance and electrolyte composition is required to maximize cardiac function. Bleeding may be worsened by underlying coagulopathy due to clotting factor deficiencies, thrombocytopenia, dilution, and the degree of portal hypertension.

Stage II may have a profound effect on the patient's cardiovascular system depending on the surgical technique used. In stage I, the diseased liver may be removed with preservation of the intrahepatic vena cava (piggyback dissection), or by resection of the suprahepatic and infrahepatic vena cava. The latter technique may be performed with or without venovenous bypass (VVB). In all approaches, the portal vein, hepatic artery, and common bile duct must be transected. The piggyback technique requires partial occlusion of the intrahepatic vena cava at the level of hepatic venous inflow. The degree of caval occlusion necessary to isolate the hepatic veins and anastomose the suprahepatic donor vena cava to the recipient hepatic vein cuff often contributes to hemodynamic instability. If the diseased liver is removed along with the intrahepatic vena cava, vascular clamping of the suprahepatic and infrahepatic vena cava is required. This may lead to significant hemodynamic instability if VVB is not used. Venous return to the heart will decrease by over 50%, owing to the lack of blood return from below the diaphragm, which may lead to hypotension and tachycardia, and require inotropic support. Vascular engorgement with increased venous pressure to the splanchnic bed and kidneys may lead to intestinal edema and contribute to the development of renal insufficiency. When VVB is not used, excessive volume loading should be avoided as blood pooled in the lower extremities and splanchnic system will be returned to the systemic circulation acutely with reperfusion of the graft, which may result in right heart failure. Problems also occur with VVB. Venous inflow to the bypass pump may be inadequate because of problems positioning the venous inflow cannula, thrombus formation may occur as patients are usually not heparinized, and air embolization can occur. Near the end of the vascular anastomosis phase (stage II), the donor graft's vascular system is flushed retrogradely from the infrahepatic through the portal vein with cold lactated Ringer's solution, normal saline, or albumin. This removes the preservative solution and accumulated ischemic metabolites, which would be harmful to the recipient. Occasionally the patient's own blood is used to flush the donor organ, particularly if the ischemic period was prolonged or if hyperkalemia on reperfusion is a particular concern. Bleeding may worsen during stage II owing to consumption and dilution of clotting factors and platelets, an inability to clear circulating plasminogen activators, and decreased levels of plasminogen activator inhibitors, leading to fibrinolysis.

Each phase of hepatic transplantation is associated with distinct pathophysiological effects.

Reperfusion, or stage III, commences with removal of the vascular clamps at the portal, then the infrahepatic and suprahepatic anastomotic sites. When the suprahepatic clamp is removed blood flow to the heart is fully restored, and significant hemodynamic changes may occur. Transient slowing of the heart rate may occur due to the cold, acidotic, hyperkalemic effluent blood from the liver. Electrocardiographic changes, including ST-segment elevation and T-wave peaking, may be seen because of a transient increase in K^+ (up to 12–15 mEq/L), which may lead to a sinusoidal electrocardiogram and asystole. These changes are usually temporary, but can lead to cardiac arrest, requiring temporary cardiac support and rescue with chest compressions and small intravenous boluses of epinephrine (10–100 μg) or calcium chloride (500 mg–1 g) if there is evidence of ionized hypocalcemia. Hypotension occurring within the first 5 minutes of reperfusion and lasting more than 1 minute may occur in up to 30% of patients and is referred to as the post-reperfusion syndrome (PRS). Optimization of acid–base balance, ventilation, volume, and electrolyte status prior to reperfusion may decrease the adverse effects of PRS. The onset of stage III may be marked by the development of fibrinolysis, which is noted in up to 80% of patients, requiring treatment (with ε-aminocaproic acid or aprotinin) in 20% of patients because of diffuse bleeding. In addition, the release of heparin-type substances and hypothermia owing to perfusion of the cold/ischemic donor organ may worsen coagulopathy. If necessary, these may be treated with small doses of protamine and warming the patient.

HEPATIC TOXICITY

Hepatotoxic drug reactions can be divided into predictable (dose dependent), idiosyncratic (dose independent), and bile duct injury reactions. Several drug reactions, the type of hepatic injury, and their cell targets are described in Table 64.3. Liver disease predisposes to drug toxicity, and for this reason appropriate dose adjustments are necessary. Because patients with chronic liver diseases have low albumin levels, toxicity may be enhanced for drugs that are protein bound.

Hepatotoxicity is often accompanied by symptoms of malaise, anorexia, abdominal pain, and fever, a clinical scenario that resembles viral hepatitis. A four- to fivefold increase in ALT and AST indicates hepatotoxicity in a patient with previously normal tests. Elevation of alkaline phosphatase and bilirubin predominates in cholestatic syndromes. For patients with prior elevated transaminases there are no specific guidelines for what constitutes a significant increase, but greater vigilance will help to detect early injury.

Acetaminophen toxicity may occur after attempted suicide, or unintentionally. This is the most common etiology of acute liver failure in the United States, accounting for 39% of cases. Chronic alcohol abuse or concomitant treatment with phenytoin or isoniazid can worsen the liver injury due to acetaminophen. Enzyme inducers, together with substrate competition, have a dynamic role in enhancing acetaminophen hepatotoxicity. During metabolism of acetaminophen, *N*-acetyl-*p*-benzoquinone-imine (NAPQI) formation is diminished when alcohol is present, because alcohol competes with acetaminophen for the cytochrome P450 2E1 enzyme. During the next 24 hours, after the cessation of alcohol consumption, NAPQI formation is enhanced, resulting in increased hepatic injury. *N*-acetylcysteine (NAC) given for 36–72 hours replenishes glutathione levels and prevents injury if the treatment is initiated within 12–24 hours after the ingestion of acetominophen.

In patients with liver disease, hypoalbuminemia may play a role in aspirin-induced hepatic damage. There is an increase in unbound plasma concentration of aspirin that is inversely proportional to the serum albumin, and directly related to the rise in transaminases. Aspirin is metabolized to salicyl-CoA, which impairs mitochondrial β-oxidation of fatty acids, with the subsequent development of microvesicular steatosis as described in Reye's syndrome.

The etiology of halothane-induced hepatic dysfunction is controversial. In a metabolic model, a reductive metabolite of halothane is formed rather than the normal oxidative metabolite, producing fluorinated compounds under hypoxic conditions. Other mechanisms suggest that several prior exposures to halothane induce an immune-mediated sensitization to the compound. The fluorinated metabolite of halothane has been linked with a humoral antibody response.

Table 64.3 Drug-induced hepatotoxicity

Type of reaction	Effect on hepatic cells	Drugs
Hepatocellular	Cell and membrane dysfunction, cytotoxic T-cell response	Isoniazid, trazodone, diclofenac, nefazodone, venlafaxine, lovastatin
Cholestasis	Injury to canalicular membrane and transporters	Chlorpromazine, estrogen, erythromycin
Immunoallergic	Enzyme – drug adducts on cell surface induce Ig E	Halothane, phenytoin, sulfamethoxazole
Granulomatous	Macrophages, lymphocytes infiltrate hepatic lobule	Diltiazem, sulfa drug, quinidine
Microvesicular fat	Altered mitochondrial respiration	Didanosine, tetracycline, acetylsalicylic acid, valproic acid
Steatohepatitis	Multifactor	Amiodarone, tamoxifen, alcohol
Autoimmune	Cytotoxic lymphocyte response directed at hepatocyte membrane	Nitrofurantoin, methydopa, lovastatin, minocycline activation of stellate cells
Fibrosis	Activation of stellate cells	Methotrexate, vitamin A intoxication
Vascular collapse	Ischemic or hypoxic injury	Nicotinic acid, cocaine, methylenediomethamphetamine
Oncogenesis	Tumor formation (adenoma)	Oral contraceptive, androgens
Mixed	Cytoplasmatic and canalicular injury, direct damage to bile ducts	Amoxicillin–clavulanate, carbamazepine, herbs, ciclosporin, methimazole, troglitazone

(With permission from Lee WM. New Engl J Med 2003;349: 474–85.)

Key references

Gelman S. Anesthesia and the liver. In: Barash PG, Cullen BF, Stoelting RK, eds. Clinical anesthesia, 3rd edn. Baltimore: Lippincott Williams & Wilkins; 1997:1003-21.

Luxon BA. Anatomy and physiology of the liver and biliary tree. In: Bacon BR, Di Bisceglie AM, eds. Liver disease: diagnosis and management. Edinburgh: Churchill Livingstone; 2000:3–15.

Merritt WT, Gelman S. Anesthesia for liver surgery. In: Rogers MC, Tinker JH, Covino BG, Longnecker DE, eds. Principles and practice of anesthesiology. Vol 2. Chicago: Mosby Year Book; 1993:1991–2034.

Parks D, Skinner KA, Gelman S, Maze M. Hepatic physiology. In: Miller RD, ed. Anesthesia, 5th edn. Edinburgh: Churchill Livingstone; 2000:647–61.

Rosen HR, Keefe EB. Evaluation of abnormal liver enzymes, use of liver tests and the serology of viral hepatitis. In: Bacon BR, Di Bisceglie AM, eds. Liver disease: diagnosis and management. Edinburgh: Churchill Livingstone; 2000:24–35.

Further reading

Crawford JM. Development of the intrahepatic biliary tree. Semin Liver Dis. 2002;22:213–26.

Deshpande RR, Heaton ND, Rela M. Surgical anatomy of segmental liver transplantation. Br J Surg. 2002;89:1078–88.

Hardy KJ. The dorsal liver: an analysis. Aust NZ J Surg. 1999;69:167–9.

Huet PM, Villeneuve JP, Fenyves D. Drug elimination in chronic liver disease. J Hepatol. 1997;26(Suppl):63–72.

Lee WM. Medical progress: drug-induced hepatotoxicity. New Engl J Med. 2003;349:474–85.

Lewis M, Howdle PD. The neurology of liver failure. Quant J Med. 2003;96:623–33.

Limdi JK, Hyde GM. Evaluation of abnormal liver function tests. Postgrad Med J. 2003;79:307–12.

Pannen BHJ. New insights into the regulation of hepatic blood flow after ischemia and reperfusion. Anesth Analg. 2002;94:1448–57.

Schenker S, Ralston MR, Anastacio HM. Antecedent liver disease and drug toxicity. J Hepatol. 1999;31:1098–105.

Chapter 65

Regulation of intermediary metabolism

Iain T Campbell

TOPICS COVERED IN THIS CHAPTER

- **Bioenergetics**
  - Adenosine triphosphate
- **Carbohydrate metabolism**
  - Glucose metabolism
  - Tricarboxylic acid cycle
  - The adenosine triphosphate balance sheet
  - Aerobic and anaerobic metabolism
  - The pentose monophosphate shunt
  - Glycogen metabolism
  - The endocrine pancreas
- **Fat metabolism**
  - Fat as a metabolic fuel
- **Protein metabolism**
  - Amino acid metabolism
  - Gluconeogenesis
  - Regulation of protein metabolism
- **Whole-body protein and energy metabolism**
  - Measurement of energy expenditure
  - Heat and energy
  - Factors that affect respiratory exchange ratio
  - Energy expenditure in humans
  - Measurement of 24-hour energy expenditure
- **Energy and nutrient intake**
  - Assessment of nutrient intake

BIOENERGETICS

The body obtains its energy from the oxidation of carbohydrate, fat, and protein. Glucose is an immediate source of energy, fat the major store, and protein forms the structure of the body itself. Fat and carbohydrate are the principal energy substrates, but 10–15% of energy is normally derived from protein oxidation. Protein synthesis and breakdown take place simultaneously, so that lean tissue mass is in a dynamic equilibrium. In the healthy individual, protein oxidation occurs at a rate equal to that of protein intake, usually around 1 g/kg/day.

Adenosine triphosphate

The energy derived from oxidation of these complex organic molecules is taken up by the formation of high-energy phosphate bonds, mainly in adenosine triphosphate (ATP). This ubiquitous molecule is the immediate energy supply for most energy-requiring processes in the body. The hydrolysis of ATP into adenosine diphosphate (ADP) releases energy for immediate use in processes such as muscle contraction, membrane transport, protein synthesis, etc. At any one moment the body contains only about 1 g of ATP, but the 24-hour turnover rate is in the region of 45 kg. Thus, mechanisms for the replenishment of ATP need to be integrated intimately with those of ATP utilization.

Some ATP is formed directly by chemical reactions that incorporate a phosphate group. This is known as *substrate-level phosphorylation* and does not involve oxygen, but most ATP is created by a more complex process known as *oxidative phosphorylation* (Fig. 65.1).

'Oxidation' means loss of electrons, but organic molecules do not give up electrons easily and oxidation of a complex molecule such as glucose involves the loss of an entire atom, usually hydrogen. Thus oxidation (dehydrogenation) of a compound such as glucose involves the production of the low-energy compound carbon dioxide, acceptance of electrons (H atoms) ultimately by oxygen to produce water, and the release of energy, which is 'captured' in ATP.

Highly reduced compounds such as glucose (i.e. containing many hydrogen atoms) are high-energy compounds, whereas oxidized compounds with few or no hydrogen atoms (CO_2 and H_2O) are of relatively low energy. As hydrogen ions are released in various parts of the glucose oxidation pathway they are taken up temporarily by *coenzymes*, most commonly nicotinamide adenine dinucleotide (NAD^+) and flavine adenine dinucleotide (FAD), which are converted into NADH and $FADH_2$, respectively. They are then passed on to the flavoprotein–cytochrome system, a series of enzymes situated in the inner membrane of the mitochondrion, known also as the respiratory chain, where the process of oxidative phosphorylation takes place (see Fig. 65.1). Each enzyme in the respiratory chain has a greater affinity for electrons than the one before, which facilitates the passage of electrons from one enzyme to the next, with the release of free energy at each step. Each enzyme is reduced and then reoxidized as electrons pass down the chain. The final enzyme in

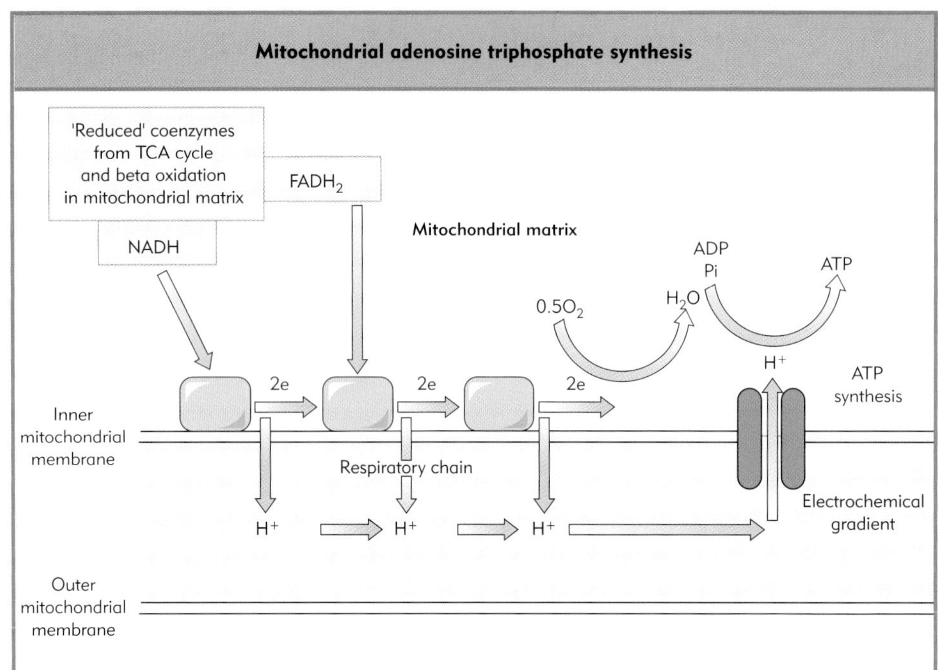

Figure 65.1 Mitochondrial ATP synthesis. Hydrogen atoms are transferred on to the flavoprotein–cytochrome (respiratory) chain, which moves protons through the inner mitochondrial membrane and subsequently generates ATP. Protons transferred into the intermembrane space create an electrochemical gradient that drives ATP synthesis by the H^+ ATPase. TCA, tricarboxylic acid; NADH, reduced nicotinamide adenine dinucleotide; $FADH_2$, reduced flavine adenine dinucleotide, Pi, inorganic phosphate.

the chain is cytochrome oxidase, which transfers hydrogen to oxygen to form water.

Enough free energy is released to synthesize a molecule of ATP at three sites in the respiratory chain, and so three molecules of ATP are synthesized for each molecule of NADH that is oxidized, i.e. that donates a hydrogen atom. The electrons from $FADH_2$ enter the chain at the second electron transfer step, so two molecules of ATP are synthesized for each hydrogen atom donated. This makes a total of four for each molecule of $FADH_2$ oxidized (see Fig. 65.1).

ATP is not synthesized directly: the energy released drives hydrogen ions (protons) across the inner mitochondrial membrane into the intermembrane space to create an electrochemical gradient across the inner membrane. The protons then pass back down this gradient, passively, into the mitochondrion and drive a reversible ATPase in the membrane; it is this protein ATPase that generates ATP from ADP (see Fig. 65.1).

CARBOHYDRATE METABOLISM

The principal product of the digestion and absorption of complex carbohydrate is glucose, but other monosaccharides include fructose and galactose. Glucose passes via the portal system through the liver (where some is stored as glycogen) into the systemic circulation, where it may also be stored as glycogen in muscle, or metabolized to give carbon dioxide and water, with the release of energy and the synthesis of ATP.

Carbohydrate normally provides about 40–50% of the body's energy requirements. Some tissues (such as skeletal and cardiac muscle) can function without glucose, and obtain their energy from fatty acid oxidation should their supply of glucose cease, but others (such as nervous tissue and blood cells) are obligatory users of glucose and cannot survive without it.

Glucose is transported into the cytoplasm of cells via a family of glucose transporters – GLUT 1–5. Glucose is transported down a concentration gradient. GLUT 1–3 and GLUT 5 are independent of insulin and are found in erythrocytes (GLUT 1), liver and kidney (GLUT 2), brain (GLUT 3), and jejunum (GLUT 5). GLUT 4 is insulin dependent and is found in muscle – probably the largest glucose 'sink' in the body – and in adipose tissue.

Glucose metabolism

Glucose is metabolized via two sequential metabolic pathways, the Embden–Meyerhof pathway (or glycolysis) and the Krebs or tricarboxylic acid (TCA) cycle (Fig. 65.2).

Glycolysis is the first stage of glucose breakdown; most of the steps in this pathway are reversible. Glucose (6C) is metabolized via six discrete steps to give two molecules of pyruvic acid (3C). At the start of the glycolytic pathway glucose is phosphorylated by hexokinase to give glucose-6-phosphate (not shown in Fig. 65.2); this step, in contrast to most others, is irreversible. Glucose-6-phosphate in liver or muscle can either be converted into glycogen (see later) or enter the glycolytic pathway. In the third step of the pathway, a second phosphorylation occurs by phosphofructokinase to give fructose-1,6-bisphosphate. This step is also irreversible; its regulation is related to the energy status of the cell (i.e. the availability of ATP). Fructose-1,6-bisphosphate (6C) is split into dihydroxyacetone phosphate (3C) and glyceraldehyde-3-phosphate (3C). Dihydroxyacetone phosphate undergoes isomerization to glyceraldehyde-3-phosphate, which is eventually metabolized to pyruvate.

In the liver, dihydroxyacetone phosphate can also be synthesized from glycerol via glycerol-3-phosphate, thus providing a link with fat metabolism and a route whereby glycerol from triglycerides can enter the glycolytic pathway. Two molecules of ATP are used in glycolysis and four are produced. In addition, two molecules of NAD^+ are reduced to NADH, which provides the potential for ATP production in the respiratory chain within the mitochondrion. The net gain of ATP to the cell directly from glycolysis of one molecule of glucose is thus only two molecules of ATP, which is not very efficient, but as substrate-level

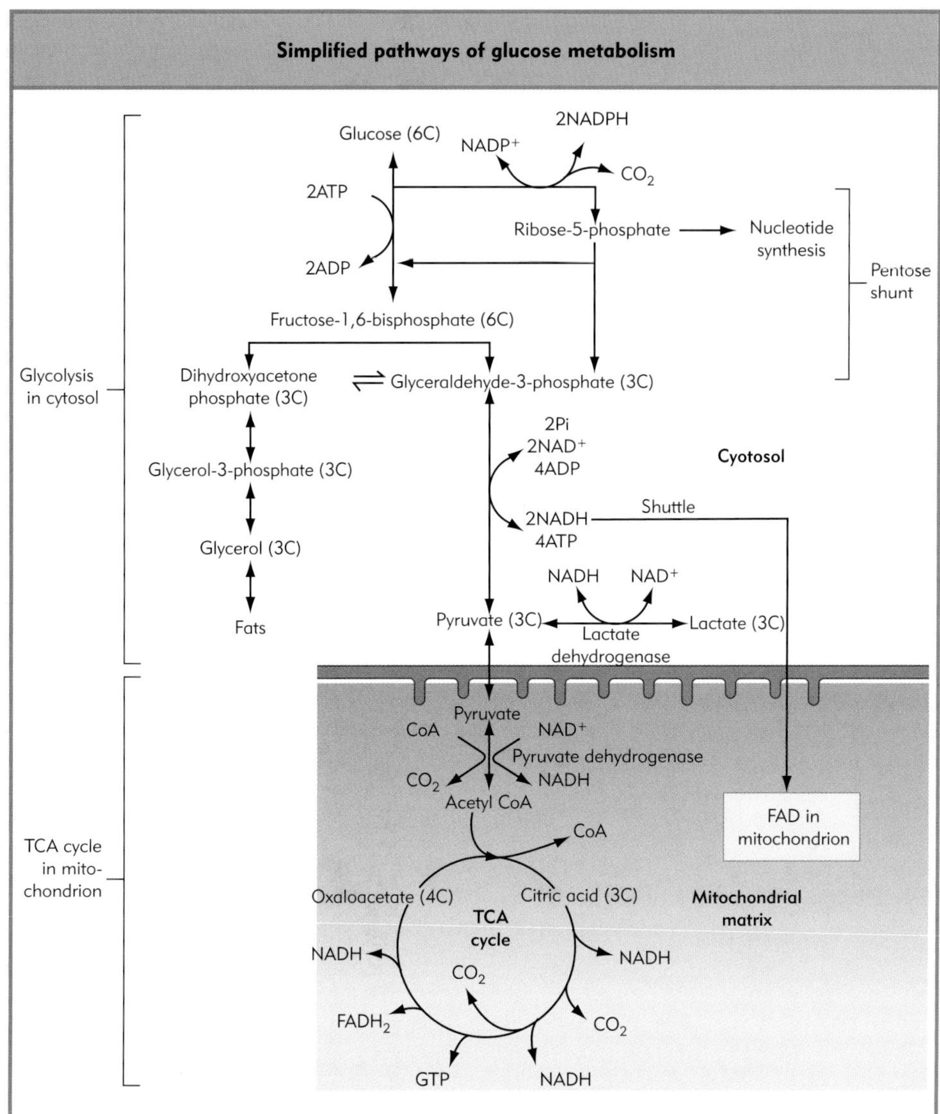

Figure 65.2 Simplified pathways of glucose metabolism. Reduced coenzymes and some ATP are generated by glycolysis. Most ATP is generated in the TCA cycle.

oxidation it occurs in the absence of oxygen. The free-energy yield from glucose at this stage is about 84 kJ/mol (20 kcal/mol), compared with 2827 kJ/mol (673 kcal/mol) when glucose is fully oxidized to carbon dioxide and water. Thus only 3% of the total energy available in the molecule is released by glycolysis.

When NADH is oxidized in the mitochondrion, three molecules of ATP are produced for each molecule of NADH that enters the respiratory chain. The mitochondrial membrane, however, is impermeable to NADH; when NADH is produced in the cytosol by glycolysis, as described above, a shuttle mechanism transfers protons and electrons to FAD within the mitochondrion. For each hydrogen ion, FAD produces only two molecules of ATP, so the two molecules of NADH produced in glycolysis result eventually in a gain of four molecules of ATP instead of six, and this only in the presence of oxygen.

Tricarboxylic acid cycle

Under aerobic conditions, pyruvate now crosses from the cytosol into the mitochondrial matrix and enters the TCA cycle. In a reaction catalyzed by pyruvate dehydrogenase, a two-carbon acetyl group is transferred from pyruvate to the reduced form of coenzyme A (CoA). The third carbon of pyruvate is lost as carbon dioxide via the lungs. It is as acetyl CoA that the two atoms from pyruvate enter the TCA cycle, which is the final common pathway for the breakdown of all intracellular substrate molecules. All two-carbon acetyl groups ($CH_3COO–$) enter the TCA cycle in this fashion, coupled to the terminal SH group of CoA as acetyl CoA ($CH_3COOCoA$).

In the first part of the cycle the acetyl group is transferred to oxaloacetic acid (4C) to form citric acid and free CoA (see Fig. 65.2). There are a further eight steps in the cycle, which generate a number of other intermediate compounds, such as 2-oxoglutarate (5C) and malate (4C), before the regeneration of oxaloacetic acid ready for another round. Two molecules of carbon dioxide are produced for every (2C) acetyl group that enters the cycle; the carbon atoms lost as carbon dioxide in one round of the cycle are those that entered as an acetyl group in the previous round. The oxidation of each of these acetyl groups to carbon dioxide is coupled to the reduction of NAD^+ and FAD, and each round of the cycle generates three molecules of NADH and one of $FADH_2$, as well as one high-energy phosphate bond in guanosine triphosphate (GTP), which is used to phosphorylate a molecule of ADP to give ATP.

The adenosine triphosphate balance sheet

The net gain during glycolysis is two molecules of ATP, and a further four are gained from the NAD^+–FAD mitochondrial shuttle mechanism. Conversion of pyruvic acid into acetyl CoA yields two molecules of NADH per molecule of glucose (i.e. one per molecule of pyruvate – six ATP molecules altogether) and a further six NADH (18 ATP) molecules are produced by two rounds of the TCA cycle, along with two $FADH_2$ (four ATP) molecules and two ATP molecules via GTP. Thus, 36 molecules of ATP are produced from the complete oxidation of one glucose molecule.

Aerobic and anaerobic metabolism

Molecular oxygen is not needed in the TCA cycle itself but is essential for the oxidation of reduced coenzymes in the mitochondrial electron-transport chain. The regeneration (reduction) of oxidized coenzyme is vital and requires oxygen. Metabolism in the absence of oxygen stops in the cytosol. Available NAD is converted into NADH, so NAD^+ is not available, and hence glycolysis and ATP production cease. Pyruvate, however, can accept hydrogen from NADH to form lactic acid and release some NAD^+, a reaction catalyzed by lactate dehydrogenase. This allows glycolysis to continue until NAD^+ really is exhausted. When the oxygen supply resumes and NAD^+ once more becomes available, lactic acid is converted back into pyruvic NADH, which ultimately transfers its hydrogen to the cytochrome chain.

The pentose monophosphate shunt

An alternative pathway to glycolysis is the pentose monophosphate pathway or shunt (see Fig. 65.2), which is also situated in the cytosol. Its main function is to provide a supply of pentose sugars, essential in the synthesis of nucleotides and nucleic acids, and the reduced form of nicotinamide adenine dinucleotide phosphate (NADPH), a phosphorylated form of NADH used in a variety of biosynthetic pathways. The pathway starts with glucose-6-phosphate and ultimately forms two molecules of NADPH and one molecule of ribose-5-phosphate. Excess ribose-5-phosphate, not needed in nucleotide synthesis, is shunted back into the glycolytic pathway as fructose-6-phosphate and glyceraldehyde-3-phosphate. The pentose phosphate pathway does not use ATP or oxygen; whether glucose is metabolized by this route or via the glycolytic pathway seems to depend on whether the cell is engaged in biosynthesis. It is particularly important in the liver.

Glycogen metabolism

LIVER

Glucose is absorbed, via the portal vein, from the gastrointestinal tract into the liver. Systemic glucose concentrations average 5 mmol/L (90 mg/100 mL), but after a meal portal blood glucose can rise to 10 mmol/L (180 mg/100 mL). Glucose enters cells by carrier-mediated diffusion via specialized proteins in the membrane. The glucose transporter for the liver is GLUT-2, which is not responsive to insulin. Glucose is absorbed into the liver down a diffusion gradient. Hexokinase phosphorylates the glucose to give glucose-6-phosphate, which is also normally independent of insulin. When more glucose is present than required, it is stored as glycogen, a process stimulated and controlled by insulin and by the presence of glucose itself, and mediated by glycogen synthase via glucose-1-phosphate (Fig. 65.3).

Hepatic glycogen is the body's glucose buffer. Glucose is stored in the liver at times of excess – normally following a meal – and maintains blood glucose in the absence of glucose intake. With a prolonged fast, hepatic glycogen stores become exhausted within 24–48 hours. Glucose can be mobilized from liver glycogen when required. Glycogen is broken down via glucose-1-phosphate into glucose-6-phosphate, and glucose is formed from glucose-6-phosphate by glucose-6-phosphatase. The usual stimulus to glycogen breakdown is a fall in blood glucose, and it is mediated by glycogen phosphorylase and brought about by a

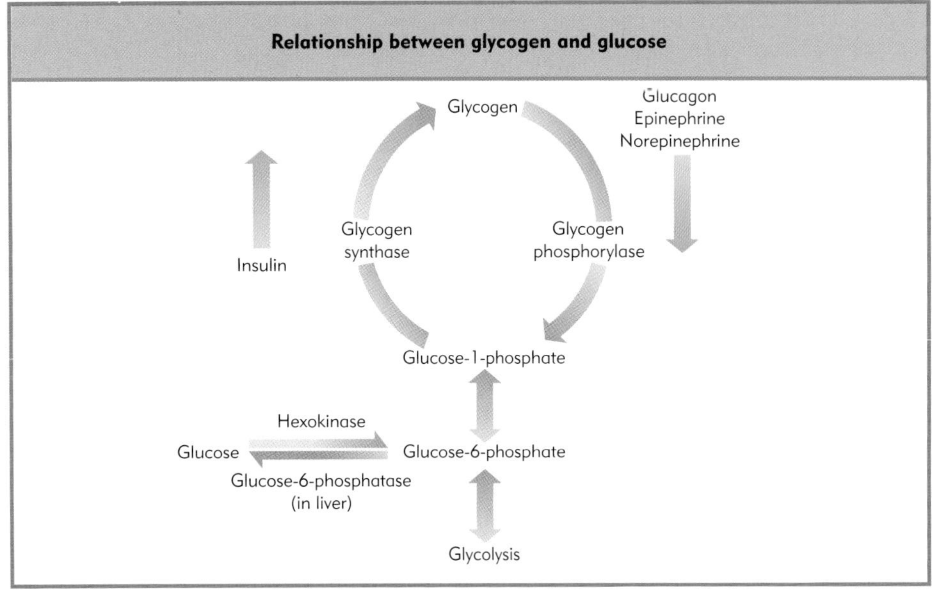

Figure 65.3 Glycogen, its relation to glucose, and the factors that drive its synthesis and breakdown.

change in the balance of the hormones insulin and glucagon; insulin secretion falls and glucagon secretion rises. This stimulates phosphorylation of glycogen phosphorylase by phosphorylase kinase, changing it from its inactive *b* form into its active *a* form, which acts on glycogen to release one molecule of glucose as glucose-1-phosphate. The action of glucagon is mediated by cyclic AMP (cAMP). Other hormones that stimulate glycogenolysis are the catecholamines epinephrine (adrenaline) and norepinephrine (noradrenaline). Their role is important in stress, with the acute mobilization of energy substrate, but probably not in the day-to-day control of blood glucose concentration.

MUSCLE

Muscle is the other major store of glycogen, which is broken down into glucose-6-phosphate with activation of phosphorylase *b* into phosphorylase *a*, as it is in liver. The stimulus on this occasion is usually a nerve impulse that releases Ca^{2+} from the sarcoplasmic reticulum, which results ultimately in the activation of phosphorylase and the formation of glucose-6-phosphate. The other stimulus to glycogenolysis is epinephrine, a process that occurs in stress, such as 'shock' or severe exercise. Muscle does not express glucose-6-phosphatase, and so glucose is not released into the bloodstream but is metabolized via the glycolytic pathway. If the demand for oxygen is greater than the supply, as it may be in 'shock' or severe exercise, lactic acid accumulates and diffuses into the general circulation. This produces a metabolic acidosis, usually buffered by hyperventilation and corrected when the balance of oxygen demand and delivery is restored. Lactate also passes to the liver, where it is synthesized to give glucose via gluconeogenesis.

The endocrine pancreas

Glucose metabolism is largely under the control of insulin and glucagon, hormones secreted by the pancreas. Most of the pancreatic cells are concerned with the exocrine functions of digestion in the small intestine, but insulin and glucagon are both secreted by the islets of Langerhans, little groups of cells that are scattered throughout the pancreas. About a million islets constitute around 1–2% of the pancreatic mass and consist of three cell types, A, B, and D. The A cells secrete glucagon, the B cells insulin, and the D cells somatostatin. Each islet is supplied by a branch of the pancreatic artery, and the venous drainage, via the pancreatic vein, enters into the portal vein just before it enters the liver. Thus, the liver is the first organ on which insulin and glucagon exert their effects before being diluted by the general circulation.

Insulin consists of two peptide chains linked by two disulfide bonds (Fig. 65.4). The A chain has 21 amino acids and the B chain 30. Insulin is synthesized as a single polypeptide chain (proinsulin), and the connecting peptide, C peptide, is removed before secretion. Insulin is internalized and hydrolyzed by the cells it acts upon, so that circulating concentrations are a function of both rates of utilization and rates of secretion. As C peptide is not utilized it can be used as an indicator of insulin secretion. The stimulus to insulin secretion, and to its synthesis, is the plasma glucose concentration. Secretion is stimulated when plasma glucose rises above 5 mmol/L (90 mg/100 mL). It circulates freely in the bloodstream, not attached to any carrier proteins, and binds to specific receptors on its target cells. The intracellular action of insulin is mediated ultimately by dephosphorylation or sometimes phosphorylation of specific enzymes.

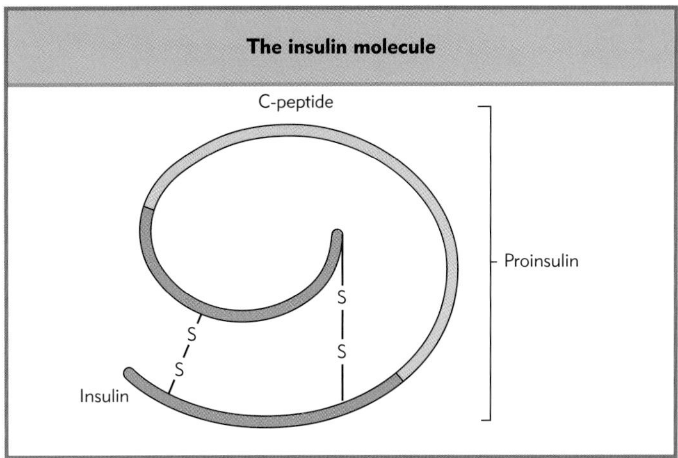

Figure 65.4 The insulin molecule. Insulin in synthesized as proinsulin, which is cleaved to insulin and C peptide.

Only about 50% of the insulin secreted by the pancreas reaches the general circulation; the rest is taken up by the liver after its initial secretion into the portal vein. This close relationship with the liver is a major regulatory factor in the control of glucose metabolism.

Glucagon is a polypeptide of 29 amino acids. Its major action is to elevate blood glucose by stimulating glycogenolysis in the liver. Secretion is stimulated by a fall and suppressed by an increase in blood glucose. Glucagon, like insulin, is also partially removed on its first pass through the liver, but in smaller quantities. It acts on receptors in the membrane of its target cells; the receptors are coupled to stimulation of adenylyl cyclase via G proteins. Glucagon and insulin thus have reciprocal roles in glucose homeostasis.

In addition, glucagon and insulin secretion are both controlled by the sympathetic nervous system. β-Adrenergic stimulation of the islets of Langerhans stimulates insulin secretion, whereas α-adrenergic stimulation inhibits it. Following a stressful stimulus, such as trauma, the α or inhibiting effect is predominant. Sympathetic activation stimulates glucagon secretion.

FAT METABOLISM

Fat is an integral part of the cell membrane and lipids of various sorts are fundamental to the structure of the central nervous system. It is as adipose tissue, however, that fat (triacylglycerol (TAG) or triglyceride) forms the major energy store of the body. Formed of glycerol and three fatty acids, TAG is absorbed from the gastrointestinal tract via the lymphatics in chylomicrons, the largest of the lipoprotein particles that transport lipids in the plasma, and so it does not pass through the liver. In the tissues, lipoprotein lipase hydrolyzes TAG in the chylomicron to release free fatty acids, which mostly pass into adipose tissue (Fig. 65.5). Lipoprotein lipase is synthesized in adipocytes, but in adipose tissue it is attached to the capillary endothelium. It is activated by insulin, which rises rapidly after a meal in response to glucose, but the maximum action of insulin on lipoprotein lipase is 2–3 hours after the meal.

The mobilization of FFAs from adipose tissue is known as *lipolysis*, which releases them (bound to albumin) into the circulation for use as energy substrate. The hydrolysis of TAG to

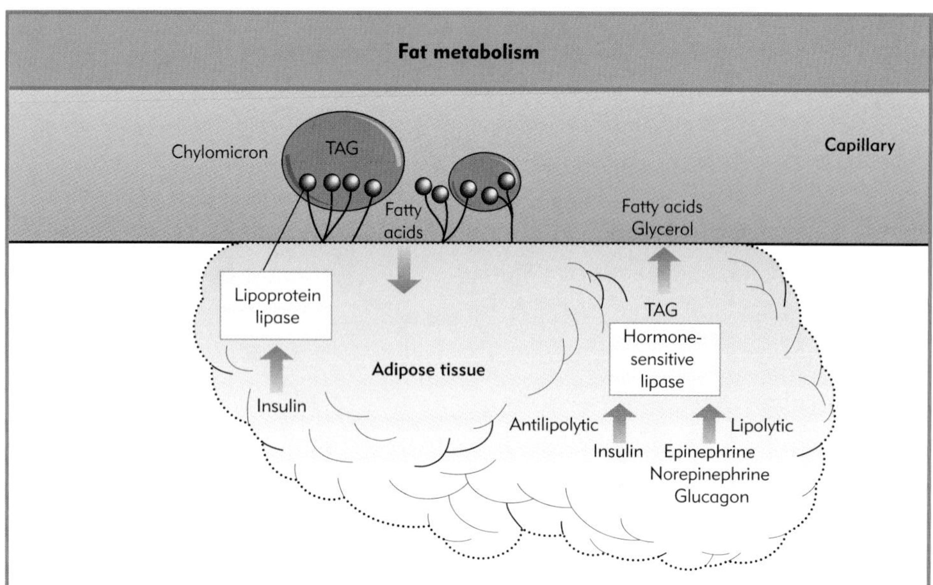

Figure 65.5 Fat metabolism. The take-up of free fatty acids (FFSs) into adipose tissue and the factors that control their release into the circulation. Lipoprotein lipase hydrolyzes TAG molecules in the chylomicron to release fatty acids and glycerol. The process is stimulated by insulin and reversed by hormone-sensitive lipase, which is stimulated by the 'stress' or counterregulatory hormones.

give FFAs and glycerol is controlled by the enzyme hormone-sensitive lipase, situated within the adipocyte, which is stimulated by the catecholamines epinephrine and norepinephrine and inhibited by insulin. Glucagon stimulates lipolysis in vitro, but it is unclear whether it is active in vivo. It may have a role by virtue of its reciprocal activity with insulin, rising and stimulating lipolysis when blood glucose and insulin levels fall.

Fat as a metabolic fuel

Fatty acids are used as a metabolic fuel by peripheral tissues, including skeletal muscle and myocardium. They arise from lipolysis of TAG in adipose tissue in the form of FFAs or from TAG circulating in lipoprotein particles. As TAG cannot be taken up directly by the cell, it is first hydrolyzed to FFAs and glycerol. This is carried out by lipoprotein lipase attached to the capillary endothelium, as described previously in relation to fatty acid uptake (see Fig. 65.5). The FFAs are taken up across the cell membrane, possibly by a specific transport mechanism, at a rate closely related to their concentration in the plasma, and oxidized in the cell in accordance with their rate of uptake. The glycerol moiety is transported to the liver, where it is converted into dihydroxyacetone phosphate, a component of the glycolysis pathway, and is either oxidized via pyruvate and acetyl CoA or converted into glucose (see Fig. 65.2).

β OXIDATION AND CARNITINE

Fatty acids are oxidized in mitochondria by β oxidation, which results in the formation of acetyl CoA. Two carbon fragments are cleaved from the end of the fatty acid molecule by a process that involves dehydrogenation and hydration, with hydrogen atoms transferred to a flavoprotein to form acetyl CoA. Most of the metabolically important fatty acids have an even number of carbon atoms, so the whole molecule is converted into acetyl CoA, which can then enter the TCA cycle. The longer-chain fatty acids, however, are unable to penetrate mitochondria unless linked to carnitine, a substance synthesized from methionine and lysine in the liver and kidneys. It is only as acyl carnitine that the longer-chain FFAs gain access to the β oxidation system in mitochondria. Shorter, so-called medium-chain (8–12C) fatty acids do not need carnitine to gain access to the mitochondrion.

KETONE BODIES

In the absence of exogenous energy substrate, glycogen stores are exhausted within 24–48 hours. The glucose requirements of nervous tissue, including the brain, which can oxidize nothing else are met initially by glucose formed by gluconeogenesis, which inevitably involves an undesirable breakdown of lean tissue (see later). After 4–10 days of simple starvation the brain adapts (in part) to obtain about a half to two-thirds of its requirements from ketone bodies. These substances – acetoacetate and β-hydroxybutyrate – are synthesized in the liver from FFAs. Acetone is formed from acetoacetate by loss of carbon dioxide, but is not metabolized further and is excreted on the breath.

FAT STORES

Fat is the main storage tissue in the body. In the last 10 years it has been recognized that the size of the fat store appears to be regulated by leptin. This is a polypeptide hormone secreted by adipocytes. Circulating concentrations are proportional to adipose tissue mass. Leptin acts on the hypothalamus; high circulating leptin concentrations reduce energy (food) intake and lower leptin levels increase it. In small animals leptin also increases energy expenditure via an action on the sympathetic nervous system.

PROTEIN METABOLISM

Proteins are made up of amino acid chains connected by amide bonds (see Chapter 1), and are digested in the small intestine and absorbed as amino acids and dipeptides. They are incorporated into different proteins in the body in a continual cycle of replacement and renewal, but in the process some are oxidized and about 10–15% of the body's energy requirements are derived from protein oxidation. The nitrogen in proteins is excreted as urea.

Amino acid metabolism

The first step in the catabolism of an amino acid is removal of the NH_2 group and its replacement with a C=O group (deamination) to form a keto or oxo acid. The various oxo acids are metabolic intermediates in, or closely related to, the metabolic pathways already described (glycolysis, TCA cycle, etc.) and can be oxidized to give carbon dioxide and water. Thirteen of them, derived from the so-called glucogenic amino acids, can be synthesized into glucose only (a process called gluconeogenesis), one can be synthesized into fat (ketogenic), and the remainder can be synthesized into either glucose or fat.

The conversion of amino acids into glucose is important in the absence of glucose intake, particularly as a means of maintaining a supply of glucose for the CNS. Gluconeogenesis occurs in both the liver and the kidney. The removal of the NH_2 group from an amino acid produces ammonia, which is toxic. It is metabolized, however, as soon as it is formed, and blood concentrations of ammonia itself are normally very low. In the liver, ammonia forms urea via the urea cycle (see below), but in peripheral tissues NH_2 groups are transferred (transaminated) to keto acids, principally α-ketoglutarate, an intermediate in the TCA cycle, to form glutamate (one NH_2 group) and glutamine (two NH_2 groups). They are also transferred to pyruvate, the corresponding keto acid to alanine; it is principally as alanine and glutamine that NH_2 groups are transported from the periphery to the liver and kidney. As well as being a precursor for renal gluconeogenesis, glutamine also helps to buffer excess acid secretion. Alanine is the major precursor of hepatic gluconeogenesis.

THE UREA CYCLE

Urea synthesis takes place in the liver via a cyclic pathway. The key compound is ornithine, on which the urea molecule is 'built'; intermediates in the process include citrulline and arginine. Ammonia is released from amino acids, largely glutamine and alanine (as described earlier), and incorporated, along with carbon dioxide and ATP, into carbamoyl phosphate in the mitochondrion of the hepatocyte. Urea synthesis and its 'release' take place in the cytosol. The whole process is stimulated by glucagon, which is also important in regulating the uptake of amino acids by the liver.

Gluconeogenesis

In times of nutrient shortage, such as simple starvation and the undernutrition that usually complicates sepsis and trauma, the body maintains its glucose requirements by synthesizing glucose from a number of smaller molecules, mainly glycerol, lactate, and amino acids. Essentially, the process is a reversal of glycolysis except that there are three irreversible steps in glycolysis; in gluconeogenesis, these are bypassed. Most of the amino acids are deaminated and enter the TCA cycle at a variety of points. Pyruvate, the corresponding oxo acid to alanine, is the main precursor and is, of course, closely related to lactate. It is carboxylated to give oxaloacetate (a constituent of the TCA cycle), and then converted into phosphoenolpyruvate by the enzyme phosphoenolpyruvate carboxykinase (PEPCK). Phosphoenolpyruvate is a constituent of the second part of the glycolytic pathway, which is reversed to form glucose. Stages of glycolysis that are otherwise irreversible – the conversion of fructose-6-phosphate into fructose-1,6-bisphosphate by phosphofructokinase, and the formation of glucose from glucose-6-phosphatase – are bypassed by fructose-1,6-bisphosphatase and glucose-6-phosphatase, respectively. Glycerol, the third main precursor, is converted into glycerol-3-phosphate and dihydroxyacetone, which are also constituents of the second part of the glycolytic pathway (see Fig. 65.2).

Gluconeogenesis is controlled by the rate of arrival of the precursors at the liver from peripheral tissue, and by the activity of PEPCK, fructose-l,6 bisphosphatase, and glucose-6-phosphatase. The delivery of gluconeogenic precursors to the liver is controlled by events in peripheral tissues, such as the production of lactate from muscle during exercise (or shock), glycerol from lipolysis in starvation or after adrenergic stimulation, and amino acids in starvation or injury, brought about by inhibition of insulin release or resistance to its action. The activity of the various enzymes is stimulated principally by glucagon, but cortisol and lack of insulin has some effect as well.

Regulation of protein metabolism

In the normal individual who has a stable body mass, protein intake, protein synthesis, and protein degradation are in balance. Insulin normally stimulates protein synthesis and maintains protein balance, although other hormones are important, particularly in skeletal muscle (the largest depot of protein in the body). These include growth hormone, insulin-like growth factor-l (IGF-l), glucocorticoids, and thyroxine. Insulin secretion is stimulated by amino acids, but protein taken in excess of requirements is not stored and so does not lead to an increase in lean body mass. Exogenous stimuli that increase lean body mass include exercise and anabolic steroids, and also growth hormone and IGF-l. In animals, β_2-adrenergic stimulants are anabolic, but such an effect has not yet been convincingly shown in humans. However, during recovery from a wasting illness, such as trauma, sepsis, or malnutrition, the body avidly retains ingested nitrogen by mechanisms that remain unclear.

In trauma and sepsis the balance between protein synthesis and breakdown is disturbed. In relatively mild trauma, such as elective surgery, protein synthesis is depressed but degradation may be normal, so the net effect is a loss of lean body mass. In severe sepsis and multiple injury both are elevated; in absolute terms breakdown is elevated more than synthesis, so lean tissue is lost. The situation is also affected by feeding, in that an increase in nutrient intake elevates both breakdown and synthesis, but in a complex fashion that depends on the level of feeding.

An increase in gluconeogenesis occurs in starvation and following sepsis and trauma. The use of amino acids as gluconeogenic precursors is of concern because they arise from the breakdown of lean tissue mass. In the normal individual glucose infusion suppresses gluconeogenesis completely. In the septic or injured patient gluconeogenesis is suppressed, but only by about 50%. The most that can be achieved by feeding the severely septic or injured individual is to attenuate the rate of loss of lean tissue, not prevent it.

The stimulus to this catabolism of protein in trauma and sepsis is considered to be the counterregulatory hormones –

catecholamines, cortisol, glucagon, and growth hormone – but infusion of these substances into normal volunteers does not reproduce a catabolic state of the severity seen after injury or sepsis. Cytokines are probably involved as well. They are certainly involved centrally in terms of stimulating the counter-regulatory hormone output, but the extent to which they affect peripheral protein metabolism, either directly or via an effect on hepatic protein metabolism, is not known.

WHOLE-BODY PROTEIN AND ENERGY METABOLISM

Measurement of energy expenditure

The energy released by the oxidation of carbohydrate, fat, and protein is taken up to produce high-energy phosphate compounds, which are used in various energy-requiring processes. Two methods of measuring energy expenditure are to measure either the energy liberated *(direct calorimetry)* or the oxygen consumed *(indirect calorimetry)*. The latter technique requires assumptions about the amount of energy liberation that the consumption of a given quantity of oxygen denotes.

Heat and energy

The terms heat and energy have so far been used interchangeably; heat, however, is a form of energy. Because the early metabolic measurements in humans were of heat output, the units used in energy metabolism are usually those of heat, the calorie or kilocalorie (kcal), and the techniques of biologic energy measurement are referred to as *calorimetry*. The calorie is defined as the amount of heat required to raise the temperature of 1 g of water by 1°C. The unit of energy or work is the Joule; this is the work done when a force of 1 Newton moves through a distance of 1 m. The two are interrelated by a constant known as the *mechanical equivalent of heat*: 1 calorie = 4.2 Joules (J).

With the arrival of the SI system of units nearly 40 years ago, it was deemed more correct to report metabolic measurements in Joules, or more conveniently kiloJoules (kJ), as this was the true unit of energy, but the kilocalorie is still in common use.

INDIRECT CALORIMETRY

Direct calorimetry is a tedious and cumbersome technique and is not discussed here.

The traditional method, and probably still the simplest way of measuring oxygen consumption, is the use of a spirometer, such as the Benedict–Roth. This consists of a volume of oxygen in a spirometer bell and a closed circuit through which the subject breathes. Carbon dioxide is absorbed and the rate of decrease of the bell's volume over a given period is calculated. The design of the circuit bears a remarkable resemblance to some of the more commonly used (closed) anesthetic circuits. Gas volumes in indirect calorimetry are conventionally reported at standard temperature and pressure dry (STPD; i.e. at 32°F 0°C) and 101.3 kPa (760 mmHg)).

The energy value of oxygen consumed depends on the substrate metabolized. Equations 65.1–65.3 summarize energy values for carbohydrate (65.1), fat (65.2), and amino acid (65.3) oxidation; Equation 65.4 shows the synthesis of fat from carbohydrate, which consumes energy and results in a respiratory quotient greater than 1. The respiratory quotient (RQ) is the ratio of carbon dioxide produced to oxygen consumed.

■ Equation 65.1

$$1\text{ glucose} + 6O_2 \rightarrow 6CO_2 + 6H_2O + 673\text{ kcal }(2827\text{ kJ})$$
$$\text{i.e. } 5.03\text{ kcal }(21.1\text{ kJ})/\text{L } O_2$$
$$RQ = 1.0$$

■ Equation 65.2

$$1\text{ palmitate} + 23O_2 \rightarrow 16CO_2 + 16H_2O + 2398\text{ kcal }(10\,072\text{ kJ})$$
$$\text{i.e. } 4.68\text{ kcal }(19.7\text{ kJ})/\text{L } O_2$$
$$RQ = 0.7$$

■ Equation 65.3

$$1\text{ amino acid} + 5.1O_2 \rightarrow 4.1CO_2 + 0.7\text{urea} + 28H_2O + 475\text{ kcal}(1995\text{ kJ})$$
$$\text{i.e. } 4.18\text{ kcal }(17.4\text{ kJ})/\text{L } O_2$$
$$RQ = 0.8$$

■ Equation 65.4

$$45\text{ glucose} + 4O_2 \rightarrow 1\text{ palmitoyl} — [11CO_2 + 11H_2O + 630\text{ kcal}(2646\text{ kJ})]$$
$$\text{i.e. } 7.06\text{ kcal }(29.7\text{ kJ})/\text{L } O_2$$
$$RQ = 2.75$$

It can be seen that the relationships between oxygen consumed, carbon dioxide produced, and energy released vary. At STPD, in the oxidation of fat the calorific value of 1 L of oxygen is 19.7 kJ (4.68 kcal) and in the oxidation of carbohydrate it is 21.1 kJ (5.03 kcal). An RQ in excess of 1.0 denotes net fat synthesis from carbohydrate. The RQ, however, is a biochemical concept and is impossible to measure in the whole body. What can be measured is the pulmonary exchange of oxygen and carbon dioxide, but this is affected by factors other than substrate oxidation. It is more correctly known as the respiratory exchange ratio (RER). For RER to approximate RQ, the subject has to be in a steady state and the measurement has to be made over at least 30 minutes.

The RQ of protein depends on the precise make-up of the protein and is generally in the region of 0.80–0.85, but protein is not oxidized completely into carbon dioxide and water; a variety of other nitrogen- and energy-containing products of protein metabolism are excreted in the urine. The relationship between protein oxidation and urinary nitrogen is fairly constant; on average, 1 g of urinary nitrogen denotes oxidation of 6.3 g of protein. The amount of protein used as an energy substrate over a given period can thus be quantified purely from a measure of urinary nitrogen collected over that period, with a correction made as necessary for alterations in the body urea pool (estimated from changes in blood urea). In practice, urinary nitrogen is rarely measured because of technical difficulties; it is more usual to measure urinary urea. Of the urinary nitrogen, 80% is excreted as urea, although this is highly variable (both between and within individuals) and has a range of 60–100%. Also, during starvation more nitrogen is excreted in the form of ammonia. As a technique to assess protein metabolism for research purposes urea measurement is not really acceptable, but for clinical purposes it is probably adequate.

Excretion of 1 g of nitrogen also denotes the consumption of 5.94 L of oxygen and the production of 4.76 L of carbon dioxide; thus the gas exchange associated with protein metabolism can be calculated and subtracted from total gas exchange as measured, to give the gas exchange associated with fat and carbohydrate oxidation only. The RQ so calculated and associated with only fat and carbohydrate oxidation is called the *nonprotein* RQ and, assuming RQ and RER to be equivalent, allows the proportions of energy expenditure derived from fat and carbohydrate oxidation to be calculated. This, in combination with the oxygen consumption figure, also enables values for total quantities of fat and carbohydrate to be calculated. Equations 65.5 and 65.6 can also be used to quantify fat and carbohydrate oxidation, in which C and F are carbohydrate and fat oxidation in grams, $\dot{V}O_2$ and $\dot{V}CO_2$ are expressed in liters (at STPD), and N represents urinary nitrogen excretion in grams.

■ Equation 65.5

$$C = 4.14\dot{V}CO_2 - 2.908\dot{V}O_2 - 2.543N$$

■ Equation 65.6

$$F = 1.689\ (\dot{V}O_2 - \dot{V}CO_2) - 1.943N$$

The problem with using the spirometer to measure oxygen consumption is that it has to be 'driven' by the subject, who interfaces with the instrument via a mouthpiece and nose clip. This works for a trained volunteer, but seriously ill patients tolerate it poorly.

An alternative technique is to measure inspired ($\dot{V}I$) and expired $\dot{V}E$) air volumes and the concentrations of oxygen and carbon dioxide in each, either via a mouthpiece and nose clip or face mask, or by drawing a measured volume of air past the subject's face and collecting the mixed expired air for analysis. Equations 65.7 and 65.8 are used, in which (FI) and (FE) are the fractional concentrations of oxygen and carbon dioxide in inspired and mixed expired air, respectively. The concentration of carbon dioxide in inspired air is usually ignored.

■ Equation 65.7

$$\dot{V}O_2 = (\dot{V}I \times (FIO_2)) - (\dot{V}E \times (FEO_2))$$

■ Equation 65.8

$$\dot{V}CO_2 = \dot{V}E \times (FECO_2)$$

Inspired and expired volume are measured separately as they are usually unequal – less carbon dioxide is normally expired than oxygen is consumed, as the RQ is usually in the range 0.7–1.0. To measure both inspired and expired volumes is complex and probably introduces more errors than would exist if the difference between the two volumes were ignored completely. The conventional procedure is for one of these two volumes to be measured and the other calculated using the inspired and expired nitrogen concentrations, as in Equation 65.9, in which NI and NE are the concentrations of nitrogen in the inspired and mixed expired air, respectively.

■ Equation 65.9

$$\dot{V}E = \dot{V}I \times \left(\frac{NI}{NE}\right)$$

This is known as the Haldane transformation and assumes that the net ventilatory exchange of nitrogen is zero (i.e. the subject is in a steady state). Nitrogen is not normally measured, but is taken to be the nonoxygen, noncarbon dioxide gas in the inspired and expired gas volumes.

This works well when the subject breathes air and the nitrogen concentration in the system is high, but in the presence of a high FIO_2 as in ventilated patients, the concentration of nitrogen is diminished; with an inspired oxygen concentration of 100%, no nitrogen is in the system and so the Haldane transformation is not applicable. In practice, with most indirect calorimeters that use the Haldane transformation, the system ceases to function at an FIO_2 of about 0.7.

There are essentially two ways around the problem: one is to measure the inspired and expired volumes separately, but this is complex and demands a very high degree of accuracy from the volume measuring devices. The other is to calculate $\dot{V}CO_2$ from measurement of $\dot{V}E$ and the mixed expired carbon dioxide concentration alone, then assume RQ and calculate $\dot{V}O_2$ and energy expenditure accordingly. This can introduce an error of up to about 15%, but for clinical purposes is not unreasonable. In a critically ill patient in multiple organ failure it is certainly better than not to make the measurement at all.

Factors that affect respiratory exchange ratio

Factors other than substrate oxidation also affect RER, and include hyperventilation (or hypoventilation), which produces a transient rise (or fall) in RER until a new steady state is achieved, and metabolic acidosis (or alkalosis) in which carbon dioxide is excreted (or retained) to compensate. As a result of the different solubilities of the two gases in the body, a change in body temperature produces a differential retention of carbon dioxide should temperature fall, or a rise in carbon dioxide excretion should temperature rise. All of these limitations need to be borne in mind when interpreting measurements of RER as an indicator of substrate oxidation.

Energy expenditure in humans

The principal components of energy expenditure in humans are basal energy expenditure, dietary-induced thermogenesis, activity, nonshivering thermogenesis, and hormonal control of metabolic rate.

BASAL ENERGY EXPENDITURE

Basal energy expenditure is the energy expended when the body is totally at rest in such processes as the maintenance of cell membrane potentials, ventilation, and the action of the heart. It is the largest single component of 24-hour energy expenditure and is conventionally measured at rest, after an overnight fast, and with the subject thermoneutral (i.e. neither hot enough to stimulate heat loss nor cold enough to stimulate heat generation).

Although ideally basal metabolism is measured, it is possible to predict it using a number of formulae. One such is the Harris–Benedict formula, in which B is 24-hour basal energy expenditure (kcal), W is body weight (kg), H is height (cm), and A is age (years). Equation 65.10 is for men, and Equation 65.11 is for women.

■ Equation 65.10

$$B = 66.47 + 13.75W + 5.003H - 6.750A$$

■ Equation 65.11

$$B = 655.1 + 9.563W + 1.850H - 4.676A$$

The more recent Schofield analysis gives a series of equations of the form $y = mx + c$ (x is weight) for various age groups. The factors common to these formulae and to others of the same type are *body size* (i.e. height and/or weight), *age* (metabolic rate decreases steadily from the age of 6 months, with a minor rise at puberty), and *gender* (women generally have more body fat than men; this is metabolically less active than lean tissue and is a better insulator).

DIETARY-INDUCED THERMOGENESIS

Dietary-induced thermogenesis, formerly called specific dynamic action, is the rise in metabolic rate associated with the ingestion of food and is said to represent the energy cost of digestion and assimilation. The argument for this centered on whether the rise in expenditure is related only to the size and timing of a discrete meal, or whether it is related more to the general 'level of nutrition', that is, whether a means exists for humans to oxidize food eaten in excess of requirements, perhaps by mechanisms such as nonshivering thermogenesis. Certainly, starvation is associated with a decrease in basal metabolism, but the conventional view is that a mechanism to metabolize energy eaten in excess of requirements probably does not exist.

ACTIVITY

Energy expenditure rises with activity. In hospital practice the addition of 10–30% to basal expenditure (measured or calculated) is usually enough to take activity into account. For a very active individual, such as a manual laborer or a professional sportsperson, a figure closer to 100% is more appropriate.

NONSHIVERING THERMOGENESIS

Nonshivering thermogenesis is a mechanism of heat production that occurs in hibernating animals and in humans in the first 6 months of life, whereby neonates thermoregulate and hibernating animals warm themselves up after winter. It is associated with a special type of fat called *brown adipose tissue*. In rodents this is found in depots in the back (between the scapulae), and in human neonates in the suprarenal fat, in axillary fat, and around the great vessels of the heart and vertebral arteries. The tissue appears brown because of large numbers of mitochondria, which can be uncoupled; that is, instead of ATP being generated when foodstuffs are metabolized to carbon dioxide and water, free energy is released to serve as a direct heat source. This is associated with the presence of a specific *uncoupling protein* in the walls of the mitochondria, formerly called thermogenin. Thermogenin is now called uncoupling protein 1 (UCP1). Over the last 10 years other uncoupling proteins (UCP2–4) have been described. UCP2 is expressed widely in many types of cells and UCP3 and 4 in skeletal muscle and brain, respectively. Their precise role is uncertain, but they may be involved in fatty acid transport out of the mitochondrion. The protons that pass down the electrochemical gradient and across the inner membrane of the mitochondrion release free energy instead of generating ATP. The process is under the control of the sympathetic nervous system, and brown adipose tissue is richly innervated with sympathetic nerve endings.

This is the principal means available for varying heat production that does not involve muscle contraction. It has been unclear whether the mechanism exists in adult humans as a means of body weight control, as referred to earlier, or to raise body temperature and heat output in response to a pyrogen. The consensus at the moment is that brown adipose tissue probably does not act in this way.

HORMONAL CONTROL OF METABOLIC RATE

Overall control of metabolic rate in the body is via the thyroid hormones. Thyrotoxicosis is associated with a high metabolic rate and myxedema with a reduced one. The catecholamines also increase metabolism, certainly when given in pharmacologic doses, and probably also in response to stimulation of endogenous catecholamine output, possibly secondary to a stimulation of glycolysis, lipolysis, an increase in myocardial contractility, and an increase in muscle tone.

Measurement of 24-hour energy expenditure

INDIRECT CALORIMETRY

The classic method to assess an individual's 24-hour energy expenditure is to keep a record of their activity and measure the energy cost of each type of activity using indirect calorimetry.

Heart rate is also a useful index of energy expenditure and is monitored by telemetry or a portable monitor, and energy expenditure is measured simultaneously by indirect calorimetry and at various levels of expenditure for discrete periods. A regression line is then constructed for an individual that relates heart rate to energy expenditure. If heart rate is measured over 24 hours, expenditure over that period can be predicted from the regression line. This technique is also reasonably accurate for the population, but individual errors are large.

Doubly labeled water is now the standard method of measuring energy expenditure in the free-living individual. A mixture of two isotopes of water (^2H_2O and $H_2{}^{18}O$) is drunk; ^2H_2O equilibrates with the body water pool and $H_2{}^{18}O$ with both the body water and the bicarbonate pools. The (logarithmic) rate of decline of ^2H_2O in the body is a function of whole-body water turnover, and the rate of decline of $H_2{}^{18}O$ is a function of both body water and carbon dioxide turnover, so the difference between the two is a function of carbon dioxide output. A value can be assumed for RQ and energy expenditure calculated, or a dietary record can be kept and RQ derived from the food intake.

The application of this technique is limited by the length of time it takes for isotope enrichment in the body to decline such that a reasonable assessment of carbon dioxide production over that period can be made. This is usually 10–15 days, but obviously varies with the intensity of the activity. Also, only an average measure of energy expenditure is obtained for the period of measurement; if energy expenditure varies widely from day to day, this variability is not identified. Obviously, the longer the period of measurement the smaller the errors. Other limitations are the expense of the isotopes and the specialized nature of the analysis (mass spectrometry).

Rates of decline in isotope enrichment are measured by monitoring body water in blood, urine, or saliva. These can be measured every day for accuracy, but one assessment 10–15 days after administration and mathematic assumptions about the rate of isotope excretion are most convenient.

ENERGY AND NUTRIENT INTAKE

Foodstuffs in the body are metabolized to give carbon dioxide and water, or in the case of protein to give carbon dioxide, water, and urea, creatinine, uric acid, and ammonia. With fat and carbohydrate there is no difference in terms of waste products and energy released when these substrates are oxidized via the numerous biochemical pathways described earlier, or if they are merely burnt (the energy content of fat and carbohydrate can be determined by doing just that in a *bomb calorimeter*). The substance under investigation, in this case food, is dried (either freeze dried or dried in an oven) and ground into a fine powder. A weighed quantity is burnt in oxygen under pressure, which ensures its complete combustion (oxidation). Heat output is measured either in absolute quantities by absorption into a water jacket of known thermal capacity or, in a simpler type of instrument that measures relative heat production, the heat emitted is absorbed by a steel jacket that surrounds the sample. The temperature of this jacket rises transiently to a value that is a function of the total amount of heat emitted, which is compared with the heat emitted by combustion of a known quantity of a standard substance, such as glucose.

The heat energy released from foodstuffs by combustion is the 'gross energy' (GE). For carbohydrate and fat this is the same as the 'metabolizable energy' (ME; i.e. the energy available to the body for metabolic purposes). Equation 65.12 can be used to calculate ME from GE.

■ Equation 65.12

$$ME = 0.95GE - 0.075\%N$$

Equation 65.12 assumes 95% absorption of all foodstuffs – an average value for a standard, mixed western diet (this is somewhat nearer 90% for a high-roughage or high-fiber diet) – and allows for the incomplete oxidation of protein in the body. Products of protein metabolism, mainly urea, still contain energy. A sample has to be analyzed for its nitrogen content.

Assessment of nutrient intake

Methods to assess an individual's energy and nitrogen intake include:

- collecting a duplicate sample of everything the individual eats over a period and subjecting it to the bombing and nitrogen analysis procedures described above;
- collecting a duplicate sample and analyzing it for carbohydrate, fat, and protein content; standard factors are used to convert the figures obtained into energy (carbohydrate, 16.8 kJ/g (4 kcal/g); fat, 37.8 kJ/g (9 kcal/g), and protein,16.8 kJ/g (4.0 kcal/g)); these nutrient conversion factors are average figures – the precise values depend on the particular carbohydrate, fat, or protein being eaten. Other factors commonly used are 9.3 kcal for fat, 4.3 kcal for protein, and 3.75 kcal for carbohydrate (glucose).
- in clinical practice the patient keeps a record of what they eat, either weighing their food or describing portion size, or food intake may be assessed by interview, usually with a dietician. Nutrient analysis is then performed using food composition tables (see Holland et al. for further reading). Many of these are now computerized.

Key references

Frayn KN. Metabolic regulation. A human perspective. Oxford: Blackwell Science; 2003.

Frayn KN. Calculation of substrate oxidation rates in vivo from gaseous exchange. J Appl Physiol. 1989;55:628–34.

Hinkle PL, McCarty RE. How cells make ATP. Sci Am. 1978;238:104–23.

Pilkus SI, El-Maghrahi MR. Hormonal regulation of hepatic gluconeogenesis and glycolysis. Annu Rev Biochem. 1988;57:755–83.

Schofield WN. Predicting basal metabolic rate, new standards and review of previous work. Hum Nutr Clin Nutr. 1985; 39(suppl1):5–41.

Further reading

Bender DA. Introduction to nutrition and metabolism, 2nd edn. London: Taylor & Francis; 1997.

Burzstein S, Elwyn DH, Askanazi J, Kinney JM. Energy metabolism, indirect calorimetry and nutrition. London: Williams & Wilkins; 1989.

Girardier L, Stock MJ. Mammalian thermogenesis. London: Chapman & Hall; 1983.

Holland B, Welch AA, Unwin ID, Buss DH, Paul AA, Southgate DAT. McCance and Widdowson's the composition of foods, 5th edn. London: Royal Society of Chemistry and Ministry of Agriculture, Fisheries and Food; 1991.

Kinney JM, ed. Assessment of energy metabolism in health and disease. Columbus: Ross Laboratories; 1981.

Kleiber M. The fire of life: an introduction to animal energetics. Huntington: Robert Kreiger Publishing Company; 1975.

Matthews HR, Freedland RA, Miesfield RL. Biochemistry. A short course. New York: Wiley-Liss; 1997.

Stryer L. Biochemistry, 4th edn. San Francisco: Freeman & Co; 1995.

Wilmore DW The metabolic management of the critically ill. New York: Plenum Medical Book Company; 1977.

Chapter 66

Endocrinology

Franco Carli, Maria G Annetta and Thomas Schricker

Conceptually the nervous system and the endocrine system have functional similarities in the sense that both operate in a stimulus–response manner and transmit signals. The incoming stimuli and the response are integrated, with changes occurring in the internal and external milieu. Both neurons and endocrine cells can secrete into the bloodstream and generate electrical potential. There are four types of hormonal signaling:

1. endocrine, where the molecular signal is transmitted from an endocrine cell through the bloodstream to a distant target cell;
2. neurocrine, where a molecular signal is transmitted from a neuron, first down its axon and then into bloodstream to a distant target cell;
3. paracrine, where a molecular signal is transmitted from one cell type to a different cell type by diffusion through intercellular fluid channels; and
4. autocrine, where the molecular signal released is transmitted into the intercellular fluid back to the cell of origin or to neighboring identical cells.

There are three chemical classes of hormone: steroids, amines, and peptides/proteins. The amines are synthesized from tyrosine, the steroids from cholesterol, and the peptides/proteins through transcription and specific messenger RNA in the rough endoplasmic reticulum. The secretion of hormones can occur through different feedback mechanisms, which can be either negative or positive. In the former type the excessive secretion of one hormone limits the output of another (e.g. the relationship between the hormones of the pituitary gland and its target glands). With positive feedback the secretion of a target hormone is amplified. Many hormones are secreted in pulses according to a certain pattern. For example, the secretion of cortisol occurs in pulses with a 12-hour variation or circadian rhythm.

The action of a hormone on a target cell occurs through three successive processes: hormone and receptor form a complex, the conformation of the receptor is changed, and the message is generated. Factors such as hormone concentration, receptor number, duration of exposure, and intracellular concentration of rate-limiting enzymes, cofactors, and substrates influence the hormonal effect. The signal (second messenger) causes intracellular changes by modifying the concentration of proteins and enzymes. The second messenger can be either an adenylyl cyclase–cAMP system, a calcium–calmodulin system, or a membrane phospholipase–phospholipid system. The dose–response curve for the action of a hormone exhibits a sigmoidal shape. Sensitivity is expressed as the concentration of the hormone that produces 50% response. Hormones undergo hepatic metabolic degradation by enzymatic processes that include oxidation, reduction, proteolysis, hydroxylation, decarboxylation, and methylation, and are cleared by the kidney.

HYPOTHALAMUS AND PITUITARY GLAND

Anatomy and physiology

The hypothalamus is part of the diencephalon and is located in the area of the third ventricle. It is anatomically and functionally related to the pituitary gland (Fig. 66.1). The entire pituitary gland is situated in a socket of the sphenoid bone called the sella turcica. It consists of two parts, the anterior or adenohypophysis, and the posterior or neurohypophysis. The two lobes are clearly

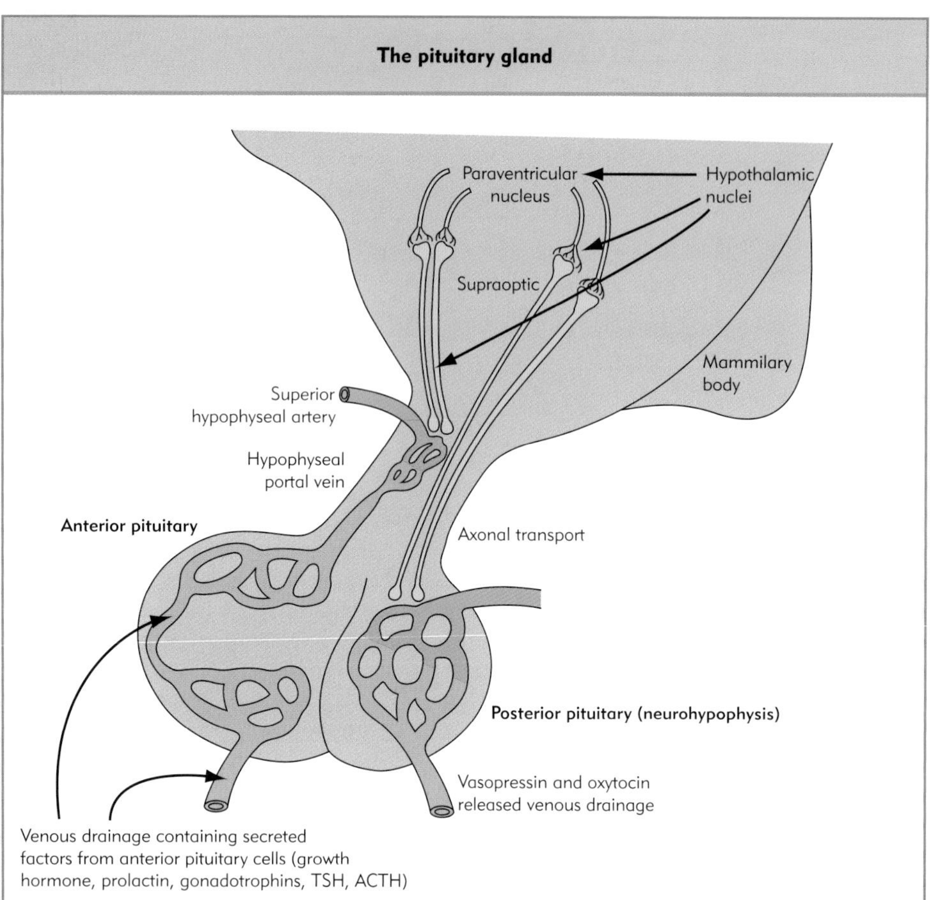

Figure 66.1 The pituitary gland. The hypothalamopituitary axis, showing the hypophyseal portal venous system for delivery of releasing factors.

demarcated and distinguishable. The anterior lobe constitutes 80% of the gland, and is composed of three sections: the pars distalis, or the largest, which is the site of the hormone-producing cells, the intermediate pars, and the tuberalis attached to the pituitary stalk. The posterior pituitary consists of the median eminence of the tuber cinereum, the infundibular stem, and the infundibular process.

The neurohypophysis represents a collection of axons whose cell bodies lie in the hypothalamus. Peptide hormones synthesized in the cell bodies of these hypothalamic neurons travel down their axons in neurosecretory granules to be stored in the nerve terminals, which have neurosecretory vesicles, lying in the posterior pituitary gland. When cell bodies are stimulated the granules are released from the axon terminals by exocytosis, and the peptide hormones enter the peripheral circulation via the capillary plexuses of the inferior hypophyseal artery. This implies that a single cell synthesizes, stores, and releases hormones (neurocrine hormones). Two peptides are synthesized in the cell bodies of hypothalamic neurons and secreted from the posterior pituitary gland: oxytocin, and antidiuretic hormone (ADH) or arginine vasopressin (VAP). Oxytocin's role is to facilitate the ejection of milk from the lactating mammary gland. ADH or VAP has a role to conserve body water and regulate the tonicity of body fluids (Chapter 59).

The anterior pituitary gland or adenohypophysis is a collection of endocrine cells that are regulated by bloodborne stimuli originating in the neural tissue. Hypothalamic neurons synthesize releasing and inhibiting hormones that travel down the axons at the level of the median eminence and are stored as neurosecretory granules in the nerve terminals. Under stimulation of these cells, the releasing and inhibiting hormones are discharged and enter the capillary plexus of the superior hypophyseal artery, and then are transported down the portal veins to reach their specific endocrine target cells in the adenohypophysis. The output of tropic hormones from these cells is increased or decreased in response to the releasing and inhibiting hormones. The tropic hormones released enter a second capillary plexus and then the peripheral circulation. Anterior pituitary hormones are under feedback regulation via the hormones secreted by the target glands on which the pituitary hormones act (Table 66.1). Thus signals from the brain and the periphery interact to regulate pituitary hormone secretions and maintain a normal endocrine state (positive and negative feedback). The hypothalamic–pituitary unit regulates growth, lactation, and the function of the thyroid gland, adrenal glands, and gonads.

Hypothalamic dysfunction

Hypopituitarism (failure to produce hormones) and hyperpituitarism (excess production of hormones) occur as a result of diseases that affect brain tissue, such as primary tumors and metastatic deposits, and of trauma, surgery, radiotherapy, and vascular accidents.

Table 66.1 Hypothalamic releasing or inhibiting hormones and target pituitary hormones

Hypothalamic	Pituitary
Thyrotropin-releasing hormone (TRH)	Thyrotropin (TSH)
Gonadotropin-releasing hormone (GnRH)	Luteinizing hormone (LH) Follicle-stimulating hormone (FSH)
Corticotropin-releasing hormone (CRH)	Adrenocorticotropin (ACTH)
Growth hormone-releasing hormone (GHRH)	Growth hormone (GH)
Growth hormone-inhibiting hormone (somatostatin)	Growth hormone (GH), prolactin
Prolactin-releasing factor (PRF)	Prolactin
Prolactin-inhibiting factor (PIF)	Prolactin

ADH deficiency, called also diabetes insipidus, is caused by the destruction or dysfunction of the supraoptic and paraventricular nuclei of the hypothalamus. This syndrome is characterized by the inability to concentrate urine, resulting in urine osmolality as low as 100 mmol/kg and large volumes of urine (>10 L/day). Administration of fluids and desmopressin (DDAVP) is a standard treatment.

Inappropriate secretion of ADH can be the result of intracranial tumors, hypothyroidism, and carcinoma of the lung. Hyponatremia and low plasma osmolarity need to be monitored to reduce the risk of cerebral edema and seizures. Restriction of oral fluids and administration of demeclocycline are recommended.

THYROID GLAND

Anatomy and physiology

The thyroid is the largest endocrine gland in the human body, weighing about 20–30 g. The adult size is usually reached at age 15. The normally developed thyroid is a bilobed structure lying next to the thyroid cartilage, in a position anterior and lateral to the junction between the larynx and the trachea. The two lobes are joined at the midline by an isthmus which encircles about 75% of the diameter of the junction betweeen the larynx and upper trachea. A feedback loop between hypothalamus, pituitary, and thyroid regulates the secretion of thyroid hormone. The hypothalamus generates thyrotropin-releasing hormone (TRH), which in turn stimulates the production and release of thyrotropin or thyroid-stimulating hormone (TSH) from thyrotropic cells in the anterior pituitary gland. TSH stimulates thyroid hormonal output, which feeds back on both hypothalamus and pituitary to complete the circle. Changes in thyroid hormone levels produce inverse logarithmic changes in thyrotropin secretion. When there is a change in thyroxine levels by a factor of 2, there will be a reflex inverse change in thyrotropin by a factor of 100. This close relationship is the rationale for obtaining thyrotropin serum levels as first-line testing for thyroid dysfunction.

The secretory products of the thyroid gland are *thyroxine* (T_4), *triiodothyronine* (T_3) and *calcitonin*. T_4 is produced only by the thyroid gland, and its daily production ranges between 80 and 100 μg. In contrast, 20% of T_3 is derived directly from thyroid secretion and 80% from peripheral T_4 conversion. The daily T_3 production is 30–40 μg.

In physiologic conditions, thyroid hormone production (Fig. 66.2) requires normal levels of TSH and an adequate supply of iodine. In the thyroid cell, iodide is rapidly oxidized and enzymatically incorporated via thyroid peroxidase into tyrosine molecules to finally form iodotyrosines, either in a single confirmation (monoiodothyrosine, MIT) or in a coupled confirmation (diiodotyrosine, DIT). These forms are stored within the follicle as thyroglobulin. The formation of DIT and MIT is dependent on thyroid peroxidase. Antithyroid medications such as propylthiouracil (PTU) and methimazole inhibit the thyroid peroxidase enzyme, thus decreasing thyroid hormone formation. In normal circumstances, the formation of T_4 is the major pathway. T_3 and T_4 are both bound to thyroglobulin (a 660 kDa lipoprotein) and stored within colloid in the center of the follicular unit. This process results in the storage of about a 2 weeks' supply of thyroid hormone within the organism under normal circumstances.

Reverse T_3 (rT_3) is a thyroid hormone identified only in humans and differs from normal T_3 by the location of iodine on the molecule. The actual source of rT_3 is not precisely known, although it seems that 95–98% is produced in similar fashion to T_3, by deiodination of circulating T_4. Although its exact function and purpose are not known, rT_3 increases in hyperthyroidism and decreases in hypothyroidism. Interestingly, rT_3 increases in several nonthyroid disease states, such as in cirrhosis, in some neoplastic diseases, after major surgery, and with prolonged fasting. Reverse T_3 inhibits the thermogenic activity of T_4 and T_3. T_4 and T_3 exist in plasma in free and protein-bound forms. There are three major thyroid hormone-binding proteins in human serum: thyroxine-binding globulin (TBG), transthyretin (TTR), and albumin. Normally, T_4 is strongly protein bound and only 0.03% is free, whereas 0.3% of T_3 is in free form. TBG binds about 70% of circulating T_4 and T_3, TTR 10–20%, and albumin about 10–20%. A minor fraction of T_3 and T_4 is carried by lipoproteins. The functional status of the hypothalamopituitary axis is usually tested by TRH stimulation. After an intravenous dose of TRH, the normal response should be an elevation in TSH that peaks within 15–35 minutes. In pituitary insufficiency there is a subnormal response to TRH, whereas patients with primary hypothyroidism demonstrate an enhanced TSH release from the anterior pituitary.

Free T_4 and T_3 are hydrophobic and readily pass through cell membranes. In the cell cytoplasm T_4 is converted to T_3, which passes into the nucleus where it binds to nuclear T_3 receptors. Unbound T_3 receptors repress expression of a range of genes, whereas bound T_3 receptors promote gene expression. The actions of thyroid hormone are widespread and complex. Thyroid hormone is important for growth and development, the regulation of intermediary metabolism, and has effects on the cardiovascular system. The importance of normal thyroid function is, however, perhaps appreciated by considering the effects of thyroid dysfunction

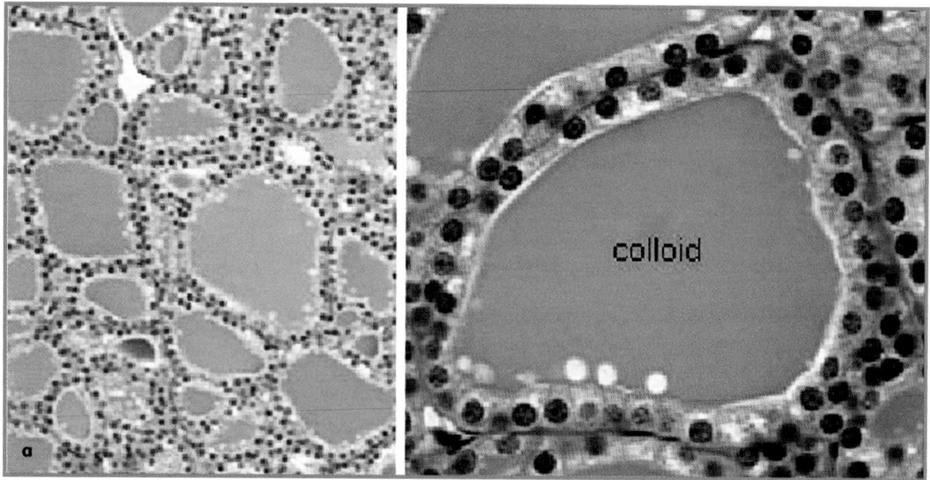

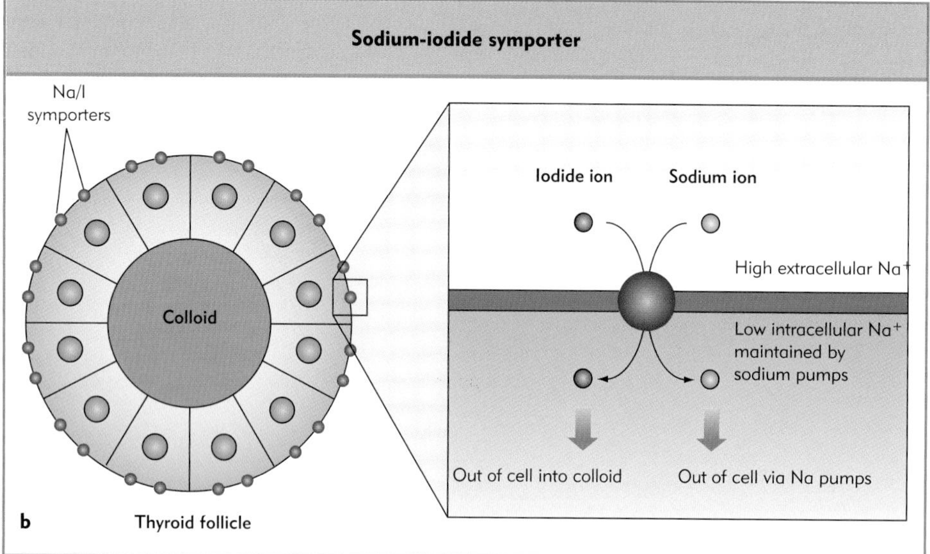

Figure 66.2 Production of thyroid hormones. The thyroid gland consists of follicles of thyroid epithelial cells enclosing colloidal thyroglobulin. (a) Histological section of thyroid gland under low (left) and high (right) magnification. Thyroid hormones require iodintion of tyrosine. Iodine is actively taken up from plasma into thyroid epithelial cells by the sodium–iodide symporter (b).

Continued

Thyroid dysfunction

HYPOTHYROIDISM

Hypothyroidism is the clinical syndrome that results from decreased secretion of thyroid hormone from the thyroid gland. It most frequently reflects a disease of the gland itself (primary hypothyroidism), but can also be caused by pituitary disease (secondary hypothyroidism) or hypothalamic disease (tertiary disease). Hypothyroidism leads to a slowing of metabolic processes, and in its most severe form to the accumulation of mucopolysaccharides in the skin, causing a nonpitting edema termed *myxedema*.

Primary hypothyroidism occurs approximately in 1–2% of the general population. It occurs in women 14 times more often than in men, and is the most common disorder of thyroid function. In many underdeveloped countries the most common cause of hypothyroidism is iodine deficiency, whereas in more developed countries the most common cause of adult hypothyroidism is chronic autoimmune thyroiditis (Hashimoto's thyroiditis). The second most common causes are silent and postpartum thyroiditis, overaggressive radioactive iodine therapy, surgical ablation, and drug-related altered thyroid function, such as occurs with the use of the cardiac antiarrhythmic drug amiodarone.

The diagnosis of hypothyroidism is divided into four categories, based on laboratory studies. *Overt hypothyroidism* is defined by low T_4 and T_3 levels and elevated thyrotropin levels (> 20 mU/L). *Subclinical hypothyroidism* is defined by normal T_4, normal T_3, and mildly elevated thyrotropin levels (5–20 mU/L). Less common, secondary/tertiary or *central hypothyroidism* is defined by low T_4, low T_3, and low thyrotropin plasma levels. *Peripheral tissue resistance* to thyroid hormone is associated with high T_4 and TSH levels, and is possibly caused by an altered receptor mechanism.

Hypothyroidism involves most organ systems to varying degrees. The levels of involvement of each target organ correlates with the duration and amount of decrease in circulating T_4. Most affected are the integument and cardiovascular, gastrointestinal, musculoskeletal, hemopoietic, endocrine, and neuropsychiatric function. Typical complaints of hypothyroid patients include increased tiredness, increased sleep requirement, depressed mood, feeling cold, gaining weight on the same diet, constipation, increased forgetfulness, increased time needed to fulfil a task, and reduced exercise tolerance associated with muscle

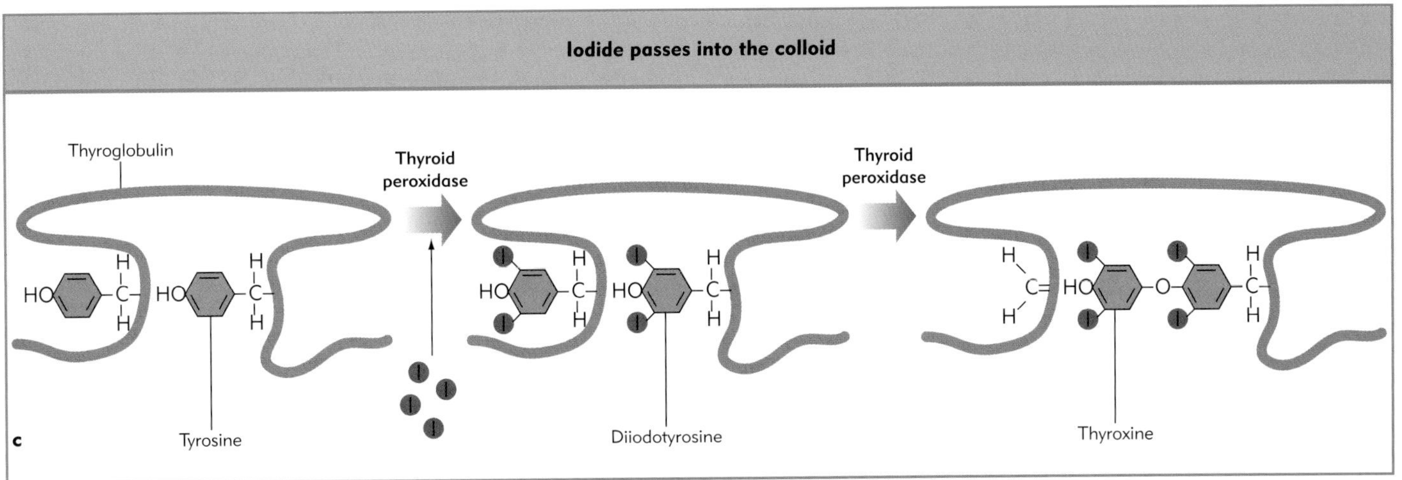

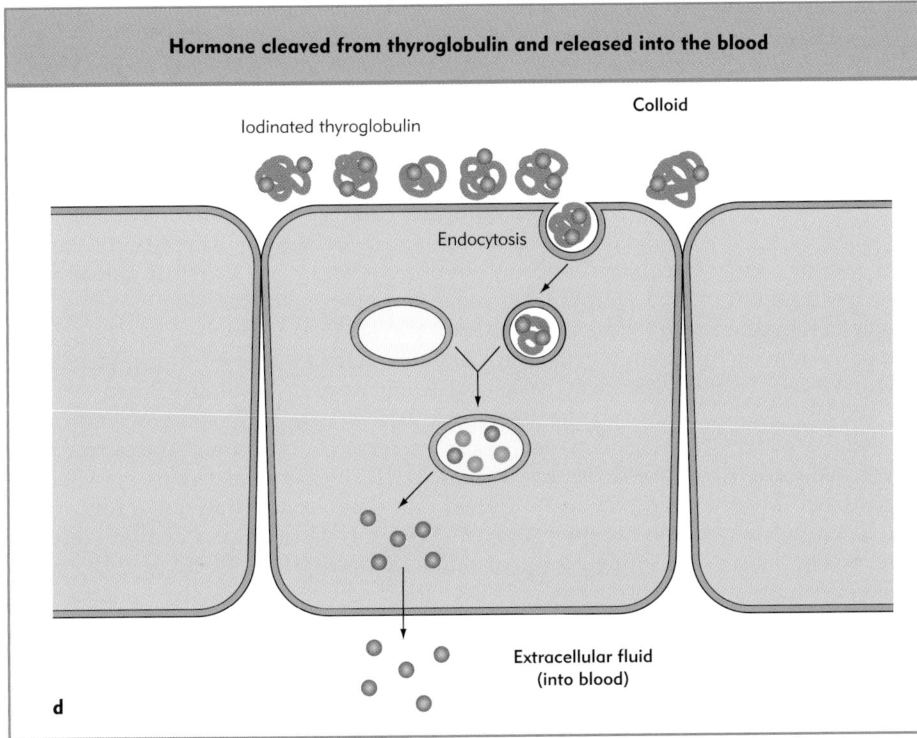

Figure 66.2, cont'd The iodide passes into the colloid, where it is combined with tyrosine (bound to thyroglobulin) by the action of thyroid peroxidase (c). Thyroid hormones bound to thyroglobulin are taken up into lysosomes of the epithelial cells by endocytosis; the hormone is cleaved from thyroglobulin by hydrolytic enzymes and subsequently released into the blood (d).

cramps on strenuous exercise. The facial appearance is dull and apathetic, with puffiness around the eyes and loss of lateral eyebrows. The skin appears cold, dry, and rough, with nonpitting edema (myxedema).

The most important adverse effects of hypothyroidism, possibly associated with a poor surgical outcome, are those affecting cardiac and respiratory function.

Cardiovascular effects of hypothyroidism include impaired cardiac contractility with decreased cardiac output, increased peripheral vascular resistance, decreased systolic blood pressure, increased diastolic blood pressure, and bradycardia. Pericardial effusion occurs in up to 50% of individuals, and cases of torsades de pointes have been reported. A decrease of 60% in left ventricular ejection time and a prolongation of the pre-ejection period by 40% can been seen in cases of severe hypothyroidism. The causes underlying these cardiac abnormalities are multifactorial. Myxedematous infiltration of the myocardial tissue, alterations in calcium handling in the cytoplasmic reticulum, and a depression of myosin ATP-ase activity are important causes of myocardial contractility depression.

Anemia is often associated with hypothyroidism (25–50% of patients) and can contribute to angina symptoms. Iron and folic acid absorption are both reduced in hypothyroidism, and pernicious anemia may result from gastric mucosal atrophy because of the presence of antibodies against the gastric mucosa.

Several abnormalities of the respiratory function have been described in hypothyroidism. Pulmonary function is characterized by shallow and slow breathing, and impairment of both hypoxic and hypercapneic ventilatory drive. One of the major respiratory features of hypothyroidism is sleep apnea and all its complications, which can adversely influence surgical outcome or make postoperative extubation problematic.

L-thyroxine replacement, even in the absence of obesity, may improve respiratory function. Hypothyroid patients have slowed drug metabolism and are very sensitive to sedatives or anesthetic agents that can precipitate respiratory failure. The use of tranquilizers, narcotics, and hypnotics should be avoided, or reduced to a minimum. Gastrointestinal motility is markedly decreased and can lead to paralytic ileus and the megacolon of myxedema. Coagulation disorders may be associated with bleeding diathesis in the hypothyroid patient.

Hypothyroidism is preferentially treated with L-thyroxine (T_4), with doses ranging from 0.05 to 0.2 mg/day. In patients with coronary artery disease replacement therapy should be cautious because it may precipitate angina or myocardial infarction. In these patients, coronary revascularization may be required before starting the therapy.

It is important to establish the euthyroid state before surgery. In severe untreated hypothyroidism elective surgery must be postponed. In emergency surgery, mortality is very high. Anesthetic requirements in the hypothyroid patient are diminished. Moreover, emergence from anesthesia may be prolonged and hypothermia may occur readily.

Hypothyroid patients have slowed drug metabolism and are very sensitive to sedatives and anesthetics.

HYPERTHYROIDISM

The term hyperthyroidism indicates an increased secretion and release of thyroid hormones, which results from an increased function of the thyroid gland. The clinical syndrome of a hypermetabolic state which results from the increased plasma concentration of thyroid hormones is usually named thyrotoxicosis.

Increased thyroid secretion can be caused by primary alteration within the gland (Graves' disease, toxic nodular goiter, toxic thyroid adenoma) or central nervous system disorders and increased TSH-produced stimulation of the thyroid. Most patients are women between the ages of 20 and 40 years. Men experience one-tenth of the occurrence in women. The most frequent cause of thyrotoxicosis is Graves' disease, accounting for 60–90% of cases. Silent and postpartum thyroiditis is the next most common. When thyrotoxicosis occurs acutely it is most often caused by thyroiditis, whereas Graves' disease has a more insidious course, evolving over a more protracted period. Symptoms in younger individuals are usually the result of sympathoadrenal activity. At clinical presentation patients complain of sweating, weight loss, heat intolerance, thirst, tremor, palpitations, and altered menstrual cycle to the point of amenorrhea. Cardiac signs include high-output cardiac failure and congestive heart failure with peripheral edema. Arrhythmias include ventricular tachycardia, increased sleeping pulse rate, or atrial fibrillation, atrial flutter, paroxysmal supraventricular tachycardia, and premature ventricular beats. There may be thyroid swelling and exophthalmos. Sometimes a goiter may cause tracheal compression. Clinically overt myopathy is infrequent, but there is some degree of EMG abnormality in 90% of thyrotoxic patients and serum creatine kinase concentrations are often raised. Gastrointestinal signs include increased bowel frequency to the point of diarrhea and electrolyte wasting. Psychiatric signs may include altered sleep patterns, emotional mood swings, anxiety, fatigue, excitability, and agitation. In older patients, the manifestations of thyrotoxicosis can be considerably modified. Affected patients may appear apathetic rather than nervous. Cardiovascular signs, general muscle weakness, and weight loss are more prominent. Cardiac arrhythmias in elderly hyperthyroid patients may be refractory to conventional treatment. An enlarged smooth thyroid mass and signs and symptoms of thyrotoxicosis suggest the diagnosis. Elevated levels of T_3 and T_4 with reduced or undetectable levels of TSH confirm the diagnosis. Thyroid antibodies are usually detected in elevated quantities. A ^{123}I radionuclide scan should demonstrate diffuse uptake throughout an enlarged gland. An ultrasound or CT scan of the neck may be used to evaluate clinical landmarks.

The most frequent anesthetic problems in the perioperative period are caused by the adrenergic and metabolic abnormalities of hyperthyroidism. Adrenergic effects place hyperthyroid patients at great risk during surgery. Increased numbers of β-adrenergic receptors in the heart of hyperthyroid animals have been reported, but the most important effect is the direct inotropic and chronotropic actions of T_3 and T_4 on cardiac muscle. Cardiac hypertrophy is common, and atrial fibrillation occurs in 10–15% of hyperthyroid patients. A basal increase in cardiac output in hyperthyroidism significantly limits cardiac reserve during surgery. Cardiovascular symptoms of anesthesiologic interest include resting tachycardia, wide pulse pressure, exercise intolerance, and dyspnea on exertion. Decreased peripheral resistance, decreased cardiac filling times, increased blood volume, and fluid retention are also of interest. Increased basal oxygen consumption, cardiac arrhythmias, mild anemia, and vitamin B_6 deficiency secondary to increased coenzyme requirements may contribute to cardiac decompensation. Signs and symptoms of congestive heart failure are common in young and old individuals with thyrotoxicosis. The response to digoxin is often inadequate, and may reflect increased drug metabolism. Dependent peripheral edema, especially of the lower extremities and the sacral area, occurs frequently and is secondary to the aldosterone-related increase in sodium and water retention caused by the decreased effective arterial circulating volume. Because high thyroid hormone concentrations result in β-adrenoceptor upregulation, tachyarrhythmias require therapy with high doses of β-blockers (propranolol) and may represent unsuspected coronary artery disease. Pulmonary edema may develop intraoperatively, with cyanosis, tachycardia, and respiratory distress. It is caused by a combination of hypertension, tachycardia, and increased blood volume.

A euthyroid state should be achieved before surgery. Therapy should be aimed at decreasing thyroid hormone formation and secretion. Three different therapeutic approaches are used: antithyroid medications, radioactive iodine ablation, and surgery. The most frequently used treatment modalities are antithyroid drugs or radioactive iodine, and the choice depends on the phase and severity of disease, the specific situation of the patient, and the preference and experience of clinicians. Only a minority of patients require surgery. Treatment of patients with severe thyrotoxicosis initially starts with β-blockers such as propranolol, which is very effective in treating the peripheral effects of the thyroid hormones (i.e. tachycardia). Propranolol 40–120 mg/day is given for 2–3 weeks, with the addition of potassium iodide (Lugol solution) for the last 10 days. Esmolol can be used to control the tachycardia in severe thyrotoxicosis that is refractory to the treatment previously described. Propylthiouracil, carbimazole, and methimazole may then be added, with close monitoring of T_4 and TSH levels. All these medications should be continued up to the time of surgery.

Thyroid overactivity not properly controlled before surgery may precipitate a thyroid crisis, which can be life threatening.

Thyrotoxic crisis is a severe exacerbation of hyperthyroidism which may be precipitated by infections, labor, trauma, a major surgical procedure, acute medical illness, and stress. Perioperatively it occurs within 6–18 hours after surgery, but can also occur intraoperatively, presenting as a hypermetabolic state that resembles malignant hyperthermia.

Clinical signs of thyrotoxic crisis are fever with a temperature of 41°C (or even higher), mental disorientation, anorexia, extreme anxiety and restlessness, agitation, tremor, and tachycardia. Hypotension with congestive heart failure and signs of acute abdomen can develop. The diagnosis is made clinically. Treatment is both specific and supportive. Antithyroid drugs such as carbimazole 60–120 mg or propylthiouracil 600–1200 mg should be given orally or by nasogastric tube. This usually starts to act within 1 hour of administration. Potassium or sodium iodide acts immediately to inhibit further release of thyroid hormone, but it should not be given until 1 hour after the antithyroid drug. The use of β-adrenoceptor antagonists includes oral propranolol 20–80 mg 6-hourly or IV 1–5 mg 6-hourly. Esmolol infusion can be used for short-term control in an emergency if propranolol fails to work. High-dose corticosteroids may be administered to block the release of thyroid hormone from the thyroid gland, as well as the peripheral conversion of T_4 to T_3. Hydrocortisone 100 mg every 8 hours is the steroid of choice to treat thyroid storm.

PARATHYROID GLAND

Anatomy and physiology

The parathyroids are a group of pea-sized glands derived embryologically from the third and fourth pharyngeal pouches. They are typically four in number, lying on the dorsal face of the thyroid gland. Approximately 2–5% of glands may be located intrathyroid. The average weight of a parathyroid is 35–40 mg. The blood supply to the parathyroids is predominantly by way of the inferior thyroid artery (ITA) system. Parathyroid glands, through the release of parathyroid hormone (PTH) from the chief cells, are important regulators of serum Ca^{2+} levels. Direct determination of serum Ca^{2+} and PTH is the best test of parathyroid function. The primary target tissues for PTH action are bone, kidneys, and intestines. PTH increases extracellular calcium through a direct effect on bone resorption by osteoclasts and through renal Ca^{2+} resorption, and indirectly enhancing gastrointestinal absorption by activating the enzyme in the kidney (1α-hydroxylase) that converts vitamin D to its active form (calcitriol, or 1,25 dihydroxycholecalciferol). Additionally, parathyroid hormone reduces serum phosphate by increasing renal excretion. Calcitonin, secreted by the thyroid gland, counteracts the effect of PTH on Ca^{2+} levels. PTH secretion is regulated by the serum Ca^{2+} concentration, with low levels stimulating PTH secretion and elevated level inhibiting it.

Parathyroid dysfunction

HYPERPARATHYROIDISM

Primary hyperparathyroidism is characterized by hypersecretion of parathyroid hormone (PTH), which leads to hypercalcemia. In about 85% of cases hyperparathyroidism is caused by a sporadic, solitary adenoma, but 2–5% of patients may have adenomas in two glands (double adenoma). Hyperplasia of all four glands occurs in about 10% of cases and is more often familial, in the context of three distinct autosomal dominant inherited diseases: multiple endocrine neoplasia (MEN) types I and II, and familial hypocalciuric hypercalcemia. Parathyroid carcinoma is a slow-growing neoplasm of the parenchymal cells that is responsible for 0.5–2% of cases of primary hyperparathyroidism.

Primary hyperparathyroidism is the third most common endocrine disorder, after diabetes mellitus and thyroid disease. Its incidence increases with age, with an average age at diagnosis of 55 years. Women are affected about twice as often as men. The diagnosis is made by demonstrating an elevated serum Ca^{2+} level, elevated PTH level, and normal or increased urinary calcium concentration in the setting of normal renal function.

Secondary hyperparathyroidism occurs as a compensatory mechanism to hypocalcemia in the setting of chronic renal failure or intestinal malabsorptive disorders.

Clinical manifestations of hypercalcemia include the classic pentad of painful bones, kidney stones, abdominal groans, psychic moans, and fatigue overtones (*'bones, stones, groans, moans and overtones'*). Hypertension has been noted in about one-third of patients with hyperparathyroidism. Neurologic manifestations include confusion, lethargy, weakness, and hyporeflexia. Gastrointestinal manifestations include constipation with nausea and vomiting, anorexia, epigastric discomfort, and peptic ulceration. Effects on the kidneys lead to polyuria and polydipsia. Nephrolithiasis with or without renal colic is commonly seen in hyperparathyroid patients. Neuromuscular abnormalities include proximal muscle weakness affecting the lower limbs. Cardiovascular risk may be higher in patients with hyperparathyroidism secondary to hypertension, cardiomyopathy, and left ventricular hyperthrophy (LVH) leading to congestive heart failure. Echocardiograms of patients with primary hyperparathyroidism have demonstrated calcification of myocardium, increased LVH, and aortic and mitral valve calcifications. Cardiovascular risk may be not reduced by surgery, although a certain degree of regression in left ventricular hypertrophy has been shown. Prolonged PR interval, wide QRS complexes, and shortened QT interval may be seen on the ECG. Surgery is the treatment of choice for patients with symptomatic disease.

Preoperative evaluation should include volume status assessment to avoid hypotension during the induction phase of anesthesia. Hydration with normal saline and diuresis with furosemide may be helpful in decreasing the serum Ca^{2+} to more acceptable levels. Phosphate should be given to correct hypophosphatemia. More rarely, aggressive therapy with mithramycin, glucocorticoids, and calcitonin may be necessary. Hypoventilation should be avoided because acidosis increases ionized Ca^{2+} levels. Elevated calcium levels may precipitate cardiac arrhythmias. A calcium channel blocker (i.e. verapamil) may be used to treat supraventricular dysarrhythmias. Hemodialysis remains the treatment of choice in case of severe hypercalcemia. The response to muscle relaxants may be altered in patients with pre-existing muscle weakness, but there is no evidence that one drug has any advantage over another. Careful titration of muscle relaxants and appropriate monitoring is recommended. Osteoporosis predisposes patients to vertebral compression and bone fractures during positioning or transport.

HYPOPARATHYROIDISM

Hypoparathyroidism is an uncommon endocrine disorder characterized by an insufficiency of PTH (true hypoparathyroidism) or resistance to the action of the hormone (pseudohypoparathyroidism). The most common cause of true hypoparathyroidism is surgical damage to the parathyroid glands during thyroidectomy, parathyroidectomy, and radical surgery for head and neck malignancy. Postoperative hypoparathyroidism may be transient (secondary to compromise of blood supply to the parathyroids), or can develop many years after neck surgery. Less frequently hypoparathyroidism may be caused by genetic abnormalities that impair the synthesis, secretion, or function of PTH, either alone or in association with other endocrinopathies.

Clinically, the most important signs and symptoms of hypoparathyroidism are related to the reduction of plasma ionized Ca^{2+}, which leads to increased neuromuscular excitability. The earliest manifestations are numbness and tingling in the circumoral area, the fingers, and the toes. Tetany may develop, with muscle cramps, carpopedal spasm, laryngeal stridor, tonic–clonic convulsions, and choreoathetosis. Cramps, paresthesias, and stridor may be precipitated by exercise. Mental symptoms are common and the patient appears anxious, depressed, or confused. On physical examination, contraction of the facial muscles is elicited by tapping on the facial nerve anterior to the ear (Chvostek's sign). Trousseau's sign is elicited by occluding blood flow to the forearm for 3 minutes. The development of carpal spasm indicates hypocalcemia. The electrocardiograph (ECG) may show prolongation of the QT interval. Hypotension and congestive heart failure may be present. Treatment of symptomatic hypocalcemia consists of intravenous administration of calcium gluconate or calcium chloride. Vitamin D and oral calcium are used for long-term management. Anesthetic drugs that depress the myocardium should be avoided. There is concern regarding the manifestations of neuromuscular irritability (e.g. laryngospasm). Alkalosis due to hyperventilation and sodium bicarbonate administration will further reduce ionized Ca^{2+}. Decreased Ca^{2+} levels potentiate responses to nondepolarizing neuromuscular drugs. Citrate-containing blood products should be administered slowly in patients with pre-existing hypocalcemia, as well as 5% albumin solution (which might bind the ionized Ca^{2+}). Coagulopathy may be present.

ADRENAL GLAND

The adrenal glands are situated in the retroperitoneum and are composed of an outer cortex, which comprises 80% of the gland, and an inner medulla. They are complex, multifunctional endocrine organs.

Adrenal cortex

ANATOMY AND PHYSIOLOGY

The cortex is composed of an outermost zone, the zona glomerulosa, which is very thin and consists of small cells with numerous elongated mitochondria, the middle zone, the zona fasciculata, with columnar cells, and the innermost zone, the zona reticularis, which contains interconnecting cells.

The major hormones of the cortex are the glucocorticoids, cortisol and corticosterone; a mineralcorticoid, aldosterone; and precursors to the sex steroids, androgens and estrogens. All hormones represent chemical modifications of the steroid nucleus (Fig. 66.3). The precursor is free cholesterol, which is actively taken up from the plasma by adrenal cells via endocytosis and becomes esterified and stored in cytoplasmic vacuoles. Most of the reactions from cholesterol to active hormones involve cytochrome P450 enzymes, which are mixed oxygenases that catalyze steroid hydroxylation.

The synthesis of glucocorticoids occurs largely in the zona fasciculata. Cortisol is the dominant glucocorticoid for humans; however, if the latter's synthesis is blocked, synthesis of corticosterone provides the necessary glucocorticoid activity.

The secretion of cortisol by the zona fasciculata, with a smaller contribution from the zona reticularis, is under the exclusive control of the hypothalamopituitary CRH–ACTH axis. It circulates in plasma 75–80% bound to a specific corticosteroid-binding α_2-globulin. The vast majority of cortisol is metabolized in the liver, and the reduced metabolites are conjugated and excreted in the urine as glucuronides. As long as hepatic and renal function is normal, the measurement of urinary metabolites provides a reliable index of cortisol secretion. Cortisol maintains glucose production from protein (gluconeogenesis), facilitates fat metabolism, supports vascular responsiveness, and modulates central nervous system function, skeletal turnover, muscle function, and immune responses. Plasma cortisol levels are increased by the stress of surgery, burns, infection, fever, psychosis, electroconvulsive therapy, acute anxiety, prolonged and strenuous exercise, and hypoglycemia.

The synthesis of sex steroid precursors occurs largely in the zona reticularis, whereas that of aldosterone is carried out exclusively by the zona glomerulosa. The principal function of aldosterone, the major mineralocorticoid, is to sustain extracellular fluid volume by conserving body sodium. Aldosterone is largely secreted in response to signals arising from the kidney when a reduction in circulating fluid volume is sensed. Activation of the renin–angiotensin system in response to hypovolemia is the predominant stimulus to aldosterone production. Elevation of plasma potassium is the other major stimulus. ACTH, in doses and in a manner similar to those that increase cortisol secretion from the zona fasciculata, also stimulates aldosterone secretion. Aldosterone binds to mineralocorticoid receptors in target cells, with complex transcriptional changes. The kidney is the major site of mineralocorticoid activity. Aldosterone stimulates active reabsorption of sodium from the tubular urine by the cells of the collecting ducts and late distal convoluted tubules. Sodium is then transported into capillary blood. The net urinary sodium excretion is decreased and water is passively reabsorbed with the sodium. Concurrently with sodium reabsorption, aldosterone also stimulates the active secretion of potassium out of tubular cells and into the urine, and enhances tubular secretion of hydrogen ions as sodium is reabsorbed (Chapter 57).

As with T_3, the steroid hormones act by binding to intracellular receptors. These are polypeptides that contain hormone-binding and DNA-binding domains. When the steroid hormone binds to the receptor, the complex binds to recognition sites in the promoter regions of a range of genes. Once bound, the amino terminal of the steroid receptor can interact with other transcription factors regulating gene expression (Chapter 3).

Adrenocortical dysfunction

ADRENOCORTICAL EXCESS

Glucocorticoid excess or Cushing's syndrome can be the result of pituitary tumors producing excess ACTH (70–90%) or adrenal hyperplasia. Clinical characteristics include truncal obesity with thin extremities, muscle wasting, thin skin, osteopenia, hypertension, diabetes, and signs of hyperandrogenicity. Treat-

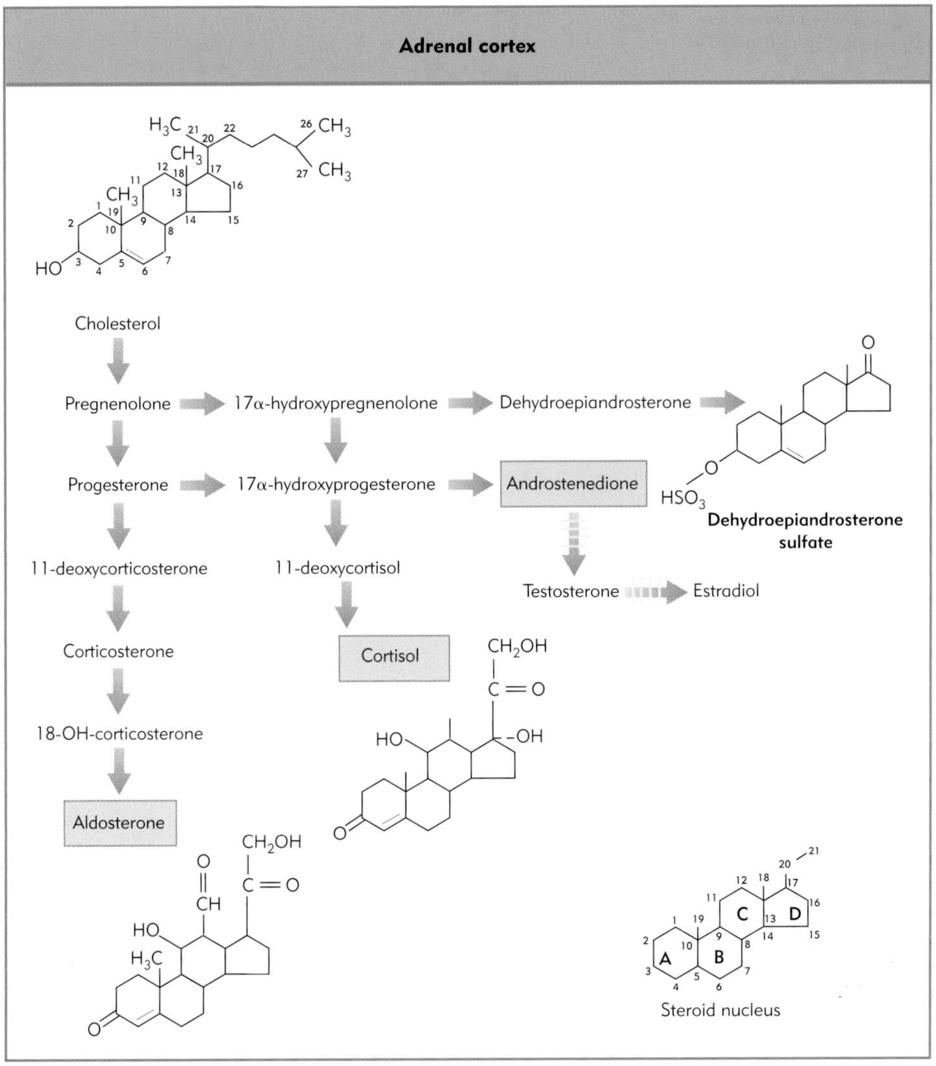

Adrenal cortex

Cholesterol

Pregnenolone → 17α-hydroxypregnenolone → Dehydroepiandrosterone →

Progesterone → 17α-hydroxyprogesterone → Androstenedione

Dehydroepiandrosterone sulfate

11-deoxycorticosterone

11-deoxycortisol

Testosterone → Estradiol

Corticosterone

Cortisol

18-OH-corticosterone

Aldosterone

Steroid nucleus

Figure 66.3 The adrenal cortex. Principal pathways for human adrenal steroid hormone synthesis.

ment of Cushing's syndrome where pituitary tumor is the main cause includes transsphenoidal tumor resection. Preoperative correction of diabetes, hypertension, and hypokalemic alkalosis is recommended. If glucocorticoid excess is due to adrenal adenomas or carcinomas, these can be resected surgically or the secretion can be suppressed by inhibitors of steroid biosynthesis, such as metapyrone or mitotane, or glucocorticoid receptor antagonists such as mifepristone. Perioperatively, during resection, and postoperatively, steroid supplementation is necessary.

ADRENOCORTICAL INSUFFICIENCY

Addison's disease or primary autoimmune disorder of the adrenals causes both glucocorticoid and mineralocorticoid deficiency. All zones of the adrenal cortex are involved. Patients complain of tiredness, fatigue, orthostatic hypotension, hypoglycemia, hyponatremia, hyperkalemia, and skin hyperpigmentation. The diagnosis of Addison's disease is confirmed by low plasma cortisol levels and decreased urinary excretion of 17-hydroxycorticoids. Plasma levels of ACTH are elevated. Secondary adrenal insufficiency results from insufficient ACTH secretion, pituitary or hypothalamic tumor, or is associated with chronic steroid therapy. The clinical symptoms do not include hyperkalemia and hyperpigmentation. Treatment of acute adrenal insufficiency consists of large doses of intravenous hydrocortisone phosphate (100–200 mg) and isotonic sodium chloride solutions. Perioperative cover with hydrocortisone phosphate (25–100 mg) is recommended empirially in patients with chronic steroid therapy undergoing moderate to major surgery.

Mineralocorticoid excess or primary hyperaldosteronism (Conn's syndrome) and secondary hyperaldosteronism are associated with hypokalemia, sodium retention, muscle weakness, hypertension, polyuria, and hypokalemic alkalosis. Conn's syndrome often results from unilateral adenoma or bilateral hyperplasia. Spironolactone is highly indicated to correct the preoperative hypertension, and hemodynamic monitoring is advised in those patients with ischemic heart disease.

Mineralocorticoid deficiency or hypoaldesteronism is characterized by hyperkalemic acidosis, hypertension, and hyponatremia. It can be the result of unilateral adrenalectomy, chronic diabetes, or renal failure, or can be congenital. Administration of 0.5–1 mg/day of 9α-fluorocortisol is the chosen treatment.

Adrenal medulla

ANATOMY AND PHYSIOLOGY

The inner zone of the adrenal gland, or medulla, is derived from neuroectodermal cells of the sympathetic ganglia and is the source of circulating catecholamines, epinephrine, and, to a lesser extent, norepinephrine. The neuronal cell bodies do not have axons and discharge the hormones directly into the bloodstream. They are organized in cords and clumps in close relationship with venous drainage from the adrenal cortex, and with nerve endings from cholinergic preganglionic fibers of the sympathetic nervous system. The adrenal medulla is activated in association with the rest of the sympathetic nervous system. All circulating epinephrine derives from adrenal medullary secretion, whereas norpinephrine derives from nerve terminal endings. The hormones are synthesized from tyrosine (Fig. 66.4) and stored within the chromaffin cells, an energy-requiring process. Their half-life is 1–3 minutes and they are metabolized in the liver and kidney (Fig. 66.4). The activity of the adrenal medulla can only be assessed by measuring urinary free epinephrine or plasma epinephrine concentrations. Anxiety, fear, pain, hypovolemia, hypotension, hypoxia, hypercapnia, extreme of temperature, hypoglycemia, and severe exercise are some of the conditions initiating the stimulation of sympathetic nervous system, with responses activated in the hypothalamus and brainstem. Both catecholamines exert their effects on a group of plasma membrane receptors, β_1, β_2, α_1 and α_2 resulting in specific actions (Chapter 34).

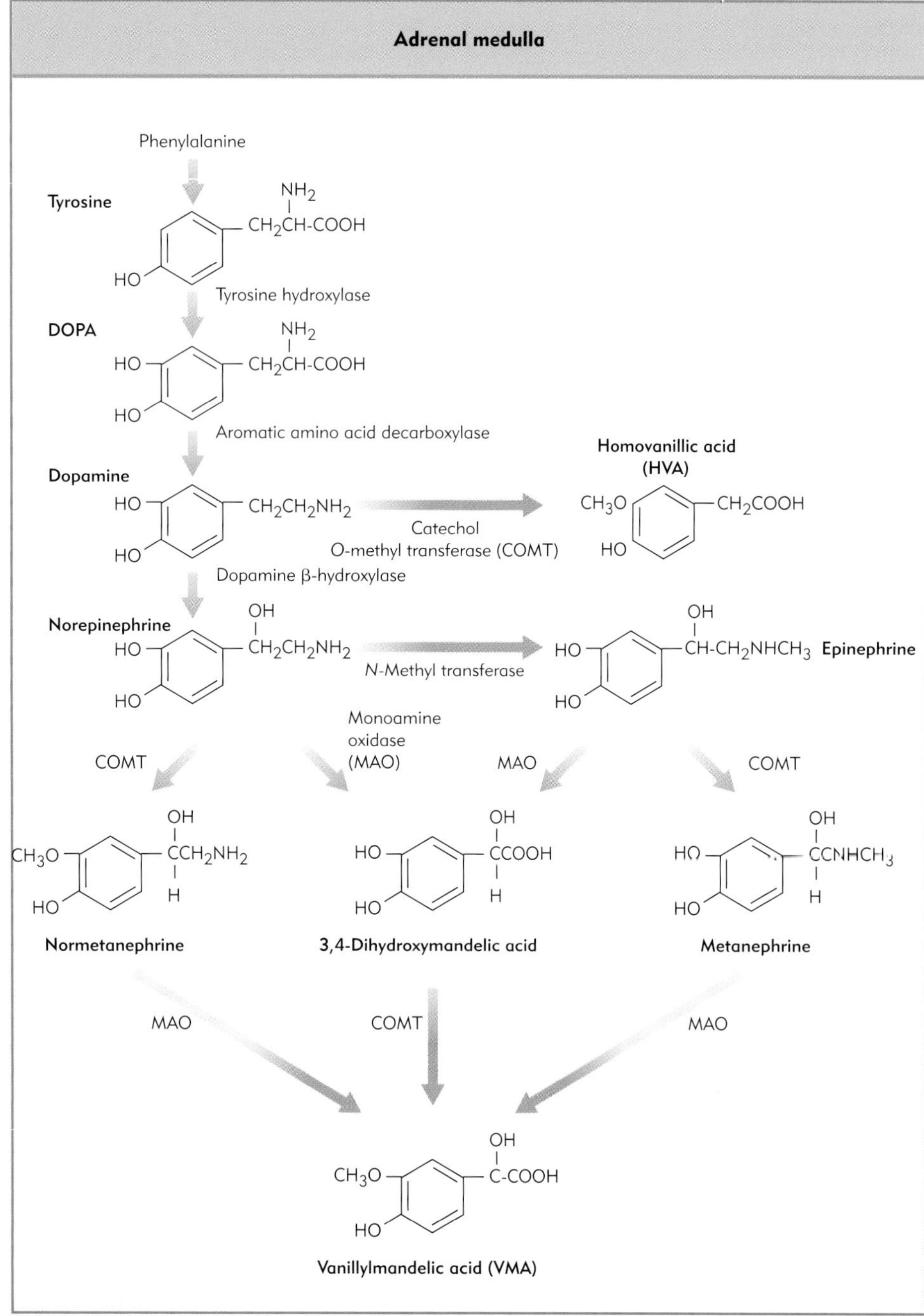

Figure 66.4 The adrenal medulla. Metabolic pathways for catecholamines. DOPA, dihydroxyphenylalanine

Adrenal medulla dysfunction

PHEOCHROMOCYTOMA

This is a tumor of the chromaffin cells usually involving the adrenal medulla (>90% cases). Extra-adrenal tumors are rare (10%) and can be located in the abdomen or mediastinum. Pheochromocytoma is occasionally inherited as an autosomal dominant trait and may be part of a pluriglandular neoplastic syndrome (MEN). Clinical symptoms include excessive sweating, headache, palpitations, severe hypertension, orthostatic hypotension, and tachycardia. Other features include orthostatic hypotension caused by reduced plasma volume, ischemic cardiac disease, cardiomyopathy, and hyperglycemia.

Diagnosis is obtained by measuring plasma and urinary catecholamines. Plasma levels of epinephrine and norepinephrine at rest are very high. Similarly, urinary excretion of metanephrines, free catecholamines, and vanillylmandelic acid (VMA) is increased. Radiological imaging (MRI, CT) and radionuclide scanning are used for tumor localization.

The preoperative use of α-adrenergic receptor blockade with prazocin or phenoxybenzamine is indicated before surgery to counteract the intense vasoconstriction and hypertensive crises that occur during the intraoperative manipulation of the tumor. In addition, the α-blockers allow re-expansion of intravascular space. β-blockers are also indicated for those patients who have persistent tachycardia and dysrhythmias, but these should be introduced only after α-blockade is effective.

THE ENDOCRINE PANCREAS

Anatomy and physiology

The islets of Langerhans are the anatomic units that determine the endocrine function of the pancreas. They are composed of four types of cell, each of which synthesizes and secretes a distinct polypeptide hormone: glucagon in the α (A) cell, insulin in the β (B) cell, somatostatin in the δ (D) cell, and pancreatic polypeptide in the PP or F cell. D_1 and G cells secreting vasoactive intestinal peptide (VIP) and gastrin are rare. The amount of somatostatin and gastrin normally secreted by the islets is too small to be of any physiologic significance.

GLUCAGON

Glucagon plays a role in the regulation of glucose and ketone metabolism. By reducing the concentration of fructose-2, 6-biphosphate glucagon diminishes the activity of phosphofructokinase 1, the rate-limiting enzyme in glycolysis. Glucagon stimulates phosphorylase, the rate-limiting step in glycogenolysis, and increases lipolysis in adipose tissue. Although glucagon is an important regulator of glucose homeostasis in humans, its absence has not been shown to cause clinical disease.

INSULIN

The β cells of the islets are the only source of insulin in the body. They synthesize insulin from a single-chain precursor of 110 amino acids (preproinsulin). After translocation through the membrane of the rough endoplasmic reticulum, the 24-amino acid N-terminal peptide of insulin is cleaved off to form proinsulin. In the Golgi complex, the proteolytic removal of the connecting peptide gives rise to the C-peptide and insulin, which are secreted into the circulation in equimolar amounts. Therefore, the C-peptide can be used to determine the degree of native insulin production in type 2 diabetic patients receiving insulin (Chapter 65).

The insulin molecule consists of two peptide chains (A and B) with one intrasubunit and two intersubunit disulfide bonds. Under fasting conditions the islet cells secrete about 1 unit (U) of insulin per hour into the portal vein. Because most of the insulin that reaches the liver via the portal vein is destroyed, the concentration of insulin in the peripheral circulation (12 μU/mL) is much smaller than in the portal blood (50–100 μU/mL). Glucose is the principal stimulus to insulin secretion in humans. Amino acids, fatty acids, ketone bodies, gastrointestinal hormones (gastrointestinal inhibitory peptide, glucagon-like peptide, gastrin, secretin, cholecystokinin, VIP, gastrin-releasing peptide, enteroglucagon), β_2-adrenergic receptor agonists, and vagal nerve stimulation also enhance insulin release, whereas α_2-adrenergic receptor agonists inhibit insulin secretion. Any stressful condition, including hypoxia, hypothermia, surgical trauma, injury, or burns, suppresses the secretion of insulin by stimulation of α_2-adrenergic receptors.

Mechanisms of insulin action

Insulin is the primary hormone responsible for controlling the uptake, utilization, and storage of cellular nutrients in humans. These purposes are accomplished by:

- stimulating the transport of substrates into the cells;
- promoting the translocation of proteins between cellular components;
- activating specific enzymes;
- altering the rate of transcription of specific genes.

Insulin interacts with target cells that have transmembrane insulin receptors. Important target tissues are liver, muscle, and fat, although receptors have been demonstrated in virtually all mammalian cells. Glucose enters the cell by facilitated diffusion through glucose transporters, which are integrated in the cell membrane (GLUT). To date, six distinct transporters have been identified. Insulin promotes the synthesis and translocation of intracellular vesicles that contain GLUT 4 and GLUT 1 to the plasma membrane. The facilitated diffusion of glucose into cells along a downhill gradient is assured by glucose phosphorylation. The conversion of glucose to glucose-6-phosphate is accomplished by one of a family of hexokinases. Two (II and IV) of the four hexokinases (I–IV) are regulated by insulin. Hexokinase IV, commonly known as glucokinase, is found in association with GLUT 2 in liver and pancreatic β cells. Hexokinase II is found in association with the insulin sensitive GLUT 4 in skeletal and cardiac muscle, and in adipose tissue. Insulin also influences the transcription of specific enzymes. It has been shown to inhibit the transcription of phosphoenolpyruvate carboxykinase, one of the key enzymes in gluconeogenesis. This may explain why the liver overproduces glucose in insulin-resistant states.

Classic insulin function

The classic hormonal function of insulin is based on two principal types of action:

- anabolic, i.e. favoring synthetic pathways by directing substrates into glycogen, protein, and lipid synthesis; and
- anticatabolic, i.e. inhibiting catabolic processes such as the degradation of glycogen, fat, and protein.

Although insulin acts on the whole of intermediary metabolism, its chief control is exerted on the glucose system. At concentrations below those required to affect glucose metabolism, insulin inhibits the hormone-sensitive lipase in adipose tissue and thus decreases the hydrolysis of triglycerides stored in the adipocytes. Insulin stimulates amino acid uptake, enhances protein synthesis, and inhibits protein degradation in muscle and other tissues, thereby decreasing the plasma concentrations of most amino acids. The circulating concentration of glucose, unlike those of lipids or amino acids, is a strongly homeostatic variable, the excursions of which are confined to the very narrow range of 60–120 mg/dL, independent of the nutritional state.

Fed state

Following the ingestion of carbohydrate blood glucose concentration rises, but normally does not exceed 120 mg/dL, as a result of increased secretion of insulin. Carbohydrates more effectively provoke insulin secretion when taken orally than when administered intravenously, because the ingestion of glucose induces the release of gastrointestinal hormones and increases vagal activity. Insulin prevents hyperglycemia by inhibiting hepatic glucose production and by stimulating the uptake and metabolism of glucose by muscle and adipose tissue. These two effects occur at different concentrations of insulin. Production of glucose is inhibited half-maximally by an insulin concentration of about 20 μU/mL, whereas glucose utilization is stimulated half-maximally at about 50 μU/mL. The average peak plasma insulin response to a high-carbohydrate meal in normal individuals typically rises 10-fold from a fasting value of 5 μU/mL to a peak of about 50 μU/mL. Under physiological conditions, plasma insulin concentrations rarely increase above 100 μU/mL in humans.

Fasting state

Two mechanisms operate to keep fasting blood glucose concentration in the normal range. Initially, hepatic glycogen is mobilized. After 12–18 hours of fasting, peripheral tissues, particularly muscle, begin to use free fatty acid for fuel, thereby sparing glucose. Controlled ketosis occurs with prolonged fasting. Insulin levels fall sufficiently to permit the release of fatty acids and the activation of the hepatic enzymes of ketogenesis. Ketoacids can substitute for glucose as energy source in muscle (up to 100%) and in the brain (up to 50%).

Nonclassic insulin function

More recently a number of newer actions of insulin have been delineated. In sensitive individuals insulin inhibits platelet aggregation. Hence, in the presence of insulin resistance dyslipidemia, hyperaggregation, and antifibrinolysis may create a prothrombotic milieu. Preliminary evidence suggests that insulin also has pro-oxidant, thermogenic, and vasodilatory effects. In the kidney, insulin spares sodium and uric acid from excretion. Thus chronic hyperinsulinemic states may lead to hypertension and hyperuricemia.

Pancreatic dysfunction

DIABETES MELLITUS

Failure of adequate secretion of insulin causes diabetes mellitus. Once relative or absolute insulin deficiency occurs energy substrates flood the system, resulting in hyperglycemia, osmotic dehydration, protein wasting, and ketoacidosis. The chronic complications of diabetes affect the micro- and macrovasculature, mainly in the cardiovascular system, with hypertension, ischemic heart disease, and peripheral vascular disease; the kidney, with renal failure; the nervous system, with peripheral and autonomic polyneuropathies; and the eyes, causing retinopathy and blindness.

An additional problem relevant for anesthesiologists is the stiff joint syndrome affecting the cervical spine, which may cause difficulty with intubation.

The most recent criteria for the diagnosis of diabetes mellitus are given in Table 66.2. Whereas the determination of blood glucose concentration and glucose tolerance provides information about the patient's glucose metabolism only at the time of the test, the glycosylated hemoglobin (HbA_{1C}) level can be used to assess the quality of long-term glucose control. Because the level of HbA_{1C} depends on the serum glucose concentration, and because HbA_{1C}, once formed, remains in the erythrocyte for its 120-day lifespan, HbA_{1C} levels indicate blood glucose elevations in the previous 2–3 months. Normal HbA_{1C} is around 6% of total hemoglobin.

The vast majority of cases of diabetes fall into two broad etiopathogenetic categories (Table 66.3).

Table 66.2 Criteria for the diagnosis of diabetes mellitus

Symptoms of diabetes[a] plus casual[b] plasma glucose concentration ≥200 mg/dL (11.1 mmol/L)
or
Fasting[c] plasma glucose concentration ≥126 mg/dL (7.0 mmol/L)
or
Two-hour plasma glucose concentration ≥200 mg/dL during an oral glucose tolerance test[d]

[a] Polyuria, polydipsia, unexplained weight loss.
[b] Any time of the day without regard to time since last meal.
[c] No caloric intake for at least 8 hours.
[d] Performed as described by the WHO using a glucose load containing the equivalent of 75 g anhydrous glucose dissolved in water.

Table 66.3 General characteristics of type 1 and type 2 diabetes mellitus

	Type 1	Type 2
Incidence (% of cases of primary diabetes mellitus)	15	85
Age (years)	<30	>40
Body habitus	Normal	Obese
Genetic predisposition	Weak	Strong
Association with HLA system	Yes	No
Acute complication	Ketoacidosis Hyperosmolar coma	
Plasma insulin	Low to absent	Normal to high
Classic symptoms	Common	Rare

Type 1 diabetes encompasses cases primarily caused by pancreatic islet cell destruction due to autoimmune or unknown mechanisms. It does not include those forms of β-cell failure for which other causes can be assigned (e.g. pancreatitis, cystic fibrosis, hemochromatosis). Patients with early disease show lymphocytic infiltrates in the islet ('insulinitis'), which is thought to be the autoimmune response to mild viral β-cell injury. Islet cell autoantibodies are present in 90% of newly diagnosed cases.

The rate of β-cell destruction is quite variable. Some patients, particularly children and adolescents, may present with ketoacidosis as the first manifestation of the disease. Others have modest fasting hyperglycemia, which can rapidly change to severe hyperglycemia and ketoacidosis in the presence of infection or surgical stress. Insulin is required for treatment of all patients with type 1 diabetes.

HLA-linked immune response genes may explain the genetic susceptibility, which is shown by the history of diabetes in about 20% of first-degree relatives. In the United States, similar to the United Kingdom, the incidence of type 1 diabetes is 17 per 100 000 inhabitants. The incidence in Europe varies with latitude, with highest rates in Finland (43 per 100 000) and the lowest in the south (France and Italy, 8 per 100 000).

Patients with type 2 diabetes have two physiologic defects: abnormal insulin secretion and resistance to insulin action in target tissues. β-cell mass is intact and basal insulin secretion normal, but postprandial release of insulin is impaired. Insulin secretion can be therapeutically stimulated by oral administration of sulfonylureas. Although insulin resistance is associated with decreased numbers of insulin receptors, the bulk of the resistance is postreceptor in type. Furthermore, the α-cell population is increased, accounting for an excess glucagon/insulin ratio. Tissue insulin sensitivity can be improved pharmacologically (thiazolidinediones, i.e. so-called insulin sensitizers, biguanides) or by changes in lifestyle (diet, exercise, weight loss). Exogenous insulin is therefore not essential in treatment.

No HLA relationship has been identified in type 2 diabetes, and autoimmune destruction of β cells does not occur. Most patients are obese, and obesity itself causes some degree of insulin resistance. Ketoacidosis seldom occurs spontaneously. This form of diabetes frequently goes undiagnosed for many years because hyperglycemia develops gradually and is often not severe enough to cause any of the classic symptoms of diabetes polyuria, polydipsia, and weight loss. Whereas most patients develop type 2 diabetes in adult life, a subgroup of patients develops disease at a young age. They were formerly referred to as maturity onset diabetes of the young (MODY), and are characterized by impaired insulin secretion with minimal defects in insulin action.

In the United States about 90% of all diabetic patients have type 2 diabetes. The genetic factor is very strong, with a history of type 2 diabetes present in about 50% of first-degree relatives. Incidence rates increase with age, with a mean rate of about 440 per 100 000 per year by the sixth decade in males. Unlike that for type 1 diabetes the incidence rate of type 2 diabetes is lower in northern Europe (100–250 per 100 000) than in the south (800 per 100 000).

Perioperative considerations

The prevalence of diabetes mellitus has been steadily rising over recent decades. Inevitably, diabetic patients have become an increasing burden on anesthetic and surgical services worldwide. Diabetic patients have a worse outcome after coronary artery bypass grafting (CABG) surgery and stay in hospital longer. They are more likely to develop postoperative renal failure and to suffer delayed stroke. Wound infection rates are higher, and mortality is reported to be greater than in nondiabetics. This increased susceptibility to complications after elective surgery cannot be explained by the greater prevalence of comorbidity in the diabetic patient population (coronary artery disease, congestive heart failure, kidney dysfunction, polyneuropathy), but may be a result of poor perioperative metabolic control.

DIABETES OF INJURY

The metabolic and endocrine alterations observed in patients with type 2 diabetes mellitus are similar to those induced by surgical tissue trauma per se, i.e. in the absence of diabetes. The endocrine milieu after surgery is characterized by increased plasma levels of the so-called counterregulatory hormones cortisol, glucagon, epinephrine, and norepinephrine. All these hormones directly inhibit insulin secretion and/or counteract its peripheral action through perturbations in the insulin-stimulated GLUT 4 transport system, leading to hyperglycemia ('diabetes of injury'). Owing to further reduction of an already reduced tissue insulin sensitivity, this hyperglycemic response is pronounced in type 2 diabetics.

MAINTENANCE OF PERIOPERATIVE NORMOGLYCEMIA

In the past, fear of undetected hypoglycemia during general anesthesia and the technical difficulty of measuring blood glucose in the operating room led to the practice of 'permissive hyperglycemia'. However, growing awareness of the adverse effects of acute hyperglycemia in surgical patients (Table 66.4) and the availability of accurate portable glucose monitoring devices make this practice unacceptable, particularly in diabetic patients. Better glucose control in diabetics has been shown to reduce mortality, and deep sternal wound infections in diabetics undergoing CABG. In nondiabetic patients the avoidance of

Table 66.4 Clinical and biochemical consequences of acute hyperglycemia

Clinical
↑ mortality after cardiopulmonary resuscitation
↑ risk of neurological deficit after head injury, hypothermic cardiac arrest, cerebral ischemia
Independent predictor of prognosis after myocardial infarction and the need for CABG
Impaired anastomotic healing
↑ portal vein pressure
Biochemical
Immunosuppression Impaired phagocytic capacity of polymorphonuclear leukocytes Dysfunction of the complement system
↑ risk of hyperglycemia, hyperosmolar dehydration, hypokalemia, hypophosphatemia
↑ CO_2 production

hyperglycemia improved recovery after CABG. In critically ill surgical patients, mostly after cardiac surgery, aggressive maintenance of normoglycemia (72–108 mg/dL) reduced mortality during intensive care by 40% compared to a control group (mean blood glucose concentration 153 mg/dL). Consequently, tight perioperative glucose control has been integrated into the ACC/AHA Guidelines for Coronary Artery Bypass Grafting and the Guidelines for Prevention of Surgical Site Infection.

ANESTHESIA AND PERIOPERATIVE GLUCOSE CONTROL

Anesthetic techniques, particularly neural blockades using spinal and epidural local anesthetics, modulate the catabolic response to surgery. The perioperative increase in circulating concentrations of counterrgulatory hormones and glucose has been shown to be blunted or inhibited in nondiabetic patients receiving epidural anesthesia for abdominal surgery. Postoperative insulin sensitivity was better preserved in the presence of epidural anesthesia. Type 2 diabetics undergoing cataract surgery under local anesthesia experienced better glucose control than with general anesthesia. Routine dilution of drugs in normal saline instead of dextrose 5% further avoids unnecessary increases in blood glucose during major surgery. Simple measures such as the avoidance of long preoperative fasting periods and postoperative immobilization may also prevent the development of insulin resistance after surgery.

Hyperfunction

In most cases, hyperfunction of the pancreatic islet cells is restricted to the oversecretion of one hormone; rarely, two or more hormones are involved.

INSULIN

Seventy per cent of cases of hyperinsulinism are caused by solitary β-cell adenomas (insulinomas), 10% by multiple adenomas, 10% by carcinomas, and 10% by islet cell hyperplasia. Clinical features include hypoglycemia precipitated by fasting or exercise, prompt relief of symptoms after glucose administration, and plasma glucose levels under 40 mg/dL (Whipple's triad).

GLUCAGON

Hyperfunction of α cells is rare and thought to be caused by an islet cell neoplasm (glucagonoma). Clinically patients have mild diabetes mellitus and a typical erythematous necrotizing skin eruption.

GASTRIN

Gastrin hypersecretion is second in frequency to hyperinsulinism among this group of diseases. Seventy per cent of gastrinomas are malignant. Secretion of large amounts of gastrin leads to Zollinger–Ellison syndrome, characterized by continuous hypersecretion of gastric juices. Unrelenting peptic ulcers occur in the stomach, duodenum, esophagus, and jejunum in 90% of patients.

SOMATOSTATIN

D-cell neoplasms of the pancreas are very rare. Mild diabetes mellitus due to impaired release of insulin is the most constant clinical feature

VIP

Watery diarrhea, hypokalemia and alkalosis (WDHA syndrome; Verner–Morrison syndrome) are the typical symptoms of D_1-cell neoplasms of the islets (VIPomas).

Key references

Gavin JR, Alberti KG, Davidson MB, DeFronzo RA. Report of the Expert Committee on the Diagnosis and Classification of Diabetes Mellitus. Diabetes Care 1997;20:1183–97.

Kinney MAO, Bradly JN, Warner MA. Perioperative management of pheochromocytoma. J Cardiothorac Vasc Anesth. 2002;16:359–69.

Krempl GA, Medina JE, Bouknight AL. Surgical management of the parathyroids. Otolaryngol Clin North Am. 2003;36:217–28.

Langley RW, Burch HB. Perioperative management of the thyrotoxic patient. Endocrinol Metab Clin. 2003;32:519–32.

McAnulty GR, Robertshaw HJ, Hall GM. Anesthetic management of patients with diabetes mellitus. Br J Anaesth. 2000;85:80–90.

Stathatos N, Wartofsky L. Perioperative management of patients with hypothyroidism. Endocrinol Metab Clin. 2003;32:503–18.

Further reading

Affleck BD, Swartz K, Brennan J. Surgical considerations and controversies in thyroid and parathyroid surgery. Otolaryngol Clin North Am. 2003;36:159–87.

Chrousos GP. The hypothalamic–pituitary–adrenal axis and immune-mediated inflammation. New Engl J Med. 1995;332:1351–62.

Kehlet H. Modifications of responses to surgery and anesthesia by neural blockade: clinical implications. In: Cousins M, Bridenbaugh P, eds. Neural blockade in clinical anesthesia and management of pain. Philadelphia: JB Lippincott; 1998:129–75.

Van den Berghe G, Wouters P, Weekers F et al. Intensive insulin therapy in critically ill patients. New Engl J Med. 2001;345:1359–67.

Wilson GR. Thyroid disorders. Clin Fam Pract. 2002;4:667–701.

Young JB, Landsberg L. Catecholamines and the adrenal medulla. In: Wilson JD, Foster DW, Kronenberg HM, Larsen PR, eds. Williams' Textbook of endocrinology. Philadelphia: WB Saunders; 1998:705–28s.

Chapter 67

Thermoregulation

Mary Doherty and Donal J Buggy

TOPICS COVERED IN THIS CHAPTER

- **Physiology**
  - The compartment model
  - Heat production
  - Heat loss
  - Physiological control
  - Control of vasoconstriction: cutaneous arteriovenous shunts
  - Shivering
  - Perioperative shivering
  - Nonshivering thermogenesis
  - Sweating
  - Vasodilatation
- **Measurement of temperature**
- **Effects of anesthesia**
  - General anesthesia
  - Regional anesthesia
  - Combined general and regional anesthesia
- **Consequences of perioperative hypothermia**
  - Perioperative hypothermia and drug metabolism
- **Prevention and treatment of perioperative hypothermia**
  - Minimizing heat redistribution
  - Cutaneous warming during anesthesia
  - Internal warming
- **Pediatric considerations**
- **Cardiopulmonary bypass**
- **Hyperthermia**
  - Mechanism of fever
  - Malignant hyperthermia

Thermoregulation is the process by which thermal homeostasis is maintained. Mammals, including humans, are *homeothermic*, i.e. core body temperature is actively maintained within tight limits. In contrast, the body temperature of *poikilothermic* reptiles and amphibians fluctuates with changes in ambient temperature. 'Normal' core body temperature is actively maintained within 0.5–0.8°C, typically 36.5–37.3°C, with slight diurnal, gender, and individual variations. This tight range is sometimes referred to as the 'set-point range'. If core body temperature moves outside this narrow range, physiological effector mechanisms are activated which restore temperature to the set-point range.

Anesthesia presents a considerable challenge to thermoregulatory mechanisms. Thermoregulation is an aspect of homeostasis that is often neglected in anesthetic practice, leading to inadvertent perioperative hypothermia. This has significant adverse consequences, mandating careful attention to maintenance of normothermia during anesthesia to optimize patient outcome. Simple, consistently applied measures can largely eradicate inadvertent postoperative hypothermia. Effective prevention and treatment require an understanding of thermoregulatory physiology and its modulation by general and regional anesthesia.

PHYSIOLOGY

In a large series of normal adults, morning oral temperature averaged 36.9 ± 0.2°C (standard deviation). Therefore, 95% of the population is expected to have a morning oral temperature of 36.5–37.3°C. This relatively narrow range is essential to the integrity of cellular chemical reactions, which have a narrow temperature range for optimal function. There is a circadian fluctuation of body temperature of 0.5–0.8°C. Temperature is lowest when one is asleep, higher when awake, and rises further with activity. Rectal temperature can reach 40.0°C during exercise. There is also a monthly variation in menstruating women, with an increase of up to 1°C at the time of ovulation owing to the effect of luteinizing hormone.

The compartment model

Body heat is not uniformly distributed: various parts of the body have different temperatures. The body may be considered to consist of two principal compartments: a central *core* compartment, comprising the major trunk organs and brain, accounts for two-thirds of body heat content and is maintained within a narrow temperature range (36.5–37.3°C). The second *peripheral* compartment consists of the limbs and the skin and subcutaneous tissues. This compartment contains about one-third of total body heat content and may undergo wide temperature variability, ranging from close to 0°C in extreme cold conditions to 40°C in conditions of extreme heat. Under room conditions,

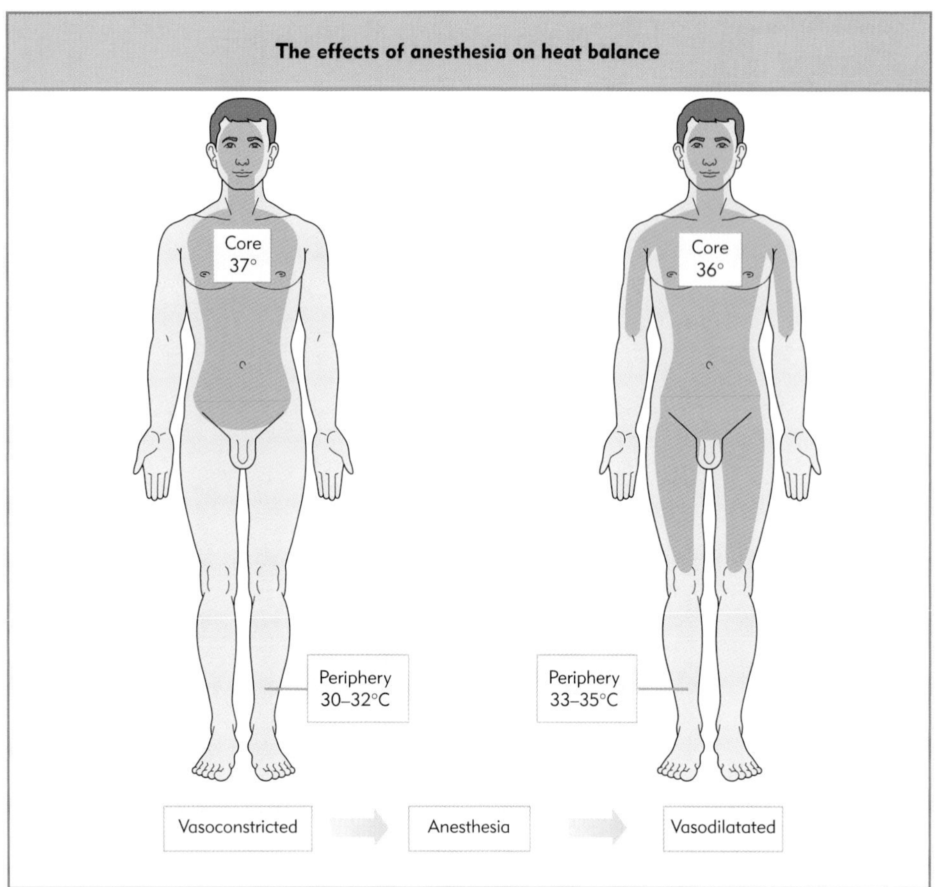

Figure 67.1 The effects of anesthesia on heat balance. In a simplified model, the human body is composed of two compartments, the core and the periphery. Under baseline conditions, the core is considerably warmer than the periphery. By decreasing vasomotor tone, both regional and general anesthesia decrease core temperature by redistribution of heat, whereby heat flows from the core to the peripheral thermal compartment. This effect decreases core temperature by about 1°C (1.8°F) in the first 30–60 minutes following induction of anesthesia. This redistribution predisposes to further hypothermia, as an increased temperature gradient results between the skin surface and the surrounding environment.

peripheral compartment temperature is typically 30–32°C, with a gradient of 5–7°C between core and peripheral compartments. This gradient is maintained by tonic vasoconstriction in the blood vessels leading to the peripheral tissues. During anesthesia, vasodilatation occurs and heat is transferred down the temperature gradient from the core to the peripheral compartment, reducing core body temperature by approximately 1°C and increasing peripheral body temperature to 33–35°C (Fig. 67.1).

Heat production

Total body heat content is the balance between heat production and heat loss (Table 67.1). Heat is produced by metabolism, shivering, and exercise. Basal metabolic rate (BMR), which is defined as the energy cost of maintaining homeostasis at rest, amounts to 40 kcal/m^2/h, or approximately 1700 kcal/day for an average 70 kg adult. BMR is independent of thermoregulatory mechanisms, is higher in children, and is increased by hormones such as thyroxine and growth hormone.

The amount of heat produced by cellular metabolism is dependent on the metabolic substrate. Metabolism of glucose and amino acids produce 4.1 kcal/kg, compared with fat, which releases 9.3 kcal/kg. Approximately two-thirds of the energy available from the metabolism of glucose, amino acids, or fat is dissipated as heat, the remainder being stored as chemical energy, primarily in the form of adenosine triphosphate (ATP). Heat is also produced by exercise, shivering, and nonshivering thermogenesis. The principal autonomic mechanisms whereby body heat is preserved and heat production increased are vasoconstriction and shivering. Shivering increases heat production up to sixfold. Nonshivering thermogenesis, whereby the energy of metabolism is dissipated as heat and none stored as ATP, is due to uncoupling of oxidative phosphorylation in brown adipose tissue. Nonshivering thermogenesis is particularly important in

Table 67.1 Mechanisms of heat production and heat loss

Heat production	Heat loss
Basal metabolism (40 kcal/M^2/h)	Radiation (60%) Increased in vasodilatation; depends on $(T_1–T_2)^4$
Shivering; can increase heat production sixfold	Evaporation of sweat (17%) 0.58 kcal lost per kg sweat
Nonshivering thermogenesis (neonates); can increase heat production threefold	Convection (20%)
Exercise; can increase heat production 20-fold	Conduction (1%)
Behavior (e.g. use of warm clothing, taking shelter, move towards heat source, etc.)	Behavior (e.g. reduce clothing, reduce activity, seek shade, etc.)

neonates, and can increase heat production threefold. Exercise can increase heat production by up to 20-fold at maximal intensity.

Anesthesia impairs the tonic peripheral vasoconstriction that maintains the normal thermal gradient between the central core compartment and the cooler peripheral compartment.

Unless actively warmed, most surgical patients become hypothermic owing to substantial heat loss. For example, a 3°C decrease in mean body temperature corresponds to a debt of approximately 175 kcal in a 70 kg patient, equivalent to basal heat production for 3 hours.

Heat loss

Heat loss occurs by radiation, conduction, convection and evaporation (Table 67.1). Radiation is the transfer of heat by infrared electromagnetic waves from a warm object to a cooler one. It depends on the fourth power of the temperature difference. Therefore, if the ambient temperature of an operating room is increased by 2°C, reducing the difference between it and body temperature by 2°C, radiation heat loss is decreased by a factor of 16 (2^4). Radiation can account for 60% of heat loss. Convective heat loss occurs when the layer of air next to the skin moves or is disturbed, thereby removing its insulative properties, and can account for 25% of heat loss. Evaporative heat loss normally accounts for <10%, but is increased during surgery as there is substantial loss of heat from large surgical incisions and evaporation of skin-preparation solutions. Each gram of sweat that evaporates dissipates 0.58 kcal of heat from the body. Evaporative heat loss through the skin is significant in premature neonates because of their increased skin permeability. Conduction via direct contact with a cooler object accounts for only 1–2% of heat loss.

Skin temperature determines the degree to which body heat is lost or gained. The amount of heat reaching the skin from deep tissues is varied by alterations in skin blood flow via arterio-venous anastamoses. Vasoconstriction is the main physiological means of preventing heat loss. A layer of air is normally trapped next to the skin, which contributes to insulation. Heat transfer across this layer is reduced by horripilation, the well-known effect of cold-induced contraction of piloerector muscles that causes 'goose pimples'. Clothing also increases this layer, and the magnitude of heat transfer is a function of the texture and thickness of the material.

Physiological control

Similar to many physiological control systems, the thermoregulatory control system consists of an afferent signaling input, an integrating mechanism in the central nervous system (CNS), and an efferent response capability, which works to restore core body temperature to normal (Fig. 67.2).

Temperature sense organs are naked nerve endings located in the skin and subcutaneous tissue that respond to changes in temperature by changing the rate at which afferent impulses are sent to the CNS. There are two types of temperature-sensitive neuron: warm receptors and cold receptors. They respond maximally to temperatures slightly above and slightly below core temperature, respectively. Cold receptors predominate over warm receptors in the peripheral compartment by a factor of 10:1, and respond to temperatures ranging from 10 to 36°C. Most cold afferent input comes from the skin and peripheral compartment.

Warm receptors, by contrast, respond from 30 to 45°C. Thermally sensitive cells exist throughout the body and the skin provides only 20% of total thermal afferent information. The remaining afferent input comes from deep tissues. Cold signals are mediated by Aδ fibers and warm signals by unmyelinated C-fibers, but some overlap exists. The peripheral sense organs are located in the subepithelium; therefore, it is the temperature of the subcutaneous tissue that determines the response.

Thermally sensitive neurons are subject to adaptation, which occurs between 20 and 40°C. The sensation of heat or cold produced by a temperature change gradually fades to one of thermal neutrality. For example, if the hands are placed separately into cold and hot water for a few minutes and then

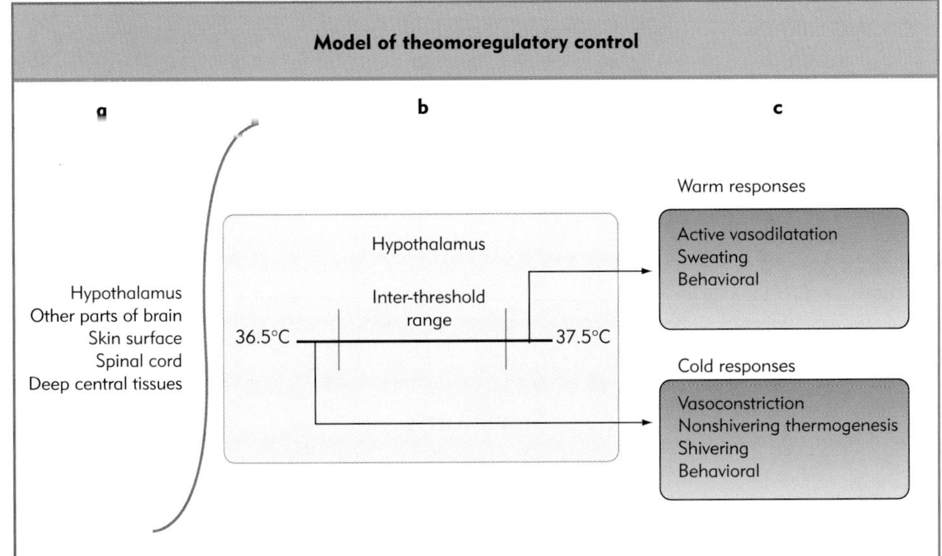

Figure 67.2 A model of thermoregulatory control. The three components of the thermoregulatory system are (a) afferent temperature input, (b) central processing of this information, and (c) the efferent responses that control heat balance. Afferent thermal information is derived from tissues throughout the body, including the brain, skin surface, spinal cord, and deep tissues. Central processing occurs in the preoptic area of the hypothalamus. A mean body temperature below or above the set point initiates the efferent cold or warm responses respectively. (Modified with permission from Sessler DI. Temperature monitoring. In: Miller RD, ed. Anesthesia, 3rd edn. New York: Churchill Livingstone; 1990:315–17.)

together into tepid water, the temperature will feel different in each hand. Cold metal objects seem colder than wood at the same temperature because metal conducts heat away from skin more rapidly, cooling the subcutaneous tissue more. As temperature rises to above 45°C tissue damage ensues and the warm sensation changes to pain.

Most ascending thermal information travels in the lateral spinothalamic tracts in the anterior spinal cord. It appears that signals are modified in the spinal cord and some responses effected from this level, as patients with high spinal cord transections regulate temperature better than expected. The entire anterior spinal cord must be destroyed to ablate thermoregulatory responses completely.

The hypothalamus is the key center where afferent thermal inputs from the skin and deep tissues are integrated and compared with the predetermined set-point temperature range (typically 36.5–37.3°C). Afferent input is integrated in the preoptic area of the anterior hypothalamus, which itself contains thermally sensitive cells. Cold afferent input is primarily received from the periphery, whereas heat-sensitive responses are mainly received from centrally located heat-sensitive neurons. The posterior hypothalamus compares the aggregate afferent thermal input with the set-point temperature and instigates appropriate effector responses, if necessary. Human thermoregulation is in fact a multiple-input multiple-level control system, and many centers below the hypothalamus are also capable of integrating thermal messages and instigating effector responses. Examples include the spinal cord, the nucleus raphe magnus, and the periaqueductal gray matter area in the pons.

Autonomic thermoregulatory effector responses to cold are vasoconstriction and shivering, and are controlled by the posterior hypothalamus. Responses to warmth are sweating and vasodilatation, which are controlled primarily from the anterior hypothalamus, although some thermoregulation against heat still occurs after decerebration at the level of the rostral midbrain. Thermoregulatory effectors have three characteristics: threshold, gain, and maximal response intensity.

The *threshold* of a thermoregulatory effector is the temperature at which the response is triggered. Threshold temperatures may be altered by diurnal rhythm, gender, exercise, food intake, infection, hypo-/hyperthyroidism, and certain drugs. Normally, the threshold for thermoregulatory vasoconstriction is 36.5°C and shivering commences at 36.0–36.2°C. General anesthesia reduces these thresholds by 2–3°C, but gain and maximal response intensity are unaffected. Each thermoregulatory effector mechanism has its own threshold, gain, and maximum intensity, which leads to an energy-efficient progression of responses. Maximal vasoconstriction is reached after a relatively small decrease in core temperature, i.e. the gain is high, whereas maximal shivering intensity is reached more slowly and a larger change in temperature is required. The interthreshold range is the range of core temperatures at which no thermoregulatory response is necessary or triggered. This is normally only 0.2–0.5°C. Sweating occurs at the upper end and vasoconstriction at the lower end of the range. General anesthesia increases the interthreshold range by up to 10 times, to 5.0°C (Fig. 67.3). Cold and warm adaptation also alter threshold temperatures.

The *gain* of a thermoregulatory effector is the rate of change of its response with a given change in temperature, i.e. the slope of the response curve. For example, the gain of shivering is the rate of increased shivering as core temperature continues to decrease below the shivering threshold.

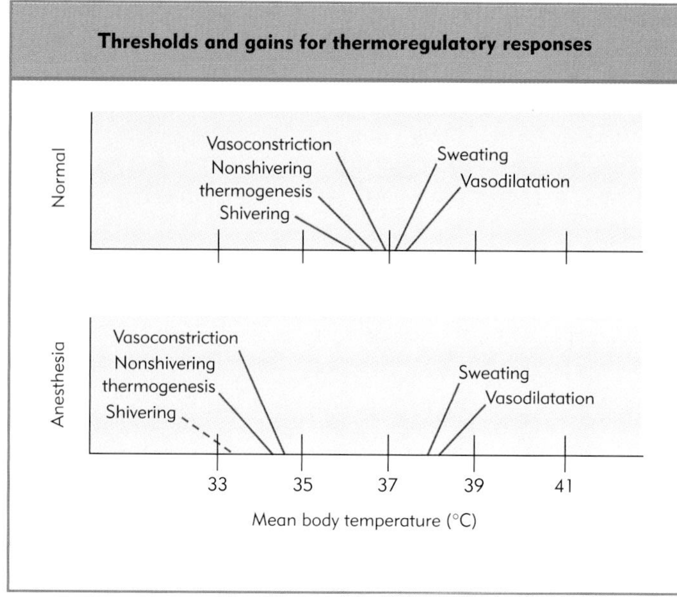

Figure 67.3 Threshold temperature for initiation of thermoregulatory effector responses. Thresholds and gains for thermoregulatory responses in awake and anesthetized humans. For each individual thermoregulatory response the threshold is indicated by the intersection with the x-axis and the gain is represented by the slope of the intersecting line. The interthreshold range is shown as the range of temperatures that do not trigger a response. This range (between sweating and vasoconstriction) is expanded approximately 10-fold in the anesthetized patient. This effect of general anesthesia renders patients 'poikilothermic', and body temperature drifts towards environmental temperature. (a) Normal: Note that the temperature range within which no autonomic effector is activated is about 0.5°C. (b) Anesthesia: The threshold temperature for activation of cold responses (vasoconstriction and shivering) is shifted to the left, and for warm responses (vasodilation and sweating) is shifted to the right. Therefore, the temperature range within which no thermoregulatory effector is activated is increased up to 5.0°C. (Adapted with permission from Sessler DI. Temperature monitoring. In: Miller RD, ed. Anesthesia, 3rd edn. New York: Churchill Livingstone; 1990:1227–42.)

The *maximal response intensity* is the upper limit (plateau) of the effector response.

In the awake state, *behavioral* responses have the greatest effect in preventing hypothermia in response to a cold environment. In extreme cold, vasoconstriction and shivering are of limited efficacy compared with behavioral measures such as taking shelter and wearing protective clothing. Similarly, behavioral adaptation to extremely warm conditions has quantitatively the greatest impact.

The range of ambient temperatures that can be tolerated is decreased if any effector mechanisms are inhibited. For example, low muscle mass or neurological disease may reduce shivering, or it may be prevented by neuromuscular blockade. This has the effect of raising the minimum tolerable temperature. Conversely, anticholinergic drugs inhibit sweating, thereby lowering the maximum tolerable temperature.

Control of vasoconstriction: cutaneous arteriovenous shunts

The first autonomic thermoregulatory response to cold is cutaneous vasoconstriction. Skin blood flow consists of nutritional and thermoregulatory components. Heat loss is regulated by varying skin blood flow via arteriovenous shunts located in

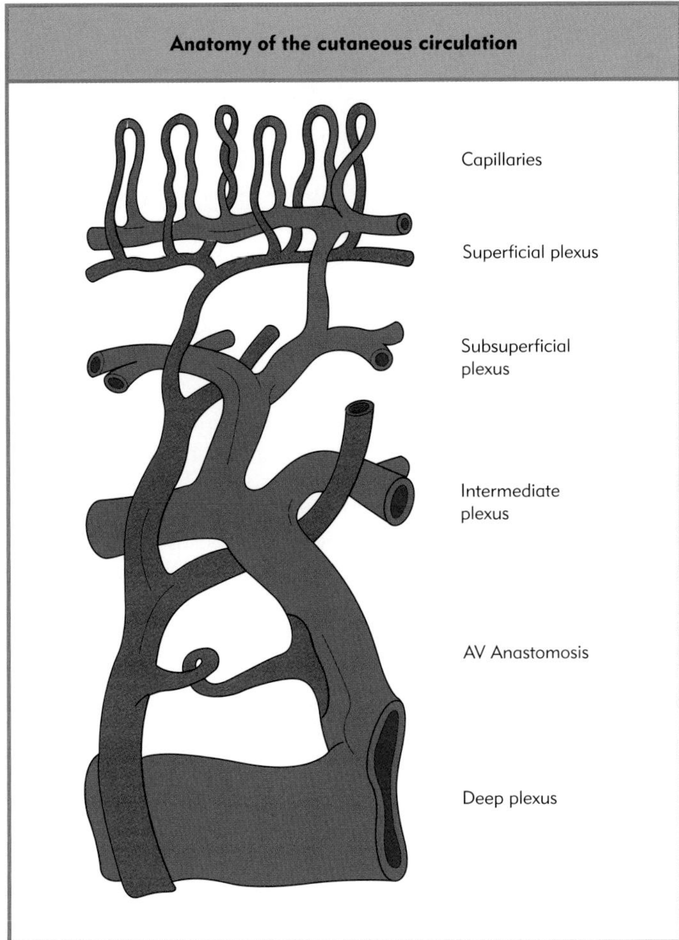

Figure 67.4 Anatomy of the cutaneous circulation. A special feature of the cutaneous vasculature is the presence of arteriovenous (AV) anastomoses, which are most numerous in the palmar surfaces of the hands and feet, but are also present in the nose and ears. The AV anastomoses are coiled vessels with thick, muscular, highly innervated walls that connect the arterioles and venules in the dermis. Under steady-state conditions most heat exchange occurs in the terminal capillary loops that are closest to the external environment and have the greatest surface-to-volume ratio. Blood flow through the AV anastomoses serves as a backup mechanism when capillary flow is inadequate to control heat exchange. Although their surface area is small, AV anastomoses can dramatically alter flow and thus heat exchange. (Adapted with permission from Conrad MC. Functional anatomy of the circulation to the lower extremities. Chicago: Mosby Year Book; 1971.)

fingers, toes, palms, and earlobes (Fig. 67.4). These well-innervated anastomotic connections between arterioles and venules are anatomically and functionally distinct from the nutritional capillary network, ensuring that thermoregulatory vasoconstriction does not compromise the circulatory needs of peripheral tissues. Shunts are controlled by local α-adrenergic sympathetic innervation; flow is minimally affected by circulating catecholamines. The thermoregulatory system has a high capacity compared to the nutritional capillary network: blood flow can vary from 1 mL/100 g of skin per minute to as much as 150 mL/100 g of skin per minute. Although up to 10% of cardiac output flows through these shunts, systemic hemodynamic changes are usually not seen because larger arterioles controlling blood pressure are not influenced.

Shivering

Shivering is an involuntary, oscillatory pattern of skeletal muscle activity that occurs once the cold core temperature threshold is reached (typically 35.9°C). Vigorous shivering can increase metabolic heat production briefly up to sixfold, but sustained shivering doubles heat production. Thermoregulatory shivering consists of two components: a rapid-frequency component of 200 Hz and a slow-frequency (4–8 Hz) synchronous waxing and waning of muscle contraction that is centrally mediated. A motor center for shivering exists between the anterior and the posterior hypothalamus. It is normally inhibited by impulses from the heat-sensitive area in the anterior hypothalamus. The efferent pathway makes multiple connections with the reticular formation in the mesencephalon, pons, and medulla before ending on spinal α motor neurons. Initially muscle tone is increased, then shivering is observed.

Perioperative shivering

Postanesthetic shivering is common, distressing for the patient, and often remembered as the worst aspect of the perioperative experience. It increases pain by movement-induced shearing forces on surgical incisions. Perioperative shivering is a complex response that remains poorly understood, but is probably thermoregulatory in origin. It is unlikely to be associated with adverse outcomes, even though oxygen consumption is increased. Those at risk, i.e. frail and elderly patients, generally do not shiver because of age-related impairment of thermoregulatory control. Shivering is not associated with significant hypoxemia, because the response is actually inhibited by hypoxemia. However, it does cause difficulties with monitoring techniques. Prevention of inadvertent hypothermia is the best treatment option. Other options exist, of which the most commonly used is meperidine (pethidine) (Table 67.2). It is not clear how meperidine exerts its anti-shivering action. Pharmacological ablation of shivering will reduce physiological heat production, therefore active warming must be instituted.

Perioperative shivering increases oxygen consumption but is rarely associated with significant hypoxemia, which itself inhibits the response.

Table 67.2 Drugs effective in treating postanesthetic shivering
Meperidine (pethidine) 0.33 mg/kg IV or epidural
Other opioids, e.g. fentanyl 1 μg/kg
Doxapram 1.5 mg/kg
Clonidine 2 μg/kg
Methylphenidate 0.1 mg/kg
Physostigmine 0.04 mg/kg
Ondansetron 0.1 mg/kg

Nonshivering thermogenesis

This occurs in specialized *brown adipose tissue*, which consists of multinucleated cells with numerous mitochondria and an abundant blood and autonomic nerve supply. Its metabolism is mediated by catecholamines and the substrate used for heat production is mainly fatty acids. Cold stimuli induce norepinephrine release, which uncouples oxidative phosphorylation. Therefore, the energy of glucose metabolism is released as heat rather than stored as ATP. Nonshivering thermogenesis increases metabolic heat production without producing mechanical work. It can double heat production in neonates but has minimal effect in adults.

Sweating

Sweating is an active process of dissipating body heat by the evaporation of fluid released on to the body surface. It is mediated by sympathetic postganglionic cholinergic nerves and prevented by nerve block or atropine administration. It is the only mechanism by which heat can be dissipated at an environmental temperature that exceeds core temperature. The specific latent heat of vaporization of water from the skin and mucous membranes is 0.58 kcal/kg. Heat loss by water vaporization can vary from 30 to 900 kcal/h. Sweating rates can reach >1 L/h for a short time, resulting in heat loss of up to 15 times BMR. During exercise in hot environments, sweat secretion can reach 1.6 L/h in trained individuals.

Vasodilatation

Active vasodilatation is mediated by the arteriovenous shunts, which also control vasoconstriction. Maximum cutaneous vasodilatation usually occurs at a temperature above that which provokes maximum sweating intensity. During extreme heat stress, blood flow through the top millimeter of skin can reach 7.5 L/min, equaling entire resting cardiac output.

MEASUREMENT OF TEMPERATURE

Core body temperature can be measured at a number of sites. Measuring blood temperature in the pulmonary circulation using a pulmonary artery catheter is the gold standard, but is invasive and rarely justified. Tympanic membrane temperature is accurate, but the thermometer probe requires careful positioning to avoid damage to the tympanum and is more suited to single measurements than continuous monitoring. Indirect measures of tympanic membrane temperature (infrared thermometers) are increasingly being used. Axillary temperature reflects core temperature if the thermistor probe is placed near the axillary artery and the arm adducted.

Core temperature may be measured reliably in the nasopharynx or the lower esophagus. Ideally, the thermistor should be placed in the lower third of the esophagus to avoid falsely low readings caused by gas flowing in the trachea. An esophageal stethoscope with an integral thermistor is ideal, and is in optimal position behind the left atrium where the heart sounds are best heard. Rectal and bladder temperatures lag behind changes in core temperature because these organs are not sufficiently well perfused to reflect rapid changes in body heat content. Simultaneous nasopharyngeal and rectal temperature monitoring is often used during cardiopulmonary bypass to demonstrate completion of rewarming (see below).

Simultaneous monitoring of core and peripheral temperature sites serves as an indirect monitor of cardiac output. A decrease in cardiac output elicits a compensatory increase in systemic vascular resistance and hence vasoconstriction. Vasoconstriction in turn decreases peripheral (skin) temperature, and therefore the core–peripheral temperature gradient increases.

EFFECTS OF ANESTHESIA

General anesthesia

General anesthesia precludes behavioral responses and also significantly impairs autonomic thermoregulation. Warm response thresholds are increased and cold response thresholds are reduced, thereby increasing the interthreshold range 10–20-fold. Cold response thresholds are decreased by all anesthetic agents in a dose-dependent manner. Gain and maximum intensity remain unchanged. General anesthesia typically results in mild, inadvertent core hypothermia (34.0–36.4°C), which occurs in a characteristic three-phase pattern (Fig. 67.5).

Phase 1 is a rapid reduction in core temperature of 1.0–1.5°C within the first 30–45 minutes after induction. This is attributable to core-to-peripheral redistribution of body heat. General anesthetic-induced vasodilatation, in addition to a shift of the vasoconstriction threshold, inhibits normal tonic vasoconstriction, resulting in a core-to-peripheral temperature gradient and redistribution of body heat from core to peripheral tissues. Core temperature becomes much lower before the reset vasoconstrictor response can occur.

Phase 2 is a more gradual, linear reduction in core temperature of a further 1°C over the next 2–3 hours of anesthesia due

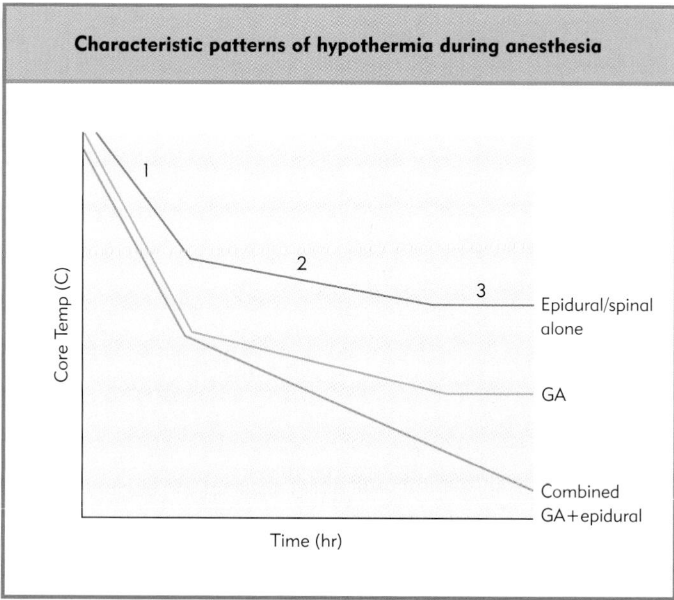

Figure 67.5 Characteristic patterns of hypothermia during anesthesia. Characteristic patterns of hypothermia during general anesthesia alone, epidural or spinal anesthesia alone, and combined general and epidural anesthesia. Patients in this last category are more likely to develop profound hypothermia than others.

to heat loss exceeding heat production. Basal metabolic rate during anesthesia is reduced by 20–40%. Radiation and convective heat losses in this phase are determined by the fourth power of the difference between peripheral and ambient temperature. Evaporative heat loss is exacerbated during major surgery, where a greater surface area of tissue may be exposed to the environment, e.g. during major laparotomy or thoracotomy.

Phase 3 is a 'plateau' phase where heat loss is matched by metabolic heat production. This occurs when anesthetized patients become sufficiently hypothermic to reach the lower threshold for vasoconstriction, which restricts further core-to-peripheral heat transfer.

Regional anesthesia

As with general anesthesia, redistribution of body heat during spinal or epidural anesthesia is the main cause of hypothermia. Because redistribution during spinal or epidural anesthesia is usually confined to the lower half of the body, the initial core hypothermia is not as pronounced as in general anesthesia (approximately 0.5°C; see Fig. 67.4). Otherwise, the pattern of hypothermia during spinal or epidural anesthesia is similar to that of general anesthesia for the first two phases. The major difference with neuraxial anesthesia is that the plateau phase may not emerge because vasoconstriction is blocked. A passive plateau may emerge in well-insulated patients undergoing minor procedures, but in patients undergoing long procedures the potential for serious hypothermia exists.

Redistribution of body heat is the main cause of hypothermia during regional anesthesia, but is less pronounced than in general anesthesia owing to the restricted vasodilation.

Altered thermoregulation during regional anesthesia results from the effect of the regional block on afferent signals, i.e. decreased cold afferent input from the legs. Vasoconstriction and shivering thresholds are reduced by regional anesthesia, and further reduced by adjuvant sedative drugs and advanced age. When triggered, shivering is less effective because it is confined to the upper body, and the gain and maximum response intensity are about half normal. The patient may not perceive cold impulses and may shiver while denying feeling cold. If core temperature is not monitored in these patients significant hypothermia can go undetected.

Combined general and regional anesthesia

Patients undergoing long procedures with combined general and regional anesthesia are at the greatest risk of inadvertent perioperative hypothermia. The major difference with combined general and neuraxial anesthesia is that the plateau phase does not emerge. The reduction in vasoconstriction threshold caused by neuraxial block is superimposed on that due to general anesthesia. Also, vasoconstriction, which would be activated at a lower threshold in general anesthesia alone, is prevented by peripheral nerve block. Even when vasoconstriction is triggered at the lower threshold it less effective and core temperature continues to decline.

CONSEQUENCES OF PERIOPERATIVE HYPOTHERMIA

Irrefutable evidence clearly demonstrates significant adverse outcomes associated with mild inadvertent perioperative hypothermia.

Evidence from multiple prospective randomized controlled trials demonstrates that perioperative hypothermia of 1–2°C can be detrimental. All the adverse outcomes listed in Table 67.3 resulted from core hypothermia of 34.5–35.9°C.

Perioperative hypothermia of 1–2°C increases the incidence of multiple adverse outcomes: cardiac, hemostatic, and infectious.

In a randomized controlled trial (RCT) involving 300 patients with known coronary artery disease, a hypothermic group, which received only standard care and reached a mean core temperature of 35.7°C, was three times more likely to have a morbid cardiac event (myocardial infarction, life-threatening arrhythmia) in the first 30 days postoperatively. The mechanism by which mild hypothermia induces myocardial ischemia and arrhythmias may be increased plasma catecholamine concentrations resulting in hypertension and myocardial irritability.

In an RCT of 60 patients undergoing hip arthroplasty, patients randomized to receive standard therapy, which resulted in a mean core temperature of 35.4°C by the end of surgery, had a 30% increase in blood loss (500 mL) and significantly increased allogenic transfusion requirements compared to normothermic patients who received active warming.

Increases in intraoperative blood loss and requirements for blood transfusion are attributable to hypothermia-induced impairment of platelet function and clotting factor enzyme function. Although platelet numbers remain normal, hypothermia seriously impairs platelet function owing to the reduced release of thromboxane A_2. During hypothermic coagulopathy, standard tests of coagulation, the prothrombin and partial thromboplastin times, remain normal, as they are usually performed at 37°C regardless of the actual patient temperature. Fibrinolysis remains normal during mild hypothermia, but is increased during hyperthermia. Thromboelastographic data suggest that hypothermia impairs clot formation rather than facilitates clot lysis.

Mild inadvertent hypothermia also predisposes to surgical wound infection and poor wound healing. The incidence of surgical wound infection is directly related to subcutaneous wound tissue oxygen tension (PtO_2), which is compromised by hypothermia-induced vasoconstriction. Moreover, mild hypothermia directly impairs immune function, including B cell-mediated antibody production and nonspecific oxidative bacterial killing by neutrophils.

In an RCT of 200 patients undergoing colon surgery hypothermia caused a threefold increase in surgical wound infection compared to the actively warmed group. Hypothermia also increased the duration of hospitalization in the noninfected hypothermic patients owing to impaired healing. This is consistent with the finding that hypothermia is associated with increased postoperative protein catabolism, and that maintaining normothermia can reduce urinary nitrogen excretion, suggesting a decrease in postoperative catabolism.

Table 67.3 Major adverse consequences of inadvertent perioperative hypothermia (values shown are mean ± SD)

Adverse outcome	Normothermic group	Hypothermic group	Reference
Myocardial ischemia or arrhythmias	1%	6%	Frank et al. JAMA 1997;277:1127–34
Intraoperative blood loss	1.7±0.3 L	2.2±0.5 L	Schmied et al. Lancet 1996;347:289–92
Allogeneic blood transfusion requirement	1 unit	8 units	Schmied et al. Lancet 1996;347:289–92
Surgical wound infection	6%	19%	Kurz et al. New Engl J Med 1996;334:1209–15
Urinary nitrogen excretion	982 mmol/day	1,798 mmol/day	Carli et al. Br J Anaesth 1989;63:276–82
Duration of action of neuromuscular blockers	44±4 min	68±7 min	Leslie et al. Anesth Analg 1995;80:1007–14
Duration of postanesthetic recovery	53±36 min	94±65 min	Lenhardt et al. Anesthesiology 1997;87:1318–23
Duration of hospitalization	12.1±4.4 days	14.7±6.5 days	Kurz et al. New Engl J Med 1996;334:1209–15

Perioperative hypothermia and drug metabolism

Because the enzyme systems that metabolize most drugs are temperature sensitive, drug metabolism is altered in hypothermia. The duration of action of vecuronium is more than doubled in patients with a core temperature <35.0°C, even exceeding the duration of action of pancuronium in a normothermic patient. Atracurium is less temperature dependent than vecuronium: the duration of action is increased by only 60% with a 3°C core temperature reduction.

Hypothermia slows drug metabolism and increases volatile anesthetic potency.

Volatile anesthetic agents exhibit increased tissue solubility with hypothermia. The minimum alveolar concentration (MAC) of halothane and isoflurane decreases about 5% per 1°C reduction in core temperature. At a brain temperature of 20°C no anesthesia is necessary. Hypothermia increases plasma concentrations of propofol by 30% with 3°C hypothermia, and fentanyl by 5% per 1°C decrease in core temperature. These effects contribute to prolonged recovery from anesthesia with hypothermia. In a randomized controlled trial involving 150 patients, mild inadvertent hypothermia significantly delayed discharge from the postanesthesia care unit, even when return to normothermia was not required for discharge. The duration of recovery room stay and overall hospitalization is reduced by the avoidance of mild perioperative hypothermia, which has significant healthcare cost implications.

PREVENTION AND TREATMENT OF PERIOPERATIVE HYPOTHERMIA

There are three basic strategies for the prevention and treatment of mild perioperative hypothermia (Table 67.4).

Table 67.4 Prevention and management of inadvertent perioperative hypothermia

Minimize body heat redistribution	Preoperative peripheral warming with forced-air warmer over 30–60 min Preoperative pharmacological vasodilatation
Active peripheral warming during anesthesia	Forced convective air warming Radiant heat
Passive peripheral warming during anesthesia	Space blanket
Internal warming during anesthesia	Fluid warming Airway gases humidification Invasive internal warming (e.g. cardiopulmonary bypass, central venous infusion of fluids, etc.) Metabolic stimulation (e.g. amino acid infusion)

Minimizing heat redistribution

This may be achieved by (a) preoperative warming of peripheral tissue, and (b) preoperative pharmacological vasodilatation. Preoperative warming of peripheral tissue reduces the normal core-to-peripheral temperature gradient so that the induction of anesthesia does not result in the sudden core hypothermia seen in phase 1. To be effective, this requires over 1 hour of exposure to radiant heat preoperatively; rapid warming is ineffective, as sweating must be avoided. The use of a forced-air convective warmer, placed adjacent to the skin for 30–60 minutes, is an effective prewarming technique to reduce core-to-peripheral redistribution soon after the induction of anesthesia. Preoperative pharmacological vasodilatation facilitates core-to-peripheral redistribution of heat before anesthesia; it does not compromise core temperature because patients are not anesthetized and their thermoregulatory responses are intact. Oral nifedipine, taken preoperatively, reduces the extent of the initial redistribution hypothermia by 50%.

Cutaneous warming during anesthesia

Passive insulation, for example a single layer of any insulator (e.g. a space blanket), reduces cutaneous heat loss by approximately 30% because it traps a layer of still air between it and the skin. Additional layers of passive insulation do little to preserve core temperature.

Active warming systems maintain normothermia much more effectively than passive insulation. Once heat has been redistributed to the peripheral compartment, the major means by which the core may be rewarmed is by heating the skin and peripheral compartment above core temperature, creating a reverse temperature gradient and allowing heat to transfer from the peripheral to the core compartment. This is most effectively achieved by use of a forced-air convective warmer (e.g. Bair-Hugger). The electrically powered air heater-fan and disposable patient cover is effective because it replaces cool room air with warmed air, and also because convection increases heat gain when the forced air is warmer than skin. It must be directly next to the patient's skin, with no intervening layers. The rate of heat transfer depends on the amount of body surface covered. Various shapes and sizes of cover are available, and in certain circumstances, e.g. abdominal surgery, two separate covers should be used for the legs and upper body. Lower body warming should be temporarily switched off during procedures that cut off lower limb blood supply (e.g. aortic clamping) to minimize the effects of distal ischemia.

Active warming by a circulating water mattress is relatively ineffective because heat is applied only to the patient's back, where relatively little heat is lost. It has been superseded by forced-air warming devices. Active warming by resistive heating (electric) blankets is a recent development. It is as effective as the forced-air warming technique and may be particularly suitable in preventing hypothermia in out-of-hospital trauma situations.

Internal warming

The administration of 1 L of fluid at room temperature reduces core temperature by ~0.25°C. Fluid warming devices should be used when large amounts of fluid or blood replacement are anticipated. This is critical in the context of exsanguinating hemorrhage, where massive transfusion will lead to a dilutional coagulopathy that will be compounded by hypothermic coagulopathy if not aggressively managed. A rapid infuser system with high heat transfer capacity should be used in such cases. Fluid warming alone will not prevent core hypothermia and should be used in combination with active warming.

One liter of intravenous fluid can reduce core temperature by 0.25°C.

Airway humidification contributes little to preservation of core temperature because less than 10% of metabolic heat loss occurs via the respiratory tract.

Cardiopulmonary bypass transfers heat at a rate and magnitude not seen in any other situation (see below). Peritoneal dialysis is also very effective but not relevant to mild perioperative hypothermia. Amino acid infusion during anesthesia increases metabolic rate and patients are less hypothermic than those given the same volume of crystalloid. This technique has not gained widespread acceptance because of doubts about the effect on cardiac outcome of increased metabolic rate during anesthesia.

PEDIATRIC CONSIDERATIONS

Thermal control is critical in pediatric anesthetic practice and warrants special consideration.

Thermoregulatory responses are well developed in full-term neonates, but hypothermia develops rapidly when compensatory mechanisms are overwhelmed. A neonate has minimal insulating subcutaneous fat. Moreover, it has a body surface area to volume ratio 2.5 times that of an adult, so it can quickly become severely hypothermic.

Because infants under the age of 3 months do not shiver, the principal mechanism for heat production is nonshivering thermogenesis. Physiological responses to hypothermia compromise the sick infant. A chronically hypoxemic infant, e.g. with cyanotic congenital heart disease, decompensates rapidly if hypothermic. Nonshivering thermogenesis increases the metabolic rate and oxygen consumption may double, thereby putting additional strain on the cardiopulmonary system. The release of norepinephrine causes vasoconstriction, leading to lactic acidosis, which may increase right-to-left shunting and hypoxemia. Thus, a positive feedback loop of acidosis and hypoxemia occurs. Protective airway reflexes are obtunded, increasing the risk of aspiration of gastric contents. Sick infants should be maintained normothermic in a thermoneutral environment throughout the perioperative period.

Infants under 3 months do not shiver; nonshivering thermogenesis is their principal mechanism of heat production.

Avoiding environmental exposure is important to prevent heat loss. Adjusting the ambient temperature to 24°C or above, ideally for several hours preoperatively, will reduce radiant heat loss to cold walls. The infant should be kept wrapped and transported in an incubator until ready for induction, then placed on a heating blanket and under an overhead radiant heater set at the correct distance away. The head should be kept covered. Using warmed fluids, warmed humidified gases, and warmed skin preparation solution (drying off any excess to prevent cooling by evaporation) will help to reduce heat loss. A forced-air warming blanket should be used during the procedure, and the overhead radiant heater used again during emergence and recovery until the infant is ready to return to the incubator.

Temperature should be monitored in all pediatric patients. A thermistor in the axilla will usually suffice, but an esophageal stethoscope with a thermistor probe is ideal. For major surgery esophageal or rectal monitoring is mandatory.

CARDIOPULMONARY BYPASS

In contrast to the adverse consequences of inadvertent mild hypothermia, deliberate hypothermia is a widely used technique for myocardial and cerebral protection during cardiac and neurosurgery. Oxygen consumption is reduced by 5–7% per 1°C decrease in core temperature. At 28°C, brain metabolism is reduced by 50%. Moderate hypothermia also protects the spinal cord against ischemia.

Heat exchange during cardiopulmonary bypass (CPB) is on a different scale from any other method of heat transfer. The rate of heat exchange is such that heat cannot be distributed evenly throughout the core compartment during rapid cooling and rewarming, and the two-compartment model is inadequate. An 'intermediate' compartment, defined as the bladder and rectum, is described in CPB. Changes in core temperature eventually occur in this compartment with a time delay that reflects the extent to which redistribution of heat has been successful.

During the rewarming phase of CPB, heat is transferred to the core faster than it can be redistributed to the periphery and a substantial core–peripheral gradient develops. The subsequent reduction in core temperature after discontinuation of CPB (known as 'afterdrop') is due to redistribution to the periphery. Although hypothermia to 20–28°C is protective to myocardium, brain, and spinal cord during the period of cardiac asystole and CPB, once normal circulation is restored, mild hypothermia (34.5–36.5°C), such as occurs in 'afterdrop', is detrimental, as in all other circumstances. Therefore, measures to treat afterdrop by rewarming to normothermia should be as vigorous as in other clinical situations. Postoperative return to normothermia can take 2–5 hours in general surgical patients, and longer still in patients after cardiac surgery and CPB.

HYPERTHERMIA

Mechanism of fever

Pyrogens (e.g. bacterial lipopolysaccharides) are released by infecting organisms. Cytokines, such as interleukin (IL)-1, are released in response to this, which in turn generate prostaglandin E_2 (PGE_2) synthesis in the hypothalamus. PGE_2 increases the set-point range at which thermoregulatory effectors are active, causing pyrexia. Iatrogenic hyperthermia from excessive heating of patients during anesthesia with active warming is extremely rare, especially since the introduction of routine use of temperature monitoring during anesthesia. Thyrotoxicosis and thyroid storm may rarely cause hyperthermia. Thyroid storm occurs in thyrotoxic patients who have not been diagnosed preoperatively, or who have been inadequately treated prior to thyroidectomy. Tachycardia, hypertension, and hyperthermia (core temperature >38.0°C), despite adequate depth of anesthesia and analgesia, are typical presenting features. In contrast to malignant hyperthermia, there is no muscle rigidity and metabolic acidosis is unusual. Also, normocapnia is easy to maintain without increasing minute ventilation parameters. Hyperthermia may also occur in association with a rare condition, *osteogenesis imperfecta*, a metabolic bone disease characterized by frequent pathological bone fractures and blue sclerae. Septic patients frequently present with fever, which may persist or be aggravated during anesthesia, particularly if there is surgical manipulation of infected tissue.

Hyperthermia is a late sign in malignant hyperthermia.

Malignant hyperthermia

Malignant hyperthermia (MH) is a rare congenital autosomal dominant condition in which a life-threatening reaction to certain general anesthetic agents occurs. Presentation is characterized first by unexplained hypercapnia, followed by tachycardia, tachypnea, hypertension, sweating, muscle rigidity, and bronchospasm. Temperature elevation is a late sign. This disorder is discussed in more detail in Chapters 10 and 35.

SUMMARY

Physiological thermoregulation is a multi-input, multilevel control system. The spinal cord and a number of brainstem centers integrate afferent thermal signals and can also attenuate descending efferent responses. The normal autonomic response to cold begins with vasoconstriction, followed by shivering if core temperature continues to decrease. Both of these responses have a threshold temperature at which they are activated. Anesthesia decreases the threshold temperature of these thermoregulatory responses, facilitating core hypothermia. Hypothermia during general anesthesia develops with a characteristic three-phase pattern: an initial rapid reduction caused by redistribution of heat from core to peripheral tissues, because anesthesia inhibits tonic vasoconstriction; a more gradual decrease in core temperature determined by the difference between continuing heat loss and metabolic heat production; and vasoconstriction at its new lower threshold to prevent further heat loss.

Mild perioperative hypothermia is associated with serious adverse outcomes, including morbid cardiac events, increased blood loss, surgical wound infection, and increased duration of hospitalization. Anesthetists are uniquely placed to positively influence postoperative patient outcome by meticulous attention to maintenance of normothermia (36.5–37.0°C) during anesthesia.

Key references

Frank SM, Fleisher LA, Breslow MJ et al. Perioperative maintenance of normothermia reduces the incidence of morbid cardiac events. JAMA 1997;277:1127–34.

Kurz A, Sessler DI, Lenhardt RA. Perioperative normothermia to reduce the incidence of surgical wound infection and shorten hospitalization. New Engl J Med. 1996;334:1209–15.

Schmied H, Kurz A, Sessler DI, Kozek S, Reiter A. Mild intraoperative hypothermia increases blood loss and allogeneic transfusion requirements during total hip arthroplasty. Lancet 1996;347:289–92.

Further reading

Buggy D. Can anaesthetic management influence surgical wound healing? Lancet 2000;356:355–7.

Buggy DJ, Crossley AW. Thermoregulation, mild perioperative hypothermia and post-anaesthetic shivering. Br J Anaesth. 2000;84:615–28.

Buggy DJ. Metabolism, the stress response and thermoregulation during anaesthesia. In: Aitkinhead A, Rowbotham DJ, Smith G, eds. A textbook of anaesthesia, 4th edn. Edinburgh: Churchill Livingstone; 2002.

Kirkbride DA, Buggy DJ. Thermoregulation and inadvertent perioperative hypothermia. Br J Anaesth. 2003;3:24–8.

Sellden E, Brundin T, Wahren J. Augmented thermic effect of amino acids under general anaesthesia: a mechanism useful for prevention of anaesthesia-induced hypothermia. Clin Sci. 1994;86:611–18.

Sessler DI. Perioperative heat balance. Anesthesiology 2000;92:578–96.

Sessler DI. Complications and treatment of mild hypothermia. Anesthesiology 2001;95:531–43.

Sessler DI. Perioperative shivering. Anesthesiology 2002;96:467–84.

SECTION 9

Adaptive physiology

Chapter 68

Pregnancy

Richard M Smiley and Norman L Herman

TOPICS COVERED IN THIS CHAPTER

- **Maternal physiologic alterations**
  - Cardiovascular
  - Respiratory system
  - Central nervous system and anesthetic sensitivity
  - Renal system
  - Gastrointestinal system
  - Coagulation
  - Endocrine system
  - Uterus
- **Pharmacology in pregnancy**
  - Uteroplacental pharmacology
  - Maternal pharmacokinetics
  - Local anesthetic sensitivity and toxicity
  - Drug effects on uterine activity
- **Pre-eclampsia/eclampsia**
- **Regional analgesia and labor**
- **Complications of pregnancy**
  - Nonobstetric surgery during pregnancy
  - Amniotic fluid embolism
  - Hemorrhage

Pregnancy is, and is the most common altered physiologic state to which human beings are subject. During pregnancy, significant changes occur in the size and shape of a woman's body, the rapidity and pathways of drug and nutrient transport and metabolism, the regulation of blood pressure and cardiac function, the anatomy of the airway and neurological control of respiratory function, and even the level of neurologic functioning, consciousness, and reaction to consciousness-altering drugs. Finally, the pregnant woman carries a fetus with its own continuing physiologic growth, changes, and adaptations, which need to be considered in a variety of clinical circumstances.

This chapter covers the major organ system alterations that occur in the pregnant woman, and the changes in pharmacokinetics and pharmacodynamics specific to pregnancy. The focus is on those aspects of pregnancy physiology, pharmacology, or clinical situations that alter the way anesthesiologists assess or treat patients, or on new concepts in the physiology and pathophysiology of pregnancy, rather than on a general overview of obstetric anesthesia per se.

MATERNAL PHYSIOLOGIC ALTERATIONS

Cardiovascular

Pregnancy involves alterations in multiple components of the cardiovascular system. New blood vessels, even new organs (i.e. the placenta) develop, cardiac structural changes occur, blood volume and blood cell mass increase, and the response of the vasculature to endogenous hormones and transmitters and exogenous drugs is significantly altered.

The development and enlargement of the uteroplacental circulation necessitates enormous cardiovascular changes in the pregnant woman. Plasma volume increases by 50% by the end of pregnancy, with the majority of the increase complete by week 20. Red cell mass increases in parallel with body weight, but only by about 15%, resulting in the relative anemia of pregnancy (Fig. 68.1). This increase in volume at the expense of hemoglobin concentration increases the woman's tolerance of the obligate

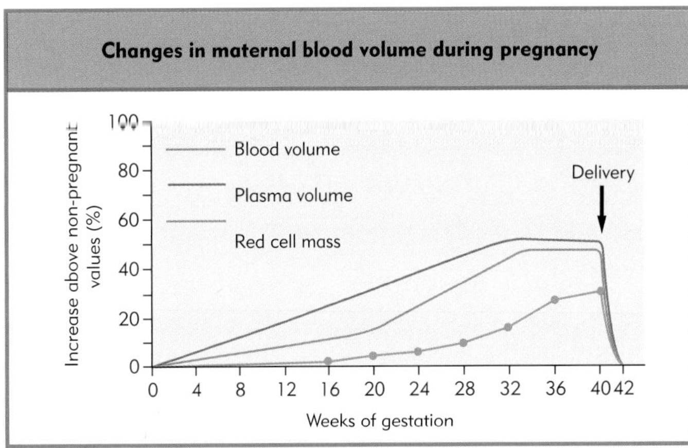

Figure 68.1 Changes in maternal blood volume during pregnancy. A plot depicting the increases in blood volume, plasma volume, and red cell mass during gestation. (British Medical Journal 1991;302:719-722, with permission from the BMJ Publishing Group.)

hemorrhage at delivery. Plasma protein concentrations are decreased by dilution, decreasing colloid osmotic pressure and predisposing the woman to peripheral and pulmonary edema.

Cardiac output increases beginning week 8 of gestation to about 40% at week 20, as a result of increases in both heart rate and stroke volume. At term the increment is 50%, with a further increase of 30–50% with the onset and progress of labor. Following delivery, involution of the uterus results in a further 50–100% augmentation of cardiac output in the absence of major hemorrhage at delivery. The need for physiological changes of such magnitude, sometimes within seconds or minutes, illustrates why lesions limiting increases in cardiac output (e.g. mitral stenosis, pulmonary hypertension, cardiomyopathies) are poorly tolerated in pregnancy. Similarly, there is frequent structural deterioration of indwelling bioprosthetic valves in pregnancy, presumably owing to increased flow and turbulence. Most of these hyperdynamic cardiovascular changes are magnified with multiple gestations.

Cardiovascular signs associated with normal pregnancy include basilar pulmonary râles, S3 gallop, systolic flow murmur, peripheral edema, cardiomegaly on by chest radiography, and electrocardiographic alterations (axis deviation, premature atrial and ventricular contractions). Symptoms may include dyspnea on exertion, palpitations, orthopnea, and even chest pain. Echocardiography may reveal increases in mitral and tricuspid valve areas, increased left ventricular wall thickness, tricuspid, pulmonary and/or mitral regurgitation, mild pericardial effusion, and altered systolic and diastolic function even in healthy women. Most of these changes resolve by 16–24 weeks postpartum.

Despite the increased blood volume, blood pressure decreases during pregnancy, especially during the first two trimesters, with a return toward prepregnancy levels by term. A decrease in systemic vascular resistance probably results from the low-resistance placental circulation and actual decreases in maternal vascular tone. A blunting of maternal responses to vasoactive drugs occurs in pregnancy (Fig. 68.2). The precise molecular nature of these alterations in signal transduction is unclear. Blood pressures above prepregnancy values often indicate a pathophysiological process (gestational hypertension, or pre-eclampsia) and may represent a failure of these adaptive vasodilatory mechanisms. Women who do not make these adaptations and develop hypertension are at higher risk of hypertension and cardiovascular disease in later life, so pregnancy may unmask an underlying tendency towards cardiovascular disease.

Multiple cardiovascular changes occur in pregnancy, including increased cardiac output and blood volume, and decreased systemic vascular resistance.

The increase in size of the uterus results in complete occlusion of the inferior vena cava in a majority of pregnant women in the supine position at term. However, only 15% demonstrate symptoms of the 'supine hypotensive syndrome', as most develop alternative pathways of venous return via the lumbosacral venous plexus and azygous system. The increased blood flow in this system, which includes the epidural veins, may speed the elimination of drugs from the epidural space and may increase the risk of venous entry of epidural catheters and needles.

Response to vasoactive drugs during pregnancy

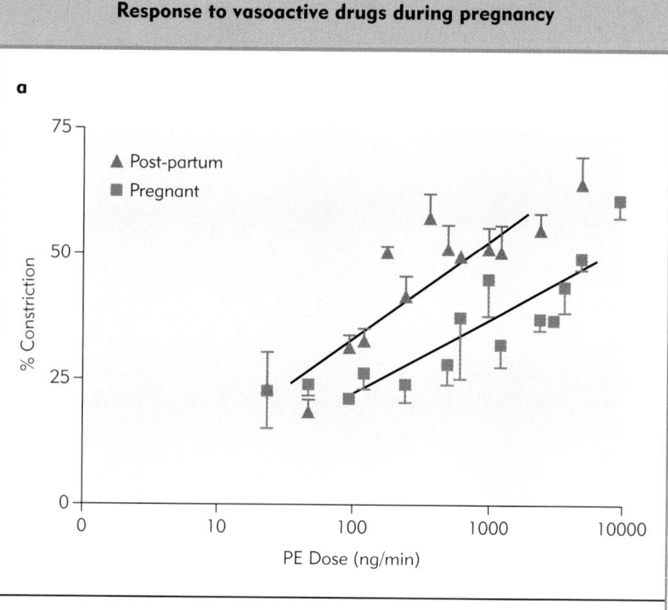

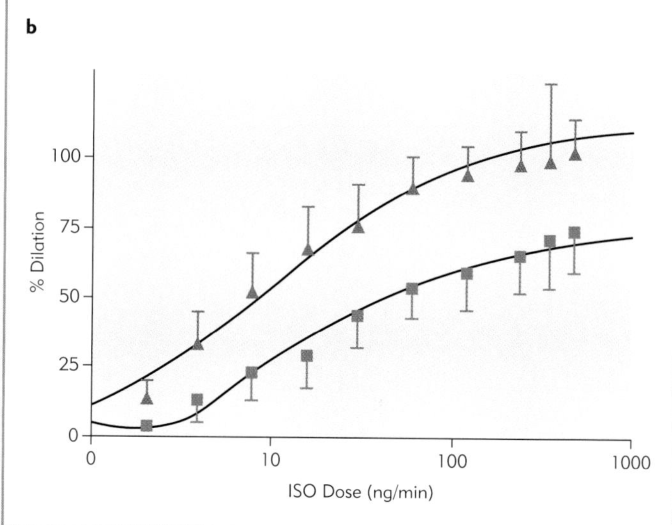

Figure 68.2 Response to vasoactive drugs during pregnancy. (a) Phenylephrine (PE) dose–response curve. Graph shows the linear portion of the dose response of hand veins to a local infusion of phenylephrine in women during (squares) and after pregnancy (triangles). The pregnant response is significantly shifted to the right, indicating a blunting of the constrictive effect of the α_1-adrenoceptor agonist. (b) Isoproterenol (ISO) dose–response curve. Hand veins were preconstricted with phenylephrine to 50% of original size. Graph of the complete dose–response curve of hand veins to a local infusion of isoproterenol in women during (squares) and after pregnancy (triangles). The pregnant response is significantly shifted to the right, indicating a blunting of the vasodilating effect of the β-adrenoceptor agonist. (Adapted with permission from Landau et al. Disproportionate decrease in the α-compared with β-adrenergic sensitivity in the dorsal hand vein in pregnancy favors vasodilation. Circulation 2002; 106: 1116–20.)

Respiratory system

Minute ventilation increases by 45% during pregnancy, mostly because of an increase in tidal volume. Early in pregnancy progesterone increases carbon dioxide sensitivity, leading to relative hyperventilation and respiratory alkalosis, with normal maternal P_aCO_2 decreasing to 30–32 mmHg. At this level of hypocarbia,

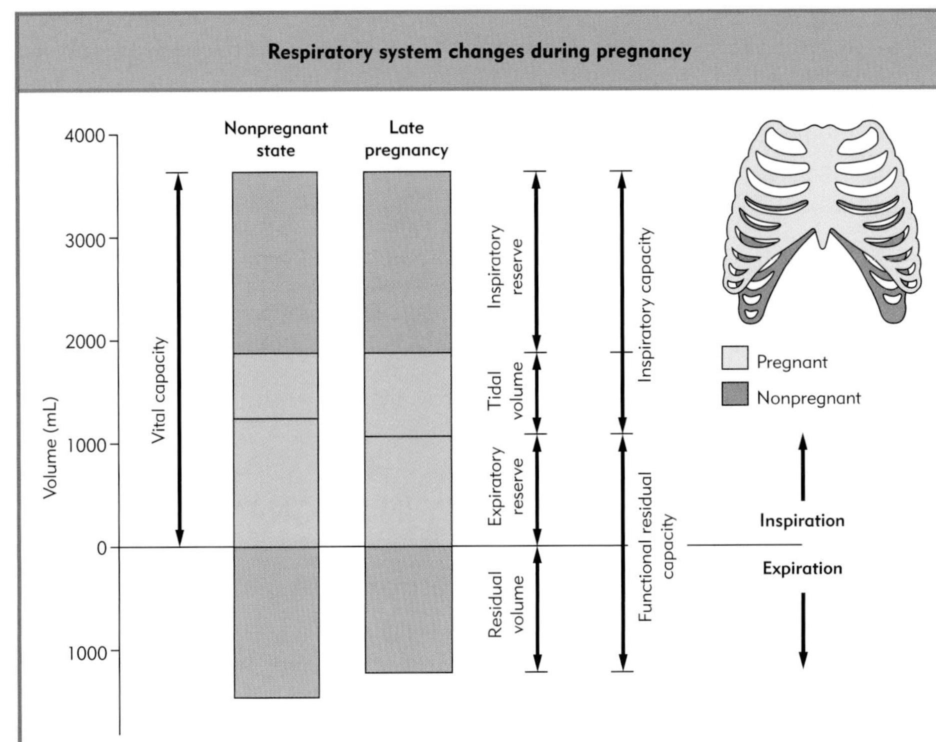

Figure 68.3 Changes in the respiratory system during pregnancy. Changes in inspiratory and expiratory volumes lead to significant reductions in functional residual capacity during pregnancy. The inset illustrates changes in thoracic dimensions. (British Medical Journal 1991;302:719-722, with permission from the BMJ Publishing Group.)

theoretically, maternal P_aO_2 should be 100 mmHg or more. However, the increase in P_aO_2 is offset by an increase in ventilation–perfusion mismatching as pregnancy progresses, which reaches 12–15% by term compared to 3–5% in nonpregnant women. Increased renal excretion of bicarbonate partially compensates for the alkalosis, and maternal pH is maintained only slightly above normal. Later in pregnancy the expanding uterus causes flaring of the ribs, with an average increase in thoracic circumference of 5–7 cm and elevation of the diaphragm by 4 cm. Expiratory reserve and residual volume decrease, reducing functional residual capacity (FRC) by 10–25% (Fig. 68.3). There are conflicting reports regarding pulmonary diffusing capacity for CO (DLCO) in pregnancy: most recent studies report little change. The decrease in FRC and the increase in oxygen consumption in pregnancy result in a rapid decline in arterial oxygen saturation during periods of apnea (e.g. during rapid-sequence induction of general anesthesia). There appears to be moderate bronchial relaxation with some protection from bronchospasm in asthmatics, although the course of asthma in individual patients is quite variable. Interestingly, these anatomic and physiologic pulmonary changes do not appear to be greater in twin than in singleton pregnancies.

The upper airway is moderately reduced in caliber in pregnancy owing to capillary engorgement and mild edema. These processes are exacerbated in labor, and may contribute to the increased difficulty in visualizing the larynx in pregnant women during attempted tracheal intubation.

Central nervous system and anesthetic sensitivity

Pregnancy induces structural, physiological, and pharmacological changes in the CNS. There is substantial evidence from both objective testing and subjective testimony that mental functioning and memory decrease mildly but noticeably during pregnancy. The brain decreases in size during pregnancy, and even more so with pre-eclampsia, although the clinical and physiological meaning or consequences of this anatomic change is unknown. The MAC (ED_{50}) of volatile anesthetics is reduced by 25–30%, and it appears that the effective doses of intravenous sedatives and hypnotics are similarly reduced. This increased sensitivity to anesthetics, and perhaps the cognitive effects, have been attributed to the sedative/anesthetic effect of progesterone. MAC values return to normal nonpregnant levels within several days of delivery.

Sensitivity to sedatives and hypnotics increases in pregnancy, probably owing to progesterone effects.

Renal system

Glomerular filtration rate increases with cardiac output; tubular reabsorption increases in parallel, maintaining fluid and electrolyte balance. Increased filtration results in a 40% decrease in plasma creatinine and urea concentrations. The clinical implication is that renally cleared drugs are more rapidly eliminated in pregnancy. More importantly for clinical diagnosis, a creatinine level that would be normal in a nonpregnant patient may indicate significant impairment of renal function in a pregnant woman.

Gastrointestinal system

Gastric volume and acidity increase early in pregnancy in response to placental gastrin. It has been taught for years that gastric emptying is slowed in pregnancy by anatomic factors and the effect of progesterone, but recent studies measuring gastric emptying indicate that normal pregnancy does not increase gastric emptying time. Labor pain and opioid administration do slow gastric emptying, and the lower esophageal sphincter is relaxed during pregnancy, so the pregnant woman is at somewhat increased risk of regurgitation and aspiration.

Coagulation

Pregnancy is a hypercoagulable state, with increased activity of coagulation factors and platelets. This affords some protection against hemorrhage with delivery, but also results in an increased risk of thromboembolism (approximately fivefold compared to the nonpregnant state) and, paradoxically, of hemorrhage, owing to a state of disseminated intravascular coagulation from the activated coagulation system. Platelet counts tend to decrease during pregnancy owing to increased consumption. The HELLP syndrome variant of pre-eclampsia (hemolysis, elevated liver enzymes, low platelets) can reduce platelets further to dangerously low levels. A variety of coagulation abnormalities, usually genetic abnormalities affecting the function or concentration of coagulation factors, are associated with early and late pregnancy loss and pre-eclampsia. The risk of coagulation-related complications leads to fairly frequent intervention with anticoagulants (e.g. low molecular weight heparin) and antiplatelet drugs (e.g. aspirin) in pregnancy, which has implications for the execution of obstetric and anesthetic plans for delivery.

Endocrine system

Enormous changes in hormone levels occur with pregnancy. The most clinically significant change involves glucose handling. Insulin resistance develops with pregnancy, starting in the mid to late second trimester. At 12–14 weeks' gestation there is an increase in insulin sensitivity, and some women with type 1 diabetes mellitus may suffer hypoglycemic episodes secondary to insulin therapy. Sensitivity to insulin declines throughout the rest of pregnancy, and leads to glucose intolerance or gestational diabetes in 2–4% of women. The development of gestational diabetes mellitus may be a 'marker' for later development of type 2 diabetes, much as the development of gestational hypertension may indicate a susceptibility to essential hypertension. Insulin resistance ends abruptly with delivery of the placenta, pointing strongly to a placental hormonal etiology. Classically, human placental lactogen was thought to be the prime agent responsible, but current evidence suggests a multifactorial etiology, with contributions from human placental growth hormone, cortisol, tumor necrosis factor-α, leptin, and some newer candidates. Insulin therapy should stop with delivery to avoid maternal hypoglycemia, as rapid resensitization is expected.

Uterus

Uterine blood flow increases from 50 mL/min to 1 L/min or more at term. Almost 90% of the flow is directed to the placental intervillous spaces for transplacental exchange with the fetus. Approximately 200 spiral arteries underlie the developing placenta. This area is invaded by trophoblastic cells, which erode the elastic and muscular components of the arteries, exposing them to systemic blood pressure. The pressure results in dilation of the spiral arteries into funnel-shaped sacs that lose most responsiveness to vasoconstrictors, although the vasoconstrictor responsiveness of the larger feeding uterine arteries is less clear. The result is a low-resistance pathway shunting blood from maternal circulation into the intervillous space (Fig. 68.4). Maternal systemic arterial blood pressure is the major determinant of intervillous flow, and thus is the target of most cardiovascular monitoring and strategies to optimize fetal condition.

Uterine blood flow ceases or is greatly diminished with contraction of the uterus, much as myocardial blood flow ceases during cardiac systole. Therefore, excessive or prolonged uterine contraction can impair uteroplacental flow and fetal oxyenation. For this reason, there are clinical situations where uterine relaxation (e.g. β-adrenoceptor agonists, nitroglycerin, volatile anesthetics) may be the appropriate response to impaired placental perfusion when uterine hypercontractility is suspected or demonstrated.

PHARMACOLOGY IN PREGNANCY

Uteroplacental pharmacology

The placenta was once believed to provide a protective barrier against fetal drug and toxin exposure. In fact, no significant barrier exists to the placental transfer of most pharmacologic agents. Gases (O_2, CO_2, anesthetics) and most small ions and molecules cross the placenta by simple diffusion, with facilitated diffusion systems existing for glucose and lactate. There is active transport of amino acids, calcium, phosphate, and some vitamins, and endocytotic mechanisms for the transfer of immunoglobulins to the fetus. A general equation for placental transport is:

$$Q_t = K \times A \times ([M] - [F])/D$$

where Q_t is the flux (amount transferred over time), A is the surface area of the placenta, D is the thickness of the fetal–maternal barrier, and [M] and [F] refer to the fetal and maternal concentrations of the substance of interest. The constant, K, is a function of the specific substance of interest, and depends predominantly on molecular weight (larger molecules cross the placenta less readily) and lipid solubility (charged or highly polar molecules do not cross as well). Lipid-soluble drugs freely cross the placenta up to a molecular weight of 600 Da, which includes most drugs commonly used by anesthesiologists. Familiar drugs that do not cross the placenta to any large extent include glycopyrrolate, nondepolarizing muscle relaxants (charged, i.e. highly polar), heparin, low-molecular weight heparin, insulin, and dextrans (high molecular weight). Much of the literature about placental transport and maternofetal distribution of drugs consists of single measurements made at the time of delivery comparing umbilical vein to maternal plasma concentrations, resulting in reports of maternal/fetal (M/F) ratios of drugs. Such studies are limited by their static nature and the implicit assumption that they are performed under equilibrium conditions, which is rarely true. Most local anesthetic drugs and opioids have been reported to have M/F ratios of 0.3–0.9. The difficulties inherent in interpreting these studies are well illustrated by the range of values reported for fentanyl (0.05–0.7).

No significant barrier exists to the placental transfer of most lipophilic low molecular weight drugs.

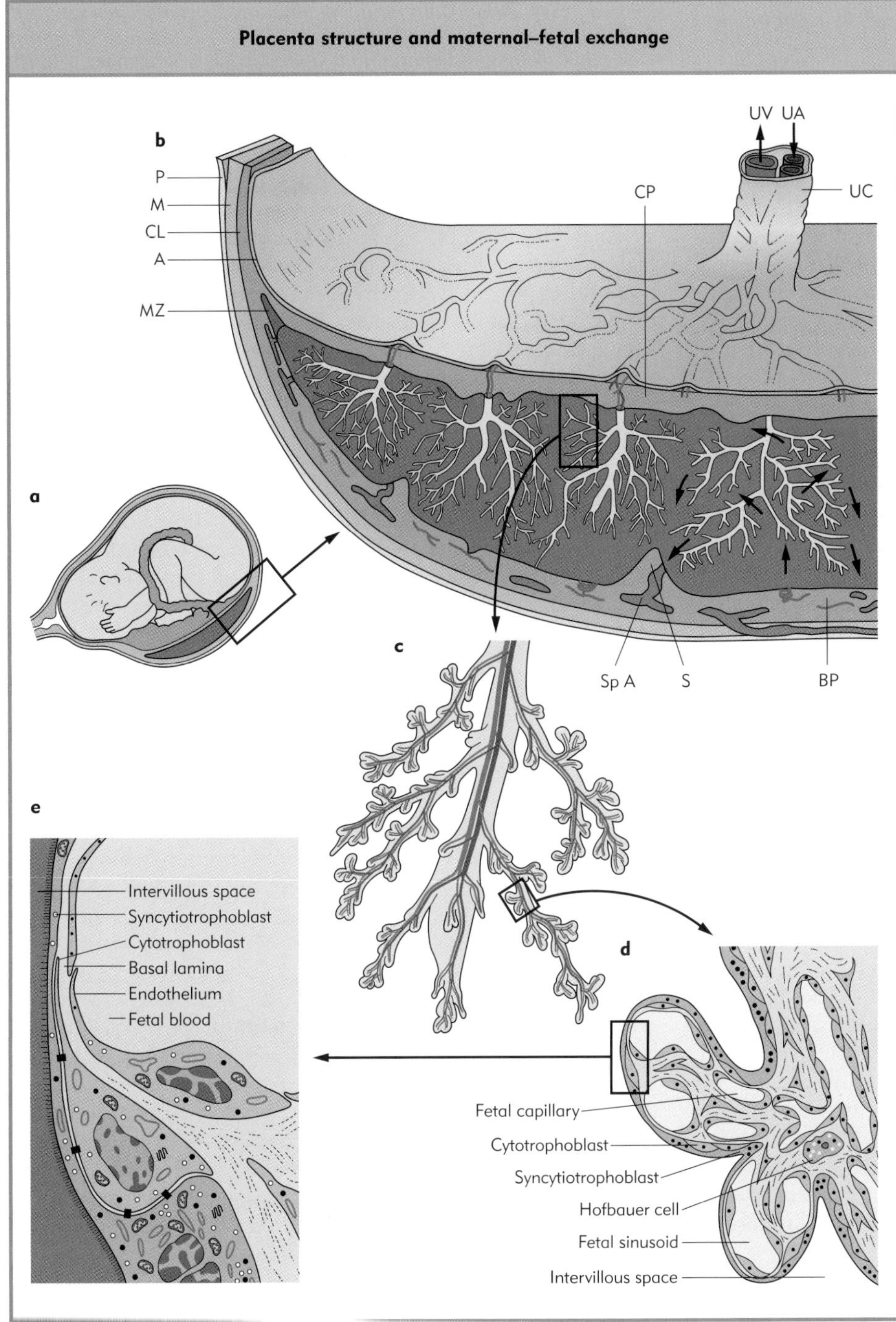

Figure 68.4 Structure of the human placenta. (a) Fetus and placenta in utero. (b) The placenta brings the maternal and fetal circulations into close apposition for exchange of solutes. The arrows illustrate the flow characteristics of maternal blood around the villous trees that contain the fetal vessels. A, amnion; BP, basal plate; CP, chorionic plate; CL, chorionic leaves; M, myometrium; MZ, marginal zone; P, perimetrium; S, septum; SpA, spiral artery; UA, umbilical artery; UC, umbilical cord; UV, umbilical vein. (c) The villi branch into multiple generations, with the terminal branches shown. (d) Light microscopic view through a terminal villous illustrating the fetal sinusoids, enlarged fetal capillaries that increase surface area for transfer. (e) Simplified electron micrograph of the 'placental barrier' where maternofetal exchange occurs. (Adapted with permission from Kaufman P, Schaffen I. Placental development. In: Polin RA, Fox WW, eds. Fetal and neonatal physiology. Philadelphia: WB Saunders; 1998:59–66; and Kaufman P. Basic morphology of the fetal and maternal circuits in the human placenta. Contrib Gynecol Obstet. 1985;13:5–17. Karger AG, Basel: S.)

Maternal pharmacokinetics

The increased cardiac output characteristic of pregnancy results in more rapid uptake of drugs from peripheral depots (intramuscular, subcutaneous, and epidural/spinal). Volume of distribution is increased for most drugs, whether lipophilic or hydrophilic, as all compartments are increased in size. Plasma concentrations of α_1-glycoprotein, an important drug binding protein, and plasma cholinesterase, the enzyme responsible for hydrolysis of succinylcholine and 2-chloroprocaine, are decreased, but the magnitude or consistency of any clinical effects of these alterations is unclear.

Local anesthetic sensitivity and toxicity

Pregnant women are more sensitive to the effects of local anesthetics. The reduced capacities of the epidural and intrathecal spaces as a result of epidural vein engorgement increase the physical spread of injected solutions. The sensitivity of nervous tissue to blockade by local anesthetics is also increased in pregnancy. Median nerve blockade with lidocaine (lignocaine) requires less drug in pregnant subjects. In isolated vagus nerve the onset of bupivacaine block is much faster in nerves from pregnant rats.

Nerve blockade by local anesthetics is enhanced in pregnancy.

Systemic toxicity with local anesthetics is usually the result of accidental injection into the circulation of doses meant for epidural or peripheral nerve blockade. An early target of local anesthetic toxicity is the brain, where increasing concentrations first block inhibitory pathways, leading to the well-described symptoms of perioral numbness and paresthesiae, metallic taste, tinnitus, and seizures. Coma and respiratory arrest follow if concentrations are increased further. With lidocaine, cardiovascular collapse occurs at about twice the seizure-inducing concentration in plasma. With bupivacaine and other long-acting local anesthetics, potentially fatal cardiac arrhythmias (ventricular fibrillation or tachycardia) may ensue near the plasma concentration that produces seizures. The difference in cardiac electrophysiologic effects may result from the relatively slow dissociation of bupivacaine, compared to lidocaine, from cardiac Na^+ channels, as well as differential CNS effects producing bradycardia, hypotension, and arrhythmias. The evidence that pregnancy enhances bupivacaine cardiotoxicity is based primarily on studies in sheep, but more recent information from this model suggests that pregnancy may not significantly increase susceptibility to a given dose or concentration of local anesthetic. However, the *consequences* of an intravascular injection are probably greater in pregnancy, as seizures with periods of hypoxemia may harm the fetus, and the risk of aspiration during such an event is greater. Ventilation and cardiopulmonary resuscitation may be more difficult in pregnancy owing to anatomic considerations. In addition, the *likelihood* of an intravascular injection of local anesthetic meant for the epidural space is increased in pregnancy because of increased vascularity. The newer local anesthetics ropivacaine, which is produced and marketed only as the S-enantiomer, and the S-enantiomer of bupivacaine, levobupivacaine, may be less likely to cause cardiac arrhythmias upon inadvertent intravascular injection, although there is controversy about whether the comparison of these drugs has been at equivalent anesthetic doses. Current strategies of dosing for labor epidural analgesia with low or moderate concentrations of bupivacaine (0.05–0.125%) combined with opioids are very unlikely to result in toxic systemic concentrations of any local anesthetic, even if all or part of the dose is administered intravenously.

Drug effects on uterine activity

A pharmacologic concern specific to pregnancy is the effect of drugs on uterine activity. Drugs are given to increase contractions (uterotonics) or to stop or diminish them (tocolytics). The effect of neuraxial analgesia (as opposed to a direct effect of drugs) on the progress and outcome of labor is discussed briefly in the next section.

Whereas local anesthetics and opioids do not appear to have a consistent direct effect on the frequency or strength of uterine contractions, volatile anesthetics cause dose-dependent uterine relaxation. Concentrations of 1 MAC or above are necessary to produce clinically significant uterine relaxation, such as that needed to stop a tetanic contraction, for placental removal after delivery, or in cases of uterine inversion. Lower concentrations typically administered during general anesthesia for cesarean section may have mild uterine relaxing activity, but do not detectably increase bleeding at operation.

Drugs given specifically to relax the uterus are utilized for preterm labor and contractions, hypercontractility in labor (usually a result of relative overdose of oxytocics), and in external cephalic version or fetal surgery. The β-adrenergic agonists (terbutaline and ritodrine in North America, hexaprenaline and salbutamol in Europe) are commonly used tocolytic agents, although the use of alternatives is increasing because of their high incidence of side effects. The β_1-adrenoceptor effects of these drugs (especially ritodrine and terbutaline) result in tachycardia, increases in cardiac contractility, and tachyarrythmias. The β_2-adrenergic effects include venous and arteriolar dilation, and a further contribution to tachycardia. Other β-adrenoceptor-related effects include hyperglycemia and hypokalemia. β-Adrenoceptor agonist therapy can lead to pulmonary edema, often in the context of infection or aggressive hydration. Hydration status must be carefully monitored, and precipitants of tachycardia or arrhythmias (halothane, additional β-adrenergic drugs, ketamine, light anesthesia) should be avoided. The calcium channel antagonist nifedipine, the oxytocin receptor antagonist atisoban, and nonsteroidal anti-inflammatory drugs (e.g. indomethacin) are equally or more efficacious as tocolytics as β-agonists, with fewer hemodynamic side effects and probably fewer anesthetic implications.

Magnesium sulfate ($MgSO_4$) is widely used for tocolysis and for the treatment and prevention of eclampsia. Multicenter trials demonstrate that $MgSO_4$ is the drug of choice for prevention of seizures in pre-eclampsia or eclampsia. Mg^{2+} competes directly with Ca^{2+} for binding and uptake, and also increases intracellular cyclic AMP, both of which decrease smooth muscle intracellular Ca^{2+} concentration and the actin–myosin interaction. $MgSO_4$ also has major effects on neuromuscular signal transmission by inhibiting acetylcholine release at the neuromuscular junction, desensitizing the motor endplate, and altering muscle membrane excitability. Patients receiving $MgSO_4$ are profoundly sensitive to nondepolarizing neuromuscular blockers and require significantly reduced doses and close monitoring of neuromuscular function. The response to succinylcholine is variable, but of less clinical significance as succinylcholine block will dissipate by the end of most procedures.

Nitroglycerin has been reported effective for uterine relaxation in numerous case reports, at doses ranging from 50 to 500 μg intravenously, but clear scientific evidence of its efficacy, dose response, indications, or limitations is lacking.

Oxytocin is the most common uterotonic drug given by continuous infusion for the induction or augmentation of labor. This nonapeptide hormone released from the posterior pituitary stimulates specific oxytocin receptors (OXTR) in the myometrium that couple to Gq and phospholipase C, increasing intramyometrial Ca^{2+} and contractility. The OXTR is up- and downregulated such that the amount in the uterus increases 100-fold during pregnancy to increase receptivity. The receptor appears to be internalized and downregulated by agonist exposure, perhaps explaining why postpartum uterine atony is more common in women having received oxtocin in high doses for long periods. The OXTR is also present in vascular endothelial cells, where it is coupled to nitric oxide release. This may be the mechanism of the hypotension seen when high-dose oxytocin is administered to induce postpartum uterine contraction/involution.

A variety of prostaglandins are utilized for uterine 'ripening', labor induction, and to treat postpartum hemorrhage. As would be expected from this class of drugs, side effects are varied and common and include fever, nausea/vomiting, hypercontraction of the uterus, bronchospasm, and cardiovascular alterations.

PRE-ECLAMPSIA/ECLAMPSIA

Pre-eclampsia is a complex, multisystem hypertensive disorder of pregnancy that affects up to 10% of parturients. Current classification systems (Table 66.1) differentiate conditions associated with hypertension alone and those involving proteinuria, which indicates the multisystem immunologic or inflammatory syndrome of pre-eclampsia. The increased blood pressure of pre-eclampsia is important more because it reflects underlying disease rather than because it is inherently dangerous; few of the serious consequences of pre-eclampsia actually result from increased blood pressure. Organs affected by pre-eclampsia include the vasculature, kidneys, liver, brain, heart, platelets, and the developing fetus (intrauterine growth restriction). When neurologic involvement progresses to seizures, thought to result from either cerebrovascular involvement or brain edema, the syndrome is classified as *eclampsia*. The cause is unknown, although it is clear that pre-eclampsia is a placental disease, related to placental ischemia and consequent reactions. Multiple associations with plasma markers, ethnic, genetic, and other epidemiologic factors have been reported. Long intervals between pregnancies, a new partner, or short intervals of cohabitation and sexual relations, or the use of barrier contraceptives before pregnancy all appear to increase risk, pointing towards an immunologic etiology. Risk factors include nulliparity, extremes of maternal age (although the association with young mothers may be due to the effect of first pregnancies), pre-existing hypertension, collagen vascular disorders or thrombophilias, family (maternal or paternal) history of pre-eclampsia, black race, obesity, insulin resistance, and diabetes mellitus. Conditions with increased placental or trophoblastic tisse (e.g. molar pregnancy, multiple gestation) increase the risk, which reaches 20–30% in triplet pregnancies. There are interesting similarities between the histology of the pre-eclamptic placenta and allograft rejection of transplants, further suggesting an immunologic mechanism.

Some aspects of the pathophysiology are understood. The first step appears to be the failure of trophoblastic cells to produce vascular remodeling in the placental bed. The resultant narrow, constrictable spiral arteries provide inadequate perfusion to the intervillous space as the placenta enlarges, leading to placental and potentially fetal ischemia. The next steps are less clear, but the ischemic fetoplacental unit releases mediators that result in a multisystem disorder. Current evidence suggests that the primary target is the endothelial cell. Markers of endothelial activation and damage are detectable well before the clinical signs of hypertension and proteinuria are evident, confirming that it is not hypertension per se that causes the pathologic changes. Recently, a specific tyrosine kinase (sFlt1) has been identified that may be a major factor in producing the pathologic lesions seen in women with pre-eclampsia, which may improve our understanding of the disease and possible treatments. When administered to rats, this protein produces the classic renal histology of pre-eclampsia, glomerular endotheliosis, suggesting that an animal model of the disease could finally be developed.

Preclampsia is a placental disease, with effects on the vasculature, kidneys, liver, brain, heart, and platelets – and the fetus.

Table 68.1 Classification of hypertension in pregnancy (Reprinted with permission from Elsevier. (The Lancet 2000;356:1260–5.))

Pre-existing hypertension (3-5% of pregnancies)
Hypertension existing before pregnancy or detected before 20 weeks' gestation, or persisting after the pregnancy ends. Many of these patients have essential hypertension; some have renal disease or other disorders
Pregnancy-associated hypertension
Hypertension occurring de novo after 20 weeks'gestation and resolving within 6 weeks of delivery. Two groups: Gestational hypertension (6–7%): hypertension without proteinuria or other associated features Pre-eclampsia (5–6%): hypertension with proteinuria of at least 0.3 g/24 h
Superimposed pre-eclampsia (25% of women with pre-existing hypertension)
Signs and symptoms of pre-eclampsia in women with pre-existing hypertension
Eclampsia
Convulsions in any woman who has or who later presents with hypertension in pregnancy of any cause

Peripheral vascular resistance is moderately – sometimes severely – elevated, resulting in increased maternal blood pressure and relative hypovolemia. An imbalance between vasoconstrictors (e.g. thromboxane, angiotensin II) and vasodilators (prostacyclin, nitric oxide) has been a target of research, but has not led to mechanistic breakthroughs. There is an exaggerated response to vasoconstrictors, especially angiotensin II, compared to the usual blunted response in pregnancy. There is generalized activation of the sympathetic nervous system, with elevated peripheral neural signaling detected in pre-eclamptic women compared to healthy pregnant women (Fig. 68.5).

Several strategies for prevention and treatment have been tried, none with notable success. There is some evidence that prophylactic aspirin therapy may benefit some women at high risk. Other anti-inflammatory drugs, antioxidants, and anticoagulants are occasionally tried. Treatment is largely symptomatic, and the definitive treatment is delivery of the fetus. Blood pressure has classically been treated with α-methyldopa or hydralazine; current therapy involves β-adrenergic blockade, combined α- and β-blockade with labetalol, or calcium channel antagonists. Blood pressure treatment, though necessary in some cases to avoid complications directly related to blood flow or pressure, does not alter the course and progression of disease. Decisions regarding specific antihypertensive drugs are based on similar hemodynamic and pharmacologic criteria as in nonpregnant women, with the exception that angiotensin inhibitors are contraindicated in pregnancy. Maternal hemodynamic changes may affect the fetus; therefore, fetal monitoring is essential when maternal hemodynamics are manipulated.

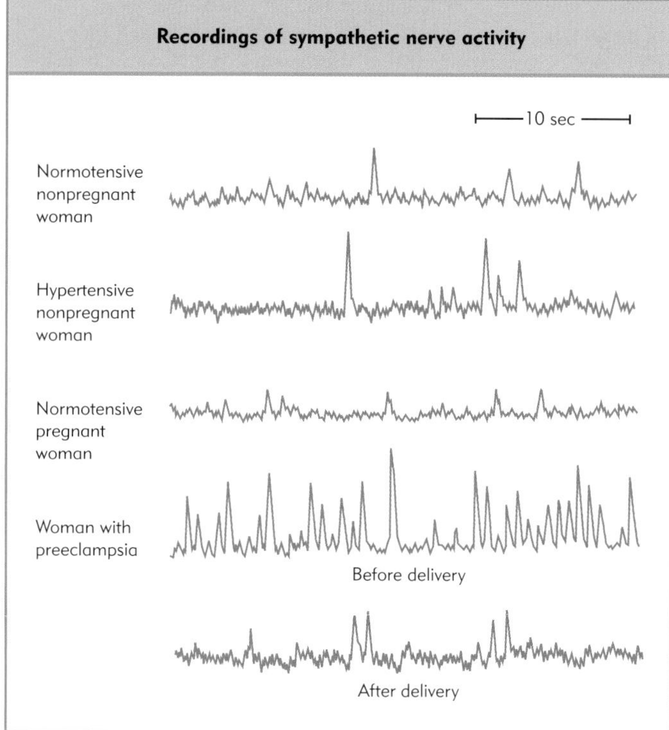

Figure 68.5 Recordings of sympathetic nerve activity. Representative recordings of sympathetic nerve activity from tungsten microelectrodes inserted into peroneal nerve. Representative recordings from normotensive nonpregnant, hypertensive pregnant, normotensive pregnant, and pre-eclamptic women. The rate of sympathetic discharge is similar in the first three, but significantly higher in women with pre-eclampsia. Blood pressure and sympathetic nerve activity returned to normal after delivery. (Adapted from Schobel et al. Pre-eclampia – a state of sympathetic overactivity. New Engl J Med. 1996; 335: 1480–5).

REGIONAL ANALGESIA AND LABOR

Controversy has existed for years regarding the effect (if any) of epidural (and now spinal) analgesia on the speed and success of vaginal delivery. Most studies on the effect of epidural (or spinal) analgesia on the progress of labor suffer from avoidable and unavoidable design flaws and selection bias. There is an *association* of neuraxial analgesia with longer, more difficult labors, and an increased incidence of instrumental vaginal and cesarean delivery. The controversy concerns whether the association is causal, or whether women who opt for epidural analgesia are those experiencing difficult labor, such that women with rapidly progressing uncomplicated labors are selected out by not requesting or receiving neuraxial analgesia. This topic has been the subject of several recent reviews and meta-analyses, and will be discussed only briefly here.

Several randomized trials of epidural (almost exclusively bupivacaine with or without fentanyl) versus systemic analgesia (usually intravenous meperidine) suggest that epidural analgesia per se does not increase the cesarean section rate, but may increase the instrumental vaginal delivery rate and slightly prolong labor (Table 68.2). Recent studies have attempted to avoid the potential selection bias in even randomized studies by utilizing a population-based 'catastrophe analysis' strategy, examining whether the introduction of a labor analgesia service at a given institution increases the cesarean section percentage. These studies strongly (unanimously) suggest that there is no increase.

The widespread adoption of lower doses of local anesthetics for epidural analgesia over the past decade and a half, and one of the rationales for the introduction of spinal analgesia using opioids with or without low-dose local anesthetics, was the hope that decreasing motor block would decrease any effects on fetal malrotation and dystocia. Some studies suggest that spinal analgesia may result in more rapid labors or more rapid cervical dilation than with epidural or systemic analgesia. It has proved very difficult to demonstrate differences between anesthetic doses, drugs, or techniques (e.g. combined spinal–epidural versus epidural) in their effects on labor outcome. This is perhaps not surprising, as there is still considerable controversy about the magnitude or indeed the existence of any effect.

COMPLICATIONS OF PREGNANCY

Nonobstetric surgery during pregnancy

Each year about 50 000 (~1%) of pregnant women in the United States undergo nonobstetric surgery. In a large series, 42% of operations during pregnancy occurred during the first trimester, 35% during the second trimester, and 23% during the third trimester.

Surgery during pregnancy exposes the fetus to drugs (including anesthetics), potential impairment of uteroplacental blood flow by surgical manipulation or maternal cardiovascular changes, and preterm labor and delivery or spontaneous abortion. No anesthetic agent has ever been shown to be directly teratogenic (or to cause fetal loss or intrauterine death) in humans. Alterations in blood flow, oxygenation, and temperature, or the effects of surgery and associated events (e.g. infection), are probably much more important than specific perioperative drugs. However, no studies have been or will be done that are large enough to detect a small risk to fetuses of anesthetic exposure.

The greatest risk of pregnancy loss appears to be when the surgical field is close to the uterus, especially with an infectious process (e.g. perforated or ruptured appendix). Uterine contraction is usually monitored perioperatively, either during the operative period itself or limited to the preoperative and postoperative periods. Some anesthesiologists omit nitrous oxide because of its possible effects on DNA synthesis, and many attempt to omit or limit benzodiazepines because of a 1975 FDA warning suggesting an association with long-term benzodiazepine use and cleft lip and palate. There is no convincing evidence favoring regional versus general anesthesia, or any specific drugs. Despite this, anesthesiologists and patients often prefer local or regional anesthesia for surgery during pregnancy owing to fears, rational or not, about drug effects on the fetus. If general anesthesia is chosen, precautions similar to those taken at the time of cesarean section should be employed, especially after 18–20 weeks' gestation. These would include aspiration prophylaxis and cricoid pressure at time of induction and intubation. Maintenance of left uterine displacement is also important by the third trimester, and is sometimes forgotten outside the labor suite. Hyperventilation should be avoided unless clearly indicated, because decreased arterial $P\text{CO}_2$ reduces uterine blood flow.

There are no universally accepted guidelines or standards for the management of nonobstetric surgery during pregnancy. Fetal

Table 68.2 Effect of epidural analgesia versus systemic opioids on cesarean section rate. Overall cesarean rate from randomized studies comparing epidural analgesia with systemic (intramuscular or intravenous) opioid for labor analgesia. First column, author's name and year of publication; second column, number of cesarean sections performed over the total number of subjects randomized to epidural group; third column, number of cesarean sections performed over the total number of subjects randomized to opioid group; fourth column, graphic display of odds ratio for effect of epidural versus systemic analgesia on cesarean risk. The center of the diamond indicates the odds ratio, bars indicate 95% confidence interval (CI); fifth column, numerical odds ratio and 95% CI. (Leighton BL, Halpern SH. Am J Ob Gyn 2002;186:S69–S77, with permission from Elsevier.)

Study	Epidural (n/N)	IM/IV opioid (n/N)	OR (95% CI random)	OR (95% CI random)
Clark 1998	15/156	22/162		0.68 (0.34, 1.36)
Sharma 2000	11/70	15/172		0.72 (0.32, 1.63)
Sharma 1997	13/358	16/357		0.80 (0.38, 1.70)
Howell 2001	13/175	16/178		0.81 (0.38, 1.74)
Loughan 2000	36/304	40/310		0.91 (0.56, 1.47)
Muir 2000	11/97	9/88		1.12 (0.44, 2.85)
Ramin 2000	43/664	37/666		1.18 (0.75, 1.85)
Muir 1996	3/28	2/22		1.20 (0.18, 7.89)
Philipsen 1989, 1990	10/57	6/54		1.70 (0.57, 5.06)
Bofill 1997	5/49	3/51		1.82 (0.41, 8.06)
Thorp 1993	12/48	1/45		14.67 (1.82,118.23)
Robinson (2) 1980	0/17	0/18		Not estimable
Robinson (1) 1980	0/28	0/30		Not estimable
Nikkola 1997	0/10	0/10		Not estimable
Total (95% CI)	172/2161	167/2136		1.00 (0.77, 1.28)

.001 .02 1 50 1000
Favors Epidural Favors IV/IM opioid

heart rate (FHR) monitoring intraoperatively is sometimes – but not universally – recommended. The problem with assessing such changes perioperatively is that volatile anesthetics, opioids, and other drugs administered during surgery may significantly decrease FHR variability and have mild effects on heart rate in the absence of fetal hypoxia. Still, gross changes in variability that occur without changes in drug delivery should be investigated, and tachycardia or bradycardia should prompt a rapid search for a reversible cause.

Amniotic fluid embolism

The incidence of this frequently fatal complication has been reported as 1:8000–1:80 000 pregnancies; the wide range reflects problems in diagnosis. Mortality for amniotic fluid embolism (AFE) is as high as 90% in some series, but population-based surveys and the recognition of milder cases suggest mortality rates in the 10–30% range. This complication can occur at any time in pregnancy, from first-trimester abortions to the postpartum period. As the name implies, the syndrome was thought to result from embolism of material into the pulmonary circulation, with subsequent pulmonary hypertension and cardiovascular collapse. This is almost certainly a minor part of the pathophysiology, and humoral factors are much more important. The symptoms of cardiovascular collapse, respiratory failure, and severe disseminated intravascular coagulopathy and hemorrhage suggest a similarity with anaphylactoid or septic shock. AFE has been associated with a history of atopy and allergy and with male fetuses, further implying an immunologic basis. Most current theories suggest that the entry of amniotic fluid into the maternal circulation in susceptible women results in the activation of mast cells and/or complement factors, and the syndrome is usually now referred to as anaphylactoid syndrome of pregnancy.

Therapy is almost completely supportive. Intensive care is usually required for inotropic support, fluid and blood replacement, ventilatory management, and other treatment of multisystem organ failure. Early aggressive intervention decreases mortality; a high index of suspicion should be present whenever a pregnant woman presents with any of the classic symptoms. No specific therapy has been demonstrated to be useful. Case reports recommend hemofiltration and other kinds of plasma exchange to help remove circulating factors (e.g. cytokines) that keep the syndrome active.

Hemorrhage

Blood loss following vaginal or operative delivery is normal, expected, and usually well tolerated. Tolerance for this obligatory hemorrhage is an obvious advantage, but this adaptation and the relative health of most pregnant women may hide the true extent of postpartum hemorrhage until blood loss is large and the woman presents with cardiovascular collapse. Hemorrhage is still one of the leading causes of maternal death worldwide, including the developed world. This potential for blood loss and the potential for coagulopathy due to disseminated intravascular coagulation remain central concerns for the obstetric anesthesiologist.

PLACENTA PREVIA

Placenta previa is the cause of one-third of cases of vaginal bleeding in the second and third trimesters. It literally means 'placenta going ahead', and involves implantation of the placenta near or over the internal cervical os. Diagnosis is now almost always made by ultrasound. The blood that is lost is maternal, except for the rare cases of vasa previa, where fetal blood is lost and fetal compromise can be rapid and catastrophic. Placenta previa may lead to excessive bleeding upon placental detachment after delivery, as the lower uterine segment is more fibrous and less muscular than the fundus and thus does not contract as well around the spiral arteries, the major mechanism that halts uterine bleeding postpartum. Risk factors for placenta previa include multiparity, previous cesarean section, and uterine anatomic abnormalities. Anesthetic implications of a placenta previa are the necessity for cesarean section, the potential for increased bleeding, and potentially a longer and more complicated operation. Bleeding from a simple placenta previa is usually not catastrophic, but can be if the placenta is also a placenta accreta (below).

PLACENTAL ABRUPTION

Abruptio placentae is the premature separation of the placenta from the basalis membrane of the uterus, with resultant bleeding from the exposed spiral arteries; it occurs in 0.2–0.4% of pregnancies. This separation, most commonly after 30 weeks' gestation, can be complete or partial. Abruption can result in the formation of a hematoma which pushes the placenta further away from its attachment, setting up a 'vicious cycle' of continued disruption of the placental–myometrial interface. The consequences are twofold: maternal bleeding and loss of placental function. If the abruption is contained within the placental margins, it is possible that no external blood will be detected (retroplacental hematoma), although significant blood loss (>2 L can be sequestered in the uterus) and severe fetal consequences can result. As pressure rises from trapped blood behind the placenta, tissue thromboplastins, prostaglandins, amniotic fluid, and other factors may be forced into the myometrium, leading to uterine spasm, and into the maternal circulation, leading to disseminated intravascular coagulation.

The classic signs are abdominal pain and vaginal bleeding, but both may be absent, and the presenting sign in modern labor suites is often a deteriorating fetal heart rate tracing. Hypertension is the most common risk factor, with prolonged rupture of the fetal membranes, smoking, increased age (> 35 years), alcohol, and especially cocaine use all implicated, suggesting a vascular etiology. Treatment, as in all pregnancy-related hemorrhage, is based on the degree of blood loss and fetal condition. Delivery is usually by cesarean section, and the anesthesiologist must be prepared to replace volume lost before surgery and expect excessive intraoperative blood losses from poor uterine contraction and/or coagulopathy.

PLACENTA ACCRETA, INCRETA, PERCRETA

When the placenta implants into the uterus beyond the decidua basalis it becomes abnormally adherent. This can result in incomplete separation at delivery and/or tearing of the uterus, with severe maternal hemorrhage. Placenta accreta is related to both placenta previa and to prior cesarean section or other surgical procedures involving the lower uterine segment. Approximately 10% of placenta previas will have some portion of accreta, and the incidence of accreta is about 1 in 20 000 in the absence of a previa (relative risk > 2000). The incidence of placenta accreta in the context of a previa increases with the number of prior cesarean sections, reaching almost 40% in the presence of a previa and more than two previous cesareans. Given the current trends in cesarean incidence, more placenta previas and accretas should be expected. The abnormal implantation is categorized according to the degree of penetration into the myometrium. With placenta accreta, the synctiotrophoblasts anchor the placenta on to the myometrium. Invasion into the myometrium is denoted by the term placenta increta, and a placenta that penetrates to the serosal layer or even into the abdominal cavity is a placenta percreta. The risk of bleeding is significant, because the adherent placenta acts as a stent, preventing the uterus from contracting and leading to significant bleeding from the placental bed that has detached. Alternatively, if the adherent placenta is removed, severe uterine trauma may result, with resultant catastrophic hemorrhage. Ultrasound with color Doppler studies and magnetic resonance imaging improves detection and guides risk assessment, but no imaging technique is sufficiently sensitive or specific to completely guide clinical management. Vessel embolization and/or placement of intra-arterial occlusive balloon catheters are only moderate successful at reducing the magnitude of hemorrhage. Cesarean hysterectomy is common, and monitoring and vascular access should be established that is appropriate for surgery involving potentially massive blood replacement.

UTERINE RUPTURE

Uterine rupture may or may not involve significant hemorrhage. Rupture is a rare event in the absence of previous uterine surgery (0.01–0.05%), but has an incidence of ~1% in women attempting vaginal birth after a previous low transverse cesarean (VBAC). The risk is greater if labor is induced or augmented, particularly with prostaglandins. The classic symptom of uterine rupture is either continuous pain (rather than with contractions) or increasing abdominal pain, but many ruptures now present with evidence of fetal compromise. Lack of descent or recession of the presenting part, vaginal bleeding, or maternal hemodynamic instability in a patient with a previous cesarean should suggest the diagnosis. The treatment is usually surgical delivery.

Key references

Maynard SE, Min J-Y, Merchan J et al. Excess placental soluble fms-like tyrosine kinase 1 (sFlt1) may contribute to endothelial dysfunction, hypertension, and proteinuria in pre-eclampsia. J Clin Invest. 2003;111:649–58.

McAuliffe F, Kametas N, Costello J, Rafferty GF, Greenough A, Nicolaides K. Respiratory function in singleton and twin pregnancy. Br J Obstet Gynaecol. 2002;109:765–9.

Sadaniantz A, Kocheril AG, Emaus SP et al. Cardiovascular changes in pregnancy evaluated by two-dimensional and Doppler echocardiography. Am J Soc Echocardiogr. 1992;5:253–8.

Schnobel BP, Fischer T, Heuszer K, Geiger H, Schmieder RE. Pre-eclampia – a state of sympathetic overactivity. New Engl J Med. 1996;335:1480–5.

Segal S, Su M, Gilbert P. The effect of a rapid change in availability of epidural analgesia on the cesarean delivery rate: A meta-analysis. Am J Obstet Gynecol. 2000;183:974–8.

Further reading

Herman NL. Surgery during pregnancy. In: Norris MC, ed. Obstetric anesthesia, 2nd edn. Philadelphia: JB Lippincott; 1999:161–85.

Landau R, Xie H-G, Dishy V, Wood AJJ, Stein CM, Smiley RM. Disproportionate decrease in α- compared to β-adrenergic sensitivity in the dorsal hand vein in pregnancy favors vasodilation. Circulation 2002;106:1116–20.

Leighton BL, Halpern SH. The effects of epidural analgesia on labor, maternal, and neonatal outcomes: A systematic review. Am J Obstet Gynecol. 2002;186:S69–S77.

Lieberman E, O'Donoghue C. Unintended effects of epidural analgesia during labor: a systematic review. Am J Obstet Gynecol. 2002;186:S31–S68.

Miller DA, Chollet JA, Goodwin TM. Clinical risk factors for placenta previa–placenta accreta. Am J Obstet Gynecol. 1997;177:210–14.

Mone SM, Sanders SP, Colan SD. Control mechanisms for the physiological hypertrophy of pregnancy. Circulation 1996;94:667–72.

Roberts JM, Pearson G, Cutler J, Lindheimer M. Summary of the NHLBI Working Group on Research on Hypertension During Pregnancy. Hypertension 2003;41:437–45.

Thacker SB, Stroup DF. Methods and interpretation in systematic reviews: Commentary on two parallel reviews of epidural analgesia during labor. Am J Obstet Gynecol. 2002;186:S78–S80.

Tuffnell DJ. Amniotic fluid embolism. Curr Opin Obstet Gynecol. 2003;15:119–22.

Chapter 69

Geriatrics

Jeffrey H Silverstein and Michael Zaugg

TOPICS COVERED IN THIS CHAPTER
- Theories of aging
- Neurological system
- Cardiovascular system
- Respiratory system
- Drug disposition
- Other effects

In 1927, an age of 50 years was considered a relative contraindication to surgical repair of an inguinal hernia. By 1994, 31 000 patients over the age of 65 were discharged from US hospitals following inguinal hernia repair, and another 114 000 had the same procedure done on an ambulatory basis. Two parallel phenomena underlie this change. Anesthesia developed from an adjunct of surgery into a complicated, and much safer, medical specialty. Simultaneously, the 20th century witnessed the greatest increase in longevity in recorded history (Fig. 69.1). Improvements in public health and the introduction of antibiotics in the middle of the last century, followed by a significant decrease in mortality from cardiovascular disease in the 1970s and 1980s, have been primarily responsible for the increase in life expectancy (75.8 years in 1995 in the USA).

As a result of increased longevity, the population of older people continues to grow. From 2000 to 2030, it is projected that there will be an increase from 35 million to 74 million persons over the age of 65 in the US; by 2030, people over 65 will constitute 20% of the total population. Patients over 65 already represent approximately 35% of the workload of most anesthetic practices. Roughly 50% of people over 65 will have at least one operation before death.

Aging might be described as the composite of all changes that occur in an organism with the passage of time, incorporating the findings that functional impairment and the likelihood of death increase with aging. Aging has also been characterized as a progressive loss of those physiologic processes necessary to maintain homeostasis, death being the ultimate failure of these mechanisms. Senescence may be defined as the progressive deterioration of physiological functions with aging. Much of the apparent loss of function is noted as loss of reserve function in specific organs, as opposed to evident deterioration of function. Longevity, then, is the summation of forces that avoid or retard senescence. Aging clearly progresses at different rates in

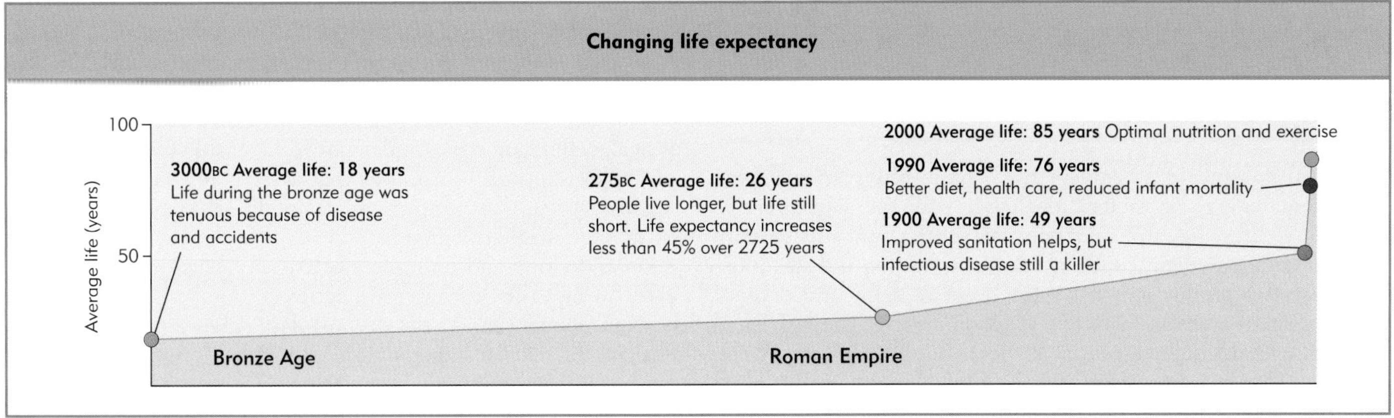

Figure 69.1 Changing life expectancy. The 20th century has seen the greatest increase in life expectancy in recorded history, primarily owing to improvements in public health and an associated decrease in infant mortality. (Reprinted from Putting Aging on Hold, an official report to the 1995 White House Conference on Aging. American Federation of Aging Research and the Alliance for Aging Research.)

different individuals: the physiologic age of older patients is more relevant than their chronologic age. This variability represents a key modulating concept in aging; the balance between senescence and longevity provides the basis for this variability.

Human aging is divided into three patterns: a pattern that involves the accumulation of disease and disability; a pattern referred to as usual or normal aging that describes individuals free of identifiable disease but nonetheless manifesting evident signs of senescence; and 'successful aging', in which individuals reach advanced age with relatively minimal impairment. A balance in favor of longevity over senescence defines successful aging. Successful aging includes a low probability of disease and related disability, high physical and cognitive function, and active engagement with life. This highlights a singularly difficult aspect of aging research: that of defining the population to be included in any study of aging phenomena. Modern gerontology now eschews the previous assumption that in the absence of disease other age-related alterations, such as modest cognitive deterioration or changes in blood glucose metabolism, are normal.

The balance between senescence and longevity provides the basis for variability in individual rates of aging.

It is becoming increasingly clear that there are important interactions between age-related changes and specifically identifiable disease processes. In recent years, attempts have been made to distinguish a syndrome of frailty as a multisystem physiologic dysregulation of aging. The systems at the core of this syndrome are endocrine and immune/inflammatory function, as well as other effects on muscle (sarcopenia), bone (osteoporosis), and brain. There is extensive evidence that loss of physiologic reserve for a specific biological system is particularly manifest in the presence of stressors. Many of the areas compromised in the frail patient involve multisystemic dynamics. To date, a unifying hypothesis of frailty that captures this concept in a manner useful for either research or clinical care remains elusive.

Research into the aging process and its implications has been extensive over the last five decades. An important limitation for anesthesiologists is that relatively little of this research is focused on perioperative care of geriatric patients, leaving both scientist and clinician to interpret and extrapolate from published data. This chapter attempts to provide a foundation of the science underlying geriatric anesthetic care; a few areas have been selected for more extensive treatment as examples of the depth and breadth of knowledge.

THEORIES OF AGING

Theories of aging must explain three basic observations: why organisms undergo physiologic decline in later life; why there is variation in lifespan within and between species; and why certain experimental paradigms, such as caloric restriction and selection for delayed reproduction, delay the onset of aging and extend the lifespan of animals. Caloric restriction involves the provision of a diet with adequate essential nutrients but 30–70% of normal calories. This consistently slows the rate of aging in rats and mice, and delays many phenotypic characteristics of aging and the occurrence and progression of age-associated disease. Lifespan can increase by more than 50% compared to a normally fed cohort.

Theories to explain how or why we age can be divided into those taking an evolutionary approach on the one hand, and those focused more on biological mechanisms such as molecular theories, cellular theories, and those that propose dysfunction in systems physiology. The application of general evolution theory to aging has been utilized to provide a sense of unification. Although it is intellectually intriguing, it is nonetheless clear that aging is a stochastic process in which a genetic program provides direction which is subject to environmental influence.

Three theories involving population genetic or evolutionary mechanisms have been invoked to describe aging. The first, *mutation accumulation*, posits that alleles with neutral early effects are not eliminated by natural selection despite deleterious effects in later life. The frequency of the allele will be determined by genetic drift, and will therefore not be present in high frequency in large populations. Continuous damage occurs to DNA, but is rapidly eliminated by a number of repair enzymes. In mutation accumulation, levels of mutation would be expected to correlate with lifespan. Genetic diseases associated with higher levels of DNA damage or a marked deficiency in DNA repair should manifest premature aging. Genetic defects in helicases – enzymes that unwind the DNA double helix – are responsible for Bloom syndrome and Werner syndrome. Werner syndrome is a rare disorder that includes bilateral cataracts, progeria, hypogonadism, and a tendency toward type II diabetes mellitus. The exponential increase in the risk of cancer with age, which in many cases is associated with a series of mutations, is consistent with mutation accumulation.

The second population genetic theory is called antagonistic pleiotropy. In contrast to mutation accumulation, *antagonistic pleiotropy* predicts that alleles that may cause physiologic decline at later ages become fixed in populations because they may have beneficial effects early in life. That is, early beneficial effects lead to selection and accumulation, even though the subsequent effects are deleterious. This mechanism suggests that there is a means to determine lifespan – a biologic clock of sorts. Such a 'clock' has yet to be detected. There are a very few disease entities which are consistent with antagonistic pleiotropy, that is, genetic disorders that have late-life onset, such as Huntington's chorea and idiopathic hemochromatosis. Both mechanisms and their associated predictions have been supported by experimentation in animal models, including *Drosophila* (fruit fly) and *Caenorhabditis elegans* (roundworm).

The third evolutionary theory is the *disposable soma* theory, which argues that organisms are maintained primarily only for reproductive success; after reproductive success the soma is disposable. Inherent in this idea is that resources utilized in promoting reproduction are not available to promote longevity.

Mechanistic theories of aging are divided into system physiological, cellular, and molecular categories (Table 69.1). A systems physiology approach proposes that aging is related to decline in organ systems that control and maintain other systems, and/or those that enable the organism to adapt to the environment. The neuroendocrine and immune systems are suggested to play this role, owing to their integrative actions.

Neuroendocrine theories postulate that aging is due to changes in neural and endocrine functions crucial for coordinating and programming physiological responses to external stimuli and maintaining optimal states for reproduction and survival. The idea of a 'biological clock' is most easily incorporated into neuroendocrine theories. The hypothalamus is a candidate because of its role in the control of numerous physiologic

Table 69.1 Some theories of aging (Modified from Weinert BT, Timiras PS. Physiology of aging, invited review: theories of aging. J Appl Physiol. 2003;95:1706–16)

Systems physiology	Cellular	Molecular
Neuroendocrine	Wear and tear	Gene regulation
Immunologic	Limited cellular replication/telomere shortening	Codon restriction
Rate of living	Free radicals Apoptosis	Somatic mutation Error/catastrophe Dysdifferentiation

systems, including growth, metabolic homeostasis, sympathetic balance, and sexual function. Hormonal dysregulation, particularly of glucocorticoids, has been implicated in normal aging. An ancestral insulin pathway that controls stress responsiveness and longevity involves many genes that are conserved through humans (IGF-I, *Daf*-2, *Daf*-16, among others), thus supporting the potential importance of the neuroendocrine theory of aging.

Immunosenescence is manifested by a decrease in resistance to infections, an increased incidence of cancers, and an increase in autoimmune pathology. The components of the immune system age differently. The thymus reaches is peak in size and function in early puberty, whereas most lymphocyte and complement functions are preserved in centenarians.

Wear and tear theories propose that death is the result of cumulative damage to vital body components. Although this was originally conceived in terms of organs or organisms, at the level of DNA the question again becomes one of the balance between damage and repair capacity. At the physiological level senescence can be correlated with metabolic rate: the higher the metabolic rate per unit of body mass, the shorter the lifespan. Manipulation by persistent exercise has shown no effect on lifespan. In certain species, reproductive exhaustion can be seen to have dramatic effects. For example, the lifespan of a salmon, which spawns and then dies, can be dramatically extended by castration.

The idea that cells possess a limited capacity to divide was initially developed by Hayflick, working with human fibroblasts. There is a limited number of 'passages' in cultured cells that is related to the lifespan of the source of the cells, i.e. a cell has the capacity to divide a limited number of times. The broader concept of the Hayflick limit is sometimes used to represent the theoretical upper limit of survivability of a given species. Replicative senescence is a subgrouping of general cell senescence that results from the loss of telomeres. Telomeres are repeated sequences of DNA at the ends of each chromosome that maintain the integrity of the chromosomes. They protect chromosomes from degradation or fusion with other chromosomes. Telomere length is shortened each time a cell divides, and a mutation in yeast that shortens telomeres causes early senescence. Once the telomeres reach a critically short length, the cell stops dividing. Expression of telomerase, an enzyme that replaces telomeric DNA, nearly eliminates telomeric shortening and extends the cell's replicative span. Regulation of telomere length was thought to represent another form of biological clock, but experiments in rodents provide little support for this mechanism.

Telomerase deficient mice do not age rapidly and only start to manifest an early aging phenotype after many generations. Deficiency of the tumor suppressor p53 suppresses the early aging phenotype in late-generation telomerase-deficient mice and represents a new front for investigation in this area. Examination of patients with dyskeratosis congenita suggests that telomeres may contribute to human aging, but the overall role of telomere shortening in normal aging is likely to be limited.

Forces both natural and unnatural can damage cells by either somatic mutation, altered genetic expression, or both. Agents that can damage DNA, enzymes, other proteins, and lipids include free radicals, infectious diseases (viruses, prions), temperature, and radiation. Free radicals are highly reactive species that are continuously produced in living organisms. Organisms have developed extensive antioxidant defense systems, such as superoxide dismutase, catalase, and glutathione peroxidase. The administration of antioxidants has been reported to increase lifespan, but alterations in other aspects of metabolism cannot be excluded in interpreting these experiments. Proponents of these theories suggest that persistent minor damage accumulates over time, resulting in the changes observed as aging (i.e. mutation accumulation). Support for this theory includes the observations that overexpression of antioxidant enzymes can extend the lifespan of *Drosophila*, that the rate of mitochondrial superoxide formation is inversely correlated with longevity, and that caloric restriction is associated with a decrease in oxidative stress.

Mammalian cells have a limited capacity to divide, determined in part by telomere length.

Theoretic considerations have generally followed extensive descriptive evaluation of the aged and aging. Folkow and Svanbourg focused on four general manifestations of aging: 1) a slow progressive reduction of both peripheral and central neuronal networks; 2) a slow decline in muscle cell number, strength, and speed of contraction; 3) a slow decline in tissue compliance or distensibility; and 4) a modest decline in basal metabolic rate and oxygen consumption per unit body weight.

NEUROLOGICAL SYSTEM

Central neurological changes are among the most profound of those associated with aging, accounting for approximately 50% of disability after age 65. Major deficits occur in both the central and peripheral neurological systems. Clinically, hearing, vision, olfaction, memory, and learning are variously affected. Neuronal loss was long thought to be a hallmark of aging, although the mechanism of neuronal attrition was not understood. Extensive neuroanatomical studies identified a 48% decrease in neuronal density in the visual cortex from the third to the ninth decade of life. Similar losses were reported in the cortex, hippocampus, anterior thalamus, and locus ceruleus. This well accepted concept was challenged when advanced screening methods were used to eliminate patients with signs of Alzheimer's disease. Although studies have found age-related decrements in brain weight, cortical thickness in the midfrontal and superior temporal areas, large neurons in all three areas, and the neuron:glia ratio in the midfrontal and inferior parietal areas, the total number of neurons, percentage of cell area, and neuronal density do not appear to change significantly. The number of small neurons in the midfrontal cortex and glia in the midfrontal and superior temporal areas increased with age. Recent studies of brain plasticity have contradicted the notion that individuals are born with a full compliment of neurons and that none are produced subsequently. The brains of adult mammals retain neural stem cells that perpetuate neurogenesis for the life of the animal. These findings have been limited to specific brain regions, and the local environment in which neurogenesis occurs is highly specific and complicated. The idea that the aging nervous system retains the capacity to generate new neurons suggests at least the possibility of treating age-related cognitive dysfunction. Glial cells, long thought to be purely supportive structures for the real work of neurons, have emerged as important mediators of CNS function. Their role in aging is just beginning to be discovered.

Mitochondria, in addition to providing the main source of energy for the cell, also play a key role in determining cell viability, senescence, and death. They modulate intracellular Ca^{2+} concentrations, heat production, and the balance between pro- and antiapoptotic signals, thus controlling programmed cell death. Therefore, mitochondrial dysfunction has become a major focus of research into aging.

Extensive evaluation of all types of receptor on both neurons and glia has produced a catalogue of contradictory age-related alterations that so far defy a clear pattern. An exciting aspect which has generated intensive research is the role of steroids (neurosteroids) that act at the level of the central nervous system. These substances affect neural activity by acting on both classic steroid receptors (i.e. receptors for androgens, estrogens, and progestagens) and NMDA and GABA receptors. It appears that the CNS produces de novo or locally metabolizes steroids produced in peripheral sites. There is a strong suggestion that one such steroid (pregnenolone sulfate) influences cognitive processes in aging animals by modulating cerebral plasticity and acetylcholine metabolism.

Age-related changes in general anesthetic potency and effects may be related to parallel changes in their molecular targets.

Age-related alterations in γ-aminobutyric acid (GABA) and opioid receptors are particularly relevant to anesthesia (Chapter 24). Early studies described a 20–30% decrease in $GABA_A$ receptor benzodiazepine-binding sites in cerebral cortex, hippocampus, and cerebellum. More recently, $GABA_A$ receptor benzodiazepine sites were found to be maintained in both number and affinity in the hippocampus, whereas alterations in GABA binding were present in frontal cortex. Alterations in mRNA of specific subunits of the $GABA_A$ receptor have been reported in the inferior colliculus (associated with hearing). This is interesting, given the correlation between auditory evoked potentials and anesthetic potency. Preliminary findings suggest a correlation between altered $GABA_A$ receptors and age-related alterations in anesthetic potency.

The change in perception of patterns of neuronal loss and reactive gliosis in the brain has yet to be evaluated to the same extent in the spinal cord. Reports of loss of small neurons in the intermediate zone of the ventral horn associated with preservation of larger neurons in the medial and lateral nuclei suggest a lack of generalized neuron loss. The conduction velocities of spinal nerves decrease to a clinically insignificant extent. The clinical result is not necessarily apparent from these alterations. In a series of experiments evaluating the effects of aging on spinal opioid-induced antinociception, aging animals responded more rapidly to painful stimuli and required higher doses of intrathecal opioid agonists to produce significant increases in tail-flick latency (time to nocifensive response).

Aging is a significant risk factor for postoperative cognitive dysfunction.

The routine mental status examination in the elderly should be normal. Although complaints of subjective memory loss and cognitive deficits are common and neuropsychological evaluation shows slowing of central processing time, the acquisition of new information, and a decline in 'fluid intelligence', these changes are below the threshold of detectability of most clinical mental state examinations. Clear abnormalities in mental state should not be attributed to aging, but should lead to consideration of a differential diagnosis. Aging appears to be a significant risk factor for cognitive dysfunction following anesthesia (postoperative cognitive dysfunction). A study of 1218 patients over 60 years of age found a 9.8% incidence of cognitive dysfunction after major surgery under general anesthesia at 3 months following the operation; age was significantly correlated with this effect. Follow-up studies using a similar testing battery suggest that a similar pattern is not found in younger (40–60-year-old) subjects, and that minor surgical procedures do not incur a similar risk. An evaluation of general versus regional anesthesia subsequently suggested that choice of anesthetic is not an important variable. However, very preliminary reports suggest the potential of volatile anesthetic agents to increase the production of β-amyloid, a key proteinin dementing illness.

CARDIOVASCULAR SYSTEM

Hypertension and atherosclerosis are the most common disorders of the elderly, and more than 50% have significant coronary artery disease, often without symptoms. The chemical and ultrastructural changes of the aging myocardium have been studied quite extensively. Two major areas of research are of particular interest in anesthesiology: age-related alterations in β-adrenergic function, and structural alterations to the heart and vessels. Both areas have expanded our understanding of cardiovascular function in the elderly.

In healthy humans in the absence of coronary artery disease, hypertension, or severe deconditioning, resting cardiovascular performance is not significantly altered (Fig. 69.2; Table 69.2). However, during significant exercise there is less of an increase in heart rate although stroke volume is maintained or increased, a pattern similar to that in younger individuals who undergo exercise in the presence of β-adrenergic blockade. This is particularly intriguing given that circulating levels of norepinephrine, but not epinephrine, increase progressively with age. Extensive studies in myocardium as well as other tissues have failed to identify a decrease in β-adrenergic receptor density. The β-adrenergic receptors are G-protein linked and exist in at least two states, described as high and low affinity (Chapter 3). β-Adrenergic agonist-binding affinity is significantly decreased with aging in rat myocardium, associated primarily with a decrease in

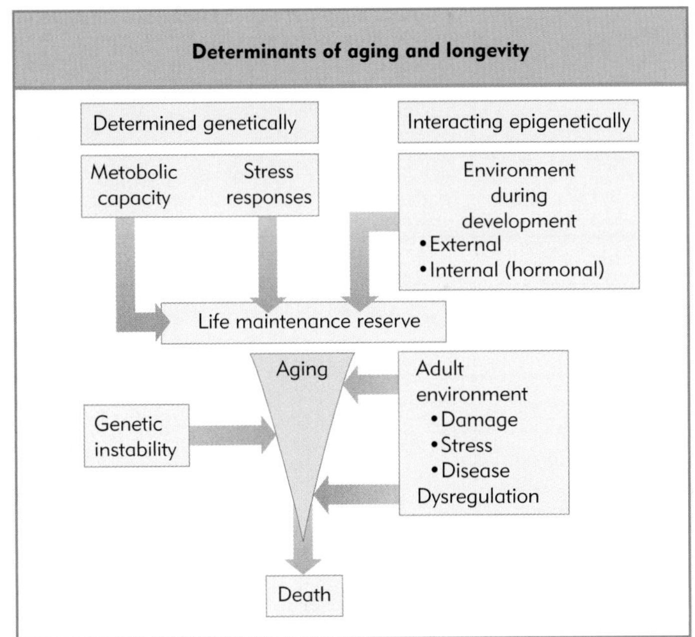

Figure 69.2 Determinants of aging and longevity. Rather than molecular mechanisms, physiologic mechanisms of aging are described. Environment, metabolic capacity, and stress responses all contribute to the life maintenance reserve. Genetic instability is influenced by environmental factors. The essential concept is that aging functions at all levels of biological organization; it is not possible to separate cellular changes from organism aging. (Reprinted from Jazwinski SM. Longevity, Genes, and Aging. Science 1996;273:57. Copyright © 1999 AAAS.)

the proportion of receptors in the high-affinity state. Affinity for β-adrenergic antagonists, however, is not altered with age.

Myocardial contractile response to either β_1- or β_2-adrenergic stimulation is reduced with aging. This is due to a failure of β-adrenergic agonists to increase $Ca^{2+}{}_i$ to the same extent in senescent as in younger heart cells. This effect results from a limited capacity to increase L-type sarcolemmal Ca^{2+} channel availability, which limits the increase in Ca^{2+} influx. The well studied reduction in response to β-adrenergic stimulation found in aging myocardial cells appears to be the result of multiple alterations in biochemical and molecular pathways. The principal limiting factor in rat myocardium appears to be the coupling of β-adrenergic receptors to the adenylyl cyclase catalytic unit by means of the G_s protein. In addition, age-related changes in adenylyl cyclase protein reduce the capacity to augment cellular cAMP and to activate protein kinase A that drives the phosphorylation of key proteins involved in myocardial contractility. The desensitization of β-adrenergic signaling is not mediated by β-adrenergic kinase (β-ARK) or increased G_i activity.

In contrast to β-adrenergic system function, α_1-adrenergic function appears to be preserved in aging, whereas α_2-adrenergic responses appear to be decreased. Vagal cholinergic tone increases in aging rats. Finally, there is a suggestion that thyroid hormone can compensate for age-related alterations in adrenergic tone.

Table 69.2 Changes in cardiac output regulation between ages 20 and 80 years. At rest cardiac index is not changed with aging as a result of a 10% decrease in heart rate and an increase in stroke volume. With exercise, peak cardiac index is 25% less than in the young subject. The mechanisms and limits of adaptation of the aging heart are easily translated to clinical use

	Rest	Exhaustive exercise
Cardiac index	No change	Decrease 25%
Heart rate	Decrease 10%	Decrease 25%
Stroke volume	Increase 10%	No change
Preload – EDV	Increase 12%	Increase 30%
Afterload – PVR	Increase	Increase 30%
Contractility	No change	Decrease 60%
Ejection fraction	No change	Decrease 15%

Structural changes in the heart and major vessels lead to altered physiology with age.

Structural changes in the heart and major vessels contribute greatly to the altered physiology of the aging cardiovascular system. Although initially described as a separate entity, long-term follow-up from the Baltimore Longitudinal Study on Aging indicates that the structural changes described below play an integral role in the development of diseases for which age is a principal factor, such as hypertension and atherosclerosis. Aging is associated with a decrease in connective tissue compliance and distensibility, primarily due to increasing cross-bridging between elastin and collagen filaments. One result is the well known elongation, stiffening, and widening of the aorta. Stiffening of the aorta results in a higher peak systolic pressure, which considerably increases afterload. In addition to systemic vascular resistance, pulse wave reflection from the periphery is integrated into the overall pressure characteristics that constitute the afterload of the left ventricle. When the ventricle contracts, a pulse wave is transmitted and at least partially reflected back into the great vessels. Pulse wave velocity increases two- to threefold with aging. In young cardiovascular systems the reflected pulse wave tends to arrive following systole, but in the elderly this component is appended to the end-systolic afterload. Standard measurement of blood pressure by forearm sphygmomanometry fails to discern this aspect of pressure, as the reflected wave is not retransmitted significantly down the arterial tree.

Age-related increases in aortic–arterial stiffness are one of the most serious changes affecting the cardiovascular system.

Age-related alteration in aortic–arterial stiffness is one of the most serious changes to affect the normal aging human cardiovascular system. Figure 69.3 depicts the essential alterations of the aging heart as a response to increased afterload. The heart is unusual in that it does not decrease in size with age as do most other organs. Although fewer myocytes are present, there is a general hypertrophy of the cells and a marked increase in connective tissue. Cardiac structural alterations in the human are not well represented by rat models, but are well described in humans. The two primary alterations noted in elderly hearts, *in the absence of disease states and severe deconditioning,* are concentric left ventricular hypertrophy and a substantial decline in diastolic compliance. Left ventricular wall thickness increases with age secondary to myocardial hypertrophy and increases in connective tissue components, including fibrous tissue, lipids,

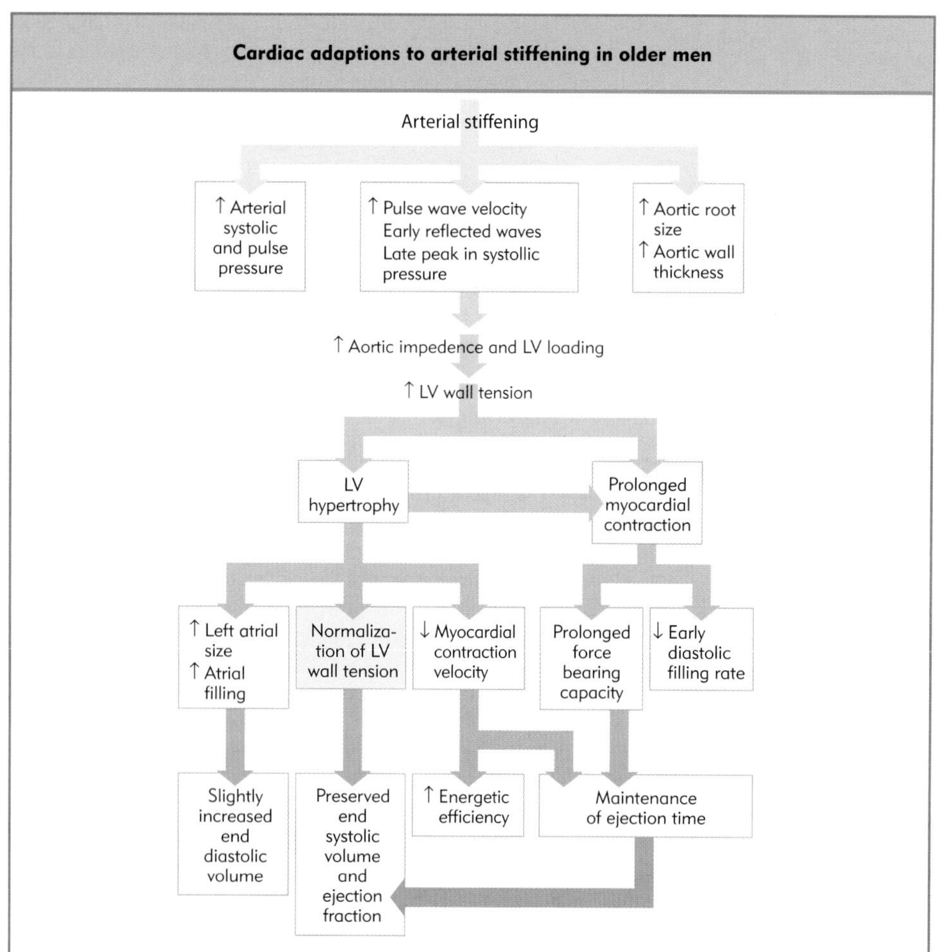

Figure 69.3 Cardiac adaptations to arterial stiffening in older men. Most changes in the aging heart result from alterations in stiffness of the aorta. LV, left ventricle. (From Lakkata E. In: Merck manual of geriatrics, Whitehouse Station: Merck Research Laboratories; 1995:433.)

and collagen. Echocardiographic measurements describe a 30% increase in LV thickness, with interventricular septal thickness increasing to the greatest extent.

Alterations in diastolic compliance are seen primarily in humans and not in elderly rats. Ca^{2+} is removed from the myocardial cytoplasm to the sarcoplasmic reticulum during diastole, a process requiring substantial energy (Chapter 39). Relaxation is dependent on this process, which is substantially impaired during aging. There is also a suggestion of decreased oxygen utilization by mitochondria. Finally, a prolonged action potential and isovolemic relaxation time in senescent hearts delays diastolic filling. The result is a 50% decline in early diastolic ventricular filling in the aged. The importance of atrial contraction to ventricular filling increases from 10% to 30% in elderly subjects. A decrease in early diastolic filling has been described in a group of older male athletes. From a comparison of these conditioned individuals to a sedentary cohort, it was concluded that diastolic dysfunction is intrinsic to aging rather than the result of a reduction in aerobic capacity.

Left ventricular end-diastolic pressure is increased, both at rest and during exercise, secondary to altered diastolic relaxation. Higher pressure is needed to achieve the same stroke volume. The upper limit of pressure at which hydrostatic forces are overcome is not altered with age. Thus the aged heart can be exquisitely sensitive to alterations in ventricular preload, particularly loss of the atrial systole. Cardiac output, despite multiple reports of a progressive decline with age, is essentially maintained in subjects who are carefully screened for occult disease.

The response to exercise in the elderly as an index of organ reserve has long been of interest to anesthesiologists. Although cardiac performance at rest may not be altered, major limitations occur during strenuous exercise. Maximum aerobic capacity decreases with age. Conditioning and the presence of even occult coronary artery disease play an important limiting role. Although $\dot{V}O_2$max declines with age, this is not entirely due to the alterations in the central circulation. It is possible that an age-related difference in muscle mass, oxidation capacity per unit muscle, and/or inability to shunt blood to exercising muscles could also contribute.

The nature of the aging cardiac physiology predicts the clinical implications. Diastolic-based cardiac dysfunction has been distinguished from systolic dysfunction as a cause of heart failure (Chapter 42). A number of studies indicate a significant and increasing prevalence of coronary artery disease in elderly patients. Thus, although pure age related alterations in the cardiovascular system have been well delineated, it is clear that these changes are integrally related to the development of clinical disease.

RESPIRATORY SYSTEM

The loss of respiratory function with aging is extremely variable between persons of the same chronological age. In general, the elderly have a greater predisposition to pulmonary dysfunction during the perioperative period. The primary age-related alterations are: 1) progressive (20–30%) loss of alveolar surface area;

2) a reduction in the elastic recoil of lung tissue combined with stiffening of the chest wall; 3) decreased strength of the respiratory muscles; and 4) impaired nervous control of ventilation.

Chronic oxidative damage to lung tissue by environmental factors, including oxygen free radicals, is thought to be responsible for the tissue alterations typically found in the aged lung. Antioxidant consumption (e.g. vitamins C and E) can improve lung function in elderly patients. Microscopically, aged respiratory bronchioles and alveolar ducts are dilated and the pores of Kohn become larger and more numerous. Whole alveolar septa may be eliminated by this process, known as interalveolar fenestration, or duct ectasia. In contrast to emphysematous lung tissue, no signs of destruction or inflammation can be demonstrated in this process. However, marked fibrosis is frequently present. The direct consequences of the reduced alveolar surface area are a slightly increased alveolar dead space and a decreased oxygen diffusing capacity. From youth to age 80, maximal diffusing capacity can decrease up to 50%.

Compliance of the chest wall falls and that of lung parenchyma increases with age, with profound effects on respiratory function.

The elastic properties of lung tissue and the thoracic wall gradually change with aging. The chest wall becomes stiffer (calcification of the ribs, arthritic changes in rib and vertebral joints) and less compliant, whereas the lung parenchyma loses elastic recoil and becomes more compliant secondary to modified protein crosslinking, rearrangement of collagen fibrils and elastin, and an altered surfactant composition. Clinically, this results in a barrel-shaped chest with a flattened diaphragm. The new equilibrium of the opposing thoracic and pulmonary forces increases the interpleural pressure by 2–4 cmH_2O and has a significant impact on static and dynamic lung volumes, as well as on the respiratory mechanics (Fig. 69.4; see Chapter 49). The application of Laplace's law to diaphragmatic contraction demonstrates that the flattened diaphragm of old people must generate more power to achieve the necessary transpulmonary pressure. The diaphragmatic efficacy is additionally impaired by a significant age-related loss of motor neurons, particularly type II fast twitch fibers. Although the work of breathing at rest is unchanged with age, vigorous exercise may elevate the work of breathing by 30%.

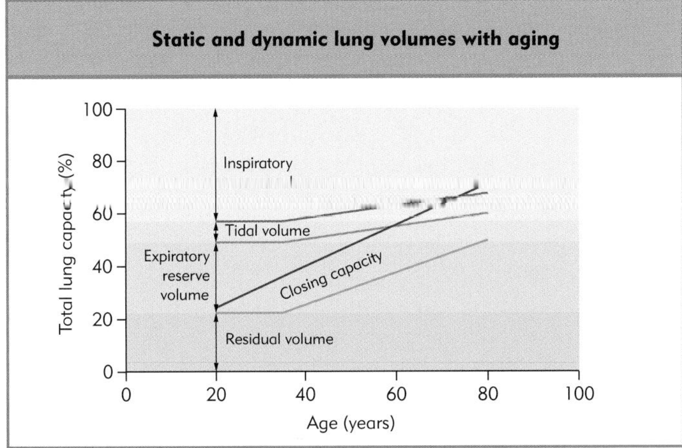

Figure 69.4 Static and dynamic lung volumes with aging. Residual volume (RV) (+5–10% per decade) and functional residual capacity (FRC = ERV + RV) (+1–3% per decade) gradually increase with aging, while expiratory and inspiratory reserve volumes (ERV, IRV) and hence vital capacity (VC = ERV + IRV) decrease.

Arterial oxygen tension falls approximately 5 mmHg per decade from 20 years of age. This is primarily due to an increased ventilation/perfusion maldistribution, with shunt rather than decreased diffusing capacity. Alterations in hypoxic pulmonary vasoconstriction and hypocapnic bronchoconstriction may also contribute to age-related ventilation/perfusion maldistribution. The magnitude of shunting can be markedly increased by atelectasis following the induction of anesthesia. Unfortunately, positive end-expiratory pressure has a limited impact on atelectasis, as the elastic recoil curves of atelectatic and nonatelectatic lung units can be quite different (zones of different time constants). Finally, an increased tendency for upper airway collapse, decreased tonic activity of upper airway muscles (pharyngeal collapse), and decreased ventilatory response to both hypercapnia and hypoxia are present in the elderly. Thus there is a dangerous predisposition to hypoxemia in the perioperative period. The loss of protective reflexes also increases the risk of aspiration. Finally, both hypercapnic and hypoxemic respiratory drive are decreased to a greater degree in older people by both sedative drugs and analgesic medications.

DRUG DISPOSITION

Essentially, all clinically relevant data on drug disposition in the elderly can be summarized by stating that elderly patients require smaller doses of intravenous anesthetics. The essential concepts of pharmacokinetics are discussed in Chapter 8. A number of age-related physiologic changes alter the pharmacokinetics of many anesthetic agents: reduced total body water, blood volume, and skeletal muscle mass; altered protein binding; and increased body fat. Pharmacodynamic changes result in increased sensitivity to opioids, benzodiazepines, and volatile anesthetics (e.g. MAC decreases ~4% per decade after age 40). Animal models have limited applicability in determining age-related alterations in humans to drug actions, and each drug must be treated individually. Renal mass, renal blood flow, glomerular blood flow, and number of glomeruli (cortical > medullary) all decrease with age. Glomerular filtration rate decreases approximately 1 mL/min/year after age 40. Because there is a decline in muscle mass and creatinine production, serum creatinine concentration is not a useful indicator of glomerular filtration in the elderly. Creatinine clearance (C_{cr}) can be estimated from the serum creatinine (S_{cr}) by the following formula:

$$C_{cr} = (140 - \text{age [yrs]}) \times (\text{weight[kg]}/72) \times S_{cr}\ [\text{mg/dL}]$$

Apart from clearance issues, changes in body composition prove important in the alterations seen and expected in the elderly patient's response to pharmaceutical agents. Aging humans manifest a decrease in total body water and lean body mass, whereas total body fat increases. Whereas this may be expected to increase the volume of distribution at steady state for lipophilic drugs, the volume of the central compartment is reduced, which increases initial serum concentrations. For example, the principle drug-binding proteins, albumin and α_1-acid glycoprotein, are affected differently by the aging process. Albumin decreases, whereas α_1-acid glycoprotein levels typically increase. Alterations in free fraction and hence the clearance and volume of distribution of a given drug depend on which protein is the principal binding site for that drug.

Table 69.3 summarizes the observed alterations for various drugs in aged patients. Figure 69.5 illustrates a recent examination of the pharmacokinetics and pharmacodynamics of the opioid remifentanil. The necessary initial bolus dose for an 80-year-old is 50% that for a 20-year-old, and the infusion rate is approximately two-thirds less.

OTHER EFFECTS

Loss of hearing with age affects more than 30% of adults between the ages of 65 and 74, and about 50% of individuals between the ages of 75 and 80. Presbyacusis is the bilaterally symmetric sensorineural hearing loss that is associated with aging. Hearing loss is 2.5–5 times more frequent in men than in women, and is likely to be more severe. Presbyacusis can be divided into sensory, neural, metabolic, and cochlear conductive defects. High frequencies are much more affected than lower frequencies. Acute sensorineural hearing loss can occur after general anesthesia (not ear surgery) or spinal anesthesia. This 10–20 dB hearing loss appears to be more common in the elderly and is generally transient; the cause is still unknown. Postoperative hearing deficits can exacerbate postoperative confusion or simply impair communication.

Elderly patients are more prone to hypothermia because of reduced basal metabolic rate (about 11% per year), causing decreased heat production and a lower threshold for cold-induced peripheral vasoconstriction.

Table 69.3 Age-related pharmacologic changes of anesthetics and drugs in anesthesia practice

Anesthetic/drug	Pharmacodynamics	Pharmacokinetics	Anesthetic management
Inhalational anesthetics	Sensitivity of the brain ↑ (cerebral metabolic rate ↓)	Ventilation/perfusion mismatch with slow rise of alveolar/inspired ratio of inhaled gases; maximal cardiac output ↓; volume of distribution ↑	Minimum alveolar concentration (MAC) down 30%; slower induction and emergence; delayed but more profound onset of anesthesia
Hypnotics			
Thiopental	No changes	Central volume of distribution ↓; intercompartmental clearance ↑	Induction dose reduced by 15% (20-year-old patient: 2.5–5.0 mg/kg IV; 80-year-old patient: 2.1 mg/kg IV). Maintenance dose: same requirements 60 minutes after starting a continuous infusion. Emergence: slightly faster
Propofol	No changes	Central volume of distribution ↓; intercompartmental clearance ↑	Induction dose reduced by 20% (slower induction requires lower doses) (20-year-old: 2.0–3.0 mg/kg IV; 80-year-old: 1.7 mg/kg IV). Maintenance dose: same requirements 120 minutes after starting a continuous infusion. Emergence: slightly faster (?)
Midazolam	Sensitivity of the brain ↑	Clearance ↓	Sedation/induction dose reduced by 50% (20-year-old: 0.07–0.15 mq/kq IV; 80-year-old: 0.02–0.03 mg/kg IV). Maintenance dose reduced by 25%. Recovery: delayed (hours)
Etomidate	No changes	Central clearance ↓; volume of distribution ↓	Induction dose reduced by 20% (20-year-old: 0.3 mg/kg IV; 80-year-old: 0.2 mg/kg IV). Emergence: slightly faster (?)
Ketamine	?	?	Use with caution: hallucinations, seizures, mental disturbance, release of catecholamines: avoid in combination with levodopa (tachycardia, arterial hypertension)
Opioids			
Fentanyl, alfentanil, sufentanil	Sensitivity of the brain ↑	No changes	Induction dose reduced by 50%. Maintenance doses reduced by 30–50%. Emergence: may be delayed

Table 69.3 Age-related pharmacologic changes of anesthetics and drugs in anesthesia practice—cont'd

Anesthetic/drug	Pharmacodynamics	Pharmacokinetics	Anesthetic management
Opioids—cont'd			
Remifentanil	Sensitivity of the brain ↑	Central volume of distribution ↓; intercompartmental clearance ↓	Induction dose reduced by 50%. Maintenance dose reduced by 70%. Emergence: may be delayed
Muscle relaxants			
Mivacurium Succinylcholine	No changes	Plasma cholinesterase ↓; muscle blood flow ↓; cardiac output ↓; intercompartmental clearance ↓	Onset time ↑. Maintenance dose requirements ↓. Duration of action ↑ Clinically indistinguishable from mivacurium. Differences: no changes in initial dose, prolonged block with metoclopramide
Pancuronium, doxacuronium, pipecuronium, vecuronium, rocuronium	No changes	Muscle blood flow ↓; cardiac output ↓; intercompartmental clearance ↓; clearance ↓; (volume of distribution ↓)	Onset time ↑. Maintenance dose requirements ↓. Duration of action ↑. Recommended dose reduced by 20%
Atracurium	No changes	No changes	No changes
Reversal agents			
Neostigmine, pyridostigmine	No changes	Clearance ↓	Duration of action ↑↑; because muscle relaxants have a markedly prolonged duration of action, larger doses of reversal agents are needed in elderly patients
Edrophonium	No changes	No changes	No change
Local anesthetics	Sensitivity of the nervous tissue ↑ (?)	Hepatic microsomal metabolism of amide local anesthetics (lidocaine (lignocaine), bupivacaine ↓); plasma protein binding ↓; cephalad spread ↑	Epidural (and spinal) dose requirements ↓. Duration of spinal and epidural anesthesia seems clinically independent of age, toxicity ↑ (percent free drug ↑)

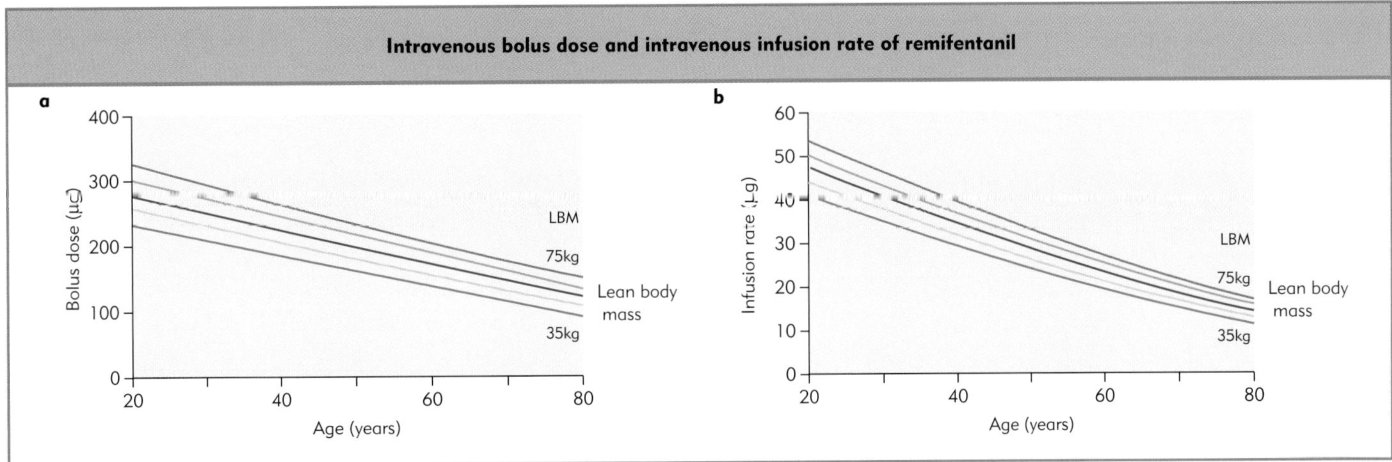

Figure 69.5 Nomogram for calculating intravenous bolus dose (a) and intravenous infusion rate (b) of remifentanil required to cause 50% of the maximum effect as a function of age and lean body mass. Note that the principal effect of age is altered significantly by the relative lean body mass. This highlights some of the many factors to consider when choosing drug dosages for elderly patients. Center lines show mean values with outer lines showing one and two standard deviations from the mean. (Reprinted from Minto CF, Schnider TW, Shafer SL. Pharmacokinetics and pharmacodynamics of remifentanil. II. Model application. Anesthesiology 1997; 86:24–33.)

Key references

Jazwinski SM. Longevity, genes, and aging. Science 1996;273:54–9.

Lakatta EG, Levy D. Arterial and cardiac aging: major shareholders in cardiovascular disease enterprises. Part I: aging arteries: a 'set up' for vascular disease. Circulation 2003;107:139–46.

Lakatta EG, Levy D. Arterial and cardiac aging: major shareholders in cardiovascular disease enterprises. Part II: The aging heart in health: links to heart disease. Circulation 2003;107:346–54.

Lakatta EG. Arterial and cardiac aging: major shareholders in cardiovascular disease enterprises. Part III: Cellular and molecular clues to heart and arterial aging. Circulation 2003;107:490–7.

Shafer SL. Pharmacokinetics and pharmacodynamics of the elderly. In: McLeskey CH, ed. Geriatric anesthesiology. Baltimore: Williams & Wilkins; 1997:123–42.

Weinert BT, Timiras PS. Physiology of aging, invited review: theories of aging. J Appl Physiol. 2003;95:1706–16.

Xiao RP, Lakatta EG. Deterioration of beta-adrenergic modulation of cardiovascular function with aging. Ann NY Acad Sci. 1992; 673:293–310.

Further reading

Alvarez-Buylla A, Lim DA. For the long run: maintaining germinal niches in the adult brain. Neuron 2004;41:683–6.

Bertoni-Freddari C, Fattoretti P, Giorgetti B, Solazzi M, Balietti M, Meier-Ruge W. Role of mitochondrial deterioration in physiological and pathological brain aging. Gerontology 2004;50:187–92.

Fleg JL, Schulman SP, O'Connor FC et al. Cardiovascular responses to exhaustive upright cycle exercise in highly trained older men. J Appl Physiol. 1994;77:1500–6.

Folkow B, Svanborg A. Physiology of cardiovascular aging. Physiol Rev. 1993;73:725–64.

Minto CF, Schnider TW, Shafer SL. Pharmacokinetics and pharmacodynamics of remifentanil. II. Model application. Anesthesiology 1997;86:24–33.

Muravchick S. Geroanesthesia. Principles for management of the elderly patient. St. Louis: Mosby; 1997.

Rowe JW, Kahn RL. Successful aging. Gerontologist 1997;37:433–40.

Ruano D, Araujo F, Bentareha R, Vitorica J. Age-related modifications on the $GABA_A$ receptor binding properties from Wistar rat prefrontal cortex. Brain Res. 1996;738:103–8.

Sapolsky RM, Krey LC, McEwen BS. The neuroendocrinology of stress and aging: the glucocorticoid cascade hypothesis. Endocrine Rev. 1986;7:284–301.

Sohal RS, Weindruch R. Oxidative stress, caloric restriction, and aging. Science 1996;273:59–63.

Chapter 70

Neonatology

Ian G Wilson and Jane E Sellors

TOPICS COVERED IN THIS CHAPTER

- **Respiratory physiology**
  - Control of ventilation
  - Apnea and periodic breathing
  - Gas transport
- **Cardiovascular physiology**
  - The fetal circulation
  - The transition to extrauterine life
- **Nervous system**
  - Retinopathy of prematurity (ROP)
- **Renal physiology**
- **Liver function and pharmacology**
- **Thermoregulation**
- **Evaluation and resuscitation of the newborn**
- **Anesthetic considerations**
  - Ventilation
  - Temperature regulation
  - Fluid balance
  - Clinical pharmacology

The neonatal period is defined as the first 28 days of life following delivery. For a baby born at term (40 weeks post conception), many of the immature physiological systems begin their progress to maturity during this period. The advances in neonatal and reproductive medicine have resulted in the survival of babies born after 24 weeks' gestation, a time at which many systems are extremely immature. In these babies the neonatal period should be considered to last until 44 weeks post conception. Thus the concept of postconceptional age is important for anyone involved in the management of these patients.

One cannot fail to marvel at the resilience and adaptability required to complete the transition from intrauterine to extrauterine life. A reduction in the time allowed to prepare for this transition results in increased morbidity and mortality. The basic science described in this book applies in the vast majority of situations to the neonate. This chapter focuses on situations where there are important differences relevant to the practice of anesthesia. Some of the important pathophysiologic aspects of the premature neonate are summarized in Table 70.1 and discussed below.

Table 70.1 Problems associated with the premature infant

The following have an increased incidence or are specific to the premature infant
Respiratory
Respiratory distress syndrome – surfactant deficiency
Bronchopulmonary dysplasia – chronic lung disease
Apnea and periodic breathing
Persistent pulmonary hypertension
Cardiac
Patent ductus arteriosus – premature ductus less responsive to oxygen
Nervous system
Intraventricular/periventricular hemorrhages – reduced cerebral autoregulation
Retinopathy of prematurity– exposure to high FiO_2
Gastrointestinal
Gastroesophageal reflux
Necrotizing enterocolitis – association with hypoxia
Metabolic
Hypoglycemia – low glycogen stores
Hypocalcemia – immature parathyroid action, low vitamin D stores
Jaundice – poor hepatic conjugation and increased bilirubin load
Skin
Fluid losses – large insensible losses due to thin epidermis
Infection – immature immune system

RESPIRATORY PHYSIOLOGY

The neonate has a metabolic rate and oxygen consumption per kilogram approximately twice that of adults. To meet these higher demands neonates need relatively higher minute ventilation (100–150 mL/kg/min, compared to 60 mL/kg/min in the adult). This, coupled with the immaturity of the respiratory system at birth, makes the neonate more vulnerable to hypoxia and respiratory failure, especially if it is placed under any further physiological stress

The lungs develop early in fetal life and by 16 weeks' gestation the airways are relatively formed. It is only at 24 weeks that the fetus starts to develop primitive alveoli, along with a blood supply that will enable gas exchange. A full-term neonate is born with fewer alveoli than an adult; their number continues to increase until the age of 8. Therefore, at birth the neonate has a much smaller area over which gas exchange can take place. Surfactant is produced by type 2 alveolar cells from 24 to 25 weeks, but reaches normal concentrations at 34 weeks. Surfactant is important in reducing surface tension in the alveoli (Chapter 47). Any infant born before 24 weeks post conception has poorly compliant lungs and is at risk of developing respiratory distress syndrome (RDS; Fig. 70.1). The incidence of RDS has been reduced dramatically by maternal administration of glucocorticoids to accelerate fetal lung maturation. Steroids appear to increase the number of type 2 pneumocytes and lamellar bodies, and the size of alveoli.

The diaphragm is the primary muscle of respiration in the neonate, but is less efficient than the adult diaphragm for a number of reasons. It has a lower proportion of type 1 respiratory fibers, as well as a lower muscle mass. The type 1 fibers (slow twitch, high oxidative) are more resistant to fatigue. The diaphragm of a premature baby has about 10% of such fibers, whereas a full-term neonate has 25%, compared to an adult who has 50% of type 1 fibers. Diaphragmatic descent is limited by the contents of the abdominal cavity, and ventilation can be drastically compromised by situations where it is increased, such as air in the stomach or organomegaly. At birth the neonatal ribcage is cylindrical rather than the ellipsoidal shape of adults, and the ribs run horizontally rather than obliquely. Thus the neonate has less ability to increase its intrathoracic volume and hence its tidal volume during inspiration. The ribs themselves are soft and pliable, which is important to allow compression of the chest wall through the birth canal. However, this also means that the chest wall offers little resistance to collapse at the end of expiration. This contributes to the relatively small functional residual capacity (FRC) and intrathoracic volume in the newborn. The FRC in the adult is a buffer against hypoxia, but its smaller size in the neonate, coupled with the higher oxygen consumption, means that the oxygen reserves in the neonatal FRC are consumed more rapidly.

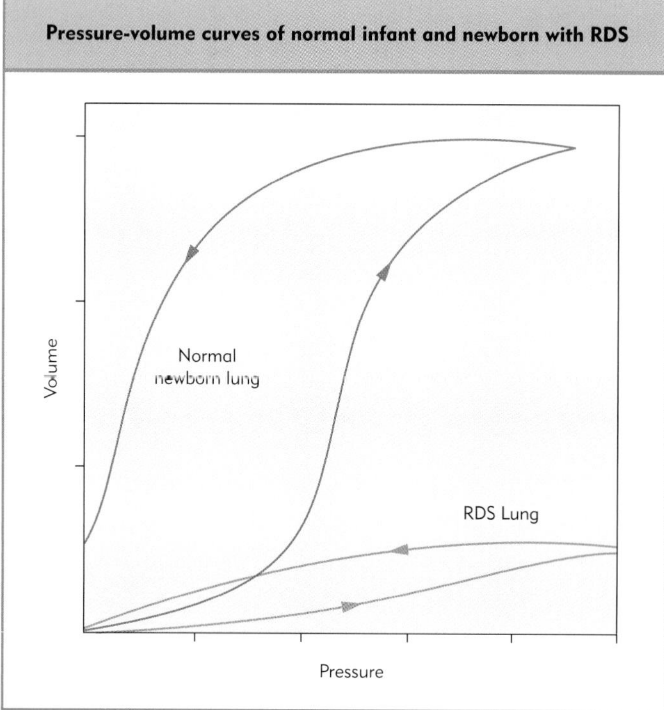

Figure 70.1 Comparison of the pressure volume curve of a normal infant compared to that of a newborn with hyaline membrane disease and respiratory distress syndrome. Note the lack of hysteresis in the RDS lung due to deficient surfactant. (After Goldsmith JP and Karotkin EH, Assisted ventilation of the neonate. 3rd edition, W. B. Saunders Company, 1996.)

The relatively smaller FRC of the neonate, coupled with a higher oxygen consumption, leads to move rapid depletion of oxygen reserves during apnea.

Neonates can maintain their FRC by a number of mechanisms. When awake, the intercostals muscles have normal phasic tone, which helps stabilize the chest wall, but this is abolished in REM sleep. Expiratory braking (grunting), in which upper airway resistance is increased by adduction of the vocal cords, also helps preserve FRC. Closing volume in neonates – and indeed in children of 5 or under – is equal to or even higher than FRC when they are supine, and can encroach on tidal volume even when the neonate is awake.

The arterial Po_2 in the neonate (60–80 mmHg; 8–10.6 kPa) is lower than in adults (95–100 mmHg; 12.6–13.3 kPa). The A–ao_2 difference in neonates is approximately 4 kPa (30 mmHg) compared to 1 kPa (7.5 mmHg) in adults. This is due in part to the continued right-to-left shunting of blood, and in part to blood flow through nonventilated capillaries.

Control of ventilation

Breathing movements begin in utero at approximately 11 weeks. They are intermittent but become continuous at birth. The low Pao_2 in utero may inhibit continuous breathing. The chemoreceptors are active before birth, but are not fully developed. At birth both premature and full-term neonates show a biphasic response to hypoxemia. They initially increase their ventilation for about 1 minute before returning to baseline, and then develop depressed ventilation. In a cold environment even the transient hyperventilation on exposure to hypoxia is abolished (Fig. 70.2). By 3 weeks the full-term neonate develops an adult response to hypoxemia.

Mechanoreceptors play an important role in ventilation in the neonate, especially the premature infant. Stretch receptors in the airways are stimulated by lung inflation and deflation, and have a role in regulating lung volume and FRC. These are known as the Hering–Breuer reflexes and are not found in the adult.

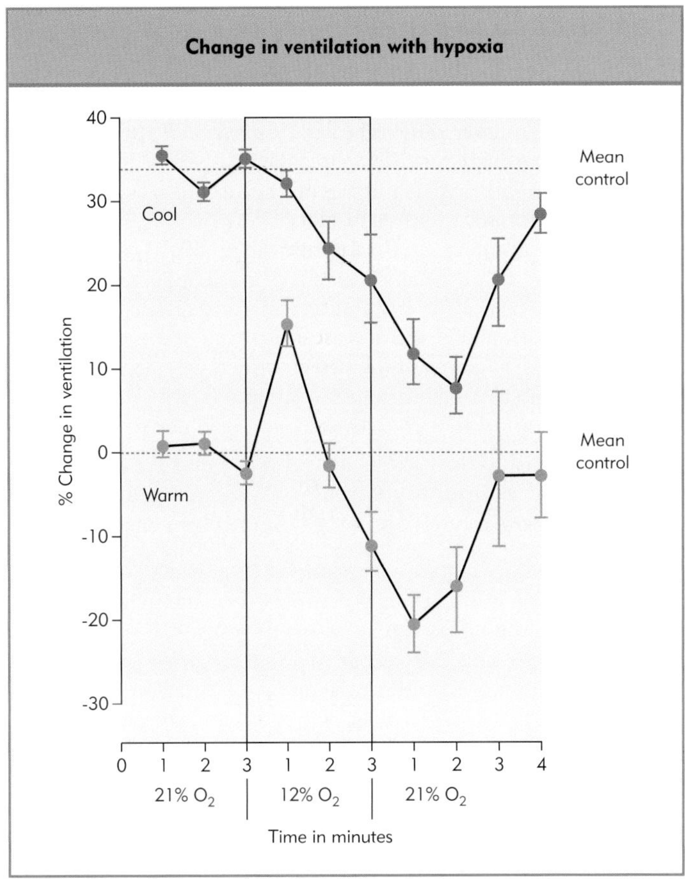

Figure 70.2 Change in ventilation in response to breathing 12% oxygen in normal full term infants in warm and cool temperatures. (From Ceruti E. Chemoreceptor reflexes in the newborn infant, effect of cooling on the response to hypoxia. Pediatrics. 1966; 37(4) 556–64.)

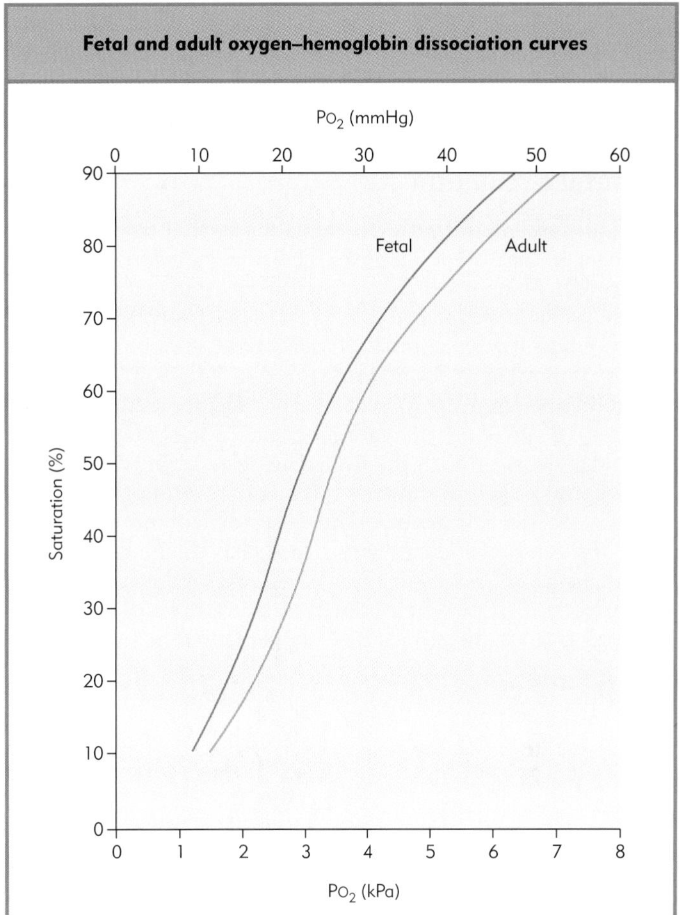

Figure 70.3 Oxygen–hemoglobin dissociation curves for fetal and adult hemoglobin. (From Darling R, Smith C, Assmussen El. Some properties of human fetal and maternal blood. J Clin Invest. 1941;20;739–47.)

Apnea and periodic breathing

Periodic breathing is defined as regular respiration of 20 seconds or more followed by periods of apnea of 10 seconds or less occurring at least three times in a row. Periodic breathing can be normal and occurs in approximately 75% of neonates, although the incidence increases markedly with prematurity. Pathological apnea is defined as an episode of apnea lasting for 20 seconds or longer, or less than 20 seconds if accompanied by oxygen desaturation or bradycardia. Apnea of prematurity is defined as periodic breathing with pathologic apnea in a premature infant. Causes of apnoea may be central, owing to immaturity of respiratory control mechanisms, obstructive, or a combination of the two. The incidence of apnea is increased during REM sleep, or with prematurity. It may be indicative of number of pathological processes, such as respiratory infection, sepsis, intracranial hemorrhage, patent ductus arteriosus, gastroesphageal reflux, anemia, acidosis, or drugs.

Gas transport

As oxygen tension is much lower in fetal than in maternal blood, the fetus has developed a mechanism to improve oxygen carriage. Fetal hemoglobin (HbF) reacts poorly with 2,3-diphosphoglycerate (2,3-DPG), which binds to deoxyhemoglobin and not oxyhemoglobin. This has the effect of increasing the affinity of HbF for oxygen. The oxyhemoglobin dissociation curve is shifted to the left and thus the P_{50} is reduced. The P_{50} is the partial pressure of oxygen at which the oxygen saturation is 50% (Fig. 70.3). The adult value for P_{50} is 27 mmHg (3.6 kPa), whereas in the neonate it is 20 mmHg (2.7 kPa) and for HbF it is 18 mmHg (2.4 kPa). At birth between 50 and 85% of hemoglobin is HbF, and even higher in premature infants. From 32 weeks' gestation onwards HbA is synthesized and HbF concentrations gradually decline; by 4 months HbF accounts for only 5–10% of hemoglobin. As HbF levels decline, the P_{50} increases to the adult value by 3 months.

The higher affinity of HbF for oxygen facilitates oxygen transfer from the placenta to the fetus. In the neonate HbF may be a disadvantage, as its increased affinity for O_2 impairs release to peripheral tissues. Higher neonatal Hb (18–19 g/dL) and cardiac output help compensate for this. If a neonate is hypoxic and anemic (Hb less than 12 g/dL), blood transfusion may improve tissue oxygenation

CARDIOVASCULAR PHYSIOLOGY

Whereas the lungs take a back seat to the placenta, the fetal heart must function from an early stage to ensure survival. Fetal lungs only require enough of the cardiac output to supply nutrition, and not for gas exchange. Thus the fetus must have shunts to minimize pulmonary flow and maximize the supply of oxygen to brain and heart. These shunts are the foramen ovale (FO), the ductus arteriosus (DA), and the ductus venosus (DV).

The fetal circulation

An understanding of the fetal circulation is vital to understand the changes that occur at birth. The fetal circulation is characterized by high pulmonary vascular resistance (PVR), low systemic vascular resistance (SVR), and right-to-left shunting via the FO and DA. The umbilical vein carries oxygenated blood (Po_2 = 35 mmHg (4.7 kPa)) from the placenta to the fetus via the umbilical vein. At this point the flow divides and about 50% bypasses the liver in the inferior vena cava (IVC), and the remainder flows through the liver. The more highly oxygenated blood from the IVC is directed by the crista terminalis through the FO into the left atrium. This ensures that the blood perfusing the cerebral and coronary arteries has the highest oxygen content.

The portion of blood entering the right atrium that stays on the right side of the circulation joins blood from the superior vena cava and is ejected into the pulmonary artery. Here, because of high resistance to flow, only a small amount enters the pulmonary veins, and about 90% is shunted across the huge ductus arteriosus into the descending aorta (Fig. 70.4). The majority of the flow from the descending aorta returns to the placenta via the umbilical artery for reoxygenation.

The transition to extrauterine life

The changes required at birth are dramatic. Some occur almost instantaneously, but others take much longer, and so the neonate has what is accurately referred to as a *transitional circulation* for some time after birth.

The first breath and clamping of the umbilical cord reduce right atrial pressure. Pulmonary blood flow increases as a result of decreased pulmonary vascular resistance (PVR), so that left atrial pressure rises. This reversal of the pressure difference closes the foramen ovale, and the fetal circulation shifts from the parallel circulation that existed in utero to a series circulation. PVR decreases as a result of direct effects of increased oxygenation and local mediators such as bradykinin.

Pulmonary blood flow increases with the first breath owing to decreased pulmonary vascular resistance produced by lung expansion, oxygen, and local pulmonary vasodilators.

The initiation of breathing is complex. During vaginal delivery fluid within the lungs is squeezed out as a result of pressure on the thorax; when this pressure is released, air enters the airways passively. Removal of the placental circulation decreases prostaglandin E_2 (PGE_2) levels, which inhibits respiration, and rising oxygen tensions stimulate breathing. The first few breaths rapidly establish the FRC (Fig. 70.5). Surprisingly high inspiratory pressures are required at first (>50 cmH_2O) to overcome

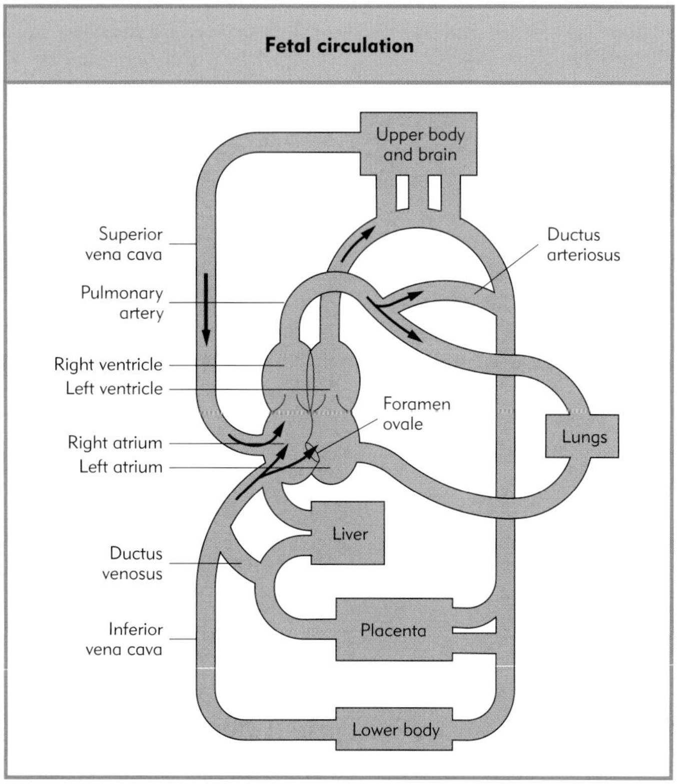

Figure 70.4 Schematic representation of the fetal circulation. The arrows show the preferential flow through the fetal shunts to avoid the lungs. Also shown is the diversion of deoxygenated blood from the superior vena cava, via the right ventricle, to avoid the brain.

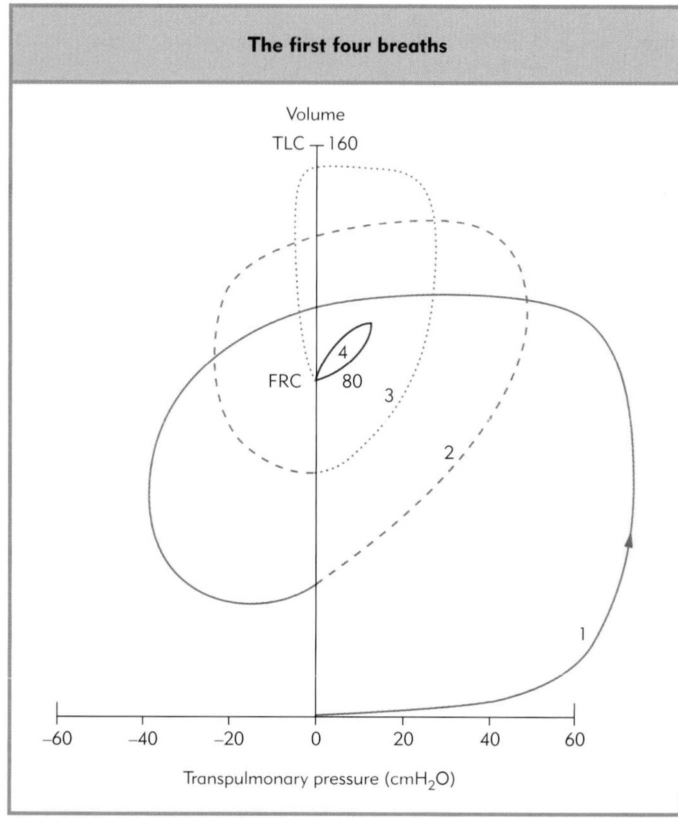

Figure 70.5 The first four breaths. Each successive breath requires less pressure and increases the FRC. (From Hatch D, Sumner E, Hellmann J, eds. The surgical neonate: anaesthesia and intensive care. London: Edward Arnold; 1995.)

viscous forces; these pressures decrease over the first four or five breaths. Hypercarbia is reduced within 5 minutes, and acidemia resolves over the first day of life.

The clamping of the cord removes the low-resistance placental unit and this, in combination with the decrease in PVR, leads to a reversal of flow across the ductus arteriosus, which begins to close in response to increasing PaO_2 and decreasing prostaglandins. The spiral smooth muscle constricts and cushions of mucoid protrude into the lumen. This initial physiological closure occurs in the first 12 hours, but permanent closure takes 2–4 weeks in term infants. Closure takes longer in premature infants, and the DA may not even close at all, as its responsiveness to oxygen is reduced. Hypoxia and PGE_1 and PGE_2 maintain potency in utero, and can continue to do so after birth.

As these shunts do not close anatomically at first, they can open in response to physiologic challenges, most importantly hypoxia, hypercarbia, and acidemia. Reversion of the transitional circulation to the fetal circulatory pattern can occur at this stage. Pulmonary vessels in the neonate are very reactive, and pulmonary arteriolar constriction can be precipitated by hypoxemia, acidemia, or an increase in pulmonary blood volume. In addition, hypoxia dilates the DA (just as increased O_2 constricts it).

Pulmonary vessels in the neonate are highly reactive to hypoxia, hypercarbia, and acidosis, which can cause pulmonary arteriolar constriction and increase right-to-left shunting.

The rise in PVR will worsen right-to-left shunting with increased flow across the FO and DA, which leads to hypoxia and a further increase in PVR, thus creating a vicious cycle. This condition is known as persistent pulmonary hypertension of the neonate (PPHN). In addition to the dangerous triad of hypoxia, hypercarbia, and acidosis, PPHN may result from excessive muscularization of the pulmonary arterioles, hypoplastic lungs, or reduced flow due to increased blood viscosity or a congenital defect. Those neonates who are more at risk of PPHN include those with congenital diaphragmatic hernia, infection, meconium aspiration, and polycythemia. A diagnosis of PPHN will be supported by blood measurements taken simultaneously from the pre- and postductal arteries. A difference of greater than 20 mmHg (2.6 kPa) is abnormal. This scenario is not unusual in neonates presenting for anesthesia. PVR is manipulated by adjusting mechanical ventilation to produce alkalosis and hyperoxia (temporarily), with vasodilators, and with inhaled nitric oxide.

Neonatal cardiac output (per kg) is approximately twice that of adults (in order to meet the increased O_2 demands), but the heart is less contractile and thus has less ability to increase stroke volume. Cardiac output is maintained by and dependent on heart rate (around 120–160 beats/min in the newborn). The activities of the baroreflexes are reduced, and there is less ability to mount a physiological response to hemorrhage than in the adult.

The autonomic nervous system is incompletely developed at birth. α-Adrenergic control is virtually complete at term, but β-adrenergic control is still incomplete. Therefore, sympathetic responses, although present at birth, are diminished. In contrast, the cholinergic system (vagal) is complete at birth. Thus anything leading to stimulation of the autonomic nervous system can lead to bradycardia rather than tachycardia.

THE NERVOUS SYSTEM

The brain has a different rate of growth from other organs. There are two spurts: neuronal cells multiply at 15–20 weeks' gestation and glial cells from 25 weeks to 2 years. Myelination is incomplete at birth and continues until the third year of life. The brain is relatively large at birth, representing 10% of total body weight, and it has about a quarter of the number of brain cells of the adult. Poor nutrition during these rapid growth spurts severely impairs brain development.

Immature reflexes (such as the Moro and grasp reflexes) are dependent on cutaneous stimuli and owe their presence to immature myelination. Neurological development and gestational age can be estimated by examining these reflexes.

Neonates feel pain; at 28 weeks the density of nociceptive nerve endings in the skin is similar to that of adults. Myelination may not be complete in the premature infant, and this may have an effect on the central processing of pain. However, it is now well established that even preterm babies can respond to a painful stimulus by withdrawal, autonomic stimulation, and stress hormone release. Neonates undergoing surgery who do not receive adequate anesthesia to prevent them mounting a stress response are more likely to have adverse events postoperatively. Early pain experience in this age group can alter subsequent nociceptive responses owing to CNS plasticity (Chapter 23). Several studies indicate that noxious stimuli without adequate analgesia can lead to hypersensitivity in later life. There may also be long-term effects of opioid drugs given to neonates undergoing intensive care. These exogenous opioids may change the proportion of opioid receptors and alter subsequent responses to opioids.

Loss of cerebral autoregulation in the neonate due to hypoxia, acidosis, or hypercarbia increases the risk of peri- and intraventricular hemorrhage.

Cerebral autoregulation is present in the neonate but its range is narrower than in adults, and reduced even further in the premature infant. Autoregulation can be abolished by hypoxemia, acidosis, and hypercarbia; in the absence of autoregulation cerebral blood flow will become dependent on blood pressure. The loss of autoregulation together with surges in cerebral blood flow can increase the risk of periventricular or intraventricular hemorrhage in the premature neonate. Risk appears to be maximal in the first 72 hours of life. Hemorrhages occur in the delicate capillaries in the germinal matrix, which is an area of the developing brain that regresses at term. Thus factors that may alter either autoregulation or cerebral blood flow should be avoided.

Retinopathy of prematurity (ROP)

This condition was previously referred to as retrolental fibroplasia. The vessels in the retina are formed from the nasal side to the temporal side by 44 weeks of gestation. Exposure to high oxygen concentrations during the process, especially early on, causes vascular spasm. The retinal tissue necroses and heals with fibrosis. New vessels proliferate in the fibrosed area and can cause retinal detachment. Those most at risk are the premature, those on high inspired oxygen, and those receiving adult blood (the dissociation curve is shifted to the right). Maintaining the $Pa\text{O}_2$ at 45–60 mmHg (6–8 kPa) is the best preventative measure.

RENAL PHYSIOLOGY

Despite the fact that the fetus maintains metabolic homeostasis through the placenta, the kidney is remarkably well developed by 34 weeks of gestation. At this stage all nephrons have formed but growth continues well into childhood, particularly in tubule length. Nevertheless, the fetal kidney has an important role in maintaining amniotic fluid volume. Although the neonatal kidney is pressed into action straight from birth it has different demands from that of the adult. Around 50% of nitrogen intake is utilized by growth, such that growth is known as the infant's 'third kidney'. Nitrogen is used to make new tissue and protein, and not metabolized to produce urea.

Renal vascular resistance (RVR) is initially high, but after birth there is a fall in RVR and the percentage of cardiac output the kidney receives increases from about 5% to the adult value of 25% by 24 months. The glomerular filtration rate (GFR) is only 15–30% that of the adult in the first few days, but reaches 50% by the tenth day. Renal tubular function is reduced, and this limits the ability of the newborn to handle solute (e.g. Na^+ and glucose) and fluid loads. Concentrating ability (to a maximum of 800 mmol/L, or about half that of the adult) is reduced by fewer and shorter loops of Henle, but there is also a lower concentration of urea in the medulla. The 'physiological acidemia' of infancy extends beyond the immediate respiratory and metabolic load of the stress of delivery, and is largely due to a low renal threshold for bicarbonate. That is, HCO_3^- appears in the urine at low serum concentrations. Serum HCO_3^- may be lower in the term neonate (around 20 mm) and as low as 12 mm in the premature infant. Most newborns secrete HCO_3^- at maximum levels, so conditions that produce acidosis are compensated for and more likely to produce a change in pH.

The normal situation for a neonate is a restricted fluid intake for the first few days while lactation is established. During this time weight is lost. Total body water is high in the neonate, mainly because extracellular fluid exceeds intracellular in the neonatal period. Insensible water loss from the respiratory tract (30%) and the skin (70%) is relatively high in the neonate, but becomes huge in the very premature (200 mL/kg/day at 26 weeks' gestation, compared to 10 mL/kg/day at term). This is because the thin epidermis and virtually absent fat offer much less resistance to the diffusion of water.

LIVER FUNCTION AND PHARMACOLOGY

The liver also takes over essential functions from the placenta at birth. The liver is well developed and relatively large compared to that in the adult (4% of body weight in the neonate, 2% in the adult). However, many of the enzyme systems are deficient. Microsomal cytochrome P450 activity is half that of the adult. Phase I reactions, which produce more polar metabolites, are reduced in effectiveness but less so than the phase II conjugation reactions. This is clinically significant, in that neonates clear drugs such as morphine more slowly, and drug doses and dosing intervals must be adjusted accordingly. However, hepatic enzyme systems develop quickly, reaching adult levels by 3 months in both premature and term infants.

The neonate has a reduced capacity to excrete Na^+, water, and drugs.

Physiological neonatal jaundice is common and appears by 48 hours, peaking on the fourth day. The causes include reduced uptake of bile by the liver, reduced conjugation of bilirubin, and increased bilirubin availability. Increased availability results from reabsorption of bilirubin from the gut, rapid red cell breakdown, and hematomas from trauma at delivery, which easily overload the immature liver. The danger is the formation of bilirubin–membrane complexes in the basal ganglia and brainstem, which cause serious neurological damage. This process (kernicterus) is more likely to occur in sick premature infants. The problem is avoided by treatment with phototherapy. Unconjugated bilirubin in the skin is degraded and photoisomerized by blue light (425–475 nm) to nontoxic products, which are more easily excreted.

The neonate, especially preterm, is at risk of hypoglycemia. This is due in part to the higher metabolic rate and in part to low glycogen stores (which limits glycogenolysis) and immature liver function (gluconeogenesis develops after birth). Blood glucose can drop rapidly after birth owing to high circulating catecholamines.

Drug action in the neonate is affected by more systems than hepatic enzyme systems. Both quantitative plasma protein concentrations and qualitative plasma protein binding are reduced. Many drugs that bind to plasma proteins such as α_1 acidic glycoprotein or albumin have an increased unbound fraction of the drug and increased potential for toxicity. This reduced plasma protein concentration protects the fetus from placental transfer of drugs to a certain extent, as fetal protein binding is less than maternal.

It is often held that the blood–brain barrier is poorly developed in the neonate. In practice this may have more to do with reduced protein binding and the lipid content of the neonatal brain, rather than changes in the permeability of the blood–brain barrier.

Neonates have a greater percentage of total body water than adults and a lower percentage of fat and muscle. The fluid is differently distributed, with a greater proportion in the extracellular compartment. There is a greater volume of distribution for water-soluble drugs, which may increase the duration of action (Chapter 8). Renal tubular function and GFR are reduced, which can lead to the accumulation of renally excreted drugs and active metabolites.

Gastric pH is high in neonates. After oral administration, basic drugs such as penicillins have high bioavailability, and acidic drugs such as phenobarbital and phenytoin show reduced absorption.

Increased surface to volume ratio, increased skin water content, and less keratin all predispose the neonate to greater percutaneous drug absorption. This has caused problems with methemoglobinemia following the use of EMLA (the eutectic mixture of lidocaine and prilocaine) in neonates.

The result of the complex interactions of hepatic, renal, and other physiological variables is that the loading dose of many drugs is increased in the neonate to account for the increased volume of distribution, whereas the longer elimination half-lives require less frequent doses.

THERMOREGULATION

Humans are homeothermic, which means they can maintain a stable core temperature in the face of changes in ambient temperature. However, neonates are especially prone to heat loss. Radiation is the major source of loss, as newborns have a larger surface area to volume ratio, although convection and evaporation are also very important (Chapter 67).

To maintain body temperature in cold environments, the homeotherm must be able to produce heat. Three mechanisms are available: voluntary muscle activity, involuntary muscle activity (shivering), and nonshivering thermogenesis.

Shivering is poorly developed in the neonate and voluntary activity is inadequate. Thus nonshivering thermogenesis is vital. Although heat production can occur in muscle, liver, and brain, the metabolism of brown fat is by far the most important mechanism. Brown fat, differentiating between 26 and 30 weeks' gestation, comprises around 11% of the total body fat of the neonate. It is found between the scapulae, in the axillae and the mediastinum, around major blood vessels in the neck, and around the kidneys. It is well vascularized and well innervated by the sympathetic nervous system. The many mitochondria in brown fat cells are packed with cristae. The stress of cold stimulates the release of norepinephrine, which metabolizes brown fat to free fatty acids and glycerol. This mechanism of thermogenesis can be inhibited by surgical or pharmacological sympathetic block.

Nonshivering thermogenesis is vital to neonatal thermoregulation.

The range over which a neonate can thermoregulate is considerably more limited than in an adult. The lower limit in adults is 0°C, whereas that of the neonate is 22°C. However, a more useful concept is that of the neutral thermal environment. This is the range of temperatures at which body temperature can be maintained at minimum oxygen expenditure. In the first few days of life this range is narrow and the temperature surprisingly high (Fig. 70.6). The importance of maintaining body temperature cannot be overemphasized. The metabolism required to increase temperature rapidly is very energy expensive. If not treated promptly, hypothermia results in hypoxia and hypoglycemia.

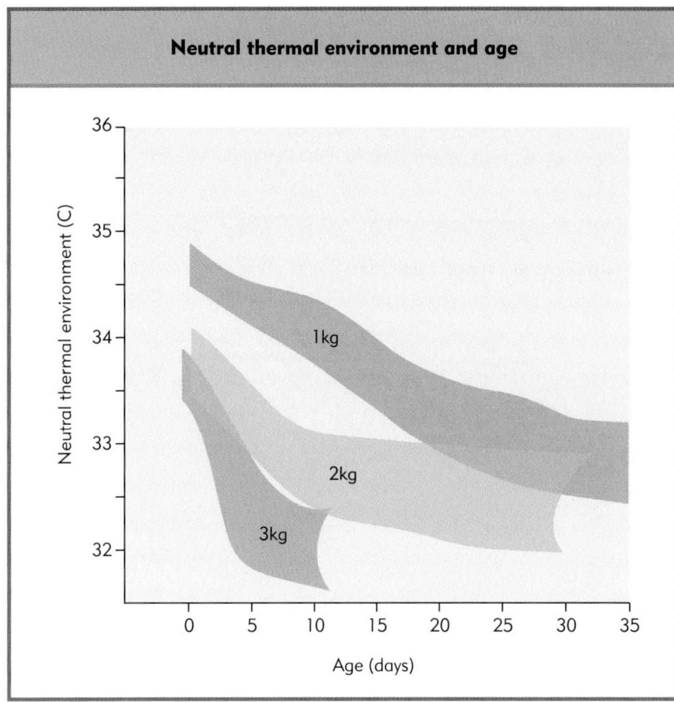

Figure 70.6 Neutral thermal environment for babies of various birth weights in the first month of life. (From Hey EN, Katz G. Optimal thermal environment of naked babies. Arch Dis Child. 1970;45:328–34.)

EVALUATION AND RESUSCITATION OF THE NEWBORN

Mild hypoxia occurs with each contraction during labor, and the fetus has protective responses to this. Blood is diverted to major organs, and the lining reflex results in bradycardia and increased mean arterial pressure. The pattern of heart rate responses to uterine contractions is used to interpret the degree of fetal distress. When the cord is clamped and the newborn is removed from the placental oxygen supply, breathing should begin within 60–90 seconds. Should this fail to happen, the asphyxiated fetus will respond initially with tachypnea, tachycardia, and hypertension (Fig. 70.7). This rapidly progresses to bradycardia and primary apnea as the respiratory center fails. If hypoxia continues, primitive spinal centers initiate gasping, which fades to secondary or terminal apnea. The heart will usually remain active until all respiratory activity ceases, which can take 20 minutes. Spontaneous recovery usually occurs if the baby is stimulated before secondary apnea. However, once secondary apnea is established the baby will succumb without active intervention. As it may be difficult to distinguish primary from secondary apnea, every apneic neonate must be treated aggressively.

Traditionally Apgar scores were used to evaluate the newborn. The current emphasis is on prompt evaluation and the initiation of resuscitation (Fig. 70.8), rather than enumerating a score, which may be more useful in retrospect.

It is still vital to evaluate respiration, color, heart rate, and tone in the initial examination, as well as assessing the presence of meconium and the gestational age of the infant, and institute treatment accordingly.

The familiar sequence of airway, breathing, and circulation (ABC) is appropriate, with the simple maneuvers of drying, warming, suctioning, and stimulating being performed in *all* babies. Temperature control is of the utmost importance, as hypothermia exacerbates the effects of acidosis, impairs myocardial function, and reduces the production of surfactant.

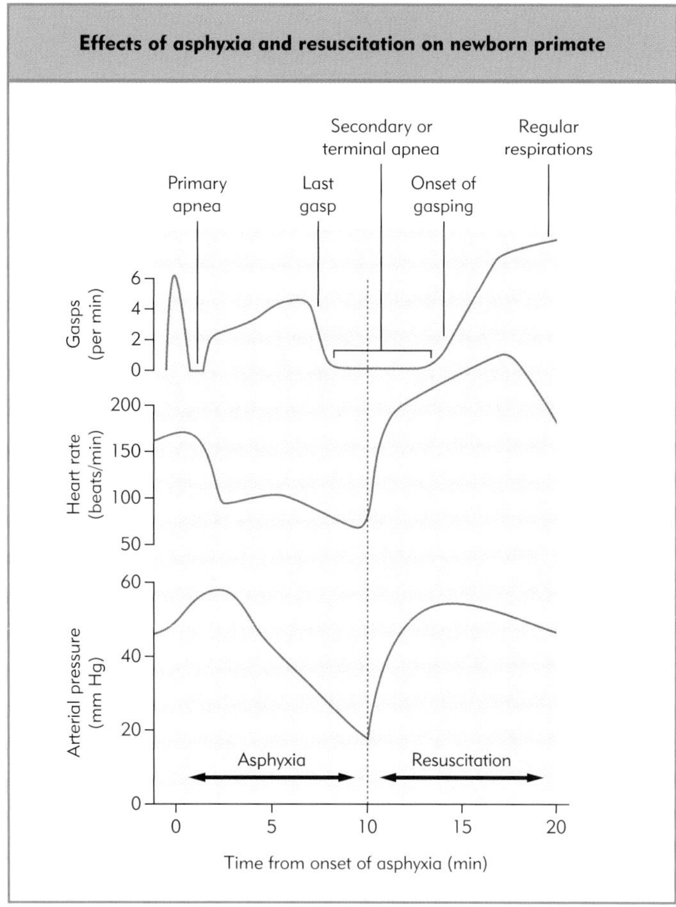

Figure 70.7 Effects of asphyxia and resuscitation on the newborn primate. (Klaus MH, Fanaroff AA. Care of the high risk neonate. 4th edition, W.B. Saunders Company, 1993)

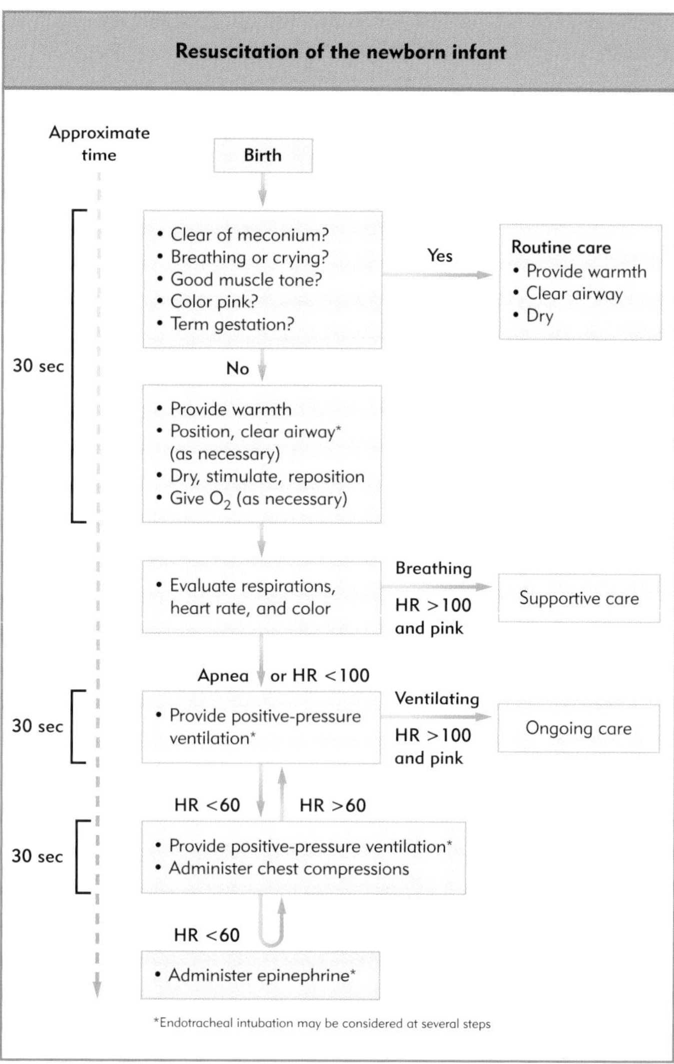

Figure 70.8 Algorithm for the resuscitation of the newborn infant. (From International Guidelines for Neonatal Resuscitation, with permission.)

ANESTHETIC CONSIDERATIONS

Neonates who require surgery and hence anesthesia usually have significant medical problems. Operations in this age group are usually required to correct a congenital malformation or a disease process related to prematurity, such as necrotizing enterocolitis or inguinal hernia. This is at a time when the infant is undergoing dramatic changes in physiology, particularly cardiovascular, in adapting to extrauterine life. An appreciation of the scientific principles involved in these changes is vital to the safe delivery of anesthetic care to these babies.

Ventilation

General anesthesia in a neonate can increase the risk of respiratory failure. Sedation or anesthesia can depress ventilation and increase the risk of apnea. Anesthesia inhibits intercostal muscle activity and reduces the already limited ability of the neonate to stabilize the ribcage during respiration.

The FRC is reduced by sedation and airways may close, with normal tidal breathing leading to increased V/Q mismatch and decreased $Pa\text{O}_2$. In most cases controlled ventilation is employed, and PEEP should be used to minimize the fall in FRC. The size of anesthetic circuits and filters should be chosen carefully, as they can increase V_D dramatically in a small infant. Oxygen levels should be optimized to prevent hypoxemia but minimize the risk of ROP. Oxygen saturations of 95% are considered adequate in the neonate.

Temperature regulation

The neonate is vulnerable to hypothermia. Not only does hypothermia increase oxygen consumption, it also delays recovery from anesthesia and increases the risk of apnea. It is vital to minimize heat loss and maintain a neutral thermal environment.

Fluid balance

The principles of fluid management in the neonate are not so different from those in the adult, but the margin for error is small. For example, the volume of drugs and flushes needs to be taken into account when calculating the fluid balance. It is useful starting point to calculate the hourly fluid requirement, which is approximately 100 mL/kg/day in a neonate. Preoperative and intraoperative losses can be estimated from information such as the length of starvation and the type of surgery, and corrected as appropriate.

It is important to be aware of the risk of hypoglycemia in the fasting neonate. They often need glucose in IV infusions if their own stores are insufficient, but it is also important to avoid hyperglycemia, which can act as an osmotic diuretic. Hyperglycemia can exacerbate neurological damage and should be avoided in high-risk cases.

Neonatal blood volumes are higher in than adults owing to increased plasma volume. Values of 80–90 mL/kg and 90–100 mL/kg are considered normal for term and preterm neonates, respectively.

Clinical Pharmacology

INHALATION AGENTS

Neonates are particularly susceptible to cardiorespiratory depression by volatile anesthetics. The uptake and time to equilibration are more rapid in infants (Chapter 27) because alveolar ventilation is greater in relation to FRC, blood gas solubilities are lower, and the distribution of cardiac output to brain and heart is greater. Baroreceptor responses are depressed by volatile agents to a greater degree in neonates. These effects combine to reduce the therapeutic ratio between satisfactory anesthesia and myocardial depression.

Neonates are exquisitely sensitive to cardiorespiratory depression by volatile anesthetics.

Minimal alveolar concentration (MAC) for all agents is low at birth and increases to a maximum at around 6 months, before gradually declining throughout life. Many theories have been put forward to explain this, including reduced response to pain and low blood gas solubility.

MUSCLE RELAXANTS

Larger doses of succinylcholine per kilogram are required in neonates owing to a combination of increased volume of distribution and immature acetylcholine receptors. Infants have lower plasma cholinesterase activity. As extracellular fluid and surface area have a constant relationship throughout life, doses calculated on this basis are more constant. The duration of action is similarly reduced.

Neonates have long been held to be sensitive to nondepolarizing neuromuscular blockers, and this is certainly true of tubocurarine. Vecuronium seems to have a longer duration of action in neonates, whereas atracurium is generally less effective and may have a shorter duration of action. The message is that these drugs are unpredictable in this age group, and great care should be taken. It is perfectly possible to monitor neuromuscular blockade in this age group.

Key references

Anand KJS, Brown MJ, Causon RC, Christofides ND, Bloom SR, Aynsley-Green A. Can the human neonate mount an endocrine and metabolic response to surgery? J Pediatr Surg. 1985;20:41–8.

Contributors and reviewers for the Neonatal Resuscitation Guidelines: International guidelines for neonatal resuscitation: An excerpt from the guidelines 2000 for cardiopulmonary resuscitation and emergency cardiovascular care. International consensus on science. Pediatrics 2000;106:e29.

Han VKM. Neonatal anatomy, physiology and development. Curr Opin Pediatr. 1990;2:275–81.

Hatch D, Sumner E, Hellmann J. Perinatal physiology and medicine. In: Hatch et al's The surgical neonate: anaesthesia and intensive care. London: Edward Arnold; 1995:1–97.

Krishna G, Emhardt JD. Anesthesia for the newborn and ex-preterm infant. Semin Pediatr Surg. 1992;1:32–44.

Motoyama EK, Davis PJ. Basic principles in pediatric anesthesia. In: Smith's Anesthesia for infants and children. Chicago: Mosby Year Book; 1996:1– 212.

Further reading

Aynsley-Green A, Ward Platt MP, Lloyd-Thomas AR. Clinical paediatrics: stress and pain in infancy and childhood. London: Baillière Tindall; 1995.

Berde CB, Sethna NF. Analgesics for the treatment of pain in children. New Engl J Med. 2002;347:1094–103.

Hatch DJ. Respiratory physiology in neonates and infants. Curr Opin Anaesthesiol. 1995;8:224–9.

Levine MI, Tudehope D, Thearle MJ. Essentials of neonatal medicine. Oxford: Blackwell Science; 1993.

Parkin KJ, Poets CF, O'Brien LM, Stebbings VA, Southall DP. Effects of exposure to 15% oxygen on breathing patterns and oxygen saturation in infants: interventional study. BMJ 1998;316:887–94.

Taddio A, Goldbach M, Ipp M, Stevens B, Koren G. Effect of neonatal circumcision on pain responses during vaccination in boys. Lancet 1995;345:291–2.

Useful websites

eMedicine www.emedicine.com

Neonatology On The Web www.neonatology.org

The Virtual Children's Hospital www.vh.org/VCH/Providers/Information.html

Chapter 71

The pathophysiology of obesity and its implications for anesthesia

Paul G Murphy and John P Adams

TOPICS COVERED IN THIS CHAPTER

- **Definitions**
- **Epidemiology**
  - Mortality
  - Etiology
  - Distribution of body fat and health risk
- **Medical therapy for obesity**
- **Surgical treatment of obesity**
- **Obesity and the heart**
  - Hypertension
  - Ischemic heart disease
  - Blood volume
  - Cardiac arrhythmias
  - Obesity cardiomyopathy
  - Clinical features
  - Anesthetic implications
- **Obesity and the respiratory system**
  - Lung volumes
  - Oxygen consumption and carbon dioxide production
  - Gas exchange
  - Lung compliance and resistance
  - Work of breathing
  - Ventilatory control
  - Anesthetic implications
  - Laparoscopy and anesthesia
- **Obesity and other medical conditions**
  - Hiatus hernia and gastroesophageal reflux
  - Diabetes mellitus and other metabolic considerations
  - Thromboembolic disease
- **Altered drug handling in obesity**
  - Volume of distribution
  - Drug clearance
  - Inhalational anesthetics
- **General perioperative management of the morbidly obese**
- **Postoperative outcomes in the morbidly obese**

It has been known since ancient times that obesity is associated with increased morbidity and premature death. Hippocrates wrote: 'Those naturally fat are more liable to sudden death than the thin'. Contemporary actuarial data support the view that obesity is the commonest nutritional disorder of the civilized world, and its prevalence continues to increase. Much of our current knowledge of the pathophysiology of obesity comes from studies on morbidly obese patients undergoing bariatric (weight reduction) surgery, and justifiably centers on the cardiovascular, respiratory, and metabolic consequences of the condition. It should be understood that this is a selected group of (younger) patients who represent the fittest examples of their type, and that (older) individuals presenting with other medical or surgical conditions may provide attending physicians with far greater challenges than those faced by anesthesiologists involved in anesthesia for surgical correction of severe obesity.

DEFINITIONS

Obesity is a condition of excessive body fat (from the Latin *obesus*, meaning 'fattened by eating'). The difference between normality and obesity is arbitrary, but an individual must be considered obese when the amount of fat tissue is increased to such an extent that physical and mental health are affected and life expectancy reduced. Examples of body fat contents in adults from affluent Westernized societies are shown below:

Average female	20–30%
Average male	18–25%
Professional soccer player	10–12%
Marathon runner	7%

Accurate measurement of body fat content is difficult and requires sophisticated imaging techniques such as computed tomography (CT) or magnetic resonance imaging (MRI). Useful estimates, however, can be obtained by evaluating weight for a given height and then comparing that figure with an ideal weight. The concept of ideal body weight (IBW) originates from life insurance studies, such as those presented by the Metropolitan Life Insurance Company in 1959 and 1979, which describe the weight associated with the lowest mortality rate for a given height and gender (and in some studies body frame size). Although such study populations are highly selective (North

Table 71.1 Definitions of obesity

Definition	Weight related to ideal body weight (IBW)	Body mass index
Normal		15–25
Overweight	110–119% IBW	27
Obesity	120–199% IBW	30
Morbid obesity	>200% IBW or IBW + 100 lb (45.5 kg)	35
Supermorbid obesity	IBW + 200 lb (90 kg)	50

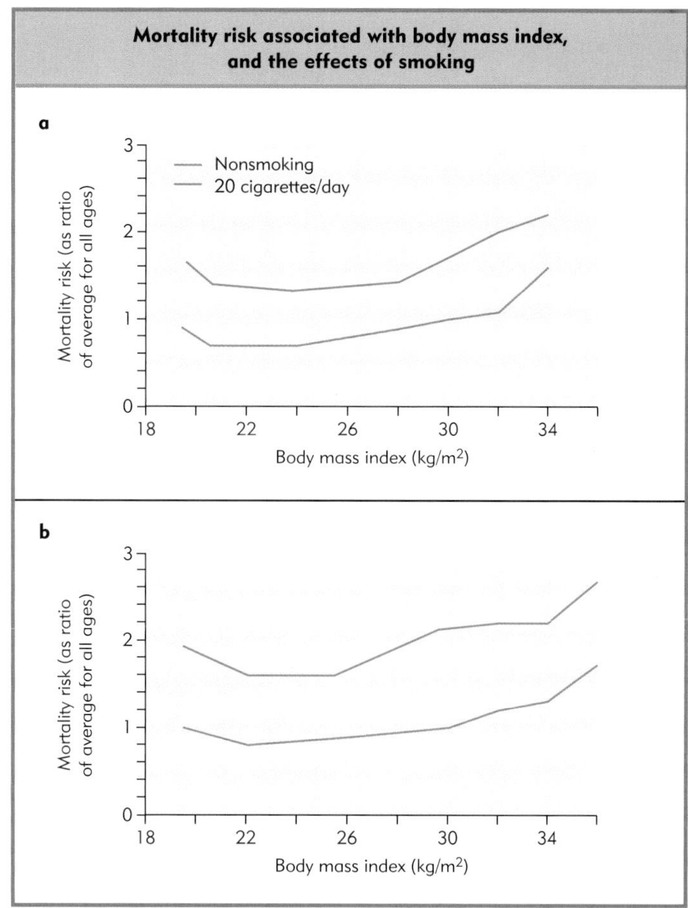

Figure 71.1 Relationship between body mass index and mortality risk in (a) men and (b) women, and the effects of coincident cigarette smoking.

American individuals holding life insurance policies) the population size is impressive (>4 million) and the findings have been confirmed in more robust population studies, particularly when the sample size has been sufficient, the follow-up period has been long enough, and other influences such as tobacco usage have been eliminated (e.g. that of the American Cancer Society, published in 1979). For most day-to-day clinical purposes IBW can be estimated from the following:

Adult males: IBW (kg) = height (cm) - 100
Adult females: IBW (kg) = height (cm) - 105

The *body mass index* (BMI) is a more robust assessment of weight for height, and has gained widespread use in most clinical and epidemiological studies of obesity. The BMI (weight/height^2 in kg/m^2) correlates reasonably well with measures of body fat content (r >0.5).

Definitions of obesity in terms of IBW and BMI are given in Table 71.1.

Although it is a very robust and practical assessment of obesity, the BMI does have its limitations. For instance, heavily muscled individuals would be classified as overweight. It is now thought that other factors, such as young age and the pattern of adipose tissue distribution, may be better predictors of health risk.

EPIDEMIOLOGY

Most epidemiological studies use a BMI of 30 kg/m^2 to define obesity, because mortality risk rises sharply at this level. Using such a definition, many studies have detailed a worldwide increase in the prevalence of obesity, which has been attributed largely to the widespread adoption of Western lifestyles and dietary habits in the developing world.

The prevalence of obesity continues to increase at an alarming rate. In 2002, 70% of adult males and 63% of adult females in the UK were considered overweight or obese. Unfortunately, this worrying trend also appears to be occurring in children.

Mortality

A wealth of epidemiological and actuarial studies have linked obesity to increased mortality.

Although there is little evidence suggest that being moderately overweight (actual body weight of 110–120% IBW) carries much excess risk in young adults, morbidity and mortality rise sharply when BMI exceeds 30 kg/m^2, particularly with concomitant cigarette smoking (Fig. 71.1). Morbid obesity (BMI >35 kg/m^2) is associated with a twofold increase in overall mortality, a 13-fold increase in sudden unexplained female deaths, and a severalfold increase in mortality from diabetes, respiratory, cerebrovascular and cardiovascular diseases, and certain forms of cancer.

In the Framingham study, being overweight was associated with a mortality rate nearly four times that of the normal weight group.

The risks of obesity are proportional to its duration, that is, young adults who are obese are far more at risk than older individuals, in whom the acceptable weight for height is higher. Continued weight gain in obese individuals is associated with a higher risk than in obese individuals whose weight is constant. For a given degree of obesity, males are more at risk than females, but for both groups weight loss reduces the risk associated with previous obesity. Despite this, weight reduction immediately before surgery has not been shown to reduce perioperative morbidity and mortality.

Etiology

Obesity is a complex and multifactorial disease, but in simple terms it occurs when net energy intake exceeds net energy expenditure over a prolonged period. It is not, however, always easy to identify a single explanation as to why this occurs in some individuals and not others. There does, however, appear to be a genetic predisposition, with children of two obese parents having about a 70% chance of becoming obese themselves, compared with a 20% risk for children of nonobese parents, even after diet and lifestyle influences have been taken into account. However, the rapid increase in the prevalence of obesity over the last 30 years, and the fact that the gene pool has remained relatively constant, suggests that environmental factors are much more important determinants.

The total number of calories consumed and the dietary fat content are the prime determinants of obesity (the proportion of fat in the UK diet has increased from 20% to 40% over the last 50 years). Alcohol appears to play a key role too, by influencing the site of fat deposition and encouraging central fat to be laid down.

Contrary to popular belief, obese people have a greater energy expenditure than thin people as it takes more energy to maintain their increased body size. Inactivity is usually the result – but not necessarily the cause – of the obesity. Individuals who remain active in their adult life do best at maintaining healthy weight levels.

Distribution of body fat and health risk

There is increasing evidence that the risks of obesity are determined as much by the distribution of body fat as by the extent of its excess. Two different types of obesity are recognized. In the central or *android* type, which is more common in males, the distribution is predominantly upper body, and it may also be associated with increased proportions of intra-abdominal or visceral fat. In the peripheral or *gynecoid* type, fat is located predominantly around the hips, buttocks, and thighs; this is the more usual female pattern of distribution. Central adipose tissue is metabolically more active than fat in the peripheral distribution and is associated with more metabolic complications, such as dyslipidemias, glucose intolerance, and diabetes mellitus, and a higher incidence of mortality from ischemic heart disease. Morbidly obese individuals with a high proportion of visceral fat are also at a greater risk from cardiovascular disease, left ventricular dysfunction, and stroke. The mechanism for this increased risk with intra-abdominal fat is unclear, but one widely held theory implicates the products of the breakdown of visceral fat being delivered directly into the portal circulation and thereby inducing secondary metabolic imbalances (e.g. dyslipidaemia, glucose intolerance and hyperinsulinaemia, elevated plasma triglycerides, low plasma high-density lipoprotein (HDL) levels).

MEDICAL THERAPY FOR OBESITY

There are currently two drugs licensed for adjunctive management of obesity in the UK. Both are recommended only in individuals with a BMI >30 kg/m^2 or those with a BMI >27 kg/m^2 with obesity-related medical complications. Orlistat is a lipase inhibitor and reduces the absorption of dietary fat. Its main side effects are gastrointestinal complaints induced by fat malabsorption. Patients taking warfarin may experience an increased anticoagulant effect because of the decreased absorption of vitamin K. Sibutramine is a norepinephrine (noradrenaline) and serotonin reuptake inhibitor and acts centrally as an appetite suppressant. Its side effects include dry mouth, insomnia, constipation, and dose-related increases in blood pressure and heart rate.

SURGICAL TREATMENT OF OBESITY

Surgical methods used to treat obesity are classified as restrictive or malabsorptive. Restrictive procedures include vertical banded gastroplasty and gastric banding; the malabsorptive methods include jejunal–ileal bypass and biliopancreatic bypass. The Roux-en-Y gastric bypass combines gastric resection with a minimal degree of malabsorption and is considered by most to be the 'gold standard' bariatric procedure. It involves anastomosing a gastric pouch to a segment of proximal jejunum, so bypassing most of the stomach and the entire duodenum. Patients can expect to lose approximately 50% of their excess weight in the first 1–2 years. The procedure can be performed laparoscopically, and in experienced hands this technique has a reduced complication rate and improved cost-effectiveness compared with an open procedure. Specific complications include anastomotic leak, gastric outlet obstruction, gallstones, incisional hernia, and a 'dumping' syndrome.

OBESITY AND THE HEART

Cardiovascular disease figures prominently among the causes of morbidity and mortality in the obese. Specifically, obesity is considered to be a significant risk factor for hypertension, ischemic heart disease, and a form of ventricular impairment unique to severe obesity, so-called obesity cardiomyopathy. Right-sided heart failure may result from coexisting respiratory disease and add to the cardiovascular problems.

Hypertension

The link between obesity and hypertension has been well established in several large epidemiological studies. The Framingham study showed that a 10% gain in body fat was associated with a 6 mmHg rise in systolic and 4 mmHg rise in diastolic blood pressure. The proportion of individuals requiring antihypertensive therapy increases steadily with body weight. In individuals who have a BMI of 30 kg/m^2 or more, 60% will be hypertensive, and in one in six the hypertension will be severe.

An expansion of the extracellular volume, resulting in hypervolemia, and an increase in cardiac output are characteristic of obesity-induced hypertension. The exact mechanism for hypertension in the obese is not known, and probably represents an interaction between genetic, hormonal, renal, and hemodynamic factors. Hyperinsulinemia, which is characteristic of obesity, can contribute by activating the sympathetic nervous system and by causing sodium retention. In addition, insulin resistance may be responsible for the enhancement of the pressor activity of norepinephrine and angiotensin II.

Hypertension leads to concentric left ventricular (LV) hypertrophy and a progressively noncompliant LV which, when added to the increased blood volume, increases the risk of cardiac failure.

Weight loss has been shown to reduce hypertension in the obese.

Ischemic heart disease

Epidemiological studies have demonstrated a clear association between obesity and sudden death, acute myocardial infarction, and coronary insufficiency. Although previously controversial, it is now generally accepted that this increased risk is independent of confounding influences such as hypertension, hypercholesterolemia, reduced HDL levels, and diabetes mellitus, all of which are more common in the obese. Ischemic heart disease is particularly common in individuals who have a central or visceral distribution of excess body fat: for any given degree of obesity, a visceral distribution approximately doubles cardiac risk.

Blood volume

Total blood volume is increased in the obese, but on a weight/volume basis is less than in lean individuals (50 mL/kg compared to 75 mL/kg), with most of the extra volume being distributed to the fat organ. Splanchnic blood flow is increased by 20%, whereas renal and cerebral blood flow are normal.

Cardiac arrhythmias

Arrhythmias may be precipitated in the obese by a number of factors: hypoxia, hypercapnia, electrolyte disturbance caused by diuretic therapy, coronary artery disease, increased circulating catecholamine concentrations, obstructive sleep apnea (OSA), myocardial hypertrophy, and fatty infiltration of the conducting system.

Obesity cardiomyopathy

In 1933, Smith and Willius reported a systematic autopsy study of heart morphology in 135 severely obese individuals. They demonstrated a more or less linear relationship between heart weight and body weight up to 105 kg, beyond which the heart continued to increase in weight but in a decreasing manner. In contrast to early ideas, founded on the Victorian belief in the 'fatty heart' (*cor adiposum*), this and later studies demonstrated that the increased heart weight was largely a consequence of dilatation and eccentric hypertrophy of the LV, and to a lesser extent the right ventricle (RV). Although increases in epicardial fat were often noted, fatty infiltration of the myocardium (previously believed to account for sudden death by causing arrhythmias) was uncommon and restricted to the RV. Although many of the patients studied in these reports appeared both clinically and post mortem to have suffered a cardiac death (most notably congestive cardiac failure), the nature of the underlying cause remained unclear.

Functional studies have added considerable clarity to our understanding of the cardiovascular consequences of obesity, particularly by identifying a form of cardiomyopathy specific to severe obesity and by showing its interaction with systemic hypertension. In the 1960s, Alexander described a striking relationship between the degree of obesity and both circulating blood volume and resting cardiac output (Fig. 71.2), which in a 170 kg individual are approximately double those found in a subject weighing 70 kg. These increases are mostly attributable to an increased blood flow to the (enlarged) fat organ (which requires 2–3 mL/min/100 g tissue at rest). Radionuclide and echocardiographic studies in normotensive morbidly obese individuals undergoing weight-reduction surgery have elaborated our understanding of the hemodynamic response to obesity.

The increased cardiac output is achieved largely through an increase in stroke volume resulting from an increase in LV cavity size. As predicted by LaPlace's law, LV wall stress increases as

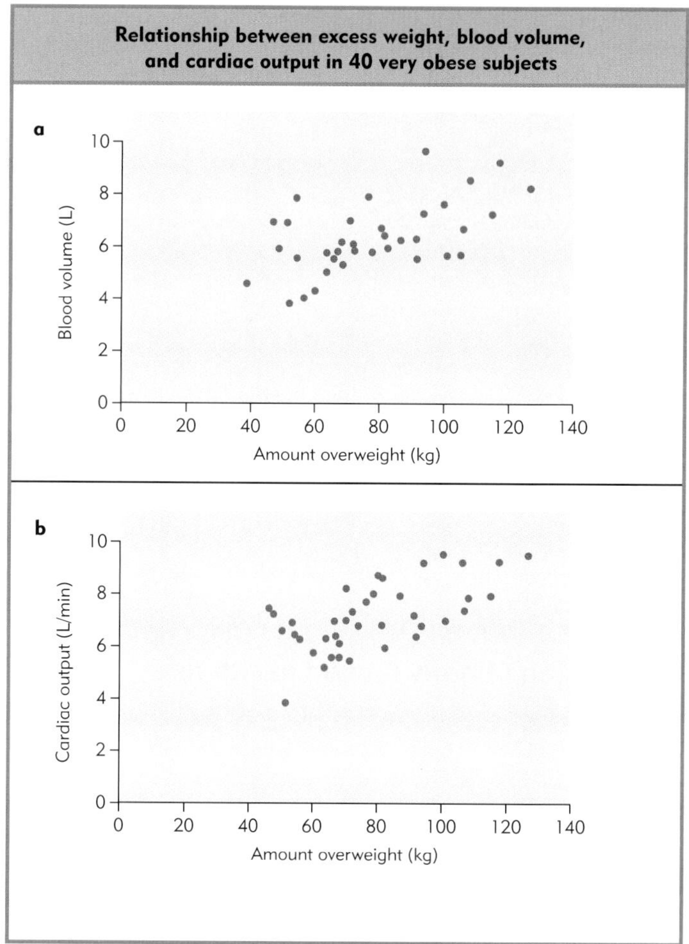

Figure 71.2 Changes in blood volume (a) and cardiac output (b) in obesity. Relationships between excess weight, blood volume, and cardiac output in 40 very obese subjects.

the cavity dilates, and the ventricular wall hypertrophies as a result. Such *eccentric* hypertrophy (as opposed to the *concentric* pattern seen in nonobese hypertensive individuals, in which increased LV wall thickness is associated with a reduction in cavity size) serves to reduce LV wall stress. Eccentric hypertrophy is associated with diastolic LV dysfunction, with higher LV end-diastolic pressures at rest, during exercise, or in response to increased venous return; pulmonary edema may therefore develop under such circumstances. The capacity of the dilated ventricle to hypertrophy is limited, whereupon *systolic* dysfunction ensues. Superimposed systemic hypertension compounds these problems. The adverse changes in LV cavity size, wall thickness, and stress, and adverse changes in function in both systole and diastole worsen with increasing duration of obesity and improve with weight loss. Morbidly obese individuals tolerate exercise badly. Consequently, they exhibit a lower than anticipated increase in cardiac output in response to graded work. In these individuals, an increase in cardiac output is achieved solely by an increase in heart rate, without any increase in stroke volume or ejection fraction, and often at the expense of rises in filling pressures; this may cause pulmonary edema. The obstructive sleep apnea/obesity hypoventilation syndrome occurs in 5% of morbidly obese individuals. Recurrent hypoxemia and hypercapnia lead to chronic pulmonary hyper-

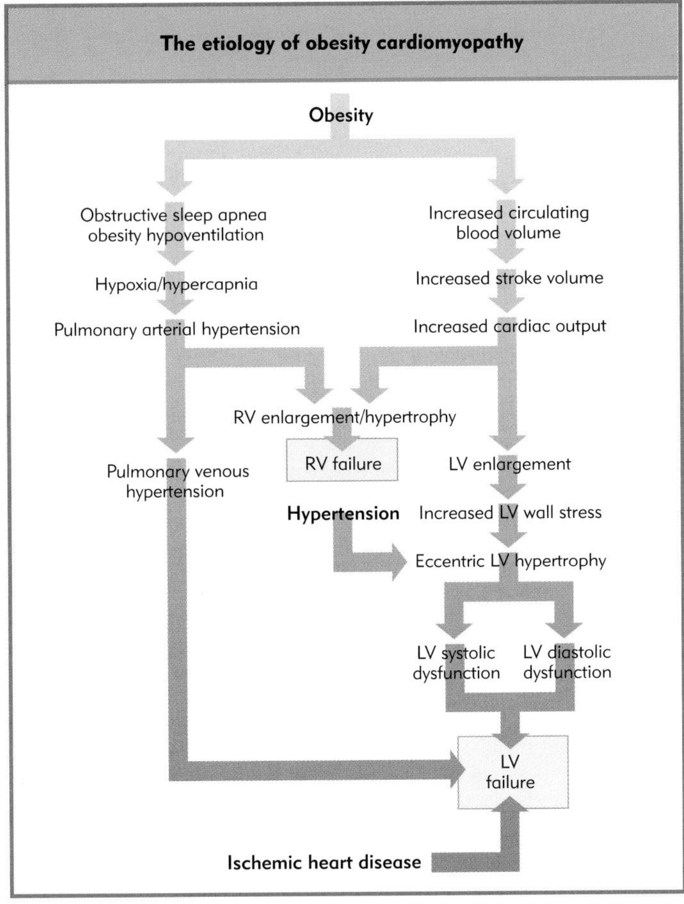

Figure 71.3 The etiology of obesity cardiomyopahty, and its interaction with hypertension, ischemic heart disease, and respiratory impairment.

tension, and eventually to RV failure. It is invariably the case in such patients that the LV is also impaired, heart failure then being biventricular.

The etiology of obesity cardiomyopathy and its interaction with hypertension, ischemic heart disease, and respiratory impairment is illustrated in Figure 71.3.

Clinical features

Patients with severe obesity often have very limited mobility, and may therefore appear asymptomatic in the face of significant ventricular impairment. The earliest symptoms include exertional dyspnea and orthopnea, although many individuals sleep sitting in a chair and therefore rarely, if ever, lie supine. Symptoms may be episodic and initially associated with good systolic but reduced diastolic function. Accelerated weight gain may indicate decompensating ventricular function before peripheral edema becomes clinically obvious; it may be precipitated by the onset of the sleep apnea/obesity hypoventilation syndrome or accelerated hypertension. Clinical examination may be difficult, although the signs of congestive cardiac failure (added heart sounds, pulmonary crepitations, elevated jugular venous pressure, hepatomegaly, ascites, and peripheral edema) have the usual significance. Placing the patient in the supine position and observing the effect on cardiorespiratory function should be a routine part of the clinical examination; acute decompensation and cardiac arrest have been reported. Systemic blood pressure may be overestimated if a standard sized, rather than large, blood pressure cuff is employed.

The electrocardiogram is frequently of low voltage and significantly underestimates the severity of RV and LV hypertrophy. Axis deviation and atrial tachyarrhythmias are relatively common. Cardiomegaly may be seen on chest X-ray, although it is often normal. Echocardiography can be very informative: eccentric LV hypertrophy suggests significant obesity-induced changes even if LV function appears good. Although such examinations may be difficult in inexperienced hands, studies can be improved if nonstandard echocardiographic windows are used in recognition of the distorted architecture of the intrathoracic contents.

Anesthetic implications

The severity of ventricular impairment is often underestimated by standard clinical evaluation; in experienced hands, transthoracic echocardiography adds considerably to the preoperative assessment. Ventricular impairment is inevitable in patients who have coexisting respiratory failure, and such patients should be considered as extremely high risk. Sudden weight gain may indicate fluid retention and biventricular failure. Intraoperative ventricular failure may develop for several reasons: increased venous return associated with rapid intravenous fluid administration, supine or Trendelenburg positions; negative inotropic effects of anesthetic agents; or pulmonary hypertension caused by hypoxia and hypercapnia. It is good practice to have a range of inotropes and vasodilators immediately to hand so as to be able to respond quickly in the event of difficulties.

A large cuff will be required for noninvasive measurement of arterial pressure; however, this can often disturbed by external compression of the cuff by arm supports or members of the surgical team. Invasive arterial pressure monitoring is recommended because it avoids these problems and allows regular estimation of blood gas and acid–base status. Central venous pressure monitoring is more debatable, although it does provide secure venous access in patients who might otherwise present difficulties, and allows cardiovascular support to be instituted if necessary. In our experience placement of right internal jugular lines does not present undue difficulty. The recent introduction of ultrasound scanning techniques for line placement may improve success rates. Patients with clinical evidence of heart failure who are undergoing major surgery may benefit from the use of a pulmonary artery flotation catheter. Monitoring should be extended into the postoperative period.

OBESITY AND THE RESPIRATORY SYSTEM

Most of our understanding of the respiratory consequences of obesity comes from studies on individuals undergoing bariatric surgery and can be considered under the headings of lung volumes, oxygen consumption and carbon dioxide production, gas exchange, lung compliance and resistance, work of breathing, and ventilatory control. The respiratory consequences of severe obesity are summarized in Table 71.2.

Lung volumes

Morbid obesity is associated with reductions in the expiratory reserve volume (ERV), functional residual capacity (FRC), and

Table 71.2 Pulmonary abnormalities in severe obesity

Lung volumes	Reduced expiratory reserve volume, reduced functional residual capacity, reduced total lung capacity, increased residual volume
Lung mechanics	Reduced lung compliance, reduced chest wall compliance, increased airway resistance, increased work of breathing, reduced respiratory muscle efficiency
Gas exchange	Increased O_2 consumption, increased CO_2 production, increased ventilation/perfusion abnormalities, particularly during anesthesia, limited maximum lung capacity (inability to increase ventilation in response to increased demand), increased sensitivity to respiratory depressant drugs
Respiratory control	Obstructive sleep apnea, obesity hypoventilation syndrome, high risk of airway and intubation difficulties at induction of anesthesia

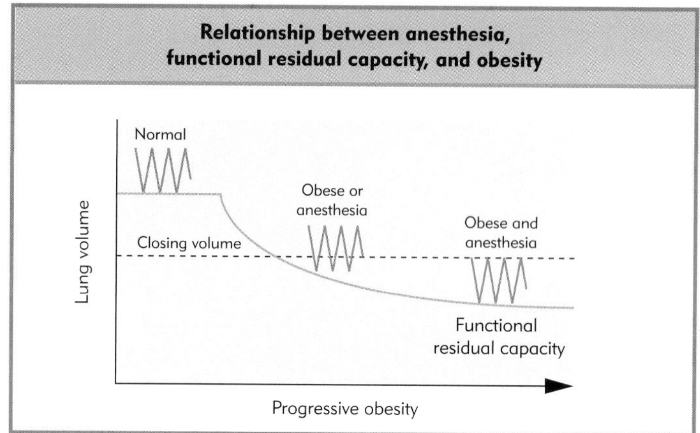

Figure 71.4 Relationship between anesthesia, functional residual capacity (FRC), and closing volume in obese patients. Obesity is associated with a progressive fall in FRC, so that tidal ventilation increasingly encroaches on the lung closing volume. anesthesia also results in a fall in FRC, adding to the intrapulmonary shunt suffered by patients who have severe obesity.

total lung capacity, with FRC declining exponentially as BMI increases. These changes have been attributed to mass loading and splinting of the diaphragm. FRC may be reduced in the upright obese patient to the extent that it falls within the range of the closing capacity, with subsequent small airway closure, ventilation/perfusion mismatch, right-to-left shunting, and arterial hypoxemia. Anesthesia compounds these problems, such that a 50% reduction in observed FRC occurs in the obese anesthetized patient, compared to a 20% fall in anesthetized nonobese subjects (Fig. 71.4). One investigator found an intrapulmonary shunt of 10–25% in anesthetized obese subjects and of 2–5% in lean individuals. FRC can be increased by ventilating with large tidal volumes (15–20 mL/kg), although this has been shown to improve arterial oxygen tension only minimally. In contrast, the addition of positive end-expiratory pressure (PEEP) achieves an improvement in both FRC and arterial oxygen tension, but only at the expense of cardiac output and oxygen delivery. Santesson detailed these perioperative changes in oxygenation in patients undergoing bariatric surgery (Table 71.3). A modest defect in gas exchange and increased shunt fraction preoperatively deteriorate dramatically following the induction of anesthesia and intubation.

The reduction in FRC impairs the capacity of the obese patient to tolerate periods of apnea. Obese individuals desaturate rapidly after induction of anesthesia, despite preoxygenation. This is a result of having a smaller oxygen reservoir in their reduced FRC and an increase in oxygen consumption.

Usually FRC is reduced as a consequence of a reduction in ERV, with residual volume (RV) remaining within normal limits. However, in some obese patients RV is increased, suggesting gas trapping and coexisting obstructive airways disease. Forced expiratory volume in 1 second (FEV_1) and forced vital capacity are usually within the predicted range, but 6–7% improvements have been demonstrated after weight loss. Obese males appear to be at greater risk of airflow limitation than females.

Oxygen consumption and carbon dioxide production

Oxygen consumption and carbon dioxide production are increased in the obese as a result of the metabolic activity of the excess fat and the increased workload on supportive tissues. Basal metabolic activity as related to body surface area is usually within normal limits. Normocapnia is maintained usually by an increase in the minute ventilation, which in turn leads to an increased cost of breathing. However, most obese patients retain the normal response to hypoxemia and hypercapnia. In exercise, oxygen consumption rises more sharply than in nonobese subjects, which implies respiratory muscle inefficiency.

Table 71.3 Perioperative changes in oxygenation and the influence of PEEP in patients undergoing bariatric surgery. IPPV, intermittent positive pressure ventilation; PEEP, positive and expiratory pressure; Do_2, oxygen delivery; Q_T, cardiac output; Q_S/Q_T, shunt fraction; $P(A\text{-}a)o_2$, alveolar arterial oxygen difference

	Pao_2 (kPa)	$Paco_2$ (kPa)	$P(A\text{-}a)o_2$ (kPa)	Q_t (L/min)	Q_s/Q_t (%)	DO_2 (mL/min)
Preoperative air	10.9 ± 1.1	4.6 ± 0.3	3.5 ± 1.1	7.3 ± 1.1	10 ± 4	1346 ± 222
IPPV, zero PEEP, $FiO_2 = 0.5$	14.0 ± 2.7	4.5 ± 0.5	28.4 ± 2.6	5.5 ± 1.1	21 ± 5	1039 ± 239
IPPV, 10 cmH_2O PEEP, $FiO_2 = 0.5$	15.8 ± 3.0	4.5 ± 0.3	26.7 ± 3.0	5.2 ± 0.9	17 ± 3	996 ± 210
IPPV, 15 cmH_2O PEEP, $FiO_2 = 0.5$	21.5 ± 7.2	4.3 ± 0.3	21.2 ± 7.1	4.4 ± 0.6	13 ± 4	863 ± 170

Gas exchange

Morbidly obese individuals usually have only a modest defect in gas exchange preoperatively, with a reduction in PaO_2 and increases in alveolar-to-arterial oxygen difference and shunt fraction. These deteriorate markedly on induction of anesthesia, and high inspired fractions of oxygen are required to maintain adequate arterial oxygen tensions. As previously stated, PEEP improves the PaO_2, but only at the expense of cardiac output and oxygen delivery.

Lung compliance and resistance

Increasing BMI is associated with an exponential decline in respiratory compliance; in several cases, total compliance can fall to 30% of predicted normal. Although accumulation of fat tissue in and around the chest wall leads to a modest reduction in chest wall compliance, recent work suggests that the decrease in total compliance is principally a consequence of a reduction in lung compliance, this in turn being a result of an increased pulmonary blood volume. Reduced compliance is associated with a decrease in the FRC, encroachment on the closing volume, and impairment of gas exchange. Significant obesity is also associated with an increase in total respiratory resistance; once again this is largely a result of an increase in lung resistance. This derangement of lung compliance and resistance results in a shallow and rapid pattern of breathing, increases the work of breathing, and limits the maximum ventilatory capacity. As might be anticipated, these changes are even more marked upon assumption of the supine position.

Work of breathing

The combination of increased mechanical pressure from the abdomen, reduction in pulmonary compliance, and increase in the metabolic demands of the respiratory musculature results in respiratory muscle inefficiency and an increase in the work of breathing. In normocapnic obese individuals at rest, this may be reflected in a modest 30% increase in the work of breathing, although such respiratory muscle inefficiency may limit the maximum ventilatory capacity and lead to relative hypoventilation at times of high metabolic activity. In the obese individual with established daytime hypoventilation syndrome, the work of breathing may approach four times that predicted.

Ventilatory control

Severe obesity is associated with two disorders of ventilatory control: obstructive sleep apnea (OSA), and obesity hypoventilation syndrome. Because the two often coexist, they can be considered together.

The occurrence of OSA is a common and potentially serious medical problem characterized by frequent episodes of apnea and/or hypopnea during sleep. Its consequences include repeated arousal from sleep, along with recurrent episodes of hypoxemia and hypercapnia. It occurs because during sleep the pharyngeal muscles relax, promoting upper airway collapse under the influence of the subatmospheric intrathoracic pressure generated during inspiration. Total occlusion becomes more likely when the pharyngeal soft tissues are expanded, if the airway morphology is abnormally narrowed, or if pharyngeal muscle tone is further reduced by drugs, alcohol, etc. The airway only reopens when the pharyngeal muscle tone is restored; this occurs when the individual is aroused from sleep in response to the hypoxemia/hypercapnia. An obstructive apneic episode is defined arbitrarily as a total cessation of airflow for 10 seconds or more despite continued respiratory efforts against an obstructed pharyngeal airway, whereas hypopnea is defined as a 50% reduction in airflow or a reduction sufficient to lead to 4% or greater reduction in arterial oxygen saturation. The precise definition of significant OSA is disputed, and relies as much on the incidence of clinical sequelae as the precise number of apneic/hypopneic episodes, although a frequency of five or more episodes per hour of sleep, or more than 30 episodes per night, is often quoted. In extreme cases there may be 300–400 obstructive episodes per night.

SNORING

Snoring occurs that is typically *crescendo* snoring, which gets louder as the airway obstruction worsens, followed by silence when airflow ceases altogether, and finally gasping or choking as the patient is aroused and airway patency is restored. The patient himself may be completely unaware of his snoring until a partner or even the neighbors make complaints!

DAYTIME SOMNOLENCE

Frequent arousals each night severely fragment sleep and cause marked daytime sleepiness. This is associated with memory problems, poor attention and concentration skills, personality changes, and a high incidence of accidents (sufferers are 10 times more likely to be involved in road traffic accidents than normal individuals).

PHYSIOLOGICAL RESPONSES

The physiological responses to recurrent apnea include hypoxemia and hypercapnia, as well as pulmonary and systemic vasoconstriction. Repeated episodes of hypoxemia lead to secondary polycythemia, whereas recurrent pulmonary vasoconstriction leads to right ventricular impairment.

OBESITY HYPOVENTILATION SYNDROME

A further response to long term severe OSA is a progressive alteration in the central control of breathing. These changes are limited initially to sleep, and are manifested by a reduction in respiratory drive leading to *central* apneic events (i.e. apnea without respiratory effort) and are accompanied by altered chemoreceptor sensitivity to carbon dioxide. Eventually, however, there is a loss of normal respiratory control during the day, and daytime respiratory failure develops – the so-called obesity hypoventilation syndrome.

OTHER FEATURES

Features that help to identify significant OSA include BMI >30 kg/m^2, hypertension, observed apneic episodes during sleep, collar size greater than 16.5, polycythemia, hypoxemia/hypercapnia, and right ventricular strain/impairment on electrocardiography and echocardiography. Overnight oximetry is also a practical assessment in many institutions.

Anesthetic implications

Preoperative assessment should include lung function tests, arterial blood gases, overnight pulse oximetry, and full blood count (to exclude polycythemia). Patients who have symptoms of significant OSA may benefit from full polysomnography, and even from preoperative treatment for such airway problems.

Induction of anesthesia a particularly hazardous time, for a number of reasons. Although BMI per se is a poor predictor of perioperative airway difficulties, the same factors that promote OSA in obese patients (fatty infiltration of the soft tissues of the neck) make airway maintenance and intubation more difficult. All patients who have OSA are at risk of airway obstruction on induction of anesthesia and should be considered to be a potentially difficult intubation.

Obese patients tolerate periods of apnea badly, even if an adequate period of preoxygenation has been used. Bag/mask ventilation is likely to be very difficult because of the upper airway obstruction and the low chest compliance. The risk of regurgitation and inspiration of stomach contents will be increased to by gastric insufflation during ineffective mask ventilation.

Awake fiberoptic intubation should be considered in patients likely to present airway or intubation difficulties. Otherwise, a rapid-sequence induction technique with succinylcholine (suxamethonium) following a period of preoxygenation will provide the best conditions in which to intubate the trachea as quickly and as safely as possible. It is particularly important under these circumstances to have skilled and physically strong anesthetic assistance, along with a comprehensive range of aids for a difficult intubation.

Episodes of hypoxemia and hypercapnia may increase pulmonary vascular resistance and may precipitate right-sided heart failure. Hypoventilation is likely to occur if obese patients are allowed to breath spontaneously under anesthesia. The lithotomy or Trendelenburg positions may further impair respiratory function. Intubation and mechanical ventilation with high inspired oxygen fractions should be employed in all but the briefest of cases, and PEEP may be required to maintain adequate oxygenation. Care must be taken to ensure that a sufficiently powerful and sophisticated mechanical ventilator is available. End-tidal capnography may significantly underestimate arterial carbon dioxide because of an increased alveolar to arterial carbon dioxide difference, and it is therefore a poor guide to ventilation. Adequacy of minute ventilation is best assessed by frequent arterial blood gas measurements, particularly in those patients at risk of pulmonary hypertension and right-sided heart failure.

The postoperative period is often the time of greatest danger. Whether or not a period of postoperative ventilation is employed, such patients should be monitored closely. Patients may be very sensitive to the effects of sedatives, opioids, and anesthetic drugs, all of which may further worsen upper airway control and ventilatory drive. Postoperative ventilation may be indicated in such circumstances in order to safely allow the elimination of residual sedative agents; regional analgesic techniques should be used if at all possible.

Anesthesia abolishes rapid eye movement (REM) sleep in the first 2–3 postoperative nights, which leads to a compensatory increase in REM sleep in subsequent nights. Because OSA episodes are worse during REM sleep, obstructive airway problems may be worse on the third to fifth postoperative nights. High-risk patients may therefore require appropriate monitoring (e.g. continuous pulse oximetry) for longer periods than might otherwise be anticipated from the surgery alone.

Laparoscopy and anesthesia

As many of the surgical procedures carried out on obese patients are now undertaken using laparoscopic techniques, specific consideration needs to be given to the physiological effects of a pneumoperitoneum in the obese patient.

Pneumoperitoneum and increased intra-abdominal pressure (IAP) lead to significant physiological changes that may be detrimental to the obese patient with already compromised cardiorespiratory reserve. IAP >20 mmHg causes inferior vena cava compression, decreased venous return, and a reduction in cardiac output as well as an increase in renal vascular resistance, with a consequent drop in renal blood flow.

It would be expected that the Trendelenburg and reverse Trendelenburg positions during laparoscopy would have marked effects upon respiratory mechanics, ventilation, and arterial oxygen tension. It appears, however, that arterial oxygen tension is adversely affected only by increased body weight, whereas respiratory mechanics are affected by both obesity and pneumoperitoneum but vary little with body position. Pneumoperitoneum and Trendelenburg positioning can lead to a reduction in femoral blood flow and an increased risk of deep vein thrombosis.

OBESITY AND OTHER MEDICAL CONDITIONS

The diverse medical consequences of obesity are listed in Table 71.4. The increased incidence of surgical pathologies such as neoplasia, osteoarthritis, gallstones, incontinence, and infertility means that obese individuals present for anesthesia more frequently than their lean peers. The medical consequences of obesity mean that this group of patients may be more difficult to manage in the perioperative period. Although most of the conditions listed in Table 71.4 require no specific consideration here, a number merit some attention.

Hiatus hernia and gastroesophageal reflux

It is commonly believed that the combination of increased intra-abdominal pressure, high volume and low pH of gastric contents, delayed gastric emptying, and an increased incidence of hiatus hernia and gastroesophageal reflux places the obese patient at a higher risk of regurgitation and aspiration. Recent work has challenged this contention, and it appears that obese patients without symptoms of reflux have a resistance gradient between the stomach and the gastroesophageal junction similar to that in nonobese subjects in both lying and sitting positions.

Similarly, it appears that gastric emptying is actually faster in the obese, although residual gastric volume is larger. However, opinion remains divided and many physicians continue to take precautions against acid aspiration with the use of H_2 receptor antagonists, proton pump inhibitors, antacids, and prokinetics.

Diabetes mellitus and other metabolic considerations

In one perioperative series more than 10% of patients undergoing bariatric surgery had an abnormal glucose tolerance test. There is a clear causal relationship between obesity and type 2 or maturity-onset diabetes mellitus (DM), so much so that it is now considered to be a surgically correctable disease in the

Table 71.4 Medical and surgical conditions associated with obesity

Cardiovascular
Sudden (cardiac) death
Obesity cardiomyopathy
Hypertension
Ischemic heart disease
Hyperlipidemia
Cor pulmonale
Cerebrovascular disease
Peripheral vascular disease
Varicose veins
Deep vein thrombosis and pulmonary embolism
Respiratory
Restrictive lung disease
Obstructive sleep apnea
Obesity hypoventilation syndrome
Endocrine
Diabetes mellitus
Cushing's disease
Hypothyroidism
Infertility
Gastrointestinal
Hiatus hernia
Gallstones
Inguinal hernia
Genitourinary
Menstrual abnormalities
Female urinary incontinence
Renal calculi
Musculoskeletal
Osteoarthritis of weightbearing joints
Back pain
Malignancy
Breast
Prostate
Colorectal
Cervical and endometrial

morbidly obese. The catabolic response to (surgical) trauma or sepsis may worsen glucose intolerance to the extent that insulin becomes necessary to control blood sugar perioperatively. The preoperative work-up of morbidly obese individuals should include a random blood sugar and, if necessary, a glucose tolerance test.

Patients who return for further surgery after an initial weight-reduction procedure may have metabolic abnormalities such as vitamin B_{12}, folate, iron, and calcium deficiencies. Rapid weight loss may result in protein depletion, and there may be electrolyte disturbance if the patient is acutely unwell. Clotting studies should be checked, as chronic vitamin K deficiency may lead to a prolonged prothrombin time.

Thromboembolic disease

The incidence of deep vein thrombosis following nonmalignant abdominal surgery in obese individuals, as revealed by iodine-labeled fibrinogen uptake scans, is twice that of lean patients (48% vs 23%), and there is a similar increased risk of pulmonary embolus in patients weighing more than 91 kg. Furthermore, it is the most serious nonsurgical complication of bariatric surgery, with an incidence as high as 4.5%. The higher incidence of thromboembolic disease in obese patients overall is likely to be multifactorial in origin, including venous stasis owing to reduced mobility, increased pressure on the deep venous channels of the lower limb, and global reductions in cardiac output because of ventricular impairment; the occurrence of prolonged surgery; increased blood viscosity resulting from polycythemia; and reduced fibrinolysis.

There is no general agreement as to how to reduce the risk of perioperative thromboembolism. Approaches include the use of anticoagulant regimens such as subcutaneous heparin (including low molecular weight preparations such as enoxaparin), elasticated stockings, intermittent calf compression devices, axial sympathetic blockade to increase lower limb blood flow, and prompt postoperative mobilization.

ALTERED DRUG HANDLING IN OBESITY

Obesity is associated with alterations in the distribution, binding, and elimination of many drugs; the resulting pharmacokinetic consequences may be of considerable importance to the anesthesiologist. The implications for the use of specific anesthetic drugs are summarized in Table 71.5.

Volume of distribution

Factors that influence the volume of distribution (V_D) of a drug in obesity include increased size of the fat organ, increased lean body mass, increased blood volume and cardiac output, reduced total body water, and alterations in blood concentrations of species that alter protein binding, such as free fatty acids and α_1-acid glycoprotein.

The consequences of these changes on the clinical effectiveness of a drug will depend on its lipid solubility, its route of administration, and whether the effect is achieved at bolus or steady-state concentrations. Any increase in the volume of distribution will reduce the elimination half-life unless the clearance is increased. The altered kinetics of thiopental (thiopentone) illustrate these effects. Because of an increased blood volume, cardiac output, and muscle mass there is an increase in its central volume of distribution; therefore, the absolute dose should be increased: up to 1 g may be required, although on a weight per weight basis (mg/kg) the dose required is less than in nonobese patients. As with other highly lipid-soluble drugs, the terminal disposition and steady-state volumes of distribution for thiopental are three to four times greater than normal; as a result, the elimination of thiopental can be expected to be

Table 71.5 Influence of obesity on the pharmacokinetics of anesthetic drugs (Adapted from Shenkman et al., 1993.)

Drug	Altered pharmacokinetics	Clinical implications
Hypnotics		
Thiopental (thiopentone)	Increased central volume of distribution, prolonged elimination half-life	Increased absolute dose, reduced dose/unit body weight, prolonged duration of action
Propofol	Little known	Increased absolute dose, reduced dose/unit body weight
Midazolam, diazepam	Central volume of distribution increases in line with body weight, prolonged elimination half-life	Increased absolute dose, same dose/unit body weight, prolonged duration of action, particularly after infusion
Muscle relaxants		
Succinylcholine	Plasma cholinesterase activity increases in proportion to body weight	Increased absolute dose, reduced dose/unit body weight, doses of 120–140 mg appear satisfactory
Atracurium	No change in absolute clearance, absolute volume of distribution and absolute elimination half-life	Unchanged dose/unit body weight
Vecuronium	Impaired hepatic clearance and increased volume of distribution lead to delayed recovery time	Give according to estimated lean body weight
Rocuronium	Faster onset and longer duration of action	Give according to estimated LBW
Pancuronium	Low lipid solubility	Unchanged dose/unit body weight
Dimethyl tubocurarine	Elimination half-life increases in proportion with degree of obesity	Give according to estimated LBW
Opioids		
Fentanyl	No change in elimination following 10 μg/kg	Dose/unit body weight unchanged
Alfentanil	Elimination may be prolonged	Adjust dose to LBW
Remifentanil	Pharmacokinetics similar in obese and nonobese patients	Dose according to age and estimated LBW
Morphine	No information available	
Local anesthetics		
Lidocaine	Increased absolute V_D, unchanged V_D adjusted for body weight, increased epidural fat content and epidural venous engorgement	IV dose unchanged/unit body weight, extradural dose 75% of dose calculated according to TBW
Bupivacaine	No information available	High segmental level following subarachnoid blockade
Inhalational anesthetics		
Nitrous oxide	Little information	Decreased F_IO_2, limits practical usefulness, intestinal distension may contribute to perioperative difficulties
Halothane	Considerable deposition in adipose tissue, increased risk of reductive hepatic metabolism	Possible risk of halothane hepatitis
Enflurane	Blood:gas partition coefficient falls with increasing obesity, inorganic fluoride levels rise twice as fast in obese individuals	Possibly lower MAC, increased risk of fluoride nephrotoxicity following prolonged administration
Sevoflurane	No difference in fluoride levels between obese and nonobese patients	
Desflurane	Little information available	Improved immediate postoperative recovery compared to isoflurane or propofol anesthesia

delayed. This is of particular clinical importance following the administration of benzodiazepines, when the effects may persist for some days after discontinuation.

Remifentanil is unusual in that although it is a highly lipophilic drug, there does not appear to be a systematic relationship between its degree of lipophilicity and its V_D. Its V_D remains relatively consistent between obese and nonobese individuals, and the dose should be calculated according to ideal body weight.

Drugs with weak or moderate lipophilicity (e.g. nondepolarizing muscle relaxants) can be dosed on the basis of lean body mass (LBM). This is not the same as IBW, as 20–40% of an obese patient's excess weight can be attributed to an increase in LBM. Adding 20% to the dose calculated for IBW is usually sufficient to take into account the extra lean mass.

Drug clearance

Renal clearance increases in obesity because of the increased renal blood flow and glomerular filtration rate. The effects on liver metabolism are more unpredictable, although reduction in liver blood flow in patients who have congestive cardiac failure may slow the elimination of drugs with a rapid hepatic elimination such as lidocaine (lignocaine) and midazolam.

Inhalational anesthetics

It has been traditionally held that the slow emergence from anesthesia often experienced by obese patients results from the delayed release of the highly lipid-soluble volatile agents from the excessive amount of adipose tissue. This is probably not the case, because reductions in fat blood flow may limit the delivery of volatile agents to such fat stores, and the slow emergence is more likely to result from increased central sensitivity to anesthetic drugs.

Obese patients may be more at risk from ill effects as a consequence of changed hepatic metabolism of volatile agents. For example, plasma bromide levels – a marker of both oxidative and reductive metabolism of halothane – are higher in obese patients. Increased reductive metabolism of halothane is considered to be an important factor in the etiology of liver injury following halothane exposure, and may be more likely in obese individuals at risk of hypoxemia and reduced hepatic blood flow. The hepatic metabolism of the halogenated volatile agents may also result in increased plasma concentrations of inorganic fluoride ions, which are potentially nephrotoxic if levels exceed 95 mg/dL (50 mmol/L). Plasma fluoride levels following methoxyflurane, halothane, and enflurane are all higher in obese patients, although this appears not to occur with sevoflurane. The increased levels following enflurane may be of practical importance, fluoride concentrations being up to 60% higher in obese patients. Desflurane appears to be the most attractive inhalational agent in the obese, with a more rapid and consistent immediate postoperative recovery compared to isoflurane or propofol anesthesia, and a reduced incidence of desaturation episodes.

Little is known about the effects of nitrous oxide in the obese. The need to use higher inspired oxygen fractions in obese patients limit its use as an adjunct to anesthesia, and its harmful effects on a compromised myocardium should also be borne in mind. Intestinal distension following prolonged anesthesia may contribute to the perioperative difficulties.

GENERAL PERIOPERATIVE MANAGEMENT OF THE MORBIDLY OBESE

The technical difficulties associated with the hospital care of morbidly obese subjects should not be underestimated. Standard hospital beds, transportation trolleys, and operating tables may be neither big enough nor strong enough to support such patients. Particular care should be taken to protect pressure areas when positioning the obese, as they are at high risk for pressure sores and neural injuries. Diabetes further increases the risk. Compression of the inferior cava in the supine position can be a problem and may require a degree of left lateral tilt or the placement of a wedge under the patient. The grossly obese may be at risk from compartment syndrome during prolonged periods of immobilization because of excessive load on weight-bearing areas causing local ischemia. The perioperative implications of the patient's size require particular attention. As a general principle, the number of transfers should be kept to an absolute minimum, particularly once the patient is anesthetized. Transportation to the operating room is best carried out on the patient's bed. Wherever possible the patient should transfer themselves on to the operating table. Occasionally it is necessary to place two operating tables side by side, with the obvious potential dangers that result. If a regional neural blockade is to be used as part of a general anesthetic technique this should be performed before induction in order to allow the patient to position themselves. Given the cramped nature of many anesthetic rooms, anesthesia may be best induced in the operating room. Large-bore intravenous access should be established prior to induction of anesthesia. There should be enough personnel present at the induction to turn the patient immediately if necessary. Once the patient is anesthetized, attention should be paid to positioning, with particular care given to potential nerve compression injuries.

POSTOPERATIVE OUTCOMES IN THE MORBIDLY OBESE

It is traditionally held that severe obesity is associated with higher rates of postoperative morbidity and mortality, although the data are conflicting. For instance, although obesity does not influence mortality after hysterectomy or open cholecystectomy, in a survey of more than 2000 patients undergoing duodenal ulcer surgery the mortality rate was 6.6% in obese patients and 2.7% in the nonobese. Mortality rates following renal transplantation are considerably higher in obese patients. Furthermore, life insurance statistics have associated obesity with a two- to threefold increase in mortality from appendicitis and cholelithiasis. The most common causes of death following surgery for severe obesity are pulmonary embolism and anastomotic breakdown.

Logistic regression analysis of more than 3000 patients undergoing surgery for severe obesity suggests that postoperative complications are related to age, preoperative BMI, and male gender. Respiratory problems are the most common postoperative complication in obese patients. The reduced lung volumes observed during anesthesia persist for some days postoperatively, particularly following abdominal surgery, and correlate with hypoxemia. In one series of obese individuals undergoing bariatric surgery there was a 22% incidence of postoperative lung collapse. Wound infections are also more common, and presumably result from longer incisions, extended operative times, difficulty in obliterating tissue dead space, and the inability of adipose tissue to resist infection. The morbidly obese parturient represents a particularly high-risk group. Compared to nonobese parturients they carry a higher risk of premature labor, emergency cesarean section (with longer operative times), and failed epidural analgesia. There may also be a higher incidence of accidental dural puncture.

Key references

Adams JP, Murphy PG. Obesity in anaesthesia and intensive care. Br J Anaesth. 2000;85:91–108.

Ogunnaike BO, Jones SB, Jones DB, Provost D, Whitten CW. Anesthetic considerations for bariatric surgery. Anesth Analg. 2002;95:1793–805.

Shenkman Z, Shir Y, Brodsky JB. Perioperative management of the obese patient. Br J Anaesth. 1993;70:349–59.

Williams JM, Hanning CD. Obstructive sleep apnoea. Br J Anaesth CEPD Rev. 2003;3:75–8.

Further reading

Alpert MA, Hashimi MW. Obesity and the heart. Am J Med Sci. 1993;306:117–23.

Caterson ID (ed) Obesity. Baillière's Clin Endocrinol Metab. 1994; 8. Several articles of interest, including Hodge AM, Zimmet PZ. The epidemiology of obesity. 577–600; Després J-P. Dyslipidaemia and obesity. 629–60; Grunstein RR, Wilcox I. Sleep-disordered breathing and obesity. 601–28.

Millman RP, Meyer TJ, Eveloff SE. Sleep apnea in the morbidly obese. Rhode Island Med. 1992;75:483–6.

Chapter 72

Physiologic responses to surgery and trauma

Joan P Desborough

TOPICS COVERED IN THIS CHAPTER

- **Hormonal and metabolic responses to surgery**
- **Autonomic system**
  - Pituitary hormones
  - Insulin and glucagon
  - Thyroid hormones
  - Gonadotropins
- **Metabolic sequelae**
  - The glycemic response
  - Protein catabolism
  - Fat metabolism
  - Renal effects
- **Cytokines**
- **Effect of anesthesia on the endocrine response**
  - Nerve blockade
  - Regional analgesia
  - Opioids
  - Intravenous and inhalational agents
  - Multimodal therapy
  - Influence of inhibition of hormonal responses on surgical outcome
- **Physiologic reponses to hemorrhage and anemia**
  - Immediate changes
  - Effects of blood loss
  - Longer-term compensatory mechanisms
  - Fluid therapy
- **Burns**
  - Resuscitative measures and fluid therapy
  - Hypermetabolism

Surgery and trauma evoke a range of physiologic responses, which are part of a widespread systemic inflammatory reaction to injury. These responses include endocrinologic, immunologic, and hematologic changes and the release of inflammatory mediators such as cytokines (Fig. 72.1). This so-called 'stress response' is seen after all major systemic disturbances, including traumatic injury, burns, and major infection, as well as surgery. The aim of the response is to restore homeostasis by activating defense mechanisms, mobilizing substrates, and promoting healing and repair.

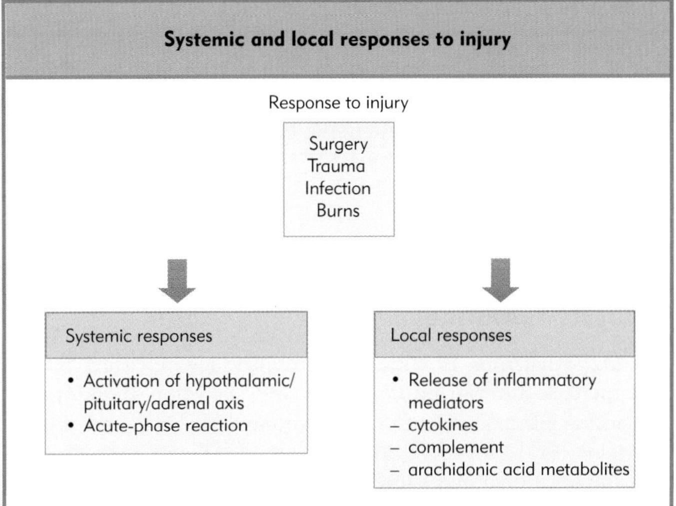

Figure 72.1 Systemic and local responses to injury.

The hormonal and metabolic changes are initiated by activation of the hypothalamopituitary–adrenal (HPA) axis, which leads to increased secretion of pituitary hormones and cortisol. As a result, catabolism of stored body fuels occurs, with an increase in metabolic rate and oxygen consumption. In addition to alterations in endocrine secretion, other characteristic changes occur that are known as the 'acute-phase response' (Table 72.1).

Table 72.1 Acute-phase responses to surgery and trauma

Acute-phase protein production in the liver (e.g. C-reactive protein, fibrinogen)
Decreased hepatic synthesis of albumin and transferrin
Decreased circulating concentrations of divalent cations
Neutrophil leukocytosis
Lymphocyte proliferation and differentiation
Increased body temperature

HORMONAL AND METABOLIC RESPONSES TO SURGERY

Afferent neuronal impulses from the site of the operation activate the sympathetic nervous system and stimulate hormonal secretion from the hypothalamus and pituitary gland. Both autonomic and somatic nerve pathways are involved. In addition to neural activation, many substances are released from cells as a result of tissue injury. These mediators, which include cytokines, augment the acute-phase reaction and have both local and systemic effects.

The magnitude and duration of the hormonal and metabolic response to surgery depends largely on the severity of the surgical stimulus. As discussed below, the responses can be modified by local and general anesthesia. The principal hormonal and metabolic sequelae are shown in Figure 72.2.

AUTONOMIC SYSTEM

The sympathetic nervous system is activated and epinephrine (adrenaline) is released from the adrenal medulla. Norepinephrine is released at adrenergic nerve terminals and may spill over into the circulation. Therefore, the concentrations of circulating catecholamines become elevated, which leads to tachycardia, hypertension, and increased systemic vascular resistance, although these effects are often obtunded by general or local anesthesia.

Pituitary hormones

The hypothalamus is stimulated to produce releasing factors that increase anterior pituitary hormone secretion. β-endorphin, prolactin, adrenocorticotropic hormone (ACTH), and growth hormone (GH) are secreted, of which ACTH and GH have significant hormonal and metabolic effects. Much of the research on hormonal responses to surgery is centered on changes in catecholamines, cortisol production, and the glycemic responses. Changes in thyroid hormone and gonadotropin secretion also occur, but have received less attention. Overall, the endocrine response is characterized by an increase in catabolic hormone secretion, which is usually accompanied by suppression of the release of the anabolic hormones testosterone and insulin (Fig. 72.3).

Increased amounts of arginine vasopressin are secreted from the posterior pituitary, with a resultant conservation of salt and water by the kidney.

Insulin and glucagon

Insulin is secreted from the β cells of the islets of Langerhans in the pancreas in response to increases in blood glucose (Chapter 66). Insulin is an anabolic hormone; it promotes the uptake of glucose and its storage as glycogen, and it inhibits the mobilization of fat and muscle protein. After the onset of surgery, circulating concentrations of insulin may increase or decrease, but occasionally do not change. However, insulin secretion fails to increase appropriately for the hyperglycemia that is provoked by surgery.

The exact mechanism(s) for the relative lack of insulin remains unclear. It is possible that secretion may be inhibited by anesthesia, either directly or through decreased blood flow. It is widely assumed that sympathetic stimulation and circulating epinephrine inhibit insulin secretion through α-adrenoceptors. In addition to the relative hyposecretion of insulin in the perioperative period, insulin appears to be less effective metabolically; this is known as insulin resistance.

Glucagon is released from the α cells of the pancreas. This hormone increases blood glucose concentrations by glycogenolysis in the liver and gluconeogenesis. It stimulates lipolysis and ketone body formation. Secretion of glucagon changes little after surgical stimulation.

Thyroid hormones

The influence of surgery on thyroid hormone concentrations is well defined. For example, in one study of abdominal surgery,

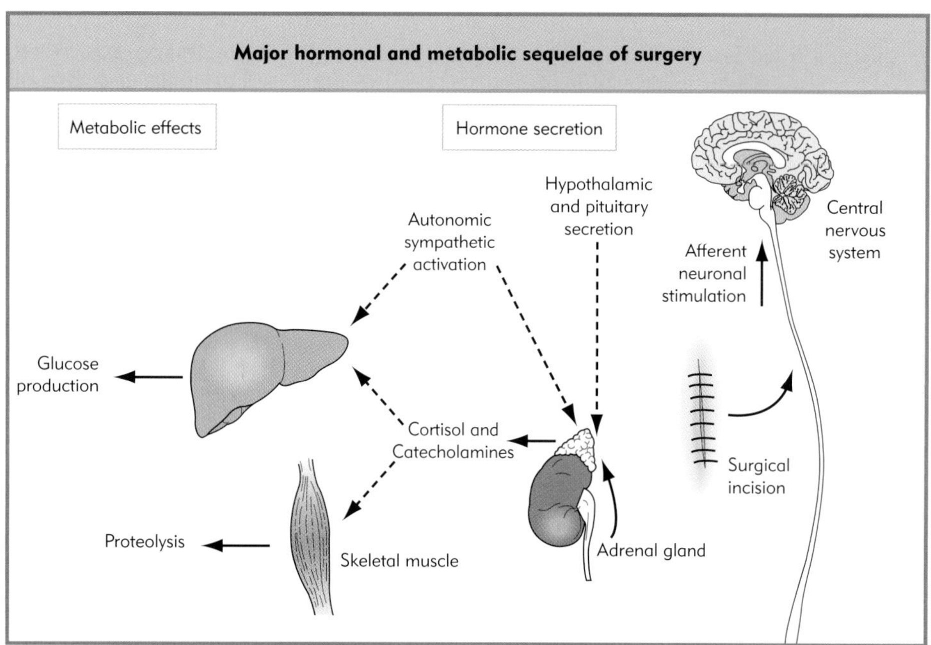

Figure 72.2 Major hormonal and metabolic sequelae of surgery.

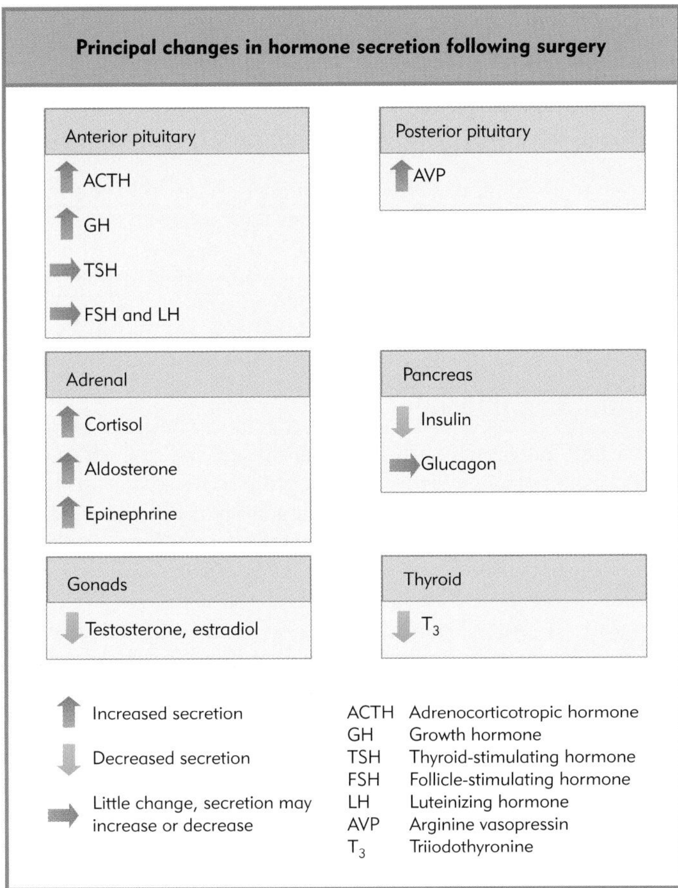

Figure 72.3 Principal changes in hormone secretion following surgery.

total and free triiodothyronine (T_3) values decreased markedly during surgery, returning to normal after about 7 days. Free thyroxine (T_4) concentrations increased during surgery itself and remained constant during the postoperative period, despite a slight postoperative decrease in total T_4. Thyroid-stimulating hormone (TSH) values showed a profound decrease during the first 24 hours postoperatively and returned to preoperative levels. Such changes, the cause of which remains unclear, suggest that production of TSH and T_3 is suppressed in the early postoperative period. A relationship between thyroid hormones, cortisol, and catecholamines after surgery and other trauma has been suggested. Thus, hyperadrenocortisolism may suppress T_3. An alternative theory is that because thyroid hormones have a stimulatory effect on metabolism, suppression of these hormones guards against excessive catabolism in the presence of high concentrations of catecholamines.

Gonadotropins

Pituitary secretion of leuteinizing hormone increases during surgery, returning close to preoperative values by the first postoperative day. Serum values of follicle-stimulating hormone show no significant changes in the perioperative period. Circulating concentrations of testosterone and estradiol are decreased following surgery, reaching minimum values around the fourth and fifth postoperative days.

METABOLIC SEQUELAE

The effect of catabolic hormone secretion is substrate mobilization. In evolutionary terms, this probably represents a survival mechanism that allows injured animals to sustain themselves using their own stored body fuel. Hyperglycemia occurs during surgery as a result of increased hepatic glycogenolysis and gluconeogenesis. This is facilitated by catecholamines and cortisol, together with a relative suppression of insulin secretion. Protein catabolism releases amino acids, which are used in the synthesis of acute-phase proteins by the liver, and in gluconeogenesis. Production of free fatty acids from triglyceride breakdown is stimulated by catecholamines.

The glycemic response

Blood glucose values vary with the intensity of surgical stimulation. For example, concentrations of blood glucose may reach up to 180 mg/dL (10 mmol/L) in cardiac surgery, but are much lower after cataract surgery. The changes are closely associated with increases in catecholamine secretion, which suggests that catecholamines have a key role in the glycemic response. Interestingly, the feedback mechanisms that usually restore normoglycemia are ineffective after surgery, so that hyperglycemia continues unabated until the stimulus subsides.

Evidence that prolonged hyperglycemia may be harmful is increasing, particularly in diabetic patients. In diabetic subjects, poor glycemic control is associated with an increased incidence of diabetic complications. Potential risks of perioperative hyperglycemia include impaired wound healing and wound infection. In addition, ischemic damage to the myocardium and nervous system is worsened by the presence of hyperglycemia.

Protein catabolism

Following major surgery, muscle protein is catabolized. Considerable weight loss up to 0.5 kg of lean body mass per day can occur after major surgery or trauma. The amino acids mobilized are used in gluconeogenesis and the formation of new acute-phase proteins in the liver. The stimulus for protein breakdown is likely to be a combination of factors, which include catabolic hormone secretion, low insulin concentrations, and cytokines.

Fat metabolism

The effects of surgical trauma on fat metabolism have received much less attention than the glycemic changes – there are few changes, unless starvation is an important feature. In cardiac surgery, heparinization leads to marked increases in circulating nonesterified (or free) fatty acids (NEFA) values. Heparin activates lipoprotein lipase, which acts on triglycerides, ultimately releasing NEFAs.

Renal effects

The neuroendocrine control of the kidney and the regulation of blood volume and electrolyte concentrations are described in Chapters 57 and 59. In response to surgery, a number of hormonal changes occur that influence salt and water metabolism and allow the preservation of an adequate circulating blood volume. The release of vasopressin from the posterior pituitary leads to water retention and the production of concentrated urine by a direct action on the kidney. Increased vasopressin release may last for 3–5 days, depending on the severity of surgery and the development of complications such as sepsis. Renin secretion is increased, partly as a result of sympathetic stimulation of the juxtaglomerular cells of the kidney, which promotes the production of angiotensin II. This has a number of important effects, including stimulation of the release of aldosterone from the adrenal cortex, which promotes Na^+ and water reabsorption from the distal tubules in the kidney.

CYTOKINES

Cytokines are low molecular weight (up to 80 kDa) proteins produced from activated white blood cells, in particular monocytes, and from activated fibroblasts and endothelial cells. These proteins, together with other inflammatory mediators, are released as an early cellular response to tissue injury. The cytokines act on surface receptors of many different target cells (Chapter 54), and their effects ultimately result from an influence on protein synthesis within these target cells. Cytokines play a major role in the inflammatory responses to trauma and infection, but they also have longer-term effects on cells as regulators of cell growth and differentiation.

The main cytokine produced after major surgery is interleukin-6 (IL-6). Other cytokines released after surgical stimuli are tumor necrosis factor-α and IL-1. Under normal circumstances in healthy individuals circulating values of cytokines are low, if at all detectable. Increased circulating values of IL-6 are found within 30–60 minutes of the start of surgery, with significant increases after 2–4 hours. The response reflects the degree of tissue trauma, so that cytokine production is lowest with minimally invasive and laparoscopic procedures. The largest increases in IL-6 concentrations are found after procedures such as joint arthroplasty, vascular reconstruction, and colorectal surgery. Following these operations, cytokine values are elevated for 48–72 hours. Peak values occur at about 24 hours. If complications such as sepsis arise in the postoperative period, concentrations of cytokines remain elevated until the stimulus subsides.

It is now recognized that acute-phase responses that cannot be explained by activation of the HPA axis are stimulated by cytokines. Although IL-1 was thought initially to be responsible for inducing the fever that follows surgery, IL-6 is likely to be involved in this response. One of the principal effects of IL-6 is to stimulate the manufacture in the liver of acute-phase proteins (one of the early names for IL-6 was hepatocyte-stimulating factor). The acute-phase proteins act as inflammatory mediators in scavenging and in tissue repair. They include C-reactive protein (CRP), fibrinogen, and α_2-macroglobulin and other antiproteinases. The changes in circulating CRP values lag behind the changes in IL-6, and CRP acts as a nonspecific opsonin to augment the phagocytosis of bacteria.

Another key action of cytokines is their effect on the immune system. The production and maturation of B and T lymphocytes and the maturation of hemopoietic stem cells are stimulated by IL-6. The cytokines also interact with the neuroendocrine system (e.g. IL-6 stimulates pituitary hormone secretion). Conversely, glucocorticoids have anti-inflammatory actions, and in large doses have inhibitory actions on cytokine production and the subsequent synthesis of acute-phase proteins.

EFFECT OF ANESTHESIA ON THE ENDOCRINE RESPONSE

Nerve blockade

Complete afferent and efferent nerve blockade will prevent the hormonal and metabolic responses to surgery. Such total blockade is possible if there is a specific nerve supply to the operative site. For example, the hormonal responses to cataract surgery can be abolished with retrobulbar or peribulbar block of the optic nerve.

Regional analgesia

Extradural analgesia with local anesthetic agents effectively inhibits the hormonal and metabolic consequences of surgery in the pelvis or lower limbs. The blockade must be extensive, from dermatomal levels T4 to S5. Afferent impulses from the operative site to the brain and efferent autonomic pathways to the liver and adrenal gland are blocked. Thus, the cortisol and glycemic responses to surgery are abolished. Less extensive blockade does not completely prevent the hormonal and metabolic changes.

For surgery in the upper abdomen and the chest, extensive blockade with local anesthetic modifies the glycemic responses. In a classic study, Bromage showed that despite extensive block (up to the C6 dermatomal level in some cases), the hypercortisolemia of surgery was unaffected. Bromage suggested that afferent impulses were able to pass through the vagus nerve. Thus, the hypothalamus and pituitary were stimulated, with subsequent release of ACTH and cortisol. The glycemic response was inhibited because the extradural block effectively inhibited the efferent sympathetic supply to the liver and adrenal gland. Other investigators suggest that in upper abdominal and thoracic surgery afferent impulses might also pass via diaphragmatic or peritoneal innervation. The failure of regional anesthesia to prevent endocrine responses in this type of surgery is caused by incomplete neural blockade.

Epidural analgesia with opioid alone has little effect on hormonal or metabolic responses to surgery. Conduction blockade can be achieved only with local anesthetics, and epidural opioid administration alone has an insignificant effect on surgical stress responses.

Opioids

Opioids suppress hypothalamic and pituitary hormone secretion. It was demonstrated many years ago that morphine inhibited ACTH release from the pituitary gland, with subsequent suppression of cortisol secretion by an effect at hypothalamic level. High-dose intravenous opioids have been used to suppress the endocrine changes that occur during surgery. Although these techniques are valuable in elucidating hormonal responses, they are of limited use in clinical practice because of the associated ventilatory depression.

Fentanyl (50 μg/kg) abolishes the endocrine and metabolic changes found during pelvic surgery, but larger doses are needed to inhibit responses to surgery in the upper abdomen. In a study using a dose of 100 μg/kg fentanyl the hormonal responses to cholecystectomy (via laparotomy) were suppressed, but postoperative ventilation of the lungs was required.

Morphine (4 mg/kg) and fentanyl (50–100 μg/kg) suppress the hormonal responses to cardiac surgery until the onset of cardiopulmonary bypass (CPB). At the beginning of CPB, intense afferent stimulation results from sudden and profound hemodilution, hypothermia, and the perturbations associated with flow through the bypass circuit. The consequent hormonal changes cannot be suppressed by high-dose opioids.

Intravenous and inhalational agents

Etomidate directly inhibits corticosteroid production in the adrenal gland by inhibition of the enzyme 11β-hydroxylase – the synthesis of both cortisol and aldosterone are blocked. Following a single dose of etomidate, production of these two hormones is inhibited for 6–12 hours. In healthy patients undergoing routine elective surgery no deleterious effects seem to result from this adrenal suppression. However, in the early 1980s an audit of the use of etomidate in the sedation of critically ill patients found the drug to be associated with increased mortality. As a result, it is no longer licensed to be used in long-term sedation.

Benzodiazepines inhibit hormone production from adrenocortical cells in vitro. In clinical studies, midazolam decreased the cortisol response in both minor surgery and cholecystectomy. In one of these studies cortisol secretion was enhanced by the administration of exogenous ACTH, which demonstrates that the effect is at the level of the hypothalamus and pituitary, although a direct effect on the adrenal cortex may occur.

The volatile anesthetic agents have little influence on hormonal and metabolic responses to surgery. In high inspired concentrations these agents may obtund the responses to minor surface operations, but were found to be ineffective in inhibiting the hormonal changes associated with pelvic surgery.

Multimodal therapy

Although regional techniques with local anesthetics and opioids provide excellent analgesia, they are ineffective in suppressing completely the hormonal responses to abdominal surgery. Combinations of other analgesics have been used with regional analgesia in an attempt to enhance pain relief after surgery. The addition of a nonsteroidal anti-inflammatory drug to a regimen of extradural bupivacaine and morphine gave very good postoperative analgesia following conventional cholecystectomy. However, it was no more effective in hormonal blockade than the extradural analgesia alone. The addition of high-dose corticosteroid (methylprednisolone 30 mg/kg) to the combined regimen was associated with a small decrease in the acute-phase and IL 6 responses. Inflammatory responses to surgery can be minimized using minimally invasive techniques.

Influence of inhibition of hormonal responses on surgical outcome

It is clear that extensive regional blockade with local anesthesia is most effective in suppressing the hormonal response to surgery, and it is also the most effective method of providing dynamic pain relief. Evidence to directly link the effect of regional anesthesia on the suppression of surgical stress responses with improved surgical outcome is lacking. However, it is well known that epidural anesthesia has beneficial effects on many aspects of surgical outcome. These include a reduced incidence of deep venous thrombosis and pulmonary embolism, and decreased blood loss. There is evidence also to show that epidural anesthesia has beneficial effects in terms of reduced incidence of postoperative respiratory and cardiac complications.

PHYSIOLOGIC RESPONSES TO HEMORRHAGE AND ANEMIA

Immediate changes

Loss of circulating volume by hemorrhage decreases cardiac filling and cardiac output falls, which activates numerous compensatory mechanisms (Table 72.2). Arterial baroreceptors are situated in the carotid sinus and aortic arch; cardiopulmonary baroreceptors are located in the pulmonary circulation and left ventricle. The rate of afferent discharge from these receptors depends on the degree of stretch to which the baroreceptor tissue is subjected. As circulating volume decreases, afferent nerve discharge decreases and sympathetic activity increases, thereby stimulating the cardiovascular system. The sympathetic reflexes are activated within 30 seconds of the onset of hemorrhage. Tachycardia helps maintain cardiac output, and intense vasoconstriction maintains arterial pressure by an increase in total peripheral resistance.

Vasoconstriction is most intense in the skin (causing pallor), viscera, and kidneys. Reflex venoconstriction also helps maintain cardiac filling pressure. Blood is shifted out of venous reservoirs in the skin, and from the pulmonary veins and the visceral circulation into the systemic circulation. Contraction of the spleen also mobilizes a small volume of blood. Vasoconstriction spares the coronary and cerebral circulations, but not the kidneys. In the brain and heart, local autoregulation allows maintenance of blood flow at near-normal levels, provided mean arterial pressure is >70 mmHg (9.3 kPa). Both afferent and efferent arterioles of the kidney are constricted, the efferent to a greater degree. Glomerular filtration is decreased and blood is shunted away from the cortical glomeruli. Urine output is decreased, which conserves circulating blood volume.

Table 72.2 Immediate physiologic responses to hemorrhage

Cause	Effect
Reduced cardiac filling	Reduced cardiac output
Decreased baroreceptor activity	Increased sympathetic stimulation Tachycardia, peripheral vasoconstriction
Fluid redistribution	Venoconstriction, decreased ECF volume
Increased pituitary and adrenal hormone secretion	Increased circulating catecholamines Oliguria
Increased chemoreceptor stimulation	Tachypnea

ECF, extracellular fluid.

The decrease in cardiac output and vasoconstriction reduces tissue perfusion, with consequent anaerobic cell metabolism and increased production of lactic acid. Blood lactate levels may increase markedly from the normal value of about 1 mmol/L. The metabolic acidosis can cause myocardial depression. Fluid is redistributed from the interstitial spaces into the intravascular compartment, which helps to maintain circulating blood volume. The pressure in the capillary beds is decreased because arterioles are constricted, and the venous pressure is decreased by reduced blood volume. According to the Starling forces that govern fluid transfer across capillary membranes, fluid moves into the capillaries from the interstitial spaces. Subsequently, the interstitial fluid volume is decreased and fluid moves out of cells.

Hemorrhage stimulates the release of catecholamines through increased sympathetic activity. Adrenal medullary secretion of epinephrine increases, and circulating values of norepinephrine also increase as a result of release from sympathetic noradrenergic nerve terminals. The circulating catecholamines make a small contribution to the stimulus for vasoconstriction.

Other hormones are also secreted as a result of hemorrhage. Increased secretion of angiotensin II results from increased renin activity – angiotensin II is a very powerful vasoconstrictor and its release contributes to the maintenance of blood pressure. Arginine vasopressin, released from the posterior pituitary, also has an important role in maintaining blood pressure, as well as in promoting the preservation of water in the kidneys. Anterior pituitary hormone secretion increases in response to the stress of hemorrhage. Together with angiotensin, ACTH increases the release of aldosterone from the adrenal cortex. Aldosterone and vasopressin act on the kidney to conserve salt and water, which helps to maintain circulating blood volume. This mechanism takes at least 30 minutes to have an effect; the immediate decrease in urine output and Na^+ excretion is caused by the hemodynamic changes in the kidney.

During hemorrhage, anemia and stagnant hypoxia stimulate the chemoreceptors in the carotid and aortic bodies. Metabolic acidosis may also stimulate the chemoreceptors. Increased afferent nerve activity stimulates respiration, and also adds to the stimulus for vasoconstriction.

The osmoreceptors in the hypothalamus of the brain are sensitive to changes in the osmolarity of the extracellular fluid and decreases in extracellular fluid volume. Increased afferent neural activity leads to the sensation of thirst in conscious patients.

Effects of blood loss

Circulatory shock is the term used when inadequate blood flow results in damage to body tissues. Provided that sympathetic reflexes are intact, about 10% of the blood volume can be lost with little change in either arterial pressure or cardiac output. At this stage, shock is reversible. With larger amounts of blood loss cardiac output starts to decrease, followed by arterial pressure. The reflex compensatory mechanisms allow systemic arterial pressure to be maintained at an adequate level with blood volume losses of up to about 30–35%. Without intervention, losses greater than 35–45% are not likely to be compatible with survival. In such circumstances, cardiac output declines progressively. Coronary blood flow decreases, which damages the myocardium and further reduces cardiac output. Blood flow to the vasomotor area of the brain falls so that the center becomes inactive and sympathetic output fails. Tissue hypoxia ensues as the circulation to the capillary beds becomes inadequate for cell survival.

Longer-term compensatory mechanisms

In the longer term, changes occur to restore body fluid volume and blood components that have been lost. Most of the fluid that moves into the intravascular compartment is protein free. Albumin moves into capillaries from stores in the skin and other sites. Plasma protein production in the liver is increased to replace the losses over a period of 3–4 days. Secretion of erythropoietin increases, which stimulates the formation of new red blood cells. The reticulocyte count increases, and peaks at about 10 days after the hemorrhagic event. The red cell mass is restored to normal in 4–8 weeks.

Fluid therapy

The basis of fluid replacement is to maintain circulating fluid volume and ensure blood flow to the vital organs. Blood may be required to replace losses. Usually, a combination of concentrated red blood cells and plasma or plasma substitutes is infused to replace lost blood and maintain intravascular volume. Plasma substitutes are colloidal solutions that contain particles of such a molecular size that they stay in the intravascular space for a useful period of time. Thus they provide more rapid and effective circulatory support than do crystalloid solutions. When crystalloid solutions are infused, the water is distributed throughout the extracellular fluid space; if used alone, large volumes are required. However, some crystalloid solutions are needed to replace fluid that has been lost from the intracellular and interstitial fluid spaces.

Allogeneic blood transfusion is associated with a number of adverse effects, high costs, and occasional blood shortages. Although red cell transfusion is essential in major trauma and other cases of massive blood loss, it is appropriate to avoid transfusion if possible in less extreme circumstances.

BURNS

Burn injury is associated with a widespread systemic disturbance that involves endocrinologic, metabolic, physiologic, and immunologic changes.

Burn injury results in significant fluid losses because of local and systemic increases in capillary permeability. Edema occurs in the burn wound, and also in unburned tissue. The loss of fluid into the tissues reduces the extracellular and circulating volume, which leads to a decline in cardiac output. Hypovolemic shock follows unless fluid resuscitation is prompt.

In addition to the gross systemic disturbance, many local changes occur. Inflammatory mediators are released at the burn site and contribute to the increased vascular permeability and a hypermetabolic state, with the potential for wound infection, sepsis, and multiorgan failure. Increased plasma concentrations of the cytokines IL-1β and IL-6 are found in many patients following burn injury. Although these mediators are beneficial, very high cytokine concentrations may exacerbate tissue damage. Prostaglandins and leukotrienes are vasoactive products of arachidonic acid metabolites that are released at the burn site, with a variety of effects. They increase permeability in the microvascular circulation, and prostaglandin E_2 allows the accumulation of neutrophils at the burn site, but not all of the mediators contribute to tissue repair and healing. For example, some of the thromboxanes cause local tissue ischemia and can lead to decreased perfusion of the gut and the kidneys. Sepsis and multiorgan failure may develop, even if the initial fluid resuscitation is adequate.

Resuscitative measures and fluid therapy

The mainstay of the initial management of burn injury is adequate fluid resuscitation. Most regimens are derived from retrospective data on fluid requirements and are based on the size of the burn. Many formulae now use similar volumes of fluid, and no single regimen has been shown to be superior to any other. One example is an infusion of crystalloid 4 mL/kg multiplied by the percentage of body size affected by the burn during the first 24 hours. Other regimens differ in the type of fluid that is given. The use of colloid reduces the total volume required, although its use has declined because controlled trials have shown it to provide no advantage. In adults, an hourly urine output >0.5 mL/kg is a useful guide to adequate tissue perfusion.

The use of hypertonic fluid, such as crystalloid that contains sodium 250 mmol/L, can decrease the total fluid volume requirements. This may theoretically be beneficial in patients who have poor cardiopulmonary function, as the risks of volume overload are lessened. However, the safety of hypertonic saline is unclear, so very careful patient monitoring is required. One study reported that the use of hypertonic saline in burns increased the incidence of renal failure and death.

Hypermetabolism

Increased circulating concentrations of cortisol, catecholamines, and glucagon occur after burn injury. Patients become hypermetabolic, with proteolysis, lipolysis, and gluconeogenesis. Massive protein catabolism may occur, with severe weight loss and muscle wasting. The release of inflammatory mediators, including cytokines, from the injured tissue contributes to the hypermetabolic state. The metabolic rate is also increased because of the fluid and heat losses from burned skin. Early nutritional support is provided, using the gut whenever possible.

Many strategies have been used to ameliorate the catabolic changes that occur after burns. Early closure of burn wounds and raised environmental temperature have been used to decrease fluid losses and metabolic rate in thermally injured rats, although clinical studies of large burns show that early wound closure alone does not suppress the metabolic response. Efforts to modify the physiological state have not been particularly successful. Essential amino acids, growth hormone, insulin, IGF-1, anabolic steroids and β-adrenergic drugs have all been used in clinical trials, but none has become a standard part of burn management.

Key references

Bruttig SP, Calgani DE. Hemorrhage and its treatment. Curr Opin Anaesthesiol. 1997;10:124–9.

Desborough JP. The stress response to trauma and surgery. Br J Anaesth. 2000;85:109–17.

Kao CC, Garner WL. Acute burns. Plast Reconstruct Surg. 2000;105:2482–93.

Kehlet H, Holte K. Effect of postoperative analgesia on surgical outcome. Br J Anaesth. 2001;87:67–72.

Lin E, Calvano SE, Lowry SF. Inflammatory cytokines and the cell response in surgery. Surgery 2000;127:117–26.

Ramsey G. Intravenous volume replacement: indications and choices. Br Med J. 1988;196:1422–3.

Further reading

Holte K, Kehlet H. Epidural anaesthesia and analgesia – effects on surgical stress responses and implications for postoperative nutrition. Clin Nutr. 2002;21:199–206.

Pearl RG, Sibbald WJ (eds) Anemia and blood management in critical care. Crit Care Med. 2003;31(Suppl):S649–720

Sheeran P, Hall GM. Cytokines in anaesthesia. Br J Anaesth. 1997;78:201–19.

Sheridan RL. Burn care: Results of technical and organizational progress. JAMA 2003;290:719–22.

Wilmore DW. From Cuthbertson to fast-track surgery: 70 years of progress in reducing stress in surgical patients. Ann Surg. 2002;236:643–8

Chapter 73

Sepsis

Nigel R Webster and Helen F Galley

TOPICS COVERED IN THIS CHAPTER
- **Definitions**
- **Pathophysiology**
- **Cytokines**
- **Process of the inflammatory response**
  - Nitric oxide
- **Multiorgan failure**
- **Treatment**
  - Immunotherapy
  - Activated protein C
- **Genetic studies**
  - Future immunogenetic therapy

Sepsis and septic shock are the most common causes of death in the intensive care unit (ICU). An estimated 400 000–500 000 patients develop sepsis each year in both European and American ICUs, and some 50% of these demonstrate signs of shock. Sepsis often leads to multiorgan dysfunction and failure, with an associated high mortality rate. Of those patients developing septic shock, some 50–60% will die despite the best of currently available treatment. The incidence of sepsis in the ICU is increasing. This is most likely a consequence of our ability to sustain life through better organ support techniques and because of the more widespread use of invasive procedures in patients, more of whom are now immunocompromised.

DEFINITIONS

Definitions of sepsis and shock were agreed at a recent consensus meeting of the American Thoracic Society and the American Society of Critical Care Medicine.

- *Infection* is an inflammatory response to the presence of microorganisms or the invasion of normally sterile host tissue by those organisms.
- *Bacteremia* is the presence of viable bacteria in the blood.
- *Septicemia is* a clinical term, the use of which is now discouraged.
- *Sepsis* is the systemic response to infection, manifest by two or more of the following conditions as a result of infection: temperature $>$100.4°F ($>$38.8°C) or $<$96.8°F ($<$36.8°C); heart rate $>$90 bpm; respiratory rate $>$20 breaths/min or a requirement for artificial ventilation; and white blood cell count $>$12 000/mm^3 or $<$4000/mm^3 ($>12 \times 10^9$ cells/L or $<4 \times 10^9$ cells/L).
- *Severe sepsis* is sepsis associated with organ dysfunction, hypoperfusion, or hypotension.
- *Septic shock* is sepsis-induced hypotension (systolic blood pressure $<$90 mmHg) or a requirement for vasoconstrictors despite adequate fluid resuscitation.
- *Multiple organ dysfunction syndrome* (MODS) is the presence of altered organ function such that homeostasis cannot be maintained without intervention.

In addition, it is now appreciated that no source of infection is found in many patients demonstrating all the classic signs of sepsis. This condition is referred to as the *systemic inflammatory response syndrome* (SIRS), and it is thought that it results when inflammatory mediators (probably identical to those found in bacteremic patients) are released from ischemic and infarcted tissue.

Other terms have recently been added to this list to reflect the growing understanding of the relationship of the two counter systems that regulate the inflammatory response, namely, the proinflammatory and anti-inflammatory processes. It is now thought that there is a carefully maintained balance between these two processes, with *compensatory anti-inflammatory response syndrome* (CARS) and *mixed anti-inflammatory response syndrome* (MARS) suggested as suitable titles to describe this. These phases of the inflammatory response occur at differing intervals from the initial insult, as depicted in Figure 73.1.

PATHOPHYSIOLOGY

Much evidence supports the hypothesis that molecules released from bacteria (called either *exotoxins* (secreted from live bacteria) or *endotoxins* (present in the cell wall of bacteria and usually released on bacterial death)) are responsible for the altered physiology seen in sepsis. These molecules are complexes of

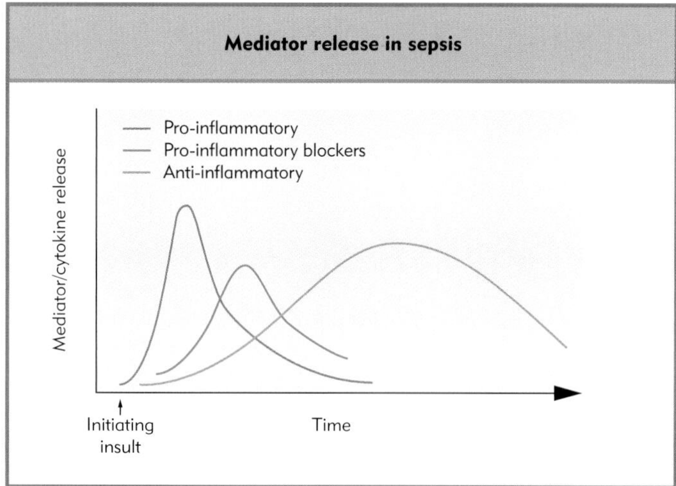

Figure 73.1 The time course of mediator release in sepsis. An early proinflammatory response is mounted (e.g. TNF-α and IL-1β), followed by a later release of proinflammatory blockers (e.g. IL-1 receptor antagonist) and anti-inflammatory cytokines (e.g. IL-10).

polysaccharide and fatty acids, with endotoxin commonly being called lipopolysaccharide (LPS). Examples of exotoxins include tetanus and botulinus toxins, and the toxins seen in toxic shock syndrome. All of the signs and symptoms of sepsis can be reproduced by the injection of endotoxin into human volunteers. These subjects display an increased heart rate and cardiac output, with a fall in blood pressure owing to vasodilatation and a decreased systemic vascular resistance. Respiratory rate increases, with a decreased arterial carbon dioxide partial pressure; although arterial oxygenation is maintained initially, it eventually falls because of an increased alveolar to arterial oxygen gradient caused by ventilation/perfusion mismatch. In addition, there is an accumulation of edema fluid because of increased capillary permeability. The endotoxin also causes changes in white blood cell and capillary endothelial function. A cascade of inflammatory mediators is released that will activate and recruit white cells to the affected region. It is against this inflammatory mediator cascade that most of the current research to improve treatment is directed.

Outcome from sepsis is determined not only by the infection but also by the intensity of the immunoinflammatory response. This response is essential for the resolution of infection but may occur in an uncontrolled manner, causing damage to the host. The pronounced synergy and interaction of the components of the immune system dictate that modulation may result in either immunostimulation or immunosuppression. Coordination is therefore vital for an optimum response. Mediators of immunity and inflammation (families of protein and lipid molecules) are part of an intricate intercellular signaling system that enables cells, tissues, and organs to produce a response to an insult. This response may be modified if previous exposure to the insult has occurred.

The body possesses a range of barriers to prevent microorganisms from entering, including the skin, mucus secretion, ciliary action, and gastric acid. If these barriers are crossed, microorganisms are destroyed by soluble factors such as lysozyme and by phagocytosis with intracellular digestion (termed innate immunity). The complement system is a multicomponent triggered enzyme cascade that attracts phagocytes to microorganisms, increasing capillary permeability and neutrophil chemotaxis and adhesion. Specific acquired immunity in the form of antibodies inactivates microorganisms that are not destroyed by the innate immune system. Microorganisms evading the innate system fail to either activate the complement pathway or to prevent the activation of phagocytes. Acquired immune defense against specific microorganisms (antigen) forms the second component of the immune response. Antibodies activate the complement system, stimulate phagocytic cells, and specifically inactivate microorganisms (Chapter 54).

CYTOKINES

Cytokines are low molecular weight proteins produced by a variety of cells; they regulate the amplitude and duration of the inflammatory response (described in detail in Chapter 54). Cytokines have numerous effects on growth and differentiation in a variety of cell types, with considerable overlap and redundancy between different cytokines, partially accounted for by their shared ability to induce the synthesis of several proteins. Cytokines are transiently active and tightly regulated; they interact with specific high-affinity cell surface receptors to regulate gene expression. Interactions between cytokines may occur in a variety of ways: a cascade system in which one cytokine induces another; modulation of the receptor of another cytokine; synergism or antagonism between two cytokines acting on the same cell; release of receptor antagonists; and release of soluble receptors that bind cytokine without causing biologic actions.

The local balance of cytokine effects is an important determinant of immune response. Specific induction of each subset of T-helper cells causes the production of a distant and specific range of cytokines and inflammatory mediators, which may have important implications for outcome in patients who have sepsis.

Not all of the effects of the inflammatory response are deleterious; indeed, the inflammatory response is a normal host defense mechanism. Nitric oxide and oxygen-derived free radicals are released by activated white cells, forming peroxynitrite and preventing patients progressing to a systemic inflammatory response.

Several studies have shown that infusion of endotoxin or tumor necrosis factor-α (TNF-α) in animal models effectively mimics severe sepsis syndrome, with ensuing organ dysfunction, and leads to the appearance of other proinflammatory cytokines (Table 73.1). Elevated circulating TNF-α concentrations are not found in all patients who have sepsis, but are higher than in nonseptic critically ill patients (and the highest levels are associated with the development of shock and lung injury).

Several studies of patients who have severe sepsis have shown that peak TNF-α concentrations are higher in those patients who die than in those who survive; they also fail to decrease in patients who die. However, other studies have found no association with outcome. It is possible that tissue or local concentrations of mediators are important for their actions rather than their circulating levels, which may be too low to be measured in the peripheral circulation (Fig. 73.2).

Interleukin (IL)-6 concentrations are also increased in patients who have sepsis and are associated with the onset of shock. High levels have been linked to increased mortality in some studies, although again other studies have not found such a correlation. Levels of IL-1β are raised in some patients who have sepsis and

Table 73.1 Metabolic responses to tumor necrosis factor are implicated in septic shock syndrome (Reproduced with permission from Tracey and Cerami, 1992.)

System	Effects
Cardiovascular	Hypotension, myocardial suppression, decreased peripheral vascular resistance, capillary leakage syndrome
Pulmonary	Adult respiratory distress syndrome, capillary leakage with edema, leukocyte margination, respiratory arrest
Renal	Acute renal tubular necrosis
Gastrointestinal	Hemorrhagic necrosis, decreased motility, absorption
Hematologic	Neutrophilia or neutropenia, increased procoagulant activity, diffuse intravascular coagulopathy, endothelial activation
Central nervous	Fever, increased sympathetic outflow, anorexia, altered hypothalamopituitary outflow
Metabolic	Lactic acidosis, catabolic stress hormone release (catecholamines, glucagon, adrenocorticotropic hormone, cortisol), hyperglycemia followed by hypoglycemia, hyperaminoacidemia
Musculoskeletal	Myalgia, decreased resting membrane potential in skeletal muscle, increased skeletal muscle amino acid release

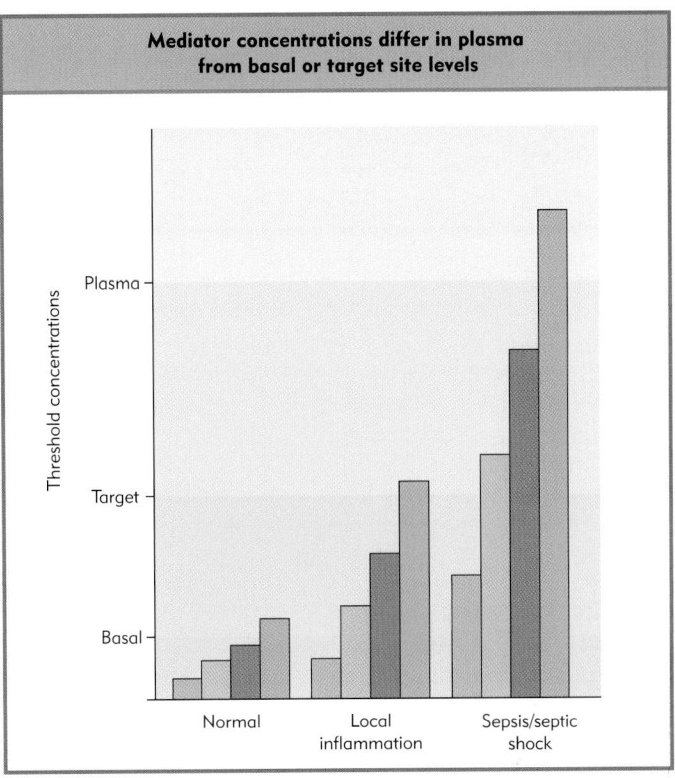

Figure 73.2 The difference between mediator concentrations basally, at the target cell site, and in plasma. Different bars represent different mediators or tissue sites during sepsis, in local inflammation, and normally. Plasma concentrations may therefore not represent either target cell or tissue levels, and may have little bearing on outcome from sepsis.

are reported to be higher in nonsurvivors, although this difference is not found in all studies. In addition, a combined cytokine score encompassing endotoxin, TNF-α, IL-1β, and IL-6 concentrations was also found to correlate with mortality. Therapeutic administration of antibodies to TNF-α has been successful in increasing survival in primate models of sepsis, but human studies showed no effect on mortality, although TNF-α and IL-6 levels were attenuated and cardiac function improved. Concentrations of the anti-inflammatory cytokine IL-10 are also elevated in sepsis, and are highest in those patients who have shock. Elevated IL-10 correlated with the subsequent development of sepsis in trauma patients, and was highest in those septic patients who did not survive. Although there are no human studies, administration of IL-10 after cecal ligation and puncture in mice blunted the rise in TNF-α and improved survival.

The biologic activities of cytokines are regulated by specific cellular receptors. Soluble receptors, released either as unique proteins or from shedding of cell surface-expressed receptors, compete with membrane-bound receptors and appear in response to stimuli as part of a naturally occurring independent regulatory process to limit the deleterious effects of the cytokine. Soluble receptors for TNF-α are elevated in patients who have severe sepsis, particularly in nonsurvivors. Circulating concentrations of the endogenous antagonist to the IL-1 receptor (IL-1RA) are elevated in patients who have sepsis, but the relationship with outcome is unclear.

PROCESS OF THE INFLAMMATORY RESPONSE

Severe infection leads to the appearance of LPS in the bloodstream, which triggers innate immune responses such as the activation of phagocytic cells and the complement cascade, and leads to the production of the primary proinflammatory mediators TNF and IL-1. Secondary mediators, including other cytokines, prostaglandins, and platelet-activating factor (PAF), are then released, with further activation of complement, the initiation of the acute-phase response, expression of adhesion molecules, T-cell selection, antibody production, and the release of oxygen-derived free radicals. Other toxins and cellular debris must also trigger such a systemic inflammatory response, as this process can occur in the absence of LPS release.

Prolonged systemic exposure to high concentrations of cytokines and other components of the immunoinflammatory cascade may contribute to the development of MODS. Damage to and activation of the endothelium, which plays a pivotal role in the regulation of hemostasis, vascular tone, and fibrinolysis, has profound consequences. The endothelium produces several substances that regulate inflammation and regional perfusion, including nitric oxide, vasoactive arachidonic acid metabolites, and cytokines. Changes in the balance of concentrations of these substances may contribute to the pathogenesis of the inflammatory response during sepsis and injury. Phagocytic cells are in constant contact with the endothelium, and disturbance of the relationship between these two cell types may result in direct tissue damage through local production of oxygen-derived free radicals, hypochlorous acid, and proteolytic enzymes.

Nitric oxide

Nitric oxide has many potential roles in the inflammatory process. Besides its vasodilatory effects (see Chapter 38), it reduces platelet aggregation, prevents monocyte chemotaxis, and inhibits leukocyte adhesion to the endothelium. Trials are currently ongoing using nitric oxide synthase (NOS) inhibitors to increase blood pressure in sepsis (Fig. 73.3). However, nitric oxide also reduces cytokine-induced expression of a number of effector molecules important in sepsis. Nitric oxide donors inhibit cytokine-induced vascular cell adhesion molecule (VCAM) expression and monocyte adhesion. This effect is more interesting because it appears that it is not caused by the usual activation of guanylyl cyclase, but most likely by inhibition of the transcription factor nuclear factor-κB (NF-κB) (Fig. 73.4). This transcription factor regulates the expression of adhesion molecules and various inflammatory cytokines such as IL-6 and IL-8. Because the activation of NF-κB by TNF-α is thought to occur via reactive oxygen species, nitric oxide may inhibit NF-κB by scavenging and inactivating superoxide anion. Nitric oxide has also been found to stabilize the inhibitory subunit of NF-κB (IκB).

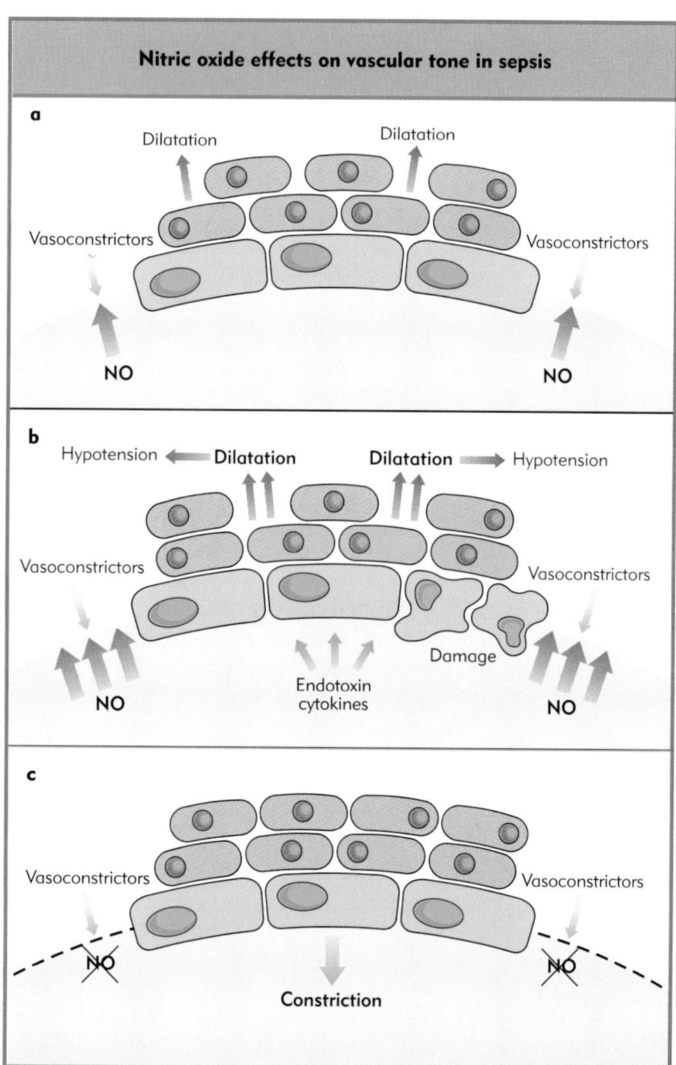

Figure 73.3 Nitric oxide effects on vascular tone in sepsis. Constitutively produced nitric oxide usually maintains a state of constant vasodilatation (a). During septic shock, large quantities of nitric oxide are produced in response to endotoxin and cytokines, resulting in excessive vasodilatation and hypotension (b). Inhibition of nitric oxide synthase in septic shock blocks the production of nitric oxide and results in vasoconstriction and reversal of shock (c).

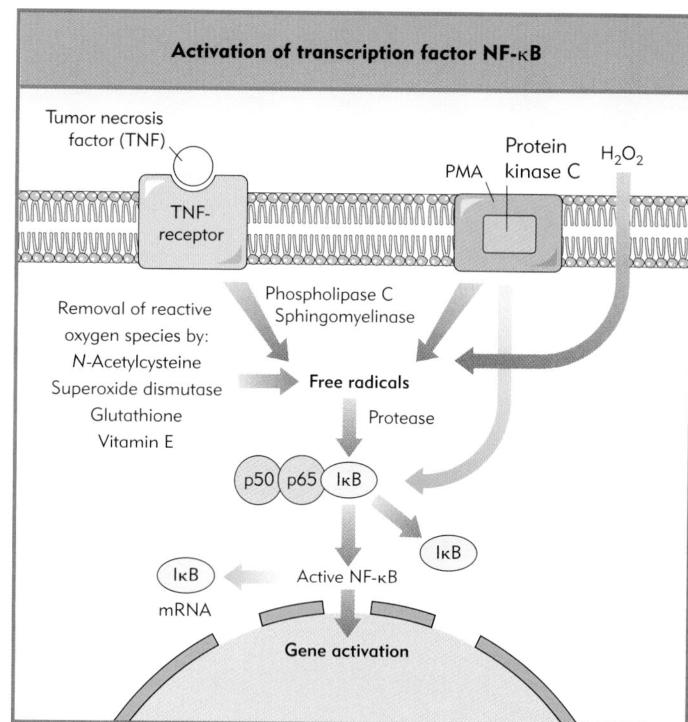

Figure 73.4 Schematic representation of the activation of the transcription factor nuclear factor-κB (NF-κB). Activation of NF-κB occurs by a common route involving free radicals and leading to removal of the inhibitory subunit IκB. The active NF-κB, consisting of the two subunits p50 and p65, then moves into the cell nucleus and binds to target DNA, leading to gene activation and transcription of mRNA for adhesion molecules, cytokines, NOS, and other inflammatory proteins. Antioxidants such as *N*-acetylcysteine block NF-κB activation by removing reactive oxygen species.

In alveolar cells grown in culture, nitric oxide has been shown to modulate the cytotoxic effects of superoxide anion. Basal rates of cytolysis and superoxide-dependent oxidative damage to the cells was attenuated either by enhanced rates of endogenous nitric oxide production following cytokine stimulation or by exogenous nitric oxide administration using either nitric oxide itself or the potentially more biologically important nitrosothiol compounds. In this model, nitric oxide alone was not cytotoxic. When control and cytokine-stimulated cells were treated with L-*N*-monomethylarginine (L-NMMA), a competitive inhibitor of NOS, cell injury was significantly increased, suggesting a protective role for endogenously produced nitric oxide.

MULTIORGAN FAILURE

Once the inflammatory response has been activated, many organ systems can be adversely affected. Of prime importance are the effects on the cardiovascular system that characterize severe sepsis. There is a marked fall in systemic vascular resistance resulting from arterial and venous dilatation; this is accompanied by leakage of plasma into the extravascular space, leading to relative hypovolemia. With adequate fluid resuscitation, the cardiac output is usually elevated. Despite this, myocardial performance is below normal, possibly because of the occurrence of circulating factors with myocardial depressant properties. Myocardial contractility is decreased and the left ventricular ejection fraction reduced, with high cardiac output being maintained by an increase in heart rate. The microcirculation is adversely affected, with maldistribution of blood flow (Fig. 73.5). Measurements of arteriovenous oxygen content difference and mixed venous saturations suggest that oxygen is neither reaching nor being effectively extracted by the cells. The reason for this is not fully understood, but may be related to arteriovenous shunting or abnormalities in cellular metabolism. It has recently been demonstrated that nitric oxide can irreversibly inhibit enzymes involved in the electron transport chain of oxidative phosphorylation. Most patients have a raised blood lactate level and are acidotic.

Pulmonary manifestations of sepsis are common, ranging from mild hypoxemia to adult respiratory distress syndrome (ARDS). Hyperventilation occurs at first, probably because of the fall in arterial oxygen partial pressure, which is a consequence of ventilation/perfusion mismatch. This progresses to acute lung injury, with severe abnormalities in pulmonary gas exchange and the appearance of pulmonary edema that can be seen on chest X-ray. The edema results from margination of activated polymorphonuclear leukocytes within the pulmonary vascular bed and the release of mediators that increase vascular leakage.

Coagulation abnormalities are common, ranging from mild derangement of clotting times to disseminated intravascular coagulation (DIC) and thrombocytopenia. Decreased synthesis by the liver is one possible explanation. However, the vascular endothelium has an important role in the synthesis and release of antithrombotic and antiplatelet agents, and these are altered by the presence of inflammatory mediators.

Blood flow is altered to other organ systems in the presence of sepsis; this is particularly noticeable in the CNS, the kidneys, and the gastrointestinal system. Despite increased total hepatosplanchnic perfusion in sepsis and an accompanying rise in oxygen extraction across the gut wall, oxygen demand frequently outstrips supply, leading to inadequate oxygenation of the splanchnic bed.

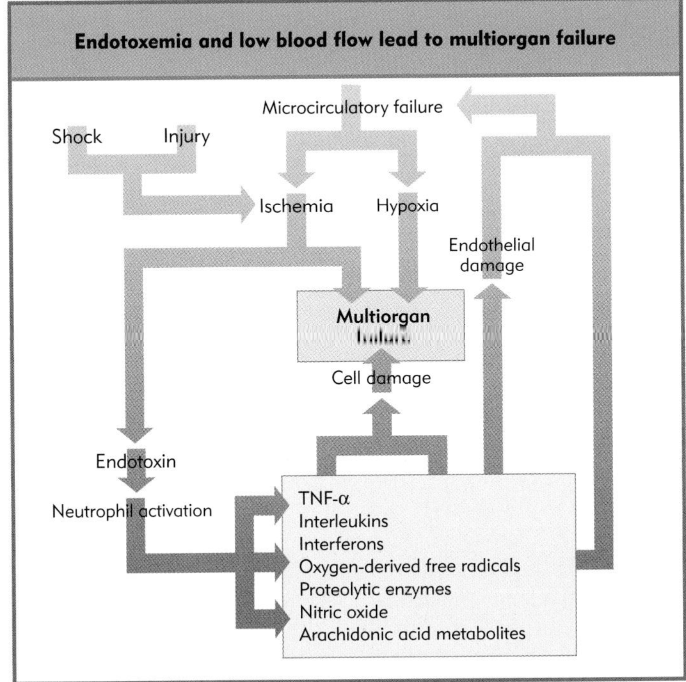

Figure 73.5 Endotoxemia and low blood flow in critically ill patients, resulting in multiorgan dysfunction syndrome.

TREATMENT

The recognition of sepsis often requires a high index of suspicion: whereas some cases will be obvious, with fever and an identifiable source of sepsis, others will be much more subtle, particularly in the elderly and immunocompromised. A full microbiologic screen is imperative. Further investigations, including sophisticated imaging techniques to identify possible sources of infection, can be guided by the findings on initial clinical assessment. Because bacteriologic confirmation of the responsible organism is not usually immediately available, two or more antibiotics are often administered empirically. These should provide coverage against a broad spectrum of organisms, but can often be targeted at likely organisms based on the site of infection and the local patterns of sensitivity of common organisms. Vigorous steps should be taken to eradicate any source of infection; collections of pus must be drained (either surgically or using radiologically guided drain insertion) and nonviable tissue excised. Resuscitative measures are then instituted.

Oxygen is administered, and many patients may require ventilatory support. Fluid resuscitation is commenced in an attempt to reverse the hypotension and tissue hypoperfusion. Septic patients often require large amounts of fluids to attain a reasonable cardiac preload. The choice of fluid used is a matter of some controversy, and the type may be of little significance, but it must be remembered that almost three times as much crystalloid as colloid will be required to achieve an equal expansion of the intravascular space. It would seem logical to transfuse blood if the hemoglobin is less than 10 g/dL in order to facilitate tissue oxygen delivery. Frequent monitoring of the cardiovascular status is required. Central venous pressure rarely gives an accurate assessment of left ventricular preload in sepsis because of myocardial dysfunction, and pulmonary artery catheterization is currently recommended. Fluids are given to optimize both cardiac output and blood pressure, and a Frank–Starling curve can readily be estimated by measuring cardiac output as fluid resuscitation continues. Inotropes and vasoconstrictors, including dopamine, dobutamine, epinephrine (adrenaline), phenylephrine, and norepinephrine (noradrenaline), are given to elevate cardiac output and systemic vascular resistance as appropriate (Chapters 41–43).

Immunotherapy

Steroids are well known immunomodulators and have been shown to alter the production of TNF by a specific effect on TNF messenger ribonucleic acid (mRNA). However, clinical studies have not universally shown that the use of steroids is beneficial. The use of high-dose steroids has been shown to be associated with excess mortality in patients with sepsis. However, lower and more physiological replacement doses are known to reverse insensitivity to vasoconstrictors in patients with septic shock. There is currently still controversy about whether this is associated with an improved outcome, either in these more severely ill patients or in the broader group of all patients with sepsis. Similarly, pentoxyphylline (oxpentifylline) alters TNF production but has not been proved to be useful clinically. Both soluble receptors and monoclonal antibodies directed against receptors can be used to block the interaction of a cytokine with its receptor. This prevents transduction of the relevant biologic signal in the target cell. Use of a recombinant soluble receptor might also prevent the deleterious effect of excessive cytokine production. Administration of a recombinant form of the human IL-1RA to a heterogeneous group of patients who had sepsis was unsuccessful in reducing mortality. In addition to soluble receptors, monoclonal antibodies that block cellular cytokine receptors can be used as anticytokine therapy. However, it has been shown that cytokine complexed to such binding proteins is still available for receptor binding and will act as an agonist. Another approach to minimize the deleterious effects of the uncontrolled inflammatory process is to blunt the final common pathways of damage (i.e. using either agents that decrease free radical production, or antioxidants that inactivate free radicals as they are produced). Monoclonal antibodies to TNF-α have been used in both clinical and animal studies. The use of soluble TNF receptors has also been evaluated in sepsis. The naturally occurring IL-1RA has been studied in two large clinical trials. Specific chemical antagonists, for example against PAF, have also been evaluated in patients who have sepsis.

Blockade of any single inflammatory mediator or a combination of mediators may not be successful for a number of reasons. First, the immunoinflammatory process is a normal response to infection and is essential not only for the resolution of infection, but also for the initiation of other adaptive stress responses required for host survival (e.g. acute-phase and heat-shock responses). Second, the profound redundancy of action of many cytokines means that there are many overlapping pathways for cellular activation and further mediator release. Third, the synergy of actions and effects of many cytokines suggests that balance in the process of the immune response may be adversely affected by inhibition of a single agent. Fourth, exogenously administered anticytokine therapy may have hitherto unrecognized effects because of its interaction with other immunomodulators or their receptors. Finally, the timing of any potential anticytokine therapy is clearly crucial. Strategies designed to predict the activation of specific components of the inflammatory response may therefore be useful. It is also possible that specific cellular targeting of such therapy may be more beneficial than global inhibition. Preliminary animal studies suggest that the therapeutic use of anti-inflammatory cytokines such as IL-10 and IL-13 may be beneficial in sepsis, although as yet there have been no confirmatory clinical studies.

Activated protein C

A number of small studies and case reports have suggested a possible beneficial effect of protein C in patients with severe sepsis. The rationale for using protein C originated because of the coagulopathy often seen in sepsis and the quite significant risk of tissue loss associated with intravascular thrombosis, particularly in meningococcal sepsis. Activated protein C has both antithrombotic and profibrinolytic activity. A phase III study of recombinant human activated protein C was halted at an interim analysis because of efficacy in the study group – mortality was decreased from 30.83% to 24.72% ($p = 0.0054$). Although activated protein C has its well known effects within the coagulation system as an antithrombotic and profibrinolytic agent, it is now becoming acknowledged that it also has anti-inflammatory actions. In the phase III study patients who received activated protein C had lower plasma IL-6 concentrations, and there is now laboratory evidence that it can alter NF-κB activation and hence the production of a range of cytokines.

GENETIC STUDIES

Polymorphisms are gene variations that occur in a population (Chapter 4). They can be either single nucleotide base substitutions – point mutations – or repeated units of two nucleotides called dinucleotide repeats. Polymorphisms may be functional, such that the occurrence of a specific allele may lead to, for example, greater protein expression or increased disease susceptibility.

Polymorphisms have been identified for genes for several cytokines and their receptors. In postoperative patients who have sepsis, homozygotes for the TNFB2 allele had higher TNF-α levels than heterozygotes and were more likely to die from sepsis, strongly suggesting that regulatory polymorphisms of the gene for TNF-α can affect outcome from severe infection. An allele of polymorphism in the gene for the IL-1RA is associated with raised IL-1RA concentrations in patients who have sepsis. The gene for the anti-inflammatory cytokine IL-10 has been assigned to chromosome 1q31, and a functional dinucleotide repeat polymorphism has been identified in the promoter region. The relationship with levels of IL-10 in sepsis is not known. Low-frequency polymorphisms for the IL-6 receptor (IL-6R) gene have been reported in a small group of healthy subjects, but there have been no studies of the genetics of these mediators in sepsis. The soluble form of IL-6R, which binds IL-6 and mediates IL-6 signaling through interaction with gp130, may modulate the biologic activity of IL-6 in a range of pathologic conditions. Outcome in sepsis has been linked to levels of IL-6, IL-10, and IL-1RA, but there have been no studies investigating the role of these polymorphisms in the outcome from sepsis.

Studies of mice that have been rendered genetically deficient in TNF receptors (TNFR) or in intercellular cell adhesion molecule 1 (ICAM-1) have revealed the critical role of these molecules in septic shock. These and other experiments suggest that there are differences in the molecular and cellular mechanisms underlying shock induced by endotoxins and exotoxins. Results from these experiments are, however, occasionally different from those generated in experiments that use blocking antibodies against the same inflammatory mediators. Also, mice are relatively resistant to bacterial toxins, and septic shock in mice may not represent the situation in humans. Nevertheless, a high dose of toxin in mice (the 'high-dose endotoxin' model) might correlate with a substantially lower dose in human shock. Furthermore, it is possible to sensitize mice dramatically to low doses of toxin by impairing their liver metabolism with D-galactosamine (D-Gal) (the 'low-dose endotoxin' model). This model could be relevant to the human situation when recurrent episodes of sepsis are combined with organ failure.

Deficiency of the gene encoding ICAM-1 renders mice resistant to the lethal effects of high-dose LPS. Because levels of TNF and IL-1 after LPS injection are similar to those in the wildtype mice, the protection appears to be distal to the event triggering cytokine production. $TNFR_1$-deficient mice are not protected against lethality, which suggests the involvement of other TNF–TNFR signaling pathways (the same is true of $TNFR_2$-deficient mice). Mice incapable of making IL-1 are markedly protected in the high-dose LPS model.

The increased susceptibility of rodents to TNF-induced lethality after pretreatment with D-Gal was shown to be largely a consequence of a relative and selective liver failure. D-Gal acts as a specific transcriptional inhibitor in hepatocytes. This sensitizes the hepatocyte to the cytotoxic action of TNF and induces death by apoptosis. Transcriptionally arrested primary hepatocytes from $TNFR_1$-deficient mice were found to be protected from TNF-induced apoptosis, and these mice showed no signs of liver failure in in vivo experiments. Mice deficient in ICAM-1 and IL-1 are not resistant to low doses of LPS after D-Gal pretreatment, and ICAM deficiency does not reduce macrophage activation as reflected by normal TNF production. These experiments highlight the importance of TNF in this process.

Future immunogenetic therapy

Because cytokines are potent bioactive molecules, it is not surprising that their production is tightly regulated at several steps. Cytokines exert their effects by binding to their membrane receptors and activating intracellular signal transduction pathways, leading to alterations in targeted cells. Each of these steps may be a target for therapeutic manipulation. In addition, there are soluble receptors and receptor antagonists that modulate cytokine effects. Future therapeutic options for modulating the inflammatory response include neutralizing antibodies to block cytokine inducers, proinflammatory cytokines, and their cell-surface receptors; blocking the interaction between cytokines and cell-surface receptors with naturally expressed molecules; enhancing protective activities in target cells; and the intracellular blockade of cytokine-induced responses.

Gene therapy is a therapeutic approach by which a recombinant gene is introduced into the cells of patients. These genes can then synthesize a novel or missing/defective gene product in vivo. The use of genes as drugs, or in combination with drug therapy, to enhance anti-inflammatory responses has tremendous potential in critical care. The first step is to introduce the gene of interest into the target cell. Two general categories of gene transfer vector have been developed: viral and nonviral. In viral vectors, adenovirus or retrovirus DNA is modified to incorporate the therapeutic gene. The virus then acts as a shuttle for the gene; because the virus can self-replicate, this can be a very efficient mode of transfection. Nonviral vectors include liposomes and molecular conjugates, which exploit endogenous transport systems to permit efficient delivery of the therapeutic gene into the cell. Examples of gene transfers tested in sepsis models include IL-10, soluble TNFR, the antioxidant enzymes superoxide dismutase and catalase, the antiprotease α_1-antitrypsin, and heat-shock proteins (particularly HSP72).

Identification and targeting of those patients likely to benefit from modulation of the inflammatory response may be possible through analysis of polymorphisms of genes of relevant mediators, cytokines, receptors, and antagonists. The future may present a scenario of full genetic screening on admission to the ICU in order to determine the most appropriate therapeutic strategy.

Key references

Bernard GR, Vincent JL, Laterre PF et al. Efficacy and safety of recombinant human activated protein C for severe sepsis. New Engl J Med. 2001;344:699–709.

Bone RC, Balk RA, Cerra FB et al. American College of Chest Physicians/Society of Critical Care Medicine Consensus Conference: definitions for sepsis and organ failure and guidelines for the use of innovative therapies in sepsis. Crit Care Med. 1992;20:864–74.

Galley HF, Webster NR. The immuno-inflammatory cascade. Br J Anaesth. 1996;77:11–16.

Goode HF, Webster NR. Free radicals and antioxidants in sepsis. Crit Care Med. 1993;21:1770–6.

Lamy M, Thijs LG, eds. Mediators of sepsis. Berlin: Springer-Verlag; 1992:124–35.

Liu M, Slutsky AS. Anti-inflammatory therapies: application of molecular biology techniques in intensive care medicine. Int Care Med. 1997;23:718–31.

Parillo JE. Pathogenic mechanisms of septic shock. New Engl J Med. 1993;328:1471–7.

Tracey KJ, Cerami A. Tumor necrosis factor and regulation of metabolism in infection: role of systemic versus tissue levels. Proc Soc Exp Biol Med. 1992;200:233–9.

Further reading

Tracey KJ, Cerami A. Tumor necrosis factor: a pleiotropic cytokine and therapeutic target. Annu Rev Med. 1994;45:491–503.

van der Poll T, Lowry SF. Tumor necrosis factor in sepsis; mediator of multiple organ failure or essential part of host defense? Shock 1995;3:1–12.

Index

A

B

C

D

F

G

H

N

O

P

Q

R

S

W

X

Y

Z

ELSEVIER CD-ROM LICENCE AGREEMENT

PLEASE READ THE FOLLOWING AGREEMENT CAREFULLY BEFORE USING THIS PRODUCT. THIS PRODUCT IS LICENSED UNDER THE TERMS CONTAINED IN THIS LICENCE AGREEMENT ('Agreement'). BY USING THIS PRODUCT, YOU, AN INDIVIDUAL OR ENTITY INCLUDING EMPLOYEES, AGENTS AND REPRESENTATIVES ('You' or 'Your'), ACKNOWLEDGE THAT YOU HAVE READ THIS AGREEMENT, THAT YOU UNDERSTAND IT, AND THAT YOU AGREE TO BE BOUND BY THE TERMS AND CONDITIONS OF THIS AGREEMENT. ELSEVIER LIMITED ('Elsevier') EXPRESSLY DOES NOT AGREE TO LICENSE THIS PRODUCT TO YOU UNLESS YOU ASSENT TO THIS AGREEMENT. IF YOU DO NOT AGREE WITH ANY OF THE FOLLOWING TERMS, YOU MAY, WITHIN THIRTY (30) DAYS AFTER YOUR RECEIPT OF THIS PRODUCT RETURN THE UNUSED PRODUCT AND ALL ACCOMPANYING DOCUMENTATION TO ELSEVIER FOR A FULL REFUND.

DEFINITIONS As used in this Agreement, these terms shall have the following meanings:

'Proprietary Material' means the valuable and proprietary information content of this Product including without limitation all indexes and graphic materials and software used to access, index, search and retrieve the information content from this Product developed or licensed by Elsevier and/or its affiliates, suppliers and licensors.

'Product' means the copy of the Proprietary Material and any other material delivered on CD-ROM and any other human-readable or machine-readable materials enclosed with this Agreement, including without limitation documentation relating to the same.

OWNERSHIP This Product has been supplied by and is proprietary to Elsevier and/or its affiliates, suppliers and licensors. The copyright in the Product belongs to Elsevier and/or its affiliates, suppliers and licensors and is protected by the copyright, trademark, trade secret and other intellectual property laws of the United Kingdom and international treaty provisions, including without limitation the Universal Copyright Convention and the Berne Copyright Convention. You have no ownership rights in this Product. Except as expressly set forth herein, no part of this Product, including without limitation the Proprietary Material, may be modified, copied or distributed in hardcopy or machine-readable form without prior written consent from Elsevier. All rights not expressly granted to You herein are expressly reserved. Any other use of this Product by any person or entity is strictly prohibited and a violation of this Agreement.

SCOPE OF RIGHTS LICENSED (PERMITTED USES) Elsevier is granting to You a limited, non-exclusive, non-transferable licence to use this Product in accordance with the terms of this Agreement. You may use or provide access to this Product on a single computer or terminal physically located at Your premises and in a secure network or move this Product to and use it on another single computer or terminal at the same location for personal use only, but under no circumstances may You use or provide access to any part or parts of this Product on more than one computer or terminal simultaneously.

You shall not (a) copy, download, or otherwise reproduce the Product or any part(s) thereof in any medium, including, without limitation, online transmissions, local area networks, wide area networks, intranets, extranets and the Internet, or in any way, in whole or in part, except for printing out or downloading nonsubstantial portions of the text and images in the Product for Your own personal use; (b) alter, modify, or adapt the Product or any part(s) thereof, including but not limited to decompiling, disassembling, reverse engineering, or creating derivative works, without the prior written approval of Elsevier; (c) sell, license or otherwise distribute to third parties the Product or any part(s) thereof; or (d) alter, remove, obscure or obstruct the display of any copyright, trademark or other proprietary notice on or in the Product or on any printout or download of portions of the Proprietary Materials.

RESTRICTIONS ON TRANSFER This Licence is personal to You, and neither Your rights hereunder nor the tangible embodiments of this Product, including without limitation the Proprietary Material, may be sold, assigned, transferred or sublicensed to any other person, including without limitation by operation of law, without the prior written consent of Elsevier. Any purported sale, assignment, transfer or sublicense without the prior written consent of Elsevier will be void and will automatically terminate the Licence granted hereunder.

TERM This Agreement will remain in effect until terminated pursuant to the terms of this Agreement. You may terminate this Agreement at any time by removing from Your system and destroying the Product and any copies of the Proprietary Material. Unauthorized copying of the Product, including without limitation, the Proprietary Material and documentation, or otherwise failing to comply with the terms and conditions of this Agreement shall result in automatic termination of this licence and will make available to Elsevier legal remedies. Upon termination of this Agreement, the licence granted herein will terminate and You must immediately destroy the Product and all copies of the Product and of the Proprietary Material, together with any and all accompanying documentation. All provisions relating to proprietary rights shall survive termination of this Agreement.

LIMITED WARRANTY AND LIMITATION OF LIABILITY Elsevier warrants that the software embodied in this Product will perform in substantial compliance with the documentation supplied in this Product, unless the performance problems are the result of hardware failure or improper use. If You report a significant defect in performance in writing to Elsevier within ninety (90) calendar days of your having purchased the Product, and Elsevier is not able to correct same within sixty (60) days after its receipt of Your notification, You may return this Product, including all copies and documentation, to Elsevier and Elsevier will refund Your money. In order to apply for a refund on your purchased Product, please contact the return address on the invoice to obtain the refund request form ('Refund Request Form'), and either fax or mail your signed request and your proof of purchase to the address indicated on the Refund Request Form. Incomplete forms will not be processed. Defined terms in the Refund Request Form shall have the same meaning as in this Agreement.

YOU UNDERSTAND THAT, EXCEPT FOR THE LIMITED WARRANTY RECITED ABOVE, ELSEVIER, ITS AFFILIATES, LICENSORS, THIRD PARTY SUPPLIERS AND AGENTS (TOGETHER 'THE SUPPLIERS') MAKE NO REPRESENTATIONS OR WARRANTIES, WITH RESPECT TO THE PRODUCT, INCLUDING, WITHOUT LIMITATION THE PROPRIETARY MATERIAL. ALL OTHER REPRESENTATIONS, WARRANTIES, CONDITIONS OR OTHER TERMS, WHETHER EXPRESS OR IMPLIED BY STATUTE OR COMMON LAW, ARE HEREBY EXCLUDED TO THE FULLEST EXTENT PERMITTED BY LAW.

IN PARTICULAR BUT WITHOUT LIMITATION TO THE FOREGOING NONE OF THE SUPPLIERS MAKE ANY REPRESENTIONS OR WARRANTIES (WHETHER EXPRESS OR IMPLIED) REGARDING THE PERFORMANCE OF YOUR PAD, NETWORK OR COMPUTER SYSTEM WHEN USED IN CONJUNCTION WITH THE PRODUCT, NOR THAT THE PRODUCT WILL MEET YOUR REQUIREMENTS OR THAT ITS OPERATION WILL BE UNINTERRUPTED OR ERROR-FREE.

EXCEPT IN RESPECT OF DEATH OR PERSONAL INJURY CAUSED BY THE SUPPLIERS' NEGLIGENCE AND TO THE FULLEST EXTENT PERMITTED BY LAW, IN NO EVENT (AND REGARDLESS OF WHETHER SUCH DAMAGES ARE FORESEEABLE AND OF WHETHER SUCH LIABILITY IS BASED IN TORT, CONTRACT OR OTHERWISE) WILL ANY OF THE SUPPLIERS BE LIABLE TO YOU FOR ANY DAMAGES (INCLUDING, WITHOUT LIMITATION, ANY LOST PROFITS, LOST SAVINGS OR OTHER SPECIAL, INDIRECT, INCIDENTAL OR CONSEQUENTIAL DAMAGES ARISING OUT OF OR RESULTING FROM: (I) YOUR USE OF, OR INABILITY TO USE, THE PRODUCT; (II) DATA LOSS OR CORRUPTION; AND/OR (III) ERRORS OR OMISSIONS IN THE PROPRIETARY MATERIAL.

IF THE FOREGOING LIMITATION IS HELD TO BE UNENFORCEABLE, OUR MAXIMUM LIABILITY TO YOU IN RESPECT THEREOF SHALL NOT EXCEED THE AMOUNT OF THE LICENCE FEE PAID BY YOU FOR THE PRODUCT. THE REMEDIES AVAILABLE TO YOU AGAINST ELSEVIER AND THE LICENSORS OF MATERIALS INCLUDED IN THE PRODUCT ARE EXCLUSIVE.

If the information provided in the Product contains medical or health sciences information, it is intended for professional use within the medical field. Information about medical treatment or drug dosages is intended strictly for professional use, and because of rapid advances in the medical sciences, independent verification of diagnosis and drug dosages should be made.

The provisions of this Agreement shall be severable, and in the event that any provision of this Agreement is found to be legally unenforceable, such unenforceability shall not prevent the enforcement or any other provision of this Agreement.

GOVERNING LAW This Agreement shall be governed by the laws of England and Wales. In any dispute arising out of this Agreement, you and Elsevier each consent to the exclusive personal jurisdiction and venue in the courts of England and Wales.